BRITISH PHARMACEUTICAL CODEX

1973

ANNOUNCEMENT

The Council of the Pharmaceutical Society of Great Britain recommends that the British Pharmaceutical Codex 1973 come into force in the United Kingdom on December 1, 1973. It is open to overseas authorities to fix such a date as is convenient to them.

ACKNOWLEDGEMENT

Information from the British Pharmacopoeia is used with permission of the Controller of Her Majesty's Stationery Office.

BRITISH PHARMACEUTICAL CODEX

1973

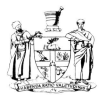

Prepared in the Department of Pharmaceutical Sciences
of the Pharmaceutical Society of Great Britain
and published by direction of the Society's Council

LONDON
THE PHARMACEUTICAL PRESS
17 BLOOMSBURY SQUARE WC1A 2NN

ISBN 0 85369 084 7

Made and printed in Great Britain by
William Clowes & Sons, Limited, London, Beccles and Colchester

CONTENTS

Page

CODEX REVISION COMMITTEE

PREFACE

In 1903 the Council of the Pharmaceutical Society of Great Britain adopted a resolution to produce a book of reference for those engaged in prescribing and dispensing medicines and the first British Pharmaceutical Codex, published in 1907, gave effect to this resolution. Subsequent revisions of the Codex were published in 1911, 1923, 1934, 1949, 1954, 1959, 1963, and 1968. Significant changes were made both in the scope of the book and the method of presenting information in each edition until the fifth. Since 1949, however, the general format of the Codex has remained unchanged until this, the tenth edition, although its scope has continued to extend.

Changes that have been made in the later editions include the introduction of a large number of detailed analytical standards (from 1949), the use of authentic specimens in analytical procedures (from 1963), the reorganisation of the information on drug actions to give due prominence to adverse effects (1968), the introduction of more monographs giving standards for pharmaceutical adjuvants (1968), and the abandonment of the Imperial system of weights and measures in favour of the metric system; this process, which began with the solid dosage forms in the 1963 Codex, continued with the conversion of formulae for liquid preparations in 1968, and is completed in 1973 by changes in the dimensions of surgical dressings.

With each succeeding edition, it has become increasingly difficult to accommodate all the required information within the confines of a volume of convenient size, while retaining the general format so long familiar to users of the Codex. On this occasion, therefore, the opportunity has been taken to reconsider the general lay-out of the text and the Codex is now presented in an entirely redesigned form. Had the old format been retained, the text of this new edition would have occupied some 1850 pages and increased the thickness of the book beyond easily manageable proportions. By modifying the typographical style, increasing the page size, and adopting a double-column format, it has been possible not only to improve the legibility of the text but almost to halve the number of pages required, thus improving the proportions of the book and allowing ample scope for the further expansion of subsequent editions, as necessitated by the continuing progress in the development and use of medicinal products.

At the request of the British Pharmacopoeia Commission, the Council of the Pharmaceutical Society agreed in 1959 that the publication of the Codex should coincide with that of the British Pharmacopoeia, so that new versions of the two books could come into effect on the same dates. This arrangement makes it possible to provide continuing current standards for those drugs and preparations that cease to be the subjects of monographs in the Pharmacopoeia and become the subjects of monographs in the Codex, and *vice versa*. Close co-operation between the British Pharmacopoeia Commission and the Codex Revision Committee has been necessary to provide comparable standards for simultaneous publication, but it is considered that the additional effort involved is justified, as the transition between editions should now be more convenient for users of the two books.

ix

The Codex is also closely linked with the British National Formulary, for which it provides formulae and standards, and arrangements have been made for the new edition of the Formulary to come into effect on the same date as the Pharmacopoeia and the Codex.

This tenth British Pharmaceutical Codex has been prepared by the Codex Revision Committee at the direction of the Council of the Pharmaceutical Society, which acknowledges its great indebtedness to all members of the Committee and its sub-committees for the expert knowledge they have contributed and the valuable time they have so freely given. The membership of the Codex Revision Committee is given on page viii, and that of its sub-committees is set out below.

ACTIONS AND USES SUBCOMMITTEE

Chairman: T. D. Whittet, PH.D., B.SC., F.P.S., F.R.I.C., D.SC., D.B.A.

G. Bryan, F.P.S.

N. C. Cooper, M.SC., M.P.S.

F. Dudley Hart, M.D., F.R.C.P.

Professor P. C. Elmes, B.M., F.R.C.P.

S. J. Hopkins, F.P.S.

A. P. Launchbury, B.SC., M.P.S.

P. A. Parish, M.D., M.R.C.G.P.

F. Prescott, PH.D., M.SC., M.R.C.P., F.R.I.C.

L. Priest, M.SC., B.PHARM., F.P.S.

Professor H. Schnieden, M.D., M.SC.

Elizabeth J. Stokes, M.B., B.S., F.R.C.P.

Professor P. Turner, M.D., B.SC., M.R.C.P.

Professor D. W. Vere, M.D., M.B., B.S., F.R.C.P.

Professor A. W. Woodruff, M.D., PH.D., F.R.C.P., F.R.C.P.E., D.T.M. and H.

Secretary to the Committee: G. R. Brown

BIOLOGICAL PRODUCTS SUBCOMMITTEE

Chairman: D. Jack, PH.D., B.SC., F.P.S., F.R.I.C.

R. D. Andrews, M.B., B.S., B.SC., PH.D.

A. J. Beale, M.D., DIP.BACT., F.R.C.PATH.

A. B. Christie, M.A., M.D., D.P.H., D.C.H.

A. H. Griffith, M.D., D.P.H.

J. A. Holgate, M.B., CH.B., M.SC.

W. d'A. Maycock, M.V.O., M.D., F.R.C.PATH.

F. T. Perkins, B.SC., M.SC., PH.D.

C. H. Smith, M.D., F.R.C.PATH.

A. F. B. Standfast, M.A., SC.D., DIP.BACT.

P. B. Stones, M.B., B.S., F.R.C.PATH.

L. Vallet, M.A.

Secretary to the Committee: G. R. Brown

FORMULARY STANDARDS SUBCOMMITTEE A

Chairman: D. C. Garratt, D.SC., PH.D., F.R.I.C., M.CHEM.A.

A. S. Beidas, B.SC., F.R.I.C., M.PH.A.

P. Cleevely, B.SC., F.R.I.C., M.PH.A.

L. E. Coles, B.PHARM., PH.D., F.P.S., F.R.I.C., M.PH.A., M.CHEM.A.

R. E. King, F.R.I.C.

C. A. Macdonald, B.SC., F.R.I.C., M.CHEM.A.

M. J. de Faubert Maunder, B.SC., A.R.I.C.

A. J. Middleton, B.PHARM., M.P.S., F.R.I.C., M.PH.A.

*W. Mitchell, B.SC., PH.D., F.R.I.C.

A. W. C. Peacock, B.PHARM., F.P.S.

Secretary to the Committee: E. S. Greenfield

* Resigned, August 1971

Formulary Standards Subcommittee B

Chairman: D. C. Garratt, D.SC., PH.D., F.R.I.C., M.CHEM.A.

T. M. Blackwood, B.SC.
A. C. Caws, B.SC., A.R.I.C.
A. E. Corker, F.P.S., F.R.I.C.
D. H. Dorken, B.PHARM., M.P.S., F.R.I.C.
M. J. de Faubert Maunder, B.SC., A.R.I.C.
C. Radford, F.P.S.

R. Sinar, B.PHARM., B.SC., F.P.S., F.R.I.C.
D. O. Singleton, B.SC., F.R.I.C.
W. H. Stephenson, F.P.S., F.R.I.C., D.B.A., M.PH.A., M.CHEM.A.
W. R. Thompson, M.SC., F.R.I.C., M.CHEM.A.

Secretary to the Committee: E. S. Greenfield

Ligatures and Sutures Subcommittee

Chairman: K. R. Capper, PH.D., B.PHARM., F.P.S., D.I.C., F.R.I.C.

J. S. Amor, B.SC.
C. Buckler
R. B. Christie, M.P.S.
J. Owen Dawson, B.SC., F.P.S.
Professor H. Ellis, D.M., M.CH., F.R.C.S.

J. A. Holgate, M.B., CH.B., M.SC.
H. V. Rosewarn
D. J. Smith, PH.D., B.SC.
D. G. Thompson
C. C. Yates, A.R.I.C.

Secretary to the Committee: K. B. K. Davis

Pharmaceutical Chemistry Subcommittee

Chairman: Professor A. H. Beckett, D.SC., PH.D., F.P.S., F.R.I.C.

A. J. Badby, B.SC., F.R.I.C.
A. C. Caws, B.SC., A.R.I.C.
G. Drewery, B.SC., F.R.I.C., M.CHEM.A.
A. Holbrook, F.R.I.C., M.CHEM.A.
G. F. Phillips, M.SC., F.R.I.C.

H. T. Searle, M.A., B.SC.
J. E. Shinner, F.P.S.
W. H. Stephenson, F.P.S., F.R.I.C., D.B.A., M.PH.A., M.CHEM.A.
W. R. Thompson, M.SC., F.R.I.C., M.CHEM.A.

Secretary to the Committee: E. S. Greenfield

Pharmacognosy Subcommittee A

Chairman: Professor J. W. Fairbairn, D.SC., PH.D., B.SC., F.P.S., F.L.S.

W. E. Court, M.PHARM., PH.D., F.P.S., F.L.S.
D. F. Cutler, PH.D., B.SC., F.L.S., D.I.C.
W. C. Evans, B.PHARM., PH.D., D.SC., F.P.S.
F. Fish, B.PHARM., PH.D., F.P.S.
Betty P. Jackson, B.PHARM., PH.D., B.SC., F.P.S., F.L.S.
G. B. Pickering, M.A., B.SC., D.PHIL., A.R.I.C.

M. H. Ransom, B.PHARM., M.P.S.
Professor E. J. Shellard, B.PHARM., PH.D., F.P.S., F.R.I.C., F.L.S.
G. R. A. Short, F.P.S., F.L.S.
A. A. Williams
A. J. Woodgate, B.SC., A.R.I.C.

Secretary to the Committee: K. B. K. Davis

Pharmacognosy Subcommittee C

Chairman: D. C. Garratt, D.SC., PH.D., F.R.I.C., M.CHEM.A.

D. Holness, B.A.
A. M. Humphrey, B.SC., A.R.C.S.
P. A. Linley, PH.D., B.PHARM., M.P.S.
C. A. Macdonald, B.SC., F.R.I.C., M.CHEM.A.
*W. Mitchell, B.SC., PH.D., F.R.I.C.

N. Nix, B.SC., F.R.I.C.
R. A. Rabnott
M. H. Ransom, B.PHARM., M.P.S.
Professor E. J. Shellard, B.PHARM., PH.D., F.P.S., F.R.I.C., F.L.S.

Secretary to the Committee: E. S. Greenfield

* Resigned, August 1971

PHARMACY SUBCOMMITTEE A

Chairman: J. W. Hadgraft, F.P.S., F.R.I.C.

C. F. Abbott, B.PHARM., B.SC., F.P.S., F.R.I.C.
C. W. Barrett, M.PHARM., M.P.S.
Professor J. E. Carless, B.PHARM., M.SC., PH.D., F.P.S.
C. L. J. Coles, B.PHARM., F.P.S.
A. E. Davis, B.PHARM., F.P.S.
D. N. Gore, F.P.S., F.R.I.C.

W. H. Howarth, M.P.S.
Christobel E. Mozley-Stark, M.B.E., F.P.S.
A. W. Newberry, F.P.S.
J. R. Phillips, F.P.S.
G. Smith, PH.D., B.SC., F.P.S.
F. H. Tresadern

Secretary to the Committee: K. B. K. Davis

FORMULATION PANEL. G. Smith (*Chairman*), A. E. Davis, A. W. Newberry, and F. H. Tresadern. *Secretary:* W. Lund

DISPENSING PANEL. J. R. Phillips (*Chairman*), W. H. Howarth, J. G. Iles, B.SC., M.P.S., A. King, F.P.S., and C. McArdle, F.P.S. *Secretary:* K. B. K. Davis

PHARMACY SUBCOMMITTEE B

Chairman: J. W. Hadgraft, F.P.S., F.R.I.C.

A. W. Baker, F.P.S., D.B.A.
H. S. Bean, PH.D., B.PHARM., F.P.S.
W. R. L. Brown, B.PHARM., PH.D., F.P.S.
J. P. Curtis, F.P.S.
A. E. Davis, B.PHARM., F.P.S.
D. J. Drain, B.A., F.R.I.C.

J. Flint, F.P.S.
Professor D. A. Norton, B.SC., F.P.S., D.B.A., A.C.T., F.I.BIOL.
W. J. W. Price, F.P.S.
G. Smith, PH.D., B.SC., F.P.S.

Secretary to the Committee: K. B. K. Davis

SURGICAL DRESSINGS SUBCOMMITTEE

Chairman: L. B. Tansley, M.C., M.A., M.SC., F.R.I.C.

F. Carus
R. Crabtree
J. Flint, F.P.S.
D. C. Harrod, B.SC., F.P.S., F.L.S.
H. A. Hunt, B.SC.
E. Jones, B.SC., F.R.I.C.
R. Lant, B.SC., A.R.I.C.
K. Lunn, B.SC.
R. Maxwell-Savage, PH.D., M.A., F.R.I.C.

B. W. Mitchell, B.A., B.SC., F.R.I.C.
Christobel E. Mozley-Stark, M.B.E., F.P.S.
J. A. Myers, B.PHARM., F.P.S., LL.B., D.P.A., A.C.I.S.
P. J. Perry
R. Robinson, B.SC.
J. T. Scales, F.R.C.S., L.R.C.P.
T. D. Turner, M.PHARM., M.P.S., F.L.S.

Secretary to the Committee: E. S. Greenfield

PANEL ON PERFORMANCE OF SURGICAL DRESSINGS. T. D. Turner (*Chairman*), K. J. Harkiss, M.SC., PH.D., M.P.S., K. Lunn, B. W. Mitchell, P. J. Perry, and J. T. Scales.

PANEL ON STERILITY TESTING OF SURGICAL DRESSINGS. P. E. Harbord, A.I.M.L.T., E. Jones, A. Keale, B.SC., A. F. Lott, B.SC., R. Maxwell-Savage, and G. Sykes, M.SC., F.R.I.C.

K. B. K. Davis, M.P.S., and E. S. Greenfield, members of the staff of the Department of Pharmaceutical Sciences, have acted as secretaries to the committees and assisted with editorial work. In the laboratories of the Department of Pharmaceutical Sciences, formulation problems were investigated by W. Lund, F.P.S., assisted by A. A.

Chalmers, B.SC., M.P.S., Mary Neil, M.P.S., Veronica Russell, B.SC., M.P.S., I. E. Williams, B.PHARM., M.P.S., and Elma J. W. Young, B.SC., A.R.C.S.T., M.P.S., while analytical problems were investigated by J. D. Edmond, B.SC., A.R.I.C., assisted by D. Glencorse and Margaret Scott, B.SC.

Dorothy E. Aimes, Susan Cross, B.PHARM., M.P.S., H. C. Happold, M.P.S., D. A. Kennedy, Wendy Oliver, B.PHARM., M.P.S., and Gwyneth Wass also assisted in the preparation of the text and in reading the proofs.

The Codex Revision Committee gratefully acknowledges the invaluable assistance and advice it has received from government departments, professional institutions, and other organisations, including the Association of the British Pharmaceutical Industry, the British Standards Institution, the Commissioners of Customs and Excise, the Department of Health and Social Security, the Faculty of Ophthalmologists, the Home Office (drugs branch), the Laboratory of the Government Chemist, the Medical Research Council, the National Pharmaceutical Union, the Royal Botanic Gardens, Kew, and the Society for Analytical Chemistry.

Valuable advice has also been received from various overseas authorities, particularly the Department of Health, Australia, the Department of Health and Welfare, Canada, and the Directorate General of Health Services, India, and this advice has been of great assistance to the committee in ensuring that the statements in the Codex are acceptable in many countries.

Numerous experts have provided information and advice on specific points, especially the following: A. G. Allnutt, G. Ansell, E. H. Fagg, R. Goulding, J. P. Griffin, S. F. Hall, C. A. Johnson, G. R. Kitteringham, K. W. Lovel, D. E. Lovett, D. Mansel-Jones, J. P. Nicholson, S. Powlson, G. A. Rose, A. J. P. Shearlaw, A. D. Thornton-Jones, and A. Wade. The continued co-operation of the British Pharmacopoeia Commission and the help of numerous pharmaceutical manufacturers and of pharmacists in hospital and general practice are also gratefully acknowledged.

The Codex Revision Committee has also co-operated with the World Health Organisation in the preparation and revision of relevant standards of the International Pharmacopoeia and has also advised the British Delegation to the European Pharmacopoeia Commission on various monographs.

INTRODUCTION

The British Pharmaceutical Codex fulfils two important functions, namely, to give information on drugs, other pharmaceutical substances, and formulated products, and to provide standards for a range of substances and materials that are not included in the British Pharmacopœia. It provides authoritative information on the actions and uses of drugs and on their pharmaceutical properties. As new monographs are added to the Codex, it is necessary to omit monographs on older and less frequently used drugs and pharmaceutical adjuvants in order to keep the size of the book within reasonable limits, but the policy, introduced in the last edition, of including any substance which is in sufficiently wide use for a published standard to be desirable has been continued in this edition.

The work of revision has been influenced by the coming into effect in the United Kingdom of various sections of the Medicines Act 1968 which has resulted in the manufacture of medicinal products being controlled by a system of licensing. By virtue of section 65 of the Act the British Pharmaceutical Codex standards are recognised for relevant medicinal products, and the standards of the European Pharmacopoeia and of the British Pharmacopoeia are applicable where stated in the monographs.

The most important aspects of this revision are discussed briefly in the following pages.

Part 1. Drugs and Pharmaceutical Adjuvants

Monographs have been added on a variety of substances including aminobenzoic acid (which has sun-screening properties), calcium, magnesium, and potassium acetates (used in the preparation of haemodialysis solutions), chlorpromazine (for the preparation of suppositories), coconut oil (used as an ointment basis), and hydrocortisone sodium phosphate (used in the preparation of the injection). Other additions include antibiotics, β-adrenergic blocking agents, local anaesthetics, cytotoxic agents, and radiopharmaceuticals, including the important diagnostic material, sodium pertechnetate (^{99m}Tc). Monographs are included on all the substances of the British Pharmacopoeia 1973 with the exception of Alprenolol Hydrochloride. The Committee considered that at the time of preparation of the text there was not enough experience of the use of this substance to enable a sufficiently authoritative monograph to be prepared.

In this revision, particular attention has been paid to extending the information on the pharmaceutical properties of Codex substances and preparations and on their stability, incompatibility, storage, and sterilisation.

Earlier editions of the Codex were accompanied by a pamphlet containing names that were not recognised as synonyms for the Codex substances but that were sometimes applied to these substances or their preparations. For convenience in reference, these names have now been appended to the monographs and included in the index.

xiv

They comprise both proprietary and non-proprietary names and they have been placed, after the subheading "OTHER NAMES", at the foot of the monographs to which they refer so as to distinguish them from the synonyms at the head of the monographs, which have the same status as the main titles. The synonyms have been revised to include the Latin titles used in volumes I and II of the European Pharmacopoeia; other Latin titles, formerly widely used, have been omitted except in certain instances where they differ significantly from the English titles.

Part 2. Immunological Products and Related Preparations
The information on these products has been revised and considerable rearrangement of the monographs has been necessary as a result of the coming into effect in the United Kingdom of the standards of the European Pharmacopoeia. The recommendations on the immunisation of children and of travellers have been amended to conform to current practice, and, where appropriate, to the latest recommendations of the Department of Health and Social Security.

Part 3. Preparations of Human Blood
The information in this section has been revised to conform to modern practice; in particular, precautions to minimise the risk of transmitting serum hepatitis have been strengthened as a result of the development of tests to detect Australia (hepatitis-associated) antigen.

Part 4. Surgical Ligatures and Sutures
In this edition the former B.P.C. gauge numbers have been omitted and only the metric size designations, first introduced in the 1968 Codex, have been retained. These metric size designations and the standards, except those for stainless steel sutures, have been modified to conform to the requirements of the European Pharmacopoeia.

Part 5. Surgical Dressings
Many changes in points of detail have been made in the monographs. A test for colour fastness has been introduced and the sterility test has been completely revised.

Part 6. Formulary
Close co-operation with the Joint Formulary Committee, responsible for the revision of the British National Formulary, has been continued and further monographs have been added to this edition to provide standards for and other information on preparations included in the British National Formulary 1973; examples of such preparations are Betamethasone Valerate Scalp Application, Clioquinol Cream, Betamethasone Eye-drops, Hydrocortisone Sodium Phosphate Injection, and Betamethasone Valerate Lotion. Development work was undertaken by members of the pharmacy subcommittees and the Society's laboratories to establish the formula for Isoniazid Elixir; patient acceptability tests were carried out at several hospitals.

The introduction of a monograph on Diamorphine and Cocaine Elixir provides a standard formula for the preparation used for the relief of pain in terminal carcinoma and the last stages of other painful and fatal illnesses; the formula is capable of adjustment to the needs of the patient and if the prescriber so indicates the strength can be varied and morphine can be used instead of diamorphine. This monograph also provides for the inclusion of chlorpromazine in the elixir.

The formula for Aminobenzoic Acid Lotion is based on the reports of M. A. Pathak, T. B. Fitzpatrick, and E. Frenk, *New Engl. J. Med.*, 1969, **280**, 1459 and I. Willis and A. M. Kligman, *Archs Derm.*, 1970, **102**, 405 who have shown that it is an effective preparation for the protection of the skin of light-sensitive persons. The formula was selected after investigation of published information by the Society's laboratories and members of the subcommittees.

Investigations in the Society's laboratories have resulted in the addition to the monograph on idoxuridine of information on the preparation of solutions for injection. Such solutions are occasionally required for the treatment of life-threatening systemic viral infections, and formulation must take into consideration that the breakdown products are toxic and that idoxuridine has its optimum stability and lowest solubility at the same pH. The method given is based on the practical examination of published methods and reduces idoxuridine breakdown to an acceptable level. The formulation of eye-drops and an eye ointment of idoxuridine is under investigation with a view to the publication of monographs at a later date.

Work on the formulation of eye-drops has been continued and the range of formulae has been extended. The requirement that multiple-dose containers of eye-drops issued for domiciliary treatment should bear a statement that the drops should not be used for more than one month after first opening the container has been abandoned, following representations from the Faculty of Ophthalmologists that some patients continued to misinterpret such directions and discontinued the treatment, a practice that is more likely to harm them than the possible risk of infection due to using old eye-drops. However, the volume limit of 10 ml per container has been retained and thus in most cases there will be insufficient solution supplied for the contents to be used for a prolonged period.

A working party appointed by the Central Health Services Council is reviewing recommendations for the use of eye-drops in hospitals. The statements in this edition of the Codex are believed to be in accord with the views of the working party but may need to be reviewed when the working party has published its report.

In revising the formulae of mixtures and similar preparations account has been taken of the findings of the Public Health Laboratory Service Working Party (*Pharm. J.* 1971, **207**, 96), which showed that alkaline mixtures are especially liable to microbial growth. Mixtures are now required to be prepared with water of low bacterial content, and most formulae include a preservative such as chloroform. Peppermint oil is added, if required, in the form of a concentrated emulsion. Most of the mixtures contain 0·25 per cent v/v of chloroform, incorporated in the form of double-strength chloroform water. Water of low bacterial count is also required for other aqueous preparations in which bacterial growth is liable to occur, and suitable water is defined in the introduction to the Formulary Section (page 642).

In this edition general standards for pessaries and suppositories have been added. The policy of adding tests for the presence of active ingredients of medicinal products, begun in the last edition, has been continued.

Appendixes

The information provided in appendixes has been greatly extended. Details of ultra-violet absorption spectra required for identification purposes have been collected together in an appendix instead of being given in the monographs. Other appendixes describe general methods of ascending paper chromatography, the determination of distillation range and boiling-point, and the determination of water.

For the determination of alcohol in preparations described in the Codex the traditional distillation method is still used; this method is considered to be the most convenient when dealing with isolated samples. The gas-liquid chromatographic method may be advantageous when dealing with a large series of samples, and analysts may use such a method provided they are satisfied that the method they adopt gives equivalent results.

The appendix on thin-layer chromatography has been expanded and includes a large number of individual identification tests and tests for specific impurities in substances and medicinal products. Many of these tests have been specially developed in the laboratories of the Pharmaceutical Society at the instigation of the analytical sub-committees. In addition, general methods for the identification of certain steroids in preparations and for the identification of phenothiazine derivatives have been included. The scheme for the identification of alkaloids in medicinal products, originally included in the last edition of the Codex, has been reorganised to avoid the need for extensive cross referencing.

The quantitative tests for arsenic and lead in Appendixes 6 and 7 have been entirely rearranged to improve legibility and ease of reference.

In the appendix on powders and suspensions (page 911), the designation of sieve sizes has been amended to conform to British Standard 410:1969.

Appendix 28 (page 917) is an interpretation of the test for sterility of the European Pharmacopoeia designed to make the test applicable to surgical dressings and non-absorbable sutures.

European Pharmacopoeia

The Codex Revision Committee has co-operated with other authorities in the preparation of a European Pharmacopoeia published under a convention signed by the governments of Belgium, France, West Germany, Italy, Luxembourg, the Netherlands, Switzerland, and the United Kingdom. From the date of coming into effect of any volume of the European Pharmacopoeia, the standards in its monographs on any article become the standards in the United Kingdom for that article when used in the practice of medicine, surgery, or midwifery.

For the convenience of users of the Codex, those monographs in the 1973 Codex on substances for which a standard was formerly set by the Codex and is now (1973) set by the European Pharmacopoeia have been brought into agreement with the requirements of the European Pharmacopoeia. In order that these monographs shall conform to the style of the other Codex monographs it has been necessary to reword to some extent the pharmacopoeial standards and in certain cases to place an interpretation upon those pharmacopoeial statements which are ambiguous. Every care has been taken to ensure that the wording in the Codex monographs does not change the intentions of the European Pharmacopoeia Commission, but it must be emphasised that the requirements of that book are the legal standards in the United Kingdom and that in any case of dispute it is necessary to refer to the original text.

There has been insufficient time during the current revision to treat in the same way those monographs in the 1973 Codex on substances for which a standard was formerly set by the British Pharmacopoeia and is now set by the European Pharmacopoeia. For those monographs there is now a simple statement under the side-heading "Standard" to the effect that the substance must comply with the requirements of the European Pharmacopoeia in the same way that reference is made in monographs on substances for which the British Pharmacopoeia provides the standard. This has resulted in a few anomalies, which will be noted if, for example, the Codex monographs on Senna Leaf and Senna Fruit and on Sterilised Surgical Catgut and Non-absorbable Surgical Sutures are compared.

ADDITIONS

The following monographs of the British Pharmaceutical Codex 1973 were not included in the British Pharmaceutical Codex 1968 as amended by the Supplement 1971.

Part 1. Drugs and Pharmaceutical Adjuvants

Aluminium Phosphate Gel
Dried Aluminium Phosphate Gel
Aminobenzoic Acid
Calcium Acetate
Capreomycin Sulphate
Carbenoxolone Sodium
Cardamom Oil
Cephalexin
Chlorpromazine
Clomiphene Citrate
Coconut Oil
Danthron
Deslanoside
Dextran 70 Injection
Dextrose Monohydrate for Parenteral Use
Fenfluramine Hydrochloride
Framycetin Sulphate
Fusidic Acid
Hydrocortisone Sodium Phosphate
Isoprenaline Hydrochloride
Light Kaolin (Natural)
Lanatoside C
Levodopa

Macrisalb (^{131}I) Injection
Macrogol 1540
Magnesium Acetate
Meglumine Diatrizoate Injection
Melarsoprol Injection
Fractionated Palm Kernel Oil
Potassium Acetate
Practolol
Prilocaine Hydrochloride
Propanidid
Propicillin Potassium
Salbutamol Sulphate
Secbutobarbitone
L-Selenomethionine (^{75}Se) Injection
Sodium Methyl Hydroxybenzoate
Sodium Pertechnetate (^{99m}Tc) Injection
Sodium Propyl Hydroxybenzoate
Tetracosactrin Acetate
Tropicamide
Vincristine Sulphate
Xenon (^{133}Xe) Injection
Xylose

ADDITIONS (*continued*)

Part 2. Immunological Products and Related Preparations

Adsorbed Diphtheria Vaccine
Adsorbed Diphtheria and Tetanus Vaccine
Adsorbed Diphtheria, Tetanus, and
   Pertussis Vaccine
Eltor Vaccine

Rubella Vaccine (Live Attenuated)
Dried Smallpox Vaccine
Adsorbed Tetanus Vaccine
Typhoid Vaccine
Typhoid and Tetanus Vaccine

Part 3. Preparations of Human Blood

Human Albumin
Dried Human Albumin
Dried Human Antihaemophilic Fraction

Dried Human Fibrinogen for Isotopic
   Labelling
Human Tetanus Immunoglobulin
Human Vaccinia Immunoglobulin

Part 4. Surgical Ligatures and Sutures

Polyamide 6 Suture
Sterile Polyamide 6 Suture

Polyamide 6/6 Suture
Sterile Polyamide 6/6 Suture

Part 5. Surgical Dressings

Cotton Conforming Bandage
Absorbent Ribbon Gauze, X-ray-detectable

Absorbent Viscose Wadding

Part 6. Formulary

Betamethasone Valerate Scalp Application
*Paromomycin Capsules
Clioquinol Cream
Ipecacuanha Emetic Draught, Paediatric
*Cascara Elixir
Chlorpromazine Elixir
Diamorphine and Cocaine Elixir
Isoniazid Elixir
Propicillin Elixir
Peppermint Emulsion, Concentrated
*Hyoscyamus Dry Extract
*Hyoscyamus Liquid Extract
Betamethasone Eye-drops
Chloramphenicol Sodium Succinate
   Injection
Hydrocortisone Sodium Phosphate
   Injection
Procyclidine Injection
*Suramin Injection
Aminobenzoic Acid Lotion

Betamethasone Valerate Lotion
Cephalexin Mixture
Co-trimoxazole Mixture
Fusidic Acid Mixture
Indomethacin Mixture
Betamethasone Valerate with
   Chlortetracycline Ointment
Gentamicin Ointment
Hydrocortisone and Clioquinol Ointment
Nystatin Ointment
*Paraffin Ointment
*Kaolin Poultice
*Calcium Hydroxide Solution
Chlorhexidine Solution, Dilute
*Morphine Hydrochloride Solution
Chlorpromazine Suppositories
*Tolu Syrup
*Carbromal Tablets
*Gentian Tincture, Compound

In addition to the above individual monographs there are also additions in the form of short introductions to various groups of products included in the Formulary.

* A monograph for a preparation of similar or identical composition was included in the British Pharmacopoeia 1968.

ADDITIONS (*continued*)

The following monographs were added to the British Pharmaceutical Codex 1968 by means of amendments and of the Supplement 1971.

Part 1. Drugs and Pharmaceutical Adjuvants

Allopurinol
Aminocaproic Acid
Amitriptyline Embonate
Amphotericin
Azathioprine
Beclomethasone Dipropionate
Bethanidine Sulphate
Bupivacaine Hydrochloride
Carbamazepine
Carbenicillin Sodium
Cephalothin Sodium
Chlormerodrin (^{197}Hg) Injection
Clofibrate
Desferrioxamine Mesylate
Diazepam
Diphenoxylate Hydrochloride
Doxycycline Hydrochloride
Dydrogesterone
Ecothiopate Iodide
Ethambutol Hydrochloride
Ethynodiol Diacetate
Fluocortolone Hexanoate
Fluocortolone Pivalate
Fluphenazine Hydrochloride
Gentamicin Sulphate
Haloperidol
Hydroxyprogesterone Hexanoate
Idoxuridine
Indomethacin
Inulin
Iodinated (^{125}I) Human Albumin Injection

Lincomycin Hydrocholoride
Lithium Carbonate
Mefenamic Acid
Megestrol Acetate
Melphalan
Metformin Hydrochloride
Methacycline Hydrochloride
Methaqualone
Methotrexate
Metyrapone
Mexenone
Nitrazepam
Pentagastrin
Phenformin Hydrochloride
Prothionamide
Protriptyline Hydrochloride
Riboflavine Phosphate (Sodium Salt)
Salbutamol
Selenium Sulphide
Sodium Cromoglycate
Sodium Iodide (^{125}I) Solution
Sorbitol
Sulphamethoxazole
Thiabendazole
Thiacetazone
Thiotepa
Tolnaftate
Trimethoprim
Trimipramine Maleate
Vinblastine Sulphate

Part 6. Formulary

Aerosol Inhalations
Ergotamine Aerosol Inhalation
Isoprenaline Aerosol Inhalation
Isoprenaline Aerosol Inhalation, Strong
Orciprenaline Aerosol Inhalation
Salbutamol Aerosol Inhalation
Selenium Sulphide Scalp Application
Mexenone Cream
Cloxacillin Elixir
Digoxin Elixir, Paediatric
Orciprenaline Elixir
Phosphates Enema

Prednisolone Enema
Physostigmine and Pilocarpine Eye-drops
Hydrocortisone and Neomycin Eye Ointment
Lignocaine Gel
Sodium Aminosalicylate and Isoniazid
    Granules
Corticotrophin Carboxymethylcellulose
    Injection
Dextromoramide Injection
Phenytoin Injection
Codeine Linctus, Diabetic
Zinc Sulphide Lotion

ADDITIONS *(continued)*

Part 6. Formulary *(continued)*

Amphotericin Lozenges
Amitriptyline Mixture
Nalidixic Acid Mixture
Trimethoprim and Sulphamethoxazole
Mixture, Paediatric
Hexachlorophane Solution, Concentrated
Ethambutol Tablets
Prothionamide Tablets
Thiabendazole Tablets

Thiacetazone Tablets
Trimethoprim and Sulphamethoxazole
Tablets
Trimethoprim and Sulphamethoxazole
Tablets, Paediatric
Troxidone Tablets, Paediatric
Opium Tincture, Concentrated Camphorated
Camphor Water, Concentrated

DELETIONS

The following monographs, which were included in the British Pharmaceutical Codex 1968, as amended by the Supplement 1971, are not included in the British Pharmaceutical Codex 1973.

Part 1. Drugs and Pharmaceutical Adjuvants

Acepromazine Maleate
Aminacrine Hydrochloride
Bacitracin
Bemegride
Benzalkonium Bromide Solution
Butacaine Sulphate
Caffeine and Sodium Iodide
Calcium Cyclamate
Caramiphen Hydrochloride
Chloramphenicol Cinnamate
Chromium Trioxide
Prepared Coffee
Cottonseed Oil
Cyclamic Acid
Diethanolamine Fusidate
Disulphamide
Dyflos
Ergot
Prepared Ergot
Erythromycin Ethyl Carbonate
Ethyl Biscoumacetate
Furazolidone
Hexamethonium Bromide
Hexoestrol
Ispaghula
Lobeline Hydrochloride
Lucanthone Hydrochloride
Mebhydrolin Napadisylate
Mecamylamine Hydrochloride
Melarsoprol
Mercuric Oxycyanide

Mesulphen
Methylpentynol
Naphazoline Hydrochloride
Nealbarbitone
Nitrofurazone
Octyl Nitrite
Oestradiol
Fresh Bitter-orange Peel
Oxyphenisatin Acetate
Pempidine Tartrate
Potassium Perchlorate
Prednisone Acetate
Sesame Oil
Silver Protein
Mild Silver Protein
Sodium Antimonylgluconate
Anhydrous Sodium Carbonate
Sodium Cyclamate
Solapsone
Spermaceti
Spike Lavender Oil
Stibophen
Sulphadiazine Sodium
Sulphanilamide
Sulphaphenazole
Terpin Hydrate
Tretamine
Triacetyloleandomycin
Tricyclamol Chloride
Trimetaphan Camsylate
Tryparsamide

DELETIONS (*continued*)

Part 2. Immunological Products and Related Preparations

Diphtheria and Pertussis Vaccine
Measles Vaccine (Inactivated)

Staphylococcus Antitoxin
Staphylococcus Toxoid

Part 4. Surgical Ligatures and Sutures

Monofilament Polyamide Suture
Sterile Monofilament Polyamide Suture

Plaited Polyamide Suture
Sterile Plaited Polyamide Suture

Part 5. Surgical Dressings

Rayon and Rubber Elastic Bandage

Part 6. Formulary

Calcium Aminosalicylate Cachets
Alum and Zinc Dusting-powder, Paediatric
Zinc and Salicylic Acid Dusting-powder
Diamorphine and Terpin Elixir
*Cetomacrogol Emulsifying Wax
Sodium Bicarbonate Eye Lotion
Atropine and Cocaine Eye Ointment
Zinc Gelatin
*Kanamycin Injection
Lobeline Injection
*Lymecycline and Procaine Injection
Mephenesin Injection
Morphine and Hyoscine Injection
Pituitary (Posterior Lobe) Injection
*Potassium Chloride and Dextrose Injection
Solapsone Injection, Strong
Aconite Liniment
Aconite, Belladonna, and Chloroform
  Liniment
Belladonna Liniment
Camphor Liniment, Ammoniated
Betamethasone Lozenges
Fusidate Mixture
Saline Mixture
*Cetomacrogol Emulsifying Ointment
*Cetrimide Emulsifying Ointment
Iodine Ointment, Non-staining
Iodine Ointment, Non-staining, with
  Methyl Salicylate
Ginger Oleoresin
Iodine Paint, Compound
Ichthammol Pessaries
Silver Nitrate, Mitigated
Benzylpenicillin Solution-tablets, Buffered

Isoprenaline Spray
Isoprenaline Spray, Compound
*Aminophylline Suppositories
Chloral Syrup
Ferrous Phosphate Syrup, Compound
Ferrous Phosphate, Quinine and
  Strychnine Syrup
Acepromazine Tablets
Aspirin and Opium Tablets, Compound
Aspirin and Phenacetin Tablets
Aspirin with Ipecacuanha and Opium
  Tablets
Atropine Sulphate Tablets, Soluble,
  Paediatric
*Dihydrocodeine Tablets
Disulphamide Tablets
Ergot Tablets
*Ethambutol Tablets
Ethyl Biscoumacetate Tablets
Furazolidone Tablets
Hexoestrol Tablets
Mebhydrolin Tablets
Pentolinium Tablets
Phenacetin Tablets
Phenacetin and Caffeine Tablets
Potassium Tablets, Effervescent
Potassium Iodide Tablets
Potassium Perchlorate Tablets
Sulphaphenazole Tablets
*Trimethoprim and Sulphamethoxazole
  Tablets
Octyl Nitrite Vitrellae
Camphor Water

* A monograph for a preparation of similar or identical composition is included in the British Pharmacopoeia 1973.

ALTERATIONS IN TITLE

Part 1. Drugs and Pharmaceutical Adjuvants

Present Name	*Former Name*
Caramel	Burnt Sugar
Cineole	Eucalyptol
Corticotrophin Zinc Injection	Corticotrophin Zinc Hydroxide Injection
Demeclocycline Hydrochloride	Demethylchlortetracycline Hydrochloride
Anhydrous Dextrose	Dextrose
Dextrose	Dextrose Monohydrate
Dihydrocodeine Tartrate	Dihydrocodeine Acid Tartrate
Glycerol	Glycerin
Iodinated (^{125}I) Human Albumin Injection	Iodinated (^{125}I) Human Serum Albumin Injection
Macrogol 300	Liquid Macrogol
Macrogol 4000	Hard Macrogol
Sterilisable Maize Starch	Absorbable Dusting-powder

Part 2. Immunological Products and Related Preparations

Present Name	*Former Name*
Gas-gangrene Antitoxin (Perfringens)	Gas-gangrene Antitoxin (Welchii)

Part 3. Preparations of Human Blood

Present Name	*Former Name*
Human Albumin Fraction (Saline)	Human Plasma Protein Fraction
Dried Human Albumin Fraction (Saline)	Dried Human Plasma Protein Fraction
Dried Human Fibrinogen	Human Fibrinogen
Dried Human Thrombin	Human Thrombin

Part 5. Surgical Dressings

Present Name	*Former Name*
Absorbent Cotton Gauze (13 Light)	Absorbent Gauze

Part 6. Formulary

Present Name	*Former Name*
Selenium Sulphide Scalp Application	Selenium Sulphide Application
Prednisolone Eye-drops	Prednisolone Sodium Phosphate Eye-drops
Co-trimoxazole Mixture, Paediatric	Trimethoprim and Sulphamethoxazole Mixture, Paediatric
Co-trimoxazole Tablets, Paediatric	Trimethoprim and Sulphamethoxazole Tablets, Paediatric
Vitamin B Tablets, Compound	Thiamine Tablets, Compound
Vitamin B Tablets, Compound, Strong	Thiamine Tablets, Compound, Strong

CHANGES IN STANDARDS

The following standards which were given in the British Pharmaceutical Codex 1968 by reference to the British Pharmacopoeia are now given by reference to the European Pharmacopoeia.

Part 1. Drugs and Pharmaceutical Adjuvants

Acacia
Adrenaline Acid Tartrate
Alum
Amethocaine Hydrochloride
Aminophylline
Ammonium Chloride
Amylobarbitone Sodium
Ascorbic Acid
Aspirin
Atropine Sulphate
Barium Sulphate
Belladonna Herb
Prepared Belladonna Herb
Benzocaine
Benzylpenicillin
Betamethasone
Borax
Boric Acid
Butobarbitone
Caffeine
Caffeine Hydrate
Calcium Aminosalicylate
Calcium Carbonate
Calcium Chloride
Calcium Gluconate
Carbon Dioxide
Cascara
Cetrimide
Chloral Hydrate
Chloramphenicol
Chlortetracycline Hydrochloride
Cocaine Hydrochloride
Codeine Phosphate
Cortisone Acetate
Cyanocobalamin
Cyclobarbitone Calcium
Demeclocycline Hydrochloride
Deoxycortone Acetate
Anhydrous Dextrose
Digitoxin
Digoxin
Dimercaprol
Ergometrine Maleate
Ergotamine Tartrate

Erythromycin
Ethinyloestradiol
Ferrous Sulphate
Gallamine Triethiodide
Gentian
Griseofulvin
Hydrochloric Acid
Hydrocortisone
Hydrocortisone Acetate
Hydrogen Peroxide Solution, Strong
Hyoscine Hydrobromide
Hyoscyamus
Imipramine Hydrochloride
Iodine
Ipecacuanha
Prepared Ipecacuanha
Isoniazid
Lactose
Laevulose
Lignocaine Hydrochloride
Liquorice
Heavy Magnesium Carbonate
Light Magnesium Carbonate
Light Magnesium Oxide
Magnesium Sulphate
Methyl Salicylate
Methyltestosterone
Morphine Hydrochloride
Neomycin Sulphate
Neostigmine Bromide
Nicotinamide
Nikethamide
Nitrous Oxide
Noradrenaline Acid Tartrate
Oestradiol Benzoate
Oxygen
Oxytetracycline Dihydrate
Oxytetracycline Hydrochloride
Papaverine Hydrochloride
Paraldehyde
Phenacetin
Phenobarbitone
Phenoxymethylpenicillin
Phenylbutazone

CHANGES IN STANDARDS (*continued*)

Part 1. Drugs and Pharmaceutical Adjuvants (*continued*)

Phosphoric Acid
Physostigmine Salicylate
Pilocarpine Nitrate
Polymyxin B Sulphate
Potassium Bromide
Potassium Chloride
Potassium Iodide
Potassium Permanganate
Prednisolone
Prednisone
Procaine Hydrochloride
Progesterone
Pyridoxine Hydrochloride
Quinalbarbitone Sodium
Quinine Hydrochloride
Riboflavine
Senna Fruit
Silver Nitrate
Sodium Aminosalicylate
Sodium Bicarbonate
Sodium Chloride

Sodium Iodide
Sodium Phosphate
Sodium Sulphate
Starch
Stramonium
Streptomycin Sulphate
Succinylsulphathiazole
Sucrose
Sulphadimidine
Suxamethonium Chloride
Testosterone Propionate
Theophylline
Theophylline Hydrate
Thiamine Hydrochloride
Thiopentone Sodium
Tolbutamide
Tubocurarine Chloride
Purified Water
Zinc Oxide
Zinc Sulphate

Part 2. Immunological Products and Related Preparations

Bacillus Calmette-Guérin Vaccine
Botulinum Antitoxin
Cholera Vaccine
Diphtheria Antitoxin
Gas-gangrene Antitoxin (Oedematiens)
Gas-gangrene Antitoxin (Perfringens)
Gas-gangrene Antitoxin (Septicum)
Mixed Gas-gangrene Antitoxin
Influenza Vaccine

Measles Vaccine (Live Attenuated)
Pertussis Vaccine
Poliomyelitis Vaccine (Inactivated)
Poliomyelitis Vaccine (Oral)
Rabies Antiserum
Smallpox Vaccine
Tetanus Antitoxin
Old Tuberculin
Tuberculin Purified Protein Derivative

Part 3. Preparations of Human Blood

Human Normal Immunoglobulin Injection

Part 4. Surgical Ligatures and Sutures

Sterilised Surgical Catgut

Standards for the following substances which were included in the British Pharmacopoeia 1968 are now given in the British Pharmaceutical Codex 1973.

Part 1. Drugs and Pharmaceutical Adjuvants

Atropine
Chlorinated Lime
Ichthammol
Heavy Kaolin
Paromomycin Sulphate

Phenolsulphonphthalein
Proflavine Hemisulphate
Suramin
Tolu Balsam

CHANGES IN STANDARDS (*continued*)

Part 3. Preparations of Human Blood

Human Fibrin Foam

Standards for the following substances which were included in the British Pharmaceutical Codex 1968 are now given in the British Pharmacopoeia 1973.

Part 1. Drugs and Pharmaceutical Adjuvants

Bacitracin Zinc
Cetomacrogol 1000
Coconut Oil, Fractionated
Dihydrocodeine Tartrate
Ethacrynic Acid
Kanamycin Sulphate

Lymecycline
Macrogol 300
Macrogol 4000
Phenazocine Hydrobromide
Phenylpropanolamine Hydrochloride
Pseudoephedrine Hydrochloride

Standards for the following substances which were included in the British Pharmaceutical Codex 1968 have been modified to conform to the requirements of the European Pharmacopoeia.

Part 1. Drugs and Pharmaceutical Adjuvants

Aluminium Sulphate
Bismuth Carbonate
Senna Leaf
Sodium Carbonate

Anhydrous Sodium Sulphate
Theobromine
Zinc Chloride

Part 4. Surgical Ligatures and Sutures

Sterile Linen Suture
Sterile Plaited Polyester Suture

Sterile Plaited Silk Suture

Part 5. Surgical Dressings

Absorbent Cotton Wool

Absorbent Cotton Gauze (13 Light)

TRANSFERS

Monograph of Part 1 of the British Pharmaceutical Codex 1968 transferred to Part 6 of the British Pharmaceutical Codex 1973:

Hamamelis Water

Monograph of Part 6 of the British Pharmaceutical Codex 1968 transferred to Part 1 of the British Pharmaceutical Codex 1973:

Dilute Sulphuric Acid

SIGNIFICANT ALTERATION IN COMPOSITION

The composition of Potassium Chlorate and Phenol Gargle has been changed to include Patent Blue V (Colour Index No. 42051) in place of Sulphan Blue.

EUROPEAN PHARMACOPOEIA

Monographs included in the European Pharmacopoeia, Volumes I and II, but not otherwise referred to in the British Pharmaceutical Codex 1973.

Acidum Phosphoricum Dilutum
Aminophenazonum
Barbitalum
Codeinum
Fila Collagenis Resorbilia Aseptica
Frangulae Cortex
Hydrogenii Peroxidum Dilutum
Hyoscyami Pulvis Normatus
Immunoglobulinum Humanum
 Antimorbillorum
Menadionum

Methylphenobarbitalum
Natrii Carbonas Monohydricus
Oestronum
Ratanhiae Radix
Stramonii Pulvis Normatus
Tela Gossypii Absorbens★
Tela Gossypii Absorbens Aseptica★
Vaccinum Cholerae Cryodesiccatum
Vaccinum Influenzae Adsorbatum
Vaccinum Pertussis Adsorbatum
Vaccinum Typhoidi Cryodesiccatum

★ Except for Gauge 13 (Light).

GENERAL NOTICES

Legal Aspects

Substances and their preparations described in monographs of the British Pharmaceutical Codex may be subject to legal control in the United Kingdom or in other parts of the world in which the British Pharmaceutical Codex is effective. This control may be concerned with preparation, labelling, and standards.

In the United Kingdom, regulations under the Medicines Act 1968 require the licensing of the manufacture of medicinal products and the examination of new products by the Committee on Safety of Medicines before they are marketed. It should not be assumed that medicinal products prepared in accordance with the requirements of the British Pharmaceutical Codex will necessarily have been approved by the Committee on Safety of Medicines.

Licence to manufacture substances protected by Letters Patent is neither conveyed nor implied by the inclusion of monographs on such substances in the British Pharmaceutical Codex.

Titles and Synonyms

The following have the same status as the main titles: the names and abbreviated names appearing at the head of monographs after the side-heading SYNONYM(S), and inversions of main titles and their synonyms; the letter "f" may be substituted for "ph" in any title or synonym containing the syllable "sulph".

The names appearing after the heading OTHER NAME(S) at the foot of monographs in Part 1 of the Codex are names known to be used for the substances described in the monographs or for medicinal products prepared from those substances. Such names printed in *italic* type followed by the symbol ® are or have been used as proprietary names in the United Kingdom. These "other names" are included for information only. They are not to be regarded as official synonyms and their inclusion does not imply that they are the only other names used for the substances, or preparations of those substances, to which they refer.

In the Formulary the use of capital initial letters for the names of ingredients implies that these ingredients must comply with the appropriate requirements of the British Pharmacopoeia or of the British Pharmaceutical Codex.

Names in the text printed in *italic* type, other than those that are proprietary names or the names of plants, animals, and micro-organisms, refer to reagents, details of which are given in the relevant appendixes.

Latin Synonyms

Many of the Latin synonyms given in previous editions of the Codex have been omitted from this edition. Now, only those Latin synonyms are retained which (1) form the Latin titles of the corresponding monographs in the European Pharmacopoeia or (2) differ significantly from the English titles.

The following Latin synonyms for the various types of medicinal product described in the general monographs in the Formulary section of the Codex have also been omitted, although some of these terms are retained in Latin synonyms for individual products.

Applicatio (application)
Aqua Aromatica (water, aromatic)
Auristillae (ear-drops)
Capsulae (capsules)
Capsulae Amylaceae (cachets)
Cataplasma (poultice)
Collodium (collodion)
Collutorium (mouth-wash)
Collyrium (eye lotion)
Conspersus (dusting-powder)
Cremor (cream)
Emulsio (emulsion)
Extractum (extract)
Gargarisma (gargle)
Glycerinum (glycerin)
Guttae Ophthalmicae (eye-drops)
Guttae pro Auribus (ear-drops)
Haustus (draught)
Infusum (infusion)
Injectio (injection)
Insufflatio (insufflation)
Linimentum (liniment)
Liquor (solution)

Lotio (lotion)
Mistura (mixture)
Mucilago (mucilage)
Naristillae (nasal drops)
Nebula (spray)
Oblata (cachets)
Oculentum (eye ointment)
Pasta (paste)
Pastilli (pastilles)
Pessi (pessaries)
Pigmentum (paint)
Pilulae (pills)
Pulvis (powder)
Solvellae (solution-tablets)
Spiritus (spirit)
Suppositoria (suppositories)
Syrupus (syrup)
Tabellae (tablets)
Tinctura (tincture)
Trochisci (lozenges)
Unguentum (ointment)
Vapor (inhalation)

Chemical Formulae and Nomenclature

When the subject of a monograph is a chemical of known composition, structural and molecular formulae are included at the head of the monograph and a chemical name is given. This information refers to the chemically pure compound and should not be regarded as an indication of the purity of the material.

In structural formulae containing a ring system, each junction of two or more straight lines represents a carbon atom; each line represents a valency bond, and any valency not accounted for is assumed to be satisfied by a hydrogen atom. Unsaturation is represented in the conventional manner.

The chemical nomenclature is generally in accordance with the definitive rules issued by the International Union of Pure and Applied Chemistry, 1971, as accepted and interpreted by The Chemical Society, London.

Atomic and Molecular Weights

Molecular weights, which are given to four significant figures, are based on the Table of Relative Atomic Weights 1969, with 1971 amendments, published by the International Union of Pure and Applied Chemistry and based on the ^{12}C scale. Values for selected elements are given in Appendix 32 (page 932).

Methods of Manufacture

CHEMICAL SUBSTANCES. Methods of preparing chemical substances are given only if the composition of the substance is governed by the process employed or if the information may assist in an understanding of the chemistry of the compound and of the impurities that may occur in it. If a statement is made that a substance may be prepared by a certain method, this does not imply that other methods are not permitted. Whatever method of manufacture is used, the resulting substance must conform to the requirements given in the monograph under the side-heading "Standard".

FORMULATED MEDICINAL PRODUCTS. When making products in accordance with the recipes given in the Formulary, the ingredients must, unless otherwise indicated, comply with the requirements of the British Pharmacopoeia or of the British Pharmaceutical Codex. When an ingredient is described as "of commerce", it must be of good commercial quality suitable for medicinal and pharmaceutical use; when described as "food grade of commerce" or "nitration grade of commerce", it must comply with the appropriate specification of the British Standards Institution.

The instructions given for compounding medicinal products described in the Formulary (pages 641–825) are suitable when relatively small quantities, such as those specified in the recipe, are made by a pharmacist in general practice. Deviations from these instructions are permitted, provided that the products do not differ significantly from those produced when the methods of the British Pharmaceutical Codex are applied to the quantities in the recipe.

COLOURING AND FLAVOURING. The addition of colouring and flavouring agents is not permitted except where permission or a direction to the contrary is expressly given. When colouring is permitted in a medicinal product, any dye used must be of food grade of commerce and it must be one that is permitted for colouring food in the country in which the product is intended to be used.

ADDED SUBSTANCES. When the addition of substances acting as binders, disintegrants, preservatives, antoxidants, etc., is permitted, the substances used must have no significant adverse influence on the efficacy of the active ingredients and must not interfere with the assays and tests. Care should be taken that starches and other inert substances used in the products are free from harmful organisms.

Temperatures

Unless otherwise indicated, temperatures are expressed in degrees Celsius (centigrade).

Measures

Unless otherwise indicated, measurements are intended to be made at 20°. Measures are to be graduated at 20°.

Percentage Strengths

Percentage strengths are expressed as w/w, w/v, v/v, or v/w, and represent the number of grams or millilitres of substance in 100 g or 100 ml of the product. Unless otherwise stated, solutions of solids in liquids are expressed as percentage w/v, of liquids in liquids as percentage v/v, of liquids in solids as percentage v/w, and of gases in liquids as percentage w/w.

Solubility

Statements of solubility, except those given under the side-heading "Standard", are intended as information on approximate solubility only and should not be regarded as part of the standard for a substance. Where no temperature is given, statements of solubility apply at ordinary room temperature.

When the word "parts" is used in expressing the solubility of a substance, it means, unless otherwise stated, parts by weight (grams) of a solid in parts by volume (millilitres) of the solvent, or parts by volume (millilitres) of a liquid in parts by volume (millilitres) of the solvent, or parts by weight (grams) of a gas in parts by weight (grams) of the solvent.

Generally, when a substance is soluble in less than 1000 parts of solvent a figure is given; a solubility of about 1 in 1000 to 1 in 2000 is indicated by the expression "slightly soluble", and lower solubilities are indicated by the expressions "very slightly soluble" and "insoluble".

In statements of solubility the word "water" refers to purified water, the word "ether" to solvent ether, and the word "alcohol", without qualification, to alcohol (95 per cent).

Quality

A substance, medicinal product, or device not the subject of a monograph in the British Pharmacopoeia is of British Pharmaceutical Codex quality, provided that it is of the nature or composition specified in the monograph and complies with all the requirements stated in the section headed "Standard". In addition, a drug of biological origin must be derived from the biological source or sources stated in the first paragraph of the monograph.

The standards are designed to take account of impurities likely to occur in substances obtained from natural sources or to be introduced during manufacture, but the tests do not provide against all possible contaminants. Impurities not precluded by tests given in the standards are not tolerated should rational consideration and good pharmaceutical practice require them to be absent. In formulated products, impurities due to the use of unsuitable methods of manufacture, or to ingredients not of the required standard, are not tolerated.

Application of Standards

The standards stated in the monographs are intended to apply to articles supplied for medicinal use, but not necessarily to articles that may be supplied under the same name for other purposes.

The standards given in the general monographs on Antisera in Part 2, on Nonabsorbable Surgical Sutures in Part 4, and on the various types of medicinal product in Part 6 are intended to be applied primarily to the individual products of that type included in the Codex, and they are not necessarily applicable to other similar products.

Standards

UPPER LIMIT OF CONTENT. Where no upper limit is specified in the standard for content of a substance, a limit of 100·5 per cent is implied.

FORMULATED PRODUCTS PREPARED WITH TAP WATER. The specified limits in the standards for the medicinal products described in the Formulary section (Part 6, pages 641 to 825) apply to products made with purified water, and in appropriate instances when potable water has been used analysts should make an additional allowance to cover impurities likely to be contributed by the local water supply.

INTERPRETATION OF LIMITS. The number of significant figures given in expressing the permissible limits of quantitative determinations is related to the accuracy that may be expected from the specified analytical procedure. The analyst should calculate his results and reduce them to the required number of figures by rounding-off in the usual manner; thus analytical results falling in the range 24·95 to 26·04 per cent satisfy a requirement of 25·0 to 26·0 per cent.

CRUDE DRUGS. These are required to be as free as practicable from moulds, foreign insects and other animal matter, and from animal excreta.

Unless otherwise stated, the limits in the monographs are calculated with reference to the air-dry drug.

The term "foreign organic matter" refers to any organic matter not included by the definition of the drug given in the first sentence of the monograph, but excludes structures for which specific limits are given under "Standard".

Tests and Assays

IDENTIFICATION. Identification tests given in the monographs in Part 1 are not necessarily sufficient to establish the identity of the substance, but when used in conjunction with the other tests and quantitative determinations in the monograph, they generally suffice to distinguish the compound from others likely to be encountered in pharmaceutical practice. Further tests, such as mixed melting-points with authentic samples, may be necessary to provide a final proof of identity. Reference should be made to the British Pharmacopoeia for details of tests for certain basic and acidic radicals.

Whenever possible, suitable tests for the presence of active ingredients, even if not included in the Standard, should be applied to dosage forms, such as cachets, capsules, injections, and tablets, to establish the identity of the active ingredients of these products.

INFRA-RED ABSORPTION SPECTRA. Identification tests involving infra-red spectroscopy are included for a number of substances in the British Pharmaceutical Codex, and authentic specimens of these substances (see page xxxv) are available for use as standards of comparison. The technique described in Appendix IV (I) of the British Pharmacopoeia 1973 should be used. Experience in the interpretation of infra-red spectra is essential when carrying out these tests, as peaks and inflexions may occur which can be attributed to impurities but which can be disregarded for identification purposes.

USE OF PHARMACOPOEIAL METHODS. Where a method of determination is not described, the appropriate method of the British Pharmacopoeia or of the European Pharmacopoeia should be used.

Methods and tests, which are not described in the Codex and to which no direct cross-reference is made in the text, will be found as follows.

In the European Pharmacopoeia:

Test for sterility   Test for pyrogens

In the British Pharmacopoeia:

Acid-insoluble ash	Optical rotation
Acid value	Refractive index
Alcohol-soluble extractive	Saponification value
Ash	Specific gravity
Chloride limit test	Specific rotation
Complete extraction of alkaloids	Sulphate limit test
Continuous extraction of drugs	Sulphated ash
Determination of pH values	Total solids
Ester value	Unsaponifiable matter
Foreign organic matter	Viscosity
Iodine value	Water-soluble extractive
Iron limit test	Weight per millilitre
Melting-point	

The British Pharmacopoeia also describes the qualitative reactions characteristic of acetates, aluminium, primary aromatic amines, ammonium salts, antimony, bicarbonates, bromides, calcium, carbonates, chlorides, ferrous salts, iodides, magnesium, nitrates, phosphates, potassium, sodium, sulphates, tartrates, and zinc.

ALTERNATIVE METHODS OF ANALYSIS AND TESTING. Alternative methods, including micro-analytical techniques, may be used in place of those described, provided that they are of equivalent accuracy. In the event of doubt or dispute, the methods prescribed by the British Pharmaceutical Codex must be used.

QUANTITIES TO BE WEIGHED OR MEASURED. In quantitative tests, where an approximate quantity is directed to be taken and accurately weighed, the weight taken must be within 10 per cent of the quantity specified, and the result calculated from the exact weight. Volumes of liquid samples and of volumetric solutions must be measured accurately by means of standardised pipettes or burettes. In other instances the accuracy required in weighing or measuring materials for the tests may be inferred from the number of significant figures given in the text; in no case should the quantity taken deviate by more than 10 per cent from the specified amount.

All measurements involved in analytical operations are intended to be carried out at 20°, unless otherwise indicated. Graduated glass apparatus used in the analytical operations should have been calibrated at 20° and should comply with Class A requirements of the appropriate specification issued by the British Standards Institution.

REAGENTS AND SOLUTIONS. Reagents and volumetric solutions are described in the Appendixes or in those of the British Pharmacopoeia.

Titles of reagents are printed in *italic* type throughout the standards of the British Pharmaceutical Codex.

NEUTRALITY OF SOLVENTS USED IN TESTS AND ASSAYS. In appropriate instances, when a blank test is not prescribed, solvents must be previously neutralised to the indicator used in the test or assay concerned.

INDICATORS. Unless otherwise stated, the quantity of an indicator solution appropriate for use in acid-base titrations is 0·1 ml.

CRUDE DRUG ASSAYS. In the alkaloidal and other assays of crude drugs and their preparations, the quantities of solvent used may be varied to overcome difficulties that may be encountered.

LOSS ON DRYING. Unless otherwise indicated the determination is carried out by drying about 1 gram, accurately weighed, under the specified conditions.

Crude Drugs

VARIETIES. The description of a crude drug is designed to include those commercial varieties suitable for medicinal use. Frequently these commodities have distinctive names related to their country of origin or to some individual peculiarity. In order to provide useful information about commodities that are acceptable for medicinal use, they are named and briefly described in the paragraph headed "Varieties", and their quality is governed by the standard given in the monograph. In this context the term "variety" is not necessarily equivalent to the botanical "varietas".

SUBSTITUTES AND ADULTERANTS. Substances referred to under this heading do not comply with the description and standards given in the monograph. Substances are described that have occurred in admixture with the genuine drug or as a complete counterfeit. They may contain active principles related to those in the drug that is the subject of the monograph, but more frequently are useless or dangerous materials.

CONSTITUENTS. The information given under this heading relates to commercially available drugs, but it is not intended to be regarded as a standard.

POWDERING. When a batch of a crude drug is ground and sifted no portion of the drug shall be rejected. However, the final tailings may be withheld if an approximately equal weight of tailings from a previous batch has been added before grinding.

Essential Oils

Certain essential oils are liable to deteriorate on keeping. This deterioration is accompanied by increase in viscosity, and by changes in the quality of the odour and in other properties. Oils that have deteriorated are not regarded as being of the quality required by the British Pharmaceutical Codex.

Syrup

When Syrup is used for the dilution of elixirs, linctuses, and mixtures, as described in the relevant general monographs, there is the possibility of incompatibility between these preparations and any preservatives used in the Syrup. Preliminary investigations in the Laboratories of the Pharmaceutical Society have provided indications of incompatibility between the following preparations and Syrup preserved with hydroxybenzoate esters: Cloxacillin Elixir, Methadone Linctus, Noscapine Linctus, Paediatric Opiate Squill Linctus, Paediatric Belladonna and Ephedrine Mixture, Paediatric Belladonna and Ipecacuanha Mixture, Ferrous Sulphate Mixture, Paediatric Ferrous Sulphate Mixture, Paediatric Ipecacuanha Mixture, Paediatric Opiate Ipecacuanha Mixture, and Sodium Citrate Mixture. In these cases, and in any case of doubt, Syrup containing no preservative should be used.

Authentic Specimens

An authentic specimen of a substance is a sample, the identity of which has been established and which may be used to identify other samples of the same substance or to establish the presence of that substance in a product by comparative methods. In some instances, the purity and/or the proportion of certain impurities has been established, so that the specimen may be used in a comparative assay method or limit test.

For the assay of a few medicinal products, a sample of the unformulated substance of British Pharmaceutical Codex quality is required as a standard for comparison, and in certain instances the unformulated substance is a proprietary article which is not obtainable from the usual source of supply. In these cases an authentic specimen is available.

The authentic specimens required for tests of the British Pharmaceutical Codex are listed in Appendix 1C (page 852); they should be ordered from the relevant supplier specified in the Appendix.

British Chemical Reference Substances

A British Chemical Reference Substance is a sample which has been purified as far as is practically and economically feasible, any remaining impurities having been identified and a limit set on their presence.

The British Chemical Reference Substances required for the tests of the British Pharmaceutical Codex are listed in Appendix 1C (page 853).

Doses

Dosage schemes for specific purposes are given in the paragraphs on "Actions and uses". Where it appears to be useful to do so, this information is summarised in the form of a statement of the usual dose range under the heading "Dose". Unless otherwise stated or implied in the context, such doses are suitable for adults. When doses for children are expressed as a range of doses applying within specified age limits, the lower dose applies at the lower age and the higher dose at the higher age limit.

The doses are based on the opinions of medical and pharmaceutical experts and are intended for general guidance, but they should not be regarded as binding upon the prescriber. When an unusually large dose appears to have been prescribed, it is the duty of the pharmacist to ensure that the prescriber's intention has been correctly interpreted.

Storage

Substances and preparations should be stored under conditions which prevent contamination and, as far as possible, deterioration. The statements under the side-heading "Storage" in the monographs draw attention to the precautions that should be taken in specific cases. Further precautions may be necessary when some materials are stored under conditions of extreme temperature and/or high humidity.

Containers

WELL-CLOSED CONTAINER. This container protects the contents from contamination with extraneous solids and does not allow the contents to be released unintentionally under ordinary conditions of handling, storage, and transport.

AIRTIGHT CONTAINER. This container protects the contents from contamination with extraneous solids, liquids, and vapours, from loss of volatile constituents, and from changes due to efflorescence, deliquescence, and evaporation under ordinary conditions of handling, storage, and transport.

SECURELY CLOSED CONTAINER. This is an airtight container fitted with some means of preventing the unintentional displacement of the closure.

HERMETICALLY SEALED CONTAINER. This container is impervious to air and other gases under ordinary conditions of handling, storage, and transport. It is usually a glass ampoule sealed by fusion of the glass.

LIGHT-RESISTANT CONTAINER. For protection against light, a container should be made of materials which do not transmit more than 10 per cent of incident radiation at any wavelength between 290 nm and 450 nm.

SINGLE-DOSE CONTAINER. This container is a hermetically sealed container which is used to hold a quantity of an injection solution intended to be administered as a single dose and which, once opened, cannot be resealed.

MULTIPLE-DOSE CONTAINER. This container is a well-closed container which as far as possible prevents access of moisture and which is fitted with a closure, usually a rubber cap, that prevents the access of micro-organisms and allows the withdrawal of successive doses of an injection solution.

PLASTIC CONTAINERS AND CLOSURES. Containers and closures made of plastic material or rubber must not yield any harmful substance to the substance or preparation with which they are in contact. Similarly, dropper teats must not yield any harmful substance to the preparation with which they are used.

NOTE. The terms *well-closed package* and *sealed package* relating to surgical dressings are defined on page 610.

Labelling

The label on the container states, in addition to any statements required by the monographs (1) the name of the article, and (2) a reference, which consists of either figures, or letters, or a combination of figures and letters, by which the history of the article may be traced.

Statements required to appear on the label of a container may be on a label fastened to the immediate container or in indelible writing in or on the body of the container. Statements required to appear on the label of the package may appear on a label adherent to the package or on the package itself. Labelling requirements do not necessarily apply to bulk containers or to the containers of products supplied in compliance with a medical prescription, but otherwise they are intended to apply to the containers in which the products are issued for use.

PRODUCTS CONTAINING ASPIRIN. Unless the word "aspirin" appears in the name used on the label, the label on the container must state that the product contains aspirin. This requirement does not apply in countries where exclusive rights in the name "aspirin" are claimed.

Drug Interactions

The effect of one medicinal substance administered to a patient may be modified as a result of the concurrent administration of another. There are many possibilities for interaction and only a few of the more important ones have been singled out for mention in the monographs. A few of the commoner mechanisms involved are outlined below.

1. ALTERATION IN ALIMENTARY ABSORPTION OF MEDICINAL SUBSTANCES ADMINISTERED BY MOUTH
   (a) Decreased absorption as a result of decreased intestinal mobility.
   (b) Decreased absorption as a result of the formation of insoluble complexes.
       Example: tetracyclines in the presence of calcium compounds.
   (c) Increased absorption as a result of the presence of solubilising agents.

2. DISPLACEMENT OF ONE DRUG BY ANOTHER AT PROTEIN BINDING SITES IN THE PLASMA OR TISSUES
   Examples: (a) phenylbutazone displaces coumarin anticoagulants and enhances the anticoagulant effect;
   (b) sulphonamides displace tolbutamide and enhance the hypoglycaemic effect;
   (c) salicylates, sulphonamides, and thiazide diuretics displace methotrexate to give rise to toxic effects.

3. COMPETITION BETWEEN DRUGS AT THE SITE OF ACTION OR AT PHYSIOLOGICALLY RELATED SITES
   Example: imipramine competes with guanethidine and reduces the antihypertensive effect.

4. MODIFICATION OF THE METABOLIC INACTIVATION OF A DRUG BY THE ACTION OF ANOTHER DRUG
   Examples: (a) barbiturates accelerate metabolic inactivation of many drugs (such as warfarin) and so reduce their effects;

(b) monoamine-oxidase inhibitors enhance the effects of certain sympathomimetic amines by inhibiting an enzyme responsible for their metabolism. Similarly, anticholinesterases enhance the effect of suxamethonium compounds.

5. MODIFICATION OF EXCRETION THROUGH THE KIDNEY
Examples: (a) weakly acidic substances such as salicylates and phenobarbitone are excreted more rapidly when the urine is alkaline; weakly basic substances such as pethidine and amphetamine are more rapidly excreted when the urine is acid;
(b) certain diuretics, by increasing the urinary excretion of potassium ions, increase the sensitivity of the heart to digitalis.

6. INACTIVATION OF BIOLOGICAL PRODUCTS
Example: antibacterial substances when given concurrently with live bacterial vaccines prevent the growth of bacteria and so interfere with the development of immunity. Similarly, antiviral substances interfere with immunisation by live viral vaccines.

7. SUMMATION OF A MAIN OR SIDE EFFECT OF ONE DRUG WITH A MAIN OR SIDE EFFECT OF ANOTHER
Examples: (a) aspirin increases the danger of haemorrhage in patients being treated with anticoagulants;
(b) alcohol increases the depressant action of hypnotic and sedative drugs and antihistamines.

Substances that affect the Central Nervous System

Medicinal substances such as those used as analgesics, hypnotics, antihistamines, travel-sickness remedies, and psychiatric drugs have different actions on the central nervous system. Some affect reaction time and some cause dizziness or drowsiness, and others distort perception. Most of these effects are increased if alcohol is taken. These different influences on the co-ordination mechanism of the nervous system may severely impair the skill and judgement necessary to drive a motor vehicle or operate moving machinery.

Attention has been drawn to these effects in the monographs on the substances most likely to produce them, but they should be borne in mind whenever drugs having a central action are used.

Use of Medicinal Substances in Pregnancy

Where it has been established that a medicinal substance has a teratogenic or other undesirable effect in pregnancy, this has been mentioned in the appropriate monograph. However, the absence of such a statement should not be taken to imply that any drug may be used without associated risk during pregnancy, as in many cases the effects on the foetus have not been established. Caution should always be exercised in prescribing drugs during the first three months of pregnancy. Unless the patient's illness is likely to produce marked morbidity, the desirability of postponing treatment should be considered.

Explanation of Terms Used

WATER. The term *water* used in analytical procedures and for preparing reagents refers to Purified Water. The term *water* is used in recipes with the meaning given on page 642.

OVERNIGHT. This term means a period of 16 hours.

IN VACUO. This term means a pressure not exceeding 5 mm of mercury.

CALCULATED WITH REFERENCE TO THE DRIED OR ANHYDROUS SUBSTANCE. The expression "calculated with reference to the dried substance" implies that the method of drying is that specified for the determination of the loss on drying. The expression "calculated with reference to the anhydrous substance" implies that allowance is made for the content of water, as determined in the test headed "Water".

ODOURLESS. When a substance is described as "odourless", the test given in the British Pharmacopoeia should be applied.

WATER-BATH. This term means a bath of boiling water, unless water at some other temperature is indicated by the context.

CONSTANT WEIGHT. The term "constant weight" used in relation to drying and ignition procedures means that two consecutive weighings do not differ by more than 0·5 mg per g of substance taken for the determination, the second weighing being made after an additional hour of drying, or after further ignition, at the stated temperature.

COOL PLACE. This is a space in which the temperature does not exceed 15°.

DATE OF MANUFACTURE. The expression "date of manufacture" used in connection with products subject to biological testing means either the date of completion of the biological assay, or the date on which the substance was removed from cold storage, after having been kept there continuously at a temperature not exceeding 6° for a period not exceeding two years from the time the biological assay was completed. The date of manufacture should be stated as the month and year.

APPROPRIATE PHARMACEUTICAL ADJUVANTS. This term means additives such as antoxidants, and buffering, dispersing, suspending, wetting and preserving agents, but it does not include flavouring and colouring agents.

POLARS. This term is used to embrace all polarising devices suitable for use in microscopy, including calcite prisms and manufactured polarising disks.

ROOM TEMPERATURE. This is a temperature between 15° and 25°.

PART 1

Drugs
and Pharmaceutical Adjuvants

ACACIA

SYNONYMS: Acac.; Acaciae Gummi; Gum Acacia; Gum Arabic

Acacia is the air-dried gummy exudation from the stem and branches of *Acacia senegal* (L.) Willd. (Fam. Leguminosae), a small tree widely distributed in North, East, and West Africa. It may also be derived from certain other species of *Acacia*.

Varieties. Many varieties of acacia occur in commerce, but the most esteemed is that collected in Kordofan, the best varieties of which are sun-bleached and yellowish-white in colour.

The best qualities of Nigerian and Senegal gum are also suitable for pharmaceutical use. They are more transparent than the bleached Kordofan gum and contain occasional pieces of vermiform shape.

Constituents. Acacia is composed chiefly of the calcium, potassium, and magnesium salts of arabic acid, which on hydrolysis with sulphuric acid (2 per cent v/v) yields L-rhamnopyranose, D-galactopyranose, L-arabofuranose, and an aldobionic acid, 6-β-D-glucuronosido-D-galactose. It also contains small amounts of 4-O-methyl-D-glucuronic acid, diastase, and an oxidase system. It yields about 2·7 to 4 per cent of ash, which consists chiefly of the carbonates of calcium, potassium, and magnesium.

Solubility. Almost entirely soluble in 2 parts of water, forming a slightly acid solution or mucilage which is not glairy; insoluble in alcohol.

Standard

It complies with the requirements of the European Pharmacopoeia.

UNGROUND DRUG. Rounded or ovoid tears, about 0·5 to 4 cm in diameter; tears yellowish-white to pale amber, sometimes with a pinkish tint; either brittle and opaque from the presence of numerous minute fissures, often broken into angular fragments with glistening surfaces, or transparent, breaking with difficulty, and exhibiting a conchoidal fracture. Almost odourless; taste bland and mucilaginous. The loss on drying at 100° to 105° is not more than 15·0 per cent.

A 10 per cent solution in water is laevorotatory.

A 5 per cent solution in water develops a deep blue or bluish-green colour when shaken with 0·5 ml of *diluted hydrogen peroxide solution* and 0·5 ml of *guaiacum tincture* and allowed to stand for a few minutes.

Acacia, in powder, is not stained red with *ruthenium red solution* (distinction from sterculia and agar).

A solution in water does not become cloudy after shaking with *lead acetate solution* and when 0·02N iodine is added to acacia, in powder, the mixture does not acquire a crimson or olive-green colour (distinction from agar and tragacanth).

A solution in water, previously boiled and cooled, does not develop a blue or reddish brown colour with 0·1N iodine (absence of starch and dextrin).

POWDERED DRUG: Powdered Acacia. A white or yellowish-white powder possessing the odour, taste, and characteristic reactions of the unground drug.

Adulterants and substitutes. Many dark-coloured kinds of gum arabic occur in commerce and are used for various industrial purposes.

Gum acacia of Indian origin is obtained from numerous species of *Acacia* and from plants of other families unrelated to Leguminosae; the commercial article collected locally is therefore of a very mixed character and consists of tears of different sizes and colours, the majority being dark brown.

Hygroscopicity. At relative humidities between about 25 and 65 per cent, the equilibrium moisture content of powdered acacia at 25° is between about 8 and 13 per cent, but at relative humidities above about 70 per cent, it absorbs substantial amounts of moisture.

Storage. It should be stored in a cool dry place. Powdered Acacia should be stored in airtight containers.

Uses. Acacia forms viscous solutions with water and is used as a suspending agent, usually with tragacanth, in mixtures containing resinous tinctures or powders which do not readily disperse. A mucilage is prepared by dissolving 40 g of acacia tears, previously rinsed, in 60 ml of chloroform water. The mucilage deteriorates rapidly on storage.

Acacia is an effective emulsifying agent and the powdered gum is used for emulsifying fixed and volatile oils and liquid paraffin; in the case of fixed oils and liquid paraffin, one part of powdered acacia may first be incorporated with four parts of the oil, the subsequent addition of 2 parts of water producing the primary emulsion; volatile oils require twice the proportion of gum and water.

Acacia is a strong binding agent and is used as such in the preparation of lozenges and pastilles, for which it provides slow disintegration and a mucilaginous sensation in the mouth. It is occasionally used in tablets, but care must be taken to avoid prolonging the disintegration time.

Acacia is used chiefly for preparations administered by mouth; it is not suitable for injectable solutions and acacia emulsions or suspensions are usually too sticky for use on the skin.

Preparation

COMPOUND TRAGACANTH POWDER, B.P. It contains 20 per cent of acacia, with tragacanth, starch, and sucrose. It should be stored in airtight containers.

ACETARSOL

SYNONYM: Acetarsone

$C_8H_{10}AsNO_5 = 275·1$

Acetarsol is 3-acetamido-4-hydroxyphenylarsonic acid.

Solubility. Very slightly soluble in cold water; slightly soluble in boiling water; insoluble in alcohol and in dilute acids; soluble in dilute alkalis.

Standard

It complies with the requirements of the British Pharmacopoeia.

It is a white, crystalline, odourless powder and contains not less than 99·0 and not more than the equivalent of 101·0 per cent of $C_8H_{10}AsNO_5$, calculated with reference to the dried substance. The loss on drying under the prescribed conditions is not more than 0·5 per cent. It melts with decomposition at about 240°.

Actions and uses. Acetarsol is used in the treatment of amoebiasis and *Trichomonas vaginalis* vaginitis.

For intestinal amoebiasis, 250 milligrams is given by mouth twice daily for ten days; it is used chiefly for chronic infection and to supplement treatment with emetine or other amoebicides. Acetarsol is excreted slowly after oral administration and care must be taken to allow adequate periods between courses of treatment to avoid accumulation.

Vincent's angina has been treated by the oral administration of 250 to 500 milligrams daily, combined with local application of a paste containing acetarsol.

For *T. vaginalis* vaginitis, acetarsol is applied locally in pessaries or as a powder containing 12·5 per cent of acetarsol in a mixture of equal parts of light kaolin and sodium bicarbonate, a single vaginal insufflation of 4 grams being given. It should not be used during menstruation as toxic amounts may be absorbed.

UNDESIRABLE EFFECTS. Gastro-intestinal disturbances, urticaria, and erythema may occur.

CONTRA-INDICATIONS. It is contra-indicated in liver disease and kidney disease.

POISONING. For the treatment of anaphylactoid reactions, injections of a pressor drug such as adrenaline should be given.

The toxic effects of arsenic, such as exfoliative dermatitis and arsenical encephalopathy, may be treated by intramuscular injections of dimercaprol.

Dose. See above under **Actions and uses.**

Preparations
ACETARSOL PESSARIES, B.P.C. (page 772)
ACETARSOL TABLETS, B.P.C. (page 805)

OTHER NAME: *Stovarsol*®

ACETAZOLAMIDE

$C_4H_6N_4O_3S_2 = 222\cdot2$

Acetazolamide is 5-acetamido-1,3,4-thiadiazole-2-sulphonamide.

$$CH_3\cdot CO\cdot NH \overbrace{}^{S} SO_2\cdot NH_2$$
$$N {=\!=} N$$

Solubility. Slightly soluble in water; soluble, at 20°, in 400 parts of alcohol and in 100 parts of acetone; insoluble in ether, in chloroform, and in carbon tetrachloride.

Standard
It complies with the requirements of the British Pharmacopoeia.
It is a fine, white or yellowish-white, crystalline, odourless powder and contains not less than 99·0 per cent of $C_4H_6N_4O_3S_2$, calculated with reference to the dried substance. The loss on drying under the prescribed conditions is not more than 0·5 per cent.

Actions and uses. Acetazolamide is a specific inhibitor of carbonic anhydrase. It is used as a diuretic and to reduce intra-ocular pressure. It acts on the renal tubules, and when the rate at which carbonic acid is formed is reduced by the inhibition of carbonic anhydrase, hydrogen- and sodium-ion exchange is greatly reduced. As a result, bicarbonate resorption is incomplete and there is an increased volume of alkaline urine. Because of this loss of bicarbonate and water a metabolic acidosis may result.

Acetazolamide is of limited value in the treatment of oedema because, if it is given continuously, the decrease of bicarbonate ion in the extracellular fluid has the effect of decreasing the tubular load. Most of the filtered bicarbonate is then resorbed and the diuresis ceases, but a mild degree of metabolic acidosis may persist. Carbonic anhydrase is inhibited for six hours by a single dose of 250 milligrams of acetazolamide. Renal compensation for the disturbed acid–base balance occurs in the subsequent eighteen hours and the composition of the extracellular fluid is thereby restored to normal. The effect of subsequent doses on consecutive days diminishes and diuresis ceases by the sixth day.

Both acetazolamide and the organic mercurial diuretics alter the acid–base balance, the mercurials causing metabolic alkalosis and acetazolamide an acidosis. In combination, one may correct the disturbance in acid–base balance caused by the other.

As a diuretic, 250 to 500 milligrams of acetazolamide is given by mouth once daily or every other day.

In glaucoma, the initial dose is 500 milligrams, followed by 250 milligrams every six hours; when the intra-ocular tension is normal, the maintenance dosage is 250 milligrams two or three times daily.

UNDESIRABLE EFFECTS. Large doses of acetazolamide may cause drowsiness and numbness and tingling of the face and extremities. If potassium bicarbonate is given with acetazolamide, renal stone formation may occur.

Dose. See above under **Actions and uses.**

Preparation
ACETAZOLAMIDE TABLETS, B.P. Unless otherwise specified, tablets each containing 250 mg of acetazolamide are supplied.

OTHER NAMES: *Acetazide*®; *Diamox*®

ACETIC ACID

Acetic Acid may be prepared by diluting 1 part by weight of Glacial Acetic Acid with 2 parts by weight of Purified Water or by suitably diluting a pure commercial acetic acid, usually one containing 80 per cent of $C_2H_4O_2$.

Solubility. Miscible with water, with alcohol, and with glycerol.

Standard
It complies with the requirements of the British Pharmacopoeia.
It is a clear colourless pungent liquid and contains 32·5 to 33·5 per cent w/w of $C_2H_4O_2$. It has a weight per ml at 20° of 1·040 g to 1·042 g.

Actions and uses. Acetic acid has a mild expectorant action. It is administered by mouth, usually in linctuses, as Oxymel or Squill Oxymel. Applied externally, it has an irritant action and has been used in liniments.

Preparations
ACETIC ACID, DILUTE, B.P. It contains 6·0 per cent w/w of $C_2H_4O_2$.

OXYMEL, B.P.C. (page 764)

SQUILL OXYMEL, B.P.C. (page 765)

GLACIAL ACETIC ACID

SYNONYM: Glac. Acet. Acid $CH_3 \cdot CO_2H$

$C_2H_4O_2 = 60·05$

Glacial Acetic Acid may be readily supercooled. Its vapour burns with a blue flame; the flash-point is about 111°F. Commercial varieties include a technical acid containing not less than 98 per cent of $C_2H_4O_2$.

Solubility. Miscible with water, with alcohol, with chloroform, and with most fixed and volatile oils.

Standard
DESCRIPTION. A translucent crystalline mass or, at temperatures above its crystallising-point, a clear colourless liquid; odour pungent.

IDENTIFICATION TESTS. 1. It is strongly acid, even when freely diluted with water.
2. It boils at about 117°, determined by the method given in Appendix 9B, page 888.
3. When diluted with water and neutralised, it gives the reactions characteristic of acetates.

CRYSTALLISING-POINT. Not lower than 14·8°, determined by Method II of the British Pharmacopoeia for freezing-point.

WEIGHT PER ML. At 20°, 1·048 g to 1·051 g.

ARSENIC. It complies with the test given in Appendix 6, page 877 (2 parts per million).

LEAD. It complies with the test given in Appendix 7, page 881 (3 parts per million).

CHLORIDE. 5 ml complies with the limit test for chlorides (70 parts per million).

SULPHATE. 2·5 ml complies with the limit test for sulphates (240 parts per million).

CERTAIN ALDEHYDIC SUBSTANCES. Not more than 0·05 per cent w/w, calculated as C_2H_4O, determined by the following method:
To about 10 g, accurately weighed, add 50 ml of water and 10 ml of a 1·25 per cent w/v solution of *sodium metabisulphite* in water, allow to stand for 30 minutes, and titrate the excess of sodium metabisulphite with 0·1N iodine. Repeat the procedure omitting the sample. The difference between the two titrations represents the amount of sodium metabisulphite required by the sample; each ml of 0·1N iodine is equivalent to 0·002203 g of C_2H_4O.

FORMIC ACID AND OXIDISABLE IMPURITIES. Mix 5 ml with 10 ml of water and reserve 5 ml for the test for readily oxidisable impurities; to a further 5 ml add 6 ml of *sulphuric acid*, cool, add 2 ml of 0·1N potassium dichromate, allow to stand for one minute, add 25 ml of water and 1 ml of freshly prepared *potassium iodide solution*, and titrate the liberated iodine with 0·1N sodium thiosulphate, using *starch mucilage* as indicator; not less than 1 ml of 0·1N sodium thiosulphate is required.

READILY OXIDISABLE IMPURITIES. To 5 ml of the solution reserved in the determination of formic acid and oxidisable impurities add 20 ml of water and 0·2 ml of 0·1N potassium permanganate and allow to stand for half a minute; the colour is not entirely discharged.

ODOROUS IMPURITIES. Dilute 1·5 ml to 5 ml with water and neutralise to *litmus paper* with *sodium hydroxide solution*; not more than a faint acetous odour is apparent.

NON-VOLATILE MATTER. Not more than 0·01 per cent w/w, the residue being dried at 105°.

CONTENT OF $C_2H_4O_2$. Not less than 99·0 per cent w/w, determined by the following method:
To about 2 g, accurately weighed, add 50 ml of water and titrate with 1N sodium hydroxide, using *phenolphthalein solution* as indicator; each ml of 1N sodium hydroxide is equivalent to 0·06005 g of $C_2H_4O_2$.

Storage. It should be stored in airtight containers.

Uses. Glacial acetic acid is used to prepare dilute acetic acids and Strong Ammonium Acetate Solution. It has been used for the destruction of warts.

POISONING. A stomach tube or emetics should not be used. The acid must be neutralised as quickly as possible. Calcium hydroxide in water and Magnesium Hydroxide Mixture are good antidotes; carbonates should be avoided if possible, as they lead to the liberation of carbon dioxide and the consequent risk of perforation.
After neutralisation of the acid, demulcents such as milk, raw eggs, or a vegetable oil, such as olive oil, should be given, and shock should be treated by warmth and an intravenous infusion if required. Morphine should be given for the relief of pain.
Glacial acetic acid burns should be treated immediately by flooding with water, followed by the application of sodium bicarbonate or chalk in powder, or by sodium bicarbonate or saline packs.

ACETOMENAPHTHONE

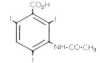

SYNONYM: Acetomenaph.

$C_{15}H_{14}O_4 = 258.3$

Acetomenaphthone is 1,4-diacetoxy-2-methylnaphthalene.

Solubility. Very slightly soluble in water; slightly soluble in cold alcohol; soluble in 3·3 parts of boiling alcohol; soluble in acetic acid.

Standard
It complies with the requirements of the British Pharmacopoeia.
It is a white crystalline powder which is odourless or has a slight odour of acetic acid and contains not less than 98·0 per cent of $C_{15}H_{14}O_4$, calculated with reference to the dried substance. The loss on drying under the prescribed conditions is not more than 0·5 per cent. It has a melting-point of 112° to 115°.

Actions and uses. Acetomenaphthone has actions, uses, and undesirable effects similar to those described under Phytomenadione (page 381), but it acts more slowly and phytomenadione is therefore preferred.

Dose. As a prophylactic against neonatal haemorrhage: 5 to 10 milligrams daily for one week before delivery.
For the pre-operative treatment of obstructive jaundice: 10 to 20 milligrams daily for one week.
For haemorrhagic disease of the newborn: a total of 1 milligram over a period of twenty-four hours; for premature babies, a total of 0·5 milligram over a period of twenty-four hours.

Preparations
ACETOMENAPHTHONE TABLETS, B.P. Unless otherwise specified, tablets each containing 5 mg are supplied. Tablets containing 10 mg are also available.

ACETONE

$C_3H_6O = 58.08$

$CH_3 \cdot CO \cdot CH_3$

Acetone is dimethyl ketone.

Solubility. Miscible with water, with alcohol, with methyl alcohol, with ether, and with chloroform.

Standard
DESCRIPTION. A clear, colourless, inflammable, mobile, volatile liquid; odour characteristic.

IDENTIFICATION TESTS. 1. To 1 ml of a 0·5 per cent v/v solution in water add 1 ml of *sodium nitroprusside solution*, 2 ml of 1N sodium hydroxide, and a slight excess of *acetic acid*; a deep red colour is produced which changes to violet on dilution with water.
2. To 10 ml of a 0·1 per cent v/v solution in *alcohol (50 per cent)* add 1 ml of *2-nitrobenzaldehyde solution*, followed by 1 ml of *sodium hydroxide solution*, allow to stand for about 2 minutes, and acidify with *acetic acid*; a bluish-green colour is produced.

ACIDITY. To 20 ml add 20 ml of *carbon dioxide-free water*, cool, and titrate with 0·1N sodium hydroxide, using *phenolphthalein solution* as indicator; not more than 0·2 ml is required.

ALKALINITY. Add 10 ml to 10 ml of *carbon dioxide-free water*, previously neutralised to 0·05 ml of *methyl red solution*; no change in colour occurs.

DISTILLATION RANGE. Determine by the method given in Appendix 9A, page 887; the temperature at which the first drop falls from the condenser (initial boiling-point) is not lower than 55·7° and the temperature at which the last drop evaporates (dry-point) is not higher than 56·7°.

WEIGHT PER ML. At 20°, 0·789 g to 0·791 g.

READILY OXIDISABLE SUBSTANCES. To 30 ml add 0·1 ml of 0·1N potassium permanganate and allow to stand in the dark for 2 hours at 15°; the colour is not completely discharged.

RESIDUE ON EVAPORATION. Not more than 0·005 per cent w/v, the residue being dried to constant weight at 105°.

WATER-INSOLUBLE MATTER. Mix 1 ml with 19 ml of water; no opalescence is produced.

Storage. It should be stored in airtight containers, in a cool place.

Uses. Acetone is used as a solvent for organic substances, including resins, fats, and pyroxylin, and in some solutions used for film coating tablets. It should not be used as a solvent for iodine, with which it forms a volatile compound which is extremely irritating to the eyes. On account of its low boiling-point it is a suitable menstruum for extracting thermolabile substances from crude drugs. It is an ingredient of some preparations for cleansing the skin before operations.

ACETRIZOIC ACID

$C_9H_6I_3NO_3 = 556.9$

Acetrizoic Acid is 3-acetamido-2,4,6-tri-iodobenzoic acid.

Solubility. Very slightly soluble in water, in ether, and in chloroform; soluble, at 20°, in 20 parts of alcohol; soluble in solutions of alkali hydroxides.

Standard
It complies with the requirements of the British Pharmacopoeia.

It is a white or almost white odourless powder and contains not less than 99·0 and not more than the equivalent of 101·0 per cent of $C_9H_6I_3NO_3$, calculated with reference to the dried substance. The loss on drying under the prescribed conditions is not more than 0·5 per cent.

Sterilisation. Solutions for injection are sterilised by heating in an autoclave or by filtration.

Storage. It should be protected from light.

Actions and uses. Acetrizoic acid, in the form of Sodium Acetrizoate Injection, may be used in radiography as a contrast medium with general properties and dosage similar to those described under Sodium Diatrizoate (page 450). It has, however, been almost entirely replaced by the newer tri-iodo-compounds such as sodium diatrizoate, because they less frequently cause undesirable effects. A 40 per cent viscous solution containing dextran is used for hysterosalpingography and

urethrography. A 30 per cent solution was formerly used for peripheral arteriography, cerebral angiography, cholangiography, and retrograde pyelography, a 50 per cent solution for intravenous pyelography, and a 70 per cent solution for translumbar arteriography and for angiocardiography.

UNDESIRABLE EFFECTS. These are described under Sodium Diatrizoate (page 450), but in addition acetrizoic acid frequently causes pain along the injected vessel and severe vascular spasm.

Preparation

SODIUM ACETRIZOATE INJECTION, B.P. It consists of a sterile solution of sodium acetrizoate in Water for Injections. It may contain suitable buffering and stabilising agents. The strength of the solution should be specified by the prescriber. It should be protected from light.

OTHER NAMES: *Diaginol®*; *Salpix®*

ACONITE

SYNONYM: Aconite Root

Aconite is the dried root of *Aconitum napellus* L. (agg.) (Fam. Ranunculaceae). It is obtained chiefly from plants growing wild in central and southern Europe and is imported mainly from Yugoslavia and Spain. The roots are dried either entire or after being split longitudinally.

Constituents. Aconite contains the alkaloids aconitine (acetylbenzoylaconine), benzoylaconine, aconine, mesaconitine, hypaconitine, neopelline, napelline, and neoline. Traces of ($-$)-ephedrine and sparteine have been reported to be present, but it is to the aconitine only that the toxic action of the root is due. The total amount of alkaloid present varies from 0·2 to 1·5 per cent. The ether-soluble alkaloids (chiefly aconitine) vary in amount, the root usually containing from 0·2 to 0·6 per cent. Other constituents are starch and aconitic acid.

Standard for unground drug

DESCRIPTION. *Macroscopical:* root dark brown, 4 to 10 cm long and 1 to 3 cm wide at crown, bearing numerous rootlets or the scars left by them; smaller daughter roots frequently attached laterally; aerial shoot remains or bud present at crown; fracture short; smoothed, transversely cut surface at about one-third of length from crown showing wide bark separated from inner part by a darker stellate cambium with 5 to 8 projecting angles. Odour faint; taste at first slight, followed by persistent sensation of tingling and numbness.

Microscopical: the diagnostic characters are: Root: *suberised cells* of outer layers, tabular rectangular, about 34 to 55 μm wide with length to breadth ratio of about 4 or 5 to 1, walls brown; *sclereids* occasional, usually isolated, with moderately thick walls, in parenchyma of cortex and pericycle; *cortex* with abundant parenchyma containing small *starch* granules, simple or compound with 2 to 6 components, individual granules 2 to **8** to **16** to 30 μm in diameter; *xylem* vessels with reticulate or bordered pitted walls, or spiral thickenings; *pith* composed of rounded parenchymatous cells; *fibres* and *crystals* of calcium oxalate absent. Stem base present on second year roots: *epidermal cells* with thick outer and thin anticlinal walls; *cortex* narrow, parenchymatous; *vascular bundles* collateral, 30 to 60 arranged in a ring next to the cortex; *fibres* present as pericyclic bundle caps, these frequently fused laterally to form a cylinder with few gaps; *pith* aerenchymatous, with hollow centre; *crystals* of calcium oxalate absent.

ACID-INSOLUBLE ASH. Not more than 1·5 per cent.

AERIAL STEM. Not more than 5·0 per cent.

FOREIGN ORGANIC MATTER. Not more than 2·0 per cent.

CONTENT OF TOTAL ALKALOIDS. Not less than 0·50 per cent, calculated as aconitine, $C_{34}H_{47}NO_{11}$, determined by the following method:
Introduce about 20 g of the root, accurately weighed, and 5 g of acid-washed sand, both in No. 250 powder, into a pear-shaped separator of about 400-ml capacity, add 200 ml of a mixture of 3 volumes of *solvent ether* and 1 volume of *chloroform*, and shake for 15 minutes; add 10 ml of *dilute ammonia solution* and shake occasionally during 1½ hours. Insert a plug of cotton wool into the stem of the separator and allow the liquid to percolate into another separator; when the liquid ceases to flow, pack the drug firmly and continue the percolation with the mixture of solvent ether and chloroform until complete extraction of the alkaloids is effected.
Acidify the percolate in the separator with 1N sulphuric acid and extract with successive quantities of 0·1N sulphuric acid until complete extraction of the alkaloids is effected. Wash the mixed acidic liquids with 10 ml of *chloroform*, and run off the chloroform into a second separator containing 20 ml of 0·1N sulphuric acid, shake, allow to separate, and discard the chloroform; continue the washing with two further successive 5-ml portions of *chloroform*, transferring each to the second separator and washing with the same acidic aqueous liquid as before. Transfer the acidic aqueous washings to the first separator containing the mixed acidic liquids, make alkaline with *dilute ammonia solution*, and shake with successive quantities of *chloroform* until complete extraction of the alkaloids is effected, washing each chloroform solution with the same 20 ml of water.
Remove the chloroform at as low a temperature as possible, add to the residue 2 ml of *alcohol (95 per cent)*, remove the alcohol by evaporation, and dry the residue at 60° for one hour. Dissolve the residue in 2 ml of *alcohol (95 per cent)*, add 20 ml of 0·02N sulphuric acid and titrate with 0·02N sodium hydroxide, using *methyl red solution* as indicator; each ml of 0·02N

sulphuric acid is equivalent to 0.01291 g of $C_{34}H_{47}NO_{11}$.

Standard for powdered drug: Powdered Aconite
DESCRIPTION. A pale greyish-brown powder, possessing the diagnostic microscopical characters, odour, and taste of the unground drug.

ACID-INSOLUBLE ASH; FOREIGN ORGANIC MATTER; CONTENT OF TOTAL ALKALOIDS. It complies with the requirements for the unground drug.

Adulterants and substitutes. Japanese aconite is said to be obtained from *A. japonicum* Thunb. and possibly other species of *Aconitum*; it is distinguished by its dark greyish colour, smaller size, smoother surface, and circular cambium; the root of *A. japonicum* contains japaconitine, which has an action similar to that of aconitine and may be identical with it.
Indian aconite is derived from *A. chasmanthum* Stapf and contains indaconitine. Another Indian (Nepal) aconite (bikh or bish) consists of the root of *A. deinorrhizum* Stapf and of *A. spicatum* Stapf; the larger size and less tapering character sufficiently distinguish it from the official drug. The root of *A. spicatum* contains bikhaconitine; that of *A. deinorrhizum* contains pseudaconitine (acetylveratroylpseudaconine), which is about twice as active as aconitine.
Soviet aconite is derived from *A. tianschanicum* Rupr. and consists of pieces which are composed of 2 to 5 seasons' growth to form a kind of rhizome; it contains about 1.5 to 2 per cent of total alkaloids.
Atis root (*A. heterophyllum* Wall. ex Royle) and the roots of certain other species of *Aconitum* occur in commerce; they contain non-poisonous alkaloids and may be distinguished by their failure to produce a tingling sensation on being chewed.

Actions and uses. The actions of aconite are due to the aconitine it contains. When preparations containing the drug are applied to unbroken skin, they produce tingling followed by numbness, and hence its former use in liniments in the treatment of neuralgia, sciatica, and rheumatism.

UNDESIRABLE EFFECTS. When taken by mouth, aconite affects both the heart and the central nervous system and is one of the most potent and quick-acting of poisons; the heart is first slowed through the vagus centre, but it is also affected directly, its excitability is increased and its co-ordination disturbed so that the blood ebbs and flows without effective circulation. Eventually the heart stops, often suddenly. Respiration is depressed progressively by large doses.

PRECAUTIONS AND CONTRA-INDICATIONS. Because of the danger of absorption, liniments containing aconite should never be used on wounds or even abraded surfaces and the use of aconite in dental periostitis or as a febrifuge is unjustifiable.

POISONING. The stomach should be emptied by gastric lavage, or apomorphine hydrochloride (6 milligrams) should be given subcutaneously. An emetic of mustard or zinc sulphate has been recommended. Atropine should be given, and if there is respiratory depression, artificial respiration should be applied and analeptics given. The patient should be kept lying down and warm.

ADRENALINE

SYNONYMS: Adren.; Epinephrine

$C_9H_{13}NO_3 = 183.2$

$$CH_3 \cdot NH \cdot CH_2 \cdot CH \cdot OH$$

Adrenaline, $(-)$-1-(3,4-dihydroxyphenyl)-2-methylaminoethanol, is an active principle of the medulla of the suprarenal gland and may be obtained from the glands of certain animals or prepared synthetically.

Solubility. Slightly soluble in water; insoluble in alcohol, in ether, in chloroform, in liquid paraffin, and in many other organic solvents; readily soluble in solutions of mineral acids and of alkali hydroxides, but not in solutions of ammonia or of alkali carbonates.

Standard
It complies with the requirements of the British Pharmacopoeia.
It is a white or creamy-white, sphaerocrystalline, odourless powder and contains not less than 98.5 and not more than the equivalent of 101.0 per cent of $C_9H_{13}NO_3$, calculated with reference to the dried substance. The loss on drying under the prescribed conditions is not more than 1.0 per cent. It melts with decomposition at about $212°$. A solution in water is alkaline to litmus.

Stability. It darkens on exposure to air and light. Neutral or alkaline solutions are unstable and rapidly become red on exposure to air.

Incompatibility. It is incompatible with oxidising agents.

Storage. It should be stored in airtight containers, protected from light, preferably in an atmosphere of nitrogen.

Actions and uses. Adrenaline acts on the effector cells of the sympathetic system. Some effector cells that respond to sympathetic-nerve stimulation are stimulated by adrenaline; others are inhibited. At these sites two kinds of receptors are assumed and called, for convenience, alpha and beta.
The alpha receptors are concerned generally with the excitatory effects, including vasoconstriction, dilatation of the pupil, inhibition of the movements of the stomach, intestine, and bladder, and the liberation of glucose from the liver. These effects are usually blocked by adrenergic-blocking agents such as phentolamine, tolazoline, and phenoxybenzamine.
The beta receptors are generally concerned with inhibitory effects, an important exception being the stimulatory effect on the heart; the effects include vasodilatation of the blood vessels of voluntary muscle, acceleration of

the heart rate, increase of the heart output, and relaxation of the uterus and bronchial muscle. The beta receptors can be blocked by propranolol and similar drugs.

Adrenaline and ephedrine show both alpha- and beta-receptor effects, noradrenaline almost entirely alpha-receptor effects, and isoprenaline, orciprenaline, and salbutamol mostly beta-receptor effects. Salbutamol acts mainly on the beta-receptors in the bronchi and the respiratory tract and the cardiac beta-receptors are relatively little affected.

Adrenaline is particularly effective in the treatment of bronchial asthma and may be life-saving in status asthmaticus. It relaxes the constricted bronchial musculature and also reduces bronchial oedema by inducing local vasoconstriction. It is of value in allergic states, such as angioneurotic oedema and urticaria, in anaphylactic shock of any origin, and often in serum sickness. When extrasystoles are present, adrenaline should not be used because of the risk of inducing ventricular fibrillation.

The vasoconstrictor action of adrenaline is used to diminish the absorption and localise the effects of local anaesthetics and to reduce local haemorrhage. For these purposes a concentration of 1 in 200,000 of adrenaline should not be exceeded if more than 50 millilitres is to be injected; higher concentrations such as 1 in 100,000 or 1 in 50,000 are used in dentistry, but the total quantity of adrenaline injected should not exceed 500 micrograms. Solutions of local anaesthetics containing adrenaline should not be used for producing anaesthesia in digits, because the profound ischaemia produced may lead to gangrene. Adrenaline should not be used with cocaine.

For the control of capillary bleeding the local application of a 1 in 5000 solution is usually effective.

Applied to mucous membranes, adrenaline produces ischaemia by constricting the peripheral vessels; it therefore relieves turgescence and is of value in hay fever and laryngeal, nasal, and ophthalmic inflammations; for these purposes, however, phenylephrine is usually preferred.

Noradrenaline or metaraminol is to be preferred to adrenaline as a vasoconstrictor for restoring peripheral vascular collapse.

Adrenaline is usually administered by subcutaneous or intramuscular injection, or by inhalation of a fine mist through the mouth; it is almost ineffective when swallowed. In extreme emergency it may be given intravenously in dilute solution and in reduced dosage. It is usually administered as the acid tartrate.

UNDESIRABLE EFFECTS. In therapeutic doses, adrenaline may cause toxic effects, such as anxiety, fear, tremor, headache, and palpitations. It should not be used in hyperthyroidism or coronary insufficiency, or in the presence of ventricular hyperexcitability produced by chloroform, halothane, cyclopropane, digitalis, mercurial diuretics, or quinidine.

Dose. 200 to 500 micrograms by subcutaneous injection as a single dose.

Preparation
NEUTRAL ADRENALINE EYE-DROPS, B.P.C. (page 688)

ADRENALINE ACID TARTRATE

SYNONYMS: Adren. Tart.; Adrenaline Tartrate; Adrenalinii Tartras; Epinephrine Bitartrate

$C_9H_{13}NO_3,C_4H_6O_6 = 333\cdot3$

Adrenaline Acid Tartrate is the hydrogen tartrate of $(-)$-1-(3,4-dihydroxyphenyl)-2-methylaminoethanol.

Solubility. Soluble, at 20°, in 3 parts of water and in 520 parts of alcohol; very slightly soluble in ether and in chloroform.

Standard
It complies with the requirements of the European Pharmacopoeia.
It is a white to greyish-white, crystalline, odourless powder and contains not less than 99·0 per cent of $C_9H_{13}NO_3,C_4H_6O_6$, calculated with reference to the dried substance. The loss on drying under the prescribed conditions is not more than 0·5 per cent. It melts with decomposition at about 150°. A 5 per cent solution in water has a pH of 3·0 to 4·0.

Stability. It slowly darkens on exposure to air and light. Aqueous solutions have their optimum stability at about pH 3·6.

Incompatibility. It is incompatible with oxidising agents.

Sterilisation. Solutions are sterilised by heating in an autoclave or by filtration.

Storage. It should be stored in airtight containers, protected from light, preferably in an atmosphere of nitrogen.

Actions and uses. Adrenaline acid tartrate has the actions, uses, and undesirable effects described under Adrenaline; 1·8 milligrams of adrenaline acid tartrate is approximately equivalent to 1 milligram of adrenaline.

Dose. 0·4 to 1 milligram by subcutaneous injection as a single dose.

Preparations
ZINC SULPHATE AND ADRENALINE EYE-DROPS, B.P.C. (page 696)
ADRENALINE INJECTION, B.P. (*Syn.* Adrenaline Tartrate Injection). It consists of a sterile solution containing adrenaline acid tartrate equivalent to adrenaline 1 in 1000. It should be protected from light. Dose: 0·2 to 0·5 millilitre by subcutaneous injection as a single

dose; for status asthmaticus and other allergic emergencies, this is followed by 0·05 millilitre per minute by subcutaneous injection.

LIGNOCAINE AND ADRENALINE INJECTION, B.P. It consists of a sterile solution of lignocaine hydrochloride and adrenaline acid tartrate in Water for Injections containing 0·1 per cent of sodium metabisulphite. The percentage w/v of lignocaine hydrochloride and the proportion of adrenaline base in the injection should be stated on the label. It should be protected from light.

PROCAINE AND ADRENALINE INJECTION, B.P. (*Syn.* Strong Procaine and Adrenaline Injection). It consists of a sterile solution containing 2 per cent of procaine hydrochloride and Adrenaline Solution equivalent to adrenaline 1 in 50,000. It should be protected from light.

ADRENALINE SOLUTION, B.P. (*Syn.* Adrenaline Tartrate Solution). It contains adrenaline acid tartrate equivalent to adrenaline 1 in 1000. It should be stored in well-filled containers, protected from light.

ADRENALINE AND ATROPINE SPRAY, COMPOUND, B.P.C. (page 794)

ALCOHOL (95 PER CENT)

Alcohol (95 per cent) is a mixture of ethyl alcohol, $CH_3 \cdot CH_2OH$ (ethanol), and water.

Solubility. Miscible with water, with ether, and with chloroform; when mixed with water, contraction of volume and rise of temperature occur.

Standard
It complies with the requirements of the British Pharmacopoeia.
It is a clear, colourless, mobile, volatile liquid with a characteristic spirituous odour and contains 94·7 to 95·2 per cent v/v or 92·0 to 92·7 per cent w/w of C_2H_6O. It boils at about 78° and is readily inflammable, burning with a blue smokeless flame. It has a specific gravity (20°/20°) of 0·8119 to 0·8139.

Dilute alcohols. Dilute alcohols of various strengths may be prepared by diluting Alcohol (95 per cent) with Purified Water in the proportions stated below. Before the final adjustment of volume is made, the mixture is cooled to the same temperature, about 20°, as that at which the alcohol (95 per cent) was measured. The dilute alcohols comply with the chemical tests for purity of the British Pharmacopoeia given under Alcohol (95 per cent) and with specified limits for specific gravity and refractive index.

Alcohol (90 per cent) (*Syn.* Rectified Spirit). Dilute 947 ml of alcohol (95 per cent) to 1000 ml with purified water. It contains 89·6 to 90·5 per cent v/v of C_2H_6O.

Alcohol (80 per cent). Dilute 842 ml of alcohol (95 per cent) to 1000 ml with purified water. It contains 79·5 to 80·3 per cent v/v of C_2H_6O.

Alcohol (70 per cent). Dilute 737 ml of alcohol (95 per cent) to 1000 ml with purified water. It contains 69·5 to 70·4 per cent v/v of C_2H_6O.

Alcohol (60 per cent). Dilute 632 ml of alcohol (95 per cent) to 1000 ml with purified water. It contains 59·7 to 60·2 per cent v/v of C_2H_6O.

Alcohol (50 per cent). Dilute 526 ml of alcohol (95 per cent) to 1000 ml with purified water. It contains 49·6 to 50·2 per cent v/v of C_2H_6O.

Alcohol (45 per cent). Dilute 474 ml of alcohol (95 per cent) to 1000 ml with purified water. It contains 44·7 to 45·3 per cent v/v of C_2H_6O.

Alcohol (25 per cent). Dilute 263 ml of alcohol (95 per cent) to 1000 ml with purified water. It contains 24·6 to 25·4 per cent v/v of C_2H_6O.

Alcohol (20 per cent). Dilute 210 ml of alcohol (95 per cent) to 1000 ml with purified water. It contains 19·5 to 20·5 per cent v/v of C_2H_6O.

Proof spirit. Proof spirit (Spiritus Tenuior) is defined legally as "that which at the temperature of 51° by Fahrenheit's thermometer weighs exactly twelve-thirteenth parts of an equal measure of distilled water". It has a specific gravity (60°/60°F) of 0·9198 and contains about 57·1 per cent v/v or 49·2 per cent w/w of C_2H_6O. Spirits are described in terms of so many degrees over or under proof (O.P. or U.P.), according to the quantity of distilled water which must be added to, or deducted from, 100 volumes of the sample in order to produce spirit of proof strength. The "Proof Gallon" is the unit of alcohol for revenue purposes.

Bulk gallons of "over proof" alcohol may be converted into "proof gallons" by multiplying by the factor

$$\frac{100 + \text{the number of degrees over proof}}{100},$$

and "under proof" alcohol by the factor

$$\frac{100 - \text{the number of degrees under proof}}{100}.$$

An alternative method of indicating spirit strength is sometimes used on the labels of alcoholic beverages. The strength is given as a number of degrees, proof spirit being taken as 100°; for example, a spirit stated to be "70°" would be 30° under proof and would contain 70 per cent of proof spirit. Alcohol (95 per cent) corresponds to about 66° over proof, and 100 volumes thus contain about as much C_2H_6O as 166 volumes of proof spirit. If 100 volumes of alcohol (95 per cent) are diluted to 166 volumes with water, the resulting spirit is of approximately proof strength.

Sterilisation. Alcohol is sterilised by heating in sealed ampoules in an autoclave or by filtration.

Storage. It should be stored in airtight containers, in a cool place.

Actions and uses. The action of alcohol on the central nervous system is depressant and is most marked on the cerebral cortex and on its inhibitory functions. By masking hesitancy, circumspection, and self-criticism, alcohol in small doses may appear initially to stimulate, especially in surroundings which are conducive to excitement; without such an environment its action is usually hypnotic. The effect of small amounts may be to postpone the onset of fatigue and to increase the work done, as long as the task involved is simple.

Alcohol is rapidly absorbed when taken by mouth, but only 10 to 15 millilitres is metabolised per hour; this and the action of alcohol on the central nervous system limit its food value, but it is useful in illness and convalescence when appetite is deficient and the assimilation of ordinary food is impaired. It also produces peripheral vasodilatation which increases heat loss.

Preparations containing high concentrations of alcohol irritate the stomach and produce gastritis if taken habitually, but small amounts adequately diluted help digestion by inhibiting emotions such as anxiety and anger. Any alcohol which is not metabolised has a diuretic action and is excreted mainly in the urine, but traces can be detected in the breath.

Concentrations of 80 per cent or more are sometimes injected into ganglia or around nerve trunks to destroy them and to relieve severe and chronic pain.

Solutions containing from 2·5 to 10 per cent of alcohol, with about 5 per cent of dextrose, in Water for Injections are used by intravenous drip as a source of calories in malnutrition and post-operatively. The rate of administration should not exceed the equivalent of 15 millilitres of alcohol per hour.

Alcohol is a valuable solvent and preservative. In appropriate strengths it is used in the manufacture of tinctures, spirits, and many other galenical preparations. For external use, industrial methylated spirit and Surgical Spirit may be used.

Alcohol has some antibacterial action, but it is not a reliable bactericide.

UNDESIRABLE EFFECTS. The consumption of small amounts of alcohol impairs the ability of an individual to carry out tasks involving discrimination or selection; accuracy is diminished and the amount of work done may be reduced, even though the subject feels particularly efficient. Such loss of efficiency is important when the control of mechanically propelled vehicles is concerned.

A limited tolerance to the action of alcohol on the brain may develop, and addiction to alcohol usually involves tolerance to other aliphatic narcotics and anaesthetics.

Alcohol increases, sometimes dangerously, the intensity and duration of action of barbiturates, and increases the sedative action of antihistamine drugs.

DEPENDENCE. Dependence of the barbiturate–alcohol type is described under Phenobarbitone (page 366).

POISONING. In acute alcoholic poisoning the stomach should be washed out and respiration sustained, if depressed, by analeptics and artificial respiration.

Preparations
SPIRIT EAR-DROPS, B.P.C. (page 666)
LEAD LOTION, EVAPORATING, B.P.C. (page 728)

DEHYDRATED ALCOHOL

SYNONYMS: Absolute Alcohol; Ethanol

$C_2H_6O = 46·07$

$CH_3·CH_2OH$

Solubility. Miscible with water, with ether, and with chloroform; when mixed with water, contraction and rise of temperature occur.

Standard
It complies with the requirements of the British Pharmacopoeia.
It is a clear, colourless, mobile, volatile, very hygroscopic liquid with a characteristic spirituous odour and contains 99·4 to 100·0 per cent v/v or 99·0 to 100·0 per cent w/w of C_2H_6O. It is readily inflammable, burning with a blue smokeless flame. It has a specific gravity (20°/20°) of 0·7904 to 0·7935.

Storage. It should be stored in airtight containers, in a cool place.

Uses. Dehydrated alcohol is used as a solvent and dehydrating agent and for the destruction of nerve tissue.

ALGINIC ACID

Alginic Acid is a polyuronic acid composed of residues of D-mannuronic and L-guluronic acids and is obtained chiefly from algae belonging to the Phaeophyceae, mainly species of *Laminaria*.

The algae from which alginic acid is obtained grow in large quantities off the west coasts of Scotland and Ireland. A small proportion of the acid groups of alginic acid may be neutralised with sodium carbonate in order to produce a more granular and less bulky material. Alginic acid has an equivalent weight of about 200.

Solubility. Insoluble in water and in organic solvents; soluble in solutions of alkali hydroxides.

Standard
DESCRIPTION. A white to pale yellowish-brown powder; odourless or almost odourless.

IDENTIFICATION TESTS. 1. To 5 mg add 5 ml of water, 1 ml of a freshly prepared 1 per cent w/v solution of *naphthoresorcinol* in *alcohol (95 per cent)* and 5 ml of *hydrochloric acid*; boil for 3 minutes, cool, add 5 ml of water, and extract with 15 ml of *isopropyl ether*. Repeat the test without the sample; the isopropyl ether extract from the sample exhibits a deeper purple colour than that from the blank.

2. To 5 ml of a 0·5 per cent solution in 0·1N sodium hydroxide add 1 ml of *calcium chloride solution*; a voluminous gelatinous precipitate is formed.

ARSENIC. It complies with the test given in Appendix 6, page 877 (3 parts per million).

IRON. Ignite 1·66 g, cool, dissolve the residue in 3 ml of *hydrochloric acid FeT*, and dilute to 50 ml with water; 4 ml of this solution complies with the limit test for iron (300 parts per million).

LEAD. It complies with the test given in Appendix 7, page 881 (10 parts per million).

LOSS ON DRYING. Not more than 18·0 per cent, determined by drying to constant weight at 105°.

SULPHATED ASH. Not more than 7·0 per cent.

ACID VALUE. Not less than 230, calculated with reference to the substance dried under the prescribed conditions, determined by the following method:

Suspend about 1 g, accurately weighed, in a mixture of 50 ml of water and 30 ml of 0·25M calcium acetate, shake thoroughly, allow to stand for one hour, and titrate the liberated acetic acid with 0·1N sodium hydroxide, using *phenolphthalein solution* as indicator. Repeat the procedure omitting the sample. Calculate the acid value from the following formula:

$$\text{Acid value} = \frac{(A - B) \times 5 \cdot 61 \times 100}{W(100 - L)},$$

where A = volume, in ml, of 0·1N sodium hydroxide used in the titration with the sample,

B = volume, in ml, of 0·1N sodium hydroxide used in the blank titration,
W = weight, in g, of the sample taken, and
L = percentage loss on drying of the sample.

Sterilisation. It is sterilised by heating in an autoclave. Solutions of soluble alginates may be similarly sterilised. Some loss of viscosity usually occurs in solutions prepared from sterilised alginic acid and in sterilised alginate solutions to an extent which varies according to the nature of the other substances present.

Uses. Alginic acid is used as a tablet disintegrant and binder; it is preferably incorporated by a dry-mixing process.

ALLOPURINOL

$C_5H_4N_4O = 136 \cdot 1$

Allopurinol is 1*H*-pyrazolo[3,4-*d*]pyrimidin-4-ol.

Solubility. Very slightly soluble in water and in alcohol; insoluble in ether and in chloroform; soluble in solutions of alkali hydroxides.

Standard
It complies with the requirements of the British Pharmacopoeia.
It is a white or almost white, microcrystalline, odourless powder and contains not less than 98·0 and not more than the equivalent of 101·0 per cent of $C_5H_4N_4O$, calculated with reference to the dried substance. The loss on drying under the prescribed conditions is not more than 0·5 per cent.

Actions and uses. Allopurinol, by inhibiting xanthine oxidase, reduces the formation of uric acid from mono- and di-substituted purines. Serum levels of hypoxanthine and xanthine, however, remain low because of their high renal clearance rates and because of their re-entry into purine metabolic processes. Serum and urine levels of uric acid therefore fall and are maintained at normal levels so long as therapy is continued regularly.
Acute attacks of gout may be precipitated in the early stages of therapy, particularly if the drug is started in full dosage, but after some weeks or months attacks become infrequent and finally stop altogether; tophi also gradually diminish in size and may finally disappear.
Allopurinol is useful, not only in reducing the incidence of attacks of gout, lessening tophi, and rendering plasma uric acid levels normal, but also in reducing the incidence of urinary calculi and possibly in preventing damage to the kidneys. Impaired renal function is therefore not a contra-indication, but rather an added indication in suitable cases, whereas uricosuric agents may become ineffective in advanced renal failure. The kidneys of patients about to undergo treatment for conditions likely to release large amounts of uric acid into the circulation, such as deep X-ray or cytotoxic therapy for lymphosarcoma, polycythaemia, or leukaemia, are best protected by allopurinol started before such therapy commences and continued throughout it.

Allopurinol will prevent elevation of plasma uric acid levels in thiazide-treated patients and allow such treatment to be given to patients with gout and congestive heart failure when diuresis is an essential part of treatment. If allopurinol alone is not enough to restore normal levels of plasma uric acid, a uricosuric agent, such as probenecid or sulphinpyrazone, may be given in addition, but this should only occasionally be necessary.
Treatment is continuous and it is best to start with small doses such as 50 milligrams two or three times a day to prevent precipitation of acute attacks of gout and to increase the dose by 50 milligrams daily every week until the serum uric acid level is in the normal range. An effective final dosage is usually between 300 and 600 milligrams daily in divided doses. To prevent acute attacks of gout in the early stages of treatment a suitable analgesic such as 500 micrograms of colchicine may be given two or three times a day.
Allopurinol may be used for the prevention of uric acid nephropathy due to excessive nucleoprotein catabolism in neoplastic disease, especially during treatment with X-rays or cytotoxic drugs. The usual dosage is 600 milligrams daily in divided doses for adults or 8 milligrams per kilogram body-weight for children, beginning two or three days before the X-irradiation or cytotoxic treatment and reducing to about half these doses if prolonged treatment is necessary to control the serum uric acid level.

UNDESIRABLE EFFECTS. Toxic effects are uncommon and are rarely severe. They include maculopapular rashes, pruritus, nausea, and, very rarely, vomiting, diarrhoea, abdominal pain, malaise, fever, and headaches.

Dose. See above under **Actions and uses.**

Preparation
ALLOPURINOL TABLETS, B.P. Unless otherwise specified, tablets each containing 100 mg of allopurinol are supplied.

OTHER NAME: *Zyloric*®

ALMOND OIL

Synonym: Oleum Amygdalae

Almond Oil is the fixed oil obtained by cold expression from the seeds of *Prunus amygdalus* Batsch. var. *dulcis* (DC.) Koehne (sweet almond) or of *P. amygdalus* Batsch. var. *amara* (DC.) Focke (bitter almond) (Fam. Rosaceae). Both varieties are cultivated in countries bordering on the Mediterranean Sea; supplies are derived mainly from bitter almond.

Constituents. Almond oil consists of glycerides, the fatty acid constituents of which are chiefly oleic acid and smaller amounts of linoleic, palmitic, and myristic acids.

Solubility. Very slightly soluble in alcohol; miscible with ether, with chloroform, and with light petroleum.

Standard
It complies with the requirements of the British Pharmacopoeia.
It is a pale yellow oil with a slight characteristic odour. It has a weight per ml at 20° of 0·910 g to 0·915 g. Almond Oil remains clear after exposure to a tem-

perature of −10° for three hours and does not congeal until the temperature has been reduced to about −18°.

Sterilisation. It is sterilised by dry heat.

Storage. It should be stored in well-filled airtight containers.

Actions and uses. Almond oil has properties similar to those of olive oil (page 336). It is used in emollient preparations for the skin and as a vehicle for oily injections.

Dose. 15 to 30 millilitres.

ALOES

Synonym: Aloe

Aloes is the solid residue obtained by evaporating the liquid which drains from the leaves cut from various species of *Aloë* (Fam. Liliaceae). The juice is concentrated by spontaneous evaporation, or more generally by boiling, and poured into boxes or other suitable receptacles; on cooling, it solidifies.

Varieties. Cape aloes is prepared in Cape Province from *A. ferox* Mill. and possibly from hybrids of *A. ferox* with other species. Curaçao aloes is obtained from *A. barbadensis* Mill. on the islands of Curaçao, Aruba, and Bonaire; it was formerly produced on the island of Barbados and is still frequently, but improperly, called Barbados aloes.

Constituents. Aloes contains the pale yellow crystalline substance barbaloin, a 10-glucopyranosyl derivative of aloe-emodin anthrone (10-deoxyglucosyl-9,10-dihydro-1,8-dihydroxy-3-hydroxymethyl-9-oxoanthracene). In Curaçao aloes this is accompanied by isobarbaloin, little or none of which is found in Cape aloes; there is also present in Cape aloes an amorphous β-barbaloin and aloinosides A and B. Aloinoside B is an 11-mono-α-L-rhamnoside of barbaloin.
Other constituents of aloes are resin and aloe-emodin (9,10-dihydro-1,8-dihydroxy-3-hydroxymethyl-9,10-dioxoanthracene). The resin of Cape aloes may partly consist of capaloresinotannol combined with *p*-coumaric acid; the resin of Curaçao aloes contains also barbaloresinotannol combined with cinnamic acid; these resins may be associated with condensation products of anthraquinones and anthranols.
Good Curaçao aloes may yield up to 30 per cent of crystallisable aloins; Cape aloes may yield nearly 10 per cent of crystallisable aloins and about 40 per cent of amorphous aloin.

Solubility. Almost entirely soluble in alcohol (60 per cent).

Standard
It complies with the requirements of the British Pharmacopoeia.
Cape aloes contains not less than 15 per cent and Curaçao aloes not less than 30 per cent of anhydrous barbaloin, both calculated with reference to the air-dried drug.

Unground drug. *Macroscopical characters:* Cape aloes: dark brown or greenish-brown glassy masses; thin fragments transparent, exhibiting a yellowish or

reddish-brown tinge; fracture clean and glassy; odour distinctive, somewhat acid.
Curaçao aloes: dark chocolate-brown, usually in opaque masses; fracture dull, waxy, uniform, and frequently conchoidal; occasional specimens vitreous; penetrating characteristic odour reminiscent of iodoform.
Taste nauseous and bitter.

Microscopical characters: mounted in *lactophenol*: Cape aloes composed of fragments, usually amorphous but sometimes having crystals embedded; Curaçao aloes appearing as fragments composed of numerous small acicular crystals.

Powdered drug: Powdered Aloes. A yellowish-brown to dark reddish-brown powder, possessing the diagnostic microscopical characters, odour, and taste of the unground drug.
The following tests may be used to identify aloes and distinguish the varieties.
Shake 0·1 g, in powder or small pieces, with 10 ml of *ferric chloride solution* mixed with 5 ml of *hydrochloric acid*, and immerse in a water-bath for about 10 minutes; filter immediately, cool the filtrate, and extract with 10 ml of *carbon tetrachloride*; separate the carbon tetrachloride layer, wash with 5 ml of water, and shake with 5 ml of *dilute ammonia solution*; a rose-pink to cherry-red colour is produced in the ammoniacal layer (presence of anthraquinone derivatives).
Prepare a 1 per cent solution by boiling aloes with water until nearly dissolved, adding *kieselguhr*, and filtering until clear. Add 0·2 g of *borax* to 5 ml of the filtrate, and dissolve by boiling; a few drops of the resulting solution gives a green fluorescence when added to water (presence of anthranols). Another portion of the filtrate gives a copious, pale yellow precipitate when mixed with an equal volume of freshly prepared *bromine solution* (presence of aloin). Mix 5 ml of the filtrate with 2 ml of *nitric acid*; that prepared from Cape aloes gives a yellowish-brown colour, passing rapidly to a vivid green; with Curaçao aloes, the colour is a deep brownish-red (distinction from Socotrine aloes, which gives a pale brownish-yellow colour,

and from Zanzibar aloes, which gives a yellowish-brown colour). Dilute 1 ml of the filtrate to 10 ml with water, add 0·05 ml of *copper sulphate solution*, 0·5 ml of *brine*, and 1 ml of *alcohol* (*95 per cent*), and warm gently; Curaçao aloes gives a reddish-violet colour and Cape aloes a faint evanescent violet tint (presence of isobarbaloin, and distinction from Zanzibar and Socotrine aloes).

Adulterants and substitutes. Socotrine aloes occurs in hard dark-brown or nearly black opaque masses, with an uneven porous fracture and an unpleasant cheesy odour. It is prepared to a certain extent on the island of Socotra, but probably more largely on the African and possibly also on the Arabian mainland, from the leaves of *A. perryi* Baker; it is imported usually in a pasty condition in kegs, and subsequent drying is necessary.
Zanzibar aloes is livery-brown and has a nearly smooth, slightly porous fracture; its odour is slight and not disagreeable. It was usually imported in masses partly covered with leaves, or in skins.
Natal aloes, believed to be derived from *A. spectabilis* Reynolds, has been imported; it resembles Cape aloes in odour, but is opaque; when the powder is mixed with *sulphuric acid* and the vapour of *nitric acid* blown over it, a deep blue coloration is produced.

Actions and uses. Aloes is a purgative; it is administered by mouth and after absorption is excreted partly into the colon and partly in the urine. A dose of 125 to 200 milligrams takes from eight to twelve hours to produce an effect. Antispasmodics may be added to prevent griping. It colours alkaline urine red.

UNDESIRABLE EFFECTS. Aloes causes some pelvic congestion.

PRECAUTIONS AND CONTRA-INDICATIONS. Aloes should not be given when there is intestinal irritation, or to pregnant women. In nursing mothers, it may be excreted in the milk.

Dose. 100 to 300 milligrams.

Preparation
BENZOIN TINCTURE, COMPOUND, B.P.C. (page 820)

ALOIN

Aloin is a crystalline substance obtained chiefly from Curaçao aloes, but also from Cape aloes. It may be extracted from aloes by means of hot acidified water and subsequently purified and crystallised.

Constituents. Aloin consists almost entirely of crystalline barbaloin, a 10-glucopyranosyl derivative of aloe-emodin anthrone (10-deoxyglucosyl-9,10-dihydro-1,8-dihydroxy-3-hydroxymethyl-9-oxoanthracene).

Solubility. Almost entirely soluble, at 20°, in 130 parts of water; soluble in alcohol and in acetone; very slightly soluble in ether and in chloroform.

Standard
DESCRIPTION. A pale or dull yellow crystalline powder; odourless or almost odourless.

IDENTIFICATION TESTS. 1. To 5 mg add 5 ml of *dilute ammonia solution*; a yellow colour is produced which changes to green and finally to brown. The solution gives a yellow fluorescence in ultraviolet light (distinction from aloes and amorphous aloin).

2. When mounted in *cresol* and examined microscopically the material does not dissolve and shines brightly on a dark field when viewed between crossed polars (distinction from amorphous aloin).

ACIDITY OR ALKALINITY. A saturated solution in *carbon dioxide-free water* is neutral or not more than slightly acid to *litmus solution*.

LIGHT ABSORPTION. The extinction of a 1-cm layer of a 0·0025 per cent w/v freshly prepared solution in water, calculated with reference to the substance dried to constant weight at 60°, at 298 nm is about 0·55, and at 354 nm, about 0·61; the ratio of the extinction at 354 nm to that at 298 nm is greater than 1·0 (absence of amorphous aloin).

WATER-INSOLUBLE MATTER. Not more than 1·5 per cent, determined by the following method:
Shake frequently during 2 hours about 1 g, accurately weighed, with 120 ml of water, maintaining the temperature at 25°, and filter through a sintered-glass filter; wash the residue with 25 ml of water and dry to constant weight at 105°.

ASH. Not more than 0·5 per cent.

Adulterants and substitutes. Amorphous aloin is obtained from Cape aloes; it is distinguished by its ready solubility in water and in *cresol*, by its invisibility on a dark field when viewed between crossed polars, and by the blue fluorescence in ultra-violet light of its solution in *dilute ammonia solution*.

Actions and uses. Aloin has actions and uses similar to those of aloes.

Dose. 15 to 60 milligrams.

Preparation
PHENOLPHTHALEIN PILLS, COMPOUND, B.P.C. (page 774)

ALUM

SYNONYMS: Alumen; Potash Alum; Potassium Aluminium Sulphate

$KAl(SO_4)_2,12H_2O = 474\cdot4$

Solubility. Very soluble in water and in glycerol; insoluble in alcohol.

Standard
It complies with the requirements of the European Pharmacopoeia.
It occurs as odourless, colourless, transparent, crystalline masses or a granular powder and contains not less than 99·0 per cent of $KAl(SO_4)_2,12H_2O$. A 10 per cent solution in water has a pH of 3·0 to 3·5.

When heated, it melts, and at about 200° loses its water of crystallisation with the formation of the anhydrous salt.

Actions and uses. Alum precipitates proteins and is a powerful astringent. It is now seldom given by mouth.
Dilute solutions (1 to 4 per cent) have been

used as astringent mouth-washes and gargles; a 2 per cent solution has been used for application to the skin to reduce excessive perspiration. Stronger solutions (5 or 10 per cent) are used to harden the skin, especially of the feet.

Alum, diluted with 6 parts of purified talc, has been used as a foot powder.

ALUMINIUM HYDROXIDE GEL

SYNONYM: Alum. Hydrox. Gel

Aluminium Hydroxide Gel is an aqueous suspension of hydrated aluminium oxide containing varying quantities of basic aluminium carbonate.

Aluminium Hydroxide Gel may be prepared by the interaction in aqueous solution of an aluminium salt and a suitable alkali such as ammonium carbonate or sodium carbonate and washing the precipitate. A suitable preservative, such as 0·5 per cent w/w of Sodium Benzoate, and, as a flavouring agent, 0·015 per cent v/v of Peppermint Oil are added; Saccharin Sodium may be added as a sweetening agent.

Standard
It complies with the requirements of the British Pharmacopoeia.
It is a white viscous suspension from which small amounts of clear liquid may separate on standing; it may exhibit thixotropic properties. It contains 3·5 to 4·4 per cent w/w of Al_2O_3. A 50 per cent dilution in water has a pH of not more than 7·5.

Storage. It should be stored at a temperature not exceeding 25°, but should not be allowed to freeze.

Actions and uses. Aluminium hydroxide gel is a useful slow-acting antacid; it is mildly astringent and may therefore cause constipation. It adsorbs small quantities of phosphate and vitamins from the gastro-intestinal tract, but this is probably of little significance unless the diet is low in these substances.

Aluminium hydroxide gel is used in the treatment of peptic ulcer and hyperchlorhydria; it may be administered diluted with water or milk. In peptic ulcer it is given every two hours just after food; during convalescence it is given every four hours.

Aluminium hydroxide gel, diluted with 2 to 3 parts of water, may also be given by intragastric drip, the rate of flow being from 15 to 20 drops a minute throughout the day.

UNDESIRABLE EFFECTS. Aluminium hydroxide gel diminishes the absorption of the tetracyclines from the gut and is therefore pharmacologically incompatible with them.

Dose. 7·5 to 15 millilitres, repeated in accordance with the needs of the patient.

Preparation
ALUMINIUM HYDROXIDE AND BELLADONNA MIXTURE, B.P.C. (page 735)

OTHER NAMES: *Aludrox®*; Aluminium Hydroxide Mixture

DRIED ALUMINIUM HYDROXIDE GEL

SYNONYM: Dried Alum. Hydrox. Gel

Dried Aluminium Hydroxide Gel consists mainly of hydrated aluminium oxide, together with varying quantities of basic aluminium carbonate.

Dried Aluminium Hydroxide Gel may be prepared by drying under suitable conditions the precipitate formed by the interaction in aqueous solution of an aluminium salt with ammonium carbonate or sodium carbonate.

Solubility. Insoluble in water and in alcohol; soluble in dilute mineral acids and in excess of caustic alkalis.

Standard
It complies with the requirements of the British Pharmacopoeia.
It is a fine, white, odourless powder containing some aggregates. It contains not less than 47·0 per cent of Al_2O_3. A 4 per cent suspension in water has a pH of not more than 10·0.

Stability. Heating to temperatures much in excess of 30° results in gradual dehydration and loss of therapeutic value; partial loss of neutralising activity may occur during tabletting.

Hygroscopicity. At relative humidities between about 15 and 70 per cent, the equilibrium moisture content at 25° is between about 17 and 20 per cent, but at relative humidities above 75 per cent, the powder absorbs substantial amounts of moisture.

Storage. It should be stored in airtight containers at a temperature not exceeding 25°.

Actions and uses. Dried aluminium hydroxide gel has the actions, uses, and undesirable effects described under Aluminium Hydroxide Gel.

Dose. 0·5 to 1 gram, repeated in accordance with the needs of the patient.

Preparations
ALUMINIUM HYDROXIDE TABLETS, B.P. Each tablet contains 500 mg of dried aluminium hydroxide gel, with peppermint oil. They should be stored in airtight containers at a temperature not exceeding 25°. Dose: 1 or 2 tablets; they should be chewed before being swallowed.
MAGNESIUM TRISILICATE TABLETS, COMPOUND, B.P.C. (page 812)

OTHER NAMES: *Alocol-P®*; *Aludrox®*; Aluminium Hydroxide Powder

ALUMINIUM MAGNESIUM SILICATE

Aluminium Magnesium Silicate is a native colloidal hydrated aluminium magnesium silicate (saponite) freed from gritty particles.

A number of different grades of aluminium magnesium silicate are available which are distinguished by the degree of alkalinity and the viscosity of an aqueous dispersion. With an average pharmaceutical grade, the pH of a 4 per cent dispersion in water is about 9 and the viscosity of a 5 per cent dispersion is about 250 centipoises.

Solubility. Insoluble in water, but swells to form a colloidal dispersion; insoluble in organic solvents.

Standard
DESCRIPTION. *Macroscopical:* Small creamy-white flakes or a creamy-white powder; odourless or almost odourless.
Microscopical: Aluminium magnesium silicate consists of a powder or of flakes varying in shape and in size from about 0·3 by 0·4 mm to 1·0 by 2·0 mm and about 25 to 240 μm thick; many of the flakes are perforated by scattered circular holes about 20 to **50** to 120 μm in diameter. Between crossed polars on a dark field innumerable bright specks are seen scattered over the flakes.

IDENTIFICATION TEST. Fuse 1 g with 2 g of *anhydrous sodium carbonate*, warm the residue with water, filter, acidify the filtrate with *hydrochloric acid*, evaporate to dryness, and warm the residue with *dilute hydrochloric acid*; a residue of silica is obtained, and the solution, after filtration and neutralisation with *dilute ammonia solution*, gives the reactions characteristic of aluminium and of magnesium.

ALKALINITY. Disperse 1·0 g in 50 ml of water and titrate with 0·1N hydrochloric acid until the pH of the dispersion has been reduced to pH 4·0; not more than 10·0 ml of 0·1N hydrochloric acid is required.

ARSENIC. It complies with the test given in Appendix 6, page 877 (3 parts per million).

LOSS ON DRYING. Not more than 10·0 per cent, determined by drying to constant weight at 105°.

RESIDUE ON IGNITION. Not less than 83·0 per cent, determined by igniting to constant weight at about 800°.

Uses. Aluminium magnesium silicate is available in a number of different grades, all of which are used, usually at a concentration of 0·5 to 2·5 per cent, for their suspending, thickening, and emulsion-stabilising properties. Dispersions in water are thixotropic and at a concentration of 10 per cent a firm gel is formed. The viscosity of dispersions is increased by heating, by the addition of electrolytes, and, at higher concentrations, by ageing.
When used in conjunction with other suspending agents such as methylcellulose and sodium carboxymethylcellulose, the dispersions produced have an enhanced viscosity; it can also be used in conjunction with natural gums such as acacia.
Aluminium magnesium silicate is also used as a binder and disintegrant in tablets.

OTHER NAME: *Veegum®*

ALUMINIUM PHOSPHATE GEL

SYNONYM: Alum. Phos. Gel

Aluminium Phosphate Gel is an aqueous suspension of aluminium orthophosphate.

Aluminium Phosphate Gel may be prepared by precipitation from a solution of an aluminium salt by the addition of a suitable alkali phosphate such as sodium phosphate. A suitable preservative is added and Peppermint Oil, 0·01 per cent v/v, is added as a flavouring agent; Saccharin Sodium may be added as a sweetening agent.

Standard
It complies with the requirements of the British Pharmacopoeia.
It is a white viscous suspension, from which small amounts of clear liquid may separate on standing, and contains not less than 7·0 and not more than 8·0 per cent w/w of $AlPO_4$. A 50 per cent dilution with carbon dioxide-free water has a pH of 5·0 to 6·0.

Storage. It should be stored at a temperature not exceeding 30°; it should not be allowed to freeze.

Actions and uses. Aluminium phosphate gel has the actions, uses, and undesirable effects described under Aluminium Hydroxide Gel to which it is a useful alternative for patients on restricted diets low in phosphates because, unlike the Hydroxide Gel, it does not interfere with the absorption of phosphates.

Dose. 5 to 15 millilitres, repeated in accordance with the needs of the patient.

OTHER NAME: *Aluphos Gel®*

DRIED ALUMINIUM PHOSPHATE GEL

SYNONYM: Dried Alum. Phos. Gel

Dried Aluminium Phosphate Gel consists largely of hydrated aluminium orthophosphate.

Dried Aluminium Phosphate Gel may be prepared by drying under suitable conditions the product of interaction in aqueous solution of an aluminium salt with an alkali phosphate such as sodium phosphate.

Solubility. Insoluble in water and in alcohol; soluble in dilute mineral acids; insoluble in solutions of alkali hydroxides.

Standard
It complies with the requirements of the British Pharmacopoeia.
It is a white odourless powder containing some friable aggregates. It contains not less than 80·0 per cent of $AlPO_4$. A 4 per cent suspension in water has a pH of 5·5 to 6·5.

Storage. It should be stored at a temperature not exceeding 30°.

Actions and uses. Dried aluminium phosphate gel has the actions, uses, and undesirable effects of aluminium phosphate gel.

Dose. 400 to 800 milligrams, repeated in accordance with the needs of the patient.

Preparation
ALUMINIUM PHOSPHATE TABLETS, B.P. Each tablet contains dried aluminium phosphate gel, equivalent to 400 mg of aluminium phosphate, $AlPO_4$, with peppermint oil. They should be stored at a temperature not exceeding 30°. Dose: 1 or 2 tablets; they should be chewed before being swallowed.

OTHER NAME: *Aluphos®*

ALUMINIUM POWDER

Al = 26·98

Aluminium Powder consists principally of metallic aluminium in the form of very small flakes and may be prepared by hammering aluminium in a suitable mill.

In addition to metallic aluminium, the powder usually contains an appreciable proportion of aluminium oxide. Aluminium Powder is lubricated with stearic acid during manufacture and this lubricant serves to protect the material from oxidation during storage.

Solubility. Almost completely soluble, with evolution of hydrogen, in dilute acids and in solutions of caustic alkalis; insoluble in water and in alcohol.

Standard
DESCRIPTION. A silvery-grey powder; odourless or almost odourless.

IDENTIFICATION TEST. A solution in *dilute hydrochloric acid* gives the reactions characteristic of aluminium.

LEAD. It complies with the test given in Appendix 7, page 881 (100 parts per million).

FOREIGN METALS. Dissolve 2·0 g in 40 ml of *dilute hydrochloric acid.*
Metals other than iron. Dilute 20 ml of the solution to 100 ml with water, make alkaline to *litmus paper* with *dilute ammonia solution,* boil, and filter; evaporate the filtrate to dryness, add 0·05 ml of *sulphuric acid,* and ignite; the residue weighs not more than 0·002 g (0·2 per cent).
Iron. Dilute 16 ml of the solution to 100 ml with water; 0·5 ml complies with the limit test for iron (1 per cent).

LUBRICANT. Weigh 2·0 g into a 600-ml beaker, add 100 ml of hot water, cover, and add a mixture of equal volumes of *hydrochloric acid* and water, dropwise, until the metal has almost completely dissolved; heat to complete solution, cool, filter through a hardened filter paper, and wash the beaker and paper thoroughly with cold water; drain as much water as possible from the beaker and allow the paper to drain well; finally dry both beaker and paper at room temperature. Extract the paper with three successive 100-ml portions of boiling freshly distilled *acetone,* using the original beaker to contain the solvent and collecting the filtrate in a 600-ml beaker; wash the paper finally with five successive 10-ml portions of freshly distilled

acetone and rinse the tip of the funnel; evaporate the combined filtrate and washings to about 30 ml on a water-bath, transfer to a tared platinum or glass basin, and complete the evaporation to dryness; dry the residue at 105° for 30 minutes, cool, and weigh; the residue weighs not more than 0·06 g and not less than 0·01 g.
When the basin containing the residue is floated in a beaker of water suitably heated and stirred, the residue melts between 40° and 60°.
The residue is almost completely soluble, with effervescence, in hot *sodium carbonate solution.*

VOLATILE MATTER. Not more than 0·5 per cent, determined by heating to constant weight at 105°.

SURFACE-COVERING POWER. Not less than 4000 cm² per g, determined by the following method:
Fill with water a shallow trough, measuring approximately 60 × 12 × 1·5 cm, fitted with a movable partition so constructed that it is a sliding fit and can be used to divide the trough into two rectangular areas. Place the movable partition near one end; sprinkle about 0·05 g of the sample, accurately weighed, on the surface of the liquid confined in the smaller area. By means of a glass rod, spread the aluminium evenly over the liquid surface until an unbroken film covers the entire confined surface. Move the partition so as to increase the area confined and again spread the powder to cover the increased surface. Continue this process and determine the maximum unbroken surface area obtained.
The surface-covering power is the area covered by 1 g of the powder at the breaking-point of the film.

CONTENT OF METALLIC ALUMINIUM. Not less than 86·0 per cent, calculated as Al, with reference to the substance freed from lubricant and volatile matter, determined by the following method:
Transfer about 0·2 g, accurately weighed, to a 500-ml flask fitted with a rubber stopper carrying a 150-ml separating funnel, an inlet tube connected to a cylinder of carbon dioxide, and an outlet tube dipping into a water-trap. Add 60 ml of freshly boiled and cooled water and disperse the sample; replace the air by carbon dioxide and add, by the separating funnel, 100 ml of a solution containing 56 g of *ferric ammonium*

sulphate and 7·5 ml of *sulphuric acid* in freshly boiled and cooled water. While maintaining an atmosphere of carbon dioxide in the flask, heat to boiling and boil for 5 minutes after the sample has dissolved, cool rapidly to 20°, and dilute to 250 ml with freshly boiled and cooled water; to 50 ml add 15 ml of *phosphoric acid* and titrate with 0·1N potassium permanganate; each ml of 0·1N potassium permanganate is equivalent to 0·0008994 g of Al.

Storage. It should be stored in airtight containers.

Actions and uses. Aluminium powder has

been used for dusting on the skin around an ileostomy, caecostomy, or colostomy as a protection against proteolytic or irritant discharges. Compound Aluminium Paste is used similarly by applying it thickly round a fistula or sinus.

Preparation
ALUMINIUM PASTE, COMPOUND, B.P.C. (page 767)

ALUMINIUM SULPHATE

SYNONYM: Aluminii Sulfas

Aluminium Sulphate is a hydrated mixture of the normal salt, $Al_2(SO_4)_3$, with a small proportion of basic aluminium sulphate. It contains a variable quantity of water of crystallisation.

Aluminium Sulphate may be prepared by dissolving freshly precipitated aluminium hydroxide in diluted sulphuric acid and allowing to crystallise.

Solubility. Soluble, at 20°, in 1 part of water, giving a solution which may be slightly turbid; insoluble in alcohol.

Standard
Material which complies with this standard meets the requirements of the European Pharmacopoeia.
DESCRIPTION. Colourless lustrous crystals or crystalline masses; odourless.

IDENTIFICATION TESTS. A solution in water gives the reactions characteristic of aluminium and of sulphates.

APPEARANCE OF SOLUTION. A 5·0 per cent w/v solution in water complies with the following tests:
(i) The solution is clear or not more opalescent than a reference solution prepared by mixing, without vigorous shaking, 0·15 ml of *0·0004M sodium chloride*, 0·65 ml of water, 1·0 ml of *2M nitric acid*, and 0·2 ml of *dilute silver nitrate solution*, the comparison being made, 5 minutes after preparation of the reference solution, by viewing 2 ml of the liquids in matched, colourless, transparent, neutral glass tubes, 12 mm internal diameter, in darkness and with a beam of light being passed laterally through the liquids from an electric lamp giving a luminosity of 1000 lux at a distance of 1 m.
(ii) The solution has no colour when compared with water, the comparison being made by viewing vertically 10 ml of the liquids in matched, colourless, transparent, neutral glass tubes, 16 mm internal diameter and with a flat base, against a white background in diffused daylight.

ACIDITY. pH of a 2·0 per cent w/v solution in *carbon dioxide-free water*, 3·0 to 4·0.

HEAVY METALS. It complies with the test given in Appendix 8, page 887 (50 parts per million as Pb).

IRON. Dissolve 0·1 g in 10 ml of water, add 2 ml of a 20 per cent w/v solution of *citric acid FeT* in water and 0·3 ml of *thioglycollic acid*, mix, make alkaline with *strong ammonia solution*, dilute to 20 ml with water, and allow to stand for 5 minutes; any pink colour produced is not more intense than that produced when 10 ml of *weak iron standard solution* is treated in the same manner (100 parts per million).

ALKALIS AND ALKALINE EARTHS. Not more than 0·4 per

cent, determined by the following method:
Dissolve 1·0 g in 120 ml of water, warm the solution, add 0·1 ml of *methyl red solution* followed by sufficient *dilute ammonia solution* to change the colour of the indicator to yellow, dilute to 150 ml with water, heat to boiling, and filter, taking care to minimise losses by evaporation; evaporate 75 ml of the filtrate to dryness on a water-bath, ignite the residue, allow to cool, and weigh.

AMMONIUM. Dilute 0·4 ml of a 5·0 per cent w/v solution in water to 14 ml with water, make alkaline by the addition of *dilute sodium hydroxide solution*, dilute to 15 ml with water, add 0·3 ml of *potassium mercuri-iodide solution*, and allow to stand for half a minute; any yellow colour which develops is not more intense than that produced by a reference solution prepared at the same time by mixing 10 ml of *ammonium standard solution*, 5 ml of water, and 0·3 ml of *potassium mercuri-iodide solution*.

CONTENT OF $Al_2(SO_4)_3$. Not less than 51·0 and not more than 59·0 per cent, determined by the following method:
Dissolve about 0·6 g, accurately weighed, in a mixture of 2 ml of 1N hydrochloric acid and 50 ml of water, add 50 ml of 0·05M disodium edetate, neutralise the solution to *methyl red solution* by the addition of 1N sodium hydroxide, and heat to boiling; allow to stand on a water-bath for 10 minutes, cool rapidly, add 0·05 g of *xylenol orange mixture* and 5 g of *hexamine*, and titrate the excess of disodium edetate with 0·05M lead nitrate to a red end-point; each ml of 0·05M disodium edetate is equivalent to 0·00855 g of $Al_2(SO_4)_3$.

Actions and uses. Aluminium sulphate has actions similar to those described under Alum (page 14), but is more astringent than alum. A saturated solution is employed as a mild caustic. Solutions (5 to 10 per cent) have been used as local applications to ulcers and to arrest foul discharges from mucous surfaces.

Aluminium sulphate is also employed in the preparation of Aluminium Acetate Solution, which is used as astringent ear-drops.

Preparation
ALUMINIUM ACETATE SOLUTION, B.P.C. (page 780)

AMETHOCAINE HYDROCHLORIDE

SYNONYMS: Tetracaine Hydrochloride; Tetracainii Chloridum

$C_{15}H_{25}ClN_2O_2 = 300\cdot8$

Amethocaine Hydrochloride is 2-dimethylaminoethyl *p*-butylaminobenzoate hydrochloride.

Solubility. Soluble, at 20°, in 7·5 parts of water and in 40 parts of alcohol; insoluble in ether.

Standard

It complies with the requirements of the European Pharmacopoeia.

It is a white, crystalline, odourless powder and contains not less than 99·0 per cent of $C_{15}H_{25}ClN_2O_2$, calculated with reference to the dried substance. The loss on drying under the prescribed conditions is not more than 1·0 per cent. It has a melting-point of about 148° or may occur in either of two polymorphic modifications which melt at about 134° and about 139°; mixtures of the forms may melt within the range 134° to 147°. A 1·0 per cent solution in water has a pH of 4·5 to 6·5.

Sterilisation. Solutions are sterilised by heating with a bactericide or by filtration.

Storage. It should be protected from light.

Actions and uses. Amethocaine is a local anaesthetic which is suitable for infiltration, surface, or spinal anaesthesia. Although it is several times more toxic than either procaine by injection or cocaine by application, it is relatively safer because its local anaesthetic action is greater and it can therefore be used in lower concentrations than are normally employed with procaine or cocaine; in addition, it does not produce the idiosyncratic reactions that may arise after the administration of cocaine.

The risk of toxic effects may be reduced by the addition of adrenaline, which delays absorption; solutions containing adrenaline should not, however, be used for inducing anaesthesia in digits, because the profound ischaemia produced may lead to gangrene.

In infiltration and spinal anaesthesia, the action of amethocaine is slower in onset than that of procaine, but is of longer duration.

In ophthalmology, amethocaine hydrochloride is usually employed as a 0·25 per cent solution; the use of solutions stronger than 1 per cent should be avoided as they may result in damage to the cornea. As an analgesic in oto-rhinolaryngology, a 0·5 to 2 per cent solution is employed; stronger solutions are sometimes used, but it is doubtful whether they are necessary. A 0·5 per cent solution may be used as a throat spray before the introduction of a gastroscope, and a 0·1 per cent solution may be injected into the urethra before the introduction of a catheter or cystoscope. A 1 to 3 per cent ointment or suppository is useful in painful conditions of the anus and rectum.

For spinal anaesthesia, 5 to 20 milligrams may be administered as a 0·1 to 0·5 per cent solution. Solutions having a higher density than that of cerebrospinal fluid may be prepared by dissolving the dose in a 6 per cent Dextrose Injection. Solutions having a density approximately equal to that of cerebrospinal fluid are also used; these are prepared by dissolving 1 per cent of amethocaine hydrochloride in Sodium Chloride Injection or occasionally by dissolving the dose in cerebrospinal fluid. For techniques in which a solution of relatively low density is required, a suitable preparation is a 0·066 per cent solution of amethocaine hydrochloride in Water for Injections containing 0·5 per cent of sodium chloride.

For infiltration anaesthesia, up to 4 milligrams per kilogram body-weight, with a maximum of 250 milligrams, administered as a 0·03 to 0·1 per cent solution in Sodium Chloride Injection, may be used.

POISONING. The procedure described under Cocaine (page 120) should be adopted.

Preparation

AMETHOCAINE EYE-DROPS, B.P.C. (page 688)

OTHER NAME: *Anethaine*®

AMINOBENZOIC ACID

SYNONYM: *p*-Aminobenzoic Acid

$C_7H_7NO_2 = 137\cdot1$

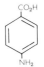

Solubility. Soluble, at 20°, in 200 parts of water and in 8 parts of alcohol; soluble in solutions of alkali hydroxides and carbonates.

Standard

DESCRIPTION. White or slightly yellow crystals or crystalline powder, gradually darkening on exposure to air and light; odourless or almost odourless.

IDENTIFICATION TESTS. 1. Dissolve 0·1 g in 2 ml of *dilute hydrochloric acid* with the aid of heat if necessary, cool in ice, add 4 ml of a 1 per cent w/v solution of *sodium nitrite* in water and pour the mixture into 2 ml of *2-naphthol solution* containing 1 g of *sodium acetate*; a bright red precipitate is produced.

2. It complies with the thin-layer chromatographic test given in Appendix 5A, page 858.

3. The ultraviolet absorption spectrum exhibits the characteristics given in Appendix 3, page 855.

4. The infra-red absorption spectrum exhibits maxima

which are only at the same wavelengths as, and have similar relative intensities to, those in the spectrum of *p-aminobenzoic acid A.S.*

MELTING-POINT. 186° to 189°.

IRON. Ignite 1·0 g with 1 g of *anhydrous sodium carbonate* and dissolve the residue in 15 ml of *dilute hydrochloric acid*; the solution complies with the limit test for iron (40 parts per million).

p-NITROBENZOIC ACID. It complies with the test given in Appendix 5A, page 858 (0·2 per cent).

WATER. Not more than 0·5 per cent w/w, determined by the method given in Appendix 16, page 895.

SULPHATED ASH. Not more than 0·2 per cent.

CONTENT OF $C_7H_7NO_2$. Not less than 98·5 per cent, calculated with reference to the anhydrous substance, determined by the following method:

Dissolve about 0·3 g, accurately weighed, in 60 ml of water and titrate with 0·1N sodium hydroxide, using *phenolphthalein solution* as indicator; each ml of 0·1N sodium hydroxide is equivalent to 0·01371 g of $C_7H_7NO_2$.

Incompatibility. Incompatible with ferric salts and oxidising agents.

Storage. It should be stored in airtight containers, protected from light.

Actions and uses. Aminobenzoic acid has sun-screening properties and is used as an ingredient of topical preparations for the prevention of sunburn.

Preparation
AMINOBENZOIC ACID LOTION, B.P.C. (page 727)

AMINOCAPROIC ACID

$C_6H_{13}NO_2 = 131·2$ $NH_2 \cdot [CH_2]_5 \cdot CO_2H$

Aminocaproic Acid is 6-aminohexanoic acid.

Solubility. Soluble, at 20°, in 1·5 parts of water.

Standard
It complies with the requirements of the British Pharmacopoeia.
It occurs as odourless colourless crystals or white crystalline powder and contains not less than 98·5 per cent of $C_6H_{13}NO_2$, calculated with reference to the dried substance. The loss on drying under the prescribed conditions is not more than 0·5 per cent. It melts with decomposition at about 204°. A 20 per cent solution in water has a pH of 7·5 to 8·0.

Sterilisation. Solutions for injection are sterilised by filtration.

Actions and uses. Aminocaproic acid inhibits plasminogen activation in blood and urine and so reduces fibrinolysis and increases the stability of clots when they have been formed. As there are potent plasminogen activators in urine, saliva, and endometrial secretions, aminocaproic acid may be expected to reduce haemorrhage after dental extraction and urinary surgery and in menorrhagia; it may also stabilise internal thrombi once they have been formed.
Aminocaproic acid should only be used where there is free haemorrhage on a mucous surface or as an antagonist to streptokinase. It may be used in haemophilia to reduce bleeding after tooth extraction by preventing lysis of the first formed clot, so avoiding exhaustion of depleted coagulation factors. For this purpose the sockets are rinsed with a sterile 10 per cent solution and plugs moistened with the solution are inserted in the sockets.
Aminocaproic acid may also be useful in limiting the action of streptokinase. It has not been found of established benefit in menorrhagia and most other conditions in which it

might be expected to be of value; spontaneous bleeding in haemophilia is not significantly reduced and organising clots may persist in joints and serous cavities. It apparently increases clot colic and retention when the bleeding is in the urinary tract.
Aminocaproic acid is administered by mouth; sachets containing effervescent powder equivalent to 3 grams of aminocaproic acid and a mixture containing 300 milligrams per millilitre are available. It may also be administered by slow intravenous injection or by intravenous infusion of a solution diluted with Sodium Chloride Injection or with Dextrose Injection (5 per cent w/v).

UNDESIRABLE EFFECTS. Nausea, diarrhoea, and dizziness may occur, but these disappear when the dose is reduced.

CONTRA-INDICATIONS. Aminocaproic acid should not be given when there is renal impairment, which increases the risk of overdosage, or to patients taking contraceptive steroids, as this may increase the risk of blood-clot formation.

Dose. By mouth or by slow intravenous injection, 100 milligrams per kilogram body-weight five times a day.
In menorrhagia, 3 grams by mouth four to six times daily for three to six days.

Preparation
AMINOCAPROIC ACID INJECTION, B.P. It consists of a sterile solution of aminocaproic acid in Water for Injections, the pH of the solution being adjusted to 6·6. Unless otherwise specified, a solution containing 400 mg in 1 ml is supplied.

OTHER NAMES: EACA; *Epsikapron*®; Epsilon Aminocaproic Acid

AMINOPHYLLINE

SYNONYMS: Theophylline and Ethylenediamine; Theophyllinum et Ethylenediaminum

Aminophylline may be prepared by dissolving theophylline in ethylenediamine hydrate and evaporating to dryness. Its composition is approximately represented by the formula $(C_7H_8N_4O_2)_2,C_2H_4(NH_2)_2,2H_2O$.

Solubility. Soluble, at 25°, in 5 parts of water, the solution usually becoming turbid on standing; insoluble in dehydrated alcohol and in ether.
In order to effect complete solution in water the addition of ethylenediamine or ammonia solution may be necessary.

Standard
It complies with the requirements of the European Pharmacopoeia.
It occurs as a white or slightly yellowish powder or granules with a slightly ammoniacal odour and contains 78·0 to 84·0 per cent of anhydrous theophylline, $C_7H_8N_4O_2$, and 13·0 to 14·0 per cent of ethylenediamine, $C_2H_4(NH_2)_2$. It contains a variable proportion of water.

Stability. It absorbs carbon dioxide from the air with liberation of theophylline. Aqueous solutions absorb carbon dioxide from the air with precipitation of theophylline.

Sterilisation. Solutions for injection are sterilised by heating in an autoclave or by filtration, exposure to carbon dioxide and contact with metals being avoided throughout.

Storage. It should be stored in small, well-filled, airtight containers, protected from light.

Actions and uses. Aminophylline has actions and uses similar to those described under Theophylline (page 501), but with the advantage of greater solubility. It relaxes involuntary muscle and relieves bronchial spasm and is used in the treatment of asthma, bronchopneumonia, and bronchitis. It is given for its diuretic action in the treatment of cardiac or renal oedema.
Aminophylline is effective when given by intravenous injection or by rectum; the intra-venous injection should be given very slowly. It may be given by mouth, but it is a gastric irritant and may cause nausea and vomiting; choline theophyllinate is therefore preferred.

Aminophylline Suppositories are of value when a prolonged prophylactic effect is desired and may be used at bedtime to abort attacks of paroxysmal dyspnoea or asthma.

Dose. 100 to 300 milligrams by mouth; 250 to 500 milligrams by slow intravenous injection; 360 milligrams once or twice daily by rectum.

Preparations
AMINOPHYLLINE INJECTION, B.P. (*Syn.* Theophylline and Ethylenediamine Injection). It consists of a sterile solution of aminophylline in Water for Injections free from carbon dioxide. For intravenous injection, unless otherwise specified, a solution containing 250 mg in 10 ml is supplied. A solution containing 500 mg in 2 ml is also available.

AMINOPHYLLINE SUPPOSITORIES, B.P. (*Syn.* Theophylline and Ethylenediamine Suppositories). They may be prepared by incorporating aminophylline in theobroma oil or other suitable fatty basis. Approximately 1·5 g of aminophylline displaces 1 g of theobroma oil. Unless otherwise specified, suppositories each containing 360 mg of aminophylline and prepared in a 2-g mould are supplied. Suppositories containing 25, 100, and 150 mg are also available.

AMINOPHYLLINE TABLETS, B.P. (*Syn.* Theophylline and Ethylenediamine Tablets). Unless otherwise specified, tablets each containing 100 mg of aminophylline are supplied. They should be stored in airtight containers, protected from light.

OTHER NAME: *Cardophylin*®

AMITRIPTYLINE EMBONATE

$C_{63}H_{62}N_2O_6 = 943·2$

Amitriptyline Embonate is 5-(3-dimethyla-minopropylidene)-10,11-dihydro-5*H*-dibenzo[*a,d*]cycloheptene 4,4′-methylenebis(3-hydroxynaphthalene-2-carboxylate).

Solubility. Insoluble in water; soluble, at 20°, in 8 parts of chloroform and in 6 parts of acetone; slightly soluble in alcohol.

Standard
DESCRIPTION. A pale yellow to brownish-yellow powder; odourless or almost odourless.

IDENTIFICATION TESTS. 1. It complies with the thin-layer chromatographic test given in Appendix 5A, page 859.
2. The ultraviolet absorption spectrum exhibits the characteristics given in Appendix 3, page 855.

LEAD. It complies with the test given in Appendix 7, page 881 (20 parts per million).

CHLORIDE. Not more than 0·2 per cent, calculated as Cl, determined by the following method:
Dissolve about 1 g, accurately weighed, in a mixture of 50 ml of *acetone* and 50 ml of water, add 2 ml of *nitric acid*, and titrate by the method given in Appendix 11, page 891, using 0·01N silver nitrate instead of 0·1N silver nitrate; each ml of 0·01N silver nitrate is equivalent to 0·0003545 g of Cl.

KETONE. It complies with the test given in Appendix 5A, page 859 (500 parts per million).

WATER. Not more than 5·0 per cent w/w, determined by the method given in Appendix 16, page 895.

SULPHATED ASH. Not more than 0·3 per cent.

CONTENT OF $C_{63}H_{62}N_2O_6$. Not less than 97·0 and not more than the equivalent of 103·0 per cent, calculated with reference to the anhydrous substance, determined by the following method:
Dissolve about 0·6 g, accurately weighed, in 50 ml of *dioxan* with the aid of gentle heat, cool, and titrate the solution by Method I of the British Pharmacopoeia for non-aqueous titration; repeat the procedure omitting the sample. The difference between the two titrations represents the amount of 0·1N perchloric acid required by the sample; each ml of 0·1N perchloric acid is equivalent to 0·04716 g of $C_{63}H_{62}N_2O_6$.

Actions and uses. Amitriptyline embonate has the actions of amitriptyline, as described under Amitriptyline Hydrochloride. Because it is insoluble in water it is almost tasteless and is therefore preferred to the hydrochloride for preparing liquid medicines for oral administration; 1·5 grams of amitriptyline embonate is approximately equivalent to 1 gram of amitriptyline hydrochloride.

UNDESIRABLE EFFECTS. As for Amitriptyline Hydrochloride.

PRECAUTIONS AND CONTRA-INDICATIONS. As for Amitriptyline Hydrochloride.

Preparation
AMITRIPTYLINE MIXTURE, B.P.C. (page 736)

OTHER NAME: *Tryptizol®*

AMITRIPTYLINE HYDROCHLORIDE

$C_{20}H_{24}ClN = 313·9$

Amitriptyline Hydrochloride is 5-(3-dimethylaminopropylidene)-10,11-dihydro-5*H*-dibenzo-[*a,d*]cycloheptene hydrochloride.

Solubility. Soluble, at 20°, in 1 part of water, in 1·5 parts of alcohol, in 1·2 parts of chloroform, and in 1 part of methyl alcohol; insoluble in ether.

Standard
It complies with the requirements of the British Pharmacopoeia.
It occurs as odourless or almost odourless colourless crystals or white or almost white powder and contains not less than 99·0 and not more than the equivalent of 101·0 per cent of $C_{20}H_{24}ClN$, calculated with reference to the dried substance. The loss on drying under the prescribed conditions is not more than 0·5 per cent. It has a melting-point of about 197°. A 1 per cent solution in water has a pH of 4·5 to 6·0.

Sterilisation. Solutions for injection are sterilised by filtration.

Actions and uses. Amitriptyline is an antidepressant drug with anticholinergic activity, but which does not inhibit monoamine oxidase. It is used in the treatment of depression, anxiety tension, and psychosomatic disorders, particularly those affecting the gastro-intestinal tract.
The initial daily dosage varies between 30 and 150 milligrams; 25 milligrams three times daily is usually adequate for the treatment of depression and 10 milligrams three or four times daily for mild anxiety states associated with depression and for mild psychosomatic disorders. In elderly or agitated patients, treatment may be initiated by the intramuscular or intravenous injection of 50 to 100 milligrams daily in divided doses. When a satisfactory response has been achieved, usually in seven to ten days, the dosage should be reduced to the smallest amount that will control the symptoms; this maintenance dosage is usually 20 to 100 milligrams daily in divided doses.

UNDESIRABLE EFFECTS. The most frequently occurring reactions are dryness of the mouth, drowsiness, constipation, and blurred vision.
Amitriptyline may cause a reversal of the effect of antihypertensive drugs and may give rise to hypertension in patients being given local anaesthetics containing adrenaline or noradrenaline.

PRECAUTIONS AND CONTRA-INDICATIONS. Because of its anticholinergic activity amitriptyline should not be given to patients with glaucoma or to those who might develop urinary retention.
Caution should be exercised when giving amitriptyline to patients who are being treated with a monoamine-oxidase inhibitor, such as isocarboxazid, nialamide, phenelzine, or tranylcypromine, or who have been so treated within the previous ten days.
Amitriptyline should be avoided in patients with ischaemic heart disease, especially when there is evidence of rhythm disturbance.

Dose. See above under **Actions and uses.**

Preparations
AMITRIPTYLINE INJECTION, B.P. It consists of a sterile solution of amitriptyline hydrochloride. Unless otherwise specified, a solution containing 10 mg in 1 ml is supplied.
AMITRIPTYLINE TABLETS, B.P. Unless otherwise specified, tablets each containing 25 mg of amitriptyline hydrochloride are supplied. They are film coated or sugar coated. Tablets containing 10 and 50 mg are also available.

OTHER NAMES: *Laroxyl®*; *Lentizol®*; *Saroten®*; *Tryptizol®*

STRONG AMMONIA SOLUTION

SYNONYM: Liquor Ammoniae Fortis

Strong Ammonia Solution is an aqueous solution of ammonia, NH_3, which is usually prepared by synthesis from atmospheric nitrogen or may be obtained from the ammoniacal liquors from gas works by distillation with slaked lime.

Solubility. Miscible with water.

Standard

DESCRIPTION. A clear colourless liquid; odour strongly pungent and characteristic.

IDENTIFICATION TESTS. 1. It is strongly alkaline, even when freely diluted with water.

2. When the vapour is brought into contact with gaseous hydrochloric acid, dense white fumes are produced.

WEIGHT PER ML. At 20°, 0·892 g to 0·901 g.

ARSENIC. It complies with the test given in Appendix 6, page 877 (0·4 part per million).

LEAD. It complies with the test given in Appendix 7, page 881 (1 part per million).

TARRY MATTER. In 5 ml, diluted with 10 ml of water, dissolve 6 g of powdered *citric acid*; no tarry or unpleasant odour is produced.

NON-VOLATILE MATTER. Not more than 0·01 per cent w/v, determined by evaporating 100 ml to dryness on a water-bath and drying the residue to constant weight at 105°.

CONTENT OF NH_3. 27·0 to 30·0 per cent w/w, determined by the following method:
To 50 ml of 1N hydrochloric acid add about 2 g, accurately weighed, taking precautions during the addition to avoid loss of ammonia, and titrate the excess of acid with 1N sodium hydroxide, using *methyl red solution* as indicator; each ml of 1N hydrochloric acid is equivalent to 0·01703 g of NH_3.

Storage. It should be stored in airtight containers, in a cool place.

Actions and uses. Ammonia, when inhaled, irritates the mucosa of the upper respiratory tract and reflexly, through the medulla, causes stimulation of respiration, acceleration of the heart, and rise of blood pressure; the rationale of smelling-salts depends upon these effects. As a restorative in cases of fainting and collapse it is usually administered as Aromatic Ammonia Spirit.

Applied externally, solutions of ammonia have rubefacient and counter-irritant actions and have been used as ingredients of liniments. Strong Ammonia Solution is used in the preparation of Strong Ammonium Acetate Solution, which is used as a mild expectorant, diuretic, and diaphoretic.

PRECAUTIONS. Great care should be taken in handling strong solutions of ammonia, as the vapour may inflame the respiratory tract and cause tracheitis, bronchitis, and pneumonia. Spasm of the glottis with resulting asphyxia may occur. Ammonia burns of the eye should be treated by irrigation with water, followed by drops of liquid paraffin.

Ammonia burns have resulted from treating insect bites and stings with the strong solution and even with the dilute solution, especially if a dressing is subsequently applied.

POISONING. Vinegar, or any suitable mineral acid well diluted, should be given, followed by demulcent drinks or olive oil. Morphine may be necessary for the relief of pain and the patient should be treated for shock.

Preparations
AMMONIA SOLUTION, AROMATIC, B.P.C. (page 780)
AMMONIA SOLUTION, DILUTE, B.P.C. (page 780)
AMMONIUM ACETATE SOLUTION, STRONG, B.P.C. (page 780)
AMMONIA SPIRIT, AROMATIC, B.P.C. (page 793)

AMMONIUM BICARBONATE

SYNONYM: Ammon. Bicarb.

$NH_4HCO_3 = 79·06$

Solubility. Soluble, at 20°, in 5 parts of water; insoluble in alcohol.

Standard

DESCRIPTION. Slightly hygroscopic white crystals, white fine crystalline powder, or colourless glassy solid; odour slightly ammoniacal.

IDENTIFICATION TESTS. It gives the reactions characteristic of ammonium salts and of bicarbonates.

ARSENIC. It complies with the test given in Appendix 6, page 877 (2 parts per million).

IRON. 1·0 g dissolved in 40 ml of water and boiled until all the ammonia has been removed complies with the limit test for iron (40 parts per million).

LEAD. It complies with the test given in Appendix 7, page 881 (5 parts per million).

CHLORIDE. 5·0 g dissolved in water and boiled until all the ammonia has been removed complies with the limit test for chlorides (10 parts per million).

SULPHATE. 5·0 g dissolved in water and boiled until all the ammonia has been removed complies with the limit test for sulphates (120 parts per million).

SULPHIDE. Dissolve 5·0 g in 50 ml of freshly boiled and cooled water and add 2 ml of *potassium plumbite solution*; no darkening in colour is produced.

TARRY MATTER. Mix 5·0 g with 15 ml of water and 5 g of *citric acid*; no tarry odour is detectable.

NON-VOLATILE MATTER. Not more than 0·01 per cent, determined by heating to constant weight at 300°.

CONTENT OF NH_4HCO_3. Not less than 98·0 and not more than the equivalent of 101·0 per cent, determined by the following method:
Dissolve about 2 g, accurately weighed, in 40 ml of 1N

hydrochloric acid diluted with 50 ml of water, boil, cool, and titrate the excess of acid with 1N sodium hydroxide, using *methyl red solution* as indicator; each ml of 1N hydrochloric acid is equivalent to 0·07906 g of NH_4HCO_3.

Stability. It volatilises rapidly at 60°, with dissociation into ammonia, carbon dioxide, and water; the volatilisation takes place slowly at ordinary temperatures if the substance is slightly moist.

Storage. It should be stored in airtight containers, in a cool place.

Actions and uses. Ammonium bicarbonate is irritant to mucous membranes and in small doses it is used as a reflex expectorant. Large doses produce nausea and vomiting.

NOTE. When Ammonium Carbonate or Ammonii Carbonas is prescribed or demanded, Ammonium Bicarbonate is dispensed or supplied.

Dose. 300 to 600 milligrams.

Preparations
AMMONIA AND IPECACUANHA MIXTURE, B.P.C. (page 736)
AMMONIUM CHLORIDE AND MORPHINE MIXTURE, B.P.C. (page 736)
IPECACUANHA AND AMMONIA MIXTURE, PAEDIATRIC, B.P.C. (page 745)
OPIUM MIXTURE, CAMPHORATED, COMPOUND, B.P.C. (page 749)
POTASSIUM IODIDE MIXTURE, AMMONIATED, B.P.C. (page 751)
RHUBARB AND SODA MIXTURE, AMMONIATED, B.P.C. (page 752)
AMMONIA SOLUTION, AROMATIC, B.P.C. (page 780)
AMMONIUM ACETATE SOLUTION, STRONG, B.P.C. (page 780)
AMMONIA SPIRIT, AROMATIC, B.P.C. (page 793)

AMMONIUM CHLORIDE

SYNONYMS: Ammon. Chlor.; Ammonii Chloridum

$NH_4Cl = 53·49$

Solubility. Soluble, at 20°, in 2·7 parts of water and in 100 parts of alcohol.

Standard
It complies with the requirements of the European Pharmacopoeia.
It occurs as odourless colourless crystals or white crystalline powder and contains not less than 99·5 per cent of NH_4Cl, calculated with reference to the dried substance. The loss on drying under the prescribed conditions is not more than 1·0 per cent.

Sterilisation. Solutions are sterilised by heating in an autoclave or by filtration.

Storage. It should be stored in airtight containers.

Actions and uses. Ammonium chloride is rapidly absorbed from the gastro-intestinal tract. The ammonium ion is converted into urea in the liver; the anion thus liberated into the blood stream and extracellular fluids causes a metabolic acidosis and decreases the pH of the urine; this is followed by transient diuresis.

A mild acidosis is produced by the administration of ammonium chloride by mouth in a single dose of 2 grams. This is used to increase the diuretic effect of mercurial diuretics and in the treatment of urinary tract infections when a low urinary pH is required. In smaller doses, ammonium chloride is an ingredient of expectorant cough mixtures, but it is doubtful whether its irritant action on the

gastric mucous membrane contributes to any expectorant action.

Large doses should be given in tablets, coated to prevent disintegration in the stomach; Liquorice Liquid Extract may be used to disguise its taste in liquid medicines.

UNDESIRABLE EFFECTS. Large doses of ammonium chloride may cause nausea, vomiting, thirst, headache, hyperventilation, progressive drowsiness, mental confusion, and hyperchloraemic acidosis. It is contra-indicated in the presence of renal or hepatic disease.

POISONING. Acidosis and electrolyte loss should be corrected by sodium bicarbonate or sodium lactate given intravenously, and hypokalaemia prevented by potassium gluconate or other suitable source of potassium given by mouth.

Dose. 0·3 to 2 grams.
Before the administration of Mersalyl Injection, 3 to 6 grams daily in divided doses.

Preparations
WHITE LINIMENT, B.P.C. (page 726)
AMMONIUM CHLORIDE MIXTURE, B.P.C. (page 736)
AMMONIUM CHLORIDE AND MORPHINE MIXTURE, B.P.C. (page 736)
AMMONIUM CHLORIDE TABLETS, B.P.C. (page 805)

AMODIAQUINE HYDROCHLORIDE

$C_{20}H_{24}Cl_3N_3O,2H_2O = 464·8$

Amodiaquine Hydrochloride is 7-chloro-4-(3-diethylaminomethyl-4-hydroxyanilino)quinoline dihydrochloride dihydrate.

2HCl. 2H₂O

Solubility. Soluble, at 20°, in 22 parts of water and in 70 parts of alcohol; very slightly soluble in ether and in chloroform.

Standard
It complies with the requirements of the British Pharmacopoeia.

It is a yellow, odourless or almost odourless, crystalline powder and contains not less than 98·0 and not more than the equivalent of 101·5 per cent of $C_{20}H_{24}Cl_3N_3O$, calculated with reference to the dried substance. The loss on drying under the prescribed conditions is 6·0 to 10·0 per cent. It has a melting-point of about 158°. A 2·0 per cent solution in water has a pH of 4·0 to 4·6.

Actions and uses. Amodiaquine hydrochloride is an antimalarial drug which has actions and uses similar to those described under Chloroquine Phosphate (page 101). A dose equivalent to 200 to 400 milligrams of the base given by mouth once a week is usually adequate for the suppression of malaria in an adult; 130 milligrams of the hydrochloride is approximately equivalent to 100 milligrams of the base. A single dose equivalent to 600 milligrams of the base is often sufficient to control a malarial attack, although the equiva-lent of 400 to 600 milligrams of the base daily for three days may be necessary.

Amodiaquine is also used for the treatment of chronic discoid lupus erythematosus; a single dose equivalent to 200 milligrams of the base is given daily until the condition is controlled, and thereafter 200 milligrams is given three or four times a week for maintenance.

UNDESIRABLE EFFECTS. Undesirable effects are rare with antimalarial doses. Long-continued use of the drug may result in blue-grey deposits in the cornea, fingernails, and hard palate.

Dose. See above under **Actions and uses.**

Preparation
AMODIAQUINE TABLETS, B.P. Unless otherwise speci-fied, tablets each containing amodiaquine hydrochloride equivalent to 200 mg of amodiaquine base are supplied.

OTHER NAME: *Camoquin*®

AMPHETAMINE SULPHATE

SYNONYM: Amphet. Sulph.

$C_{18}H_{28}N_2O_4S = 368·5$

$[C_6H_5 \cdot CH_2 \cdot CH(NH_2) \cdot CH_3]_2 H_2SO_4$

Amphetamine Sulphate is $(\pm)$-α-methylphenethylamine sulphate.

Solubility. Soluble, at 20°, in 9 parts of water and in 515 parts of alcohol; insoluble in ether and in chloro-form.

Standard
It complies with the requirements of the British Pharmacopoeia.
It is a white odourless powder and contains not less than 99·0 per cent of $C_{18}H_{28}N_2O_4S$, calculated with reference to the dried substance. The loss on drying under the prescribed conditions is not more than 1·0 per cent.

Hygroscopicity. It absorbs insignificant amounts of moisture at 25° at relative humidities of up to about 90 per cent.

Incompatibility. It is incompatible with alkalis and with calcium salts.

Sterilisation. Solutions for injection are sterilised by heating in an autoclave or by filtration.

Actions and uses. Amphetamine is a sympathomimetic drug with marked central stimulant effects. Like ephedrine, it produces vasoconstriction, inhibition of the gastro-intestinal tract and bladder, and dilatation of the pupil. It is less effective than ephedrine in relaxing bronchial muscle and less liable to increase the heart rate.

Its principal actions are stimulation of the cerebral cortex and the respiratory and vaso-motor centres. These actions produce in-creased motor activity and mental alertness, euphoria, diminished sense of fatigue, and increased wakefulness. In some patients the drug produces insomnia, headache, hyper-excitability, and cardiac and gastro-intestinal disturbances. Large doses are followed by fatigue and mental depression; a rise in blood pressure may also occur.

Amphetamine sulphate is administered by mouth. It was formerly used in narcolepsy and depressive states but has now been re-placed by other drugs. It has also been used in the treatment of certain types of obesity.

PRECAUTIONS AND CONTRA-INDICATIONS. Am-phetamine sulphate should not be given to patients who are being treated with a mono-amine-oxidase inhibitor, such as isocar-boxazid, nialamide, phenelzine, or tranylcy-promine, or within about ten days of the discontinuation of such treatment.

The indiscriminate use of amphetamine in attempts to increase capacity for work or to overcome fatigue is undesirable, as it may lead to dependence (see below).

Amphetamine is contra-indicated in patients with cardiovascular disease and thyrotoxi-cosis, and in those showing anxiety, hyper-excitability, and restlessness. It may cause a reversal of the effect of antihypertensive drugs. It is advisable not to administer the drug later than the early afternoon as it may cause insomnia.

DEPENDENCE. The characteristics of drug de-pendence of the amphetamine type are: (i) strong psychic dependence; (ii) a high degree of tolerance; (iii) no readily evident physical dependence and consequently no characteris-tic abstinence syndrome, although with-drawal will be followed by a state of mental and physical depression as the stimulatory effect of the drug diminishes.

POISONING. An intermediate-acting barbi-turate, such as quinalbarbitone sodium or cyclobarbitone, should be given by mouth or, if necessary, thiopentone sodium should be administered by intravenous injection.

A suitable acidic salt such as ammonium chloride should be administered in a sufficient quantity to render the patient's urine acid, so as to increase the rate of excretion of amphetamine.

Dose. 5 to 10 milligrams two or three times daily.

Preparation
AMPHETAMINE SULPHATE TABLETS, B.P. Unless otherwise specified, tablets each containing 5 mg are supplied.

AMPHOTERICIN

Amphotericin is a mixture of antifungal substances produced by the growth of certain strains of *Streptomyces nodosus* or by any other means.

Solubility. Very slightly soluble in water, in alcohol, and in ether; soluble, at 20°, in 625 parts of dehydrated methyl alcohol, in 20 parts of dimethyl sulphoxide, and in 200 parts of dimethylformamide; soluble in propylene glycol.

Standard
It complies with the requirements of the British Pharmacopoeia.
It is a yellow to orange, odourless or almost odourless powder and contains not less than 750 Units per mg, calculated with reference to the dried substance. The loss on drying under the prescribed conditions is not more than 5·0 per cent. It contains not more than 15·0 per cent of amphotericin A. A 3 per cent suspension in water has a pH of 6·0 to 8·0.

Stability. It is inactivated at low pH values and dilute solutions are sensitive to light.

Storage. It should be stored in airtight containers, protected from light, at a temperature between 2° and 10°. Under these conditions it may be expected to retain its potency without significant deterioration for at least one year.

Actions and uses. Amphotericin is a polyene antibiotic related to nystatin. It has an antifungal action against a wide range of yeasts and fungi. It is used in the treatment of infections by yeast-like organisms, such as cryptococcosis, candidiasis, blastomycosis, and histoplasmosis.

For the treatment of local infections it is used in the form of a mixture containing 100 milligrams per millilitre, tablets containing 100 milligrams, cream, lotion, and ointment containing 3 per cent, lozenges containing 10 milligrams, and pessaries containing 50 milligrams.

For the treatment of systemic infections a special grade of amphotericin is usually administered by slow intravenous infusion of a solution containing 100 micrograms per millilitre in the form of a water-soluble complex with sodium deoxycholate dissolved in Dextrose Injection (5 per cent w/v). In meningeal infections an aqueous solution containing the equivalent of 250 micrograms per millilitre may be mixed with cerebrospinal fluid in the syringe and given intrathecally if intravenous infusion is not effective. Solutions should be protected from light before and during administration.

The usual dose by intravenous infusion is the equivalent of 0·25 to 1 milligram of amphotericin per kilogram body-weight daily, beginning with the smaller quantity and increasing gradually to the maximum possible without causing toxic effects. Since the compound is excreted slowly, the larger doses are best given on alternate days until the patient's reaction is ascertained. Treatment may need to be continued for some months. In view of its toxicity, amphotericin should be given by injection only in susceptible types of infection.

UNDESIRABLE EFFECTS. Unpleasant and potentially dangerous side-effects of systemic treatment are common because dosage must be as high as possible. Headache, anorexia, and fever occur frequently at the beginning of treatment but usually pass off in a few days. The main toxic effect is disturbance of renal function, which should be tested at intervals, and administration of amphotericin should be stopped if progressive deterioration occurs.

PRECAUTIONS. The injection is irritant to the endothelium of the vein and may be painful. The risk of thrombophlebitis is reduced by frequently changing the site of the injection, by reducing the rate of administration, and by the addition of a soluble hydrocortisone derivative to the infusion.

Dose. See above under **Actions and uses.**

Preparation
AMPHOTERICIN LOZENGES, B.P.C. (page 731)

OTHER NAMES: *Fungilin®; Fungizone®*

AMPICILLIN

SYNONYM: Anhydrous Ampicillin

$C_{16}H_{19}N_3O_4S = 349·4$

Ampicillin is D(−)-6-(α-amino-α-phenylacetamido)penicillanic acid.

Solubility. Soluble, at 20°, in 170 parts of water; very slightly soluble in alcohol, in ether, in chloroform, in acetone, and in fixed oils.

Standard
It complies with the requirements of the British Pharmacopoeia.

It is a white, microcrystalline, odourless or almost odourless powder and contains not less than 95·0 per cent of $C_{16}H_{19}N_3O_4S$, calculated with reference to the anhydrous substance. It contains not more than 1·5 per cent w/w of water. A 0·25 per cent solution in water has a pH of 3·5 to 5·5.

Hygroscopicity. It absorbs insignificant amounts of moisture at 25° at relative humidities up to about 80 per cent, but under damper conditions it absorbs significant amounts.

Storage. It should be stored in airtight containers at a temperature not exceeding 25°.

Actions and uses. Ampicillin is a semisynthetic penicillin which is acid resistant and can therefore be given orally, while the sodium salt may be given parenterally. It is destroyed by most bacterial penicillinases but it is more effective against non-penicillinase-producing Gram-negative organisms than benzylpenicillin. It is particularly useful against *Haemophilus influenzae* infections but its effectiveness against *Proteus* species and coliform organisms may be slowly diminishing because of replacement of sensitive strains by resistant ones.

Ampicillin is inappropriate for the treatment of staphylococcal infections because it is destroyed by staphylococcal penicillinase and because the minimum inhibitory concentration is higher than that of benzylpenicillin.

The usual oral dose is 1 to 6 grams daily in divided doses every six hours or 1 gram twice daily by intramuscular injection as the sodium salt. Larger doses are painful when given by intramuscular injection and should be given by slow intravenous injection of a solution of the sodium salt containing the equivalent of 250 to 500 milligrams of ampicillin in 20 to 40 millilitres.

UNDESIRABLE EFFECTS. Ampicillin carries a relatively high risk of morbilliform drug rashes appearing ten to twenty days after the initiation of treatment even though the medication has been discontinued.

PRECAUTIONS. The precautions against allergy described under Benzylpenicillin (page 51) should be observed. Patients allergic to other penicillins must be assumed to be allergic to ampicillin.

Dose. See above under **Actions and uses.**

Preparations
AMPICILLIN CAPSULES, B.P. Unless otherwise specified, capsules each containing 250 mg of ampicillin or an equivalent amount of ampicillin trihydrate are supplied. Capsules containing 500 mg of ampicillin, or an equivalent amount of ampicillin trihydrate, are also available.
AMPICILLIN MIXTURE, B.P.C. (page 737)
AMPICILLIN TABLETS, PAEDIATRIC, B.P.C. (page 805)

OTHER NAME: *Penbritin*®

AMPICILLIN SODIUM

$C_{16}H_{18}N_3NaO_4S = 371·4$

Ampicillin Sodium is the sodium salt of D(−)-6-(α-amino-α-phenylacetamido)penicillanic acid.

Solubility. Soluble, at 20°, in 2 parts of water and in 50 parts of acetone; slightly soluble in chloroform; insoluble in ether, in liquid paraffin, and in fixed oils.

Standard
It complies with the requirements of the British Pharmacopoeia.
It is a white, crystalline, odourless powder and contains not less than the equivalent of 85·0 per cent of $C_{16}H_{19}N_3O_4S$, calculated with reference to the anhydrous substance. It contains not more than 2·0 per cent w/w of water. A 10 per cent solution in water has a pH of 8·0 to 10·0.

Stability. Aqueous solutions decompose on storage; when stored at 5°, 90 per cent of the potency may be expected to be retained for 7 days for solutions containing 1 per cent and for 24 hours for solutions containing 5 per cent; solutions containing 10 and 25 per cent may be expected to retain 80 per cent of their original potency for 24 hours and 6 hours respectively.

Hygroscopicity. It is deliquescent, substantial amounts of moisture being absorbed even at low relative humidities.

Labelling. If the material is not intended for parenteral administration, the label on the container states that the contents are not to be injected.

Storage. It should be stored in airtight containers at a temperature not exceeding 25°. If it is intended for parenteral administration the containers should be sterile and should be sealed to exclude micro-organisms.

Actions and uses. Ampicillin sodium has the actions described under Ampicillin and on account of its solubility it is used for the preparation of injections; 1·06 grams of ampicillin sodium is approximately equivalent to 1 gram of ampicillin.

UNDESIRABLE EFFECTS; PRECAUTIONS. As for Ampicillin.

Dose. By intramuscular injection, the equivalent of 1 to 3 grams of ampicillin daily in divided doses.

Preparation
AMPICILLIN INJECTION, B.P. It consists of a sterile solution prepared by dissolving the sterile contents of a sealed container in Water for Injections. The quantity of ampicillin sodium in each container, in terms of the equivalent amount of ampicillin, should be specified by the prescriber. Vials containing the equivalent of 100, 250, and 500 mg are available. Ampicillin Injection containing 10 per cent w/v or more of ampicillin sodium deteriorates rapidly on storage and should be used immediately after preparation; weaker solutions are more stable.

OTHER NAME: *Penbritin*®

AMPICILLIN TRIHYDRATE

$C_{16}H_{19}N_3O_4S,3H_2O = 403.5$

Ampicillin Trihydrate is the trihydrate of D(−)-6-(α-amino-α-phenylacetamido)penicillanic acid.

Solubility. Soluble, at 20°, in 150 parts of water; very slightly soluble in alcohol, in ether, in chloroform, in acetone, and in fixed oils.

Standard
It complies with the requirements of the British Pharmacopoeia.
It is a white, microcrystalline, odourless or almost odourless powder and contains not less than 95.0 per cent of $C_{16}H_{19}N_3O_4S$, calculated with reference to the anhydrous substance. It contains 12.0 to 15.0 per cent w/w of water. A 0.25 per cent solution in water has a pH of 3.5 to 5.5.

Hygroscopicity. It absorbs insignificant amounts of moisture at 25° at relative humidities up to about 80 per cent but under damper conditions it absorbs significant amounts.

Storage. It should be stored in airtight containers at a temperature not exceeding 25°.

Actions and uses. Ampicillin trihydrate has the actions described under Ampicillin and is used for the same purposes; 1.15 grams of ampicillin trihydrate is approximately equivalent to 1 gram of ampicillin. It is administered by mouth.

UNDESIRABLE EFFECTS; PRECAUTIONS. As for Ampicillin.

Dose. The equivalent of 1 to 6 grams of ampicillin daily in divided doses.

Preparations
AMPICILLIN CAPSULES, B.P. Unless otherwise specified, capsules each containing 250 mg of ampicillin or an equivalent amount of ampicillin trihydrate are supplied. Capsules containing 500 mg of ampicillin, or an equivalent amount of ampicillin trihydrate, are also available.
AMPICILLIN MIXTURE, B.P.C. (page 737)
AMPICILLIN TABLETS, PAEDIATRIC, B.P.C. (page 805)

OTHER NAME: *Penbritin*®

AMYL NITRITE

Amyl Nitrite is a liquid consisting of the nitrites of 3-methylbutan-1-ol, $(CH_3)_2CH \cdot CH_2 \cdot CH_2OH$, and 2-methylbutan-1-ol, $CH_3 \cdot CH_2 \cdot CH(CH_3) \cdot CH_2OH$, with other nitrites of the homologous series.

Amyl Nitrite may be prepared by treating amyl alcohol, or the fraction of fusel oil that boils between 128° and 132°, with sodium nitrite and sulphuric acid.

Solubility. Insoluble in water; miscible with alcohol and with ether.

Standard
DESCRIPTION. A clear, yellow, volatile, inflammable liquid; odour fragrant.

IDENTIFICATION TESTS. 1. To 0.2 ml add a mixture of 2 ml of *ferrous sulphate solution* and 5 ml of *dilute hydrochloric acid*; a greenish-brown colour is produced.
2. To 0.2 ml add 0.5 ml of *aniline* and 5 ml of *glacial acetic acid*; a deep orange-red colour is produced.
3. To 0.1 ml add 0.1 ml of water and 2 ml of *sulphuric acid*, and dilute to 10 ml with water; the odour of amyl valerate is produced.

ACIDITY. Shake 5 ml with 9 ml of water, 1 ml of 1N sodium hydroxide and 0.05 ml of *phenolphthalein solution*, and allow to stand for one minute; the aqueous layer remains alkaline.

DISTILLATION RANGE. Determine by the method given in Appendix 9A, page 887; not less than 85 per cent v/v distils between 90° and 100°.

WEIGHT PER ML. At 20°, 0.868 g to 0.878 g.

RESIDUE ON EVAPORATION. Not more than 0.1 per cent w/v, the residue being dried at 105°.

CONTENT OF NITRITES. Not less than 90.0 per cent w/w, calculated as $C_5H_{11}NO_2$, determined by the following method:
Dilute 5 ml to 100 ml with *alcohol (95 per cent)*; introduce 2 ml of this solution into a brine-charged nitrometer, rinsing the nitrometer funnel with small quantities of *alcohol (95 per cent)*; add 2 ml of *potassium iodide solution* and 2 ml of *dilute sulphuric acid*, shake briskly at intervals for 5 minutes, and measure the volume of nitric oxide produced; each ml of moist nitric oxide, at 20° and normal pressure, is equivalent to 0.0048 g of $C_5H_{11}NO_2$. Determine the weight per ml of the sample, and calculate the percentage of $C_5H_{11}NO_2$, weight in weight.

Stability. Amyl nitrite is liable to decompose with evolution of nitrogen, particularly if it has become acid in reaction. In the preparation of vitrellae, amyl nitrite should be tested immediately before filling in order to ensure that it complies with the test for acidity.

Storage. It should be stored in airtight containers, protected from light, in a cool place.

Actions and uses. Amyl nitrite, when inhaled, has actions similar to those described under Glyceryl Trinitrate Solution (page 212). After inhalation it is rapidly absorbed, so that the onset of its effect is immediate; its actions last for four to eight minutes.
The chief use of amyl nitrite is in the treatment of an attack of angina of effort, when it affords relief by the dilatation of the coronary vessels; it is contra-indicated, however, in coronary thrombosis. It is also used for the relief of renal and gall-bladder colic.
It is employed in the immediate treatment of cyanide poisoning to induce the formation of methaemoglobin, which combines with the cyanide to form the non-toxic cyanmethaemoglobin.

POISONING. As for Glyceryl Trinitrate Solution (page 212).

Dose. 0.12 to 0.3 millilitre by inhalation.

Preparation
AMYL NITRITE VITRELLAE, B.P.C. (page 824)

AMYLOBARBITONE

SYNONYMS: Amylobarb.; Amobarbital

$C_{11}H_{18}N_2O_3 = 226.3$

Amylobarbitone is 5-ethyl-5-isopentylbarbituric acid.

Solubility. Slightly soluble in water; soluble, at 20°, in 5 parts of alcohol, in 6 parts of ether, and in 20 parts of chloroform; readily soluble in solutions of alkali hydroxides and carbonates.

Standard
It complies with the requirements of the British Pharmacopoeia.
It is a white, crystalline, odourless powder. The loss on drying at 105° is not more than 0.5 per cent. It has a melting-point of 155° to 158°.

Hygroscopicity. It absorbs insignificant amounts of moisture at 25° at relative humidities of up to about 90 per cent.

Actions and uses. Amylobarbitone is an intermediate-acting barbiturate, the actions and uses of which are described under Phenobarbitone (page 366). It is given by mouth in a single dose of 100 to 200 milligrams as a hypnotic. Up to 600 milligrams daily may be given in divided doses as a sedative, the usual dose, however, being 30 to 60 milligrams three times daily.

UNDESIRABLE EFFECTS; CONTRA-INDICATIONS; PRECAUTIONS; DEPENDENCE. These are as described under Phenobarbitone (page 366).

POISONING. The procedure as described under Phenobarbitone (page 366) should be adopted but haemodialysis is not effective.

Dose. See above under **Actions and uses.**

Preparation
AMYLOBARBITONE TABLETS, B.P. (*Syn.* Amobarbital Tablets). The quantity of amylobarbitone in each tablet should be specified by the prescriber. Tablets containing 15, 30, 50, 100, and 200 mg are available.

OTHER NAME: *Amytal®*

AMYLOBARBITONE SODIUM

SYNONYMS: Amylobarb. Sod.; Amobarbital Sodium; Amobarbitalum Natricum; Soluble Amylobarbitone

$C_{11}H_{17}N_2NaO_3 = 248.3$

Amylobarbitone Sodium is sodium 5-ethyl-5-isopentylbarbiturate.

Solubility. Soluble, at 20°, in less than 1 part of water and in 2 parts of alcohol; insoluble in ether and in chloroform.

Standard
It complies with the requirements of the European Pharmacopoeia.
It is a white, granular, hygroscopic, odourless powder and contains not less than 98.5 and not more than the equivalent of 102.0 per cent of $C_{11}H_{17}N_2NaO_3$, calculated with reference to the dried substance. The loss on drying under the prescribed conditions is not more than 5.0 per cent. A 10 per cent solution in water has a pH of not more than 11.

Storage. It should be stored in airtight containers.

Actions and uses. Amylobarbitone sodium is an intermediate-acting barbiturate, the actions and uses of which are described under Phenobarbitone (page 366) and the oral dosage of which is described under Amylobarbitone.
It is valuable as a pre-operative sedative when given the night before an operation and it can be used as a basal anaesthetic. As it may sometimes cause increased restlessness, it is no longer given to patients in labour.
It may be given by intravenous injection in the treatment of convulsions; the dose is 300 to 1000 milligrams, adjusted according to the response; usually 500 milligrams is given slowly and this dose is repeated if necessary.

UNDESIRABLE EFFECTS; CONTRA-INDICATIONS; PRECAUTIONS; DEPENDENCE. These are as described under Phenobarbitone (page 366).

POISONING. The procedure as described under Phenobarbitone (page 366) should be adopted but haemodialysis is not effective.

Dose. See above under **Actions and uses.**

Preparations
AMYLOBARBITONE SODIUM CAPSULES, B.P. (*Syn.* Soluble Amylobarbitone Capsules; Amobarbital Sodium Capsules). The quantity of amylobarbitone sodium in each capsule should be specified by the prescriber. Capsules containing 60 and 200 mg are available.
AMYLOBARBITONE INJECTION, B.P. It consists of a sterile solution prepared immediately before use by dissolving the sterile contents of a sealed container in Water for Injections free from carbon dioxide. The quantity of amylobarbitone sodium in each container should be specified by the prescriber. Ampoules containing 125, 250, 500 and 1000 mg are available.
AMYLOBARBITONE SODIUM TABLETS, B.P. (*Syn.* Soluble Amylobarbitone Tablets; Amobarbital Sodium Tablets). The quantity of amylobarbitone sodium in each tablet should be specified by the prescriber. They should be stored in airtight containers. Tablets containing 60 and 200 mg are available.

OTHER NAME: *Sodium Amytal®*

ANISE OIL

SYNONYMS: Aniseed Oil; Oleum Anisi

Anise Oil is obtained by distillation from the dried fruits of star anise, *Illicium verum* Hook. f. (Fam. Illiciaceae), a tree indigenous to south-western China, or from anise, the dried fruits of *Pimpinella anisum* L. (Fam. Umbelliferae), an annual plant cultivated chiefly in Spain, southern Russia, and Bulgaria; star anise is the chief commercial source.

Constituents. Anise oil contains about 80 to 90 per cent of anethole. It also contains chavicol methyl ether, an isomeride of anethole, which it resembles in odour but not in taste, and *p*-methoxyphenylacetone (anise ketone).

Solubility. Soluble, at 20°, in 3 parts of alcohol (90 per cent), sometimes with a slight opalescence.

Standard
It complies with the requirements of the British Pharmacopoeia.
It is a colourless or pale yellow, highly refractive liquid, with the characteristic odour of the crushed fruit. It has a weight per ml at 20° of 0·978 g to 0·992 g.
When cooled it solidifies at about 15° to a white crystalline mass, but it can be cooled considerably below this temperature without becoming solid provided it is undisturbed; the supercooled liquid immediately solidifies if slightly agitated or if a crystal of anethole is introduced. The crystalline mass melts at about 17°.

Stability. Exposure to air causes polymerisation and some oxidation also takes place with the formation of *p*-methoxybenzaldehyde (anisaldehyde) and anisic acid.

Storage. It should be stored in well-filled containers, protected from light, in a cool place. If it has solidified, it should be completely melted and mixed before use.

Actions and uses. Anise oil is a carminative and mild expectorant. It is used in mixtures and cough lozenges, often in combination with liquorice.

Dose. 0·05 to 0·2 millilitre.

Preparation
ANISE WATER, CONCENTRATED, B.P.C. (page 824)

ANTAZOLINE HYDROCHLORIDE

$C_{17}H_{20}ClN_3 = 301·8$

Antazoline Hydrochloride is 2-(*N*-benzylanilinomethyl)imidazoline hydrochloride.

Solubility. Soluble, at 20°, in 50 parts of water and in 16 parts of alcohol; slightly soluble in chloroform; very slightly soluble in ether.

Standard
It complies with the requirements of the British Pharmacopoeia.
It is a white or almost white, odourless or almost odourless, crystalline powder and contains not less than 99·0 and not more than the equivalent of 101·0 per cent of $C_{17}H_{20}ClN_3$, calculated with reference to the dried substance. It melts with decomposition at about 240°. A 1 per cent solution in water has a pH of 5·0 to 6·5.

Sterilisation. Solutions are sterilised by heating in an autoclave or by filtration.

Storage. It should be stored in airtight containers, protected from light.

Actions and uses. Antazoline has the actions and uses of the antihistamine drugs, as described under Promethazine Hydrochloride (page 409); it is one of the weakest of these compounds. It is about fifteen times less active than promethazine hydrochloride and the duration of action is shorter.

Antazoline hydrochloride is administered by mouth; it is also applied as a 0·5 per cent solution to the skin and to the mucous membrane of the eye and nose. A 2 per cent cream or ointment is used as an antipruritic, but it is less effective than preparations containing corticosteroids and it may give rise to skin sensitisation.

UNDESIRABLE EFFECTS. Nausea and drowsiness occur in some patients.

POISONING. As for Promethazine Hydrochloride (page 409).

Dose. 100 to 300 milligrams daily in divided doses.

Preparation
ANTAZOLINE TABLETS, B.P. Unless otherwise specified, tablets each containing 100 mg of antazoline hydrochloride are supplied. They should be stored in airtight containers, protected from light.

OTHER NAME: *Antistin*®

ANTAZOLINE MESYLATE

SYNONYM: Antazoline Methanesulphonate

$C_{17}H_{19}N_3,CH_3SO_3H = 361·5$

Antazoline Mesylate is 2-(*N*-benzylanilinomethyl)imidazoline methanesulphonate.

Solubility. Soluble, at 20°, in 6 parts of water, in 7 parts of alcohol, and in 12 parts of chloroform; insoluble in ether.

Standard
DESCRIPTION. A white or almost white powder; odourless or almost odourless.

IDENTIFICATION TESTS. 1. Dissolve 0·5 g in 30 ml of water, add 1 ml of *sodium hydroxide solution*, extract with 20 ml of *chloroform*, wash the extract with 5 ml of water, and evaporate off the chloroform; the residue, after drying over *phosphorus pentoxide* in vacuo, melts at about 121°.

2. Dissolve 0·05 g in 5 ml of water, and add 0·5 ml of *nitric acid*; a red colour is produced, which rapidly becomes green.

3. The ultraviolet absorption spectrum exhibits the characteristics given in Appendix 3, page 855.

4. Mix 0·1 g with 0·5 g of *anhydrous sodium carbonate*, heat strongly, dissolve the residue in an excess of *hydrochloric acid*, and dilute to 50 ml with water; the solution gives the reactions characteristic of sulphates.

ACIDITY. pH of a 1·0 per cent w/v solution in *carbon dioxide-free water*, 4·0 to 6·5.

MELTING-POINT. 165° to 168°.

LOSS ON DRYING. Not more than 2·5 per cent, determined by drying to constant weight over *phosphorus pentoxide* in vacuo.

SULPHATED ASH. Not more than 0·1 per cent.

CONTENT OF $C_{17}H_{19}N_3,CH_3SO_3H$. Not less than 98·0 per cent, calculated with reference to the substance dried under the prescribed conditions, determined by the following method:

Dissolve about 0·5 g, accurately weighed, in 30 ml of water, add 2 ml of *sodium hydroxide solution*, and extract with five successive 25-ml portions of *chloroform*; wash the combined extracts with two successive 5-ml portions of water and evaporate to low bulk; add 20 ml of 0·1N hydrochloric acid, warm to remove the remainder of the chloroform, cool, and titrate the excess of acid with 0·1N sodium hydroxide, using *methyl red solution* as indicator; each ml of 0·1N hydrochloric acid is equivalent to 0·03615 g of $C_{17}H_{19}N_3,CH_3SO_3H$.

Hygroscopicity. It is slightly hygroscopic, significant amounts of moisture being absorbed at 20° at relative humidities above about 70 per cent.

Storage. It should be stored in airtight containers, protected from light.

Actions and uses. Antazoline mesylate has the actions, uses, and undesirable effects described under Antazoline Hydrochloride. It is usually given by injection in a solution containing 50 mg in 1 ml.

POISONING. As for Promethazine Hydrochloride (page 409).

Dose. 50 to 100 milligrams by intramuscular or slow intravenous injection.

ANTIMONY POTASSIUM TARTRATE

SYNONYMS: Antim. Pot. Tart.; Potassium Antimonyltartrate; Tartar Emetic

$C_4H_4KO_7Sb = 324·9$

Antimony Potassium Tartrate may be prepared by mixing antimonious oxide and potassium acid tartrate into a paste with water, allowing to stand until combination has taken place, and purifying by crystallisation from water.

Antimony Potassium Tartrate may occur as the hemihydrate with about 2·7 per cent of moisture, but the salt effloresces in dry air, and the commercial material rarely contains more than 1 per cent of moisture. The salt becomes anhydrous at 100° and does not readily rehydrate on exposure to the atmosphere.

A less pure "tartar emetic" is prepared for use as a mordant in the dyeing industry.

Solubility. Soluble, at 20°, in 13 parts of water and in 20 parts of glycerol; soluble in 3 parts of boiling water; insoluble in alcohol.

Standard

DESCRIPTION. Colourless transparent crystals or white granular powder; odourless or almost odourless.

IDENTIFICATION TESTS. It gives the reactions characteristic of antimony and of potassium and, after the removal of antimony, of tartrates.

ACIDITY OR ALKALINITY. Dissolve 1·0 g in 50 ml of *carbon dioxide-free water* and titrate with 0·01N hydrochloric acid or with 0·01N sodium hydroxide, using *bromocresol green solution* as indicator; not more than 2·0 ml is required.

ARSENIC. It complies with the test given in Appendix 6, page 877 (8 parts per million).

LEAD. It complies with the test given in Appendix 7, page 881 (20 parts per million).

CONTENT OF $C_4H_4KO_7Sb$. Not less than 98·5 per cent and not more than the equivalent of 101·0 per cent, determined by the following method:
Dissolve about 0·5 g, accurately weighed, in 50 ml of water, add 5 g of *sodium potassium tartrate* and 2 g of *borax*, and titrate with 0·1N iodine, using *starch mucilage*, added towards the end of the titration, as indicator; each ml of 0·1N iodine is equivalent to 0·01625 g of $C_4H_4KO_7Sb$.

Sterilisation. Solutions for injection are sterilised by heating in an autoclave or by filtration.

Storage. It should be stored in airtight containers.

Actions and uses. Antimony potassium tartrate has the actions, uses, and undesirable effects described under Antimony Sodium Tartrate and is used in similar dosage. It is less soluble and more irritant than the sodium salt, which is therefore more suitable for intravenous injection. The emetic dose is 30 to 60 milligrams.

PRECAUTIONS. As for Antimony Sodium Tartrate.

POISONING. As for Antimony Sodium Tartrate.

Dose. See above under **Actions and uses.**

ANTIMONY SODIUM TARTRATE

SYNONYMS: Antim. Sod. Tart.; Sodium Antimonyltartrate

$C_4H_4NaO_7Sb = 308.8$

Antimony Sodium Tartrate may be prepared by mixing antimonious oxide and sodium hydrogen tartrate into a paste with water, allowing to stand until combination has taken place, and purifying by crystallisation from water.

Solubility. Soluble, at 20°, in 1·5 parts of water; insoluble in alcohol.

Standard
It complies with the requirements of the British Pharmacopoeia.
It occurs as colourless or whitish, odourless, hygroscopic scales or powder and contains not less than 98·0 and not more than the equivalent of 101·0 per cent of $C_4H_4NaO_7Sb$, calculated with reference to the dried substance. The loss on drying under the prescribed conditions is not more than 6·0 per cent.

Sterilisation. Solutions for injection are sterilised by heating in an autoclave or by filtration.

Storage. It should be stored in airtight containers.

Actions and uses. Antimony sodium tartrate has an irritant action on mucous membranes and when given by mouth causes nausea and vomiting.
In the treatment of schistosomiasis it is given intravenously thrice weekly. The initial dose is 60 milligrams, and the second and third doses 90 and 120 milligrams respectively. Thereafter, doses of 120 milligrams are given up to a total of at least 1·2 grams.

UNDESIRABLE EFFECTS. Undesirable effects frequently occur and include cough, anorexia, nausea, vomiting, diarrhoea, and abdominal, thoracic, muscle and joint pains. Acute vascular collapse resembling an anaphylactic response sometimes occurs. Changes in the electrocardiogram are usually observed during treatment, the most common being flattening or inversion of the T-wave. This effect is a property of all organic trivalent antimony derivatives.

PRECAUTIONS. Antimony sodium tartrate should never be given by intramuscular or subcutaneous injection because it causes severe pain and tissue necrosis; great care should be taken not to inject solutions outside the vein.

POISONING. In antimony poisoning persistent vomiting and diarrhoea occur, followed by muscular weakness, suppression of urine, collapse, and convulsions.
Treatment should be designed to remove the poison; if the drug has been taken by mouth and vomiting has not occurred, the stomach should be washed out. Tannic acid, calcium hydroxide, or magnesium oxide may be given to precipitate the antimony in the stomach. Respiratory stimulants and warmth are useful. In poisoning caused by intravenous injection of antimony salts, the heart is frequently affected and artificial cardiac stimulation or the use of a pacemaker may be required for a while; the patient must be kept warm and a high fluid intake ensured. Injections of dimercaprol should be given.

Dose. See above under **Actions and uses.**

Preparation
ANTIMONY SODIUM TARTRATE INJECTION, B.P. (*Syn.* Sodium Antimonyltartrate Injection). It consists of a sterile solution of antimony sodium tartrate in Water for Injections. Unless otherwise specified, a solution containing 60 mg in 1 ml is supplied.

APOMORPHINE HYDROCHLORIDE

SYNONYM: Apomorph. Hydrochlor.

$C_{17}H_{18}ClNO_2,\tfrac{1}{2}H_2O = 312.8$

Apomorphine Hydrochloride is the hemihydrate of the hydrochloride of an alkaloid, apomorphine, which may be obtained from morphine by the abstraction of the elements of a molecule of water.

Solubility. Soluble, at 20°, in 50 parts of water and in 50 parts of alcohol; slightly soluble in chloroform and in ether.

Standard
It complies with the requirements of the British Pharmacopoeia.
It is a colourless or greyish-white, odourless, glistening, microcrystalline powder which becomes green on exposure to air and light. It contains not less than 98·0 and not more than the equivalent of 101·0 per cent of $C_{17}H_{18}ClNO_2$, calculated with reference to the dried substance. The loss on drying under the prescribed conditions is 2·5 to 4·0 per cent. A 1 per cent solution in water has a pH of 4·5 to 5·5.

Stability. Aqueous solutions are colourless when freshly prepared, but readily decompose and become green on exposure to air; the change may be retarded by the addition of dilute hydrochloric acid or sodium metabisulphite.
Apomorphine Hydrochloride should not be used if it at once gives an emerald-green solution when one part is shaken with 100 parts of water.

Incompatibility. It is incompatible with alkaline substances.

Sterilisation. Solutions for injection are sterilised by heating in an autoclave in an atmosphere of nitrogen or other suitable gas.

Storage. It should be stored in airtight containers, protected from light.

Actions and uses. Apomorphine hydrochloride causes vomiting as a result of central stimulation. A dose of 2 to 8 milligrams by subcutaneous or intramuscular injection can produce vomiting in a few minutes, but the same dose taken by mouth may act merely as an expectorant. Following its emetic action, it commonly induces sleep. Apomorphine is used in aversion therapy.

Dose. 2 to 8 milligrams by subcutaneous or intramuscular injection.

Preparation
APOMORPHINE INJECTION, B.P. (*Syn.* Apomorphine Hydrochloride Injection). It consists of a sterile solution of apomorphine hydrochloride in Water for Injections free from dissolved air, and containing 0·1 per cent of sodium metabisulphite. Unless otherwise specified, a solution containing 3 mg in 1 ml is supplied.

ARACHIS OIL

SYNONYMS: Groundnut Oil; Oleum Arachis; Peanut Oil

Arachis Oil is the refined fixed oil obtained from the seeds of *Arachis hypogaea* L. (Fam. Leguminosae), a tree native to Brazil and widely cultivated in Africa, the Indian subcontinent, China, and America.

Constituents. Arachis oil consists of glycerides, the fatty acid constituents of which are chiefly oleic and linoleic acids with smaller amounts of palmitic, arachidic, lignoceric, and stearic acids. The proportion of arachidic and lignoceric acids taken together is usually about 5 per cent and their low solubility in alcohol (70 per cent) is used in testing for arachis oil. The unrefined oil may sometimes contain toxic substances.

Solubility. Very slightly soluble in alcohol; miscible with ether, with chloroform, and with light petroleum.

Standard
It complies with the requirements of the British Pharmacopoeia.
It is a pale yellow oil with a faint odour. It has a weight per ml at 20° of 0·911 g to 0·915 g.

Stability. On exposure to air it thickens very slowly and may become rancid.

Sterilisation. It is sterilised by dry heat.

Storage. It should be stored in well-filled airtight containers. It becomes cloudy at about 3° and partly solidifies at lower temperatures. If it has solidified it should be completely remelted and mixed before use.

Actions and uses. Arachis oil has properties similar to those of olive oil (page 336) and is used for the same purposes. Emulsions containing 10 per cent of arachis oil and 40 per cent of dextrose have been used by intragastric drip as a nitrogen-free diet.

ARROWROOT

SYNONYM: Maranta

Arrowroot consists of the starch granules of the rhizome of *Maranta arundinacea* L. (Fam. Marantaceae). The plant is a native of central America; it is cultivated in tropical and subtropical countries, chiefly in the West Indies, and is imported mainly from St. Vincent.

Varieties. Several grades of St. Vincent or West Indian arrowroot are found in commerce and are usually sold on the basis of colour and general appearance. The mucilages formed from these varieties differ slightly in viscosity, which may form an additional criterion of quality.

Constituents. Arrowroot consists chiefly of amylose and amylopectin and contains about 14 to 17 per cent of moisture.

Standard
DESCRIPTION. *Macroscopical:* a white powder, much of which may cohere to form small irregular masses up to about 8 mm in length; it crepitates slightly when pressed.
Odourless; tasteless.

Microscopical: the diagnostic characters are: *starch* granules ovoid or ellipsoid, simple, frequently with small local enlargements or tuberosities; hilum well marked, generally situated near the broader end of the granules, usually in the form of a 2-rayed cleft; striations concentric, clearly marked but very fine; granules ranging from 7 to **30** to **50** to 75 μm in their greatest dimension and exhibiting a well marked cross when viewed between crossed polars.

IDENTIFICATION TESTS. 1. Boil 1 g with 15 ml of water and cool; a translucent whitish gelatinous mass is formed. Add 0·2 ml of *iodine solution*; a deep blue colour is produced which disappears on warming and reappears on cooling.

2. Add to a sample on a microscope slide 0·2 ml of a 0·9 per cent w/v solution of *potassium hydroxide* in water, apply a cover-glass, and examine under a 4-mm objective; the granules are not gelatinised (distinction from potato starch).

LOSS ON DRYING. Not more than 16·0 per cent, determined by drying to constant weight at 100°.

ASH. Not more than 0·3 per cent.

Adulterants and substitutes. Many starches have been described as arrowroots and are sometimes substituted for arrowroot; the most important of these substitutes are the following:
The starch of potato, *Solanum tuberosum* L. ("English" arrowroot), which is described under Starch.

Manihot (Manioc) starch ("Brazilian" or "Rio" arrowroot), often known as cassava or tapioca starch, obtained from *Manihot esculenta* Crantz (Fam. Euphorbiaceae), has subspherical and muller-shaped granules, the smaller ones being about 5 to **12** to 25 μm and the larger ones about 25 to 35 μm in diameter.

Sweet potato starch ("Brazilian" arrowroot), obtained from *Ipomoea batatas* (L.) Poir. (Fam. Convolvulaceae), has rounded, polyhedral and muller-shaped granules, the smaller ones being about 15 to 22 μm and the larger ones about 25 to **50** to 55 μm in diameter.

"Queensland" arrowroot or "tous-les-mois" starch, from *Canna edulis* Edwards (Fam. Cannaceae), has flattened ovoid granules about 30 to **70** to **100** to 130 μm in diameter.

Sago starch, from *Metroxylon rumphii* Mart., *M. sagu* Rottb., and *M. laeve* Mart. (Fam. Palmae), has ovoid, subspherical and muller-shaped granules, the smaller ones being about 10 to 20 μm and the larger ones about 50 to **60** to 80 μm in diameter.

"Indian" or "Bombay" arrowroot, from *Curcuma angustifolia* Roxb., and "East Indian" arrowroot, from *C. leucorrhiza* Roxb. (Fam. Zingiberaceae), have scitaminaceous granules, about 30 to **60** to 140 μm long, 25 to 35 μm wide and 7 to 8 μm thick.

Actions and uses. Arrowroot has the general properties of starch and is used as a gruel in the treatment of diarrhoea. It has been employed as a suspending agent in the preparation of barium meals and is sometimes preferred to starch for use in tablet-making.

ASCORBIC ACID

SYNONYMS: Acidum Ascorbicum; Vitamin C

$C_6H_8O_6 = 176 \cdot 1$

$$\overset{\displaystyle\overset{O}{\rule{3cm}{0.4pt}}}{CO \cdot C(OH) : C(OH) \cdot CH \cdot CH(OH) \cdot CH_2OH}$$

Ascorbic Acid is the enolic form of 3-oxo-L-gulofuranolactone and may be prepared synthetically or extracted from various vegetable sources in which it occurs naturally, such as rose hips, black currants, the juice of citrus fruits, and the ripe fruit of *Capsicum annuum* L. (Fam. Solanaceae).

Solubility. Soluble, at 20°, in 3·5 parts of water, in 25 parts of alcohol, and in 10 parts of methyl alcohol; insoluble in ether and in light petroleum.

Standard
It complies with the requirements of the European Pharmacopoeia.
It occurs as almost odourless, colourless crystals or white or very pale yellow crystalline powder and contains not less than 99·0 per cent of $C_6H_8O_6$. It melts with decomposition at about 190°. A 5 per cent solution in water has a pH of 2·2 to 2·5.

Stability. It is unstable, especially in alkaline solution, readily undergoing oxidation even by atmospheric oxygen, the change being accelerated by light and heat; it exhibits maximum stability in solution at about pH 5·4. The first stage in the oxidation is reversible and results in the formation of dehydroascorbic acid.

Sterilisation. Solutions for injection are sterilised by heating with a bactericide in an atmosphere of nitrogen or other suitable gas, or by filtration.

Storage. It should be stored in airtight containers, free from contact with metal and protected from light.

Actions and uses. Ascorbic acid is essential for the formation of collagen and intercellular material, and hence for the development of cartilage, bone, and teeth, and for the healing of wounds. It is also essential for the conversion of folic acid to folinic acid. It facilitates the absorption of iron from the gut, 5 milligrams of ascorbic acid being required for each milligram of iron. It also influences the formation of haemoglobin and erythrocyte maturation.

The minimal daily requirement of ascorbic acid is probably about 20 milligrams; this requirement is increased during pregnancy and lactation, in adolescence, in hyperthyroidism, during infections, and after surgery.

Ascorbic acid is used primarily for the prophylaxis and treatment of scurvy. Although this condition is now seldom seen, it may occur in the undernourished and in bottle-fed infants. To prevent infantile scurvy, bottle-fed infants should have their feed supplemented by 2·5 to 5 milligrams of ascorbic acid daily. It is also used to prevent scurvy in patients on restricted diets and in alcoholics. Supplements of the vitamin may also be necessary to promote healing of wounds and fractures and in those conditions where vomiting, diarrhoea, or diuresis are likely to interfere with its absorption and utilisation. Some types of hypochromic anaemia respond to treatment with ascorbic acid and iron, as ascorbic acid facilitates the absorption of ferrous iron.

Large doses of ascorbic acid are often administered therapeutically, but there is little evidence to show that a daily intake of more than 30 to 50 milligrams has any beneficial effect except in the treatment of methaemoglobinaemia, for which 200 milligrams is given thrice daily; in this dosage ascorbic acid has a diuretic action.

Ascorbic acid is usually administered by mouth; it may also be given parenterally, but since it is absorbed efficiently when taken by mouth parenteral administration is necessary only when absorption from the gastrointestinal tract is unsatisfactory.

Dose. Prophylactic, 25 to 75 milligrams daily; therapeutic, 200 to 600 milligrams daily.

Preparations
VITAMINS CAPSULES, B.P.C. (page 654)
ASCORBIC ACID INJECTION, B.P.C. (page 709)
VITAMINS B AND C INJECTION, B.P.C. (page 720)

Ascorbic Acid Tablets, B.P. (*Syn.* Vitamin C Tablets). Unless otherwise specified, tablets each containing 25 mg of ascorbic acid are supplied. They should be stored in airtight containers, free from contact with metal, and protected from light. Tablets containing 50, 100, 200, and 500 mg are also available.

Other Name: *Redoxon®*

ASPIRIN

Synonyms: Acetylsal. Acid; Acetylsalicylic Acid; Acidum Acetylsalicylicum

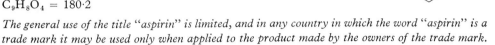

$C_9H_8O_4 = 180 \cdot 2$

The general use of the title "aspirin" is limited, and in any country in which the word "aspirin" is a trade mark it may be used only when applied to the product made by the owners of the trade mark.

Aspirin is *o*-acetoxybenzoic acid.

Solubility. Soluble, at 20°, in 300 parts of water, in 7 parts of alcohol, in 20 parts of ether, and in 17 parts of chloroform; soluble in solutions of acetates and citrates and, with decomposition, in solutions of alkali hydroxides and carbonates.

Standard
It complies with the requirements of the European Pharmacopoeia.
It occurs as odourless or nearly odourless colourless crystals or white crystalline powder and contains not less than 99·5 per cent of $C_9H_8O_4$, calculated with reference to the dried substance. The loss on drying under the prescribed conditions is not more than 0·5 per cent. It has a melting-point of 141° to 144°.

Stability. It is stable in dry air but in contact with moisture it gradually hydrolyses into acetic and salicylic acids.

Storage. It should be stored in airtight containers.

Actions and uses. Aspirin has analgesic, anti-inflammatory, and antipyretic actions. It is rapidly absorbed from the upper gastro-intestinal tract and its effects are apparent within a few minutes. It is eliminated by the kidneys, excretion beginning shortly after it is administered.
Aspirin is given by mouth in a dose of 300 to 900 milligrams for the relief of minor pain and symptoms of inflammation. Up to 3·6 grams may be given daily in divided doses.
Aspirin is also used in the treatment of acute and chronic rheumatic states. For acute episodes, 3·6 to 7·2 grams is given daily in divided doses; for the control of chronic rheumatic disease, 300 to 900 milligrams is administered every four hours over long periods.
Aspirin is relatively ineffective for most pains of visceral origin.
Mixtures of aspirin with other analgesics have not been shown to be superior in analgesic effect to the use of only one drug, and some of the mixtures have been shown to induce dependence.
Aspirin should not be given to children under one year of age except under medical supervision. The usual dosage as an analgesic for a child from one to two years is 75 to 150 milligrams not more than four times daily, from three to five years 225 to 300 milligrams not more than three times daily, and from six to twelve years 300 milligrams not more than four times daily. These doses should not be given for more than two days except under medical supervision.
The use of aqueous preparations of aspirin, such as mixtures, should be avoided because they decompose rapidly with the liberation of acetic and salicylic acids.
Symptoms of gastric irritation may be reduced by taking aspirin after food or with plenty of fluid.

Undesirable effects. Small and occasional doses of aspirin rarely produce serious gastric irritation, but some patients are unable to tolerate it even in low dosage. After large or repeated doses haemorrhage may occur and blood may be present in the stools, although usually in small amounts.
Aspirin produces reactions in hypersensitive patients; skin eruptions and swelling of the mucous membranes of the nose and throat with an asthma-like attack are the most common symptoms. It decreases platelet adhesiveness and increases the coagulation time of the blood. It may give rise to angioneurotic oedema, urticaria, and myocarditis.

Precautions. The use of aspirin in conjunction with anticoagulant drugs should be avoided as it may increase the risk of haemorrhage. Aspirin may increase the toxic effects of methotrexate.

Poisoning. The stomach should be washed out with a 5 per cent sodium bicarbonate solution, and intravenous injections of saline with sodium bicarbonate may be required to correct dehydration and metabolic disturbances.

Dose. See above under **Actions and uses.**

Preparations
Aspirin Tablets, B.P. (*Syn.* Acetylsalicylic Acid Tablets). Unless otherwise specified, tablets each containing 300 mg are supplied. They should be stored in airtight containers.
Aspirin Tablets, Compound, B.P.C. (page 806)

ASPIRIN TABLETS, SOLUBLE, B.P. (*Syn.* Soluble Acetylsalicylic Acid Tablets). Each tablet contains 300 mg of aspirin, with calcium carbonate, anhydrous citric acid, and saccharin sodium. They should be stored in airtight containers. Dose: up to 12 tablets daily in divided doses; for acute rheumatism, 12 to 24 tablets daily in divided doses.
When Calcium Aspirin Tablets are ordered or prescribed, Soluble Aspirin Tablets are supplied.

ASPIRIN TABLETS, SOLUBLE, PAEDIATRIC, B.P.C. (page 806)

ASPIRIN, PHENACETIN, AND CODEINE TABLETS, B.P.

(*Syn.* Compound Codeine Tablets). Each tablet contains 250 mg of aspirin and of phenacetin and 8 mg of codeine phosphate. They should be stored in airtight containers, protected from light. Dose: 1 or 2 tablets.

ASPIRIN, PHENACETIN, AND CODEINE TABLETS, SOLUBLE, B.P. (*Syn.* Soluble Compound Codeine Tablets). Each tablet contains 250 mg of aspirin and of phenacetin and 8 mg of codeine phosphate with calcium carbonate, anhydrous citric acid, and saccharin sodium. They should be stored in airtight containers, protected from light. Dose: 1 or 2 tablets.

ATROPINE

$C_{17}H_{23}NO_3 = 289.4$

Atropine is $(\pm)$-hyoscyamine and may be prepared by racemisation of $(-)$-hyoscyamine, an alkaloid extracted from *Duboisia* species, *Hyoscyamus muticus* L., and other solanaceous plants, or by synthesis.

Solubility. Soluble, at 20°, in 400 parts of water, in 3 parts of alcohol, in 60 parts of ether, and in 1 part of chloroform.

Standard

DESCRIPTION. Colourless crystals or a white crystalline powder; odourless or almost odourless.

IDENTIFICATION TESTS. 1. Dissolve 0.05 g in a mixture of 5 ml of water and 0.05 ml of *hydrochloric acid* and add 5 ml of *gold chloride solution*; a lemon-yellow, oily precipitate is produced which rapidly crystallises. This precipitate, after recrystallisation from 3 ml of boiling water containing 0.05 ml of *hydrochloric acid*, has a minutely crystalline character, is dull and pulverulent when dry, and has a melting-point of about 136° (distinction from hyoscyamine).

2. Add 1 mg to 0.2 ml of *fuming nitric acid* and evaporate to dryness on a water-bath; a yellow residue is obtained. Cool the residue and add 2 ml of *acetone* and 0.2 ml of a 3 per cent w/v solution of *potassium hydroxide* in *methyl alcohol*; a deep violet colour is produced. (Hyoscyamine and hyoscine produce the same colour as atropine; the presence of other alkaloids masks the reaction.)

3. To 10 mg in a porcelain basin add 1.5 ml of a 2 per cent w/v solution of *mercuric chloride* in *alcohol (60 per cent)*; a yellow colour is produced which changes to red on gently warming (distinction from most other alkaloids except homatropine and hyoscyamine).

ALKALINITY. A saturated solution in water is alkaline to *phenolphthalein solution*.

MELTING-POINT. 115° to 118°.

OPTICAL ROTATION. $-0.25°$ to $+0.05°$, determined in a 10 per cent w/v solution in *alcohol (90 per cent)*, in a 2-dm tube.

READILY OXIDISABLE SUBSTANCES. To 5 ml of a 1.0 per cent w/v solution in 0.05N hydrochloric acid add 0.25 ml of 0.1N potassium permanganate; the solution does not become decolorised in less than 5 minutes.

SULPHATED ASH. Not more than 0.1 per cent.

CONTENT OF $C_{17}H_{23}NO_3$. Not less than 99.0 per cent, determined by the following method:
Dissolve about 0.25 g, accurately weighed, in 5 ml of *alcohol (95 per cent)* previously neutralised to *methyl red solution*, add 20 ml of 0.1N hydrochloric acid and titrate the excess acid with 0.1N sodium hydroxide, using *methyl red solution* as indicator; each ml of 0.1N hydrochloric acid is equivalent to 0.02894 g of $C_{17}H_{23}NO_3$.

Actions and uses. Atropine has central and peripheral actions. It may initially stimulate the central nervous system, causing excitement and restlessness, and in larger doses it produces depression with drowsiness, delirium, and, later, coma. It also acts on the lower motor centres and diminishes the muscular rigidity and salivation of parkinsonism. It antagonises the muscarinic actions of acetylcholine and of similarly acting drugs. It diminishes the secretions of the salivary and sweat glands and of the bronchial and gastrointestinal tract. It also relaxes spasmodic contraction of involuntary muscle, increases the heart rate, and produces vasodilatation. It dilates the pupil, paralyses the muscles of accommodation, and increases intra-ocular pressure.

When given by mouth, atropine, administered as the sulphate or methonitrate, is slowly absorbed and takes effect after about three-quarters of an hour; after subcutaneous injection the effect of the drug is maximal within about half an hour.

Atropine is given before the administration of a volatile anaesthetic to prevent excessive bronchial secretion, but hyoscine is often preferred for this purpose. It is also used in the treatment of renal and biliary colic and of asthma to prevent or relieve spasm of involuntary muscle; this action may also explain some of the beneficial effects which follow its use in the treatment of incontinence of urine in children.

Small doses of atropine are often used to prevent excessive peristalsis and colicky pains produced by irritant purgatives or by anticholinergic drugs.

As it diminishes gastric and intestinal motility it is frequently used in conjunction with other measures in the treatment of gastric and duodenal ulcer.

In the treatment of postencephalitic parkinsonism large doses of atropine salts are used, although this treatment has been largely replaced by the use of other parasympatholytics such as benzhexol; the dryness of the mouth which is often associated with these large doses may be relieved by the oral administration of pilocarpine nitrate.

In the treatment of severe anticholinesterase poisoning, for example with organophosphorus compounds, atropine sulphate may be given intramuscularly in doses of 2 milligrams at intervals of ten to thirty minutes.

In ophthalmology, atropine has been used to dilate the pupil prior to retinoscopy, but homatropine is to be preferred for this purpose because of its shorter duration of action and the fact that its effect is more easily reversed by physostigmine. Atropine is also applied locally to the conjunctiva to immobilise the ciliary muscle and iris; for this purpose atropine sulphate may be used as 1 per cent aqueous eye-drops or eye ointment; an oily solution of atropine is also used as eye-drops.

The disadvantage of atropine in ophthalmology is that its effect is very persistent and may last for several days and the rise in intra-ocular pressure may precipitate a case of latent glaucoma into an acute attack. In general it is not used in cases of increased intra-ocular tension, and in the treatment of adults, homatropine is usually preferred. In hypersensitive individuals, atropine gives rise to irritation of the conjunctiva; for these patients, lachesine chloride may be a suitable alternative.

PRECAUTIONS. Atropine should not be given to patients who are being treated with a monoamine-oxidase inhibitor, such as isocarboxazid, nialamide, phenelzine, or tranylcypromine, or within about ten days of the discontinuation of such treatment.

POISONING. Poisoning by atropine is characterised in the early stages by marked excitement, delirium, dilated pupils, a rapid pulse, and a hot, flushed, dry skin. Belladonna fruits are sometimes a cause of poisoning in children, and gastric lavage with saline or a solution of tannic acid should be employed.

When atropine or belladonna fruit has been taken by mouth, the stage of excitement should be treated by administration of an intermediate-acting barbiturate, which may be repeated when necessary. In the later stages of central depression, artificial respiration or inhalation of carbon dioxide and oxygen may be necessary to restore respiration.

ATROPINE METHONITRATE

SYNONYM: Atrop. Methonit.

$C_{18}H_{26}N_2O_6 = 366.4$

$$\left[\begin{array}{c} H_2C\text{---}CH\text{---}CH_2 \quad C_6H_5 \\ \quad | \quad CH_3\cdot N\cdot CH_3 \quad CH\cdot O\cdot CO\cdot CH\cdot CH_2OH \\ H_2C\text{---}CH\text{---}CH_2 \end{array}\right]^+ NO_3^-$$

Atropine Methonitrate is the methonitrate of the alkaloid atropine, (±)-hyoscyamine.

Solubility. Soluble, at 20°, in less than 1 part of water, and in 13 parts of alcohol; insoluble in ether and in chloroform.

Standard
It complies with the requirements of the British Pharmacopoeia.
It occurs as colourless odourless crystals and contains not less than 99.0 and not more than the equivalent of 101.0 per cent of $C_{18}H_{26}N_2O_6$, calculated with reference to the dried substance. The loss on drying under the prescribed conditions is not more than 0.5 per cent. It has a melting-point of 166° to 168°.

Stability. Aqueous solutions are unstable; stability is enhanced in acid solutions of pH below 6. Solutions should be protected from alkali.

Actions and uses. Atropine methonitrate has the actions described under Atropine. It has less effect on the central nervous system and is less toxic than atropine.

It is used mainly in the treatment of congenital hypertrophic pyloric stenosis; 2 millilitres of a freshly prepared 0.01 per cent aqueous solution, or a solution of similar strength prepared by dilution of a 0.6 per cent alcoholic solution with water, is given by mouth half an hour before food, seven times during twenty-four hours. Thereafter the dose is increased by 1 millilitre daily to a maximum of 6 millilitres per dose, and treatment is continued until ten days after vomiting has ceased. If the patient is in a dehydrated condition it is important to correct this before treatment.

When atropine methonitrate is given as an alcoholic solution the danger of concentration by evaporation should be guarded against; it has been given in this form in the treatment of whooping-cough in infants.

Atropine methonitrate is an ingredient of compound spray solutions used in the treatment of asthma and hay fever.

PRECAUTIONS. As for Atropine.

POISONING. As for Atropine.

Dose. For congenital hypertrophic pyloric stenosis of infants: 200 to 600 micrograms, half an hour before meals.

Preparation
ADRENALINE AND ATROPINE SPRAY, COMPOUND, B.P.C. (page 794)

OTHER NAME: *Eumydrin®*

ATROPINE SULPHATE

SYNONYMS: Atrop. Sulph.; Atropini Sulfas

$(C_{17}H_{23}NO_3)_2,H_2SO_4,H_2O = 694.8$

Atropine Sulphate is the sulphate of the alkaloid atropine, ($\pm$)-hyoscyamine.

Solubility. Soluble, at 20°, in less than 1 part of water and in 4 parts of alcohol; insoluble in ether and in chloroform.

Standard
It complies with the requirements of the European Pharmacopoeia.
It occurs as odourless colourless crystals or white crystalline powder and contains not less than 98.5 per cent of $(C_{17}H_{23}NO_3)_2,H_2SO_4$, calculated with reference to the dried substance. The loss on drying under the prescribed conditions is not more than 4.0 per cent. It melts with decomposition at about 190°, after drying at 135° for 15 minutes. A 2 per cent solution in water has a pH of 4.5 to 6.2.

Incompatibility. Atropine salts are incompatible with alkalis, tannic acid, and salts of mercury.

Sterilisation. Solutions are sterilised by heating in an autoclave or by filtration.

Actions and uses. Atropine sulphate has the actions and uses described under Atropine.

PRECAUTIONS. As for Atropine.

POISONING. As for Atropine.

Dose. 0.25 to 2 milligrams daily in single or divided doses by mouth; 0.25 to 2 milligrams by subcutaneous, intramuscular, or intravenous injection.

Preparations
ATROPINE SULPHATE EYE-DROPS, B.P.C. (page 688)

ATROPINE EYE OINTMENT, B.P. Unless otherwise specified, an eye ointment containing 1.0 per cent of atropine sulphate is supplied.

ATROPINE SULPHATE INJECTION, B.P. It consists of a sterile solution of atropine sulphate in Water for Injections. Unless otherwise specified, a solution containing 1 mg in 1 ml is supplied.

MORPHINE AND ATROPINE INJECTION, B.P.C. (page 715)

ATROPINE SULPHATE TABLETS, B.P. Unless otherwise specified, tablets each containing 500 µg of atropine sulphate are supplied. Tablets containing 600 µg are also available.

AZATHIOPRINE

$C_9H_7N_7O_2S = 277.3$

Azathioprine is 6-(1-methyl-4-nitroimidazol-5-ylthio)purine.

Solubility. Insoluble in water; very slightly soluble in alcohol and in chloroform; soluble in dilute mineral acids; soluble in dilute solutions of alkali hydroxides but decomposes in stronger solutions.

Standard
It complies with the requirements of the British Pharmacopoeia.
It is a pale yellow odourless powder and contains not less than 98.0 and not more than the equivalent of 102.0 per cent of $C_9H_7N_7O_2S$, calculated with reference to the dried substance. The loss on drying under the prescribed conditions is not more than 1.0 per cent. It melts with decomposition at about 238°.

Storage. It should be protected from light.

Actions and uses. Azathioprine is a cytotoxic and immunosuppressive agent. Its actions partly depend upon its steady conversion into another cytotoxic drug, mercaptopurine, thus providing a prolonged therapeutic effect unobtainable by the use of mercaptopurine itself. The effects of azathioprine appear within two to four days of administration and about half the dose is excreted in the urine in the first day either as unchanged drug or as its metabolites.
Azathioprine is used as a cytotoxic drug in the treatment of acute leukaemia and as an immunosuppressive agent in organ transplantation to suppress the homograft reaction.

For this purpose it is often used with other immunosuppressive drugs such as the corticosteroids and other cytostatic agents such as actinomycin.
Azathioprine has also been used for the treatment of some diseases thought to have an immunological mechanism, such as lupus erythematosus and polyarteritis nodosa, and to reduce the dose of corticosteroids in patients with very severe rheumatoid arthritis, ulcerative colitis, Crohn's disease, and various kinds of nephritis.

UNDESIRABLE EFFECTS. Azathioprine causes hypoplasia of the bone marrow, the blood cell mainly affected being the granulocyte. Haematological control is therefore essential when the drug is being administered.
Other toxic effects are anorexia, nausea, and malaise; hepatotoxicity has also been observed. It may cause foetal damage.
The toxicity of azathioprine is dose dependent.

Dose. For immunosuppressive therapy: 2 to 5 milligrams per kilogram body-weight daily, reduced to half as a maintenance dose. On organ transplantation the dose may be temporarily increased and another immunosuppressive agent added if the graft shows signs of rejection.

For the treatment of leukaemia: 1·5 to 4 milligrams per kilogram body-weight daily.

Preparation
AZATHIOPRINE TABLETS, B.P. The quantity of aza-thioprine in each tablet should be specified by the prescriber. They should be protected from light. Tablets containing 50 mg are available.

OTHER NAME: *Imuran®*

AZURESIN

SYNONYM: Azure A Carbacrylic Resin

Azuresin is a cation-exchange compound and consists of a carbacrylic cation-exchange resin containing about 6 per cent of 3-amino-7-dimethylaminophenazathionium chloride (Azure A).

Standard
DESCRIPTION. Moist, irregular, dark blue or purple granules; odour slightly pungent.

IDENTIFICATION TEST. Shake 2 g with 50 ml of water, and allow to stand; the supernatant solution is not more than slightly blue. Add 2 ml of *hydrochloric acid*; the supernatant solution becomes deep blue.

ELUTION. Transfer 1·00 g to each of two flasks; add to the first flask 100 ml of water adjusted to pH 1·5 with *hydrochloric acid* and to the second flask 100 ml of water adjusted to pH 3·0 with *hydrochloric acid*, shake for one hour, and measure the pH; the pH does not change by more than 0·10.
Dilute 5 ml of each of the supernatant solutions to 500 ml with 0·1N hydrochloric acid and measure the extinction of a 1-cm layer of these solutions at the maximum at about 630 nm; the extinction of the solution initially adjusted to pH 3·0 is not more than 0·1A, and that of the solution initially adjusted to pH 1·5 is not less than 0·3A, where A is the extinction of a 1-cm layer at the maximum at about 690 nm of the solution prepared for the determination of 3-amino-7-dimethylaminophenazathionium chloride.

LOSS ON DRYING. 18·0 to 35·0 per cent, determined by drying for 18 hours at 38° in vacuo.

CONTENT OF 3-AMINO-7-DIMETHYLAMINOPHENAZA-THIONIUM CHLORIDE. 5·0 to 7·0 per cent, calculated with reference to the substance dried under the

prescribed conditions, determined by the following method:
Shake for 4 hours about 0·50 g, accurately weighed, with a mixture of 1 volume of *hydrochloric acid* and 2 volumes of *alcohol (50 per cent)*, dilute to 1000 ml with the mixture, and allow to stand for 16 hours; dilute 10 ml of the supernatant solution to 50 ml with the acid–alcohol mixture, and measure the extinction of a 1-cm layer at the maximum at about 690 nm.
For the purposes of calculation use a value of 1360 for the E(1 per cent, 1 cm) of 3-amino-7-dimethylamino-phenazathionium chloride. Calculate the percentage of 3-amino-7-dimethylaminophenazathionium chloride in the sample.

Storage. It should be stored in airtight containers.

Actions and uses. Azuresin is used for the detection of free hydrochloric acid in the gastric juice. In the presence of the free acid in the stomach the dye component of the resin is displaced by hydrogen ions and is subsequently excreted in the urine, to which it imparts a green or blue colour. The amount of dye present in the urine is determined by matching the colour against that of the control urine containing a known amount of the dye.

Dose. 2 grams as a single dose.

OTHER NAME: *Diagnex Blue®*

BACITRACIN ZINC

Bacitracin Zinc is a zinc salt of bacitracin, one or more of the antimicrobial polypeptides produced by certain strains of *Bacillus licheniformis* and by *B. subtilis* var. *Tracy* and yielding on hydrolysis the amino-acids L-cysteine, D-glutamic acid, L-histidine, L-isoleucine, L-leucine, L-lysine, D-ornithine, D-phenylalanine, and DL-aspartic acid.

Solubility. Soluble, at 20°, in 250 parts of water and in 500 parts of alcohol; very slightly soluble in ether; insoluble in chloroform.

Standard
It complies with the requirements of the British Pharmacopoeia.
It is a white or pale buff, odourless or almost odourless, hygroscopic powder and contains not less than 55 Units per mg, calculated with reference to the dried substance. The loss on drying under the prescribed conditions is not more than 5·0 per cent. A 10 per cent solution in water has a pH of 6·0 to 7·0.

Storage. It should be stored in airtight containers.

Actions and uses. Bacitracin is an antibiotic which is active against a wide range of Gram-positive organisms and against spirochaetes and some Gram-positive cocci.
It is used in the form of its zinc salt in lozenges,

ointments, dusting-powders, and aerosol sprays, often in conjunction with other antibiotics such as neomycin or polymyxins, or with hydrocortisone, in the treatment of local infections by susceptible organisms.
In dentistry it may be used as an ingredient of preparations for treating infections of the root canal.

UNDESIRABLE EFFECTS. Absorption from open wounds or the use of aerosol sprays over the site of abdominal operation may give rise to signs of renal toxicity.

Preparation
NEOMYCIN AND BACITRACIN OINTMENT, B.P.C. (page 762)

BARBITONE SODIUM

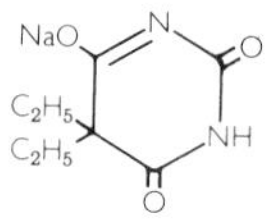

SYNONYMS: Barbital Sodium; Soluble Barbitone

$C_8H_{11}N_2NaO_3 = 206.2$

Barbitone Sodium is sodium 5,5-diethylbarbiturate.

Solubility. Soluble, at 20°, in 5 parts of water and in 600 parts of alcohol; insoluble in ether and in chloroform.

Standard
It complies with the requirements of the British Pharmacopoeia.
It is a white, crystalline, odourless powder and contains not less than 98.5 per cent of $C_8H_{11}N_2NaO_3$, calculated with reference to the dried substance. The loss on drying under the prescribed conditions is not more than 1.0 per cent. It has a melting-point of about 190°.

Stability. A solution in water slowly decomposes, the rate of decomposition increasing with rise of temperature.

Hygroscopicity. It absorbs insignificant amounts of moisture at 25° at relative humidities of up to about 80 per cent.

Incompatibility. It is incompatible with acids, acidic salts such as ammonium bromide, acidic syrups such as lemon syrup, and with chloral hydrate.

Storage. It should be stored in airtight containers.

Actions and uses. Barbitone sodium is a long-acting barbiturate, the actions and uses of which are described under Phenobarbitone (page 366).

It is usually given by mouth in a single dose of 300 to 600 milligrams as a hypnotic; up to 900 milligrams daily may be given in divided doses as a sedative. It may be given as a 10 per cent solution by intramuscular injection; it has been administered rectally as a 5 per cent solution. As it is only slowly excreted, accumulation may occur.

UNDESIRABLE EFFECTS; PRECAUTIONS; CONTRA-INDICATIONS; DEPENDENCE. These are as described under Phenobarbitone (page 366).

POISONING. The procedure as described under Phenobarbitone (page 366) should be adopted.

Dose. See above under **Actions and uses.**

Preparation
BARBITONE SODIUM TABLETS, B.P. (*Syn.* Soluble Barbitone Tablets; Barbital Sodium Tablets). The quantity of barbitone sodium in each tablet should be specified by the prescriber. They should be stored in airtight containers. Tablets containing 300 and 450 mg are available.

BARIUM SULPHATE

SYNONYM: Barii Sulfas

$BaSO_4 = 233.4$

Barium Sulphate is prepared by the interaction of a soluble barium salt and a soluble sulphate.

Solubility. Insoluble in water; very slightly soluble in hydrochloric acid, in nitric acid, and in solutions of many salts.

Standard
It complies with the requirements of the European Pharmacopoeia.
It is a fine, heavy, white, odourless powder free from gritty particles. The loss on ignition at 600° is not more than 2.0 per cent.

Actions and uses. Barium sulphate is used as a contrast medium for the X-ray examination of the gastro-intestinal tract. It is administered as a suspension and is not absorbed.

BECLOMETHASONE DIPROPIONATE

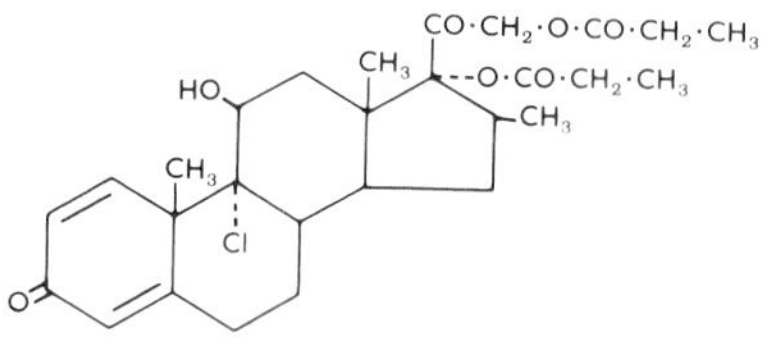

$C_{28}H_{37}ClO_7 = 521.0$

Beclomethasone Dipropionate is 9α-chloro-11β-hydroxy-16β-methyl-17α,21-dipropionyloxypregna-1,4-diene-3,20-dione.

Solubility. Insoluble in water; soluble, at 20°, in 60 parts of alcohol and in 8 parts of chloroform.

Standard
It complies with the requirements of the British Pharmacopoeia.
It is a white to creamy-white odourless powder and contains not less than 96.0 and not more than the equivalent of 104.0 per cent of $C_{28}H_{37}ClO_7$, calculated with reference to the dried substance. The loss on drying under the prescribed conditions is not more than

0.5 per cent. It melts with decomposition at about 212°.

Storage. It should be protected from light.

Actions and uses. Beclomethasone dipropionate is a corticosteroid for topical application with an action that is more potent than that of hydrocortisone (page 224); it should not be given by mouth. It has marked vasoconstrictor and anti-inflammatory activity. Its effectiveness is increased by dissolving it in propylene glycol before incorporation in an ointment basis.

It is suitable for use when local corticosteroid treatment is required, and is applied as an ointment or cream containing up to 0·025 per cent.

Beclomethasone applications may be used with or without conventional dressings, or under an occlusive dressing such as polythene when a more intensive effect is required, as in chronic psoriasis. However, if large areas are treated under occlusive dressings, sufficient of the drug may be absorbed to give rise to systemic effects.

PRECAUTIONS. It should not be used on infected skin without the simultaneous application of a suitable antibacterial agent.

OTHER NAME: *Propaderm®*

WHITE BEESWAX

SYNONYM: Cera Alba

White Beeswax is obtained by bleaching yellow beeswax. The bleaching may be effected by exposure of the wax in thin layers to the action of air, sunlight, and moisture, or by treatment with chemicals such as potassium dichromate and sulphuric acid.

Solubility. Insoluble in water; slightly soluble in alcohol; soluble in warm ether, in chloroform, and in fixed and volatile oils.

Standard
It complies with the requirements of the British Pharmacopoeia.
It is a yellowish-white solid with a faint characteristic odour; in thin layers it is translucent. It has a melting-point of 62° to 64°.
Adulterants and substitutes. Stearic acid, Japan wax, hard paraffin, and tallow have all been reported as adulterants.

Uses. White beeswax is used chiefly to stiffen ointments and occasionally to adjust the melting-point of suppositories. It has been used, often in conjunction with borax or spermaceti, in the preparation of water-in-oil creams.

YELLOW BEESWAX

SYNONYM: Cera Flava

Yellow Beeswax is a secretion formed by the hive bee, *Apis mellifera* L., and possibly other species of *Apis* (Fam. Apidae), and is used by the insect to form the cells of the honeycomb. After extraction of the honey, the wax is melted with water, separated, and strained.

Constituents. Yellow beeswax contains about 70 per cent of esters, the chief of which is myricyl palmitate, together with free wax acids, hydrocarbons, lactones, cholesteryl esters, and pollen pigments.

Solubility. Insoluble in water; slightly soluble in alcohol; soluble in warm ether, in chloroform, and in fixed and volatile oils.

Standard
DESCRIPTION. A yellowish-brown solid, somewhat brittle when cold, but becoming plastic when warm; odour agreeable and honey-like; fracture dull and granular.

ACID VALUE. 17 to 23, determined by the following method: dissolve about 5 g, accurately weighed, in 20 ml of boiling *dehydrated alcohol*, previously neutralised to *phenolphthalein solution*, and titrate with 0·5N alcoholic potassium hydroxide using *phenolphthalein solution* as indicator.

ESTER VALUE. 70 to 80, calculated by subtracting the acid value from the saponification value. The saponification value is determined by boiling about 5 g, accurately weighed, for 75 minutes with 25 ml of 1N potassium hydroxide in dehydrated alcohol, and titrating the excess of alkali, while hot, with 1N sulphuric acid, using *phenolphthalein solution* as indicator.

MELTING-POINT. 62° to 65°, determined by method V of the British Pharmacopoeia, Appendix IVA.

RATIO NUMBER. 3·3 to 4·2, calculated by dividing the ester value by the acid value.

FATS, FATTY ACIDS, JAPAN WAX AND RESIN. Boil 5·0 g for 10 minutes with 40 ml of *sodium hydroxide solution* and 40 ml of water, replacing the water lost by evaporation, cool, filter the solution through glass wool or asbestos, and acidify to *litmus paper* with *hydrochloric acid*; no turbidity is produced.

CERESIN, PARAFFIN, AND CERTAIN OTHER WAXES. Transfer 3·0 g to a 100-ml round-bottom flask, add 30 ml of *potassium hydroxide solution in aldehyde-free alcohol*, and boil the mixture gently for 2 hours under a reflux condenser. Remove the condenser and immediately insert a thermometer, place the flask in a bath of water at 80°, and allow to cool, swirling the solution continuously; the solution shows no cloudiness or globule formation before the temperature reaches 65°.

Adulterants and substitutes. Colophony, hard paraffin, various fats and waxes, stearic acid, soap, and foreign colouring matters have all been reported as adulterants.

Uses. Yellow beeswax is used in the preparation of ointments in which the yellow colour is not objectionable. A preparation of 10 per cent of phenol in a mixture of olive oil and yellow beeswax is known as Horsley's wax and is used to control haemorrhage in bone in cranial surgery.

BELLADONNA HERB

SYNONYMS: Bellad. Leaf; Belladonna Leaf; Belladonnae Folium

Belladonna Herb consists of the dried leaves, or leaves and other aerial parts, of *Atropa belladonna* L. (Fam. Solanaceae), collected when the plants are in flower. The plant is a tall branching herbaceous perennial, indigenous to and cultivated in Great Britain and other European countries.

Constituents. Belladonna herb contains the alkaloid (−)-hyoscyamine, the total quantity of alkaloid present in dried herb of good quality being about 0·4 to 1 per cent. The herb also contains β-methylaesculetin, which gives a blue fluorescence in ultraviolet light, and small quantities of hyoscine, belladonnine and other alkaloids. Further constituents are variable amounts of volatile bases, including pyridine, N-methylpyrroline, and N-methylpyrrolidine.

Standard
It complies with the requirements of the European Pharmacopoeia.
It contains not less than 0·30 per cent of alkaloids, calculated as hyoscyamine, $C_{17}H_{23}NO_3$, with reference to the substance dried at 100° to 105°.

UNGROUND DRUG. *Macroscopical characters:* Leaves thin, brittle, yellowish-green, alternate but arranged in pairs on upper stems, each pair consisting of a larger and a smaller leaf, simple; petiole up to 4 cm long; lamina broadly ovate, usually from 5 to 25 cm long and 3 to 12 cm broad, margin entire, apex acuminate, base somewhat decurrent down the petiole; venation pinnate, secondary veins leaving midrib at angle of about 60° and anastomosing near the margin; surface slightly hairy.
Flowers borne singly upon short drooping pedicels arising in axils of paired leaves; calyx gamosepalous forming a cup about 5 mm deep and bearing 5 triangular lobes about 1·25 cm long; corolla campanulate, livid purple, about 2·0 cm long and 1·5 cm wide, with 5 small reflexed lobes; stamens 5, epipetalous; ovary superior, bilocular, ovules numerous, placentation axile.
Fruit, a berry, when ripe purplish-black, up to about 12 mm in diameter, bearing persistent inferior calyx with widely spreading lobes; seeds numerous, brown, reticulate.
Odour slight; taste unpleasant, bitter.

Microscopical characters: the diagnostic characters are: Leaf: *epidermal cells* with slightly sinuous anticlinal walls, *cuticle* striated; *stomata* anisocytic, occurring on both surfaces, stomatal index (abaxial surface) 20 to **22** to 23; *trichomes* (a) *non-glandular*, occasional, uniseriate, (b) *glandular*, either short, clavate, with multicellular heads, or less frequently long, with uniseriate stalks and unicellular heads; *mesophyll* with one layer of palisade parenchyma, the palisade ratio varying from 5 to 7 (mean of 20 observations); *idioblasts* containing microsphenoidal *crystals* of calcium oxalate present in mesophyll; *phloem* intraxylary in midrib and petiole vascular bundles.
Stem: *fibres* present in pericycle and xylem; *phloem* intraxylary; *xylem* with wide vessels; microsphenoidal *crystals* of calcium oxalate present in idioblasts of parenchyma.
Pollen grains subspherical, 37 to 50 μm in diameter, containing minute starch granules and droplets of oil, *extine* marked with rows of fine pits radiating from the poles to the equator where they number about 84, 3 *pores* about 8 mm in diameter, 3 *germinal furrows* extending nearly to the poles.

POWDERED DRUG: Powdered Belladonna Herb. A green powder possessing the diagnostic microscopical characters, odour, and taste of the unground drug.

Adulterants and substitutes. Indian belladonna, from *A. acuminata* Royle ex Lindley, has leaves which are usually brownish-green, oblong-elliptical, tapering both at the apex and the base of the lamina; the flowers have a yellowish-brown corolla. The microscopical characters are similar to those of belladonna herb, but the stomatal index is 16·5 to **17·5** to 19·0.
The leaves of *Phytolacca americana* L. (*P. decandra* L.) and of other species of *Phytolacca* (Fam. Phytolaccaceae), of *Scopolia carniolica* Jacq., and *Solanum nigrum* L. (Fam. Solanaceae), and of *Ailanthus altissima* (Mill.) Swingle (Fam. Simarubaceae), occur at times as substitutes for belladonna herb. They are best distinguished by their microscopical features: phytolacca leaves contain idioblasts with acicular raphides of calcium oxalate; scopolia leaves possess stomata on the under surface only and the palisade ratio varies from 3 to 5, occasionally 6, while the fruit, a nearly spherical pyxis, is usually present; ailanthus leaves have cluster crystals of calcium oxalate near the veins, and unicellular thick-walled trichomes; leaves of *S. nigrum* have a palisade ratio varying from 2 to 4.

Storage. It should be stored in a cool dry place, protected from light.

Actions and uses.
The actions of preparations of belladonna herb are chiefly due to the atropine they contain. Belladonna is therefore used to decrease secretions of the sweat, salivary, and gastric glands. It acts as a powerful spasmolytic in intestinal colic and, given with purgatives, allays griping. It is also used for the relief of spasm associated with biliary and renal colic.

NOTE. When Belladonna Herb, Belladonna Leaf, Belladonnae Folium, Powdered Belladonna Herb, or Belladonnae Herbae Pulvis is prescribed, Prepared Belladonna Herb is dispensed.

POISONING. In cases of poisoning by belladonna herb or its alkaloids, the procedure described under Atropine (page 36) should be adopted.

Preparations
BELLADONNA HERB, PREPARED (page 43).
BELLADONNA DRY EXTRACT, B.P. It contains 1 per cent of alkaloids. It should be stored in small wide-mouthed airtight containers, in a cool place. Dose: 15 to 60 milligrams.
ALUMINIUM HYDROXIDE AND BELLADONNA MIXTURE, B.P.C. (page 735)
BELLADONNA MIXTURE, PAEDIATRIC, B.P.C. (page 737)
BELLADONNA AND EPHEDRINE MIXTURE, PAEDIATRIC, B.P.C. (page 737)
BELLADONNA AND IPECACUANHA MIXTURE, PAEDIATRIC, B.P.C. (page 738)
CASCARA AND BELLADONNA MIXTURE, B.P.C. (page 738)
MAGNESIUM TRISILICATE AND BELLADONNA MIXTURE, B.P.C. (page 747)
PHENOLPHTHALEIN PILLS, COMPOUND, B.P.C. (page 774)
BELLADONNA AND PHENOBARBITONE TABLETS, B.P.C. (page 807)
BELLADONNA TINCTURE, B.P. It contains 0·03 per cent of alkaloids. Dose: 0·5 to 2 millilitres.

PREPARED BELLADONNA HERB

SYNONYMS: Belladonnae Pulvis Normatus; Prep. Bellad.; Prepared Belladonna

Prepared Belladonna Herb is obtained by reducing Belladonna Herb to a fine powder and adjusting, if necessary, to the required alkaloidal content. When adjustment is necessary, powdered Lactose or Powdered Belladonna Herb of lower alkaloidal content is added.

Standard
It complies with the requirements of the European Pharmacopoeia.
It is a fine greyish-green powder with a slightly nauseous odour and a slightly bitter taste. It contains 0·3 per cent of alkaloids, calculated as hyoscyamine, $C_{17}H_{23}NO_3$ (limits, 0·28 to 0·32 per cent), with reference to the substance dried at 100° to 105°. It possesses the diagnostic microscopical characters of Powdered Belladonna Herb.

Storage. It should be stored in airtight containers, protected from light, in a cool place.

Actions and uses. Prepared belladonna herb has the actions and uses described under Belladonna Herb.

POISONING. As for Atropine (page 36).

Dose. 30 to 200 milligrams.

BELLADONNA ROOT

SYNONYM: Bellad. Root

Belladonna Root is the dried root, or root and rootstock, of *Atropa belladonna* L. (Fam. Solanaceae), entire or longitudinally divided. The plant is a tall branching herbaceous perennial, indigenous to and cultivated in Great Britain and other European countries.

Constituents. Belladonna root contains the alkaloid (−)-hyoscyamine and traces of hyoscine. The drug also contains β-methylaesculetin, which gives a blue fluorescence in ultraviolet light. The total amount of alkaloid in the root varies from about 0·3 to 0·8 per cent.

Standard for unground drug
DESCRIPTION. *Macroscopical:* Root simple or occasionally branched, subcylindrical, occurring entire or split longitudinally, the pieces being about 10 to 30 cm long and up to about 4 cm wide at crown; external covering of cork, thin pale greyish-brown, longitudinally wrinkled; fracture short; smoothed, transversely cut surface whitish to brownish showing dark cambium line separating the narrow bark, devoid of fibres, from the mainly parenchymatous xylem containing scattered groups of vessels; vessels most numerous and inconspicuously radiate just to inner side of cambium; root crown exhibiting a central pith, a markedly radiate xylem, and a bark with few phloem fibres.
Odour slight; taste starchy and faintly bitter.

Microscopical: the diagnostic characters are: Root: *cork* cells in several layers; *phloem fibres* and *sclereids* absent; *parenchyma* abundant, containing *starch* as simple or occasional 2- to 5-compound granules, individual granules 3 to **8** to **16** to 30 μm in diameter; *idioblasts* containing microsphenoidal *crystals* of calcium oxalate, about 1 to 7 μm; *vessels* about 20 to **60** to **120** to 180 μm in diameter, individual elements about 50 to **145** to **175** to 410 μm long, their walls with closely arranged bordered pits; *xylem fibres* thin-walled; *intraxylary phloem* in small, scattered groups; primary xylem and a little secondary xylem forming a compact diarch or occasionally triarch strand.
Rootstock: similar in most particulars to the root, except for presence of occasional *phloem fibres*, lignified *xylem parenchyma*, and occasional *fibres* in intraxylary phloem.

ACID-INSOLUBLE ASH. Not more than 2·0 per cent.

FOREIGN ORGANIC MATTER. Not more than 2·0 per cent.

CONTENT OF TOTAL ALKALOIDS. Not less than 0·40 per cent, calculated as hyoscyamine, $C_{17}H_{23}NO_3$, determined by the following method:
Mix about 10 g, finely powdered and accurately weighed, with 50 ml of a mixture containing 4 volumes of *solvent ether* and 1 volume of *alcohol (95 per cent)*, shake, allow to stand for 10 minutes, add a mixture of 1·5 ml of *dilute ammonia solution* and 2 ml of water and shake for 1 hour.

Transfer the mixture to a small percolator, previously lightly plugged with cotton wool just above the tap, and, when the liquid ceases to flow, pack firmly and continue the percolation with 25 ml of the ether-alcohol mixture followed by successive portions of *solvent ether* until complete extraction of the alkaloids is effected; the total time of percolation should not exceed 3 hours.
Reduce the volume of the percolate to about 20 ml by distillation on a water-bath, transfer the solution to a separating funnel using three successive 10-ml portions of *chloroform* to wash the distillation flask, and extract the combined solution and washings with 20 ml of 0·5N sulphuric acid, followed by successive 10-ml portions of a mixture containing 3 volumes of 0·1N sulphuric acid and 1 volume of *alcohol (95 per cent)* until complete extraction of the alkaloids is effected; wash the combined acid extractions with 10-, 5-, and 5-ml portions of *chloroform*, extracting each chloroform wash with the same 20 ml of 0·1N sulphuric acid, discard the chloroform washes, combine the acid solutions, neutralise to *litmus paper* with *dilute ammonia solution* and add 5 ml in excess, and extract with successive 25-ml portions of *chloroform* until complete extraction of the alkaloids is effected, washing each extract with the same 10 ml of water and subsequently filtering each extract through a plug of cotton wool previously moistened with *chloroform*.
Distil the combined filtrates to a small volume, transfer to a shallow open dish, carefully evaporate to dryness without the use of a current of air, heat the residue in an oven at 100° for 15 minutes, dissolve in a little *chloroform*, evaporate to dryness, again heat in an oven at 100° for 15 minutes, dissolve the residue in 2 ml of *chloroform*, add 5 ml of 0·05N sulphuric acid, warm to evaporate the chloroform, cool, and titrate the excess of acid with 0·05N sodium hydroxide, using *methyl red solution* as indicator; each ml of 0·05N sulphuric acid is equivalent to 0·01447 g of $C_{17}H_{23}NO_3$.

Standard for powdered drug: Powdered Belladonna Root
DESCRIPTION. A grey to light-brown powder possessing the diagnostic microscopical characters and odour of the unground drug.

ACID-INSOLUBLE ASH; FOREIGN ORGANIC MATTER; CONTENT OF TOTAL ALKALOIDS. It complies with the requirements for the unground drug.

Adulterants and substitutes. Indian belladonna root, derived from *A. acuminata* Royle ex Lindley, closely resembles belladonna root; the secondary xylem is yellowish in colour and is arranged in 1 to 4 concentric cylinders separated by narrow cylinders of parenchyma and sieve-tissue, the whole being traversed radially by numerous medullary rays; the rootstock has a similarly constructed xylem. The content of total alkaloid is usually low and includes an excessive amount of volatile bases.

Phytolacca, or poke root, from *Phytolacca americana* L. (*P. decandra* L.) (Fam. Phytolaccaceae), is sometimes substituted for belladonna and may be detected by the presence of concentric cylinders of separate vascular bundles alternating with cylinders of parenchyma, and, in powder, by the presence of acicular crystals of calcium oxalate.

Scopolia, the dried rhizome of *Scopolia carniolica* Jacq. (Fam. Solanaceae), has also occurred as a substitute and can be recognised by its yellowish-brown colour, the numerous cup-shaped stem-scars on the upper surface, the horny central pith, and microscopically by the preponderance of reticulate vessels.

Storage. It should be stored in a cool dry place.

Actions and uses. Belladonna root has actions similar to those described under

Belladonna Herb. It is used chiefly in preparations for external application, but there is no reliable evidence that belladonna, when applied externally, is absorbed in sufficient amount to produce systemic effects.

Liniments containing belladonna are sometimes used as counter-irritants but the efficacy of these preparations is not due to belladonna.

Although there is little evidence that belladonna has any analgesic action, belladonna glycerin and belladonna plaster have been used locally to allay pain. Belladonna suppositories have been used to relieve the painful spasm of anal fistula.

POISONING. The procedure as described under Atropine (page 36) should be adopted.

Preparation
BELLADONNA LIQUID EXTRACT, B.P.C. (page 682)

BENDROFLUAZIDE

$C_{15}H_{14}F_3N_3O_4S_2 = 421 \cdot 4$

Bendrofluazide is 3-benzyl-3,4-dihydro-7-sulphamoyl-6-trifluoromethyl-2*H*-benzo-1,2,4-thiadiazine 1,1-dioxide.

Solubility. Very slightly soluble in water; soluble, at 20°, in 17 parts of alcohol, in 500 parts of ether, and in 1·5 parts of acetone; insoluble in chloroform.

Standard
It complies with the requirements of the British Pharmacopoeia.

It is a white or almost white, crystalline, odourless powder and contains not less than 98·0 and not more than the equivalent of 102·0 per cent of $C_{15}H_{14}F_3N_3O_4S_2$, calculated with reference to the dried substance. The loss on drying under the prescribed conditions is not more than 0·5 per cent.

Actions and uses. Bendrofluazide is a non-mercurial diuretic which has actions and uses similar to those described under Chlorothiazide (page 103); it is effective in smaller doses than chlorothiazide and produces a

more prolonged diuresis, which continues for about eighteen hours.

The initial dosage is 5 to 20 milligrams by mouth once a day and this may be reduced to 2·5 to 10 milligrams daily or on alternate days for maintenance.

UNDESIRABLE EFFECTS; PRECAUTIONS. As for Chlorothiazide (page 103).

Dose. See above under **Actions and uses.**

Preparation
BENDROFLUAZIDE TABLETS, B.P. Unless otherwise specified tablets each containing 2·5 mg of bendrofluazide are supplied. Tablets containing 5 mg are also available.

OTHER NAMES: *Aprinox®*; Bendroflumethiazide; *Berkozide®*; *Centyl®*; *Neo-Naclex®*

BENETHAMINE PENICILLIN

SYNONYM: Beneth. Penicil.

$C_{15}H_{17}N, C_{16}H_{18}N_2O_4S = 545 \cdot 7$

Benethamine Penicillin is the *N*-benzylphenethylamine salt of benzylpenicillin. One mega unit of penicillin is contained in approximately 1 gram of benethamine penicillin.

Solubility. Soluble, at 20°, in 1500 parts of water, in 50 parts of chloroform, in 100 parts of acetone (50 per cent), and in 50 parts of methyl alcohol (75 per cent).

Standard
DESCRIPTION. A white or almost white crystalline powder; odourless or almost odourless.

IDENTIFICATION TESTS. 1. Dissolve 5 mg in 2 ml of *acetone* (*50 per cent*), dilute to 20 ml with sterile *solution of standard pH 7·4*, add an excess of *penicillinase*

solution to inactivate an equivalent amount of penicillin, and maintain at 37° for 2 hours; the solution shows no activity in the determination of potency.

2. Shake 1 g for 2 minutes with 5 ml of *dilute sodium hydroxide solution*, extract with two successive 10-ml portions of *solvent ether*, evaporate the combined extracts to dryness, dissolve the residue in 5 ml of *alcohol* (*95 per cent*), warm with 5 ml of a saturated solution of *picrolonic acid* in *alcohol* (*95 per cent*), and

cool; a precipitate is formed which, after recrystallising from *alcohol (95 per cent)* and drying, melts at about 230°.

ACIDITY. pH of a 1·5 per cent w/v suspension in *carbon dioxide-free water*, 5·5 to 7·0.

SPECIFIC ROTATION. $+120°$ to $+125°$, calculated with reference to the substance dried under the prescribed conditions, determined, at 20°, in a 1·0 per cent w/v solution in *chloroform*.

WATER-SOLUBLE IMPURITIES. Not more than 2·5 per cent, determined by the following method:
Shake 2·5 g with 50 ml of water for one hour and filter; evaporate 25 ml of the filtrate to dryness on a water-bath, dry the residue to constant weight at 60° in vacuo, cool, and weigh. From the weight of residue, subtract 0·0225 g to correct for the solubility of benethamine penicillin in water.

LOSS ON DRYING. Not more than 0·5 per cent, determined by drying to constant weight at 105°.

SULPHATED ASH. Not more than 0·2 per cent.

STERILITY. It complies with the test for sterility of the European Pharmacopoeia.

PYROGENS. It complies with the test for pyrogens of the European Pharmacopoeia.
A quantity equivalent to not less than 2 mg per kg of the rabbit's weight suspended in not more than 5 ml of *water for injections* is used.

CONTENT OF $C_{15}H_{17}N$. 36·5 to 39·0 per cent, calculated with reference to the substance dried under the prescribed conditions, determined by the following method:
Shake thoroughly about 0·1 g, accurately weighed, with 20 ml of a 5 per cent w/v solution of *anhydrous sodium sulphate* in water, 5 ml of *sodium carbonate solution*, and 20 ml of *anaesthetic ether*, allow to separate, and extract the aqueous layer with two further successive 20-ml portions of *anaesthetic ether*; wash the combined ethereal extracts with three successive 5-ml portions of water, extract the combined ethereal extracts with 25 ml of 0·01N sulphuric acid, wash the ethereal layer with three successive 5-ml portions of water, and titrate the excess of acid in the combined aqueous extract and washings with 0·01N borax, using *methyl red and methylene blue solution* as indicator; each ml of 0·01N sulphuric acid is equivalent to 0·002113 g of $C_{15}H_{17}N$.

CONTENT OF TOTAL PENICILLINS. Not less than 95·0 and not more than the equivalent of 102·0 per cent, calculated as $C_{15}H_{17}N,C_{16}H_{18}N_2O_4S$ and with reference to the substance dried under the prescribed conditions, determined by the following method:
Suspend 0·150 g, finely powdered and accurately weighed, in a mixture of 90 ml of water and 50 ml of 1N sodium hydroxide, dilute to 150 ml with water, mix, and allow to stand for 20 minutes; transfer 15 ml of this solution to a stoppered flask, add 20 ml of a freshly prepared buffer solution containing 5·44 per cent w/v of *sodium acetate* and 2·40 per cent w/v of

glacial acetic acid, 5 ml of 1N hydrochloric acid, and 25 ml of 0·02N iodine, close the flask with a wet stopper, and allow to stand for 20 minutes, protected from light. Titrate the excess of iodine with 0·02N sodium thiosulphate, using *starch mucilage*, added towards the end of the titration, as indicator.
To a further 0·150 g, finely powdered and accurately weighed, add 100 ml of water, shake vigorously for 2 minutes, filter, and, using 10 ml of the filtrate, repeat the procedure above beginning at the words "add 20 ml of a freshly prepared buffer solution . . ." but omitting the 5 ml of 1N hydrochloric acid.
The difference between the two titrations represents the volume of 0·02N iodine equivalent to the total penicillins in the sample.
Calculate the content of total penicillins from the difference obtained by repeating the procedure with *benzylpenicillin sodium B.C.R.S.* in place of the sample; each mg of *benzylpenicillin sodium B.C.R.S.* is equivalent to 1·531 mg of total penicillins, calculated as $C_{15}H_{17}N,C_{16}H_{18}N_2O_4S$.

Only Benethamine Penicillin intended for use in the preparation of injections is required to comply with the tests for sterility and pyrogens.

Labelling. If the material is intended for the preparation of injections, the label states "Benethamine Penicillin for Injection".

Storage. It should be stored in airtight containers in a cool place. If it is intended for parenteral administration the containers should be sterile and sealed to exclude micro-organisms.

Actions and uses. Benethamine penicillin has antibacterial actions similar to those described under Benzylpenicillin (page 51). As it is only slightly soluble in water, it releases penicillin slowly into the circulation after intramuscular injection; a single dose of 300 to 600 milligrams will maintain an effective concentration of penicillin in the blood for three or four days.

Like benzathine penicillin it can be added to preparations containing benzylpenicillin and procaine penicillin to give an injection producing immediate and prolonged antibacterial effect.

Dose. 300 to 600 milligrams (approximately 300,000 to 600,000 Units of penicillin) by intramuscular injection every three or four days.

Preparation
BENETHAMINE PENICILLIN INJECTION, FORTIFIED, B.P.C. (page 709)

BENTONITE

Bentonite is a native colloidal hydrated aluminium silicate, the principal constituent being montmorillonite, $Al_2O_3,4SiO_2,H_2O$. Materials suitable for pharmaceutical purposes are generally obtained from Wyoming; African and Italian bentonites are used for packing and other non-pharmaceutical purposes.

Solubility. Insoluble in water, but swells into a homogeneous mass; insoluble in organic solvents.

Standard
It complies with the requirements of the British Pharmacopoeia.

DESCRIPTION. *Macroscopical:* A very fine, pale buff or cream-coloured, odourless powder, which is free from gritty particles.

Microscopical: Bentonite consists of particles about 50 to 150 μm and numerous smaller particles about 1 to 2 μm; the larger particles have rounded corners and an uneven surface with frequent cracks; mounted in *safranine solution* or *alcoholic methylene blue solution*, the particles are strongly stained red or blue respectively; mounted in *alcohol (95 per cent)* and irrigated with water, the larger fragments, as they come in contact with the water, rapidly swell to give a jelly-like matrix in which numerous minute particles are embedded; mounted in *cresol* it becomes nearly invisible, but shines brightly on a dark field between crossed polars.

A 2 per cent suspension in water has a pH of 9 to 10·5. The loss on drying to constant weight at 105° is 5 to 12 per cent.

Sterilisation. It is sterilised by dry heat, after previously drying at 100°; aqueous suspensions are sterilised by heating in an autoclave.

Uses. Bentonite absorbs water readily to form either sols or gels, depending upon its concentration, a preparation containing about 7 per cent of bentonite being just pourable. The sols are suitable for suspending powders in aqueous preparations such as calamine lotion, and the gels for ointment and cream bases; these preparations have a pH of about 9.

The gelling property of bentonite is much reduced in the presence of acid and increased by the addition of such alkaline substances as magnesium oxide. In aqueous sols and gels bentonite particles are negatively charged and flocculation occurs when electrolytes or positively charged suspensions are added.

Because of this property bentonite is sometimes used in clarifying turbid liquids.

Sols and gels may conveniently be prepared by sprinkling the bentonite on the surface of hot water and allowing to stand for about twenty-four hours, stirring occasionally when the bentonite has become thoroughly wetted. Water should not be added to bentonite alone, but a satisfactory dispersal in water may be effected if the bentonite is first triturated with glycerol or if it is intimately mixed with powders such as calamine or zinc oxide.

For suspending powders in aqueous preparations and for the preparation of cream bases containing suitable proportions of oil-in-water emulsifying agents such as emulsifying wax and self-emulsifying monostearin, 2 per cent of bentonite is adequate. A preparation containing 10 to 20 per cent of bentonite and 10 per cent of glycerol is also suitable as a basis. A sol containing 5 per cent is convenient for dispensing purposes.

Bentonite should be sterilised before it is used for preparations intended for application to open wounds.

BENZALDEHYDE

$C_7H_6O = 106·1$

$C_6H_5 \cdot CHO$

Solubility. Soluble, at 20°, in 350 parts of water; miscible with alcohol and with ether.

Standard

DESCRIPTION. A clear colourless liquid; odour characteristic of bitter almonds.

REFRACTIVE INDEX. At 20°, 1·544 to 1·546.

WEIGHT PER ML. At 20°, 1·043 g to 1·049 g.

FREE ACID. Not more than 1·0 per cent w/v, calculated as benzoic acid, $C_7H_6O_2$, determined by the following method:

To 10 ml add 20 ml of *alcohol (95 per cent)*, previously neutralised to *phenolphthalein solution*, and titrate with 0·1N sodium hydroxide, using *phenolphthalein solution* as indicator; each ml of 0·1N sodium hydroxide is equivalent to 0·01221 g of $C_7H_6O_2$.

CHLORINATED COMPOUNDS. Not more than 0·05 per cent w/v, calculated as Cl, determined by the following method:

To 5 ml add 50 ml of *amyl alcohol* and 3 g of *sodium* and boil under a reflux condenser for one hour; cool, add 50 ml of water and 15 ml of *nitric acid*, cool, add 5 ml of 0·1N silver nitrate, shake, and titrate the excess

of silver nitrate with 0·1N ammonium thiocyanate, using *ferric ammonium sulphate solution* as indicator. Repeat the procedure omitting the sample.

The difference between the two titrations represents the amount of silver nitrate required by the chlorine; each ml of 0·1N silver nitrate is equivalent to 0·003545 g of Cl.

CONTENT OF C_7H_6O. Not less than 98·0 per cent w/w, determined by the method given in Appendix 14 (page 893) for the determination of aldehydes in volatile oils, about 0·5 g, accurately weighed, being used; each ml of 0·5N potassium hydroxide is equivalent to 0·05348 g of C_7H_6O.

Storage. It should be stored in well-filled airtight containers, protected from light, in a cool place.

Uses. Benzaldehyde is used as a flavouring agent. A syrup containing 0·2 per cent v/v of Benzaldehyde Spirit may be used as an alternative to Wild Cherry Syrup.

Preparation

BENZALDEHYDE SPIRIT, B.P.C. (page 793)

BENZALKONIUM CHLORIDE SOLUTION

Benzalkonium Chloride Solution is an aqueous solution containing a mixture of alkylbenzyldimethylammonium chlorides, equivalent to 50 per cent w/v of $C_6H_5 \cdot CH_2 \cdot N(CH_3)_2(C_{13}H_{27}) \cdot Cl$. The alkyl groups contain eight to eighteen carbon atoms.

Solubility. Miscible with water and with alcohol.

Standard

It complies with the requirements of the British Pharmacopoeia.

The solution is a clear colourless to pale yellow syrupy liquid with an aromatic odour and contains 49·0 to

51·0 per cent w/v of alkylbenzyldimethylammonium chlorides, calculated as $C_{22}H_{40}ClN$.

Incompatibility. It is incompatible with soaps and similar anionic compounds and with alkali hydroxides.

Sterilisation. Solutions are sterilised by heating in an autoclave or by filtration.

Preparation and storage of solutions. See statement on aqueous solutions of antiseptics, under Solutions (page 779).

Actions and uses. Benzalkonium chloride has the actions and uses of the quaternary ammonium compounds, as described under Cetrimide (page 88).

Benzalkonium Chloride Solution may be used, in a dilution of 1 in 500, for the pre-operative preparation of unbroken skin, but for application to mucous membranes and denuded skin the dilution should not be stronger than 1 in 1000. In obstetrics and for application to wounds and burns, dilutions of 1 in 500 to 1 in 1000 may be used. Dilutions of 1 in 10,000 are employed for irrigation of the bladder, urethra, and vagina, and a concentration not exceeding 1 in 20,000 for retention lavage.

Rubber articles should not be stored in benzalkonium solutions.

Benzalkonium Lozenges are used to relieve painful infections of the mouth and throat.

A 0·02 per cent v/v dilution of Benzalkonium Chloride Solution is used as a preservative for eye-drops.

PRECAUTIONS. Benzalkonium chloride should not be applied repeatedly and wet dressings should not be left in contact with the skin, as hypersensitivity may develop.

Preparation
BENZALKONIUM LOZENGES, B.P.C. (page 732)

OTHER NAMES: *Empiquat BAC®*; *Hyamine 3500®*; *Marinol®*; *Silquat B50®*; *Vantoc CL®*

BENZATHINE PENICILLIN

SYNONYM: Benzathine Penicillin G

$C_{16}H_{20}N_2,(C_{16}H_{18}N_2O_4S)_2 = 909·1$

Benzathine Penicillin is the *NN'*-dibenzylethylenediamine salt of benzylpenicillin, free from added substances and containing a variable amount of water of crystallisation.

Solubility. Very slightly soluble in water, in ether, and in chloroform; slightly soluble in alcohol; soluble, at 20°, in 10 parts of formamide and in 7 parts of dimethylformamide.

Standard
It complies with the requirements of the British Pharmacopoeia.
It is a white, odourless or almost odourless, hygroscopic powder and contains not less than 96·0 per cent of total penicillins, calculated as $C_{16}H_{20}N_2,(C_{16}H_{18}N_2O_4S)_2$, and 25·0 to 26·5 per cent of $C_{16}H_{20}N_2$, both calculated with reference to the anhydrous substance. It contains 5·0 to 8·0 per cent w/w of water.
1·2 mega Units of penicillin are contained in approximately 900 milligrams of benzathine penicillin; this weight of benzathine penicillin is approximately equivalent to 720 milligrams of benzylpenicillin.

Stability. Aqueous suspensions are most stable when buffered to pH 6·0 to 7·0 and stored at low temperatures. Such buffered aqueous suspensions containing 25 to 50 mg per ml may be expected to retain 90 per cent of their original potency for two years when stored at a temperature not exceeding 25°.

Labelling. If the material is not intended for parenteral administration, the label on the container states that the contents are not to be injected.

Storage. It should be stored in airtight containers in a cool place. If it is intended for parenteral administration the containers should be sterile and sealed to exclude micro-organisms.

Actions and uses. Benzathine penicillin is relatively stable in the presence of gastric juice or serum and penicillin is slowly released when the compound is given either by mouth or by intramuscular injection.

When given by mouth, the maximum concentration of penicillin in the blood is obtained less rapidly than after a comparable dose of a soluble salt of penicillin by injection, but the level is maintained for a longer period, and doses of 225 milligrams usually give an effective concentration for six hours; absorption of the penicillin from the gastro-intestinal tract is not affected by the food intake.

When given by intramuscular injection, benzathine penicillin forms a depot from which penicillin is released over several days, and following a single dose of 450 milligrams an effective concentration in the blood may be maintained for a week or even longer.

Benzathine penicillin injections are used to provide a prolonged effect and avoid the need for repeated injections after an initial dose of benzylpenicillin, especially in infants and children with acute streptococcal infections when oral therapy is unreliable because of a lack of parental co-operation.

Fortnightly injections of benzathine penicillin may be used to prevent relapses of rheumatic fever in patients who cannot be relied upon to take the drug regularly by mouth.

Dose. See above under **Actions and uses.**

Preparation
BENZATHINE PENICILLIN INJECTION, FORTIFIED, B.P.C. (page 710)

OTHER NAME: *Penidural®*

BENZHEXOL HYDROCHLORIDE

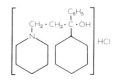

SYNONYM: Trihexyphenidyl Hydrochloride

$C_{20}H_{32}ClNO = 337.9$

Benzhexol Hydrochloride is 1-cyclohexyl-1-phenyl-3-piperidinopropan-1-ol hydrochloride.

Solubility. Soluble, at 20°, in 100 parts of water, in 22 parts of alcohol, in 15 parts of chloroform, and in 10 parts of methyl alcohol.

Standard
It complies with the requirements of the British Pharmacopoeia.
It is a white or creamy-white, crystalline, almost odourless powder and contains not less than 98.0 and not more than the equivalent of 101.0 per cent of $C_{20}H_{32}ClNO$, calculated with reference to the dried substance. The loss on drying under the prescribed conditions is not more than 0.5 per cent. A saturated solution in water has a pH of 5.0 to 6.0.

Actions and uses. Benzhexol antagonises some of the actions of acetylcholine in a manner similar to that described under Atropine (page 36), although it is less active; it diminishes salivation, increases the heart rate, dilates the pupil, and reduces the spasm of involuntary muscle, particularly of the intestine. In small doses it depresses the central nervous system, but larger doses cause cerebral excitement.
Benzhexol is used in the treatment of post-encephalitic, arteriosclerotic, and idiopathic types of parkinsonism. In all types of parkinsonism, benzhexol usually increases mobility and decreases rigidity, but it has only a

limited effect on the tremors; the frequency and duration of oculogyric crises are also diminished.
Treatment is usually begun with a dosage of 1 to 2 milligrams of benzhexol hydrochloride by mouth three times daily and this is gradually increased to 20 milligrams daily in divided doses. Post-encephalitic patients as a rule tolerate and require higher doses, sometimes as much as 100 milligrams daily.
Benzhexol is sometimes given in conjunction with solanaceous alkaloids or other drugs used for the relief of parkinsonism.

UNDESIRABLE EFFECTS. Giddiness, dryness of the mouth, nausea, vomiting, and blurred vision occur occasionally, but readily disappear when the dose is reduced.

CONTRA-INDICATION. It is contra-indicated in closed-angle glaucoma.

Dose. See above under **Actions and uses.**

Preparation
BENZHEXOL TABLETS, B.P. Unless otherwise specified, tablets containing 2 mg of benzhexol hydrochloride are supplied. Tablets containing 5 mg are also available.

OTHER NAMES: *Artane®*; *Pipanol®*; *Trinol®*

BENZOCAINE

SYNONYMS: Benzocainum; Ethyl Aminobenzoate

$C_9H_{11}NO_2 = 165.2$

Benzocaine is ethyl *p*-aminobenzoate.

Solubility. Very slightly soluble in water; soluble, at 20°, in 8 parts of alcohol, in 4 parts of ether, in 2 parts of chloroform, and in 50 parts of fixed oils.

Standard
It complies with the requirements of the European Pharmacopoeia.
It occurs as colourless crystals or a white crystalline powder and contains not less than 99.0 per cent of $C_9H_{11}NO_2$, calculated with reference to the dried substance. The loss on drying under the prescribed conditions is not more than 0.5 per cent. It has a melting-point of 89° to 92°.

Storage. It should be stored in airtight containers, protected from light.

Actions and uses. Benzocaine is a sparingly soluble local anaesthetic with a toxicity about one-tenth that of cocaine. It may be given by mouth to relieve the pain of gastric carcinoma and is used, as an insufflation or as a 2 per cent solution in equal parts of alcohol and

water, in the symptomatic treatment of tuberculous laryngitis.
Benzocaine has been given by injection into the submucous and subcutaneous tissues in the treatment of pruritus ani and anal fissure.
Compound Benzocaine Lozenges, allowed to dissolve slowly in the mouth, produce a local anaesthetic effect and are used to prevent nausea and vomiting during such procedures as the taking of impressions for, or the fitting of, dentures, and the passing of instruments for laryngoscopy, bronchoscopy, or gastroscopy. These lozenges may also be used to relieve the pain arising from lacerations of the tongue or cheek, acute pharyngitis, tonsillectomy, or carcinoma of the mouth.
Compound Benzocaine Ointment may be applied to burns and cancerous ulcerations

and is of value for the relief of intractable pruritus.

Benzocaine has also been used in suppositories and pessaries containing 500 milligrams and in the form of a dusting-powder containing 10 per cent.

POISONING. As for Procaine Hydrochloride (page 404).

Preparations
BENZOCAINE LOZENGES, COMPOUND, B.P.C. (page 732)
BENZOCAINE OINTMENT, COMPOUND, B.P.C. (page 758)

BENZOIC ACID

$C_7H_6O_2 = 122 \cdot 1$

$C_6H_5 \cdot CO_2H$

Solubility. Soluble, at 20°, in 350 parts of water and in 3 parts of alcohol; readily soluble in ether, in chloroform, and in fixed and volatile oils.

Standard
It complies with the requirements of the British Pharmacopoeia.
It occurs as almost odourless, colourless, light, feathery plates or needles or white powder and contains not less than 99·5 per cent of $C_7H_6O_2$. It has a melting-point of 121·5° to 123·5°, forming a feathery sublimate. A solution in water is acid to methyl red.

Actions and uses. Benzoic acid has anti-

bacterial and antifungal properties. In a concentration of 0·1 per cent it is a moderately effective preservative for acid preparations, but is much less effective in neutral or alkaline media. Compound Benzoic Acid Ointment is used in the treatment of fungous infections of the skin.

Preparations
BENZOIC ACID OINTMENT, COMPOUND, B.P.C. (page 758)
BENZOIC ACID SOLUTION, B.P.C. (page 781)

BENZOIN

Benzoin is a balsamic resin obtained from the incised stem of *Styrax benzoin* Dryand. and of *S. paralleloneurus* Perkins (Fam. Styracaceae) and known in commerce as Sumatra benzoin.

Constituents. Benzoin contains various resinous esters of benzoic and cinnamic acids, together with free benzoic, cinnamic, siaresinolic (19-hydroxyoleanolic acid) and sumaresolinolic (6-hydroxyoleanolic acid) acids. The proportion of total cinnamic acid is usually about twice that of total benzoic acid.

Standard
DESCRIPTION. Hard, brittle masses consisting of whitish tears embedded in a greyish-brown to reddish-brown translucent matrix; odour agreeable and balsamic.

IDENTIFICATION TESTS. 1. Heat 0·5 g gently in a dry test-tube; it melts and evolves white fumes, which form a white crystalline sublimate.

2. Warm gently 1 g, in powder, with 5 ml of *potassium permanganate solution*; a distinct odour of benzaldehyde is produced (distinction from Siam benzoin).

3. Triturate 0·1 g, in powder, with 5 ml of *alcohol (95 per cent)*, filter, and to the filtrate add 0·5 ml of a 5 per cent w/v solution of *ferric chloride* in *alcohol (95 per cent)*; no bright green colour is produced (distinction from Siam benzoin).

ALCOHOL (90 PER CENT)-INSOLUBLE MATTER. Not more than 20·0 per cent, determined by the following method:
Warm about 2 g, in coarse powder, accurately weighed, with 25 ml of *alcohol (90 per cent)*, filter, wash the residue with hot *alcohol (90 per cent)* until extraction is complete, and dry to constant weight at 100°.

LOSS ON DRYING. Not more than 10·0 per cent, determined by the following method: spread evenly about 2 g, accurately weighed, in coarse powder, in a flat-bottomed dish, 9 cm in diameter and 1·5 cm deep, and dry over *phosphorus pentoxide* for 4 hours in vacuo.

ASH. Not more than 2·0 per cent.

CONTENT OF TOTAL BALSAMIC ACIDS. Not less than 25·0 per cent, calculated as cinnamic acid and with reference to the material dried under the prescribed conditions, determined by the following method:
Boil about 1·25 g, accurately weighed, with 25 ml of 0·5N alcoholic potassium hydroxide under a reflux condenser for 1 hour; evaporate off the alcohol, dis-

perse the residue in 50 ml of hot water, cool, add 80 ml of water and 1·5 g of *magnesium sulphate* dissolved in 50 ml of water, mix thoroughly, and allow to stand for 10 minutes.
Filter, wash the residue on the filter with 20 ml of water, acidify the combined filtrates with *hydrochloric acid*, and extract with four successive 40-ml portions of *solvent ether*; discard the aqueous solution, combine the ether extracts and extract with successive 20-, 20-, 10-, 10-, and 10-ml portions of a 5 per cent w/v solution of *sodium bicarbonate* in water, washing each aqueous extract with the same 20 ml of *solvent ether*.
Discard the ethereal liquids, acidify the mixed aqueous extracts with *hydrochloric acid*, and extract with successive 30-, 20-, 20-, and 10-ml portions of *chloroform*, filtering each chloroform extract through a layer of *anhydrous sodium sulphate* supported on a pledget of cotton wool; evaporate the combined filtrates to dryness in a current of air, taking care to stop the evaporation immediately the last trace of chloroform has been removed.
Dissolve the residue, with the aid of gentle heat, in 10 ml of *alcohol (95 per cent)* previously neutralised to *phenol red solution*, cool, and titrate with 0·1N sodium hydroxide, using *phenol red solution* as indicator; each ml of 0·1N sodium hydroxide is equivalent to 0·01482 g of total balsamic acids, calculated as cinnamic acid.

Adulterants and substitutes. Penang or "glassy" Penang benzoin, from Sumatra, has a greyish vitreous appearance and no aromatic odour.
Palembang benzoin, also from Sumatra, consists of a reddish resinous mass in which are embedded a few scattered tears, and has a slight odour.
Siam benzoin from *Styrax tonkinensis* Craib (Fam. Styracaceae) occurs in tears and blocks having a slight odour of vanillin; the surface is brownish-red with a varnished appearance; the tears are milky-white internally and occur also embedded in the brownish-red resinous matrix of the block variety. When it is warmed with potassium permanganate solution it yields no odour of benzaldehyde.

Storage. It should be stored in a cool place.

Actions and uses. Benzoin is an ingredient of inhalations which are used, by adding 5 millilitres of the inhalation to 500 millilitres of hot water and inhaling the vapour, in the treatment of catarrh of the upper respiratory tract.

Preparations

BENZOIN INHALATION, B.P.C. (page 705)

MENTHOL AND BENZOIN INHALATION, B.P.C. (page 705)

BENZOIN TINCTURE, B.P.C. (page 820)

BENZOIN TINCTURE, COMPOUND, B.P.C. (page 820)

OTHER NAMES: Gum Benjamin; Gum Benzoin

BENZTROPINE MESYLATE

$C_{22}H_{29}NO_4S = 403.5$

Benztropine Mesylate is 3-(diphenylmethoxy)tropane methanesulphonate.

$$\left[\begin{array}{c} H_2C - CH - CH_2 \quad C_6H_5 \\ | \quad N \cdot CH_3 \quad CH \cdot O \cdot CH \\ H_2C - CH - CH_2 \quad C_6H_5 \end{array} \right] CH_3 \cdot SO_3H$$

Solubility. Soluble, at 20°, in less than 1 part of water and in 1·5 parts of alcohol; insoluble in ether.

Standard
It complies with the requirements of the British Pharmacopoeia.
It is a white, crystalline, odourless powder and contains not less than 98·0 per cent of $C_{22}H_{29}NO_4S$, calculated with reference to the dried substance. The loss on drying under the prescribed conditions is not more than 5·0 per cent. It has a melting-point of 142° to 144°.

Sterilisation. Solutions for injection are sterilised by heating in an autoclave or by filtration.

Storage. It should be stored in airtight containers.

Actions and uses. Benztropine depresses the motor cortex and also has antihistamine and atropine-like actions. It reduces spasm and tremor of voluntary muscle and is used in the treatment of parkinsonism, usually in conjunction with other drugs.

The initial daily dosage is 500 micrograms of benztropine mesylate by mouth, gradually increased according to the response of the patient; the effective dosage is usually from 2 to 6 milligrams daily in divided doses.

UNDESIRABLE EFFECTS. The usual undesirable effects are dryness of the mouth, nausea, blurring of vision, and dizziness.

Dose. See above under **Actions and uses.**

Preparation
BENZTROPINE TABLETS, B.P. Unless otherwise specified, tablets each containing 2 mg of benztropine mesylate are supplied. They should be stored in airtight containers.

OTHER NAMES: Benztropine Methanesulphonate; *Cogentin*®

BENZYL ALCOHOL

$C_7H_8O = 108.1$

$C_6H_5 \cdot CH_2OH$

Solubility. Soluble, at 20°, in 25 parts of water; miscible with alcohol, with ether, and with chloroform.

Standard
It complies with the requirements of the British Pharmacopoeia.
It is a colourless, almost odourless liquid and contains not less than 97·0 per cent w/w of C_7H_8O. It has a weight per ml at 20° of 1·043 g to 1·046 g and a boiling-point not lower than 200°, not less than 95 per cent v/v distilling between 203° and 208°.

Sterilisation. Solutions for injection are sterilised by heating in an autoclave.

Actions and uses. Benzyl alcohol is a weak local anaesthetic with antiseptic properties. Occasionally, therefore, 1 per cent of benzyl alcohol is included in injections. It is almost non-toxic and non-irritant, but strong solutions may cause oedema and pain when injected.

BENZYL BENZOATE

$C_{14}H_{12}O_2 = 212.2$

$C_6H_5 \cdot CO \cdot O \cdot CH_2 \cdot C_6H_5$

Solubility. Insoluble in water and in glycerol; soluble in alcohol, in chloroform, and in ether.

Standard
It complies with the requirements of the British Pharmacopoeia.
It occurs as colourless crystals or oily liquid with a faintly aromatic odour and contains not less than 99·0 per cent w/w of $C_{14}H_{12}O_2$. It has a weight per ml at 20° of 1·116 g to 1·120 g. It has a freezing-point not lower than 17·0°, but is liable to become supercooled.

Actions and uses. Benzyl benzoate is an acaricide used in the treatment of scabies. The patient is scrubbed with soft soap in a hot bath to open up the burrows and, immediately after drying, Benzyl Benzoate Application is applied over the affected area; a second application is made on the following day.

Although more than one course of treatment may be necessary, benzyl benzoate is more efficient, cleaner, and easier to use than sulphur preparations.

Preparation
BENZYL BENZOATE APPLICATION, B.P. It contains 25 per cent of benzyl benzoate.

BENZYLPENICILLIN

SYNONYMS: Crystalline Penicillin G; Penicillin; Penicillin G

$C_{16}H_{17}N_2NaO_4S = 356·4$

$C_{16}H_{17}KN_2O_4S = 372·5$

Benzylpenicillin is either the potassium salt (Benzylpenicillin Potassium; Benzylpenicillinum Kalicum) or the sodium salt (Benzylpenicillin Sodium; Benzylpenicillinum Natricum) of an antimicrobial acid produced by growing certain strains of *Penicillium notatum* or related organisms under appropriate conditions in a suitable culture medium, or produced by any other means. Non-specific impurities are removed as completely as possible, and when the material is required for the preparation of injections the purified salts of benzylpenicillin are obtained from solution under conditions that yield a sterile product.

The penicillins are based on an unstable ring structure known as the β-lactam structure, with various side-chains in position 6, this being a phenylacetamido-group in benzylpenicillin. The ring structure may be defined as 4-thia-1-azabicyclo[3,2,0]heptane or azeto[2,1-*b*]thiazole; the systematic name of benzylpenicillin is therefore sodium (or potassium) 3,3-dimethyl-7-oxo-6-phenylacetamido-4-thia-1-azabicyclo[3,2,0]heptane-2-carboxylate or sodium (or potassium) 2,2-dimethyl-5-oxo-6-phenylacetamidoazeto-[2,1-*b*]thiazole-3-carboxylate.

Solubility. Very soluble in water; insoluble in fixed oils and in liquid paraffin.

Standard

It complies with the requirements of the European Pharmacopoeia.

Both salts are white, finely crystalline powders with a faint characteristic odour and contain not less than 96 per cent of total penicillins. They contain not more than 1·0 per cent w/w of water. A 10 per cent solution in water has a pH of 5·5 to 7·5.

Stability. The stability of benzylpenicillin depends mainly on its moisture content; provided that it contains less than 0·5 per cent, it can be stored at room temperature for two to three years without significant loss of potency.

For maximum stability, aqueous solutions of benzylpenicillin should be buffered at pH 6·0 to 7·0 and kept at a low temperature. Dilute solutions are more stable than concentrated ones, probably because less penicilloic acid is produced on hydrolysis with the lower concentration.

Hygroscopicity. Both salts are hygroscopic, but the potassium salt is less so. At relative humidities up to 55 per cent, they absorb insignificant amounts of moisture at 25°; at relative humidities between 55 and 80 per cent, the amounts absorbed by the potassium salt are larger but still small (e.g. about 0·4 per cent in 12 days at a relative humidity of 70 per cent), but with the sodium salt significant amounts are absorbed at relative humidities between 55 and 70 per cent; under damper conditions, both salts absorb substantial amounts of moisture.

Incompatibility. In addition to acids, alkalis, and penicillinase, numerous other substances inactivate benzylpenicillin at varying rates. Traces of heavy metals (copper, lead, zinc, or mercury) have a deleterious action on penicillin solutions. Although high concentrations of ethyl alcohol should be avoided, rigorous exclusion of alcohol from preparations is unnecessary and it can be used to wipe caps of bottles containing either the dry powder or its solutions for injection.

Low concentrations of glycerol (say 10 per cent) have little effect on the deterioration of aqueous solutions of benzylpenicillin, but high concentrations increase the loss of activity; impurities in the glycerol may be responsible for some of the inactivation. Similar effects occur with propylene glycol.

Benzylpenicillin in slightly alkaline solution is rapidly inactivated by cysteine and other aminothiol compounds.

Benzylpenicillin salts are incompatible with sympathomimetic amines and hydrochlorides of the tetracyclines, the degree of incompatibility being dependent on concentrations, pH of vehicles, and time.

Other substances with an adverse effect on benzylpenicillin include compounds leached from vulcanised rubber, oxidising agents (especially in the presence of trace metals), organic peroxides, thiomersal, wool alcohols, cetostearyl alcohol, paraffins, macrogols, cocoa butter, and many ionic and non-ionic surface-active agents.

Benzylpenicillin should not be given by intravenous drip in Dextrose Injection because the acidity of the sugar solution will bring about rapid decomposition, up to half its activity being lost in a few hours; this loss is likely to be increased if sodium bicarbonate is added in an attempt to neutralise the acidity; it may, however, be safely injected into the drip tubing after being well diluted with Sodium Chloride Injection, normal doses being administered over one to two minutes and larger doses more slowly.

Labelling. The label on the container states whether the contents are the sodium or the potassium salt. If the material is not intended for parenteral administration, the label also states that the contents are not to be injected.

Storage. It should be stored in airtight containers at a temperature not exceeding 30°. If it is intended for parenteral administration, the containers must be sterile and sealed to exclude micro-organisms.

Actions and uses. Benzylpenicillin is a highly potent antibiotic from which a group of semisynthetic penicillins have been derived for special clinical purposes. These penicillins share the following characteristics and many of them release benzylpenicillin in the tissues and share the same mode of excretion.

They act mainly by interfering with the synthesis of the bacterial cell wall and are therefore more effective when the bacterial cell is dividing. Penicillins may give rise to cell-wall-free variants of certain species of bacteria. The mammalian cell wall is only affected at high dose levels exceeding 12 grams (20 mega Units) daily which may cause haemolysis. The penicillins have additional bactericidal effects within the bacterial cell which occur at high dose levels and may affect dormant bacteria.

The penicillins are readily absorbed through the intestinal mucosa into the blood stream and diffuse into all body fluids but varying proportions are carried bound to protein. Only free penicillin is active but the protein-bound material acts as a reservoir which replaces the free material as the latter is excreted. The cerebrospinal fluid contains a relatively low concentration of total penicillin in the normal patient because it contains only the free component. When there is inflammation of the meninges and a proteinous exudate the levels are the same as in blood.

Free penicillin is rapidly excreted having a half-life of about three hours; it can be prolonged by the administration of probenecid which blocks the tubular component of the excretion. Most of the penicillin is excreted active and unchanged but some is degraded in the liver and kidneys through various pathways and excreted in inactive forms.

Benzylpenicillin is mainly used to treat infections by the Gram-positive pyogenic organisms, species of *Neisseria* and *Actinomyces*, *Bacillus anthracis*, species of *Clostridium*, *Corynebacterium*, and *Erysipelothrix*, and *Spirillum minus* and the spirochaetes. However, it would probably be effective against many of the Gram-negative bacteria as well as the "resistant" staphylococci were it not for strains and species which produce a variety of penicillinases. These are enzymes which are excreted by the bacteria and destroy the penicillin by opening the β-lactam ring. The production of these enzymes is an inherited characteristic which seldom (if ever) results from mutation. The spread of "resistant" strains particularly of staphylococci through the community is largely a result of replacement of sensitive by naturally resistant strains.

Benzylpenicillin is sometimes given orally to prevent streptococcal reinfection after rheumatic fever but acid-resistant penicillins such as phenoxymethylpenicillin are to be preferred. Oral benzylpenicillin is inappropriate for the treatment of infection because adequate blood levels are unlikely to be attained. In most acute illnesses 300 milligrams (500,000 Units) twice daily by intramuscular injection is sufficient.

Doses up to 300 milligrams (500,000 Units) of benzylpenicillin may be dissolved in 1 millilitre of Water for Injections, and larger doses in 2 millilitres. As all except the weakest solutions are hypertonic, Sodium Chloride Injection should not be used as the solvent. When a high dose is needed as may be the case in many cases of subacute bacterial endocarditis due to *Streptococcus viridans* or *S. faecalis* a continuous intravenous infusion may be preferred to avoid the painful sites caused by large volumes of hypertonic injections. When such infusions are given over long periods there is a danger of fungal infections occurring at the injection site.

The effect of intramuscular doses of benzylpenicillin may be prolonged by the use of procaine penicillin suspensions from which penicillin is released for up to twelve hours. They are not suitable for high dosage levels.

Benzylpenicillin may be used with streptomycin or other bactericidal drugs in the treatment of bacterial endocarditis but synergy with other antibiotics is believed not to occur and many consider that the synchronous use of a bacteriostatic agent is a disadvantage.

UNDESIRABLE EFFECTS. A cell-wall-damaging effect in high concentrations, limits the intrathecal dose to a maximum of 12 milligrams (20,000 Units) of benzylpenicillin in an adult. All penicillins carry a risk of hypersensitivity which develops most readily as a result of topical application. It is possible that pure penicillin is not the cause of the allergy in many cases but degradation products appearing during manufacture or storage or during metabolism of the penicillins in the body are responsible. Some but not all of the allergic responses may be avoided by using specially purified preparations.

These allergies are common to the whole group and penicillins should be avoided or used with great caution in patients with a history of allergy to any form of penicillin. The reaction usually develops during the second week of the first course of treatment and consists of an urticarial rash and fever. Subsequent administration can lead to more serious reactions of the serum sickness type and deaths have occasionally resulted from anaphylaxis.

Encephalopathy may occasionally follow the intravenous administration of high doses of benzylpenicillin in patients with renal failure.

PRECAUTIONS. As with all antibiotics, penicillin should not be used either prophylactically or for an established infection unless there is a positive indication that it is necessary. Otherwise penicillin will become useless both because of replacement of bacterial flora by resistant strains and the presence in the community of many individuals allergic to this group of drugs.

Benzylpenicillin should only be given to patients thought to be allergic to it if there is no satisfactory alternative and the infection is life-threatening. Preparations should be made to deal with anaphylactic shock before the first dose is given.

Benzylpenicillin should not be used topically either on the skin or mucous membranes. When high doses are given the effect of the associated sodium or potassium ions should be taken into account and the appropriate salt or mixture of salts should be used. It should not be given in a dose greater than 12 milligrams (20,000 Units) intrathecally in an adult and the equivalent dose in infants and children. A freshly prepared solution containing not more than 2 milligrams (3,500 Units) per millilitre should be used.

Dose. 125 to 500 milligrams (approximately 200,000 to 800,000 Units) by mouth every four hours; 150 to 600 milligrams (approximately 250,000 to 1,000,000 Units) by intramuscular injection twice to four times daily.

Doses up to 20 grams (approximately 35,000,000 Units) daily may be given by intravenous infusion.

Preparations

BENZYLPENICILLIN INJECTION, B.P. (*Syn.* Penicillin Injection). It consists of a sterile solution of benzylpenicillin prepared by dissolving the contents of a sealed container, which may also contain a suitable buffering agent, in Water for Injections. Unless otherwise specified, a solution containing 150 mg (approximately 250,000 Units) in 1 ml is supplied. It should be used within 7 days of its date of preparation, which is stated on the label, or within 14 days if a buffering agent is present, provided that it is stored during this period at 2° to 10°; at temperatures approaching 20° it should be used within 24 hours of preparation, or within 4 days if a buffering agent is present.

PROCAINE PENICILLIN INJECTION, FORTIFIED, B.P. It consists of a sterile suspension of 5 parts of procaine benzylpenicillin in Water for Injections containing 1 part of benzylpenicillin in solution. It is prepared by adding Water for Injections to the contents of a sealed container, which contains suitable dispersing agents and may also contain a suitable buffering agent. Unless otherwise specified, an injection containing 300 mg of procaine penicillin (equivalent to approximately 300,000 Units of penicillin) and 60 mg (approximately 100,000 Units) of benzylpenicillin in 1 ml is supplied. It should be used within 7 days of its date of preparation, which is stated on the label, or within 14 days if a buffering agent is present, provided that it is stored during this period at 2° to 10°; at temperatures approaching 20° it should be used within 24 hours of preparation, or within 4 days if a buffering agent is present.

PENICILLIN LOZENGES, B.P.C. (page 733)

BENZYLPENICILLIN TABLETS, B.P. (*Syn.* Penicillin Tablets). Unless otherwise specified, tablets each containing 250 mg (approximately 400,000 Units) of benzylpenicillin are supplied. They may be film coated or sugar coated. They should be stored in airtight containers, at a temperature not exceeding 30°. Tablets containing 125 mg are also available.

OTHER NAMES: *Crystapen®*; *Falapen®*; *Solupen®*; *Tabillin®*

BEPHENIUM HYDROXYNAPHTHOATE

$C_{28}H_{29}NO_4 = 443.5$

$$\left[\begin{array}{c} CH_3 \\ | \\ C_6H_5 \cdot CH_2 \cdot N \cdot [CH_2]_2 \cdot O \cdot C_6H_5 \\ | \\ CH_3 \end{array} \right]^+ \quad \text{(naphthalene ring with } CO_2^- \text{ and } OH)$$

Bephenium Hydroxynaphthoate is benzyldimethyl(2-phenoxyethyl)ammonium 3-hydroxynaphthalene-2-carboxylate.

Solubility. Insoluble in water; soluble in 50 parts of alcohol.

Standard

DESCRIPTION. A yellow crystalline powder; odourless or almost odourless.

IDENTIFICATION TESTS. 1. Dissolve 0·2 g in 10 ml of warm *dehydrated alcohol*, add 15 ml of *trinitrophenol solution*, and allow to stand; a precipitate is formed which, after washing with *alcohol (95 per cent)* and then with water, and drying at 105°, melts at about 134°, with decomposition.

2. Examine under screened ultraviolet light; a green fluorescence is produced.

3. It melts at about 170°, with decomposition.

4. The infra-red absorption spectrum exhibits maxima which are only at the same wavelengths as, and have similar relative intensities to, those in the spectrum of *bephenium hydroxynaphthoate A.S.*

SURFACE AREA. Not less than 7000 cm² per g, determined by the method given in Appendix 25, page 911.

CHLORIDE. Boil 1·25 g with 50 ml of water, cool in ice, and filter. To 20 ml of the filtrate, add 10 ml of *dilute nitric acid*, shake, and filter; the filtrate complies with the limit test for chlorides (700 parts per million).

SULPHATE. To a further 20 ml of the filtrate obtained in the test for chloride, add 10 ml of *dilute hydrochloric acid*, shake, and filter; the filtrate complies with the limit test for sulphates (0·12 per cent).

RELATED COMPOUNDS. It complies with the test given in Appendix 5A, page 860.

LOSS ON DRYING. Not more than 1·0 per cent, determined by drying to constant weight at 105°.

CONTENT OF $C_{28}H_{29}NO_4$. Not less than 99·0 per cent, calculated with reference to the substance dried under the prescribed conditions, determined by the following method:
Titrate about 1 g, accurately weighed, by Method I of the British Pharmacopoeia for non-aqueous titration; each ml of 0·1N perchloric acid is equivalent to 0·04435 g of $C_{28}H_{29}NO_4$.

Actions and uses. Bephenium hydroxynaphthoate is an anthelmintic which is effective against a variety of intestinal nematodes. It is sparingly soluble, and only a small fraction of the dose given by mouth is absorbed from the gastro-intestinal tract.

Bephenium hydroxynaphthoate in a single dose of 5 grams by mouth is usually effective in removing hookworms of the species *Ancylostoma duodenale* and roundworms (*Ascaris*). The dose should be given on an empty stomach and food withheld for one hour afterwards. The drug is less effective against *Necator americanus* and single doses on several successive days may be needed to remove all the worms. It is also effective against intestinal trichostrongyles and has a slight effect against whipworms (*Trichuris*).

UNDESIRABLE EFFECTS. It may occasionally cause transient diarrhoea and the bitter taste may cause nausea and sometimes vomiting.

Dose. 5 grams as a single dose.

Preparation

BEPHENIUM GRANULES, B.P.C. (page 702)

OTHER NAME: *Alcopar®*

BETAMETHASONE

SYNONYMS: Betameth.; Betamethasonum

$C_{22}H_{29}FO_5 = 392.5$

Betamethasone is 9α-fluoro-11β,17α,21-trihydroxy-16β-methylpregna-1,4-diene-3,20-dione, and may be prepared by partial synthesis.

Solubility. Very slightly soluble in water; soluble, at 20°, in 75 parts of alcohol and in 1100 parts of chloroform.

Standard
It complies with the requirements of the European Pharmacopoeia.
It is a white to creamy-white, odourless powder and contains not less than 96.0 and not more than the equivalent of 104.0 per cent of $C_{22}H_{29}FO_5$, calculated with reference to the dried substance. The loss on drying under the prescribed conditions is not more than 0.5 per cent. It melts with decomposition at about 240°.

Preparation of solid dosage forms. In order to achieve a satisfactory rate of dissolution betamethasone in the form of an ultra-fine powder should be used.

Storage. It should be protected from light.

Actions and uses. Betamethasone has actions and uses similar to those of prednisolone and is effective in much lower dosage. It may be used in the treatment of all conditions for which cortisone acetate is indicated (page 132), except adrenocortical deficiency states, for which its lack of sodium-retaining properties makes it less suitable than cortisone.

In rheumatoid arthritis, 0.5 to 2 milligrams daily may be given by mouth in divided doses, the dosage being modified according to the response; as Cushing's syndrome may occur after a few weeks at the full dosage level it is usual to give the lowest dose that controls symptoms adequately, preferably not more than 1 milligram daily. In disseminated disorders of connective tissue, such as polyarteritis nodosa and systemic lupus erythematosus, much larger doses are often necessary. In the treatment of asthma 1 to 5 milligrams may be given daily in divided doses.

Betamethasone may also be given by intra-articular injection, a dose suitable for a knee-joint being 1 to 5 millilitres of a preparation containing in each millilitre 4 milligrams of betamethasone in suspension with the equivalent of 1 milligram of betamethasone, in the form of betamethasone sodium phosphate, in solution.

UNDESIRABLE EFFECTS; PRECAUTIONS AND CONTRA-INDICATIONS. As for Cortisone Acetate (page 132).

Dose. 0.5 to 5 milligrams by mouth daily in divided doses.

Preparation
BETAMETHASONE TABLETS, B.P. Unless otherwise specified, tablets each containing 500 μg of betamethasone are supplied. Tablets containing 250 μg are also available.

OTHER NAME: *Betnelan*®

BETAMETHASONE SODIUM PHOSPHATE

SYNONYM: Betameth. Sod. Phos.

$C_{22}H_{28}FNa_2O_8P = 516.4$

Betamethasone Sodium Phosphate is the disodium salt of the 21-phosphate ester of 9α-fluoro-11β,17α,21-trihydroxy-16β-methylpregna-1,4-diene-3,20-dione.

Solubility. Soluble, at 20°, in 2 parts of water and in 350 parts of dehydrated alcohol; insoluble in chloroform.

Standard
It complies with the requirements of the British Pharmacopoeia.
It is a white or almost white, hygroscopic, odourless powder and contains not less than 96.0 and not more than the equivalent of 103.0 per cent of $C_{22}H_{28}FNa_2O_8P$, calculated with reference to the anhydrous substance. It contains not more than 8.0 per cent w/w of water. A 0.5 per cent solution in water has a pH of 7.5 to 9.0.

Stability. Aqueous solutions having a pH of about 8.0 are stable if protected from light. Particular care must be taken to prevent microbial contamination of the solutions so as to avoid hydrolysis of the ester by phosphatase which is a common product of microbial metabolism.

Sterilisation. Solutions for injection are sterilised by filtration.

Storage. It should be stored in airtight containers, protected from light.

Actions and uses. Betamethasone sodium phosphate has the actions and uses described under Betamethasone; 1.3 g of betamethasone sodium phosphate is equivalent to 1 g of betamethasone. It is soluble in water, and is used as an anti-inflammatory agent in preparations for local application to the ear and eye.

It is also given by intra-articular or intra-bursal injection in rheumatoid arthritis to relieve local pain and swelling in affected joints, and by intramuscular injection for systemic effect.

UNDESIRABLE EFFECTS; PRECAUTIONS AND CONTRA-INDICATIONS. As for Cortisone Acetate (page 132).

Dose. The equivalent of 0·5 to 5 milligrams of betamethasone by mouth daily in divided doses.

Preparations
BETAMETHASONE EYE-DROPS, B.P.C. (page 688)
BETAMETHASONE SODIUM PHOSPHATE INJECTION, B.P. It consists of a sterile solution of betamethasone sodium phosphate in Water for Injections with suitable stabilising agents. Unless otherwise specified, a solution containing the equivalent of 4 mg of betamethasone in 1 ml is supplied. It should be stored at a temperature below 30°, protected from light.
BETAMETHASONE SODIUM PHOSPHATE TABLETS, B.P. Unless otherwise specified, tablets each containing the equivalent of 500 µg of betamethasone are supplied. Tablets containing the equivalent of 250 µg are also available.

OTHER NAME: *Betnesol*®

BETAMETHASONE VALERATE

SYNONYM: Betameth. Valerate

$C_{27}H_{37}FO_6 = 476·6$

Betamethasone Valerate is 9α-fluoro-11β,21-dihydroxy-16β-methyl-17α-valeryloxypregna-1,4-diene-3,20-dione.

Solubility. Very slightly soluble in water and in light petroleum; soluble, at 20°, in 12 parts of alcohol and in 2 parts of chloroform.

Standard
It complies with the requirements of the British Pharmacopoeia.
It is a white to creamy-white, odourless powder and contains not less than 96·0 and not more than the equivalent of 104·0 per cent of $C_{27}H_{37}FO_6$, calculated with reference to the dried substance. The loss on drying under the prescribed conditions is not more than 0·5 per cent.

Stability. Aqueous solutions have their maximum stability at pH 5·0. In neutral and alkaline solutions the substance is converted to betamethasone 21-valerate which has only about one-tenth of the clinical activity of the 17-valerate. Betamethasone valerate is inactivated by coal tar, salicylic acid, and many other substances.

Storage. It should be protected from light.

Actions and uses. Betamethasone valerate is a corticosteroid for topical application and is applied as an ointment, cream, or lotion.

The affected area of skin is treated once or twice daily. The anti-inflammatory effect is enhanced by covering with an occlusive dressing, but if large areas are treated in this way sufficient of the drug may be absorbed to give rise to systemic effects.

UNDESIRABLE EFFECTS. Sensitisation occurs occasionally.

PRECAUTIONS. It should not be used on infected skin without the simultaneous application of a suitable antibacterial agent.

Preparations
BETAMETHASONE VALERATE SCALP APPLICATION, B.P.C. (page 648)
BETAMETHASONE VALERATE CREAM, B.P.C. (page 656)
BETAMETHASONE VALERATE LOTION, B.P.C. (page 727)
BETAMETHASONE VALERATE OINTMENT, B.P.C. (page 759)
BETAMETHASONE VALERATE WITH CHLORTETRACYCLINE OINTMENT, B.P.C. (page 759)

OTHER NAME: *Betnovate*®

BETHANIDINE SULPHATE

$C_{20}H_{32}N_6O_4S = 452·6$

Bethanidine Sulphate is *N*-benzyl-*N'N"*-dimethylguanidine sulphate.

Solubility. Soluble, at 20°, in 1 part of water and in 30 parts of alcohol; insoluble in ether.

Standard
It complies with the requirements of the British Pharmacopoeia.
It is a white odourless powder and contains not less than 98·0 and not more than the equivalent of 101·0 per cent of $C_{20}H_{32}N_6O_4S$, calculated with reference to the dried substance. The loss on drying under the prescribed conditions is not more than 1·0 per cent.

Actions and uses. Bethanidine is a hypotensive agent which reduces blood pressure

by selectively blocking transmission at the post-ganglionic adrenergic nerve endings. In tissue concentrations reached with oral therapeutic doses it prevents release of noradrenaline at the nerve ending without producing noradrenaline depletion, but in higher concentrations depletion may occur. Parenteral administration causes an initial increase in blood pressure, probably due to release of noradrenaline from adrenergic nerve endings.

Bethanidine is used to control hypertension. It causes a greater fall in blood pressure in the erect than in the supine position. The effect of a single oral dose reaches a maximum in four hours and is complete within twelve hours. Treatment is started with an oral dosage of 5 to 10 milligrams of bethanidine sulphate twice daily, increasing to four times daily and then by increments of 10 to 20 milligrams daily in divided doses until the optimum dosage is reached.

After bethanidine is discontinued, pretreatment levels of blood pressure are reached in twenty-four hours. Tolerance to bethanidine may occur, making necessary a progressive increase in dose. A thiazide diuretic may be given with bethanidine to enhance the antihypertensive effect.

UNDESIRABLE EFFECTS. Severe postural hypotension and interference with sexual function in the male may occur. Diarrhoea occurs more rarely than when other similar drugs are used.

PRECAUTIONS AND CONTRA-INDICATIONS. Since bethanidine may enhance the effects of circulating catecholamines, it is contraindicated in phaeochromocytoma. It should be used with caution in patients with renal failure.

Dose. Initial dose, 10 to 20 milligrams daily in divided doses; maintenance dose, up to 200 milligrams daily in divided doses, in accordance with the needs of the patient.

Preparation
BETHANIDINE TABLETS, B.P. Unless otherwise specified, tablets each containing 10 mg of bethanidine sulphate are supplied. Tablets containing 50 mg are also available.

OTHER NAME: *Esbatal*®

BISACODYL

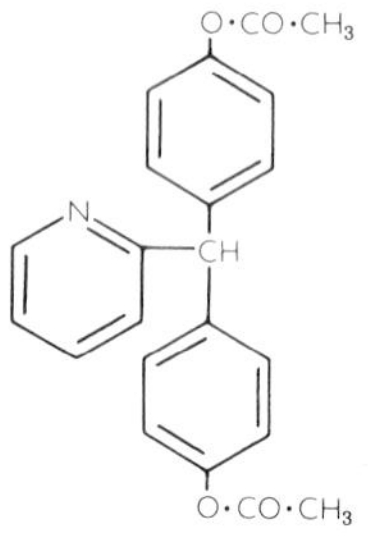

$C_{22}H_{19}NO_4 = 361.4$

Bisacodyl is 2-(*pp'*-diacetoxydiphenylmethyl)pyridine.

Solubility. Very slightly soluble in water; soluble, at 20°, in 100 parts of alcohol, in 170 parts of ether, and in 35 parts of chloroform.

Standard
It complies with the requirements of the British Pharmacopoeia.
It is an odourless white or almost white crystalline powder and contains not less than 98.0 and not more than the equivalent of 101.0 per cent of $C_{22}H_{19}NO_4$, calculated with reference to the dried substance. The loss on drying under the prescribed conditions is not more than 1.0 per cent. It has a melting-point of 133° to 135°.

Storage. It should be stored in airtight containers, protected from light.

Actions and uses. Bisacodyl is a laxative used for the treatment of constipation, for evacuation of the colon before radiological examination of the abdomen, or endoscopy, and before or after surgical operations. It has little or no action on the small intestine and is not absorbed. It acts within six to twelve hours when given by mouth and within one hour when given by rectum.

UNDESIRABLE EFFECTS. Occasionally severe abdominal cramps may occur. Suppositories sometimes cause local rectal irritation.

Dose. 5 to 10 milligrams daily by mouth or by rectum.

Preparations
BISACODYL SUPPOSITORIES, B.P. Unless otherwise specified, suppositories each containing 10 mg of bisacodyl are supplied. Suppositories containing 5 mg are also available.
BISACODYL TABLETS, B.P. Unless otherwise specified, tablets each containing 5 mg of bisacodyl are supplied. They are enteric coated and sugar coated.

OTHER NAME: *Dulcolax*®

BISMUTH CARBONATE

SYNONYMS: Bism. Carb.; Bismuth Subcarbonate; Bismuthi Subcarbonas

Bismuth Carbonate is a basic carbonate which may be prepared by the interaction of a solution of bismuth nitrate and of an alkaline carbonate.

The composition of bismuth carbonate varies with the conditions under which it is precipitated, but corresponds approximately to the formula $(BiO)_2CO_3,\frac{1}{2}H_2O$. The bulk density also varies considerably, depending upon the conditions of precipitation.

Solubility. Insoluble in water and in neutral organic solvents; completely soluble with effervescence in mineral acids.

Standard
Material which complies with this standard meets the requirements of the European Pharmacopoeia.

DESCRIPTION. A white or creamy-white powder; odourless; tasteless.

IDENTIFICATION TESTS. It gives the reactions characteristic of bismuth (Appendix 2, page 854) and of carbonates.

APPEARANCE OF SOLUTION. Dissolve 1 g in 50 ml of *dilute hydrochloric acid* with the aid of gentle heat. This solution complies with the following tests:
(i) The solution is clear or not more opalescent than a reference solution prepared by mixing 0·25 ml of *0·00002M sodium chloride*, 3·75 ml of water, 5·0 ml of *2M nitric acid*, and 1·0 ml of *dilute silver nitrate solution*, the comparison being made, 5 minutes after preparation of the reference solution, by viewing vertically 10 ml of the liquids in matched, colourless, transparent, neutral glass tubes, 16 mm internal diameter and with a flat base, against a black background in diffused light.

(ii) The solution has no colour when compared with water, the comparison being made by viewing vertically 10 ml of the liquids in matched, colourless, transparent, neutral glass tubes, 16 mm internal diameter and with a flat base, against a white background in diffused daylight.

ARSENIC. It complies with the test given in Appendix 6, page 877 (5 parts per million).

COPPER. Dissolve 0·5 g in 20 ml of *dilute hydrochloric acid* with the aid of gentle heat and make alkaline with *dilute ammonia solution*; no blue colour is produced.

LEAD. It complies with the test given in Appendix 8, page 886 (80 parts per million).

SILVER. Dissolve 2·5 g in 10 ml of *hydrochloric acid* with the aid of heat; the solution is clear. Allow to cool, and add 0·1 ml of *potassium iodide solution*; no opalescence is produced within 5 minutes.

CHLORIDE. Dissolve 0·35 g in a mixture of 30 ml of water and 6 ml of *nitric acid* and dilute to 50 ml with water; 15 ml of this solution complies with the test for Chloride given under Sodium Carbonate, page 445 (500 parts per million).

NITRATE. Dissolve 25 mg in 20 ml of *sulphuric acid* (*50 per cent v/v*) with the aid of heat and cool. To 2 ml of the solution add 4 ml of water, 0·15 ml of *sodium chloride solution*, and 6 ml of *diphenylamine solution*, and allow to stand for 15 minutes. Any blue colour which develops is not more intense than that produced when 1 ml of *nitrate standard solution* and 5 ml of water are used in place of the test solution and 4 ml of water (0·4 per cent).

ALKALIS AND ALKALINE EARTHS. Not more than 1·0 per cent, determined by the following method:
Boil about 1 g, accurately weighed, with 10 ml of *acetic acid* and 10 ml of water for 2 minutes; cool, filter and wash the residue with 20 ml of water. To the combined filtrate and washings add 2 ml of *dilute hydrochloric acid* and 20 ml of water, boil, and pass *hydrogen sulphide* through the boiling solution until no further precipitate is formed; filter, wash the residue with water, and evaporate the combined filtrate and washings to dryness; add 0·5 ml of *sulphuric acid*, ignite the residue gently, allow to cool, and weigh.

LOSS ON DRYING. Not more than 1·0 per cent, determined by drying to constant weight at 105°.

CONTENT OF Bi. 80·0 to 82·5 per cent, calculated with reference to the substance dried under the prescribed conditions, determined by the following method:
Dissolve about 0·2 g, accurately weighed, in just sufficient *dilute nitric acid*, add 50 ml of water and adjust the pH to 1 to 2 by the dropwise addition of *2M nitric acid* or *dilute ammonia solution*. Add about 30 mg of *xylenol orange mixture*, and titrate slowly with *0·05M disodium edetate* until the colour changes from red to yellow; each ml of 0·05M disodium edetate is equivalent to 0·01045 g of Bi.

Storage. It should be protected from light.

Actions and uses. Bismuth carbonate is a very weak antacid which has been used to treat dyspepsia. It is uncertain whether it has any other useful action on the mucosa of the gut.

Dose. 0·6 to 2 grams.

Preparations
BISMUTH LOZENGES, COMPOUND, B.P.C. (page 732)
BISMUTH POWDER, COMPOUND, B.P.C. (page 775)

BISMUTH SUBGALLATE

SYNONYMS: Basic Bismuth Gallate; Bism. Subgall.; Bismuth Oxygallate

Bismuth Subgallate may be prepared by the action of gallic acid on freshly precipitated bismuth hydroxide.

Solubility. Insoluble in water, in ether, and in dehydrated alcohol; readily soluble in hot mineral acids, with decomposition, and in solutions of alkali hydroxides, forming clear yellow solutions which rapidly become dark red.

Standard
DESCRIPTION. A citron-yellow powder; odourless or almost odourless.

IDENTIFICATION TESTS. 1. Suspend 0·1 g in water, saturate with *hydrogen sulphide*, filter, boil the filtrate to expel the excess gas, cool, and add 0·05 ml of *ferric chloride test-solution*; a bluish-black colour is produced.
2. Ignite; the residue gives the reactions characteristic of bismuth (Appendix 2, page 854).

ARSENIC. It complies with the test given in Appendix 6, page 877 (2 parts per million).

COPPER. It complies with the test described under Bismuth Subnitrate, 2·0 g ignited and re-ignited after the addition of 0·2 ml of *nitric acid* being used in place of the sample.

LEAD. It complies with the test given in Appendix 8, page 887 (30 parts per million).

SILVER. Ignite 2·5 g, add 0·2 ml of *nitric acid*, re-ignite, dissolve the residue in 10 ml of *hydrochloric acid*, and add 0·1 ml of *potassium iodide solution*; no opalescence is produced.

NITRATE. Dissolve 0·01 g in a cold mixture of 1 ml of water and 5 ml of *nitrogen-free sulphuric acid*, carefully overlay with 5 ml of *ferrous sulphate solution*, and allow to stand for 5 minutes; no brown ring is produced at the interface.

ALKALIS AND ALKALINE EARTHS. It complies with the test described under Bismuth Carbonate.

FREE GALLIC ACID. Not more than 0·25 per cent, determined by the following method:
Shake for one minute about 1 g, accurately weighed, with 20 ml of *alcohol (95 per cent)*, filter, wash the residue with 5 ml of *alcohol (95 per cent)*, evaporate the combined filtrate and washings to dryness on a water-bath, and dry the residue to constant weight at 105°.

LOSS ON DRYING. Not more than 7·0 per cent, determined by drying to constant weight at 105°.

CONTENT OF Bi. 46·0 to 52·0 per cent, calculated with reference to the substance dried under the prescribed conditions, determined by the following method:
Moisten about 0·8 g, accurately weighed, with *sulphuric acid*, ignite at a temperature not exceeding 500°, and continue by the method for Bismuth Subnitrate, using the residue in place of the sample.

Storage. It should be stored in airtight containers, protected from light.

Actions and uses. Bismuth subgallate is used in the form of suppositories for the treatment of haemorrhoids and as an ingredient of dusting-powders.

Preparations
BISMUTH SUBGALLATE SUPPOSITORIES, B.P.C. (page 796)
BISMUTH SUBGALLATE SUPPOSITORIES, COMPOUND, B.P.C. (page 796)

BISMUTH SUBNITRATE

SYNONYMS: Bism. Subnit.; Bismuth Oxynitrate

Bismuth Subnitrate is a basic salt and may be prepared by the interaction of a solution of bismuth nitrate with sodium hydroxide solution. It corresponds approximately in composition to the formula $6Bi_2O_3,5N_2O_5,9H_2O$.

Solubility. Insoluble in water and in alcohol; readily soluble in dilute nitric acid and in dilute hydrochloric acid.

Standard
DESCRIPTION. A white microcrystalline powder; odourless or almost odourless.

IDENTIFICATION TESTS. 1. Heat; brown fumes of nitrogen oxides are evolved and a yellow residue remains which gives the reactions characteristic of bismuth (Appendix 2, page 854).
2. Boil with *sodium carbonate solution* and filter; the filtrate gives the reactions characteristic of nitrates.
3. A suspension in water is slightly acid to *litmus solution*.

ARSENIC. It complies with the test given in Appendix 6, page 877 (2 parts per million).

COPPER. Dissolve 1·5 g in 2 ml of warm *nitric acid* and 1 ml of *hydrochloric acid*, pour into 50 ml of water, and filter; wash the residue with water, evaporate the combined filtrate and washings to 15 ml on a water-bath, and filter.
To 1 ml of the filtrate add 4 ml of water, neutralise to *litmus paper* with *dilute ammonia solution*, and add a further 5 ml; filter and wash the residue with 20 ml of water; to the combined filtrate and washings add 5 ml of *sodium diethyldithiocarbamate solution* and dilute to 50 ml with water; any colour which develops is not deeper than that produced by 0·5 ml of *dilute copper sulphate solution* when similarly treated, beginning with the words "add 4 ml of water . . ." (50 parts per million).

LEAD. It complies with the test given in Appendix 8, page 887 (30 parts per million).

SILVER. Dissolve 2·5 g in 10 ml of *hydrochloric acid* and add 0·1 ml of *potassium iodide solution*; no opalescence is produced.

CHLORIDE. 0·25 g dissolved in water with the addition of 6 ml of *nitric acid* complies with the limit test for chlorides (0·14 per cent).

SULPHATE. Dissolve 1·0 g in 4 ml of *hydrochloric acid*, dilute to 20 ml with water, boil, cool, add 0·5 ml of *barium chloride solution*, and allow to stand for 5 minutes; no turbidity is produced.

ALKALIS AND ALKALINE EARTHS. It complies with the test described under Bismuth Carbonate.

CARBONATE. Mix 1·0 g with 1 ml of water, add 2 ml of *nitric acid*, and warm; not more than a slight effervescence is produced.

LOSS ON DRYING. Not more than 2·0 per cent, determined by drying to constant weight at 105°.

CONTENT OF Bi. 71·0 to 75·0 per cent, calculated with reference to the substance dried under the prescribed conditions, determined by the following method:
Dissolve about 0·5 g, accurately weighed, in 2 ml of *nitric acid* and 4 ml of water, add 50 ml of water, 20 ml of *glycerol*, and 0·2 g of *sulphamic acid*, allow to stand for one minute, and add 200 ml of water and 0·3 ml of *catechol violet solution*; if a violet colour is produced add *dilute ammonia solution*, dropwise, until a blue colour is produced; titrate with 0·05M disodium edetate until a yellow colour is produced; each ml of 0·05M disodium edetate is equivalent to 0·01045 g of Bi.

Incompatibility. It is incompatible with carbonates, bicarbonates, iodides, tannin, and sulphur.

Actions and uses. Bismuth subnitrate is used with iodoform in the preparation of an antiseptic paste.

Preparation
RESORCINOL OINTMENT, COMPOUND, B.P.C. (page 763)

BLACK CURRANT

SYNONYM: Ribes Nigrum

Black Currant consists of the fresh ripe fruits of *Ribes nigrum* L. (Fam. Grossulariaceae), together with their pedicels and rachides. The plant is cultivated in temperate regions, especially in Europe, Australia, and Canada.

Constituents. Black currant contains invert sugar (about 6 to 8 per cent), citric, malic, and ascorbic acids (giving an acidity equivalent to about 3 per cent of citric acid), pectin, and colouring matter. The ascorbic acid content of the fruit varies from 100 to 300 mg per 100 g.

Standard
DESCRIPTION. *Macroscopical:* berries globose, ranging in diameter from about 7 to 15 mm, occurring in pendulous racemes; epicarp shiny black externally, enclosing a yellowish-green translucent pulp containing numerous flattened ovoid seeds, about 2·5 mm long, 1·25 mm wide, and 1 mm thick; berry crowned with withered remains of 5-cleft calyx; pedicels thin, up to about 10 mm long, attached to a rachis of varying length.
Odour strong, characteristic; taste pleasantly acidic.

Microscopical: The diagnostic characters are: Epicarp: *glands* yellow, disk-shaped, roughly circular or broadly elliptical, varying in diameter from about 140 to 240 μm, each consisting of a single layer of cells attached in the centre to the epicarp by means of a short multiseriate stalk.
Calyx: *trichomes* unicellular, blunt-ended, with thin, crooked walls, about 10 to 14 μm wide and averaging about 350 μm in length.
Seed: testa with *pigment layer* composed of small cells with horse-shoe-shaped wall thickenings as seen in cross section, each cell containing 1 or 2 prismatic *crystals* of calcium oxalate; *endosperm* cells with irregularly thickened walls.

Uses. Black currant is rich in ascorbic acid and is used in the form of a syrup as a dietary supplement, particularly for children. The syrup is also used as a flavouring agent in cough mixtures.

Preparation
BLACK CURRANT SYRUP, B.P.C. (page 799)

BORAX

SYNONYMS: Sodium Borate; Sodium Tetraborate

$Na_2B_4O_7,10H_2O = 381·4$

Solubility. Soluble, at 20°, in 20 parts of water and in 1 part of glycerol; soluble in less than 1 part of boiling water; insoluble in alcohol.

Standard
It complies with the requirements of the European Pharmacopoeia.
It occurs as odourless colourless crystals or white powder and contains not less than 99·0 and not more than the equivalent of 103·0 per cent of $Na_2B_4O_7$, $10H_2O$. A 5 per cent solution in water has a pH of 9·0 to 9·6.

Stability. It effloresces on exposure to air and on ignition it loses its water of crystallisation.

Incompatibility. It precipitates many alkaloids, including cocaine, from solutions of their salts.

Sterilisation. Solutions are sterilised by heating in an autoclave or by filtration.

Storage. It should be stored in airtight containers, in a cool place.

Actions and uses. Borax has a feeble antibacterial action similar to that of boric acid. It has been used in a lotion in the treatment of inflammatory conditions of the eye, and in gargles and mouth-washes. Lozenges of borax have been used for their astringent action.

UNDESIRABLE EFFECTS. Excessive use of preparations containing borax may lead to toxic effects due to absorption, as described under Boric Acid, and they should therefore be used sparingly.

POISONING. The procedure described under Boric Acid should be adopted.

Preparation
THYMOL GLYCERIN, COMPOUND, B.P.C. (page 702)

BORIC ACID

SYNONYMS: Acidum Boricum; Boracic Acid

$H_3BO_3 = 61·83$

Boric Acid is a weak acid, and its alkali salts, which are hydrolysed, particularly in dilute solution, are alkaline. It volatilises in steam. When heated to 100°, boric acid loses water and is slowly converted into metaboric acid, HBO_2; at 140° tetraboric acid, $H_2B_4O_7$, is formed and at higher temperatures, boron trioxide, B_2O_3.

Solubility. Soluble, at 20°, in 20 parts of water, in 16 parts of alcohol, and in 4 parts of glycerol; soluble in 3 parts of boiling water.

Standard
It complies with the requirements of the European Pharmacopoeia.
It occurs as odourless, white, unctuous, shining scales, crystals, or powder and contains not less than 99·5 per cent of H_3BO_3. A 3 per cent solution in water has a pH of 3·8 to 4·8.

Sterilisation. Solutions are sterilised by heating in an autoclave or by filtration.

Actions and uses. Boric acid has feeble antibacterial and antifungal properties. Aqueous solutions have been used as mouth-washes, eye lotions, and skin lotions, and as douches for irrigating the bladder and vagina and hot fomentations for ulcers, whitlows, boils, and carbuncles.

UNDESIRABLE EFFECTS. Because boric acid is excreted very slowly, repeated doses, by whatever route they are given, have a cumulative effect. When ingested it causes gastrointestinal irritation with loss of appetite and a toxic action on the kidneys.

Toxic effects may result from absorption and fatal cases of poisoning have been recorded in infants following the application of strong ointments of boric acid to extensive raw areas;

deaths have also occurred from the absorption arising from the lavage of body cavities with solutions of boric acid.

POISONING. If the boric acid has been ingested, gastric lavage or an emetic should be employed, and a purgative dose of magnesium sulphate given. The patient should be kept warm and treated for shock.

Preparations
CHLORINATED LIME AND BORIC ACID SOLUTION, B.P.C. (page 782)
CHLORINATED SODA SOLUTION, SURGICAL, B.P.C. (page 782)

BRILLIANT GREEN

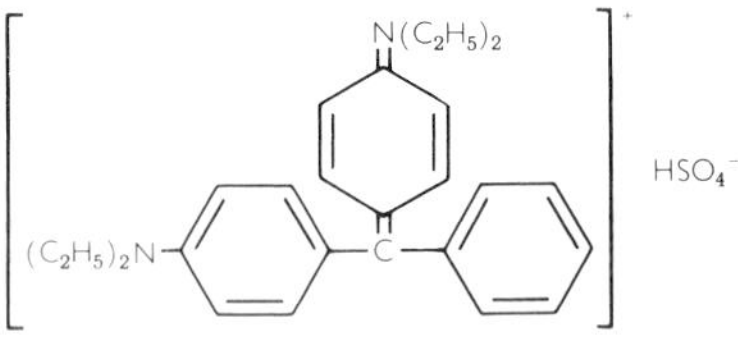

SYNONYM: Viride Nitens

$C_{27}H_{34}N_2O_4S = 482.6$

Brilliant Green (Colour Index No. 42040) is anhydrodi(p-diethylamino)triphenylmethanol hydrogen sulphate.

Solubility. Soluble, at 20°, in 5 parts of water and in 12 parts of alcohol.

Standard
It complies with the requirements of the British Pharmacopoeia.
It occurs as small, glistening, golden crystals and contains not less than 96.0 per cent of $C_{27}H_{34}N_2O_4S$, calculated with reference to the dried substance. The loss on drying under the prescribed conditions is not more than 3.5 per cent.

Actions and uses. Brilliant green is an antiseptic which is used in the treatment of infected wounds and burns. It is applied as a

0.05 to 0.1 per cent solution in water or hypertonic saline. A solution containing 0.5 per cent each of brilliant green and crystal violet has been used for sterilising the skin.

A paint containing 0.5 per cent each of brilliant green and mercuric chloride in industrial methylated spirit is used for the treatment of paronychia.

Preparation
BRILLIANT GREEN AND CRYSTAL VIOLET PAINT, B.P.C. (page 765)

BUPIVACAINE HYDROCHLORIDE

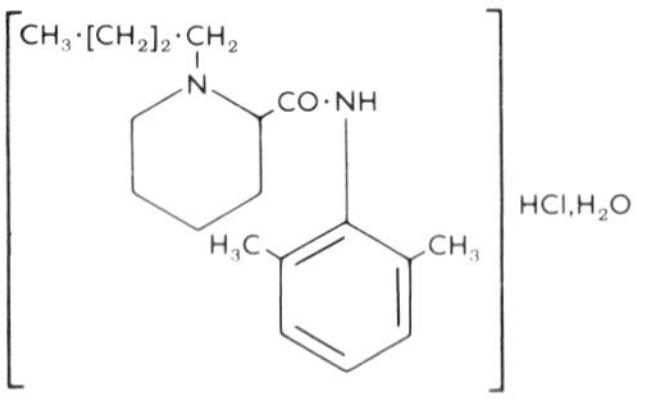

$C_{18}H_{29}ClN_2O,H_2O = 342.9$

Bupivacaine Hydrochloride is (±)-1-butyl-2-(2,6-xylylcarbamoyl)piperidine hydrochloride monohydrate.

Solubility. Soluble, at 20°, in 25 parts of water and in 8 parts of alcohol; slightly soluble in ether and in chloroform.

Standard
It complies with the requirements of the British Pharmacopoeia.
It is a white, crystalline, odourless powder and contains not less than 98.5 and not more than the equivalent of 101.0 per cent of $C_{18}H_{29}ClN_2O$, calculated with reference to the dried substance. The loss on drying under the prescribed conditions is 4.5 to 6.0 per cent. It has a melting-point of about 250°. A 1 per cent solution in water has a pH of 4.5 to 6.0.

Sterilisation. Solutions are sterilised by heating in an autoclave or by filtration.

Storage. It should be stored in airtight containers.

Actions and uses. Bupivacaine is a local

anaesthetic with an action similar to lignocaine, but of longer duration. Its laevoisomer has an even more prolonged action than bupivacaine.

Bupivacaine is used in local and spinal anaesthesia and may also be used to produce surface anaesthesia. It is usually administered as a solution containing 0.5 per cent of bupivacaine hydrochloride with adrenaline 1 in 200,000 or 0.25 per cent with adrenaline 1 in 400,000. Local anaesthesia lasting up to seven hours may be obtained with these solutions, but the total quantity administered over a period of four hours should not contain more than 2 milligrams of bupivacaine hydrochloride per kilogram body-weight; this is approximately equivalent to 40 to 60 millilitres of the 0·25 per cent solution or 20 to 30 millilitres of the 0·5 per cent solution for an adult.

Like other local anaesthetics, bupivacaine may have a quinidine-like action on the heart, but it is not used as an antiarrhythmic agent. Bupivacaine is cleared rapidly from the blood.

UNDESIRABLE EFFECTS. The toxic effects of bupivacaine are similar to those of other local anaesthetics. Hypotension, muscular twitching, respiratory depression, and convulsions may occur with overdosage.

PRECAUTIONS. Special care, including the recording of the foetal heart rate, should be taken when using bupivacaine to produce paracervical block in labour, as serious foetal bradycardia may be produced; if this condition occurs the intravenous administration of atropine sulphate may be required.

Dose. See above under **Actions and uses.**

OTHER NAME: *Marcain®*

BUSULPHAN

$C_6H_{14}O_6S_2 = 246·3$

$$CH_3 \cdot SO_2 \cdot O \cdot [CH_2]_4 \cdot O \cdot SO_2 \cdot CH_3$$

Busulphan is 1,4-di(methanesulphonyloxy)butane.

CAUTION. *Busulphan is irritant, and contact with the skin or inhalation of dust should be avoided.*

Solubility. Soluble, at 20°, in 750 parts of water and in 25 parts of acetone; slightly soluble in alcohol.

Standard
It complies with the requirements of the British Pharmacopoeia.
It is a white, crystalline, almost odourless powder and contains not less than 98·5 per cent of $C_6H_{14}O_6S_2$, calculated with reference to the dried substance. The loss on drying under the prescribed conditions is not more than 2·0 per cent. It has a melting-point of 115° to 118°

Storage. It should be stored in airtight containers, protected from light.

Actions and uses. Busulphan is a cytotoxic agent. Its pharmacological actions are ascribed to its ability to react with unknown cell components which are essential for normal division. It produces radiation-like effects with suppression of proliferating germinal tissues. This cytotoxic action is, when therapeutic doses are given, mainly exerted on the bone marrow and especially on the production of granulocytes. Platelet production is very liable to be depressed, with resultant thrombocytopenia.
Busulphan is given by mouth in the treatment of chronic myeloid leukaemia. In most cases it produces early symptomatic relief and reduction in the size of the spleen. A dosage of 2 to 4 milligrams daily for several weeks will usually produce a prolonged remission. Busulphan may also be used for maintenance therapy, the usual daily dosage being 0·5 to 2 milligrams.

In exceptional circumstances, doses of 6 milligrams or more daily may be given for short periods; this, however, increases the risk of irreversible bone-marrow damage. After large doses of busulphan, a rapid fall in the granulocyte count occurs, but with small repeated doses this may not commence for several weeks. A rise in the haemoglobin level and in the red-cell count is associated with a favourable response.

Busulphan is also useful in the treatment of polycythaemia vera and myelosclerosis.

UNDESIRABLE EFFECTS. Prolonged therapy with busulphan can cause fibrosing alveolitis. Other undesirable effects are hyperpigmentation and amenorrhoea.

PRECAUTIONS. Weekly examinations of the blood are necessary during busulphan therapy; the platelet count reaches a minimum several weeks after the granulocyte count has reached a stable level.

Dose. See above under **Actions and uses.**

Preparation
BUSULPHAN TABLETS, B.P. The quantity of busulphan in each tablet should be specified by the prescriber. They are compression coated or sugar coated. Tablets containing 0·5 and 2 mg are available.

OTHER NAME: *Myleran®*

BUTOBARBITONE

SYNONYMS: Butobarb.; Butobarbital; Butobarbitalum

$C_{10}H_{16}N_2O_3 = 212·2$

Butobarbitone is 5-butyl-5-ethylbarbituric acid.

Solubility. Soluble, at 20°, in 250 parts of water, in 1 part of alcohol, in 10 parts of ether, and in 3 parts of chloroform; readily soluble in solutions of alkali hydroxides and carbonates.

Standard
It complies with the requirements of the European Pharmacopoeia.
It occurs as colourless crystals or white crystalline

powder with a very slight odour and contains not less than 98·5 and not more than the equivalent of 102·0 per cent of $C_{10}H_{16}N_2O_3$, calculated with reference to the dried substance. The loss on drying under the prescribed conditions is not more than 0·5 per cent. It has a melting-point of 122° to 127°. A saturated solution in water is acid to litmus.

Hygroscopicity. It absorbs insignificant amounts of moisture at 25° at relative humidities up to about 90 per cent.

Actions and uses. Butobarbitone is an intermediate-acting barbiturate, the actions and uses of which are described under Phenobarbitone (page 366).

When given by mouth in doses of 100 to 200 milligrams it produces sleep in about half an hour. It may also be given by rectum in doses of 200 to 300 milligrams.

UNDESIRABLE EFFECTS; CONTRA-INDICATIONS; PRECAUTIONS; DEPENDENCE. These are as described under Phenobarbitone (page 366).

POISONING. The procedure as described under Phenobarbitone should be adopted.

Dose. 100 to 200 milligrams.

Preparation
BUTOBARBITONE TABLETS, B.P. The quantity of butobarbitone in each tablet should be specified by the prescriber. Tablets containing 100 mg are available.

OTHER NAMES: Butethal; *Soneryl*®

BUTYLATED HYDROXYANISOLE

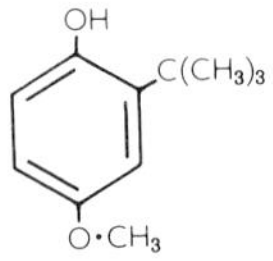

SYNONYM: BHA

$C_{11}H_{16}O_2 = 180·2$

Butylated Hydroxyanisole is 4-methoxy-2-t-butylphenol.

Solubility. Insoluble in water; soluble, at 20°, in 4 parts of alcohol, in 3 parts of arachis oil, in 100 parts of liquid paraffin, in 4 parts of lard, and in 1 part of propylene glycol; soluble in solutions of alkali hydroxides.

Standard
It complies with the requirements of the British Pharmacopoeia.
It is a white or almost white, crystalline powder with an aromatic odour. It has a melting-point of 62° to 65°.

Storage. It should be protected from light.

Uses. Butylated hydroxyanisole is used as an antioxidant for preserving oils and fats. It may be used for this purpose either alone or with propyl, octyl, or dodecyl gallate; an antioxidant synergist such as citric acid or phosphoric acid is sometimes added.

Butylated hydroxyanisole may be dissolved in many oils at room temperature, or by warming slightly; it dissolves readily in molten fats. Care should be taken not to incorporate air in the oil or fat while dissolving the antioxidant.

Up to 200 parts per million of butylated hydroxyanisole or of butylated hydroxytoluene, or of a mixture of these, may be used in pharmaceutical practice for the preservation of fixed oils, fats or vitamin oil concentrates; up to 1000 parts per million may be added to essential oils used in foods, but inclusion of antioxidants is not permitted in essential oils of the British Pharmacopoeia and the British Pharmaceutical Codex.

BUTYLATED HYDROXYTOLUENE

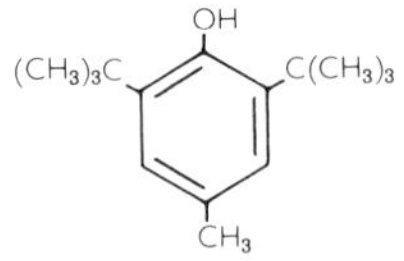

SYNONYM: BHT

$C_{15}H_{24}O = 220·4$

Butylated Hydroxytoluene is 2,6-di-t-butyl-*p*-cresol.

Solubility. Insoluble in water, in glycerol, and in propylene glycol; soluble, at 20°, in 4 parts of alcohol, in 0·5 part of ether, in 3 parts of fixed oils, and in 5 parts of liquid paraffin; very slightly soluble in solutions of alkali hydroxides.

Standard
It complies with the requirements of the British Pharmacopoeia.

It occurs as odourless colourless crystals or white crystalline powder. It has a freezing-point not lower than 69·2°.

Uses. Butylated hydroxytoluene is used for the same purposes as butylated hydroxyanisole.

CADE OIL

SYNONYMS: Juniper Tar Oil; Oleum Cadinum

Cade Oil is obtained by the destructive distillation of the branches and wood of *Juniperus oxycedrus* L. (Fam. Cupressaceae), a tree common in the Mediterranean areas of North Africa, France, and Spain.

Constituents. Cade oil contains guaiacol, together with ethylguaiacol, creosol, the sesquiterpene cadinene, and a varying amount of non-volatile material.

Solubility. Very slightly soluble in water; partly soluble in cold alcohol (90 per cent); almost entirely soluble in hot alcohol (90 per cent); soluble, at 20°, in 3 parts of ether; soluble in chloroform.

Standard
DESCRIPTION. A dark reddish-brown or almost black oily liquid; odour empyreumatic.

IDENTIFICATION TESTS. The filtrate prepared in the test for colour and acidity of an aqueous solution complies with the following tests:
1. To 5 ml add 0·2 ml of a 0·1 per cent w/v solution of *ferric chloride* in water; a red colour is produced.
2. Boil 5 ml with 2 ml of *potassium cupri-tartrate solution*; a red precipitate is formed.

COLOUR AND ACIDITY OF AN AQUEOUS SOLUTION. Shake 5 ml with 100 ml of water, allow to separate, and filter the aqueous layer; the filtrate is almost colourless and is acid to *litmus solution*.

REFRACTIVE INDEX. At 20°, 1·510 to 1·530.

WEIGHT PER ML. At 20°, 0·970 g to 1·010 g.

PINE TAR OIL. Shake 1 ml with 15 ml of *light petroleum* (*boiling-range, 40° to 60°*) and filter; shake 10 ml of the filtrate with 10 ml of *strong copper acetate solution*, allow to separate, and to 10 ml of the upper layer add 20 ml of *solvent ether*; no green colour and not more than a pale brown colour is produced.

Adulterants and substitutes. Pine tar oil, obtained as a tarry fraction in the destructive distillation of the wood of various species of *Pinus*, *Larix*, and *Abies*.

Actions and uses. Cade oil has been used in local applications for the treatment of psoriasis but has now been almost completely replaced by coal tar preparations.

Preparation
RESORCINOL OINTMENT, COMPOUND, B.P.C. (page 763)

CAFFEINE

SYNONYMS: Anhydrous Caffeine; Coffeinum

$C_8H_{10}N_4O_2 = 194·2$

Caffeine is 1,3,7-trimethylxanthine and is obtained chiefly from tea waste or coffee or from the dried leaves of *Camellia sinensis* (L.) O. Kuntze; it may also be prepared synthetically. When crystallised from water, caffeine contains one molecule of water of crystallisation, but it is anhydrous when crystallised from alcohol, chloroform, or ether.

Solubility. Soluble, at 20°, in 60 parts of water and in 130 parts of alcohol; slightly soluble in ether; soluble in chloroform.

Standard
It complies with the requirements of the European Pharmacopoeia.
It occurs as odourless, white, silky crystals or white crystalline powder. The loss on drying at 100° to 105° for one hour is not more than 0·5 per cent. It has a melting-point of 234° to 239°.

Stability. It is a very weak base and is decomposed by strong solutions of caustic alkalis; its salts are decomposed by water.

Storage. It should be stored in airtight containers.

Actions and uses. Caffeine has a stimulating effect on the central nervous system and a weak diuretic action. It may increase renal blood flow or the proportion of functioning glomeruli, but its main action is due to the reduction of the normal tubular resorption. It is less effective as a diuretic than theobromine, which has less central stimulant effect.

Dose. 100 to 300 milligrams.

Preparations
CAFFEINE IODIDE ELIXIR, B.P.C. (page 667)
ASPIRIN TABLETS, COMPOUND, B.P.C. (page 806)

CAFFEINE HYDRATE

SYNONYMS: Caffeine Monohydrate; Coffeinum Monohydricum

$C_8H_{10}N_4O_2,H_2O = 212 \cdot 2$

Caffeine Hydrate is the monohydrate of 1,3,7-trimethylxanthine. When crystallised from water, caffeine contains one molecule of water of crystallisation, but it is anhydrous when crystallised from alcohol, chloroform, or ether.

Solubility. Soluble, at 20°, in 60 parts of water and in 110 parts of alcohol; slightly soluble in ether; soluble in chloroform, with separation of water.

Standard
It complies with the requirements of the European Pharmacopoeia.
It occurs as odourless, white, silky crystals or white crystalline powder. The loss on drying at 100° to 105° for one hour is from 5·0 to 9·0 per cent. It has a melting-point of 234° to 239°.

Stability. It effloresces on exposure to dry air and loses its water of crystallisation when heated, becoming anhydrous at 100°; it sublimes at about 180°.

Storage. It should be stored in airtight containers.

Actions and uses. Caffeine hydrate has the actions and uses described under Caffeine.

Dose. 100 to 300 milligrams.

CAJUPUT OIL

SYNONYM: Oleum Cajuputi

Cajuput Oil is obtained from the fresh leaves and twigs of certain species of *Melaleuca*, such as *M. cajuputi* Powell and *M. leucadendron* (L.) L. (Fam. Myrtaceae), trees indigenous to Northern Australia and the Malay Archipelago. The oil is distilled mainly in the Molucca Islands and rectified by steam distillation.

Constituents. The chief constituents of cajuput oil are cineole, terpineol (both free and esterified), terpenes, and sesquiterpenes.

Solubility. Soluble, at 20°, in 2 parts of alcohol (80 per cent), becoming less soluble with age; miscible with alcohol (90 per cent).

Standard
DESCRIPTION. A colourless, yellow, or green liquid; odour agreeable and camphoraceous.

OPTICAL ROTATION. At 20°, +1° to −4°.

REFRACTIVE INDEX. At 20°, 1·464 to 1·472.

WEIGHT PER ML. At 20°, 0·910 g to 0·923 g.

CONTENT OF CINEOLE. Carry out the method of the British Pharmacopoeia, Appendix IXD, for the determination of cineole; the freezing-point of the mixture lies between 27·4° and 38·9°, corresponding to 50 to 65 per cent w/w of cineole.

Storage. It should be stored in well-filled airtight containers, protected from light, in a cool place.

Actions and uses. Cajuput oil is a mild counter-irritant and is a constituent of some ointments and liniments.

Preparation
METHYL SALICYLATE OINTMENT, COMPOUND, B.P.C. (page 762)

CALAMINE

SYNONYM: Prepared Calamine

Calamine is a basic zinc carbonate suitably coloured with ferric oxide.

Solubility. Insoluble in water; almost completely soluble in hydrochloric acid, with effervescence.

Standard
It complies with the requirements of the British Pharmacopoeia.
It is an amorphous impalpable pink or reddish-brown powder, the shade depending upon the variety and amount of ferric oxide present and the process by which it is incorporated. When ignited, it loses water and carbon dioxide, leaving 68·0 to 74·0 per cent of a residue composed of oxides of zinc and iron.

Actions and uses. Calamine has a mild astringent action on the skin and is used in dusting-powders, lotions, and ointments to relieve the discomfort of dermatitis.

Oily Calamine Lotion is a soothing appli-cation for the treatment of eczema; Calamine Lotion cools the skin by evaporation and is useful for allaying the pain and swelling of sunburn.

Preparations
CALAMINE APPLICATION, COMPOUND, B.P.C. (page 648)
CALAMINE CREAM, AQUEOUS, B.P.C. (page 656)
CALAMINE LOTION, B.P. It contains 15 per cent of calamine and 5 per cent of zinc oxide, with bentonite, sodium citrate, Liquified Phenol, and glycerol, in Purified Water.
CALAMINE LOTION, OILY, B.P.C. (page 727)
CALAMINE OINTMENT, B.P.C. (page 759)
CALAMINE AND COAL TAR OINTMENT, B.P.C. (page 760)

CALCIFEROL

SYNONYMS: Ergocalciferol; Vitamin D$_2$

$C_{28}H_{44}O = 396.7$

Calciferol is 9,10-secoergosta-5,7,10(19),22-tetraen-3β-ol and may be prepared by the ultraviolet irradiation of ergosterol.

Solubility. Insoluble in water; soluble, at 20°, in 2 parts of alcohol, in 2 parts of ether, in less than 1 part of chloroform, in 10 parts of acetone, and in 50 to 100 parts of fixed oils.

Standard
It complies with the requirements of the British Pharmacopoeia.
It occurs as odourless or almost odourless colourless crystals or white crystalline powder and contains 40,000 Units of antirachitic activity (vitamin D) per mg. It has a melting-point of 115° to 118°.

Storage. It should be stored in hermetically sealed glass containers in which the air has been replaced by an inert gas, and protected from light in a cool place.

Actions and uses. Calciferol has the actions and uses of naturally occurring vitamin D, which is necessary for the absorption of calcium and phosphorus.

Deficiency of vitamin D results in rickets in children and osteomalacia in adults. Children and infants require relatively more vitamin D than adults, their daily requirement being about 400 Units (10 micrograms) but it is important that infants should not be given more than 800 Units daily because of the danger of causing hypercalcaemia. The daily requirement of the mother in pregnancy and lactation is also of the order of 400 Units (10 micrograms).

In the treatment of vitamin-D-deficiency rickets the minimum daily dose is 1000 Units (25 micrograms) but 3000 to 4000 Units (75 to 100 micrograms) may be given for rapid healing; cases of vitamin-D-resistant rickets may require as much as 20,000 Units (500 micrograms) daily. Even higher doses are required for the treatment of hypoparathyroidism and vitamin-D resistance due to steatorrhoea, chronic renal failure, or hypophosphataemia, and in these cases the regime is similar to that described under Dihydrotachysterol (page 164).

Vitamin D$_3$ (cholecalciferol) is obtained by the ultraviolet irradiation of 7-dehydrocholesterol. It occurs in various fish-liver oils and it is responsible for the antirachitic action of cod- and other fish-liver oils. Hence it is sometimes described as "natural" vitamin D. Its chemical structure and physiological action are similar to those of calciferol, although there is some evidence of a difference in antirachitic activity in man.

UNDESIRABLE EFFECTS. Excessive doses, that is, 150,000 Units (3.75 milligrams) or more daily, may give rise to anorexia, nausea, vomiting, diarrhoea, loss of weight, headache, polyuria, thirst, vertigo, and eventually a raised blood urea. The urinary excretion of calcium is raised, and metastatic calcification may occur, particularly in the arteries and kidneys.

Treatment consists in withdrawing the calciferol, reducing the dietary calcium intake, and increasing the fluid intake.

PRECAUTIONS. There is danger of overdosage of calciferol in infants and in patients with chronic renal failure. Liquid preparations for infants and children should be particularly carefully measured.

Calciferol appears to take slightly longer to act and slightly longer to cease acting than dihydrotachysterol, and it is therefore even more important to avoid overdosage with calciferol than with dihydrotachysterol.

Dose. Prophylactic, 400 Units (10 micrograms) daily; therapeutic, see above under **Actions and uses.**

Preparations

CALCIFEROL INJECTION, B.P.C. (page 711)

CALCIFEROL SOLUTION, B.P. (*Syn.* Vitamin D$_2$ Solution). It consists of a solution of calciferol in a suitable vegetable oil containing 75 µg (3000 Units of antirachitic activity) in 1 ml. It should be stored in well-filled airtight containers, protected from light, in a cool place. Dose: prophylactic, not more than 0.25 millilitre (approximately 800 Units) daily, allowance being made for vitamin D obtained from other sources; therapeutic, 1.5 to 16 millilitres (approximately 5000 to 50,000 Units) daily.

CALCIFEROL TABLETS, STRONG, B.P. (*Syn.* Strong Vitamin D$_2$ Tablets). Each tablet contains 1.25 mg of calciferol (50,000 Units of antirachitic activity). They are sugar coated. They should be stored in well-closed containers, in a cool place. Dose: for hypoparathyroidism, 1 to 4 tablets (50,000 to 200,000 Units) daily. When Calciferol Tablets are ordered, Strong Calciferol Tablets should not be supplied unless it is confirmed that these are intended.

CALCIUM WITH VITAMIN D TABLETS, B.P.C. (page 809)

CALCIUM ACETATE

$(CH_3 \cdot CO_2)_2Ca$

$C_4H_6CaO_4 = 158 \cdot 2$

Solubility. Soluble, at 20°, in 3 parts of water; slightly soluble in alcohol.

Standard

DESCRIPTION. A white hygroscopic powder; odourless or almost odourless.

IDENTIFICATION TESTS. It gives the reactions characteristic of calcium and of acetates.

ALKALINITY. pH of a 5·0 per cent w/v solution in *carbon dioxide-free water*, 7·2 to 8·2.

ARSENIC. It complies with the test given in Appendix 6, page 877 (2 parts per million).

BARIUM. Not more than 50 parts per million, determined by the following method:
Dissolve 5·0 g in sufficient water to produce 100 ml and determine by emission spectroscopy at a wavelength of 455·5 nm with a nitrous oxide–acetylene flame, using Method II of the British Pharmacopoeia, Appendix XIA; use *barium solution FP*, diluted if necessary with water, for the standard solution.

LEAD. It complies with the test given in Appendix 7, page 881 (10 parts per million).

MAGNESIUM. Not more than 500 parts per million, determined by the following method:
Dissolve 0·2 g in sufficient water to produce 100 ml and determine by atomic absorption spectroscopy at a wavelength of 285·2 nm, using Method II of the British Pharmacopoeia, Appendix XIA; use *magnesium solution FP*, diluted if necessary with water, for the standard solution.

POTASSIUM. Not more than 0·1 per cent, determined by the method given under Magnesium Acetate (page 275).

SODIUM. Not more than 0·5 per cent, determined by the method given under Magnesium Acetate (page 275).

STRONTIUM. Not more than 500 parts per million, determined by the following method:
Dissolve 2·0 g in sufficient water to produce 100 ml and determine by atomic absorption spectroscopy at a wavelength of 460·7 nm, using Method II of the British Pharmacopoeia, Appendix XIA; use *strontium solution FP*, diluted if necessary with water, for the standard solution.

CHLORIDE. 1·0 g complies with the limit test for chlorides (350 parts per million).

NITRATE. It complies with the test given under Magnesium Acetate (page 275).

SULPHATE. 1·0 g complies with the limit test for sulphates (0·12 per cent).

READILY OXIDISABLE SUBSTANCES. It complies with the test given under Magnesium Acetate (page 275).

WATER. Not more than 8·0 per cent w/w, determined by the method given in Appendix 16, page 895, about 0·8 g, accurately weighed, being used and 20 ml of *glacial acetic acid* being added to the titration vessel in addition to the 20 ml of methyl alcohol.

CONTENT OF $C_4H_6CaO_4$. Not less than 98·0 per cent, calculated with reference to the anhydrous substance, determined by the following method:
Dissolve about 0·6 g, accurately weighed, in 15 ml of *ammonia-ammonium chloride solution* and titrate with 0·1M disodium edetate, using *methyl thymol blue solution* as indicator; each ml of 0·1M disodium edetate is equivalent to 0·01582 g of $C_4H_6CaO_4$.

Storage. It should be stored in airtight containers.

Uses. Calcium acetate is a source of calcium ions and may be used to adjust the calcium content of solutions for haemodialysis.

CALCIUM ALGINATE

Calcium Alginate consists chiefly of the calcium salt of alginic acid. It may contain a small proportion of sodium alginate in order to give a product which, although insoluble in water, is more easily absorbed by the body tissues.

Solubility. Insoluble in water and in organic solvents; soluble in solutions of sodium citrate.

Standard

DESCRIPTION. A white to pale yellowish-brown powder or fibres; odourless or almost odourless.

IDENTIFICATION TESTS. 1. It complies with test 1 described under Alginic Acid (page 11).
2. Boil 0·1 g with 5 ml of water; the sample does not dissolve. Add 2 ml of *sodium carbonate solution* and boil for 1 minute; a white precipitate is formed. Centrifuge and acidify the clear solution; a gelatinous precipitate is formed.
3. Ignite a suitable quantity, dissolve the residue in *dilute hydrochloric acid*, and filter; the filtrate gives the reactions characteristic of calcium.

ARSENIC. It complies with the test given in Appendix 6, page 877 (3 parts per million).

IRON. Ignite 0·75 g, cool, dissolve the residue in 3 ml of *hydrochloric acid FeT*, and dilute to 50 ml with water; 5 ml of this solution complies with the limit test for iron (530 parts per million).

LEAD. It complies with the test given in Appendix 7, page 881 (10 parts per million).

LOSS ON DRYING. Not more than 22·0 per cent, determined by drying to constant weight at 105°.

SULPHATED ASH. 31·0 to 34·0 per cent, calculated with reference to the substance dried under the prescribed conditions.

Sterilisation. Solutions are sterilised as described under Alginic Acid (page 11).

Uses. Calcium alginate is used as an absorbable haemostatic. Fibres of calcium alginate are prepared in a form resembling gauze or wool and this is used to cover lacerated wounds or burns.

Calcium alginate dressings, frequently soaked in sodium alginate solution, are used to pack sinuses, fistulas, and bleeding tooth sockets; the dressings are also used similarly to cover surgical incisions and sites from which skin grafts have been removed. Sterile powder consisting of a mixture of calcium and sodium alginates is used in place of talc in glove powders.

Calcium alginate is also used as a tablet disintegrant.

CALCIUM AMINOSALICYLATE

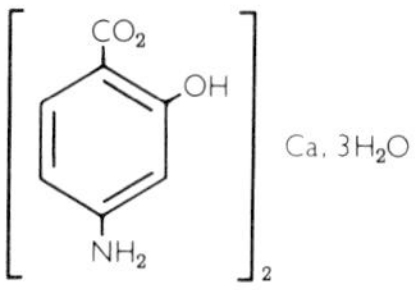

SYNONYMS: Calc. Aminosal.; Calcii Aminosalicylas;
Calcium Para-aminosalicylate

$C_{14}H_{12}CaN_2O_6,3H_2O = 398\cdot4$

Calcium Aminosalicylate is calcium 4-amino-2-hydroxybenzoate trihydrate.

Solubility. Soluble, at 20°, in 10 parts of water; slightly soluble in alcohol.

Standard
It complies with the requirements of the European Pharmacopoeia.
It is a white or slightly yellow, crystalline, hygroscopic, odourless powder and contains not less than 98·0 and not more than the equivalent of 101·0 per cent of $C_{14}H_{12}CaN_2O_6$ and 11·3 to 11·8 per cent of Ca, both calculated with reference to the anhydrous substance. It contains 12·0 to 14·0 per cent w/w of water. A 2·0 per cent solution in water has a pH of 6·0 to 8·0.

Stability. Aqueous solutions decompose slowly and darken in colour.

Storage. It should be stored in airtight containers, protected from light.

Actions and uses. Calcium aminosalicylate has actions, uses, and undesirable effects similar to those described under Sodium Aminosalicylate (page 442).

PRECAUTIONS. As for Sodium Aminosalicylate (page 442).

Dose. 10 to 15 grams daily in divided doses.

Preparation
CALCIUM AMINOSALICYLATE TABLETS, B.P.C. (page 807)

OTHER NAME: Calcium PAS

CALCIUM CARBONATE

SYNONYMS: Calc. Carb.; Calcii Carbonas

$CaCO_3 = 100\cdot1$

Solubility. Very slightly soluble in water; slightly soluble in water containing carbon dioxide.

Standard
It complies with the requirements of the European Pharmacopoeia.
It is a white odourless powder and contains not less than 98·5 per cent of $CaCO_3$, calculated with reference to the dried substance. The loss on drying under the prescribed conditions is not more than 2·0 per cent.

Hygroscopicity. It absorbs insignificant amounts of moisture at 25° at relative humidities up to about 90 per cent.

Sterilisation. It is sterilised by heating in a closed container at a temperature not lower than 160° for sufficient time to ensure that the whole of the powder is maintained at this temperature for one hour.

Actions and uses. Calcium carbonate is an antacid which tends to cause constipation and is usually given with other antacid substances in mixtures, powders, and tablets. It is also used as a basis for dentifrices.

Dose. 1 to 5 grams, repeated in accordance with the needs of the patient.

Preparations
BISMUTH LOZENGES, COMPOUND, B.P.C. (page 732)
CALCIUM CARBONATE MIXTURE, COMPOUND, PAEDIATRIC, B.P.C. (page 738)
BISMUTH POWDER, COMPOUND, B.P.C. (page 775)
CALCIUM CARBONATE POWDER, COMPOUND, B.P.C. (page 775)
MAGNESIUM CARBONATE POWDER, COMPOUND, B.P.C. (page 778)
MAGNESIUM CARBONATE TABLETS, COMPOUND, B.P.C. (page 812)

OTHER NAME: Precipitated Calcium Carbonate

CALCIUM CHLORIDE

SYNONYMS: Calc. Chlor.; Calcii Chloridum; Calcium Chloride Dihydrate

$CaCl_2,2H_2O = 147\cdot0$

NOTE. *The name Calcium Chloride has also been applied to the hexahydrate, $CaCl_2,6H_2O = 219\cdot1$, and to the anhydrous salt, $CaCl_2 = 111\cdot0$.*

Solubility. Soluble, at 20°, in less than 1 part of water and of alcohol.

Standard
It complies with the requirements of the European Pharmacopoeia.
It is a white, crystalline, odourless, hygroscopic powder and contains not less than 97·0 per cent and not more than the equivalent of 103·0 per cent of $CaCl_2,2H_2O$.

Storage. It should be stored in airtight containers at a temperature not exceeding 25°.

Actions and uses. Calcium chloride has the actions of soluble calcium salts, as described under Calcium Gluconate, and is used in the preparation of solutions for injection, although calcium gluconate is now usually preferred for this purpose. It is irritant when given by intramuscular or subcutaneous injection and should therefore be given intravenously, from 6 to 10 millilitres of a 5 to 10 per cent solution (340 to 680 millimoles, or 680 to 1360 milliequivalents, of Ca^{2+} per litre) being given by slow infusion.

Dose. See above under **Actions and uses.**

Preparation
SODIUM LACTATE INJECTION, COMPOUND, B.P. (*Syn.*

Hartmann's Solution for Injection; Ringer-Lactate Solution for Injection). It consists of a sterile solution containing sodium lactate, prepared from 2·4 ml of lactic acid and 1·15 g of sodium hydroxide, with sodium chloride, potassium chloride, and calcium chloride, in Water for Injections to 1000 ml. This solution provides approximately 2 millimoles, or 4 milliequivalents, of Ca^{2+}, 131 millimoles, or milliequivalents, of Na+, 5 millimoles, or milliequivalents, of K+, 111 millimoles, or milliequivalents, of Cl−, and the equivalent of 29 millimoles, or milliequivalents, of HCO_3^- per litre. On storage, this solution may cause separation of small solid particles from glass containers; solutions containing such particles must not be used.

CALCIUM GLUCONATE

SYNONYMS: Calc. Glucon.; Calcii Gluconas

$C_{12}H_{22}CaO_{14},H_2O = 448·4$

$$[CH_2OH \cdot [CH(OH)]_4 \cdot CO_2]_2 Ca, H_2O$$

Solubility. Slowly soluble, at 20°, in 30 parts of water; soluble in 5 parts of boiling water; insoluble in dehydrated alcohol, in ether, and in chloroform.

Standard
It complies with the requirements of the European Pharmacopoeia.
It is an odourless, white, crystalline powder or granules and contains not less than 98·5 per cent and not more than the equivalent of 102·0 per cent of calcium D-gluconate monohydrate.

Sterilisation. Solutions for injection are sterilised by heating in an autoclave.

Actions and uses. Calcium is an essential element of the tissues and of the blood, which contains approximately 10 milligrams per 100 millilitres; of this, about 7 milligrams is in ionised form and the remainder is in colloidal form united with proteins. The average daily requirement of calcium is 500 milligrams, but larger amounts are necessary during periods of growth, pregnancy, and lactation.

Inadequate calcium absorption in infancy leads to rickets, which is characterised by malformation and imperfect calcification of bones and teeth; the demand by the infant upon the mother during pregnancy and lactation may cause depletion of calcium from the maternal bones, resulting in osteomalacia. These deficiencies are more often caused by lack of vitamin D in the diet than by lack of calcium, but both calcium salts and vitamin D should be employed in their treatment.

Calcium balance is influenced by the parathyroid hormone, excess of which mobilises calcium from the bones, increases the calcium level and the proportion of ionic, compared with bound, calcium in the blood, and increases the excretion of this ion. Deficiency of parathyroid hormone reverses these effects. An abnormally low level of ionic calcium in the blood causes increased excitability of muscle and nerve tissues and may produce tetany or even convulsions; conversely, a high level of ionic calcium decreases muscular and nervous excitability. Calcium gluconate by mouth or by intravenous injection, or calcium chloride

by intravenous injection, is therefore used in the treatment of tetany arising in association with parathyroid deficiency, rickets, chronic renal disease, uraemia, and coeliac disease in children, and to check hypocalcaemic convulsions in children.

A high-calcium diet has been used in the treatment of lead poisoning, in which it causes the deposition of lead in bone in the form of an insoluble double salt. In the treatment of lead colic, calcium gluconate intravenously gives prompt relief from the acute pain. Conversely, a low-calcium diet, together with the administration of ammonium chloride, accelerates the excretion of lead, but caution is necessary because the rapid mobilisation of the lead may provoke severe symptoms of plumbism.

Calcium gluconate, being tasteless and non-irritant to the stomach, is a more acceptable salt for oral administration than the chloride or lactate. As it does not cause pain or necrosis, it is also given by intramuscular injection, the usual dose being 1 gram. In urgent cases, 1 to 2 grams (4·5 to 9 milliequivalents of Ca^{2+}) may be given by intravenous injection. Injections of calcium salts should not be given during digitalis therapy.

Calcium gluconate is also administered in suppositories containing 1 gram.

Dose. 1 to 6 grams (2·25 to 13·5 millimoles, or 4·5 to 27 milliequivalents, of Ca^{2+}) by mouth, repeated in accordance with the needs of the patient; 1 to 2 grams (2·25 to 4·5 millimoles, or 4·5 to 9 milliequivalents, of Ca^{2+}) by intravenous or intramuscular injection.

Preparations
CALCIUM GLUCONATE INJECTION, B.P. It consists of a sterile solution of calcium gluconate in Water for Injections. Not more than 5 per cent of the calcium gluconate may be replaced by calcium (+)-saccharate, or other suitable harmless calcium salt, as a stabiliser. Unless otherwise specified, a solution containing 10 per cent of calcium gluconate (225 millimoles, or 450

milliequivalents, of Ca^{2+} per litre) is supplied. The injection must not be used if separation of crystals has occurred.

CALCIUM GLUCONATE TABLETS, B.P.C. (page 808)
CALCIUM GLUCONATE TABLETS, EFFERVESCENT, B.P.C. (page 808)

CALCIUM HYDROXIDE

$Ca(OH)_2 = 74 \cdot 09$

Solubility. Almost completely soluble in 600 parts of water; less soluble in hot water; more soluble in aqueous solutions of glycerol and of sugars. It dissolves in solutions of sucrose with the formation of calcium saccharosates.

Standard
It complies with the requirements of the British Pharmacopoeia.
It is a soft white powder and contains not less than 90·0 per cent of $Ca(OH)_2$. A solution in water is alkaline to phenolphthalein and readily absorbs carbon dioxide.

Sterilisation. It is sterilised by heating at a temperature not lower than 160° for sufficient time to ensure that the whole of the powder is maintained at this temperature for one hour.

Storage. It should be stored in airtight containers.

Actions and uses. Calcium hydroxide is an antacid and astringent. It is given by mouth as the solution, which, when added to milk, prevents the formation of large clots of curd in the stomach; however, it dilutes the milk unduly, and sodium citrate, which is used in a more concentrated solution, is preferable.

Preparation
CALCIUM HYDROXIDE SOLUTION, B.P.C. (page 781)

CALCIUM LACTATE

$C_6H_{10}CaO_6,5H_2O = 308 \cdot 3$

$(C_3H_5O_3)_2Ca,5H_2O$

Solubility. Soluble, at 25°, in 20 parts of water; readily soluble in hot water; slightly soluble in alcohol; insoluble in ether.

Standard
It complies with the requirements of the British Pharmacopoeia.
It is a white powder with a slight and not unpleasant odour and contains not less than 98·0 and not more than the equivalent of 101·0 per cent of $C_6H_{10}CaO_6$, calculated with reference to the anhydrous substance. It contains 26·0 to 30·0 per cent of water.
It effloresces on exposure to air and becomes anhydrous when heated at 100°.

Storage. It should be stored in airtight containers.

Actions and uses. Calcium lactate has the actions of soluble calcium salts, as described under Calcium Gluconate.

Dose. 1 to 5 grams, repeated in accordance with the needs of the patient.

Preparation
CALCIUM LACTATE TABLETS, B.P. Unless otherwise specified, tablets each containing 300 mg of calcium lactate are supplied. They should be stored in airtight containers.

CALCIUM PHOSPHATE

Calcium Phosphate consists chiefly of tricalcium diorthophosphate $Ca_3(PO_4)_2$, together with calcium phosphates of more acidic or basic character. Calcium Phosphate is sometimes supplied as "tribasic calcium phosphate", but the pure compound, $Ca_3(PO_4)_2$, has not been obtained.

Solubility. Very slightly soluble in water; soluble in dilute mineral acids.

Standard
DESCRIPTION. A white amorphous powder; odourless or almost odourless.

IDENTIFICATION TESTS. It gives the reactions characteristic of calcium and of phosphates.

ARSENIC. It complies with the test given in Appendix 6, page 877 (4 parts per million).

IRON. 0·10 g dissolved in a mixture of 5 ml of water, 0·5 ml of *hydrochloric acid FeT* and 1 g of *citric acid FeT* and the solution diluted to 40 ml with water complies with the limit test for iron (400 parts per million).

LEAD. It complies with the test given in Appendix 7, page 881 (5 parts per million).

CARBONATE. 5·0 g, suspended in 30 ml of freshly boiled and cooled water, dissolves with not more than a slight effervescence on the addition of 10 ml of *hydrochloric acid*.

CHLORIDE. 0·10 g dissolved in water with the addition of 1 ml of *nitric acid* complies with the limit test for chlorides (0·35 per cent).

SULPHATE 0·10 g dissolved in water with the addition of 3 ml of *dilute hydrochloric acid* complies with the limit test for sulphates (0·6 per cent).

FLUORINE. Not more than 50 parts per million, determined by the method given in Appendix 20, page 902.

HYDROCHLORIC ACID-INSOLUBLE MATTER. Not more than 0·3 per cent, determined by the following method: Dissolve about 5 g, accurately weighed, in 30 ml of water and 10 ml of *hydrochloric acid*, filter, wash the residue with water, and dry to constant weight at 105°.

WATER. Not more than 2·5 per cent w/w, determined by the method given in Appendix 16, page 895.

CONTENT OF CALCIUM PHOSPHATES. Not less than 90·0 per cent, calculated as $Ca_3(PO_4)_2$, determined by the following method:
Dissolve, by heating on a water-bath, about 1 g, accurately weighed, in 10 ml of *hydrochloric acid*, add 50 ml of water, cool, and dilute to 250 ml with water; to 25 ml of this solution add 30 ml of 0·05M disodium edetate, 10 ml of *ammonia buffer solution*, and 100 ml

of water, and titrate the excess of disodium edetate with 0·05M zinc chloride, using *mordant black 11 solution* as indicator; each ml of 0·05M disodium edetate is equivalent to 0·005170 g of $Ca_3(PO_4)_2$.

Hygroscopicity. At relative humidities between about 15 and 65 per cent, the equilibrium moisture contents at 25° are about 2 per cent, but at relative humidities above about 75 per cent, it absorbs small amounts of moisture.

Uses. Calcium phosphate is a useful non-hygroscopic diluent for powders and vegetable extracts, but it should not be used as a diluent or excipient in calciferol preparations because it may considerably modify the results of the administration of high doses of the vitamin.

It is not a satisfactory source of calcium or phosphorus for therapeutic use owing to its insolubility and limited absorption.

CALCIUM SODIUM LACTATE

SYNONYM: Calc. Sod. Lact.

$C_{12}H_{20}CaNa_2O_{12},4H_2O = 514·4$

$2C_3H_5NaO_3,(C_3H_5O_3)_2Ca,4H_2O$

Calcium Sodium Lactate may be prepared by dissolving two equal parts of calcium lactate separately in water, adding to one portion the required amount of sodium carbonate, filtering off the precipitated calcium carbonate, and then mixing the two clear solutions; the double salt is obtained on evaporation.

It melts when heated above 100°, and loses water of crystallisation on further heating.

Solubility. Soluble, at 20°, in 14 parts of water; soluble in 25 parts of boiling alcohol; insoluble in ether.

Standard

DESCRIPTION. White, deliquescent powder or granules; odour slight and characteristic.

IDENTIFICATION TESTS. 1. Heat gently 1 g with *dilute sulphuric acid* and 0·1 g of *potassium permanganate*; the odour of acetaldehyde is produced.

2. It gives the reactions characteristic of calcium and of sodium.

ACIDITY OR ALKALINITY. Dissolve 5·0 g in 100 ml of hot *carbon dioxide-free water*; the solution is not alkaline to *phenolphthalein solution* and requires not more than 0·5 ml of 0·5N sodium hydroxide to render the solution alkaline.

ARSENIC. It complies with the test given in Appendix 6, page 877 (2 parts per million).

IRON. 0·50 g complies with the limit test for iron (80 parts per million).

LEAD. It complies with the test given in Appendix 7, page 881 (10 parts per million).

CHLORIDE. 0·50 g dissolved in water with the addition of 1·5 ml of *nitric acid* complies with the limit test for chlorides (700 parts per million).

SULPHATE. 0·25 g dissolved in water with the addition of 3 ml of *dilute hydrochloric acid* complies with the limit test for sulphates (0·24 per cent).

REDUCING SUGARS. Dissolve 1·0 g in 10 ml of water, add 5 ml of *potassium cupri-tartrate solution*, and boil; not more than the slightest trace of a red precipitate is formed.

CONTENT OF Ca. 7·5 to 8·5 per cent, determined by the following method:
Dissolve about 0·5 g, accurately weighed, in 50 ml of water, add 5 ml of 0·05M magnesium sulphate and 10 ml of *ammonia buffer solution*, and titrate with 0·05M disodium edetate, using *mordant black 11 solution* as indicator; each ml of 0·05M disodium edetate, after deduction of the volume of 0·05M magnesium sulphate added, is equivalent to 0·002004 g of Ca.

CONTENT OF Na. 8·5 to 10·0 per cent, determined by the following method:
Gently ignite until carbonised about 2 g, accurately weighed, cool, boil the residue with 50 ml of water and 50 ml of 0·5N hydrochloric acid, and filter; wash the residue with water and titrate the excess of acid in the combined filtrate and washings with 0·5N sodium hydroxide, using *methyl orange solution* as indicator; each ml of 0·5N hydrochloric acid, after deduction of an amount equal to one-fifth of the amount of 0·05M disodium edetate which would be required by the calcium in the weight of sample taken, is equivalent to 0·01149 g of Na.

Storage. It should be stored in airtight containers.

Actions and uses. Calcium sodium lactate has the actions of soluble calcium salts, as described under Calcium Gluconate (page 68).

Dose. 0·3 to 2 grams.

Preparations
CALCIUM SODIUM LACTATE TABLETS, B.P.C. (page 808)
CALCIUM WITH VITAMIN D TABLETS, B.P.C. (page 809)

DRIED CALCIUM SULPHATE

SYNONYMS: Exsiccated Calcium Sulphate; Plaster of Paris

$CaSO_4,\frac{1}{2}H_2O = 145·1$

Dried Calcium Sulphate is prepared by heating powdered gypsum, $CaSO_4,2H_2O$, at about 150° until three-quarters of the water of crystallisation is lost.

When dried calcium sulphate is mixed with a little water it forms a smooth paste which rapidly sets to a hard mass, but if completely dehydrated or heated above 200°, or if much atmospheric moisture has been absorbed, it loses this property. The setting-time is retarded by adding a colloid such as dextrin, acacia, or glue, or any substance which will decrease the solubility, such as alcohol or a citrate; it is accelerated by adding substances such as gypsum, sodium chloride, alum, or potassium sulphate.

It rapidly deteriorates in the presence of moisture. Deterioration is indicated either by too rapid setting or by very slow setting, the set mass being more or less weakened and friable according to the degree of deterioration.

Solubility. Slightly soluble in water; more soluble in dilute mineral acids; insoluble in alcohol.

Standard
DESCRIPTION. A white hygroscopic powder; odourless or almost odourless.

IDENTIFICATION TESTS. It gives the reactions characteristic of calcium and of sulphates.

ACIDITY OR ALKALINITY. pH of a 20 per cent w/w slurry in water, 6·5 to 7·5.

SETTING PROPERTIES. 20 g mixed with 10 ml of water at 15° to 20° in a cylindrical mould, about 2·4 cm in diameter, sets in 4 to 8 minutes. The mass thus formed, after standing for 3 hours, possesses sufficient hardness to resist pressure of the fingers at the edges, which retain their sharpness of outline and do not crumble.

LOSS ON IGNITION. 4·5 to 8·0 per cent, determined by igniting to constant weight at red heat.

Storage. It should be stored in airtight containers.

Uses. Dried calcium sulphate, consisting of a mixture of amorphous and crystalline forms, is used in the preparation of Plaster of Paris Bandage (page 614).

Bandages may be prepared extemporaneously by applying dried calcium sulphate thickly to a material such as check muslin or book muslin before rolling; after rolling, the bandage is thoroughly wetted and wound round the limb.

Alternatively, the dried calcium sulphate may be mixed to a thin cream in a basin and the unrolled bandaging material passed through the cream immediately before applying to the limb; 1½ to 2 parts of water to 1 part of dried calcium sulphate is a suitable proportion for the cream; a 5 per cent solution of dextrin may be used in place of water.

The plaster will set and a splint form in fifteen to twenty minutes. The bulk of the mass increases slightly as the plaster sets; interstices are thus filled and close application obtained.

Dried calcium sulphate is also employed in dental practice for making plaster casts.

OTHER NAME: Calcined Gypsum

CAMPHOR

$C_{10}H_{16}O = 152·2$

Camphor is a crystalline ketonic substance obtained from the wood of *Cinnamomum camphora* (L.) T. F. Nees and Eberm. (Fam. Lauraceae), a tree growing abundantly in Formosa, Japan, and China, or by synthesis. Natural camphor is dextrorotatory; synthetic camphor is optically inactive.

In preparing natural camphor, the wood of *C. camphora*, in small pieces, is subjected to a process of steam distillation; the crude natural camphor obtained contains a variable quantity of camphor oil and is purified by sublimation. Synthetic camphor may be prepared from pinene of turpentine oil by converting through camphene to isoborneol, which is then oxidised.

Solubility. Soluble, at 20°, in 700 parts of water, in 1 part of alcohol, and in less than 1 part of chloroform; very soluble in ether and in fixed oils.

Standard
It complies with the requirements of the British Pharmacopoeia.
It is a colourless crystalline solid with a characteristic penetrating aromatic odour. According to the manner of condensation, it is obtained as "bells" or "flowers" of camphor; "blocks" and "tablets" are obtained by compression of the powder or by sublimation. It has a melting-point of 174° to 181°. It may readily be powdered by trituration with a few drops of alcohol or other volatile organic solvent.

Storage. It should be stored in airtight containers, in a cool place.

Actions and uses. Applied externally, camphor is a mild analgesic and rubefacient and is used in liniments, such as Camphor Liniment, as a counter-irritant in the treatment of fibrositis and neuralgia.

POISONING. Poisoning has occurred through the accidental administration of Camphor Liniment to young children in mistake for castor oil. The symptoms are nausea, vomiting, colic, disturbed vision, delirium, and epileptiform convulsions. Recovery is the rule, but in rare cases death may occur from respiratory failure.

The stomach should be evacuated by stomach tube or by injecting apomorphine and the delirium and convulsions controlled by a short-acting barbiturate, given intravenously if necessary.

Preparations
CAMPHOR LINIMENT, B.P. (*Syn.* Camphorated Oil). It contains 20 per cent w/w of camphor in arachis oil. It should be stored in airtight containers, in a cool place.

SOAP LINIMENT, B.P.C. (page 726)
TURPENTINE LINIMENT, B.P. It contains about 5 per cent of camphor with turpentine oil and soft soap.
CAMPHORATED OPIUM TINCTURE, B.P. (*Syn.* Paregoric). It contains 0·3 per cent of camphor and 5 per cent of Opium Tincture in alcohol (60 per cent). Dose: 2 to 10 millilitres.
CAMPHORATED OPIUM TINCTURE, CONCENTRATED, B.P.C. (page 822)
CAMPHOR WATER, CONCENTRATED, B.P.C. (page 825)

CAPREOMYCIN SULPHATE

Capreomycin Sulphate is a mixture of the sulphates of the antimicrobial substances produced by certain strains of *Streptomyces capreolus*.

Solubility. Soluble, at 20°, in 1 part of water; very slightly soluble in alcohol; insoluble in ether and in chloroform.

Standard
It complies with the requirements of the British Pharmacopoeia.
It is a white or almost white odourless or almost odourless solid and contains not less than 700 Units per mg, calculated with reference to the dried substance. The loss on drying under the prescribed conditions is not more than 10·0 per cent. A 3 per cent solution in water has a pH of 4·5 to 7·5.

Labelling. If the material is not intended for parenteral administration, the label on the container states that the contents are not to be injected.

Storage. It should be stored in airtight containers. If it is intended for parenteral administration, the containers should be sterile and sealed to exclude micro-organisms.

Actions and uses. Capreomycin is an antibiotic which is effective against *Mycobacterium tuberculosis*. It is bactericidal but, like other members of the aminoglycoside group of antibiotics, it should not be used alone because of the rapid emergence of drug resistance.
Capreomycin is used in treatment of tuberculosis as a second-line or reserve drug for patients who cannot tolerate certain other drugs or whose tuberculous infection is not sensitive to them. It is less effective, even in conjunction with other drugs, than streptomycin, rifampicin, ethambutol, or prothionamide, and should be used together with at least one of these substances, the choice depending on bacterial sensitivity and the patient's tolerance. It is preferable to kanamycin because the incidence of serious undesirable effects at effective dosage is lower. Capreomycin sulphate is administered by intramuscular injection as it is not absorbed from the gastro-intestinal tract. The usual dose is 1 mega Unit, equivalent to approximately 1 gram of capreomycin daily. It shows marked cross-resistance to kanamycin, but not to streptomycin, and no allergy is shared with streptomycin.

UNDESIRABLE EFFECTS. Progressive renal damage, nitrogen retention, and disturbances of calcium and potassium metabolism may occur. Vertigo, tinnitus, and sometimes deafness occur as a result of a selective toxic action similar to but independent of the action of streptomycin and kanamycin, and these changes may be irreversible. Allergic skin rashes rarely occur.

PRECAUTIONS. As the excretion of capreomycin is related to the creatinine clearance, the dose should be reduced when this test shows that renal function is impaired.

Dose. See above under **Actions and uses.**

Preparation
CAPREOMYCIN INJECTION, B.P. It consists of a sterile solution prepared by dissolving the contents of a sealed container in Water for Injections. It may be used up to 14 days after preparation provided it is stored at a temperature between 2° and 10°; at temperatures approaching 20° it should be used within forty-eight hours of preparation. Vials containing 1 mega Unit of capreomycin are available.

OTHER NAME: *Capastat*®

CAPSICUM

SYNONYM: Chillies

Capsicum consists of the dried ripe fruits of *Capsicum annuum* var. *minimum* (Miller) Heiser and small-fruited varieties of *C. frutescens* L. (Fam. Solanaceae), small erect shrubs cultivated in central and east Africa and in other tropical countries. In commerce, all small-fruited varieties are referred to as chillies and the larger less pungent varieties as capsicums.

Varieties. Numerous varieties of chillies occur in commerce. Mombasa chillies, grown and collected in Uganda and on the mainland of Tanzania, are dull in colour; the pods are broad and short, and the stalk is present. Zanzibar chillies are more attractive in appearance. Central African chillies (Zambian chillies), with somewhat slender pods, are brighter in colour and almost free from stalk.

Constituents. Capsicum contains about 0·5 to 0·9 per cent of the colourless crystalline pungent principle capsaicin (8-methyl-*N*-vanillylnon-6-enamide), which melts at about 65° and is volatile at higher temperatures, the vapour being extremely irritating. The carotenoid pigments, capsanthin, capsorubin, zeaxanthin, cryptoxanthin, lutein, and carotene are also present, together with thiamine and ascorbic acid.

Capsicum also contains a fatty oil (about 4 to 16 per cent) and protein. It yields to alcohol (60 per cent) from 20 to 30 per cent of extractive and to acetone about 10 per cent.

Standard for unground drug

DESCRIPTION. *Macroscopical:* Fruit dull orange-red or red, oblong conical with an obtuse apex, 2-celled, length about 12 to 25 mm, diameter up to 7 mm at widest part, occasionally attached to a 5-toothed inferior calyx and a straight pedicel about 1 mm thick; calyx and pedicel together measuring about 2 to 3 cm. Pericarp somewhat shrivelled, glabrous and translucent, enclosing about 10 to 20 flat, reniform seeds. Seeds 3 to 4 mm long, either loose or attached to a reddish dissepiment. Odour characteristic, not powerful; taste extremely pungent. The pungency is not destroyed by boiling with a 2 per cent w/v solution of sodium hydroxide in water (distinction from ginger) but is destroyed by potassium permanganate solution.

Microscopical: the diagnostic characters are: Pericarp: *outer epidermis* with cells often arranged in rows of 5 to 7, anticlinal walls straight, moderately and evenly thickened, *cuticle* uniformly striated; parenchymatous cells frequently containing droplets of *red oil*, occasionally containing microsphenoidal *crystals* of calcium oxalate; *inner epidermis* with characteristic island groups of *sclerenchymatous cells* having somewhat wavy, moderately thick, pitted and lignified anticlinal walls, groups separated by thin-walled parenchyma. Seeds: *epidermis* composed of large, sinuous cells with thin outer walls but strongly thickened, pitted, radial and inner walls; *endosperm* parenchymatous, cells with drops of *fixed oil* and *aleurone grains* 3 to 6 μm in diameter. Calyx: *outer epidermis* with anisocytic *stomata*, *inner epidermis* with many trichomes but no stomata; *trichomes* glandular, with uniseriate stalks and multicellular heads; mesophyll with many idioblasts containing microsphenoidal *crystals* of calcium oxalate. Pedicel: *epidermis* of somewhat axially elongated subrectangular cells, with numerous *stomata* and scattered glandular *trichomes*; *cortex* of 7 to 8 layers of thin-walled cellulosic parenchyma with occasional idioblasts containing microsphenoidal *crystals* of calcium oxalate; *fibres* in isolated groups 2 to 3 cells wide and 1 cell thick, to outer side of narrow cylinder of phloem; *intraxylary phloem*, with *fibres* to inner side; *pith* parenchymatous, with large central cavity.

CALYCES AND PEDICELS. Not more than 3·0 per cent.

FOREIGN ORGANIC MATTER. Not more than 1·0 per cent.

ASH. Not more than 8·0 per cent.

CONTENT OF CAPSAICIN. Not less than 0·50 per cent, determined by the following method: Transfer about 5 g, in No. 500 powder, accurately weighed, to an apparatus for the continuous extraction of drugs, extract with *dehydrated methyl alcohol* for not less than 6 hours, or until the sample is exhausted, and dilute the extract to 100 ml with *dehydrated methyl alcohol*; to 10 ml of this solution add 15 ml of *dehydrated methyl alcohol*, 15 ml of water, 2 g of *sodium chloride* and 5 ml of 0·1N sodium hydroxide, mix, and extract with three successive 10-ml portions of *light petroleum* (*boiling-range, 80° to 100°*); wash the combined extracts with two successive 5-ml portions of *methyl alcohol* (*60 per cent*) and discard the light-petroleum extract; filter the combined aqueous solution and washings through cotton wool, washing the filter with 10 ml of *methyl alcohol* (*60 per cent*), evaporate the combined filtrate and washings on a water-bath until the volume is reduced to about 5 ml, dilute the solution to about 50 ml with water, adjust the pH to 7·0 to 7·5 with 0·1N hydrochloric acid, using either a pH meter or *phenol red solution* as indicator, extract with six successive 20-ml portions of redistilled

anaesthetic ether, wash the combined extracts with 10 ml of water, and discard the aqueous solution and washings; add 20 ml of *dehydrated methyl alcohol*, evaporate on a water-bath in a fume cupboard until the volume is reduced to about 1 ml, dilute to 100 ml with *dehydrated methyl alcohol*, add 0·05 g of *decolorising charcoal*, shake, and filter through a fine-grade filter paper, discarding the first 20 ml of filtrate. To 10 ml of this solution add 5 ml, accurately measured, of 0·1N sodium hydroxide, cool, and dilute to 25 ml with *dehydrated methyl alcohol*; to a further 10 ml add 5 ml, accurately measured, of 0·05N hydrochloric acid, cool, and dilute to 25 ml with *dehydrated methyl alcohol*; measure the extinction of a 1-cm layer of the alkaline solution against the acid solution at the maxima at about 248 and 296 nm. Using *dehydrated methyl alcohol* as solvent, dilute 5 ml, accurately measured, of 0·1N sodium hydroxide to 25 ml, and 5 ml, accurately measured, of 0·05N hydrochloric acid to 25 ml; measure the extinction of a 1-cm layer of the alkaline solution against the acid solution at the maxima at about 248 and 296 nm. From the extinctions at these maxima given by the solutions containing the sample deduct the corresponding extinctions given by the blank solutions. For purposes of calculation, use a value of 313 for the E(1 per cent, 1 cm) of capsaicin at 248 nm under these conditions, and 127 for that at 296 nm; calculate the proportion of capsaicin in the sample from the extinctions at each wavelength. If the two results so obtained differ by not more than 5 per cent, the content of capsaicin is given by the mean of the two results.

Standard for powdered drug: Powdered Capsicum DESCRIPTION. An orange to brownish-red powder possessing the diagnostic microscopical characters, odour, and taste of the unground drug; strongly sternutatory.

Adulterants and substitutes. Japanese chillies possess about one-quarter of the pungency of the African varieties, but are valued for their bright colour. They are derived from an unnamed species of *Capsicum*; they are free from stalk and are distinguished by their somewhat larger size and very bright reddish colour; the cells of the epidermis of the pericarp have a smooth cuticle, strongly thickened anticlinal walls, and a radiate lumen; the cells of the single-layered hypoderm have somewhat thick pitted cuticularised walls.

Paprika is extensively grown and used in central and southern Europe and is derived from mild races of *C. annuum*; the fruits are large and more or less tetrahedral and have a conspicuous green calyx. Other varieties commonly occurring in commerce include East African capsicums, originating from Malawi and Tanzania, Ethiopian capsicums, Nigerian chillies, and Chinese chillies and capsicums. Varieties occasionally seen include chillies from Thailand, Indonesia, Sierra Leone, Natal, and India. Ground Cayenne pepper of commerce is normally a blend of any of the varieties mentioned.

Storage. It should be stored in a cool dry place, protected from light.

Actions and uses. Capsicum, usually as the tincture, is given by mouth as a carminative. It is used externally as a counter-irritant for the treatment of rheumatism, lumbago, and neuralgia.

Preparations

CAPSICUM OINTMENT, B.P.C. (page 760)
CAPSICUM OLEORESIN, B.P.C. (page 764)
CAPSICUM TINCTURE, B.P.C. (page 821)

CARAMEL

SYNONYMS: Burnt Sugar; Saccharum Ustum

Caramel may be prepared by heating a suitable water-soluble carbohydrate with a suitable accelerator until a black viscid mass is formed. It is then adjusted to the required standard by the addition of water and strained.

Solubility. Miscible with water, with dilute alcohols (up to about 60 per cent v/v), with dilute mineral acids, and with sodium hydroxide solution; immiscible with chloroform and with ether; it is precipitated by strong alcohol.

Standard
DESCRIPTION. A thick but free-flowing, dark brown liquid; odour slight.

ACIDITY. pH of a 10·0 per cent w/v solution in *carbon dioxide-free water*, 3·0 to 5·5.

WEIGHT PER ML. A 10·0 per cent w/v solution in water has a weight per ml, at 20°, of 1·023 g to 1·025 g.

ARSENIC. It complies with the test given in Appendix 6, page 878 (5 parts per million).

COPPER. Not more than 30 parts per million, determined by the following method:
To 4·0 g add 15 ml of water, 5 ml of *nitric acid*, and 5 ml of *sulphuric acid*, and heat gently in a long-necked flask until the mixture is colourless, adding, dropwise, more of the nitric acid if necessary; cool, add 25 ml of water, boil until white fumes are evolved, cool, add a further 25 ml of water, and again boil until white fumes are evolved; cool and dilute to 100 ml with water. All subsequent operations be carried out in subdued light. To 25 ml of this solution, add 10 ml of *edetate–citrate solution*, 0·1 ml of *thymol blue solution*, and sufficient *dilute ammonia solution* to give a green or bluish-green colour, and cool; add 15 ml, accurately measured, of *dithiocarbamate solution*, shake for 2 minutes, and allow to separate; filter the carbon tetrachloride layer through cotton wool and measure the extinction of a 1-cm layer at the maximum at about 436 nm.

The extinction is not greater than that produced when a 0·00047 per cent w/v solution of *copper sulphate* in *dilute sulphuric acid* is similarly treated, beginning with the words "To 25 ml of this solution . . .".

IRON. Evaporate 0·40 g to dryness, add 0·2 ml of *nitric acid*, ignite, and dissolve the residue in 1 ml of *dilute nitric acid*; the solution complies with the limit test for iron (100 parts per million).

LEAD. It complies with the test given in Appendix 7, page 881 (5 parts per million).

COLOUR INTENSITY OF AQUEOUS DILUTION. The colour of a 0·13 per cent w/v solution in water, when viewed in a 1-cm cell, is equivalent to 1·5 to 4·0 Lovibond Red Units and 5·0 to 10·0 Lovibond Yellow Units.

STABILITY. Mix 1 g separately with 300 ml of a 2·0 per cent w/v solution of *citric acid* in water, with 300 ml of a 2·0 per cent w/v solution of *sodium carbonate* in water, and with 300 ml of *alcohol (60 per cent)*, and allow to stand for one week at 20°; no precipitate is formed in any of these solutions.

SULPHATED ASH. Not more than 2·0 per cent.

Uses. Caramel is used as a colouring agent and is capable of producing a range of colours from a pale straw colour to dark brown. It is usually employed as a 50 per cent solution in Chloroform Water, 2 millilitres of which is sufficient to colour 100 millilitres of most liquid preparations.
Caramel has no calorific value.

CARAWAY

SYNONYM: Carum

Caraway consists of the dried ripe fruits of *Carum carvi* L. (Fam. Umbelliferae), an erect biennial herb indigenous to and cultivated in central and northern Europe, chiefly in Holland. The plant is cut when the fruit is ripe and the fruits are obtained by threshing.

Constituents. Caraway contains 2·5 to 6 per cent of volatile oil, containing about 55 per cent of carvone; it also contains fixed oil and about 20 per cent of protein. It yields to cold water from 20 to 26 per cent of non-volatile extractive.

Standard
It complies with the requirements of the British Pharmacopoeia.
It contains not less than 3·5 per cent v/w and Powdered Caraway not less than 2·5 per cent v/w of volatile oil.

UNGROUND DRUG. *Macroscopical characters:* cremocarp oblong-ellipsoidal, laterally compressed; mericarps glabrous, brown, usually detached from pedicel and carpophores, up to about 7 mm long and 1 to 2 mm broad, tapered to curved ends, with 5 narrow, slightly yellow primary ridges; pericarp thin; endosperm oily, not grooved on commissural surface.
Odour and taste characteristic, aromatic.

Microscopical characters: the diagnostic characters are: *epidermis* of polygonal cells with outer walls thickened, *cuticle* striated, *stomata* anomocytic; *vittae* 4 dorsal and 2 commissural; *vascular strands* 1 in each ridge, with narrow vessels and a sclerenchyma cap of *fibres* and

sclereids; *parenchyma* of mesocarp without reticulate wall thickening, endosperm cells with thick cellulose walls, cells containing *oil* and numerous *aleurone grains* up to 10 μm in diameter containing minute rosette *crystals* of calcium oxalate.

POWDERED DRUG. Powdered Caraway. A fawn to brown powder possessing the diagnostic microscopical characters, odour, and taste of the unground drug.

Adulterants and substitutes. Fruits from which the volatile oil has been partially removed are sometimes offered; they may be recognised by their dark colour, shrivelled appearance, lack of aroma, and low yield of aqueous extractive (less than 15 per cent).
Levant or Mogador caraway is light brown, the mericarps usually united, about 5 to 6 mm long, the pedicels often being present; the odour and taste are similar to those of caraway; it yields about 1·5 per cent of volatile oil.
Indian dill, a variety of *Anethum graveolens* L. (*A. sowa* Roxb. ex Flem.) (Fam. Umbelliferae), has been substituted for caraway; it consists usually of entire cremocarps which often have the pedicel attached; they are oval, dorsally compressed, pale brown with

narrow yellowish wings; each mericarp is straight with three yellowish dorsal ridges and is about 4 to 6 mm long, 2 mm wide, and 1 mm thick, the ratio of length to breadth being about 2·5 to 1.

Storage. It should be stored in a cool dry place.

Powdered Caraway should be stored in airtight containers, in a cool place.

Actions and uses. Caraway is a carminative and a flavouring agent.

OTHER NAMES: Caraway Fruit; Caraway Seed

CARAWAY OIL

SYNONYMS: Oleum Cari; Oleum Carui

Caraway Oil is obtained by distillation from freshly crushed caraway.

Constituents. Caraway oil contains about 60 per cent w/w of (+)-carvone; it also contains (+)-limonene.

Standard
DESCRIPTION. A colourless or pale yellow liquid; odour that of caraway.

OPTICAL ROTATION. At 20°, +74° to +80°.

REFRACTIVE INDEX. At 20°, 1·485 to 1·492.

SOLUBILITY IN ALCOHOL. Soluble, at 20°, in 7 volumes of *alcohol (80 per cent)*.

WEIGHT PER ML. At 20°, 0·902 g to 0·912 g.

CONTENT OF KETONES. 53·0 to 63·0 per cent w/w, calculated as carvone, determined by the method given in Appendix 14, page 893.

Storage. It should be stored in well-filled airtight containers, protected from light, in a cool place.

Actions and uses. Caraway oil is a carminative and a flavouring agent.
Caraway Water is used in the treatment of flatulence and is a suitable vehicle for children's medicines.

Dose. 0·05 to 0·2 millilitre.

Preparation
CARAWAY WATER, CONCENTRATED, B.P.C. (page 825)

CARBACHOL

$C_6H_{15}ClN_2O_2 = 182·6$

Carabachol is *O*-carbamoylcholine chloride.

$$[NH_2 \cdot CO \cdot O \cdot CH_2 \cdot CH_2 \cdot N(CH_3)_3]^+ Cl^-$$

Solubility. Very soluble in water; soluble, at 20°, in 55 parts of alcohol; very slightly soluble in dehydrated alcohol, in ether, and in acetone.

Standard
It complies with the requirements of the British Pharmacopoeia.
It occurs as very hygroscopic, colourless, prismatic crystals or white crystalline powder with a faint fishy odour resembling that of an aliphatic amine and contains not less than 99·5 and not more than the equivalent of 101·0 per cent of $C_6H_{15}ClN_2O_2$, calculated with reference to the dried substance. The loss on drying under the prescribed conditions is not more than 1·0 per cent. It melts with decomposition at about 210°.

Stability. Aqueous solutions are most stable to autoclaving when buffered to pH 3·5. Up to 5 per cent decomposition may occur when unbuffered solutions are heated in an autoclave and the decomposition increases the pH of the solutions; such autoclaved solutions should not be stored for more than one year.

Sterilisation. Solutions are sterilised by heating in an autoclave or by filtration.

Storage. It should be stored in airtight containers.

Actions and uses. Carbachol has the muscarinic and nicotinic actions of acetylcholine, as described under Physostigmine Salicylate (page 380). Whereas acetylcholine is rapidly inactivated by cholinesterase enzymes, carbachol is not and its action is therefore more prolonged. Since it is also resistant to the action of the digestive enzymes, it is effective when administered by mouth in a dose of 2 to 4 milligrams. It is, however, usually given by subcutaneous injection.
Carbachol may be used where the effects of

parasympathetic stimulation are required. It is of value in the treatment of post-operative intestinal atony and post-operative retention of urine, for which it is given by subcutaneous injection in a dose of 250 micrograms; this dose may be repeated two or three times at intervals of thirty minutes. It is also used to stop paroxysmal tachycardia when all other measures have failed, but methacholine is usually preferred.
Carbachol has a miotic action and a 0·8 per cent aqueous solution has been used to lower intraocular pressure in glaucoma, sometimes in conjunction with other miotics such as physostigmine.

UNDESIRABLE EFFECTS. Sweating, nausea, faintness, and abdominal pain occur; these are seldom serious and, if necessary, may be readily controlled or prevented by injection of atropine.

CONTRA-INDICATIONS. Carbachol is contra-indicated in patients with acute cardiac failure.

Dose. 250 to 500 micrograms by subcutaneous injection.

Preparations
CARBACHOL EYE-DROPS, B.P.C. (page 689)
CARBACHOL INJECTION, B.P. It consists of a sterile solution of carbachol in Water for Injections containing 5 per cent of dextrose. Unless otherwise specified, a solution containing 250 µg in 1 ml is supplied.

CARBAMAZEPINE

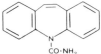

$C_{15}H_{12}N_2O = 236.3$

Carbamazepine is dibenz[b,f]azepine-5-carboxamide.

Solubility. Very slightly soluble in water and in ether; soluble, at 20°, in 10 parts of alcohol and in 10 parts of chloroform.

Standard
It complies with the requirements of the British Pharmacopoeia.
It is a white or yellowish-white, crystalline, almost odourless powder and contains not less than 97·0 and not more than the equivalent of 103·0 per cent of $C_{15}H_{12}N_2O$, calculated with reference to the dried substance. The loss on drying under the prescribed conditions is not more than 0·5 per cent. It has a melting-point of 189° to 193°.

Actions and uses. Carbamazepine has marked anticonvulsant properties. It is used, particularly in conjunction with other drugs, in the treatment of grand mal epilepsy with temporal lobe features and of temporal lobe epilepsy, the usual dosage being 200 milligrams daily in divided doses, increasing to 1·2 grams daily in divided doses.
Carbamazepine is sometimes effective in the treatment of trigeminal neuralgia, for which purpose an initial dose of 100 milligrams daily may be given and gradually increased until a suitable response is obtained; the average dosage required is 200 milligrams three or four times a day.

UNDESIRABLE EFFECTS. Dizziness, dryness of the mouth, diarrhoea, nausea, diplopia, and rashes may occur and, rarely, aplastic anaemia and jaundice.

PRECAUTIONS AND CONTRA-INDICATIONS. Carbamazepine should not be given to patients who are being treated with a monoamine-oxidase inhibitor, such as isocarboxazid, nialamide, phenelzine, or tranylcypromine, or within about ten days of the discontinuation of such treatment. It should not be administered during the first three months of pregnancy unless specifically indicated.

Dose. See above under **Actions and uses.**

Preparation
CARBAMAZEPINE TABLETS, B.P. Unless otherwise specified, tablets each containing 200 mg of carbamazepine are supplied.

OTHER NAME: *Tegretol®*

CARBENICILLIN SODIUM

$C_{17}H_{16}N_2Na_2O_6S = 422.4$

Carbenicillin Sodium is the disodium salt of 6-(α-carboxy-phenylacetamido)penicillanic acid.

Solubility. Soluble, at 20°, in 1·2 parts of water and in 25 parts of alcohol; insoluble in ether and in chloroform.

Standard
It complies with the requirements of the British Pharmacopoeia.
It is a white or almost white, hygroscopic, odourless powder and contains not less than 89·0 per cent of $C_{17}H_{16}N_2Na_2O_6S$, calculated with reference to the anhydrous substance. It contains 2·5 to 5·5 per cent w/w of water. A 10 per cent solution in water has a pH of 6·0 to 8·0.

Storage. It should be stored in sterile containers, sealed to exclude micro-organisms and as far as possible moisture, protected from light, at a temperature not exceeding 5°.

Actions and uses. Carbenicillin is a semi-synthetic penicillin which resembles ampicillin (page 27). It is decomposed by staphylococcal penicillinase, but it is active against *Pseudomonas* species and some ampicillin-resistant strains of *Proteus*. To prevent the development of resistance by these species, for which at present there are few effective drugs, the use of carbenicillin should be limited to serious generalised infections by these organisms. Blood levels may be raised by blocking tubular excretion, and high levels must be attained if treatment is to succeed. To prevent the development of resistance during treatment carbenicillin is given in conjunction with gentamicin.
The usual initial dose is the equivalent of 5 grams of carbenicillin by intramuscular injection, followed by the intravenous injection of 20 to 30 grams in divided doses over a period of twenty-four hours, usually by injection into the tubing of a saline infusion apparatus.

PRECAUTIONS. The precautions against allergy described under Benzylpenicillin (page 51) should be observed. Carbenicillin should not be used topically or for infections that would respond to other more active penicillins.

Dose. See above under **Actions and uses.**

Preparation
CARBENICILLIN INJECTION, B.P. It consists of a sterile solution prepared by dissolving the sterile contents of a sealed container in Water for Injections. The quantity of carbenicillin sodium in each container should be specified by the prescriber. It should be used immediately after preparation. Vials containing the equivalent of 1 and 5 g of carbenicillin are available.

OTHER NAME: *Pyopen®*

CARBENOXOLONE SODIUM

$C_{34}H_{48}Na_2O_7 = 614 \cdot 7$

Carbenoxolone Sodium is the disodium salt of 3β-(3-carboxypropionyloxy)-11-oxo-olean-12-en-30-oic acid.

Solubility. Soluble in 6 parts of water and in 30 parts of alcohol; very slightly soluble in chloroform and in ether.

Standard
It complies with the requirements of the British Pharmacopoeia.
It is a white or pale cream-coloured hygroscopic powder and contains not less than 97·0 and not more than the equivalent of 103·0 per cent of $C_{34}H_{48}Na_2O_7$, calculated with reference to the anhydrous substance. It contains not more than 4·0 per cent w/w of water. A 10 per cent solution in water has a pH of 7·9 to 8·7.

Storage. It should be stored in airtight containers.

Actions and uses. Carbenoxolone sodium increases the rate of healing of benign gastric ulcers. This is most marked in ambulant patients, but patients who are treated with bed rest do not seem to gain any further obvious benefit from the use of the drug. Its mechanism of action is unknown, and its therapeutic effects on duodenal ulcer have not been proved. Carbenoxolone also has aldosterone-like actions, giving rise to weight gain, sodium and chloride retention, and hypokalaemia and anti-inflammatory activity in animals, which is reduced by adrenalectomy.
An oral dose is absorbed from the stomach, the rate of absorption depending on presence or absence of food in the stomach. Maximum blood levels are obtained within one hour after administration in the fasting state, but may be delayed for several hours if the dose is given after food. A second peak blood level is reached after a further two or three hours,

and is probably due to intestinal resorption of biliary-excreted metabolites, the major route of excretion in man being in the bile.
Treatment is started with 50 milligrams of carbenoxolone sodium by mouth three times daily after food, increasing to 100 milligrams three times daily if required, and is continued for four to six weeks. A thiazide diuretic with potassium supplements may be given to reduce signs of fluid retention, but spironolactone should not be used as it antagonises the healing properties as well as the unwanted effects of carbenoxolone.

UNDESIRABLE EFFECTS. Weight gain frequently occurs, with hypertension, and the associated sodium and water retention may precipitate cardiac failure in patients with heart disease. Hypokalaemic paresis may occur rarely, and severe muscle damage with myoglobinuria has been described. Marked increases in hepatocellular enzymes are common; they return to normal after stopping treatment.

PRECAUTIONS. It should be used with care in patients with heart disease or hypertension, and treatment should not be continued for more than four to six weeks. A potassium supplement is usually required.

Dose. See above under **Actions and uses.**

Preparation
CARBENOXOLONE TABLETS, B.P. Unless otherwise specified, tablets each containing 50 mg of carbenoxolone sodium are supplied. They contain peppermint oil as a flavouring agent.

OTHER NAME: *Biogastrone*®

CARBIMAZOLE

$C_7H_{10}N_2O_2S = 186 \cdot 2$

Carbimazole is ethyl 3-methyl-2-thio-4-imidazoline-1-carboxylate.

Solubility. Soluble, at 20°, in 500 parts of water, in 50 parts of alcohol, in 330 parts of ether, in 3 parts of chloroform, and in 17 parts of acetone.

Standard
It complies with the requirements of the British Pharmacopoeia.
It is a white or creamy-white crystalline powder with a characteristic odour and contains not less than 98·5 per cent of $C_7H_{10}N_2O_2S$, calculated with reference to the dried substance. The loss on drying under the prescribed conditions is not more than 0·5 per cent. It has a melting-point of 122° to 125°.

Storage. It should be stored in airtight containers.

Actions and uses. Carbimazole is an antithyroid substance which depresses the formation of thyroid hormone and so lowers the basal metabolic rate. It reduces the uptake and concentration of inorganic iodine by the thyroid, but its main effect is to reduce the formation of di-iodotyrosine and thyroxine, although, once formed, their action is not antagonised.
Carbimazole is absorbed rapidly from the gastro-intestinal tract and is widely distributed

throughout the body. It readily crosses the placental barrier; it also attains a high concentration in the milk of lactating patients. Excretion in the urine is rapid, being almost complete within twenty-four hours; the remainder is destroyed in the body.

Carbimazole is used to control hyperthyroidism. It is given by mouth in a dosage of 10 to 60 milligrams daily in divided doses, according to the severity of the disorder. The dosage is then gradually reduced to the smallest amount that will control the disease, usually 5 to 20 milligrams daily. Marked thyroid enlargement is an indication of excessive dosage; occasionally eye signs worsen as the condition comes under control. After prolonged administration of carbimazole for many months or years, the disorder may abate spontaneously, but it may recur and signs of hyperthyroidism may reappear within some weeks or months of withdrawal of the drug.

Carbimazole is also used in the preparation of patients for thyroidectomy. Under the influence of this therapy, the patient is rendered euthyroid, and the metabolic rate returns to normal. The drug is usually then discontinued and iodine or iodides substituted for ten or twelve days before operation to render the gland firmer and less vascular.

Carbimazole is useless in the treatment of thyroid crisis or for the rapid control of a severe fulminating case, for which iodine or iodide is required.

UNDESIRABLE EFFECTS. Granulocytopenia and swelling of the joints rarely occur; rashes may occasionally occur.

PRECAUTIONS. Patients should be told to report sore throats, fever, or rashes, as these may precede by several days abnormal findings in the circulating blood.

Carbimazole may be given during pregnancy to a thyrotoxic patient, but care should be taken lest overdosage adversely affects the foetus. In thyrotoxic heart failure, carbimazole therapy should be supplemented by treatment with digitalis and diuretics.

Carbimazole should be given with the utmost caution, or not at all, if there is any degree of tracheal obstruction, as high dosage may produce thyroid enlargement and obstructive symptoms may become marked.

Dose. See above under **Actions and uses.**

Preparation

CARBIMAZOLE TABLETS, B.P. Unless otherwise specified, tablets each containing 5 mg of carbimazole are supplied. They should be stored in airtight containers.

OTHER NAMES: *Bimazol*®; *Neo-Mercazole*®

CARBON DIOXIDE

SYNONYM: Carbonei Dioxidum

$CO_2 = 44\cdot01$

Carbon Dioxide may be obtained from naturally occurring carbonates, particularly the carbonates of calcium and magnesium, by treatment with an acid, but is more commonly obtained as a by-product of alcoholic fermentation; it is also obtained by the combustion of fuels. It does not support combustion and is about 1·5 times as heavy as air. A solution in water has weakly acidic properties and reddens blue litmus. Carbon dioxide can be liquified by pressure at a temperature of 31° or lower; at 31° a pressure of 72 atmospheres is required. It is supplied liquefied in metal cylinders.

LIQUID CARBON DIOXIDE is a limpid colourless liquid, which is immiscible with water, but readily dissolves in alcohol, ether, and volatile oils; at atmospheric pressure it boils at about −78°.

SOLID CARBON DIOXIDE, "dry ice", is obtainable commercially and is widely used in refrigeration; owing to its low thermal conductivity it is more stable than liquid carbon dioxide. It has a temperature of −80°. A less compact form, "carbon dioxide snow", may be obtained by suddenly releasing liquid carbon dioxide from a cylinder fitted with an internal tube.

Solubility. One volume, measured at normal temperature and pressure, dissolves, at 20°, in 1·2 volumes of water.

Standard

It complies with the requirements of the European Pharmacopoeia.

It is a colourless odourless gas and contains not less than 99·0 per cent v/v of CO_2.

Storage, labelling, and colour markings. Carbon dioxide for inhalation should be stored in metal cylinders in a special storage room, which should be cool and free from materials of an inflammable nature.

The whole of the cylinder should be painted grey and the name of the gas or the chemical symbol "CO_2" should be stencilled in paint on the shoulder of the cylinder. The name or chemical symbol should be clearly and indelibly stamped on the cylinder valve.

Carbon dioxide for "snow"-making should be stored under similar conditions, but in metal cylinders with an internal tube.

Actions and uses. Carbon dioxide, when given by mouth in solution or as carbonates or bicarbonates, promotes the absorption of liquids by the mucous membranes. For this reason aerated waters rapidly relieve thirst, hasten the action of alcohol, and soon cause diuresis. Carbon dioxide in the stomach increases the secretion of gastric juice, particularly its hydrochloric acid. Effervescing waters are useful for masking the unpleasant taste of saline aperients.

Carbon dioxide is important for regulating the acid–base balance of the blood and tissues. Increased metabolic activity results in a corresponding increase in the proportion of carbon dioxide in the tissues and a decrease in the proportion of oxygen.

As carbon dioxide is a natural direct stimulant of the respiratory centre, an increase in the proportion of carbon dioxide inhaled will cause deeper and more frequent respiration. Air normally contains about 0·04 per cent of carbon dioxide; if this concentration is increased to 3 per cent the depth of respiration in the normal subject is doubled; if it is increased to 5 per cent, the depth is almost trebled and the rate of respiration may increase; if it is further raised to 7 per cent, the rate and depth of respiration may be further increased. Higher concentrations cause dyspnoea, raised blood presure, headache, mental confusion and eventually (with 10 per cent or more) unconsciousness.

Withdrawal of carbon dioxide after prolonged inhalation commonly produces pallor, lowered blood pressure, severe headache, and nausea or vomiting.

For therapeutic purposes a mixture of 5 or 7 per cent of carbon dioxide in oxygen may be administered. The mixtures are usually available in cylinders or may be prepared by mixing the gases from separate cylinders. They are used to induce or improve respiration in newborn infants, in drowning persons, and in the treatment of poisoning by carbon monoxide, morphine, hypnotics, and other depressants. For many of these purposes, however, oxygen combined with artificial respiration is adequate, and carbon dioxide may be dangerous in some circumstances.

Mixtures of oxygen and carbon dioxide may be used to accelerate excretion of inhalation anaesthetics by the lungs and so to reduce the risk of bronchitis and vomiting. Carbon dioxide inhalations may relieve persistent hiccup.

Solid carbon dioxide has a destructive action on tissues and is used to destroy warts and naevi, being applied with light pressure for five to six seconds. The application is almost painless, but the surrounding tissues should be covered with soft paraffin and the solid shaped, by compressing in a mould or trimming to a point, to suit the part to be treated. A weal is afterwards formed, followed by a vesicle, but very little scarring occurs. If a second application is necessary, the inflammation from the first must be allowed to subside.

CARBROMAL

$C_7H_{13}BrN_2O_2 = 237·1$

$$Br \cdot C(C_2H_5)_2 \cdot CO \cdot NH \cdot CO \cdot NH_2$$

Carbromal is (α-bromo-α-ethylbutyryl)urea.

Solubility. Slightly soluble in water; soluble, at 20°, in 18 parts of alcohol, in 25 parts of ether, and in 2 parts of chloroform.

Standard
It complies with the requirements of the British Pharmacopoeia.
It is a white, crystalline, odourless or almost odourless powder and contains not less than 98·0 and not more than the equivalent of 101·0 per cent of $C_7H_{13}BrN_2O_2$. It has a melting-point of 117° to 120°. A saturated solution in water is neutral to litmus.

Actions and uses. Carbromal has sedative and hypnotic properties. It is given as a hypnotic by mouth in doses of 0·3 to 1 gram or in doses of 250 milligrams, together with an intermediate-acting barbiturate.

UNDESIRABLE EFFECTS. Rashes may occur. Carbromal may release sufficient bromide ions to affect persons hypersensitive to bromides.

Preparation
CARBROMAL TABLETS, B.P.C. (page 809)

CARDAMOM FRUIT

SYNONYM: Cardamomi Fructus

Cardamom Fruit consists of the dried, nearly ripe fruits of *Elettaria cardamomum* Maton var. *minuscula* Burkill (Fam. Zingiberaceae), a plant growing in southern India and produced on the Malabar coast, in Ceylon, in Guatemala, and in Tanzania.

Varieties. Alleppey cardamoms are elongated ovoid in shape, three-sided, varying from about 8 to 20 mm in length and 4 to 10 mm in breadth, green to pale buff in colour, and strongly striated longitudinally.
Mangalore cardamoms, both full-bleached and half-bleached, are about 20 mm long and 15 mm wide, somewhat globular, and with a roughish, somewhat scurfy surface.
"Ceylon greens" resemble Alleppey fruits, but are generally greener, larger, and more elongated.
Guatemalan cardamoms resemble Alleppey cardamoms.

The Tanzanian variety resembles Alleppey cardamoms in shape but is pale to dark buff in colour and more strongly striated longitudinally. Ripe, split fruits are frequently present.

Constituents. Cardamom seeds contain from about 3 to 8 per cent of a volatile oil; much starch is also present. They yield to alcohol (45 per cent) about 7 per cent of extractive.

Standard
It complies with the requirements of the British Pharmacopoeia.
The seeds of Cardamom Fruit contain not less than 4·0 per cent v/w of volatile oil.
Macroscopical characters: Fruit a trilocular inferior capsule, up to about 2 cm long, ovoid or oblong, dull green to pale buff, plump or slightly shrunken, obtusely triangular in section, nearly smooth or longitudinally striated; apex with beak formed by flower remains, base rounded or with remains of the stalk.
Seeds: in 2 rows in each loculus, forming an adherent mass attached to the axile placenta; seeds pale to dark reddish-brown, about 4 mm long and 3 mm broad, irregularly angular, hard, transversely rugose, with 6 to 8 rugae, raphe contained in longitudinal channel, each seed enveloped by a colourless, membranous aril; transversely cut surface of seed showing a brown testa, white starchy perisperm grooved on one side, yellowish endosperm, and a paler embryo.
Odour and taste agreeable, strongly aromatic.

Microscopical characters: the diagnostic characters are: seed: *aril* composed of flattened, thin-walled, parenchymatous cells; *outer epidermis* of the testa composed of thick-walled, narrow, axially elongated cells, followed by one layer of collapsed parenchyma and one layer (2 to 3 layers near raphe) of large, thin-walled *rectangular cells* containing *volatile oil*; the layer of conspicuously dark-brown *stegmata*, each cell about

35 or 40 μm long and about 20 μm wide, lumina narrow, bowl-shaped, each containing a warty *silica-body*; inner epidermis consisting of flattened cells; *vessels* few, narrow, with spiral wall thickening; *perisperm* cells thin-walled, containing numerous *starch* granules in adherent polyhedral masses, individual granules up to 6 μm in diameter; each starch mass with 1 to 7 prismatic *crystals* of calcium oxalate embedded in it.

Substitutes. Ceylon fruits, known as Long Wild Natives, derived from *E. cardamomum* var. *major* Thwaites, are an article of commerce and are readily distinguished by their elongated shape, shrivelled appearance, and rather dark greyish-brown colour; the seeds have about 4 rugae only in their length.
Cluster cardamoms, derived from *Amomum kepulaga* Sprague and Burkill (Fam. Zingiberaceae), have seeds with a camphoraceous taste and with about 14 interrupted rugae in the length of the seed.
The seeds, imported loose, are usually inferior and less aromatic; they are often more fully ripe and hence contain more fixed oil.

Storage. It should be stored in a cool dry place; the seeds should not be stored after removal from the fruit.

Actions and uses. Cardamom is a carminative and a flavouring agent.
In making preparations of cardamom, only the seed is used. The seeds are removed from the capsules, immediately powdered or bruised, and used without delay.

Preparation
CARDAMOM TINCTURE, COMPOUND, B.P. It is prepared from cardamom seed, 1·4 per cent, caraway, cinnamon, cochineal, glycerol, and alcohol (60 per cent). Dose: 2 to 5 millilitres.

CARDAMOM OIL

Cardamom Oil is obtained by distillation from crushed Cardamom Fruit.

Constituents. Cardamom oil contains cineole, terpineol, mainly as the acetic ester, and limonene.

Solubility. Soluble, at 20°, in 6 parts of alcohol (70 per cent).

Standard
DESCRIPTION. A colourless or pale yellow liquid; odour pungent and aromatic.
OPTICAL ROTATION. At 20°, +20° to +44°.
REFRACTIVE INDEX. At 20°, 1·461 to 1·467.
WEIGHT PER ML. At 20°, 0·917 g to 0·940 g.

ESTER VALUE. 90 to 156.

Storage. It should be stored in well-filled airtight containers, protected from light, in a cool place.

Actions and uses. Cardamom oil has carminative properties. It is sometimes used as a flavouring agent.

Dose. 0·03 to 0·2 millilitre.

Preparation
CARDAMOM TINCTURE, AROMATIC, B.P.C. (page 821)

CARMINE

Carmine is the aluminium lake of the colouring matter of cochineal, the dried female insect *Dactylopius coccus* Costa.

Carmine may be prepared by treating an aqueous infusion of cochineal with alum. It contains about 50 per cent of carminic acid. Unless precautions are taken during manufacture and transport to prevent contamination, carmine may be infected with salmonellae. It must be pasteurised or treated in some other appropriate manner to ensure the

destruction of any viable salmonella organisms present.

Solubility. Insoluble in water and in dilute acids; readily soluble in dilute ammonia solution and in other dilute alkaline liquids, forming a dark purplish-red solution.

Standard
DESCRIPTION. Light bright-red pieces, readily reducible to powder.

IDENTIFICATION TEST. Gently ignite 0·1 g until the organic matter is destroyed; an odour of burnt feathers is produced and the residue gives the reactions characteristic of aluminium.

COLOUR INTENSITY OF AQUEOUS SOLUTION. Dissolve an amount equivalent to 0·20 g of the substance dried under the prescribed conditions in 5 ml of *dilute ammonia solution* and dilute to 200 ml with water; to 5 ml of this solution add 5 ml of *dilute ammonia solution*, dilute to 200 ml with water, and measure the extinction of a 1-cm layer at the maximum at about 518 nm; the extinction is not less than 0·40.

ARSENIC. It complies with the test given in Appendix 6, page 878 (5 parts per million, calculated with reference to the substance dried under the prescribed conditions).

LEAD. It complies with the test given in Appendix 7, page 882 (10 parts per million, calculated with reference to the substance dried under the prescribed conditions).

MATTER INSOLUBLE IN DILUTE AMMONIA SOLUTION. Not more than 1·0 per cent, calculated with reference to the substance dried under the prescribed conditions, determined by the following method:
Dissolve about 0·25 g, accurately weighed, in 2·5 ml of *dilute ammonia solution*, and dilute to 100 ml with water; the solution is clear. Filter the solution through a sintered-glass filter (British Standard Grade No. 3), wash the filter with a solution containing 0·1 per cent w/w of NH_3, and dry to constant weight at 105°.

LOSS ON DRYING. 10·0 to 21·0 per cent, determined by drying to constant weight at 105°.

ASH. Not more than 13·0 per cent, calculated with reference to the substance dried under the prescribed conditions.

ABSENCE OF SALMONELLAE. Add 25 g, in powder, to 50 ml of sterile *saline solution* and incubate at 37° for 2 hours. Add approximately half the incubated solution to 25 ml of *double-strength selenite F broth* and the remainder to 25 ml of *double-strength Rappaport's medium* and incubate both mixtures at 37°. After 24 and 48 hours, plate out each mixture on *bismuth sulphite medium* (*Wilson and Blair*) and on *desoxycholate citrate agar* and incubate the inoculated plates at 37°. Examine the incubated plates after 24- and 48-hours' incubation; no colonies characteristic of salmonella organisms are visible.

Sterilisation. It may be sterilised by heating in an autoclave; if necessary, it should be subsequently dried at 80°.

Storage. It should be stored in airtight containers.

Uses. Carmine is used for colouring ointments, tooth powders, mouth-washes, dusting-powders, medicines, and other preparations. If it is used in solid form, prolonged trituration with a powder is necessary to obtain a good colour and an even distribution. To obtain the maximum colour carmine should be dissolved in a small quantity of strong ammonia solution before triturating with the powder. The colouring matter is precipitated in acid solution.

Carmine passes unchanged through the gastro-intestinal tract and is used as a "marker" in metabolism experiments in a dose of 200 to 500 milligrams, administered in a cachet or gelatin capsule.

CASCARA

SYNONYMS: Cascara Sagrada; Rhamni Purshianae Cortex

Cascara is the dried bark of *Rhamnus purshiana* DC. (Fam. Rhamnaceae), a small tree growing in North California, Oregon, Washington, and British Columbia.

The bark is collected in the spring and early summer and dried, the collection being made at least one year before the bark is used. It is available as quilled, channelled, or nearly flat pieces, known commercially as "natural" cascara, but is often processed into small, nearly flat, uniform fragments, known commercially as "evenised", "processed", or "compact" cascara bark.

Constituents. Cascara contains about 6 to 9 per cent of anthraquinone glycosides; the most important are cascarosides A and B [glucosides of barbaloin, a 10-glucopyranosyl derivative of aloe-emodin anthrone (10-glucopyranosyl-9,10-dihydro-1,8-dihydroxy-3-hydroxymethyl-9-oxoanthracene)] and cascarosides C and D [glucosides of chrysaloin (11-deoxybarbaloin, 10-glucopyranosyl-9,10-dihydro-1,8-dihydroxy-3-methyl-9-oxoanthracene)].
Several glycosides of emodin (9,10-dihydro-1,6,8-trihydroxy-3-methyl-9,10-dioxoanthracene), of emodin oxanthrone (9,10-dihydro-1,6,8,10-tetrahydroxy-3-methyl-9-oxoanthracene, of aloe-emodin (9,10-dihydro-1,8-dihydroxy-3-hydroxymethyl-9,10-dioxoanthracene), and of chrysophanol (9,10-dihydro-1,8-dihydroxy-3-methyl-9,10-dioxoanthracene) are also present.
Small quantities of breakdown products from these glycosides occur, including barbaloin, chrysaloin, aloe-emodin, chrysophanol, and emodin. The cascarosides are almost tasteless, but barbaloin and chrysaloin are extremely bitter.

The bark yields to water from 23 to 28 per cent of extractive.

Standard
It complies with the requirements of the European Pharmacopoeia.
It contains not less than 8 per cent of hydroxyanthracene derivatives, calculated as cascaroside A, of which not less than 60 per cent consists of cascarosides, calculated as cascaroside A.

UNGROUND DRUG. *Macroscopical characters:* quilled, channelled or nearly flat pieces from 1 to 4 mm thick, varying greatly in length and breadth, usually broken into small, nearly flat, uniform fragments; outer surface nearly smooth, cork dark purplish-brown and bearing scattered lenticels; usually more or less completely covered by a whitish coat of lichens and some pieces of bark with many small mosses and foliaceous liverworts growing epiphytically on the outer surface; mussel-scale insects also often present; inner surface yellow to reddish-brown or nearly black, with longitudinal striations and faint transverse corrugations; fracture short, somewhat fibrous near inner surface; smoothed, transversely cut surface exhibiting a narrow, purplish cork, a yellowish-grey cortex with darker translucent groups of sclerenchymatous cells, and a brownish-yellow phloem traversed by slightly wavy medullary rays.
Odour characteristic and nauseous; taste persistently bitter.
Cascara responds to the following test:
Shake 0·1 g, in powder or small pieces, with 10 ml of *ferric chloride solution* mixed with 5 ml of *hydrochloric*

acid and immerse in a water-bath for about 10 minutes; filter immediately, cool the filtrate, and extract with 10 ml of *carbon tetrachloride*; separate the carbon tetrachloride layer, wash with 5 ml of water, and shake with 5 ml of *dilute ammonia solution*; a rose-pink to cherry-red colour is produced in the ammoniacal layer (presence of anthraquinone derivatives).

Microscopical characters: The diagnostic characters are: *sclereids* in groups in cortex and phloem; *phloem fibres* slender, in bundles accompanied by *crystal sheaths* with prisms of calcium oxalate; *sieve tubes* thin-walled, with well defined sieve plates on the oblique end walls; cluster *crystals* of calcium oxalate scattered throughout the parenchyma, the cells of which contain a yellow substance coloured violet by *sodium hydroxide solution*; when bryophytic epiphytes are present the powder may contain either the leaves of liverworts, entire or in fragments, exhibiting a lamina one cell thick, composed of isodiametric cells and having no midrib, or the leaves of mosses, having a lamina one cell thick composed of somewhat elongated cells and possessing a midrib several cells thick, or both.

POWDERED DRUG: Powdered Cascara. A light yellowish-brown to olive-brown powder possessing the diagnostic microscopical characters, odour, and taste of the unground drug.

Adulterants and substitutes. The bark of *R. californica* Eschscholz is occasionally substituted for the official drug. The bark of *R. cathartica* L. is glossy, reddish-brown and has very distinct lenticels.
Frangula bark, the young bark of *Frangula alnus* Mill. (Fam. Rhamnaceae), occurs as single or double quills, about 1 to 2 cm wide, with an outer surface of smooth dark-purplish cork bearing numerous transversely elongated whitish lenticels; when gently scraped, the deep crimson colour of the inner layers of cork be-comes evident; fracture short in the cork and cortex and fibrous in the phloem; the older bark is rougher externally, thicker, usually occurring in single quills or channelled pieces; taste sweetish or slightly bitter. The microscopical characters resemble those of cascara, from which it is distinguished by the absence of groups of sclereids.

Storage. It should be stored in a cool dry place. Powdered Cascara should be stored in airtight containers, in a cool place.

Actions and uses. Cascara is an anthraquinone purgative with actions and uses similar to those of senna fruit. It is used as the dry extract in tablets, as the liquid extract, or as the more pleasant-tasting elixir.

Preparations
CASCARA ELIXIR, B.P.C. (page 668)
LIQUID PARAFFIN EMULSION WITH CASCARA, B.P.C. (page 680)
CASCARA DRY EXTRACT, B.P. A dry aqueous extract containing not less than 13·0 per cent of the total hydroxyanthracene derivatives, of which not less than 40 per cent consists of cascarosides, both calculated as cascaroside A. It should be stored in airtight containers.
CASCARA LIQUID EXTRACT, B.P. Dose: 2 to 5 millilitres.
CASCARA AND BELLADONNA MIXTURE, B.P.C. (page 738)
FIGS SYRUP, COMPOUND, B.P.C. (page 800)
CASCARA TABLETS, B.P. They contain cascara dry extract and may be sugar coated. Each tablet contains 17 to 23 mg of total hydroxyanthracene derivatives of which not less than 50 per cent consists of cascarosides, both calculated as cascaroside A. Unless otherwise specified sugar-coated tablets are supplied. Dose: 1 or 2 tablets.

CASTOR OIL

SYNONYM: Oleum Ricini

Castor Oil is the fixed oil obtained by cold expression from the seeds of *Ricinus communis* L. (Fam. Euphorbiaceae). The expressed oil is steamed to coagulate proteins and, after filtration, is usually bleached by exposure to the sun or by chemical means.

Constituents. Castor oil consists chiefly of the triglyceride of ricinoleic acid (12-hydroxyoleic acid), which is present to the extent of about 80 per cent. It also contains small amounts of other glycerides, the fatty acid constituents of which include oleic, linoleic, stearic, and 9,10-dihydroxystearic acids.

Solubility. Soluble, at 20°, in 2·5 parts of alcohol (90 per cent); miscible with dehydrated alcohol, with ether, and with glacial acetic acid.

Standard
It complies with the requirements of the British Pharmacopoeia.
It is a nearly colourless or faintly yellow viscous oil with a slight odour. It has a weight per ml at 20° of 0·953 g to 0·964 g. It gives a clear solution with half its volume of light petroleum (boiling-range, 40° to 60°); it is only partially soluble in two volumes. On cooling to 0° it remains bright, but on cooling to −18° it congeals to a yellowish mass.
The most distinctive features of the oil are its high density, the highest of any natural fatty oil, its behaviour with light petroleum, its solubility in alcohol (90 per cent), its high acetyl value, and its high viscosity.

Sterilisation. It is sterilised by dry heat.

Storage. It should be stored in well-filled airtight containers.

Actions and uses. Castor oil is a purgative, its action being exerted in four to eight hours. It is best administered in milk or fruit juice.
Castor oil is emollient and is used in preparations such as Zinc and Castor Oil Ointment. Sterilised castor oil is a soothing application when dropped into the eye after removal of foreign bodies; is used as an oily vehicle for eye-drops.

Dose. 5 to 20 millilitres.

Preparation
ZINC AND CASTOR OIL OINTMENT, B.P. (*Syn.* Zinc and Castor Oil Cream; Zinc and Castor Oil). It contains 7·5 per cent of zinc oxide and 50 per cent w/w of castor oil.

CATECHU

SYNONYMS: Pale Catechu; Gambier

Catechu is a dried aqueous extract prepared from the leaves and young shoots of *Uncaria gambier* (Hunter) Roxb. (Fam. Rubiaceae), a climbing shrub indigenous to and cultivated in the Malay Archipelago.

Constituents. Catechu contains about 7 to 33 per cent of (+)-catechin, which may be obtained as a tetrahydrate consisting of white silky needles having a melting-point of about 95°.

On drying over sulphuric acid catechin forms a monohydrate having a melting-point of 175°; on drying at 100° it becomes anhydrous and melts at about 177°. It is sparingly soluble in cold water (1 in 1100 to 1200), but freely soluble in boiling water and in alcohol, and produces with ferric salts a deep green colour.

Other constituents are 22 to 50 per cent of catechutannic acid, which is coloured dirty green by ferric salts, and small amounts of (+)-epicatechin, quercetin, wax, fixed oil, catechu red, and a fluorescent substance, gambier-fluorescein, and occasionally traces of indole alkaloids.

Catechu also contains mineral matter (about 3 to 5 per cent) and vegetable debris.

Standard for unground drug
DESCRIPTION. *Macroscopical:* cubes, usually irregular and agglutinated and mixed with fragments of broken cubes; friable and porous, measuring about 2·5 cm in each direction, larger cubes and brick-shaped pieces up to 5 cm long, sometimes broken into angular fragments; external surface light brown to black, freshly broken surface pale cinnamon brown, occasionally showing darker streaks.

Odourless; taste at first bitter and very astringent but subsequently sweetish.

Microscopical: the diagnostic characters are: *crystals,* acicular, numerous in abundant yellowish-brown masses, composed of catechin and soluble in hot water; varying amounts of fragments from the leaves and shoots of the plant also present, including: *trichomes,* unicellular, non-glandular, occurring singly or in groups attached to pieces of epidermis, mostly about 250 to 540 μm long, lignified, with 1 or 2 thin, transverse septa, base pitted, also a few smaller, about 25 to 45 μm long, conical, with unlignified, warty walls; *epidermis of leaves,* cells thin-walled, slightly sinuous and polygonal, *cuticle* finely striated, *stomata* paracytic, on abaxial surface only; *epidermis of corolla* reddish-brown, with numerous non-glandular *trichomes,* these sometimes broken off leaving characteristic pitted and lignified cicatrices; *parenchymatous cells* containing cluster and microsphenoidal *crystals* of calcium oxalate; *cork* present as occasional fragments; *pollen grains* subspherical, about 11 to 18 μm in diameter with 3 pores and 3 furrows, extine covered with minute scattered pits.

IDENTIFICATION TEST. Warm 0·3 g with 2 ml of *alcohol (95 per cent),* cool, and filter; to the filtrate add 2 ml of *sodium hydroxide solution,* shake, add 2 ml of *light petroleum (boiling-range, 40° to 60°),* shake, and allow to separate; a brilliant greenish fluorescence is produced in the upper layer (distinction from black catechu).

ALCOHOL (95 PER CENT)-INSOLUBLE MATTER. Not more than 34·0 per cent, calculated with reference to the dried material, determined by the following method:
Macerate about 5 g, accurately weighed, in coarse powder, with 100 ml of *alcohol (95 per cent),* shaking frequently during 6 hours and allowing to stand for 18 hours; filter, wash the residue with *alcohol (95 per cent),* and dry to constant weight at 100°.

STARCH. The residue obtained in the test for alcohol (95 per cent)-insoluble matter contains not more than an occasional starch granule.

WATER-INSOLUBLE MATTER. Not more than 28·0 per cent, calculated with reference to the dried material, determined by the method for alcohol (95 per cent)-insoluble matter, water being used in place of alcohol (95 per cent).

LOSS ON DRYING. Not more than 13·0 per cent, determined by drying to constant weight at 105°.

ASH. Not more than 8·0 per cent.

Standard for powdered drug: Powdered Catechu
DESCRIPTION. A pale brown powder possessing the diagnostic microscopical characters and taste of the unground drug; odourless.

IDENTIFICATION TEST; ALCOHOL (95 PER CENT)-INSOLUBLE MATTER; STARCH; WATER-INSOLUBLE MATTER; LOSS ON DRYING; ASH. It complies with the requirements for the unground drug.

Adulterants and substitutes. Black catechu (cutch) is the dried aqueous extract prepared from the heartwood of *Acacia catechu* Willd. and possibly other species of *Acacia* (Fam. Leguminosae). It occurs in irregular dark brown to almost black masses, frequently having pieces of brownish-buff leaves attached to them; it contains acacatechin, which is an optically inactive form of catechin, 25 to 50 per cent of catechutannic acid, quercetin, and catechu red.

Incompatibility. It is incompatible with iron salts and with gelatin.

Actions and uses. Catechu is an astringent and is used in conjunction with other astringents in the symptomatic treatment of diarrhoea.

Preparations
CHALK WITH OPIUM MIXTURE, AROMATIC, B.P.C. (page 739)
CATECHU TINCTURE, B.P.C. (page 821)

CELLACEPHATE

SYNONYM: Cellulose Acetate Phthalate

Cellacephate consists of cellulose in which about half of the hydroxyl groups are acetylated and about one quarter are esterified with one of the two acid groups of phthalic acid. It is prepared by reacting a partial acetate ester of cellulose with phthalic anhydride.

Solubility. Insoluble in water; soluble, at 20°, in 6 parts of a mixture of equal volumes of ethyl acetate and isopropyl alcohol and in 4 parts of acetone containing 0·4 per cent v/v of water (the solution may be slightly turbid if less water is present); very slightly soluble in alcohol and in chloroform.

Standard

DESCRIPTION. A white hygroscopic powder; odourless or almost odourless.

IDENTIFICATION TESTS. 1. Mix 0·01 g with 0·5 ml of *alcohol (95 per cent)* and 0·5 ml of *sulphuric acid*; the odour of ethyl acetate is produced.

2. Mix 0·05 g with 2 ml of *dilute sodium hydroxide solution* and 2 ml of water, warm to dissolve, boil to form a gel, and cool; add 3 ml of *dilute hydrochloric acid*, extract with 5 ml of *solvent ether*, allow to separate, and evaporate the ether layer to dryness. Heat the residue with 0·01 g of *resorcinol* and 0·5 ml of *sulphuric acid*, allow the reaction to subside, cool, dilute the greenish-brown mixture with 10 ml of water, and make alkaline with *strong ammonia solution*; a reddish-brown solution is produced which, on dilution, has an intense green fluorescence.

3. Dissolve 0·1 g in 1 ml of *acetone* and allow to evaporate in a glass dish; a clear glossy film is produced.

RESISTANCE OF FILM TO DIGESTION. The film produced in Identification test 3 remains undissolved for at least one hour when immersed in 0·06N hydrochloric acid at 36° to 38°, but dissolves completely in less than one hour when immersed in *solution of standard pH 6·8* at 36° to 38°.

LOSS ON DRYING. Not more than 5·0 per cent, determined by drying to constant weight at 105°.

SULPHATED ASH. Not more than 0·1 per cent.

FREE ACID. Not more than 6·0 per cent, calculated as $C_8H_6O_4$, determined by the following method: Dissolve about 3 g, accurately weighed, in 100 ml of a mixture of 3 parts of *alcohol (95 per cent)* and 2 parts of *dichloromethane*, add 150 ml of water with shaking, extract with 100 ml of *hexane*, and reserve the aqueous layer; wash the hexane extract with 100 ml of water, and titrate the combined aqueous layer and washings with 0·1N sodium hydroxide, using *phenolphthalein solution* as indicator; repeat the procedure omitting the sample. The difference between the two titrations represents the amount of 0·1N sodium hydroxide required by the free acid in the sample; each ml of 0·1N sodium hydroxide is equivalent to 0·008307 g of $C_8H_6O_4$.

CONTENT OF COMBINED PHTHALYL GROUPS. 30·0 to 40·0 per cent, calculated as $C_8H_5O_3$ and with reference to the acid-free ester, determined by the following method: Dissolve about 1 g of the previously dried material, accurately weighed, in 50 ml of a mixture of 3 parts of *alcohol (95 per cent)* and 2 parts of *dichloromethane*, add 25 ml of *alcohol (95 per cent)* and *phenolphthalein solution* as indicator, and titrate with 0·1N sodium hydroxide to the first distinct end-point; repeat the procedure omitting the sample. The difference between the two titrations represents the amount of 0·1N sodium hydroxide required by the unesterified phthalyl in the sample; each ml of 0·1N sodium hydroxide is equivalent to 0·01491 g of $C_8H_5O_3$, and hence

calculate the apparent total combined phthalyl in the sample.

Determine the free acid, calculate its equivalent in terms of combined phthalyl by multiplying by 1·795, and subtract it from the apparent total combined phthalyl obtained in the above assay. From the content of combined phthalyl so found, calculate the content of combined phthalyl with reference to the acid-free ester.

CONTENT OF COMBINED ACETYL GROUPS. 19·0 to 23·5 per cent, calculated as CH_3CO and with reference to the acid-free ester, determined by the following method: Dissolve about 0·5 g of the previously dried material, accurately weighed, in 50 ml of a mixture of equal parts of *pyridine* and *acetone*, add alternate 10-ml portions of water and 0·5N sodium hydroxide, with shaking, until 50 ml of each has been added, the additions being made at such a rate that the ester remains in solution as long as possible; allow to stand overnight and titrate with 0·5N hydrochloric acid, using *phenolphthalein solution* as indicator; repeat the procedure omitting the sample.

The difference between the two titrations represents the amount of 0·5N sodium hydroxide required by the apparent acetyl content of the sample; each ml of 0·5N sodium hydroxide is equivalent to 0·02152 g of CH_3CO, and hence calculate the apparent acetyl content.

Determine the free acid and the combined phthalyl in the sample, and calculate the content of combined acetyl in the acid-free ester from the following formula:

$$\frac{a - 0·5182b}{d} - 0·5773c$$

where a = apparent acetyl content,
b = free acid content,
c = combined phthalyl content, and
d = acid-free ester content.

Stability. Cellacephate hydrolyses fairly rapidly if its moisture content is above about 6 per cent.

Hygroscopicity. It is rather hygroscopic, its equilibrium moisture content at room temperature and a relative humidity of 50 per cent being about 5 per cent and at a relative humidity of 75 per cent, about 9 per cent.

Storage. It should be stored in airtight containers.

Uses. Cellacephate is used in the form of a solution in a suitable solvent, such as acetone or a mixture of ethyl acetate and isopropyl alcohol, for the enteric coating of tablets and capsules. It is generally used in conjunction with plasticisers, such as diethyl phthalate, castor oil, or triacetin, and waxes such as carnauba wax are often incorporated to retard the penetration of water from acid media.

MICROCRYSTALLINE CELLULOSE

Microcrystalline Cellulose is partially depolymerised cellulose and is prepared by acid hydrolysis of purified wood cellulose. It has a molecular weight of about 36,000.

There are two pharmaceutical grades of microcrystalline cellulose commercially available, one being a colloidal water-dispersible powder having a much smaller average particle size than the other non-dispersible powder. The colloidal type may contain a small percentage of sodium carboxymethylcellulose to aid its dispersion.

Solubility. Both types of powder are insoluble in water, but the colloidal type is dispersible, forming

colloidal suspensions at low concentrations and thixotropic gels at higher concentrations. Both types are partially soluble in dilute alkalis with swelling; insoluble in acids and in most organic solvents.

Standard

DESCRIPTION. A fine white or almost white powder; odourless or almost odourless.

Microscopical: Mounted in *lactophenol* the non-dispersible type exhibits particles of various sizes and irregular shapes, many pieces about 100 to 150 μm long and 20 to 30 μm wide, showing numerous cracks and a rather irregular outline and also many minute particles about 10 to 50 μm in width or length and marked with short irregular lines.

The particles of the colloidal type are similar in appearance but smaller, most being about 12 to 15 μm or occasionally up to 18 μm, and some rather square, about 40 μm, or somewhat elongated, about 50 μm by 10 to 20μm.

Between crossed polars on a dark field the material shines brightly.

Crystalline structures are absent.

IDENTIFICATION TESTS. 1. To 1 mg add 1 ml of *phosphoric acid*, heat on a water-bath for 30 minutes, add 4 ml of a 0·2 per cent solution of *catechol* in *phosphoric acid*, and heat for a further 30 minutes; a red colour is produced.

2. Soak in *iodine water* for a few minutes and remove the excess of reagent; it is not stained blue (distinction from starch). Add one or two drops of *sulphuric acid* (*66 per cent v/v*); it is stained blue (distinction from certain other cellulose derivatives).

3. Treat with *phloroglucinol solution* followed by *hydrochloric acid*; no red colour is produced.

ACIDITY. Shake 5 g with 40 ml of *carbon dioxide-free water* for 20 minutes and centrifuge; pH of the supernatant liquid, 5·5 to 7·0.

ARSENIC. It complies with the test given in Appendix 6, page 878 (2 parts per million).

LEAD. It complies with the test given in Appendix 7, page 882 (10 parts per million).

CHLORIDE; SULPHATE. Boil 2 g with 20 ml of water, filter, and divide the filtrate into two equal portions; one portion complies with the limit test for chlorides (350 parts per million) and the other portion complies with the limit test for sulphates (600 parts per million).

LOSS ON DRYING. Not more than 5·0 per cent, determined by drying to constant weight at 105°.

SULPHATED ASH. Not more than 0·1 per cent.

Labelling. The label on the container indicates whether the material is intended for use in tabletting or as a suspending agent.

Uses. The non-dispersible type of microcrystalline cellulose is used as a binder, filler, disintegrant, and lubricant in tablets. Water-soluble active ingredients can be adsorbed on to the material before compression.

The colloidal type of powder is used, either alone or in conjunction with other cellulose derivatives such as sodium carboxymethyl-cellulose and hypromellose, as a suspending agent for pharmaceutical preparations.

OTHER NAME: *Avicel*®

CEPHALEXIN

$C_{16}H_{17}N_3O_4S,H_2O = 365·4$

Cephalexin is D-7-(α-amino-α-phenylacetamido)-3-methyl-8-oxo-5-thia-1-azabicyclo[4,2,0]oct-2-ene-2-carboxylic acid monohydrate.

Solubility. Soluble, at 20°, in 100 parts of water and in 30 parts of diluted hydrochloric acid (0·2 per cent w/v); very slightly soluble in alcohol, in ether, in chloroform, and in acetone.

Standard
It complies with the requirements of the British Pharmacopoeia.
It is a white to cream-coloured crystalline powder with a characteristic odour and contains not less than 95·0 per cent of $C_{16}H_{17}N_3O_4S$, calculated with reference to the anhydrous substance. It contains 4·0 to 8·0 per cent w/w of water. A 0·5 per cent solution in water has a pH of 3·5 to 5·5.

Stability. Aqueous solutions and suspensions decompose on storage but have their optimum stability at pH 4·5.

Hygroscopicity. It absorbs insignificant amounts of moisture at 20° at relative humidities up to about 20 per cent but under damper conditions it absorbs substantial amounts.

Storage. It should be stored in airtight containers, protected from light, at a temperature not exceeding 30°.

Actions and uses. Cephalexin is one of the cephalosporin antibiotics and has the same mode of action, antigenicity, and spectrum of activity as cephaloridine (page 86) and cephalothin (page 87). Minor differences in sensitivity to penicillinases are not of clinical importance and, in general, organisms resistant to the other cephalosporins will not respond to cephalexin. Blood levels may be

increased by blocking the tubular excretion with probenecid.

Cephalexin differs from other cephalosporins in that it is well absorbed by mouth and adequate therapy can usually be maintained by an oral dose of 500 milligrams every six hours. The usual dose for children is 25 to 50 milligrams per kilogram body-weight daily in divided doses.

UNDESIRABLE EFFECTS. Cephalexin may cause abdominal discomfort and diarrhoea in some patients but otherwise its side-effects are similar to those of cephalothin sodium (page 87).

PRECAUTIONS. It should be used with caution in allergic patients, especially when there is a history of penicillin allergy.

Dose. 1 to 4 grams daily in divided doses.

Preparations
CEPHALEXIN CAPSULES, B.P. Unless otherwise specified, capsules each containing 250 mg of cephalexin are supplied. Capsules containing 500 mg are also available.
CEPHALEXIN MIXTURE, B.P.C. (page 738)
CEPHALEXIN TABLETS, B.P. Unless otherwise specified, tablets each containing 250 mg of cephalexin are supplied. Tablets containing 500 mg are also available.

OTHER NAMES: Cefalexin; *Ceporex*®; *Keflex*®

CEPHALORIDINE

$C_{19}H_{17}N_3O_4S_2 = 415.5$

Cephaloridine is 8-oxo-3-(pyrid-1-ylmethyl)-7-(α-thien-2-ylacetamido)-5-thia-1-azabicyclo-[4,2,0]oct-2-ene-2-carboxylic acid betaine (α-form or δ-form).

Solubility. Soluble, at 20°, in 12 parts of water and in 1000 parts of alcohol; very slightly soluble in ether and in chloroform.

Standard
It complies with the requirements of the British Pharmacopoeia.
It is a white or almost white crystalline powder, odourless or with a slight odour of pyridine, and contains not less than 95.0 per cent of $C_{19}H_{17}N_3O_4S_2$, calculated with reference to the anhydrous solvent-free substance. It contains not more than 0.5 per cent (α-form) or 3.0 per cent (δ-form) w/w of water. A 10 per cent solution in water has a pH of 4.0 to 6.0.

Stability. Solutions containing 1 gram in 500 ml of Ringer's Solution, Hartmann's Solution, Darrow's Solution, Sodium Chloride and Dextrose Injection, Calcium Gluconate Injection, or dextran injections, may be expected to retain their activity when stored for twenty-four hours at room temperature.
Cephaloridine is unstable in solutions which contain both dextrose and sodium bicarbonate.

Labelling. The label on the container states whether the contents are the α-form or the δ-form.

Storage. It should be stored in sterile airtight containers, sealed to exclude micro-organisms, in a cool dry place.

Actions and uses. Cephaloridine is one of the cephalosporin antibiotics which have a molecular structure and mode of action on the bacterial cell wall similar to penicillin. These antibiotics are bactericidal and tend to promote allergy especially in patients already allergic to penicillin. They have a broader spectrum than benzylpenicillin, being relatively resistant to staphylococcal penicillinase and to some of the penicillinases produced by *Proteus mirabilis* and other coliform species. Therefore, although the cephalosporin antibiotics have a wide spectrum, resistance may occur in many bacterial species and successful use is dependent upon careful bacteriological assessment.

Cephaloridine is given by intramuscular injection in doses of 0.5 to 1 gram every eight to twelve hours, or 20 to 40 milligrams per kilogram body-weight daily in children. The dose should be reduced in patients with poor renal function. The administration of probenecid does not significantly increase the blood level of cephaloridine. It is not absorbed by mouth and diffuses poorly into the cerebrospinal fluid. It may be given intrathecally, in a dose of 50 milligrams daily in 2 to 10 millilitres of Sodium Chloride Injection for an adult; for children under five years the dose is 500 micrograms per kilogram body-weight and over five years 750 micrograms per kilogram body-weight daily. Larger doses cause meningism.

UNDESIRABLE EFFECTS. As for Cephalothin Sodium.

PRECAUTIONS. It should be used with care in patients with an allergic diathesis, especially those already sensitised to penicillin. The dose should be reduced in patients with poor renal function, as otherwise further increases in blood urea and tubular damage may occur. The concurrent use of diuretics is potentially dangerous because it enhances the toxicity of cephaloridine.

Preparation
CEPHALORIDINE INJECTION, B.P. It consists of a sterile solution prepared by dissolving the sterile contents of a sealed container in Water for Injections. It should be used within 4 days of its date of preparation, which is stated on the label, provided that it is stored during this period at 2° to 10°; at temperatures not exceeding 20° it should be used within 24 hours of preparation. The quantity of cephaloridine in each container should be specified by the prescriber. Vials containing 250 and 500 mg and 1 g are available.

OTHER NAME: *Ceporin*®

CEPHALOTHIN SODIUM

$C_{16}H_{15}N_2NaO_6S_2 = 418.4$

Cephalothin Sodium is the sodium salt of 3-acetoxymethyl-8-oxo-7-(α-thien-2-ylacetamido)-5-thia-1-azabicyclo[4,2,0]oct-2-ene-2-carboxylic acid.

Solubility. Soluble, at 20°, in 3.5 parts of water and in 700 parts of alcohol; insoluble in ether and in chloroform.

Standard
It complies with the requirements of the British Pharmacopoeia.
It is a white or almost white, crystalline, almost odourless powder and contains not less than 90.0 per cent

of $C_{16}H_{16}N_2O_6S_2$, calculated with reference to the dried substance. The loss on drying under the prescribed conditions is not more than 1.5 per cent. A 10 per cent solution in water has a pH of 4.5 to 7.0.

Stability. Aqueous solutions may be expected to retain their potency for two days when stored at 2° to 10° or for at least six hours at room temperature.

Labelling. If the material is not intended for

parenteral administration, the label on the container states that the contents are not to be injected.

Storage. It should be stored in airtight containers, protected from light, at a temperature not exceeding 25°. If it is intended for parenteral administration, the containers should be sterile and sealed to exclude micro-organisms.

Actions and uses. Cephalothin is an antibiotic with actions and uses similar to those described under Cephaloridine, but it is less likely to cause renal damage and may therefore be preferred for the treatment of patients with renal failure or those being dialysed.

The principal use of cephalothin is in the treatment of serious infections due to organisms that have become resistant to benzylpenicillin and ampicillin. It does not cross the blood–brain barrier in effective quantities even in purulent meningitis. It is the most active of the cephalosporins against staphylococci.

Cephalothin sodium may be administered in a dosage equivalent to 2 to 6 grams of cephalothin daily, in divided doses, by intramuscular or intravenous injection or by intravenous infusion; in life-threatening infections, doses of up to 6 grams may be administered every four hours. The usual dose for children is the equivalent of 50 milligrams of cephalothin per kilogram body-weight daily and the dose should not exceed the equivalent of 80 milligrams per kilogram body-weight daily.

UNDESIRABLE EFFECTS. High concentrations of cephalothin in the blood may give rise to renal damage, convulsions, and an auto-immune type of haemolytic anaemia. At lower blood levels the development of a positive Coombs test may interfere with cross-matching procedures. Neutropenia may occur. Allergic rashes may also occur, especially in patients hypersensitive to penicillin.

PRECAUTIONS. It should be used with caution in penicillin-sensitive patients. To prevent renal damage during prolonged periods of use, as in the treatment of bacterial endocarditis, the glomerular filtration rate should be estimated regularly and the dose varied accordingly.

The concurrent use of diuretics is potentially dangerous because it enhances the toxicity of cephalothin.

Solutions for intravenous administration should be suitably diluted as concentrated solutions may cause thrombophlebitis.

Dose. See above under **Actions and uses.**

Preparation

CEPHALOTHIN INJECTION, B.P. It consists of a sterile solution prepared by dissolving the sterile contents of a sealed container in Water for Injections. The equivalent quantity of cephalothin in each container should be specified by the prescriber. It should be used within forty-eight hours of preparation and should be stored during this period at a temperature between 2° and 10°. Vials containing the equivalent of 1 g of cephalothin are available.

OTHER NAMES: Cefalotin Sodium; *Keflin*®

CETOMACROGOL 1000

Cetomacrogol 1000 may be prepared by condensing cetyl or cetostearyl alcohol with ethylene oxide under controlled conditions. It may be represented by the formula $CH_3 \cdot [CH_2]_m \cdot [O \cdot CH_2 \cdot CH_2]_n \cdot OH$, where m is 15 or 17 and n is 20 to 24.

Solubility. Soluble in water, in alcohol, and in acetone; insoluble in light petroleum.

Standard

It complies with the requirements of the British Pharmacopoeia.

It is an almost odourless, cream-coloured, waxy, unctuous mass melting, when heated, to a clear brownish-yellow liquid. It has a melting-point not lower than 38°.

Incompatibility. It is incompatible with phenols and it reduces the antibacterial activity of quaternary ammonium compounds. When solutions are added to strong solutions of electrolytes, the cetomacrogol may separate.

Sterilisation. It is sterilised by dry heat.

Storage. It should be stored in airtight containers.

Uses. Cetomacrogol 1000 is a non-ionic emulsifying agent and is used in the preparation of Cetomacrogol Emulsifying Wax, which can be employed as an emulsifying agent for producing oil-in-water creams which are

stable over a wide pH range and suitable for the incorporation of many anionic, cationic, and non-ionic medicaments.

Cetomacrogol 1000 is used to disperse volatile oils in water, producing transparent sols; a proportion of 10 parts of cetomacrogol 1000 to 1 part of volatile oil is suitable in most cases.

Preparations

CETOMACROGOL CREAM, B.P.C. (page 657)

CETOMACROGOL EMULSIFYING OINTMENT, B.P. It consists of cetomacrogol emulsifying wax 30 per cent, liquid paraffin 20 per cent, and white soft paraffin 50 per cent. It may be prepared by melting the ingredients together and stirring until cold.

CETOMACROGOL EMULSIFYING WAX, B.P. (*Syn.* Non-ionic Emulsifying Wax). It consists of 20 per cent of cetomacrogol 1000 and 80 per cent of cetostearyl alcohol. It may be prepared by melting the ingredients together and stirring until cold.

OTHER NAME: Polyethylene Glycol 1000 Monocetyl Ether

CETOSTEARYL ALCOHOL

Cetostearyl Alcohol is a mixture of solid aliphatic alcohols and consists chiefly of stearyl alcohol, $CH_3 \cdot [CH_2]_{16} \cdot CH_2OH$, and cetyl alcohol, $CH_3 \cdot [CH_2]_{14} \cdot CH_2OH$, with small amounts of other alcohols, mainly myristyl alcohol, $CH_3 \cdot [CH_2]_{12} \cdot CH_2OH$.

Cetostearyl alcohol usually consists of about 50 to 70 per cent of stearyl alcohol and about 20 to 35 per cent of cetyl alcohol, but the proportions may vary considerably. Material which is known in commerce as "cetyl alcohol", unless specified as pure, is a cetostearyl alcohol usually containing about 60 to 70 per cent of cetyl alcohol and 20 to 30 per cent of stearyl alcohol. Pure cetyl alcohol, containing not less than 98 per cent of $CH_3 \cdot [CH_2]_{14} \cdot CH_2OH$, is also available.

Solubility. Insoluble in water; soluble in ether; less soluble in alcohol and in light petroleum.

Standard

It complies with the requirements of the British Pharmacopoeia.

It occurs as a white or cream-coloured, unctuous mass, or almost white flakes or granules, with a faint characteristic odour. It has a solidifying-point of 45° to 53°. When heated, it melts to a clear colourless or pale yellow liquid which is free from cloudiness or suspended matter.

Uses. Cetostearyl alcohol is strongly hydrophobic and when used alone has little value as an emulsifying agent. Oil-in-water emulsions produced by hydrophilic substances, such as sulphated fatty alcohols or cetomacrogol, are stabilised over a wide pH range when cetostearyl alcohol is included.

It may be used to increase the viscosity of oil-in-water and water-in-oil emulsions, thereby improving their stability, and may be added to paraffin ointments to improve their emollient properties.

Preparations

CETOMACROGOL EMULSIFYING WAX, B.P. (*Syn.* Nonionic Emulsifying Wax). It consists of 20 per cent of cetomacrogol 1000 and 80 per cent of cetostearyl alcohol. It may be prepared by melting the ingredients together and stirring until cold.

CETRIMIDE EMULSIFYING WAX, B.P.C. (page 678)

EMULSIFYING WAX, B.P. (*Syn.* Anionic Emulsifying Wax). It contains cetostearyl alcohol and sodium lauryl sulphate or similar sodium salts of sulphated higher primary aliphatic alcohols. A suitable preparation may be prepared from 90 g of cetostearyl alcohol, 10 g of sodium lauryl sulphate, and 4 ml of water.

CETRIMIDE

SYNONYM: Cetrimidum

Cetrimide consists chiefly of tetradecyltrimethylammonium bromide, together with smaller amounts of dodecyl- and hexadecyl-trimethylammonium bromide.

Cetrimide may be prepared from a suitable mixture of alkyl bromides and trimethylamine.

Solubility. Soluble, at 20°, in 2 parts of water; very soluble in alcohol.

Standard

It complies with the requirements of the European Pharmacopoeia.

It is a white to creamy-white, voluminous, free-flowing powder with a faint characteristic odour and contains not less than 96.0 per cent of alkyltrimethylammonium bromides, calculated as $C_{17}H_{38}BrN$, with reference to the dried substance. The loss on drying under the prescribed conditions is not more than 2.0 per cent. A 2 per cent solution in water is clear or not more than faintly opalescent.

Hygroscopicity. At 20°, at relative humidities of 40 to 50 per cent, it absorbs sufficient moisture to cause caking of the powder.

Incompatibility. It is incompatible with soaps and similar anionic compounds, with iodine, and with alkali hydroxides.

Sterilisation. Solutions are sterilised by heating in an autoclave or by filtration.

Preparation and storage of solutions. See statement on aqueous solutions of antiseptics, under Solutions, (page 779).

Stock solutions containing up to 40 per cent w/v of cetrimide may be stored and subsequently diluted; as a precaution against contamination with *Pseudomonas* species they should contain at least 7 per cent v/v of ethyl alcohol or 4 per cent v/v of isopropyl alcohol.

Actions and uses. Cetrimide is a quaternary ammonium compound. It is a relatively non-toxic antiseptic with detergent properties. Like other quaternary ammonium compounds it is active against Gram-positive organisms, but it is less effective against Gram-negative organisms (especially *Pseudomonas*) and is inactive against acid-fast bacilli and bacterial spores.

Aqueous solutions and creams containing 0.1 to 1 per cent have been used for the treatment of wounds and burns, for pre-operative cleansing of the skin, and for the removal of scabs and crusts in skin diseases. Solutions containing 1 to 3 per cent are used in seborrhoea of the scalp.

For the cleansing and disinfection of utensils, vessels, and apparatus, solutions containing 0.5 to 1 per cent may be used; rubber articles are adversely affected by prolonged or repeated immersion, and polythene tubing and catheters and articles made of plastics should not remain immersed for more than thirty minutes.

The activity of quaternary compounds is greatly reduced in the presence of organic matter, soap, and anionic compounds.

Cetrimide is used in the preparation of Cetrimide Emulsifying Wax, which can be used as an emulsifying agent for producing oil-in-water creams, suitable for the incorporation of cationic and non-ionic medicaments. For anionic medicaments, Emulsifying Wax and Cetomacrogol Emulsifying Wax should be used.

PRECAUTIONS. Cetrimide should not be applied repeatedly to and wet dressings should not be left in contact with the skin as hypersensitivity may occur.

Preparations
CETRIMIDE CREAM, B.P.C. (page 657)
CETRIMIDE EMULSIFYING WAX, B.P.C. (page 678)
CETRIMIDE EMULSIFYING OINTMENT, B.P. It consists of centrimide 3 per cent, cetostearyl alcohol 27 per cent, liquid paraffin 20 per cent, and white soft paraffin 50 per cent. It may be prepared by melting the ingredients together and stirring until cold.
CETRIMIDE SOLUTION, B.P.C. (page 781)
CETRIMIDE SOLUTION, STRONG, B.P.C. (page 781)

OTHER NAMES: *Cetavlon®*; *Cycloton V®*; *Morpan CHSA®*

CETYLPYRIDINIUM CHLORIDE

$C_{21}H_{38}ClN,H_2O = 358 \cdot 0$

Cetylpyridinium Chloride is 1-hexadecylpyridinium chloride monohydrate.

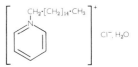

Solubility. Soluble, at 20°, in 20 parts of water.

Standard
It complies with the requirements of the British Pharmacopoeia.
It is a white powder with a slight characteristic odour and contains not less than 98·0 per cent of $C_{21}H_{38}ClN,H_2O$. It contains 4·5 to 5·5 per cent w/w of water. A 1 per cent solution in water has a pH of 5·0 to 5·4. It has a melting-point of 79° to 83°.

Incompatibility. It is incompatible with soaps and similar anionic compounds.

Storage. It should be stored in airtight containers.

Preparation and storage of solutions. See statement on aqueous solutions of antiseptics, under Solutions (page 779).

Actions and uses. Cetylpyridinium chloride has actions similar to those of Cetrimide. It is used as a 0·1 per cent solution for minor wounds and burns, and as a 1 per cent solution for pre-operative cleansing of the skin. More dilute solutions (0·01 to 0·02 per cent) should be used for application to mucous membranes or to large areas of exposed tissue. Its activity is greatly reduced by the presence of soap or serum.

Lozenges containing 4 milligrams of cetylpyridinium chloride are used for the treatment of superficial infections of the mouth and throat.

CHALK

SYNONYMS: Creta; Creta Praeparata; Prepared Chalk

$CaCO_3 = 100 \cdot 1$

Chalk is native calcium carbonate freed from most of its impurities by elutriation and dried.

Solubility. Almost insoluble in water; slightly soluble in water containing carbon dioxide; soluble in mineral acids with effervescence.

Standard
It complies with the requirements of the British Pharmacopoeia.
It contains not less than 97·0 per cent of $CaCO_3$, calculated with reference to the dried substance. The loss on drying under the prescribed conditions is not more than 1·0 per cent.

DESCRIPTION. *Macroscopical:* odourless, white or greyish-white, amorphous, earthy, friable masses or powder, soft to the touch.

Microscopical: chalk consists of the shells of cretaceous fossil foraminifera belonging to several genera, including *Globigerina*, about 35 to 80 μm in diameter, and *Textularia*, about 50 to 180 μm long by 40 to 100 μm across the base, accompanied by large numbers of fossil remains of small algae belonging to the Coccolithophoridaceae and having the appearance of small disks or rings, about 1 to 2 μm in diameter; small amounts of detritus of echinoderms and of molluscs are also present; when mounted in alcohol and irrigated with acetic acid, it dissolves with effervescence.

Actions and uses. Chalk is absorbent and antacid and is an ingredient of mixtures and powders used in the treatment of diarrhoea.

Dose. 1 to 5 grams, repeated in accordance with the needs of the patient.

Preparations
CHALK MIXTURE, PAEDIATRIC, B.P.C. (page 739)
CHALK WITH OPIUM MIXTURE, AROMATIC, B.P.C. (page 739)
CHALK POWDER, AROMATIC, B.P.C. (page 776)
CHALK WITH OPIUM POWDER, AROMATIC, B.P.C. (page 776)
MAGNESIUM TRISILICATE POWDER, COMPOUND, B.P.C. (page 778)

CHARCOAL

SYNONYMS: Carbo; Medicinal Charcoal

Charcoal may be prepared from vegetable matter such as sawdust, peat, cellulose residues and coconut shells. The raw material is carbonised and subsequently activated at a high temperature, with or without the addition of inorganic salts, in a stream of activating gases such as steam and carbon dioxide. Alternatively, raw vegetable matter may be treated with a chemical activating agent such as phosphoric acid, zinc chloride, or potassium thiocyanate, the mixture carbonised at a suitable temperature, and the chemical agent removed by washing.

A combination of both processes may also be employed. Further treatment, such as acid extraction, may be employed to improve the purity of the finished product.

Commercial varieties of charcoal differ widely in their characteristics, depending largely upon the method of manufacture.

The adsorptive power of charcoal depends upon the total available surface area, which may include external and internal surfaces. Charcoals showing high adsorptive power for gases may be relatively inactive in liquid-phase systems, and charcoals showing high adsorptive power in liquid media may be relatively inactive for gases.

Technical grades of activated charcoal are widely used as purifying and decolorising agents, for the removal of residual gases in low-pressure apparatus, and in respirators as a protection against toxic gases.

Solubility. Insoluble in water and in alcohol.

Standard

DESCRIPTION. A black, very fine powder, free from grittiness; odourless; tasteless.

IDENTIFICATION TESTS. 1. Heat in the absence of air; it is unchanged in properties and appearance.

2. Burn in the presence of air; carbon dioxide and carbon monoxide are produced.

ACIDITY OR ALKALINITY. pH of the filtrate obtained in the test for water-soluble matter, 5·0 to 8·0.

ARSENIC. It complies with the test given in Appendix 6, page 878 (2 parts per million).

COPPER. It complies with the test given in Appendix 8, page 886 (50 parts per million).

LEAD. It complies with the test given in Appendix 8, page 886 (30 parts per million).

ZINC. It complies with the test given in Appendix 8, page 886 (50 parts per million).

TARRY MATTER. Boil 2 g with 20 ml of *sodium hydroxide solution* for 20 minutes, cool, and filter; the colour of the filtrate is not deeper than that of the sodium hydroxide solution.

CYANOGEN COMPOUNDS. Add 5·0 g to a solution of 2 g of *tartaric acid* in 50 ml of water contained in a distillation flask; attach the flask to an efficient condenser with the outlet tube dipping below the surface of 10 ml of 1N sodium hydroxide, and distil about 25 ml; to the liquid in the receiver add 2 ml of *ferrous sulphate*

solution and acidify to *litmus paper* with *hydrochloric acid*; no blue colour or precipitate is produced.

HIGHER AROMATIC HYDROCARBONS. Boil under reflux 10 g of the dried material with 100 ml of *cyclohexane* for 2 hours, filter, and allow to cool.
Examine the filtrate under filtered ultraviolet radiation; any fluorescence is not greater than that of a freshly prepared solution containing 0·1 part per million of *quinine sulphate* in 0·1N sulphuric acid.
Evaporate the solution to dryness on a water-bath and dry the residue to constant weight at 105°; the residue weighs not more than 1 mg.

SULPHIDE. Boil 0·50 g with 25 ml of *dilute hydrochloric acid*; the vapour does not blacken *lead paper*.

WATER-SOLUBLE MATTER. Not more than 1·0 per cent, determined by the following method:
Boil about 2 g, accurately weighed, with 40 ml of *carbon dioxide-free water* for one minute and filter; evaporate 20 ml of the filtrate to dryness and dry the residue to constant weight at 105°.

LOSS ON DRYING. Not more than 15·0 per cent, determined by drying to constant weight at 105°.

ASH. Not more than 10·0 per cent.

ADSORPTIVE CAPACITY. (a) Adsorbs from solution not less than 30·0 per cent of its weight of phenazone, calculated with reference to the substance dried at 105°, determined by the following method:
Add about 0·3 g, accurately weighed, of the charcoal, previously dried to constant weight at 105°, to 50 ml of a 0·4 per cent w/v solution of *phenazone* in water contained in a stoppered flask and shake at frequent intervals for 20 minutes; filter through a dry filter paper, discarding the first 15 ml of the filtrate; to 25 ml of the filtrate in a stoppered flask add 2 g of *sodium acetate* and 30 ml of 0·1N iodine and shake occasionally for 20 minutes; add 10 ml of *chloroform*, shake until the precipitate is dissolved, and titrate the excess of iodine with 0·1N sodium thiosulphate. Repeat the procedure omitting the sample. Twice the difference between the two titrations represents the amount of iodine required by the phenazone adsorbed by the charcoal; each ml of 0·1N iodine is equivalent to 0·009405 g of phenazone.

(b) 1 g adsorbs not less than 0·4 g of chloroform from air saturated with chloroform vapour at 16° to 20°, calculated with reference to the substance dried at 105°, determined by the following method:
Weigh accurately about 1 g of the charcoal, previously dried to constant weight at 105°, in a shallow glass dish fitted with a ground-in stopper; place the dish, with stopper removed, in a closed vessel containing *chloroform* in an open dish and allow to stand for 24 hours at 16° to 20°; withdraw the dish, insert the stopper, and weigh.

Storage. It should be stored in airtight containers.

Uses. Charcoal will adsorb certain substances from solution and when dry is an efficient adsorbent of gases. It is sometimes given by mouth to adsorb gases in the treatment of flatulence and intestinal distension, but it is doubtful if it is of much value in these circumstances. It is also given in the treatment of poisoning by alkaloids and similar drugs to adsorb the poison. Charcoal is used to indicate the passage of intestinal contents.

Charcoal is administered in powder, granules, and tablets, sometimes with light kaolin.

Dose. 4 to 8 grams.

CHLORAL HYDRATE

SYNONYM: Chlorali Hydras

$C_2H_3Cl_3O_2 = 165{\cdot}4$ $CCl_3{\cdot}CH(OH)_2$

Chloral Hydrate is 2,2,2-trichloroethane-1,1-diol.

Solubility. Soluble, at 20°, in less than 1 part of water, of alcohol, and of ether, and in 3 parts of chloroform; soluble in fixed and volatile oils.

Standard
It complies with the requirements of the European Pharmacopoeia.
It occurs as colourless transparent crystals with a pungent but not acrid odour and contains not less than 98·5 per cent of $C_2H_3Cl_3O_2$. It volatilises slowly on exposure to air, and when heated it liquefies between 50° and 58°.

Incompatibility. It is incompatible with alkalis, alkaline earths, alkali carbonates, and soluble barbiturates.
It forms a liquid mixture when triturated with many organic compounds such as camphor, menthol, thymol, phenol, and phenazone.

Storage. It should be stored in airtight containers.

Actions and uses. Chloral hydrate is a hypnotic which is particularly useful for children and elderly patients. When given by mouth it is rapidly absorbed and acts within half an hour, the effect lasting for about eight hours. It is excreted in the urine in combination with glycuronic acid and sulphuric acid.

UNDESIRABLE EFFECTS. Headache, nausea, giddiness, rashes, and blood dyscrasias may occur.

PRECAUTIONS AND CONTRA-INDICATIONS. Chloral hydrate is a gastric irritant and must be well diluted before administration. It is contra-indicated in patients with severe cardiac disease or marked hepatic or renal dysfunction.

DEPENDENCE. It may give rise to dependence of the barbiturate–alcohol type as described under Phenobarbitone (page 366) and it may also enhance the effects of alcohol.

Dose. 0·5 to 2 grams.

Preparations
CHLORAL ELIXIR, PAEDIATRIC, B.P.C. (page 668)
CHLORAL MIXTURE, B.P.C. (page 739)

CHLORAMBUCIL

$C_{14}H_{19}Cl_2NO_2 = 304{\cdot}2$

Chlorambucil is γ-[p-di(2-chloroethyl)aminophenyl]butyric acid.

Solubility. Insoluble in water; soluble, at 20°, in 1·5 parts of alcohol, in 2·5 parts of chloroform, and in 2 parts of acetone.

Standard
It complies with the requirements of the British Pharmacopoeia.
It is a white crystalline powder with a slight odour and contains not less than 98·5 per cent of $C_{14}H_{19}Cl_2NO_2$, calculated with reference to the anhydrous substance. It contains not more than 0·5 per cent w/w of water. It has a melting-point of 64° to 67°.

Storage. It should be stored in airtight containers.

Actions and uses. Chlorambucil is a cytotoxic agent. It is radiomimetic, damaging cells by fragmentation of the nuclear chromosomes.
In the normal dosage, chlorambucil acts mainly on the lymphocytes and to a lesser extent on neutrophils and platelets. Large doses given over prolonged periods can, however, produce severe neutropenia and thrombocytopenia and irreversible damage to the bone marrow, with subsequent failure of haemopoiesis.
The best results have been obtained in the treatment of those conditions associated with proliferation of white blood cells, particularly lymphocytes, and in the treatment of follicular lymphoma, lymphocytic lymphoma with or without leukaemia, and some cases of Hodgkin's disease and reticulum-cell sarcoma. It is also effective in the treatment of lymphosarcoma, carcinoma of the breast and ovary, chronic lymphocytic and chronic myelocytic leukaemias, and the macroglobulinaemia of Waldenström.

Chlorambucil is better tolerated than mustine or tretamine and, if the dosage is kept low, repeated courses can be given without depression of haemopoiesis.

Chlorambucil is administered by mouth, the usual dosage being 0·2 milligram per kilogram body-weight, which corresponds to 10 to 12 milligrams, for the average patient, given as a single dose daily for three to six weeks. This dose should be halved if there is lymphocytic infiltration of the bone marrow or if the bone marrow is hypoplastic, as in cases of long standing and in patients who have undergone extensive treatment. Absorption is more consistent than with tretamine and is not related to food intake, whilst the effect on the bone marrow is more easily controlled. In general, chlorambucil should not be used within a month of therapeutic irradiation or chemotherapy, as these may have caused some bone-marrow damage. If, however, low doses of radiation have been given to parts remote from the bone marrow and the neutrophil and platelet-cell counts are not depressed, treatment with chlorambucil is permissible. If these cell counts are depressed, they should be allowed to reach normal levels before chlorambucil therapy is begun.

Improvement, if it occurs, is usually apparent by the third week of treatment. If the drug is well tolerated and the blood picture is satisfactory, a daily maintenance dose of 0·03 to 0·1 milligram per kilogram body-weight, which corresponds to about 2 to 5 milligrams for the average adult patient, may be given. Alternatively, short interrupted courses of treatment may be given.

During treatment, total and differential white-cell counts and haemoglobin estimations should be made weekly and skin and mucous membranes examined for signs of haemorrhage.

UNDESIRABLE EFFECTS. A slowly progressive leucopenia may develop during treatment, but this is reversible on withdrawing the drug. A fall in the neutrophil count may continue for ten days after the last dose of chlorambucil. As the total dose of drug approaches 6·5 milligrams per kilogram body-weight (about 400 to 450 milligrams) there is grave risk of irreversible bone-marrow damage.

Dose. See above under **Actions and uses.**

Preparation
CHLORAMBUCIL TABLETS, B.P. The quantity of chlorambucil in each tablet should be specified by the prescriber. They are sugar coated or compression coated. They should be stored in a cool place. Tablets containing 2 and 5 mg are available.

OTHER NAME: *Leukeran®*

CHLORAMINE

SYNONYMS: Chloraminum; Chloramine-T

$C_7H_7ClNNaO_2S,3H_2O = 281·7$

Chloramine is toluene-*p*-sulphonsodiochloroamide trihydrate.

Solubility. Soluble, at 20°, in 7 parts of water and in 12 parts of alcohol, with slow decomposition; soluble in 2 parts of boiling water; insoluble in ether and in chloroform.

Standard
DESCRIPTION. A white or slightly yellow efflorescent crystalline powder; odour that of chlorine.

IDENTIFICATION TESTS. 1. A solution in water turns *red litmus paper* blue and then bleaches it.

2. Dissolve 0·5 g in 10 ml of water and add 10 ml of *diluted hydrogen peroxide solution*; a white precipitate is formed which dissolves on heating the solution. Filter the hot solution and allow to cool; a white crystalline precipitate is formed which, after washing with water and drying at 105°, melts at about 137°.

3. Ignite; sudden decomposition occurs, and the residue gives the reactions characteristic of sodium and of sulphates.

APPEARANCE OF SOLUTION. Dissolve 1·0 g in 20 ml of water. This solution complies with the following tests:
(i) The solution is clear or not more opalescent than a reference solution prepared by mixing 0·75 ml of *0·00002M sodium chloride*, 0·05 ml of water, 1·0 ml of *2M nitric acid*, and 0·2 ml of *dilute silver nitrate solution*, the comparison being made 5 minutes after preparation of the reference solution by viewing 2 ml of the liquids in matched, colourless, transparent, neutral glass tubes, 12 mm internal diameter, in darkness, and with a beam of light being passed laterally from an electric lamp giving a luminosity of 1000 lux at a distance of 1 m.

(ii) The solution has no colour when compared with water, the comparison being made by viewing horizontally 2 ml of the liquids in matched, colourless, transparent, neutral glass tubes, 12 mm internal diameter, against a white background in diffused daylight.

MATTER INSOLUBLE IN ALCOHOL. Not more than 2·0 per cent, determined by the following method:
Shake 1·00 g with 20 ml of *dehydrated alcohol* for 30 minutes, filter, wash the residue with *dehydrated alcohol*, allow to dry, and weigh.

CONTENT OF $C_7H_7ClNNaO_2S,3H_2O$. Not less than 98·0 and not more than the equivalent of 103·0 per cent, determined by the following method:
Dissolve about 0·3 g, accurately weighed, in 100 ml of water, add 1 g of *potassium iodide* and 1 ml of *hydrochloric acid*, allow to stand for 3 minutes, and titrate the liberated iodine with 0·1N sodium thiosulphate, using *starch mucilage* as indicator; each ml of 0·1N sodium thiosulphate is equivalent to 0·01409 g of $C_7H_7ClNNaO_2S,3H_2O$.

Storage. It should be stored in airtight containers, protected from light, in a cool place.

Actions and uses. Chloramine is a bactericide and in aqueous solution is almost neutral and non-irritant. A 2 per cent solution may be used in the irrigation of wounds.

The stability of solutions may be improved by buffering at pH 9.

CHLORAMPHENICOL

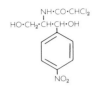

SYNONYMS: Chloramphen.; Chloramphenicolum

$C_{11}H_{12}Cl_2N_2O_5 = 323.1$

Chloramphenicol is D-*threo*-2-dichloroacetamido-1-*p*-nitrophenylpropane-1,3-diol and is produced by the growth of *Streptomyces venezuelae*, or prepared synthetically.

Solubility. Soluble, at 20°, in 400 parts of water, in 2·5 parts of alcohol, and in 7 parts of propylene glycol; soluble in acetone and in ethyl acetate; slightly soluble in ether.

Standard
It complies with the requirements of the European Pharmacopoeia.
It occurs as a fine, white to greyish-white or yellowish-white, crystalline powder, or crystals, needles, or elongated plates. The loss on drying at 100° to 105° is not more than 0·5 per cent. It has a melting-point of 149° to 153°. A 0·5 per cent suspension in water has a pH of 5·0 to 7·5. Solutions in ethyl acetate are laevorotatory and solutions in dehydrated alcohol are dextrorotatory.

Sterilisation. Solutions in propylene glycol are sterilised by filtration.

Storage. It should be protected from light.

Actions and uses. Chloramphenicol is an antibiotic which has a wide range of antimicrobial activity similar to that described under Tetracycline Hydrochloride (page 498) but including also *Salmonella typhi* and *S. paratyphi*. It is active when administered by mouth, being rapidly absorbed from the gastro-intestinal tract. It enters the bile, cerebrospinal fluid, and urine and passes the placental barrier in therapeutically effective amounts.

It is the antibiotic of choice for the treatment of typhoid and paratyphoid fevers, but it does not eliminate the typhoid carrier state. It is also used in the treatment of *Haemophilus influenzae* meningitis, chronic infections of the urinary tract with a sensitive strain of *Proteus vulgaris* that is resistant to other antibiotics, and rickettsial infections which do not respond to treatment with other drugs.

Chloramphenicol is usually administered by mouth in a dosage of 500 milligrams every six hours. A higher initial dosage, with the object of obtaining rapidly a high concentration in the blood, should not be given in the treatment of typhoid fever because of the release of endotoxins from the infecting organisms.

Treatment should be continued for two or three days after the patient's temperature has returned to normal so as to minimise the risk of relapse, but it is inadvisable to continue the course for more than ten days or to exceed a total dose of 26 grams. For a child, the usual daily dosage is 25 to 50 milligrams per kilogram body-weight, given in divided doses at intervals of six hours.

Chloramphenicol is usually administered in capsules; patients unable to swallow the capsules may be given the antibiotic by mouth

as a suspension of the palmitate. Chloramphenicol may be given to seriously ill patients by injection of aqueous solutions of chloramphenicol sodium succinate.

Chloramphenicol is of value when applied to the skin and mucous membranes in the treatment of infections due to sensitive organisms. The ear-drops are used in chronic otorrhoea and are often effective even when such organisms as *P. vulgaris* and *Pseudomonas aeruginosa*, which are resistant to many antibacterial agents, are present.

Chloramphenicol is used in the treatment of a wide variety of infections of the eye, and for treatment of superficial infections of the skin such as impetigo, sycosis barbae, and furunculosis.

UNDESIRABLE EFFECTS. The most serious toxic effect caused by chloramphenicol is that occasionally exerted on the haemopoietic system, resulting in agranulocytosis, thrombocytopenic purpura, or aplastic anaemia. Fatal cases of aplastic anaemia following the administration of chloramphenicol have occurred, and other antibiotics, such as the tetracyclines, are preferred whenever the infecting organism is sensitive to them. Other serious effects may include renal toxicity, optic neuritis, jaundice, and the Stevens–Johnson syndrome.

Topical or systemic use of chloramphenicol may give rise to allergic skin rashes and more serious allergic reactions may occur in sensitised patients.

Other toxic reactions, which may occur in a small proportion of patients, include dryness of the mouth, nausea, vomiting, diarrhoea, and urticarial skin rashes. Disturbance of the normal bacterial flora of the mouth and gastro-intestinal tract produced by chloramphenicol may be followed by excessive growth of *Candida albicans* and other fungi on the mucous membrane, producing stomatitis, sore tongue, rectal or vaginal irritation and, rarely, pneumonia.

The occurrence of the more serious toxic effects is usually associated with high dosage or prolonged administration or with repeated courses of treatment, but blood dyscrasias have also occurred with relatively low dosage. Several months may elapse between the completion of treatment and the onset of aplastic anaemia, and although frequent blood counts are advisable they cannot be relied upon to give adequate warning.

PRECAUTIONS AND CONTRA-INDICATIONS. Chloramphenicol should not be used for its systemic effect in the treatment of any infection which can be treated with a less toxic antibiotic or a sulphonamide. Its use by mouth is therefore virtually limited to the treatment of typhoid and paratyphoid fevers.

Dose. For an adult, 1·5 to 3 grams daily in divided doses; for a child, 25 to 50 milligrams per kilogram body-weight daily in divided doses.

Preparations
CHLORAMPHENICOL CAPSULES, B.P. Unless otherwise specified, capsules each containing 250 mg are supplied.
CHLORAMPHENICOL EAR-DROPS, B.P.C. (page 664)
CHLORAMPHENICOL EYE-DROPS, B.P.C. (page 689)
CHLORAMPHENICOL EYE OINTMENT, B.P.C. (page 698)

OTHER NAMES: *Chloromycetin®*; *Clorcetin®*; *Kemicetine®*

CHLORAMPHENICOL PALMITATE

SYNONYM: Chloramphen. Palm.

$C_{27}H_{42}Cl_2N_2O_6 = 561·6$

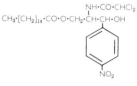

Chloramphenicol Palmitate is the 3-palmitic ester of chloramphenicol

Chloramphenicol Palmitate exists in several polymorphic forms. In making preparations which contain chloramphenicol palmitate in solid form, any polymorph may be used, but the manufacturing process must be such as to ensure that the final product contains the desired polymorph B.

Solubility. Insoluble in water; soluble, at 20°, in 45 parts of alcohol, in 14 parts of ether, and in 6 parts of chloroform.

Standard
DESCRIPTION. A fine, white, unctuous powder; odour faint.

IDENTIFICATION TESTS. 1. It melts at about 89°.

2. The ultraviolet absorption spectrum exhibits the characteristics given in Appendix 3, page 855.

3. To 0·05 g add 2 ml of *alcoholic potassium hydroxide solution* and heat on a water-bath for 15 minutes; the solution gives the reactions characteristic of chlorides.

ACIDITY. Dissolve 1·0 g by warming to 35° with 5 ml of a mixture of equal volumes of *alcohol (95 per cent)* and *solvent ether*, previously neutralised to *phenolphthalein solution*, and titrate the solution with 0·1N sodium hydroxide, using *phenolphthalein solution* as indicator, until, on gentle shaking, a pink colour persists for 30 seconds; not more than 0·4 ml is required.

SPECIFIC ROTATION. +22·5° to +25·5°, calculated with reference to the substance dried under the prescribed conditions, determined, at 20°, in a 5·0 per cent w/v solution in *dehydrated alcohol*.

FREE CHLORAMPHENICOL. Not more than 450 parts per million, determined by the following method:
Dissolve, with the aid of gentle heat, 1·0 g in 80 ml of *xylene*, cool, and extract with three successive 15-ml portions of water; discard the xylene, and dilute the combined aqueous extracts to 50 ml with water; extract the solution with 10 ml of *carbon tetrachloride*, allow to separate, discard the carbon tetrachloride, centrifuge a portion of the aqueous solution, and measure the extinction of a 1-cm layer of the clear aqueous solution at the maximum at about 278 nm, using as the blank a solution prepared by repeating the procedure without the sample; the extinction of this blank solution must not be greater than 0·05.
For purposes of calculation use a value of 298 for the E(1 per cent, 1 cm) of chloramphenicol. Calculate the concentration of free chloramphenicol in the sample.

LOSS ON DRYING. Not more than 0·5 per cent, determined by drying to constant weight over *phosphorus pentoxide* in vacuo.

SULPHATED ASH. Not more than 0·1 per cent.

CONTENT OF $C_{27}H_{42}Cl_2N_2O_6$. Not less than 98·0 and not more than the equivalent of 102·0 per cent, calculated with reference to the substance dried under the prescribed conditions, determined by the following method:
Using *dehydrated alcohol* as solvent, dissolve about 0·03 g, accurately weighed, and dilute to 100 ml; dilute 10 ml of this solution to 100 ml, and measure the extinction of a 1-cm layer at the maximum at about 271 nm. For purposes of calculation, use a value of 178 for the E(1 per cent, 1 cm) of $C_{27}H_{42}Cl_2N_2O_6$. Calculate the percentage of $C_{27}H_{42}Cl_2N_2O_6$ in the sample.

Storage. It should be protected from light.

Actions and uses. Chloramphenicol palmitate has the actions, uses, and undesirable effects described under Chloramphenicol, to which it is hydrolysed in the gastro-intestinal tract.

Because it is insoluble in water, it is almost tasteless and is therefore preferred to chloramphenicol for oral administration to children and to adults when capsules cannot be swallowed; 174 milligrams of chloramphenicol palmitate is equivalent to 100 milligrams of chloramphenicol.

PRECAUTIONS AND CONTRA-INDICATIONS. As for Chloramphenicol.

Dose. For an adult, the equivalent of 1·5 to 3 grams of chloramphenicol daily in divided doses; for a child, the equivalent of 25 to 50 milligrams of chloramphenicol per kilogram body-weight daily in divided doses.

Preparation
CHLORAMPHENICOL MIXTURE, B.P.C. (page 740)

OTHER NAME: *Chloromycetin Palmitate®*

CHLORAMPHENICOL SODIUM SUCCINATE

SYNONYM: Chloramphen. Sod. Succ.

$C_{15}H_{15}Cl_2N_2NaO_8 = 445·2$

Chloramphenicol Sodium Succinate is the sodium salt of the 3-monosuccinic ester of chloramphenicol.

NH·CO·CHCl₂
NaO₂C·[CH₂]₂·CO·O·CH₂·CH·CH·OH

NO₂

Solubility. Soluble, at 20°, in less than 1 part of water and in 1 part of alcohol; almost insoluble in ether and in chloroform.

Standard
DESCRIPTION. A hygroscopic, white or yellowish-white powder; odourless or almost odourless.

IDENTIFICATION TESTS. 1. To 0·05 g add 5 ml of *pyridine* and 5 ml of *sodium hydroxide solution*, mix well, and heat on a water-bath for a few minutes; a deep red colour develops in the pyridine layer.
2. To 0·1 g add 0·2 g of *resorcinol* and 0·2 ml of *sulphuric acid*, heat gently until a deep red solution is produced, and then pour the solution carefully into a large volume of water; an orange-yellow solution with an intense green fluorescence is produced.
3. The ultraviolet absorption spectrum exhibits the characteristics given in Appendix 3, page 855.
4. To 0·05 g add 2 ml of *alcoholic potassium hydroxide* and heat on a water-bath for 15 minutes; the solution gives the reactions characteristic of chlorides.
5. It gives the reactions characteristic of sodium.

ACIDITY. pH of a 25 per cent w/v solution in water, 6·4 to 7·0.

SPECIFIC ROTATION. $+5·0°$ to $+8·0°$, calculated with reference to the anhydrous substance, determined, at 20°, in a 5·0 per cent w/v solution in water.

FREE CHLORAMPHENICOL. Not more than 2·0 per cent, determined by the following method:
Dissolve about 0·1 g, accurately weighed, in 20 ml of *buffer solution pH 9* and extract with two successive 40-ml portions of *ethyl acetate*, washing each extract with 10 ml of *buffer solution pH 9* followed by two 10-ml portions of water; discard the aqueous solution and washings, combine the ethyl acetate extracts, and filter through a layer of *anhydrous sodium sulphate*, supported on a glass-fibre filter paper, the prepared filter having previously been washed with *ethyl acetate*; after filtration, wash the filter with *ethyl acetate*, dilute the combined filtrate and washings to 100 ml with *ethyl acetate*, and measure the extinction of a 1-cm layer at the maximum at about 274 nm, using *ethyl acetate* as the blank.
For purposes of calculation use a value of 320 for the E(1 per cent, 1 cm) of chloramphenicol. Calculate the concentration of free chloramphenicol in the sample.

WATER. Not more than 1·0 per cent w/w, determined by the method given in Appendix 16, page 895.

OTHER NAME: *Chloromycetin Succinate®*

CONTENT OF $C_{15}H_{15}Cl_2N_2NaO_8$. Not less than 98·0 and not more than the equivalent of 102·0 per cent, calculated with reference to the anhydrous substance, determined by the following method:
Using water as solvent, dissolve about 0·2 g, accurately weighed, and dilute to 500 ml; dilute 5 ml of this solution to 100 ml and measure the extinction of a 1-cm layer at the maximum at about 276 nm.
For purposes of calculation, use a value of 216 for the E(1 per cent, 1 cm) of $C_{15}H_{15}Cl_2N_2NaO_8$. Calculate the percentage of $C_{15}H_{15}Cl_2N_2NaO_8$ in the sample.

Storage. It should be stored in airtight containers, protected from light.

Actions and uses. Chloramphenicol sodium succinate has the actions, uses, and undesirable effects described under Chloramphenicol, but being soluble in water it is suitable for administration by injection. Solutions containing 25 to 40 per cent are given by deep intramuscular injection and a 10 per cent solution by subcutaneous or intravenous injection. The usual dose for adults is the equivalent of 1 gram of chloramphenicol every six to eight hours; 1·4 grams of chloramphenicol sodium succinate is approximately equivalent to 1 gram of chloramphenicol. Larger doses may be necessary in the treatment of meningitis. For children, the usual dose is the equivalent of 50 milligrams of chloramphenicol per kilogram body-weight daily in divided doses, but up to 100 milligrams per kilogram body-weight may be given daily in whooping cough, septicaemia, or meningitis.

PRECAUTIONS AND CONTRA-INDICATIONS. As for Chloramphenicol.

Dose. See above under **Actions and uses.**

Preparation
CHLORAMPHENICOL SODIUM SUCCINATE INJECTION, B.P.C. (page 712)

CHLORBUTOL

SYNONYM: Chlorbutanol

$C_4H_7Cl_3O,\frac{1}{2}H_2O = 186·5$

$CCl_3·C(CH_3)_2·OH, \frac{1}{2}H_2O$

Chlorbutol is 2,2,2-trichloro-1,1-dimethylethanol hemihydrate.

Solubility. Soluble, at 20°, in 130 parts of water, in less than 1 part of alcohol, and in 8 parts of glycerol; soluble in ether, in chloroform, and in volatile oils.

Standard
It complies with the requirements of the British Pharmacopoeia.
It occurs as colourless crystals with a characteristic musty and somewhat camphoraceous odour and con-

tains not less than 98·0 and not more than the equivalent of 101·0 per cent of $C_4H_7Cl_3O,\frac{1}{2}H_2O$. It has a melting-point, without previous drying, not lower than 77°. A freshly prepared solution in water is neutral to litmus.

Storage. It should be stored in airtight containers.

Actions and uses. Chlorbutol is a mild sedative and local analgesic. Its sedative action resembles that of chloral hydrate (page 91), but it is less hypnotic and less irritant to mucous membranes. It has been used in the treatment of motion-sickness, but it is less effective for this purpose than hyoscine and the antihistamine drugs.

Chlorbutol has antibacterial and antifungal properties. It is used at a concentration of 0·5 per cent as a preservative in eye-drops and injections. At this concentration it is close to its solubility limit at low temperatures and crystallisation from solutions may occur.

Chlorbutol is unstable in alkaline solution, and although it is more stable in acid solution at room temperatures, it decomposes appreciably on steaming or autoclaving. It may also be lost from aqueous solutions by volatilisation.

Dose. 0·3 to 1·2 grams.

CHLORCYCLIZINE HYDROCHLORIDE

$C_{18}H_{22}Cl_2N_2 = 337·3$

Chlorcyclizine Hydrochloride is (±)-1-(p-chlorodiphenylmethyl)-4-methylpiperazine hydrochloride.

Solubility. Soluble, at 20°, in 2 parts of water, in 11 parts of alcohol, and in 4 parts of chloroform; very slightly soluble in ether.

Standard
It complies with the requirements of the British Pharmacopoeia.
It is a white, odourless or almost odourless, crystalline powder and contains not less than 98·0 and not more than the equivalent of 101·0 per cent of $C_{18}H_{22}Cl_2N_2$, calculated with reference to the dried substance. The loss on drying under the prescribed conditions is not more than 2·5 per cent.

Actions and uses. Chlorcyclizine has the actions and uses of the antihistamine drugs, as described under Promethazine Hydrochloride (page 409). It has a prolonged action and is given by mouth in a dosage of 50 to 100 milligrams of chlorcyclizine hydrochloride once or twice daily.

UNDESIRABLE EFFECTS. Drowsiness and dizziness may occur in some patients.

POISONING. See under Promethazine Hydrochloride (page 409).

Dose. 50 to 200 milligrams daily.

Preparation
CHLORCYCLIZINE TABLETS, B.P. These tablets may be sugar coated. Unless otherwise specified, sugar-coated tablets each containing 50 mg of chlorcyclizine hydrochloride are supplied.

OTHER NAMES: *Di-Paralene®*; *Histantin®*

CHLORDIAZEPOXIDE HYDROCHLORIDE

$C_{16}H_{15}Cl_2N_3O = 336·2$

Chlordiazepoxide Hydrochloride is 7-chloro-2-methylamino-5-phenyl-3H-1,4-benzodiazepine 4-oxide hydrochloride.

Solubility. Soluble, at 20°, in 10 parts of water and in 40 parts of alcohol; very slightly soluble in chloroform and in ether.

Standard
It complies with the requirements of the British Pharmacopoeia.
It is a white crystalline powder with a slight odour and contains not less than 99·0 and not more than the equivalent of 101·0 per cent of $C_{16}H_{15}Cl_2N_3O$, calculated with reference to the dried substance. The loss on drying under the prescribed conditions is not more than 0·5 per cent. A 10 per cent solution in water has a pH of 2·0 to 2·5.

Storage. It should be stored in airtight containers, protected from light.

Actions and uses. Chlordiazepoxide is a tranquillising drug which relieves nervous tension and anxiety states. It has slight muscle-relaxant properties similar to those of mephenesin.

Dosage depends on the clinical conditions and response of the patient, varying from 30 milligrams of chlordiazepoxide hydrochloride daily in divided doses for mild anxiety states to 100 milligrams daily in divided doses in severe conditions. The daily dosage is reduced to 5 to 20 milligrams in children and elderly and debilitated patients.

Chlordiazepoxide may be given by intramuscular injection for the rapid relief of acute conditions; it must not be given intravenously. Patients receiving injections should be kept under observation, preferably in bed.

UNDESIRABLE EFFECTS. Drowsiness and ataxia occur, especially with high dosage. Treatment with chlordiazepoxide in the severely disturbed patient sometimes results in paradoxical reactions, provoking excitement instead of sedation.

Chlordiazepoxide may give rise to dependence of the barbiturate-alcohol type as described under Phenobarbitone (page 366). It may add to the effects of alcohol and reduce ability to drive motor cars and operate moving machinery.

Rashes, blood dyscrasias and hepatic dysfunction have occasionally been reported.

PRECAUTIONS. Caution should be exercised in using chlordiazepoxide in conjunction with other drugs that act on the central nervous system.

Dose. See above under **Actions and uses**.

Preparation

CHLORDIAZEPOXIDE CAPSULES, B.P. Unless otherwise specified, capsules each containing 5 mg of chlordiazepoxide hydrochloride are supplied. Capsules containing 10 mg are also available.

OTHER NAMES: *Librium®*; *Tropium®*

CHLORHEXIDINE ACETATE

$C_{26}H_{38}Cl_2N_{10}O_4 = 625 \cdot 6$

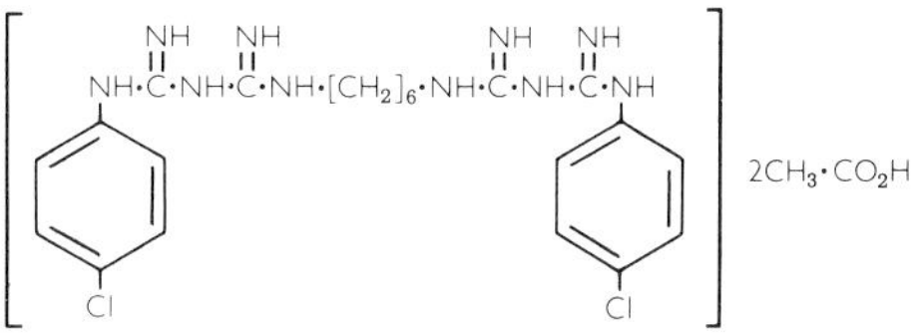

Chlorhexidine Acetate is 1,6-di(*N-p*-chlorophenyldiguanido)hexane diacetate.

Solubility. Soluble, at 20°, in 55 parts of water and in 15 parts of alcohol; very slightly soluble in glycerol and in propylene glycol.

Standard

DESCRIPTION. A white to pale cream microcrystalline powder; odourless or almost odourless.

IDENTIFICATION TESTS. 1. Dissolve 0·1 g in 5 ml of a 20 per cent w/v solution of *cetrimide* in water by gently warming and add 1 ml of *bromine* and 1 ml of *sodium hydroxide solution*; a deep red colour is produced.

2. Dissolve 0·1 g in 10 ml of water and add, while shaking, 0·1 to 0·2 ml of *ammoniacal copper chloride solution*; a purple precipitate is formed immediately which changes to blue on the addition of a further 0·5 ml of *ammoniacal copper chloride solution*.

3. The ultraviolet absorption spectrum exhibits the characteristics given in Appendix 3, page 855.

4. It gives the reactions characteristic of acetates.

CHLOROANILINE. Not more than 0·05 per cent, determined by the following method:

Dissolve 0·20 g in 30 ml of water and add in rapid succession, with mixing between each addition, 5 ml of 1N hydrochloric acid, 1 ml of 0·5M sodium nitrite, and 2 ml of a 5 per cent w/v solution of *ammonium sulphamate* in water. Add 5 ml of a 0·1 per cent w/v solution of N-(*1-naphthyl*)*ethylenediamine hydrochloride* in water, 1 ml of *alcohol (95 per cent)*, and sufficient water to produce 50 ml, and allow to stand for 30 minutes. Any magenta colour that develops is not deeper than that produced by treating in the same manner 10·0 ml of a 0·001 per cent w/v solution of *4-chloroaniline* in water, diluted to 30 ml with water slightly acidified with *hydrochloric acid*.

RELATED COMPOUNDS. It complies with the test given in Appendix 5A, page 860 (2·0 per cent).

LOSS ON DRYING. Not more than 3·5 per cent, determined by drying to constant weight at 105°.

SULPHATED ASH. Not more than 0·2 per cent determined on 1 g.

CONTENT OF $C_{26}H_{38}Cl_2N_{10}O_4$. Not less than 97·5 per cent, calculated with reference to the substance dried under the prescribed conditions, determined by the following method:

Titrate about 0·45 g, accurately weighed, by Method I of the British Pharmacopoeia for non-aqueous titration, using *α-naphtholbenzein solution* as indicator; each ml of 0·1N perchloric acid is equivalent to 0·01564 g of $C_{26}H_{38}Cl_2N_{10}O_4$.

Stability. It is stable at ordinary temperatures but when heated it decomposes with the production of trace amounts of 4-chloroaniline. Aqueous solutions slowly decompose with the formation of trace amounts of 4-chloroaniline.

Hygroscopicity. It absorbs insignificant amounts of moisture at temperatures up to 37° at relative humidities up to about 80 per cent.

Incompatibility. It is incompatible with soaps and similar anionic compounds.

Sterilisation. Solutions are sterilised by heating in an autoclave at 115° for 30 minutes. The solutions should not be alkaline or contain other ingredients that affect the stability of chlorhexidine. If glass containers are used they should be of neutral glass.

Storage. It should be stored in airtight containers, protected from light, in a cool place.

Preparation and storage of solutions. The directions given under Chlorhexidine Gluconate Solution should be followed.

Actions and uses. Chlorhexidine acetate has the actions and undesirable effects described under Chlorhexidine Gluconate Solution. It is used as an antibacterial agent in eye-drops.

OTHER NAME: *Hibitane®*

CHLORHEXIDINE GLUCONATE SOLUTION

Chlorhexidine Gluconate Solution is a 20 per cent aqueous solution of 1,6-di(N-p-chlorophenyldiguanido)hexane digluconate, $C_{22}H_{30}Cl_2N_{10},2C_6H_{12}O_7 = 897\cdot8$.

Solubility. Miscible with water, with up to 5 parts of alcohol, and with up to 3 parts of acetone.

Standard
It complies with the requirements of the British Pharmacopoeia.
It is an almost colourless to pale straw coloured, odourless or almost odourless liquid and contains 19·0 to 21·0 per cent w/v of $C_{34}H_{54}Cl_2N_{10}O_{14}$. It has a weight per ml at 20° of 1·06 g to 1·07 g. A 5 per cent solution in water has a pH of 5·5 to 7·0.

Incompatibility. It is incompatible with soaps and similar anionic compounds.

Sterilisation. Solutions are sterilised by heating in an autoclave at 115° for 30 minutes. The solutions should not be alkaline or contain other ingredients that affect the stability of chlorhexidine. If glass containers are used they should be of neutral glass.

Storage. It should be stored at a temperature not exceeding 25° and protected from light.

Preparation and storage of solutions. See statement on aqueous solutions of antiseptics, under Solutions (page 779).
As a precaution against contamination with *Pseudomonas* species, stock solutions should contain at least 7 per cent v/v of ethyl alcohol or 4 per cent v/v of isopropyl alcohol.

Actions and uses. Chlorhexidine is an antiseptic which is relatively non-toxic and is active against Gram-positive and Gram-negative organisms. Species of *Proteus* and *Pseudomonas* are relatively less susceptible, and it is inactive against acid-fast bacilli and bacterial spores and fungi.

Solutions containing 0·02 to 0·05 per cent are used for treatment of wounds and burns, and solutions containing 0·05 to 0·5 per cent for the disinfection of the hands. A 0·02 per cent solution is used for irrigation of the bladder and serous surfaces. A 0·5 per cent solution in alcohol (70 per cent) may be used for pre-operative disinfection of the skin.

Cetrimide and other cationic detergents may be added to chlorhexidine solutions when additional detergency is required.

UNDESIRABLE EFFECTS. Strong solutions may cause irritation of the conjunctiva and other sensitive tissues.

Preparations
CHLORHEXIDINE CREAM, B.P.C. (page 657)
CHLORHEXIDINE SOLUTION, DILUTE, B.P.C. (page 782)

OTHER NAME: *Hibitane*®

CHLORHEXIDINE HYDROCHLORIDE

$C_{22}H_{32}Cl_4N_{10} = 578\cdot4$

Chlorhexidine Hydrochloride is 1,6-di(N-p-chlorophenyldiguanido)hexane dihydrochloride.

Solubility. Soluble, at 20°, in 1700 parts of water, in 450 parts of alcohol, and in 50 parts of propylene glycol.

Standard
It complies with the requirements of the British Pharmacopoeia.
It is a white or almost white, crystalline, odourless powder and contains not less than 98·0 and not more than the equivalent of 101·0 per cent of $C_{22}H_{32}Cl_4N_{10}$, calculated with reference to the dried substance. The loss on drying under the prescribed conditions is not more than 2·0 per cent.

Stability. It is stable at ordinary temperatures but when heated it decomposes with the formation of trace amounts of 4-chloroaniline. It is less readily decomposed than chlorhexidine acetate and may be heated at 150° for one hour without appreciable production of 4-chloroaniline.

Hygroscopicity. It absorbs significant amounts of moisture at temperatures up to 37° and relative humidities up to about 80 per cent.

Incompatibility. It is incompatible with soaps and similar anionic compounds.

Sterilisation. It is sterilised by dry heat.

Storage. It should be stored in airtight containers, protected from light, in a cool place.

Preparations and storage of solutions. The directions given under Chlorhexidine Gluconate Solution should be followed.

Actions and uses. Chlorhexidine hydrochloride has the actions of chlorhexidine, as described under Chlorhexidine Gluconate Solution. As the hydrochloride is sparingly soluble in water, it is used when a prolonged action is required. It is used in dusting-powders, creams, and ointments containing 0·1 to 1 per cent, in lozenges containing 5 mg, and as an antiseptic in surgical dressings.

A cream containing 0·1 per cent of chlorhexidine hydrochloride and 0·5 per cent of neomycin sulphate is used for the treatment of nasal carriers of staphylococci.

Preparation
CHLORHEXIDINE DUSTING-POWDER, B.P.C. (page 662)

OTHER NAME: *Hibitane*®

CHLORINATED LIME

SYNONYM: Calx Chlorinata

Chlorinated Lime may be prepared by exposing slaked lime to chlorine until absorption ceases; it is sometimes known as "chloride of lime".

Solubility. Partly soluble in water and in alcohol.

Standard

DESCRIPTION. A dull white powder; odour characteristic.

IDENTIFICATION TESTS. 1. It evolves chlorine copiously on the addition of *dilute hydrochloric acid.*

2. Shake a suitable quantity with water and filter; the filtrate gives reactions A and B characteristic of calcium and reaction B characteristic of chlorides given in the British Pharmacopoeia, Appendix V.

CONTENT OF AVAILABLE CHLORINE. Not less than 30·0 per cent, calculated as Cl, determined by the following method:

Triturate about 4 g, accurately weighed, with successive small portions of water, dilute the combined triturates to 1000 ml with water, and shake thoroughly; mix 100 ml of the suspension with a solution containing 3 g of *potassium iodide* in 100 ml of water, add 5 ml of *acetic acid,* and titrate the liberated iodine with 0·1N sodium thiosulphate; each ml of 0·1N sodium thiosulphate is equivalent to 0·003545 g of Cl.

Stability. On exposure to air it becomes moist and gradually decomposes, carbon dioxide being absorbed and chlorine evolved. It is decomposed by hydrochloric acid with evolution of "available chlorine", upon which its value depends. The stability of chlorinated lime in tropical climates is increased by admixture with quicklime.

Storage. It should be stored in airtight containers.

Actions and uses. Chlorinated lime is a powerful, rapidly acting bactericide and deodorant. Its action is brief because the available chlorine is soon exhausted by combination with organic material. It is used to disinfect faeces, urine and other infected organic material and as a cleansing agent for closets, drains and effluents. It is a powerful bleaching agent and will decolorise most dyes.

Chlorinated lime is also used to disinfect swimming baths; it should be added in such an amount that the free chlorine, after combining with any organic matter in the water, is left in a concentration of 0·25 to 1 part per million parts of water.

A concentration of 1 part of free chlorine per million parts of water, maintained for thirty minutes, is an efficient disinfectant for drinking water; the taste of chlorine can be removed by adding a small crystal of sodium thiosulphate to a tumblerful of water.

Hypochlorite solutions have been advocated for the irrigation of wounds and burns and for removing dead tissue and preparing an area for skin grafting. Infected wounds treated by the Carrel–Dakin method of continuous or frequent irrigation with Surgical Chlorinated Soda Solution containing 0·5 per cent of available chlorine are rapidly cleansed and disinfected, but the solution must be renewed at least every two hours. The solution is irritating to the surrounding skin, which should be protected by smearing with soft paraffin. Electrolytically prepared solutions are used similarly, but at the same pH they are no more stable than Surgical Chlorinated Soda Solution, although the salt concentration is usually lower.

Surgical Chlorinated Soda Solution is also a valuable cleansing antiseptic for superficial infected wounds and burns, when applied as a lotion or on gauze as a wet dressing. Diluted with 3 or 4 parts of water, it may be used as a gargle for the treatment of tonsillitis and, with 20 to 40 parts of water or normal saline, as an irrigation solution for infections of the bladder and vagina; it is also used as a foot-bath for the prophylaxis of fungous infections of the feet.

Preparations

CHLORINATED LIME AND BORIC ACID SOLUTION, B.P.C. (page 782)

CHLORINATED SODA SOLUTION, SURGICAL, B.P.C. (page 782)

CHLORMERODRIN (^{197}Hg) INJECTION

SYNONYM: Chlormerodrin (^{197}Hg) Inj.

This material is radioactive and any regulations in force must be complied with.

Chlormerodrin (^{197}Hg) Injection is a sterile solution of 3-chloromercuri-2-methoxypropylurea (^{197}Hg) made isotonic with blood by the addition of sodium chloride.

Mercury-197 is a radioactive isotope of mercury which emits γ- and X-radiation and has a half-life of 65 hours; it may be prepared by the neutron irradiation of mercury isotopically enriched in mercury-196 so that the mercury-203 activity is not more than 0·2 per cent of the total activity, expressed as disintegrations

per second, at the date and hour stated on the label.

Standard

It complies with the requirements of the British Pharmacopoeia.

It is a clear colourless solution and contains not less than 85·0 and not more than 115·0 per cent of the quantity of mercury-197 stated on the label at the date and hour stated on the label. The specific activity is not less than 200 millicuries per gram of chlormerodrin at the date and hour stated on the label. It has a pH of 6·0 to 8·0.

Because of the short half-life of mercury-197 the tests for sterility cannot be completed until after the injection has been issued for use but the tests are carried out to keep the method of preparation under surveillance.

Sterilisation. It is sterilised by filtration.

Labelling. The label on the container states:
(1) the content of mercury-197 expressed in millicuries at a given date and hour;
(2) the volume;
(3) the amount of chlormerodrin in the stated volume;
(4) that the injection is radioactive; and
(5) either that the injection does not contain a bactericide, or the name and proportion of any added bactericide.

Storage. It should be stored in an area assigned for the purpose. The storage conditions should be such that the maximum radiation-dose-rate to which persons may be exposed is reduced to an acceptable level.

Actions and uses. Chlormerodrin (^{197}Hg) is used in a test of renal function. After intravenous injection radioactive chlormerodrin is concentrated in the renal tubular cells, the amount reaching a maximum from one to six hours after administration, the rate of accumulation depending upon the renal blood flow and the efficiency with which the tubules concentrate the substance; the presence of viable renal tissue may then be shown by scanning the area of the kidneys with a radiation detector. The usual dose for this purpose is 150 microcuries.

Chlormerodrin (^{197}Hg) is discharged slowly from the kidneys and is therefore preferred to sodium iodohippurate (^{131}I), which is discharged too quickly to allow satisfactory scanning.

Chlormerodrin (^{197}Hg) is also used for localisation of the kidneys for biopsy and other purposes. It is also administered by intravenous injection, in doses of about 700 microcuries, for the localisation of brain tumours by scanning procedures, but Sodium Pertechnetate (^{99m}Tc) Injection is generally preferred for this purpose.

Dose. See above under **Actions and uses.**

CHLOROCRESOL

$C_7H_7ClO = 142·6$

Chlorocresol is 4-chloro-3-methylphenol.

Solubility. Soluble, at 20°, in 260 parts of water and in less than 1 part of alcohol; soluble in ether, in terpenes, in fixed oils, and in solutions of alkali hydroxides.

Standard
It complies with the requirements of the British Pharmacopoeia.
It occurs as colourless or faintly coloured crystals with a characteristic phenolic odour. It has a melting-point of 64° to 66°; it is volatile in steam.

Preparation and storage of solutions. See statement on aqueous solutions of antiseptics, under Solutions (page 779).

Actions and uses. Chlorocresol is a powerful bactericide and fungicide of low toxicity which exerts its action in acid solution and, to a lesser degree, in alkaline solution. It is used in a concentration of 0·2 per cent in the process of sterilisation by heating with a bactericide and in a concentration of 0·1 per cent as a bacteriostat. It should not be used in solutions intended for intrathecal, intracisternal, or peridural injection, since it may damage delicate tissues; neither should it be used in solutions for intravenous injection where the dose exceeds 15 millilitres.

It is used as a preservative in creams and other preparations for external use which contain water, but its effectiveness is reduced if oils, fats, or non-ionic surface-active agents are present.

OTHER NAME: Parachlorometacresol

CHLOROFORM

$CHCl_3 = 119·4$

Chloroform is trichloromethane to which 1 to 2 per cent by volume of dehydrated alcohol has been added.

Chloroform is non-inflammable, but the strongly heated vapour may be ignited; it burns with a green flame with production of noxious vapours. On exposure to air and light, trichloromethane is gradually oxidised, becoming contaminated with the very poisonous carbonyl chloride (phosgene) and with chlorine. The decomposition is greatly retarded by the addition of the small percentage of alcohol; the alcohol serves also to decompose any carbonyl chloride that may have been formed.

Solubility. Soluble, at 20°, in 200 parts of water;

miscible with dehydrated alcohol, with ether, with most other organic solvents, and with fixed and volatile oils.

Standard
It complies with the requirements of the British Pharmacopoeia.
It is a colourless, heavy, volatile liquid with a characteristic odour. It has a weight per ml at 20° of 1·474 g to 1·479 g. On heating, not more than 5 per cent v/v distils below 60° and the remainder distils between 60° and 62°.

Storage. It should be stored in airtight containers, with glass stoppers or other suitable closures, protected from light.

Actions and uses. Chloroform is a volatile anaesthetic with a pleasant odour. It is one of the most potent, but also one of the most toxic, anaesthetics. The vapour is non-inflammable and relatively non-irritant, although the liquid is irritant to both skin and mucous membranes and may cause burns if spilt on them.
Chloroform sensitises the heart to adrenaline and is liable to lead to ventricular fibrillation with sudden cardiac arrest; this is more likely to occur in patients who are excited, and it may be avoided by adequate premedication.
During anaesthesia with chloroform the blood pressure falls, the respiratory centre is depressed and severe anoxia may occur; this is more likely to occur in exhausted, dehydrated, semi-starved, or toxic patients.
Chloroform is used as an emergency anaesthetic for major first-aid field surgery and for the symptomatic control of convulsions. A concentration of 2 to 3 per cent of the vapour is adequate for induction and 1 to 2 per cent for maintenance of anaesthesia. It is usually administered by open mask or by the semi-closed method, but the use of chloroform in major surgery has been largely discontinued in favour of less toxic drugs.
When taken by mouth, chloroform has an agreeable taste and causes a sensation of warmth. It is used as a carminative and as a flavouring agent and preservative.
Externally, chloroform has a rubefacient action and is used as a counter-irritant. It is also used as a solvent for resins, alkaloids, fats, fixed and volatile oils, gutta percha, and rubber.
Chloroform in a concentration of 0·2 per cent is a useful preservative for aqueous extracts of vegetable and animal tissues.

UNDESIRABLE EFFECTS. Delayed chloroform poisoning occurs from six to twenty-four hours after the administration of the anaesthetic and is characterised by abdominal pain, vomiting and, at a later stage, jaundice. The prolonged use of preparations such as Chloroform and Morphine Tincture which contain substantial amounts of chloroform may give rise to liver damage, especially in children.

CONTRA-INDICATIONS. Chloroform should not be administered to patients with renal, hepatic, or cardiovascular disease.

POISONING. The patient should be kept warm and artificial respiration applied. If necessary, oxygen and carbon dioxide (5 per cent) may be administered. Where poisoning occurs from swallowing chloroform, gastric lavage should be used.

Dose. 0·06 to 0·3 millilitre.

Preparations
CHLOROFORM SPIRIT, B.P. It contains 5 per cent of chloroform, in alcohol (90 per cent). Dose: 0·25 to 2 millilitres.
CHLOROFORM AND MORPHINE TINCTURE, B.P.C. (page 821)
CHLOROFORM WATER, B.P. It contains 0·25 per cent of chloroform.
CHLOROFORM WATER, DOUBLE-STRENGTH, B.P.C. (page 825)

CHLOROQUINE PHOSPHATE

$C_{18}H_{32}ClN_3O_8P_2 = 515.9$

Chloroquine Phosphate is 7-chloro-4-(4-diethylamino-1-methylbutylamino)quinoline diphosphate.

Solubility. Soluble, at 20°, in 4 parts of water; very slightly soluble in alcohol, in ether, and in chloroform.

Standard
It complies with the requirements of the British Pharmacopoeia.
It is a white or almost white, odourless or almost odourless powder and contains not less than 98·0 per cent of $C_{18}H_{32}ClN_3O_8P_2$, calculated with reference to the dried substance. The loss on drying under the prescribed conditions is not more than 1·5 per cent. A 10 per cent solution in water has a pH of 3·5 to 4·5.

Stability. Solutions of pH 4·0 to 6·0 are stable when heated but sensitive to light.

Hygroscopicity. It absorbs insignificant amounts of moisture at temperatures up to 37° at relative humidities up to about 80 per cent.

Sterilisation. Solutions for injection are sterilised by heating in an autoclave or by filtration.

Storage. It should be protected from light.

Actions and uses. Chloroquine kills malaria schizonts at all stages of development. It does not affect the sporozoites inoculated by the mosquito or the forms of the parasite that develop in the cells of the human liver. Chloroquine therefore prevents or terminates the clinical symptoms of malaria by suppressing erythrocytic parasites; it does not necessarily eliminate the infection, and overt malaria may develop when the drug is withdrawn.

When given by mouth as the phosphate or sulphate, it is rapidly absorbed from the gastro-intestinal tract and is slowly excreted. A considerable proportion of a dose is retained in the liver, spleen, lungs, and kidneys, and chloroquine may be detected in the tissues for more than a week after a dose has been given.

Chloroquine is more active and more rapid in action than mepacrine; it causes fewer toxic side-effects and does not stain the skin yellow.

Chloroquine is used for the suppression and treatment of malaria. A total dose equivalent to 1·5 grams of chloroquine base by mouth is usually sufficient to terminate an acute attack of malaria caused by *Plasmodium vivax*, *P. falciparum*, or *P. malariae*; 1 gram of chloroquine phosphate is approximately equivalent to 600 milligrams of chloroquine base. An initial dose equivalent to 600 milligrams of the base is followed by the equivalent of 300 milligrams of the base after six to eight hours, and a further dose equivalent to 300 milligrams of the base is given on each of the two following days. A single dose equivalent to 450 milligrams of the base is usually sufficient to terminate an attack in a partially immune patient.

For the treatment of cerebral malaria in an adult, a condition in which the patient is unable to swallow, chloroquine may be given in a dose equivalent to 200 to 300 milligrams of the base by intramuscular or intravenous injection as the phosphate or sulphate and repeated if necessary on two or three occasions at intervals of four to twelve hours.

For children suffering from severe malaria, with or without cerebral manifestations, chloroquine may be given intravenously. It is best diluted in 250 ml or more of isotonic saline or dextrose saline and given slowly, each dose being run into a vein over a period of not less than thirty minutes. A single dose of 5 milligrams of chloroquine base per kilogram body-weight is usually given and this dose may be repeated after six to eight hours, if necessary.

For the suppression of malaria, the equivalent of 300 milligrams of chloroquine base is given regularly by mouth once a week during exposure to the risk and for three weeks after leaving a malarious area. This dosage will in most cases suppress all species of the malaria parasite and will cure malaria due to *P. falciparum*.

Chloroquine may be given together with primaquine, pyrimethamine, or proguanil.

Chloroquine has no action on malarial sporozoites or on the tissue forms of *P. vivax*, *P. ovale*, and *P. malariae*. Recrudescences may therefore occur in infections due to these species during the year following the cessation of treatment; to prevent these recrudescences, a single dose equivalent to 600 milligrams of chloroquine base is given by mouth to kill erythrocytic parasites and this is followed by a course of treatment with primaquine.

Malarial infections that are resistant to chloroquine should be treated with quinine, pyrimethamine, proguanil, or chlorproguanil, or with pyrimethamine together with a sulphonamide or sulphone.

Chloroquine is of value in the treatment of hepatic amoebiasis, but it has no effect in intestinal amoebiasis. For the treatment of hepatic amoebiasis and liver abscess, the equivalent of 300 milligrams of chloroquine base is given by mouth twice a day for two days or longer and then once a day for a further two or three weeks.

Chloroquine is also used for the treatment of giardiasis, but mepacrine is more effective. For this purpose, the equivalent of 150 milligrams of chloroquine base is given daily by mouth.

Chloroquine is of value in the treatment of systemic lupus erythematosus, particularly when the skin is involved, and of discoid lupus erythematosus and rheumatoid arthritis. Dosage in these conditions lies within a range equivalent to 120 to 900 milligrams of the base daily. For lupus erythematosus, treatment is usually begun with the equivalent of 300 to 450 milligrams of the base daily by mouth, and this is subsequently reduced to the equivalent of 150 milligrams daily. In the treatment of rheumatoid arthritis, remission of symptoms has been obtained after two or three months by giving the equivalent of 75 to 300 milligrams of chloroquine base daily by mouth.

UNDESIRABLE EFFECTS. Chloroquine is well tolerated and toxic effects from antimalarial doses are rare. Pruritus is the most common side-effect; occasionally headache and visual or gastro-intestinal disturbances have been observed. None of these effects is serious and they disappear when administration of the drug is discontinued.

Administration of large doses for periods exceeding one to two years, or occasionally, shorter periods, may produce permanent retinal degeneration and corneal opacities; depigmentation of the skin and hair, wasting of muscle, and acute psychoses may also occur. For this reason, the daily dose for long-term therapy should not exceed 300 milligrams.

PRECAUTIONS. Chloroquine should not be given to patients who are being treated with a monoamine-oxidase inhibitor, such as iso-carboxazid, nialamide, phenelzine, or tranylcypromine, or within about ten days of the discontinuation of such treatment.

Dose. For the treatment of malaria: suppressive, 500 milligrams weekly; therapeutic, initial dose, 1000 milligrams, subsequent doses, 500 milligrams by mouth daily, or, for an adult, the equivalent of 200 to 300 milligrams of chloroquine base by intravenous or intramuscular injection daily.

For the treatment of lupus erythematosus or rheumatoid arthritis: see above under **Actions and uses.**

For the treatment of giardiasis: 250 milligrams daily.

For the treatment of hepatic amoebiasis: 0·5 to 1 gram daily.

Preparations

CHLOROQUINE PHOSPHATE INJECTION, B.P. It consists of a sterile solution of chloroquine phosphate in Water for Injections. Unless otherwise specified, a solution containing the equivalent of 40 mg of chloroquine base in 1 ml is supplied.

CHLOROQUINE PHOSPHATE TABLETS, B.P. These tablets may be sugar coated. Unless otherwise specified, tablets each containing 250 mg of chloroquine phosphate are supplied.

OTHER NAMES: *Aralen®*; *Avloclor®*; *Bemaphate®*; *Resochin®*

CHLOROQUINE SULPHATE

$C_{18}H_{26}ClN_3,H_2SO_4,H_2O = 436·0$

Chloroquine Sulphate is 7-chloro-4-(4-diethylamino-1-methylbutylamino)quinoline sulphate monohydrate.

Solubility. Soluble, at 20°, in 3 parts of water; very slightly soluble in alcohol; slightly soluble in ether and in chloroform.

Standard

It complies with the requirements of the British Pharmacopoeia.

It is a white or almost white, crystalline, odourless powder and contains not less than 98·0 per cent of $C_{18}H_{26}ClN_3,H_2SO_4$, calculated with reference to the dried substance. The loss on drying under the prescribed conditions is 3·0 to 5·0 per cent. A 10 per cent solution in water has a pH of 4·0 to 5·0.

Sterilisation. Solutions for injection are sterilised by heating in an autoclave or by filtration.

Actions and uses. Chloroquine sulphate has the actions, uses, and undesirable effects described under Chloroquine Phosphate; 1 gram of chloroquine sulphate is approximately equivalent to 750 milligrams of chloroquine base.

PRECAUTIONS. As for Chloroquine Phosphate.

Dose. For the treatment of malaria: suppressive, 400 milligrams weekly; therapeutic,

initial dose, 800 milligrams, subsequent doses, 400 milligrams by mouth daily, or, for an adult, the equivalent of 200 to 300 milligrams of chloroquine base by intravenous or intramuscular injection daily.

For the treatment of lupus erythematosus or rheumatoid arthritis: see above under **Actions and uses** of Chloroquine Phosphate.

For the treatment of giardiasis: 200 milligrams daily.

For the treatment of hepatic amoebiasis: 400 to 800 milligrams daily.

Preparations

CHLOROQUINE SULPHATE INJECTION, B.P. It consists of a sterile solution of chloroquine sulphate in Water for Injections. Unless otherwise specified, a solution containing the equivalent of 40 mg of chloroquine base in 1 ml is supplied.

CHLOROQUINE SULPHATE TABLETS, B.P. Unless otherwise specified, tablets each containing 200 mg of chloroquine sulphate are supplied. These may be compression coated.

OTHER NAMES: *Bemasulph®*; *Nivaquine®*

CHLOROTHIAZIDE

$C_7H_6ClN_3O_4S_2 = 295·7$

Chlorothiazide is 6-chloro-7-sulphamoyl-2*H*-benzo-1,2,4-thiadiazine 1,1-dioxide.

Solubility. Very slightly soluble in water; soluble, at 20°, in 650 parts of alcohol and in 100 parts of acetone; insoluble in ether and in chloroform.

Standard

It complies with the requirements of the British Pharmacopoeia.

It is a white or almost white, crystalline, odourless powder and contains not less than 98·0 per cent of $C_7H_6ClN_3O_4S_2$, calculated with reference to the dried substance. The loss on drying under the prescribed conditions is not more than 1·0 per cent.

Storage. It should be stored in airtight containers.

Actions and uses. Chlorothiazide is a non-mercurial diuretic which reduces the resorption of electrolytes by the proximal renal tubules, thereby increasing the excretion of sodium, potassium, and chloride ions, and consequently of water. It also reduces carbonic anhydrase activity so that bicarbonate excretion is slightly increased, but this effect is small compared with the effect on chloride excretion and does not appreciably alter the acid–base balance.

Chlorothiazide is rapidly absorbed when given by mouth and produces a response in about two hours; the diuresis is maintained for six to twelve hours. Tolerance does not develop and the therapeutic efficacy of chlorothiazide is maintained when administered over long periods, but patients may not respond if their glomerular filtration rate is markedly reduced. The usual initial dosage is 1 to 2 grams each morning for two to three days, followed by 1 gram daily for a further two days. Thereafter, continuous therapy is unnecessary and undesirable; the maintainance dose is adjusted to keep the patient free from oedema, the usual practice being to give the drug every second, third, or fourth day. Chlorothiazide and mersalyl may be given together in the management of resistant oedema.

Chlorothiazide is used for the treatment of oedema and of the toxaemias of pregnancy. It enhances the effect of antihypertensive agents and is used, usually in doses of 250 to 500 milligrams, in conjunction with hypotensive drugs in the treatment of hypertension.

Prolonged regular administration of chlorothiazide may produce hypokalaemia. This intensifies the effect of digitalis on cardiac muscle, and administration of digitalis or its glycosides may have to be temporarily suspended.

UNDESIRABLE EFFECTS. Toxic effects such as hypochloraemic alkalosis, acute pancreatitis, and blood dyscrasias such as agranulocytosis and thrombocytopenia, are rare; allergies, epigastric pain, and nausea occur occasionally and acute episodes may be precipitated in gouty subjects. Chlorothiazide may precipitate hepatic coma in patients with impaired liver function and should be used with great caution when there is renal or hepatic dysfunction. It may aggravate existing diabetes or precipitate the condition from a prediabetic state.

PRECAUTIONS. During prolonged treatment with chlorothiazide, supplements of potassium in the form of chloride, citrate, or gluconate should be given. Some patients also show a chloride deficiency and should preferably receive their potassium supplement in the form of potassium chloride. Supplements should be given after meals several hours after the drug or preferably on the days when chlorothiazide is not given, as otherwise much of the potassium is rapidly excreted under the influence of the drug; the usual amount required is 40 to 80 millimoles, or 3 to 6 grams of potassium chloride, daily in divided doses.

Dose. See above under **Actions and uses.**

Preparation
CHLOROTHIAZIDE TABLETS, B.P. Unless otherwise specified, tablets each containing 500 mg of chlorothiazide are supplied.

OTHER NAME: *Saluric*®

CHLOROTRIANISENE

$C_{23}H_{21}ClO_3 = 380\cdot9$

Chlorotrianisene is 1-chloro-1,2,2-tri(*p*-methoxyphenyl)ethylene.

CAUTION. *Chlorotrianisene is a powerful oestrogen. Contact with the skin or inhalation of the dust should be avoided. Rubber gloves should be worn when handling the powder and, if the powder is dry, a face mask should also be worn.*

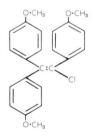

Solubility. Slightly soluble in water; soluble, at 20°, in 360 parts of alcohol, in 28 parts of ether, in 1·5 parts of chloroform, in 7 parts of acetone, and in 100 parts of fixed oils.

Standard
It complies with the requirements of the British Pharmacopoeia.
It occurs as odourless, small, white crystals or crystalline powder and contains not less than 98·0 and not more than the equivalent of 102·0 per cent of $C_{23}H_{21}ClO_3$, calculated with reference to the dried substance. The loss on drying under the prescribed conditions is not more than 1·0 per cent. It has a melting-point of about 118°.

Actions and uses. Chlorotrianisene is a synthetic oestrogen which is stored in body fat, from which it is gradually released. It has the general actions of the oestrogens, as described under Oestradiol Benzoate (page 335).

Chlorotrianisene is given by mouth for the treatment of menopausal disturbances in a dosage of 12 to 24 milligrams daily, for relief in prostatic carcinoma in a dosage of 24 milligrams daily, and for suppression of lactation in a dosage of 48 milligrams daily for seven days.

UNDESIRABLE EFFECTS. Withdrawal bleeding, nausea, and vomiting are rare.

Dose. See above under **Actions and uses.**

Preparations
CHLOROTRIANISENE CAPSULES, B.P. Unless otherwise specified, capsules each containing 12 mg of chlorotrianisene in maize oil are supplied.
CHLOROTRIANISENE TABLETS, B.P. Unless otherwise specified, tablets each containing 24 mg of chlorotrianisene are supplied.

OTHER NAMES: *Tace*®; Tri-*p*-anisylchloroethylene

CHLOROXYLENOL

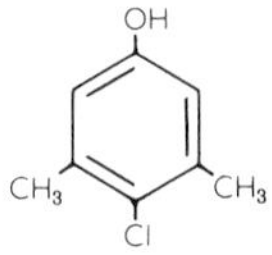

SYNONYM: Parachlorometaxylenol

$C_8H_9ClO = 156.6$

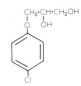

Chloroxylenol is 4-chloro-3,5-xylenol. It is volatile in steam.

Solubility. Soluble, at 20°, in 3000 parts of water and in 1 part of alcohol; soluble in ether, in terpenes, in fixed oils, and in solutions of alkali hydroxides.

Standard
DESCRIPTION. White or creamy-white crystals or crystalline powder; odour characteristic.

IDENTIFICATION TESTS. 1. To 5 ml of a saturated solution in water add 0·5 ml of *ferric chloride test-solution*; no bluish colour is produced (distinction from chlorocresol).
2. Fuse 0·05 g with 0·5 g of *anhydrous sodium carbonate*, boil the residue with 5 ml of water, acidify to *litmus paper* with *nitric acid*, and filter; the filtrate gives the reactions characteristic of solutions of chlorides.

MELTING-POINT. 114° to 116°.

SULPHATED ASH. Not more than 0·1 per cent.

Preparation and storage of solutions. See statement on aqueous solutions of antiseptics, under Solutions (page 779).

Actions and uses. Chloroxylenol is a relatively non-toxic and non-irritant antiseptic. Because it is only slightly soluble in water it is used chiefly as Chloroxylenol Solution, in which its solubility is increased by the presence of soap and which contains other substances such as terpineol and alcohol.

Chloroxylenol Solution is active against Gram-positive and Gram-negative organisms, but species of *Staphylococcus* and *Pseudomonas*, particularly the latter, are relatively less susceptible; it is inactive against bacterial spores.

Chloroxylenol Solution is used as an antiseptic for the skin in surgical and obstetrical practice, and also for cuts, wounds, and abrasions. For general purposes a 5 per cent v/v dilution is used, but twice this concentration should be used in adverse conditions or when excessive amounts of blood, serum or pus are present, as, in common with all bactericides, its activity is reduced by organic matter.

PRECAUTIONS. Solutions should not be applied repeatedly to and wet dressings should not be left in contact with the skin, as hypersensitivity may occur.

Preparation
CHLOROXYLENOL SOLUTION, B.P.C. (page 783)

CHLORPHENESIN

$C_9H_{11}ClO_3 = 202.6$

Chlorphenesin is 3-*p*-chlorophenoxypropane-1,2-diol.

Solubility. Soluble, at 20°, in 200 parts of water and in 5 parts of alcohol; soluble in ether; slightly soluble in fixed oils.

Standard
It complies with the requirements of the British Pharmacopoeia.
It occurs as white or pale cream-coloured crystals or crystalline aggregates with a slightly phenolic odour and contains not less than 99·0 per cent of $C_9H_{11}ClO_3$, calculated with reference to the dried substance. The loss on drying under the prescribed conditions is not

more than 1·0 per cent. It has a melting-point of 78° to 81°.

Actions and uses. Chlorphenesin has antibacterial, antifungal, and trichomonicidal properties and is used for the prophylaxis and treatment of fungous infections of the skin.

Preparations
CHLORPHENESIN CREAM, B.P.C. (page 657)
CHLORPHENESIN DUSTING-POWDER, B.P.C. (page 663)

OTHER NAME: *Mycil*®

CHLORPHENIRAMINE MALEATE

$C_{20}H_{23}ClN_2O_4 = 390.9$

Chlorpheniramine Maleate is (3-*p*-chlorophenyl-3-pyrid-2'-ylpropyl)dimethylamine hydrogen maleate.

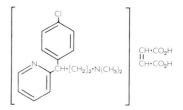

Solubility. Soluble, at 20°, in 4 parts of water, in 10 parts of alcohol, and in 10 parts of chloroform; slightly soluble in ether.

Standard
It complies with the requirements of the British Pharmacopoeia.
It is a white, crystalline, odourless powder and contains not less than 98·5 and not more than the equivalent of 101·0 per cent of $C_{20}H_{23}ClN_2O_4$, calculated with reference to the dried substance. The loss on drying under the prescribed conditions is not more than 0·5 per cent. It has a melting-point of 132° to 135°. A 1 per cent solution in water has a pH of 4·0 to 5·0.

Sterilisation. Solutions for injection are sterilised by heating in an autoclave in an atmosphere of nitrogen or other suitable gas.

Storage. It should be protected from light.

Actions and uses. Chlorpheniramine has the actions and uses of the antihistamine drugs, as described under Promethazine Hydrochloride (page 409) and it is effective in smaller doses than promethazine but it has no marked anti-emetic effect. The usual dose for an adult is 2 to 4 milligrams of chlor-pheniramine maleate by mouth, and for a child 1 to 2 milligrams. In severe allergies it may be given by intramuscular, subcutaneous, or slow intravenous injection in doses of 10 to 20 milligrams; the total dose given by injection in twenty-four hours should not normally exceed 40 milligrams.

UNDESIRABLE EFFECTS. Slight drowsiness and dizziness may occur in some patients.

POISONING. As for Promethazine Hydrochloride, page 409.

Dose. See above under **Actions and uses.**

Preparations
CHLORPHENIRAMINE ELIXIR, B.P.C. (page 668)
CHLORPHENIRAMINE INJECTION, B.P. It consists of a sterile solution of chlorpheniramine maleate in Water for Injections free from dissolved air. Unless otherwise specified, a solution containing 10 mg in 1 ml is supplied. It should be protected from light.
CHLORPHENIRAMINE TABLETS, B.P. Unless otherwise specified, tablets each containing 4 mg of chlorpheniramine maleate are supplied.

OTHER NAMES: Chlorprophenpyridamine Maleate; *Piriton*®

CHLORPROGUANIL HYDROCHLORIDE

$C_{11}H_{16}Cl_3N_5 = 324.6$

Chlorproguanil Hydrochloride is N^1-(3,4-dichlorophenyl)-N^5-isopropyldiguanide hydrochloride.

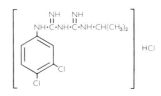

Solubility. Soluble, at 20°, in 140 parts of water and in 50 parts of alcohol; insoluble in ether and in chloroform.

Standard
It complies with the requirements of the British Pharmacopoeia.
It is a white, crystalline, odourless powder and contains not less than 99·0 and not more than the equivalent of 101·0 per cent of $C_{11}H_{16}Cl_3N_5$, calculated with reference to the dried substance. The loss on drying under the prescribed conditions is not more than 0·5 per cent.

Actions and uses. Chlorproguanil is an anti-malarial drug with a mode of action similar to that described under Proguanil Hydrochloride (page 408). It is more active than proguanil and has a longer duration of action. As a prophylactic, 20 milligrams of chlorproguanil hydrochloride is given by mouth at weekly or fortnightly intervals, and administration should be continued for three weeks after leaving a malarious area. It may be given together with chloroquine.

UNDESIRABLE EFFECTS. These very rarely occur during the administration of prophylactic doses.

Dose. 20 milligrams as a single dose.

Preparation
CHLORPROGUANIL TABLETS, B.P. Unless otherwise specified, tablets each containing 20 mg of chlorproguanil hydrochloride are supplied.

OTHER NAME: *Lapudrine*®

CHLORPROMAZINE

$C_{17}H_{19}ClN_2S = 318.9$

Chlorpromazine is 2-chloro-10-(3-dimethylaminopropyl)phenothiazine.

CAUTION. *Chlorpromazine may cause severe dermatitis in sensitised persons, and pharmacists, nurses, and others who handle the drug frequently should wear masks and rubber gloves.*

Solubility. Insoluble in water; soluble, at 20°, in 2 parts of alcohol, in 1 part of ether, and in less than 1 part of chloroform.

Standard

DESCRIPTION. A white or creamy-white powder or waxy solid; odourless or almost odourless.

IDENTIFICATION TESTS. 1. Dissolve 5 mg in 5 ml of *sulphuric acid*; a cherry-red colour is produced which darkens slowly on standing. Warm a portion of the solution; the colour changes to red and finally to magenta. To the remainder of the solution add 0·2 ml of 0·1N potassium dichromate; the colour changes to brownish-red.

2. It complies with the thin-layer chromatographic test given in Appendix 5C, page 873.

3. The ultraviolet absorption spectrum exhibits the characteristics given in Appendix 3, page 855.

4. The infra-red absorption spectrum exhibits maxima which are only at the same wavelengths as, and have similar relative intensities to, those in the spectrum of *chlorpromazine A.S.*

MELTING-POINT. 56° to 58°.

RELATED COMPOUNDS. It complies with the test given in Appendix 5A, page 861 (0·5 per cent).

LOSS ON DRYING. Not more than 0·5 per cent determined by drying to constant weight over *phosphorus pentoxide* in vacuo.

SULPHATED ASH. Not more than 0·1 per cent.

CONTENT OF $C_{17}H_{19}ClN_2S$. Not less than 99·0 and not more than the equivalent of 101·0 per cent, calculated with reference to the substance dried under the prescribed conditions, determined by the following method:

Dissolve about 0·8 g, accurately weighed, in 300 ml of *acetone*, and titrate the solution by Method I of the British Pharmacopoeia for non-aqueous titration, using 3 ml of a saturated solution of *methyl orange* in *acetone* as indicator; each ml of 0·1N perchloric acid is equivalent to 0·03189 g of $C_{17}H_{19}ClN_2S$.

Actions and uses. The actions, uses, and undesirable effects of chlorpromazine are described under Chlorpromazine Hydrochloride.

Chlorpromazine is used in the preparation of suppositories.

PRECAUTIONS AND CONTRA-INDICATIONS. As for Chlorpromazine Hydrochloride.

Preparation

CHLORPROMAZINE SUPPOSITORIES, B.P.C. (page 796)

OTHER NAME: *Largactil*®

CHLORPROMAZINE HYDROCHLORIDE

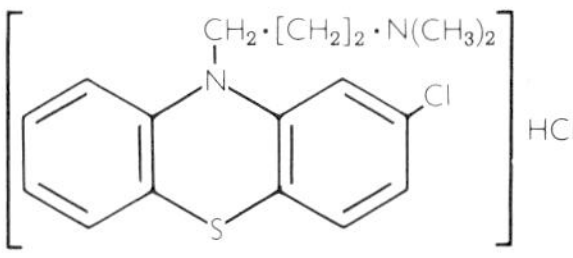

$C_{17}H_{20}Cl_2N_2S = 355.3$

Chlorpromazine Hydrochloride is 2-chloro-10-(3-dimethylaminopropyl)phenothiazine hydrochloride.

CAUTION. *Chlorpromazine may cause severe dermatitis in sensitised persons, and pharmacists, nurses, and others who handle the drug frequently should wear masks and rubber gloves.*

Solubility. Soluble, at 20°, in less than 1 part of water, in 1·3 parts of alcohol, and in 1 part of chloroform; insoluble in ether.

Standard

It complies with the requirements of the British Pharmacopoeia.

It is a white or cream-coloured powder with a slight odour and contains not less than 99·0 and not more than the equivalent of 101·0 per cent of $C_{17}H_{20}Cl_2N_2S$, calculated with reference to the dried substance. The loss on drying under the prescribed conditions is not more than 0·5 per cent. It has a melting-point of 194° to 197°. A freshly prepared 10 per cent solution in water has a pH of 4·0 to 5·0.

Incompatibility. It is incompatible in aqueous solution with benzylpenicillin potassium, pentobarbitone sodium, and phenobarbitone sodium.

Sterilisation. Solutions for injection are sterilised by heating in an autoclave in an atmosphere of nitrogen or other suitable gas.

Storage. It should be protected from light.

Actions and uses. Chlorpromazine is a central nervous depressant which especially inhibits autonomic nervous activity without appreciable action on the spinal cord. It is closely related chemically to promethazine, but it has a much weaker antihistamine action and a stronger local anaesthetic action.

Chlorpromazine reduces the efficiency of the heat-regulating centre so that the patient tends to acquire the temperature of his environment. It produces vasodilatation and a fall in blood pressure, but does not reduce cardiac output. It may induce tachycardia. It reduces salivary and gastric secretions and has a transient anti-adrenaline effect. It causes the skin to become warm, dry, and pale, and it may relieve itching. It induces changes in the electroencephalogram which resemble those of natural sleep more closely than those induced by barbiturates. Chlorpromazine enhances the action of other central nervous depressants, especially barbiturates and analgesics.

In psychiatry, chlorpromazine is used successfully in the treatment of severe psycho-motor excitement and anxiety states. Patients previously aggressive and confused become quiet and co-operative. Within an hour of an oral dose of chlorpromazine and half an hour or less after subcutaneous or intramuscular injection, the patient becomes drowsy, apathetic, less anxious, and occasionally euphoric. A very high proportion of manic depressives in the manic phase have benefited from chlorpromazine. It is not excreted in the milk in significant amounts. Like other sedatives it should be used with care in elderly and debilitated patients, and withdrawn if the depression deepens. It has proved useful in the treatment of addiction to alcohol, barbiturates, morphine, and pethidine.

Chlorpromazine is a valuable adjunct in the treatment of advanced malignant disease; it may be used to reduce the dose of analgesic required and to delay the need to increase the dose, and it may permit the use of a less potent and less dangerous analgesic. Chlorpromazine relieves the nausea and vomiting associated with malignant disease or with the therapy used in its treatment. It not only spares the patient much discomfort, but also helps to maintain his nutrition. It also improves the mental outlook beyond what can be expected from the relief of pain and vomiting. The usual dosage is 25 to 50 milligrams of chlorpromazine hydrochloride by mouth three times a day, or about half this amount by subcutaneous or intramuscular injection. The dosage may need to be increased as tolerance develops.

In anaesthesia, a mixture of 50 milligrams each of chlorpromazine hydrochloride and promethazine hydrochloride and 100 milligrams of pethidine hydrochloride is sometimes given to render the patient tranquil, free from pain, and easily anaesthetised.

Chlorpromazine is effective in the relief of hiccup and of vomiting provoked by morphine and apomorphine. It also reduces the incidence of post-anaesthetic vomiting, but is less effective than certain antihistamines in the control of motion-sickness.

Chlorpromazine hydrochloride has been used in doses of 50 to 100 milligrams four times daily in conjunction with antitoxin in the treatment of tetanus.

UNDESIRABLE EFFECTS. Pallor, postural hypotension, tachycardia, arrhythmias, hypotonia of voluntary muscle, drowsiness, indifference, dryness of the mouth, nightmares, insomnia, depression, and, rarely, agitation may occur but rarely necessitate discontinuation of treatment.

Chlorpromazine may also give rise to amenorrhoea, galactorrhoea, gynaecomastia, blurred vision, corneal and lens opacity, and pigmentation of the cornea, conjunctiva, skin, and retina. High doses may cause the body temperature to fall but sometimes there may be a rise in temperature; cholestatic hepatitis, blood dyscrasias, contact skin sensitisation, rashes, photosensitivity, and megacolon may occur.

Chlorpromazine may cause parkinsonism and other dystonias.

PRECAUTIONS AND CONTRA-INDICATIONS. It is contra-indicated in coma due to direct central nervous depressants such as alcohol, barbiturates, or opiates, and in patients with liver dysfunction or a low leucocyte count. It should not be used in conjunction with drugs such as thiouracil derivatives, amidopyrine, and phenylbutazone that depress leucopoiesis.

Caution should be exercised when treating patients suffering from tachycardia or cardiac insufficiency and those being treated with drugs that may give rise to hypotension. Patients on prolonged therapy should be examined for abnormal skin pigmentation on exposed areas of the body and for ocular changes, and if necessary the drug should be withdrawn.

POISONING. In acute poisoning the stomach should be washed out. If there is acute hypotension the patient should be placed in the prone position with the feet raised, and noradrenaline administered by intravenous drip. The central nervous system depression should be allowed to recover naturally. The body temperature should be allowed to return to normal without active warming, unless the temperature approaches levels at which cardiac arrhythmias may be feared.

Dose. As an anti-emetic: 25 to 50 milligrams by mouth or by intramuscular injection.

For psychiatric states: 75 to 800 milligrams daily in divided doses.

Preparations

CHLORPROMAZINE ELIXIR, B.P.C. (page 669)

CHLORPROMAZINE INJECTION, B.P. It consists of a sterile solution of chlorpromazine hydrochloride in Water for Injections free from dissolved air. It should be protected from light. The strength of the solution should be specified by the prescriber. Solutions containing 25 mg in 1 ml, 50 mg in 2 ml, and 50 mg in 5 ml are available.

CHLORPROMAZINE TABLETS, B.P. The quantity of chlorpromazine hydrochloride in each tablet should be specified by the prescriber. They are film coated or sugar coated. Tablets containing 10, 25, 50, and 100 mg are available.

OTHER NAME: *Largactil*®

CHLORPROPAMIDE

$C_{10}H_{13}ClN_2O_3S = 276.7$

Chlorpropamide is N-p-chlorobenzenesulphonyl-N'-propylurea.

$SO_2 \cdot NH \cdot CO \cdot NH \cdot [CH_2]_2 \cdot CH_3$

Solubility. Insoluble in water; soluble, at 20°, in 12 parts of alcohol, in 200 parts of ether, in 9 parts of chloroform, and in 5 parts of acetone; soluble in solutions of alkali hydroxides.

Standard
It complies with the requirements of the British Pharmacopoeia.
It is a white, crystalline, odourless or almost odourless powder and contains not less than 99.0 and not more than the equivalent of 101.0 per cent of $C_{10}H_{13}ClN_2O_3S$, calculated with reference to the dried substance. The loss on drying under the prescribed conditions is not more than 1.5 per cent. It has a melting-point of 126° to 130°.

Actions and uses. Chlorpropamide is a hypoglycaemic agent which is effective when given by mouth. It probably acts by making more insulin available to the tissues as it has no action on muscle-glucose metabolism. Its only advantage over insulin is that it may be given by mouth; it is not a substitute for insulin, as it is effective only in the presence of functioning islet tissue. It is excreted slowly, the effect of a single dose lasting for twenty-four hours, and the higher blood concentrations which can be maintained with chlorpropamide may make it effective in patients whose blood-sugar levels cannot be controlled adequately with tolbutamide. Hypoglycaemic attacks may, however, be provoked, and may cause prolonged disorientation, especially in elderly patients.
Chlorpropamide is used in the treatment of mild diabetes; it is unsuitable for the treatment of diabetics with more than a trace of ketonuria or with diabetic ketosis, and should not be used in the obese to replace dietetic therapy. The initial daily dosage is 100 to 500 milligrams by mouth. The dose should be adjusted to a suitable maintenance level as soon as the diabetic condition allows, otherwise hypoglycaemic attacks and undesirable effects, such as vertigo, headache, and confusion, may occur. The maximum effect of chlorpropamide may not be evident for four to seven days and adequate control may not be achieved for several weeks. In cases inadequately controlled with chlorpropamide, metformin or phenformin may be administered in addition.
If the patient is taking less than 20 Units of insulin daily, it is usually possible to change to oral treatment with chlorpropamide without admission to hospital. After some weeks or months chlorpropamide may fail to control some diabetics, who then require insulin therapy. During periods of stress, such as pregnancy, infection, or operation, insulin therapy may be necessary for a time.

UNDESIRABLE EFFECTS. Skin sensitisation, gastro-intestinal disturbances, leucopenia, intolerance to alcohol, and jaundice may occur. Such effects are comparatively rare with a daily dosage of less than 500 milligrams. In the event of sore throat or fever, repeated white-cell counts should be carried out, because abnormalities in the circulating blood may not appear for several days.

CONTRA-INDICATIONS. It is contra-indicated when liver function is impaired.

Dose. 100 to 500 milligrams daily.

Preparation
CHLORPROPAMIDE TABLETS, B.P. Unless otherwise specified, tablets each containing 100 mg of chlorpropamide are supplied. Tablets containing 250 mg are also available.

OTHER NAME: *Diabinese®*

CHLORTETRACYCLINE HYDROCHLORIDE

SYNONYMS: Chlortetracyclini Hydrochloridum; Aureomycin Hydrochloride; Aureomycin

$C_{22}H_{24}Cl_2N_2O_8 = 515.3$

NOTE. *The names Aureomycin Hydrochloride and Aureomycin may be used freely in some countries, including Great Britain and Northern Ireland, but in other countries exclusive proprietary rights in these names are claimed.*

Chlortetracyline Hydrochloride is the hydrochloride of 7-chloro-4-dimethylamino-1,4,4a,5,5a, 6,11,12a-octahydro-3,6,10,12,12a-pentahydroxy-6-methyl-1,11-dioxonaphthacene-2-carboxy-amide, an antimicrobial substance produced by the growth of *Streptomyces aureofaciens*, or by any other means.

Solubility. Soluble, at 20°, in 110 parts of water and in 250 parts of alcohol; insoluble in propylene glycol.

Standard
It complies with the requirements of the European Pharmacopoeia.
It occurs as yellow odourless crystals and contains not less than 950 Units per mg, calculated with reference to the dried substance. The loss on drying under the prescribed conditions is not more than 2·0 per cent. A 1 per cent solution in water has a pH of 2·3 to 3·3.

Storage. It should be stored in airtight containers, protected from light.

Actions and uses. Chlortetracycline hydrochloride has the actions and uses described under Tetracycline Hydrochloride (page 498), and is given in similar dosage. The usual dose for children is 20 to 40 milligrams per kilogram body-weight.

Salts of aluminium, calcium, iron, and magnesium, which may decrease the absorption of tetracyclines from the gut, should not be given with chlortetracycline.

UNDESIRABLE EFFECTS; PRECAUTIONS AND CONTRA-INDICATIONS. These are as described under Tetracycline Hydrochloride (page 498).

Dose. For an adult, 1 to 3 grams daily in divided doses.

Preparations
CHLORTETRACYCLINE CAPSULES, B.P. Unless otherwise specified, capsules each containing 250 mg of chlortetracycline hydrochloride are supplied.
BETAMETHASONE VALERATE WITH CHLORTETRACYCLINE OINTMENT, B.P.C. (page 759)
CHLORTETRACYCLINE EYE OINTMENT, B.P.C. (page 698)
CHLORTETRACYCLINE OINTMENT, B.P.C. (page 760)

CHLORTHALIDONE

$C_{14}H_{11}ClN_2O_4S = 338·8$

Chlorthalidone is 3-(4-chloro-3-sulphamoylphenyl)-3-hydroxy-isoindolin-1-one.

Solubility. Very slightly soluble in water; soluble, at 20°, in 150 parts of alcohol, in 650 parts of chloroform, and in 25 parts of methyl alcohol; slightly soluble in ether; soluble in solutions of alkali hydroxides.

Standard
It complies with the requirements of the British Pharmacopoeia.
It is a white or creamy-white, crystalline, odourless or almost odourless powder and contains not less than 98·0 and not more than the equivalent of 102·0 per cent of $C_{14}H_{11}ClN_2O_4S$, calculated with reference to the dried substance. The loss on drying under the prescribed conditions is not more than 0·5 per cent. It melts with decomposition at about 220°.

Actions and uses. Chlorthalidone is a non-mercurial diuretic which has the actions and uses described under Chlorothiazide (page 103). It is effective in smaller doses than chlorothiazide and, as it is more slowly absorbed from the gastro-intestinal tract, its diuretic effect is much more prolonged. It produces diuresis in about two hours and this

may continue for up to forty-eight hours. It does not greatly increase bicarbonate excretion. The usual dosage is 100 to 200 milligrams by mouth on alternate days, but for severe cases the initial dose may be 400 milligrams.

UNDESIRABLE EFFECTS. As for Chlorothiazide (page 103).

PRECAUTIONS. When treatment is prolonged, loss of potassium ions may be sufficient to produce hypokalaemia; potassium supplements should therefore be given as described under Chlorothiazide (page 103).

Dose. See above under **Actions and uses.**

Preparation
CHLORTHALIDONE TABLETS, B.P. Unless otherwise specified, tablets each containing 50 mg of chlorthalidone are supplied. Tablets containing 100 mg are also available.

OTHER NAME: *Hygroton®*

CHOLINE THEOPHYLLINATE

$C_{12}H_{21}N_5O_3 = 283·3$

Choline Theophyllinate is the choline salt of theophylline and may be prepared by the interaction of choline bicarbonate and theophylline.

Solubility. Soluble, at 20°, in less than 1 part of water and in 10 parts of alcohol; very slightly soluble in ether and in chloroform.

Standard
It complies with the requirements of the British Pharmacopoeia.

It is a white crystalline powder which is odourless or has a faint amine-like odour and contains not less than 98·5 and not more than the equivalent of 101·0 per cent of $C_{12}H_{21}N_5O_3$, calculated with reference to the dried substance. The loss on drying under the prescribed conditions is not more than 0·5 per cent. It has a melting-point of 187° to 192°.

Storage. It should be stored in airtight containers, protected from light, at a temperature not exceeding 25°.

Actions and uses. Choline theophyllinate has the pharmacological actions of theophylline and is administered by mouth for its bronchodilator effect in the treatment of bronchial asthma and pulmonary emphysema. It is also used as a mild diuretic for the relief of oedema secondary to congestive heart failure and as a vasodilator in the management of angina pectoris.

The usual dosage is 200 milligrams two or three times a day.

When given by mouth in therapeutically effective doses, choline theophyllinate causes substantially less gastric irritation or nausea than aminophylline.

Dose. 0·4 to 1·6 grams daily in divided doses.

Preparation

CHOLINE THEOPHYLLINATE TABLETS, B.P. Unless otherwise specified, tablets each containing 200 mg of choline theophyllinate are supplied. They are compression coated. They should be protected from light and stored at a temperature not exceeding 25°. Tablets containing 100 mg are also available.

OTHER NAME: *Choledyl*®

CINCHOCAINE

$C_{20}H_{29}N_3O_2 = 343.5$

Cinchocaine is 2-butoxy-*N*-(2-diethylaminoethyl)quinoline-4-carboxyamide.

Solubility. Very slightly soluble in water; soluble in ether.

Standard

DESCRIPTION. A white powder; odourless or almost odourless.

IDENTIFICATION TEST. Dissolve 0·25 g in 8 ml of 0·1N hydrochloric acid and add 10 ml of a saturated solution of *potassium perchlorate* in water; a precipitate is formed which, after recrystallising from water and drying, melts at about 132°.

ALKALINITY. Shake 1·0 g with 50 ml of *carbon dioxide-free water* for 5 minutes and filter; the filtrate is not alkaline to *phenolphthalein solution*.

CLARITY OF SOLUTION. 1. 0·5 g dissolves readily and completely on warming with 5 ml of *light petroleum* (*boiling-range, 40° to 60°*).
2. 0·2 g dissolves completely in 10 ml of 0·1N hydrochloric acid on warming to 50°.
3. 0·2 g dissolves in 40 ml of *liquid paraffin* on warming to 70° to 80°, with occasional shaking; the solution, allowed to stand for 16 hours in the dark at a temperature not below 15°, does not become fluorescent and shows no turbidity or precipitate.

MELTING-POINT. 63·5° to 65·5°.

CHLORIDE. 1·0 g dissolved in 20 ml of water with the addition of 1 ml of *nitric acid* complies with the limit test for chlorides (350 parts per million).

LOSS ON DRYING. Not more than 1·0 per cent, determined by drying for 24 hours over *phosphorus pentoxide* in vacuo.

SULPHATED ASH. Not more than 0·1 per cent.

CONTENT OF $C_{20}H_{29}N_3O_2$. Not less than 98·0 per cent, calculated with reference to the substance dried under

the prescribed conditions, determined by the following method:
Dissolve about 0·3 g, accurately weighed, in 20 ml of 0·1N hydrochloric acid and titrate the excess of acid with 0·1N sodium hydroxide, using *methyl red solution* as indicator; each ml of 0·1N hydrochloric acid is equivalent to 0·03435 g of $C_{20}H_{29}N_3O_2$.

Actions and uses. Cinchocaine has the local anaesthetic properties described under Cinchocaine Hydrochloride and, because of its solubility in oils, it is employed in the preparation of ointments and oily solutions. It is used as a 1 per cent ointment for the treatment of irritant and painful conditions of the skin and mucous membranes. A similar preparation has been incorporated in paraffin gauze dressings and used for dressing burns and raw or granulating surfaces.

An oily solution containing 0·5 per cent of cinchocaine is employed in the injection treatment of haemorrhoids, anal fissure, and pruritus ani and for relieving spasm of the anal sphincter. The prolonged analgesia produced by such a solution is especially valuable in the relief of pain following operations on the anus and rectum.

Oily solutions for injection are prepared by an aseptic technique with a suitable oil which has been previously sterilised by heating at 150° for one hour.

POISONING. The procedure as described under Cocaine (page 120) should be adopted.

CINCHOCAINE HYDROCHLORIDE

$C_{20}H_{29}N_3O_2,HCl = 379.9$

Cinchocaine Hydrochloride is 2-butoxy-N-(2-diethylaminoethyl)quinoline-4-carboxyamide hydrochloride.

Solubility. Soluble, at 20°, in less than 1 part of water; soluble in alcohol, in chloroform, and in acetone; insoluble in ether and in oils.

Standard
It complies with the requirements of the British Pharmacopoeia.
It occurs as fine, white, hygroscopic, odourless crystals and contains not less than 99.0 and not more than the equivalent of 101.0 per cent of $C_{20}H_{29}N_3O_2,HCl$, calculated with reference to the dried substance. The loss on drying under the prescribed conditions is not more than 2.5 per cent. A 2 per cent solution in water has a pH of 5.0 to 6.0.

Sterilisation. Solutions for injection are sterilised by heating in an autoclave or by filtration.

Storage. It should be stored in airtight containers.

Actions and uses. Cinchocaine is a local anaesthetic which is suitable for infiltration, surface, or spinal anaesthesia. Although it is several times more toxic than procaine by injection or cocaine by surface application, it is relatively safer because its local anaesthetic action is greater and it can therefore be used in lower concentrations than are normally employed with procaine or cocaine; in addition it does not produce the idiosyncratic reactions that may arise after the administration of cocaine.

The risk of toxic effects may be reduced by the inclusion of adrenaline, which delays absorption. Solutions containing adrenaline should not, however, be used for inducing anaesthesia in digits, because the profound ischaemia produced may lead to gangrene.

In infiltration anaesthesia, the action of cinchocaine is more prolonged than that of procaine.

For surface application in otorhinolaryngology, cinchocaine hydrochloride is used as a 0.5 or 2 per cent solution. In ophthalmology, a 0.1 per cent solution produces an analgesic effect comparable to that produced by a 3 per cent solution of cocaine hydrochloride. Water-soluble jellies containing 1 to 5 per cent have been employed as anaesthetic lubricants for the passage of bronchoscopes and nasal and urethral instruments. Cinchocaine suppositories have been used for the relief of pain in anal fissure and haemorrhoids.

Lozenges containing 1 milligram may be used for anaesthetising the larynx and pharynx prior to laryngoscopy, bronchoscopy, or gastroscopy, and a 0.1 per cent solution may be injected into the intact urethra before passing a catheter or cystoscope. The onset of analgesia may be preceded by irritation.

For infiltration anaesthesia a 0.03 to 0.1 per cent solution may be used.

For spinal anaesthesia, cinchocaine hydrochloride is usually administered as a 0.1 to 0.5 per cent solution having a higher density than that of cerebrospinal fluid; this solution is prepared by dissolving the requisite dose in Dextrose Injection (6 per cent). Solutions having a density approximately equal to that of cerebrospinal fluid are also used; these are prepared by dissolving 1 per cent of cinchocaine hydrochloride in Sodium Chloride Injection or by dissolving the requisite dose in cerebrospinal fluid. For techniques in which a solution of relatively low density is required, a suitable preparation is a 0.066 per cent solution of cinchocaine hydrochloride in Water for Injections containing 0.5 per cent of sodium chloride.

POISONING. The procedure as described under Cocaine (page 120) should be adopted.

Preparation
CINCHOCAINE SUPPOSITORIES, B.P.C. (page 797)

OTHER NAMES: *Nupercainal®*; *Nupercaine®*

CINEOLE

SYNONYM: Eucalyptol

$C_{10}H_{18}O = 154.3$

Cineole is the anhydride of p-menthane-1,8-diol, and may be obtained from eucalyptus oil, cajuput oil, and other oils.

Solubility. Miscible with alcohol and with light liquid paraffin.

Standard
DESCRIPTION. A colourless liquid; odour aromatic and camphoraceous.

FREEZING-POINT. Not lower than 0°, determined by Method II of the British Pharmacopoeia, Appendix IVB.

OPTICAL ROTATION. At 20°, $-1°$ to $+1°$.

REFRACTIVE INDEX. At 20°, 1.456 to 1.460.

SOLUBILITY IN ALCOHOL. Soluble, at 20°, in 2 parts of *alcohol (70 per cent)*.

WEIGHT PER ML. At 20°, 0.922 g to 0.924 g.

Storage. It should be stored in airtight containers, protected from light, in a cool place.

Actions and uses. Cineole has the actions and uses described under Eucalyptus Oil (page 193), but it is less irritating to mucous membranes. It is used with other counter-irritants in some ointments. It is also used as an antiseptic (0·25 per cent) in dentifrices and as a softening agent to adapt gutta percha fillings and cones to cavities and root canals of teeth. Cineole has been used as an ingredient of oily nasal drops and throat sprays, but oily solutions are unsuitable for these purposes because they inhibit ciliary action and may cause lipoid pneumonia.

Dose. 0·05 to 0·2 millilitre.

Preparation
METHYL SALICYLATE OINTMENT, COMPOUND, B.P.C. (page 762)

CINNAMIC ACID

$C_9H_8O_2 = 148·2$

Cinnamic Acid is *trans-β-phenylacrylic* acid.

Solubility. Very slightly soluble in water; soluble, at 20°, in 6 parts of alcohol and in 15 parts of ether and of chloroform.

Standard
DESCRIPTION. Colourless crystals; odour faint and balsamic.

IDENTIFICATION TESTS. 1. Warm 0·1 g with 0·1 g of *potassium permanganate* and 5 ml of *dilute sulphuric acid*; an odour of benzaldehyde is produced.

2. A saturated solution in *carbon dioxide-free water* is acid to *methyl red solution*.

MELTING-POINT. 132° to 134°.

ALCOHOL-INSOLUBLE MATTER. A 10·0 per cent w/v solution in *alcohol (95 per cent)* is clear.

$$C_6H_5—CH$$
$$\|$$
$$CH—CO_2H$$

SULPHATED ASH. Not more than 0·1 per cent.

CONTENT OF $C_9H_8O_2$. Not less than 99·0 per cent, determined by the following method:
Dissolve about 2·5 g, accurately weighed, in 15 ml of warm *alcohol (95 per cent)*, previously neutralised to *phenolphthalein solution*, and titrate with 0·5N sodium hydroxide, using *phenolphthalein solution* as indicator; each ml of 0·5N sodium hydroxide is equivalent to 0·07408 g of $C_9H_8O_2$.

Uses. Cinnamic acid is used with benzoic acid as an ingredient of Opiate Squill Pastilles to simulate the flavour of tolu.

CINNAMON

SYNONYMS: Cinnamomi Cortex; Cinnamon Bark

Cinnamon consists of the dried inner bark of the shoots of coppiced trees of *Cinnamomum zeylanicum* Blume (Fam. Lauraceae), a small tree indigenous to and cultivated in Ceylon. It is known in commerce as Ceylon cinnamon.

The trees are cut down to form stools, from which adventitious shoots arise; these are cut off when about one or two metres in length, the bark is stripped, and the epidermis and cortex removed by scraping; the strips are then packed, the smaller within the larger, and dried to form compound quills.

Varieties. "Quillings" consist of pieces of broken quills obtained during the manipulation of the quills; they yield about 0·9 to 1·3 per cent of volatile oil.

Constituents. Cinnamon contains about 1 to 2 per cent of volatile oil, with tannin and mucilage. It yields to alcohol (90 per cent) about 14 to 16 per cent of extractive and gives 26 to 36 per cent of crude fibre.

Standard
It complies with the requirements of the British Pharmacopoeia.
It contains not less than 1·0 per cent v/w and Powdered Cinnamon not less than 0·7 per cent v/w of volatile oil.

UNGROUND DRUG. *Macroscopical characters:* single or double, closely packed compound quills, up to about 1 m or more in length and about 1 cm in diameter; outer surface dull yellowish-brown, marked with pale longitudinal lines and often with small scars or holes, cork patches rare; inner surface darker and striated longitudinally; bark about 0·5 mm thick, brittle, fracture splintery.
Odour fragrant; taste warm, sweet, and aromatic.
Microscopical characters: the diagnostic characters are:

sclereids present in the outer phloem, mostly isodia-metric, but sometimes slightly elongated tangentially, usually with the inner and radial walls thicker than the outer walls; some sclereids containing starch granules; inner phloem narrow, mainly consisting of tangential bands of sieve tissue alternating with parenchyma, but containing some axially elongated cells filled with *volatile oil* or *mucilage*; *fibres* thick-walled, up to 30 μm in diameter, solitary or in short tangential rows; total length of fibres per gram 230 to 265 to 290 m; *medullary rays* mostly 2 cells wide, consisting of isodiametric cells; simple or 2- to 4-compound *starch* granules mostly 4 to 8 and rarely more than 10 μm in diameter; minute acicular *crystals* of calcium oxalate also present in some parenchymatous cells.

POWDERED DRUG: Powdered Cinnamon. A dull yellowish-brown powder possessing the diagnostic microscopical characters, odour, and taste of the unground drug.

Adulterants and substitutes. Jungle cinnamon is obtained from wild plants; the bark is darker, coarser, less carefully trimmed and less aromatic than the cultivated bark.
Cinnamon chips consist of small pieces of untrimmed bark; they can be distinguished by their lower yield to alcohol (90 per cent) and, microscopically, by the abundance of cork. A similar material to "chips", but of a better quality, is known as "featherings".
Saigon cinnamon is referred to *C. loureirii* Nees; the quills are thicker than those of Ceylon cinnamon and of a greyish-brown colour with lighter patches, warty and ridged externally, and have a sweeter taste.

Java cinnamon is obtained from *C. burmanni* Blume. It may be distinguished by its low yield of extractive to alcohol (90 per cent) and, microscopically, by the presence in the medullary rays of small tabular crystals of calcium oxalate. The odour is less delicate than that of Ceylon cinnamon.

Seychelles cinnamon, which is inferior in aroma and flavour, is obtained from plants of *C. zeylanicum* introduced into the Seychelles, where they have become wild. It occurs in broken pieces or as rolled quills.

Cassia bark is known as Chinese cinnamon; it is the dried bark of *C. cassia* Blume, a tree indigenous to Indo-China and southern China. It occurs in single quills or channelled pieces, 5 to 40 cm long, 12 to 18 mm in diameter, and 1 to 3 mm thick; colour dark earthy brown, except where patches of thin greyish cork persist; fracture short and granular in the outer part, but slightly fibrous in the inner part; odour resembling that of cinnamon, but less delicate; taste more mucilaginous and astringent. The chief microscopical characters which distinguish it are the presence of cork in alternating layers of thick- and thin-walled cells, the phloem fibres up to about 40 μm in width, the somewhat larger starch granules, often more than 10 μm in diameter. Cassia bark contains about 1 to 2 per cent of volatile oil. The total length of fibres present is characteristic, being 27 to **40** to 55 m per gram.

Storage. It should be stored in a cool dry place. Powdered Cinnamon should be stored in airtight containers, in a cool place.

Actions and uses. Cinnamon is a carminative and is slightly astringent.

Preparation
CHALK POWDER, AROMATIC, B.P.C. (page 776)

CINNAMON OIL

SYNONYM: Oleum Cinnamomi

Cinnamon Oil is obtained by distillation from cinnamon.

Constituents. Cinnamon oil contains about 70 per cent w/w of cinnamic aldehyde, together with eugenol, phellandrene, and other terpenes.

Standard
DESCRIPTION. A yellow liquid when freshly distilled, gradually becoming reddish-brown with age; odour that of cinnamon.

OPTICAL ROTATION. At 20°, 0° to −2°.

REFRACTIVE INDEX. At 20°, 1·573 to 1·595.

SOLUBILITY IN ALCOHOL. Dissolve, at 20°, 1 ml in 3 ml of *alcohol (70 per cent)*; any opalescence produced is not greater than that produced when 0·5 ml of 0·1N silver nitrate is added to a mixture of 0·5 ml of 0·02N sodium chloride and 50 ml of water.

WEIGHT PER ML. At 20°, 1·000 g to 1·035 g.

CONTENT OF ALDEHYDES. 60·0 to 75·0 per cent w/w, calculated as cinnamic aldehyde, C_9H_8O, determined by the method given in Appendix 14, page 893; each ml of 0·5N potassium hydroxide in *alcohol (60 per cent)* is equivalent to 0·06661 g of C_9H_8O.

Adulterants and substitutes. Cassia oil is obtained from the leaves and twigs of *Cinnamomum cassia* Blume (Fam. Lauraceae); it has a much less delicate odour and taste than cinnamon oil and has a cinnamic aldehyde content of 80 per cent or more, a weight per ml at 20° of about 1·06 g, and a refractive index of about 1·61.

Cinnamon-leaf oil contains about 80 per cent of eugenol, has a weight per ml at 20° of about 1·05 g, and a refractive index of about 1·53.

Adulteration with cassia oil or with cinnamic aldehyde increases the weight per ml and the cinnamic aldehyde content. Adulteration with cinnamon-leaf oil diminishes the cinnamic aldehyde content and increases the eugenol content and may be detected by the blue-green colour produced on the addition of 0·25 ml of a 5 per cent alcoholic solution of *ferric chloride* to 10 ml of a 20 per cent alcoholic solution of the oil.

Storage. It should be stored in well-filled airtight containers, protected from light, in a cool place.

Actions and uses. Cinnamon oil is a carminative and is used largely as a flavouring agent and sometimes as a preservative.

Dose. 0·05 to 0·2 millilitre.

Preparation
CINNAMON WATER, CONCENTRATED, B.P.C. (page 825)

CITRIC ACID

$C_6H_8O_7,H_2O = 210\cdot1$

$$CH_2(CO_2H) \cdot C(OH)(CO_2H) \cdot CH_2 \cdot CO_2H, H_2O$$

Citric Acid may be obtained by the growth, under suitable conditions, of *Aspergillus* species on a medium containing glucose, or from the juice of lemons or other citrus fruits.

Solubility. Soluble, at 20°, in less than 1 part of water, in 1·5 parts of alcohol, and in 2 parts of glycerol; slightly soluble in ether.

Standard
It complies with the requirements of the British Pharmacopoeia.

It occurs as odourless colourless prismatic crystals or white powder and contains not less than 99·5 and not more than the equivalent of 101·0 per cent of $C_6H_8O_7,H_2O$.

Stability and hygroscopicity. At relative humidities lower than about 65 per cent, it effloresces at 25°, the anhydrous acid being formed at relative humidities lower than about 40 per cent; at relative humidities between about 65 and 75 per cent it absorbs insignificant amounts of moisture, but under damper conditions it absorbs substantial amounts. At 75° it begins to lose water; at 135° it becomes anhydrous; at about 153° it fuses, and at about 175° it is decomposed into water and aconitic acid.

Storage. It should be stored in airtight containers.

Actions and uses. Citric acid is absorbed from the gastro-intestinal tract, oxidised, and eliminated in the urine as bicarbonate. The alkali citrates increase the secretion of urine and render it less acid.

Citric acid is used in the preparation of effervescent granules. Effervescent draughts may be prepared with citric acid and carbonates or bicarbonates; they are more agreeable if they contain a slight excess of acid.

The following substances form approximately neutral solutions when mixed in the proportions stated with 10 parts of citric acid: ammonium bicarbonate $7\frac{1}{2}$ parts, magnesium carbonate 7 parts, potassium bicarbonate $14\frac{1}{2}$ parts, and sodium bicarbonate 12 parts.

A 7 per cent solution of citric acid is approximately equal in acidity to lemon juice.

Dose. 0·3 to 2 grams.

Preparations
SIMPLE LINCTUS, B.P.C. (page 724)
SIMPLE LINCTUS, PAEDIATRIC, B.P.C. (page 725)

ANHYDROUS CITRIC ACID

$C_6H_8O_7 = 192\cdot1$

$$CH_2(CO_2H)\cdot C(OH)(CO_2H)\cdot CH_2\cdot CO_2H$$

Solubility. Soluble, at 20°, in less than 1 part of water and in 1·5 parts of alcohol; slightly soluble in ether.

Standard
It complies with the requirements of the British Pharmacopoeia.
It occurs as odourless colourless crystals or white powder and contains not less than 99·0 per cent of $C_6H_8O_7$.

Hygroscopicity. At relative humidities between about 25 and 50 per cent, it absorbs insignificant amounts of moisture at 25°; at relative humidities between 50 and 75 per cent it absorbs significant amounts, the monohydrate being formed at relative humidities in the upper part of this range; under damper conditions it absorbs substantial amounts of moisture.

Storage. It should be stored in airtight containers.

Actions and uses. Anhydrous citric acid has the actions described under Citric Acid. It is used for the preparation of effervescent tablets.

CITRONELLA OIL

SYNONYM: Oleum Citronellae

Citronella Oil is obtained by distillation from *Cymbopogon nardus* Rendle or *C. winterianus* Jowitt (Fam. Gramineae) or from varietal or hybrid forms of these species; producing countries include Ceylon, Indonesia, Taiwan, and other tropical countries.

There are two main types of Citronella Oil in commerce which differ in odour and composition and are known as Ceylon oil and Java oil; Formosa oil closely resembles the latter.

Constituents. The chief constituents of citronella oil are geraniol and citronellal. Java oil contains about 35 per cent of citronellal and 21 per cent of geraniol and Ceylon oil contains about 10 per cent of citronellal and 18 per cent of geraniol.

Standard
DESCRIPTION. A pale to deep yellow oil; odour pleasant and characteristic.

OPTICAL ROTATION. At 20°, Ceylon oil, $-9°$ to $-18°$; Java oil, $-5°$ to $+2°$.

REFRACTIVE INDEX. At 20°, Ceylon oil, 1·480 to 1·485; Java oil, 1·468 to 1·473.

SOLUBILITY IN ALCOHOL. Shake 1 volume with 4 volumes of *alcohol (80 per cent)*; a clear or slightly opalescent solution is produced. Allow to stand for 24 hours at 20° to 30°; no globules on the surface are visible to the naked eye.

WEIGHT PER ML. At 20°, Ceylon oil, 0·895 g to 0·905 g; Java oil, 0·880 g to 0·895 g.

ESTER VALUE AFTER ACETYLATION. Ceylon oil not less than 175·0, Java oil not less than 250·0, determined by the following method:
Acetylate the oil and determine the ester value of the acetylated oil by the method given in the British Pharmacopoeia, Appendix IXC, for the determination of free menthol.

Storage. It should be stored in well-filled airtight containers, protected from light, in a cool place.

Uses. Citronella oil is used as a constituent of insect repellents, but is ineffective for this purpose. It is used as a perfume for soaps and brilliantines and is included in Dicophane Application (page 648).

CLEFAMIDE

$C_{17}H_{16}Cl_2N_2O_5 = 399\cdot2$

Clefamide is $\alpha\alpha$-dichloro-N-2-hydroxyethyl-N-p-(p-nitrophenoxy)benzylacetamide.

Solubility. Insoluble in water; soluble, at 20°, in 100 parts of alcohol, in 80 parts of chloroform, and in 40 parts of ethyl acetate.

Standard
DESCRIPTION. A lemon-yellow crystalline powder; odourless or almost odourless.

IDENTIFICATION TESTS. 1. Dissolve 0·01 g in 1 ml of *alcohol (95 per cent)*, add 5 ml of water, 0·5 ml of *sulphuric acid (60 per cent v/v)*, and 0·05 g of *zinc powder*, and allow to stand for 10 minutes; decant the supernatant liquid, cool in ice, add 0·5 ml of *sodium nitrite solution*, allow to stand for 2 minutes, and add 1 g of *urea* followed by 1 ml of a 5 per cent solution of β-*naphthol* in a 7 per cent w/v solution of *sodium hydroxide* in water and 2 ml of a 30 per cent w/v solution of *sodium hydroxide* in water; a red colour is produced.

2. The ultraviolet absorption spectrum exhibits the characteristics given in Appendix 3, page 855.

3. The infra-red absorption spectrum exhibits maxima which are only at the same wavelengths as, and have similar relative intensities to, those in the spectrum of *clefamide A.S.*

4. Mix 0·05 g with 2 ml of a 10 per cent w/v solution of *sodium hydroxide* in *alcohol* (95 *per cent*) and heat on a water-bath for 15 minutes; add 20 ml of water and 5 ml of a 65 per cent w/w solution of *nitric acid* in water and filter; the filtrate gives the reactions characteristic of chlorides.

MELTING-POINT. 134° to 137°.

LEAD. It complies with the test given in Appendix 7, page 882 (10 parts per million).

IONISABLE CHLORINE. Dissolve 0·5 g in a mixture of 50 ml of *acetone* and 25 ml of water, and add a mixture of 0·5 ml of *silver nitrate solution* and 0·05 ml of *nitric acid*; no immediate opalescence or precipitate is produced.

SULPHATE. Shake 1 g with 20 ml of water, and filter; the filtrate complies with the limit test for sulphates (600 parts per million).

TERTIARY BASE. To 2·0 g add 30 ml of *glacial acetic acid* and 5 ml of *acetic anhydride* and titrate with 0·1N perchloric acid, using *crystal violet solution* as indicator; not more than 1·2 ml of 0·1N perchloric acid is required.

LOSS ON DRYING. Not more than 2·0 per cent, determined by drying to constant weight at 105°.

SULPHATED ASH. Not more than 0·1 per cent.

CONTENT OF $C_{17}H_{16}Cl_2N_2O_5$. Not less than 97·0 per cent, calculated with reference to the substance dried under the prescribed conditions, determined by the following method:

Burn about 0·05 g, accurately weighed, by the oxygen flask method of the British Pharmacopoeia, using a mixture of 20 ml of water and 1 ml of *hydrogen peroxide solution* as the absorbing liquid. Titrate the resulting solution by the method given in Appendix 11, page 891, but using 0·02N silver nitrate in place of 0·1N silver nitrate; each ml of 0·02N silver nitrate is equivalent to 0·003992 g of $C_{17}H_{16}Cl_2N_2O_5$.

Actions and uses. Clefamide is an amoebicide with a mode of action similar to that of diloxanide furoate (page 166). It is of particular value in the treatment of chronic intestinal amoebiasis.

The usual dosage is 1·5 grams daily in divided doses for ten days; the daily dose may be increased if necessary to 2·25 grams for a further five to ten days. Doses for children are reduced in proportion to body-weight.

Clefamide is poorly absorbed from the intestine and therefore has no effect in amoebic hepatitis.

Dose. See above under **Actions and uses.**

Preparation
CLEFAMIDE TABLETS, B.P.C. (page 810)

OTHER NAME: *Mebinol*®

CLIOQUINOL

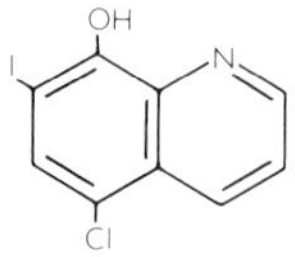

SYNONYM: Iodochlorhydroxyquin

$C_9H_5ClINO = 305·5$

Clioquinol is 5-chloro-8-hydroxy-7-iodoquinoline.

Solubility. Very slightly soluble in water and in alcohol; soluble in dimethylformamide and in pyridine.

Standard
It complies with the requirements of the British Pharmacopoeia.
It is a yellowish-white to brownish-yellow, voluminous powder with a faint characteristic odour and contains not less than 97·0 and not more than the equivalent of 103·0 per cent of total phenols and not less than 90·0 per cent of C_9H_5ClINO, both calculated with reference to the dried substance. The loss on drying under the prescribed conditions is not more than 0·5 per cent.

Storage. It should be protected from light.

Actions and uses. Clioquinol is an antiseptic and amoebicide. It is used in the treatment of intestinal amoebiasis, bacillary dysentery, and ulcerative colitis, the usual dose being 0·75 to 1·5 grams daily in divided doses. For intestinal amoebiasis, treatment should be given initially for ten days and the course repeated after an interval of seven to ten days.

Clioquinol is also used in lotions, creams, and ointments, usually in a concentration of 3 per cent, for the treatment of skin infections.

UNDESIRABLE EFFECTS. Clioquinol stains skin yellow and occasionally causes hypersensitivity.

Preparations
CLIOQUINOL CREAM, B.P.C. (page 658)
HYDROCORTISONE AND CLIOQUINOL OINTMENT, B.P.C. (page 761)

OTHER NAME: *Vioform*®

CLOFIBRATE

$C_{12}H_{15}ClO_3 = 242.7$

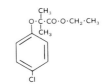

Clofibrate is ethyl α-p-chlorophenoxy-α-methylpropionate.

Solubility. Very slightly soluble in water; miscible with alcohol, with ether, and with chloroform.

Standard
It complies with the requirements of the British Pharmacopoeia.
It is a clear, almost colourless liquid with a characteristic, faintly acrid odour. It has a weight per ml at 20° of 1·138 g to 1·144 g.

Actions and uses. Clofibrate reduces elevated plasma cholesterol, triglyceride, and phospholipid levels, reduces platelet stickiness, and increases fibrinolysis. The mechanism of action is not known.
Clofibrate is used in lipidaemia and other conditions characterised by high blood cholesterol levels, tuberous xanthomatosis,

and diabetic exudative lipaemic retinopathy. There is, however, no conclusive evidence that it improves survival rates in patients with ischaemic heart disease.

UNDESIRABLE EFFECTS. Transient nausea and diarrhoea may occur.

PRECAUTIONS. Clofibrate prolongs thrombin time when anticoagulants are being given and careful control of anticoagulant dosage is therefore necessary.

Dose. 1·5 to 2 grams daily in divided doses.

Preparation
CLOFIBRATE CAPSULES, B.P. Unless otherwise specified, capsules each containing 500 mg are supplied.

OTHER NAME: *Atromid-S*®

CLOMIPHENE CITRATE

$C_{32}H_{36}ClNO_8 = 598.1$

Clomiphene Citrate is a mixture of the cis and trans isomers of 1-chloro-2-[4-(2-diethylaminoethoxy)phenyl]-1,2-diphenyl-ethylene citrate.

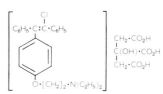

Solubility. Soluble, at 20°, in 900 parts of water, in 40 parts of alcohol, and in 800 parts of chloroform; insoluble in ether.

Standard
It complies with the requirements of the British Pharmacopoeia.
It is a white to pale yellow odourless powder and contains not less than 97·0 and not more than the equivalent of 101·0 per cent of $C_{32}H_{36}ClNO_8$, calculated with reference to the anhydrous substance. It contains not more than 1·0 per cent w/w of water.

Storage. It should be protected from light.

Actions and uses. Clomiphene stimulates the production of pituitary gonadotrophins. It is used to induce fertility by the stimulation of ovulation in anovulatory patients. For this purpose doses of 50 to 100 milligrams of clomiphene citrate are given daily for five days, starting on the fifth day of the menstrual cycle. In patients with amenorrhoea, treatment can be started at any time. If pregnancy has not occurred after six courses of treatment

it is unlikely to do so after further courses and treatment should be discontinued.
Clomiphene has also been used in daily doses of 50 to 200 milligrams for the stimulation of spermatogenesis, but its value for this purpose has not been established.

UNDESIRABLE EFFECTS. Hot flushes, abdominal disturbances, ovarian enlargement, and visual blurring may occur.

PRECAUTIONS AND CONTRA-INDICATIONS. Clomiphene should not be given to patients with ovarian cysts or endometrial carcinoma or during pregnancy and it is inadvisable to continue treatment for prolonged periods. Patients should be advised of the possible occurrence of multiple pregnancy.

Preparation
CLOMIPHENE TABLETS, B.P. The quantity of clomiphene citrate in each tablet should be specified by the prescriber. They should be stored in airtight containers, protected from light, at a temperature not exceeding 25°. Tablets containing 50 mg are available.

OTHER NAME: *Clomid*®

CLOVE

SYNONYMS: Caryophyllum; Cloves

Clove consists of the dried flower-buds of *Eugenia caryophyllus* (Spreng.) Bullock and Harrison (Fam. Myrtaceae), an evergreen tree indigenous to Amboyna and other Molucca Islands, but now cultivated chiefly in Zanzibar and Pemba, Malagasy, and Penang.

The flower-buds are white when young, becoming green and then crimson during ripening; they are collected when ripe and dried in the sun.

Varieties. The bulk of the supplies of clove comes from Zanzibar and Malagasy; these cloves are somewhat shrunken and are smaller, darker in colour, and less fragrant than Penang cloves which are plump and bright reddish-brown in colour.

Constituents. Clove contains about 15 to 20 per cent of volatile oil of which about 85 to 92 per cent consists of eugenol. The drug also contains about 13 per cent of tannins, up to 10 per cent of fatty oil, resin, and a crystalline substance, caryophyllin, which is odourless and appears to be a phytosterol.

Clove yields about 6 to 10 per cent of crude fibre.

Standard for unground drug

DESCRIPTION. *Macroscopical:* from 10 to 17·5 mm long, reddish-brown, heavier than water; lower portion consisting of a slightly flattened 4-sided hypanthium containing in its upper part 2 loculi with numerous ovules on axile placentae; calyx with 4 thick, acute, divergent sepals surrounding a dome-shaped head consisting of 4 paler, unexpanded, membranous imbricate petals enclosing numerous incurved stamens and a single stiff erect style; indentation of the hypanthium with the finger-nail causes oil to extrude.

Odour strong, aromatic, and spicy; taste pungent.

Microscopical: the diagnostic characters are: *epidermis* of hypanthium and calyx teeth composed of straight-walled cells about 8 to **10** to **15** to 25 μm, with thick cuticle; *stomata* anomocytic, circular, 30 to 35 μm in diameter; *glands* ovoid, schizolysigenous, up to 200 μm long, found in all parts; phloem *fibres* occasional, isolated; spongy tissue of the hypanthium; *stamens* each with an oil gland in the apex of the connective; anther walls with a *fibrous layer*; *pollen grains* triangularly lenticular, 15 to 20 μm in diameter; cluster *crystals* of calcium oxalate, 6 to 20 μm in diameter; *starch* absent.

A small number of *sclereids* and prismatic *crystals* of calcium oxalate from the stalk.

ACID-INSOLUBLE ASH. Not more than 1·0 per cent.

ASH. Not more than 7·0 per cent.

FOREIGN ORGANIC MATTER. Not more than 1·0 per cent.

STALKS. Not more than 5·0 per cent.

VOLATILE OIL. Not less than 15·0 per cent v/w, determined by the method given in Appendix 13, page 893.

Standard for powdered drug: Powdered Clove

DESCRIPTION. A brown powder possessing the diagnostic microscopical characters, odour, and taste of the unground drug.

ACID-INSOLUBLE ASH; ASH; FOREIGN ORGANIC MATTER; STALKS. It complies with the requirements for the unground drug.

VOLATILE OIL. Not less than 12·0 per cent v/w, determined by the method given in Appendix 13, page 893.

Adulterants and substitutes. "Blown" cloves are the expanded flowers from which the petals and stamens have become detached. Clove "dust" often consists largely of broken stamens, petals, etc.

Clove stalks are up to about 3·5 cm in length with opposite and decussate branching, the ultimate branches being about 3 mm thick; they are brownish and woody and break with a short fracture; they contain about 5 to 7 per cent of volatile oil, which is less aromatic and somewhat different from that of clove. Clove stalks are said to be used for adulterating powdered clove, in which their presence is easily detected by means of the isodiametric sclereids, by the higher proportion of ash, and by the prisms of calcium oxalate; they yield about 13·6 to 18·7 per cent of crude fibre.

The nearly ripe fruits are also exported under the name "mother cloves" (anthophylli); they contain very little volatile oil and their presence may be detected in powdered clove by the large starch granules which the seeds contain.

Exhausted cloves, from which the oil has been removed by distillation, yield no oil when indented with the finger-nail; they are sometimes artificially coloured.

Storage. It should be stored in a cool dry place. Powdered Clove should be stored in airtight containers, in a cool place.

Actions and uses. Clove is a carminative and a flavouring agent. Infusions of clove have been used as vehicles for mixtures.

Preparation

CHALK POWDER, AROMATIC, B.P.C. (page 776)

CLOVE OIL

SYNONYM: Oleum Caryophylli

Clove Oil is obtained by distillation from clove. It is prepared in Great Britain and also imported from Zanzibar.

Constituents. The chief constituent of clove oil is eugenol (about 85 to 90 per cent v/v). It also contains the sesquiterpene caryophyllene, furfural, which is probably the cause of the oil darkening on storage, methyl pentyl ketone, which gives the much valued fruity odour to the oil, vanillin, methyl salicylate, and up to about 10 per cent of acetyleugenol.

Solubility. Soluble, at 20°, in 2 parts of alcohol (70 per cent); miscible with alcohol (90 per cent) and with ether.

Standard

It complies with the requirements of the British Pharmacopoeia.

When freshly distilled it is a colourless or pale yellow liquid with the odour of clove. It has a weight per ml at 20° of 1·041 g to 1·054 g.

Adulterants and substitutes. The oils, containing 90 per cent or more of eugenol, distilled from clove stems are less fragrant and are used chiefly as a source of eugenol.

Stability. It darkens with age or on exposure to air, becoming reddish-brown in colour.

Storage. It should be stored in well-filled airtight containers, protected from light, in a cool place; contact with iron or zinc should be avoided.

Actions and uses. Taken by mouth, clove oil is carminative. Applied externally to skin and mucous membranes, it is irritant, rubefacient, and slightly analgesic.

Clove oil is used to flavour dentifrices, to which it imparts feebly antiseptic properties.

It is used as a local analgesic for hypersensitive dentine, carious cavities, or exposed tooth pulps, but should be used with caution as repeated application may damage the gingival tissues. A mixture of clove oil with zinc oxide is used as a temporary analgesic filling for deep cavities, but eugenol is often preferred to clove oil for this purpose.

Clove oil has useful preservative properties.

Dose. 0·05 to 0·2 millilitre.

CLOXACILLIN SODIUM

$C_{19}H_{17}ClN_3NaO_5S,H_2O = 475·9$

Cloxacillin Sodium is the monohydrate of the sodium salt of 6-(3-o-chlorophenyl-5-methylisoxazole-4-carboxyamido)penicillanic acid.

Solubility. Soluble, at 20°, in 2·5 parts of water, in 30 parts of alcohol, and in 500 parts of chloroform.

Standard

It complies with the requirements of the British Pharmacopoeia.

It is a white, crystalline, odourless, hygroscopic powder and contains not less than 95·0 per cent of $C_{19}H_{17}ClN_3NaO_5S,H_2O$ and 7·0 to 7·5 per cent of Cl. It contains not more than 4·5 per cent w/w of water. A 10 per cent solution in water has a pH of 5·0 to 7·0.

Stability. Solutions containing 2·5 to 20 per cent w/v may be expected to lose about 5 per cent of their activity when stored for seven days in a refrigerator. At room temperature, losses of up to 15 per cent may be expected over four days, and thereafter the rate of decomposition may be accelerated. The use of buffering agents is of little advantage.

Labelling. If the material is not intended for parenteral administration, the label on the container states that the contents are not to be injected.

Storage. It should be stored in airtight containers at a temperature not exceeding 25°. If it is intended for parenteral administration the containers should be sterile and sealed to exclude micro-organisms.

Actions and uses. Cloxacillin is a semisynthetic penicillin which is not decomposed by staphylococcal penicillinase but which has a considerably reduced antibiotic potency compared with benzylpenicillin. It is destroyed by other penicillinases.

It is stable in acid media and may be administered orally or parenterally. The proportion bound to protein in the blood and tissue

fluids is high so that the level of free cloxacillin in the cerebrospinal fluid is low.

Cloxacillin is mainly of value in the treatment of penicillinase-producing staphylococcal infections. The usual adult dose is 250 milligrams, dissolved in 1·5 millilitres of Water for Injections, by intramuscular injection or 500 milligrams by mouth, taken before meals to ensure maximum absorption, every six hours. In serious infections this can be increased to 2 grams by injection every six hours.

Strains of cloxacillin-resistant staphylococci have been reported.

PRECAUTIONS. The same precautions against allergic reactions should be taken as for benzylpenicillin (page 52). It should not be used topically.

Preparations

CLOXACILLIN CAPSULES, B.P. Unless otherwise specified, capsules each containing the equivalent of 250 mg of cloxacillin are supplied.

CLOXACILLIN ELIXIR, B.P.C. (page 669)

CLOXACILLIN INJECTION, B.P. It consists of a sterile solution of cloxacillin sodium prepared by dissolving the sterile contents of a sealed container in Water for Injections. It should be used within 4 days of its date of preparation, which is stated on the label, provided that it is stored during this period at 2° to 10°; at temperatures approaching 25° it should be used within 24 hours of preparation. The equivalent quantity of cloxacillin in each container should be specified by the prescriber. Vials containing 250 mg are available.

OTHER NAME: *Orbenin*®

COCAINE

$C_{17}H_{21}NO_4 = 303.4$

Cocaine is methyl benzoylecgonine, an alkaloid occurring in coca together with variable proportions of other alkaloids of closely related structure.

Coca consists of the dried leaves of *Erythroxylum coca* Lam. (Bolivian or Huanuco leaf) or of *E. truxillense* Rusby (Peruvian or Truxillo leaf) (Fam. Erythroxylaceae).

The mixed alkaloids of coca are extracted from the powdered leaves by mixing with lime and percolating with naphtha or other similar solvent. Cocaine is either obtained directly from the crude mixture of alkaloids by suitable methods of purification or the mixed alkaloids may be hydrolysed with acid to yield ecgonine, from which, after purification, cocaine may be synthesised.

Solubility. Very slightly soluble in water; soluble, at 20°, in 7 parts of alcohol, in 4 parts of ether, in less than 1 part of chloroform, in 30 parts of arachis oil, and in 120 parts of liquid paraffin; insoluble in glycerol.

Standard
It complies with the requirements of the British Pharmacopoeia.
It occurs as odourless colourless crystals or white crystalline powder and contains not less than 98·0 and not more than the equivalent of 101·0 per cent of $C_{17}H_{21}NO_4$, calculated with reference to the dried substance. The loss on drying under the prescribed conditions is not more than 0·5 per cent. It is slightly volatile and has a melting-point of 96° to 98°. A saturated solution in water is alkaline to phenolphthalein.

Sterilisation. Sterile oily solutions are prepared by an aseptic technique.

Actions and uses. Cocaine is the oldest local anaesthetic, but, because of systemic toxic effects and the danger of causing dependence, its use is now almost entirely restricted to local administration in ophthalmic and ear, nose, and throat surgery.
In low concentrations cocaine affects the nerve fibres and endings concerned with touch and pain more readily than those serving the senses of temperature and pressure, and sensory paralysis may be produced while motor fibres are still active. It should never be applied in an unnecessary high concentration, as, in addition to risks following absorption, it may produce lasting local damage.
When a suitable concentration of cocaine hydrochloride is applied to the mucous membrane, surface anaesthesia develops in five to ten minutes and persists for twenty to thirty minutes or longer, depending on the concentration used and the vascularity of the tissue.
Cocaine differs from other local anaesthetics in that it behaves as a vasoconstrictor, so that adrenaline should not be added to the solution to intensify and prolong its action.
When instilled into the eye, cocaine blanches the conjunctiva and dilates the pupil.

Cocaine is used chiefly as the hydrochloride, but the alkaloid is more convenient for the preparation of oily solutions, suppositories, and ointments. A 5 to 10 per cent spray solution may be used for anaesthetising the nose and throat; concentrations up to 20 per cent may be used for the larynx. The drug may be applied to the urethra as a 0·5 per cent solution before cystoscopy, but even this concentration may prove dangerous if there is any lesion in the urethra.
When taken by mouth, cocaine causes a sensation of exhilaration and well-being, due to stimulation of the cerebral cortex. There is also an increased power to work and overcome fatigue, but large doses cause restlessness, tremors, and hallucinations. The general action of cocaine is used in its administration with morphine or diamorphine for the relief of pain in patients suffering from advanced malignant disease.

UNDESIRABLE EFFECTS. Some people have a distinct cocaine idiosyncrasy and may become dangerously ill after quite small doses; the symptoms are headache, faintness, and collapse, and these may occur with alarming rapidity and terminate fatally. The toxic effects of cocaine are more persistent than is usual with other local anaesthetics, as cocaine is less readily broken down and excreted.
The repeated use of cocaine may lead to dependence (see below); cocaine addicts inject it subcutaneously or use it in the form of a snuff. The addict suffers from extreme stimulation, loss of memory, and an intolerable craving for the drug; loss of weight is usually marked and there is mental deterioration, leading ultimately to a state of permanent moral degeneracy with lack of social responsibility.

PRECAUTIONS. Cocaine solutions should never be administered by injection for local or regional anaesthesia; other local anaesthetics are equally effective and much safer for such use. In particular, cocaine is much too dangerous for administration as a spinal anaesthetic.

DEPENDENCE. The characteristics of drug dependence of the cocaine type are (i) strong psychic dependence, (ii) no development of physical dependence and therefore absence of a characteristic abstinence syndrome when the drug is withdrawn, (iii) absence of tolerance and sensitisation to the drug's effects in some cases, and (iv) a strong need for rapid repetition of the dose.

POISONING. In acute cocaine poisoning, convulsions should be treated by the intravenous injection of a short-acting barbiturate and respiratory depression may necessitate the use of artificial respiration.

COCAINE HYDROCHLORIDE

SYNONYM: Cocaini Hydrochloridum

$C_{17}H_{21}NO_4$,HCl = 339·8

Cocaine Hydrochloride is the hydrochloride of the alkaloid cocaine (methyl benzoylecgonine).

Solubility. Soluble, at 20°, in less than 1 part of water, in 4·5 parts of alcohol, in 18 parts of chloroform, and in 3 parts of glycerol; very slightly soluble in ether; insoluble in fixed oils.

Standard
It complies with the requirements of the European Pharmacopoeia.
It occurs as odourless, hygroscopic, colourless crystals or white crystalline powder and contains not less than 98·0 per cent of $C_{17}H_{21}NO_4$,HCl, calculated with reference to the dried substance. The loss on drying under the prescribed conditions is not more than 0·5 per cent. It melts with decomposition at about 197°.

Incompatibility. It is incompatible with borax, but a clear aqueous solution may be made by dissolving equal weights of borax and boric acid and adding the cocaine salt in solution. It is also incompatible with alkali hydroxides and carbonates, mercuric chloride, phenol, tannic acid, and soluble silver salts.

Sterilisation. Solutions are sterilised by heating with a bactericide or by filtration.

Storage. It should be stored in airtight containers.

Actions and uses. Cocaine hydrochloride has the actions described under Cocaine and is used for the administration of cocaine in aqueous solution.
For ophthalmic use, cocaine hydrochloride is employed in solutions containing 1 to 4 per cent, alone or with homatropine hydro-bromide. The use of eye-drops containing concentrations of cocaine hydrochloride higher than 5 per cent should be avoided, as it may cause desiccation of the cornea.
Pastilles and lozenges containing 1·5 to 10 milligrams are used to relieve throat irritation and hoarseness.
Solutions containing 2 to 20 per cent of cocaine hydrochloride are applied locally to mucous surfaces prior to operation. These solutions are liable to develop fungoid growths and should therefore contain a preservative such as chlorbutol or chlorocresol.

UNDESIRABLE EFFECTS; PRECAUTIONS; DEPENDENCE. These are as described under Cocaine.

POISONING. The procedure as described under Cocaine should be adopted.

Dose. 8 to 16 milligrams.

Preparations
DIAMORPHINE AND COCAINE ELIXIR, B.P.C. (page 669)
COCAINE EYE-DROPS, B.P.C. (page 690)
COCAINE AND HOMATROPINE EYE-DROPS, B.P.C. (page 690)

COCHINEAL

SYNONYMS: Coccus; Coccus Cacti

Cochineal is the dried female insect, *Dactylopius coccus* Costa (Fam. Coccidae), containing eggs and larvae.

The insects are indigenous to central America and Mexico, but the drug is now chiefly obtained from Peru and also from the Canary Islands, where the insects are reared upon the branches of various species of *Nopalea* (Fam. Cactaceae). After fecundation the insects increase in size and develop an abundance of red colouring matter. They are then brushed off the plant, killed by the fumes of burning sulphur or charcoal, or by heat, and dried in the sun.

Varieties. "Black-brilliant" cochineal is uniformly purplish-black and consists of insects of which the waxy secretion has been melted by the heat applied during preparation for the market. "Silver-grey" cochineal is greyish-white and retains some or all of the waxy covering in its original condition.

Constituents. Cochineal contains about 10 per cent of the anthraquinone glycoside 6-D-glucopyranosyl-9,10-dihydro-2,5,7,8-tetrahydroxy-4-methyl-9,10-dioxoanthracene-1-carboxylic acid (carminic acid), which occurs as small red prismatic crystals, soluble in water, in alcohol, and in alkaline solutions.
About 10 per cent of fat and 2 per cent of wax are also present, as well as albuminoids and inorganic matter. The fat consists almost entirely of free oleic, linoleic, and myristic acids.

Standard
It complies with the requirements of the British Pharmacopoeia.

Macroscopical characters: purplish-black or purplish-grey in colour, about 3·5 to 5·5 mm long and 3 to 4·5 mm broad, oval in outline; dorsal surface convex, transversely wrinkled, and showing about 11 segments; ventral surface flat or slightly concave, whole insects carrying upon anterior part two 7-jointed straight

antennae, about 0·3 mm long, 3 pairs of short legs, each about 1 mm long, terminating in a single claw, and a mouth from which projects the remains of a filiform proboscis; drug readily reduced to red or puce-coloured powder.
Odour and taste characteristic.

Microscopical characters: the diagnostic characters are: numerous short tubular *wax glands* scattered over the dermis, either singly or in groups; the insect has two *eyes*, each composed of a single lens; numerous *larvae*, usually about 150, present in each insect; each larva about 0·75 mm long with *proboscides* appearing as two circular coils, one in each side of head; *muscle fibre* abundant.

Adulterants and substitutes. Cochineal has been artificially weighted with inorganic matter. In the case of the "silver-grey" variety, barium or lead carbonate or sulphate has been used, while the "black-brilliant" variety has been "faced" with graphite, ivory black, or manganese dioxide, and has been mixed with very dark grains of magnetic sand containing iron.

Storage. It should be stored in a dry place.

Uses. Cochineal, in the form of a tincture or solution, is used as a colouring agent, but its colouring properties are modified in acid solution.

COCILLANA

SYNONYMS: Grape Bark; Guapi Bark

Cocillana is the dried bark from *Guarea rusbyi* (Britton) Rusby and closely related species (Fam. Meliaceae). The tree is indigenous to South America, growing on the eastern slopes of the Andes in Bolivia.

Constituents. Cocillana contains about 2·3 per cent of resins, about 2·5 per cent of fixed oil, and tannin; traces of an alkaloid and possibly a glycoside are also present. The bark yields about 7·5 per cent of ash.

Standard for unground drug
DESCRIPTION. *Macroscopical:* large flattish or curved pieces up to about 60 cm long and 15 cm wide and from 5 to 20 mm in thickness; outer surface showing shallow or deep longitudinal fissures according to age, colour grey-brown or orange-brown where cork has been removed, and often bearing whitish patches of lichens; inner surface longitudinally striated with straight or slightly wavy striae and easily detachable fibre strands; fracture short and granular in outer part, coarsely splintery, fibrous, and soft in the much thicker inner part; tranversely cut surface showing a narrow outer corky region and wider inner region with dark-coloured, narrow, wavy medullary rays.
Odour slight and characteristic; taste slightly astringent and slightly nauseous.

Microscopical: the diagnostic characters are: *cork* cells in layers alternating with parenchyma containing yellowish *sclereids*, angular or irregular in shape and up to 150 μm long; *fibres* straight, in numerous tangentially elongated groups alternating with tangential bands of dark-coloured *parenchyma* and *sieve tubes*, each fibre group surrounded by a *crystal sheath* with prisms of calcium oxalate from 10 to 25 μm long; *medullary rays* 1 to 3 cells wide; cells of medullary rays and parenchyma with red-brown contents and single sphaeroidal 2- to 4-compound *starch* granules, individual granules 5 to 20 μm in diameter.

ALCOHOL (60 PER CENT)-SOLUBLE EXTRACTIVE. Not less than 3·5 per cent.

Standard for powdered drug: Powdered Cocillana DESCRIPTION. A greyish-brown powder possessing the diagnostic microscopical characters, odour, and taste of the unground drug.

ALCOHOL (60 PER CENT)-SOLUBLE EXTRACTIVE. It complies with the requirement for the unground drug.

Adulterants and substitutes. The barks of *G. bangii* Rusby and of species of *Nectandra* (Fam. Lauraceae) have been reported as adulterants.
The bark of *G. bangii* is roughly striate and peels in long thin fibrous strips; it has a more reddish cork; its fracture is tougher and more fibrous, the fibres projecting throughout the inner bark; the sclereids are smaller and the crystals less numerous; the powdered bark is light chocolate-brown.
Bark of *Nectandra* species contains oil cells and has a camphoraceous odour.

Actions and uses. Cocillana is an expectorant and, in large doses, an emetic. It has been used as an alternative to ipecacuanha in the treatment of coughs. It is administered as the liquid extract in conjunction with other expectorants.

Dose. 0·5 to 1 gram.

Preparation
COCILLANA LIQUID EXTRACT, B.P.C. (page 682)

COCONUT OIL

Coconut Oil is the oil obtained by expression from the dried solid part of the endosperm of *Cocos nucifera* L. (Fam. Palmae), a tree cultivated throughout the tropics.

Constituents. Coconut oil contains triglycerides, the fatty acid constituents of which are mainly lauric and myristic acids with smaller proportions of capric, caproic, caprylic, oleic, palmitic, and stearic acids.

Solubility. Soluble, at 60°, in 2 parts of alcohol, less soluble at lower temperatures; very soluble in ether and in chloroform.

Standard
DESCRIPTION. A white or pearl-white unctuous mass; odourless or with the odour of coconut.

REFRACTIVE INDEX. At 40°, 1·448 to 1·450.

MELTING-POINT. 23° to 26°, determined by Method IV of the British Pharmacopoeia, Appendix IVA.

ACID VALUE. Not more than 0·2, determined on 20 g.

IODINE VALUE. 7·0 to 11·0.

PEROXIDES. Dissolve 5·0 g in 15 ml of *chloroform*, add 20 ml of *acetic acid* and 0·5 ml of a saturated solution of *potassium iodide* in water, mix, and allow to stand in the dark for exactly 1 minute. Add 30 ml of water and titrate with 0·01N sodium thiosulphate, using *starch mucilage* as indicator; not more than 0·5 ml is required.

SAPONIFICATION VALUE. 250 to 264.

UNSAPONIFIABLE MATTER. Not more than 0·8 per cent.

Stability. On exposure to the air, the oil readily becomes rancid, acquiring an unpleasant odour and a strong, acrid taste.

Storage. It should be stored in well-filled, airtight containers, protected from light, in a cool place.

Uses. Coconut oil is used as an ointment basis, particularly in preparations intended for application to the scalp. It is also used to prepare soaps with a high solubility in water.

FRACTIONATED COCONUT OIL

SYNONYM: Thin Vegetable Oil

Fractionated Coconut Oil is the fixed oil, subsequently fractionated and refined, obtained from the dried solid part of the endosperm of *Cocos nucifera* L. (Fam. Palmae), a tree cultivated throughout the tropics.

Constituents. It consists of a mixture of triglycerides containing only short- and medium-chain saturated fatty acids, mainly octanoic and decanoic acids.

Solubility. Almost insoluble in water; miscible with alcohol, with ether, and with chloroform.

Standard

It complies with the requirements of the British Pharmacopoeia.

It is a clear, pale yellow, odourless or almost odourless liquid. It has a weight per ml at 20° of 0·940 g to 0·950 g.

It solidifies at about 0° and has a low viscosity even at temperatures near its solidification point.

Storage. It should be stored in well-filled containers, protected from light, in a cool place.

Uses. Fractionated coconut oil is used as a non-aqueous vehicle for oral preparations. Because of its oily nature, the addition of suitable colouring or flavouring agents presents difficulties.

Flavouring agents are limited to imitation ground-almond flavour and imitation olive-oil flavour. Only two oil-soluble colours are permitted in the United Kingdom and these are both shades of yellow, but the lakes of suitable water-soluble food dyes may be dispersed in the oil; sweetening agents such as saccharin may be added in a similar manner.

CODEINE PHOSPHATE

SYNONYM: Codeinii Phosphas

$C_{18}H_{24}NO_7P,\frac{1}{2}H_2O = 406·4$

Codeine Phosphate is the phosphate of the 3-methyl ether of morphine.

Solubility. Soluble, at 20°, in 4 parts of water and in 450 parts of alcohol; very slightly soluble in ether and in chloroform.

Standard

It complies with the requirements of the European Pharmacopoeia.

It occurs as odourless, small, colourless crystals or white crystalline powder and contains not less than 98·0 per cent of $C_{18}H_{24}NO_7P$, calculated with reference to the dried substance. The loss on drying under the prescribed conditions is not more than 3·0 per cent. A 4 per cent solution in water has a pH of 4·2 to 5·0.

Sterilisation. Solutions for injection are sterilised by heating in an autoclave or by filtration.

Storage. It should be stored in airtight containers, protected from light.

Actions and uses. Codeine has moderate analgesic and weak cough-suppressant effects. It is also used to check diarrhoea. It is less depressant to the respiratory centre and causes much less nausea and vomiting than morphine.

UNDESIRABLE EFFECTS. Constipation commonly occurs.

POISONING. The procedure described under

Morphine Hydrochloride (page 314) should be adopted.

Dose. 10 to 60 milligrams.

Preparations

CODEINE LINCTUS, B.P.C. (page 722)

CODEINE LINCTUS, DIABETIC, B.P.C. (page 722)

CODEINE LINCTUS, PAEDIATRIC, B.P.C. (page 722)

CODEINE PHOSPHATE SYRUP, B.P.C. (page 799)

ASPIRIN, PHENACETIN, and CODEINE TABLETS, B.P. (*Syn.* Compound Codeine Tablets). Each tablet contains 250 mg of aspirin and of phenacetin and 8 mg of codeine phosphate. They should be stored in airtight containers, protected from light. Dose: 1 or 2 tablets.

ASPIRIN, PHENACETIN, and CODEINE TABLETS, SOLUBLE, B.P. (*Syn.* Soluble Compound Codeine Tablets). Each tablet contains 250 mg of aspirin and of phenacetin and 8 mg of codeine phosphate with calcium carbonate, anhydrous citric acid, and saccharin sodium. They should be stored in airtight containers, protected from light. Dose: 1 or 2 tablets.

CODEINE PHOSPHATE TABLETS, B.P. Unless otherwise specified, tablets each containing 30 mg of codeine phosphate are supplied. They should be stored in airtight containers, protected from light. Tablets containing 15 and 60 mg are also available.

COD-LIVER OIL

SYNONYM: Oleum Morrhuae

Cod-liver Oil is the fixed oil obtained from the fresh liver of the cod, *Gadus morhua* (= *G. callarius* L.) (Fam. Gadidae), and other species of *Gadus*, by the application of low-pressure steam at a temperature not exceeding 85°. The oil is cooled to about 0° and filtered to remove the separated fat.

Constituents. The vitamin-A activity varies very widely in different samples, but an average sample contains about 1000 Units per g. The vitamin-D content varies from about 50 to 250 Units of antirachitic activity (vitamin D) per g, the average being about 100 Units. The fatty acid constituents of the glycerides of cod-liver oil are largely unsaturated and consist chiefly of docosahexaenoic acid and a highly unsaturated acid containing 18 to 20 carbon atoms; glycerides of oleic acid are probably absent, but those of palmitic and stearic acids occur in small quantities. The unsaponifiable matter consists chiefly of cholesterol with small amounts of batyl alcohol, squalene, and the vitamins A and D. Cod-liver oil may contain a trace of iodine.

Solubility. Very slightly soluble in alcohol; miscible with ether, with chloroform, and with light petroleum.

Standard
It complies with the requirements of the British Pharmacopoeia.
It is a pale yellow liquid with a slightly fishy but not rancid odour and contains in 1 g not less than 600 Units of vitamin-A activity and not less than 85 Units of antirachitic activity (vitamin D). It may contain up to 100 parts per million of dodecyl gallate, or propyl gallate, or any mixture of these substances, as an antioxidant. It has a weight per ml at 20° of 0·917 g to 0·924 g.
When maintained at 0° for three hours, it remains bright (limit of stearin).

Adulterants and substitutes. Other liver oils such as those of the seal (*Phoca* species), haddock (*Melanogrammus aeglefinus*), shark (*Carcharias* species), and coal fish (*Pollachius carbonarius*).

Stability. If properly stored, cod-liver oil retains its potency and characters for many years. Inferior or old oils are liable to be dark in colour, acrid or bitter, unduly acid, and somewhat rancid. On exposing the oil to sunlight the vitamin A is rapidly destroyed; on exposure to air the oil absorbs oxygen and becomes thicker, but does not dry to a hard varnish.

Storage. It should be stored in well-filled airtight containers, protected from light, in a cool place.

Actions and uses. Cod-liver oil is a valuable source of vitamins A and D and of readily digestible fat. Because of its vitamin-D content, cod-liver oil promotes absorption of calcium and phosphorus from the gut and prevents rickets. Cod-liver oil also contains several unsaturated fatty acids which are essential food factors. These are absent from vitamin A and D concentrates, which are often given in place of cod-liver oil.

The antirachitic activity of cod-liver oil is believed to be due to vitamin D_3 (cholecalciferol), which occurs in various fish-liver oils and may be obtained by the ultraviolet irradiation of 7-dehydrocholesterol; there is some evidence that vitamin D_2 (calciferol) differs from vitamin D_3 in antirachitic activity in man.

Cod-liver oil is used as a dietary supplement for infants and children to prevent the occurrence of rickets and to improve nutrition and calcification of bones in undernourished children and in patients with rickets. It is administered alone, in capsules, and in Malt Extract with Cod-liver Oil.

Cod-liver oil is also used externally as an application for the treatment of burns, wounds, and ulcers, but there is no evidence that such treatment is beneficial.

Dose. As a prophylactic against rickets, not more than 10 millilitres daily, allowance being made for vitamin D obtained from other sources.

Preparation
MALT EXTRACT WITH COD-LIVER OIL, B.P.C. (page 684)

COLCHICINE

$C_{22}H_{25}NO_6 = 399·4$

Colchicine is an alkaloid obtained from colchicum corm and seeds.

Solubility. Soluble in water, in alcohol, and in chloroform; soluble, at 15·5°, in 160 parts of ether; almost insoluble in light petroleum.
Moderately concentrated aqueous solutions may deposit crystals of a sesquihydrate, which is almost insoluble in cold water.

Standard
It complies with the requirements of the British Pharmacopoeia.
It occurs as pale yellow odourless crystals, amorphous scales, or powder. It has a hay-like odour when

damped and warmed and darkens on exposure to light. The loss on drying over phosphorus pentoxide at a pressure not exceeding 5 mmHg is not more than 2·0 per cent.

Sterilisation. Solutions for injection are sterilised by heating in an autoclave or by filtration.

Storage. It should be stored in airtight containers protected from light.

Actions and uses. Colchicine is used for the relief of pain in acute gout.

For the treatment of acute episodes, it is administered by mouth in a dosage of 1 milligram initially, followed by 500 micrograms every two hours until relief is obtained or gastro-intestinal symptoms such as vomiting and diarrhoea make its further use undesirable; the total amount given during a course of treatment should not exceed 6 milligrams. When a rapid response is required or gastro-intestinal upset precludes oral administration, 2 to 4 milligrams in Sodium Chloride Injection can be given by intravenous injection. For the prevention of acute episodes, colchicine may be given for long periods in smaller

doses such as 0·5 to 1 milligram by mouth each night.

UNDESIRABLE EFFECTS. In large doses, after a latent period of one to three hours, colchicine has a marked action on involuntary muscle, especially that of the intestine, and causes severe diarrhoea. Liver damage may occur.

Dose. See above under **Actions and uses.**

Preparation
COLCHICINE TABLETS, B.P. Unless otherwise specified, tablets each containing 500 μg of colchicine are supplied. They should be protected from light. Tablets containing 250 μg are also available.

COLCHICUM CORM

Colchicum Corm is the corm of the meadow saffron, *Colchicum autumnale* L. (Fam. Liliaceae), a plant widely distributed over central and southern Europe and common in parts of England.

Colchicum Corm is collected in early summer after the leaves have died down, and is prepared by removing the scale leaves, slicing transversely, and drying at a temperature not higher than 65°.

Constituents. Colchicum corm contains about 0·08 to 0·15 per cent of the alkaloid colchicine, together with closely related alkaloids; it also contains starch, gum, sugar, tannin, colouring matter, and fat. It yields about 4 per cent of ash.

Standard
It complies with the requirements of the British Pharmacopoeia.
It contains not less than 0·25 per cent of alkaloids.

UNGROUND DRUG. *Macroscopical characters:* slices, about 2 to 5 mm thick, sub-reniform or ovate in outline, a few subconical or plano-convex, edges yellowish-brown; fracture short, mealy; transversely cut surfaces white and starchy with numerous scattered vascular bundles showing as small greyish points; cut surface immediately coloured yellow by *hydrochloric acid* or *sulphuric acid (20 per cent v/v).* Odourless; taste bitter and acrid.

Microscopical characters: the diagnostic characters are: *epidermal cells* brown, rectangular to polygonal, 40 to **60** to 90 μm wide, anticlinal walls slightly wavy and indistinctly pitted; *stomata* anomocytic, occasional; *ground tissue* of very thin-walled, polygonal, parenchymatous cells about 50 to 100 μm in diameter; cells pitted, containing simple or usually 2- to 3-compound *starch* granules, individual granules spherical, polyhedral, or muller-shaped, about 3 to **12** to **16** to 30 μm in diameter, usually with a triangular or stellate central hilum; numerous slender *vascular bundles* with *vessels*

up to 30 μm wide, wall thickening spiral or annular; *crystals* of calcium oxalate absent.

POWDERED DRUG: Powdered Colchicum Corm. A pale buff powder possessing the diagnostic microscopical characters, odour, and taste of the unground drug.

Adulterants and substitutes. Indian colchicum corm consists of the corms of *C. luteum* Baker; they are small, usually entire, and often semi-translucent owing to gelatinisation of the starch. It contains only traces of colchicine.
Colchicum seeds are subspherical, about 2 to 3 mm in diameter, with a projection at the hilum and a strophiole extending along about one-quarter of the circumference; testa reddish-brown, dull, somewhat rough; endosperm hard, oily and yellowish; embryo straight, about 0·5 mm long, placed radially; odourless, taste unpleasant and bitter; they contain about 0·3 to 0·6 per cent of alkaloids, calculated as colchicine.

Actions and uses. Preparations of colchicum corm relieve the pain and inflammation of acute gout; their use for long periods is not recommended. They may cause considerable gastro-intestinal irritation with vomiting and purging.

Preparations
COLCHICUM LIQUID EXTRACT, B.P. It contains 0·3 per cent of alkaloids.

COLCHICUM AND SODIUM SALICYLATE MIXTURE, B.P.C. (page 740)

COLCHICUM TINCTURE, B.P. It contains 0·03 per cent of alkaloids. Dose: 0·5 to 2 millilitres; up to 6 millilitres daily in divided doses.

COLISTIN SULPHATE

Colistin Sulphate is a mixture of the sulphates of the antimicrobial substances produced by the growth of a selected strain of *Bacillus polymyxa* var. *colistinus.*

Solubility. Soluble, at 20°, in less than 2 parts of water and in 300 parts of alcohol; insoluble in ether, in chloroform, in acetone, and in propylene glycol.

Standard
It complies with the requirements of the British Pharmacopoeia.
It is a white to cream-coloured powder with a faint

odour and contains not less than 17,500 Units per mg, calculated with reference to the dried substance. The loss on drying under the prescribed conditions is not more than 3·5 per cent. A 1 per cent solution in water has a pH of 4·0 to 5·8.

Stability. Aqueous solutions may be expected to retain their potency for four weeks when stored at room temperature or for eight weeks when stored at 2° to 4°.

Storage. It should be stored in airtight containers, protected from light.

Actions and uses. Colistin is an antibiotic with a range of activity similar to polymyxin B (page 388), being active against a wide variety of Gram-negative bacteria, with the exception of strains of *Proteus*. It is poorly absorbed from the gastro-intestinal tract and so is of no value in systemic infections, but may be useful when antibiotic treatment of gastro-

enteritis is thought necessary. Overgrowth of non-susceptible organisms, particularly species of *Proteus*, may occur.

UNDESIRABLE EFFECTS. Rashes may occur.

Dose. 9 to 18 mega Units daily in divided doses.

Preparation

COLISTIN TABLETS, B.P. Unless otherwise specified, tablets each containing 1·5 mega Units of colistin sulphate are supplied. They should be stored in airtight containers, protected from light. Tablets containing 250,000 Units are also available.

OTHER NAME: *Colomycin*®

COLISTIN SULPHOMETHATE SODIUM

Colistin Sulphomethate Sodium may be prepared from colistin sulphate by the action of form-aldehyde and sodium bisulphite, whereby amino-groups are sulphomethylated.

Solubility. Soluble, at 20°, in less than 2 parts of water and in 500 parts of alcohol; insoluble in de-hydrated alcohol, in ether, in chloroform, in acetone, and in propylene glycol.

Standard
It complies with the requirements of the British Pharmacopoeia.
It is a cream-coloured powder with a faint odour and contains not less than 11,500 Units per mg, calculated with reference to the dried substance. The loss on drying under the prescribed conditions is not more than 1·5 per cent. A 1 per cent solution in water has a pH of of 6·2 to 7·5.

Stability. Aqueous solutions containing 0·5 or 1·0 per cent may be expected to retain their potency for one week when stored at room temperature or eight weeks in the frozen state.

Storage. It should be stored in airtight containers, protected from light. If it is intended for parenteral administration, the containers should be sterile and sealed to exclude micro-organisms.

Actions and uses. Colistin sulphomethate sodium is a compound of colistin which is suitable for administration by injection. It has a range of activity similar to polymyxin B (page 388) and sulphomyxin (page 486) and is used in the treatment of Gram-negative infections, particularly those due to species of *Pseudomonas* and *Aerobacter*, that have failed to respond to other antibiotics. It is administered by intramuscular injection for the treatment of septicaemia and urinary tract infections and by intrathecal injection for meningitis.

The usual dosage for an adult is 3 to 4·5 mega Units daily by intravenous infusion, or by intramuscular injection in divided doses, and for children 50,000 Units per kilogram body-weight daily in divided doses. Doses of 500 to 1000 Units per kilogram body-weight daily may be given by intrathecal injection.

UNDESIRABLE EFFECTS. Allergy may develop and the drug should not be used again in patients showing allergy to it. If the stated dose is exceeded or the excretion delayed by renal insufficiency, vertigo, perioral paraesthesia, and migraine-like syndromes may develop.
Colistin sulphomethate sodium may also give rise to renal toxicity, hypokalaemia, neuromuscular block, and neurotoxic reactions such as ataxia and apnoea.

Dose. 3 to 9 mega Units daily by intravenous infusion, or by intramuscular injection in divided doses.

Preparation

COLISTIN SULPHOMETHATE INJECTION, B.P. It consists of a sterile solution of colistin sulphomethate sodium prepared by dissolving the sterile contents of a sealed container in Sodium Chloride Injection. It should be used within 48 hours of its preparation and should be stored during this period at 2° to 10°. The quantity of colistin sulphomethate sodium in each container should be specified by the prescriber. Vials containing 0·5 and 1 mega Unit are available.

OTHER NAME: *Colomycin*®

COLOPHONY

SYNONYM: Resin

Colophony is the residue left after removal, by distillation, of the oil of turpentine from the crude oleoresin obtained from various species of *Pinus* (Fam. Pinaceae), including *P. palustris* Mill., *P. elliottii* Engelm., and *P. caribaea* Mor. in North America and *P. pinaster* Ait. in southern Europe.

Constituents. Colophony contains about 90 per cent of resin acids, of which about one-third is abietic acid. The remaining 10 per cent of the resin consists principally of esters of oleic acid, of other fatty acids, and of resin acids. The resin acids appear to undergo change when exposed to air. The composition of colophony varies according to its source, age, and method of storage.

Solubility, Insoluble in water; soluble in alcohol, in ether, in carbon disulphide, and in many fixed and volatile oils; partly soluble in light petroleum.

Standard
It complies with the requirements of the British Pharmacopoeia.
It occurs as translucent, pale yellow or brownish-yellow, angular, brittle, glassy masses which are readily fusible and have a faint terebinthinate odour and taste.

Adulterants and substitutes. An opaque resin results when water is not entirely removed during the preparation of colophony.
Black resin is the resin obtained from the later runnings from the incisions into the trees, or it may result from long-continued application of heat to the amber-coloured colophony.

Storage. It should be stored in the unground condition.

Uses. Colophony is an ingredient of certain plaster-masses and collodions.

CONGO RED

SYNONYM: Rubrum Congoensis

$C_{32}H_{22}N_6Na_2O_6S_2 = 696 \cdot 7$

Congo Red (Colour Index No. 22120) is disodium 4,4′-di(1-amino-4-sulphonaphth-2-ylazo)biphenyl. It usually contains sodium chloride.

Solubility. Soluble in water; partly and sparingly soluble in alcohol.

Standard
DESCRIPTION. A reddish-brown powder.

IDENTIFICATION TESTS. 1. Dissolve 0·1 g in 10 ml of water and add 5 ml of *dilute hydrochloric acid*; a blue precipitate is formed and the supernatant solution is blue.

2. To 0·1 g add 2 ml of *sulphuric acid*; a blue solution is produced. Dilute with water; a blue precipitate is formed.

3. Ignite; the residue gives the reactions characteristic of sodium.

ARSENIC. It complies with the test given in Appendix 6, page 878 (1 part per million).

LEAD. It complies with the test given in Appendix 7, page 882 (10 parts per million).

UNDUE TOXICITY. 0·5 ml of a 1·0 per cent w/v solution in *water for injections*, when injected intravenously into each of 5 normal mice, each weighing approximately 20 g, does not cause the death of any of them within 24 hours. If 1 of the 5 mice dies, repeat the test; the sample complies if none of the second group dies within 24 hours.

PYROGENS. It complies with the test for pyrogens, 2 ml of a 1·0 per cent w/v solution in *water for injections* being used for each kg of the rabbit's body-weight.

LOSS ON DRYING. Not more than 10·0 per cent, determined by drying to constant weight at 105°.

CONTENT OF $C_{32}H_{22}N_6Na_2O_6S_2$. Not less than 90·0 per cent, calculated with reference to the substance dried under the prescribed conditions, determined by the following method:
Dissolve about 0·25 g, accurately weighed, in 150 ml of water, add 10 g of *sodium potassium tartrate*, heat to boiling, maintain a current of carbon dioxide through the flask, and titrate the hot solution with 0·1N titanous chloride; each ml of 0·1N titanous chloride is equivalent to 0·008709 g of $C_{32}H_{22}N_6Na_2O_6S_2$.

Sterilisation. Solutions for injection are sterilised by heating in a autoclave or by filtration.

Actions and uses. Congo red is used for the detection of amyloidosis. A solution containing 0·5 to 1·5 per cent is administered by intravenous injection in a dose of 0·25 millilitre per kilogram body-weight. The percentage decrease of the dye content of the plasma or serum over a period of one hour is estimated colorimetrically. The dye content decreases by less than 30 per cent per hour in normal persons and by more than 30 per cent per hour in persons with amyloid disease.

PRECAUTIONS. It is essential to ensure that the dye is completely in solution at the time it is administered, as deaths have been caused by the injection of solutions containing undissolved dye; the solution should be allowed to stand undisturbed for some time and then examined for sediment immediately before use by inverting the container. It may be necessary to warm the solution to about 40° to aid solution. In addition, the injection solution should have a pH of not less than 7·0 and should be bright red and clear. Sodium chloride should not be added as this may precipitate the dye.

The material supplied as a microscopical stain is not suitable for injection.

Dose. 1·25 to 3·75 milligrams per kilogram body-weight, with a maximum of 270 milligrams, by intravenous injection.

COPPER SULPHATE

$CuSO_4,5H_2O = 249·7$

Copper Sulphate is cupric sulphate pentahydrate.

Solubility. Soluble, at 20°, in 3 parts of water and of glycerol; very slightly soluble in alcohol.

Standard

DESCRIPTION. Blue triclinic prisms or a blue crystalline powder, slowly efflorescent in air; odourless or almost odourless.

IDENTIFICATION TESTS. 1. To 10 ml of a 2 per cent w/v solution in water add 1 ml of *dilute hydrochloric acid* and pass *hydrogen sulphide* through the solution for 2 minutes; a brownish-black precipitate is formed which is insoluble in *sodium hydroxide solution* and almost insoluble in *ammonium sulphide solution*.

2. To 10 ml of a 2 per cent w/v solution in water add *dilute ammonia solution*, dropwise; a pale blue precipitate is formed which dissolves in excess of the reagent forming a deep blue solution.

3. To 5 ml of a 2 per cent w/v solution in water add 2 ml of *potassium iodide solution*; a brown precipitate is formed and a brown liquid is produced. Dilute to 50 ml with water and add *starch mucilage*; a deep blue colour is produced.

4. It gives the reactions characteristic of sulphates.

ACIDITY AND CLARITY OF SOLUTION. Dissolve 1·0 g in 20 ml of water; a clear blue solution is produced. Add 0·1 ml of *methyl orange solution*; the solution turns green.

ARSENIC. It complies with the test given in Appendix 6, page 878 (8 parts per million).

IRON. Boil 5·0 g with 25 ml of water and 2 ml of *nitric acid*, cool, make alkaline to *litmus paper* with *strong ammonia solution*, filter, and wash the residue with a mixture of 1 volume of *dilute ammonia solution* and 4 volumes of water; dissolve the residue in a mixture of 2 ml of *hydrochloric acid* and 10 ml of water, make alkaline to *litmus paper* with *dilute ammonia solution*, filter, wash the residue with water, dry, and ignite to constant weight; the residue, after ignition, weighs not more than 7 mg (0·14 per cent).

LEAD AND ZINC. Dissolve 1·0 g in 10 ml of water, add 1 g of *citric acid* and 10 ml of *dilute ammonia solution*, followed by *potassium cyanide solution*, dropwise, until the blue colour is discharged, and 0·05 ml of *sodium sulphide solution*; not more than a slight darkening and no opalescence is produced.

CONTENT OF $CuSO_4,5H_2O$. Not less than 98·5 and not more than the equivalent of 101·0 per cent, determined by the following method:
Dissolve about 1 g, accurately weighed, in 50 ml of water, add 3 g of *potassium iodide* and 5 ml of *acetic acid*, and titrate the liberated iodine with 0·1N sodium thiosulphate, using *starch mucilage* as indicator, until only a faint blue colour remains; add 2 g of *potassium thiocyanate* and continue the titration until the blue colour disappears; each ml of 0·1N sodium thiosulphate is equivalent to 0·02497 g of $CuSO_4,5H_2O$.

Actions and uses. Copper sulphate and other soluble salts of copper have an astringent action on mucous surfaces and in strong solutions are corrosive.

Concentrated solutions irritate the gastro-intestinal tract and give rise to violent vomiting and purging. About 25 millilitres of a 1 per cent solution may be given by mouth as an emetic; the action of the solution is prompt, and very little of the salt is absorbed.

Traces of copper sulphate are sometimes administered in conjunction with iron in the treatment of microcytic anaemias, but do not significantly enhance the absorption or utilisation of iron.

Copper sulphate is used in Copper and Zinc Sulphates Lotion for the treatment of impetigo. Solutions of 0·25 to 0·5 per cent are suitable for ophthalmic use as an astringent.

Copper sulphate is a potent fungicide; in a concentration of 0·5 to 1 part per million it prevents the growth of algae in reservoirs; 5 parts per million will kill the fresh-water snails which act as intermediate hosts in the life-cycle of the parasite causing schistosomiasis.

POISONING. In cases of poisoning by salts of copper, white of egg, milk, tannic acid, or magnesia should be given. An emetic is not usually required. Morphine may be given to allay the pain.

Preparations
COPPER AND ZINC SULPHATES LOTION, B.P.C. (page 727)
FERROUS SULPHATE TABLETS, COMPOUND, B.P.C. (page 811)

CORIANDER

Coriander consists of the dried, nearly ripe fruits of *Coriandrum sativum* L. (Fam. Umbelliferae). The plant is an erect herbaceous annual, indigenous to southern Europe and naturalised throughout temperate Europe. It is cultivated chiefly in Russia, central Europe, England, and North Africa.

Varieties. English fruits average 100 fruits per gram, are a uniform brownish-buff colour, are frequently split into separate mericarps, and contain 0·3 to 0·8 per cent of volatile oil.

Moroccan fruits are larger, averaging less than 75 fruits per gram, are marked with purplish patches, are rarely split, and contain 0·3 to 0·6 per cent of volatile oil.

Russian fruits are smaller, averaging more than 130 fruits per gram, are purplish-brown in colour, are usually whole cremocarps, and contain 0·8 to 1·2 per cent of volatile oil.

Argentine fruits are rather smaller than English, deep brownish-buff in colour, include some split fruits, and contain 0·3 to 0·6 per cent of volatile oil.

Constituents. Coriander contains about 0·3 to 1·2 per cent of volatile oil and about 13 per cent of fixed oil; proteins are also present.

Standard

It complies with the requirements of the British Pharmacopoeia.

It contains not less than 0·3 per cent v/w and Powdered Coriander not less than 0·2 per cent v/w of volatile oil.

UNGROUND DRUG. *Macroscopical characters:* cremocarp glabrous, sub-globular, about 2 to 4 mm in diameter; primary ridges 10, wavy and less prominent than the 8 straight secondary ridges; mericarps usually remaining united at their margins, generally brown, brownish-yellow, or purplish-brown in colour, apex with a small stylopod and remains of sepals; transversely cut surface showing sclerenchyma in a continuous band in the dorsal part of the pericarp and 2, or rarely more, large vittae on the commissure; endosperm oily, concave on the commissural side.

Odour aromatic; taste agreeable and spicy.

Microscopical characters: the diagnostic characters are: pericarp: *epidermal cells*, if present, composed of thin-walled cells, frequently containing a small prismatic *crystal* of calcium oxalate; mesocarp differentiated into outer, middle, and inner zone; outer zone parenchymatous, containing *degenerate vittae*, 2, or rarely more, *normal vittae* containing *volatile oil* also present on commissural side of each mericarp; middle zone sclerenchymatous, composed of sinuous rows of pitted *fusiform cells* often crossing one another at right angles and forming definite longitudinal strands in the secondary ridges; inner mesocarp partially composed of thin-walled hexagonal *sclereids*; *inner epidermis* consisting of thin-walled cells with parquetry arrangement. *Endosperm* parenchymatous, with thickened cellulose walls, cells containing *fixed oil* and numerous *aleurone grains*, about 4 to 8 μm in diameter, with minute rosette *crystals* of calcium oxalate.

POWDERED DRUG: Powdered Coriander. A fawn to brown powder possessing the diagnostic microscopical characters, odour, and taste of the unground drug.

Adulterants and substitutes. Indian coriander is said to be derived from a geographical race of *C. sativum*; the cremocarps are yellowish-buff, ellipsoidal in shape, up to 8 mm in length, and contain little volatile oil.

Storage. It should be stored in a cool dry place. Powdered Coriander should be stored in airtight containers, in a cool place.

Actions and uses. Coriander is a carminative and a flavouring agent.

CORIANDER OIL

SYNONYM: Oleum Coriandri

Coriander Oil is obtained by distillation from coriander.

Constituents. Coriander oil contains about 65 to 80 per cent of alcohols, chiefly (+)-linalol, together with terpenes.

Solubility. Soluble, at 20°, in 3 parts of alcohol (70 per cent) and in less than 1 part of alcohol (90 per cent); soluble in ether and in chloroform.

Standard

It complies with the requirements of the British Pharmacopoeia.

It is a colourless or pale yellow liquid with the odour of coriander. It has a weight per ml at 20° of 0·863 g to 0·870 g.

Storage. It should be stored in well-filled airtight containers, protected from light, in a cool place.

Actions and uses. Coriander oil is a carminative and is added to purgative medicines to prevent griping.

Dose. 0·05 to 0·2 millilitre.

CORTICOTROPHIN

SYNONYM: ACTH

Corticotrophin is obtained from the anterior lobe of the pituitary gland of the pig and contains the hormone which increases the rate at which corticoid hormones are secreted by the adrenal gland.

Corticotrophin may be prepared by extracting acetone-dried powder of the anterior lobes of the pituitary gland with hot glacial acetic acid, precipitating impurities from the filtered extract by the addition of acetone, and then precipitating the active material by the addition of solvent ether and washing free from acetic acid with acetone. The active material is purified by adsorption on oxycellulose or by another suitable method.

Other methods of preparation may be used provided that they do not involve any obvious hydrolysis or degradation of the active material.

The purified material may be sterilised by a process of filtration and is dried by a suitable method.

Standard
It complies with the requirements of the British Pharmacopoeia.
It occurs as white or almost white, hygroscopic flakes or powder and contains not less than 55 Units of corticotrophin activity per mg and not more than 5 Units of pressor activity per 100 Units of corticotrophin activity. The loss on drying under the prescribed conditions is not more than 7·0 per cent.

Storage. It should be stored in airtight containers, protected from light, at a temperature not exceeding 25°. Under these conditions it may be expected to retain its potency for at least two years from the date of manufacture.

Actions and uses. Corticotrophin stimulates the adrenal cortex, producing hyperplasia and increasing the hormonal output of the adrenal gland. When thus stimulated the gland increases in weight, loses ascorbic acid and cholesterol, and undergoes histological change, mainly in the zona fasciculata. The clinical effect is therefore similar to, but not identical with, that of cortisone, the patient showing some signs of Cushing's syndrome on prolonged or intensive treatment, as described under Cortisone Acetate (page 132).

After intravenous injection, it is effective within a few minutes, and 20 Units of corticotrophin given by intravenous infusion over a period of six hours or longer causes as much adrenal cortical stimulation as about six times this dose given by intramuscular injection at four- or six-hourly intervals.

The effect of corticortophin ceases within either a few hours or one or two days of stopping treatment, depending upon the dosage and route of administration, and the symptoms may recur if the disorder is still active. Treatment with corticotrophin should therefore be withdrawn gradually.

Corticotrophin is used in the treatment of the conditions described under Cortisone Acetate (page 132), with the exception of adrenocortical states (Addison's disease, adrenalectomy). Its rapid action is particularly useful in severe asthma and allergic states; it has the disadvantage that it cannot be given by mouth.

Some patients who have failed to benefit from oral corticosteroids improve when these drugs are replaced by corticotrophin; the reverse also occurs occasionally.

Long-acting preparations of corticotrophin are available; these include preparations in which corticoptrophin is combined with zinc hydroxide, or in which the viscosity is increased by the addition of gelatin or carboxymethylcellulose. With these preparations a single intramuscular dose daily may be sufficient.

UNDESIRABLE EFFECTS. Undesirable effects of corticotrophin are similar to those described under Cortisone Acetate (page 132), but gastro-intestinal side-effects are less common, whereas hypertension and acne are more common. Allergic reactions may occur, with lessening therapeutic effect. Local reactions to the injections may sometimes occur, and may be a real drawback in bleeding states, such as thrombocytopenic purpura, owing to haematoma formation.

PRECAUTIONS AND CONTRA-INDICATIONS. Corticotrophin should not be given to patients with peptic ulceration, with active or doubtfully quiescent tuberculous lesions, or with signs of mental instability or hypertension, although in these last two instances each case must be judged on its merits. Diabetes mellitus is aggravated and insulin needs are increased by corticotrophin therapy, and the signs of infective processes may be masked, as described under Cortisone Acetate (page 132).

Dose. For maximal adrenal stimulation, 45 to 90 Units, according to the age of the patient, by slow intravenous infusion over eight to twenty-four hours, of material labelled "For intravenous use only". By subcutaneous or intramuscular injection, of material labelled "For subcutaneous or intramuscular use only", the dose is determined according to the needs of the patient.

Preparations
CORTICOTROPHIN CARBOXYMETHYLCELLULOSE INJECTION, B.P.C. (page 712)
CORTICOTROPHIN INJECTION, B.P. (*Syn.* ACTH Inj.)
It consists of a sterile solution of corticotrophin, prepared immediately before use by dissolving the sterile contents of a sealed container in Water for Injections. The strength of the solution must be specified by the prescriber. The sealed container should be protected from light and stored at a temperature not exceeding 25°.
Vials containing 10, 25, and 40 Units per ml for intramuscular or subcutaneous injection, and 30, 45, and 75 Units per ml for intravenous injection, are available.

OTHER NAMES: *Acthar*®; Adrenocorticotrophic Hormone; *Cortrophin*®

CORTICOTROPHIN GELATIN INJECTION

SYNONYM: ACTH Gel. Inj.

Corticotrophin Gelatin Injection is a sterile solution of corticotrophin in Water for Injections containing suitably hydrolysed gelatin.

Corticotrophin Gelatin Injection may be prepared by heating a 16 per cent w/w solution of gelatin in Water for Injections for sufficient time to produce a solution which is mobile at 25°, cooling, and dissolving in the solution the requisite quantity of corticotrophin. The solution may be sterilised by filtration. It is distributed aseptically into sterilised containers, which are then sealed.

Standard
It complies with the requirements of the British Pharmacopoeia.
It is a clear, pale amber, viscous liquid which may solidify at temperatures below 25° and usually contains 20 or 40 Units per ml, determined by a biological method. It has a pH of 4·5 to 7·0.

Storage. It should be protected from light and stored at 2° to 10°. Under these conditions it may be expected to retain its potency for at least eighteen months from the date of manufacture.

Actions and uses. Corticotrophin Gelatin Injection has the actions, uses, and undesirable effects described under Corticotrophin. After intramuscular or subcutaneous injection, it is absorbed only slowly, so that it has a more prolonged action than corticotrophin; therapeutically effective blood levels are maintained for twelve to twenty-four hours after a single injection. It should not be given intravenously; if a rapid therapeutic effect is required, Corticotrophin Injection should be used.

PRECAUTIONS AND CONTRA-INDICATIONS. As for Corticotrophin.

Dose. By subcutaneous or intramuscular injection, the dose is determined by the physician in accordance with the needs of the patient.

OTHER NAMES: ACTH Gelatin Injection; *Acthar Gel®*; *Cortico-Gel®*

CORTICOTROPHIN ZINC INJECTION

SYNONYMS: ACTH Zinc Inj.; Corticotrophin Zinc Hydroxide Injection

Corticotrophin Zinc Injection is a sterile aqueous suspension of corticotrophin with zinc hydroxide.

Corticotrophin Zinc Injection may be prepared by adjusting the alkalinity of a sterile aqueous solution of corticotrophin containing a suitable quantity of zinc chloride to pH 8·0 with a sterile solution of sodium hydroxide. The quantity of zinc chloride is the minimum necessary to precipitate at least 90 per cent of the total protein. The suspension is made isotonic with blood by the addition of glycerol or other suitable substance and sodium phosphate is added as a stabiliser. It is distributed aseptically into sterile containers, which are then sealed.

Standard
It complies with the requirements of the British Pharmacopoeia.
It is a fine, white or almost white suspension and usually contains 20 or 40 Units per ml, determined by a biological method. It has a pH of 7·5 to 8·5.

Storage. It should be stored at 2° to 10°. Under these conditions it may be expected to retain its potency for

at least two years from the date of manufacture. It should not be allowed to freeze.

Actions and uses. Corticotrophin Zinc Injection has the actions, uses, and undesirable effects described under Corticotrophin. After intramuscular or subcutaneous injection, it is absorbed only slowly, so that it has a more prolonged action than corticotrophin; therapeutically effective blood levels are maintained for up to forty-eight hours after a single injection. It should not be given intravenously; if a rapid therapeutic effect is required, Corticotrophin Injection should be used.

PRECAUTIONS AND CONTRA-INDICATIONS. As for Corticotrophin.

Dose. By subcutaneous or intramuscular injection, the dose is determined by the physician in accordance with the needs of the patient.

OTHER NAMES: ACTH Zinc Hydroxide Injection; *Cortrophin-ZN®*

CORTISONE ACETATE

SYNONYM: Cortisoni Acetas

$C_{23}H_{30}O_6 = 402.5$

Cortisone Acetate is 21-acetoxy-17α-hydroxypregn-4-ene-3,11,20-trione.

Solubility. Very slightly soluble in water; soluble, at 20°, in 300 parts of alcohol and in 4 parts of chloroform; soluble in ether, in acetone, and in methyl alcohol.

Standard
It complies with the requirements of the European Pharmacopoeia.
It is a white or almost white, crystalline, odourless powder and contains not less than 96·0 and not more than the equivalent of 104·0 per cent of cortisone acetate, calculated with reference to the dried substance. The loss on drying under the prescribed conditions is not more than 1·0 per cent. It melts with decomposition at about 240°.

Preparation of solid dosage forms. In order to achieve a satisfactory rate of dissolution, cortisone acetate in the form of an ultra-fine powder should be used.

Stability. Cortisone acetate exists in several polymorphic forms, and when aqueous suspensions are being prepared, all particles should be converted to the most stable of these forms as otherwise crystal growth will occur.

Storage. It should be protected from light.

Actions and uses. Cortisone acetate has the actions and uses of the naturally occurring adrenocortical hormone, hydrocortisone (page 224). It is used in adrenocortical deficiency states and as an anti-inflammatory agent in a large number of disorders. Its action is transitory, and relapse soon occurs when therapy is stopped unless the underlying disease has in the meantime spontaneously abated.

With continued therapy, endogenous pituitary secretion of corticotrophin is depressed and the adrenal cortex undergoes involution with diminution in its secretions. Electrolyte balance is affected to varying degrees in different patients; retention of sodium and water may sometimes be observed early in therapy, usually followed by spontaneous diuresis. The urinary potassium level may rise, and metabolic alkalosis, with symptoms of muscular weakness and electrocardiographic evidence of hypokalaemia, may occasionally occur. Carbohydrate metabolism may also be affected in that the blood sugar rises, and glycosuria may occur. Protein metabolism is affected in many patients, continued administration causing a negative nitrogen balance. Resistance of the patient's tissue to bacterial infection is diminished and, as the inflammatory response to infection is also diminished or absent, diagnostic signs of infection may be completely absent; granulation and fibrous growth may be inhibited, although epithelialisation usually continues normally. The main use of cortisone is therefore in those conditions which are self-limiting and where inflammation may be harmful, as in the eye.

Cortisone is rapidly effective when given by mouth, and more slowly when given by intramuscular injection. Unlike hydrocortisone acetate, it is ineffective when injected into joints or applied to the skin.

In suppressing inflammation, as in the treatment of asthma and rheumatoid arthritis, and in the treatment of disorders of the blood, it is preferable to use prednisolone or some other corticosteroid that has less sodium- and water-retaining effects. When cortisone is used in these conditions, the correct dosage is the lowest that produces the desired effect. Close watch must always be kept for signs of bacterial infections and the appropriate antibiotic given, because cortisone may mask diagnostic features of such infections.

In adrenocortical deficiency states, such as Addison's disease, a daily dosage of 25 to 50 milligrams by mouth is required for maintenance therapy; in some cases cortisone alone is inadequate and fludrocortisone must be given in addition to increase sodium retention. In Addisonian crisis intravenous injection of hydrocortisone sodium succinate is to be preferred. In hypopituitarism with secondary adrenocortical deficiency, smaller doses such as 12·5 to 37·5 milligrams daily are usually adequate.

The diseases of the eye which respond to local application of cortisone and its analogues are inflammatory lesions of the anterior segment such as allergic conjunctivitis, and keratitis, acute iritis, non-specific keratitis, and phlyctenular keratoconjunctivitis; initially, one or two drops of a 0·5 to 2·5 per cent suspension of cortisone acetate in normal saline are placed in the conjunctival sac every hour during the day, the frequency of dosage being gradually decreased as the condition improves. Alternatively, an ointment containing 1 per cent of cortisone acetate may be applied three or four times a day. Cortisone has no antibacterial action, does not control degenerative, as opposed to inflammatory, processes and does not remove organised products of inflammation.

UNDESIRABLE EFFECTS. In some cases gravitational oedema, ascites, and other signs of congestive heart failure may occur, owing to electrolyte imbalance.

Other toxic effects of therapy include features of Cushing's syndrome, such as rounding of the face, hirsuties, striae over the hips and shoulders, and acne; more serious effects are crush fractures of vertebrae, mental changes in those predisposed, hypertension, and possibly thrombo-embolic episodes.

If withdrawal of the drug be sudden and the disease still active, symptoms and signs return rapidly, sometimes with evidence of adrenal exhaustion—the so-called "withdrawal syndrome". This may sometimes prove fatal, or lead to serious progression and worsening of the disease under treatment.

PRECAUTIONS AND CONTRA-INDICATIONS. Care should be taken in treating diabetic patients, as insulin requirements are usually increased during administration of cortisone. The risk of peptic ulceration is a real one, and caution is necessary in treating patients with past symptoms of peptic ulceration, as relapse and haemorrhage or perforation may occur.

Cortisone should be used with great care in the presence of active or doubtfully quiescent tuberculosis.

It may, however, be used in conjunction with specific antituberculous therapy in certain forms of tuberculosis in an attempt to suppress inflammatory features of the disease and adhesion formation.

When cortisone is used in the eye, infections must be controlled by means of antibiotics, sulphonamides, or other antibacterial agents, as otherwise the infection may progress and cause fibrosis, scarring, and even dissolution of the structures affected; it should never be applied to dendritic ulcers, herpetic lesions, or inflammation suspected to be of viral origin, because of the risk of causing blindness. Cortisone delays regeneration of epithelial tissue and must not be used for treating corneal ulcers.

Dose. See above under **Actions and uses**.

Preparations

CORTISONE INJECTION, B.P. (*Syn.* Cortisone Acetate Injection). It consists of a sterile suspension of cortisone acetate in Water for Injections containing suitable dispersing agents. Unless otherwise specified, a suspension containing 25 mg in 1 ml is supplied. It should be stored at room temperature, protected from light.

CORTISONE TABLETS, B.P. (*Syn.* Cortisone Acetate Tablets). Unless otherwise specified, tablets containing 25 mg of cortisone acetate are supplied. Tablets containing 5 mg are also available. They should be protected from light.

OTHER NAMES: *Adreson*®; *Cortelan*®; *Cortistab*®; *Cortisyl*®

CRESOL

Cresol is a mixture of *o*-, *m*-, and *p*-cresol, $CH_3 \cdot C_6H_4 \cdot OH$, in which the *meta*-isomer predominates, and of other phenols obtained from coal tar.

The characters of the constituent isomers are as follows.

o-Cresol is a colourless, deliquescent solid with a characteristic odour; it becomes yellow on keeping, melts at about 30°, and boils at about 191°.

m-Cresol is a colourless or yellowish liquid, slightly soluble in water and readily soluble in organic solvents; it melts at about 10° and boils at about 202°.

p-Cresol is a crystalline solid, slightly soluble in water and readily soluble in alcohol and in ether; it melts at about 36° and boils at about 201°.

Solubility. Almost completely soluble in 50 parts of water; soluble in alcohol, in ether, in chloroform, in glycerol, and in fixed and volatile oils.

Standard

It complies with the requirements of the British Pharmacopoeia.

It is an almost colourless to pale brownish-yellow liquid which becomes darker on keeping or on exposure to light. It has a weight per ml at 20° of 1·029 g to 1·044 g. When heated, not more than 2 per cent v/v distils below 188° and not less than 80 per cent v/v distils between 195° and 205°. A 2 per cent solution in water is neutral to bromocresol purple.

Storage. It should be stored in airtight containers, protected from light.

Preparation and storage of solutions. See statement on aqueous solutions of antiseptics, under Solutions (page 779).

Actions and uses. Cresol has actions similar to those described under Phenol (page 367) but it is less caustic and less poisonous than phenol. Most pathogens are killed in ten minutes by exposure to solutions containing 0·3 to 0·6 per cent of cresol, but spores require higher concentrations and longer exposure times.

Cresol may be used in place of phenol in lotions and ointments. It is sometimes added, in a concentration of about 0·3 per cent, as a preservative to solutions for parenteral administration.

Cresol is an ingredient of lysol (a 50 per cent v/v solution of cresol in soap solution) which is used as a general antiseptic but which has been largely replaced by similar preparations containing other alkyl phenols; when used on the skin, these solutions may be irritant even when well diluted. Lysol and similar preparations may be used as general disinfectants at the following dilutions: for drains, 1 in 20; for heavily infected linen, 1 in 40; for floors and walls, 1 in 100.

POISONING. As for Phenol (page 367).

CROTAMITON

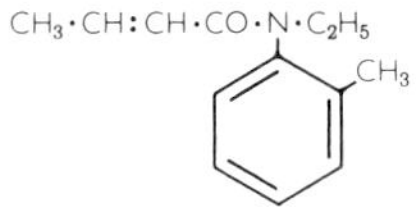

$C_{13}H_{17}NO = 203\cdot3$

Crotamiton is *N*-ethyl-*N*-*o*-tolylcrotonamide.

Solubility. Soluble, at 20°, in 400 parts of water; miscible with alcohol and with ether.

Standard
It complies with the requirements of the British Pharmacopoeia.
It is a colourless or pale yellow oily liquid with a faint odour and contains not less than 95·0 per cent w/w of $C_{13}H_{17}NO$. It has a weight per ml at 20° of 1·004 g to 1·009 g. At low temperatures, it may solidify partly or completely.

Storage. It should be stored in small containers. If it has solidified, it should be completely melted and mixed before use.

Actions and uses. Crotamiton is an antipruritic which is applied as a cream or lotion containing 10 per cent. It has also been used as an acaricide for the treatment of scabies.

UNDESIRABLE EFFECTS. Sensitivity to crotamiton is rare, but the drug may produce irritation in the presence of acute vesicular dermatitis.

OTHER NAME: *Eurax®*

CRYSTAL VIOLET

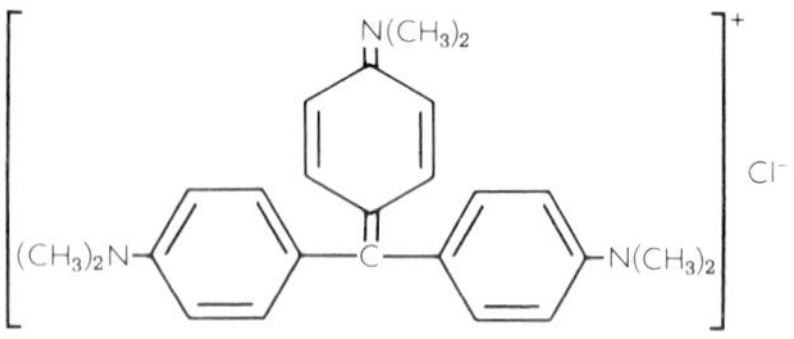

SYNONYMS: Medicinal Gentian Violet;
Viola Crystallina

$C_{25}H_{30}ClN_3 = 408\cdot0$

Crystal Violet (Colour Index No. 42555) is hexamethylpararosaniline hydrochloride.

Solubility. Soluble, at 20°, in 200 parts of water and in 30 parts of glycerol; soluble in alcohol and in chloroform; insoluble in ether.

Standard
It complies with the requirements of the British Pharmacopoeia.
It occurs as odourless or almost odourless, greenish-bronze crystals or powder and contains not less than 96·0 per cent of $C_{25}H_{30}ClN_3$, calculated with reference to the dried substance. The loss on drying under the prescribed conditions is not more than 9·0 per cent.

Actions and uses. Crystal violet is an antiseptic with a selective action on Gram-positive organisms. It does not irritate the skin. A 0·5 per cent aqueous solution is used in the treatment of burns, boils, carbuncles, and mycotic skin affections. An aqueous solution containing 0·5 per cent each of crystal violet and brilliant green has been used for sterilising the skin.

Preparations
BRILLIANT GREEN AND CRYSTAL VIOLET PAINT, B.P.C. (page 765)
CRYSTAL VIOLET PAINT, B.P.C. (page 766)
CRYSTAL VIOLET PESSARIES, B.P.C. (page 772)

CYANOCOBALAMIN

SYNONYM: Cyanocobalaminum

$C_{63}H_{88}CoN_{14}O_{14}P = 1355\cdot4$

Cyanocobalamin is α-(5,6-dimethylbenzimidazol-1-yl)cyanocobamide, a cobalt-containing substance which may be obtained from liver or separated from the products of metabolism of various micro-organisms.

Solubility. Soluble, at 20°, in 80 parts of water; soluble in alcohol; insoluble in ether, in chloroform, and in acetone.

Standard
It complies with the requirements of the European Pharmacopoeia.
It occurs as dark red, odourless, hygroscopic crystals or crystalline powder and contains not less than 96·0 per cent of $C_{63}H_{88}CoN_{14}O_{14}P$, calculated with reference to the dried substance. The loss on drying under the prescribed conditions is not more than 12·0 per cent.

Sterilisation. Solutions for injection are sterilised by heating in an autoclave or by filtration.

Storage. It should be stored in airtight containers, protected from light.

Actions and uses. Cyanocobalamin has the actions and uses described under Hydroxocobalamin (page 229) but it is more rapidly excreted and so has the disadvantage that it does not produce such a high initial serum-vitamin-B_{12} level as hydroxocobalamin and the serum level is not maintained for so long a period. Cyanocobalamin should not be given by mouth because of its variable absorption.
In the treatment of pernicious anaemia, five intramuscular injections, each of 1 milligram of cyanocobalamin, are generally given with-

in the first week, followed by 250 micrograms weekly until the blood count is normal; the usual maintenance dosage is 250 micrograms every three or four weeks. In all cases the dosage must be related to the patient's response; in patients with neurological abnormalities, the doses should be doubled.

PRECAUTIONS. Cyanocobalamin should not be given before a diagnosis of pernicious anaemia has been fully established, because of its ability to mask symptoms of subacute combined degeneration of the spinal cord.

Dose. See above under **Actions and uses.**

Preparation
CYANOCOBALAMIN INJECTION, B.P. It consists of a sterile solution of cyanocobalamin in Water for Injections, the pH of the solution being adjusted to about 4·5. Unless otherwise specified, a solution containing the equivalent of 250 micrograms of anhydrous cyanocobalamin in 1 ml are supplied. It should be protected from light. Ampoules containing 100 and 200 micrograms and 1 milligram are also available.

OTHER NAMES: *Cobastab®*; *Cytamen®*

CYANOCOBALAMIN (^{57}Co)

This material is radioactive and any regulations in force must be complied with.

Cyanocobalamin (^{57}Co) is α-(5,6-dimethylbenzimidazol-1-yl)cyano[^{57}Co]cobamide. It may be produced by the growth of certain micro-organisms on a medium containing [^{57}Co] cobaltous ions.

Cobalt-57 is a radioactive isotope of cobalt which emits γ-radiation and has a half-life of 270 days; it may be prepared by the irradiation of nickel with protons of suitable energy.

Standard
It complies with the requirements of the British Pharmacopoeia.
It is supplied as a freeze-dried solid in sealed glass containers or capsules or as a solution containing suitable stabilisers. It contains not less than 85·0 and not more than 115·0 per cent of the quantity of cobalt-57 stated on the label at the date stated on the label.
Not less than 90 per cent of the cobalt-57 is in the form of cyanocobalamin at the date stated on the label and not more than 1·0 per cent of the total activity, expressed as disintegrations per second, is due to cobalt-60 at the date stated on the label.

Stability. Cyanocobalamin (^{57}Co) decomposes with an accompanying decrease in the radiochemical purity. It should be issued in such a form that when stored under the prescribed conditions the rate of decomposition, measured in terms of radiochemical purity, does not exceed 2 per cent a month during a period of three months from the date stated on the label.

Labelling. The label on the container states:
(1) the form of the preparation;
(2) the content of cobalt-57 expressed in microcuries or millicuries at a given date; and
(3) that the preparation is radioactive.

The label on the package also states:
(1) the total quantity in the container; and
(2) the name of any added stabilising agent.

Storage. It should be stored in an area assigned for the purpose, protected from light, at a temperature not exceeding 10°. The storage conditions should be such that the maximum radiation-dose-rate to which persons may be exposed is reduced to an acceptable level.

Actions and uses. Cyanocobalamin labelled with radioactive cobalt is used to measure the absorption of orally administered cyanocobalamin in the investigation of megaloblastic anaemias and particularly for the detection of pernicious anaemia. Impaired absorption which can be corrected by the simultaneous oral administration of intrinsic factor occurs in pernicious anaemia or following total gastrectomy; impaired absorption which cannot be corrected by intrinsic factor is usually due to disease of the small bowel.

Cyanocobalamin absorption tests are especially useful in cases where haematological investigations are vitiated by premature treatment or where neurological manifestations of pernicious anaemia precede the development of abnormalities in the marrow. The procedure is also used in subjects with pernicious anaemia to standardise preparations of intrinsic factor.

Various methods of performing cyanocobalamin absorption tests are in use. As the proportion of cyanocobalamin absorbed after oral administration depends upon the quantity administered, a standard dose, for example 1 microgram, should be administered; the labelled material may be diluted if necessary with non-radioactive cyanocobalamin so that the standard dose contains a suitable amount of radioactivity for measurement in the test.

A common procedure is the Schilling test, in which a large dose of non-radioactive cyanocobalamin is given by injection to impede uptake by the liver of the absorbed oral dose; the proportion absorbed may be assessed by measuring the radioactivity of the urine.

Other methods involve (*a*) measuring the radioactivity of the plasma, (*b*) using a scintillation counter over the liver, and (*c*) determining the non-absorbed fraction in the faeces after ashing, using a conventional well-type sodium iodide scintillation counter.

Observations of the radioactivity of the urine following intravenous injection of cyanocobalamin (^{57}Co) have also been used for the determination of the glomerular filtration rate of the kidneys.

Cyanocobalamin labelled with cobalt-57 or cobalt-58 is available and both forms are used for the tests; cyanocobalamin labelled with cobalt-60 should not be used because of the long half-life of this isotope. Cyanocobalamin (^{57}Co) may be stored for a longer period and, for a given activity, provides a lower dose of radiation to the liver.

Solutions of cyanocobalamin (^{57}Co) of high specific activity are used for the estimation *in vitro* of plasma vitamin-B$_{12}$ levels.

Dose. In the investigation of the absorption and metabolism of cyanocobalamin, 1 micro-curie.

CYANOCOBALAMIN (^{58}Co)

This material is radioactive and any regulations in force must be complied with.

Cyanocobalamin (^{58}Co) is α-(5,6-dimethylbenzimidazol-1-yl)cyano[^{58}Co]cobamide. It may be produced by the growth of certain micro-organisms on a medium containing [^{58}Co] cobaltous ions.

Cobalt-58 is a radioactive isotope of cobalt which emits β- and γ-radiation and has a half-life of 71 days; it may be prepared by the neutron irradiation of nickel.

Standard
It complies with the requirements of the British Pharmacopoeia.
It is supplied as a freeze-dried solid in sealed glass containers or capsules or as a solution containing suitable stabilisers. It contains not less than 90·0 and not more than 110·0 per cent of the quantity of cobalt-58 stated on the label at the date stated on the label.
Not less than 90·0 per cent of the cobalt-58 is in the form of cyanocobalamin at the date stated on the label and not more than 1·0 per cent of the total activity, expressed as disintegrations per second, is due to cobalt-60 at the date stated on the label.

Stability. Cyanocobalamin (^{58}Co) decomposes with an accompanying decrease in the radiochemical purity. It should be issued in such a form that when stored under the prescribed conditions the rate of decomposition, measured in terms of radiochemical purity, does not exceed 2 per cent a month during a period of three months from the date stated on the label.

Labelling. The label on the container states:
(1) the form of the preparation;
(2) the content of cobalt-58 expressed in microcuries or millicuries at a given date; and
(3) that the preparation is radioactive.

The label on the package also states:
(1) the total quantity in the container; and
(2) the name of any added stabilising agent.

Storage. It should be stored in an area assigned for the purpose, protected from light, at a temperature not exceeding 10°. The storage conditions should be such that the maximum radiation-dose-rate to which persons may be exposed is reduced to an acceptable level.

Actions and uses. Cyanocobalamin (^{58}Co) is used in the investigation of megaloblastic anaemias as described under Cyanocobalamin (^{57}Co).

Dose. In the investigation of the absorption and metabolism of cyanocobalamin, 1 micro-curie.

CYCLIZINE HYDROCHLORIDE

$C_{18}H_{23}ClN_2 = 302·8$

Cyclizine Hydrochloride is 1-diphenylmethyl-4-methylpiperazine hydrochloride.

Solubility. Soluble, at 20°, in 125 parts of water and in 120 parts of alcohol; insoluble in ether.

Standard
It complies with the requirements of the British Pharmacopoeia.
It is a white, crystalline, almost odourless powder and contains not less than 98·0 and not more than the equivalent of 101·0 per cent of $C_{18}H_{23}ClN_2$, calculated with reference to the dried substance. The loss on drying under the prescribed conditions is not more than 1·0 per cent.

Sterilisation. Solutions for injection are sterilised by heating in an autoclave or by filtration.

Actions and uses. Cyclizine has the actions and uses of the antihistamine drugs, as described under Promethazine Hydrochloride (page 409). It is given by mouth for the prevention and relief of motion-sickness; it acts rapidly.
The usual dose for an adult is 50 milligrams of cyclizine hydrochloride, for a child aged six to ten years, 25 milligrams, and for a younger child, 12·5 milligrams. The first dose should be taken twenty minutes before a journey, and the dose should not be repeated more than twice in twenty-four hours.
Cyclizine has also been used for the relief of the nausea and vomiting of pregnancy and for the symptomatic treatment of vertigo and labyrinthine disorders due to Ménière's disease and other causes.

UNDESIRABLE EFFECTS. Drowsiness and dizziness may occur in some patients.

POISONING. As for Promethazine Hydrochloride (page 409).

Dose. See above under **Actions and uses.**

Preparation
CYCLIZINE TABLETS, B.P. Unless otherwise specified, tablets each containing 50 mg of cyclizine hydrochloride are supplied. They should be stored in airtight containers.

OTHER NAMES: *Marzine*® ; *Valoid*®

CYCLOBARBITONE CALCIUM

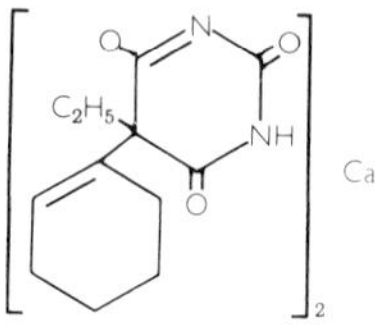

SYNONYMS: Cyclobarb. Calc.;
Cyclobarbital Calcium;
Cyclobarbitalum Calcicum

$C_{24}H_{30}CaN_4O_6 = 510.6$

Cyclobarbitone Calcium is calcium 5-cyclohex-1'-enyl-5-ethylbarbiturate.

Solubility. Soluble, at 20°, in 100 parts of water; very slightly soluble in alcohol, in ether, and in chloroform.

Standard
It complies with the requirements of the European Pharmacopoeia.
It is a white or slightly yellowish, crystalline, almost odourless powder and contains not less than 98·5 and not more than the equivalent of 102·0 per cent of $C_{24}H_{30}CaN_4O_6$, calculated with reference to the dried substance. The loss on drying under the prescribed conditions is not more than 1·0 per cent.

Actions and uses. Cyclobarbitone is an intermediate-acting barbiturate, the actions and uses of which are described under Phenobarbitone (page 366).

UNDESIRABLE EFFECTS; CONTRA-INDICATIONS; PRECAUTIONS; DEPENDENCE. These are as described under Phenobarbitone (page 366).

POISONING. The procedure described under Phenobarbitone (page 366) should be followed.

Dose. As a hypnotic, 200 to 400 milligrams.

Preparation
CYCLOBARBITONE TABLETS, B.P. (*Syn.* Cyclobarbital Calcium Tablets). The quantity of cyclobarbitone calcium in each tablet should be specified by the prescriber. They should be stored in airtight containers. Tablets containing 200 mg are available.

OTHER NAMES: *Phanodorm®*; *Rapidal®*

CYCLOMETHYCAINE SULPHATE

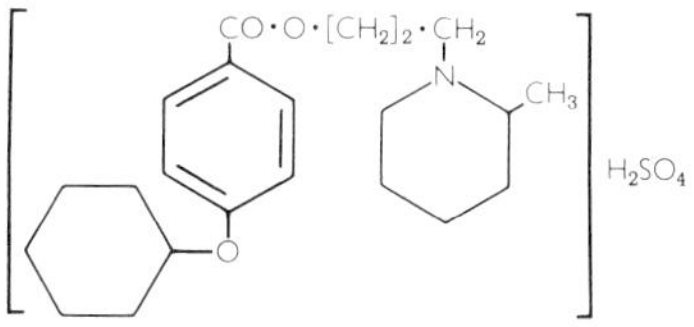

$C_{22}H_{35}NO_7S = 457.6$

Cyclomethycaine Sulphate is 3-(2-methylpiperidino)propyl *p*-cyclohexyloxybenzoate hydrogen sulphate.

Solubility. Soluble, at 20°, in 50 parts of water, in 50 parts of alcohol, and in 227 parts of chloroform; slightly soluble in dilute mineral acids.

Standard
It complies with the requirements of the British Pharmacopoeia.
It is a white, crystalline, odourless powder and contains not less than 98·0 and not more than the equivalent of 101·0 per cent of $C_{22}H_{35}NO_7S$, calculated with reference to the dried substance. The loss on drying under the prescribed conditions is not more than 1·0 per cent. It has a melting-point of 162·5° to 165·5°.

Sterilisation. Solutions for injection are sterilised by heating in an autoclave or by filtration.

Actions and uses. Cyclomethycaine sulphate is a sparingly soluble local anaesthetic which is applied for surface analgesia in cuts and abra-

sions, skin irritations, burns, pruritus ani and vulvae, haemorrhoids and anal fissure, and cracked nipples. It may be used before cystoscopy, except when injury is present. Analgesia occurs within five to ten minutes and lasts from four to eight hours.
Cyclomethycaine is not suitable for otolaryngological or ophthalmic use and should not be used on extensive areas of broken or burnt skin. It does not inactivate sulphonamides.

UNDESIRABLE EFFECTS. Cyclomethycaine occasionally causes sensitisation reactions.

POISONING. The procedure as described under Procaine Hydrochloride (page 404) should be adopted.

CYCLOPENTHIAZIDE

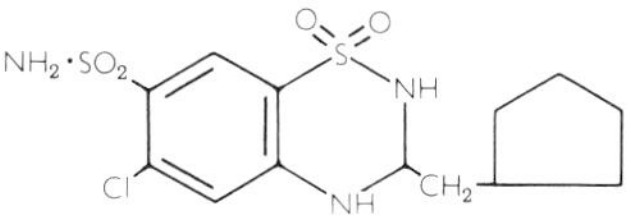

$C_{13}H_{18}ClN_3O_4S_2 = 379.9$

Cyclopenthiazide is 6-chloro-3-cyclopentylmethyl-3,4-dihydro-7-sulphamoyl-2*H*-benzo-1,2,4-thiadiazine 1,1-dioxide.

Solubility. Very slightly soluble in water; soluble, at 20°, in 12 parts of alcohol and in 600 parts of chloroform; soluble in ether.

Standard
It complies with the requirements of the British Pharmacopoeia.

It is a white odourless powder and contains not less than 98·0 and not more than the equivalent of 102·0 per cent of $C_{13}H_{18}ClN_3O_4S_2$, calculated with reference to the dried substance. The loss on drying under the prescribed conditions is not more than 0·5 per cent.

Actions and uses. Cyclopenthiazide is a non-mercurial diuretic which has actions and uses similar to those described under Chlorothiazide (page 103). The usual dose is 250 to 500 micrograms by mouth, once or twice daily.

UNDESIRABLE EFFECTS; PRECAUTIONS. As for Chlorothiazide (page 103).

Dose. See above under **Actions and uses.**

Preparation
CYCLOPENTHIAZIDE TABLETS, B.P. Unless otherwise specified, tablets each containing 500 micrograms of cyclopenthiazide are supplied.

OTHER NAME: *Navidrex®*

CYCLOPENTOLATE HYDROCHLORIDE

$C_{17}H_{26}ClNO_3 = 327.9$

Cyclopentolate Hydrochloride is 2-dimethylaminoethyl α-(1-hydroxycyclopentyl)-α-phenylacetate hydrochloride.

Solubility. Soluble, at 20°, in less than 1 part of water and in 5 parts of alcohol; insoluble in ether.

Standard
It complies with the requirements of the British Pharmacopoeia.
It is a white crystalline powder which is odourless or has a characteristic odour and contains not less than 98.5 and not more than the equivalent of 101.0 per cent of $C_{17}H_{26}ClNO_3$, calculated with reference to the dried substance. The loss on drying under the prescribed conditions is not more than 0.5 per cent. It has a melting-point of 135° to 137°. A 1 per cent solution in water has a pH of 4.5 to 5.5.

Sterilisation. Solutions are sterilised by filtration.

Actions and uses. Cyclopentolate has mydriatic and cycloplegic properties similar to those described under Atropine (page 36), but it acts more quickly and its effect lasts for a shorter time.

The usual quantity required for refraction

procedures is one drop of a 0.5 per cent solution instilled into the eye; children aged six to sixteen years usually require one drop of a 1 per cent solution and children under six years one or two drops of a 1 per cent solution. As a mydriatic one drop of a 0.5 or 1 per cent solution may be used.

Cyclopentolate is also used in the treatment of corneal ulceration, iritis, iridocyclitis, keratitis, and choroiditis, one or two drops of a 0.5 or 1 per cent solution being used as required.

PRECAUTIONS. Cyclopentolate has relatively little effect on intra-ocular tension in the normal eye, but it should be used with caution in patients with increased intra-ocular pressure.

Preparation
CYCLOPENTOLATE EYE-DROPS, B.P.C. (page 690)

OTHER NAME: *Mydrilate®*

CYCLOPHOSPHAMIDE

$C_7H_{15}Cl_2N_2O_2P,H_2O = 279.1$

Cyclophosphamide is 2-[di(2-chloroethyl)amino]-1-oxa-3-aza-2-phosphacyclohexane 2-oxide monohydrate.

Solubility. Soluble, at 20°, in 25 parts of water and in 1 part of alcohol; slightly soluble in ether.

Standard
It complies with the requirements of the British Pharmacopoeia.
It is a fine, white, crystalline, odourless or almost odourless powder and contains not less than 98.0 per cent of $C_7H_{15}Cl_2N_2O_2P$, calculated with reference to the anhydrous substance. It contains 6.0 to 7.0 per cent w/w of water. It has a melting-point of 49.5° to 53°. A freshly prepared 2 per cent solution in water has a pH of 4.0 to 6.0.

Stability. It discolours on exposure to light. Aqueous solutions may be kept for a few hours at room temperature but at temperatures above 30° hydrolysis occurs with removal of chlorine atoms.

Storage. It should be stored in airtight containers, protected from light.

Actions and uses. Cyclophosphamide is a cytotoxic drug with the actions and uses described under Mustine Hydrochloride (page

316). It is broken down, probably by phosphoramidases, at the nitrogen-phosphorus linkage, liberating an alkylating agent in the tumour cells. Unlike mustine, it has no vesicant action. It may be administered orally, intramuscularly, intravenously, or directly into body cavities.

Cyclophosphamide is used for the treatment of lymphosarcoma, Hodgkin's disease, multiple myeloma, lymphatic leukaemia, ovarian and other carcinomas, tumours of the head and neck, retinoblastoma, and malignant pleural effusions and as an adjuvant in the treatment of inoperable bronchocarcinoma and inoperable carcinoma of the breast.

Cyclophosphamide may also be used to suppress cellular auto-immune reactions in tissue transplantations, such as kidney grafts, in the nephrotic syndrome and nephritis associated with systemic lupus erythematosus, and for prolonging survival of homografts. It may be used in a dose of 3 milligrams per kilogram body-weight in the treatment of the nephrotic syndrome in children when treatment with corticosteroids has proved unsuccessful.

In the treatment of localised tumours, cyclophosphamide may be given by regional perfusion into a main artery. It can also be injected directly into tumour tissue.

The limiting factor in determining dosage and duration of treatment is depression of the white-cell count. If this is kept within the range of 2000 to 5000 white cells per cubic millimetre, treatment can be prolonged. It is started with a daily dosage of 100 milligrams intravenously, increased to 200 to 300 milligrams, or in certain circumstances to 400 milligrams, until a total dose of 6 to 8 grams has been given, the dose depending on the white-cell count. The daily dosage for maintenance therapy is 50 to 300 milligrams given orally. For a child, the initial dosage is 5 milligrams per kilogram body-weight daily by intravenous injection; this is repeated until the white-cell count has fallen as far as permissible and then 2 to 5 milligrams per kilogram body-weight daily is given by mouth as a maintenance dose. Treatment can be continued with a maintenance dose for one or two years if the white-cell count is favourable.

In the treatment of tumours by intra-arterial infusion a total dose of 40 milligrams per kilogram body-weight in Sodium Chloride Injection is slowly infused at 42°. For the treatment of malignant ascites 200 to 500 milligrams may be given intraperitoneally, and for malignant pleural effusions, 600 to 800 milligrams intrapleurally.

Cyclophosphamide is perhaps one of the safest alkylating agents because depression of the white-cell count from overdosage is readily reversed on withdrawing the drug.

UNDESIRABLE EFFECTS. Leukopenia (particularly of the neutrophil cells), loss of hair, anorexia, nausea, and vomiting may occur.

Dose. See above under **Actions and uses.**

Preparations

CYCLOPHOSPHAMIDE INJECTION, B.P. It consists of a sterile solution prepared immediately before use by dissolving the sterile contents of a sealed container in Water for Injections. The sealed container contains cyclophosphamide and sodium chloride. The quantity of cyclophosphamide in each container should be specified by the prescriber. Vials containing 100, 200, and 500 mg and 1 g are available.

CYCLOPHOSPHAMIDE TABLETS, B.P. The quantity of cyclophosphamide in each tablet should be specified by the prescriber. They are coated. Tablets containing 10 and 50 mg are available.

OTHER NAME: *Endoxana*®

CYCLOPROPANE

$C_3H_6 = 42·08$

CAUTION. *Cyclopropane is highly inflammable and mixtures of its vapour with oxygen or air at certain concentrations are explosive; it should not be used in the presence of a naked flame or of any electrical apparatus liable to produce a spark. Precautions should be taken against the production of static electrical discharge.*

Solubility. One volume, measured at normal temperature and pressure, dissolves, at 20°, in 2·85 volumes of water; soluble in alcohol, in ether, in chloroform, and in fixed oils.

Standard
It complies with the requirements of the British Pharmacopoeia.
It is a colourless inflammable gas with a characteristic odour and contains not less than 99·0 per cent v/v of C_3H_6. At a pressure of 760 mm of mercury it has a boiling-point of about −34·5°. It is supplied compressed in metal cylinders.

Storage, labelling, and colour-markings. It should be stored in metal cylinders in a special storage room, which should be cool and free from material of an inflammable nature. The whole of the cylinder should be painted orange and the name of the gas or chemical symbol "C_3H_6" should be stencilled in paint on the shoulder of the cylinder. The name or chemical symbol of the gas should be clearly and indelibly stamped on the cylinder valve.

Actions and uses. Cyclopropane is the most potent of the gaseous anaesthetics.
Its advantages are that it is non-irritant, that induction and recovery are rapid, and that it can be administered with a high percentage of oxygen. It is non-toxic to the liver and kidneys and causes only mild excitement during induction and only slight post-operative vomiting. Its disadvantages are that it is a respiratory depressant and that it has a tendency to cause cardiac irregularities and increased haemorrhage. It may also cause bronchospasm if surgical stimulation occurs under light anaesthesia, and if it is used in conjunction with thiopentone sodium, laryngospasm may occur.

Because of the risk of explosion the usual method of administration is by means of a closed circuit. It is usually administered with oxygen; a concentration of 4 per cent of cyclopropane in oxygen produces analgesia, 8 per cent produces light anaesthesia, and 20 to 25 per cent produces surgical anaesthesia.

PRECAUTIONS. Respiratory depressants in preoperative medication should be given with caution, and during cyclopropane anaesthesia the pulse must be carefully observed and the use of sympathomimetic drugs, such as adrenaline, should be avoided. A marked fall in systolic blood pressure and varying degrees of lung collapse may be occasional sequelae.

POISONING. As for Chloroform (page 100).

CYCLOSERINE

$C_3H_6N_2O_2 = 102·1$

Cycloserine is D-4-aminoisoxazolid-3-one, an antimicrobial substance produced by the growth of *Streptomyces orchidaceus* or *S. garyphalus*, or obtained by synthesis.

Solubility. Soluble, at 20°, in 10 parts of water and in 50 parts of alcohol; slightly soluble in ether and in chloroform.

Standard
It complies with the requirements of the British Pharmacopoeia.
It is a white or pale yellow, crystalline, hygroscopic, odourless or almost odourless powder and contains not less than 98·0 per cent of $C_3H_6N_2O_2$, calculated with reference to the dried substance. The loss on drying under the prescribed conditions is not more than 0·5 per cent. A 10 per cent solution in water has a pH of 5·7 to 6·3.

Storage. It should be stored in airtight containers at a temperature not exceeding 25°.

Actions and uses. Cycloserine is a water-soluble antibiotic which is active against a wide range of Gram-positive and Gram-negative bacteria, including *Mycobacterium tuberculosis*, streptococci, staphylococci, *Aerobacter aerogenes*, and *Escherichia coli*. Its antibacterial activity is lower than that of other antibiotics available for treating infections due to these micro-organisms and it is therefore used only when the infecting organism has acquired resistance to other agents or when the patient has become hypersensitive to these other agents. It is not active against *Proteus vulgaris*, *Pseudomonas* species, or gonococci.

After oral administration, cycloserine is readily absorbed from the gastro-intestinal tract and therapeutically effective concentrations in the blood are attained within four to six hours. Only a relatively small proportion of cycloserine is excreted in the urine; the fate of the remainder is not known.

The main use of cycloserine is in the treatment of pulmonary tuberculosis when an antibiotic of the streptomycin group cannot be used because the organism is resistant or the patient hypersensitive. As with streptomycin, treatment with cycloserine should be combined with the administration of isoniazid or an aminosalicylate in order to minimise the emergence of resistant strains.

Cycloserine is given by mouth in an initial dosage of 250 milligrams daily; if no toxic effects are observed in about two weeks this dose may be given twice daily, and then three time daily if no serious toxic effects have been observed.

Cycloserine is also used in urinary tract infections when other drugs are contra-indicated or ineffective.

UNDESIRABLE EFFECTS. When the dosage recommended for the treatment of tuberculosis is used, the incidence of side-effects may be as high as 30 per cent; the most common are headache and dizziness, but reflex changes, speech difficulty, convulsions, and coma may also occur. Gastro-intestinal symptoms and changes in serum transaminase may occur, but allergic reactions are uncommon.

PRECAUTIONS. The blood level of cycloserine should be maintained between 15 and 25 micrograms per millilitre by appropriate adjustment of the dose and the use of lower dosage in patients with renal impairment.

CONTRA-INDICATIONS. It should not be given to patients with a history of epilepsy or mental disturbance or with impaired renal function.

Dose. 250 to 750 milligrams daily in divided doses.

Preparations
CYCLOSERINE CAPSULES, B.P. Unless otherwise specified, capsules each containing 250 mg of cycloserine are supplied. Capsules containing 125 mg are also available.

CYCLOSERINE TABLETS, B.P. Unless otherwise specified, tablets each containing 250 mg of cycloserine are supplied.

CYPROHEPTADINE HYDROCHLORIDE

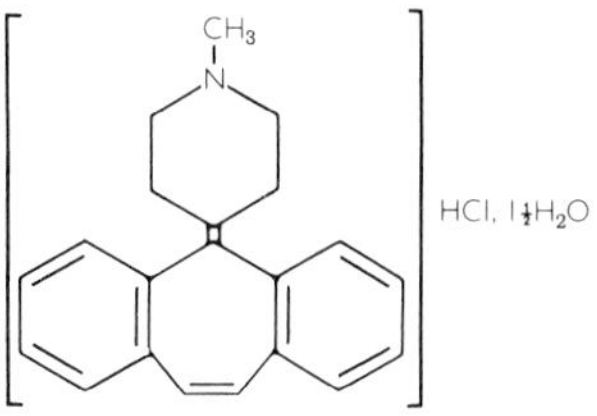

$C_{21}H_{22}ClN,1\frac{1}{2}H_2O = 350.9$

Cyproheptadine Hydrochloride is 4-(5*H*-dibenzo[*a,d*]-cyclohepten-5-ylidene)-1-methylpiperidine hydrochloride sesquihydrate.

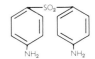

Solubility. Soluble, at 20°, in 275 parts of water, in 35 parts of alcohol, in 16 parts of chloroform, and in 1·5 parts of methyl alcohol; insoluble in ether.

Standard
It complies with the requirements of the British Pharmacopoeia.
It is a white to slightly yellow, crystalline, almost odourless powder and contains not less than 98·5 and not more than the equivalent of 101·0 per cent of $C_{21}H_{22}ClN$, calculated with reference to the dried substance. The loss on drying under the prescribed conditions is 7·0 to 9·0 per cent.

Storage. It should be stored in airtight containers.

Actions and uses. Cyproheptadine has the actions, uses, and undesirable effects of the antihistamine drugs, as described under Promethazine Hydrochloride (page 409); 1·1 g of cyproheptadine hydrochloride is approximately equivalent to 1 g of anhydrous cyproheptadine hydrochloride.

POISONING. As for Promethazine Hydrochloride (page 409).

Dose. The equivalent of 4 to 20 milligrams of anhydrous cyproheptadine hydrochloride daily in divided doses.

Preparation
CYPROHEPTADINE TABLETS, B.P. Unless otherwise specified, tablets each containing the equivalent of 4 mg of anhydrous cyproheptadine hydrochloride are supplied.

OTHER NAME: *Periactin*®

DANTHRON

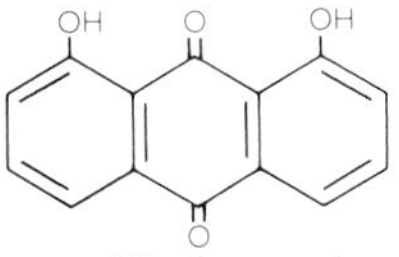

$C_{14}H_8O_4 = 240.2$

Danthron is 1,8-dihydroxyanthraquinone.

Solubility. Very slightly soluble in water; soluble, at 20°, in 2500 parts of alcohol, in 500 parts of ether, and in 30 parts of chloroform; soluble in solutions of alkali hydroxides.

Standard
It complies with the requirements of the British Pharmacopoeia.
It is an orange, crystalline, almost odourless powder and contains not less than 98·0 and not more than the equivalent of 102·0 per cent of $C_{14}H_8O_4$, calculated with reference to the dried substance. The loss on drying under the prescribed conditions is not more than 0·5 per cent.

Actions and uses. Danthron is an anthraquinone purgative which acts by stimulating the muscles of the colon. It may colour the urine pink or red.

Dose. 25 to 50 milligrams.

OTHER NAMES: Dihydroxyanthraquinone; *Dorbanex*®

DAPSONE

$C_{12}H_{12}N_2O_2S = 248.3$

Dapsone is di(*p*-aminophenyl)sulphone.

Solubility. Very slightly soluble in water; soluble, at 20°, in 30 parts of alcohol; soluble in acetone and in dilute mineral acids.

Standard
It complies with the requirements of the British Pharmacopoeia.
It is a white or creamy-white, crystalline, odourless powder and contains not less than 99·0 per cent of $C_{12}H_{12}N_2O_2S$, calculated with reference to the dried substance. The loss on drying under the prescribed conditions is not more than 1·5 per cent. It has a melting-point of 176° to 181°.

Stability. It becomes discoloured on exposure to light but this is not accompanied by significant decomposition.

Hygroscopicity. It absorbs insignificant amounts of water when stored under ordinary conditions.

Sterilisation. Dapsone is prepared as a sterile powder by the method described under Sulphadimidine (page 478). Oily suspensions are sterilised by dry heat.

Actions and uses. Dapsone is an antibacterial substance which, like the sulphonamides, probably acts by preventing the use by certain bacteria of essential metabolites, as its action is antagonised by *p*-aminobenzoic acid. Its principal use is in the treatment of leprosy, but it is also of value in unrelated diseases such as dermatitis herpetiformis, toxoplasmosis, and mycetoma (maduromycosis). It has a suppressive action on the malaria parasite.
Dapsone is usually given by mouth, the initial

dosage in leprosy being 25 milligrams twice weekly. The dose may be increased gradually over the next three to four months to a maximum of 350 milligrams twice weekly, at which stage the dosage may be changed to 100 milligrams daily if this is more convenient. However, in most cases of leprosy a dosage of 50 milligrams twice weekly is adequate and this produces fewer reactions than higher doses; a dosage of 200 milligrams per week is now rarely exceeded.

In certain circumstances, particularly in the treatment of out-patients suffering from leprosy, dapsone may be administered intramuscularly at fortnightly intervals in the form of a suspension of 1·0 to 1·2 grams in 5 millilitres of a sterile vehicle such as arachis oil, chaulmoogra oil, or ethyl esters of hydnocarpus oil, but the injections are liable to cause pain and possibly severe abscess formation.

In tuberculoid leprosy, skin lesions usually disappear in three to nine months, and in lepromatous leprosy, in one to five years; in the dimorphous (borderline) form of the disease, lesions disappear in an intermediate period of time. In lepromatous leprosy, acid-fast bacilli can be demonstrated in the skin for months or years after the disappearance of lesions, but these bacilli have undergone characteristic morphological changes, resulting in fragmentation and the appearance of granularity, and, on electron-microscopical examination, appear to be non-viable. However, viable bacilli may persist in the peripheral nervous system, so it is advisable to continue to give maintenance doses of dapsone for eighteen months after the disappearance of skin lesions in tuberculoid leprosy and for even longer periods after the disappearance of granular bacilli from the skin in lepromatous leprosy.

In dermatitis herpetiformis the initial dosage is usually 100 milligrams daily, which is gradually reduced to the lowest effective maintenance dose, usually about 25 milligrams on alternate days.

For the suppression of malaria the usual dosage is 100 milligrams of dapsone with 12·5 milligrams of pyrimethamine weekly. The same dosage of dapsone is used in conjunction with other antimalarial drugs in the treatment of chloroquine-resistant *Plasmodium falciparum* infections.

UNDESIRABLE EFFECTS. Undesirable effects are rare and include anaemia, dermatitis, and hepatitis; psychosis has been reported, but has not been proved to be caused by the drug. The anaemia is haemolytic in type and usually disappears when dapsone is withheld. Blood transfusion is required if the anaemia is severe; the administration of a ferrous salt may prove useful by correcting any underlying iron-deficiency anaemia.

Lepra reactions (reactional states), which may complicate the treatment of leprosy, are not toxic effects of dapsone as they can occur during treatment with other unrelated antileprotic drugs, or even when no treatment is being given. Antimalarial drugs, parenteral antimony compounds and corticosteroids may be of value in the management of these reactions, particularly the type known as erythema nodosum leprosum.

Dose. See above under **Actions and uses.**

Preparation
DAPSONE TABLETS, B.P. Unless otherwise specified, tablets each containing 100 mg of dapsone are supplied.

OTHER NAMES: DADPS; DDS; Diaphenylsulfone

DEMECLOCYCLINE HYDROCHLORIDE

SYNONYMS: Demeclocyclini Hydrochloridum; Demethylchlortetracycline Hydrochloride

$C_{21}H_{22}Cl_2N_2O_8 = 501·3$

Demeclocycline Hydrochloride is the hydrochloride of 7-chloro-4-dimethylamino-1,4,4a,5,5a,6,11,12a-octahydro-3,6,10,12,12a-pentahydroxy-1,11-dioxonaphthacene-2-carboxyamide, an antimicrobial substance produced by the growth of *Streptomyces aureofaciens* or by any other means.

Solubility. Soluble, at 20°, in 30 parts of water and in 45 parts of alcohol; slightly soluble in acetone; very slightly soluble in ether and in chloroform; soluble in aqueous solutions of alkali hydroxides and carbonates.

Standard
It complies with the requirements of the European Pharmacopoeia.
It is a yellow, odourless, crystalline powder and contains not less than 950 Units per mg, calculated with reference to the dried substance. The loss on drying under the prescribed conditions is not more than 2·0 per

cent. A 1 per cent w/v solution in water has a pH of 2·0 to 3·0.

Storage. It should be stored in airtight containers, protected from light.

Actions and uses. Demeclocycline has a range of activity similar to that described under Tetracycline Hydrochloride (page 498) and is used for similar purposes. As it is excreted more slowly, the concentration in the blood from the same dose is maintained for a longer period. The usual dosage for an adult is 600 milligrams by mouth daily in two to four doses; for a child it is 6 to 12 milligrams per kilogram body-weight daily.

Salts of aluminium, calcium, iron, and magnesium, which may decrease the absorption of tetracycline from the gut, should not be given with demeclocycline.

In addition to the capsules, demeclocycline is available as oral liquid preparations containing base equivalent to 75 milligrams of demeclocycline hydrochloride in 5 millilitres and base equivalent to 60 milligrams of hydrochloride per millilitre, and as an ointment containing 0·5 per cent of demeclocycline hydrochloride.

UNDESIRABLE EFFECTS; PRECAUTIONS AND CONTRA-INDICATIONS. These are as described under Tetracycline Hydrochloride (page 498); there is the additional hazard of photosensitisation which makes it desirable for patients to avoid exposure to sunlight during treatment.

Dose. For an adult, 0·6 to 1·8 grams daily, in divided doses; for a child, 6 to 12 milligrams per kilogram body-weight daily, in divided doses.

Preparation

DEMECLOCYCLINE CAPSULES, B.P. (*Syn.* Demethylchlortetracycline Capsules). Unless otherwise specified, capsules each containing 150 mg of demeclocycline hydrochloride are supplied.

OTHER NAME: *Ledermycin®*

DEOXYCORTONE ACETATE

SYNONYMS: Deoxycort. Acet.;
Desoxycorticosterone Acetate;
Desoxycortoni Acetas

$C_{23}H_{32}O_4 = 372·5$

Deoxycortone Acetate is 21-acetoxypregn-4-ene-3,20-dione.

Solubility. Very slightly soluble in water; soluble, at 20°, in 50 parts of alcohol, in 30 parts of acetone, in 170 parts of propylene glycol, in 150 parts of ethyl oleate, in 140 parts of arachis oil, and in other fixed oils.

Standard
It complies with the requirements of the European Pharmacopoeia.
It occurs as odourless, colourless crystals or white, crystalline powder and contains not less than 96·0 and not more than the equivalent of 104·0 per cent of $C_{23}H_{32}O_4$, calculated with reference to the dried substance. The loss on drying under the prescribed conditions is not more than 0·5 per cent. It has a melting-point of 157° to 161°.

Sterilisation. Oily solutions for injection are sterilised by dry heat.

Storage. It should be protected from light.

Actions and uses. Deoxycortone is a mineralocorticoid which causes sodium retention and potassium excretion. It is used in conjunction with cortisone or hydrocortisone in the treatment of Addison's disease, or after total adrenalectomy in patients in whom cortisone or hydrocortisone given alone does not prevent the development of sodium deficiency. For this purpose, however, fludrocortisone given by mouth is often preferred.

Deoxycortone acetate is given by intramuscular injection in a dosage of 2 to 5 milligrams daily or on alternate days, or as an implant of 100 to 400 milligrams every four to five months. It may also be given sublingually in a dosage of 2 to 10 milligrams daily in tablets containing 1 milligram.

UNDESIRABLE EFFECTS. Overdosage causes sodium retention with elevation of blood pressure in both normal and adrenal-deficient subjects, and oedema occasionally occurs.

Dose. See above under **Actions and uses.**

Preparations
DEOXYCORTONE ACETATE IMPLANTS, B.P. Unless otherwise specified, sterile implants each consisting of 100 mg of deoxycortone acetate are supplied. They should be protected from light. Implants consisting of 25 mg are also available.

DEOXYCORTONE ACETATE INJECTION, B.P. It consists of a sterile solution of deoxycortone acetate in ethyl oleate or other suitable ester, in a suitable fixed oil, or in any mixture of these; it may also contain suitable alcohols. Unless otherwise specified, a solution containing 5 mg in 1 ml is supplied. It should be protected from light. Solid matter may separate on standing and should be redissolved by heating before use. Ampoules containing 2 and 10 mg in 1 ml are also available.

DEOXYCORTONE PIVALATE

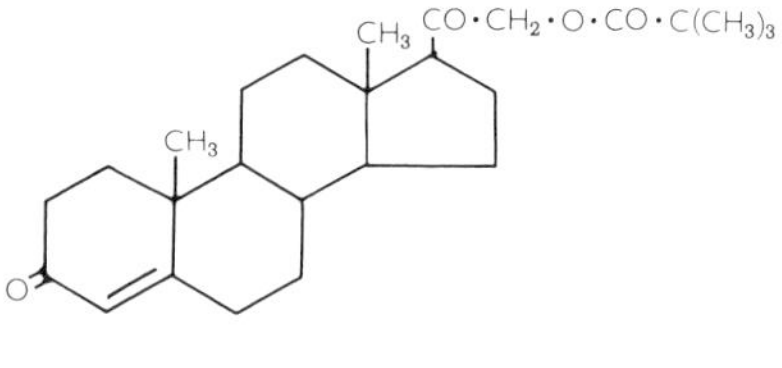

SYNONYMS: Deoxycortone Trimethylacetate;
Desoxycorticosterone Trimethylacetate

$C_{26}H_{38}O_4 = 414.6$

Deoxycortone Pivalate is 21-pivaloyloxypregn-4-ene-3,20-dione.

Solubility. Very slightly soluble in water; soluble, at 20°, in 350 parts of alcohol, in 160 parts of methyl alcohol, and in 57 parts of dioxan; slightly soluble in fixed oils.

Standard
DESCRIPTION. A white or creamy-white crystalline powder; odourless or almost odourless.

IDENTIFICATION TESTS. 1. To a warm 1 per cent w/v solution in *methyl alcohol* add an equal volume of *potassium cupri-tartrate solution*; a red precipitate is produced.

2. It complies with the thin-layer chromatographic test given in Appendix 5A, page 861.

3. The infra-red absorption spectrum exhibits maxima which are only at the same wavelengths as, and have similar relative intensities to, those in the spectrum of *deoxycortone pivalate A.S.*

MELTING-POINT. 198° to 204°.

SPECIFIC ROTATION. +153° to +161°, calculated with reference to the anhydrous substance, determined at 20° in a 1.0 per cent w/v solution in *dioxan.*

RELATED FOREIGN STEROIDS. It complies with the test given in Appendix 5A, page 862.

LOSS ON DRYING. Not more than 0.5 per cent, determined by drying to constant weight at 105°.

SULPHATED ASH. Not more than 0.1 per cent.

CONTENT OF $C_{26}H_{38}O_4$. Not less than 96.0 and not more than the equivalent of 104.0 per cent, calculated with reference to the dried substance, determined by the following method:
Using *dehydrated alcohol* as solvent, dissolve about 0.01 g, accurately weighed, and dilute to 100 ml; dilute 5 ml of this solution to 50 ml, and measure the extinction of a 1-cm layer at the maximum at about 240 nm. For purposes of calculation, use a value of 405 for the E(1 per cent, 1 cm) of $C_{26}H_{38}O_4$. Calculate the percentage of $C_{26}H_{38}O_4$ in the sample.

Storage. It should be protected from light.

Actions and uses. Deoxycortone pivalate has the actions, uses, and undesirable effects described under Deoxycortone Acetate. It is given by intramuscular injection as a microcrystalline suspension containing 25 mg per ml and is very slowly absorbed from the site of injection, the therapeutic effect being maintained over a period of two to three weeks.

Dose. 25 to 100 milligrams by intramuscular injection, repeated as required.

OTHER NAME: *Percorten-M®*

DEQUALINIUM ACETATE

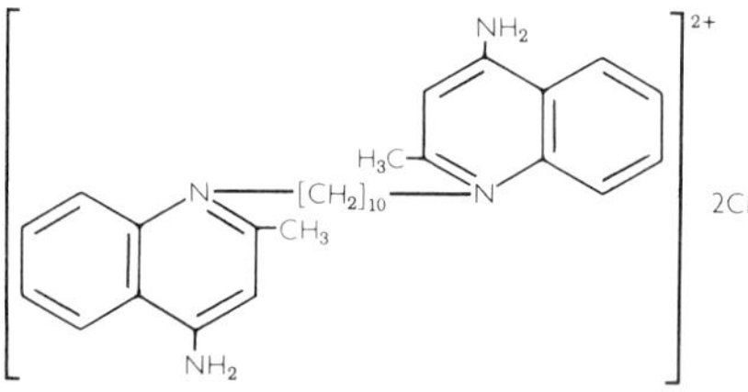

$C_{34}H_{46}N_4O_4 = 574.8$

Dequalinium Acetate is decamethylenebis-(4-aminoquinaldinium acetate).

Solubility. Soluble, at 20°, in 2 parts of water and in 12 parts of alcohol.

Standard
It complies with the requirements of the British Pharmacopoeia.
It is a white or pinkish-buff, slightly hygroscopic, odourless powder and contains not less than 97.0 and not more than the equivalent of 101.0 per cent of $C_{34}H_{46}N_4O_4$, calculated with reference to the dried substance. The loss on drying under the prescribed conditions is not more than 5.0 per cent. It melts with decomposition at about 280°. A 5 per cent solution in water has a pH of 6.0 to 8.0.

Incompatibility. It is incompatible with soaps and similar anionic compounds, with phenol, and with chlorocresol.

Storage. It should be stored in airtight containers, protected from light.

Preparation and storage of solutions. See statement on aqueous solutions of antiseptics, under Solutions (page 779).

Actions and uses. Dequalinium acetate has antibacterial and antifungal properties similar to those described under Dequalinium Chloride and is used for similar purposes.

DEQUALINIUM CHLORIDE

$C_{30}H_{40}Cl_2N_4 = 527.6$

Dequalinium Chloride is decamethylenebis(4-aminoquinaldinium chloride).

Solubility. Slightly soluble in water; soluble in 30 parts of boiling water; soluble, at 20°, in 200 parts of propylene glycol.

Standard
It complies with the requirements of the British Pharmacopoeia.
It is a creamy-white odourless powder and contains not less than 95·0 and not more than the equivalent of 101·0 per cent of $C_{30}H_{40}Cl_2N_4$, calculated with reference to the dried substance. The loss on drying under the prescribed conditions is not more than 5·0 per cent. It melts with decomposition at about 315°.

Incompatibility. It is incompatible with soaps and similar anionic compounds, with phenol, and with chlorocresol.

Storage. It should be stored in airtight containers.

Preparation and storage of solutions. See statement on aqueous solutions of antiseptics, under Solutions (page 779).

Actions and uses. Dequalinium chloride has antibacterial and antifungal properties. It is active against Gram-positive and Gram-negative bacteria and against *Borrelia vincentii*, *Candida albicans*, and several species of *Trichophyton*. Its action is little affected by the presence of serum.
Dequalinium chloride is used in the treatment of infections of the gums, mouth, and throat, for which it may be administered in lozenges containing 0·25 milligram or applied as a paint containing 0·5 per cent in propylene glycol.

OTHER NAME: *Dequadin*®

DESFERRIOXAMINE MESYLATE

$$NH_2 \cdot [CH_2]_5 N \cdot C \cdot [CH_2]_2 \cdot C \cdot NH \cdot [CH_2]_5 \cdot N \cdot C \cdot [CH_2]_2 \cdot C \cdot NH \cdot [CH_2]_5 \cdot N \cdot C \cdot CH_3 , CH_3 SO_3 H$$
$$\overset{|}{HO}\ \overset{\|}{O} \qquad \overset{\|}{O} \qquad \overset{|}{HO}\ \overset{\|}{O} \qquad \overset{\|}{O} \qquad \overset{|}{HO}\ \overset{\|}{O}$$

$C_{26}H_{52}N_6O_{11}S = 656.8$

Desferrioxamine Mesylate is 30-amino-3,14,25-trihydroxy-3,9,14,20,25-penta-azatriacontane-2,10,13,21,24-pentaone methanesulphonate.

Solubility. Soluble, at 20°, in 5 parts of water and in 20 parts of alcohol; insoluble in ether, in chloroform, and in dehydrated alcohol.

Standard
It complies with the requirements of the British Pharmacopoeia.
It is a white to cream-coloured, odourless or almost odourless powder and contains not less than 98·0 and not more than the equivalent of 102·0 per cent of $C_{26}H_{52}N_6O_{11}S$, calculated with reference to the anhydrous substance. It contains not more than 2·0 per cent w/w of water. A 10 per cent solution in water has a pH of 4·5 to 6·5.

Storage. It should be stored in airtight containers, protected from light, at a temperature not exceeding 4°.

Actions and uses. Desferrioxamine mesylate is a chelating agent with a specific affinity for iron. It combines with any available iron in the tissues and body fluids and is excreted through the kidneys as ferrioxamine B.
Desferrioxamine mesylate is used for the removal of iron in poisoning due to iron. For this purpose it is injected intramuscularly in doses of 2 grams dissolved in 8 to 12 millilitres of Water for Injections. Gastric lavage should be carried out as quickly as possible with 1 per cent sodium bicarbonate solution. Oral administration of 5 grams of desferrioxamine mesylate in 50 millilitres of fluid should then be used to bind any iron remaining in the stomach and to prevent any further absorption. Intubation may be necessary in comatose patients.

Desferrioxamine mesylate may also be administered by continuous intravenous infusion at a rate of not more than 15 milligrams per kilogram body-weight per hour to a maximum dose of 80 milligrams per kilogram body-weight in twenty-four hours; it may be added to Sodium Chloride Injection, Dextrose Injection, or blood.
Intramuscular injection may be repeated at intervals of twelve hours and if large amounts of iron have been taken it may have to be given to a maximum of 12 grams.
Desferrioxamine mesylate is also used in a variety of haemolytic anaemias to remove iron from the body. Dosage is 1 to 1·5 grams daily, given in one to three intramuscular injections. Intermittent maintenance treatment may be necessary for several months. It is used in conjunction with venesection in patients with primary haemochromatosis and is the only treatment applicable in secondary haemochromatosis. It has also been used in the treatment of thalassaemia in children.

UNDESIRABLE EFFECTS. Rapid intravenous injection of desferrioxamine mesylate may produce anaphylactic reactions and the rate of injection should never exceed 15 milligrams per kilogram body-weight per hour. There may be pain at the site of intramuscular injection.

Dose. See above under **Actions and uses**.

Preparation

DESFERRIOXAMINE INJECTION, B.P. It consists of a sterile solution of desferrioxamine mesylate prepared by dissolving the sterile contents of a sealed container in Water for Injections. The injection deteriorates on storage and should be used immediately after preparation. Cloudy solutions should be discarded. Vials containing 500 mg of desferrioxamine mesylate are available.

OTHER NAMES: *Desferal®*; Desferrioxamine Methanesulphonate

DESIPRAMINE HYDROCHLORIDE

$C_{18}H_{23}ClN_2 = 302.8$

Desipramine Hydrochloride is the hydrochloride of 10,11-dihydro-5-(3-methylaminopropyl)-5H-dibenz[b,f]azepine.

Solubility. Soluble, at 20°, in 20 parts of water, in 20 parts of alcohol, and in 4 parts of chloroform; very slightly soluble in ether.

Standard

It complies with the requirements of the British Pharmacopoeia.

It is a white or almost white, crystalline, odourless or almost odourless powder and contains not less than 99.0 and not more than the equivalent of 101.0 per cent of $C_{18}H_{23}ClN_2$, calculated with reference to the dried substance. The loss on drying under the prescribed conditions is not more than 0.5 per cent. It has a melting-point of 212° to 216°. A 10 per cent solution in water has a pH of 4.5 to 5.7.

Sterilisation. Solutions for injection are sterilised by heating in an autoclave or by filtration.

Storage. It should be stored protected from light.

Actions and uses. Desipramine has actions, uses, and undesirable effects similar to those described under Imipramine Hydrochloride (page 234), but it may produce a more rapid response, often within three or four days of the commencement of treatment.

The usual oral dosage of desipramine hydrochloride is initially 50 to 75 milligrams daily in divided doses, increasing to 150 to 200 milligrams daily over a period of about five days. When a satisfactory response has been obtained the drug should be gradually withdrawn, but prolonged maintenance therapy with a daily dosage of 100 to 150 milligrams may be necessary. The initial dosage may be given by intramuscular injection of 25 to 50 milligrams, increasing to 100 milligrams daily. As desipramine hydrochloride may produce insomnia, it should not be administered in the evening.

In addition to the tablets, desipramine hydrochloride is available as a solution for injection containing 25 milligrams in 2 millilitres.

PRECAUTIONS. Caution should be exercised when giving desipramine hydrochloride to patients who are being treated with a mono-amine-oxidase inhibitor, such as isocarboxazid, nialamide, phenelzine, or tranylcypromine, or who have been so treated within the previous ten days. It may cause a reversal of the effect of antihypertensive drugs.

Dose. See above under **Actions and uses**.

Preparation

DESIPRAMINE TABLETS, B.P. Unless otherwise specified, tablets each containing 25 mg of desipramine hydrochloride are supplied. They are sugar coated.

OTHER NAME: *Pertofran®*

DESLANOSIDE

$C_{47}H_{74}O_{19} = 943.1$

Deslanoside is deacetyl-lanatoside C, the 3-glucosyl-tridigitoxoside of digoxigenin.

Solubility. Very slightly soluble in water, in ether, and in chloroform; slightly soluble in alcohol.

Standard

It complies with the requirements of the British Pharmacopoeia.

It occurs as odourless, hygroscopic, white crystals or powder and contains not less than 96.0 and not more than the equivalent of 104.0 per cent of $C_{47}H_{74}O_{19}$, calculated with reference to the dried substance. The loss on drying under the prescribed conditions is not more than 7.0 per cent.

Storage. It should be stored in airtight containers, protected from light.

Actions and uses. Deslanoside has the actions described under Digitalis Leaf (page 161). It is derived from lanatoside C but is administered by intravenous or intramuscular injection and is usually reserved for medical emergencies such as pulmonary oedema or left ventricular failure.

The characteristic effects of deslanoside are produced in ten to thirty minutes, reaching a maximum in one to two hours, regressing between sixteen and thirty-six hours after administration, and disappearing within three to six days. The usual digitalising dose is 1 to 1·6 milligrams. When the emergency is past, a suitable oral preparation of a digitalis glycoside should be substituted for maintenance therapy.

UNDESIRABLE EFFECTS. The undesirable effects described under Digitalis Leaf (page 161) may occur and may be severe and of rapid

onset when deslanoside is given intravenously.

PRECAUTIONS. As for Digitalis Leaf (page 161). The injection should be diluted with Sodium Chloride Injection and injected slowly to minimise toxic effects.

POISONING. The procedure as described under Digitalis Leaf (page 161) should be adopted.

Dose. See above under **Actions and uses.**

OTHER NAME: *Cedilanid®*

DEXAMETHASONE

SYNONYM: Dexameth.

$C_{22}H_{29}FO_5 = 392.5$

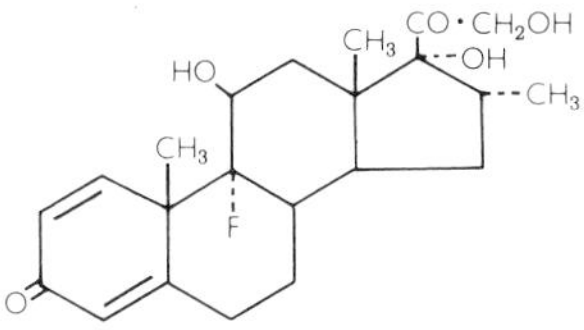

Dexamethasone is 9α-fluoro-11β,17α,21-trihydroxy-16α-methylpregna-1,4-diene-3,20-dione.

Solubility. Very slightly soluble in water; soluble, at 20°, in 42 parts of alcohol and in 165 parts of chloroform.

Standard
It complies with the requirements of the British Pharmacopoeia.
It occurs as odourless, white or almost white crystals or crystalline powder and contains not less than 96·0 and not more than the equivalent of 104·0 per cent of $C_{22}H_{29}FO_5$, calculated with reference to the dried substance. The loss on drying under the prescribed conditions is not more than 0·5 per cent.

Storage. It should be protected from light.

Actions and uses. Dexamethasone has actions and uses similar to those of prednisolone (page 399) but is effective in lower dosage.
It is used in the treatment of all conditions for which cortisone acetate (page 132) is indicated, except adrenocortical deficiency states, for

which its diminished sodium-retaining properties make it less suitable than cortisone.
It is given by mouth in a dosage of 0·5 to 2 milligrams daily in divided doses, but in potentially fatal conditions, such as leukaemia or pemphigus, up to 12 milligrams daily may be given. Soluble salts such as dexamethasone sodium phosphate may be administered by injection.

UNDESIRABLE EFFECTS; PRECAUTIONS AND CONTRA-INDICATIONS. As for Cortisone Acetate (page 132).

Dose. See above under **Actions and uses.**

Preparation
DEXAMETHASONE TABLETS, B.P. Unless otherwise specified, tablets each containing 500 µg of dexamethasone are supplied. They should be protected from light. Tablets containing 750 µg are also available.

OTHER NAMES: *Decadron®*; *Dexacortisyl®*; *Oradexon®*

DEXAMPHETAMINE SULPHATE

SYNONYMS: Dexamphet. Sulph.;
Dextro Amphetamine Sulphate

$C_{18}H_{28}N_2O_4S = 368.5$

$[C_6H_5 \cdot CH_2 \cdot CH(NH_2) \cdot CH_3]_2 H_2SO_4$

Dexamphetamine Sulphate is (+)-α-methylphenethylamine sulphate.

Solubility. Soluble, at 20°, in 9 parts of water and in 800 parts of alcohol; insoluble in ether.

Standard
It complies with the requirements of the British Pharmacopoeia.
It is a white or almost white, crystalline, odourless powder and contains not less than 99·0 per cent of $C_{18}H_{28}N_2O_4S$, calculated with reference to the dried substance. The loss on drying under the prescribed conditions is not more than 1·0 per cent.

Actions and uses. Dexamphetamine is a sympathomimetic drug which has the actions and uses described under Amphetamine Sulphate (page 25) but it is about twice as potent as the racemic compound.

Dexamphetamine is used mainly in the treatment of obesity. It has no effect on the basal metabolic rate or on nitrogen excretion, but makes a restricted food intake more acceptable to the patient, and for this purpose it is usually given by mouth in a dosage of 10 milligrams two or three times a day about half an hour before food. To avoid insomnia the last dose should be taken several hours before bedtime.

PRECAUTIONS. Dexamphetamine sulphate should not be given to patients who are being treated with a monoamine-oxidase inhibitor, such as isocarboxazid, nialamide, phenelzine, or tranylcypromine, or within about 10 days of the discontinuation of such treatment.

Its indiscriminate use in attempts to increase capacity for work or to overcome fatigue is undesirable, as it is liable to lead to dependence of the amphetamine type (see under Amphetamine Sulphate, page 25).

CONTRA-INDICATIONS. These are as described under Amphetamine Sulphate (page 25).

POISONING. As for Amphetamine Sulphate (page 25).

Dose. See above under **Actions and uses**.

Preparation
DEXAMPHETAMINE TABLETS, B.P. Unless otherwise specified, tablets each containing 5 mg of dexamphetamine sulphate are supplied.

OTHER NAMES: *Dexamed®*; *Dexedrine®*

DEXTRAN 40 INJECTION

Dextran 40 Injection is a sterile 10 per cent w/v solution, in Dextrose Injection (5 per cent w/v) or in Sodium Chloride Injection, of dextrans of weight average molecular weight about 40,000, derived from the dextrans produced by the fermentation of sucrose by means of a certain strain of *Leuconostoc mesenteroides* (National Collection of Type Cultures No. 10817).
The dextrans are polymers of glucose in which the linkages between the glucose units are almost entirely of the α-1,6 type.

Standard
It complies with the requirements of the British Pharmacopoeia.
It is an almost colourless, slightly viscous solution.

Sterilisation. It is sterilised by heating in an autoclave or by filtration.

Storage. It should not be exposed to undue fluctuations in temperature.

Actions and uses. Dextran 40 Injection, given intravenously, inhibits the intravascular aggregation of red blood cells, the so-called sludging of blood, which may occur in many pathological conditions associated with local slowing of blood flow. Sludging of the blood may also occur in normal subjects, in whom it is of no pathological significance. It is suggested that red blood cell aggregates may plug arterioles and capillaries and so diminish blood flow locally, with the production of tissue anoxia and finally necrosis. However, the clinical implications of intravascular sludging of blood are still uncertain.

As Dextran 40 Injection inhibits red-cell aggregation and lowers blood viscosity, it may improve local blood supply. It has been recommended for the treatment of a wide variety of clinical conditions where impaired blood flow results in local ischaemia.

In the doses used, Dextran 40 Injection increases plasma volume for a short time, thereby reducing blood viscosity and increasing blood flow; some of the therapeutic effects claimed for it may be the result of this. Most of a dose is excreted by the kidneys or metabolised within about twenty-four hours. It does not interfere with the cross-matching of blood, blood clotting or bleeding mechanisms, or fibrinolysis; it is compatible with heparin.

The initial dose of Dextran 40 Injection is 500 to 1000 millilitres by intravenous injection, the first 500 millilitres being injected over a period of thirty minutes. This may be followed by 1000 to 2000 millilitres daily by continuous intravenous infusion for two days, followed by 500 to 1000 millilitres daily for a further three days. In cardiovascular surgery, 20 millilitres per kilogram bodyweight may be added to the perfusion fluid. In vascular surgery, 500 millilitres may be given intravenously immediately before, and 500 millilitres during, the operation, followed post-operatively by 500 millilitres daily for three days as a continuous intravenous infusion.

Dextran 40 Injection has been recommended for use in vascular and cardiac surgery to reduce the risk of thrombosis, in oligaemic and traumatic shock, severe burns and crush injuries, fat embolism, myocardial and cerebral ischaemia, venous thrombosis, arterial embolism, pancreatitis, and peritonitis, and also in angiography.

PRECAUTIONS AND CONTRA-INDICATIONS. Dextran 40 Injection should be given with caution to patients with congestive heart failure, renal impairment, or polycythaemia, and after blood and electrolyte replacement. It should not be administered at a rate greater than 500 millilitres an hour to dehydrated patients. It is contra-indicated in patients with thrombocytopenia, as it lowers the platelet count, and in severe congestive heart failure and renal failure with anuria.

Dose. See above under **Actions and uses**.

OTHER NAMES: *Lomodex 40®*; *Rheomacrodex®*

DEXTRAN 70 INJECTION

Dextran 70 Injection is a sterile 6 per cent w/v solution, in Dextrose Injection (5 per cent w/v) or in Sodium Chloride Injection, of dextrans of weight average molecular weight about 70,000, derived from the dextrans produced by the fermentation of sucrose by means of a certain strain of *Leuconostoc mesenteroides* (National Collection of Type Cultures No. 10817).

The dextrans are polymers of glucose in which the linkages between glucose units are almost entirely of the α-1,6 type.

Standard
It complies with the requirements of the British Pharmacopoeia.
It is an almost colourless, slightly viscous solution.

Sterilisation. It is sterilised by heating in an autoclave or by filtration.

Storage. It should not be exposed to undue fluctuations in temperature.

Actions and uses. Dextran 70 Injection has actions and uses similar to those described under Dextran 110 Injection. It is also used in the prevention of post-operative thrombosis, 500 to 1000 millilitres being given over four to six hours, followed by further doses of 500 millilitres on alternate days.

PRECAUTIONS AND CONTRA-INDICATIONS. As for Dextran 40 Injection.

Dose. See above under **Actions and uses.**

OTHER NAMES: *Lomodex 70*® ; *Macrodex*®

DEXTRAN 110 INJECTION

Dextran 110 Injection is a sterile 6 per cent w/v solution, in Dextrose Injection (5 per cent w/v) or in Sodium Chloride Injection, of dextrans of weight average molecular weight about 110,000, derived from the dextrans produced by the fermentation of sucrose by means of a certain strain of *Leuconostoc mesentercides* (National Collection of Type Cultures No. 10817).

The dextrans are polymers of glucose in which the linkages between the glucose units are almost entirely of the α-1,6 type.

Standard
It complies with the requirements of the British Pharmacopoeia.
It is an almost colourless, slightly viscous solution.

Sterilisation. It is sterilised by heating in an autoclave or by filtration.

Storage. It should not be exposed to undue fluctuations in temperature.

Actions and uses. Dextran 110 Injection, given intravenously, is an effective temporary plasma substitute, because its osmotic pressure is approximately the same as that of the plasma proteins. When infused, it is retained in the circulation for two or three days, a period long enough for the normal physiological replacement of the plasma proteins. Dextran 110 Injection helps to maintain the blood volume and to increase the venous return. It raises a lowered blood pressure. The dextrans are either metabolised as a polysaccharide or excreted; none of them are retained in the body.

Dextran 110 Injection is used to restore blood volume if this has been reduced by haemorrhage, extravasation of blood or plasma, injury, shock, surgery, or burns. It is also used prophylactically in major surgery to maintain the blood pressure and prevent surgical shock during long operations or those associated with much haemorrhage.

The dose of Dextran 110 Injection and the rate of infusion depend on the condition being treated or whether it is used prophylactically. After moderate blood loss, 500 millilitres infused rapidly during ten minutes and a further 500 millilitres given during thirty to forty-five minutes may suffice. For the treatment of severe haemorrhage 1000 millilitres may be infused rapidly, with a further 500 millilitres given more slowly later if necessary. In the case of injury and shock, plasma proteins leak into the tissues and draw water osmotically from the blood. These conditions may be treated by infusing 500 millilitres or more, the rate of infusion depending on the degree of shock. Large quantities may be needed in the first few days for the treatment of burns, during which 3000 millilitres may be given; electrolytes are also required.

For prophylaxis during surgical operations associated with blood loss or shock, intravenous drip at the rate of 10 to 20 drops a minute is given as soon as the patient has been anaesthetised, and the rate adjusted to maintain a normal blood pressure during the operation.

PRECAUTIONS AND CONTRA-INDICATIONS. Blood samples for cross matching should be taken from patients before infusion with Dextran 110 Injection in case blood or packed cells need to be given later. These may be necessary after infusing large quantities of Dextran

110 Injection, which is unable to transport oxygen and dilutes the blood-clotting factors. It should not be used for the treatment of haemorrhage associated with hypofibrinogenaemia.

Dose. See above under **Actions and uses.**

OTHER NAME: *Dextraven 110*®

DEXTROMETHORPHAN HYDROBROMIDE

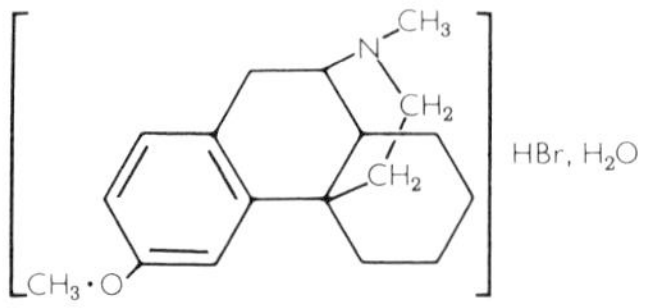

$C_{18}H_{26}BrNO,H_2O = 370 \cdot 3$

Dextromethorphan Hydrobromide is (+)-3-methoxy-*N*-methylmorphinan hydrobromide monohydrate.

Solubility. Soluble, at 20°, in 60 parts of water and in 10 parts of alcohol; freely soluble in chloroform with separation of water; insoluble in ether.

Standard
It complies with the requirements of the British Pharmacopoeia.
It is a white, crystalline, odourless powder and contains not less than 99·0 and not more than the equivalent of 101·0 per cent of $C_{18}H_{26}BrNO$, calculated with reference to the dried substance. The loss on drying under the prescribed conditions is 4·0 to 5·5 per cent. A 2 per cent solution in water has a pH of 5·2 to 6·5.

Storage. It should be stored in airtight containers.

Actions and uses. Dextromethorphan has a depressant action on the cough centre similar to that described under Codeine Phosphate (page 123), but it has no analgesic

or expectorant effect, no other depressant action on the central nervous system, nor any other established pharmacological action. Its use does not lead to addiction.

The recommended dosage is 15 to 30 milligrams by mouth once to four times a day, or half this dose for a child. Much higher doses have been used repeatedly without harm.

Dose. 15 to 30 milligrams.

Preparation
DEXTROMETHORPHAN TABLETS, B.P. Unless otherwise specified, tablets each containing 15 mg of dextromethorphan hydrobromide are supplied. They are sugar coated.

DEXTROMORAMIDE TARTRATE

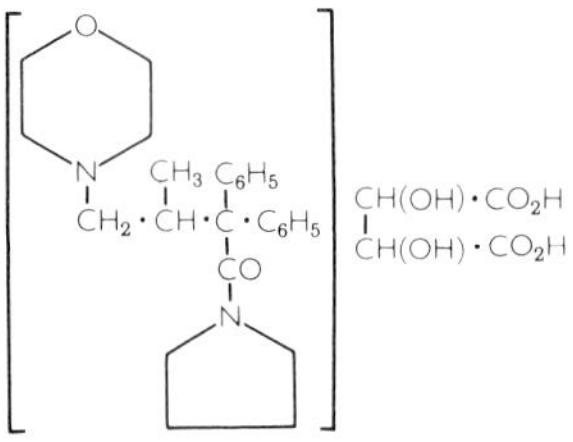

$C_{29}H_{38}N_2O_8 = 542 \cdot 6$

Dextromoramide Tartrate is (+)-1-(β-methyl-γ-morpholino-α,α-diphenylbutyryl)pyrrolidine hydrogen tartrate.

Solubility. Soluble, at 20°, in 25 parts of water and in 85 parts of alcohol; insoluble in chloroform.

Standard
It complies with the requirements of the British Pharmacopoeia.
It is a white, crystalline, odourless powder and contains not less than 99·0 and not more than the equivalent of 101·0 per cent of $C_{29}H_{38}N_2O_8$, calculated with reference to the dried substance. The loss on drying under the prescribed conditions is not more than 0·5 per cent. It melts with slight decomposition at about 190°.

Sterilisation. Solutions for injection are sterilised by heating in an autoclave or by filtration.

Actions and uses. Dextromoramide is a potent analgesic with actions and uses similar to those of methadone hydrochoride (page 297). It is used for the alleviation of severe pain.

UNDESIRABLE EFFECTS. Nausea, vomiting, dizziness, faintness, and constriction of the pupil may occur. As with morphine, many of these effects occur more often in ambulant

than in recumbent patients. When administered in therapeutic doses for prolonged periods, dextromoramide may lead to the development of tolerance, euphoria, and dependence of the morphine type (see under Morphine Hydrochloride, page 314). Dextromoramide is a powerful respiratory depressant. Cumulation occurs with repeated dosage.

POISONING. The procedure as described under Morphine Hydrochloride (page 314) should be adopted.

Dose. The equivalent of 5 milligrams of dextromoramide by mouth or by subcutaneous or intramuscular injection, repeated in accordance with the needs of the patient.

Preparations
DEXTROMORAMIDE INJECTION, B.P.C. (page 712)
DEXTROMORAMIDE TABLETS, B.P. The equivalent quantity of dextromoramide in each tablet should be specified by the prescriber. Tablets containing the equivalent of 5 mg are available.

OTHER NAME: *Palfium*®

DEXTROPROPOXYPHENE HYDROCHLORIDE

SYNONYM: Propoxyphene Hydrochloride

$C_{22}H_{30}ClNO_2 = 375.9$

$$\left[CH_3 \cdot CH_2 \cdot CO \cdot O \cdot \underset{\underset{C_6H_5 \cdot H_2C}{|}}{\overset{\overset{C_6H_5}{|}}{C}} \cdot \underset{\underset{CH_3}{|}}{CH} \cdot CH_2 \cdot N(CH_3)_2 \right] HCl$$

Dextropropoxyphene Hydrochloride is $(+)$-α-4-dimethylamino-3-methyl-1,2-diphenylbut-2-yl propionate hydrochloride.

Solubility. Soluble, at 20°, in 0·3 part of water, in 1·5 parts of alcohol, and in 0·6 part of chloroform; insoluble in ether.

Standard
It complies with the requirements of the British Pharmacopoeia.
It is a white or slightly yellow, odourless powder and contains not less than 98·5 and not more than the equivalent of 101·0 per cent of $C_{22}H_{30}ClNO_2$, calculated with reference to the dried substance. The loss on drying under the prescribed conditions is not more than 1·0 per cent. It has a melting-point of about 165°.

Sterilisation. Solutions for injection are sterilised by filtration.

Storage. It should be stored in airtight containers.

Actions and uses. Dextropropoxyphene is an analgesic of potency similar to codeine, but is less constipating. It does not have antitussive or anti-inflammatory properties. Unlike most potent analgesics its use does not appear to lead to tolerance, euphoria, or drug dependence.

Its action as an analgesic develops rapidly; a dose of 65 milligrams of dextropropoxyphene hydrochloride gives its full effect in one to two hours and lasts for five to six hours. It is frequently given in conjunction with aspirin or paracetamol.

UNDESIRABLE EFFECTS. Nausea, vomiting, drowsiness, and dizziness may occur.

POISONING. Very large doses depress respiration, but analeptics should not be given as they may provoke convulsions. Nalorphine or levallorphan should be given and, if necessary, artificial respiration should be applied.

Dose. Up to 260 milligrams daily in divided doses.

DEXTROPROPOXYPHENE NAPSYLATE

SYNONYM: Propoxyphene Napsylate

$C_{22}H_{29}NO_2,C_{10}H_8O_3S,H_2O = 565.7$

Dextropropoxyphene Napsylate is $(+)$-α-4-dimethylamino-3-methyl-1,2-diphenylbut-2-yl propionate naphthalene-2-sulphonate monohydrate.

Solubility. Very slightly soluble in water; soluble, at 20°, in 13 parts of alcohol and in 3 parts of chloroform.

Standard
It complies with the requirements of the British Pharmacopoeia.
It is a white odourless powder and contains not less than 98·0 and not more than the equivalent of 101·0 per cent of $C_{22}H_{29}NO_2,C_{10}H_8O_3S$, calculated with reference to the anhydrous substance. It contains 3·0 to 5·0 per cent w/w of water. It has a melting-point of about 160°.

Sterilisation. Solutions for injection are sterilised by filtration.

Actions and uses. Dextropropoxyphene napsylate has the actions, uses, and undesirable effects described under Dextropropoxyphene Hydrochloride, but it is less bitter and less irritant to the mucous membrane; 100 milligrams of dextropropoxyphene napsylate is approximately equivalent to 65 milligrams of dextropropoxyphene hydrochloride.

POISONING. As for Dextropropoxyphene Hydrochloride.

Dose. Up to 400 milligrams daily in divided doses.

Preparation
DEXTROPROPOXYPHENE CAPSULES, B.P. (*Syn.* Propoxyphene Capsules). The quantity of dextropropoxyphene napsylate in each capsule should be specified by the prescriber. Capsules each containing dextropropoxyphene napsylate equivalent to 65 mg of dextropropoxyphene hydrochloride are available.

OTHER NAME: *Doloxene*®

DEXTROSE

SYNONYMS: Dextrose Monohydrate; Glucose

$C_6H_{12}O_6,H_2O = 198.2$

Dextrose is the monohydrate of D-$(+)$-glucopyranose.

Solubility. Soluble, at 20°, in 1 part of water and in 200 parts of alcohol; soluble in glycerol.

Standard
It complies with the requirements of the British Pharmacopoeia.

It occurs as odourless colourless crystals or white or cream-coloured crystalline or granular powder. The loss on drying at 105° is 7·0 to 10·0 per cent.

Actions and uses. The chief use of dextrose

is as a food, and it is the substance to which carbohydrates, when given by mouth, are mainly converted. It also has an indirect food value because of the part it plays in the metabolism of fats and proteins. In the absence of sufficient glucose, the amount of fat oxidised is greatly increased and by-products such as hydroxybutyric acid and acetoacetic acid accumulate in the blood giving rise to ketosis.

Dextrose is given in all conditions associated with insufficiency of carbohydrates; it provides a rapidly available source of energy.

Aqueous solutions of dextrose are given by intravenous injection to increase the volume of the circulating blood in shock and to counteract dehydration; when it is desired to replace excessive salt loss, as in persistent vomiting, sodium chloride may be included in the solution.

Hypertonic dextrose solutions (10 to 50 per cent) are given by intravenous injection to provide temporary relief from the symptoms of increased intracranial pressure and for hypoglycaemic coma, but such solutions are liable to cause venous thrombosis at the site of injection.

Dextrose may be administered by mouth in solution or, when necessary, a 5 per cent solution may be given rectally as a retention enema.

When dextrose is required in infant feeding to supplement the carbohydrate content of cows' milk, dextrose (monohydrate) is usually employed.

UNDESIRABLE EFFECTS. Dextrose injections, and particularly hypertonic dextrose injections, may have a low pH, and such solutions when injected may irritate the venous intima near the site of the injection so causing thrombophlebitis.

NOTE. When Medicinal Glucose or Purified Glucose is prescribed or demanded, Dextrose is dispensed or supplied.

Solutions of dextrose for injection are prepared from Anhydrous Dextrose or from Dextrose Monohydrate for Parenteral Use.

ANHYDROUS DEXTROSE

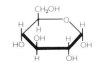

SYNONYMS: Anhydrous Dextrose for Parenteral Use; Dextrosum Anhydricum ad Usum Parenterale; Anhydrous Glucose

$C_6H_{12}O_6 = 180 \cdot 2$

Anhydrous Dextrose is D-(+)-glucopyranose.

Solubility. Soluble, at 20°, in 1 part of water and in 200 parts of alcohol; soluble in glycerol.

Standard
It complies with the requirements of the European Pharmacopoeia.
It is a white, crystalline, odourless powder. It contains not more than 1·0 per cent w/w of water.

Hygroscopicity. At relative humidities up to about 35 per cent, anhydrous dextrose absorbs insignificant amounts of moisture at 25°; at relative humidities between about 35 and 85 per cent, it absorbs significant amounts, the monohydrate being formed at relative humidities in the upper part of this range; under damper conditions it absorbs substantial amounts of moisture.

Sterilisation. Solutions for injection are sterilised, immediately after preparation, by heating in an autoclave or by filtration.

Actions and uses. Anhydrous dextrose is used for the preparation of injections of dextrose, the actions and uses of which are described under Dextrose.

NOTE. When Anhydrous Dextrose is prescribed or demanded, Anhydrous Dextrose or an equivalent amount of Dextrose Monohydrate for Parenteral Use may be dispensed or supplied.

Preparations
DEXTROSE INJECTION, B.P. It consists of a sterile solution of anhydrous dextrose in Water for Injections. Unless otherwise specified, a solution containing 5·0 per cent is supplied. It should be stored at a temperature not exceeding 25°.

DEXTROSE INJECTION, STRONG, B.P.C. (page 713)

POTASSIUM CHLORIDE AND DEXTROSE INJECTION, B.P. It consists of a sterile solution of anhydrous dextrose and potassium chloride in Water for Injections. Unless otherwise specified, a solution containing 5 per cent of anhydrous dextrose and 0·3 per cent of potassium chloride (40 millimoles, or milliequivalents, each of K+ and Cl− per litre) is supplied. On storage, this solution may cause separation of small solid particles from glass containers; solutions containing such particles must not be used. It should be stored at a temperature not exceeding 25°.

SODIUM CHLORIDE AND DEXTROSE INJECTION, B.P. It consists of a sterile solution of anhydrous dextrose and sodium chloride in Water for Injections. Unless otherwise specified, a solution containing 4·0 per cent of anhydrous dextrose and 0·18 per cent of sodium chloride (30 millimoles, or milliequivalents, each of Na+ and Cl− per litre) is supplied. On storage, this solution may cause separation of small solid particles from glass containers; solutions containing such particles must not be used. It should be stored at a temperature not exceeding 25°.

DEXTROSE MONOHYDRATE FOR PARENTERAL USE

SYNONYMS: Dextrosum Monohydricum ad Usum Parenterale; Glucose for Parenteral Use

$C_6H_{12}O_6,H_2O = 198.2$

Dextrose monohydrate for parenteral use is the monohydrate of D-(+)-glucopyranose.

Solubility. Soluble, at 20°, in 1 part of water and in 200 parts of alcohol; soluble in glycerol.

Standard
It complies with the requirements of the European Pharmacopoeia.
It is a white, crystalline, odourless powder. It contains 7.0 to 9.5 per cent w/w of water.

Sterilisation. Solutions for injection are sterilised, immediately after preparation, by heating in an autoclave or by filtration.

Actions and uses. Dextrose Monohydrate for Parenteral Use is used for the preparation of injections of dextrose, the actions and uses of which are described under Dextrose.

NOTE. When Anhydrous Dextrose is prescribed or demanded, Anhydrous Dextrose or an equivalent amount of Dextrose Monohydrate for Parenteral Use may be dispensed or supplied.

Preparations
As for Anhydrous Dextrose.

DIAMORPHINE HYDROCHLORIDE

$C_{21}H_{24}ClNO_5,H_2O = 423.9$

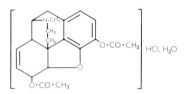

Diamorphine Hydrochloride is 3,6-O-diacetylmorphine hydrochloride monohydrate.

Solubility. Soluble, at 20°, in 1.6 parts of water, in 12 parts of alcohol, and in 1.6 parts of chloroform; insoluble in ether.

Standard
It complies with the requirements of the British Pharmacopoeia.
It is an almost white, crystalline, odourless powder and contains not less than 98.0 and not more than the equivalent of 101.0 per cent of $C_{21}H_{24}ClNO_5$, calculated with reference to the dried substance. The loss on drying under the prescribed conditions is not more than 4.5 per cent. It has a melting-point of 229° to 233°.

Stability. Diamorphine hydrolyses to 3-O- and 6-O-acetylmorphine and morphine in aqueous solutions at room temperatures to a significant extent; the rate of decomposition is minimum at about pH 4.

Incompatibility. It is incompatible with mineral acids and with alkalis. Sodium chloride precipitates diamorphine from solutions and is not suitable for adjusting the tonicity of solutions.

Storage. It should be stored in airtight containers, protected from light.

Actions and uses. Diamorphine has actions similar to those described under Morphine Hydrochloride (page 314), but it is more potent than morphine. It has less tendency to cause vomiting and constipation and is particularly effective in the relief of cough, for which purpose it is administered in a dose of 1.5 to 6 milligrams as the elixir or linctus.
Diamorphine is given by subcutaneous injection in a dose of 5 to 10 milligrams for the relief of pain and restlessness in the terminal stages of carcinoma and other fatal illnesses. It is also given by mouth in conjunction with cocaine for the same purpose.
Solutions for injection are prepared immediately before use by an aseptic technique.

UNDESIRABLE EFFECTS. Diamorphine produces dependence of the morphine type (see under Morphine Hydrochloride, page 314) more readily than morphine and the effects are worse, greater mental and moral deterioration occurring. It should be used with great caution and only when less dangerous analgesics and cough suppressants have proved inadequate or unsuitable.

POISONING. The procedure as described under Morphine Hydrochloride (page 314) should be adopted.

Dose. As an antitussive, 1.5 to 6 milligrams by mouth.
As an analgesic for terminal care, 5 to 10 milligrams, increased if necessary, by mouth or by subcutaneous or intramuscular injection.

Preparations
DIAMORPHINE AND COCAINE ELIXIR, B.P.C. (page 669)
DIAMORPHINE INJECTION, B.P. It consists of a sterile solution prepared immediately before use by dissolving the sterile contents of a sealed container in Water for Injections. The quantity of diamorphine hydrochloride in each container should be specified by the prescriber. It should be protected from light. Ampoules containing 5 and 10 mg are available.
DIAMORPHINE LINCTUS, B.P.C. (page 723)

OTHER NAME: Heroin Hydrochloride

DIAZEPAM

$C_{16}H_{13}ClN_2O = 284.7$

Diazepam is 7-chloro-2,3-dihydro-1-methyl-5-phenyl-1H-1,4-benzo-diazepin-2-one.

Solubility. Very slightly soluble in water; soluble in alcohol and in chloroform.

Standard
It complies with the requirements of the British Pharmacopoeia.
It is a white or almost white, crystalline, odourless or almost odourless powder and contains not less than 99·0 and not more than the equivalent of 101·0 per cent of $C_{16}H_{13}ClN_2O$, calculated with reference to the dried substance. The loss on drying under the prescribed conditions is not more than 0·5 per cent. It has a melting-point of 130° to 134°.

Storage. It should be stored in airtight containers, protected from light.

Actions and uses. Diazepam has tranquillising properties similar to those described under Chlordiazepoxide Hydrochloride (page 96).
It is used in the treatment of psychoneurotic disorders, when anxiety and nervous tension are present; it has also been used to relieve muscle spasm in various conditions, in the treatment of status epilepticus, in acute alcohol withdrawal, and for pre-operative medication.
Dosage depends upon the clinical condition and response of the patient, varying from 5 to 30 milligrams daily in divided doses in the treatment of anxiety and nervous tension, this dosage being reduced in elderly and debilitated patients. In anxious children the daily dose is usually 1 to 5 milligrams.
In status epilepticus and tetanus a dose of 10 milligrams of diazepam in the form of a soluble derivative may be given by intramuscular or intravenous injection. Patients should be kept under observation in the supine position in bed for at least one hour after injection.

UNDESIRABLE EFFECTS. Drowsiness, ataxia, dryness of the mouth, and hypotension may occur. In severely disturbed patients, diazepam, like chlordiazepoxide, may sometimes provoke aggressive behaviour rather than sedation. There is a danger of dependence of the barbiturate-alcohol type as described under Phenobarbitone (page 366). Rashes, blood dyscrasias, and hepatic dysfunction may rarely occur.
Diazepam may reduce the patient's ability to drive motor cars or operate moving machinery.

PRECAUTIONS AND CONTRA-INDICATIONS. Caution should be exercised in using diazepam in conjunction with alcohol and with other drugs that act on the central nervous system.
When used adjunctively in convulsive disorders, diazepam may increase the frequency and severity of grand mal seizures, necessitating an increased dosage of anticonvulsant drugs. Abrupt withdrawal may be associated with temporary increase in frequency and severity of seizures.
Diazepam should be used with caution in patients with acute narrow-angle glaucoma.

Dose. See above under **Actions and uses**.

Preparations
DIAZEPAM CAPSULES, B.P. Unless otherwise specified, capsules each containing 5 mg are supplied. They should be protected from light. Capsules containing 2 mg are also available.

DIAZEPAM TABLETS, B.P. Unless otherwise specified, tablets each containing 5 mg are supplied. They should be protected from light. Tablets containing 2 and 10 mg are also available.

OTHER NAME: *Valium*®

DIBROMOPROPAMIDINE ISETHIONATE

$C_{21}H_{30}Br_2N_4O_{10}S_2 = 722.4$

Dibromopropamidine Isethionate is 1,3-di(4-amidino-2-bromophenoxy)propane di(2-hydroxyethanesulphonate).

Solubility. Soluble, at 20°, in 2 parts of water, in 60 parts of alcohol, and in 20 parts of glycerol; insoluble in ether, in chloroform, in fixed oils, and in liquid paraffin.

Standard
It complies with the requirements of the British Pharmacopoeia.
It is a white or almost white, crystalline, odourless powder and contains not less than 97·0 and not more than the equivalent of 101·0 per cent of $C_{21}H_{30}Br_2N_4O_{10}S_2$, calculated with reference to the dried substance. The loss on drying under the prescribed conditions is not more than 2·0 per cent. A 5 per cent solution in water has a pH of 5·0 to 7·0.

Sterilisation. Aqueous solutions are sterilised by filtration.

Storage. It should be stored in airtight containers.

Actions and uses. Dibromopropamidine is an antibacterial and fungistatic agent for external use.
It is active against various streptococci and against *Staphylococcus aureus*, including forms resistant to penicillin and other antibiotics, and against certain Gram-negative bacilli, particularly *Escherichia coli*, *Proteus vulgaris*,

and some strains of *Pseudomonas aeruginosa.* Its antibacterial action is not inhibited by pus, blood, or *p*-aminobenzoic acid.
A cream containing 0·15 per cent of dibromopropamidine isethionate has been used as

a first-aid dressing for wounds, abrasions, burns, and scalds.
An eye ointment containing 0·15 per cent is used in acute infections of the conjunctiva and in blepharitis.

DICHLORALPHENAZONE

$C_{15}H_{18}Cl_6N_2O_5 = 519·0$

Dichloralphenazone is a complex of chloral hydrate and phenazone. It may be prepared by mixing strong aqueous solutions of chloral hydrate and phenazone in the correct proportions and allowing the mixture to crystallise.

Solubility. Soluble, at 20°, in 10 parts of water, in 1 part of alcohol, and in 2 parts of chloroform; soluble in dilute acids.

Standard
It complies with the requirements of the British Pharmacopoeia.
It is a white microcrystalline powder with a slight odour characteristic of chloral hydrate and contains not less than 97·0 per cent of $C_{15}H_{18}Cl_6N_2O_5$. It has a melting-point of 64° to 67°. It is decomposed by alkalis.

Storage. It should be stored in airtight containers.

Actions and uses. Dichloralphenazone has the actions of its constituents, chloral and phenazone. It is used as described under Chloral Hydrate (page 91) but is less likely to cause nausea and vomiting. A dose of 650 milligrams may be given two or three times a day as a sedative.
In domiciliary midwifery it is an effective sedative in a dose of 1·3 to 2·6 grams.
Dichloralphenazone is particularly suitable for geriatric patients, a suitable dose being 1·3 grams.

As a hypnotic, 0·65 to 2 grams may be given as a single dose.

UNDESIRABLE EFFECTS. Rashes, pruritus, nausea, headache, and lassitude may rarely occur. Dichloralphenazone may give rise to dependence of the barbiturate-alcohol type as described under Phenobarbitone (page 366) and enhance the effects of alcohol. It may increase the difficulty of controlling oral anticoagulant therapy.

CONTRA-INDICATIONS. It is contra-indicated in acute intermittent porphyria since it may precipitate an acute attack.

Dose. See above under **Actions and uses.**

Preparations
DICHLORALPHENAZONE ELIXIR, B.P.C. (page 669)

DICHLORALPHENAZONE TABLETS, B.P. Unless otherwise specified, tablets each containing 650 mg of dichloralphenazone are supplied. They should be stored in airtight containers. Tablets containing 150 mg are also available.

OTHER NAMES: *Fenzol®*; *Welldorm®*

DICHLORODIFLUOROMETHANE

SYNONYMS: Propellent 12; Refrigerant 12; Difluorodichloromethane
$CCl_2F_2 = 120·9$

Dichlorodifluoromethane is gaseous at ordinary temperatures but is liquefied by compression and is supplied in liquid form in suitable metal containers. It has a weight per ml of about 1·50 g at −35° and about 1·35 g at 15°.

Solubility. In the liquid state: immiscible with water; miscible with dehydrated alcohol.

Standard
DESCRIPTION. A clear, colourless, non-inflammable, very volatile liquid; odour faintly ethereal.

IDENTIFICATION TEST. It boils at about −29·8°.

DISTILLATION RANGE. When determined by the method given in Appendix 17A, page 896, the specified fraction distils within a range of 0·2°.

HIGH-BOILING IMPURITIES. Not more than 0·01 per cent v/v, determined by the following method:
Allow the boiling-tube containing the remaining 15 ml of sample from the determination of distillation range to stand in ice-water for 30 minutes and measure the volume of the residue.

FREE ACIDITY. Not more than 0·0002 per cent w/w,

calculated as HCl, determined by the following method:
Place 200 ml of water, previously neutralised to *bromocresol purple solution*, in a gas-washing bottle fitted with a sintered-glass distribution tube, pass 200 g of the sample through the water, and titrate with 0·02N sodium hydroxide, using *bromocresol purple solution* as indicator; each ml of 0·02N sodium hydroxide is equivalent to 0·000729 g of HCl.

CHLORIDE. Mix 5 ml with 5 ml of *methyl alcohol* and add 0·2 ml of a saturated solution of *silver nitrate* in *methyl alcohol*; no opalescence is produced.

WATER. Not more than 0·0010 per cent w/w, determined by the method given in Appendix 17B, page 896.

Storage. It should be stored in suitable metal containers, in a cool place away from any fire risk.

Uses. Dichlorodifluoromethane is used as a refrigerant and as an aerosol propellant; in aerosols it is the major source of pressure. It is sometimes used as the sole propellant, particularly if its vapour pressure is likely to be reduced by other constituents of the formulation, such as solvents. More commonly it is mixed with either trichlorofluoromethane or dichlorotetrafluoroethane to form propellant 12/11 or propellant 12/114 mixtures of lower pressure.

Typical aerosols using propellant 12/11 mixtures are spray bandages and analgesic or anaesthetic sprays. Propellant 12/114 mixtures are used mainly in antibronchitic and anti-asthmatic sprays and in nasal and dermatological sprays.

DICHLOROPHEN

$C_{13}H_{10}Cl_2O_2 = 269 \cdot 1$

Dichlorophen is di(5-chloro-2-hydroxyphenyl)methane.

Solubility. Slightly soluble in water; soluble, at 20°, in 1 part of alcohol and less than 1 part of ether.

Standard
It complies with the requirements of the British Pharmacopoeia.
It is a white to slightly cream-coloured powder with not more than a slight phenolic odour and contains not less than 98·0 per cent of $C_{13}H_{10}Cl_2O_2$, calculated with reference to the dried substance. The loss on drying under the prescribed conditions is not more than 1·0 per cent. It has a melting-point of 174° to 178°.

Actions and uses. Dichlorophen is a taenicide with a direct lethal action on the worm. After the tapeworm has been killed, the segments are partially digested in the intestine and they are therefore largely unrecognisable in the stools, so that it is impossible to be sure whether the scolex has been removed. There is no necessity for preliminary starvation or the administration of a laxative.

Dichlorophen is best given in the morning, as the dosing is usually followed in two to three hours by intestinal colic and the passing of a few loose stools.

UNDESIRABLE EFFECTS. Vomiting occurs occasionally and there is the possibility that segments or ova regurgitated into the stomach could cause cysticercosis.

CONTRA-INDICATIONS. Dichlorophen is contra-indicated when liver disease is present or when purgation is undesirable.

Dose. In divided doses on each of two successive days: for an adult, 6 grams; for a child, 2 to 4 grams.

Preparation
DICHLOROPHEN TABLETS, B.P. Unless otherwise specified, tablets each containing 500 mg of dichlorophen are supplied.

OTHER NAME: *Anthiphen*®

DICHLOROTETRAFLUOROETHANE

SYNONYMS: Propellant 114; Refrigerant 114; Tetrafluorodichloroethane $CCIF_2 \cdot CCIF_2$
$C_2Cl_2F_4 = 170 \cdot 9$

Dichlorotetrafluoroethane is 1,2-dichloro-1,1,2,2-tetrafluoroethane. It is gaseous at ordinary temperatures, but is liquefied by compression and is supplied in liquid form in suitable metal containers. It has a weight per ml of about 1·63 g at $-35°$ and about 1·49 g at 15°.

Solubility. In the liquid state: immiscible with water; miscible with dehydrated alcohol.

Standard
DESCRIPTION. A clear, colourless, non-inflammable, very volatile liquid; odour faintly ethereal.

IDENTIFICATION TEST. It boils at about 3·5°.

DISTILLATION RANGE. When determined by the method given in Appendix 17A, page 896, the specified fraction distils within a range of 0·3°.

HIGH-BOILING IMPURITIES. Not more than 0·01 per cent v/v, determined by the following method:
Allow the boiling-tube containing the remaining 15 ml of sample from the determination of distillation range to stand in a water-bath at 34° for 30 minutes and measure the volume of the residue.

FREE ACIDITY; CHLORIDE. It complies with the tests described under Dichlorodifluoromethane, page 155.

WATER. Not more than 0·0010 per cent w/w, determined by the method given in Appendix 17B, page 896.

Storage. It should be stored in suitable metal containers, in a cool place away from any fire risk.

Uses. Dichlorotetrafluoroethane is used as a refrigerant and aerosol propellant, as described under Dichlorodifluoromethane (above).

DICHLORPHENAMIDE

$C_6H_6Cl_2N_2O_4S_2 = 305 \cdot 2$

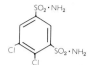

Dichlorphenamide is 4,5-dichlorobenzene-1,3-disulphonamide.

Solubility. Very slightly soluble in water and in chloroform; soluble, at 20°, in 30 parts of alcohol; soluble in solutions of alkali hydroxides.

Standard
It complies with the requirements of the British Pharmacopoeia.
It is a white or almost white crystalline powder with a slight odour and contains not less than 98·0 per cent of $C_6H_6Cl_2N_2O_4S_2$, calculated with reference to the dried substance. The loss on drying under the prescribed conditions is not more than 1·0 per cent. It has a melting-point of about 240°.

Actions and uses. Dichlorphenamide is a carbonic-anhydrase inhibitor which has an action similar to but more prolonged than that described under Acetazolamide (page 4) but which also causes an increase in chloride excretion.
Dichlorphenamide is used to effect reduction of the intra-ocular pressure in the treatment of various types of glaucoma, for which the initial dose is 100 to 200 milligrams by mouth, followed by 100 milligrams every twelve hours until the desired result is achieved, after which a maintenance dosage of 25 to 50 milligrams is given one to three times a day. Its effect begins within one hour and reaches a maximum within two to four hours.

UNDESIRABLE EFFECTS. Anorexia, nausea and vomiting, numbness and paraesthesia of the extremities, confusion, tremors, ataxia, and tinnitus may occur.

PRECAUTIONS. The concomitant use of miotics is essential when treating all types of glaucoma with dichlorphenamide. Its use over prolonged periods in chronic cases results in considerable electrolyte depletion and symptoms of potassium deficiency may develop, in which case potassium supplements should be given; such treatment does not interfere with the ocular effects of the drug.

Dose. See above under **Actions and uses.**

Preparation
DICHLORPHENAMIDE TABLETS, B.P. Unless otherwise specified, tablets each containing 50 mg of dichlorphenamide are supplied.

OTHER NAMES: *Daranide®; Oratrol®*

DICOPHANE

SYNONYMS: Chlorophenothane; DDT

$C_{14}H_9Cl_5 = 354 \cdot 5$

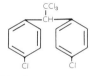

Dicophane consists chiefly of 1,1,1-trichloro-2,2-di(*p*-chlorophenyl)ethane.
It also contains variable quantities of an isomer and the carbinol resulting from condensation of one molecular proportion of chlorobenzene with chloral hydrate.

Dicophane may be prepared by treating a mixture of chlorobenzene and either chloral or chloral hydrate with sulphuric acid.

Solubility. Very slightly soluble in water; soluble in carbon tetrachloride; soluble, at 20°, in 50 parts of alcohol and in 10 parts of most fixed oils.

Standard
It complies with the requirements of the British Pharmacopoeia.
It occurs as white or almost white crystals, powder, flakes, or small granules; it is odourless or has a slight aromatic odour and contains 9·5 to 11·5 per cent of hydrolysable chlorine and not less than 70·0 per cent of 1,1,1-trichloro-2,2-di(*p*-chlorophenyl)ethane, $C_{14}H_9Cl_5$. It contains not more than 1·0 per cent w/w of water. It has a setting-point of not less than 89°.

Storage. It should be stored in airtight containers.

Actions and uses. Dicophane is an insecticide and larvicide. It is active whether ingested by the insect or absorbed through the cuticle and, because of its low volatility, retains its activity for long periods under a variety of conditions. It does not, however, have the immediate lethal effect of derris and pyrethrum.

Fleas and body lice may be eliminated by blowing a mixture of dicophane, 2 to 10 per cent, with purified talc or other inert substance, between the skin and clothing, or by wearing clothing impregnated with about 1 or 2 per cent of dicophane. Applied to the head, Dicophane Application will kill lice and persist long enough to kill larvae.
The development of resistant strains in species of insects which are normally susceptible has been reported.

UNDESIRABLE EFFECTS. In mammals, dicophane acts mainly as a peripheral nerve poison, but appears also to have an action on the central nervous system. Occasionally, hepatic insufficiency may develop without premonitory symptoms or associated nervous signs; when this happens, there is a rapid loss in body-weight and anaemia and leucocytosis develop. Kidney damage may also occur. These hepatic and renal conditions appear to be reversible.

PRECAUTIONS. Protective clothing, including

a face mask, should be worn when handling concentrated solutions of dicophane in organic solvents, as the risk of absorption is considerable. Warning of toxicity is usually given by loss of appetite, muscular weakness, and fine tremors; if at this stage further contact with dicophane is avoided, these effects usually disappear spontaneously.

The widespread use of dicophane as a general insecticide is undesirable because of the persistence of toxic residues.

POISONING. Solutions of dicophane, if swallowed, may produce vomiting, diarrhoea, and collapse; these conditions should be treated symptomatically.

Preparations
DICOPHANE APPLICATION, B.P.C. (page 648)
DICOPHANE DUSTING-POWDER, B.P.C. (page 663)

DICYCLOMINE HYDROCHLORIDE

$C_{19}H_{36}ClNO_2 = 346 \cdot 0$

Dicyclomine Hydrochloride is 2-diethylaminoethyl bi(cyclohexyl)-1-carboxylate hydrochloride.

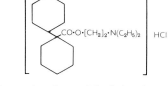

Solubility. Soluble, at 20°, in 20 parts of water, in 5 parts of alcohol, and in 2 parts of chloroform; insoluble in ether.

Standard
It complies with the requirements of the British Pharmacopoeia.
It is a white or almost white, crystalline, almost odourless powder and contains not less than 99·0 and not more than the equivalent of 101·0 per cent of $C_{19}H_{36}ClNO_2$, calculated with reference to the dried substance. The loss on drying under the prescribed conditions is not more than 1·0 per cent. It has a melting-point of 172° to 174°.

Actions and uses. Dicyclomine has peripheral actions similar to but much weaker than those of atropine (page 36). It has been given by mouth to diminish gastric secretion and to reduce gastric and intestinal motility in the treatment of peptic ulceration and pylorospasm.

Dose. 30 to 60 milligrams daily in divided doses.

Preparations
DICYCLOMINE ELIXIR, B.P.C. (page 670)

DICYCLOMINE TABLETS, B.P. Unless otherwise specified, tablets each containing 10 mg of dicyclomine hydrochloride are supplied.

OTHER NAMES: *Merbentyl*®; *Wyovin*®

DIENOESTROL

$C_{18}H_{18}O_2 = 266 \cdot 3$

Dienoestrol is 3,4-di(*p*-hydroxyphenyl)hexa-2,4-diene.

CAUTION. *Dienoestrol is a powerful oestrogen. Contact with the skin or inhalation of the dust should be avoided. Rubber gloves should be worn when handling the powder and, if the powder is dry, a face mask should be worn.*

Solubility. Very slightly soluble in water; soluble, at 20°, in 8 parts of alcohol, in 15 parts of ether, and in 5 parts of acetone; soluble in solutions of alkali hydroxides.

Standard
It complies with the requirements of the British Pharmacopoeia.
It is a white or almost white, crystalline, odourless powder and contains not less than 98·5 and not more than the equivalent of 101·5 per cent of $C_{18}H_{18}O_2$. It has a melting-point of 230° to 235°.

Storage. It should be protected from light.

Actions and uses. Dienoestrol has oestrogenic properties similar to those of Stilboestrol (page 471) but it is less potent.

Dose. For menopausal symptoms: 0·5 to 5 milligrams daily.
For suppression of lactation: 15 milligrams thrice daily for three days followed by 15 milligrams daily for six days.
For carcinoma of the prostate and mammary carcinoma: 15 to 30 milligrams daily.

Preparation
DIENOESTROL TABLETS, B.P. Unless otherwise specified, tablets each containing 1 mg of dienoestrol are supplied. They should be protected from light. Tablets containing 0·1, 0·3, and 5 mg are also available.

DIETHYL PHTHALATE

SYNONYM: Ethyl Phthalate

$C_{12}H_{14}O_4 = 222 \cdot 2$

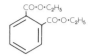

Diethyl Phthalate is ethyl *o*-benzenedicarboxylate. It boils at about 295° and has a flash-point of about 243°F (closed-cup test).

Solubility. Insoluble in water; miscible with alcohol, with ether, and with aromatic hydrocarbons.

Standard
DESCRIPTION. A clear, colourless or almost colourless, somewhat viscous liquid; odour slight.

IDENTIFICATION TESTS. 1. Gently boil 1 g for 10 minutes with 5 ml of *alcoholic potassium hydroxide solution*; add 5 ml of water, evaporate to half its volume, cool, add 1 ml of *hydrochloric acid*, and filter; melt the dried residue, add 0·5 g of *resorcinol* and 0·05 ml of *chloroform*, heat at 180° for 3 minutes, cool, add 1 ml of *sodium hydroxide solution*, and pour into water; an intense yellowish-green fluorescence is produced.
2. Boil under a reflux condenser for 2 hours with 0·5N sodium hydroxide; the product gives the reactions characteristic of ethyl alcohol, and on acidification a white precipitate is formed which, after recrystallising from water and drying, melts at about 215°.

ACIDITY. Mix 20 ml with 50 ml of *alcohol (95 per cent)*, previously neutralised to *phenolphthalein solution*, and titrate with 0·1N sodium hydroxide, using *phenolphthalein solution* as indicator; not more than 0·3 ml is required.

REFRACTIVE INDEX. At 20°, 1·500 to 1·505.

WEIGHT PER ML. At 20°, 1·115 g to 1·119 g.

WATER. Not more than 0·2 per cent w/w, determined by the method given in Appendix 16, page 895.

ASH. Not more than 0·02 per cent w/w, determined by the following method:
Heat gently about 10 g, accurately weighed, in a platinum basin until the liquid has evaporated, and ignite the residue to constant weight.

CONTENT OF $C_{12}H_{14}O_4$. Not less than 99·0 per cent w/w, determined by the following method:
Carry out the method of the British Pharmacopoeia, Appendix IXA, for the determination of esters, using about 1·5 g, accurately weighed, and 50 ml of 0·5N alcoholic potassium hydroxide; each ml of 0·5N alcoholic potassium hydroxide is equivalent to 0·05556 g of $C_{12}H_{14}O_4$.

Uses. Diethyl phthalate is used as a solvent and plasticiser for cellacephate, cellulose acetate, nitrocellulose, and rubber. It is also used as a denaturant of alcohol, for example, in surgical spirit.

UNDESIRABLE EFFECTS. It is irritant to mucous membranes and when taken in large amounts causes paralysis of the central nervous system.

DIETHYLCARBAMAZINE CITRATE

SYNONYM: Diethylcarbam. Cit.

$C_{16}H_{29}N_3O_8 = 391 \cdot 4$

Diethylcarbamazine Citrate is 1-diethylcarbamoyl-4-methylpiperazine dihydrogen citrate.

Solubility. Very soluble in water; soluble, at 20°, in 35 parts of alcohol; insoluble in ether, in chloroform, and in acetone.

Standard
It complies with the requirements of the British Pharmacopoeia.
It is a white, crystalline, odourless powder and contains not less than 98·0 and not more than the equivalent of 101·0 per cent of $C_{16}H_{29}N_3O_8$, calculated with reference to the anhydrous substance. It contains not more than 0·5 per cent w/w of water. It has a melting-point of 136° to 138°.

Storage. It should be stored in airtight containers.

Actions and uses. Diethylcarbamazine is used in the treatment of filarial infections, and is effective when given by mouth.
In the treatment of *Wuchereria bancrofti* infections the microfilariae are rapidly eliminated from the blood stream. The drug has no direct toxic action upon the larvae and it is thought that it may act by so modifying them that they are trapped by reticulo-endothelial cells in the liver sinusoids. This action upon microfilariae is important in helping to limit the spread of filariasis by the insect vector. The action of diethylcarbamazine upon the adult worms is much less rapid and they may

persist for several months, but, after they have been eliminated, microfilariae do not often reappear in the peripheral blood. Local reactions sometimes appear at the sites which commonly harbour adult worms.
In loaiasis both microfilariae and adult worms are killed; in onchocerciasis the microfilariae may be killed, but the adult parasites are less affected.
A suitable course of treatment for *Loa loa* or *W. bancrofti* infections is 6 milligrams of diethylcarbamazine citrate per kilogram body-weight by mouth daily in single or divided doses for three or four weeks. For mass treatment in endemic areas, 6 milligrams per kilogram body-weight given at weekly or monthly intervals to a total of nine doses is effective. Larger doses of 20 or 30 milligrams per kilogram body-weight have been given without serious side-effects.
Because reactions are especially prominent in *Brugia malayi* and *Onchocerca volvulus* infections, it is important in the treatment of these diseases to start with small doses; a single dose of not more than 2 milligrams of diethyl-

carbamazine citrate per kilogram body-weight should be given on the first day and the dosage should be gradually increased until the full course can be given.

UNDESIRABLE EFFECTS. Anorexia, drowsiness, headache, nausea, and vomiting sometimes occur, but are seldom serious. The release of foreign protein in the tissues by the death of adult worms or larvae often provokes allergic reactions, including fever, tender swelling, muscular pains, and skin rashes.

PRECAUTIONS AND CONTRA-INDICATIONS. It is unwise to use diethylcarbamazine for mass treatment of populations where onchocerciasis is common, because in this infection the allergic reactions may involve the eyes. If severe allergic reactions occur, treatment should be stopped and an antihistamine drug or corticosteroid administered.

Dose. See above under **Actions and uses**.

Preparation

DIETHYLCARBAMAZINE TABLETS, B.P. Unless otherwise specified, tablets each containing 50 mg of diethylcarbamazine citrate are supplied. They should be stored in airtight containers.

OTHER NAMES: *Banocide®*; *Hetrazan®*

DIGITALIS LANATA LEAF

SYNONYMS: Austrian Digitalis; Austrian Foxglove; Woolly Foxglove Leaf

Digitalis Lanata Leaf consists of the dried leaves of *Digitalis lanata* Ehrh. (Fam. Scophulariaceae). The plant is a biennial, indigenous to Austria and the Balkans, and cultivated in Great Britain and other temperate countries.

The leaves are rapidly dried, as soon as possible after collection, in a dark place, at a temperature not exceeding 60°.

Constituents. Digitalis lanata leaf contains about 1 to 1·4 per cent of a mixture of cardioactive glycosides, of which the most important is digoxin, which may be classified into five series, each based on a different steroidal aglycone.

The A series, based on digitoxigenin [3β,14-dihydroxycard-20(22)-enolide], includes the following glycosides: lanatoside A (acetylpurpurea glycoside A); purpurea glycoside A (deacetyllanatoside A), in which the hydroxyl group in position 3 of the aglycone is substituted by a chain of three digitoxose units with a terminal glucose unit and formed from lanatoside A by removal of the acetyl group; acetyldigitoxin, formed from lanatoside A by removal of the terminal glucose unit; and digitoxin, formed from lanatoside A by removal of the acetyl group and the terminal glucose unit.

The B series, based on gitoxigenin (16-hydroxydigitoxigenin), includes the analogous glycosides lanatoside B, purpurea glycoside B, acetylgitoxin, and gitoxin. Other members of this series which are also present in the leaf are: digitalinum verum (glucodigitalogitoxigenin), formed by the addition of one glucose unit and one digitalose (a deoxy sugar) unit to gitoxigenin; strospeside (digitalogitoxigenin), formed by addition of one digitalose unit to gitoxigenin; and gitorin (gluco-digitoxogitoxigenin), formed by the addition of one digitoxose (an α-deoxy sugar) unit and one glucose unit to gitoxigenin.

The C, D, and E series, based respectively on digoxigenin (12-hydroxydigitoxigenin), diginatigenin (12,16-dihydroxydigitoxigenin), and gitaloxigenin (16-formylgitoxigenin), include the following glycosides with structures analogous to those in the A and B series: deacetyllanatoside C, deacetyllanatoside D, and glucogitaloxin; acetyldigoxin, acetyldiginatin, and acetylgitaloxin; and digoxin, diginatin, and gitaloxin.

The secondary glycosides digitoxin, gitoxin, digoxin, diginatin, and gitaloxin all have in position 3 of the aglycone, a chain of three digitoxose units; removal of these sugar groups yields the corresponding, almost inactive aglycones which are present in the leaf in only small amounts. The glycosides diginin and digifolin, which are also present, are not cardioactive.

Standard for unground drug

DESCRIPTION. *Macroscopical*: leaves brittle, oblong-lanceolate, 2 to **5** to **15** to 30 cm long and 0·4 to **2** to 4·5 cm wide, sessile, margin entire and ciliate in the basal half of the leaf, becoming wavy toothed towards the apex; surface apparently glabrous; midrib strongly marked, and the main secondary veins, about 2 or 3 on each side of the basal third or quarter of the midrib, leaving it at an angle of 10° to 30° and curving towards the acute apex.

Odour slight; taste distinctly bitter.

Microscopical: the diagnostic characters are: *epidermal cells* of both surfaces with slightly sinuous and irregularly beaded anticlinal walls; *stomata* numerous, anomocytic, occurring on both surfaces; *water pores* single or in groups of **2** to 4 on the margin at intervals of about 1 to 5 mm; *trichomes*: (a) marginal, uniseriate, non-glandular, 9 to **10** to **14** to 20 cells long, (b) glandular, with bicellular heads and unicellular stalks, on both surfaces, and a few, chiefly on the adaxial surface, with 2- to 10-celled uniseriate stalks and unicellular heads; *mesophyll* with 1 to 3 rows of palisade cells; *phloem fibres* and *crystals* absent.

FOREIGN ORGANIC MATTER. Not more than 2·0 per cent.

Standard for powdered drug: Powdered Digitalis Lanata Leaf

DESCRIPTION. A green powder possessing the diagnostic microscopical characters, odour, and taste of the unground drug.

FOREIGN ORGANIC MATTER. It complies with the requirement for the unground drug.

Storage. It should be stored in airtight containers, protected from light.

Uses. Digitalis lanata leaf is a source of digoxin and certain other glycosides.

POISONING. Withdrawal of the drug is usually sufficient, but in very severe cases the administration of potassium ions orally, or even parenterally, may be required.

DIGITALIS LEAF

SYNONYMS: Digitalis; Digitalis Folium

Digitalis Leaf consists of the dried leaves of *Digitalis purpurea* L. (Fam. Scrophulariaceae), a biennial herb widely distributed and cultivated throughout Europe and indigenous to and cultivated in England.

The leaves are rapidly dried at a temperature not exceeding 60° as soon as possible after collection.

Constituents. Digitalis leaf contains about 0·2 to 0·45 per cent of a mixture of cardioactive glycosides, the majority of which can be classified into three series —the A, B, and E series described under Digitalis Lanata Leaf.

The glycosides of the A series in digitalis leaf are purpurea glycoside A and digitoxin, together with odoroside H, in which the hydroxyl group in position 3 of the aglycone digitoxigenin is substituted by a digitalose unit.

The glycosides of the B series are purpurea glycoside B, gitoxin, digitalinum verum, strospeside, and gitorin, while those of the E series are glucogitaloxin and gitaloxin, together with glucoverodoxin and verodoxin, the 16-formyl esters of digitalinum verum and strospeside respectively.

There is some evidence to show that the relative proportions of the A and B series vary with the strain of plant.

The percentages of individual glycosides in the total glycosidal mixture vary considerably; both primary and secondary glycosides are present, the latter constituting about 10 to 20 per cent of the total.

The steroidal saponins digitonin and gitonin are present in the leaf. Hydrolytic enzymes also occur and, in the presence of moisture, readily break down the primary glycosides to secondary glycosides; it is possible that such breakdowns lead to loss of therapeutic activity.

Digitalis seeds contain glucodigifucoside and gluco-digiproside (glycosides of the A series), together with digitalinum verum and other cardiac glycosides, and digitonin and gitonin.

Standard

It complies with the requirements of the British Pharmacopoeia.

UNGROUND DRUG. *Macroscopical characters:* leaf brittle, greyish-green, about 10 to 40 cm long and 4 to 15 cm wide, ovate-lanceolate to broadly ovate and petiolate; lamina with crenate, serrate, or dentate margin, decurrent base, subacute apex, and pinnate venation; petiole about one-quarter to equal in length to the lamina, winged, the lowest veins running down the wings; upper surface hairy, lower surface usually densely pubescent and marked by a reticulation of raised veinlets.

Odour slight; taste distinctly bitter.

Digitalis Leaf responds to the following test:

Boil 1 g in powder with 10 ml of *alcohol (70 per cent)* for two minutes and filter; to 5 ml of the filtrate add 10 ml of water and 5 ml of *chloroform*, separate the lower layer, and evaporate to dryness; dissolve the cooled residue in 3 ml of *glacial acetic acid* containing 0·1 ml of *ferric chloride test-solution* and transfer this solution to the surface of 2 ml of *sulphuric acid*; a reddish-brown layer forms at the interface and the upper layer gradually acquires a bluish-green colour which darkens on standing.

Microscopical characters: the diagnostic characters are: *epidermal cells* about 30 to 75 µm wide or long, with wavy anticlinal walls; *stomata* anomocytic, more numerous on abaxial than adaxial surface; *water pores* large, 1, or rarely 2, at the apex of most marginal teeth; *trichomes:* (a) usually 3 to 5 cells long, bluntly pointed, and finely warty, (b) glandular, stalk unicellular or more rarely uniseriate, head unicellular or bicellular; *midrib* strongly projecting on abaxial surface, containing an arc of radiate *xylem* and below this a narrow band of *phloem* and a narrow layer of *collen-chyma*; *endodermoid sheath* enclosing midrib bundle, containing starch; *crystals* and *sclerenchyma* absent.

POWDERED DRUG: Powdered Digitalis Leaf. A green powder possessing the diagnostic microscopical characters, odour, and taste of the unground drug.

Adulterants and substitutes. Digitalis has been known to be adulterated with *Verbascum thapsus* L. (Fam. Scrophulariaceae), *Symphytum officinale* L. (Fam. Boraginaceae), *Primula vulgaris* Huds. (Fam. Primulaceae), *Inula conyza* DC. (Fam. Compositae), *Urtica dioica* L. (Fam. Urticaceae), *D. thapsi* L., and *D. lutea* L.

Storage. It should be stored in airtight containers, protected from light.

Actions and uses. Digitalis acts mainly upon the cardiovascular system, its action being due to the glycosides it contains. It increases excitability of cardiac muscle and produces more forceful contractions. Its effect in congestive heart failure is therefore to increase cardiac output and relieve venous congestion. The consequent improvement of the circulation through the kidneys may result in diuresis and loss of oedema fluid.

Digitalis depresses conduction in the auriculoventricular bundle, producing a slower ventricular beat, which is valuable in auricular fibrillation.

Digitalis will frequently convert auricular flutter into fibrillation and, upon withdrawal of the drug, normal sinus rhythm may be restored.

The principal glycosides are metabolised slowly, and about 25 per cent of the activity of a dose is still present in the body after ten days.

The effects of digitalis in congestive heart failure may be produced rapidly or slowly according to the method of administration. If a patient is severely ill and has not recently received treatment with digitalis, rapid digitalisation is necessary and is best achieved by intravenous injection of a soluble preparation such as digoxin. Alternatively, if the patient can take the drug by mouth, a total dose of 2 grams of Prepared Digitalis is given in the first twenty-four hours. Half the total is given at once, and the other half in divided doses at six-hourly intervals, but such rapid digitalisation is rarely necessary. The patient may be digitalised more slowly by giving 200 milligrams of Prepared Digitalis three times daily for two or three days, followed by half or two-thirds of this dosage for a further two or three days. It is usually necessary to continue digitalis therapy indefinitely. The daily dosage required is usually of the order of 60 to 200 milligrams of Prepared Digitalis.

The value of digitalis in high-output failure is less evident, and it may even be contra-indicated.

UNDESIRABLE EFFECTS. Mild toxic effects, such as headache, anorexia, and nausea, are commonly associated with the therapeutic action of the drug.

More severe symptoms such as vomiting, diarrhoea, profound bradycardia, ventricular tachycardia, or the development of cardiac irregularities such as extrasystoles and coupling, are indications of overdosage.

Treatment may be temporarily withheld before continuing with a smaller dose.

PRECAUTIONS. Especial care should be taken in assessing the maintenance dose for elderly patients, particularly when they are receiving intensive diuretic therapy which may precipitate symptoms of digitalis toxicity.

POISONING. Withdrawal of the drug is usually sufficient, but in very severe cases the administration of potassium salts orally or even parenterally may be required.

NOTE. When Digitalis Leaf, Digitalis Folium, Digitalis, Powdered Digitalis Leaf, Digitalis Folii Pulvis, or Pulvis Digitalis is prescribed, Prepared Digitalis is dispensed.

Preparation
PREPARED DIGITALIS, B.P. (see below)

PREPARED DIGITALIS

SYNONYMS: Digitalis Pulverata; Powdered Digitalis; Prep. Digit.

Prepared Digitalis is obtained by reducing Digitalis Leaf to a powder not coarser than a moderately coarse powder, no portion being rejected, and determining its activity by comparison with that of the Standard Preparation on the hearts of guinea-pigs. Other methods compare the action of the preparations on the hearts of frogs, cats, or pigeons.

When adjustment is necessary, a weaker powdered digitalis leaf or powdered grass is added.

Standard
It complies with the requirements of the British Pharmacopoeia.
It is a green powder with a slight odour and a distinctly bitter taste. For therapeutic administration Prepared Digitalis must contain 10 Units in 1 g.
It possesses the diagnostic microscopical characters described under Digitalis Leaf; if powdered grass is present the structures which it exhibits are those described for this substance in the British Pharmacopoeia under Prepared Digitalis.
The loss on drying at 105° is not more than 6·0 per cent.

Labelling. The label on the container states the number of Units in 1 gram.

Storage. It should be stored in airtight containers, protected from light.

Actions and uses. Prepared digitalis has the actions, uses, and undesirable effects described under Digitalis Leaf.

PRECAUTIONS; POISONING. As for Digitalis Leaf.

Dose. Initial dose for rapid digitalisation, 1 to 1·5 grams, in divided doses; maintenance dose, 100 to 200 milligrams daily.

Preparation
PREPARED DIGITALIS TABLETS, B.P. (*Syn.* Digitalis Tablets). Unless otherwise specified, tablets each containing 60 mg of Prepared Digitalis are supplied. They should be stored in airtight containers. Tablets containing 30 and 100 mg are also available.

DIGITOXIN

SYNONYM: Digitoxinum

$C_{41}H_{64}O_{13} = 764·9$

Digitoxin is a crystalline glycoside obtained from suitable species of *Digitalis*.

Solubility. Insoluble in water; soluble at 20°, in 150 parts of alcohol and in 40 parts of chloroform; slightly soluble in ether.

Standard
It complies with the requirements of the European Pharmacopoeia.
It is a white or almost white powder and contains not less than 95·0 and not more than the equivalent of 105·0 per cent of $C_{41}H_{64}O_{13}$, calculated with reference to the dried substance. The loss on drying under the prescribed conditions is not more than 1·5 per cent.

Storage. It should be stored in airtight containers, protected from light.

Actions and uses. Digitoxin has the actions, uses, and undesirable effects described under Digitalis Leaf, it is the most potent and most cumulative of the digitalis glycosides. It is completely and readily absorbed when given by mouth, and is equally active when given by injection.

For rapid digitalisation of patients who have not been given cardiac glycosides within the preceding two weeks, 1 to 1·5 milligrams may be given by mouth in divided doses over one or two days. The maintenance dosage is 50 to 200 micrograms daily. However, digoxin is more suitable for rapid digitalisation as it has a shorter duration of action and its effect is therefore more readily controlled. When vomiting or other oral conditions prevent oral administration, digitoxin may be given by intramuscular or slow intravenous injection; the usual digitalising dosage is 1·2 milligrams daily in divided doses not exceeding 500 micrograms.

For intravenous injection, the dose is dissolved in a mixture of alcohol, glycerol, and water, and for intramuscular injection it is dissolved in propylene glycol.

If toxic effects arise, further doses of digitoxin should be withheld.

Digitoxin must be carefully distinguished from digitalin (amorphous digitalin), a standardised mixture of glycosides prepared from digitalis seeds, which does not contain digitoxin or gitoxin and is given in much larger doses.

PRECAUTIONS; POISONING. As for Digitalis Leaf.

Dose. See above under **Actions and uses.**

Preparation
DIGITOXIN TABLETS, B.P. Unless otherwise specified, tablets each containing 100 μg of digitoxin are supplied. They should be stored in airtight containers. Tablets containing 200 μg are also available.

OTHER NAMES: Digitaline Cristallisée; *Digitaline Nativelle*®

DIGOXIN

SYNONYM: Digoxinum

$C_{41}H_{64}O_{14} = 780·9$

Digoxin is a crystalline glycoside obtained from digitalis lanata leaf.

Solubility. Very slightly soluble in water, in dehydrated alcohol, and in chloroform; soluble, at 20°, in 122 parts of alcohol (80 per cent) and in 4 parts of pyridine.

Standard
It complies with the requirements of the European Pharmacopoeia.
It occurs as colourless crystals or white or almost white powder and contains not less than 95·0 and not more the equivalent of 103·0 per cent of $C_{41}H_{64}O_{14}$, calculated with reference to the dried substance. The loss on drying under the prescribed conditions is not more than 1·0 per cent.

Sterilisation. Alcoholic solutions for injection are sterilised by heating in an autoclave.

Storage. It should be stored in airtight containers, protected from light.

Actions and uses. Digoxin has the actions and uses described under Digitalis Leaf. It is excreted more rapidly than most other digitalis glycosides and its action is therefore less cumulative. Digoxin is of particular value for rapid digitalisation in the treatment of auricular fibrillation and congestive heart failure. When it is given by mouth, its characteristic effect is produced in about one hour and reaches its maximum in about six to seven hours. The usual digitalising dosage is 1 to 1·5 milligrams by mouth in single or divided doses, followed by 250 to 500 micrograms every six hours until the desired therapeutic effect is obtained. The usual maintenance dosage is 250 micrograms one to three times daily. For rapid digitalisation of

patients who have not been given cardiac glycosides within the preceding two weeks, or if the patient is unable to swallow, digoxin may be given by slow intravenous injection in a dose of 0·5 to 1 milligram; its action then begins in about five to ten minutes and reaches a maximum in one to two hours. Care should be taken to prevent any of the solution escaping into the perivenous tissues. The risk of producing toxic effects on the heart is much greater if digoxin is given intravenously. Digoxin may also be given by intramuscular injection.

UNDESIRABLE EFFECTS. The undesirable effects described under Digitalis Leaf may occur, but as digoxin is excreted more rapidly than most other cardiac glycosides it is less likely to give rise to cumulative effects.

PRECAUTIONS; POISONING. As for Digitalis Leaf.

Dose. See above under **Actions and uses.**

Preparations
DIGOXIN ELIXIR, PAEDIATRIC, B.P.C. (page 670)

DIGOXIN INJECTION, B.P. It consists of a sterile stabilised solution containing 0·025 per cent of digoxin in alcohol (80 per cent), propylene glycol, and Water for Injections. It should be protected from light. Dose: for rapid digitalisation, 2 to 4 millilitres by intramuscular or slow intravenous injection.

DIGOXIN TABLETS, B.P. Unless otherwise specified, tablets each containing 250 μg of digoxin are supplied. Tablets containing 62·5 μg are also available.

OTHER NAME: *Lanoxin*®

DIHYDROCODEINE TARTRATE

$C_{18}H_{23}NO_3,C_4H_6O_6 = 451.5$

Dihydrocodeine Tartrate is the hydrogen tartrate of dihydrocodeine.

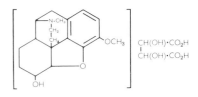

Solubility. Soluble, at $20°$, in 4·5 parts of water; slightly soluble in alcohol; insoluble in ether.

Standard
It complies with the requirements of the British Pharmacopoeia.
It occurs as odourless colourless crystals or white crystalline powder and contains not less than 98·0 and not more than the equivalent of 101·0 per cent of $C_{18}H_{23}NO_3,C_4H_6O_6$, calculated with reference to the dried substance. The loss on drying under the prescribed conditions is not more than 0·5 per cent. It has a melting-point of $190°$ to $194°$. A 10 per cent solution in water has a pH of 3·2 to 4·2.

Sterilisation. Solutions for injection are sterilised by heating in an autoclave or by filtration.

Storage. It should be protected from light.

Actions and uses. Dihydrocodeine is an analgesic intermediate in potency between codeine and morphine, and with a duration of action of about three hours. Sedation and euphoria are less marked than with morphine. Dihydrocodeine is also used as an antitussive and it has been used in conjunction with phenothiazine derivatives to relieve symptoms in terminal carcinoma.
The usual dose of dihydrocodeine tartrate as an analgesic is 30 milligrams and if this does not give relief the dose may be repeated. The response may not be enhanced by increasing the dose. Children may be given 0·5 milligram per kilogram body-weight. The usual dose as an antitussive is 10 milligrams.

UNDESIRABLE EFFECTS. Dihydrocodeine may cause constipation. It may give rise to dependence of the morphine type, as described under Morphine Hydrochloride (page 314), but this is less likely to occur than with morphine.

PRECAUTIONS. Dihydrocodeine should be used with caution in patients with asthma or impaired liver function.

Dose. See above under **Actions and uses.**

Preparations
DIHYDROCODEINE INJECTION, B.P. It consists of a sterile solution of dihydrocodeine tartrate in Water for Injections containing 0·1 per cent of sodium metabisulphite. Unless otherwise specified, a solution containing 50 mg of dihydrocodeine tartrate in 1 ml is supplied. It should be protected from light.

DIHYDROCODEINE TABLETS, B.P. Unless otherwise specified, tablets each containing 30 mg of dihydrocodeine tartrate are supplied. They should be protected from light.

OTHER NAMES: *D.F.118®*; Dihydrocodeine Acid Tartrate

DIHYDROTACHYSTEROL

$C_{28}H_{46}O = 398.7$

Dihydrotachysterol is 9,10-secoergosta-5,7,22-trien-3β-ol.

Solubility. Very slightly soluble in water; soluble, at $20°$, in 20 parts of alcohol, in less than 1 part of chloroform, in 3 parts of ether, and in 50 parts of arachis oil.

Standard
It complies with the requirements of the British Pharmacopoeia.
It occurs as odourless colourless crystals or white crystalline powder. It has a melting-point of $126°$ to $129°$; it may also occur in a lower melting form melting at about $113°$.

Storage. It should be stored in hermetically sealed glass containers, in which the air has been replaced by an inert gas, protected from light, in a cool place.

Actions and uses. The actions of dihydrotachysterol resemble those of calciferol (page 65) and vitamin D_3. It has a powerful antirachitic action in cases of steatorrhoea, chronic renal failure, and hypophosphataemia. It also has some antirachitic effect in cases of classical vitamin-D deficiency, although it is less potent than calciferol in this respect. It promotes the absorption of calcium from the intestine and the mobilisation of calcium from bone as effectively as calciferol.
Dihydrotachysterol acts more rapidly and is more rapidly eliminated than calciferol and its action is therefore more readily controlled; in practice, calciferol is generally used for the treatment of vitamin-D deficiency and dihydrotachysterol for other conditions.
Dihydrotachysterol is effective when given orally for the treatment of all forms of hypoparathyroidism with lowered plasma-calcium. A dosage of 1 to 2 milligrams daily raises the plasma-calcium to normal in five to ten days. In an emergency 8 milligrams may be given daily for two days, followed by 4 milligrams

daily for two days and 2 milligrams daily thereafter. Dosage should be adjusted in accordance with the plasma and urinary calcium. When this level becomes normal a maintenance dose of 0·5 to 2 milligrams of dihydrotachysterol is given; as dihydrotachysterol is slowly metabolised and excreted, the maintenance dose need be given only every other day. No changes in the normal dietary calcium intake are necessary.

Dihydrotachysterol is administered in cases of vitamin-D-resistant rickets and osteomalacia in the doses mentioned, until the serum-alkaline-phosphatase level returns to normal. The dose is then reduced considerably or even stopped, as the dosage that causes a reasonably rapid cure of the rickets will constitute an overdose if it is continued.

UNDESIRABLE EFFECTS. The therapeutic dose is close to that producing toxic effects. Overdosage causes decalcification of bone, increased urinary excretion of calcium, hypercalcaemia, metastatic calcification, and eventually a raised blood-urea. The symptoms are anorexia, nausea, vomiting, polyuria, vertigo, thirst, and abdominal cramps. Treatment consists in withdrawing the dihydrotachysterol, reducing the dietary calcium intake, and increasing the fluid intake.

PRECAUTIONS. Dosage may need revision in the case of patients who have undergone thyroidectomy or treatment with radioactive iodine or who are receiving a high calcium intake, as in a milk diet.

Dose. See above under **Actions and uses.**

OTHER NAME: *AT 10*®

DI-IODOHYDROXYQUINOLINE

SYNONYM: Di-iodohydroxyquin

$C_9H_5I_2NO = 397·0$

Di-iodohydroxyquinoline is 8-hydroxy-5,7-di-iodoquinoline.

Solubility. Very slightly soluble in water; slightly soluble in alcohol and in ether.

Standard

It complies with the requirements of the British Pharmacopoeia.

It is a pale yellowish to yellowish-brown, microcrystalline, odourless or almost odourless powder and contains not less than 97·0 per cent of $C_9H_5I_2NO$, calculated with reference to the dried substance. The loss on drying under the prescribed conditions is not more than 0·5 per cent.

Storage. It should be protected from light.

Actions and uses. Di-iodohydroxyquinoline is an amoebicide which is used chiefly in the treatment of chronic infections. It is less satisfactory than emetine or metronidazole for the treatment of acute amoebic dysentery, but is frequently used to supplement emetine therapy.

Di-iodohydroxyquinoline is usually administered by mouth in a dosage of 600 milligrams three times a day for twenty days. It is partly and irregularly absorbed from the small intestine, but, because of its low solubility, much of the dose reaches the large intestine,

where it is thought to act upon the amoebae living in the lumen or upon the bacteria on which they feed.

Courses of treatment with di-iodohydroxyquinoline are often supplemented by treatment with other amoebicides.

Pessaries of di-iodohydroxyquinoline are used for the treatment of trichomonal and candidal vaginitis.

UNDESIRABLE EFFECTS. Pruritus ani, furunculosis, abdominal pain with nausea, vomiting, diarrhoea, and headache may occur. Slight enlargement of the thyroid gland is common.

CONTRA-INDICATIONS. It should not be administered to iodine-sensitive persons.

Dose. See above under **Actions and uses.**

Preparations

DI-IODOHYDROXYQUINOLINE PESSARIES, B.P.C. (page 772)

DI-IODOHYDROXYQUINOLINE TABLETS, B.P. Unless otherwise specified, tablets each containing 300 mg of di-iodohydroxyquinoline are supplied. They should be protected from light. Tablets containing 650 mg are also available.

OTHER NAMES: *Diodoquin*® ; *Embequin*®

DILL OIL

SYNONYM: Oleum Anethi

Dill Oil is obtained by distillation from the dried ripe fruits of *Anethum graveolens* L. (Fam. Umbelliferae). It closely resembles caraway oil, but usually contains less carvone.

Constituents. Dill oil contains about 50 per cent of carvone, the remainder consisting chiefly of (+)-limonene.

Solubility. Soluble, at 20°, in one part of alcohol (90 per cent) and in 10 parts of alcohol (80 per cent).

Standard

DESCRIPTION. A colourless or pale yellow liquid which becomes yellowish-brown on storage; odour characteristic of the crushed fruit.

OPTICAL ROTATION. At 20°, +70° to +80°.

REFRACTIVE INDEX. At 20°, 1·481 to 1·492.

WEIGHT PER ML. At 20°, 0·895 g to 0·910 g.

CONTENT OF CARVONE. 43·0 to 63·0 per cent w/w, determined by the method given in Appendix 14, page 893.

Adulterants and substitutes. East Indian dill oil, from *Anethum sowa* Roxb. ex Hem., is distinguished by its higher weight per ml (0·945 g to 0·972 g), lower optical rotation (+48° to +57°), and by its containing dill apiole, which boils at 285° and, having a weight per ml of about 1·15 g, sinks in water. Genuine dill oil

contains no constituent boiling at so high a temperature and no portion of the distillate sinks in water.

Storage. It should be stored in well-filled airtight containers, protected from light, in a cool place.

Actions and uses. Dill oil is a carminative and is used as Dill Water in the treatment of flatulence in infants. Dill Water is a useful vehicle for children's medicines.

Dose. 0·05 to 0·2 millilitre.

Preparations

DILL WATER, CONCENTRATED, B.P.C. (page 825)

SODIUM BICARBONATE MIXTURE, PAEDIATRIC, B.P.C. (page 752)

DILOXANIDE FUROATE

$C_{14}H_{11}Cl_2NO_4 = 328·2$

Diloxanide Furoate is *p*-(*N*-methyl-αα-dichloroacetamido)-phenyl 2-furoate.

Solubility. Very slightly soluble in water; soluble, at 20°, in 100 parts of alcohol, in 130 parts of ether, and in 2·5 parts of chloroform.

Standard

It complies with the requirements of the British Pharmacopoeia.

It is a white or almost white, crystalline, odourless powder and contains not less than 98·0 and not more than the equivalent of 102·0 per cent of $C_{14}H_{11}Cl_2NO_4$, calculated with reference to the dried substance. The loss on drying under the prescribed conditions is not more than 0·5 per cent. It has a melting-point of 114° to 116°.

Storage. It should be protected from light.

Actions and uses. Diloxanide furoate is used in the treatment of amoebiasis. It has a direct effect upon the amoebae in the gut and has no antibacterial action. It is used as an alternative to di-iodohydroxyquinoline or

emetine and bismuth iodide in the treatment of chronic amoebiasis; it is also used together with chloroquine in the treatment of amoebic hepatitis.

Doses of 500 milligrams are given three times a day for ten days. The dosage for a child is 20 milligrams per kilogram body-weight daily, in divided doses, for ten days. The course of treatment may be repeated if necessary.

Dose. See above under **Actions and uses.**

Preparation

DILOXANIDE FUROATE TABLETS, B.P. Unless otherwise specified, tablets each containing 500 mg of diloxanide furoate are supplied. They should be protected from light.

OTHER NAME: *Furamide*®

DIMENHYDRINATE

SYNONYM: Diphenhydramine Theoclate

$C_{24}H_{28}ClN_5O_3 = 470·0$

Dimenhydrinate is the (2-diphenylmethoxyethyl)dimethylamine salt of 8-chlorotheophylline (theoclic acid).

Solubility. Soluble, at 20°, in 95 parts of water, in 2 parts of alcohol, and in 2 parts of chloroform; slightly soluble in ether.

Standard

It complies with the requirements of the British Pharmacopoeia.

It is a white, crystalline, odourless powder and contains not less than 97·5 and not more than the equivalent of 102·0 per cent of $C_{24}H_{28}ClN_5O_3$, calculated with reference to the dried substance. The loss on drying under the prescribed conditions is not more than 0·5 per cent. It has a melting-point of 102° to 107°.

Sterilisation. Solutions for injection are sterilised by heating with a bactericide.

Storage. It should be stored in airtight containers.

Actions and uses. Dimenhydrinate has the actions and uses of the antihistamine drugs, as described under Promethazine Hydrochloride (page 409), its activity being due to its diphenhydramine content. It is given by mouth for the prevention and relief of motion-sickness.

The usual dose for an adult is 50 milligrams, for a child aged eight to twelve years 25 milligrams, and for a younger child 12·5 milligrams. The first dose should be taken thirty minutes before a journey and the dose repeated not more than twice in twenty-four hours.

Dimenhydrinate is also used for the symptomatic treatment of irradiation sickness and of vertigo and labyrinthine disorders due to Ménière's disease.

UNDESIRABLE EFFECTS. Undesirable effects, other than drowsiness, are rare.

POISONING. As for Promethazine Hydrochloride (page 409).

Dose. 25 to 50 milligrams by mouth or by intramuscular injection.

Preparations

DIMENHYDRINATE INJECTION, B.P. It consists of a sterile solution of dimenhydrinate in a mixture of equal volumes of propylene glycol and Water for Injections containing 5 per cent v/v of benzyl alcohol. Unless otherwise specified, a solution containing 50 mg of dimenhydrinate in 1 ml is supplied.

DIMENHYDRINATE TABLETS, B.P. Unless otherwise specified, tablets each containing 50 mg of dimenhydrinate are supplied.

OTHER NAMES: *Dramamine®*; *Gravol®*

DIMERCAPROL

SYNONYMS: B.A.L.; Dimercaprolum

$C_3H_8OS_2 = 124.2$

$$CH_2(SH) \cdot CH(SH) \cdot CH_2OH$$

Dimercaprol is 2,3-dimercaptopropan-1-ol.

Solubility. Soluble, at 20°, in 20 parts of water and in 18 parts of arachis oil; miscible with alcohol and with benzyl benzoate.

Standard

It complies with the requirements of the European Pharmacopoeia.

It is a clear, colourless or slightly yellow liquid with an alliaceous odour and contains not less than 98·5 and not more than the equivalent of 101·5 per cent w/w of $C_3H_8OS_2$. It has a specific gravity at 20° of 1·239 to 1·259 corresponding to a weight per ml at 20° of 1·236 g to 1·255 g. A saturated solution in water has a pH of 5·0 to 6·5.

Sterilisation. Oily solutions for injection are sterilised by dry heat in an atmosphere of nitrogen or other suitable gas.

Storage. It should be stored in small well-filled airtight containers, in a cool place.

Actions and uses. Dimercaprol combines in the body with arsenic, mercury, and other heavy metals which inhibit the pyruvate-oxidase system by competing for the sulphydryl groups in proteins. It has a greater affinity than the proteins have for these metals and the resulting compounds are stable and rapidly excreted by the kidneys.

Dimercaprol is used in the treatment of acute poisoning by arsenic, mercury, gold, bismuth, thallium, and antimony; it should not be used in the treatment of iron, lead, and cadmium poisoning.

The toxic manifestations of arsenic therapy respond to treatment with dimercaprol, the first to disappear being haemorrhagic encephalitis, fever, agranulocytosis, and optic neuritis; exfoliative dermatitis and hyperkeratosis usually clear within twenty-one days, but aplastic anaemia shows no response. For the treatment of severe symptoms of arsenic poisoning, one scale of dosage consists in giving 3 milligrams of dimercaprol per kilogram body-weight by intramuscular injection every four hours for the first two days, four times on the third day, and twice daily for the next ten days or until recovery is complete. For milder symptoms, four doses of 2·5 milligrams per kilogram body-weight

are given daily at intervals of four hours for the first two days, followed by two doses on the third day and one or two doses daily for the next ten days or until recovery is complete. Larger doses appear to be necessary for the treatment of mercurial poisoning.

For the treatment of gold poisoning, the dosage scheme is the same as that for the milder symptoms of arsenic poisoning.

Accidental contamination of the eyes with arsenical vesicants is successfully treated by instilling a 5 to 10 per cent solution of dimercaprol into the conjunctival sac; if given within five minutes of contamination there is complete recovery.

Local applications have also proved useful in the treatment of chromium dermatitis.

UNDESIRABLE EFFECTS. In doses of 4 to 5 milligrams per kilogram body-weight, dimercaprol gives rise to malaise, nausea, vomiting, lachrymation, salivation, headache, and a burning sensation of the lips, mouth, throat, and eyes, together with a feeling of constriction in the throat and chest and an increase in systolic and diastolic blood pressure; the maximum effect is reached in about fifteen to twenty minutes. The dosage usually employed, however, seldom produces reactions severe enough to warrant cessation of treatment. Single doses of up to 8 milligrams per kilogram body-weight have been given; the toxic effects last only a few hours and are completely reversible.

Dose. In divided doses, by intramuscular injection: 400 to 800 milligrams on the first day, 200 to 400 milligrams on the second and third days, and 100 to 200 milligrams on subsequent days.

Preparation

DIMERCAPROL INJECTION, B.P. (*Syn.* B.A.L. Injection). It consists of a sterile solution containing 5 per cent of dimercaprol, with benzyl benzoate, in arachis oil. Dose: 8 to 16 ml on the first day, 4 to 8 ml on the second and third days, and 2 to 4 ml on subsequent days by intramuscular injection in divided doses.

DIMETHICONE

SYNONYMS: Dimethyl Silicone Fluid;
Dimethylsiloxane

$$CH_3 \left[\begin{array}{c} CH_3 \\ | \\ Si \cdot O \\ | \\ CH_3 \end{array} \right]_n \begin{array}{c} CH_3 \\ | \\ Si \cdot CH_3 \\ | \\ CH_3 \end{array}$$

Dimethicone is polydimethylsiloxane and may be prepared by hydrolysing a mixture of dichlorodimethylsilane, $(CH_3)_2SiCl_2$, and chlorotrimethylsilane, $(CH_3)_3SiCl$. The products of hydrolysis contain active silanol groups, $(SiOH)$, through which condensation polymerisation proceeds. By varying the proportion of chlorotrimethylsilane, which acts as a chain terminator, silicones of varying molecular weight are prepared.

As the molecular weight increases, the products become more viscous and fluids are available throughout the viscosity range of 0·65 to 3,000,000 centistokes. The various grades are distinguished by the numbers appended after the name, each number corresponding approximately to the viscosity of the product.

Solubility. Soluble in ether, in xylene, in chlorinated hydrocarbons, and in solvent naphtha; dimethicones 20, 200, 350, and 500 are also soluble in amyl acetate, in cyclohexane, in petroleum spirit, and in kerosene; dimethicones 20, 200, 350, 500, and 1000 are insoluble in water, in alcohol, in methyl alcohol, and in acetone.

Standard

DIMETHICONE 20

DESCRIPTION. A clear colourless liquid; odourless or almost odourless.

IDENTIFICATION TESTS. 1. Boil 0·3 ml with 0·3 ml of a mixture of equal parts of *sulphuric acid* and *nitric acid*; no charring occurs and a bulky white fibrous mass is produced.
2. Ignite; dense white fumes are evolved and the residue is white.
3. The infra-red absorption spectrum exhibits maxima which are only at the same wavelengths as, and have similar relative intensities to, those in the spectrum of *dimethicone A.S.*

ACIDITY. Dissolve 15·0 g in a mixture of 15 ml of *toluene* and 15 ml of *butyl alcohol*, previously neutralised to *alcoholic bromophenol blue solution*, and titrate with 0·05N alcoholic potassium hydroxide using *alcoholic bromophenol blue solution* as indicator; not more than 0·1 ml is required.

VISCOSITY. At 25°, 17·0 to 23·0 centistokes.

WEIGHT PER ML. At 20°, 0·940 g to 0·965 g.

DIMETHICONE 200

DESCRIPTION; IDENTIFICATION TESTS; ACIDITY. It complies with the requirements for Dimethicone 20.

VISCOSITY. At 25°, 190 to 210 centistokes.

WEIGHT PER ML. At 20°, 0·965 g to 0·980 g.

DIMETHICONE 350

DESCRIPTION; IDENTIFICATION TESTS; ACIDITY. It complies with the requirements for Dimethicone 20.

VISCOSITY. At 25°, 330 to 370 centistokes.

WEIGHT PER ML. At 20°, 0·965 g to 0·980 g.

DIMETHICONE 500

DESCRIPTION; IDENTIFICATION TESTS; ACIDITY. It complies with the requirements for Dimethicone 20.

VISCOSITY. At 25°, 475 to 525 centistokes.

WEIGHT PER ML. At 20°, 0·965 g to 0·980 g.

DIMETHICONE 1000

DESCRIPTION; IDENTIFICATION TESTS; ACIDITY. It complies with the requirements for Dimethicone 20.

VISCOSITY. At 25°, 950 to 1050 centistokes.

WEIGHT PER ML. At 20°, 0·965 g to 0·980 g.

Actions and uses. The dimethicones are water-repellent liquids which have a low surface tension. They are stable to heat and are resistant to most chemical substances, although they are affected by strong acids.

Dimethicones are used in industrial barrier creams for protecting the skin against irritant substances. Creams, lotions, and ointments containing 10 to 30 per cent of a dimethicone are employed for the prevention of bedsores and to protect the skin against trauma from urine or faecal discharge. Dimethicones are also used in conjunction with antacids to assist the expulsion of flatus prior to radiographic examination of the gastro-intestinal tract.

Dimethicones are used to form a water-repellent film on glass vials. A typical method is to rinse clean dry vials with a 2 per cent solution of dimethicone 1000 in xylene, drain off the excess solution, and dry the vials at 110°; the vials are then heated for three hours at 250° to 275° in order to bond the dimethicone to the glass. Solutions and suspensions can be drained completely from vials which have been so treated.

Repeated use with a dimethicone will make glass apparatus water-repellent, although cleaning with toluene after use will remove most of the polymer.

Solutions of a dimethicone in ether or light petroleum are used as syringe lubricants; for this purpose, however, a methylphenylsiloxane is sometimes preferred because of its better lubricating properties and greater stability at high temperatures.

The dimethicones are also used as antifrothing agents in manufacturing processes.

PRECAUTIONS. Dimethicone preparations should not be applied where free drainage is necessary or to inflamed or abraded skin. They may be irritant to the eye.

Preparation
DIMETHICONE CREAM, B.P.C. (page 658)

DIMETHISTERONE

$C_{23}H_{32}O_2,H_2O = 358.5$

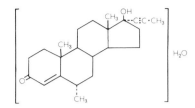

Dimethisterone is 17-hydroxy-6α-methyl-17α-prop-1'-ynylandrost-4-en-3-one monohydrate.

Solubility. Insoluble in water; soluble, at 20°, in 3 parts of alcohol, in 0·7 part of chloroform, in 1 part of pyridine, and in 80 parts of arachis oil.

Standard
It complies with the requirements of the British Pharmacopoeia.
It is a white or almost white, crystalline, odourless powder and contains not less than 97·0 and not more than the equivalent of 103·0 per cent of $C_{23}H_{32}O_2$, calculated with reference to the anhydrous substance. It contains 3·5 to 5·5 per cent w/w of water. It melts with decomposition at about 100°.

Storage. It should be protected from light.

Actions and uses. Dimethisterone is a synthetic progestogen which has actions and uses similar to those described under Progesterone (page 407).

It is active when given by mouth and is approximately as effective by this route as an equal weight of parenterally administered progesterone.

UNDESIRABLE EFFECTS. In large doses, dimethisterone may give rise to pelvic pain, breast turgidity, and vertigo.

Dose. 15 to 40 milligrams daily in divided doses.

Preparation
DIMETHISTERONE TABLETS, B.P. Unless otherwise specified, tablets each containing 5 mg of dimethisterone are supplied. They should be protected from light.

OTHER NAME: *Secrosteron®*

DIMETHYL PHTHALATE

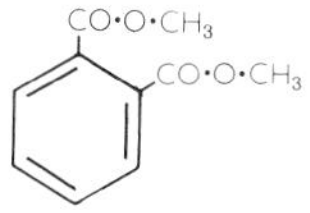

$C_{10}H_{10}O_4 = 194.2$

Dimethyl Phthalate is methyl benzene-o-dicarboxylate.

Solubility. Soluble, at 20°, in 250 parts of water; miscible with alcohol, with ether, and with most organic solvents.

Standard
It complies with the requirements of the British Pharmacopoeia.
It is a colourless or faintly coloured liquid; it is odourless or has a slight odour and contains not less than 99·0 per cent w/w of $C_{10}H_{10}O_4$. It has a weight per ml at 20° of 1·186 g to 1·192 g and boils at about 280° with decomposition.

Storage. Contact with plastic materials should be avoided.

Actions and uses. Dimethyl phthalate is an insect repellent and is very effective against mosquitoes, midges, mites, ticks, and fleas.
Owing to its low volatility it is active for three to five hours when applied to the skin,

but profuse sweating greatly reduces the effective repellent time. It is usually applied as a cream or lotion containing at least 40 per cent of dimethyl phthalate; weaker preparations are not effective as insect repellents.
Dimethyl phthalate may be used to impregnate clothing, but dibutyl phthalate is usually preferred.
It should not be allowed to come into contact with garments of rayon or other man-made fibres or with plastic spectacle frames.

UNDESIRABLE EFFECTS. Dimethyl phthalate has no serious irritant or toxic effects, although it may cause temporary smarting in tender areas of skin; it should not be applied near the eyes or to mucous surfaces.

OTHER NAMES: DMP; Methyl Phthalate

DIOCTYL SODIUM SULPHOSUCCINATE

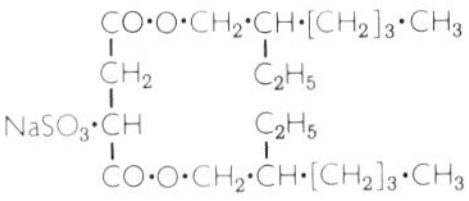

$C_{20}H_{37}NaO_7S = 444.6$

Dioctyl Sodium Sulphosuccinate is di(2-ethylhexyl) sodium sulphosuccinate.

Solubility. Soluble, at 20°, in 70 parts of water, higher concentrations forming a thick gel; soluble in 1 part of chloroform, in 1 part of ether, and in 3 parts of alcohol.

Standard

DESCRIPTION. White or almost white waxy masses or flakes; hygroscopic; odour characteristic.

IDENTIFICATION TESTS. 1. To 5 ml of a 0·1 per cent solution in water add 1 ml of *dilute sulphuric acid*, 10 ml of *chloroform*, and 0·2 ml of *dimethyl yellow solution*, and shake; the chloroform layer is coloured red. Add 0·05 g of *cetrimide* and shake; the colour of the chloroform layer changes to yellow.

2. The infra-red absorption spectrum exhibits maxima which are only at the same wavelengths as, and have similar relative intensities to, those in the spectrum of *dioctyl sodium sulphosuccinate A.S.*

LOSS ON DRYING. Not more than 3·0 per cent, determined by drying to constant weight at 105°.

SULPHATED ASH. 15·5 to 16·3 per cent, calculated with reference to the substance dried under the prescribed conditions.

CONTENT OF $C_{20}H_{37}NaO_7S$. Not less than 98·5 per cent, calculated with reference to the substance dried under the prescribed conditions, determined by the following method:

To about 3 g, accurately weighed, add 50 ml of hot water and stir until a paste is formed; add, with stirring, two further 50-ml portions of hot water, continue stirring until solution is complete, cool, and dilute to 1000 ml with water.

To 25 ml of 0·01M tetrabutylammonium iodide add a solution containing 5 g of *anhydrous sodium sulphate* and 0·5 g of *sodium carbonate* in 50 ml of water, followed by 25 ml of *chloroform* and 0·4 ml of *bromophenol blue solution*; shake well until the blue colour has passed into the chloroform layer, and titrate with the dioctyl sodium sulphosuccinate solution prepared above, shaking well and allowing to separate after each addition until the chloroform layer is colourless.

Each ml of 0·01M tetrabutylammonium iodide is equivalent to 0·004446 g of $C_{20}H_{37}NaO_7S$.

Stability. It is stable in acid solutions but it hydrolyses slowly in weak alkaline solutions and rapidly in solutions above pH 9.

Storage. It should be stored in airtight containers.

Actions and uses. Dioctyl sodium sulphosuccinate is an anionic surface-active agent. When taken by mouth it exerts a softening effect on the faeces and has a laxative action. A 1 per cent solution is used as an enema for the removal of impacted faeces. A 5 per cent solution has been used for softening wax in the ear.

Dioctyl sodium sulphosuccinate is also used as a tablet disintegrant.

Dose. 50 to 100 milligrams on alternate days.

OTHER NAMES: *Coprola*®; *Dioctyl*®; *Lancecolax*®; *Manoxol OT/P*®; *Siponol O*®

DIODONE INJECTION

Diodone Injection is a sterile aqueous solution of diodone, the diethanolamine salt of 1,4-dihydro-3,5-di-iodo-4-oxopyrid-1-ylacetic acid.

Standard

It complies with the requirements of the British Pharmacopoeia.

It is a clear colourless to pale yellow liquid with a pH of 7·0 to 8·0.

Diodone Injection is prepared in three strengths: (i) 35 per cent, containing 17·0 to 18·0 per cent w/v of I, with a weight per ml at 20° of 1·180 g to 1·200 g, (ii) 50 per cent, containing 24·2 to 25·8 per cent w/v of I, with a weight per ml at 20° of 1·260 g to 1·280 g, and (iii) 70 per cent, containing 34·0 to 36·0 per cent w/v of I, with a weight per ml at 30° of 1·355 g to 1·390 g.

Sterilisation. It is sterilised by heating in an autoclave or by filtration.

Storage. It should be stored at room temperature, protected from light; any solid matter which separates on standing should be redissolved by warming before use. It should not be allowed to come into contact with metals.

Actions and uses. Diodone is a contrast medium used mainly for retrograde pyelography. It was formerly used in intravenous pyelography and arteriography but it has been replaced for these purposes by the newer tri-iodo-compounds, such as sodium diatrizoate,

which have the advantage of giving denser shadows at comparable concentrations, of giving undesirable effects less frequently, and of being less viscous in high concentrations.

The purposes for which diodone is still used include ascending urethrography, in which the viscous solution is used, and micturating cystography, in which the 35 per cent solution is introduced by catheter to outline the bladder and urethra. If ureteric reflux occurs during cystography, the ureters and pelvicalyceal systems will be outlined.

UNDESIRABLE EFFECTS. These are as described under Sodium Diatrizoate (page 450), but some of the undesirable effects occur much more frequently. Nausea and vomiting are common and a sensation of heat is usual following intravenous injection of diodone.

Dose. The strength of solution and the dose are determined in accordance with the diagnostic procedure.

OTHER NAMES: *Periodal*®; *Vasiodone*®

DIPHENHYDRAMINE HYDROCHLORIDE

$C_{17}H_{22}ClNO = 291\cdot8$

$[(C_6H_5)_2CH\cdot O\cdot[CH_2]_2\cdot N(CH_3)_2]HCl$

Diphenhydramine Hydrochloride is (2-diphenylmethoxyethyl)dimethylamine hydrochloride.

Solubility. Soluble, at 20°, in 1 part of water, in 2 parts of alcohol, in 2 parts of chloroform, and in 50 parts of acetone; slightly soluble in ether.

Standard
It complies with the requirements of the British Pharmacopoeia.
It is a white, crystalline, odourless powder and contains not less than 98·0 and not more than the equivalent of 101·0 per cent of $C_{17}H_{22}ClNO$, calculated with reference to the dried substance. The loss on drying under the prescribed conditions is not more than 0·5 per cent. It has a melting-point of 168° to 172°.

Sterilisation. Solutions for injection are sterilised by heating in an autoclave or by filtration.

Storage. It should be stored in airtight containers, protected from light.

Actions and uses. Diphenhydramine has the actions, uses, and undesirable effects of the antihistamine drugs, as described under Promethazine Hydrochloride (page 409). It is one of the less active but more sedating of the group and is sometimes used for its sedative properties. It is usually administered by mouth, although it may be given parenterally if necessary.
Because of its mild spasmolytic properties, diphenhydramine is sometimes used as an ingredient of preparations for the relief of cough. It has also been used for the treatment of parkinsonism and for the prevention of motion-sickness; for the latter purpose the first dose should be taken before starting a journey.

POISONING. See under Promethazine Hydrochloride (page 409).

Dose. 50 to 200 milligrams by mouth daily in divided doses; 10 to 50 milligrams by intravenous or intramuscular injection, as a single dose.

Preparations
DIPHENHYDRAMINE CAPSULES, B.P. Unless otherwise specified, capsules each containing 25 mg of diphenhydramine hydrochloride are supplied. Capsules containing 50 mg are also available.

DIPHENHYDRAMINE ELIXIR, B.P.C. (page 671)

DIPHENHYDRAMINE INJECTION, B.P. It consists of a sterile solution of diphenhydramine hydrochloride in Water for Injections. Unless otherwise specified, a solution containing 10 mg in 1 ml is supplied. It should be protected from light.

OTHER NAMES: *Benadryl®*; *Histergan®*; *Histex®*

DIPHENOXYLATE HYDROCHLORIDE

$C_{30}H_{33}ClN_2O_2 = 489\cdot1$

Diphenoxylate Hydrochloride is ethyl 1-(3-cyano-3,3-diphenylpropyl)-4-phenylpiperidine-4-carboxylate hydrochloride.

Solubility. Very slightly soluble in water; soluble, at 20°, in 50 parts of alcohol, in 2·5 parts of chloroform, and in 40 parts of acetone; insoluble in ether.

Standard
It complies with the requirements of the British Pharmacopoeia.
It is a white or almost white odourless powder and contains not less than 98·0 and not more than the equivalent of 101·0 per cent of $C_{30}H_{33}ClN_2O_2$, calculated with reference to the dried substance. The loss on drying under the prescribed conditions is not more than 0·5 per cent. It has a melting-point of 221° to 226°.

Actions and uses. Diphenoxylate has an inhibitory action on intestinal mobility and is used in the symptomatic control of both acute and chronic diarrhoea, however caused. Response to treatment is usually rapid and the prompt control reduces the dehydration associated with diarrhoea. Diphenoxylate has no antibacterial properties, and its use in controlling the symptoms of diarrhoea does not remove the need for specific therapy when the diarrhoea is caused by bacterial or parasitic infection.

Diphenoxylate is also used in colostomy and ileostomy for reducing the frequency as well as the fluidity of the stools.
It is given in doses of 5 milligrams three or four times a day until the diarrhoea is controlled, when the dose may be reduced according to need to 5 milligrams daily.

UNDESIRABLE EFFECTS. Although undesirable effects are not frequent, nausea, dizziness, and sedation may occur; other side-effects include rash, pruritus, and insomnia; euphoria and abdominal distension have also been reported.

PRECAUTIONS AND CONTRA-INDICATIONS. Diphenoxylate is contra-indicated in patients with impaired liver function. The possibility that it may enhance the action of barbiturates should be borne in mind.
Although it has a structural relationship with pethidine, it has no analgesic action, but it appears to be capable of preventing withdrawal symptoms in known narcotic addicts, and the

addiction liability approximates to that of codeine.

As diphenoxylate is intended for short-term administration only, the risk of addiction is negligible, but excessive use can be discouraged by the addition of a subclinical dose of atropine.

Dose. See above under **Actions and uses.**

DIPIPANONE HYDROCHLORIDE

$C_{24}H_{32}ClNO,H_2O = 404\cdot0$

Dipipanone Hydrochloride is 4,4-diphenyl-6-piperidino-heptan-3-one hydrochloride monohydrate.

Solubility. Soluble, at 20°, in 40 parts of water, in 1·5 parts of alcohol, and in 6 parts of acetone; insoluble in ether.

Standard
It complies with the requirements of the British Pharmacopoeia.
It is a white, crystalline, almost odourless powder and contains not less than 99·0 and not more than the equivalent of 101·0 per cent of $C_{24}H_{32}ClNO$, calculated with reference to the anhydrous substance. It contains 4·0 to 5·0 per cent w/w of water. It has a melting-point of 124° to 127°, determined on the undried substance. A 2·5 per cent solution in water has a pH of 4·0 to 6·0.

Sterilisation. Solutions for injection are sterilised by heating in an autoclave or by filtration.

Actions and uses. Dipipanone has a strong analgesic action which begins about fifteen minutes after an intramuscular injection and persists for four to six hours.

Dipipanone, like methadone, has relatively little sedative and hypnotic action. It can be used to maintain relief of pain when morphine or pethidine has ceased to be effective, the usual dosage being 25 milligrams of dipipanone hydrochloride, repeated every six hours if necessary, by subcutaneous or intramuscular injection.

UNDESIRABLE EFFECTS. Nausea and vomiting may occur.

PRECAUTIONS. Dipipanone should not be given intravenously, as it may produce an alarming fall in blood pressure. Undue respiratory depression may be relieved by giving 5 to 10 milligrams of nalorphine hydrobromide intravenously.

In the presence of severe liver or kidney damage the action of dipipanone may be prolonged and it should be used with special caution in such cases.

DEPENDENCE. Prolonged administration of therapeutic doses may lead to the development of dependence of the morphine type, as described under Morphine Hydrochloride (page 314).

Dose. See above under **Actions and uses.**

Preparation
DIPIPANONE INJECTION, B.P. It consists of a sterile solution of dipipanone hydrochloride in Water for Injections, the pH of the solution being adjusted to 4·5. The strength of the solution should be specified by the prescriber. It should be protected from light. Ampoules containing 25 mg in 1 ml are available.

OTHER NAMES: *Pipadone®*; Piperidyl Methadone Hydrochloride

DISODIUM EDETATE

$C_{10}H_{14}N_2Na_2O_8,2H_2O = 372\cdot2$

Disodium Edetate is disodium dihydrogen ethylenediamine-*NNN'N'*-tetra-acetate dihydrate.

Solubility. Soluble, at 20°, in 11 parts of water; slightly soluble in alcohol; insoluble in ether and in chloroform.

Standard
It complies with the requirements of the British Pharmacopoeia.
It is a white, crystalline, odourless powder and contains not less than 98·0 per cent of $C_{10}H_{14}N_2Na_2O_8$, $2H_2O$. A 5 per cent solution in water has a pH of 4·0 to 5·5.

Actions and uses. Disodium edetate is a chelating substance which has a strong affinity for divalent and tervalent metals. It is used as a decalcifying agent in the treatment of hypercalcaemia, as the calcium ion loses its physiological properties when firmly bound in a chelate ring; the complex thus

formed is not metabolised in the body and is rapidly excreted by the kidneys.

The usual daily dosage for an adult is up to 70 milligrams per kilogram body-weight and for a child up to 60 milligrams per kilogram body-weight, given, as Trisodium Edetate Injection, diluted to about 500 millilitres with Sodium Chloride Injection or Dextrose Injection, by slow intravenous injection over a period of two to three hours; 1 gram of disodium edetate (dihydrate) is approximately equivalent to 1 gram of trisodium edetate. Rapid injection may cause a dangerous fall in the serum-calcium level, leading to convulsions and cardiac arrest, and will also damage the vein used for the injection.

Treatment is usually given for five days, followed by two days' rest; the course may be repeated as often as necessary.

Disodium edetate is used for the removal of calcium deposits from lime burns of the eye, a suitable strength of solution being 0·38 per cent with 0·1 per cent of sodium bicarbonate. For the inactivation of bacterial collagenase as an adjunct to antibiotic treatment of keratopathy caused by *Pseudomonas aeruginosa*, eye-drops containing 0·38 per cent buffered to pH 7·0 may be used. Damage to the cornea resulting from the presence of epithelial collagenase may be treated with eye-drops containing 1·9 or 3·8 per cent buffered to pH 7·0. A suitable buffer consists of sodium acid phosphate 0·42 per cent and sodium phosphate 1·43 per cent; benzalkonium chloride is a suitable preservative.

Disodium edetate is also used to remove traces of heavy metals from pharmaceutical preparations and so improve their stability.

UNDESIRABLE EFFECTS. Overdosage may lead to renal damage and haemorrhagic manifestations.

Milder undesirable effects such as nausea, diarrhoea, and cramp occur occasionally, and reactions on the skin and mucous membranes have been reported; these symptoms subside when treatment is stopped.

PRECAUTIONS. During treatment the serum-calcium level should be checked repeatedly; if signs of tetany occur the infusion rate should be reduced or treatment discontinued and, if necessary, calcium ions should be injected.

Dose. See above under **Actions and uses.**

Preparation

TRISODIUM EDETATE INJECTION, B.P. It consists of a sterile solution containing the equivalent of 20 per cent w/v of trisodium edetate in Water for Injections. It should be diluted with Sodium Chloride Injection or Dextrose Injection before administration.

DITHRANOL

SYNONYM: Dioxyanthranol

$C_{14}H_{10}O_3 = 226·2$

Dithranol is a mixture of 1,8-dihydroxy-9-anthrone and its tautomers.

CAUTION: *Dithranol is a powerful irritant and should be kept away from the eyes and tender parts of the skin.*

Solubility. Insoluble in water; slightly soluble in alcohol and in ether; soluble in chloroform, in acetone, and in fixed oils.

Standard
It complies with the requirements of the British Pharmacopoeia.
It is a yellow odourless powder with a melting-point of 176° to 181°. The loss on drying at 105° is not more than 1·0 per cent.

Storage. It should be stored in airtight containers, protected from light.

Actions and uses. Dithranol is used, in a concentration of 0·01 to 1 per cent, in external preparations for the treatment of psoriasis. It also has fungicidal properties and is used for the treatment of ringworm infections and other chronic dermatoses.

Stains on the skin may be removed with a bleaching solution such as Dilute Sodium Hypochlorite Solution and stains on the clothes may be removed with a solvent such as trichloroethylene.

PRECAUTIONS. As some patients are intolerant of the usual concentrations of dithranol, a preliminary test for sensitivity should be carried out with the ointment to guard against an excessive reaction.

Preparations
DITHRANOL OINTMENT, B.P. It consists of dithranol in yellow soft paraffin. The strength of the ointment should be specified by the prescriber.
DITHRANOL PASTE, B.P.C. (page 767)

OTHER NAME: Anthralin

DODECYL GALLATE

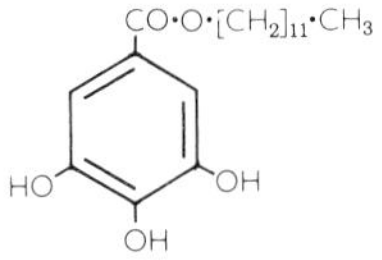

$C_{19}H_{30}O_5 = 338.4$

Dodecyl Gallate is dodecyl 3,4,5-trihydroxybenzoate.

Solubility. Insoluble in water; soluble, at 20°, in 3·5 parts of alcohol, in 4 parts of ether, in 60 parts of chloroform, in 2 parts of acetone, in 30 parts of arachis oil, in 1·5 parts of methyl alcohol, and in 60 parts of propylene glycol.

Standard
It complies with the requirements of the British Pharmacopoeia.
It is a white or creamy-white odourless powder.

The loss on drying at 70° is not more than 0·5 per cent. It has a melting-point of 96° to 97·5°.

Storage. It should be stored in airtight containers, protected from light, contact with metals being avoided.

Uses. Dodecyl gallate is used as an antoxidant for preserving oils and fats, as described under Propyl Gallate (page 413).

DOMIPHEN BROMIDE

Domiphen Bromide is a mixture of alkyldimethyl-2-phenoxyethylammonium bromides. It consists chiefly of dodecyldimethyl-2-phenoxyethylammonium bromide $\{C_6H_5 \cdot O[CH_2]_2 \cdot N(CH_3)_2(C_{12}H_{25})\}^+Br^-$ $(C_{22}H_{40}BrNO = 414.5)$.

Solubility. Soluble, at 20°, in less than 2 parts of water and of alcohol and in 30 parts of acetone.

Standard
It complies with the requirements of the British Pharmacopoeia.
It occurs as colourless or faintly yellow crystalline flakes and contains not less than 97·0 per cent of $C_{22}H_{40}BrNO$, calculated with reference to the dried substance. The loss on drying under the prescribed conditions is not more than 1·0 per cent. It melts between 106° and 116°. A 10 per cent solution in water is almost colourless and not more than slightly opalescent.

Incompatibility. It is incompatible with soaps and similar anionic detergents and with alkali hydroxides.

Storage. It should be stored in airtight containers.

Preparation and storage of solutions. See statement on aqueous solutions of antiseptics, under Solutions (page 779).

Actions and uses. Domiphen bromide has the actions and uses of the quaternary ammonium compounds, as described under Cetrimide (page 88), in addition to which it has antifungal activity.
The activity of domiphen bromide is enhanced

in alkaline media, but reduced in the presence of acid, organic matter, blood, and pus. Its activity is also reduced in the presence of soap; consequently all traces of soap should be removed from the skin before applying domiphen bromide.
A 0·02 per cent aqueous solution has been used in obstetrics, for application to wounds and burns, and for irrigation of the bladder and urethra.
Lozenges containing 0·5 milligram of domiphen bromide are used for the treatment of bacterial and fungous infections of the mouth and throat.
Domiphen bromide is used as an antiseptic in some medicated surgical dressings.

PRECAUTIONS. Continuous use may bring about defatting of the skin of the hands; protection against this may be provided by the application of a suitable cream, such as hydrous ointment, containing wool alcohols or wool fat.

OTHER NAME: *Bradosol®*

DOXYCYCLINE HYDROCHLORIDE

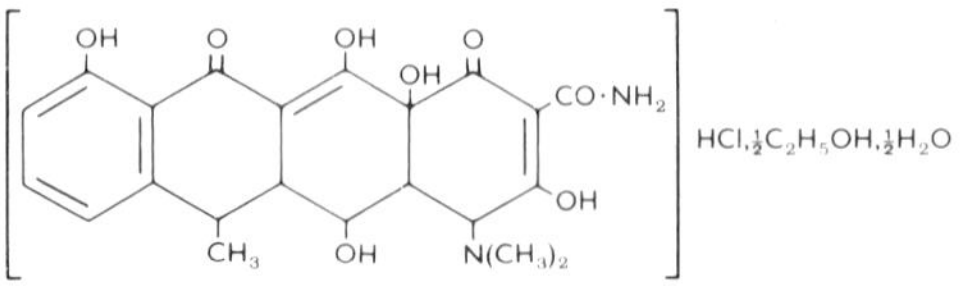

$C_{22}H_{25}ClN_2O_8, \frac{1}{2}C_2H_5OH, \frac{1}{2}H_2O = 512.9$

Doxycycline Hydrochloride is 4-dimethylamino-1,4,4a,5,5a,6,11,12a-octahydro-3,5,10,12,12a-pentahydroxy-6-methyl-1,11-dioxonaphthacene-2-carboxamide hydrochloride hemiethanolate hemihydrate, an antimicrobial substance prepared from oxytetracycline or methacycline.

Solubility. Soluble, at 20°, in 3 parts of water and in 4 parts of methyl alcohol; insoluble in chloroform.

Standard
It complies with the requirements of the British Pharmacopoeia.
It is a yellow crystalline powder with a slightly

ethanolic odour and contains not less than 822 Units per mg. It contains 4·3 to 6·0 per cent w/w of ethyl alcohol and 1·4 to 2·8 per cent w/w of water. A 1 per cent solution in water has a pH of 2·0 to 3·0.

Storage. It should be stored in airtight containers, protected from light.

Actions and uses. Doxycycline has the actions and uses described under Tetracycline Hydrochloride (page 498) but differs from tetracycline in having a high lipid solubility and a biological half-life of fifteen hours after a single dose or twenty-two hours after several daily doses.

Doxycycline is almost completely absorbed from the gut, even if taken with food, and the renal clearance rate is low; in consequence, higher concentrations are reached in secretions such as those of the bronchi and nasal sinuses than with other tetracyclines.

Salts of aluminium, calcium, iron, and magnesium, which may decrease the absorption of tetracyclines from the gut, should not be given with doxycycline.

The usual initial dose is the equivalent of 200 milligrams of doxycycline, followed by 100 milligrams daily, but this may be increased to 200 milligrams daily for the treatment of infections caused by organisms for which the minimum inhibitory concentration is greater than 0·6 microgram per millilitre; the usual dosage for children is 3 milligrams per kilogram body-weight daily; 1·15 grams of doxycycline hydrochloride is approximately equivalent to 1 gram of doxycycline.

PRECAUTIONS AND CONTRA-INDICATIONS. As for Tetracycline Hydrochloride (page 498).

Dose. See above under **Actions and uses.**

Preparation
DOXYCYCLINE CAPSULES, B.P. Unless otherwise specified, capsules each containing the equivalent of 100 mg of doxycycline are supplied.

OTHER NAME: *Vibramycin®*

DYDROGESTERONE

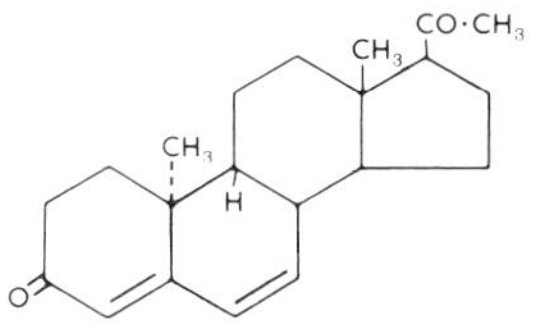

$C_{21}H_{28}O_2 = 312.5$

Dydrogesterone is 9β,10α-pregna-4,6-diene-3,20-dione.

Solubility. Insoluble in water; soluble, at 20°, in 52 parts of alcohol, in 140 parts of ether, in 2 parts of chloroform, in 17 parts of acetone, in 40 parts of methyl alcohol, and in 180 parts of fixed oils.

Standard
It complies with the requirements of the British Pharmacopoeia.
It is a white or almost white, crystalline, odourless powder and contains not less than 97·0 and not more than the equivalent of 103·0 per cent of $C_{21}H_{28}O_2$, calculated with reference to the dried substance. The loss on drying under the prescribed conditions is not more than 0·5 per cent. It has a melting-point of 167° to 171°.

Storage. It should be stored in airtight containers, protected from light.

Actions and uses. Dydrogesterone has actions similar to those of progesterone (page 407) but, being a derivative of retroprogesterone, it does not have androgenic or oestrogenic properties and does not prevent ovulation or suppress pituitary secretion of gonadotrophins. It does not raise body temperature.

Dydrogesterone is used in the differential diagnosis of amenorrhoea. It is used together with oestrogens in the treatment of mild dysfunctional menorrhagia and to prevent metrorrhagia. In doses of 5 milligrams four times daily from the fifth day of the menstrual cycle for twenty days, it may relieve pain and spasm in dysmenorrhoea. Continuous therapy for six months or more with 10 to 30 milligrams daily in divided doses may be used for the treatment of endometriosis.

Dydrogesterone may also be of value in maintaining pregnancy in threatened abortion due to progesterone deficiency; it does not lead to virilisation of the foetus. It is of no value as an oral contraceptive.

UNDESIRABLE EFFECTS. Dydrogesterone occasionally causes nausea and vomiting but this is usually mild. Uterine bleeding may occur during treatment but usually responds to reduction in dose with increased frequency of administration.

Dose. 5 to 30 milligrams daily in divided doses.

Preparation
DYDROGESTERONE TABLETS, B.P. Unless otherwise specified, tablets each containing 10 mg of dydrogesterone are supplied. They should be protected from light.

OTHER NAME: *Duphaston®*

ECOTHIOPATE IODIDE

$C_9H_{23}INO_3PS = 383.2$

$$\left[(CH_3)_3N \cdot [CH_2]_2 \cdot S \cdot \underset{\underset{O}{\parallel}}{P}(O \cdot CH_2 \cdot CH_3)_2\right]^+ \ I^-$$

Ecothiopate Iodide is *S*-2-dimethylaminoethyl diethyl phosphorothiolate methiodide.

Solubility. Soluble, at 20°, in 1 part of water, in 25 parts of alcohol, and in 3 parts of methyl alcohol; very slightly soluble in other organic solvents.

Standard
It complies with the requirements of the British Pharmacopoeia.
It is a white, crystalline, hygroscopic powder with an alliaceous odour and contains not less than 92·5 per cent of $C_9H_{23}INO_3PS$. The loss on drying under the prescribed conditions is not more than 1·0 per cent. It melts with decomposition at about 119°.

Storage. It should be stored in airtight containers, at a temperature of 2° to 10°, protected from light.

Actions and uses. Ecothiopate iodide is a powerful long-acting inhibitor of cholinesterase. It is applied locally for the reduction of intra-ocular tension.
In the treatment of glaucoma, one drop of a 0·06 per cent solution may be instilled into the conjunctival sac twice daily. Patients who have failed to respond to other miotics used in conjunction with sympathomimetics and carbonic anhydrase inhibitors may sometimes be treated successfully with a higher concentration of ecothiopate iodide, such as 0·125 or 0·25 per cent.
In the treatment of esotropia, one drop of a 0·125 per cent solution should be instilled into each eye daily at bedtime and if a satisfactory response is obtained treatment may be continued with one drop of a 0·06 per cent solution daily or one drop of a 0·125 per cent solution every other day.
Ecothiopate iodide is usually available as eye-drops containing 0·06, 0·125, and 0·25 per cent.

UNDESIRABLE EFFECTS. Systemic absorption of ecothiopate may occur during ocular treatment, and general anticholinesterase effects, including potentiation of muscle relaxants of the depolarising type, may result.

OTHER NAME: *Phospholine Iodide*®

EDROPHONIUM CHLORIDE

$C_{10}H_{16}ClNO = 201.7$

Edrophonium Chloride is ethyl(3-hydroxyphenyl)dimethylammonium chloride.

Solubility. Soluble, at 20°, in 0·5 part of water and in 5 parts of alcohol; insoluble in ether and in chloroform.

Standard
It complies with the requirements of the British Pharmacopoeia.
It is a white, crystalline, odourless powder and contains not less than 98·5 and not more than the equivalent of 101·0 per cent of $C_{10}H_{16}ClNO$, calculated with reference to the dried substance. The loss on drying under the prescribed conditions is not more than 0·5 per cent. It melts with decomposition at about 168°.

Storage. It should be stored in airtight containers, protected from light.

Actions and uses. Edrophonium chloride is an anticholinesterase drug with actions qualitatively similar to those of neostigmine methylsulphate. Its actions are rapid in onset and of short duration. It is of particular value in the diagnosis of myasthenia gravis.
It is given by intravenous injection in doses of 2 to 10 milligrams; the usual procedure is to inject 2 milligrams and, if no change in clinical signs occurs within thirty seconds, to continue with the injection of a further 8 milligrams. The dose of edrophonium chloride for a child of up to 35 kilograms bodyweight is 1 milligram, given by intravenous injection; 2 milligrams may be given by intramuscular injection when intravenous injection is difficult.

In untreated patients with myasthenia gravis, there is immediate subjective improvement and muscle strength increases. This effect usually lasts only for about five minutes, after which time the typical signs and symptoms return; because of its brief action the drug is not suitable for the routine treatment of myasthenia gravis or for use as an antagonist to curare-like drugs.
Edrophonium chloride is used in a similar way to determine whether or not a patient with severe symptoms of myasthenia gravis is suffering from the effects of inadequate or excessive treatment with anticholinesterase drugs. If treatment has been inadequate, edrophonium chloride will produce an immediate amelioration of symptoms, whereas in cholinergic crisis due to over-treatment the symptoms will be aggravated or unchanged.

Dose. See above under **Actions and uses.**

Preparation
EDROPHONIUM INJECTION, B.P. It consists of a sterile solution of edrophonium chloride in Water for Injections. Unless otherwise specified, a solution containing 10 mg in 1 ml is supplied. It should be protected from light.

OTHER NAME: *Tensilon*®

EMETINE AND BISMUTH IODIDE

SYNONYM: Emet. Bism. Iod.

Emetine and Bismuth Iodide is a complex iodide of emetine and bismuth.

Emetine and Bismuth Iodide may be prepared by mixing an aqueous solution of emetine hydrochloride with an excess of a solution prepared by dissolving bismuth carbonate and potassium iodide in hydrochloric acid.

Solubility. Insoluble in water and in alcohol; slightly decomposed by, but insoluble in, dilute acids; soluble in acetone and, with decomposition, in concentrated acids and in alkaline solutions.

Standard
It complies with the requirements of the British Pharmacopoeia.
It is a reddish-orange odourless powder and contains 25·0 to 30·0 per cent of emetine, $C_{29}H_{40}N_2O_4$, and 18·0 to 22·5 per cent of Bi, both calculated with reference to the dried substance. The loss on drying under the prescribed conditions is not more than 2·0 per cent.

Storage. It should be stored in airtight containers, protected from light.

Actions and uses. Emetine and bismuth iodide has actions similar to those described under Emetine Hydrochloride, but has the advantage that when given by mouth it is not appreciably decomposed until it reaches the small intestine, where the emetine is liberated. Emetine and bismuth iodide is given to supplement the action of injections of emetine hydrochloride in acute amoebiasis and for the treatment of chronic infections and of carriers.

A daily dosage of 60 to 200 milligrams is given by mouth for twelve consecutive days if tolerated by the patient. To minimise nausea and vomiting the dose should be given at night on an empty stomach; 200 milligrams of amylobarbitone sodium given thirty minutes before emetine and bismuth iodide is useful for patients showing intolerance. Chlorpromazine hydrochloride in doses of 25 milligrams three times daily may also be given.

Treatment with emetine and bismuth iodide is frequently supplemented with, or replaced by, other amoebicidal drugs such as metronidazole, diloxanide furoate, or acetarsol.

When the drug is dispensed in capsules it should not be suspended in an oily basis.

Dose. 60 to 200 milligrams daily.

Preparation
EMETINE AND BISMUTH IODIDE TABLETS, B.P. Unless otherwise specified, tablets each containing 60 mg of emetine and bismuth iodide are supplied. They are enteric coated and sugar coated. They should be stored in airtight containers, at a temperature not exceeding 25°.

EMETINE HYDROCHLORIDE

SYNONYM: Emet. Hydrochlor.

$C_{29}H_{42}Cl_2N_2O_4, 7H_2O = 679·7$

Emetine Hydrochloride is the hydrochloride of emetine, an alkaloid obtained from ipecacuanha or prepared by methylating cephaëline or by synthesis.

Solubility. Soluble in water and in alcohol.

Standard
It complies with the requirements of the British Pharmacopoeia.
It is a white, crystalline, odourless powder which becomes faintly yellow on exposure to light. It contains not less than 98·0 and not more than the equivalent of 101·5 per cent of $C_{29}H_{42}Cl_2N_2O_4$, calculated with reference to the dried substance. The loss on drying under the prescribed conditions is 15·0 to 19·0 per cent.

Storage. It should be stored in airtight containers, protected from light.

Actions and uses. Emetine hydrochloride is an amoebicide. It is excreted slowly and accumulates in the body during a course of treatment.

When injected subcutaneously it quickly relieves the symptoms of amoebic dysentery; it is also effective in the treatment of amoebic

hepatitis and liver abscess, but has no permanent effect in chronic amoebiasis.

Injections of emetine will not usually eradicate the intestinal infection and it is therefore necessary to give supplementary treatment by mouth with another amoebicide such as emetine and bismuth iodide, diloxanide furoate, or metronidazole. Many schedules of treatment have been devised in which alternating courses and combinations of various amoebicides are given.

Amoebic ulcers are always secondarily infected with bacteria and in some patients amoebicidal drugs have little action until the secondary infection is controlled by sulphonamides or by antibiotics.

For the treatment of acute amoebic dysentery, a daily dosage of 60 milligrams of emetine hydrochloride is administered by subcutaneous or intramuscular injection until the symptoms are controlled; three or four doses are usually sufficient, and the total dose should not exceed 750 milligrams. It should not be given intravenously.

For the irrigation of amoebic abscess cavities after the aspiration of pus, a 0·04 to 0·1 per cent solution of emetine hydrochloride in Sodium Chloride Injection has been used.

Emetine hydrochloride relieves the pain of scorpion stings when injected subcutaneously at the site of the sting; 30 milligrams is the usual dose.

UNDESIRABLE EFFECTS. When given by mouth, emetine has an irritant action upon mucous membranes. In small doses it causes increased bronchial secretion and perspiration; larger doses, of about 6 milligrams of emetine hydrochloride, cause vomiting.

Injections of emetine are sometimes painful and may cause local induration or necrosis of tissue. Prolonged administration may produce degenerative changes in the kidney tubules, liver, and muscles, and may give rise to peripheral neuritis. Its effect upon heart muscle causes changes in the electrocardiogram; rarely, acute degenerative myocarditis with cardiac irregularities and failure may occur.

CONTRA-INDICATIONS. Emetine is contra-indicated in the presence of cardiac or renal disease.

Dose. See above under **Actions and uses.**

Preparation

EMETINE INJECTION, B.P. It consists of a sterile solution of emetine hydrochloride in Water for Injections, the pH of the solution being adjusted to 3. Unless otherwise specified, a solution containing 60 mg in 1 ml is supplied. It should be protected from light.

EPHEDRINE

SYNONYMS: Ephedrinum Hydratum;
Hydrated Ephedrine

$C_{10}H_{15}NO,\frac{1}{2}H_2O = 174\cdot2$

$C_6H_5 \cdot CH(OH) \cdot CH(NHCH_3) \cdot CH_3, \frac{1}{2}H_2O$

Ephedrine is (−)-2-methylamino-1-phenylpropan-1-ol hemihydrate, an alkaloid obtained from species of *Ephedra* or prepared synthetically.

Solubility. Soluble, at 20°, in 36 parts of water, in less than 1 part of alcohol, and in 20 parts of glycerol; soluble in 25 parts of olive oil and in 100 parts of liquid paraffin with separation of water; soluble in ether and in chloroform with turbidity due to separation of water. The anhydrous alkaloid forms clear solutions in liquid paraffin.

Standard

DESCRIPTION. Colourless, hexagonal, prismatic crystals or a white crystalline powder; odourless or with a slight aromatic odour.

IDENTIFICATION TESTS. 1. Dissolve 10 mg in 1 ml of water and 0·1 ml of *strong sodium hydroxide solution* and add 0·1 ml of *copper sulphate solution*; a precipitate and a violet colour are produced. Add 1 ml of *solvent ether*, shake, and allow to separate; the ethereal layer is purple and the aqueous layer is blue.

2. Warm 0·05 g with 2 ml of 0·1N potassium permanganate; the odour of benzaldehyde is produced.

3. Dissolve 1 g in 20 ml of *carbon tetrachloride*, add a small quantity of *copper* and shake frequently; a turbidity appears followed by a copious precipitate. Allow to stand for 15 minutes and filter; the residue, after washing with three successive 5-ml portions of *carbon tetrachloride*, recrystallising from a mixture of *solvent ether* and *alcohol* (*95 per cent*), and drying at 105°, melts at about 218°.

4. A 0·05 per cent w/v solution in 0·1N hydrochloric acid exhibits maxima at about 251, 257, and 263 nm.

APPEARANCE OF SOLUTION. A 2·5 per cent w/v solution in water complies with the following tests:
(i) The solution is clear when compared with water, the comparison being made by viewing vertically 10 ml of the liquids in matched, colourless, transparent, neutral glass tubes, 16 mm internal diameter and with a flat base, against a black background in diffused light.
(ii) The solution has no colour when compared with water, the comparison being made by viewing vertically 10 ml of the liquids in matched, colourless,

transparent, neutral glass tubes, 16 mm internal diameter and with a flat base, against a white background in diffused daylight.

MELTING-POINT. 40° to 42°, determined without previous drying.

SPECIFIC ROTATION. Dissolve 2·25 g in 15 ml of *dilute hydrochloric acid* and dilute to 50 ml with water; the specific rotation of the ephedrine hydrochloride formed is −33·5° to −35·5°, calculated with reference to the anhydrous substance.

CHLORIDE. Dissolve 0·180 g in 10 ml of water, add 5 ml of *dilute nitric acid* and 0·5 ml of *silver nitrate solution*, and allow to stand for 2 minutes, protected from light; any opalescence produced is not more intense than that produced when 10 ml of *chloride standard solution* is treated in the same manner (280 parts per million).

OXALATE. Dissolve 0·50 g in 5 ml of water and 1 ml of *dilute hydrochloric acid*, make slightly alkaline to *litmus paper* with *dilute ammonia solution*, add 0·75 ml of *calcium chloride solution*, and allow to stand for 10 minutes; no opalescence is produced.

SULPHATE. Dissolve 1·0 g in a mixture of 5 ml of water and 3 ml of *acetic acid* and dilute to 20 ml with water. To 15 ml of this solution add 2·2 ml of water; this solution complies with the test for the prepared solution in the test for Sulphate given under Sodium Carbonate, page 445 (200 parts per million).

WATER. Not less than 4·5 and not more than 5·5 per cent, determined by the method given in Appendix 16, page 895.

SULPHATED ASH. Not more than 0·1 per cent.

CONTENT OF $C_{10}H_{15}NO$. Not less than 98·5 per cent, calculated with reference to the anhydrous substance, determined by the following method:
Dissolve about 0·5 g, accurately weighed, in 5 ml of *alcohol* (*95 per cent*), previously neutralised to *methyl red solution*, add 50 ml of 0·1N hydrochloric acid and

titrate with 0·1N sodium hydroxide, using *methyl red solution* as indicator; each ml of 0·1N hydrochloric acid is equivalent to 0·01652 g of $C_{10}H_{15}NO$.

Actions and uses. Ephedrine is a sympathomimetic amine which resembles adrenaline (page 8) and amphetamine (page 25) in its actions.

When given by mouth in therapeutic doses, ephedrine constricts the peripheral vessels, thus raising the blood pressure. It relaxes the bronchioles and decreases the tone and peristaltic movements of the intestine, but contracts the uterus. It contracts the sphincter but relaxes the detrusor muscle of the bladder, dilates the pupil, and stimulates the central nervous system. The prolonged administration of ephedrine has no cumulative effect but tolerance may develop.

Ephedrine has been given by intramuscular injection to combat a fall in blood pressure arising from attacks of syncope or anaphylactic shock. It is given by mouth or by subcutaneous injection to prevent attacks of bronchial spasm; its action is delayed in onset and is only fully established after about one hour, but its effect lasts for about four hours. Belladonna or atropine is often administered with ephedrine to augment its bronchodilator action.

Ephedrine is used in the treatment of allergic conditions, such as hay fever, urticaria, and serum sickness. Its action on the bladder is employed in controlling nocturnal enuresis in children. It is used in conjunction with neostigmine to decrease the fatigue of voluntary muscle in myasthenia gravis.

When applied locally to mucous membranes, ephedrine causes blanching and a reduction in the secretions of the area to which it is applied; if the mucous surface is inflamed it relieves the symptoms of painful swelling and catarrh.

UNDESIRABLE EFFECTS. A variety of undesirable effects may arise in patients with idiosyncrasy to ephedrine or as a result of overdosage. These effects include anxiety, restlessness, nausea, muscular weakness and tremors, sweating and thirst, and sometimes dermatitis. The insomnia produced in adults by ephedrine may be relieved by the administration of a barbiturate. In patients with prostatic hypertrophy ephedrine may give rise to retention of urine.

PRECAUTIONS AND CONTRA-INDICATIONS. Ephedrine should not be given to patients who are being treated with a monoamine-oxidase inhibitor, such as isocarboxazid, nialamide, phenelzine, or tranylcypromine, or within about ten days of the discontinuation of such treatment.

Because of its effects on the cardiovascular system, ephedrine is contra-indicated in coronary thrombosis, hypertension, and thyrotoxicosis.

EPHEDRINE HYDROCHLORIDE

SYNONYM: Ephed. Hydrochlor.

$C_{10}H_{15}NO,HCl = 201·7$

Ephedrine Hydrochloride is the hydrochloride of $(-)$-2-methylamino-1-phenylpropan-1-ol.

Solubility. Soluble, at 20°, in 4 parts of water and in 17 parts of alcohol; very slightly soluble in chloroform.

Standard
It complies with the requirements of the British Pharmacopoeia.
It occurs as odourless colourless crystals or white crystalline powder and contains not less than 99·0 and not more than the equivalent of 101·0 per cent of $C_{10}H_{15}NO,HCl$, calculated with reference to the dried substance. The loss on drying under the prescribed conditions is not more than 0·5 per cent. It has a melting-point of 217° to 220°. A 10 per cent solution in water is colourless and not more than very faintly opalescent.

Sterilisation. Solutions for injection are sterilised by heating in an autoclave.

Actions and uses. Ephedrine hydrochloride has the actions, uses, and undesirable effects described under Ephedrine. It is the form in which ephedrine is usually given by mouth or by injection, although great care is necessary in the parenteral administration of aqueous solutions of the drug.

Aqueous solutions containing 0·5 to 5 per cent are used for application to mucous membranes. The nasal drops may be used to reduce swelling of the turbinate bodies in hay fever and catarrhal infections.

PRECAUTIONS AND CONTRA-INDICATIONS. As for Ephedrine.

Dose. 15 to 60 milligrams.

Preparations
EPHEDRINE ELIXIR, B.P.C. (page 671)
BELLADONNA AND EPHEDRINE MIXTURE, PAEDIATRIC, B.P.C. (page 737)
EPHEDRINE NASAL DROPS, B.P.C. (page 757)
EPHEDRINE HYDROCHLORIDE TABLETS, B.P. Unless otherwise specified, tablets each containing 30 mg of ephedrine hydrochloride are supplied. Tablets containing 7·5, 15, and 60 mg are also available.

ERGOMETRINE MALEATE

SYNONYMS: Ergometrinii Maleas; Ergonovine Maleate

$C_{23}H_{27}N_3O_6 = 441·5$

Ergometrine Maleate is the hydrogen maleate of ergometrine, a water-soluble alkaloid obtained from ergot or prepared by partial synthesis.

Solubility. Soluble, at 20°, in 40 parts of water, giving a solution with a blue fluorescence, and in 100 parts of alcohol (90 per cent); insoluble in ether and in chloroform.

Standard

It complies with the requirements of the European Pharmacopoeia.
It is a white or yellowish, crystalline, odourless powder and contains not less than 98·0 per cent of $C_{23}H_{27}N_3O_6$, calculated with reference to the dried substance. The loss on drying under the prescribed conditions is not more than 2·0 per cent. A 1 per cent solution in water has a pH of 3·0 to 5·0.

Sterilisation. Solutions for injection are sterilised by heating in an autoclave in an atmosphere of nitrogen or other suitable gas.

Storage. It should be stored in an atmosphere of nitrogen, in hermetically sealed containers, protected from light, in a cool place.

Actions and uses. Ergometrine is the alkaloid responsible for the oxytocic activity of aqueous extracts of ergot.

When administered by mouth in solution, ergometrine causes contractions of the uterus, which commence about eight minutes after administration; after about an hour the contractions become less frequent. When ergometrine is administered by intramuscular injection, uterine contractions begin within two minutes; when the injection is given intravenously, they begin within one minute. Its action is more prolonged than that of oxytocin.

Ergometrine has little effect on the sympathetic nervous system, and in this respect differs from ergotamine.

Ergometrine is used mainly in the prevention and treatment of post-partum haemorrhage due to uterine atony. It may also be injected directly into the uterine muscle to control haemorrhage during Caesarean section. It may be given in conjunction with oxytocin. In emergencies, when a rapid response is needed, it may be given intravenously. It should not be given during the first or second stage of labour, as the contraction might cause the death of the foetus or rupture the uterus. Because of its powerful oxytocic action it is not generally administered before the expulsion of the placenta.

Dose. 0·5 to 1 milligram by mouth; 0·2 to 1 milligram by intramuscular injection; 100 to 500 micrograms by intravenous injection.

Preparations

ERGOMETRINE INJECTION, B.P. (*Syn.* Ergonovine Maleate Injection). It consists of a sterile solution of ergometrine maleate in Water for Injections free from dissolved air, the pH of the solution being adjusted to 3. Unless otherwise specified, a solution containing 500 µg in 1 ml is supplied. It should be protected from light.

ERGOMETRINE TABLETS, B.P. (*Syn.* Ergonovine Maleate Tablets). Unless otherwise specified, tablets each containing 500 µg of ergometrine maleate are supplied. They should be stored in airtight containers, protected from light. Tablets containing 125 and 250 µg are also available.

ERGOTAMINE TARTRATE

SYNONYM: Ergotaminii Tartras

$C_{70}H_{76}N_{10}O_{16} = 1313·4$

Ergotamine Tartrate is the tartrate of ergotamine, an alkaloid obtained from certain species of ergot. It may contain 2 molecules of methanol of crystallisation.

Solubility. Soluble in water, the solution possibly becoming turbid, but the turbidity may be removed by adding tartaric acid; soluble, at 20°, in 500 parts of alcohol (90 per cent).

Standard

It complies with the requirements of the European Pharmacopoeia.
It occurs as odourless colourless crystals or greyish-white or yellowish-white crystalline powder and contains not less than 97·0 per cent of $C_{70}H_{76}N_{10}O_{16}$, calculated with reference to the dried substance. The loss on drying under the prescribed conditions is not more than 6·0 per cent. A suspension of 5 mg in 2 ml of freshly boiled and cooled water has a pH of 3·8 to 4·8.

Sterilisation. Solutions for injection are sterilised by heating in an autoclave in an atmosphere of nitrogen or other inert gas.

Storage. It should be stored in an atmosphere of nitrogen, in hermetically sealed containers, protected from light, in a cool place.

Actions and uses. Ergotamine stimulates and, in large doses, paralyses the motor terminations of the sympathetic nerves. Prolonged administration produces gangrene due to constriction of the peripheral arterioles with consequent arrest of blood flow. When given by intravenous injection it causes contraction of involuntary muscle, including that of the uterus, and a rise in blood pressure. Ergotamine is use chiefly in the treatment of migraine. It acts most reliably when given by subcutaneous or intramuscular injection, but it is often given by mouth, preferably sublingually, or in suppositories. The most successful results are obtained when it is given before the symptoms are fully established.

UNDESIRABLE EFFECTS. Ergotamine, when used in the recommended doses for the treatment of migraine, rarely produces undesirable effects other than nausea and vomiting; occasionally, however, it produces muscular weakness and pain. In large repeated doses it can produce all the symptoms of ergot poisoning, including gangrene of the extremities and serious mental derangement.

PRECAUTIONS AND CONTRA-INDICATIONS. It should be used with caution in patients with cardiovascular disease and it should preferably not be given to such patients by injection. It should not be given during pregnancy.

Dose. 1 to 2 milligrams by mouth: 250 to 500 micrograms by subcutaneous or intramuscular injection.

Preparations
ERGOTAMINE AEROSOL INHALATION, B.P.C. (page 645)
ERGOTAMINE INJECTION, B.P. It consists of a sterile solution of ergotamine tartrate in Water for Injections, the pH of the solution being adjusted to 3·3. Unless otherwise specified, a solution containing 500 µg in 1 ml is supplied. It should be protected from light. A solution containing 250 µg in 1 ml is available.

ERGOTAMINE TABLETS, B.P. Unless otherwise specified, tablets each containing 1 mg of ergotamine tartrate are supplied. They are sugar coated.

OTHER NAMES: *Femergin®*; *Gynergen®*; *Lingraine®*

ERYTHROMYCIN

SYNONYM: Erythromycinum

$C_{37}H_{67}NO_{13} = 733·9$

Erythromycin is an antimicrobial substance produced by the growth of certain strains of *Streptomyces erythreus* Waksman.

Solubility. Soluble, at 20°, in 1000 parts of water; less soluble in hot water; soluble, at 20°, in 5 parts of alcohol and of ether and 6 parts of chloroform; soluble in dilute hydrochloric acid.

Standard
It complies with the requirements of the European Pharmacopoeia.
It occurs as slightly hygroscopic, odourless, white or slightly yellow crystals or powder and contains not less than 920 Units per mg, calculated with reference to the anhydrous substance. It contains not more than 6·5 per cent w/w of water. A saturated solution in water has a pH of 8·0 to 10·5.

Storage. It should be stored in airtight containers, protected from light, at a temperature below 30°.

Actions and uses. Erythromycin is an antibiotic which is bacteriostatic under the conditions of clinical use and is effective in the treatment of infections due to a wide range of organisms. It acts by interfering with ribosomal protein synthesis within the bacterial cell.
When given by mouth it enters all tissues of the body except the meningeal space and has a biological half-life of about four hours; it is excreted in the bile and by glomerular filtration, but more than half is metabolised in the body so that it does not accumulate very rapidly in renal failure.
Erythromycin is used mainly in the treatment of infections of patients allergic to penicillin and of infections caused by penicillinase-producing staphylococci, but it is also effective against infections due to many strains of leptospirae, of entamoebae, and of *Diplococcus pneumoniae, Streptococcus pyogenes, Streptococcus viridans, Haemophilus influenzae,* and *Bordetella pertussis.*
Its chief disadvantage is the ready induction within the bacterial cell of an alternative enzyme system which renders the drug ineffective and also produces resistance to other macrolide antibiotics and to lincomycin, leading to cross-resistance and interference, especially when these drugs are used in combination. It may also give rise to the dissemination of resistant strains in the community. Erythromycin should therefore be used only when other antibiotics cannot be used and when it has been established that the infecting organism is sensitive to its action.
As erythromycin is partially destroyed by acid

gastric juice it is administered in enteric-coated tablets. Some erythromycin compounds are better absorbed than the base when given by mouth.

UNDESIRABLE EFFECTS. Abdominal discomfort or pain and allergic drug eruptions may rarely occur.

OTHER NAMES: *Erycen®*; *Erythromid®*; *Ilotycin®*

Dose. 1 to 2 grams daily in divided doses.

Preparation
ERYTHROMYCIN TABLETS, B.P. Unless otherwise specified, tablets each containing 250 mg of erythromycin are supplied. They are enteric coated and either film coated or sugar coated. They should be stored in airtight containers. Tablets containing 100 mg are also available.

ERYTHROMYCIN ESTOLATE

$C_{40}H_{71}NO_{14},C_{12}H_{26}O_4S = 1056\cdot4$

Erythromycin Estolate is the lauryl sulphate salt of the propionyl ester of erythromycin.

Solubility. Very slightly soluble in water; soluble, at 20°, in 2 parts of alcohol; soluble in chloroform; insoluble in dilute hydrochloric acid.

Standard
It complies with the requirements of the British Pharmacopoeia.
It is a white, crystalline, odourless powder and contains not less than 610 Units per mg and 22·0 to 25·5 per cent of $C_{12}H_{26}O_4S$, both calculated with reference to the anhydrous substance. It contains not more than 4·0 per cent w/w of water. It has a melting-point of 135° to 138°.

Storage. It should be stored in airtight containers, protected from light.

Actions and uses. Erythromycin estolate has the antibacterial actions described under Erythromycin. When given by mouth, it is rapidly absorbed and, after therapeutic doses, the concentration of erythromycin in the blood is higher and a therapeutic level is maintained for a longer period than after equivalent doses of erythromycin; 144 milligrams of erythromycin estolate is approxi-

mately equivalent to 100 milligrams of erythromycin.
It is used for the treatment of pneumococcal, streptococcal, and staphylococcal infections in children.

UNDESIRABLE EFFECTS. Cholestatic jaundice may rarely occur, particularly when treatment has been continued for more than ten days.

CONTRA-INDICATIONS. It is contra-indicated in patients who develop jaundice in the course of treatment with this drug, even after the jaundice has subsided.

Dose. The equivalent of 1 to 2 grams of erythromycin daily in divided doses for not more than ten days.

Preparation
ERYTHROMYCIN ESTOLATE CAPSULES, B.P. Unless otherwise specified, capsules each containing the equivalent of 250 mg of erythromycin are supplied. Capsules containing 125 mg are also available.

OTHER NAME: *Ilosone®*

ERYTHROMYCIN STEARATE

Erythromycin Stearate is the stearate of erythromycin($C_{37}H_{67}NO_{13},C_{18}H_{36}O_2 = 1018\cdot4$), with stearic acid and sodium stearate.

Solubility. Very slightly soluble in water and in acetone; partly soluble in alcohol, in chloroform, in isopropyl alcohol, and in methyl alcohol.

Standard
It complies with the requirements of the British Pharmacopoeia.
It occurs as almost odourless, colourless or slightly yellow crystals or a white or slightly yellow powder and contains not less than 550 Units per mg, calculated with reference to the anhydrous substance. It contains not more than 4·0 per cent w/w of water, 5·0 to 18·5 per cent of free stearic acid, and not more than 6·0 per cent of sodium stearate.

Storage. It should be stored in airtight containers, protected from light.

Actions and uses. Erythromycin stearate has the actions, uses, and undesirable effects described under Erythromycin, but it is less bitter; 138 milligrams of erythromycin stearate is approximately equivalent to 100 milligrams of erythromycin.

Dose. The equivalent of 1 to 2 grams of erythromycin daily in divided doses.

Preparations
ERYTHROMYCIN MIXTURE, B.P.C. (page 741)
ERYTHROMYCIN STEARATE TABLETS, B.P. Unless otherwise specified, tablets each containing the equivalent of 250 mg of erythromycin are supplied. Tablets containing 100 mg are also available.

OTHER NAME: *Erythrocin®*

ETHACRYNIC ACID

$C_{13}H_{12}Cl_2O_4 = 303 \cdot 1$

Ethacrynic Acid is 2,3-dichloro-4-(2-ethylacryloyl)phenoxyacetic acid.

CAUTION. *Ethacrynic acid, especially in the form of dust, is irritating to the skin, eyes, and mucous membranes.*

Solubility. Very slightly soluble in water; soluble, at 20°, in 1·6 parts of alcohol, in 3·5 parts of ether, and in 6 parts of chloroform.

Standard
It complies with the requirements of the British Pharmacopoeia.
It is a white or almost white, crystalline, odourless or almost odourless powder and contains not less than 98·0 and not more than the equivalent of 102·0 per cent of $C_{13}H_{12}Cl_2O_4$, calculated with reference to the dried substance. The loss on drying under the prescribed conditions is not more than 0·5 per cent. It has a melting-point of 121° to 125°.

Actions and uses. Ethacrynic acid is a diuretic which acts by reducing resorption of sodium and chloride in the proximal renal tubule, in the ascending loop of Henle and, to a lesser extent, in the distal renal tubules; distal tubular potassium secretion is also increased to a variable degree. Urinary pH is decreased, bicarbonate excretion is diminished, ammonium excretion is increased, and serum uric acid levels may be increased. The intense initial enhancement of sodium and chloride excretion may diminish on prolonged use, but potassium and hydrogen-ion losses may be increased.
Ethacrynic acid is rapidly absorbed when given by mouth and produces an intense diuresis commencing in about thirty minutes and reaching a maximum in about two hours. The usual dosage is 50 to 200 milligrams daily in divided doses, and a daily dosage of 400 milligrams should not be exceeded. Ethacrynic acid should preferably be given with food. It is of value for the treatment of oedema and for fluid retention.
In the form of its sodium salt, ethacrynic acid may be given by intravenous injection, when it produces a rapid and intense natriuresis and diuresis; doses equivalent to 50 to 100 milligrams of ethacrynic acid may be used in the treatment of pulmonary oedema.
When a blood transfusion is administered to a chronically anaemic patient who cannot be treated by more conservative means, a dose equivalent to 12·5 to 50 milligrams of ethacrynic acid may be given separately to prevent pulmonary oedema.

UNDESIRABLE EFFECTS. Anorexia, nausea, vomiting, diarrhoea, dysphagia, headache, blurred vision, confusion, transient loss of hearing, and rashes may occur. Prolonged use may give rise to a hypochloraemic alkalosis and electrolyte imbalance; hypokalaemia may occur. Ethacrynic acid may cause hypoglycaemia and increase the blood level of urea nitrogen. Its use may occasionally precipitate an acute attack of gout, or more rarely thrombocytopenia.

PRECAUTIONS. During prolonged treatment, potassium supplements should be given, the usual amount required being about 40 to 80 millimoles, or 3 to 6 grams, of potassium chloride daily in divided doses. As ethacrynic acid may cause hypoglycaemia, its use in diabetic patients should be carefully controlled.

Dose. See above under **Actions and uses.**

Preparation
ETHACRYNIC ACID TABLETS, B.P. Unless otherwise specified, tablets each containing 50 mg of ethacrynic acid are supplied.

OTHER NAME: *Edecrin®*

ETHAMBUTOL HYDROCHLORIDE

$C_{10}H_{26}Cl_2N_2O_2 = 277 \cdot 2$

$$\left[\begin{array}{c} CH_3 \cdot CH_2 \cdot CH \cdot NH \cdot [CH_2]_2 \cdot NH \cdot CH \cdot CH_2 \cdot CH_3 \\ | \qquad\qquad\qquad\qquad\qquad | \\ CH_2OH \qquad\qquad\qquad\qquad CH_2OH \end{array} \right] 2HCl$$

Ethambutol Hydrochloride is (+)-*NN'*-di(1-hydroxymethylpropyl)ethylenediamine dihydrochloride.

Solubility. Soluble, at 20°, in 1 part of water, in 30 parts of alcohol, in 850 parts of chloroform, and in 9 parts of methyl alcohol; very slightly soluble in ether.

Standard
It complies with the requirements of the British Pharmacopoeia.
It is a white, crystalline, odourless or almost odourless powder and contains not less than 98·0 per cent of $C_{10}H_{26}Cl_2N_2O_2$, calculated with reference to the dried substance. The loss on drying under the prescribed conditions is not more than 0·5 per cent. It has a melting-point of 199° to 204°.

Actions and uses. Ethambutol is used in the treatment of mycobacterial infections, particularly tuberculosis. Peak tissue levels are achieved two to four hours after administration by mouth and excretion, which is mainly through the kidney, is complete within twenty-four hours in patients with normal renal function.
It is active against some strains of *Mycobacterium tuberculosis* that are resistant to other

drugs and cross-resistance between ethambutol and other drugs does not occur. It should always be given simultaneously with other tuberculostatic agents to delay the development of resistence.

UNDESIRABLE EFFECTS. A serious toxic effect is the insidious onset of visual loss which may be manifested as a restriction of the visual field or as a loss of colour discrimination. This effect may occur on the prolonged administration of doses of 25 milligrams per kilogram body-weight and is associated with progressive depletion of copper and zinc; it may be reversible if treatment with ethambutol is stopped promptly, and in some cases treatment may be resumed at a lower dose level.

Allergic rashes and gastro-intestinal disturbances may rarely occur.

PRECAUTIONS AND CONTRA-INDICATIONS. Dosage should be appropriately reduced in patients with impaired renal function and serum levels should not be allowed to exceed 5 micrograms per millilitre. The eyes should be examined periodically and treatment should be terminated if visual defects appear.

Dose. 25 milligrams per kilogram body-weight daily for two months, followed by 15 milligrams per kilogram body-weight daily.

Preparation
ETHAMBUTOL TABLETS, B.P. Unless otherwise specified, tablets each containing 400 mg of ethambutol hydrochloride are supplied.

OTHER NAME: *Myambutol*®

ETHAMIVAN

$C_{12}H_{17}NO_3 = 223.3$

Ethamivan is *NN*-diethylvanillamide.

Solubility. Soluble, at 20°, in 100 parts of water, in 2 parts of alcohol, in 50 parts of ether, in 1·5 parts of chloroform, and in 3 parts of acetone.

Standard
DESCRIPTION. A white crystalline powder; odourless, or almost odourless.

IDENTIFICATION TESTS. 1. Boil 0·5 g with 1 ml of *sulphuric acid (25 per cent v/v)*, cool, make alkaline with *sodium hydroxide solution*, and heat; an amine-like odour is produced.
2. Dissolve 5 mg in 1 ml of *alcohol (95 per cent)*, add 3 ml of water and 1 ml of *ferric chloride solution*; a blue colour is produced.
3. It complies with the thin-layer chromatographic test given in Appendix 5A, page 863.
4. The ultraviolet absorption spectrum exhibits the characteristics given in Appendix 3, page 855.
5. The infra-red absorption spectrum exhibits maxima which are only at the same wavelengths as, and have similar relative intensities to, those in the spectrum of *ethamivan A.S.*

ACIDITY. pH of a 1·0 per cent w/v solution in *carbon dioxide-free water*, 5·5 to 7·0.

MELTING-POINT. 96° to 99°.

RELATED COMPOUNDS. It complies with the test given in Appendix 5A, page 863.

LOSS ON DRYING. Not more than 1·0 per cent, determined by drying to constant weight over *phosphorus pentoxide* in vacuo.

SULPHATED ASH. Not more than 0·1 per cent.

CONTENT OF $C_{12}H_{17}NO_3$. Not less than 99·0 per cent, calculated with reference to the substance dried under the prescribed conditions, determined by the following method:
Dissolve about 0·2 g, accurately weighed, in 20 ml of *dimethylformamide*, and titrate with 0·1N sodium methoxide, under an atmosphere of *nitrogen* using 0·2 ml of *azo violet solution* as indicator; each ml of 0·1N sodium methoxide is equivalent to 0·02233 g of $C_{12}H_{17}NO_3$.

Actions and uses. Ethamivan is a respiratory stimulant. It increases the rate and depth of respiration by central stimulation through the respiratory centre and produces slight peripheral vasoconstriction through its action on the vasomotor centre. Its stimulant action is short and for this reason direct intravenous injection must be followed by a continuous intravenous infusion in patients with severe respiratory depression.

Ethamivan acts as an analeptic and it has been used to counteract the action of central nervous system depressants such as barbiturates. It is more effective for this purpose than leptazol or nikethamide.

In the treatment of barbiturate poisoning the dose is between 5 and 10 milligrams per kilogram body-weight given by slow intravenous injection of a 5 per cent solution, followed by continuous intravenous infusion of a 0·6 per cent solution in Sodium Chloride Injection.

In the treatment of respiratory distress of the newborn, 0·1 millilitre of a 5 per cent solution diluted to 1 millilitre with Sodium Chloride Injection should be injected into the umbilical vein, or 0·25 millilitre of Ethamivan Elixir may be given by mouth to premature infants, and 0·5 millilitre to full-term infants.

UNDESIRABLE EFFECTS. These are likely to occur only when excessively large doses have been given; they include restlessness, sneezing, muscular twitching, laryngospasm, and convulsions.

PRECAUTIONS AND CONTRA-INDICATIONS. Ethamivan should not be given to epileptic patients or to those with respiratory failure caused by a convulsant drug. It should not be given to patients who are being treated with a monoamine-oxidase inhibitor such as isocarboxazid, nialamide, phenelzine, or tranylcypromine, or within about ten days of the discontinuation of such treatment.

Dose. See above under **Actions and uses.**

Preparation
ETHAMIVAN ELIXIR, B.P.C. (page 671)

OTHER NAME: *Vandid®*

ETHANOLAMINE

SYNONYM: Monoethanolamine

C_2H_7NO = 61·08

$NH_2 \cdot CH_2 \cdot CH_2OH$

Ethanolamine is 2-aminoethanol.

Solubility. Miscible with water and with alcohol; slightly soluble in ether and in light petroleum.

Standard
DESCRIPTION. A clear colourless or pale yellow liquid; odour slight.

IDENTIFICATION TESTS. 1. It is alkaline to *litmus solution*.
2. To 0·1 ml add 0·3 g of *trinitrophenol* and 1 ml of water and evaporate to dryness on a water-bath; the residue, after crystallising from *alcohol (95 per cent)* and drying at 105°, melts at about 160°.
3. When freshly distilled and the first half of the distillate rejected, it freezes at about 10°.

REFRACTIVE INDEX. At 20°, 1·453 to 1·459.

WEIGHT PER ML. At 20°, 1·014 g to 1·023 g.

CONTENT OF C_2H_7NO. Not less than 98·0 per cent w/w, determined by the following method:
Dissolve about 2·5 g, accurately weighed, in 50 ml of 1N hydrochloric acid, and titrate the excess of acid with 1N sodium hydroxide, using *methyl red solution* as indicator; each ml of 1N hydrochloric acid is equivalent to 0·06108 g of C_2H_7NO.

Sterilisation. Solutions for injection are sterilised by heating in an autoclave; no bactericide need be added.

Actions and uses. Ethanolamine, combined with oleic acid, is given by intravenous injection as a sclerosing agent in the treatment of varicose veins. If it escapes into the perivenous tissues during injection it causes less sloughing than some other sclerosants and allergic reactions rarely follow its use.
Ethanolamine is administered as the injection, the dose of 2 to 5 millilitres being divided into three or four portions, which are injected at different sites. The treatment is usually given at intervals of about a week until the varices have been completely occluded.

CONTRA-INDICATIONS. It is contra-indicated where there is thrombosis of the deep veins of the leg or acute phlebitis.

Preparation
ETHANOLAMINE OLEATE INJECTION, B.P.C. (page 713)

ETHCHLORVYNOL

C_7H_9ClO = 144·6

$CH:C \cdot C(OH)(C_2H_5) \cdot CH:CHCl$

Ethchlorvynol is 1-chloro-3-ethylpent-1-en-4-yn-3-ol.

Solubility. Insoluble in water; miscible with alcohol, with ether, with chloroform, and with acetone.

Standard
It complies with the requirements of the British Pharmacopoeia.
It is a colourless to yellow liquid with a characteristic and pungent odour and contains not less than 97·5 per cent of C_7H_9ClO. It has a weight per ml at 20° of 1·070 g to 1·074 g. It contains not more than 0·2 per cent w/w of water.

Storage. It should be stored in airtight containers, protected from light. It should not be allowed to come into contact with metal.

Actions and uses. Ethchlorvynol has a hypnotic action resembling that of an intermediate-acting barbiturate, the actions and uses of which are described under Phenobarbitone (page 366). Sleep lasting for four to six hours is produced within about twenty minutes by oral doses of 0·25 to 1 gram. As a sedative, a dose of 100 to 250 milligrams may be given twice daily.

UNDESIRABLE EFFECTS. Dizziness, nausea, and vomiting may occur.
Ethchlorvynol may give rise to dependence of the barbiturate-alcohol type as described under Phenobarbitone (page 366). Exaggerated reactions may occur if it is taken with alcohol.

PRECAUTIONS. These are as described under Phenobarbitone (page 366).

Dose. 0·1 to 1 gram.

Preparation
ETHCHLORVYNOL CAPSULES, B.P. Unless otherwise specified, capsules each containing 500 mg of ethchlorvynol are supplied. They should be protected from light. Capsules containing 250 mg are also available.

OTHER NAMES: *Arvynol®*; *Serenesil®*

ANAESTHETIC ETHER

Synonym: Ether $C_2H_5 \cdot O \cdot C_2H_5$

$C_4H_{10}O = 74 \cdot 12$

Anaesthetic Ether is purified diethyl ether containing not more than 0·002 per cent w/v of a suitable stabiliser to retard the formation of ether peroxides. Among the substances used as stabilisers are propyl gallate and hydroquinone.

Caution. *Anaesthetic Ether is highly inflammable and mixtures of its vapour with oxygen or air at certain concentrations are explosive; it should not be used in the presence of a naked flame or of any electrical apparatus liable to produce a spark. Precautions should be taken against the production of static electrical discharge.*

Solubility. Soluble, at 20°, in 10 parts of water; miscible with alcohol, with chloroform, and with fixed and volatile oils.

Standard
It complies with the requirements of the British Pharmacopoeia.
It is a clear, colourless, very mobile liquid with a characteristic odour. It has a weight per ml at 20° of 0·7130 g to 0·7145 g and distils completely between 34·0° and 35·0°; explosive peroxides are generated by atmospheric oxidation and it is dangerous to distil a sample which contains peroxides.
It has a flash-point of about −20 F (closed-cup test).

Storage. It should be stored in dry airtight containers, protected from light, in a cool place. If the container is closed by a cork, this should be protected with metal foil.

Actions and uses. Anaesthetic ether is a volatile anaesthetic. It is much less depressant to the medullary centres than chloroform and causes less fall in blood pressure and less depression of respiration.
Ether does not lead to ventricular fibrillation in the induction stage, nor does prolonged ether anaesthesia produce a direct toxic action on the heart. It causes peripheral vasodilatation, especially of skin vessels, and this is a cause of the increased capillary oozing that may occur when ether is used. The white-cell count may rise 300 per cent after ether anaesthesia.
Although ether produces slight transient toxic effects on the liver and kidneys, it does not give rise to severe delayed poisoning and it has a wide margin of safety.
The chief disadvantage of ether as an anaesthetic is its irritant action on the mucous membrane of the respiratory tract; it stimulates the secretion of saliva and mucus from the bronchial tree. Frequently, atropine, or hyoscine, and morphine are given about one hour before the induction of anaesthesia; the atropine or hyoscine inhibits the bronchial secretion, thus reducing the risk of inhalation pneumonia, while the morphine reduces the amount of anaesthetic required.
Laryngeal spasm is an occasional complication of ether anaesthesia. Prolonged contact with ether spilt on any tissue produces necrosis.
The concentration of ether in the inspired air necessary to produce anaesthesia is normally from 6 to 7 per cent by volume, although it may be desirable to exceed this concentration, especially during induction. It is administered on an open mask or by semi-closed or closed methods. When ether is used alone in this way it requires a long time for the induction of anaesthesia, thus prolonging the stage of excitement. To reduce or obviate this, it is current practice to premedicate the patient and to employ mixtures of ether with other anaesthetics, such as nitrous oxide.

Poisoning. In the event of poisoning by ether, resulting in collapse, the procedure described under Chloroform (page 100) should be adopted. Convulsions, which are frequently fatal, occasionally occur in patients under deep ether anaesthesia, especially under hot or humid conditions, but their occurrence does not seem to be related to the presence, as impurities, of peroxides or aldehydes. The evidence seems rather to support the view that patients so affected have a predisposition to convulsions.
If ether convulsions occur, oxygen and carbon dioxide may be administered to prevent respiratory failure, and a solution of a soluble barbiturate may be given by intravenous injection.

Preparation
Ether Spirit, B.P.C. (page 793)

SOLVENT ETHER

$C_4H_{10}O = 74·12$ $C_2H_5·O·C_2H_5$

Solvent Ether is diethyl ether.

CAUTION. *Solvent Ether is highly inflammable and mixtures of its vapour with oxygen or air at certain concentrations are explosive; it should not be used in the presence of a naked flame or of any electrical apparatus liable to produce a spark. Precautions should be taken against the production of static electrical discharge.*

Solubility. Soluble, at 20°, in 10 parts of water; miscible with alcohol, with chloroform, and with fixed and volatile oils.

Standard
It complies with the requirements of the British Pharmacopoeia.
It is a clear, colourless, very mobile liquid with a characteristic odour. It has a weight per ml at 20° of 0·714 g to 0·718 g and distils completely between 34° and 36°; explosive peroxides are generated by atmospheric oxidation and it is dangerous to distil a sample which contains peroxides.
It has a flash-point of about −20°F (closed-cup test).

Storage. It should be stored in airtight containers,

protected from light, in a cool place. If the container is closed by a cork, this should be protected with metal foil.

Uses. Solvent ether is used as a solvent for oils, resins, and many other substances. It is also used, with suitable precautions against the risk of fire, for cleaning the skin before surgical operations, either alone or as Ethereal Soap Solution, and for removing adhesive plaster from the skin.

Preparation
SOAP SOLUTION, ETHEREAL, B.P.C. (page 789)

ETHINYLOESTRADIOL

SYNONYMS: Aethinyloestradiolum; Ethinyloestr.

$C_{20}H_{24}O_2 = 296·4$

Ethinyloestradiol is 19-nor-17α-pregna-1,3,5(10)-trien-20-yne-3,17-diol.

CAUTION. *Ethinyloestradiol is a powerful oestrogen. Contact with the skin or inhalation of the dust should be avoided. Rubber gloves should be worn when handling the powder and, if the powder is dry, a face mask should also be worn.*

Solubility. Very slightly soluble in water; soluble, at 20°, in 6 parts of alcohol, in 4 parts of ether, in 20 parts of chloroform, in 5 parts of acetone, and in 4 parts dioxan; soluble in solutions of alkali hydroxides.

Standard
It complies with the requirements of the European Pharmacopoeia.
It is a white or at most slightly yellowish-white, crystalline, odourless powder and contains not less than 97·0 and not more than the equivalent of 102·0 per cent of $C_{20}H_{24}O_2$, calculated with reference to the dried substance. The loss on drying under the prescribed conditions is not more than 1·0 per cent. It has a melting-point of 181° to 185°, but it may also occur in a form which melts between 141° and 146° due to polymorphism.

Storage. It should be stored in airtight containers, protected from light, in a cool place.

Actions and uses. Ethinyloestradiol has the actions and uses of the oestrogens, as described under Oestradiol Benzoate (page 335).
In the treatment of menopausal symptoms, an initial dosage of 10 to 50 micrograms is given by mouth three times a day; for maintenance, 10 micrograms once or twice a day may be sufficient.
For the treatment of primary amenorrhoea, 10 to 50 micrograms is given three times a day for two consecutive weeks in every four. Functional uterine bleeding is treated with

500 micrograms once or twice a day, or smaller doses more frequently, until the bleeding is controlled. The dosage is then reduced to 50 micrograms once to three times a day for twenty days; 5 milligrams of progesterone is sometimes given daily for the last five days.
For the inhibition of lactation, 100 micrograms is given three times a day for three days, and then 50 micrograms twice daily for two days and once daily for three more days.
For the palliative treatment of carcinoma of the prostate and of the breast, 1 to 2 milligrams is given daily, the dosage in the former condition being controlled by periodic estimations of the serum acid phosphatase.

UNDESIRABLE EFFECTS. In addition to the undesirable effects described under Oestradiol Benzoate (page 335), headache, dizziness, nausea, and vomiting may occur.

Dose. See above under **Actions and uses.**

Preparation
ETHINYLOESTRADIOL TABLETS, B.P. Unless otherwise specified, tablets each containing 20 μg of ethinyloestradiol are supplied. They should be protected from light. Tablets containing 10, 50, and 100 μg and 1 mg are also available.

OTHER NAMES: *Lynoral®; Primogyn C®*

ETHIONAMIDE

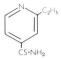

$C_8H_{10}N_2S = 166\cdot2$

Ethionamide is 2-ethylpyridine-4-carbothionamide.

Solubility. Insoluble in water; soluble, at 20°, in 30 parts of alcohol, in 600 parts of ether, and in 350 parts of chloroform.

Standard
It complies with the requirements of the British Pharmacopoeia.
It is a bright yellow crystalline powder with a slight odour and contains not less than 98·5 per cent of $C_8H_{10}N_2S$, calculated with reference to the dried substance. The loss on drying under the prescribed conditions is not more than 1·0 per cent. It has a melting-point of 161° to 165°. It darkens on exposure to light.

Storage. It should be protected from light.

Actions and uses. Ethionamide is a tuberculostatic agent with uses similar to those of sodium aminosalicylate. It is active against some strains of *Mycobacterium tuberculosis* that are resistant to other tuberculostatic drugs, although there may be cross-resistance between ethionamide and the thiosemicarbazones.
Originally sensitive strains of *M. tuberculosis* rapidly become resistant to ethionamide if it is used alone in the treatment of tuberculosis. The simultaneous administration of other tuberculostatic agents such as isoniazid, pyrazinamide, and streptomycin delays the development of resistance.
In the treatment of pulmonary and extra-pulmonary tuberculosis, the usual dosage of ethionamide by mouth is 750 to 1000 milligrams daily in divided doses, but 500 milligrams may be sufficient for some patients.

Ethionamide is broken down rapidly in the body; it has a therapeutic half-life of less than five hours and less than 1 per cent of the dose is excreted unchanged in the urine.

UNDESIRABLE EFFECTS. Disturbances of the alimentary tract, including a metallic taste, stomatitis, excessive salivation, nausea, vomiting, and diarrhoea, may occur in patients receiving more than 500 milligrams daily.
Liver damage, hypotension, convulsions, peripheral neuropathy, alopecia, gynaecomastia, impotence, menstrual disturbances, drowsiness, slight deafness, diplopia, headache, insomnia, and skin rashes have been reported. The administration of ethionamide to patients with diabetes mellitus may cause difficulty in controlling the diabetes. When it is given concurrently with other tuberculostatic drugs it may intensify their adverse effects.

CONTRA-INDICATIONS. It should not be given in early pregnancy as it may give rise to foetal malformations.

Dose. See above under **Actions and uses.**

Preparation
ETHIONAMIDE TABLETS, B.P. Unless otherwise specified, tablets each containing 125 mg of ethionamide are supplied. They may be sugar coated.

OTHER NAME: *Trescatyl*®

ETHISTERONE

SYNONYM: Ethinyltestosterone

$C_{21}H_{28}O_2 = 312\cdot5$

Ethisterone is 17-hydroxy-17α-pregn-4-en-20-yn-3-one.

Solubility. Insoluble in water; soluble, at 20°, in 1000 parts of alcohol, in 110 parts of chloroform, in 750 parts of acetone, and in 35 parts of pyridine; very slightly soluble in vegetable oils.

Standard
It complies with the requirements of the British Pharmacopoeia.
It is a white or almost white, crystalline, odourless powder and contains not less than 97·0 and not more than the equivalent of 102·0 per cent of $C_{21}H_{28}O_2$, calculated with reference to the dried substance. The loss on drying under the prescribed conditions is not more than 1·0 per cent. It has a melting-point of 272° to 276°.

Storage. It should be stored in airtight containers, protected from light.

Actions and uses. Ethisterone has the actions and uses described under Progesterone (page 407). It is effective when given by mouth, preferably sublingually; the dose is five to ten times the intramuscular dose of progesterone.

Dose. 25 to 100 milligrams daily in single or divided doses.

Preparation
ETHISTERONE TABLETS, B.P. (*Syn.* Ethinyltestosterone Tablets). Unless otherwise specified, tablets each containing 25 mg of ethisterone are supplied. They should be protected from light. Tablets containing 5 and 10 mg are also available.

OTHER NAMES: Anhydrohydroxyprogesterone; *Gestone-Oral*®; Pregneninolone

ETHOPROPAZINE HYDROCHLORIDE

$C_{19}H_{25}ClN_2S = 348.9$

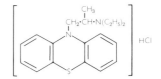

Ethopropazine Hydrochloride is 10-(2-diethylaminopropyl)-phenothiazine hydrochloride.

Solubility. Soluble, at 20°, in 225 parts of water, in 35 parts of alcohol, and in 7 parts of chloroform; insoluble in ether.

Standard
It complies with the requirements of the British Pharmacopoeia.
It is a white or slightly cream-coloured, crystalline, almost odourless powder and contains not less than 99·0 and not more than the equivalent of 101·0 per cent of $C_{19}H_{25}ClN_2S$, calculated with reference to the dried substance. The loss on drying under the prescribed conditions is not more than 0·5 per cent.

Stability. It darkens on exposure to light.

Storage. It should be stored in airtight containers, protected from light.

Actions and uses. Ethopropazine blocks both the nicotinic and muscarinic actions of acetylcholine and, to a lesser extent, antagonises the actions of histamine and adrenaline.
Ethopropazine is used for the symptomatic treatment of parkinsonism, but is less effective for this purpose than benzhexol and gives rise to undesirable effects more frequently. In most types of parkinsonism, it reduces the rigidity more than the tremor and increases the mobility of the patient; the frequency and duration of oculogyric crises are also diminished.

Treatment is usually begun with a dosage of 50 to 100 milligrams of ethopropazine hydrochloride by mouth daily in four to six divided doses. The daily dosage is then increased by 50 to 100 milligrams every few days until the optimum effect is obtained; this may require 0·5 to 1 gram daily.

Ethopropazine is sometimes given in conjunction with solanaceous alkaloids or other drugs used for the relief of parkinsonism.

UNDESIRABLE EFFECTS. Drowsiness, ataxia, giddiness, blurred vision, confusion, nausea, and vomiting may occur; these effects usually disappear when the dosage is reduced.

Dose. See above under **Actions and uses.**

Preparation
ETHOPROPAZINE TABLETS, B.P. Unless otherwise specified, tablets each containing 50 mg of ethopropazine hydrochloride are supplied. They are sugar coated.

OTHER NAMES: *Lysivane®*; Profenamine Hydrochloride

ETHOSUXIMIDE

$C_7H_{11}NO_2 = 141.2$

Ethosuximide is α-ethyl-α-methylsuccinimide.

Solubility. Soluble, at 20°, in 4·5 parts of water and in less than 1 part of alcohol, of ether, and of chloroform.

Standard
It complies with the requirements of the British Pharmacopoeia.
It is a white or almost white, odourless or almost odourless powder or waxy solid and contains not less than 98·5 per cent of $C_7H_{11}NO_2$, calculated with reference to the anhydrous substance. It contains not more than 0·5 per cent w/w of water. It has a melting-point of about 46°.

Actions and uses. Ethosuximide is an anti-convulsant used in the treatment of petit mal. Pure petit mal responds better than mixed petit mal.
Ethosuximide may be administered in combination with other anticonvulsants, such as phenobarbitone, phenytoin sodium, or primidone, to treat petit mal when it co-exists with grand mal or other forms of epilepsy. Occasionally, the use of this combined treatment may increase the frequency of the grand mal attacks in these cases and the medication used for controlling the major seizures may require adjustment. Patients with petit mal who have proved to be resistant to other anticonvulsants have been treated successfully with ethosuximide.

The initial dosage for patients under six years of age is 250 milligrams daily and, for patients six years of age and over, 500 milligrams daily in divided doses. Dosage thereafter should be adjusted by small increments, according to the response of the patient, to a maximum of 1 gram for a child of six years and of 2 grams for an adult, daily in divided doses.

UNDESIRABLE EFFECTS. Mild reactions, which are usually transient, may occur initially; these include drowsiness, headache, and gastric upset. Occasionally, skin rashes have occurred.
Haematological reactions, including leucopenia, agranulocytosis, and aplastic anaemia, have sometimes occurred with ethosuximide

therapy. Administration to patients with temporal lobe seizures may precipitate an acute psychosis.

Dose. See above under **Actions and uses.**

OTHER NAMES: *Capitus*®; *Emeside*®; *Zarontin*®

Preparations

ETHOSUXIMIDE CAPSULES, B.P. Unless otherwise specified, capsules each containing 250 mg of ethosuximide are supplied.

ETHOSUXIMIDE ELIXIR, B.P.C. (page 672)

ETHOTOIN

$C_{11}H_{12}N_2O_2 = 204·2$

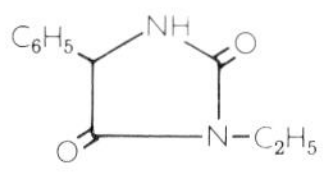

Ethotoin is 3-ethyl-5-phenylhydantoin.

Solubility. Insoluble in water; soluble, at $20°$, in 4 parts of dehydrated alcohol, in 25 parts of ether, and in 1·5 parts of chloroform.

Standard

It complies with the requirements of the British Pharmacopoeia.

It is a white, crystalline, almost odourless powder and contains not less than 98·0 per cent of $C_{11}H_{12}N_2O_2$, calculated with reference to the anhydrous substance. It contains not more than 1·0 per cent w/w of water. It has a melting-point of about $90°$.

Actions and uses. Ethotoin has an anticonvulsant action resembling that described under Phenytoin Sodium (page 378) but it is much less effective and is less liable to produce undesirable effects.

Ethotoin is usually given in conjunction with other anticonvulsant drugs, such as phenobarbitone and phenytoin, in the treatment of

grand mal epilepsy. The initial dosage for an adult is 1 gram by mouth daily, gradually increased to 2 or 3 grams daily while the dosage of the other anticonvulsant drug given at the same time is gradually reduced. The initial daily dosage for a child is 500 milligrams, which may be gradually increased to 2 grams.

UNDESIRABLE EFFECTS. Ethotoin seldom produces visual disturbances or hyperplasia of the gums, but occasionally skin rashes, nausea, vomiting, dizziness, headache, and drowsiness may occur.

Dose. See above under **Actions and uses.**

Preparation

ETHOTOIN TABLETS, B.P. Unless otherwise specified, tablets each containing 500 mg of ethotoin are supplied.

OTHER NAME: *Peganone*®

ETHYL CHLORIDE

$C_2H_5Cl = 64·51$

Ethyl Chloride is chloroethane and may be prepared by the action of hydrogen chloride on ethyl alcohol or on Industrial Methylated Spirit; in the latter case it contains a small variable proportion of methyl chloride.

Solubility. Slightly soluble in water; miscible with alcohol and with ether.

Standard

It complies with the requirements of the British Pharmacopoeia.

It is a gas at ordinary temperatures and pressures, but is liquefied by slight compression, forming a colourless, mobile, inflammable, very volatile liquid, in which form it is usually supplied. It has a pleasant ethereal odour.

Under normal pressure the liquid boils at about $12°$ and has a weight per ml at $0°$ of about 0·92 g. It has a flash-point of $-58°F$ (closed-cup test) and mixtures with 5 to 15 per cent of air are explosive.

Storage. It should be stored in a cool place, protected from light.

Actions and uses. Ethyl chloride is a volatile anaesthetic which was formerly used for the induction of general anaesthesia, but it has been largely superseded by safer agents.

Ethyl chloride has been used as a local anaesthetic, the intense cold produced by the rapid evaporation of the spray rendering the tissues insensitive by freezing, but this procedure is not recommended.

POISONING. In the event of poisoning, resulting in collapse, the procedure as described under Chloroform (page 100) should be adopted.

ETHYL OLEATE

$C_{20}H_{38}O_2 = 310.5$

$$CH_3 \cdot [CH_2]_7 \cdot CH : CH \cdot [CH_2]_7 \cdot CO \cdot O \cdot C_2H_5$$

Ethyl Oleate may be prepared by esterifying oleic acid with ethyl alcohol. It may contain a suitable antoxidant.

Solubility. Insoluble in water; miscible with alcohol, with ether, with chloroform, and with fixed oils.

Standard
It complies with the requirements of the British Pharmacopoeia.
It is a pale yellow, oily, almost odourless liquid and contains the equivalent of not less than 100·0 and not more than 105·0 per cent w/w of ethyl esters of oleic and related acids, calculated as $C_{20}H_{38}O_2$. It has a weight per ml at 20° of 0·869 g to 0·874 g.

Sterilisation. It is sterilised by dry heat.

Labelling. The label on the container states the name and proportion of any added antoxidant.

Storage. It should be stored in small, well-filled, airtight containers or in an atmosphere of nitrogen, protected from light.

Uses. Ethyl oleate has properties similar to those of certain fixed oils such as almond and arachis oils, except that it is less viscous, is a better solvent, and is more rapidly absorbed by the tissues. It is therefore sometimes used instead of fixed oils as a vehicle in injections.

ETHYLENEDIAMINE HYDRATE

$C_2H_8N_2, H_2O = 78.11$

$$NH_2 \cdot CH_2 \cdot CH_2 \cdot NH_2, H_2O$$

Ethylenediamine Hydrate may be prepared by treating 1,2-dichloroethane with ammonia.

Solubility. Miscible with water and with alcohol.

Standard
It complies with the requirements of the British Pharmacopoeia.
It is a clear, colourless or slightly yellow, strongly alkaline liquid with an ammoniacal odour and contains

not less than 97·5 and not more than the equivalent of 101·5 per cent w/w of $C_2H_8N_2, H_2O$.

Storage. It should be stored in airtight containers, protected from light.

Uses. Ethylenediamine hydrate is used in the preparation of Aminophylline Injection.

ETHYLMORPHINE HYDROCHLORIDE

SYNONYM: Ethylmorphini Hydrochloridum

$C_{19}H_{24}ClNO_3, 2H_2O = 385.9$

Ethylmorphine Hydrochloride is the dihydrate of the hydrochloride of the 3-ethyl ether of morphine.

Solubility. Soluble, at 20°, in 12 parts of water and in 25 parts of alcohol; soluble in 1 part of warm alcohol; very slightly soluble in ether and in chloroform.

Standard
DESCRIPTION. A white, minutely crystalline powder; odourless.

IDENTIFICATION TESTS. 1. Dissolve 5 mg in 5 ml of water and add 1 ml of *potassium iodobismuthate solution*; an orange or orange-red precipitate is produced.
2. To 0·01 g add 1 ml of *sulphuric acid* and 0·05 ml of *ferric chloride test-solution* and warm; a blue colour is produced. Add 0·05 ml of *nitric acid*; the colour changes to red.
3. Dissolve 0·6 g in 6 ml of water, add 15 ml of 0·1N sodium hydroxide, and induce crystallisation; a white crystalline precipitate is formed which, after washing with water, recrystallising from water, and drying in vacuo, melts at about 85°.
4. It gives the reactions characteristic of chlorides.

APPEARANCE OF SOLUTION. A 2·0 per cent w/v solution in water complies with the following tests:
(i) The solution is clear when compared with water, the comparison being made by viewing 2 ml of the liquids in matched, colourless, transparent, neutral glass tubes, 12 mm internal diameter, in darkness and with a beam of light being passed laterally through the liquids from an electric lamp giving a luminosity of 1000 lux at a distance of 1 m.

(ii) The solution is not more intensely coloured than a reference solution prepared by mixing 0·1 ml of *brownish-yellow standard solution* with 1·9 ml of *diluted hydrochloric acid (1 per cent w/v)*, the comparison being made by viewing horizontally 2 ml of the liquids in matched, colourless, transparent, neutral glass tubes, 12 mm internal diameter, against a white background in diffused daylight.

ACIDITY. pH of a 2·0 per cent w/v solution in *carbon dioxide-free water*, 4·0 to 5·4.

SPECIFIC ROTATION. $-102°$ to $-105°$, calculated with reference to the substance dried under the prescribed conditions, determined, at 20°, in a 2·0 per cent w/v solution in water.

MORPHINE. Dissolve 0·10 g in 5 ml of 0·1N hydrochloric acid, immediately add 2 ml of a 1 per cent w/v solution of *sodium nitrite* in water, allow to stand for 15 minutes, and add 3 ml of *dilute ammonia solution*; any yellow colour which develops is not more intense than that produced by 5 ml of a 0·0025 per cent w/v solution of *morphine hydrochloride* treated in the same manner (0·1 per cent).

READILY CARBONISABLE SUBSTANCES. Dissolve 0·05 g in 5 ml of *sulphuric acid* and allow to stand for 15 minutes; the solution is not more intensely coloured than a reference solution prepared by mixing 0·25 ml of *brown standard solution* with 1·75 ml of *diluted hydro-*

chloric acid (*1 per cent w/v*), the comparison being made as for test (ii) under Appearance of Solution.

LOSS ON DRYING. Not less than 8·0 and not more than 10·0 per cent, determined by drying 0·50 g to constant weight at 105°.

SULPHATED ASH. Not more than 0·1 per cent.

CONTENT OF $C_{19}H_{24}ClNO_3$. Not less than 99·0 per cent, calculated with reference to the substance dried under the prescribed conditions, determined by the following method:
Dissolve about 0·3 g, accurately weighed, in 30 ml of *glacial acetic acid*, add 20 ml of *acetic anhydride*, and titrate by Method I of the British Pharmacopoeia for non-aqueous titration; each ml of 0·1N perchloric acid is equivalent to 0·03499 g of $C_{19}H_{24}ClNO_3$.

Sterilisation. Solutions are sterilised by heating with a bactericide or by filtration.

Storage. It should be protected from light.

Actions and uses. Ethylmorphine has some of the actions of morphine and codeine but does not depress the respiratory centre to the same extent as morphine.

A 1 to 5 per cent solution of ethylmorphine hydrochloride has been used in ophthalmic practice in the treatment of corneal ulceration, iritis, and glaucoma; ethylmorphine increases the blood supply to the tissues and may provoke a sharp burning sensation and some oedema of the conjunctiva, but this soon subsides.

Ethylmorphine has also been used as an ingredient of linctuses to allay cough in bronchitis, bronchial asthma, and whooping-cough.

Dose. 6 to 30 milligrams.

ETHYNODIOL DIACETATE

$C_{24}H_{32}O_4 = 384·5$

Ethynodiol Diacetate is 3β,17-diacetoxy-19-nor-17α-pregn-4-en-20-yne.

Solubility. Very slightly soluble in water; soluble, at 20°, in 15 parts of alcohol, in 3·5 parts of ether, and in 1 part of chloroform.

Standard
It complies with the requirements of the British Pharmacopoeia.
It is a white or almost white, crystalline, odourless powder and contains not less than 97·0 and not more than the equivalent of 102·0 per cent of $C_{24}H_{32}O_4$, calculated with reference to the dried substance. The loss on drying under the prescribed conditions is not more than 0·5 per cent. It has a melting-point of 126° to 131°.

Storage. It should be stored in airtight containers, protected from light.

Actions and uses. Ethynodiol diacetate is a synthetic progestational steroid hormone which has an action similar to that of norethisterone (page 329). It is active when taken by mouth and is generally used in conjunction with oestrogens.

In the treatment of primary and secondary amenorrhoea and of functional uterine bleeding it is given daily in a dosage of 1 or 2 milligrams from the fifth day of the menstrual cycle and continuing until the twenty-fourth day; withdrawal bleeding usually occurs one to three days after discontinuing treatment.

For the treatment of endometriosis doses of 4 milligrams or more are given daily for periods of nine to twelve months.

Ethynodiol diacetate is used in conjunction with oestrogens as an oral contraceptive to inhibit ovulation. For this purpose doses of 0·5 to 2 milligrams are given daily, usually with ethinyloestradiol or mestranol, from the fifth to the twenty-fourth day of each menstrual cycle. The course is repeated after an interval of one week. Regular administration is essential.

Ethynodiol diacetate is available as tablets containing 500 micrograms together with ethinyloestradiol and as tablets containing 500 micrograms and 1 and 2 milligrams together with mestranol.

UNDESIRABLE EFFECTS; PRECAUTIONS. These are as described under Norethisterone (page 329).

Dose. 1 to 4 milligrams daily in divided doses. As an oral contraceptive, 0·5 to 2 milligrams daily.

EUCALYPTUS OIL

SYNONYM: Oleum Eucalypti

Eucalyptus Oil is obtained by rectifying the oil distilled from the fresh leaves and terminal branchlets of species of *Eucalyptus* (Fam. Myrtaceae) which yield oils containing a large proportion of cineole but little phellandrene.

Commercial sources of eucalyptus oil are Spain and Portugal, where the oil is derived from *E. globulus* Labill., and Australia, where several species of *Eucalyptus* are used.

Constituents. Eucalyptus oil contains chiefly cineole, which is also known as eucalyptol. It also contains (+)-α-pinene and other terpenes; phellandrene may also be present in small quantities.

Solubility. Soluble, at 20°, in 5 parts of alcohol (70 per cent); miscible with alcohol (90 per cent), with dehydrated alcohol, with oils, with fats, and with paraffins.

Standard
It complies with the requirements of the British Pharmacopoeia.
It is a colourless or pale yellow liquid with an aromatic camphoraceous odour and contains not less than 70·0 per cent w/w of cineole, $C_{10}H_{18}O$. It has a weight per ml at 20° of 0·904 g to 0·924 g.

Storage. It should be stored in well-filled airtight containers, protected from light, in a cool place.

Actions and uses. Eucalyptus oil has been applied to the skin in ointments and liniments as a counter-irritant. To relieve cough in chronic bronchitis and asthma it is inhaled from steam, sometimes with the addition of menthol, pine oil, and Compound Benzoin Tincture. It is an ingredient of pastilles, often with menthol, for the symptomatic relief of the common cold.
Oily solutions of eucalyptus oil should not be used as nasal drops or throat sprays because the vehicle inhibits ciliary movements and may cause lipoid pneumonia.

Dose. 0·05 to 0·2 millilitre.

Preparation
MENTHOL AND EUCALYPTUS INHALATION, B.P.C. (page 705)

EUGENOL

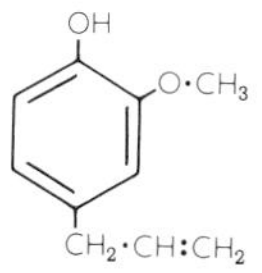

$C_{10}H_{12}O_2 = 164·2$

Eugenol is 4-allyl-2-methoxyphenol and may be obtained from clove oil.

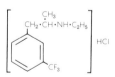

Solubility. Very slightly soluble in water; miscible with alcohol, with ether, with chloroform, and with fixed oils.

Standard
It complies with the requirements of the British Pharmacopoeia.
It is a colourless or pale yellow liquid with a characteristic odour. It has a boiling-point of about 254° and a weight per ml at 20° of 1·064 g to 1·068 g.

Stability. It darkens in colour with age or on exposure to air.

Storage. It should be stored in well-filled airtight containers, protected from light, in a cool place; contact with iron and zinc should be avoided.

Actions and uses. Eugenol has the actions and uses described under Clove Oil (page 118).

Dose. 0·05 to 0·2 millilitre.

FENFLURAMINE HYDROCHLORIDE

$C_{12}H_{17}ClF_3N = 267·7$

Fenfluramine Hydrochloride is the hydrochloride of 2-ethylamino-1-(3-trifluoromethylphenyl)propane.

Solubility. Soluble, at 20°, in 20 parts of water, in 10 parts of alcohol, and in 10 parts of chloroform; very slightly soluble in ether.

Standard
It complies with the requirements of the British Pharmacopoeia.
It is a white, crystalline, odourless powder and contains not less than 98·5 and not more than the equivalent of 101·0 per cent of $C_{12}H_{17}ClF_3N$, calculated with reference to the dried substance. The loss on drying under the prescribed conditions is not more than 0·5 per cent. It has a melting-point of 168° to 172°.

Actions and uses. Fenfluramine is an anorectic agent, chemically related to amphetamine, which is used as an aid in the treatment of obesity. Unlike amphetamine, however, fenfluramine may cause drowsiness, especially early in treatment; it does not raise the blood pressure and may increase the antihypersensitive effect of bethanidine, guanethidine, methyldopa, and reserpine, but not that of debrisoquine. Doses of up to 40 milligrams daily do not cause marked disturbance of sleep patterns, but this may occur on higher dosage, possibly accompanied by vivid or disturbing dreams.

UNDESIRABLE EFFECTS. Fenfluramine may give rise to diarrhoea. While its abuse potential appears to be low, the appearance of depressive symptoms some days after cessation of therapy may lead to a desire to recommence taking the drug.

PRECAUTIONS AND CONTRA-INDICATIONS. Fenfluramine should not be given to patients who are being treated with a monoamine-oxidase inhibitor, such as isocarboxazid, nialamide, phenelzine, or tranylcypromine, or within about ten days of the discontinuation of such treatment. It is probably best avoided in patients with a recent history of depressive illness and during the first three months of pregnancy.

Dose. Initial dose, 20 milligrams twice daily, increasing if necessary by 20 to 40 milligrams at intervals of one week to a maximum of 120 milligrams daily.

Preparation
FENFLURAMINE TABLETS, B.P. Unless otherwise specified, tablets each containing 20 mg of fenfluramine hydrochloride are supplied. They are film coated or sugar coated.

OTHER NAME: *Ponderax*®

FENNEL

SYNONYMS: Fennel Fruit; Foeniculum

Fennel consists of the dried fruits of cultivated plants of *Foeniculum vulgare* Mill. var. *vulgare* (Fam. Umbelliferae). The plant is indigenous to Europe, but commercial supplies come from India and China, with small quantities from Egypt.

Varieties. Saxon fennel fruits are about 8 to 10 mm long; they yield about 4 per cent of volatile oil of which over 20 per cent may consist of fenchone.
Russian, Galician, and Rumanian fennels closely resemble each other; they are usually shorter than the Saxon variety and yield a volatile oil containing a slightly smaller proportion of fenchone.
Indian fennel fruits are greenish-brown or yellowish-brown and 6 to 7 mm long; Chinese are slightly darker in colour.
The name bitter fennel is sometimes applied to fennel.

Constituents. Fennel yields 0·8 to 4 per cent of volatile oil, the chief constituents of which are anethole and (+)-fenchone.

Standard for unground drug
DESCRIPTION. *Macroscopical:* fruits usually entire cremocarps with pedicels attached, up to about 10 mm long and 4 mm wide; cremocarp oblong, laterally compressed, greenish-brown or yellowish-brown to brown, glabrous, with short bifid stylopod at apex; mericarps with 5 prominent yellowish primary ridges, transverse section showing in the pericarp 2 commissural vittae and 4 dorsal vittae occurring between the primary ridges, each ridge with a vascular strand; embryo small, embedded in upper end of abundant oily endosperm, commissural surface of endosperm not grooved.
Odour aromatic; taste aromatic and camphoraceous.

Microscopical: the diagnostic characters are: *outer epidermis* of pericarp composed of tetrahedral to polyhedral cells, cuticle not striated; *stomata* anomocytic, occasional; mesocarp with lignified and *reticulate parenchyma*; *inner epidermis* of pericarp with cells frequently showing a parquetry arrangement; *vittae* brown; *endosperm* composed of polyhedral, thick-walled cells containing *fixed oil* and *aleurone grains* with minute rosette *crystals* of calcium oxalate; *trichomes* and *starch* absent.

ACID-INSOLUBLE ASH. Not more than 1·5 per cent.

FOREIGN ORGANIC MATTER. Not more than 1·5 per cent.

VOLATILE OIL. Not less than 1·2 per cent v/w, determined by the method given in Appendix 13, page 893.

Standard for powdered drug: Powdered Fennel
DESCRIPTION. A greenish-yellow to yellowish-brown powder possessing the diagnostic microscopical characters, odour, and taste of the unground drug.

ACID-INSOLUBLE ASH; FOREIGN ORGANIC MATTER. It complies with the requirements for the unground drug.

VOLATILE OIL. Not less than 1·0 per cent v/w, determined by the method given in Appendix 13, page 893.

Adulterants and substitutes. The French sweet fennel, or Roman fennel [*Foeniculum vulgare* Mill. var. *dulce* (Mill.) Thellung], yields only about 2 per cent of volatile oil, which is practically free from fenchone.
Exhausted or partially exhausted fennel is deficient in oil and therefore deficient in odour.

Storage. It should be stored in a cool dry place. Powdered Fennel should be stored in airtight containers, in a cool place.

Actions and uses. Fennel is a carminative and a flavouring agent.

Preparation
LIQUORICE POWDER, COMPOUND, B.P.C. (page 777)

FERRIC AMMONIUM CITRATE

SYNONYMS: Ferr. Ammon. Cit.; Iron and Ammonium Citrate

Ferric Ammonium Citrate is a complex ammonium ferric citrate.

Ferric Ammonium Citrate may be prepared by saturating a warm aqueous solution of citric acid with freshly precipitated ferric hydroxide, adding a slight excess of a solution of ammonia, evaporating, and drying at a temperature not exceeding 40°.

Solubility. Soluble, at 20°, in less than 1 part of water; very slightly soluble in alcohol.

Standard

It complies with the requirements of the British Pharmacopoeia.

It occurs as deliquescent, dark red, thin, transparent scales or brown, shiny, granular powder and contains 20·5 to 22·5 per cent of Fe.

Stability. Aqueous solutions of ferric ammonium citrate are particularly liable to grow moulds, and chloroform or some other suitable preservative should be added.

Incompatibility. It is incompatible with mineral salts, alkali carbonates, and vegetable astringents.

Storage. It should be stored in airtight containers, protected from light.

Actions and uses. Ferric ammonium citrate has the actions and uses of iron salts, as described under Ferrous Sulphate (page 197);

100 milligrams contains approximately 20 milligrams of Fe. When given by mouth, it is better tolerated than the astringent preparations of iron. Doses of up to 9 grams daily may be needed for the treatment of iron-deficiency anaemias.

UNDESIRABLE EFFECTS. Large doses sometimes produce diarrhoea.

POISONING. As for Ferrous Sulphate (page 197).

Dose. See above under **Actions and uses.**

Preparations

FERRIC AMMONIUM CITRATE MIXTURE, B.P.C. (page 741)

FERRIC AMMONIUM CITRATE MIXTURE, PAEDIATRIC, B.P.C. (page 742)

FERRIC CITRATE (^{59}Fe) INJECTION

This material is radioactive and any regulations in force must be complied with.

Ferric Citrate (^{59}Fe) Injection is a sterile solution containing iron-59 in the ferric state, 1 per cent w/v of sodium citrate, and sufficient sodium chloride to make the solution isotonic with blood.

Iron-59 is a radioactive isotope of iron which emits β- and γ-radiation and has a half-life period of 45 days; it may be prepared by the neutron irradiation of iron-58 sufficiently low in iron-54 to ensure that the final content of iron-55 is not more than 2 per cent of the total activity; cobalt-60 is removed from the irradiated material during preparation.

Standard

It complies with the requirements of the British Pharmacopoeia.

It is a clear colourless or faintly orange-brown solution having a pH of 6·0 to 8·0. It contains not less than 90·0 and not more than 110·0 per cent of the quantity of iron-59 stated on the label at the date stated on the label. The specific activity is not less than 1 millicurie per milligram of iron at the date stated on the label.

Sterilisation. It is sterilised by heating in an autoclave.

Labelling. The label on the container states:

(1) the content of iron-59 expressed in microcuries or millicuries at a given date;

(2) that the injection is radioactive; and

(3) either that it does not contain a bactericide or the name and proportion of any added bactericide.

The label on the package also states:

(1) the total volume in the container;

(2) the content of total iron; and

(3) the calculated content of iron-55.

Storage. It should be stored in an area assigned for the purpose. The storage conditions should be such that the maximum radiation-dose-rate to which persons may be exposed is reduced to an acceptable level.

Actions and uses. Ferric Citrate (^{59}Fe) Injection is used in the investigation of iron metabolism, especially in anaemia and iron-storage disorders. For this purpose it is given by mouth or by intravenous injection. The fraction of the radioactivity absorbed after oral administration with ascorbic acid is assessed by measuring the residue in the faeces or by determining the total body radioactivity immediately after ingestion and again after an interval. A dose of about 10 microcuries is usually administered for these tests.

The rate of fall in the circulating radioactivity of the isotope following an intravenous injection of [^{59}Fe] ferric citrate may be measured to determine the turnover rate of plasma iron and red-cell iron. The incorporation of iron-59 into newly formed red cells can be measured; this may be useful in assessing marrow function in conditions associated with abnormalities of red-cell production, such as anaemias and polycythaemia. The dose usually administered for this purpose is about 5 microcuries. Iron-59 has also been used to measure red-cell life-span.

Iron-59 emits high-energy γ-rays which can be detected by a scintillation counter at the body surface. The passage of the isotope through underlying organs, including the liver, spleen, heart, and bone marrow of the lumbar or sacral regions of the vertebral column, can thus be followed. This is of value in detecting abnormalities of iron storage such as occur in primary and secondary haemochromatosis, and it may also be used to assess the distribution of sites of erythropoiesis in myeloid metaplasia.

Dose. In the investigation of haematological disorders, 5 to 10 microcuries.

FERROUS FUMARATE

$C_4H_2FeO_4 = 169 \cdot 9$

$$\left[\begin{array}{c} O_2C \cdot CH \\ \| \\ CH \cdot CO_2 \end{array}\right] Fe$$

Solubility. Slightly soluble in water; very slightly soluble in alcohol.

Standard
It complies with the requirements of the British Pharmacopoeia.
It is a fine, reddish-orange to reddish-brown, almost odourless powder and contains not less than 93·0 per cent of $C_4H_2FeO_4$, calculated with reference to the dried substance. The loss on drying under the prescribed conditions is not more than 1·0 per cent.

Hygroscopicity. It absorbs insignificant amounts of moisture at 25° at relative humidities up to about 90 per cent.

Actions and uses. Ferrous fumarate has the actions and uses of iron salts, as described under Ferrous Sulphate (page 197); 100 milligrams contains approximately 32 milligrams of Fe.

POISONING. As for Ferrous Sulphate (page 197).

Dose. Initially, 400 to 600 milligrams daily in divided doses; maintenance dosage, 200 milligrams daily.

Preparations
FERROUS FUMARATE MIXTURE, B.P.C. (page 742)
FERROUS FUMARATE TABLETS, B.P. Unless otherwise specified, tablets each containing 200 mg of ferrous fumarate are supplied.

OTHER NAMES: *Fersaday®*; *Fersamal®*; *Galfer®*

FERROUS GLUCONATE

$C_{12}H_{22}FeO_{14},2H_2O = 482 \cdot 2$

$$\left[\begin{array}{c} \quad\quad H \quad H \quad OH \quad H \\ HO \cdot CH_2 \cdot C \cdot C \cdot C \cdot C \cdot CO_2 \\ \quad\quad OH \quad OH \quad H \quad OH \end{array}\right]_2 Fe, 2H_2O$$

Solubility. Soluble, at 20°, in 8 parts of water; very slightly soluble in alcohol.

Standard
It complies with the requirements of the British Pharmacopoeia.
It occurs as grey powder or granules with a green or yellow tint and has a slight odour resembling that of burnt sugar. It contains not less than 95·0 per cent of $C_{12}H_{22}FeO_{14}$, calculated with reference to the dried substance. The loss on drying under the prescribed conditions is 7·0 to 10·0 per cent. A 5 per cent solution in water is acid to litmus.

Storage. It should be stored in airtight containers, protected from light.

Actions and uses. Ferrous gluconate has the actions and uses of iron salts, as described under Ferrous Sulphate (page 197); 100 milligrams contains approximately 12 milligrams of Fe.

POISONING. As for Ferrous Sulphate (page 197).

Dose. Initially, 1·2 to 1·8 grams daily in divided doses; maintenance dosage 600 milligrams daily.

Preparation
FERROUS GLUCONATE TABLETS, B.P. Unless otherwise specified, tablets each containing 300 mg of ferrous gluconate are supplied. They are sugar coated. They should be stored in airtight containers.

OTHER NAMES: *Cerevon®*; *Fergon®*

FERROUS SUCCINATE

Ferrous Succinate is a basic salt which may be prepared by the interaction of sodium succinate and ferrous sulphate in boiling aqueous solution.

Solubility. Very slightly soluble in water and in alcohol; soluble in dilute mineral acids.

Standard
It complies with the requirements of the British Pharmacopoeia.
It is a brownish-yellow to brown amorphous powder with a slight odour and contains 34·0 to 36·0 per cent of Fe, calculated with reference to the dried substance. The loss on drying under the prescribed conditions is not more than 1·0 per cent.

Storage. It should be stored in airtight containers, protected from light.

Actions and uses. Ferrous succinate has the actions and uses described under Ferrous Sulphate, but it produces a lower incidence of undesirable gastro-intestinal effects; 100 milligrams of ferrous succinate contains approximately 35 milligrams of iron.

Ferrous succinate should be administered between meals to obtain maximum absorption.

POISONING. As for Ferrous Sulphate.

Dose. Initially, 400 to 600 milligrams daily in divided doses; maintenance dosage 200 milligrams daily.

Preparations
FERROUS SUCCINATE CAPSULES, B.P. Unless otherwise specified, capsules each containing 100 mg of ferrous succinate are supplied. They should be protected from light.

FERROUS SUCCINATE TABLETS, B.P. Unless otherwise specified, tablets each containing 100 mg of ferrous succinate are supplied. They may be sugar coated. They should be stored in a cool place, protected from light.

OTHER NAME: *Ferromyn®*

FERROUS SULPHATE

SYNONYM: Ferrosi Sulfas

$FeSO_4,7H_2O = 278.0$

Ferrous Sulphate may be prepared by dissolving iron in dilute sulphuric acid and crystallising the product. When precipitated from a warm, concentrated, slightly acidified, aqueous solution by the addition of alcohol, it is obtained in a granular condition, in which form it is less prone to oxidation.

Solubility. Soluble, at 20°, in 1·5 parts of water; insoluble in alcohol.

Standard
It complies with the requirements of the European Pharmacopoeia.
It occurs as bluish-green crystals or pale green crystalline powder and contains not less than 98·0 and not more than the equivalent of 105·0 per cent of $FeSO_4,7H_2O$. A 5 per cent solution in water has a pH of 3·0 to 4·0.

Stability. Ferrous sulphate loses six molecules of water of crystallisation at 38°; at higher temperatures basic sulphates are produced. When exposed to moist air it is oxidised and becomes brown in colour.

Storage. It should be stored in airtight containers.

Actions and uses. Iron is essential for the formation of haemoglobin and hence for the oxidative process of living tissues. The amount of iron required daily for the formation of haemoglobin is 2 to 2·5 milligrams but, because of poor absorption, the actual intake to provide this must be greater—up to 20 milligrams. The daily requirement is raised during pregnancy and after severe or continuous haemorrhage.

Absorption of iron from food, or from iron compounds administered by mouth, takes place in the duodenum and jejunum, in amounts ranging from 1 to 50 milligrams daily, depending upon the needs of the body. The presence of free succinic acid aids the absorption of iron salts; it is decreased in the presence of antacids. Iron absorbed from the gastro-intestinal tract combines with protein and is deposited in the intestinal mucosa. Iron liberated by the destruction of red blood cells is stored in the liver and spleen. It is mobilised from these depots when required for haemoglobin formation.

Compounds of iron are used in all forms of iron-deficiency and hypochromic anaemia, anaemia of pregnancy, the nutritional anaemia of infants, anaemia due to excessive or repeated haemorrhage, and anaemia associated with infections, infestations, and malignant disease. In the treatment of macrocytic anaemia, preparations of iron given alone are of no value, but they may be of value as a supplement to vitamin-B_{12} therapy whenever the reserves of iron are depleted and the increase in haemoglobin does not parallel the rise in the number of blood cells. The soluble ferrous salts are the most satisfactory of the iron preparations for effecting haemoglobin formation; ferric salts are relatively ineffective. Since only a small proportion of the iron administered by mouth is absorbed, large doses of iron salts are necessary to produce a remission in iron-deficiency anaemia. Full doses of ferrous sulphate should be administered three or four times a day; 100 milligrams contains approximately 20 milligrams of Fe. Large doses often produce gastro-intestinal irritation with vomiting and diarrhoea and should be given after meals to reduce gastric irritation; continued administration may sometimes produce constipation. Patients intolerant of oral administration may be treated with parenteral iron preparations.

POISONING. Fatal poisoning has occurred in children after ingestion of ferrous sulphate. The procedure described under Desferrioxamine Mesylate (page 145) should be followed.

If desferrioxamine is not available the patient must be encouraged to vomit without delay and thereafter the stomach should be washed out with a 5 per cent solution of sodium bicarbonate and about 300 millilitres of the solution should be left in the stomach.

Fluid loss should be replaced by intravenous administration of Compound Sodium Lactate Injection or Sodium Chloride and Dextrose Injection. In severe cases exchange transfusion may help.

Dose. Initially, 600 to 900 milligrams daily in divided doses; maintenance dosage 300 milligrams daily.

Preparations
FERROUS SULPHATE MIXTURE, B.P.C. (page 742)

FERROUS SULPHATE MIXTURE, PAEDIATRIC, B.P.C. (page 742)

DRIED FERROUS SULPHATE

Dried Ferrous Sulphate is Ferrous Sulphate from which part of the water of crystallisation has been removed by drying at 40°.

Solubility. Slowly, but almost completely, soluble in freshly boiled and cooled water.

Standard
It complies with the requirements of the British Pharmacopoeia.
It is a greyish-white powder and contains 80·0 to 90·0 per cent of $FeSO_4$.

Storage. It should be stored in airtight containers.

Actions and uses. Dried ferrous sulphate has the actions and uses of iron salts, as described under Ferrous Sulphate; 100 milligrams contains approximately 30 milligrams of Fe.

POISONING. As for Ferrous Sulphate.

Dose. Initially, 400 to 600 milligrams daily in divided doses; maintenance dosage 200 milligrams daily.

Preparations
FERROUS SULPHATE TABLETS, B.P. Unless otherwise specified, sugar-coated tablets each containing 200 mg of dried ferrous sulphate are supplied. They should be stored in airtight containers.

FERROUS SULPHATE TABLETS, COMPOUND, B.P.C. (page 811)

OTHER NAME: Exsiccated Ferrous Sulphate

FIG

SYNONYM: Ficus

Fig is the dried succulent fruit of *Ficus carica* L. (Fam. Moraceae). The tree is indigenous to western Asia and is cultivated in most subtropical and warm climates. When the fruits are ripe, they are collected and dried in the sun.

Varieties. The varieties are known in commerce as "natural", "pulled" or "lacoum", and "layer" figs. "Natural" figs are those which are packed loose and retain to some extent their original shape. "Pulled" figs have been kneaded and pulled to make them supple. "Layer" figs have been cut into halves and closely packed, so that they are compressed and flattened.

Constituents. Fig contains about 50 per cent of sugars, consisting principally of invert sugar with some sucrose. Small quantities of citric, acetic, and malic acid and a proteolytic enzyme, ficin, are also present.

Standard
DESCRIPTION. *Macroscopical:* fruit compound, soft, fleshy, brown or yellowish-brown, sometimes covered with a saccharine efflorescence; at the summit a small opening surrounded by scales and at the base a short, stalk-like prolongation; fruit up to about 5 cm in length and breadth, consisting of a hollow receptacle bearing on the inner surface numerous druplets, each containing a stone about 1·5 to 2·0 mm long; seed containing endosperm and a curved embryo.
Odour pleasantly fruity; taste sweet.

Microscopical: the diagnostic characters are: Receptacle: *epidermal cells* polyhedral, *stomata* raised, *trichomes* unicellular and uniseriate, thick-walled, of varying length, up to about 300 μm; *hypodermis* composed of rounded polyhedral cells, some containing small rosette *crystals* of calcium oxalate; *aerenchyma*

made up of large, irregular cells, forming greater part of the receptacle, containing large rosette crystals of calcium oxalate and interspersed with numerous *latex tubes*, about 30 to 50 μm wide, and slender *vascular bundles*.
Pericarp: *epicarp* consisting of radially elongated cells with mucilaginous outer walls; *mesocarp* of delicate, often disorganised cells; *endocarp* of radially elongated *sclereids* with pitted walls.
Endosperm and embryo: small cells containing *aleurone grains* and *fixed oil*; *starch* absent.

WATER-SOLUBLE EXTRACTIVE. Not less than 60·0 per cent, determined by the following method:
To 25·0 g, minced, add 500 ml of water, boil under a reflux condenser for one hour, cool, and filter; to 20 ml of the filtrate add about 20 g, accurately weighed, of washed and ignited sand, evaporate to dryness in a tared flat-bottomed shallow dish, and dry the residue to constant weight at 100°. Subtract from the weight of residue obtained the weight of sand added and calculate the water-soluble extractive in the sample.

Storage. It should be stored in a dry place.

Actions and uses. Fig has demulcent properties and is used in confections and syrups with senna and other purgatives.

Preparation
FIGS SYRUP, COMPOUND, B.P.C. (page 800)

FLUDROCORTISONE ACETATE

SYNONYM: Fludrocort. Acet.

$C_{23}H_{31}FO_6 = 422·5$

Fludrocortisone Acetate is 21-acetoxy-9α-fluoro-11β,17α-dihydroxypregn-4-ene-3,20-dione.

Solubility. Very slightly soluble in water; soluble, at 20°, in 50 parts of alcohol, in 250 parts of ether, and in 50 parts of chloroform.

Standard
It complies with the requirements of the British Pharmacopoeia.

It occurs as an odourless or almost odourless, hygroscopic, white or almost white crystalline powder. It contains not less than 96·0 and not more than the equivalent of 104·0 per cent of $C_{23}H_{31}FO_6$, calculated with reference to the dried substance. The loss on drying under the prescribed conditions is not more than 1·0 per cent.

Storage. It should be stored in airtight containers, protected from light.

Actions and uses. Fludrocortisone has powerful glucocorticoid and mineralocorticoid actions. Given alone in adrenocortical deficiency states, its mineralocorticoid action is relatively stronger than its glucocorticoid action, and oedema and other signs of salt and water retention appear within a few days of starting treatment. With a dosage which is just enough to correct sodium loss in Addison's disease or in adrenalectomised subjects, the glucocorticoid action of fludrocortisone is insufficient to maintain the patient in normal health. For this reason fludrocortisone acetate is usually given by mouth in low dosage, such as 100 micrograms every one to five days, together with the usual maintenance replacement dose of cortisone acetate, to those adrenocortical-deficient patients who become sodium deficient on cortisone alone. In some patients adrenalectomised for metastatic carcinomatosis, symptoms of sodium deficiency may occur when the malignant process begins to extend again after the regression caused by the operation; in such cases fludrocortisone is of value. In Addisonian crisis it may be given by mouth in a dosage of 1 milligram twice daily for a few days, the dose being reduced subsequently.

UNDESIRABLE EFFECTS. Excessive dosage may result not only in Cushingoid features with oedema and electrolyte imbalance but also in marked muscle weakness and in hyperglycaemia.

Dose. For acute adrenocortical insufficiency: initial dosage, 1 to 2 milligrams daily; maintenance dosage, 100 to 200 micrograms daily.

Preparation
FLUDROCORTISONE TABLETS, B.P. Unless otherwise specified, tablets each containing 100 µg of fludrocortisone acetate are supplied. They should be protected from light. Tablets containing 1 mg are also available.

OTHER NAME: *Florinef®*

FLUOCINOLONE ACETONIDE

$C_{24}H_{30}F_2O_6 = 452·5$

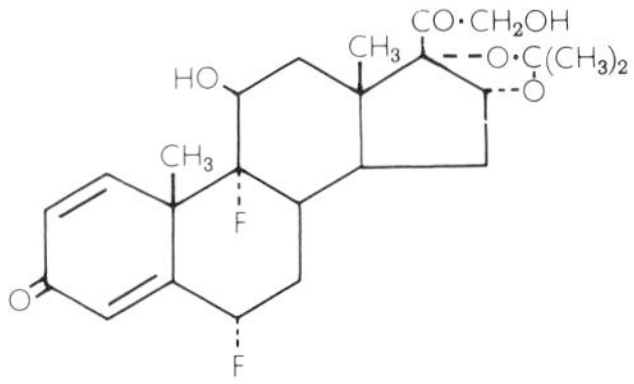

Fluocinolone Acetonide is 6α,9α-difluoro-11β,21-dihydroxy-16α,17α-isopropylidenedioxypregna-1,4-diene-3,20-dione.

Solubility. Insoluble in water; soluble, at 20°, in 26 parts of dehydrated alcohol, in 15 parts of chloroform, and in 10 parts of acetone; very slightly soluble in light petroleum.

Standard
It complies with the requirements of the British Pharmacopoeia.
It is a white or almost white, crystalline, odourless powder and contains not less than 96·0 and not more than the equivalent of 104·0 per cent of $C_{21}H_{30}F_2O_6$, calculated with reference to the dried substance. The loss on drying under the prescribed conditions is not more than 1·0 per cent.

Storage. It should be protected from light.

Actions and uses. Fluocinolone acetonide is a corticosteroid for topical application that is more potent than hydrocortisone (page 224); it should not be given by mouth.
It is applied as an ointment, lotion, or cream containing up to 0·025 per cent, and is generally used either without dressings or with conventional bandaging, but if the area is covered with a non-porous dressing such as polythene the effect is greatly enhanced. This method of application is suitable for small areas in chronic skin conditions, but if the preparation is used over large areas, sufficient of the drug may be absorbed through the skin to give rise to systemic effects.

PRECAUTIONS. It should not be used on infected skin without the simultaneous application of a suitable antibacterial agent.

Preparations
FLUOCINOLONE CREAM, B.P.C. (page 658)
FLUOCINOLONE OINTMENT, B.P.C. (page 761)

OTHER NAMES: *Synalar®*; *Synandone®*

FLUOCORTOLONE HEXANOATE

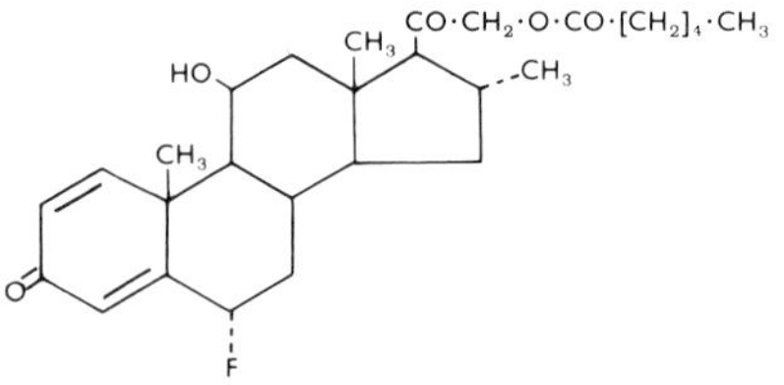

SYNONYM: Fluocortolone Caproate

$C_{28}H_{39}FO_5 = 474·6$

Fluocortolone Hexanoate is 6α-fluoro-21-hexanoyloxy-11β-hydroxy-16α-methylpregna-1,4-diene-3,20-dione.

Solubility. Insoluble in water and in ether; slightly soluble in alcohol and in methyl alcohol; soluble, at 20°, in 18 parts of chloroform.

Standard
It complies with the requirements of the British Pharmacopoeia.
It is a white to creamy-white, crystalline, odourless powder and contains not less than 97·0 and not more than the equivalent of 103·0 per cent of $C_{28}H_{39}FO_5$, calculated with reference to the dried substance. The loss on drying under the prescribed conditions is not more than 0·5 per cent. It has a melting-point of about 244°.

Storage. It should be protected from light.

Actions and uses. Fluocortolone hexanoate is a corticosteroid intended for topical application. It has the powerful anti-inflammatory action of fluocortolone, and although the onset of action is less rapid than with fluocortolone or fluocortolone pivalate, it is more prolonged. It is used, together with fluocortolone, as an ointment containing 0·25 per cent of each constituent, or as a cream or lotion with fluocortolone pivalate. Initially, it may be necessary to apply the ointment three times a day, but later a dressing once daily may be adequate. With such dressings, excessive absorption and consequent systemic effects are unlikely except in infants.
In psoriasis and other refractory conditions, the ointment should be applied thinly and covered with an occlusive dressing. Large areas of the body should not be occluded in this way because of the increased risk of systemic effects and disturbances of the heat-regulating mechanism.

PRECAUTIONS. Fluocortolone hexanoate should not be used on infected skin without the simultaneous application of a suitable antibacterial agent.

OTHER NAME: *Ultralanum®*

FLUOCORTOLONE PIVALATE

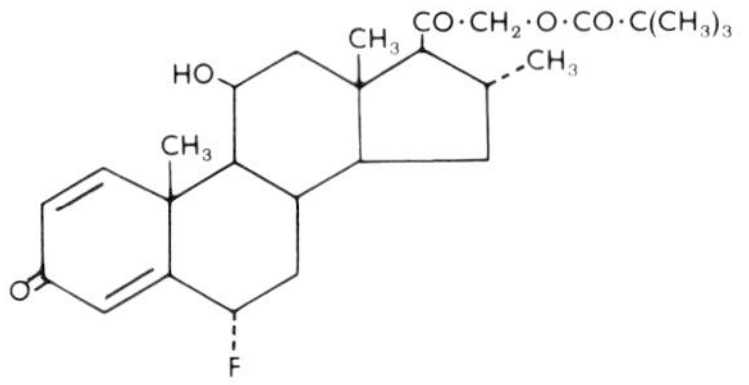

SYNONYM: Fluocortolone Trimethylacetate

$C_{27}H_{37}FO_5 = 460·6$

Fluocortolone Pivalate is 6α-fluoro-11β-hydroxy-16α-methyl-21-pivaloyloxypregna-1,4-diene-3,20-dione.

Solubility. Very slightly soluble in water; soluble, at 20°, in 36 parts of alcohol, in 3 parts of chloroform, and in 18 parts of methyl alcohol.

Standard
It complies with the requirements of the British Pharmacopoeia.
It is a white to creamy-white, crystalline, odourless powder and contains not less than 97·0 and not more than the equivalent of 103·0 per cent of $C_{27}H_{37}FO_5$, calculated with reference to the dried substance. The loss on drying under the prescribed conditions is not more than 0·5 per cent. It has a melting-point of about 187°.

Storage. It should be protected from light.

Actions and uses. Fluocortolone pivalate has the general anti-inflammatory properties of fluocortolone, as described under Fluocortolone Hexanoate.
It is used in conjunction with fluocortolone hexanoate in creams and lotions when the free alcohol would not be suitable owing to its instability.

PRECAUTIONS. Fluocortolone pivalate should not be used on infected skin without the simultaneous application of a suitable antibacterial agent.

FLUORESCEIN SODIUM

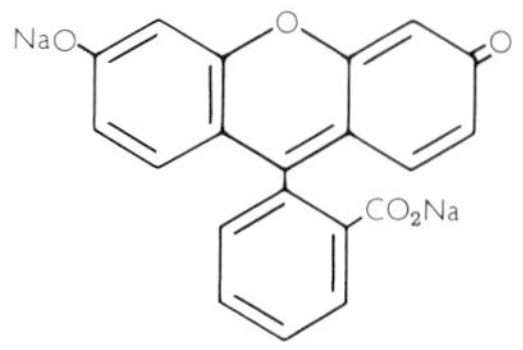

SYNONYM: Soluble Fluorescein

$C_{20}H_{10}Na_2O_5 = 376.3$

Fluorescein Sodium is disodium fluorescein.

Solubility. Soluble, at 20°, in 1·5 parts of water and in 10 parts of alcohol.

Standard
It complies with the requirements of the British Pharmacopoeia.
It is an orange-red, hygroscopic, odourless powder and contains not less than 98·5 per cent of $C_{20}H_{10}Na_2O_5$, calculated with reference to the dried substance. The loss on drying under the prescribed conditions is not more than 10·0 per cent.

Sterilisation. Solutions are sterilised by heating in an autoclave.

Storage. It should be stored in airtight containers.

Uses. Fluorescein sodium is used in ophthalmic practice as a diagnostic agent for detecting lesions and foreign bodies; a 2 per cent solution is commonly used for this purpose. When introduced into the eye it does not stain the normal cornea, but ulcers, or parts deprived of epithelium, become green, and foreign bodies are seen surrounded by a green ring. Since it is applied to abraded corneas, special care should be taken to avoid bacterial contamination.

Solutions containing 5 to 20 per cent of fluorescein sodium have been administered by intravenous injection for diagnostic purposes, such as the investigation of circulatory disorders and the differentiation of normal and malignant tissues when examined in ultraviolet light.

Preparation
FLUORESCEIN EYE-DROPS, B.P.C. (page 690)

FLUOXYMESTERONE

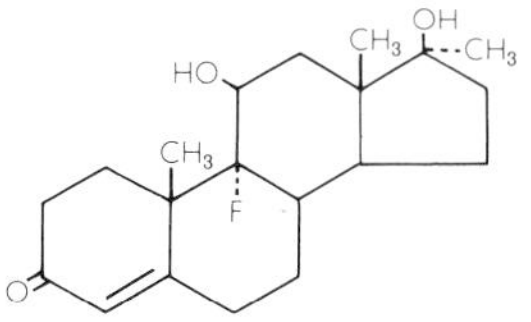

$C_{20}H_{29}FO_3 = 336.4$

Fluoxymesterone is 9α-fluoro-11β,17-dihydroxy-17α-methylandrost-4-en-3-one.

Solubility. Very slightly soluble in water; soluble, at 20°, in 70 parts of alcohol and in 200 parts of chloroform.

Standard
It complies with the requirements of the British Pharmacopoeia.
It is a white or creamy-white, crystalline, odourless powder and contains not less than 97·0 and not more than the equivalent of 103·0 per cent of $C_{20}H_{29}FO_3$, calculated with reference to the dried substance. The loss on drying under the prescribed conditions is not more than 1·0 per cent. It has a melting-point of about 278°.

Storage. It should be stored in airtight containers, protected from light.

Actions and uses. Fluoxymesterone is an androgenic hormone which has the actions and uses described under Testosterone (page 494). It is effective when given by mouth.
In the female it is given in doses of 20 milligrams in the treatment of inoperable breast cancer and in a dosage of 1 to 5 milligrams daily in functional uterine bleeding and dysmenorrhoea.

In the male it is given in the treatment of hypogonadism and eunuchoidism in a dosage of 2·5 milligrams daily.
It is administered for its anabolic effect in the treatment of osteoporosis in a dosage of 2 to 10 milligrams daily.

PRECAUTIONS AND CONTRA-INDICATIONS. The precautions described under Testosterone (page 494) should be observed; increased erythropoiesis and hypercalcaemia are rare. Salt retention and oedema may be corrected by salt restriction and administration of diuretics.
Fluoxymesterone is contra-indicated in patients with impaired liver function or prostatic carcinoma.

Dose. See above under **Actions and uses.**

Preparation
FLUOXYMESTERONE TABLETS, B.P. Unless otherwise specified, tablets each containing 5 mg of fluoxymesterone are supplied. They should be protected from light.

OTHER NAME: *Ultandren*®

FLUPHENAZINE HYDROCHLORIDE

$C_{22}H_{28}Cl_2F_3N_3OS = 510 \cdot 4$

Fluphenazine Hydrochloride is the dihydro-chloride of 10-{3-[4-(2-hydroxyethyl)pipera-zin-1-yl]propyl}-2-trifluoromethylphenothiazine.

Solubility. Soluble, at 20°, in 10 parts of water; very slightly soluble in alcohol and in ether.

Standard
It complies with the requirements of the British Pharmacopoeia.
It is a white or almost white, crystalline, odourless powder and contains not less than 98·5 and not more than the equivalent of 101·0 per cent of $C_{22}H_{28}Cl_2F_3N_3OS$, calculated with reference to the dried substance. The loss on drying under the pre-scribed conditions is not more than 1·0 per cent. A 5 per cent solution in water has a pH of 1·9 to 2·3.

Storage. It should be stored in airtight containers, protected from light.

Actions and uses. Fluphenazine is a tranquil-liser with actions similar to those of trifluo-perazine hydrochloride (page 519). It has anti-emetic properties, but little sedative and hypotensive action, and it produces less tachy-cardia than chlorpromazine.
It is used mainly in the treatment of schizo-phrenia and paranoid states and is also of value in severe anxiety disorders and for senile con-fusion.

UNDESIRABLE EFFECTS. Extrapyramidal syn-dromes are particularly likely to occur. Dystonic reactions and akathisia are common and may not be recognised when they do not resemble classical parkinsonism; dyskinesias may become irreversible. Occasionally galac-torrhoea, augmentation of epilepsy, epi-gastric pain, or jaundice may occur.
Fluphenazine may release stored catechol-amines and there is therefore a risk in cases of phaeochromocytoma.

POISONING. Heat loss should be prevented and blood pressure maintained by changing pos-ture. Drugs such as benzhexol may be re-quired for the treatment of dystonic effects.

Dose. For anxiety states: 1 to 2 milligrams daily in single or divided doses.
For schizophrenia: up to 15 milligrams daily in divided doses.

Preparation
FLUPHENAZINE TABLETS, B.P. The quantity of fluph-enazine hydrochloride in each tablet should be specified by the prescriber. They are sugar coated. Tablets containing 1, 2·5, and 5 mg are available.

OTHER NAME: *Moditen*®

FOLIC ACID

$C_{19}H_{19}N_7O_6 = 441 \cdot 4$

Folic Acid is N-p-(2-amino-4-hydroxypterid-6-ylmethylamino)benzoyl-L(+)-glutamic acid, and is identical with the liver *Lactobacillus casei* factor.
It is present, either free or combined with several L(+)-glutamic acid moieties in peptide linkages, in liver, yeast, and certain other natural products.

Solubility. Insoluble in cold water and in alcohol; soluble in 5000 parts of boiling water; soluble in dilute sodium hydroxide solution, yielding a clear orange-brown solution.

Standard
It complies with the requirements of the British Pharmacopoeia.
It is an orange-yellow, microcrystalline, almost odour-less powder and contains not less than 95·0 per cent of $C_{19}H_{19}N_7O_6$, calculated with reference to the dried substance. The loss of drying under the prescribed conditions is 5·0 to 8·5 per cent.

Sterilisation. Solutions of the sodium salt for injec-tion are sterilised by filtration.

Storage. It should be stored in airtight containers, protected from light.

Actions and uses. Folic acid is present in many foods, partly as free folic acid but mainly in the conjugated form with several glutamic acid residues. The best sources are green leafy vegetables, meat, offal, and cereals.
Without folic acid the living cell cannot divide but is halted in metaphase; this property un-derlies the use of folic acid antagonists in the treatment of neoplastic disease. Folic acid is necessary for the normal production of red blood cells, including maturation of megalo-blasts into normoblasts.
Folic acid is absorbed mainly from the proxi-mal part of the small intestine. It is enzymic-ally reduced in the body to tetrahydrofolic acid, a coenzyme that is involved in purine and pyrimidine nucleotide synthesis and some amino-acid conversions. The human require-ment is about 50 micrograms daily, the actual amount being determined by metabolic and

cell-turnover rates. The total body folic acid stores are 5 to 10 milligrams.

Symptoms of deficiency in man include megaloblastic haematopoiesis, glossitis, diarrhoea, and loss of weight. A deficiency may occur in pregnancy, in the malabsorption syndrome, after continuous administration of large doses of pyrimethamine, and in epileptics on continuous anticonvulsive treatment. In this last condition the folic acid deficiency may lead to mental deterioration, which can be prevented by giving folic acid and vitamin B_{12}. Minor variations of folic acid metabolism may occur in patients with cardiac failure and rheumatoid arthritis.

Folic acid produces a haematopoietic response in pernicious anaemia (but see precautions and contra-indications), nutritional macrocytic anaemia, megaloblastic anaemia of infancy and pregnancy, pellagra, sprue, idiopathic steatorrhoea, coeliac disease, and following gastrectomy. Folic acid is administered for the treatment of megaloblastic anaemia due to these conditions, to the malabsorption syndrome, and to the continuous use of anticonvulsants, particularly primidone and phenytoin. It is of no value in the treatment of other forms of anaemia.

Folic acid may be given by mouth in an initial dosage of 10 to 20 milligrams daily for fourteen days, or until a haematopoietic response has been obtained; the daily maintenance dosage is 2·5 to 10 milligrams. Folic acid may also be used in a dosage of 200 to 500 micrograms daily as a prophylactic for anaemia of pregnancy. It may also be administered by intramuscular injection as the sodium salt.

PRECAUTIONS AND CONTRA-INDICATIONS. Folic acid should never be given in the treatment of pernicious anaemia because it fails to prevent the onset of subacute combined degeneration of the cord; the therapy of choice in pernicious anaemia is hydroxocobalamin or cyanocobalamin.

Large and continuous doses of folic acid may lower the blood level of vitamin B_{12}.

Dose. See above under **Actions and uses.**

Preparation

FOLIC ACID TABLETS, B.P. Unless otherwise specified, tablets each containing 5 mg of folic acid are supplied. They should be stored in airtight containers, protected from light. Tablets containing 100 µg are also available.

OTHER NAME: Pteroylglutamic Acid

FORMALDEHYDE SOLUTION

SYNONYM: Formalin

NOTE. *The general use of the synonym "formalin" is limited, and in any country in which the word "formalin" is a trade mark it may be used only when applied to the product made by the owners of the trade mark.*

Formaldehyde Solution is an aqueous solution of formaldehyde, H·CHO, containing methyl alcohol to delay polymerisation of the formaldehyde to solid paraformaldehyde, $(CH_2O)_n$.

Solubility. Miscible with water and with alcohol.

Standard
It complies with the requirements of the British Pharmacopoeia.
It is a colourless liquid with a characteristic irritating odour and contains 34·0 to 38·0 per cent w/w of CH_2O.

Stability. A white deposit may form on storage; its formation occurs more rapidly if the solution is kept in a cold place.

Incompatibility. It is incompatible with ammonia, with gelatin, and with oxidising agents.

Storage. It should be stored in airtight containers in a moderately warm place.

Actions and uses. Formaldehyde Solution is a powerful antiseptic, but is very irritant to mucous membranes. It reacts with and precipitates proteins, and when applied undiluted hardens the skin. It is used in antiseptic mouth-washes and gargles. It has been used mixed with thymol, cresol, glycerol, and zinc oxide as a mummifying agent for residual dental pulp tissue and with equal parts of cresol or creosote as a dressing for septic root canals. It is used to remove the specific toxicity of bacterial toxins in the preparation of toxoids.

For the disinfection of rooms, Formaldehyde Solution may be used as a spray, or the gas may be liberated by heat. When fumigation is effected by spraying, an equal volume of industrial methylated spirit must be added to the solution in order to prevent polymerisation in the droplets and on surfaces after deposition. When vaporisation is effected by heat, 500 millilitres of Formaldehyde Solution added to 1 litre of water is boiled in a stainless steel vessel over an electric hot-plate; this volume is sufficient for 1000 cubic feet of air space. Alternatively, 170 grams of potassium permanganate added to 500 millilitres of undiluted Formaldehyde Solution will cause violent boiling within ten seconds and the production of sufficient moist formaldehyde gas to disinfect the same cubic capacity. During fumigation, the room must be effectively sealed and maintained at a temperature above 18°; contact with the vapour must continue for more than four hours, and preferably overnight.

For the disinfection of bedding and similar objects, larger quantities of Formaldehyde Solution must be vaporised to allow for the absorption of formaldehyde by the materials. Formaldehyde Solution does not damage metals or fabrics, but it should not be used for disinfection when other more reliable methods are possible.

Formaldehyde Solution is also used for the disinfection of membranes in the artificial kidney.

Diluted to ten volumes with saline solution it is used as a preservative for pathological specimens; it is not suitable for preserving urine for subsequent examination.

UNDESIRABLE EFFECTS. The vapour of formaldehyde may cause lachrymation and, if inhaled, irritation of the respiratory tract.

POISONING. Formaldehyde poisoning is characterised by severe abdominal pain, which may be followed by collapse and death; in less severe cases, acute nephritis with oliguria may result. Gastric lavage should be carried out or an emetic administered; diluted Aromatic Ammonia Spirit may be given by mouth.

FRAMYCETIN SULPHATE

$C_{23}H_{46}N_6O_{13},3H_2SO_4 = 908.9$

Framycetin Sulphate is the sulphate of O^4-(2,6-diamino-2,6-dideoxy-α-D-glucopyranosyl)-O^5-[O^3-(2,6-diamino-2,6-dideoxy-α-L-idopyranosyl)-β-D-ribofuranosyl]-2-deoxystreptamine (neomycin B), an antimicrobial base produced by certain strains of *Streptomyces fradiae* or *Streptomyces decaris* or by other means.

Solubility. Soluble, at 20°, in 1 part of water; insoluble in alcohol, in ether, and in chloroform.

Standard
It complies with the requirements of the British Pharmacopoeia.
It is a white or yellowish-white, odourless or almost odourless, hygroscopic powder and contains not less than 630 Units per mg, calculated with reference to the anhydrous substance. It contains not more than 5.0 per cent w/w of water. A 1 per cent solution in water has a pH of 6.0 to 7.0.

Storage. It should be stored in airtight containers, protected from light, at a temperature not exceeding 30°.

Actions and uses. Framycetin is an antibiotic of the neomycin group, sharing the same spectrum of bactericidal activity and cross resistance with other members of the group. It is too toxic for parenteral administration and has been used for the prevention and treatment of infections of the skin, eyes, and large bowel, as described under Neomycin Sulphate (page 320). It is available as a sterile powder and as eye ointment, eye-drops, and tablets.

PRECAUTIONS. As for Neomycin Sulphate (page 320).

Dose. See above under **Actions and uses.**

OTHER NAMES: *Framygen®*; *Soframycin®*

FRUSEMIDE

$C_{12}H_{11}ClN_2O_5S = 330.7$

Frusemide is 4-chloro-2-furfurylamino-5-sulphamoylbenzoic acid.

Solubility. Very slightly soluble in water and in chloroform; soluble, at 20°, in 75 parts of alcohol and in 850 parts of ether; soluble in solutions of alkali hydroxides.

Standard
It complies with the requirements of the British Pharmacopoeia.
It is a white or almost white, crystalline, odourless powder and contains not less than 98.5 per cent of $C_{12}H_{11}ClN_2O_5S$, calculated with reference to the dried substance. The loss on drying under the prescribed conditions is not more than 0.5 per cent.

Actions and uses. Frusemide is a diuretic which reduces the resorption of electrolytes by the proximal and distal renal tubules and by the loop of Henle. Excretion of sodium, potassium, and chloride ions is increased and as a consequence water excretion is enhanced. It has no effect on carbonic anhydrase in the renal tubular cells, and urinary pH during the phase of diuresis may be temporarily lowered; it does not appreciably alter the acid–base balance. Serum-uric-acid levels may be increased after administration of frusemide.

Frusemide is rapidly absorbed when given by mouth and provokes an intense diuresis lasting for four to six hours; this initial diuresis is greater than with equivalent dosage of the thiazide derivatives, although the total volume of fluid excreted over a period of twenty-four hours may not be greatly different.

Frusemide is used for the treatment of the same conditions as chlorothiazide. It may be effective when tolerance to thiazide diuretics has developed; its action is not enhanced by the thiazides. It is usually given by mouth in a dosage of 40 milligrams once to three times a day. As its action is intense and of short duration it is usually possible to ensure that treatment does not disturb the patient's normal sleep. Once diuresis is adequately established, frusemide may be given every other day or on three successive days in a week. In refractory cases the doses may, in exceptional circumstances, be increased to 500 milligrams a day, but careful biochemical control is necessary.

Frusemide enhances the effect of hypotensive drugs and the dose of these may have to be adjusted to suit the needs of the patient when given concurrently for the control of mild or moderate hypertension. In cerebral oedema it is given by intravenous injection and produces effects comparable with those following intravenous infusion of osmotically active substances.

UNDESIRABLE EFFECTS. Prolonged and regular administration may produce hypokalaemia. This intensifies the effect of digitalis on cardiac muscle, and the dosage of cardiac glycosides may have to be adjusted or administration temporarily suspended. It may precipitate hepatic coma in patients with impaired liver function.

PRECAUTIONS. As with chlorothiazide treatment, potassium depletion may occur when treatment with frusemide is prolonged, and potassium supplements should be given.

CONTRA-INDICATIONS. Frusemide is contra-indicated in acute nephritis, acute renal failure, and when the blood-potassium level is low; it should be used with caution in cirrhosis of the liver.

Dose. See above under **Actions and uses.**

Preparation
FRUSEMIDE TABLETS, B.P. Unless otherwise specified, tablets each containing 40 mg of frusemide are supplied. Tablets containing 20 and 500 mg are also available.

OTHER NAMES: Furosemide; *Lasix*®

FUSIDIC ACID

$C_{31}H_{48}O_6,\frac{1}{2}H_2O = 525\cdot7$

Fusidic Acid is an antimicrobial substance produced by the growth of certain strains of *Fusidium coccineum* (K. Tubaki).

Solubility. Insoluble in water; soluble, at 20°, in 5 parts of alcohol, in 60 parts of ether, and in 4 parts of chloroform.

Standard
DESCRIPTION. A white crystalline powder; odourless or almost odourless.

IDENTIFICATION TESTS. 1. It complies with the thin-layer chromatographic test given in Appendix 5A, page 864.

2. The infra-red absorption spectrum exhibits maxima which are only at the same wavelengths as, and have similar relative intensities to, those in the spectrum of *fusidic acid A.S.*

SPECIFIC ROTATION. $-7°$ to $-11°$, calculated with reference to the anhydrous substance, determined, at 20°, in a 3·0 per cent w/v solution in *chloroform*.

RELATED COMPOUNDS. It complies with the test given in Appendix 5A, page 864.

WATER. 1·4 to 2·0 per cent w/w, determined by the method given in Appendix 16, page 895.

SULPHATED ASH. Not more than 0·2 per cent.

CONTENT OF $C_{31}H_{48}O_6$. Not less than 97·5 per cent and not more than the equivalent of 101·0 per cent, calculated with reference to the anhydrous substance, determined by the following method:
Dissolve about 0·5 g, accurately weighed, in 10 ml of *alcohol (95 per cent)*, and titrate with 0·1N sodium hydroxide, using *phenolphthalein solution* as indicator; each ml of 0·1N sodium hydroxide is equivalent to 0·05167 g of $C_{31}H_{48}O_6$.

Storage. It should be stored in airtight containers, protected from light.

Actions and uses. Fusidic acid has the actions, uses, and undesirable effects described under Sodium Fusidate (page 452). It is used for the preparation of aqueous suspensions for oral administration.

Dose. For an adult, 1 to 2 grams daily in divided doses; for a child under one year 125 milligrams, from one to five years 250 milligrams, and from six to twelve years 500 milligrams, three times daily.

Preparation
FUSIDIC ACID MIXTURE, B.P.C. (page 743)

OTHER NAME: *Fucidin*®

GALLAMINE TRIETHIODIDE

SYNONYM: Gallamini Triethiodidum

$C_{30}H_{60}I_3N_3O_3 = 891.5$

Gallamine Triethiodide is 1,2,3-tri(2-diethylaminoethoxy)benzene triethiodide.

Solubility. Soluble, at 20°, in less than 1 part of water and in 115 parts of alcohol; slightly soluble in chloroform; insoluble in ether.

Standard

It complies with the requirements of the European Pharmacopoeia.

It is a white or slightly cream-coloured, odourless, hygroscopic powder and contains not less than 98.0 and not more than the equivalent of 101.0 per cent of $C_{30}H_{60}I_3N_3O_3$, calculated with reference to the dried substance. The loss on drying under the prescribed conditions is not more than 3.0 per cent.

Sterilisation. Solutions for injection are sterilised by heating in an autoclave or by filtration.

Storage. It should be stored in airtight containers, protected from light.

Actions and uses. Gallamine triethiodide has actions and uses similar to those described under Tubocurarine Chloride (page 523). It causes paralysis of voluntary muscle by blocking the transmission of impulses at the myoneural junction; this action can be counteracted by neostigmine. Gallamine also causes blockade of the cardiac vagus nerve and associated ganglia. The muscle-relaxant effect of 80 milligrams of gallamine triethiodide is approximately equivalent to that of 15 milligrams of tubocurarine chloride; muscular relaxation occurs in about four minutes after intravenous injection and the effect passes off in about twenty minutes.

Gallamine triethiodide is not broken down in the body but is largely eliminated unchanged in the urine within two hours of intravenous injection.

In conjunction with light anaesthesia, gallamine triethiodide is used to produce muscular relaxation during surgical procedures and operations and to reduce the risk of traumatic and other complications of electroconvulsive therapy. It is suitable for use with the usual anaesthetic agents, including nitrous oxide and oxygen, thiopentone sodium, ether, and cyclopropane.

Aqueous solutions of gallamine triethiodide are miscible with those of thiopentone sodium, and the two solutions may be injected simultaneously from the same syringe if desired.

For short operative procedures, 60 to 80 milligrams may be given by intravenous injection to an adult; subsequently, smaller doses, such as 40 milligrams, may be given if required, up to a total dose not exceeding 160 milligrams.

UNDESIRABLE EFFECTS. The most important undesirable effect is tachycardia, which may develop within one minute of intravenous injection and persist for longer than the relaxant effect of the drug.

PRECAUTIONS AND CONTRA-INDICATIONS. Gallamine triethiodide is contra-indicated in myasthenia gravis and should be used with care in patients with impaired renal function, hypertension, or cardiac insufficiency.

POISONING. Assisted respiration with adequate oxygenation should be instituted. Facilities for this should always be available where muscle relaxants are used. Neostigmine methylsulphate should be given intravenously in doses of 2.5 to 5 milligrams; 0.5 to 1 milligram of atropine sulphate should be given at the same time and repeated if necessary. A similar procedure may be used to terminate muscular relaxation at the end of an operation, but in this case atropine should be given fifteen minutes before neostigmine.

Dose. The dose is determined by the physician in accordance with the needs of the patient.

Preparation

GALLAMINE INJECTION, B.P. It consists of a sterile solution of gallamine triethiodide in Water for Injections containing 0.2 per cent of sodium sulphite. The strength of the solution should be specified by the prescriber. It should be protected from light. Ampoules containing 40 mg per ml are available.

OTHER NAME: *Flaxedil*®

GAMMA BENZENE HEXACHLORIDE

$C_6H_6Cl_6 = 290.8$

Gamma Benzene Hexachloride is the γ-isomer of 1,2,3,4,5,6-hexachlorocyclohexane.

Solubility. Insoluble in water; soluble, at 20°, in 19 parts of dehydrated alcohol, in 5.5 parts of ether, and in 2 parts of acetone.

Standard

It complies with the requirements of the British Pharmacopoeia.

It is a white crystalline powder with a slight odour. It has a crystallising-point not lower than 112.0°. It contains not less than 99.0 per cent of $C_6H_6Cl_6$.

Storage. It should be protected from light.

Actions and uses. Gamma benzene hexachloride is an acaricide, insecticide, and larvicide. It has a more rapid action than dicophane (page 157) and is effective in lower concentrations, but as it is more volatile it has significantly less residual action.

Used as residual sprays, solutions in kerosene and other suitable solvents containing 0·1 to 0·5 per cent are lethal to dipterous flies, including house flies. Gamma benzene hexachloride may be combined with other insecticides, such as a pyrethrum extract, to obtain a more rapid lethal effect.

A 0·2 per cent alcoholic solution or a 0·1 per cent application is effective against head lice, and a 1 per cent emulsion is employed in the treatment of scabies.

The development of resistant strains has been reported in species of insects which are normally susceptible.

UNDESIRABLE EFFECTS. Gamma benzene hexachloride is not especially toxic when applied externally in the concentrations usually employed, but when ingested it may cause convulsions.

POISONING. In cases of acute poisoning, a short-acting barbiturate should be administered to control convulsions and, as gamma benzene hexachloride is only slowly excreted, phenobarbitone should be administered for several days.

Preparation
GAMMA BENZENE HEXACHLORIDE APPLICATION, B.P.C. (page 649)

OTHER NAME: *Lorexane*®

GELATIN

Gelatin is the protein obtained by extraction from collagenous material.

Gelatin is obtained by boiling animal tissues, such as skins, tendons, ligaments, and bones, with water, skimming and straining the resulting liquid, evaporating the solution at a low temperature after purification, and drying by exposure to the air.

The viscosity of solutions and the strength and melting-point of jellies prepared from different batches of gelatin may vary. These variations are dependent on the source of the material and on the process used to prepare the gelatins.

Grading is usually by jelly strength, expressed as a "Bloom strength", which is the weight in grams which, when applied under controlled conditions to a plunger 12·7 mm in diameter, will produce a depression exactly 4 mm deep in a matured jelly containing 6·66 per cent w/w of gelatin in water.

The British Pharmacopoeia specifies a jelly strength of not less than 150 g, which is suitable for most pharmaceutical work, but grades are available giving lower and higher figures, up to 230 g. High jelly strength is preferable for gelatin capsules and for bacteriological culture media, in the latter case to allow for the inevitable lowering of the melting-point during sterilisation.

Solubility. Insoluble in cold water, but swells and softens when immersed, gradually absorbing five to ten times its own weight of water; soluble in hot water, in mixtures of glycerol and water, and in acetic acid; insoluble in alcohol, in ether, and in chloroform.

Standard
It complies with the requirements of the British Pharmacopoeia.
It occurs as colourless or pale yellowish, translucent sheets, shreds, powder, or granules, with a slight odour. A warm 5 per cent w/v solution in water is free from objectionable taste and offensive odour.

A solution of gelatin in water yields no precipitate with acids, except chromic and tannic acids, is not affected by alum, lead acetate, or ferric chloride, but gives a precipitate with trinitrophenol. When heated with soda lime, ammonia is evolved.

On the addition of *mercury nitrate solution* to a solution of gelatin in water, a white precipitate is formed which develops a brick-red colour on warming. When potassium dichromate is added to a hot aqueous solution, the jelly which forms on cooling becomes insoluble in warm water after exposure to light.

Formaldehyde renders gelatin hard and insoluble after drying.

Gelatin which has been softened by immersion in cold water dissolves when the water is heated, forming a viscous liquid which sets to a jelly on cooling; this property is much less marked after prolonged heating of the solution.

Stability. It is stable in air when dry, but putrefies rapidly when moist or in solution.

Sterilisation. It is sterilised by dry heat.

Storage. It should be stored in airtight containers.

Uses. Gelatin is an ingredient of pastilles, pastes, pessaries, bougies, and glycerol suppositories. Solutions containing 0·5 to 0·7 per cent of gelatin in an isotonic vehicle containing a suitable bactericide may be used as artifical tears.

Gelatin is used as the main constituent of hard and flexible capsule shells. It is also used for the micro-encapsulation of drugs and flavouring agents.

Highly purified and pyrogen-free grades of gelatin have been used in intravenous injections, either as a substitute for plasma or to emulsify fat ("feeding emulsions").

A solution of hydrolysed gelatin is used as a vehicle in Corticotrophin Gelatin Injection.

In the form of Absorbable Gelatin Sponge, gelatin is used as a haemostatic.

When preparations containing gelatin are to

be applied to abraded surfaces, the material should be sterilised, but prolonged heating reduces the strength of the gel.

Preparation

GLYCEROL SUPPOSITORIES, B.P. (*Syn.* Glycerin Suppositories). Each suppository contains about 14 per cent w/w of gelatin and 70 per cent w/w of glycerol.

ABSORBABLE GELATIN SPONGE

SYNONYM: Gelatin Sponge

Absorbable Gelatin Sponge is a sterile, absorbable, water-insoluble gelatin-base sponge. It may be prepared by whisking a warm solution of gelatin to a uniform foam and drying.

Solubility. Insoluble in water.

Standard

It complies with the requirements of the British Pharmacopoeia.

It is a white or almost white, tough, light, finely porous, sponge-like material which may be wetted by kneading with moistened fingers.

It is completely digested by acid solutions of pepsin.

Sterilisation. It is sterilised by dry heat.

Storage. It should be stored in containers sealed to exclude micro-organisms. It cannot be satisfactorily resterilised and, if a portion only of the contents of a container is used on any one occasion, strict aseptic precautions should be taken to avoid contamination.

Actions and uses. Absorbable gelatin sponge is a haemostatic which depends for its action upon its physical structure. Owing to its porosity it is capable of absorbing many times its weight of blood.

When absorbable gelatin sponge is applied with pressure to a bleeding surface, the blood is absorbed and rapid clotting usually occurs. The mechanically supported coagulum adheres to the tissue surface and permits the formation of fibrin plugs at the underlying capillary ends. As it is not antigenic it may be left in a wound; it is completely absorbed in four to six weeks.

Although it is an effective haemostatic in capillary oozing or venous bleeding, the sponge should not be relied upon for the control of haemorrhage from the larger vessels.

Absorbable gelatin sponge may be used either in the dry state or moistened with normal saline, a solution of an antibiotic or, to accelerate clotting in the case of a defective clotting mechanism, a solution of thrombin (100 Units per ml). If it is to be used in the moistened condition, a piece of sponge is soaked in the chosen medium, squeezed to remove air and excess of solution, moulded with the fingers to the required shape, and then applied with firm pressure to the bleeding point or area until adherent.

The absence of any but very mild cellular reaction permits the use of absorbable gelatin sponge after all types of surgical procedure. In dental and oral surgery it is of value both as a haemostatic agent and in the obliteration of "dead space".

OTHER NAME: *Sterispon*®

GELSEMIUM

SYNONYMS: Gelsemium Root; Yellow Jasmine Root

Gelsemium consists of the dried rhizome and roots of *Gelsemium sempervirens* (L.) Ait. f. (Fam. Loganiaceae). The plant is indigenous to the southern United States and is obtained chiefly from Virginia, North and South Carolina, and Tennessee.

Constituents. Gelsemium contains up to 0·5 per cent of related alkaloids of the indole type, including crystalline gelsemine and sempervirine. Smaller amounts of gelsemicine and gelsedine (crystalline substances) occur and also a non-crystalline alkaloid, gelseverine.

Gelsemium also contains β-methylaesculetin, pentatriacontane and the monomethyl ether of emodin.

Standard for unground drug

DESCRIPTION. *Macroscopical:* Rhizome usually in straight, almost cylindrical pieces 5 to 20 cm long and 3 to 30 mm thick, with attached large roots or small fibrous roots and sometimes small portions of slender aerial stems of a dark purplish colour; rhizome light yellowish-brown externally, longitudinally wrinkled, older pieces with purple reticulated lines; internally light brown or pale yellow; fracture tough and splintery; smoothed, transversely cut surface showing conspicuously and finely radiate structure of xylem in narrow yellowish wedges alternating with straight whitish medullary rays; pith small, disintegrated, bordered by 4 strands of intraxylary phloem.

Root closely resembling rhizome but somewhat tortuous, and uniformly light brown.

Surface of drug when scraped or broken exhibiting a marked blue fluorescence when exposed to filtered ultraviolet light.

Odour faintly aromatic; taste slightly bitter.

Microscopical: the diagnostic characters are: Rhizome: *cork cells* in several layers, with thin walls, *cortex* very narrow, parenchymatous, containing *starch* granules 4 to 12 μm in diameter, *pericycle* with *sclereids* singly or in groups of 2 to 12, the cells measuring about 28 to 60 μm, and unlignified *fibres*, about 350 to 400 μm long and 60 to 90 μm wide; prismatic *crystals* of calcium oxalate, up to 30 μm long, in the medullary rays of the phloem; *xylem* wide, radiate, *vessels* about 60 to 90 μm in diameter, embedded in dense mass of lignified *tracheids; medullary ray cells* with lignified walls and containing small *starch* granules 4 to 8 μm in diameter; *pith* small, with 4 groups of *intraxylary phloem*.

Root: *cork cells* in several layers, *secondary phloem* in narrow band as in rhizome, *starch* granules 4 to 8 μm in diameter present in medullary rays of xylem and all parenchymatous tissues.

Aerial stem: *cork* in up to 20 layers, cells very regular and rectangular, about 14 to 21 μm by 17 to 37 μm; *cortex* narrow, *pericycle* with unlignified *fibres* singly or in groups of 2 to about 18; *phloem* and *xylem* as in rhizome; *pith* wide.

FOREIGN ORGANIC MATTER. Not more than 2·0 per cent.

CONTENT OF TOTAL ALKALOIDS. Not less than 0·32 per cent, calculated as gelsemine, $C_{20}H_{22}N_2O_2$, determined by the following method:

Introduce about 10 g of the root, in No. 250 powder, accurately weighed, into a stoppered flask of about 300-ml capacity, add 100 ml of a mixture of 3 volumes of *solvent ether* and 1 volume of *chloroform*, shake well, and allow to stand for 10 minutes; add 5 ml of *dilute ammonia solution* and shake for one minute at 10-minute intervals during one hour.

Transfer the mixture to a small percolator plugged with cotton wool and allow the liquid to percolate into a pear-shaped separator; when the liquid ceases to flow, pack the drug firmly and continue the percolation with further portions of the solvent until extraction of the alkaloids is complete, testing the percolate for complete extraction by collecting separately 2 ml in a dish, evaporating off the solvent, dissolving the residue in 0·2 ml of 0·1N sulphuric acid and adding 0·05 ml of 0·1N iodine; in the absence of alkaloids no precipitate or turbidity is formed.

To the percolate add 30 ml of 1N sulphuric acid, shake well, allow to separate, and run off the lower layer; continue the extraction with successive 10-ml portions of 0·1N sulphuric acid until extraction is complete, as shown by the iodine test.

Wash the mixed acid solutions with 10 ml of *chloroform*, transfer the washings to a second separator containing 20 ml of 0·1N sulphuric acid, shake, allow to separate, and discard the chloroform; repeat the washing of the liquid in the first separator with two further 5-ml portions of *chloroform*, transfer each in turn to the second separator, wash with the same aqueous acid liquid, allow to separate, and discard the chloroform layer as before.

Transfer the acid liquid from the second separator to the first separator, make just alkaline to *litmus paper* with *dilute ammonia solution* and add a further 2 ml; shake with successive portions of *chloroform* until ex-

traction is complete, washing each chloroform extract with the same 20 ml of water contained in another separator.

Evaporate off the chloroform, add to the residue 2 ml of *dehydrated alcohol*, evaporate, and dry at 60° for 30 minutes.

Dissolve the residue in 2 ml of *alcohol (95 per cent)*, add 5 ml of 0·05N sulphuric acid and 10 ml of water, cool, titrate the excess of acid with 0·05N sodium hydroxide, using *methyl red solution* as indicator; each ml of 0·05N sulphuric acid is equivalent to 0·01612 g of $C_{20}H_{22}N_2O_2$.

Standard for powdered drug: Powdered Gelsemium

DESCRIPTION. A light yellowish-brown powder possessing the diagnostic microscopical characters, odour, and taste of the unground drug.

FOREIGN ORGANIC MATTER; CONTENT OF TOTAL ALKALOIDS. It complies with the requirements for the unground drug.

Actions and uses. Gelsemium depresses the central nervous system and has been used mainly in the treatment of trigeminal neuralgia and migraine. It is administered as the tincture, which may be given in admixture with other sedatives.

UNDESIRABLE EFFECTS. Large doses of gelsemium cause giddiness, double vision, and respiratory depression.

POISONING. In cases of poisoning by gelsemium or its alkaloids, gastric lavage or an emetic should be employed, followed by subcutaneous injection of atropine and administration of stimulants. Artificial respiration should be applied if necessary.

Dose. 15 to 60 milligrams.

Preparations
GELSEMIUM AND HYOSCYAMUS MIXTURE, COMPOUND, B.P.C. (page 743)
GELSEMIUM TINCTURE, B.P.C. (page 822)

GENTAMICIN SULPHATE

Gentamicin Sulphate is a mixture of the sulphates of the antimicrobial substances produced by *Micromonospora purpurea*.

Solubility. Soluble in water; insoluble in alcohol, in ether, and in chloroform.

Standard
It complies with the requirements of the British Pharmacopoeia.

It is a white to cream-coloured powder and contains not less than 590 Units per mg, calculated with reference to the anhydrous substance. It contains not more than 15·0 per cent w/w of water. A 4 per cent solution in water has a pH of 3·5 to 5·5.

Storage. It should be stored in airtight containers.

Actions and uses. Gentamicin is an antibiotic which is effective against a wide range of Gram-positive and Gram-negative bacteria, including *Staphylococcus aureus*, *Streptococcus pyogenes*, species of *Pseudomonas* and *Proteus*, and many coliform bacilli.

Resistance may develop, especially among Gram-negative organisms, and cross-resistance with other antibiotics such as kanamycin,

neomycin, and paromomycin may occur. To delay the development of resistance, gentamicin can be given in conjunction with carbenicillin for the treatment of infections that are sensitive to both these antibiotics.

As gentamicin is not absorbed when given by mouth it is administered by injection. Peak blood levels are attained about thirty minutes after administration by intramuscular injection and levels remain high for approximately two hours and fall towards zero in eight hours. Approximately 30 per cent of the dose is temporarily inactivated by protein binding. As free gentamicin is excreted through the kidney, high antibacterial concentrations are reached in the urine, but the drug cumulates where there is renal impairment.

The usual dosage is 400 to 800 Units per kilogram body-weight every eight hours by intramuscular injection; it may also be administered by intravenous injection. Serum concentrations above 10 Units per millilitre should be avoided, because of the potential toxicity of the drug, and it should only be used against organisms sensitive to much lower concentrations. Treatment should not be continued for more than seven days.

UNDESIRABLE EFFECTS. Hearing loss and vestibular damage may occur and may be permanent. Patients whose serum concentrations have exceeded 10 Units per millilitre may show acute tubular damage with impairment of renal function, which may be irreversible. Allergic rashes and fevers may occur but seldom interfere with the treatment of patients who have not received the drug previously. Topical application of gentamicin may give rise to local allergy.

PRECAUTIONS AND CONTRA-INDICATIONS. Gentamicin should only be used in pregnancy or infancy if no safer treatment is available.

Dose. See above under **Actions and uses.**

Preparations
GENTAMICIN INJECTION, B.P. It consists of a sterile solution of gentamicin sulphate in Water for Injections containing suitable stabilising agents. When gentamicin injection is prescribed for intramuscular use, unless otherwise specified, a solution containing 80,000 Units in 2 ml is supplied.

GENTAMICIN OINTMENT, B.P.C. (page 761)

OTHER NAMES: *Cidomycin®*; *Genticin®*

GENTIAN

SYNONYMS: Gentian Root; Gentianae Radix

Gentian consists of the dried rhizome and root of *Gentiana lutea* L. (Fam. Gentianaceae), a herbaceous perennial indigenous to central Europe, Yugoslavia, France, and Spain. The rhizome and root are collected from the end of May to the beginning of October. The fresh rhizome and root are yellowish-white internally, but become darker during the drying process, when partial fermentation occurs and the characteristic odour of the drug is developed.

Constituents. The fresh drug contains about 2 per cent of the bitter glycoside gentiopicroside (also known as gentiamarin and gentiopicrin), which yields on hydrolysis the lactone gentiogenin and glucose; it is decomposed during the drying of the drug. The trisaccharide gentianose and the disaccharides gentiobiose (about 2 per cent) and sucrose are present, together with pectin and fixed oil. The sugars are partially hydrolysed during slow drying into glucose and fructose. A number of enzymes, including emulsin, gentiobiase, an oxidase, and a peroxidase have been identified. The alkaloids gentianine and gentialutine [4-(2-hydroxyethyl)-3-vinylpyridine], in total amount about 0·03 per cent, are also present in the root. The dried root contains, in addition, the glycoside gentioside (3-*p*-primeverosidoisogentisin), the flavonoid gentisin (1,7-dihydroxy-3-methoxyxanthone), other xanthone colouring matters, and gentisic acid (2,5-dihydroxybenzoic acid).
Gentian yields to water 33 to 40 per cent of extractive; over-fermented gentian root may yield to cold water as little as 13 per cent of extractive.

Standard
It complies with the requirements of the European Pharmacopoeia.
It contains not less than 33 per cent of water-soluble extractive.

UNGROUND DRUG. *Macroscopical characters:* subcylindrical pieces either entire or split longitudinally, from 15 to 20 cm or more long and from 0·3 to 4·0 cm thick, occasionally up to 8 cm at the crown; outer surface of rhizome and root yellowish-brown to dark brown; root longitudinally wrinkled; rhizome occasionally branched, frequently terminating in a bud and bearing numerous encircling leaf-scars appearing as transverse annulations. When moist, tough and flexible, when dry brittle, breaking with a short fracture; smoothed, transversely cut surface reddish-yellow, well-marked cambium showing as a dark ring separating a moderately wide bark from a large, mainly parenchymatous xylem lacking a distinctly radiate structure.
Odour characteristic; taste sweet at first, afterwards intensely bitter.

Microscopical characters: the diagnostic characters are: *cork cells* yellowish-brown; *parenchyma* abundant, with moderately thickened walls, containing small *oil globules* and in some cells *crystals* of calcium oxalate either as minute needles or slender prisms about 3 to 6 μm long; *vessels* infrequent, with reticulate wall pitting or annular or spiral thickening; *starch* granules small, rounded, very infrequent; *fibres* and *sclereids* absent.

POWDERED DRUG: Powdered Gentian. A light brown or yellowish-brown powder possessing the diagnostic microscopical characters, odour, and taste of the unground drug.

Incompatibility. It is incompatible with iron salts.

Storage. It should be stored in a dry place, protected from light.

Actions and uses. Gentian is a bitter and is used to stimulate the appetite. It is usually administered as the compound infusion or compound tincture.

Preparations
GENTIAN INFUSION, COMPOUND, B.P. It contains Concentrated Compound Gentian Infusion, 1 in 10. It should be used within twelve hours of its preparation. Dose: 15 to 40 millilitres.

GENTIAN INFUSION, COMPOUND, CONCENTRATED, B.P. It is prepared from gentian, about 1 to 10, dried bitter-orange peel, dried lemon peel, and alcohol (25 per cent). Dose: 1·5 to 4 millilitres.

GENTIAN MIXTURE, ACID, B.P.C. (page 743)

GENTIAN MIXTURE, ACID, WITH NUX VOMICA, B.P.C. (page 743)

GENTIAN MIXTURE, ALKALINE, B.P.C. (page 743)

GENTIAN MIXTURE, ALKALINE, WITH NUX VOMICA, B.P.C. (page 744)

GENTIAN MIXTURE, ALKALINE, WITH PHENOBARBITONE, B.P.C. (page 744)

GENTIAN AND RHUBARB MIXTURE, B.P.C. (page 744)

GENTIAN TINCTURE, COMPOUND, B.P.C. (page 822)

GINGER

Synonym: Zingiber

Ginger consists of the rhizome of *Zingiber officinale* Roscoe (Fam. Zingiberaceae), scraped to remove the dark outer layer and dried in the sun. It is known in commerce as unbleached Jamaica ginger. The plant is indigenous to Asia, but is cultivated in the West Indies, Africa, Australia, and Taiwan.

Constituents. Ginger contains about 1 to 2 per cent of volatile oil, of which the sesquiterpene zingiberene is the principal constituent and in which many other terpenes and terpene alcohols have been reported.

The pungency of ginger is due to gingerol, a yellowish oily substance which is a mixture of homologues of zingerone (4-hydroxy-3-methoxyphenethyl methyl ketone) condensed with saturated aliphatic aldehydes, principally *n*-heptaldehyde, and to shogaol, in which the ketone is condensed with hexaldehyde to give an unsaturated side-chain.

Ginger also contains resin and much starch.

Standard
It complies with the requirements of the British Pharmacopoeia.

Unground drug. *Macroscopical characters:* rhizomes known as "races" or "hands", laterally compressed, sometimes broken, bearing short, flattened, obovate, oblique branches on upper side ("fingers"), about 2 cm in length, each having at its apex a depressed stem scar; pieces about 5 to 15 cm long, 1·5 to 6·5 (usually 3 to 4) cm wide, and 1 to 1·5 cm thick; external surface buff-coloured, longitudinally striated, and with occasional loose fibres; fracture short, with projecting fibres; smoothed, transversely cut surface exhibiting a narrow cortex separated by an endodermis from a much wider stele, numerous scattered vascular bundles and scattered oil cells with yellow contents.

Odour agreeable and aromatic; taste strongly pungent.

Microscopical characters: the diagnostic characters are: *starch* abundant in the thin-walled cells of the ground tissue, granules simple, flattened, ovate to subrectangular, with hilum frequently in a terminal projection, mostly up to 50 μm long and up to about 25 μm wide and 7 μm thick; *oil cells* with cutinised walls and yellow contents, numerous in ground tissue; *tannin cells* with dark, reddish-brown contents occurring either singly in the ground tissue or in axial rows accompanying the vascular bundles; *vessels* with spiral or reticulate thickening in the scattered *vascular bundles* showing no reaction for lignin; unlignified *fibres* with delicate transverse septa; *cork*, *sclereids*, and calcium oxalate *crystals* absent.

Powdered drug: Powdered Ginger. A light yellow powder possessing the diagnostic microscopical characters, odour, and taste of the unground drug.

Adulterants and substitutes. Jamaica ginger is sometimes limed to whiten it and is then known as "limed" ginger.

Cochin and Calicut gingers are in smaller "hands" and the branches are usually shorter and thicker; they are often imported only partly scraped ("unscraped" or "coated") and may be bleached (limed) or unbleached.

African ginger is more pungent but less aromatic; it is usually small, dark, and coated, but may also be found limed.

Nigerian ginger is obtained from *Z. officinale*; it is rather less aromatic than Jamaica ginger.

Japanese ginger is commonly in small flattened pieces; many of the starch granules are compound and the oil differs in its physical characters (weight per ml at 20° about 0·804 g; optical rotation about +9°), these particulars indicating that it is not produced by *Z. officinale*; it has been referred to *Z. mioga* Roscoe.

Ground ginger is often adulterated with exhausted ("spent") ginger, a sophistication that may be detected by a diminution in the water-soluble ash, as well as by the yields of alcohol-soluble and water-soluble extractives.

Storage. It should be stored in a cool dry place. Powdered Ginger should be stored in airtight containers, in a cool place.

Actions and uses. Ginger is a carminative and a flavouring agent.

Preparations
Rhubarb Powder, Compound, B.P.C. (page 778)
Ginger Syrup, B.P.C. (page 800)
Magnesium Carbonate Tablets, Compound, B.P.C. (page 812)
Ginger Tincture, Strong, B.P. (*Syn.* Essence of Ginger). It is prepared from ginger, 1 in 2, and alcohol (90 per cent). Dose: 0·25 to 0·5 ml.
Ginger Tincture, Weak, B.P. (*Syn.* Ginger Tincture). It contains Strong Ginger Tincture, 1 in 5, in alcohol (90 per cent). Dose: 1·5 to 3 ml.

GLUTETHIMIDE

$C_{13}H_{15}NO_2 = 217·3$

Glutethimide is α-ethyl-α-phenylglutarimide.

Solubility. Insoluble in water; soluble, at 20°, in 5 parts of alcohol, in 12 parts of ether, and in less than 1 part of chloroform; slightly soluble in light petroleum.

Standard
It complies with the requirements of the British Pharmacopoeia.

It occurs as odourless colourless crystals or white powder and contains not less than 99·0 per cent of $C_{13}H_{15}NO_2$, calculated with reference to the dried substance. The loss on drying under the prescribed conditions is not more than 1·0 per cent. It has a melting-point of 85° to 88°.

Storage. It should be stored in airtight containers, protected from light.

Actions and uses. Glutethimide has a hypnotic action closely resembling that of an intermediate-acting barbiturate, as described under Phenobarbitone (page 366). Sleep lasting for four to six hours is produced within about twenty minutes by an oral dose of 250 to 500 milligrams of glutethimide.

UNDESIRABLE EFFECTS. Glutethimide may produce nausea, dizziness, and, occasionally, skin rashes and mental excitement. It may give rise to dependence of the barbiturate-alcohol type as described under Phenobarbitone (page 366) and it may enhance the effects of alcohol.

Dose. 250 to 500 milligrams.

Preparation
GLUTETHIMIDE TABLETS, B.P. Unless otherwise specified, tablets each containing 250 mg of glutethimide are supplied. They should be stored in airtight containers, protected from light.

OTHER NAME: *Doriden*®

GLYCEROL

SYNONYM: Glycerin

$C_3H_8O_3 = 92 \cdot 09$

$$CH_2OH \cdot CH(OH) \cdot CH_2OH$$

Glycerol is propane-1,2,3-triol and may be obtained by the hydrolysis of fats and fixed oils or by synthesis.

Solubility. Miscible with water and with alcohol; insoluble in ether, in chloroform, and in fixed oils.

Standard
It complies with the requirements of the British Pharmacopoeia.
It is a clear, colourless, hygroscopic, syrupy, odourless liquid. It has a weight per ml at 20° of 1·255 g to 1·260 g, corresponding to 98·0 to 100·0 per cent of $C_3H_8O_3$. A 10 per cent solution in water is neutral to litmus.
When kept at a low temperature for some time, it solidifies to a mass of colourless crystals which melt at about 20°.

Sterilisation. It is sterilised by dry heat.

Storage. It should be stored in airtight containers.

Actions and uses. Given by mouth, glycerol is demulcent; it is an ingredient of some linctuses and pastilles and is used as a sweetening agent in mixtures. It absorbs moisture when applied undiluted to mucous membranes. It promotes peristalsis when administered by rectum, doses of 4 to 16 millilitres being given undiluted as an enema; Glycerol Suppositories are also used for this purpose. It is used as a water-retaining and emollient ingredient in dermatological preparations, toilet creams, and jellies. Glycerol, with dried magnesium sulphate, in the form of Magnesium Sulphate Paste, is used in the treatment of septic wounds and boils.

Some surgeons prefer sterile glycerol to liquid paraffin for lubricating gastroscopes and similar instruments.

Glycerol is used as a preservative in some pharmaceutical preparations, but a concentration of at least 20 per cent is needed.

Preparations
PHENOL EAR-DROPS, B.P.C. (page 665)
ICHTHAMMOL GLYCERIN, B.P.C. (page 701)
PHENOL GLYCERIN, B.P.C. (page 701)
TANNIC ACID GLYCERIN, B.P.C. (page 702)
THYMOL GLYCERIN, COMPOUND, B.P.C. (page 702)
MAGNESIUM SULPHATE PASTE, B.P.C. (page 767)
GLYCEROL SUPPOSITORIES, B.P. (*Syn.* Glycerin Suppositories). Each suppository contains about 70 per cent w/w of glycerol.

GLYCERYL TRINITRATE SOLUTION

SYNONYMS: Glyc. Trinit. Soln.; Nitroglycerin Solution; Trinitrin Solution

Glyceryl Trinitrate Solution is a solution, in alcohol (90 per cent), of glyceryl trinitrate, $CH_2(O \cdot NO_2) \cdot CH(O \cdot NO_2) \cdot CH_2(O \cdot NO_2) = 227 \cdot 1$. Glyceryl trinitrate is a colourless liquid which when undiluted explodes on rapid heating or concussion.

Standard
DESCRIPTION. A clear colourless liquid.

IDENTIFICATION TESTS. 1. Mix 10 ml with 20 ml of water; a turbid mixture is produced which deposits glyceryl trinitrate on standing.
2. Mix 5 ml with 0·5 ml of *sodium hydroxide solution*, allow to stand for one hour, and add 5 ml of *potassium iodide solution* and 5 ml of *dilute sulphuric acid*; iodine is liberated and brown fumes are evolved.
3. It is neutral to *litmus solution*.

WEIGHT PER ML. At 20°, 0·829 g to 0·838 g.

ALCOHOL CONTENT. 88 to 90 per cent v/v of ethyl alcohol, determined by the method given in Appendix 10, page 888.

CONTENT OF $C_3H_5N_3O_9$. 0·9 to 1·1 per cent w/v, determined by the following method:
Mix 5 ml with 0·5 ml of *sodium hydroxide solution* and allow to stand for one hour; introduce into a brine-charged nitrometer, rinsing the nitrometer funnel with small quantities of *alcohol (90 per cent)*, add 5 ml of *potassium iodide solution* and 5 ml of *dilute sulphuric acid*, shake briskly at intervals for 5 minutes, and measure the volume of nitric oxide produced; each ml of moist nitric oxide, at 20° and normal pressure, is equivalent to 0·0050 g of $C_3H_5N_3O_9$.

Storage. It should be stored in airtight containers, protected from light, in a cool place.

Actions and uses. Glyceryl trinitrate causes the relaxation of involuntary muscle. Its effects are most pronounced on the circulatory system; the arterioles dilate and, with therapeutic doses, the systolic blood pressure falls by 10 to 25 millimetres of mercury. The onset of its effect is delayed for three to five minutes and its action lasts for thirty to forty minutes, but preparations with a prolonged action are available. Tolerance may develop with daily use; withdrawal for a week re-establishes the original sensitivity.

Glyceryl Trinitrate Solution is used chiefly in the prophylaxis and treatment of angina of effort, in which it affords relief by the dilatation of the collateral coronary vessels; it is contra-indicated in coronary thrombosis. It is also used for the relief of renal and gall-bladder colic.

Glyceryl Trinitrate Solution is administered in tablets which should be allowed to dissolve in the mouth, since the drug is more effectively absorbed from the oral mucosa than from the stomach; long-acting tablets are, however, intended to be swallowed.

POISONING. The patient should be placed in a recumbent position with the legs elevated and oxygen, alone or with 5 per cent of carbon dioxide, given. Artificial respiration may be necessary. A sympathomimetic vasoconstrictor may be given to restore the blood pressure.

Dose. 0·05 to 0·1 millilitre, equivalent to 0·5 to 1 milligram of glyceryl trinitrate.

Preparation

GLYCERYL TRINITRATE TABLETS, B.P. (*Syn.* Nitroglycerin Tablets; Trinitrin Tablets). Unless otherwise specified, tablets each containing 500 µg of glyceryl trinitrate are supplied. They should be stored in airtight containers, protected from light, in a cool, dry place; under these conditions they may be expected to be suitable for use for at least two years from the date of preparation, which is stated on the label. The tablets should be allowed to dissolve in the mouth. Tablets containing 300 and 600 µg of glyceryl trinitrate are also available.

GOLD (^{198}Au) INJECTION

This material is radioactive and any regulations in force must be complied with.

Gold (^{198}Au) Injection is a sterile colloidal solution of gold-198 stabilised with gelatin. It may be prepared by reducing a salt of gold-198 with a suitable reducing agent, such as dextrose in alkaline solution, in the presence of gelatin.

Gold-198 is a radioactive isotope of gold which emits β- and γ- radiation and has a half-life of 2·7 days; it may be prepared by the neutron irradiation of gold.

Standard

It complies with the requirements of the British Pharmacopoeia.

It is a deep red colloidal solution and contains not less than 90·0 and not more than 110·0 per cent of the quantity of gold-198 stated on the label at the date and hour stated on the label. It has a pH of 4·0 to 8·0. About 80 per cent of the radioactivity is present in particles between 5 and 50 nm in diameter, unless a narrower range within these limits is prescribed or ordered.

Sterilisation. It is sterilised by heating in an autoclave.

Labelling. The label on the container states:
(1) the content of gold-198 expressed in microcuries or millicuries at a given date and hour;
(2) that the injection is radioactive; and
(3) that it does not contain a bactericide, or the name and proportion of any added bactericide.

The label on the package also states:
(1) the total volume in the container;
(2) the content of total gold;
(3) either that the proportion of gold-199 does not exceed 5 per cent, or the proportion of gold-199 when it exceeds 5 per cent; and
(4) the range of diameters, in nm, of the particles in which about 80 per cent of the radioactivity is present.

Storage. It should be stored in an area assigned for the purpose. The storage conditions should be such that the maximum radiation-dose-rate to which persons may be exposed is reduced to an acceptable level.

Glass containers may darken under the effects of the radiation.

Actions and uses. Gold (^{198}Au) Injection is used mainly to control malignant effusions in the peritoneal, pleural, or pericardial cavities. The usual dose is 75 millicuries for a pleural cavity or 130 millicuries for a peritoneal cavity, administered after most of the effusion has been aspirated; it is usual to attempt redistribution of the dense colloidal metal particles within the body cavity by subsequently tilting the patient.

The treatment, when successful, slows down or prevents fluid accumulation, and it may be repeated after an interval of about eight weeks. Gold (^{198}Au) Injection is also used by intralymphatic infiltration in the treatment of malignant melanoma involving the limbs or of lymph nodes involved by tumours of lymphoid tissue.

Gold (^{198}Au) Injection has also been used for diagnostic purposes such as the determination of liver blood flow, the estimation of reticuloendothelial activity, and scanning of the reticulo-endothelial system. It is also used for scanning the liver to delineate anatomical abnormalities.

Dose. In the treatment of neoplastic conditions, by intrapleural or intraperitoneal injection, 50 to 250 millicuries.

In the estimation of reticulo-endothelial activity and scanning of the reticulo-endothelial system, by intravenous injection, 10 to 100 microcuries.

For scanning the liver, by intravenous injection, 100 to 200 microcuries.

CHORIONIC GONADOTROPHIN

Chorionic Gonadotrophin is a dry sterile preparation of the gonad-stimulating substance obtained from the urine of pregnant women.

Chorionic Gonodotrophin may be prepared by the following method: the hormone is adsorbed from acidified urine on an ion-exchange resin, the resin is washed free from impurities, and the hormone is eluted from the resin with an alkaline solution and precipitated from the eluate by adjusting the acidity to pH 5 and adding sufficient dehydrated alcohol to give an alcohol concentration of about 80 per cent. The purified material obtained by this or any other suitable method is dissolved, sterilised by filtration, and dried under reduced pressure.

Solubility. Soluble in water.

Standard
It complies with the requirements of the British Pharmacopoeia.
It is a white or almost white powder and contains not less than 1500 Units per mg.

Storage. It should be stored in containers sealed to exclude micro-organisms, at a temperature not exceeding 20°, and protected from light. Under these conditions it may be expected to retain its potency for two years from the date of manufacture.

Actions and uses. The action of chorionic gonadotrophin differs from that of the gonadrotrophic hormone of the anterior pituitary gland. In the female, the action of the former is predominantly luteinising and that of the latter mainly follicle-stimulating. In the male, chorionic gonadotrophin stimulates the intersitial cells of the testes and consequently the secretion of androgens and the development of the secondary sexual characteristics.

The results of treatment with chorionic gonadotrophin are disappointing. In the female, it has been used in the treatment of metropathia haemorrhagica, in the preventive treatment of habitual abortion, and in secondary amenorrhoea. In the male, it has been used for the treatment of cryptorchidism.

Dose. 500 to 5000 Units by intramuscular injection twice weekly.

Preparation
CHORIONIC GONADOTROPHIN INJECTION, B.P. It consists of a sterile solution of chorionic gonadotrophin prepared immediately before use by dissolving the sterile contents of a sealed container in Water for Injections. The quantity of chorionic gonadotrophin in each container should be specified by the prescriber. Vials containing 100, 500, 1000, 1500 and 5000 Units are available.

OTHER NAMES: *Gonadotraphon LH®* ; *Pregnyl®*

GRISEOFULVIN

SYNONYM: Griseofulvinum

$C_{17}H_{17}ClO_6 = 352·8$

Griseofulvin is (+)-7-chloro-4,6-dimethoxycoumaran-3-one-2-spiro-1'-(2'-methoxy-6'-methylcyclohex-2'-en-4'-one), an antifungal substance produced by the growth of certain strains of *Penicillium griseofulvum*.

Solubility. Very slightly soluble in water; soluble, at 20°, in 300 parts of dehydrated alcohol, in 25 parts of chloroform, in 20 parts of acetone, in 250 parts of methyl alcohol, and in 3 parts of tetrachloroethane.

Standard
It complies with the requirements of the European Pharmacopoeia.
It is a white to pale cream, odourless or almost odourless powder, the particles of which are generally up to 5 μm in maximum dimension, although larger particles, which may occasionally exceed 30 μm may be present. It contains not less than 97·0 and not more than the equivalent of 102·0 per cent of $C_{17}H_{17}ClO_6$, calculated with reference to the dried substance. The loss on drying under the prescribed conditions is not more than 1·0 per cent. It has a melting-point of 218° to 224°.

Actions and uses. Griseofulvin is an antibiotic which when administered by mouth has an antifungal action against a wide range of dermatophytoses. After absorption from the gastro-intestinal tract, it is deposited in the keratin of the nails, hair, and skin, thus preventing fungal invasion of newly formed cells. Griseofulvin is effective against infections caused by various species of *Trichophyton*, *Epidermophyton*, and *Microsporum*, including ringworm and onychomycosis. It is ineffective against infections caused by yeasts or *Candida albicans* and against most systemic fungal infections.

The usual daily dosage is 0·5 to 1 gram for an adult and 500 milligrams for a child, in single or divided doses. For superficial forms of ringworm, treatment needs to be continued for three to six weeks, and for infections of the nails it may need to be continued for up to twelve months.

UNDESIRABLE EFFECTS. Headache, skin rashes, and gastro-intestinal disturbances may occur, but these are usually mild and transient and do not necessitate interruption of treatment.

Dose. 0·5 to 1 gram daily in single or divided doses.

Preparation

GRISEOFULVIN TABLETS, B.P. Unless otherwise specified, tablets each containing 125 mg of griseofulvin are supplied.

OTHER NAMES: *Fulcin®*; *Grisovin®*

GUAIPHENESIN

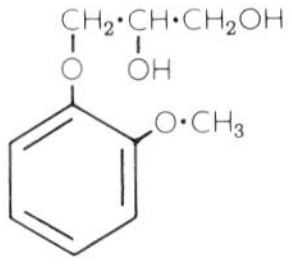

$C_{10}H_{14}O_4 = 198·2$

Guaiphenesin is 3-(*o*-methoxyphenoxy)propane-1,2-diol.

Solubility. Soluble, at 20°, in 33 parts of water, in 11 parts of alcohol, in 200 parts of ether, in 11 parts of chloroform, and in 15 parts of propylene glycol; soluble, with warming, in 15 parts of glycerol.

Standard

DESCRIPTION. White crystals or crystalline aggregates; odourless or almost odourless.

IDENTIFICATION TESTS. 1. The ultraviolet absorption spectrum exhibits the characteristics given in Appendix 3, page 855.

2. The infra-red absorption spectrum exhibits maxima which are only at the same wavelengths as, and have similar relative intensities to, those in the spectrum of *guaiphenesin A.S.*

ACIDITY. pH of a 2·0 per cent w/v solution in *carbon dioxide-free water*, 5·0 to 7·0.

MELTING-POINT. 80° to 82°.

CLARITY AND COLOUR OF SOLUTION. A 2 per cent w/v solution in water is clear and colourless.

GUAIACOL. Dissolve 0·10 g by warming with 10 ml of water. Cool, add 25 ml of water, 1 ml of *nitroaniline solution* and 0·5 ml of 0·1M sodium nitrite, and mix well; exactly 30 seconds after the addition of the sodium nitrite add 3 ml of an 8 per cent w/v solution of *sodium hydroxide* in water, mix, and dilute to 50 ml with water; the colour produced is not more intense than that produced when a mixture of 4 ml of a 0·0005 per cent w/v solution of *guaiacol* and 6 ml of water is similarly treated (200 parts per million).

LOSS ON DRYING. Not more than 0·5 per cent, determined by drying for 24 hours over *phosphorous pentoxide* in vacuo.

SULPHATED ASH. Not more than 0·1 per cent.

CONTENT OF $C_{10}H_{14}O_4$. Not less than 99·0 per cent, calculated with reference to the substance dried under the prescribed conditions, determined by the following method:

Heat about 2 g, accurately weighed, under a reflux condenser on a water-bath for 2 hours with 20 ml of a 15 per cent v/v solution of *acetic anhydride* in *pyridine*, cool, add 40 ml of water, and titrate with 1N sodium hydroxide, using a 1 per cent w/v solution of *phenolphthalein* in *pyridine* as indicator. Repeat the procedure omitting the sample.

The difference between the titrations represents the amount of acetic anhydride required by the sample; each ml of 1N sodium hydroxide is equivalent to 0·09911 g of $C_{10}H_{14}O_4$.

Actions and uses. Guaiphenesin reduces the viscosity of tenacious sputum and is used as an expectorant in cough mixtures and tablets. In large doses, it has a muscle-relaxant effect similar to that of mephenesin, but it is not used for this purpose.

Dose. 100 to 200 milligrams every two to four hours.

GUANETHIDINE SULPHATE

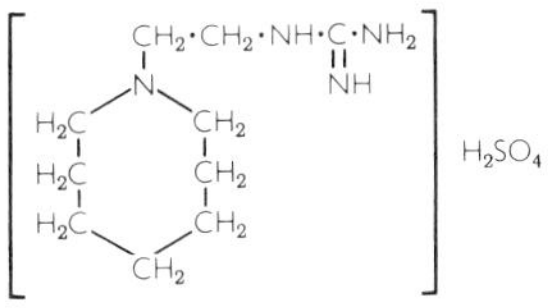

$C_{10}H_{24}N_4O_4S = 296·4$

Guaneth dine Sulphate is 1-(2-guanidinoethyl)azacyclo-octane sulphate.

Solubility. Soluble, at 20°, in 1·5 parts of water; slightly soluble in alcohol; insoluble in ether and in chloroform.

Standard

It complies with the requirements of the British Pharmacopoeia.

It is a colourless, crystalline, almost odourless powder and contains not less than 99·0 and not more than the equivalent of 101·0 per cent of $C_{10}H_{24}N_4O_4S$, calculated with reference to the dried substance. The loss on drying under the prescribed conditions is not more than 0·5 per cent. A 2 per cent solution in water has a pH of 5·0 to 6·0.

Sterilisation. Solutions for injection are sterilised by heating in an autoclave or by filtration.

Storage. It should be stored in airtight containers, protected from light.

Actions and uses. Guanethidine is a hypotensive agent which lowers the blood pressure by selectively blocking transmission in post-ganglionic adrenergic nerves, thus preventing the release of noradrenaline from the nerve endings.

It does not reduce, but may enhance, the effects of injected adrenaline and noradrenaline, and does not prevent the release of these amines from the suprarenal medulla; it may therefore cause a rise in blood pressure in patients with phaeochromocytoma.

Guanethidine is used to control hypertension. Treatment is started with an oral dosage of 10 to 30 milligrams of guanethidine sulphate daily, and this is increased by 10 milligrams every five to seven days, to a maximum which rarely exceeds 75 milligrams, until the desired reduction in blood pressure is attained.

Doses of 10 to 20 milligrams may be given by intramuscular injection to control hypertensive crises; the resulting fall in blood pressure usually reaches a maximum in one to two hours.

The effect of the drug may persist for several days after withdrawal. Tolerance rarely develops. A thiazide diuretic may be given with guanethidine to enhance the hypotensive effect.

Guanethidine is also used as eye-drops for the reduction of intra-ocular pressure and for the treatment of exophthalmos and lid retraction due to endocrine imbalance.

In addition to the tablets, guanethidine sulphate is available as a solution for injection containing 10 milligrams in 1 millilitre, and as eye-drops containing 5 per cent w/v.

UNDESIRABLE EFFECTS. Severe postural hypotension, especially with exercise, and diarrhoea may occur.

PRECAUTIONS. Guanethidine should not be given to patients who are being treated with a monoamine-oxidase inhibitor, such as isocarboxazid, nialamide, phenelzine, or tranylcypromine, or within about ten days of the discontinuation of such treatment.

Dose. See above under **Actions and uses**.

Preparation
GUANETHIDINE TABLETS, B.P. Unless otherwise specified, tablets each containing 10 mg of guanethidine sulphate are supplied. They should be stored in airtight containers, protected from light. Tablets containing 25 mg are also available.

OTHER NAME: *Ismelin*®

HALIBUT-LIVER OIL

Halibut-liver Oil is the fixed oil obtained from the fresh or suitably preserved livers of the halibut species belonging to the genus *Hippoglossus* (Fam. Pleuronectidae). It may be obtained by treatment of the livers with weak alkali and separation of the oil.

Constituents. Halibut livers yield oils with vitamin-A activities varying from about 15,000 to 250,000 Units per g. The antirachitic activity (vitamin D) is less variable, being usually between 2500 and 3500 Units per g. The composition of the fatty acids of halibut-liver oil is similar to that of the fatty acids of cod-liver oil, but the proportion of unsaturated fatty acids is lower.

Solubility. Slightly soluble in alcohol; miscible with ether, with chloroform, and with light petroleum.

Standard
It complies with the requirements of the British Pharmacopoeia.
It is a pale to golden yellow liquid with a fishy but not rancid odour and contains not less than 30,000 Units of vitamin-A activity in 1 g. It has a weight per ml at 20° of 0·915 g to 0·925 g.
Halibut-liver oil containing 30,000 Units of vitamin-A activity in 1 g contains approximately 5000 Units in 0·2 ml.

Storage. It should be stored in well-filled airtight containers, protected from light.

Actions and uses. Halibut-liver oil is used as a means of administering vitamins A and D; the proportion of vitamin A to vitamin D is usually higher in halibut-liver oil than in cod-liver oil. Gross overdosage can lead to vitamin-A and vitamin-D poisoning.

Dose. 0·2 to 0·5 millilitre daily.

Preparations
HALIBUT-LIVER OIL CAPSULES, B.P. Each capsule contains about 4500 Units of vitamin-A activity. They should be stored at a temperature not exceeding 20°, protected from light; under these conditions they may be expected to retain their potency for at least three years after the date of preparation, which is stated on the label. Dose: 1 to 3 capsules daily.
MALT EXTRACT WITH HALIBUT-LIVER OIL, B.P.C. (page 684)

HALOPERIDOL

$C_{21}H_{23}ClFNO_2 = 375·9$

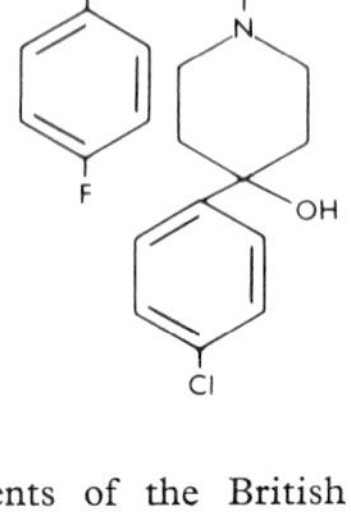

Haloperidol is γ-(4-*p*-chlorophenyl-4-hydroxypiperidino)-*p*-fluorobutyrophenone.

Solubility. Insoluble in water; soluble, at 20°, in 50 parts of alcohol, in 200 parts of ether, and in 20 parts of chloroform.

Standard
It complies with the requirements of the British Pharmacopoeia.

It is an odourless, white to faintly yellowish, amorphous or microcrystalline powder and contains not less than 98·0 and not more than the equivalent of 101·0 per cent of $C_{21}H_{23}ClFNO_2$, calculated with reference to the dried substance. The loss on drying under the prescribed conditions is not more than 0·5 per cent. It has a melting-point of 147° to 151°.

Actions and uses. Haloperidol is a selective central nervous system depressant of the butyrophenone group with properties resembling those of trifluoperazine hydrochloride (page 519). As it is almost devoid of peripheral anti-adrenergic effects, it does not cause hypotension and hypothermia is unlikely to occur; it does, however, inhibit conditioned responses and it is a powerful anti-emetic. It enhances the action of barbiturates, analgesics, and other depressants of the central nervous system.

Haloperidol is usually of more value in acute psychomotor episodes such as mania, hypomania, and acute schizophrenia than in more chronic psychoses. It is inactive in depression, but may help withdrawn apathetic patients to accept treatment. High doses may lead to abnormal wakefulness. Akathisia is a common phenomenon, especially in the elderly, even with moderate dosage. Haloperidol appears to be one of the very few drugs effective in Gilles de la Tourette's disease.

The usual initial dosage in psychiatric conditions is 6 to 12 milligrams daily, up to 15 milligrams daily in acutely disturbed patients, by mouth or by intramuscular or intravenous injection; the dosage for maintenance is usually in the range 1·5 to 3 milligrams daily. The usual dosage for anxiety neuroses is 0·5 milligram daily.

Haloperidol is used in neuroleptanalgesia, usually in combination with potent analgesics, to achieve sedation and analgesia without loss of patient co-operation and with little interference with vital functions, especially in poor-risk cases.

Haloperidol is available as the tablets, as capsules each containing 0·5 milligram, and as a solution for injection containing 3 or 5 milligrams per millilitre as a soluble salt.

UNDESIRABLE EFFECTS. Extrapyramidal syndromes are particularly likely to occur. Dystonic reactions and akathisia are common and may not be recognised when they do not resemble classical parkinsonism; dyskinesias may become irreversible. Occasionally, depression may occur during treatment and weight loss may occur during high-dosage treatment.

PRECAUTIONS AND CONTRA-INDICATIONS. Haloperidol should not be given to patients with disease of the basal ganglia. The effect of oral anticoagulants may be unpredictably reduced by haloperidol.

POISONING. Heat loss should be prevented and blood pressure maintained by changing posture. Drugs such as benzhexol may be required for the treatment of dystonic effects.

Dose. See above under **Actions and uses.**

Preparation
HALOPERIDOL TABLETS, B.P. The quantity of haloperidol in each tablet should be specified by the prescriber. Tablets containing 1·5 and 5 mg are available.

OTHER NAME: *Serenace®*

HALOTHANE

$C_2HBrClF_3 = 197·4$

CHBrCl·CF₃

Halothane is 2-bromo-2-chloro-1,1,1-trifluoroethane. It contains 0·01 per cent w/w of thymol as a preservative.

Solubility. Soluble, at 20°, in 400 parts of water; miscible with dehydrated alcohol, with ether, with chloroform, with trichloroethylene, and with fixed and volatile oils.

Standard
It complies with the requirements of the British Pharmacopoeia.
It is a colourless, mobile, heavy liquid with a characteristic odour. It has a weight per ml at 20° of 1·867 g to 1·872 g. On heating, it distils completely between 49° and 51°.

Stability. On prolonged exposure to ultraviolet radiation it is decomposed with the formation of halogen acids and free halogens.

Storage. It should be stored in airtight containers, protected from light, at a temperature not exceeding 25°.

Actions and uses. Halothane is a volatile anaesthetic which is about twice as potent as chloroform and about four times as potent as ether. It is not inflammable, is not explosive when mixed with oxygen, and is stable in contact with soda lime. It is not irritant to the skin or mucous membrane, nor does it produce necrosis when spilt on tissues.

Halothane may be administered by any of the usual methods of inducing anaesthesia, although open-mask administration is uneconomical. Because of the high vapour pressure of halothane, vapours saturated with it at 20° contain much too high a concentration, and the use of an apparatus specially calibrated for the administration of halothane is therefore recommended. The patient should be premedicated with an adequate dose of an atropine-like drug.

Anaesthesia can be induced by a concentration of 1·5 to 3 per cent v/v or more of halothane and can be maintained with 0·5 to 1·5 per cent v/v. Induction is rapid, usually without signs of excitement; ventricular tachycardia and other cardiac irregularities rarely occur. Muscular relaxation is obtained at moderately deep levels of anaesthesia with halothane.

As halothane blocks the transmission of nerve impulses through ganglia, ganglion-blocking agents, if used, should be given with caution; however, suxamethonium may be given to increase muscular relaxation if necessary.

Halothane suppresses salivary, mucous, bronchial and gastric secretions. A substantial fall in blood pressure may occasionally occur during anaesthesia. The pulse rate is usually slow and severe bradycardia is occasionally encountered; this may be controlled by reducing the dosage of the anaesthetic and by the intravenous administration of atropine.

Halothane sensitises the heart to adrenaline and noradrenaline, but to a lesser extent than cyclopropane. Respiratory depression occurs in the deeper planes of anaesthesia and should be regarded as a sign of overdosage. Both blood pressure and respiratory minute volume increase quickly if the concentration administered is decreased.

Recovery from anaesthesia is rapid, but shivering and laryngeal spasm occasionally occur; vomiting is unusual.

UNDESIRABLE EFFECTS. Liver damage may occur occasionally and caution is necessary in using this anaesthetic for patients who have previously shown this effect after halothane anaesthesia.

POISONING. Signs of overdosage with halothane are bradycardia and profound hypotension, which respond respectively to 500 micrograms of atropine and up to 10 milligrams of methoxamine hydrochloride, both by intravenous injection. Respiratory depression may also occur, and this should be treated by reducing the concentration of the anaesthetic and giving oxygen.

OTHER NAME: *Fluothane*®

HAMAMELIS

SYNONYMS: Hamamelis Leaves; Witch Hazel Leaves

Hamamelis consists of the dried leaves of *Hamamelis virginiana* L. (Fam. Hamamelidaceae), a shrub indigenous to the United States of America and to Canada and produced mainly in the eastern United States.

Constituents. Hamamelis contains tannins, principally hamamelitannin, the digalloyl ester of hamamelose (2-hydroxymethyl ribose), gallic acid, a bitter principle, and a trace of volatile oil. It yields to alcohol (45 per cent) 20 to 30 per cent of extractive.

Standard for unground drug
DESCRIPTION. *Macroscopical:* Leaves about 7 to 15 cm long, brittle, dark green or brownish-green, **broadly** oval or rhomboid-ovate; petiole about 1 to 1·5 cm long, margin coarsely crenate to sinuate, apex acute or rounded, base cordate and unequal and venation pinnate, lateral veins straight, prominent on the under surface, each ending in a marginal crenation; trichomes stellate, scattered on under surface, numerous on young leaves.

Stems and fruits present in small amounts; stems pale reddish-brown or greyish-brown, smooth or slightly warty and up to about 4 mm thick, with alternate leaf scars; fruit a woody capsule, about 15 mm long when mature, splitting at the apex into 2 halves each containing a single seed.
Odour not marked; taste bitter and astringent.

Microscopical: the diagnostic characters are: Leaf: *epidermal cells* with wavy anticlinal walls, *stomata* paracytic, numerous on abaxial surface; *trichomes* stellate, consisting of 4 to 12 slender conical cells, each about 150 to 250 and up to 500 μm long, united at their bases; *spongy mesophyll* appearing as network of cells with intercellular meshes as viewed through abaxial epidermis; *idioblastic sclereids*, large, lignified, linear or sometimes slightly branched, stretching across thickness of lamina and about 150 to 180 μm long, many with *tannin-like* contents turned black by *ferric chloride solution;* midrib prominent on abaxial surface, with a vascular strand consisting of a cylinder of *phloem* encircling a *xylem* cylinder with a central pith, a shallow adaxial arc of xylem with phloem below and a small group of *fibres* above; near leaf apex this replaced by a simple shallow arc of phloem and xylem; sclerenchyma cylinder of *fibres* surrounding the vascular strands, this in turn surrounded by an *endodermoid sheath* with many cells containing prismatic *crystals* of calcium oxalate about 10 to 35 μm long.
Stem: rounded or polygonal *sclereids* and small *vessels* and *tracheids* with bordered pits, separated by uniseriate *medullary rays.*
Fruit: large groups of fibrous *sclereids*, *epidermis* of the persistent calyx bearing numerous stellate *trichomes.*

ALCOHOL (45 PER CENT)-SOLUBLE MATTER. Not less than 20 per cent.

FOREIGN ORGANIC MATTER. Not more than 2·0 per cent.

STEMS AND FRUITS. Not more than 3·0 per cent.

Standard for powdered drug: Powdered Hamamelis
DESCRIPTION. A green to greenish-brown powder, possessing the diagnostic microscopical characters, odour, and taste of the unground drug.

ALCOHOL (45 PER CENT)-SOLUBLE MATTER; FOREIGN ORGANIC MATTER. It complies with the requirements for the unground drug.

Actions and uses. Hamamelis has astringent properties and its preparations are used in the treatment of haemorrhoids. It is used in toilet preparations.

Preparations
HAMAMELIS DRY EXTRACT, B.P.C. (page 682)
HAMAMELIS LIQUID EXTRACT, B.P.C. (page 682)
BENZOCAINE OINTMENT, COMPOUND, B.P.C. (page 758)
HAMAMELIS OINTMENT, B.P.C. (page 761)
HAMAMELIS SUPPOSITORIES, B.P.C. (page 797)
HAMAMELIS AND ZINC OXIDE SUPPOSITORIES, B.P.C. (page 797)

HELIUM

He = 4·003

Helium is obtained from natural petroleum gas by liquefaction and rectification at low temperatures.

Solubility. One volume, measured at normal temperature and pressure, dissolves, at 20°, in 72·5 volumes of water.

Standard
It complies with the requirements of the British Pharmacopoeia.
It is a light, colourless, odourless gas with a relative density not greater than 0·16 and contains not less than 98·0 per cent v/v of He. For convenience in use it is compressed in metal cylinders.

Storage, labelling, and colour-markings. It should be stored in metal cylinders in a special storage room, which should be cool and free from materials of an inflammable nature. The whole of the cylinder should be painted brown and the name of the gas or chemical symbol "He" should be stencilled in paint on the shoulder of the cylinder. The name or chemical symbol of the gas should be clearly and indelibly stamped on the cylinder valve.

Actions and uses. A mixture of 1 volume of helium and 2 volumes of air diffuses more rapidly than air itself. Breathing such a mixture requires less effort and an air–helium mixture, or a mixture of 21 volumes of oxygen and 79 volumes of helium, has been used in treating prolonged asthmatic attacks resistant to other therapy, for avoiding caisson disease, and in the treatment of oedema and spasm of the larynx.

HEPARIN

SYNONYM: Heparin Sodium

Heparin is a sterile preparation containing the sodium salt of a sulphated polysaccharide acid present in mammalian tissue and having the characteristic property of delaying the clotting of blood.

Heparin may be obtained from ox lung [Heparin (Lung); Heparin Sodium (Lung)] or intestinal mucosa of oxen, pigs, or sheep [Heparin (Mucous); Heparin Sodium (Mucous)] by enzymatic digestion, followed by purification.

Solubility. Completely soluble, at 20°, in 2·5 parts of water; soluble in saline solution, forming a clear, colourless, or straw-coloured solution.

Standard
It complies with the requirements of the British Pharmacopoeia.
It is a white or creamy-white, somewhat hygroscopic powder. Heparin (Lung) contains not less than 110 Units per mg and Heparin (Mucous) not less than 130 Units per mg, both calculated with reference to the dried substance. The loss on drying under the prescribed conditions is not more than 8·0 per cent. A 1 per cent solution in water has a pH of 6·0 to 8·0.

Sterilisation. Solutions for injection are sterilised by filtration.

Storage. It should be stored in containers sealed to exclude micro-organisms and, as far as possible, moisture.

Actions and uses. Heparin inhibits the clotting of blood *in vivo* and *in vitro* by combining with certain fractions of the plasma proteins. This action can be rapidly prevented by neutralising its electronegative charge with basic substances such as protamine. It has been shown that the heparin–protein complex inhibits the conversion of prothrombin to thrombin, antagonises thromboplastin, and prevents thrombin from reacting with fibrinogen to form fibrin. The prothrombin ratio is increased but this is not a reliable measure of the anticoagulant effect. The inhibition of the conversion of prothrombin to thrombin is probably responsible for the prevention of platelet agglutination.

Heparin is ineffective when taken by mouth and to obtain its full effect it must be given by intravenous injection or infusion.

When injected intravenously, heparin has a rapid but transient action, the extent and duration of its effect on the clotting-time depending on the dose administered. It disappears rapidly from the blood and intravenous or intramuscular injections should be given at intervals not exceeding four to six hours.

Heparin has no effect on a clot *in vitro*, but there is a more rapid resolution of a clot in a heparinised patient than in an untreated one; heparin also prevents further clotting. It is used as an anticoagulant in vascular surgery and, occasionally, in blood transfusion, but its chief use is in the treatment of arterial and venous thrombosis. In certain selected cases it may be used prophylactically after surgery to prevent thrombo-embolic complications.

The usual practice is to give an initial intravenous injection of 12,500 Units, followed by doses of about 10,000 Units at four-hourly intervals to keep the clotting-time, tested not less than three hours after the last injection of heparin, at about three times the pre-treatment figure; the intravenous dose needed to maintain this figure varies from 6000 to 12,000 Units. Regular treatment is essential, and doses must not be omitted at night; an indwelling needle is therefore frequently used.

In cases of coronary thrombosis an anti-coagulant such as warfarin sodium is commonly given by mouth at the same time as the heparin, which is discontinued after thirty-six to forty-eight hours when the action of the other anticoagulant has developed.

In an emergency, 12,500 Units of heparin may be given by intramuscular injection, although haematoma, pain, and severe bruising may occur; if necessary, a second dose should follow after an interval of six to twelve hours. Long-acting forms of heparin have been evolved which need only be given at intervals of twelve hours by deep subcutaneous or intramuscular injection.

If blood transfusions are required during anti-coagulant therapy, 3 Units of heparin per millilitre may be added to the transfused blood in addition to the dose already being administered.

Bleeding from the site of operation is unlikely if heparin therapy is started after the fourth post-operative or post-partum day.

Menstruation, unless excessive, is no contra-indication to the use of heparin.

UNDESIRABLE EFFECTS. Complications of therapy are bleeding in various sites (hae-maturia, haemothorax, retroperitoneal hae-matoma, subarachnoid haemorrhage) and, rarely, febrile or anaphylactic reactions. Occasionally there is tachyphylaxis, possibly from an endogenous antagonist. Slight epistaxis, microscopic haematuria, and bruising are signs of overdosage. More severe bleeding may be reduced by giving intravenously for each 1000 Units of heparin to be neutralised 1 millilitre of Protamine Sulphate Injection (1 per cent).

Dose. See above under **Actions and uses.**

Preparation
HEPARIN INJECTION, B.P. It consists of a sterile solution of heparin in Water for Injections. The strength of the solution should be specified by the prescriber. It should be stored, preferably in hermetically sealed containers, at a temperature not exceeding 25°; if it is stored in containers sealed by rubber closures, a satisfactory concentration of bactericide may not be maintained for more than three years.

HEXACHLOROPHANE

$C_{13}H_6Cl_6O_2 = 406·9$

Hexachlorophane is 2,2′-methylenebis(3,4,6-trichlorophenol).

Solubility. Insoluble in water; soluble, at 20°, in 3·5 parts of alcohol, in less than 1 part of ether and of acetone, and in 25 parts of chloroform; soluble in dilute solutions of alkali hydroxides.

Standard
It complies with the requirements of the British Pharmacopoeia.
It is a white or pale buff, crystalline powder, which is odourless or has a slight phenolic odour and contains not less than 98·0 per cent of $C_{13}H_6Cl_6O_2$, calculated with reference to the dried substance. The loss on drying under the prescribed conditions is not more than 1·0 per cent. It has a melting-point of about 164°.

Sterilisation. It is sterilised by dry heat.

Storage. It should be stored in airtight containers, protected from light.

Preparation and storage of solutions. See statement on aqueous solutions of antiseptics, under Solutions (page 779).

Actions and uses. Hexachlorophane has anti-bacterial properties against a wide variety of Gram-positive organisms, but it is generally less effective against Gram-negative organisms. It has the advantage over many other anti-septics of retaining its activity in the presence of soap.

Hexachlorophane is used in soaps and creams in a concentration of 1 to 3 per cent. When these preparations are used daily there is a marked diminution of the bacterial flora of the hands due to accumulation of hexa-chlorophane on the skin. Such preparations

are useful in reducing cross-infection in hospital operating theatres and wards and contamination of food during handling.

Dusting-powders containing 0·3 per cent are used for application to the umbilical stump.

The presence of serum reduces the activity of hexachlorophane, but the concentration normally used is sufficient to allow for this.

UNDESIRABLE EFFECTS. Skin sensitisation has been known to occur after the repeated use of hexachlorophane. Preparations of hexa-chlorophane are liable to contamination with Gram-negative organisms such as species of *Pseudomonas* and *Salmonella* which are resistant to its antibacterial action.

PRECAUTIONS. As hexachlorophane can be absorbed after the application of preparations of hexachlorophane to the skin, such preparations should preferably not be used for total body bathing or application to large areas of the skin. Particular caution should be exercised in applying preparations containing hex-chlorophane to infants.

Preparations
HEXACHLOROPHANE DUSTING-POWDER, B.P.C. (page 663)
HEXACHLOROPHANE SOLUTION, CONCENTRATED, B.P.C. (page 786)

OTHER NAME: Hexachlorophene

HEXYLRESORCINOL

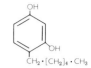

$C_{12}H_{18}O_2 = 194\cdot3$

Hexylresorcinol is 4-hexylresorcinol.

Solubility. Slightly soluble in water; readily soluble in alcohol, in ether, in chloroform, in glycerol, and in fixed oils; very slightly soluble in light petroleum.

Standard
It complies with the requirements of the British Pharmacopoeia.
It occurs as white or almost white needles, crystalline powder, plates, or plate aggregates composed of needle masses; it has a pungent odour and becomes brownish-pink on exposure to light and air. It contains not less than 98·0 and not more than the equivalent of 101·0 per cent of $C_{12}H_{18}O_2$. It has a melting-point of 66° to 68°.

Storage. It should be stored in airtight containers, protected from light.

Actions and uses. Hexylresorcinol is an anthelmintic used for the expulsion of hook-worms and dwarf tapeworms. It is administered by mouth as a single dose, which for an adult is usually 1 gram and for a child 100 milligrams for each year of age up to ten years. A saline purgative should be given two hours after the dose, and no food should be allowed for five hours. Because the drug is irritant, tablets and capsules of hexylresorcinol should not be chewed. The treatment may be safely repeated after three days, if necessary.

For the expulsion of hookworms, three courses of treatment at intervals of three days may be necessary.

For the expulsion of dwarf tapeworms, treatment may be given weekly for three weeks to ensure that autoinfection does not occur.

Dose. See above under **Actions and uses.**

HISTAMINE ACID PHOSPHATE

SYNONYM: Histamine Phosphate

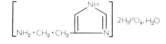

$C_5H_{15}N_3O_8P_2,H_2O = 325\cdot2$

Histamine Acid Phosphate is 4-(2-aminoethyl)imidazole di-acid phosphate monohydrate.

Solubility. Soluble, at 20°, in 4 parts of water; slightly soluble in alcohol.

Standard
It complies with the requirements of the British Pharmacopoeia.
It occurs as colourless odourless crystals and contains not less than 98·0 and not more than the equivalent of 101·0 per cent of $C_5H_{15}N_3O_8P_2$, calculated with reference to the anhydrous substance. It contains 5·0 to 6·0 per cent w/w of water. It has a melting-point of 130° to 133°, after sintering at about 127°. A solution in water is acid to litmus.

Sterilisation. Solutions for injection are sterilised by heating in an autoclave or by filtration.

Actions and uses. Histamine stimulates contraction of the involuntary muscle of the uterus, intestine, and bronchioles. It stimulates the acid-secreting cells in the gastric mucosa, producing a profuse flow of gastric juice with a high acidity but a relatively low content of pepsin; this action is unaffected by antihistamine drugs.
Histamine produces marked dilatation of the capillaries and arterioles, with a resultant fall in arterial blood pressure, which is usually followed by the onset of the characteristic histamine headache. It is rapidly absorbed when administered by injection, but is relatively inactive when given by mouth.
The therapeutic uses of histamine are limited because of its extensive systemic effects. It has been used chiefly as a diagnostic agent to test the acid-secreting function of the stomach and as a means of differentiating between the absolute achylia of pernicious anaemia and the relative achylia of carcinoma of the stomach; 0·5 to 5 milligrams of histamine acid phosphate is given by subcutaneous injection in place of a test meal. It is essential to give an antihistamine before the larger doses.
Histamine has been used for the desensitisation of patients suffering from Ménière's disease or from severe unilateral temporal headache (histamine headache) when these conditions are associated with a hypersensitivity to histamine. An intracutaneous injection of 0·05 millilitre of a 1 in 3600 solution of histamine acid phosphate is used to determine whether or not a patient is sensitive to histamine.

Dose. 0·5 to 1 milligram by subcutaneous injection; after the administration of an antihistamine drug, 5 milligrams.

Preparation
HISTAMINE ACID PHOSPHATE INJECTION, B.P. (*Syn.* Histamine Phosphate Injection). It consists of a sterile solution of histamine acid phosphate in Water for Injections. Unless otherwise specified, a solution containing 1 mg in 1 ml is supplied. It should be protected from light.

HOMATROPINE HYDROBROMIDE

Synonym: Homatr. Hydrobrom.

$C_{16}H_{22}BrNO_3 = 356.3$

$$\left[\begin{array}{c} H_2C \!\!-\!\! CH \!\!-\!\! CH_2 \\ | \quad N\!\cdot\!CH_3 \quad CH\!\cdot\!O\!\cdot\!CO\!\cdot\!CH\!\cdot\!C_6H_5 \\ H_2C \!\!-\!\! CH \!\!-\!\! CH_2 \end{array} \begin{array}{c} OH \\ \\ \end{array}\right] HBr$$

Homatropine Hydrobromide is the hydrobromide of tropyl mandelate, an alkaloid prepared by synthesis.

Solubility. Soluble, at 20°, in 6 parts of water and in 60 parts of alcohol, the solubility increasing rapidly with increase of temperature; slightly soluble in chloroform; insoluble in ether.

Standard
It complies with the requirements of the British Pharmacopoeia.
It is a colourless, crystalline, odourless powder and contains not less than 99·0 and not more than the equivalent of 101·0 per cent of $C_{16}H_{22}BrNO_3$, calculated with reference to the dried substance. The loss on drying under the prescribed conditions is not more than 0·5 per cent. It melts with decomposition at about 215°. A 2 per cent solution in water has a pH of 5·5 to 7·0.

Sterilisation. Solutions are sterilised by heating in an autoclave or by filtration.

Actions and uses. Homatropine has actions similar to those described under Atropine (page 36). It is less powerful than atropine

and is seldom used internally; its chief use is in ophthalmology to dilate the pupil. It produces mydriasis more rapidly than atropine, but its effect persists for a shorter time, passing off within twenty-four hours, and may be readily terminated by the action of physostigmine. It has less tendency than atropine to increase the intra-ocular pressure, but produces a less satisfactory mydriasis in children. Its mydriatic action may be enhanced by the simultaneous local administration of cocaine.

Poisoning. As for Atropine (page 36).

Preparations
Cocaine and Homatropine Eye-drops, B.P.C. (page 690)
Homatropine Eye-drops, B.P.C. (page 691)

PURIFIED HONEY

Synonym: Mel Depuratum

Purified Honey is obtained from the honey in the comb of the hive bee, *Apis mellifera* L. and other species of *Apis* (Fam. Apidae). The honey is melted at a temperature not exceeding 80° and allowed to stand, the impurities which rise to the surface are skimmed off, and the liquid diluted with water until the product has a weight per ml at 20° of 1·355 g.

Most of the honey of commerce is extracted from the comb by centrifugation or by pressure.

Constituents. Purified honey contains 70 to 80 per cent of glucose and fructose, the ratio of fructose to glucose usually being slightly greater than 1 to 1, together with water, sucrose, dextrin, wax, proteins, volatile oil, and formic acid.
Pollen and flocculent matter are usually present in suspension and tend to induce fermentation.

Standard
Description. A thick, syrupy, translucent, pale yellow or yellowish-brown liquid; taste sweet and characteristic, varying according to the floral origin. Odour pleasant and characteristic; when heated on a water-bath the odour becomes more pronounced but is otherwise unchanged.

Optical rotation. +0·6° to −3·0°, determined, at 20°, in a 20·0 per cent w/v solution in water containing 0·2 ml of *strong ammonia solution*, after decolorising with *decolorising charcoal* if necessary.

Weight per ml. At 20°, 1·35 g to 1·36 g.

Chloride. 10 ml of a 10·0 per cent w/v solution in water complies with the limit test for chlorides (350 parts per million).

Sulphate. 25 ml of a 10·0 per cent w/v solution in water complies with the limit test for sulphates (240 parts per million).

Commercial invert sugar. Dissolve 20 g in 20 ml of water and extract with 40 ml of *solvent ether*; evaporate the ether extract to dryness and dissolve the residue in 10 ml of *solvent ether*. To 2 ml of the ether solution at room temperature add 2 ml of *resorcinol and hydrochloric acid solution*; not more than a faint pink colour, which does not deepen to a cherry-red on standing, is

produced in the acid layer. Evaporate the remainder of the ether solution, obtained above, to dryness at room temperature and to the residue add 2 ml of *aniline acetate solution*; no pink to orange colour is produced after allowing the solution to stand for 15 minutes.

Ash. Not more than 0·3 per cent.

Adulterants and substitutes. Invert sugar is sometimes offered as honey, while sucrose and glucose may occur as adulterants. If prepared by acid hydrolysis, both invert sugar and glucose contain traces of furfuraldehyde.
Honey derived from some species of *Eucalyptus* or of *Banksia*, or of both, has a strong unpleasant aromatic odour and taste; it may be identified by finding the triangular lenticular pollen grains of *Eucalyptus* spp., measuring about 20 μm, or the sausage-shaped pollen grains of *Banksia* spp., measuring about 50 μm in length, or both these pollens.
Honey-dew honey is dark in colour, congeals with difficulty, and contains hardly any pollen, but commonly unicellular algae of the *Pleurococcus* type are present. Honey-dew does not come from flowers, but is secreted by various aphids, and occurs upon the epidermis of the leaves of conifers and other plants.

Actions and uses. Purified honey is used as a demulcent and sweetening agent, especially in linctuses and cough mixtures.

Preparations
Oxymel, B.P.C. (page 764)
Squill Oxymel, B.P.C. (page 765)

HYALURONIDASE

Hyaluronidase is a mucolytic enzyme having a specific action on the mucopolysaccharide, hyaluronic acid.

Hyaluronidase may be prepared from the testes and semen of the ox by fractional precipitation of an aqueous extract, followed by dialysis, sterilisation by a process of filtration, and freeze-drying of the resulting solution. Hydrolysed gelatin or a suitable non-protein stabilising agent may be added.

Solubility. Very soluble in water; insoluble in alcohol, in ether, and in acetone.

Standard
It complies with the requirements of the British Pharmacopoeia.
It is a white or yellowish-white odourless powder and contains not less than 300 Units per mg and not less than 10,000 Units per mg of tyrosine present. The loss on drying over phosphorus pentoxide at a pressure not exceeding 0·02 mmHg is not more than 0·5 per cent. A 0·3 per cent solution in water has a pH of 4·5 to 7·5. A 1 per cent solution in carbon dioxide-free water is clear and not more than faintly yellow.

Storage. It should be stored in single-dose containers, sealed to exclude micro-organisms, in a cool dry place.

Actions and uses. Hyaluronidase is an enzyme which breaks down the hyaluronic acid of the mucoprotein ground substance or tissue cement, thereby reducing its viscosity and rendering the tissues more readily permeable to injected fluids.

When the intravenous administration of fluids is difficult, as in infants, the addition of 500 to 1000 Units of hyaluronidase to 500 to 1000 millilitres of fluid will enable the injection to be given by the subcutaneous route at the rate of 10 millilitres per minute. Hyaluronidase may be mixed with the fluid to be injected or it may be injected into the site before the fluid is administered.

The diffusion of local anaesthetics is accelerated by the addition of 1000 Units to each 20 millilitres of the anaesthetic solution. This is of value in the reduction of fractures and in pudendal block in midwifery. Substances used in radiography, such as diodone, are rapidly absorbed from the site of intramuscular injection with the aid of hyaluronidase, thus providing an alternative to the commoner intravenous technique in pyelography. Maximum opacity in the kidney is found fifteen to forty-five minutes after the injection of diodone in conjunction with hyaluronidase. Aqueous solutions of hyaluronidase prepared by dissolving the freeze-dried material in Water for Injections are unstable. Stabilised solutions are available.

Dose. See above under **Actions and uses.**

Preparation
HYALURONIDASE INJECTION, B.P.C. (page 713)

OTHER NAME: *Hyalase*®

HYDROCHLORIC ACID

SYNONYMS: Acidum Hydrochloricum Concentratum; Concentrated Hydrochloric Acid

HCl = 36·46

Hydrochloric Acid is an aqueous solution of hydrogen chloride and may be prepared by saturating water with the hydrogen chloride evolved by the action of sulphuric acid on sodium chloride.

When hydrochloric acid is heated, hydrochloric acid gas is evolved until the strength of the solution falls to approximately 20 per cent w/w; this forms a constant-boiling mixture which boils at about 110°.

Impure hydrochloric acid of commerce is popularly known as "spirits of salt" and as "muriatic acid".

Standard
It complies with the requirements of the European Pharmacopoeia.
It is a clear, colourless, fuming liquid with a pungent odour and contains 35·0 to 38·0 per cent w/w of HCl. It has a weight per ml at 20° of about 1·18 g.

Storage. It should be stored in a stoppered or otherwise suitably closed container of glass or other inert material at a temperature below 30°.

Actions and uses. Hydrochloric acid is a powerful corrosive although less so than sulphuric acid or nitric acid. The acid is secreted in the body by the oxyntic cells of the stomach; it is essential for the activation of pepsin during the digestion of protein.

Dilute hydrochloric acid, well diluted, is given by mouth in the treatment of achlorhydria, hypochlorhydria, and gastrogenous diarrhoea. Not more than about 20 millilitres should be given during a period of twenty-four hours.

POISONING. A stomach tube or emetics should not be used. The acid must be neutralised as quickly as possible; calcium hydroxide in water and Magnesium Hydroxide Mixture are good antidotes; carbonates should be avoided if possible, as they lead to the liberation of carbon dioxide and the consequent risk of perforation.

After neutralisation of the acid, demulcents such as milk, raw eggs, or a vegetable oil such as olive oil should be given and shock should be treated by warmth and intravenous infusions if required. Morphine should be given for the relief of pain.

Hydrochloric acid burns should be treated by immediately flooding with water, followed by the application of sodium bicarbonate or chalk in powder, or by the application of sodium bicarbonate or saline packs.

Preparations

HYDROCHLORIC ACID, DILUTE, B.P. Complies with the requirements of the European Pharmacopoeia and contains 10 per cent w/w of HCl. Dose: 0·5 to 4 ml.

GENTIAN MIXTURE, ACID, B.P.C. (page 743)

GENTIAN MIXTURE, ACID, WITH NUX VOMICA, B.P.C. (page 743)

NUX VOMICA MIXTURE, ACID, B.P.C. (page 748)

HYDROCHLOROTHIAZIDE

$C_7H_8ClN_3O_4S_2 = 297·7$

Hydrochlorothiazide is 6-chloro-3,4-dihydro-7-sulphamoyl-2*H*-benzo-1,2,4-thiadiazine 1,1-dioxide.

Solubility. Very slightly soluble in water, in ether, and in chloroform; soluble, at 20°, in 200 parts of alcohol and in 20 parts of acetone; soluble in solutions of alkali hydroxides.

Standard

It complies with the requirements of the British Pharmacopoeia.

It is a white or almost white, crystalline, odourless powder and contains not less than 98·0 and not more than the equivalent of 102·0 per cent of $C_7H_8ClN_3O_4S_2$, calculated with reference to the dried substance. The loss on drying under the prescribed conditions is not more than 1·0 per cent.

Storage. It should be stored in airtight containers.

Actions and uses. Hydrochlorothiazide is a non-mercurial diuretic which has actions and uses similar to those described under Chloro-thiazide (page 103), but it is effective in smaller doses. For the treatment of oedema, the dosage is 50 to 200 milligrams by mouth daily or on alternate days, but as an adjunct to hypotensive drugs in the treatment of hypertension 25 to 50 milligrams may be sufficient.

UNDESIRABLE EFFECTS; PRECAUTIONS. These are as described under Chlorothiazide (page 103).

Dose. See above under **Actions and uses.**

Preparation

HYDROCHLOROTHIAZIDE TABLETS, B.P. Unless otherwise specified, tablets each containing 25 mg of hydrochlorothiazide are supplied. Tablets containing 50 mg are also available.

OTHER NAMES: *Direma®*; *Esidrex®*; *HydroSaluric®*

HYDROCORTISONE

SYNONYMS: Hydrocort.; Hydrocortisonum

$C_{21}H_{30}O_5 = 362·5$

Hydrocortisone is 11β,17α,21-trihydroxypregn-4-ene-3,20-dione.

Solubility. Insoluble in water; soluble, at 20°, in 40 parts of alcohol and in 80 parts of acetone; slightly soluble in chloroform; very slightly soluble in ether.

Standard

It complies with the requirements of the European Pharmacopoeia.

It is a white or almost white, crystalline, odourless powder and contains not less than 96·0 and not more than the equivalent of 104·0 per cent of $C_{21}H_{30}O_5$, calculated with reference to the dried substance. The loss on drying under the prescribed conditions is not more than 1·0 per cent. It melts with decomposition at about 214°.

Storage. It should be protected from light.

Actions and uses. Hydrocortisone is a normal secretion of the adrenal cortex in man. It has actions, uses, and undesirable effects similar to those described under Cortisone Acetate (page 132) and it is given in similar dosage.

In emergencies such as Addisonian or post-adrenalectomy crises 100 milligrams may be given by intravenous infusion over a period of four to six hours and the dose repeated when necessary; a water-soluble derivative of hydrocortisone such as hydrocortisone sodium succinate or hydrocortisone sodium phosphate is used for intravenous administration. When only an anti-inflammatory effect is required prednisolone is to be preferred.

A suspension of 100 milligrams of hydrocortisone in 120 millilitres of Sodium Chloride Solution may be used as a retention enema in the treatment of ulcerative colitis; hydrocortisone acetate and hydrocortisone sodium succinate are also used for this purpose but Prednisolone Enema is usually preferred.

Hydrocortisone may be applied externally in ointments, creams, and lotions.

PRECAUTIONS AND CONTRA-INDICATIONS. As for Cortisone Acetate (page 132).

Dose. See above under **Actions and uses.**

Preparations

HYDROCORTISONE CREAM, B.P.C. (page 659)
HYDROCORTISONE AND NEOMYCIN CREAM, B.P.C. (page 659)

HYDROCORTISONE LOTION, B.P.C. (page 728)
HYDROCORTISONE OINTMENT, B.P. It contains hydrocortisone in a base consisting of 10 per cent of wool fat in white soft paraffin. Unless otherwise specified, an ointment containing 1·0 per cent of hydrocortisone is supplied. Ointments containing 0·5 and 2·5 per cent are also available.
HYDROCORTISONE AND CLIOQUINOL OINTMENT, B.P.C. (page 761)
HYDROCORTISONE SUPPOSITORIES, B.P.C. (page 797)

OTHER NAMES: Cortisol; *Cortril*®; *Efcortelan*®; *Genacort* ®; *Hydrocortistab*®; *HydroCortisyl*®; *Hydrocortone*®

HYDROCORTISONE ACETATE

SYNONYMS: Hydrocort. Acet.; Hydrocortisoni Acetas

$C_{23}H_{32}O_6 = 404·5$

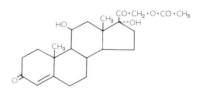

Hydrocortisone Acetate is 21-acetoxy-11β,17α-dihydroxypregn-4-ene-3,20-dione.

Solubility. Insoluble in water; soluble, at 20°, in 230 parts of alcohol and in 150 parts of chloroform.

Standard
It complies with the requirements of the European Pharmacopoeia.
It is a white or almost white, crystalline, odourless powder and contains not less than 96·0 and not more than the equivalent of 104·0 per cent of $C_{23}H_{32}O_6$, calculated with reference to the dried substance. The loss on drying under the prescribed conditions is not more than 1·0 per cent. It melts with decomposition at about 220°.

Preparation of solid dosage forms. In order to achieve a satisfactory rate of dissolution, hydrocortisone acetate in the form of an ultra-fine powder should be used.

Storage. It should be protected from light.

Actions and uses. Hydrocortisone acetate has actions, uses, and undesirable effects similar to those described under Cortisone Acetate (page 132).
It is given by intra-articular injection into joints affected by rheumatoid and other arthritic conditions; a dose of 5 to 50 milligrams, depending on the size of the joint to be injected, may relieve pain and swelling for several days or weeks. It may also be injected into painful lesions of ligaments and muscle, such as tennis elbow, and into bursae.
Hydrocortisone acetate is applied to the skin for the treatment of inflammatory conditions accompanied by irritation of the skin, such as pruritus ani. It may also be used for the treatment of inflammatory conditions of the eye, but it should be used with the utmost caution, as hydrocortisone may mask the development of infection; an antibacterial

substance, such as neomycin, may be used in conjunction with hydrocortisone to minimise this danger.
Hydrocortisone acetate is given in a retention enema in the treatment of ulcerative colitis, 100 milligrams suspended in 120 millilitres of Sodium Chloride Solution being a suitable dose; Prednisolone Enema is usually preferred for this purpose.

PRECAUTIONS AND CONTRA-INDICATIONS. As for Cortisone Acetate (page 132).

Dose. See above under **Actions and uses.**

Preparations
HYDROCORTISONE CREAM, B.P.C. (page 659)
HYDROCORTISONE AND NEOMYCIN EAR-DROPS, B.P.C. (page 665)
HYDROCORTISONE EYE-DROPS, B.P.C. (page 691)
HYDROCORTISONE AND NEOMYCIN EYE-DROPS, B.P.C. (page 691)
HYDROCORTISONE EYE OINTMENT, B.P.C. (page 699)
HYDROCORTISONE AND NEOMYCIN EYE OINTMENT, B.P.C. (page 699)
HYDROCORTISONE ACETATE INJECTION, B.P. It consists of a sterile suspension of hydrocortisone acetate, in very fine powder, in Water for Injections containing suitable dispersing agents. Unless otherwise specified, a suspension containing 25 mg in 1 ml is supplied.
HYDROCORTISONE ACETATE OINTMENT, B.P. It contains hydrocortisone acetate in a base consisting of 10 per cent of wool fat in white soft paraffin. Unless otherwise specified, an ointment containing 1·0 per cent of hydrocortisone acetate is supplied. Ointments containing 0·5 and 2·5 per cent are also available.
HYDROCORTISONE AND CLIOQUINOL OINTMENT, B.P.C. (page 761)
HYDROCORTISONE SUPPOSITORIES, B.P.C. (page 797)

OTHER NAMES: Cortisol Acetate; the other names given under Hydrocortisone are also applied to Hydrocortisone Acetate

HYDROCORTISONE HYDROGEN SUCCINATE

SYNONYM: Hydrocort. Hydrogen Succ.

$C_{25}H_{34}O_8 = 462.5$

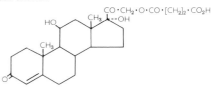

Hydrocortisone Hydrogen Succinate is 21-(β-carboxypropionyloxy)-11β,17α-dihydroxypregn-4-ene-3,20-dione.

Solubility. Very slightly soluble in water; soluble, at 20°, in 40 parts of alcohol, in 7 parts of dehydrated alcohol, and in 25 parts of sodium bicarbonate solution; soluble, with decomposition, in sodium hydroxide solution.

Standard
It complies with the requirements of the British Pharmacopoeia.
It is a white or almost white, crystalline, odourless powder and contains not less than 97.0 and not more than the equivalent of 103.0 per cent of $C_{25}H_{34}O_8$, calculated with reference to the dried substance. The loss on drying under the prescribed conditions is not more than 5.0 per cent.

Storage. It should be protected from light.

Actions and uses. Hydrocortisone hydrogen succinate has actions, uses, and undesirable effects similar to those described under Cortisone Acetate (page 132). It is used in the preparation of Hydrocortisone Sodium Succinate Injection.

PRECAUTIONS AND CONTRA-INDICATIONS. As for Cortisone Acetate (page 132).

HYDROCORTISONE SODIUM PHOSPHATE

$C_{21}H_{29}Na_2O_8P = 486.4$

Hydrocortisone Sodium Phosphate is the disodium salt of the 21-phosphate ester of 11β,17α,21-trihydroxypregn-4-ene-3,20-dione.

Solubility. Soluble, at 20°, in 4 parts of water; slightly soluble in dehydrated alcohol; insoluble in chloroform.

Standard
DESCRIPTION. A white or almost white, hygroscopic powder; odourless or almost odourless.

IDENTIFICATION TESTS. 1. Dissolve 2 mg in 2 ml of *sulphuric acid*; a yellowish-green fluorescence is immediately produced (distinction from betamethasone sodium phosphate and prednisolone sodium phosphate).

2. It complies with the thin-layer chromatographic test given in Appendix 5A, page 864.

3. Heat gently 0.04 g with 2 ml of *sulphuric acid* until fumes are evolved, add *nitric acid* dropwise until oxidation is complete, cool, add 2 ml of water, heat again until white fumes are evolved, cool, add 10 ml of water, and neutralise to *litmus paper* with *dilute ammonia solution*; the solution gives reactions A and C characteristic of sodium and reaction C characteristic of phosphates given in the British Pharmacopoeia, Appendix V.

ALKALINITY. pH of a 0.5 per cent w/v solution in *carbon dioxide-free water*, 7.5 to 9.0.

SPECIFIC ROTATION. +121° to +129°, calculated with reference to the anhydrous substance, determined, at 20°, in a 1.0 per cent w/v solution in water.

INORGANIC PHOSPHATE. Not more than 1.0 per cent, calculated as PO_4, determined by the following method: Dissolve 0.01 g, accurately weighed, in 10 ml of water, add 4 ml of *dilute sulphuric acid*, 1 ml of *ammonium molybdate solution*, and 2 ml of *methylaminophenol with sulphite solution*, allow to stand for 15 minutes, dilute to 25 ml with water, and allow to stand for a further 15 minutes. The extinction of a 4-cm layer of the resulting solution at 730 nm is not greater than the extinction at 730 nm of a 4-cm layer of a solution prepared by treating 10.0 ml of a 0.00143 per cent w/v solution of

potassium dihydrogen phosphate in a similar manner, beginning at the words "add 4 ml . . .".

FREE HYDROCORTISONE AND OTHER DERIVATIVES. It complies with the test given in Appendix 5A, page 865 (2.0 per cent, calculated with reference to the anhydrous substance).

WATER. Not more than 10.0 per cent w/w, determined by the method given in Appendix 16, page 895.

CONTENT OF $C_{21}H_{29}Na_2O_8P$. Not less than 96.0 and not more than the equivalent of 104.0 per cent, calculated with reference to the anhydrous substance, determined by the following method:
Dissolve about 0.05 g, accurately weighed, in sufficient water to produce 100 ml, dilute 10 ml of this solution to 100 ml with water, and measure the extinction of a 1-cm layer at the maximum at about 248 nm.
For purposes of calculation use a value of 333 for the E(1 per cent, 1 cm) of $C_{21}H_{29}Na_2O_8P$. Calculate the percentage of $C_{21}H_{29}Na_2O_8P$ in the sample.

Storage. It should be stored in airtight containers, protected from light.

Actions and uses. Hydrocortisone sodium phosphate has actions, uses, and undesirable effects similar to those described under Cortisone Acetate (page 132). As it is soluble in water, it is suitable for the preparation of intravenous or intramuscular injections; 134 mg of the ester is approximately equivalent to 100 mg of hydrocortisone.

PRECAUTIONS AND CONTRA-INDICATIONS. As for Cortisone Acetate (page 132).

Preparation
HYDROCORTISONE SODIUM PHOSPHATE INJECTION, B.P.C. (page 714)

OTHER NAME: *Efcortesol*®

HYDROCORTISONE SODIUM SUCCINATE

SYNONYM: Hydrocort. Sod. Succ.

$C_{25}H_{33}NaO_8 = 484.5$

Hydrocortisone Sodium Succinate is the sodium salt of 21-(β-carboxypropionyloxy)-11β,17α-dihydroxypregn-4-ene-3,20-dione.

Solubility. Soluble, at 20°, in 3 parts of water, in 34 parts of alcohol, and in 200 parts of dehydrated alcohol; insoluble in ether and in chloroform.

Standard
It complies with the requirements of the British Pharmacopoeia.
It is a white or almost white, crystalline, hygroscopic, odourless powder, and contains not less than 97·0 and not more than the equivalent of 103·0 per cent of $C_{25}H_{33}NaO_8$, calculated with reference to the dried substance. The loss on drying under the prescribed conditions is not more than 3·0 per cent.

Storage. It should be stored in airtight containers, protected from light.

Actions and uses. Hydrocortisone sodium succinate has actions, uses, and undesirable effects similar to those described under Cortisone Acetate (page 132). As it is soluble in water, it is suitable for the preparation of intravenous or intramuscular injections; 100 mg of the ester is approximately equivalent to 75 mg of hydrocortisone.

Intravenous administration of hydrocortisone may be life-saving in Addisonian crisis or severe status asthmaticus.
Hydrocortisone sodium succinate is of value in the withdrawal syndrome of long-term cortisone therapy. As an aerosol spray, it has also been used in asthma and, as lozenges, in the treatment of aphthous ulceration.

PRECAUTIONS AND CONTRA-INDICATIONS. As for Cortisone Acetate (page 132).

Preparations
HYDROCORTISONE SODIUM SUCCINATE INJECTION, B.P. It consists of a sterile solution of hydrocortisone sodium succinate prepared immediately before use by dissolving the sterile contents of a sealed container in Water for Injections. The equivalent quantity of hydrocortisone in each container should be specified by the prescriber. Vials containing the equivalent of 100 mg of hydrocortisone are available.

HYDROCORTISONE LOZENGES, B.P.C. (page 733)

OTHER NAMES: *Corlan*®; *Efcortelan Soluble*®; *Solu-Cortef*®

HYDROFLUMETHIAZIDE

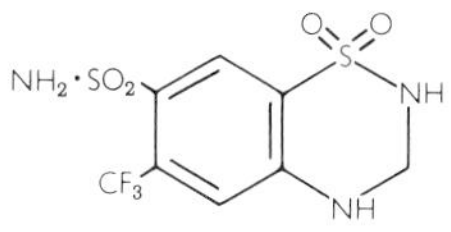

$C_8H_8F_3N_3O_4S_2 = 331.3$

Hydroflumethiazide is 3,4-dihydro-7-sulphamoyl-6-trifluoromethyl-2H-benzo-1,2,4-thiadiazine 1,1-dioxide.

Solubility. Very slightly soluble in water, in ether, and in chloroform; soluble, at 20°, in 50 parts of alcohol.

Standard
It complies with the requirements of the British Pharmacopoeia.
It occurs as white or almost white, odourless or almost odourless, glistening crystals or crystalline powder and contains not less than 98·0 and not more than the equivalent of 102·0 per cent of $C_8H_8F_3N_3O_4S_2$, calculated with reference to the dried substance. The loss on drying under the prescribed conditions is not more than 0·5 per cent.

Actions and uses. Hydroflumethiazide is a non-mercurial diuretic which has actions and uses similar to those described under Chlorothiazide (page 103), but it is effective in smaller doses.

For the treatment of oedema, the dosage is 25 to 100 milligrams by mouth once or twice daily or on alternate days, but as an adjunct to hypotensive drugs in the treatment of hypertension 25 to 50 milligrams may be sufficient.

UNDESIRABLE EFFECTS; PRECAUTIONS. These are as described under Chlorothiazide (page 103).

Dose. See above under **Actions and uses.**

Preparation
HYDROFLUMETHIAZIDE TABLETS, B.P. Unless otherwise specified, tablets each containing 50 mg of hydroflumethiazide are supplied.

OTHER NAMES: *Hydrenox*®; *NaClex*®

HYDROGEN PEROXIDE SOLUTION

SYNONYM: Hydrogen Peroxide Solution (20-volume)

Hydrogen Peroxide Solution is an aqueous solution of hydrogen peroxide, H_2O_2.

Hydrogen Peroxide Solution is prepared by diluting a strong solution, and adjusting to the appropriate acidity by the addition of

dilute phosphoric acid or dilute sulphuric acid.
Hydrogen Peroxide Solution is also known as

"20-volume", the number indicating the volume of oxygen obtainable from one volume of the solution.

Standard
It complies with the requirements of the British Pharmacopoeia.
It is a colourless, odourless liquid and contains 5·0 to 7·0 per cent w/v of H_2O_2.

Stability. It is comparatively stable in the presence of a slight excess of acid, but readily decomposes when alkaline and when in contact with oxidisable substances or certain metals. Limited amounts of a suitable stabiliser are sometimes added.

Incompatibility. It is incompatible with most organic substances and with alkalis, iodides, permanganates, and oxidisable substances.

Storage. It should be stored protected from light, in a cool place, in bottles closed with glass stoppers, paraffined corks, or plastic or protected metal screw caps.

Actions and uses. Hydrogen Peroxide Solution is an antiseptic and deodorant which owes its efficacy to the readiness with which it evolves oxygen in the presence of living or dead tissue and bacteria; however, because of the rapidity of the evolution of oxygen, its antiseptic action is brief. It does not combine with albumin and is non-poisonous.

It is useful for detaching dead tissue and bacterial nests from dirty wounds and purulent lesions, and for removing adherent blood-stained dressings.

It is used, diluted with three to eight parts of water, as a deodorant gargle or mouthwash, and as ear-drops for the removal of wax. For bleaching hair and for removing superficial stains from the teeth, it should be mixed with an equal volume of water.

UNDESIRABLE EFFECTS. Strong solutions of hydrogen peroxide produce irritating "burns" on the skin, but the pain disappears in about an hour.

NOTE. When Hydrogen Peroxide is prescribed or demanded, Hydrogen Peroxide Solution is dispensed or supplied.

Preparation
HYDROGEN PEROXIDE EAR-DROPS, B.P.C. (page 665)

STRONG HYDROGEN PEROXIDE SOLUTION

SYNONYMS: Hydrogen Peroxide Solution (100-volume); Hydrogenii Peroxidum

Strong Hydrogen Peroxide Solution is an aqueous solution of hydrogen peroxide, H_2O_2.

Strong Hydrogen Peroxide Solution is usually prepared by electrolysing a solution of ammonium sulphate and sulphuric acid, with subsequent hydrolysis and distillation. It is a strong oxidising agent which decomposes vigorously in contact with oxidisable organic matter or with certain metals and their compounds, or if rendered alkaline. Limited amounts of a suitable stabiliser are usually added. It is known as "100-volume", the number indicating the volumes of oxygen obtainable from one volume of the solution.

When used to make dilute solutions the product should be adjusted to the appropriate acidity by the addition of dilute phosphoric acid or dilute sulphuric acid.

Standard
Material which complies with this standard meets the requirements of the European Pharmacopoeia.

DESCRIPTION. A colourless liquid with a weight per ml at 20° of about 1·11 g; almost odourless.

IDENTIFICATION TESTS. 1. Cautiously make the solution alkaline; it decomposes vigorously with effervescence, evolving oxygen.
2. To 0·05 ml add 2 ml of *dilute sulphuric acid*, 2 ml of *solvent ether*, and 0·05 ml of *potassium chromate solution* and shake; the ethereal layer is coloured deep blue.

ACIDITY. To 10 ml add 100 ml of *carbon dioxide-free water* and titrate with 0·1N sodium hydroxide, using 0·25 ml of *methyl red solution* as indicator; not less than 0·05 ml and not more than 0·5 ml is required.

BARIUM. Dilute 1 ml to 10 ml with water and add 1 ml of *dilute sulphuric acid*; the solution remains clear for not less than 15 minutes when compared with water, the comparison being made by viewing vertically 10 ml of the liquids in matched, colourless, transparent, neutral glass tubes, 16 mm internal diameter and with a flat base, against a black background in diffused light.

ORGANIC PRESERVATIVES. Not more than 500 parts per million, determined by the following method:
Extract 20 ml with successive 10-, 5-, and 5-ml portions of *chloroform*; evaporate the combined chloroform extracts under reduced pressure at a temperature not exceeding 25°, dry any residue in a dessicator, and weigh.

NON-VOLATILE MATTER. Not more than 0·2 per cent w/v, determined by the following method:
Allow 25 ml to decompose in a platinum dish, cooling if necessary, evaporate the decomposed solution on a water-bath, and dry the residue to constant weight at 105°.

CONTENT OF H_2O_2. Not less than 29·0 and not more than 31·0 per cent w/v, determined by the following method:
Dilute 1·0 ml, accurately measured, to 100 ml with water; to 10 ml of this solution add a cooled mixture containing 2·5 ml of *sulphuric acid* and 20 ml of water and titrate the solution with 0·1N potassium permanganate; each ml of 0·1N potassium permanganate is equivalent to 0·001701 g of H_2O_2.

Incompatibility. It is incompatible with most organic substances and with alkalis, iodides, permanganates, and oxidisable substances.

Storage. It should be stored protected from light, in a cool place, in bottles closed with glass stoppers or suitable plastic caps and provided with a vent.

Actions and uses. Strong Hydrogen Peroxide Solution is used to prepare weaker solutions. It should never be used undiluted; if used without dilution for bleaching hair, it may produce gangrene of the scalp.

NOTE. When Hydrogen Peroxide is prescribed or demanded Hydrogen Peroxide Solution is dispensed or supplied.

HYDROXOCOBALAMIN

$C_{62}H_{89}CoN_{13}O_{15}P = 1346.4$

Hydroxocobalamin is α-(5,6-dimethylbenzimidazol-1-yl)hydroxocobamide.

Solubility. Soluble in water.

Standard
It complies with the requirements of the British Pharmacopoeia.
It occurs either as aquocobalamin chloride, $C_{62}H_{90}ClCoN_{13}O_{15}P$, or as aquocobalamin sulphate, $C_{124}H_{180}Co_2N_{26}O_{34}P_2S$. Both forms occur as dark red, almost odourless crystals or crystalline powder. Aquocobalamin chloride contains not less than 96.0 per cent of $C_{62}H_{90}ClCoN_{13}O_{15}P$ and aquocobalamin sulphate contains not less than 96.0 per cent of $C_{124}H_{180}Co_2N_{26}O_{34}P_2S$, both calculated with reference to the dried substance. The loss on drying under the prescribed conditions is 8.0 to 12.0 per cent for the chloride and 8.0 to 16.0 per cent for the sulphate; some decomposition may occur on drying.

Sterilisation. Solutions for injection are sterilised by filtration.

Storage. It should be stored in airtight containers, protected from light, in a cool place.

Actions and uses. Hydroxocobalamin is an important member of a group of similar compounds which influence erythropoiesis and which represent the "anti-pernicious anaemia principle" of purified liver extracts. It is bound more firmly to serum proteins than cyanocobalamin and hence has a longer action.
Hydroxocobalamin is effective in the treatment of pernicious anaemia and its neurological complication, subacute combined degeneration of the spinal cord. It is given by intramuscular injection, the dose depending on the clinical state of the patient and the response to treatment; it should not be given by mouth because of its variable absorption.
In uncomplicated pernicious anaemia and for patients in relapse, a weekly dose of not less than 250 micrograms will usually produce a satisfactory response, but a much higher dosage consisting of five injections, each of 1 milligram within the first week, has been recommended with the object of restoring the depleted reserve in the liver. A dose of 250 micrograms every three or four weeks is usually adequate for maintenance, but doses of 1 milligram are often given at longer intervals. In all cases the dosage must be related to the patient's response; in patients with neurological abnormalities, the doses should be doubled.
Hydroxocobalamin is also used in conjunction with folic acid in the treatment of other macrocytic anaemias associated with nutritional deficiencies and sprue. It is used in massive doses in the treatment of neuroblastoma in children.

PRECAUTIONS. Hydroxocobalamin should not be given before a diagnosis has been fully established, because of its ability to mask symptoms of subacute combined degeneration of the spinal cord.

Dose. See above under **Actions and uses.**

Preparation
HYDROXOCOBALAMIN INJECTION, B.P. It consists of a sterile solution of hydroxocobalamin in Water for Injections containing sufficient acetic acid or hydrochloric acid to adjust the pH to about 4. Unless otherwise specified, a solution containing the equivalent of 250 µg of anhydrous hydroxocobalamin in 1 ml is supplied. It should be protected from light. Ampoules containing 1 milligram in 1 ml are also available.

OTHER NAMES: *Cobalin-H®*; *Neo-Cytamen®*

HYDROXYCHLOROQUINE SULPHATE

$C_{18}H_{28}ClN_3O_5S = 433.9$

Hydroxychloroquine Sulphate is 7-chloro-4-[4-(N-ethyl-N-2-hydroxyethylamino)-1-methyl-butylamino]quinoline sulphate.

Solubility. Soluble, at 20°, in 5 parts of water; very slightly soluble in alcohol, in ether, and in chloroform.

Standard
It complies with the requirements of the British Pharmacopoeia.
It is a white or almost white, crystalline, odourless powder and contains not less than 98.0 per cent of $C_{18}H_{28}ClN_3O_5S$, calculated with reference to the dried substance. The loss on drying under the prescribed conditions is not more than 2.0 per cent. It has a melting-point of about 198° or about 240°. A 1 per cent solution in water has a pH of 3.5 to 5.5.

Storage. It should be protected from light.

Actions and uses. Hydroxychloroquine has antimalarial actions similar to those described under Chloroquine Phosphate (page 101), but is used mainly in the treatment of rheumatoid arthritis and lupus erythematosus, both discoid and the systemic form when the skin is markedly involved. The daily dosage is 0.2 to 1.2 grams of hydroxychloroquine sulphate by mouth in divided doses; the maintenance dosage is usually 200 milligrams daily, but this is adapted to the needs of the patient.
A dosage of 200 to 400 milligrams three times daily for five days has been used in the treatment of giardiasis.

The usual dosage for the suppression of malaria is 400 milligrams weekly and for treatment, 0·4 to 1·2 grams daily in divided doses.

UNDESIRABLE EFFECTS. Prolonged treatment with large doses sometimes results in nausea, diarrhoea, and intestinal cramps; if the period of administration exceeds one to two years, irreversible retinal damage may be caused.

Dose. See above under **Actions and uses.**

Preparation
HYDROXYCHLOROQUINE TABLETS, B.P. Unless otherwise specified, tablets each containing 200 mg of hydroxychloroquine sulphate are supplied. They are sugar coated.

OTHER NAME: *Plaquenil*®

HYDROXYPROGESTERONE HEXANOATE

SYNONYM: Hydroxyprogesterone Caproate

$C_{27}H_{40}O_4 = 428·6$

Hydroxyprogesterone Hexanoate is 17α-hexanoyloxy-pregn-4-ene-3,20-dione.

Solubility. Insoluble in water; soluble, at 20°, in 10 parts of alcohol, in 10 parts of ether, and in less than 1 part of chloroform; soluble in fixed oils and esters.

Standard
It complies with the requirements of the British Pharmacopoeia.
It is a white or almost white, crystalline, almost odourless powder and contains not less than 97·0 and not more than the equivalent of 103·0 per cent of $C_{27}H_{40}O_4$, calculated with reference to the dried substance. The loss on drying under the prescribed conditions is not more than 0·5 per cent. It has a melting-point of 120° to 124°.

Storage. It should be protected from light.

Actions and uses. Hydroxyprogesterone hexanoate is a synthetic progestational steroid hormone and has actions similar to those of progesterone (page 407). It is used in threatened and habitual abortion and in functional uterine disorders and amenorrhoea.

Dose. 250 to 500 milligrams once or twice weekly by intramuscular injection.

Preparation
HYDROXYPROGESTERONE INJECTION, B.P. It consists of a sterile solution of hydroxyprogesterone hexanoate in a suitable ester or in a suitable fixed oil, or in any mixture of these. Unless otherwise specified, a solution containing 250 mg in 1 ml is supplied. It should be protected from light.

OTHER NAME: *Primolut Depot*®

HYOSCINE HYDROBROMIDE

SYNONYMS: Hyoscini Hydrobromidum; Scopolamine Hydrobromide; Scopolamini Hydrobromidum

$C_{17}H_{22}BrNO_4,3H_2O = 438·3$

Hyoscine Hydrobromide is the hydrobromide trihydrate of $(-)$-hyoscine, an alkaloid obtained from various solanaceous plants, particularly species of *Datura*, *Scopolia*, and *Duboisia*.

Solubility. Soluble, at 20°, in 3·5 parts of water and in 30 parts of alcohol; very slightly soluble in ether and in chloroform.

Standard
It complies with the requirements of the European Pharmacopoeia.
It occurs as odourless, slightly efflorescent, colourless crystals or white crystalline powder and contains not less than 98·5 per cent of $C_{17}H_{22}BrNO_4$, calculated with reference to the dried substance. The loss on drying under the prescribed conditions is 10·0 to 13·0 per cent. It melts with decomposition at about 197°. A 5 per cent solution in water has a pH of 4·0 to 5·5.

Sterilisation. Solutions are sterilised by heating in an autoclave or by filtration.

Storage. It should be stored in airtight containers, protected from light, in a cool place.

Actions and uses. Hyoscine has peripheral and central actions. Like atropine, it antagonises the muscarinic effects of acetylcholine. It produces mydriasis and relaxes accommodation more quickly but for a shorter time than atropine.
The central action of hyoscine differs from that of atropine; it usually produces immediate depression of the cerebral cortex, especially of the motor areas. Hyoscine is therefore used in mania and in cerebral excitement and delirium such as occur in alcoholism, when, as a rule, it produces a sensation of fatigue and drowsiness which is quickly followed by sleep. For this purpose 1·2 milligrams of hyoscine hydrobromide and 20 milligrams of morphine sulphate may be given by subcutaneous or intramuscular injection.
For pre-operative medication, 600 micrograms of hyoscine hydrobromide and 10 to 15 milligrams of morphine sulphate or an

equivalent amount of papaveretum is given by subcutaneous injection about one hour before operation. In obstetrics, similar doses have been used for the induction of "twilight sleep"; subsequent injections containing smaller doses of hyoscine and no morphine may be sufficient. Hyoscine is similarly used in conjunction with pethidine.

Hyoscine hydrobromide is given by mouth in doses of 600 micrograms for the prevention and treatment of motion-sickness. It also reduces the tremor of paralysis agitans and chorea and relieves the salivation and, to a lesser extent, the muscular rigidity of post-encephalitic parkinsonism; for these purposes it is given by mouth, usually in a dosage of 300 to 600 micrograms three times daily; sometimes, however, the dosage may be considerably higher.

In ophthalmology, hyoscine hydrobromide may be used in eye-drops or eye ointment for its peripheral action on the eye.

Dose. See above under **Actions and uses.**

Preparations

HYOSCINE EYE-DROPS, B.P.C. (page 692)

HYOSCINE EYE OINTMENT, B.P. Unless otherwise specified, an eye ointment containing 0·25 per cent of hyoscine hydrobromide is supplied.

HYOSCINE INJECTION, B.P. It consists of a sterile solution of hyoscine hydrobromide in Water for Injections. Unless otherwise specified, a solution containing 400 µg in 1 ml is supplied. It should be protected from light. Ampoules containing 600 µg in 1 ml are also available.

HYOSCINE TABLETS, B.P. Unless otherwise specified, tablets each containing 300 µg of hyoscine hydrobromide are supplied. Tablets containing 400 and 600 µg are also available.

HYOSCYAMUS

SYNONYMS: Hyoscy.; Hyoscyami Folium; Hyoscyamus Leaf

Hyoscyamus consists of the dried leaves, or leaves and flowering tops, of *Hyoscyamus niger* L. (Fam. Solanaceae), an erect herb distributed throughout Europe and cultivated in England and elsewhere.

Varieties. Hyoscyamus occurs both as an annual and as a biennial and the corresponding leaves are available in commerce. Annual hyoscyamus is smaller than the biennial; the leaves are less hairy and less incised; the corolla is not so deeply purple-veined and the commercial drug frequently contains a large proportion of stem. The leaves of the first year's growth of the biennial plant are large, petiolate, and may be up to 30 cm or more in length; they are free from admixture with the flowers. Second year biennial hyoscyamus consists of the flowering tops of the biennial variety. These three varieties are approximately equal in alkaloidal content.

Constituents. Hyoscyamus contains the alkaloid (−)-hyoscyamine, together with smaller quantities of atropine [(±)-hyoscyamine] and (−)-hyoscine [(−)-scopolamine]. The proportion of alkaloid in the carefully dried leaf varies from 0·045 to 0·14 per cent. Larger yields of alkaloid (up to 0·27 per cent) have been reported, but these are exceptional. Volatile bases, similar to those in belladonna leaf, are also present.

Standard

It complies with the requirements of the European Pharmacopoeia.

It contains not less than 0·050 per cent of alkaloids, calculated as hyoscyamine, $C_{17}H_{23}NO_3$, with reference to the substance dried at 100° to 105°.

UNGROUND DRUG. *Macroscopical characters:* Laminae pale green, up to about 25 cm long; first year leaves of the biennial plants ovate-lanceolate, petiole flat, about 5 cm long; second year leaves shorter, sessile and ovate-oblong to triangular-ovate; margin dentately lobed, apex acute, midrib broad, yellowish, and conspicuous; secondary veins leaving midrib at a wide angle and terminating in the apices of the lobes; trichomes abundant on both surfaces, long, soft, many secreting a resinous substance rendering the leaves clammy to the touch.

Flowers crowded together, arising in the axils of large hairy bracts; calyx gamosepalous, having 5 lobes, each with an apical spine, green, hairy; corolla slightly zygomorphic, infundibuliform, yellow with purple veins; stamens 5, epipetalous, anthers purple; ovary superior, 2-celled, containing numerous ovules.

Fruit a pyxis, about 15 mm long, enclosed by the persistent calyx; seeds brownish-grey, flattened reniform-quadrangular, about 1·75 mm long; testa with wavy reticulate surface.

Odour strong and characteristic; taste bitter, slightly acrid.

Microscopical characters: the diagnostic characters are: Leaf: *epidermal cells* with wavy anticlinal walls, *cuticle* smooth; *stomata* anisocytic, on both surfaces; *trichomes* uniseriate, up to 500 µm long, of two kinds, some simple, 2- to 4-celled, the majority terminating in an ovoid multicellular gland; *crystals* of calcium oxalate either as single prisms, twin crystals, clusters of few components, or microsphenoidal sand, occurring in cells of mesophyll; *fibres* absent.

Pollen grains, when examined in chloral hydrate solution, subspherical, 35 to 48 to 56 µm diameter, *extine* marked with fine pits in a scattered arrangement, 3 *germinal furrows,* 3 *pores* each about 15 µm in diameter.

Seeds having a *testa* with *epidermal cells* about 100 to 150 µm in diameter, with lignified, wavy anticlinal walls.

POWDERED DRUG: Powdered Hyoscyamus. A green or greyish-green powder possessing the diagnostic microscopical characters, odour, and taste of the unground drug.

Adulterants and substitutes. Egyptian henbane consists of the dried leaves, flowering tops, immature fruits, and smaller stems of *H. muticus* L., a desert perennial collected chiefly in Egypt. The thick, somewhat fleshy leaves are brittle when dry, lanceolate to ovate-lanceolate, the lower and radical ones being petiolate and the upper ones sessile; the fruit is a cylindrical pyxis, about 1·5 cm long and 0·6 cm wide, enclosed by a persistent calyx, having 5 broad triangular non-spiny lobes. The drug contains about 0·6 to 1 per cent of total alkaloids, of which about 90 per cent is hyoscyamine.

H. albus L., a perennial plant growing in Mediterranean countries and in the Indian subcontinent, has leaves 5 to 10 cm long, with a slender petiole 2 to 6 cm long and a coarsely toothed margin, yellow flowers, and simple and glandular trichomes, each of the latter having a unicellular spherical head. It contains similar alkaloids to those in *H. niger*.

Some Indian henbane is derived from *H. reticulatus* L. and contains about 0·12 to 0·24 per cent of alkaloids.

Storage. It should be stored in a cool dry place, protected from light.

Actions and uses. Hyoscyamus has actions similar to those described under Belladonna Herb (page 42), but the hyoscine which it contains makes it less likely to give rise to cerebral excitement. Preparations of hyoscyamus are used to counteract the griping action of purgatives and to relieve spasm in the urinary tract.

POISONING. As for Atropine (page 36).

Preparations
HYOSCYAMUS DRY EXTRACT, B.P.C. (page 683)
HYOSCYAMUS LIQUID EXTRACT, B.P.C. (page 683)
GELSEMIUM AND HYOSCYAMUS MIXTURE, COMPOUND, B.P.C. (page 743)
POTASSIUM CITRATE AND HYOSCYAMUS MIXTURE, B.P.C. (page 751)
HYOSCYAMUS TINCTURE, B.P. It contains 0·005 per cent of alkaloids. Dose: 2 to 5 millilitres.

OTHER NAME: Henbane Leaf

HYPROMELLOSE

SYNONYM: Hydroxypropylmethylcellulose

Hypromellose is a mixed ether of cellulose in which the ether groupings are mainly methoxyl groups with a small proportion of hydroxypropoxyl groups.

Hypromellose may be prepared by reacting alkali cellulose with a mixture of methyl chloride and propylene oxide. The name "hypromellose" is followed by a number indicating the approximate viscosity of a 2·0 per cent solution.

Solubility. Soluble in cold water, forming a viscous colloidal solution; insoluble in alcohol, in ether, and in chloroform.

Standard
DESCRIPTION; IDENTIFICATION TESTS; ACIDITY OR ALKALINITY; LOSS ON DRYING; SULPHATED ASH. It complies with the tests described under Methylcellulose 20, page 307.

VISCOSITY. Determine by the method given for Methylcellulose 20, page 307. The limits for various viscosity grades and the viscometer to be used are indicated in the following table:

CONTENT OF HYDROXYPROPOXYL. 4·0 to 7·5 per cent, calculated as $C_3H_7O_2$, with reference to the substance dried under the prescribed conditions, determined by the method given in Appendix 22, page 903.

CONTENT OF METHOXYL. 27·0 to 30·0 per cent, calculated as CH_3O, with reference to the substance dried under the prescribed conditions, determined by the method given in Appendix 22, page 903.

Storage. It should be stored in airtight containers, in a cool place.

Uses. Hypromellose has properties similar to those of methylcellulose, but produces aqueous solutions having higher gel-points and greater clarity; for example, a 2 per cent solution of methylcellulose 4500 gels at about 50° and a 2 per cent solution of hypromellose 4500 gels at about 65°. Because of the greater clarity of aqueous solutions and the lower proportion of undispersed fibres, it is used in preference to methylcellulose to increase the viscosity of ophthalmic solutions; an anti-microbial agent such as benzalkonium chloride should be incorporated.

Hypromellose has also been used in the preparation of anhydrous adhesive ointments for the protection of the skin surrounding ileostomies, fistulas, and exuding ulcers. In the preparation of Plaster of Paris Bandage, hypromellose is used for the same purpose as methylcellulose.

Viscosity grade	Viscosity at 20° (centistokes)	Capillary diameter of viscometer (mm)
20	15 to 25	0·84 ± 0·02
50	40 to 60	1·15 ± 0·03
125	110 to 140	1·51 ± 0·03
450	350 to 550	2·06 ± 0·04
1500	1200 to 1800	2·74 ± 0·04
4500	3750 to 5250	3·70 ± 0·04
15,000	12,000 to 18,000	4·97 ± 0·04

ARSENIC. It complies with the test given in Appendix 6, page 878 (2 parts per million).

LEAD. It complies with the test given in Appendix 7, page 882 (5 parts per million).

Preparation
HYPROMELLOSE EYE-DROPS, B.P.C. (page 692)

ICHTHAMMOL

SYNONYM: Ammonium Ichthosulphonate

Ichthammol consists mainly of the ammonium salts of the sulphonic acids prepared by sulphonating the oily substances resulting from the destructive distillation of a bituminous schist or shale. It contains, in addition, 5 to 7 per cent of ammonium sulphate.

Solubility. Soluble in water; partly soluble in alcohol and in ether; completely soluble in a mixture of equal parts of alcohol and ether.

Standard
DESCRIPTION. An almost black, viscid liquid; odour strong and characteristic.

IDENTIFICATION TESTS. 1. Warm a small quantity with an equal volume of *sodium hydroxide solution*; ammonia is evolved.

2. Dissolve 1 g in 50 ml of water; a clear, dark brown solution is produced. Add *hydrochloric acid*; a dark resinous mass is precipitated.

SOLUBILITY IN GLYCEROL. 1 ml dissolves completely in 9 ml of *glycerol* and remains in solution for not less than 24 hours.

LOSS ON DRYING. Not more than 50·0 per cent, determined by drying to constant weight at 105°.

SULPHATED ASH. Not more than 0·3 per cent.

ORGANICALLY COMBINED SULPHUR. Not less than 10·5 per cent w/w, calculated with reference to the substance dried under the prescribed conditions, determined by the following method:

Mix in a porcelain crucible of about 50-ml capacity about 0·5 g, accurately weighed, with 4 g of *anhydrous sodium carbonate* and 3 ml of *chloroform* and warm and stir until all the chloroform has evaporated; add 10 g of coarsely powdered *copper nitrate*, mix thoroughly, heat the mixture very gently over a small flame, and, when the initial reaction has subsided, increase the temperature slightly until most of the material has blackened.

Cool, place the crucible in a large beaker, add 20 ml of *hydrochloric acid*, and, when the reaction has ceased, add 100 ml of water; boil until all the copper oxide is dissolved, filter, and to the filtrate add 400 ml of water; heat to boiling, add 20 ml of *barium chloride solution*, and allow the solution to stand for 2 hours.

Filter, wash the residue with water, dry, and ignite at a temperature of about 600°; weigh and repeat the ignition and weighing until two successive weighings do not differ by more than 0·2 per cent of the weight of the residue; each g of residue is equivalent to 0·1374 g of S.

From the percentage of total sulphur thus obtained subtract the percentage of sulphur in the form of sulphates.

SULPHUR IN THE FORM OF SULPHATES. Not more than 25·0 per cent of the total sulphur, determined by the following method:

Dissolve about 2 g, accurately weighed, in 100 ml of water, add a solution containing 2 g of *copper chloride* in 80 ml of water, dilute to 200 ml with water, shake, and filter; heat 100 ml of the filtrate nearly to boiling, add 1 ml of *hydrochloric acid* followed by 5 ml of *barium chloride solution*, dropwise, heat on a water-bath, filter, and wash the residue with water.

Ignite the residue at a temperature of about 600°, weigh, and repeat the ignition and weighing until two successive weighings do not differ by more than 0·2 per cent of the weight of the residue; each g of residue is equivalent to 0·1374 g of S present in the form of sulphates.

Incompatibility. It is incompatible with alkaloids.

Actions and uses. Ichthammol has only slight bacteriostatic properties; it is slightly irritant to the skin. It has been used in ointments and creams in the treatment of some chronic skin diseases.

Ichthammol Glycerin has been used to reduce the inflammation of lymphadenitis and of thrombophlebitis; it has also been used in pessaries and tampons for the treatment of cervicitis.

Preparations

ZINC AND ICHTHAMMOL CREAM, B.P.C. (page 661)
ICHTHAMMOL GLYCERIN, B.P.C. (page 701)
ICHTHAMMOL OINTMENT, B.P.C. (page 762)

IDOXURIDINE

$C_9H_{11}IN_2O_5 = 354·1$

Idoxuridine is 5-iodo-2′-deoxyuridine.

Solubility. Soluble, at 20°, in 500 parts of water, in 400 parts of alcohol, and in 230 parts of methyl alcohol; very slightly soluble in ether and in chloroform; slightly soluble in acetone.

Standard

It complies with the requirements of the British Pharmacopoeia.

It occurs as odourless colourless crystals or white crystalline powder and contains not less than 98·0 per cent of $C_9H_{11}IN_2O_5$, calculated with reference to the dried substance. The loss on drying under the prescribed conditions is not more than 1·0 per cent.

Stability of solutions. Aqueous solutions are most stable when the pH is adjusted to between 2 and 6; they should be freshly prepared and kept in a refrigerator. Some decomposition products are more toxic than idoxuridine and reduce its antiviral activity.

If idoxuridine is required for intravenous infusion, a 0·5 per cent w/v solution may be prepared from the following formula:

Idoxuridine	5 g
Sodium Carbonate	1 g (or a sufficient quantity)
Dilute Sulphuric Acid	a sufficient quantity
Dextrose Injection	
(5 per cent w/v)	to 1000 ml

The method is as follows:

Adjust the alkalinity of the Dextrose Injection to pH 10 by the addition of sodium carbonate and add the idoxuridine, previously ground to a fine powder. Stir mechanically, again measure the pH, and add more sodium carbonate if necessary to re-adjust to pH 10. When solution is complete, adjust the pH to 9·0, using either the dilute sulphuric acid or a further quantity of sodium carbonate, as appropriate.

Sterilise the solution by filtration, distribute, by means of an aseptic technique, into sterile containers, and seal. When stored at a temperature of 0° to 4° it should be used within six weeks of preparation. If storage at room temperature is necessary it should be used within three days. Solutions should not be used if there is evidence of deposition.

Storage. It should be stored in airtight containers, protected from light.

Actions and uses. Idoxuridine is a thymidine analogue which competes with thymidine both for incorporation into deoxyribonucleic acid and as substrate for enzymes such as thymidine kinase and thymidylate kinase. It thus acts as an antiviral agent by inhibiting the replication of deoxyribonucleic acid viruses such as herpes simplex, vaccinia, cyto-megalovirus, and adenovirus.

Idoxuridine is used in the treatment of herpetic keratitis, particularly the dendritic corneal ulcer type. Cases with deep stromal involvement respond much less satisfactorily than others.

Idoxuridine is usually applied as eye-drops containing 0·1 per cent, applications being made every hour during the day and every two hours at night; it may also be applied as an eye ointment containing 0·5 per cent. Treatment should not be continued for more than five days or the cytotoxic activity of idoxuridine may delay corneal healing.

Herpetic lesions of the skin have been treated by the local application of idoxuridine but the response is variable. Some success has been obtained in disseminated herpes zoster by injecting idoxuridine into the lesions.

In the treatment of systemic viral infections, such as herpes simplex encephalitis and con-genital cytomegalovirus infection, the intra-venous infusion of idoxuridine has been used when other methods of treatment have proved to be ineffective. Doses of up to a total of 600 milligrams per kilogram body-weight have been given over a period of five days.

UNDESIRABLE EFFECTS. Like any other cyto-toxic agent idoxuridine may be teratogenic.

POISONING. The systemic effects of idoxuri-dine may be at least partially reversed by the intravenous injection of a solution containing 50 milligrams of thymidine.

OTHER NAMES: *Dendrid®*; *Kerecid®*

IMIPRAMINE HYDROCHLORIDE

SYNONYM: Imipramini Hydrochloridum

$C_{19}H_{25}ClN_2 = 316·9$

Imipramine Hydrochloride is 5-(3-dimethylaminopropyl)-10,11-dihydro-5H-dibenz[b,f]azepine hydrochloride.

Solubility. Soluble, at 20°, in 2 parts of water and in 1·5 parts of alcohol; very slightly soluble in ether; soluble in chloroform.

Standard

It complies with the requirements of the European Pharmacopoeia.

It is a white or slightly yellow, crystalline, almost odourless powder and contains not less than 98·5 per cent of $C_{19}H_{25}ClN_2$, calculated with reference to the dried substance. The loss on drying under the pre-scribed conditions is not more than 0·5 per cent. It has a melting-point of 170° to 174°. A 10 per cent solution in water has a pH of 4·2 to 5·2.

Stability of solutions. Aqueous solutions are stable when protected from oxygen and light.

Hygroscopicity. It absorbs insignificant amounts of moisture at 23° at relative humidities up to about 60 per cent, but under damper conditions it absorbs sig-nificant amounts.

Sterilisation. Solutions for injection are sterilised by heating in an autoclave or by filtration.

Storage. It should be protected from light.

Actions and uses. Imipramine is an anti-depressant drug which does not inhibit monoamine oxidase. It has a mild atropine-like action. It is particularly valuable in the treatment of patients with endogenous de-pression, whereas a monoamine-oxidase in-hibitor, such as phenelzine, is preferred for neurotic or reactive depressive illnesses.

The usual dosage of imipramine hydrochlo-ride necessary to re-establish a normal mood varies between 25 and 75 milligrams by mouth, usually three times a day, but only 10 to 30 milligrams daily may be necessary for elderly patients. The relief of symptoms is slow in onset and the patient may show little response until after two or three weeks of treatment; sometimes, however, there is a good response within a few days.

When a satisfactory response has been ob-tained, the drug should be gradually with-drawn; prolonged maintenance therapy may, however, be necessary. In refractory cases, treatment may be combined with electro-convulsive therapy.

UNDESIRABLE EFFECTS. The most frequently occurring undesirable effects are dryness of the mouth, tachycardia, and a tendency to perspire; moderate hypotensive effects and occasional blurring of vision may occur. Imipramine increases sensitivity to alcohol, and patients should be warned of this danger. If it is given by injection, a transient increase in blood pressure may occur.

PRECAUTIONS. Caution should be exercised when giving imipramine hydrochloride to patients who are being treated with a mono-amine-oxidase inhibitor, such as isocar-boxazid, nialamide, phenelzine, or tranylcy-promine, or who have been so treated within the previous ten days. It may cause a reversal of the effect of antihypertensive drugs and may give rise to hypertension in patients being given local anaesthetics containing adrenaline or noradrenaline.

Dose. See above under **Actions and uses.**

OTHER NAMES: *Anpramine®*; *Berkomine®*; *Dimipressin®*; *Ia-pram®*; *Impamin®*; *Oppanyl®*; *Praminil®*; *Tofranil®*

Preparation

IMIPRAMINE TABLETS, B.P. Unless otherwise specified, tablets each containing 25 mg of imipramine hydrochloride are supplied. They are sugar coated. Tablets containing 10 mg are also available.

INDIGO CARMINE

$C_{16}H_8N_2Na_2O_8S_2 = 466·3$

Indigo Carmine (Colour Index No. 73015) is disodium indigotin-5,5'-disulphonate. It usually contains a considerable amount of sodium chloride.

Solubility. Soluble, at 20°, in 100 parts of water; readily soluble in warm water; very slightly soluble in alcohol.
It is precipitated from aqueous solutions by sodium chloride.

Standard
It complies with the requirements of the British Pharmacopoeia.
It occurs as almost odourless blue granules or powder with a coppery lustre and contains not less than 90·0 per cent of $C_{16}H_8N_2Na_2O_8S_2$, calculated with reference to the dried substance. The loss on drying under the prescribed conditions is not more than 10·0 per cent.

Sterilisation. Solutions for injection are sterilised by heating in an autoclave or by filtration.

Actions and uses. Indigo carmine is used as a test for renal function. Usually 10 millilitres of a 0·4 per cent solution is injected intramuscularly or intravenously. When renal function is normal the urine becomes coloured in about ten minutes. It is also used to compare the functioning of the two kidneys, the appearance of the dye at the ureteric orifices being observed by means of a cystoscope.

Dose. See above under **Actions and uses.**

OTHER NAMES: F.D. & C. Blue No. 2; Sodium Indigotindisulphonate

INDOMETHACIN

$C_{19}H_{16}ClNO_4 = 357·8$

Indomethacin is 1-*p*-chlorobenzoyl-5-methoxy-2-methylindol-3-ylacetic acid.

Solubility. Very slightly soluble in water; soluble, at 20°, in 50 parts of alcohol, in 45 parts of ether, and in 30 parts of chloroform.

Standard
It complies with the requirements of the British Pharmacopoeia.
It is a pale yellow to brownish-yellow, crystalline, odourless or almost odourless powder and contains not less than 98·5 per cent of $C_{19}H_{16}ClNO_4$, calculated with reference to the dried substance. The loss on drying under the prescribed conditions is not more than 0·5 per cent. It has a melting-point of 158° to 162°.

Storage. It should be protected from light.

Actions and uses. Indomethacin is an anti-inflammatory, antipyretic substance with analgesic properties. It is rapidly absorbed when taken by mouth and is excreted largely by the kidneys. Its action begins within two hours of ingestion.
It is effective in relieving pain and swelling in cases of gout and of rheumatoid and allied forms of arthritis and painful symptoms in other disorders of bone and joint, such as osteoarthritis and ankylosing spondylitis. It may also reduce fever and relieve symptoms in febrile inflammatory conditions such as glandular fever.

The usual dosage by mouth is 25 milligrams, two, three, or four times a day with meals, but the dose may be increased if necessary to 150 milligrams daily if the drug is well tolerated. A suppository of 100 milligrams given on retiring produces symptomatic relief through the night, and ease from pain and stiffness the following morning; 75 to 100 milligrams given by mouth with food at bedtime may prove equally effective.

UNDESIRABLE EFFECTS. The most common undesirable effects are headache and various unpleasant cerebral sensations, such as fullness and dizziness. These are dose-related and usually appear early in the course of treatment and lessen or disappear as dosage is reduced or stopped.
Dyspepsia may occur at any time during treatment and is not always dose-related; peptic ulceration with bleeding may occur and is usually, but not always, accompanied by dyspepsia. Prepyloric ulcers may sometimes be mistaken for malignant lesions on X-ray films, but they heal within three to four weeks of stopping the drug.

Rashes, including purpuric eruptions, are uncommon.

PRECAUTIONS AND CONTRA-INDICATIONS. Indomethacin should be used with caution in the presence of diminished renal function. Peptic ulceration is usually considered to be a contra-indication.

Dose. By mouth, 50 to 150 milligrams daily in divided doses; by rectum, 100 milligrams once or twice daily.

Preparations

INDOMETHACIN CAPSULES, B.P. Unless otherwise specified, capsules each containing 25 mg are supplied. Capsules each containing 50 mg are also available.

INDOMETHACIN MIXTURE, B.P.C. (page 744)

INDOMETHACIN SUPPOSITORIES, B.P. Unless otherwise specified, suppositories each containing 100 mg are supplied.

OTHER NAME: *Indocid*®

INSULIN INJECTION

SYNONYM: Insulin

Insulin Injection is a sterile solution of the protein insulin, the specific antidiabetic principle of the mammalian pancreas.

Insulin Injection may be prepared by dissolving crystalline insulin having a potency of not less than 23 Units per milligram, calculated with reference to the anhydrous material, in Water for Injections containing 1·6 per cent w/v of glycerol, sufficient hydrochloric acid to adjust the pH to 3 to 3·5, and sufficient bactericide to prevent the growth of microorganisms.

The solution is sterilised by filtration, assayed, adjusted to the required strength, and distributed aseptically into sterile containers, which are then sealed.

Insulin Injection is usually made from ox pancreas.

Standard

It complies with the requirements of the British Pharmacopoeia.

It is a colourless liquid, free from turbidity and from matter which deposits on standing, and contains 20, 40, or 80 Units per ml, the potency being determined biologically. It has a pH of 3·0 to 3·5.

Containers. The containers are glass vials, sealed so as to allow the withdrawal of successive doses on different occasions.

Storage. It should be stored at 2° to 10°; it should not be allowed to freeze. Under these conditions it may be expected to retain its potency for at least two years after the date of manufacture.

Actions and uses. Insulin is the hormone, secreted by the beta cells of the islets of Langerhans of the pancreas, that not only regulates carbohydrate metabolism but is also concerned with the synthesis of protein and fat and with the storage of the latter. Secretion of insulin is primarily regulated by the level of the blood sugar, although it is modified by other hormones such as adrenaline and hydrocortisone.

In the juvenile diabetic insulin secretion is reduced; in the middle-aged obese diabetic it is present, but largely unavailable, possibly because of the presence of insulin antagonists, or because binding prevents its access to body cells.

Insulin is bound to plasma proteins, but on release reaches and acts in all body cells. It is rapidly inactivated by the enzymes of the gastro-intestinal tract. In a normal person the fasting blood-sugar level is maintained in the region of 80 to 120 milligrams per 100 millilitres; a store of glucose, as glycogen, is maintained in the liver and muscles. As the blood-sugar level falls, the liver glycogen is mobilised and converted into glucose, which passes into the blood. If insufficient insulin is available to the tissues, as in diabetes mellitus, a rise in the blood-sugar level occurs and, when the renal threshold for sugar is exceeded, glycosuria occurs; in addition, glycogen is not stored in the liver, the respiratory quotient does not rise with increased carbohydrate intake and fat metabolism and the production of glucose from non-carbohydrate sources (gluconeogenesis) is markedly reduced. Oxidation of some of the fat is incomplete, resulting in the formation of ketones, such as acetone and acetoacetic acid, and β-hydroxybutyric acid, which appear in the urine.

When administered parenterally, insulin causes a fall in the blood-sugar level and increased storage of glycogen in the liver. In the diabetic it raises the respiratory quotient after a carbohydrate meal and prevents the formation of ketones.

Insulin is used chiefly for the control of diabetes mellitus in diabetics not responding to dietary control. It is ineffective by mouth and is usually administered by deep subcutaneous injection, although the intravenous route may be used when particularly rapid effects are required, as in diabetic coma.

The dose depends upon the patient's diabetic condition. The action of insulin begins within twenty to thirty minutes of subcutaneous injection and reaches its maximum in four to six hours. Injections are usually given twice a day, fifteen to thirty minutes before breakfast and the evening meal; a third dose may be necessary before the midday meal. The number of injections required can be reduced by the simultaneous injection of a slow-acting insulin before breakfast.

Overdosage with insulin causes hypoglycaemia. The early symptoms, such as weakness, giddiness, pallor, sweating, a sinking feeling in the stomach, palpitations, irritability and tremor, resemble those of sympathetic stimulation. Later, the higher centres may be affected, with the onset of either depression or euphoria, inability to concentrate, lack of judgment and self-control, and amnesia. Other symptoms are ataxia, diplopia, and paraesthesia. Convulsions occur if the blood-sugar level falls below 35 milligrams per 100 millilitres and if this is not corrected permanent brain damage may occur and, finally, death.

In the emergency treatment of diabetic coma, Insulin Injection, but not one of the delayed-acting preparations, is used. In the pre-comatose condition the patient should be given 20 to 50 Units of insulin every two to four hours, depending on the blood-sugar level and intensity of ketosis, although larger doses may often be needed in individual cases. Should the patient be comatose, 100 Units of insulin may be given, approximately half of it intramuscularly and half intravenously; if the insulin requirement normally exceeds 80 Units daily, or if severe infection, dehydration, or circulatory collapse is present, or if the blood-sugar level is over 600 milligrams per 100 millilitres, the initial dose should be increased up to 200 Units.

Frequent determinations of sugar in the blood and urine serve as a guide for further dosage of insulin, which may then be given subcutaneously every two to four hours. Urine estimations are less reliable as a guide than blood estimations unless specimens are obtained frequently.

Dehydration and acidosis are treated by the rapid intravenous infusion of 1000 millilitres of a solution containing 5·85 grams of sodium chloride and 3·36 grams of sodium lactate or of Sodium Chloride Injection or Sodium Bicarbonate Injection, depending upon the metabolic state; further quantities may be given if required, but at a slower rate. After diuresis has set in and the blood-sugar level has begun to fall, supplements of potassium and magnesium are frequently required. If peripheral circulatory failure has occurred, two pints of plasma may be given intravenously.

Insulin Injection may be mixed with Isophane Insulin Injection, or with Protamine Zinc Insulin Injection in the same syringe just before injection, but not with other forms of insulin.

UNDESIRABLE EFFECTS. In addition to the effects of overdosage described above, insulin may give rise to allergic reactions and atrophy of fat at the site of injection.

PRECAUTIONS. Thiazide diuretics and corticosteroids may increase insulin requirements.

POISONING. In the early stages, when the patient can swallow, three or four lumps of sugar may be given, and again in ten to fifteen minutes if there is no improvement. If consciousness is lost, food cannot be given by mouth and treatment is by the intravenous administration of 10 to 50 millilitres of Strong Dextrose Injection.

Dose. See above under **Actions and uses.**

OTHER NAME: Unmodified Insulin

BIPHASIC INSULIN INJECTION

SYNONYM: Biphasic Insulin

Biphasic Insulin Injection is a sterile buffered suspension of crystals containing the specific antidiabetic principle of the pancreas of the ox in a solution of the specific antidiabetic principle of the pancreas of the pig.

Biphasic Insulin Injection may be prepared from crystalline ox insulin, with a potency of not less than 23 Units per milligram, calculated with reference to the anhydrous material and containing about 0·8 per cent of zinc, by dissolving in a dilute hydrochloric acid, sterilising the solution by filtration, and mixing the filtrate aseptically, with constant stirring, with one third of its volume of a sterile solution containing 5·44 per cent w/v of sodium acetate, 28 per cent w/v of sodium chloride, and sufficient sodium hydroxide to produce a pH of 5·4 to 5·5 in the mixture. The stirring is continued for about twenty hours, or until the precipitated insulin is converted into rhombohedral crystals.

The suspension is then added aseptically to eight times its volume of a sterile aqueous solution of a suitable bactericide, and the mixture diluted with sufficient of a solution of sodium hydroxide to produce a preparation containing either 40 or 80 Units per ml and having a pH of about 7.

To this preparation is added a sterile solution of insulin, containing either 40 or 80 Units per millilitre, until a quarter of the insulin present is in soluble form. This sterile solution of insulin may be prepared from crystalline pig insulin with a potency of not less than 23 Units per milligram, calculated with reference to the anhydrous material, and containing about 0·8 per cent of zinc, by dissolving in a dilute hydrochloric acid, sterilising the solution by filtration, diluting the filtrate aseptically with eight times its volume of a sterile aqueous solution of a suitable bactericide and with one volume of a sterile solution containing 1·36 per cent w/v of sodium acetate, 7 per cent w/v of sodium chloride, and sufficient sodium hydroxide to produce a pH of about 7. The suspension is distributed aseptically into sterile containers which are then sealed.

Standard
It complies with the requirements of the British Pharmacopoeia.
It is an almost colourless turbid liquid in which, on examination under a microscope, the majority of the particles are seen as rhombohedral crystals with a maximum dimension greater than 10 μm but rarely exceeding 40 μm. It contains 40 or 80 Units per ml, the potency being determined biologically, and it has a pH of 6·6 to 7·2.

Containers. The containers are glass vials, sealed so as to allow the withdrawal of successive doses on different occasions.

Storage. It should be stored at 2° to 10°; it should not be allowed to freeze. Under these conditions it may be expected to retain its potency for at least two years after the date of manufacture.

Actions and uses. Biphasic Insulin Injection produces a rapid hypoglycaemic effect within half an hour of subcutaneous injection due to the soluble insulin fraction, while the insulin crystals, being slowly absorbed, produce a depot effect with an action beginning

about three hours after subcutaneous injection and reaching a maximum four to twelve hours after administration. The total duration of action is from eighteen to twenty-two hours. Biphasic Insulin Injection thus combines the properties of a quick-acting soluble insulin and the prolonged action of an insulin of intermediate duration.

Biphasic insulin is administered by subcutaneous injection twice daily, except in mild cases of diabetes when one injection daily may suffice. The first injection is usually given half an hour before breakfast to control the hyperglycaemia occurring shortly afterwards, and the second injection, which should be 30 to 50 per cent of the morning dose, is given half an hour before the evening meal. A more potent initial hypoglycaemic effect may be obtained by mixing neutral insulin with biphasic insulin; other forms of insulin should not be used for this purpose.

The usual dose is from 20 to 80 Units daily, but much more than this may be needed. When changing from another insulin to biphasic insulin it is seldom necessary to alter the total dose.

Biphasic insulin should never be given intravenously and is not suitable for the emergency treatment of diabetic coma. It is not always effective in the treatment of juvenile diabetes and brittle diabetes.

POISONING. The procedure as described under Protamine Zinc Insulin Injection (page 240) should be adopted.

Dose. See above under **Actions and uses.**

GLOBIN ZINC INSULIN INJECTION

SYNONYMS: Globin Insulin; Globin Zinc Insulin

Globin Zinc Insulin Injection is a sterile preparation of the protein insulin, the specific antidiabetic principle of the mammalian pancreas, with a suitable globin and zinc chloride.

Globin Zinc Insulin Injection may be prepared from crystalline insulin having a potency of not less than 23 Units per milligram, calculated with reference to the anhydrous material, by adding aseptically to a sterile solution in hydrochloric acid, the strength of which has been suitably adjusted, the following sterile materials: a solution of globin in the proportion of 3·6 to 4·0 milligrams of globin for each 100 Units; zinc chloride equivalent to 0·3 milligram of zinc for each 100 Units; 1·6 per cent w/v of glycerol; and sufficient bactericide to prevent the growth of micro-organisms.
The preparation is distributed aseptically into sterile containers, which are then sealed. Globin Zinc Insulin Injection is usually made from ox pancreas.

Standard
It complies with the requirements of the British Pharmacopoeia.

It is an almost colourless liquid substantially free from turbidity and from matter which deposits on standing. It contains 40 or 80 Units per ml, the potency being determined biologically, and it has a pH of 3·0 to 3·5.

Containers. The containers are glass vials, sealed so as to allow the withdrawal of successive doses on different occasions.

Storage. It should be stored at 2° to 10°; it should not be allowed to freeze. Under these conditions it may be expected to retain its potency for at least two years after the date of manufacture.

Actions and uses. Globin zinc insulin has actions which are essentially the same as those described under Insulin Injection (page 236). It has, however, a delayed action which is intermediate in onset between that of unmodified insulin and that of protamine zinc insulin. The onset of activity is two to four hours after injection, the maximum six to twelve hours, and the duration of action is eighteen to twenty-four hours.

Globin zinc insulin is used to reduce the number of injections required for the control of diabetes mellitus, as compared with the use of unmodified insulin alone, especially in patients showing hypersensitivity to protamine zinc insulin. It is usually administered by subcutaneous injection half an hour before breakfast. In some severe cases of diabetes, two injections of globin zinc insulin a day may be necessary.

Hypoglycaemic reactions, if they occur while a patient is receiving globin zinc insulin, usually take place in the late afternoon or early evening. They can be avoided by reducing the dose or redistributing the carbohydrate intake between the morning, midday, and evening meals in the proportions of one-fifth, two-fifths, and two-fifths respectively. Alternatively, or in addition, a light carbohydrate meal may be taken in the afternoon.

Globin zinc insulin should never be given by intravenous injection, and it is not suitable for the emergency treatment of diabetic coma, for which Insulin Injection should be used.

UNDESIRABLE EFFECTS. Globin zinc insulin may occasionally produce cutaneous and allergic reactions.

POISONING. The procedure as described under Protamine Zinc Insulin Injection (page 240) should be adopted.

Dose. The dose is determined by the physician in accordance with the needs of the patient.

ISOPHANE INSULIN INJECTION

SYNONYMS: Isophane Insulin; Isophane Insulin (NPH)

Isophane Insulin Injection is a sterile buffered crystalline suspension of the protein insulin, the specific antidiabetic principle of the mammalian pancreas, with a suitable protamine and zinc.

Isophane Insulin Injection may be prepared from crystalline insulin having a potency of not less than 23 Units per milligram, calculated with reference to the anhydrous material. It contains a suitable protamine in the proportion of 0·3 to 0·6 milligram of protamine sulphate for each 100 Units and a zinc salt equivalent to not more than 0·04 milligram of zinc for each 100 Units, together with 1·6 per cent w/v of glycerol, 0·15 to 0·17 per cent w/v of *m*-cresol, 0·06 to 0·07 per cent w/v of phenol, and sodium phosphate as a buffering agent. Isophane Insulin Injection is usually made from ox pancreas.

Standard
It complies with the requirements of the British Pharmacopoeia.
It is a white suspension, the particles in which, on examination under a microscope, are seen to be rod-shaped crystals about 20 μm long, free from large aggregates. It contains 40 or 80 Units per ml, the potency being determined biologically, and it has a pH of 7·1 to 7·4.

Containers. The containers are glass vials, sealed so as to allow the withdrawal of successive doses on different occasions.

Storage. It should be stored at 2° to 10°; it should not be allowed to freeze. Under these conditions it may be expected to retain its potency for at least two years after the date of manufacture.

Actions and uses. Isophane Insulin Injection has actions which are essentially the same as those described under Insulin Injection (page 236). It has a delayed action which begins about two hours after subcutaneous injection, becomes maximal after ten hours, and declines after about twenty-eight hours. Duration of action depends partly on the dosage given.

It is usually administered once a day, before breakfast. When insulin requirements are high it can be given in two doses, two-thirds of the total dose in the morning and one-third in the late afternoon. It should not be given intravenously.

Isophane Insulin Injection may be given together with unmodified insulin when the combined effect of quick-acting and slow-acting insulin is required; they may be mixed and given in the same syringe. When used in such mixtures it has the advantage over protamine zinc insulin that it does not affect the rapid action of the unmodified insulin. It may also be mixed with Neutral Insulin Injection, but not with any other forms of insulin.

POISONING. The procedure as described under Protamine Zinc Insulin Injection (page 240) should be adopted.

Dose. The dose is determined by the physician in accordance with the needs of the patient.

NEUTRAL INSULIN INJECTION

SYNONYM: Neutral Insulin

Neutral Insulin Injection is a sterile buffered solution of the protein insulin, the antidiabetic principle of the pancreas of the ox or pig.

Neutral Insulin Injection may be prepared by dissolving crystalline ox or pig insulin with a potency of not less than 23 Units per milligram, calculated with reference to the anhydrous material and containing about 0·4 per cent of zinc, in a dilute hydrochloric acid, sterilising the solution by filtration, mixing the filtrate aseptically with a sterile aqueous solution of a suitable bactericide, and adding aseptically sufficient of a sterile solution of sodium acetate, sodium chloride, and sodium hydroxide so that the final preparation contains 0·136 per cent w/v of sodium acetate, 0·7 per cent w/v of sodium chloride, and the requisite number of Units, and has a pH of about 7.

The solution is distributed aseptically into sterile containers, which are then sealed.

Standard
It complies with the requirements of the British Pharmacopoeia.
It is a colourless liquid free from turbidity and from matter which deposits on standing. It contains 40 or 80 Units per ml, the potency being determined biologically, and it has a pH of 6·6 to 7·7.

Containers. The containers are glass vials, sealed so as to allow the withdrawal of successive doses on different occasions.

Storage. It should be stored at 2° to 10°; it should not be allowed to freeze. Under these conditions it may be expected to retain its potency for at least two years after the date of manufacture.

Actions and uses. Neutral Insulin Injection has actions and uses similar to those described under Insulin Injection (page 236), but when given subcutaneously it is slightly more rapidly absorbed. The dose of Neutral Insulin Injection is the same as that of Insulin Injec-

tion, and similarly the first dose of the day is given twenty to thirty minutes before breakfast. After injection, it continues to produce a fall in the blood-sugar level for about five and a half hours and maintains its hypoglycaemic effect for eight to nine hours, or slightly longer than Insulin Injection.

Neutral Insulin Injection may be given alone or simultaneously with Biphasic Insulin Injection or Isophane Insulin Injection. It can be mixed in the same syringe with Globin Zinc Insulin Injection, Protamine Zinc Insulin Injection, Insulin Zinc Suspension, Insulin Zinc Suspension (Amorphous), or Insulin Zinc Suspension (Crystalline), but the mixture must be injected immediately after preparation. The effect of these mixtures on the blood-sugar level is very similar to that of mixtures of these preparations with Insulin Injection.

Neutral Insulin Injection should not be mixed with Insulin Injection.

Neutral insulin may be used in the emergency treatment of diabetic coma and pre-coma. Patients hypersensitive to bovine insulin may be treated with Neutral Insulin Injection prepared from pig pancreas.

UNDESIRABLE EFFECTS. These are as described under Insulin Injection (page 236).

POISONING. The procedure as described under Insulin Injection (page 236) should be followed.

Dose. The dose is determined by the physician in accordance with the needs of the patient.

PROTAMINE ZINC INSULIN INJECTION

SYNONYM: Protamine Zinc Insulin

Protamine Zinc Insulin Injection is a sterile suspension of the protein insulin, the specific antidiabetic principle of the mammalian pancreas, with a suitable protamine and zinc chloride.

Protamine Zinc Insulin Injection may be prepared from crystalline insulin having a potency of not less than 23 Units per milligram, calculated with reference to the anhydrous material, by adding aseptically to a sterile aqueous solution, the strength of which has been suitably adjusted, the following sterile materials: a suitable protamine in the proportion of 1·0 to 1·7 milligrams of protamine sulphate for each 100 Units; zinc chloride equivalent to 0·2 milligram of zinc for each 100 Units; 1·6 per cent w/v of glycerol; and

sufficient bactericide to prevent the growth of micro-organisms.

The suspension is distributed aseptically into sterile containers, and a sterile solution of sodium phosphate, containing, if necessary, either sodium hydroxide or phosphoric acid, is added so that the final mixture contains 10 to 11 milligrams of sodium phosphate for each 100 Units and has a pH of 6·9 to 7·4, within which range most of the active principle is precipitated. The containers are then sealed.

Protamine Zinc Insulin Injection is usually made from ox pancreas.

Standard
It complies with the requirements of the British Pharmacopoeia.
It is an almost colourless turbid liquid and contains 40 or 80 Units per ml, the potency being determined biologically. It has a pH of 6·9 to 7·4.

Containers. The containers are glass vials, sealed so as to allow the withdrawal of successive doses on different occasions.

Storage. It should be stored at 2° to 10°; it should not be allowed to freeze. Under these conditions it may be expected to retain its potency for at least two years after the date of manufacture.

Actions and uses. Protamine zinc insulin has actions which are essentially the same as those described under Insulin Injection (page 236). It has, however, a delayed action, which allows a slow but steady activity of insulin throughout the day.

Protamine zinc insulin is used to reduce the number of injections used in the control of diabetes mellitus, as compared with the use of unmodified insulin alone. It is usually administered once a day by subcutaneous injection thirty to sixty minutes before breakfast. A dose of unmodified insulin is often given at the same time to tide over the period until the protamine zinc insulin is absorbed; the two insulins may be mixed in the syringe immediately before the injection is given but the onset and duration of action of the resulting mixture differ from those of the two insulin preparations injected separately because some of the unmodified insulin is converted by the excess protamine in the Protamine Zinc Insulin into the latter.

The onset of action of Protamine Zinc Insulin given alone is from four to seven hours, the maximum effect is obtained in fifteen to twenty hours, and the total duration of action is twenty-four to thirty-six hours, depending on total dosage.

Intramuscular injection of protamine zinc insulin may cause pain, and it should never be given intravenously. In some patients its action following large doses is sufficiently delayed to render the next morning specimen of urine sugar-free; such patients do not require unmodified insulin.

The dose of protamine zinc insulin is adjusted to suit the needs of the patient; more than 80 Units should rarely be given, because of the severe nocturnal hypoglycaemia that may result. If the patient has previously been treated with unmodified insulin, the initial dose of protamine zinc insulin should be from two-thirds to the same number of Units. Because protamine zinc insulin lowers the blood-sugar level over a long period, a redistribution of the carbohydrate intake more evenly over the waking hours may be necessary. An increased carbohydrate intake at bedtime may prevent early morning hypoglycaemia.

Because it is slowly absorbed, protamine zinc insulin should never be given in the treatment of diabetic coma. For the same reason, hypoglycaemic attacks resulting from protamine zinc insulin are insidious and tend to occur during the night or early morning. They require immediate and continued treatment for some hours.

Protamine Zinc Insulin may be mixed with Insulin Injection or with Neutral Insulin Injection, but not with any other forms of insulin.

UNDESIRABLE EFFECTS. These are as described under Insulin Injection (page 236). Allergic reactions to the protamine may also occur.

POISONING. The treatment is the same as that for the hypoglycaemic attacks caused by overdosage of unmodified insulin, as described under Insulin Injection (page 236), except that when the patient has recovered consciousness and is able to swallow, glucose drinks and a slowly digestible form of carbohydrate, such as bread, must be given until the more prolonged action of the protamine zinc insulin has ceased.

Dose. See above under **Actions and uses.**

INSULIN ZINC SUSPENSION

SYNONYM: I.Z.S.

Insulin Zinc Suspension is a sterile buffered suspension of the protein insulin, the specific antidiabetic principle of the mammalian pancreas, with zinc chloride.

Insulin Zinc Suspension may be prepared by mixing aseptically three volumes of Insulin Zinc Suspension (Amorphous) and seven volumes of Insulin Zinc Suspension (Crystalline). The suspension is distributed aseptically into sterile containers, which are then sealed. Two forms of Insulin Zinc Suspension, one made from pig pancreas and the other from ox pancreas, are available.

Standard
It complies with the requirements of the British Pharmacopoeia.
It is an almost colourless turbid liquid in which, on examination under a microscope, the majority of the particles are seen as rhombohedral crystals with a maxi-

mum dimension greater than 10 μm but rarely exceeding 40 μm; a considerable proportion of the particles can be seen under high-power magnification to have no uniform shape and not to exceed 2 μm in maximum dimension. It contains 40 or 80 Units per ml, the potency being determined biologically, and it has a pH of 7·0 to 7·5.

Containers. The containers are glass vials, sealed so as to allow the withdrawal of successive doses on different occasions.

Storage. It should be stored at 2° to 10°; it should not be allowed to freeze. Under these conditions it may be expected to retain its potency for at least two years after the date of manufacture.

Actions and uses. Insulin zinc suspensions have actions which are essentially the same as those described under Insulin Injection (page 236). They have, however, a delayed action which varies in duration from twelve to thirty hours or longer, depending upon the amount of zinc present and the particle size of the insulin.

Insulin Zinc Suspension (Amorphous) has a relatively short duration of action; its effect begins in thirty minutes and is maximal in two to three hours and persists for twelve to sixteen hours. The effect of Insulin Zinc Suspension (Crystalline) begins a few hours after injection, is maximal seven hours after subcutaneous injection, and may persist for thirty-six hours. These two suspensions are miscible in all proportions without any modification of the one by the other, and in many diabetics good control is maintained by a single daily injection of such a mixture in the form of Insulin Zinc Suspension. Because they are free from foreign protein, these preparations are less likely than Protamine Zinc Insulin Injection and Globin Zinc Insulin Injection to produce local and allergic reactions.

For the average diabetic, Insulin Zinc Suspension gives suitable control; its onset of action is gradual, with a maximal lowering of blood-sugar level four to five hours after sub-

cutaneous injection and a total duration of action of twenty-four hours. The onset of action of the usual morning dose is sufficiently rapid to control the rise of blood-sugar level after breakfast. Most diabetics needing insulin are satisfactorily controlled by one injection a day of this preparation; a small proportion need the addition of Insulin Zinc Suspension (Amorphous) or Insulin Zinc Suspension (Crystalline) for optimal control.

These insulin zinc suspensions are not suitable for the treatment of diabetic emergencies or diabetic coma, for which Insulin Injection should be used. They should not be given intravenously or, because they are incompatible with the buffering agents, mixed with other insulin preparations; they are, however, mutually miscible. They are administered by subcutaneous injection, usually thirty to forty-five minutes before breakfast.

The dosage varies according to the condition of the patient and usually lies between 20 and 100 Units daily. The initial dose is 10 to 16 Units daily, increased by 4 Units daily until the blood sugar is controlled. Some diabetics cannot be controlled with Insulin Zinc Suspension alone. In such cases additional Insulin Zinc Suspension (Crystalline) or Insulin Zinc Suspension (Amorphous) may be added to the mixture. Alternatively, Insulin Injection may be given in the evening. Before each dose of Insulin Zinc Suspension is withdrawn from the vial it should be shaken gently; vigorous shaking may cause excessive frothing. Severe diabetes is first brought under control with Insulin Injection and an insulin zinc suspension is then substituted in the same or slightly larger daily dosage.

POISONING. The procedure as described under Protamine Zinc Insulin Injection (page 240) should be adopted.

Dose. See above under **Actions and uses.**

OTHER NAME: Insulin Lente

INSULIN ZINC SUSPENSION (AMORPHOUS)

SYNONYM: Amorph. I.Z.S.

Insulin Zinc Suspension (Amorphous) is a sterile buffered suspension of the protein insulin, the specific antidiabetic principle of the mammalian pancreas, with zinc chloride.

Insulin Zinc Suspension (Amorphous) may be prepared from crystalline insulin having a potency of not less than 23 Units per milligram, calculated with reference to the anhydrous material, by dissolving it in 0·02N hydrochloric acid containing zinc chloride equivalent to 0·01 per cent w/v of zinc; the solution is sterilised by filtration and diluted aseptically with eight times its volume of a sterile solution containing, for the 40 Units per millilitre preparation, zinc chloride equivalent to 0·00875 per cent w/v of zinc, or, for the

80 Units per millilitre preparation, zinc chloride equivalent to 0·01375 per cent w/v of zinc, together with sufficient bactericide to prevent the growth of micro-organisms in the final preparation. A sterile solution of sodium acetate, sodium chloride, and sodium hydroxide is added, with constant stirring, to give a preparation containing 0·136 per cent w/v of sodium acetate and 0·7 per cent w/v of sodium chloride and having a pH of about 7·3.

The preparation is distributed aseptically into sterile containers, which are then sealed.

Two forms of Insulin Zinc Suspension (Amorphous), one made from pig pancreas and the other from ox pancreas, are available.

Standard
It complies with the requirements of the British Pharmacopoeia.
It is an almost colourless turbid liquid in which, on examination under a microscope, the particles are seen to have no uniform shape and rarely exceed 2 μm in maximum dimension. It contains 40 or 80 Units per ml, the potency being determined biologically, and it has a pH of 7·0 to 7·5.

Containers. The containers are glass vials, sealed so as to allow the withdrawal of successive doses on different occasions.

Storage. It should be stored at 2° to 10°; it should not be allowed to freeze. Under these conditions it may be expected to retain its potency for at least two years after the date of manufacture.

Actions and uses. Insulin Zinc Suspension (Amorphous) has the actions and uses described under Insulin Zinc Suspension. It may be mixed with Insulin Zinc Suspension or with Insulin Zinc Suspension (Crystalline) but not with any other form of insulin.

POISONING. The procedure as described under Protamine Zinc Insulin Injection (page 240) should be adopted.

OTHER NAME: Insulin Semilente

INSULIN ZINC SUSPENSION (CRYSTALLINE)

SYNONYM: Cryst. I.Z.S.

Insulin Zinc Suspension (Crystalline) is a sterile buffered suspension of the protein insulin, the specific antidiabetic principle of the mammalian pancreas, with zinc chloride.

Insulin Zinc Suspension (Crystalline) may be prepared from crystalline insulin having a potency of not less than 23 Units per milligram, calculated with reference to the anhydrous material, by dissolving it in 0·02N hydrochloric acid containing, for the 40 Units per millilitre preparation, zinc chloride equivalent to 0·0133 per cent w/v of zinc, or, for the 80 Units per millilitre preparation, zinc chloride equivalent to 0·0266 per cent w/v of zinc; the solution is sterilised by filtration and is mixed aseptically, with constant stirring, with one-third of its volume of a sterile solution containing 5·44 per cent w/v of sodium acetate, 28 per cent w/v of sodium chloride, and sufficient sodium hydroxide to produce a pH of 5·4 to 5·5. The stirring is continued for about twenty hours, or until the insulin is converted into regular crystals.
The suspension is then added aseptically, with constant stirring, to nine times its volume of a sterile solution containing sufficient bactericide to prevent the growth of micro-organisms and, for the 40 Units per millilitre preparation, 0·014 per cent w/v of sodium hydroxide and zinc chloride equivalent to 0·0077 per cent w/v of zinc, or, for the 80 Units per millilitre preparation, 0·017 per cent w/v of sodium hydroxide and zinc chloride equivalent to 0·0111 per cent w/v of zinc.

The preparation is distributed aseptically into sterile containers, which are then sealed.
Insulin Zinc Suspension (Crystalline) is usually made from ox pancreas.

Standard
It complies with the requirements of the British Pharmacopoeia.
It is an almost colourless turbid liquid, the particles in which, on examination under a microscope, are seen to be rhombohedral crystals, the majority having a maximum dimension greater than 10 μm but rarely exceeding 40 μm. It contains 40 or 80 Units per ml, the potency being determined biologically, and it has a pH of 7·0 to 7·5.

Containers. The containers are glass vials, sealed so as to allow the withdrawal of successive doses on different occasions.

Storage. It should be stored at 2° to 10°; it should not be allowed to freeze. Under these conditions it may be expected to retain its potency for at least two years after the date of manufacture.

Actions and uses. Insulin Zinc Suspension (Crystalline) has the actions and uses described under Insulin Zinc Suspension. It may be mixed with Insulin Zinc Suspension or with Insulin Zinc Suspension (Amorphous) but not with any other form of insulin.

POISONING. The procedure as described under Protamine Zinc Insulin Injection (page 240) should be followed.

OTHER NAME: Insulin Ultralente

INULIN

Inulin consists of polysaccharide granules obtained from the tubers of *Dahlia variabilis* Desf. *Helianthus tuberosus* L., and other genera of the family Compositae.

Solubility. Slightly soluble in water; more soluble in hot water; slightly soluble in organic solvents.

Standard
It complies with the requirements of the British Pharmacopoeia.
It is a white, amorphous, granular, hygroscopic, odour-

less powder. The loss on drying at 105° is not more than 5·0 per cent. A 10 per cent solution in hot water is clear and colourless.

Microscopical characters: small particles, mostly spherules about 2 to 6 μm in diameter, many of them clumped into irregularly shaped granular flakes or masses about 30 to 160 μm in size; when viewed between crossed polars, it shines brightly and the rarely found larger spherules, about 20 μm in diameter, exhibit a black cross.

Sterilisation. Solutions for injection are sterilised by filtration.

Storage. It should be stored in airtight containers.

Actions and uses. Inulin is a saccharide polymer which is not degraded by any mammalian enzyme. It is excreted almost entirely in the urine and neither secreted nor resorbed by the nephron. The only pharmacological effect of inulin is an osmotic diuresis when it is given in large amounts.

Inulin is used to measure the glomerular filtration rate. A primary dose of 30 millilitres of warm Inulin Injection is injected into a forearm vein and a mixture of 70 millilitres of Inulin Injection and 500 millilitres of Sodium Chloride Injection is given by intravenous drip into the other forearm, the infusion being made at a steady rate so that the plasma level is kept as nearly constant as possible. A depot injection may be made into the subcutaneous tissue for the same purpose but is much less satisfactory than the intravenous infusion method.

The inulin content of the plasma and urine is determined after the removal of glucose and proteins. The test measures the clearance of inulin from the plasma and allows other inferences to be made. For example, substances with a clearance greater than inulin are secreted and those with a smaller clearance resorbed by the nephron.

Dose. See above under **Actions and uses.**

Preparation

INULIN INJECTION, B.P. It consists of a sterile solution of inulin 10 per cent and sodium chloride 0·8 per cent in Water for Injections. It deposits on storage, and before use solid matter should be completely redissolved by heating for not more than fifteen minutes. The solution should be cooled to a suitable temperature before administration and should not be reheated.

IODINATED (^{125}I) HUMAN ALBUMIN INJECTION

SYNONYM: IHA (^{125}I) Inj.

This material is radioactive and any regulations in force must be complied with.

Iodinated (^{125}I) Human Albumin Injection is a sterile solution in a saline solution isotonic with blood and containing a suitable bactericide, such as benzyl alcohol in a concentration of 0·9 per cent v/v, of human albumin which has been iodinated with iodine-125 and subsequently freed from ^{125}I iodide.

Iodine-125 is a radioactive isotope of iodine which emits γ- and X-radiation and has a half-life of 60 days; it may be prepared by the neutron irradiation of xenon.

Standard

It complies with the requirements of the British Pharmacopoeia.

It is a clear colourless or faintly yellow solution with a pH of 6·5 to 8·5. It contains not less than 1·0 per cent of protein. The human albumin contains not more than 5 per cent of globulins and, before the addition of carrier protein if this is added, is uniformly iodinated to an extent that does not exceed the equivalent of one atom of iodine for each molecule of albumin. The injection contains not less than 85·0 and not more than 115·0 per cent of the quantity of iodine-125 stated on the label at the date stated on the label. Not more than 1·0 per cent of the total activity, expressed as disintegrations per second, is due to iodine-126 at the date stated on the label.

Sterilisation. It is sterilised by filtration.

Labelling. The label on the container states:
(1) the content of iodine-125 expressed in microcuries or millicuries at a given date;
(2) the weight of human albumin in the container;
(3) that the injection is radioactive; and
(4) the date after which the injection should not be used.

The label on the package also states:
(1) the total volume in the container;
(2) the nature and proportion of salts and bactericide present;
(3) that the injection is not necessarily suitable for metabolic studies; and
(4) that it should be stored at a temperature between 2° and 10°.

Storage. It should be stored in an area assigned for the purpose, at a temperature between 2° and 10°. The storage conditions should be such that the maximum radiation-dose-rate to which persons may be exposed is reduced to an acceptable level.

Actions and uses. Iodinated (^{125}I) human albumin injection has actions and uses similar to those described under Iodinated (^{131}I) Human Albumin Injection.

As the radiation from iodine-125 is less penetrating than that from iodine-131 its use reduces the risk to workers carrying out diagnostic procedures and, in the estimation of blood and plasma volumes, it reduces the radiation dose to the patient, but it is of little value for techniques which depend on radiation measurements at the body surface.

PRECAUTIONS AND CONTRA-INDICATIONS. As for Iodinated (^{131}I) Human Albumin Injection.

Dose. In the determination of blood and plasma volumes, 5 microcuries.

In other investigations, up to 100 microcuries.

IODINATED (^{131}I) HUMAN ALBUMIN INJECTION

SYNONYM: IHA (^{131}I) Inj.

This material is radioactive and any regulations in force must be complied with.

Iodinated (^{131}I) Human Albumin Injection is a sterile solution in a saline solution isotonic with blood and containing a suitable bactericide, such as benzyl alcohol in a concentration of 0·9 per cent v/v, of human albumin which has been iodinated with iodine-131 and subsequently freed from ^{131}I iodide.

Iodine-131 is a radioactive isotope of iodine which emits β- and γ-radiation and has a half-life of 8 days; it may be prepared from the products of uranium fission or by the neutron irradiation of tellurium.

Standard
It complies with the requirements of the British Pharmacopoeia.
It is a clear colourless or faintly yellow solution with a pH of 6·5 to 8·5. It contains not less than 1·0 per cent of protein. The human albumin contains not more than 5 per cent of globulins and, before the addition of carrier protein if this is added, is uniformly iodinated to an extent that does not exceed the equivalent of one atom of iodine for each molecule of albumin. The injection contains not less than 90·0 and not more than 110·0 per cent of the quantity of iodine-131 stated on the label at the date and hour stated on the label, and not more than 1·5 millicuries of iodine-131 per ml at the date and hour stated on the label.

Sterilisation. It is sterilised by filtration.

Labelling. The label on the container states:
(1) the content of iodine-131 expressed in microcuries or millicuries at a given date and hour;
(2) the weight of human albumin in the container;
(3) that the injection is radioactive; and
(4) the date after which the injection should not be used.

The label on the package also states:
(1) the total volume in the container;
(2) the names and proportions of salts and bactericide present;
(3) that the injection is not necessarily suitable for metabolic studies; and
(4) that it should be stored at a temperature between 2° and 10°.

Storage. It should be stored in an area assigned for the purpose, at a temperature between 2° and 10°. The storage conditions should be such that the maximum radiation-dose-rate to which persons may be exposed is reduced to an acceptable level.
Glass containers may darken under the effects of the radiation.

Actions and uses. ^{131}I-labelled human albumin is used to estimate the blood volume and plasma volume by measuring the dilution of an injected sample, and in many respects this procedure is simpler than dye-dilution methods. The volume of fluid accumulations, such as ascites or gastric residues, can also be measured.

Circulation times, which provide an approximate measure of the velocity of blood flow between various parts of the body, have also been estimated using injected ^{131}I-labelled human albumin and a suitable detection and recording device at a distal site. Elaboration of such techniques with recording of dilution curves of radioactivity provides one method of estimating cardiac output when the other data provided by cardiac catheterisation are not required. ^{131}I-labelled human albumin is also used for the detection and localisation of venous thrombosis.

^{131}I-labelled human albumin is also used in isotope ventriculography, cisternography, and myeloscintigraphy, and for the investigation of hydrocephalus and other disorders. It may be injected intrathecally or direct into the brain cavities for this purpose.

Other uses for labelled albumin include the localisation of tumours in brain and liver by scintillation scanning; for these purposes, ^{131}I-labelled albumin has been largely replaced by other radioactive preparations. A dose of 5 microcuries per kilogram body-weight is suitable for brain scanning. In sub-arachnoid block there is no detectable spread of radioactivity after introduction of labelled albumin into the lumbar sac.

PRECAUTIONS AND CONTRA-INDICATIONS. Since iodinated(^{131}I) human serum albumin releases radioactive iodide on metabolism, it is advisable that the patient's thyroid gland should be blocked by the administration of iodide before the radioactive preparation is given.

Dose. In the determination of blood and plasma volumes, 5 microcuries.
In other investigations of the circulatory system, up to 50 microcuries.

IODINE

SYNONYM: Iodum

$I = 126·9$

Iodine is a solid non-metallic element, the chief source of which is the Chilean nitrate ore, caliche, which contains from 0·15 per cent in the form of iodates. Mother liquors obtained by lixiviation of the nitrate ore are treated with sulphides to precipitate free iodine, which is washed, and dried by pressing. Iodine is also obtained by oxidation of inorganic iodides present in some natural brine wells and in the ashes of seaweed (kelp). It is purified by sublimation.

Iodine is slowly volatile at room temperature and when heated is completely volatilised, giving off violet-coloured vapours which may be condensed as a bluish-black crystalline sublimate. A solution in alcohol, ether, or aqueous solutions of iodides is reddish-brown; in chloroform or carbon disulphide it is violet-coloured.

In contact with the skin, iodine produces a deep reddish-brown stain, which can be readily removed by dilute solutions of alkalis or sodium thiosulphate.

Standard
It complies with the requirements of the European Pharmacopoeia.
It occurs as greyish-violet, brittle plates or small crystals, with a metallic sheen and an irritant odour and contains not less than 99·5 per cent of I.

Incompatibility. It is incompatible with alkalis and alkali carbonates, turpentine oil and most volatile oils, tannin, and vegetable astringents. With acetone it forms a pungent and irritating compound.

Storage. It should be stored in glass-stoppered bottles, or in glass or earthenware containers with well-waxed bungs.

Actions and uses. When taken by mouth iodine is absorbed as iodide and is stored in the thyroid gland as thyroglobulin. In the treatment of thyrotoxicosis, iodine is given as Aqueous Iodine Solution for ten to fourteen days prior to thyroidectomy in order to produce a firm texture suitable for operation, and its administration is continued post-operatively for a few days to avert thyrotoxic crises. For these purposes 0·1 to 0·3 millilitre of the aqueous solution is administered by mouth three times a day in milk or water; larger dosages, such as 2 to 3 millilitres daily,

are given in thyrotoxic crises. The use of iodine in this way has no advantage over the use of iodides.

Iodine is an effective bactericide and is used in solution as a sterilising agent for unbroken skin.

For the pre-operative sterilisation of skin, Weak Iodine Solution or a 2 per cent solution of iodine in isopropyl alcohol or industrial methylated spirit is suitable. When industrial methylated spirit is used as the solvent it should be free from acetone, with which iodine forms an irritant and lachrymatory compound which inconveniences the surgeon. Weak Iodine Solution has been used as an antiseptic application to small wounds, but it is rapidly inactivated by combining with tissue substances and it delays healing.

Iodine ointments have been applied as counter-irritants and a compound paint (Mandl's paint) has been used as a throat paint in the treatment of pharyngitis and follicular tonsilitis.

POISONING. Large draughts of milk and a starch mucilage should be given, followed by stimulants.

Preparations
IODINE SOLUTION, AQUEOUS, B.P. (*Syn.* Lugol's Solution). It contains 10 per cent of potassium iodide and 5 per cent of iodine. It should be stored in airtight iodine-resistant containers. Dose: in the pre-operative treatment of thyrotoxicosis, 1 ml daily in divided doses.
IODINE SOLUTION, WEAK, B.P. (*Syn.* Iodine Tincture). It contains 2·5 per cent each of iodine, potassium iodide, and water, in alcohol (90 per cent). It should be stored in airtight iodine-resistant containers.

IODIPAMIDE MEGLUMINE INJECTION

$C_{34}H_{48}I_6N_4O_{16} = 1530·2$

Iodipamide Meglumine Injection is a sterile solution of the di(*N*-methylglucamine) salt of *NN'*-di(3-carboxy-2,4,6-tri-iodophenyl)adipamide.

Standard
It complies with the requirements of the British Pharmacopoeia.
It is a clear colourless to pale yellow solution and contains not less than 97·0 and not more than 103·0 per cent of the prescribed or stated amount of iodipamide meglumine. It has a pH of 6·0 to 7·1.

Sterilisation. It is sterilised by heating in an autoclave.

Actions and uses. Iodipamide meglumine injection is a radiopaque contrast medium which is available in solutions containing 30, 50, and 70 per cent w/v. The 70 per cent solution is used for hysterosalpingography and sinography. The 30 and 50 per cent solutions are used by intravenous injection for radiography of the biliary tract. The

50 per cent solution is the one usually employed, a suitable dose being 20 millilitres.

The injection should be given slowly over a period of ten minutes to minimise undesirable effects. After injection, the compound is rapidly excreted in the bile and the hepatic and common bile ducts may frequently be visualised within 20 minutes. With normal liver function, about 90 per cent of the dose is excreted in the bile and the remainder in the urine. For infusion cholangiography, the contrast medium is diluted and administered as a slow intravenous drip over a period of thirty minutes. This results in improved visualisation of the duct system and a decreased incidence of side-effects. A dose of 20 to 40 millilitres of the 50 per cent solution is commonly used in the infusion techniques; larger doses have been advocated but they are probably undesirable except in special circumstances. With the infusion technique, the common bile duct may often be satisfactorily visualised with only 10 millilitres of the 50 per cent solution.

Intravenous cholangiography is sometimes performed immediately after an oral cholangiogram. However, hepatic excretion appears to be less efficient under these circumstances and the incidence of side-effects is probably increased.

In the presence of jaundice, intravenous cholangiography is frequently disappointing, particularly if the serum bilirubin is above 3 mg per 100 ml, and the risk of the examination is also likely to be increased.

UNDESIRABLE EFFECTS. Transient restlessness, sensations of warmth, abdominal pain, nausea, and vomiting may occur, particularly if the injection has been given too rapidly. Major side-effects are as described under Sodium Diatrizoate (page 450), but the toxicity of iodipamide is approximately six times that of sodium diatrizoate.

Iodipamide has a uricosuric action similar to that of probenecid and adequate hydration is therefore advisable. Rare cases of renal failure have been reported. Predisposing factors have been liver damage, hypotensive collapse, excessive dosage, and previous oral cholangiography.

PRECAUTIONS. Caution is required in debilitated patients and in the presence of coronary artery disease. Iodipamide should not be mixed in the same syringe with antihistamines since precipitation may occur.

Dose. See above under **Actions and uses.**

OTHER NAMES: *Biligrafin®*; *Endografin®*; Iodipamide Methylglucamine Injection

IODISED OIL FLUID INJECTION

Iodised Oil Fluid Injection is a sterile iodine-addition product of the ethyl esters of the fatty acids obtained from poppy-seed oil, the oil expressed from the ripe seeds of *Papaver somniferum* L. (Fam. Papaveraceae), and may be prepared by treating these esters with hydriodic acid. It is distributed into sterile single-dose containers which are then hermetically sealed.

Solubility. Immiscible with water; miscible with ether, with chloroform, and with light petroleum.

Standard
It complies with the requirements of the British Pharmacopoeia.
It is a straw-coloured or yellow, clear, oily liquid, which is odourless or has a slightly alliaceous odour. It contains 37·0 to 39·0 per cent w/w of combined iodine. It has a weight per ml at 20° of 1·28 g to 1·30 g.

Stability. It decomposes on exposure to air and sunlight, becoming dark brown in colour.

Storage. It should be stored, protected from light, in an atmosphere of carbon dioxide or nitrogen.

Actions and uses. Iodised Oil Fluid Injection is a contrast medium which is now used almost solely for lymphography and sialography. It was formerly used in bronchography, but for this purpose it has been replaced by propyliodone.

NOTE. When Iodised Oil Injection or Iodised Oil is prescribed or demanded, Iodised Oil Fluid Injection is dispensed or supplied.

Dose. The amount required to carry out the diagnostic procedure.

OTHER NAME: *Lipiodol Ultra-Fluid®*

IOPANOIC ACID

$C_{11}H_{12}I_3NO_2 = 570·9$

Iopanoic Acid is α-(3-amino-2,4,6-tri-iodobenzyl)butyric acid.

Solubility. Insoluble in water; soluble, at 20°, in 25 parts of alcohol; soluble in acetone and in solutions of alkali hydroxides.

Standard
It complies with the requirements of the British Pharmacopoeia.

It is a white to cream-coloured odourless powder and contains not less than 98·5 and not more than the equivalent of 101·0 per cent of $C_{11}H_{12}I_3NO_2$, calculated with reference to the dried substance. The loss on drying under the prescribed conditions is not more than 0·5 per cent. It has a melting-point of about 155°.

Storage. It should be protected from light.

Actions and uses. Iopanoic acid is a radio-opaque substance which is absorbed from the gastro-intestinal tract and excreted in the bile, being eliminated in the faeces and, to some extent, in the urine. It is used as a contrast medium in radiography of the gall bladder.

Iopanoic acid is given by mouth with a light fat-free meal about ten to fifteen hours before X-ray examination, the usual dose being 3 grams. After two or three exposures have been made, an emulsion or a meal rich in fat is given and further exposures are made after ten minutes, and if necessary, after thirty minutes or one hour.

UNDESIRABLE EFFECTS. Diarrhoea is not uncommon and occasionally this may be severe enough to cause collapse. Other side-effects include nausea, vomiting, headache, dysuria, and skin rashes.

Iopanoic acid and other cholecystographic media have a uricosuric action similar to that of probenecid and adequate hydration is therefore advisable.

Rare cases of renal failure have been reported, usually associated with excess dosage in patients suffering from jaundice or liver damage.

PRECAUTIONS AND CONTRA-INDICATIONS. Pre-existing renal disease may be a contra-indication to cholecystography, particularly if liver damage is suspected. In acute gastro-intestinal disorders, the substance may not be absorbed. Caution should be exercised in patients with severe coronary artery disease.

Preparation
IOPANOIC ACID TABLETS, B.P. Unless otherwise specified, tablets each containing 500 mg of iopanoic acid are supplied. They should be protected from light.

OTHER NAME: *Telepaque*®

IOPHENDYLATE INJECTION

Iophendylate Injection is a sterile mixture of isomers of ethyl 10-(*p*-iodophenyl)undecanoate, $p\text{-}I \cdot C_6H_4 \cdot CH(CH_3) \cdot [CH_2]_8 \cdot CO \cdot O \cdot C_2H_5$ ($C_{19}H_{29}IO_2 = 416\cdot3$). It is distributed in sterile single–dose containers, which are then hermetically sealed.

Solubility. Very slightly soluble in water; soluble in 2 parts of alcohol; miscible with ether and with chloroform.

Standard
It complies with the requirements of the British Pharmacopoeia.
It is a clear, almost colourless to pale yellow, viscous liquid and contains not less than 98·0 and not more than the equivalent of 101·0 per cent w/w of $C_{19}H_{29}IO_2$. It has a weight per ml at 20° of 1·245 g to 1·260 g.

Storage. It should be protected from light.

Actions and uses. Iophendylate Injection is used as a contrast medium for myelography. It is almost completely resorbed from the spinal canal, its rate of disappearance being about 1 millilitre a year.

Iophendylate is used in the radiological diagnosis and localisation of tumours of the spinal cord, displaced intervertebral disks, and any condition in which obstructions in the cerebrospinal canal or compression of the cord are suspected.

The dose depends upon the diagnostic procedure and up to 9 millilitres may be required. The injection is usually made in the mid-lumbar region; to determine the upper level of the lesion an intracisternal injection may be necessary. Plastic syringes should not be used.

UNDESIRABLE EFFECTS. Although its toxicity is low, cases of allergic reaction and arachnoiditis have occasionally been reported.

Dose. Up to 9 millilitres depending on the diagnostic procedure.

OTHER NAMES: Ethyl Iodophenylundecanoate Injection; *Myodil*®

IOTHALAMIC ACID

$C_{11}H_9I_3N_2O_4 = 613\cdot9$

Iothalamic Acid is 3-acetamido-2,4,6-tri-iodo-5-methylcarbamoyl-benzoic acid.

Solubility. Soluble, at 20°, in 400 parts of water and in 330 parts of alcohol; very slightly soluble in chloroform; very soluble in solutions of sodium hydroxide.

Standard
It complies with the requirements of the British Pharmacopoeia.

It is a white odourless powder and contains not less than 99·0 and not more than the equivalent of 101·0 per cent of $C_{11}H_9I_3N_2O_4$, calculated with reference to the dried substance. The loss on drying under the prescribed conditions is not more than 0·5 per cent.

Sterilisation. Solutions for injection are sterilised by heating in an autoclave.

Storage. It should be protected from light.

Actions and uses. Iothalamic acid is a contrast medium for diagnostic radiology. It is used in the form of its meglumine and sodium salts, which have general properties similar to those of sodium diatrizoate (page 450) and are used in similar dosage.

Sodium iothalamate is more soluble in water than sodium diatrizoate and very concentrated solutions may be prepared without the inclusion of organic bases, thus enabling solutions of high iodine content and low viscosity to be obtained.

A 70 per cent solution is used for abdominal and intravenous aortography and an 80 per cent solution for angiography. Iothalamic acid is also used as a 35 or 60 per cent solution of meglumine iothalamate for intravenous pyelography, cerebral angiography, and peripheral aortography.

Dose. The amount necessary to carry out the diagnostic procedure.

Preparations

MEGLUMINE IOTHALAMATE INJECTION, B.P. It consists of a sterile solution of the meglumine salt of iothalamic acid; it contains suitable stabilising agents. Solutions containing 35 and 60 per cent of meglumine iothalamate are available.

SODIUM IOTHALAMATE INJECTION, B.P. It consists of a sterile solution of the sodium salt of iothalamic acid; it contains suitable stabilising agents. Solutions containing 70 and 80 per cent of sodium iothalamate are available.

IPECACUANHA

SYNONYMS: Ipecac.; Ipecacuanha Root; Ipecacuanhae Radix

Ipecacuanha consists of the dried root, or the rhizome and root, of *Cephaëlis ipecacuanha* (Brot.) A. Rich. (Fam. Rubiaceae), known in commerce as Matto Grosso (Rio) and Minas ipecacuanha, or of *C. acuminata* Karsten, known in commerce as Colombia, Nicaragua or Costa Rica ipecacuanha, or of a mixture of both species. The former is indigenous to and cultivated in Brazil; the latter is imported from Colombia and Central America.

Constituents. Ipecacuanha contains the isoquinoline alkaloids emetine and cephaëline (demethylemetine) and small proportions of psychotrine (dehydrocephaëline), methylpsychotrine, and emetamine. The root contains, in addition, ipecacuanhic acid, the glycoside ipecacuanhin, a saponin, and about 30 to 40 per cent of starch.

The total alkaloidal content of the root varies considerably, Matto Grosso ipecacuanha yielding from 2 to 2·4 per cent, of which about 60 to 75 per cent is emetine and about 26 per cent is cephaëline, while psychotrine, methylpsychotrine, and emetamine form only about 2 per cent. Colombia ipecacuanha contains 2·1 to 2·45 per cent of total alkaloids, Nicaraguan 2·65 to 3·0 per cent, and Costa Rican 2·9 to 3·5 per cent; emetine constitutes between 30 and 50 per cent of the total alkaloids in these three varieties.

Standard

It complies with the requirements of the European Pharmacopoeia.

It contains not less than 2·0 per cent of total alkaloids, calculated as emetine, $C_{29}H_{40}N_2O_4$, with reference to the drug dried at 100° to 105°.

UNGROUND DRUG. *Macroscopical characters:* Root of *C. ipecacuanha* occurring in slender somewhat tortuous pieces, rarely exceeding 15 cm in length or 6 mm in thickness and varying from dark brick-red, partly due to adhering earth, to dark brown, showing characteristic annulations resembling wedge-shaped disks, from 1 to 2 mm thick, closely applied to one another, with rounded projecting ridges; fracture short and even in the bark but splintery in the wood; smoothed, transversely cut surface showing a thick starchy grey bark and a small dense radiate wood, but no pith.
Rhizome cylindrical, up to 2 mm in diameter, with fine longitudinal wrinkles; the transverse surface showing a narrow bark, a dense xylem cylinder, and a central pith about one-sixth of the diameter of the rhizome.
Root of *C. acuminata* closely resembling that of *C. ipecacuanha*, but distinguished by its larger size, up to

9 mm in thickness, by the absence of annulations and the presence of transverse ridges only partially encircling the root by its grey or reddish-brown colour externally.
Odour faint; taste bitter.

Microscopical characters: the diagnostic characters are: *C. ipecacuanha* root: cork cells narrow, elongated; *phelloderm* composed of thin-walled parenchyma mostly filled with starch granules, but including scattered cells containing bundles of acicular *crystals* of calcium oxalate, 30 to 80 μm long; *starch* granules simple or more usually compound with 2 to 5 or up to 8 components, individual granules oval, rounded or mullershaped, rarely more than 15 μm in diameter; *xylem* with *tracheids*, narrow *vessel elements* with lateral perforations and bordered pits, and occasional *fibres*; *medullary rays* of the xylem with lignified parenchyma, this and many cells of xylem parenchyma containing starch granules.
Rhizome: thick-walled rectangular *sclereids* in the outer part of the phloem.
C. acuminata resembles in general characters *C. ipecacuanha* but the starch granules are larger, measuring up to 22 μm.

POWDERED DRUG: Powdered Ipecacuanha. A light grey to yellowish-brown powder possessing the diagnostic microscopical characters, odour, and taste of the unground drug.

Adulterants and substitutes. Ipecacuanha is now rarely adulterated, but a number of different roots have been reported from time to time as adulterants; the majority of these do not contain emetine and can be distinguished from ipecacuanha by one or more of the following characters: the presence of a violet colour in the bark, the presence of large vessels in the xylem, and the absence of starch.

Actions and uses. The actions of ipecacuanha are those of its principal alkaloids, emetine and cephaëline. In small doses it is a reflex expectorant; its action lasts several hours. Large doses are irritant to the whole gastro-intestinal tract, and produce vomiting and diarrhoea. The powdered drug is irritating to the nasal and laryngeal mucous membrane, causing violent sneezing and coughing. Ipecacuanha is used in small doses as an expectorant in acute and chronic bronchitis, and in cough when secretion is scanty. It is well tolerated by children and is used in croup and whooping-cough. For an emetic action, large doses are required.

To produce diaphoresis in the treatment of incipient colds, Ipecacuanha and Opium Powder may be given in powders or tablets, often in conjunction with aspirin.

NOTE. When Ipecacuanha, Powdered Ipecacuanha, or Ipecacuanhae Pulvis is prescribed, Prepared Ipecacuanha is dispensed.

Preparations
IPECACUANHA, PREPARED (see below)
IPECACUANHA EMETIC DRAUGHT, PAEDIATRIC, B.P.C. (page 661)
IPECACUANHA LIQUID EXTRACT, B.P. It contains 2 per cent of alkaloids. Dose: 0·025 to 0·1 ml.
IPECACUANHA AND SQUILL LINCTUS, PAEDIATRIC, B.P.C. (page 723)
AMMONIA AND IPECACUANHA MIXTURE, B.P.C. (page 736)
BELLADONNA AND IPECACUANHA MIXTURE, PAEDIATRIC, B.P.C. (page 738)
IPECACUANHA MIXTURE, PAEDIATRIC, B.P.C. (page 744)
IPECACUANHA MIXTURE, OPIATE, PAEDIATRIC, B.P.C. (page 744)
IPECACUANHA AND AMMONIA MIXTURE, PAEDIATRIC, B.P.C. (page 745)
IPECACUANHA AND MORPHINE MIXTURE, B.P.C. (page 745)
IPECACUANHA AND OPIUM POWDER, B.P.C. (page 777)
IPECACUANHA AND OPIUM TABLETS, B.P.C. (page 811)
IPECACUANHA TINCTURE, B.P. It contains 0·2 per cent of alkaloids. Dose: 0·25 to 1 millilitre.

PREPARED IPECACUANHA

SYNONYMS: Ipecacuanhae Pulvis Normatus; Prep. Ipecac.

Prepared Ipecacuanha is obtained by reducing Ipecacuanha to a fine powder and adjusting, if necessary, to the required alkaloidal content. When adjustment is necessary, powdered Lactose or Powdered Ipecacuanha of lower alkaloidal content is added.

Standard
It complies with the requirements of the European Pharmacopoeia.
It is a light grey to yellowish-brown powder with a slight odour and a nauseous and bitter taste and contains 2·0 per cent of total alkaloids, calculated as emetine, $C_{29}H_{40}N_2O_4$ (limits, 1·90 to 2·10 per cent), with reference to the substance dried at 100° to 105°.
It possesses the diagnostic microscopical characters of Powdered Ipecacuanha.

Storage. It should be stored in airtight containers, protected from light, in a cool place.

Actions and uses. Prepared ipecacuanha has the actions and uses described under Ipecacuanha.

Dose. 25 to 100 milligrams.

Preparations
IPECACUANHA AND OPIUM POWDER, B.P.C. (page 777)
IPECACUANHA AND OPIUM TABLETS, B.P.C. (page 811)

IRON

SYNONYM: Ferrum

Fe = 55·85

Iron is metallic iron in the form of fine wire.

Solubility. Insoluble in water and in alcohol; almost completely soluble in dilute mineral acids.

Standard
DESCRIPTION. Fine wire, about 0·3 mm in diameter; it is free from rust, and has a dull metallic lustre, becoming bright when freshly scratched.

IDENTIFICATION TEST. Dissolve in *hydrochloric acid*; hydrogen is evolved and the solution gives the reactions characteristic of ferrous salts.

ARSENIC. It complies with the test given in Appendix 6, page 878 (100 parts per million).

COPPER. Dissolve, as completely as possible, about 2 g, accurately weighed, by warming on a water-bath with 8 ml of *hydrochloric acid*, 4 ml of water, and 1 ml of *nitric acid*; add 1 ml of *nitric acid*, and evaporate almost to dryness on a water-bath; dissolve the residue by warming with 24 ml of *hydrochloric acid* until a clear solution is formed, add 8 ml of water, cool, and extract

with four successive 20-ml portions of *solvent ether*; discard the extracts, and evaporate the solution to dryness; dissolve the residue in 10 ml of 1N hydrochloric acid and dilute to 100 ml with water; reserve a portion of the solution for the test for zinc.
To 2 ml add 25 ml of water and 1 g of *copper-free citric acid*, make alkaline to *litmus paper* with *dilute ammonia solution*, dilute to 50 ml with water, add 1 ml of *sodium diethyldithiocarbamate solution*, and allow to stand for 5 minutes; any colour which develops is not deeper than that produced by 4 ml of *dilute copper sulphate solution* when similarly treated (0·1 per cent).

LEAD. It complies with the test given in Appendix 7, page 882 (100 parts per million).

ZINC. To 10 ml of the solution reserved in the test for copper add 10 ml of 1N sodium hydroxide and 0·2 ml of *hydrogen peroxide solution*, boil, and filter; wash the residue with water and dilute the combined filtrate and washings to 25 ml with water; add 15 ml of 1N hydrochloric acid and 2 g of *ammonium chloride*, dilute to 50 ml with water, add 1 ml of *potassium ferrocyanide solution*, and allow to stand for 15 minutes; any turbidity which develops is not greater than that produced when 1 ml of *potassium ferrocyanide solution* is added to a solution prepared from 4 ml of *dilute zinc sulphate solution*, 10 ml of 1N sodium hydroxide, 15 ml of 1N hydrochloric acid and 2 g of *ammonium chloride*, diluted to 50 ml with water, and allowed to stand for 15 minutes (500 parts per million).

CONTENT OF Fe. Not less than 99·5 per cent, determined by the following method:
Dissolve about 0·2 g, accurately weighed, by warming with 50 ml of *dilute sulphuric acid* in a flask fitted with a Bunsen valve; cool, add 25 ml of freshly boiled and cooled water, and titrate with 0·1N potassium permanganate; each ml of 0·1N potassium permanganate is equivalent to 0·005585 g of Fe.

Actions and uses. The actions and uses of iron and its compounds are described under Ferrous Sulphate (page 197). Iron wire is used in the preparation of some solutions and syrups.

Preparations
FERRIC CHLORIDE SOLUTION, B.P.C. (page 783)
FERRIC CHLORIDE SOLUTION, STRONG, B.P.C. (page 783)

IRON DEXTRAN INJECTION

Iron Dextran Injection is a sterile colloidal solution containing a complex of ferric hydroxide with dextrans of weight average molecular weight between 5000 and 7500.

Standard
It complies with the requirements of the British Pharmacopoeia.
It is a dark brown solution and contains not less than 4·75 and not more than 5·25 per cent w/v of Fe. It has a pH of 5·2 to 6·5.

Sterilisation. It is sterilised by heating in an autoclave or by filtration.

Actions and uses. Iron Dextran Injection is used for the treatment of iron-deficiency anaemia when oral administration of iron fails to correct it, when oral medication is impracticable or undesirable, in some cases of rheumatoid arthritis, and when a rapid rise of serum-iron is essential as in emergency surgery on iron-deficient patients, when iron deficiency is diagnosed in late pregnancy, and in premature iron-deficient infants. In gastro-intestinal bleeding, oral iron therapy may mask melaena, and the administration of iron parenterally may be desirable.
Absorption from the injection site is virtually complete and maximum serum levels are reached within twenty-four to forty-eight hours of administration. The iron complex is transported from the muscle to the blood and then to the liver, where the dextran fraction is removed and metabolised or excreted. The iron is then stored in the form of ferritin and haemosiderin and metabolised as required.
The usual method of administration is by deep intramuscular injection into the ventro-lateral aspect of the upper and outer quadrant of the buttock, care being taken to avoid leakage of fluid through the needle track. The initial dose is usually 1 millilitre (equivalent to 50 milligrams of iron) on the first day and then 2 millilitres is given daily or at longer intervals, according to the haemoglobin response. Up to 5 millilitres may be given as a single dose.
The total number of millilitres of Iron Dextran Injection required may be calculated from the formula $0·66WD$, in which W is the body-weight in kilograms and D the percentage haemoglobin deficiency on the Haldane scale. Alternatively, periodic intramuscular injections are given until the haemoglobin level has returned to normal. The dose for a child over 10 kilograms body-weight is up to 2 millilitres, up to 1 millilitre for a child between 4 and 10 kilograms, and up to 0·5 millilitre for a child under 4 kilograms.
Iron Dextran Injection may also be administered as a single large dose, calculated as above, given by slow intravenous infusion over a period of six to eight hours. For this treatment it is diluted with Sodium Chloride Injection or Dextrose Injection.

UNDESIRABLE EFFECTS. Iron Dextran Injection may cause staining of the skin by leakage through the needle track into subcutaneous fat. Anaphylactoid reactions have occurred after the intravenous infusion of a large dose; if these occur, administration should be stopped and treatment given for shock. Allergic reactions and transient local thrombophlebitis at the site of venepuncture, nausea, vomiting, flushing, sweating, pyrexia, leucocytosis, lymphadenopathy, dyspnoea, and circulatory collapse may occur. In cases of severe dyspnoea with collapse, an antihistamine or 0·25 to 0·5 millilitre of Adrenaline Injection may be given subcutaneously.

PRECAUTIONS. When Iron Dextran Injection is administered in large doses by intravenous infusion, measures for the treatment of anaphylactoid and allergic reactions should be at hand. If it is given by slow infusion, the patient should be kept under observation while the infusion is being given and for at least an hour afterwards.

Dose. See above under **Actions and uses.**

OTHER NAME: *Imferon*®

IRON PHOSPHATE

Iron Phosphate consists of a mixture of hydrated ferrous phosphate and ferric phosphate and some hydrated oxides of iron.

Iron Phosphate may be prepared by the interaction of ferrous sulphate, sodium phosphate, and sodium bicarbonate in aqueous solution.

Solubility. Insoluble in water; soluble in hydrochloric acid.

Standard

DESCRIPTION. A slate-blue amorphous powder.

IDENTIFICATION TEST. It gives the reactions characteristic of ferrous salts and of phosphates.

ARSENIC. It complies with the test given in Appendix 6, page 878 (4 parts per million).

LEAD. It complies with the test given in Appendix 7, page 882 (50 parts per million).

SULPHATE. 0·25 g dissolved in water with the addition of 3 ml of *dilute hydrochloric acid* complies with the limit test for sulphates (0·24 per cent).

CONTENT OF FERROUS IRON. Not less than 16·0 per cent, calculated as Fe, equivalent to not less than 47·9 per cent of $Fe_3(PO_4)_2,8H_2O$, determined by the following method:

Dissolve about 1 g, accurately weighed, in a cooled mixture of 3 ml of *phosphoric acid* and 10 ml of *sulphuric acid* (*14 per cent v/v*), add 100 ml of water, and titrate with 0·1N potassium permanganate; each ml of 0·1N potassium permanganate is equivalent to 0·005585 g of Fe.

Stability. It is liable to darken in colour on exposure to air, owing to oxidation.

Storage. It should be stored in airtight containers.

Actions and uses. Iron phosphate has the general properties of iron salts, as described under Ferrous Sulphate (page 197). It is administered in the form of syrups prepared from iron and phosphoric acid or in the tablets.

Dose. 0·3 to 2 grams.

Preparation

FERROUS PHOSPHATE, QUININE, AND STRYCHNINE TABLETS, B.P.C. (page 810)

IRON SORBITOL INJECTION

Iron Sorbitol Injection is a sterile colloidal solution of a complex of ferric iron, sorbitol, and citric acid, stabilised with dextrin and sorbitol.

Standard

It complies with the requirements of the British Pharmacopoeia.

It is a clear brown solution and contains 4·7 to 5·2 per cent w/v of Fe. It has a weight per ml at 20° of 1·17 g to 1·19 g and a pH of 7·2 to 7·9.

Sterilisation. It is sterilised by heating in an autoclave.

Storage. It should be stored at a temperature between 15° and 30°; it should not be stored at a low temperature or allowed to freeze.

Actions and uses. Iron Sorbitol Injection is used for the correction of iron deficiency when the oral administration of iron is not possible or not desirable for the reasons stated under Iron Dextran Injection. It contains in 2 millilitres the equivalent of 100 milligrams of iron. After intramuscular injection into the iron-deficient subject, half the dose of iron enters the blood stream within three-quarters of an hour, and after ten hours no significant amount remains. Some of the iron is made available almost immediately for haemoglobin synthesis in the bone marrow, the rest being stored in the liver. About 30 per cent of an injected dose appears in the urine, the actual amount depending upon the iron stores of the individual. It turns the urine a dark colour, but this is of no pathological significance and is due to chemical changes in the excreted iron. Iron Sorbitol Injection is rarely antigenic and does not cause blood haemolysis.

Iron Sorbitol Injection should be given by deep intramuscular injection into the ventro-lateral aspect of the upper and outer quadrant of the buttock, taking care to prevent leakage of the solution along the needle track. It is not suitable for intravenous injection.

The initial dose is a quantity corresponding to 1·5 milligrams of iron per kilogram body-weight for both children and adults; this corresponds to 2 millilitres of the injection for an adult of average weight. The total dose depends upon the haemoglobin level of the patient and is calculated on the basis that in women about 200 milligrams of iron and in men about 250 milligrams of iron is required to increase the haemoglobin by 1 gram per 100 millilitres of blood. Repeated haemoglobin estimations should be made to determine whether the response to treatment is satisfactory. Injections of 1 to 2 millilitres are given daily, according to body-weight. In the case of children, injections of the equivalent of 1·5 milligrams of iron per kilogram body-weight may be given daily or on alternate days. The very small volumes needed by young children may be diluted with Sodium Chloride Injection. In pregnancy, five additional injections of 2 millilitres are given after the haemoglobin has been restored to the normal level.

UNDESIRABLE EFFECTS. Nausea, vomiting, and a metallic taste or loss of taste may occur about half an hour after the injection if too high a dose is given or if iron is being erroneously given by mouth concurrently. Localised or generalised urticaria may occur but this is rare.

PRECAUTIONS AND CONTRA-INDICATIONS. At least twenty-four hours should elapse between taking iron orally and receiving an injection of iron sorbitol. Oral iron therapy should never be given concurrently. If another injectable iron preparation has been administered previously, a week should elapse between the last injection of this and the first injection of iron sorbitol.

Iron Sorbitol Injection is contra-indicated in liver disease and kidney disease, particularly pyelonephritis, and in untreated urinary tract infections.

Dose. See above under **Actions and uses.**

OTHER NAME: *Jectofer®*

ISOCARBOXAZID

$C_{12}H_{13}N_3O_2 = 231.3$

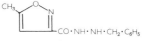

Isocarboxazid is 3-N'-benzylhydrazinocarbonyl-5-methylisoxazole.

Solubility. Slightly soluble in water; soluble, at 20°, in 150 parts of alcohol, in 50 parts of ether, and in 3 parts of chloroform.

Standard
It complies with the requirements of the British Pharmacopoeia.
It is a white or creamy-white crystalline powder with a faint characteristic odour and contains not less than 98.5 per cent of $C_{12}H_{13}N_3O_2$, calculated with reference to the dried substance. The loss on drying under the prescribed conditions is not more than 0.5 per cent. It has a melting-point of 105° to 107°.

Actions and uses. Isocarboxazid is an antidepressant drug which inhibits monoamine oxidase. It has actions and uses similar to those described under Phenelzine Sulphate (page 361).

UNDESIRABLE EFFECTS; PRECAUTIONS. These are as described under Phenelzine Sulphate (page 361). The undesirable effects can usually be controlled by reducing the dosage.

Dose. Initially, up to 30 milligrams daily in divided doses; maintenance dosage, 10 to 20 milligrams daily in single or divided doses.

Preparation
ISOCARBOXAZID TABLETS, B.P. Unless otherwise specified, tablets each containing 10 mg of isocarboxazid are supplied.

OTHER NAME: *Marplan®*

ISONIAZID

SYNONYM: Isoniazidum

$C_6H_7N_3O = 137.1$

Isoniazid is pyridine-4-carboxyhydrazide.

Solubility. Soluble, at 20°, in 8 parts of water, in 45 parts of alcohol, and in 1000 parts of chloroform; very slightly soluble in ether.

Standard
It complies with the requirements of the European Pharmacopoeia.
It occurs as odourless colourless crystals or white crystalline powder and contains not less than 99.0 per cent of $C_6H_7N_3O$, calculated with reference to the dried substance. The loss on drying under the prescribed conditions is not more than 0.5 per cent. It has a melting-point of 170° to 174°. A 5 per cent solution in water has a pH of 6.0 to 8.0.

Hygroscopicity. It absorbs insignificant amounts of moisture at 25° at relative humidities up to about 90 per cent.

Sterilisation. Solutions for injection are sterilised by heating in an autoclave or by filtration.

Storage. It should be stored in airtight containers, protected from light.

Actions and uses. Isoniazid has no significant antibacterial action against any micro-organisms except the mycobacteria; against *Mycobacterium tuberculosis* it is bacteriostatic in extremely low concentrations. When given by mouth, it is readily absorbed and diffuses freely into body tissues and fluids, including the cerebrospinal fluid; the rate of inactivation is genetically determined. It is excreted mainly by the kidneys.

Isoniazid is used mainly in the treatment of pulmonary tuberculosis, but it appears to be effective also in the treatment of extrapulmonary lesions, including meningitis and genito-urinary disease. Bacterial resistance may develop within a few weeks of commencing treatment with isoniazid alone, but when it is administered concurrently with calcium or sodium aminosalicylate, or with intramuscular injections of streptomycin, the proportion of patients in whom the infecting organisms develop resistance during six months of treatment is greatly reduced. Isoniazid therapy should, therefore, always be supplemented by the administration of calcium or sodium aminosalicylate or of streptomycin.

Isoniazid is administered by mouth, the initial dosage being usually about 4 milligrams per kilogram body-weight daily, in two or more divided doses; up to 10 milligrams per kilogram body-weight has been given daily, particularly during the first one or two weeks in the treatment of tuberculous meningitis. An effective level of isoniazid in the cerebrospinal fluid usually follows oral administration.

When isoniazid cannot be given by mouth, similar doses may be administered by intramuscular injection.

Isoniazid has been used with success in the treatment of lupus vulgaris, for which the dosage may be up to 300 milligrams or more daily in divided doses. Treatment must be continued for several months.

UNDESIRABLE EFFECTS. Peripheral neuropathy, constipation, difficulty in starting urination, dryness of the mouth, and sometimes vertigo and hyperreflexia may be troublesome with doses of 10 milligrams per kilogram body-weight. The onset of peripheral neuritis should be expected with doses of 10 milligrams per kilogram body-weight and prophy-

lactic doses of 100 milligrams of pyridoxine hydrochloride should be given daily.

Although isoniazid usually has a mood-elevating effect, mental disturbances, ranging from minor personality changes to major mental derangements, have been reported; these are usually reversed on withdrawal of the drug.

Withdrawal symptoms, which may occur on the cessation of treatment, include headache, insomnia, excessive dreaming, irritability, and nervousness.

Dose. See above under **Actions and uses.**

Preparations
SODIUM AMINOSALICYLATE AND ISONIAZID CACHETS, B.P.C. (page 650)
ISONIAZID ELIXIR, B.P.C. (page 672)
SODIUM AMINOSALICYLATE AND ISONIAZID GRANULES, B.P.C. (page 703)
ISONIAZID INJECTION, B.P.C. (page 714)
ISONIAZID TABLETS, B.P. Unless otherwise specified, tablets each containing 100 mg of isoniazid are supplied. They should be stored in airtight containers, protected from light. Tablets containing 50 mg are also available.

OTHER NAMES: Isonicotinic Acid Hydrazide; *Nicetal*®; *Pycazide*®

ISOPRENALINE HYDROCHLORIDE

$C_{11}H_{17}NO_3,HCl = 247 \cdot 7$

Isoprenaline Hydrochloride is 1-(3,4-dihydroxyphenyl)-2-isopropylaminoethanol hydrochloride.

Solubility. Soluble, at 20°, in less than one part of water and in 55 parts of alcohol; insoluble in ether and in chloroform.

Standard
DESCRIPTION. A white or almost white, crystalline powder; odourless or almost odourless.

IDENTIFICATION TESTS. 1. Dissolve 10 mg in 1 ml of water and add 0·05 ml of *ferric chloride test-solution*; an intense green colour is produced. Add, dropwise, *sodium bicarbonate solution*; the colour changes first to blue and then to red.

2. Dissolve 10 mg in 1 ml of water and add 0·05 ml of *phosphotungstic acid solution*; a white precipitate is produced which becomes brown on standing (distinction from adrenaline).

3. Dissolve 10 mg in 10 ml of water, dilute 1 ml of this solution to 10 ml with water, add 0·1 ml of 0·1N hydrochloric acid, followed by 1 ml of 0·1N iodine, allow to stand for 5 minutes, and add 2 ml of 0·1N sodium thiosulphate; a red-brown colour is produced (distinction from noradrenaline which gives no more than a faint pink colour under these conditions).

4. The ultraviolet absorption spectrum exhibits the characteristics given in Appendix 3, page 855.

5. It gives the reactions characteristic of chlorides.

MELTING-POINT. 166° to 170°.

KETONE. Extinction, at 310 nm, of a 1-cm layer of a 0·2 per cent w/v solution in water, not more than 0·2.

SULPHATE. 0·3 g complies with the limit test for sulphates (0·2 per cent).

LOSS ON DRYING. Not more than 1·0 per cent, determined by drying for 4 hours over *phosphorus pentoxide* in vacuo.

SULPHATED ASH. Not more than 0·1 per cent.

CONTENT OF $C_{11}H_{18}ClNO_3$. Not less than 98·0 and not more than the equivalent of 101·5 per cent, calculated with reference to the substance dried under the prescribed conditions, determined by the following method:
Titrate about 0·5 g, accurately weighed, by Method I of the British Pharmacopoeia for non-aqueous titration, dissolving the sample in the glacial acetic acid with the aid of a minimum of heat; each ml of 0·1N perchloric acid is equivalent to 0·02477 g of $C_{11}H_{18}ClNO_3$.

Stability. It gradually darkens in colour on exposure to air and light. Aqueous solutions become pink to brownish-pink on standing exposed to air, and almost immediately when made alkaline.

Storage. It should be stored in airtight containers, protected from light.

Actions and uses. Isoprenaline hydrochloride has the actions and undesirable effects of isoprenaline, as described under Isoprenaline Sulphate. It is usually administered in the form of slow-release tablets.

The usual initial dosage is 30 milligrams three times a day, and this may be increased until the heart rate is sufficiently accelerated. The maximum daily dosage is 750 milligrams.

PRECAUTIONS AND CONTRA-INDICATIONS. As for Isoprenaline Sulphate.

Dose. See above under **Actions and uses.**

OTHER NAME: Isoproterenol Hydrochloride

ISOPRENALINE SULPHATE

$C_{22}H_{36}N_2O_{10}S,2H_2O = 556\cdot6$

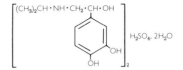

Isoprenaline Sulphate is 1-(3,4-dihydroxyphenyl)-2-isopropylaminoethanol sulphate dihydrate.

Solubility. Soluble, at 20°, in 4 parts of water; very slightly soluble in alcohol, in ether, and in chloroform.

Standard
It complies with the requirements of the British Pharmacopoeia.
It is a white or almost white odourless crystalline powder and contains not less than 98·5 per cent of $C_{22}H_{36}N_2O_{10}S$, calculated with reference to the dried substance. The loss on drying under the prescribed conditions is 5·0 to 7·5 per cent. It melts with decomposition at about 128°. A 1 per cent solution in water has a pH of 4·5 to 5·5.

Sterilisation. Solutions for injection are sterilised by heating in an autoclave or by filtration.

Storage. It should be stored in airtight containers, protected from light.

Actions and uses. Isoprenaline, like adrenaline, is a sympathomimetic amine but it acts almost exclusively on beta receptors, as described under Adrenaline (page 8), producing bronchial relaxation, peripheral vasodilatation, tachycardia, and myocardial stimulation. It is used in the treatment of bronchial asthma, but other drugs such as salbutamol, which do not markedly stimulate the heart, are usually preferred for this purpose.
Isoprenaline is such a potent cardiac stimulant that it is not usually given by injection except in cardiac surgery to combat heart block.
Isoprenaline sulphate is usually administered sublingually or by inhalation. When swallowed, its activity is markedly impaired; the tablets should therefore be allowed to dissolve under the tongue without being sucked and as little saliva as possible should be swallowed. The usual initial dosage is 10 to 20 milligrams three times a day. Very mild asthmatic spasm may require only 5 milligrams and very severe spasm up to 40 milligrams or even more; relief is felt after two to four minutes.
A more rapid effect is produced when the drug is given by inhalation of a spray containing from 0·5 to 3 per cent of isoprenaline sulphate, about 1 millilitre being inhaled. Compound sprays of similar strength and containing in addition 2·5 per cent of papaverine sulphate and 0·2 per cent of atropine methonitrate may be used when a more prolonged effect is required.
Doses of up to 1·2 milligrams may be given in the form of an aerosol inhalation and repeated if necessary after thirty minutes up to a maximum of eight doses in twenty-four hours. Doses of 15 milligrams may be administered by mouth in the treatment of heart block.
Solutions of isoprenaline sulphate should contain sodium metabisulphite as an antoxidant and should be used in an all-glass atomiser, as contact with metal causes discoloration and loss of activity.

UNDESIRABLE EFFECTS. Reactions such as tachycardia and vigorous myocardial stimulation, together with a fall in arterial pressure, may occur; these effects quickly subside on withdrawal of the drug.

PRECAUTIONS AND CONTRA-INDICATIONS. Isoprenaline should not be given simultaneously with adrenaline, but it may be used simultaneously with phenylephrine. It should not be given in hyperthyroidism.
The excessive use of sprays containing isoprenaline should be avoided as it may lead to fatal results.

Dose. See above under **Actions and uses.**

Preparations
ISOPRENALINE AEROSOL INHALATION, B.P.C. (page 645)
ISOPRENALINE AEROSOL INHALATION, STRONG, B.P.C. (page 646)
ISOPRENALINE TABLETS, B.P. Unless otherwise specified, tablets each containing 10 mg of isoprenaline sulphate are supplied. They should be protected from light. Tablets containing 20 mg are also available.

OTHER NAMES: *Aleudrin*®; Isoproterenol Sulphate; *Lomupren*®; *Medihaler Iso*®; *Meterdose-iso*®; *Neo-Epinine*®; *Norisodrine*®; *Prenomiser*®

ISOPROPYL ALCOHOL

$C_3H_8O = 60\cdot10$

$(CH_3)_2CHOH$

Isopropyl Alcohol may be prepared by the catalytic hydrogenation of acetone or by absorbing propylene in sulphuric acid and hydrolysing the resulting esters.

Solubility. Miscible with water, with ether, and with chloroform. The alcohol may be salted out from aqueous mixtures by the addition of salts or sodium hydroxide.

Standard
It complies with the requirements of the British Pharmacopoeia.
It is a clear, colourless, highly inflammable liquid with a characteristic alcoholic odour. It has a weight per ml at 20° of 0·784 g to 0·786 g. On heating, not less than 95 per cent v/v distils between 81° and 83°. It contains not more than 0·5 per cent w/w of water.
It has a flash-point of about 53°F (closed-cup test).

Storage. It should be stored in airtight containers.

Actions and uses. Isopropyl alcohol taken by mouth has an action similar to that of ethyl alcohol. Its toxicity is about twice that of ethyl alcohol and because of this and its unpleasant taste, its oral administration is inadvisable. It has a more effective antibacterial action than ethyl alcohol

Isopropyl alcohol is used extensively as a solvent, especially in perfumery and cosmetics, and externally it may be used as a substitute for industrial methylated spirit and Surgical Spirit. When mixed with a small proportion of water, it is a suitable storage fluid for surgical sutures. It is a useful non-aqueous moistening agent for tablet granulation, especially as its water content is low. It is also used in hair preparations, lotions, and liniments.

OTHER NAMES: Isopropanol; 2-Propanol

ISOPROPYL MYRISTATE

$C_{17}H_{34}O_2 = 270 \cdot 5$

$$CH_3 \cdot [CH_2]_{12} \cdot CO \cdot O \cdot CH(CH_3)_2$$

Isopropyl Myristate may be prepared by the esterification of myristic acid with isopropyl alcohol.

Solubility. Soluble, at 20°, in 3 parts of alcohol; insoluble in water, in glycerol, and in sorbitol; miscible with liquid hydrocarbons and with fixed oils.

Standard

DESCRIPTION. A colourless mobile liquid; odourless or almost odourless.

ACID VALUE. Not more than 0·5.

IODINE VALUE. Not more than 1, determined by the iodine monochloride method.

REFRACTIVE INDEX. At 20°, 1·434 to 1·437.

WEIGHT PER ML. At 20°, 0·850 g to 0·855 g.

ESTER VALUE. Not less than 205, determined by the method of the British Pharmacopoeia, Appendix IXB, about 1·1 g, accurately weighed, and 20 ml of 0·5N alcoholic potassium hydroxide being used.

Incompatibility. Isopropyl myristate is incompatible with hard paraffin, producing a granular mixture.

Uses. Isopropyl myristate may be used in external preparations in place of vegetable oils. It is resistant to oxidation and hydrolysis, does not become rancid, is free from irritant and sensitising properties, and is absorbed fairly readily by the skin.

Isopropyl myristate is used in emollient ointments and creams, giving preparations which are relatively free from greasiness. It is a solvent for many substances applied externally and is of value as a vehicle when direct contact and penetration of the medicament are required.

ISOTHIPENDYL HYDROCHLORIDE

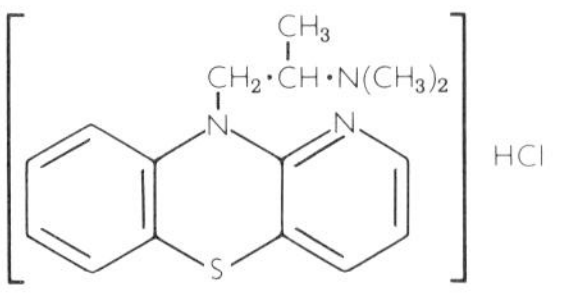

$C_{16}H_{20}ClN_3S = 321 \cdot 9$

Isothipendyl Hydrochloride is 9-(2-dimethylaminopropyl)-10-thia-1,9-diaza-anthracene hydrochloride.

Solubility. Soluble, at 20°, in 5 parts of water, in 60 parts of alcohol, and in 10 parts of chloroform; insoluble in ether.

Standard

DESCRIPTION. A fine, white, crystalline powder; odourless or almost odourless.

IDENTIFICATION TESTS. 1. Dissolve 1 mg in 10 ml of water and to 1 ml of this solution add 1 ml of a 0·1 per cent w/v solution of *ammonium persulphate* in water; a pink colour is produced.

2. It melts with decomposition at about 212°.

3. It complies with the thin-layer chromatographic test given in Appendix 5C, page 873.

4. The ultraviolet absorption spectrum exhibits the characteristics given in Appendix 3, page 855.

5. The infra-red absorption spectrum exhibits maxima which are only at the same wavelengths as, and have similar relative intensities to, those in the spectrum of *isothipendyl hydrochloride A.S.*

6. It gives the reactions characteristic of chlorides.

LOSS ON DRYING. Not more than 0·5 per cent, determined by drying to constant weight at 105°.

SULPHATED ASH. Not more than 0·1 per cent.

CONTENT OF $C_{16}H_{20}ClN_3S$. Not less than 98·0 per cent, calculated with reference to the substance dried under the prescribed conditions, determined by the following method:

Dissolve about 0·3 g, accurately weighed, in 50 ml of *chloroform*, add 50 ml of *purified acetonitrile* and 10 ml of *mercuric acetate solution*, and titrate by Method I of the British Pharmacopoeia for non-aqueous titration, using 0·1N perchloric acid in dioxan as the titrant and a 0·1 per cent w/v solution of *methyl red* in *methyl alcohol* as the indicator; each ml of 0·1N perchloric acid in dioxan is equivalent to 0·03219 g of $C_{16}H_{20}ClN_3S$.

Stability. It is affected by light. Aqueous solutions are sensitive to heat and light but are most stable at pH 4·5 to 5·0.

Sterilisation. Solutions are sterilised by filtration.

Storage. It should be protected from light.

Actions and uses. Isothipendyl has the actions, uses, and undesirable effects of the antihistamine drugs, as described under Promethazine Hydrochloride (page 409), but it is more potent than promethazine, has a shorter duration of action, and causes less sedation. It is given in a dosage of 4 to 8 milligrams three or four times a day by mouth, or 10 milligrams daily by intramuscular or slow intravenous injection.

OTHER NAME: *Nilergex®*

POISONING. As for Promethazine Hydrochloride (page 409).

Dose. See above under **Actions and uses.**

Preparation
ISOTHIPENDYL TABLETS, B.P.C. (page 812)

ISPAGHULA HUSK

Ispaghula Husk consists of the epidermis and the collapsed adjacent layers removed from the dried ripe seeds of *Plantago ovata* Forssk. (Fam. Plantaginaceae). The plant is a herbaceous annual indigenous to the Indian subcontinent and Iran.

Constituents. Ispaghula husk contains mucilage and hemicelluloses.

Standard
DESCRIPTION. *Macroscopical:* pale buff brittle flakes, more or less lanceolate, up to 2 mm long and 1 mm wide at the centre, much broken into smaller fragments; many of the flakes have a small brownish oval spot, about 0·8 to 1·0 mm long, in the centre; the drug swells rapidly in water, forming a stiff mucilage.

Microscopical: mounted in *cresol*, the particles are transparent and angular, the edges straight or curved and sometimes rolled. They are composed of polygonal prismatic cells with 4 to 6 straight or slightly curved walls; the cells vary in size in different parts of the seed-coat, being about 25 to 60 μm at the summit of the seed, that is, near and over the brown spot, to 25 to 100 μm for the remainder of the epidermis except at the edges of the seed, where the cells are again smaller, about 45 to 70μm.
Mounted in *alcohol (95 per cent)* and irrigated with water, the mucilage in the outer part of the epidermal cells swells rapidly and goes into solution, while the two inner layers of mucilage are more resistant and swell to form rounded papillae.
Mounted in *iodine water*, occasional single and 2- to 4-compound starch granules, about 2 to 10 μm, can be seen in some of the cells.
Endosperm, if present, is dark and dense.

LOSS ON DRYING. Not more than 12·0 per cent, determined by drying for 5 hours at 105°.

ASH. Not more than 4·5 per cent.

ABSORBENCY. Transfer 1·0 g to a 100-ml stoppered cylinder containing 90 ml of water, shake well for 30 seconds, and allow to stand for 24 hours, shaking gently on three occasions during this period; add water to the 100-ml mark, mix gently for 30 seconds, avoiding the entrainment of air, allow to stand for 5 hours, and measure the volume of mucilage. Repeat the determination three times; the mean of the four determinations is not less than 40 ml.

Adulterants and substitutes. Fragments of the endosperm of ispaghula seed are usually dark and dense, the cells being chiefly polyhedral with thick cellulosic walls, about 2·5 to 7·0 μm thick and perforated by simple pits; the cells are about 30 to 60 μm in diameter, a few from the radicle pocket being subcylindrical and about 18 μm in diameter. All the cells contain fixed oil and aleurone grains.

Actions and uses. Ispaghula husk has the laxative actions and uses described under Psyllium (page 418).

Dose. 3 to 5 grams.

KANAMYCIN SULPHATE

$C_{18}H_{38}N_4O_{15}S = 582·6$

Kanamycin Sulphate is the sulphate of O^4-(6-amino-6-deoxy-α-D-glucopyranosyl)-O^6-(3-amino-3-deoxy-α-D-glucopyranosyl)-2-deoxystreptamine, an antimicrobial substance produced by *Streptomyces kanamyceticus* or by any other means.

Solubility. Soluble, at 20°, in 8 parts of water; very slightly soluble in alcohol, in ether, and in chloroform.

Standard
It complies with the requirements of the British Pharmacopoeia.
It is a white or almost white, crystalline, odourless or almost odourless powder and contains not less than 735 Units per mg, calculated with reference to the dried substance. The loss on drying under the prescribed conditions is not more than 3·0 per cent. A 1 per cent solution in water has a pH of 6·0 to 8·5.

Labelling. If the material is not intended for parenteral administration, the label on the container states that the contents are not to be injected.

Storage. It should be stored in airtight containers, protected from light, at a temperature not exceeding 20°.

Actions and uses. Kanamycin is an antibiotic which is active against *Escherichia coli*, shigellae, salmonellae, neisseriae, *Proteus vulgaris, Klebsiella pneumoniae, Aerobacter aerogenes, Mycobacterium tuberculosis*, and many strains of staphylococci. It has little or no action on streptococci, brucellae, pseudomonades, clostridia, and enterococci. Bacteria do not readily develop resistance to kanamycin, but organisms resistant to it are also resistant to neomycin and *vice versa*.

Maximum blood levels are attained within about one to two hours of an intramuscular injection, and up to three-quarters of the dose is excreted within twenty-four hours. It is poorly absorbed from the gastro-intestinal tract.

Kanamycin is used in the treatment of serious systemic infections caused by strains of the organisms named above which are resistant to the more commonly used antibiotics and in the treatment of urinary tract infections caused by *P. vulgaris* and *K. pneumoniae*.

Kanamycin sulphate may be given by mouth in a dosage of the equivalent of 15 milligrams of kanamycin base per kilogram body-weight daily in divided doses for the treatment of acute enteric infections or to prepare the large bowel for surgery. However, the increasingly frequent occurrence of resistant organisms in the large bowel may decrease its effectiveness for this purpose. The daily dosage for an adult, by intramuscular injection, is the equivalent of 0·5 to 1·5 grams of kanamycin base given in divided doses every twelve hours. A child may be given a daily dosage of the equivalent of 15 milligrams of the base per kilogram body-weight; 1·2 grams of kanamycin sulphate is equivalent to 1 gram of kanamycin base.

UNDESIRABLE EFFECTS. Toxic effects occur with sufficient frequency to make kanamycin useful only when the infecting organisms are resistant to other antibiotics. Intramuscular injections are usually well tolerated in the doses given above, but they are sometimes painful, especially if the dose is increased.

Skin eruptions, nausea, and vomiting may occur, and signs of renal disturbances are relatively common but disappear when treatment is discontinued. The most serious toxic effect is that on the eighth cranial nerve; an irreversible loss of hearing may follow intramuscular injections, especially if there is impaired kidney function or when treatment is prolonged, as in tuberculosis. Treatment with kanamycin should be stopped immediately if tinnitus occurs.

The possibility of toxic reactions is greatly reduced if the dose is adjusted so that the concentration of kanamycin in the serum does not exceed 30 micrograms per millilitre and the total dose in acute infections does not exceed 15 grams spread over fourteen days, provided that the patient is not allowed to become dehydrated.

Dose. See above under **Actions and uses.**

Preparation
KANAMYCIN INJECTION, B.P. It consists of a sterile solution of kanamycin sulphate in Water for Injections containing suitable buffering and stabilising agents. The strength of the solution should be specified by the prescriber. Solutions containing 75 and 500 mg in 2 ml and 1 g in 3 ml are available.

OTHER NAME: *Kantrex*®

HEAVY KAOLIN

SYNONYM: Kaolinum Ponderosum

Heavy Kaolin is a purified native hydrated aluminium silicate, powdered, and freed from gritty particles by elutriation.

The native clay is derived from the decomposition of the felspar of granite rocks and contains about 47 per cent of silica, 40 per cent of alumina, and 13 per cent of water. It is mined in large quantities in Cornwall.

Solubility. Insoluble in water and in mineral acids.

Standard
DESCRIPTION. *Macroscopical:* a soft whitish powder, free from gritty particles; odourless or almost odourless.

Microscopical: irregularly angular particles, up to about 60 μm in width, intermixed with innumerable minute fragments, about 1 or 2 μm in width. With *alcoholic methylene blue solution*, kaolin stains deep blue, but with *safranine solution* only a very faint pink or not at all; mounted in *cresol* it is clearly visible and shines brightly on a dark field under crossed polars.

IDENTIFICATION. Fuse 1 g with 2 g of *anhydrous sodium carbonate*, warm the residue with water, filter, acidify the filtrate with *hydrochloric acid*, evaporate to dryness, and warm the residue with *dilute hydrochloric acid*; a residue of silica is obtained and the solution, after neutralisation of the free acid, gives the reactions characteristic of aluminium.

ARSENIC. It complies with the test given in Appendix 6, page 878 (2 parts per million).

LEAD. It complies with the test given in Appendix 7, page 882 (10 parts per million).

CHLORIDE. Boil 2·0 g with 80 ml of water and 20 ml of *dilute nitric acid* under a reflux condenser for 5 minutes, cool, and filter; 50 ml of the filtrate complies with the limit test for chlorides (350 parts per million).

LOSS ON DRYING. Not more than 1·5 per cent, determined by drying to constant weight at 105°.

LOSS ON IGNITION. Not more than 15·0 per cent, determined by igniting to constant weight at red heat.

SOLUBLE MATTER. Not more than 0·5 per cent, determined by the following method:
Boil 2·0 g with 100 ml of 0·2N hydrochloric acid under a reflux condenser for 5 minutes, cool, filter, evaporate 50 ml of the filtrate to dryness, and ignite the residue to constant weight at about 300°.

Uses. Heavy kaolin is used in the preparation of Kaolin Poultice.

NOTE. When Kaolin or Light Kaolin is prescribed or demanded, Light Kaolin is dispensed or supplied, unless it has been ascertained that Light Kaolin (Natural) is required.

Preparation
KAOLIN POULTICE, B.P.C. (page 774)

LIGHT KAOLIN

SYNONYM: Kaolinum Leve

Light Kaolin is a purified native hydrated aluminium silicate free from gritty particles. It may be obtained by powdering native kaolin, elutriating, and collecting the fraction which satisfies the requirements for particle size. It contains a suitable dispersing agent.

Solubility. Insoluble in water and in mineral acids.

Standard
It complies with the requirements of the British Pharmacopoeia.
It is a light, white, odourless powder free from gritty particles and unctuous to the touch. The loss on drying at 105° is not more than 1·5 per cent and the loss on ignition at red heat is not more than 15·0 per cent.

Microscopical characters: irregularly angular particles, up to about 10 μm in width, intermixed with innumerable minute fragments, about 1 to 2 μm in width. With *alcoholic methylene blue solution,* kaolin stains deep blue, but with *safranine solution* only a very faint pink or not at all; mounted in *cresol* it is clearly visible and shines brightly on a dark field under crossed polars.

Hygroscopicity. At relative humidities between about 15 and 65 per cent, the equilibrium moisture content at 25° is about 1 per cent, but at relative humidities above about 75 per cent, it absorbs small amounts of moisture.

Actions and uses. Light kaolin is an adsorbent. It is administered by mouth in the symptomatic treatment of enteritis, colitis, and dysentery associated with food poisoning and alkaloidal poisoning. It may be administered suspended in water.

Light kaolin is applied externally as a dusting-powder, either undiluted or mixed with other protectives. It is an ingredient of toilet powders and a basis of disinfectant powders. It is also used for clarification purposes.

NOTE. When Kaolin or Light Kaolin is prescribed or demanded, Light Kaolin is dispensed or supplied, unless it has been ascertained that Light Kaolin (Natural) is required.

Dose. 15 to 75 grams.

Preparations
KAOLIN MIXTURE, B.P.C. (page 745)
KAOLIN MIXTURE, PAEDIATRIC, B.P.C. (page 745)
KAOLIN AND MORPHINE MIXTURE, B.P.C. (page 746)
CALCIUM CARBONATE POWDER, COMPOUND, B.P.C. (page 775)
MAGNESIUM CARBONATE POWDER, COMPOUND, B.P.C. (page 778)
MAGNESIUM CARBONATE TABLETS, COMPOUND, B.P.C. (page 812)

LIGHT KAOLIN (NATURAL)

Light Kaolin (Natural) is a purified native hydrated aluminium silicate free from gritty particles. It differs from Light Kaolin in that it does not contain a dispersing agent.

Solubility. Insoluble in water and in mineral acids.

Standard
It complies with the requirements of the British Pharmacopoeia.
It is a light, white, odourless powder free from gritty particles and unctuous to the touch. The loss on drying at 105° is not more than 1·5 per cent and the loss on ignition at red heat is not more than 15·0 per cent.
Its microscopical characters are the same as those of Light Kaolin.

Actions and uses. Light Kaolin (Natural) may be used for the same purposes as Light Kaolin. Kaolin mixtures of the British Pharmaceutical Codex may be prepared with Light Kaolin or with Light Kaolin (Natural).

NOTE. When Kaolin or Light Kaolin is prescribed or demanded, Light Kaolin is dispensed or supplied, unless it has been ascertained that Light Kaolin (Natural) is required.

Dose. 15 to 75 grams.

LACHESINE CHLORIDE

SYNONYMS: Laches. Chlor.; Lachesine

$C_{20}H_{26}ClNO_3 = 363·9$

$$\left[HO \cdot \underset{\underset{C_6H_5}{|}}{\overset{\overset{C_6H_5}{|}}{C}} \cdot CO \cdot O \cdot [CH_2]_2 \cdot \underset{\underset{CH_3}{|}}{\overset{\overset{CH_3}{|}}{N}} \cdot C_2H_5 \right]^+ Cl^-$$

Lachesine Chloride is (2-benziloyloxyethyl)ethyldimethylammonium chloride.

Solubility. Soluble, at 20°, in 3 parts of water and in 10 parts of alcohol (90 per cent); very slightly soluble in ether, in chloroform, and in acetone.

Standard
DESCRIPTION. A white amorphous powder; odourless or almost odourless.

IDENTIFICATION TESTS. 1. Mix 0·01 g with 0·2 ml of *sulphuric acid*; an orange-red colour is produced, which quickly changes to rose-pink.
2. To a solution in water add *gold chloride solution*; a precipitate is formed which, after washing with water and drying, melts at about 148°.

MELTING-POINT. After drying at 105°, it melts at 212° to 214°, darkening and shrinking at 2° or 3° below the melting-point.

SULPHATED ASH. Not more than 0·1 per cent.

CONTENT OF $C_{20}H_{26}ClNO_3$. Not less than 99·0 and not more than the equivalent of 101·0 per cent, determined by the following method:
Titrate about 0·5 g, accurately weighed, by Method I

of the British Pharmacopoeia for non-aqueous titration; each ml of 0·1N perchloric acid is equivalent to 0·03639 g of $C_{20}H_{26}ClNO_3$.

Incompatibility. Lachesine chloride is incompatible in aqueous solution, at concentrations of 1 per cent and above, with 0·01 per cent of benzalkonium chloride; at concentrations of 2 per cent and above, it is incompatible with 0·002 per cent of phenylmercuric salts, and with 0·01 per cent of chlorhexidine acetate if the solution is boiled or autoclaved.

Sterilisation. Solutions are sterilised by heating in an autoclave or by filtration.

Actions and uses. Lachesine has mydriatic and cycloplegic actions similar to those described under Atropine (page 36). The degree and duration of the cycloplegic effect are about midway between those produced by homatropine and atropine; in old people,

however, the response to miotics is slower and less complete after lachesine than when homatropine has been used. The mydriatic action of lachesine is neither so rapid nor so prolonged as that of atropine; it reaches a maximum in about an hour and begins to subside after five or six hours.

Lachesine is particularly useful in patients with hypersensitivity to atropine and hyoscine, as it does not give rise to irritation of the conjunctiva or to eczema of the eyelids. It is usually administered as a 1 per cent aqueous solution, two drops delivered into the conjunctival sac being the usual dose.

Preparation
LACHESINE EYE-DROPS, B.P.C. (page 692)

LACTIC ACID

$C_3H_6O_3 = 90·08$

$CH_3·CH(OH)·CO_2H$

Lactic Acid consists of a mixture of α-hydroxypropionic acid and lactide, $C_6H_8O_4$, and may be prepared by the lactic fermentation of sugar.

Solubility. Miscible with water, with alcohol, and with ether.

Standard
It complies with the requirements of the British Pharmacopoeia.
It is a colourless or slightly yellow, syrupy, hygroscopic liquid which is odourless or has a slight but not unpleasant odour and contains the equivalent of not less than 87·5 per cent w/w of $C_3H_6O_3$. It is strongly acid and has a weight per ml at 20° of about 1·20 g.

Storage. It should be stored in airtight containers.

Actions and uses. Lactic acid is used in the preparation of Compound Sodium Lactate Injection and other solutions containing sodium lactate which are given by intravenous injection in the treatment of diabetic coma as described under Insulin Injection (page 236). Compound Sodium Lactate Injection is given also by mouth for infantile gastro-enteritis. Lactate is converted slowly into bicarbonate in the blood and restores diminished alkali reserve without the danger of producing alkalosis.

Lactic acid milk may be given in infantile gastro-enteritis; it may check the vomiting but not the diarrhoea. It has also been used for infant feeding when breast milk is not available. It is prepared by adding lactic acid to whole milk in the proportion of 5 to 7 millilitres to the litre; the acid should be added drop by drop to the cold milk, stirring vigorously to prevent the formation of clots. A fine floccu-

lent curd results, which will flow through an ordinary rubber teat. Sugar or honey is then added. After the addition of the acid the milk must not be unduly heated or thick clots will form.

Lactic acid, which is normally present in the vaginal secretion, is used in the treatment of leucorrhoea as a 0·5 to 2 per cent vaginal douche or in pessaries.

Preparations
SODIUM LACTATE INJECTION, B.P. It consists of a sterile solution containing sodium lactate prepared from 14·0 ml of lactic acid and 6·7 g of sodium hydroxide, in Water for Injections to 1000 ml. This solution provides approximately 167 millimoles, or milliequivalents, of Na$^+$ and the equivalent of 167 millimoles, or milliequivalents, of HCO$_3^-$ per litre. On storage, this solution may cause separation of small solid particles from glass containers; solutions containing such particles must not be used.

SODIUM LACTATE INJECTION, COMPOUND, B.P. (*Syn.* Hartmann's Solution for Injection; Ringer-Lactate Solution for Injection). It consists of a sterile solution containing sodium lactate prepared from 2·4 ml of lactic acid and 1·15 g of sodium hydroxide, with sodium chloride, potassium chloride, and calcium chloride, in Water for Injections to 1000 ml. This solution provides approximately 2 millimoles, or 4 milliequivalents, of Ca^{2+}, 131 millimoles, or milliequivalents, of Na$^+$, 5 millimoles, or milliequivalents, of K$^+$, 111 millimoles, or milliequivalents, of Cl$^-$, and the equivalent of 29 millimoles, or milliequivalents, of HCO$_3^-$ per litre. On storage, this solution may cause separation of small solid particles from glass containers; solutions containing such particles must not be used.

LACTIC ACID PESSARIES, B.P.C. (page 772)

LACTOSE

SYNONYMS: Lactosum; Milk Sugar

$C_{12}H_{22}O_{11},H_2O = 360·3$

Lactose is the monohydrate of 4-O-β-D-galactopyrano-syl-α-D-glucopyranose.

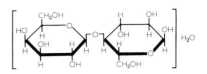

Lactose may be obtained from the whey of milk by gently evaporating it to a low bulk and allowing it to stand for a few days, when the sugar crystallises as a yellow granular mass, which is decolorised with charcoal and recrystallised.

Solubility. Soluble, at 20°, in 6 parts of water; soluble in 1 part of boiling water; very slightly soluble in alcohol, in ether, and in chloroform.

Standard
It complies with the requirements of the European Pharmacopocia.
It is a white, crystalline, odourless powder.

Hygroscopicity. It absorbs insignificant amounts of moisture at 25° at relative humidities up to about 90 per cent.

Sterilisation. It is first dried at 105° and then sterilised by dry heat.

Actions and uses. Lactose is less sweet than sucrose and less liable to cause intestinal fermentation in infants. It is added to diluted cows' milk for infant feeding to adjust the carbohydrate content to that of human milk.
Lactose is used as a diluent for standardised vegetable products and to give bulk to powders, particularly those which are to be compressed into tablets intended to dissolve completely.

LAEVULOSE

SYNONYMS: Fructose; Laevulosum

$C_6H_{12}O_6 = 180·2$

Laevulose is D-($-$)-fructopyranose.

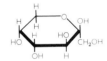

Solubility. Soluble, at 20°, in less than 1 part of water and in 15 parts of alcohol; slightly soluble in ether.

Standard
It complies with the requirements of the European Pharmacopoeia.
It is a white, crystalline, odourless powder. It contains not more than 0·5 per cent w/w of water.

Sterilisation. Solutions for injection are sterilised immediately after preparation by heating in an autoclave or by filtration.

Storage. It should be stored in airtight containers in a cool place.

Actions and uses. Laevulose is sweeter than sucrose. In contrast to dextrose it does not require insulin for its utilisation and conversion into glycogen. When administered intravenously it is metabolised nearly twice as rapidly as dextrose, but the rate of absorption after oral administration is less than half that of dextrose. Laevulose is mainly metabolised in the liver, where it is first phosphorylated and then partially converted into dextrose; it is probable that some laevulose is also metabolised in adipose tissue. Owing to its rapid metabolism by the liver, laevulose has little effect on the blood-sugar level, except in diabetics who convert it largely into dextrose. When administered intravenously in conjunction with amino-acids, laevulose has a protein-sparing action.
Laevulose accelerates the metabolism of ethyl alcohol and is used in the treatment of alcohol poisoning; for this purpose 500 millilitres of a 40 per cent solution may be given by intravenous infusion.

Laevulose is given intravenously, in preference to dextrose, as a source of carbohydrate in the treatment of renal failure, in which condition dextrose tolerance is impaired, whereas laevulose tolerance is not.
It is also useful in the management of neonatal hypoglycaemia, which may occur in newborn infants of diabetic mothers receiving large doses of insulin; laevulose given by the umbilical vein in these infants produces a more prolonged rise in blood-sugar level than an equivalent quantity of dextrose.
Laevulose offers no advantage over dextrose as a source of carbohydrate for the diabetic or in diabetic emergencies, because it is largely converted into dextrose in the diabetic liver, the degree of conversion increasing with the severity of the diabetes.
Laevulose has been used as a source of carbohydrate in debilitated patients suffering from a variety of conditions, including muscular dystrophy, vomiting of pregnancy, senility, and chronic alcoholism, but there is no evidence that it has any advantage over other carbohydrates or carbohydrate-containing foods for such patients.
Laevulose has been used as a diagnostic agent for assessing liver function.
The dosage of laevulose depends upon the condition being treated. Up to 150 grams of laevulose or even more may be given daily, in divided doses of 2 to 25 grams. It may also be given by slow intravenous infusion of a 20 or 40 per cent solution in doses up to 200 grams.

UNDESIRABLE EFFECTS. Large doses given by mouth may cause abdominal distress and diarrhoea, probably as a result of an osmotic effect. Large infusions may cause sweating, flushing, and epigastric discomfort or pain. Thrombophlebitis may occur from too rapid intravenous injection of strong solutions.

CONTRA-INDICATIONS. Laevulose should not be given to patients with familial laevulose intolerance, which is due to a congenital absence of the enzyme breaking down phos-

phorylated laevulose; in such subjects, laevulose causes hypoglycaemia and accumulation of laevulose in the liver, which may suffer damage. Sucrose produces a similar effect in such subjects.

Dose. See above under **Actions and uses.**

Preparation
LAEVULOSE INJECTION, B.P. It consists of a sterile solution of laevulose in Water for Injections. It should be stored at a temperature not exceeding 25°.

LANATOSIDE C

$C_{49}H_{76}O_{20} = 985\cdot1$

Lanatoside C is 3-(3″-acetyl-4″-β-D-glucosyltridigitoxosido)digoxigenin.

Solubility. Very slightly soluble in water and in ether; soluble, at 20°, in 20 parts of methyl alcohol.

Standard
It complies with the requirements of the British Pharmacopoeia.
It is a hygroscopic, odourless, white, crystalline powder or colourless crystals and contains not less than 96·0 and not more than the equivalent of 104·0 per cent of $C_{49}H_{76}O_{20}$, calculated with reference to the dried substance. The loss on drying under the prescribed conditions is not more than 7·5 per cent.

Storage. It should be stored in airtight containers, protected from light.

Actions and uses. Lanatoside C has the actions and uses described under Digitalis Leaf (page 161). Its rate of onset and duration of action are similar to those of oral digoxin.

The usual digitalising dose is 1 to 1·5 milligrams daily in divided doses, with a maintenance dose of 0·25 to 0·75 milligram daily when the desired therapeutic effect has been obtained.

UNDESIRABLE EFFECTS. The undesirable effects described under Digitalis Leaf (page 161) may occur, but as lanatoside C is excreted more rapidly than most other cardiac glycosides, it is less likely to give rise to cumulative effects.

PRECAUTIONS; POISONING. As for Digitalis Leaf (page 161).

Dose. See above under **Actions and uses.**

OTHER NAME: *Cedilanid*®

LAVENDER OIL

SYNONYM: Oleum Lavandulae

Lavender Oil is obtained by distillation from the fresh flowering tops of *Lavandula intermedia* Loisel. (English oil), or of *L. angustifolia* P. Miller (foreign oil) (Fam. Labiatae).

English lavender oil, which is usually considered to have the finer odour, contains little linalyl acetate. On the other hand, the fresh floral note of the French oil is enhanced in those oils having higher contents of linalyl acetate. The English oil is sometimes described as being easily distinguished from the French oil by its odour, which has a camphoraceous note.

Constituents. French lavender oil contains chiefly linalol and linalyl acetate, with small amounts of ethyl pentyl ketone, geraniol, and terpenes. English oil contains chiefly free linalol and little linalyl acetate, the total amount of linalol being similar to that in French oil. Cineole occurs in some quantity in English oil, but only in traces in French oil.

Solubility. Soluble, at 20°, English oil, in 3 parts of alcohol (30 per cent); foreign oil, in 4 parts of alcohol

(70 per cent). The solutions may be slightly opalescent and the oils become less soluble with age.

Standard
DESCRIPTION. A colourless, pale yellow, or yellowish-green liquid; odour reminiscent of the flowers.

OPTICAL ROTATION. At 20°, English oil, −5° to −13°; foreign oil, −5° to −12°.

REFRACTIVE INDEX. At 20°, English oil, 1·460 to 1·474; foreign oil, 1·457 to 1·464.

WEIGHT PER ML. At 20°, English oil, 0·875 g to 0·895 g; foreign oil, 0·878 g to 0·892 g.

ESTER VALUE. English oil, 25 to 45; foreign oil, 100 to 170.

ESTER VALUE AFTER ACETYLATION. English oil, 165 to 200; foreign oil, 220 to 280, determined by the method given in Appendix 14, page 893.

Adulterants and substitutes. Adulterants of lavender oil include spike lavender oil, lavandin oil, linalol, and synthetic esters. Spike lavender oil decreases the ester content and increases the cineole content.

Storage. It should be stored in well-filled airtight containers, protected from light, in a cool place.

Uses. Lavender oil is used largely in perfumery and occasionally to cover disagreeable odours in ointments and other preparations. It has preservative properties.

LEAD ACETATE

SYNONYM: Plumbi Acetas

$C_4H_6O_4Pb,3H_2O = 379.3$

$(CH_3 \cdot CO_2)_2Pb,3H_2O$

Solubility. Soluble, at 20°, in 2 parts of water, usually forming an opalescent solution, in 63 parts of alcohol, and in 2 parts of glycerol.

Standard

DESCRIPTION. Small, white, transparent, monoclinic prisms or heavy crystalline masses; odour acetous.

IDENTIFICATION TESTS. It gives the reactions characteristic of lead and of acetates.

COPPER, IRON, SILVER, AND ZINC. Dissolve 0.5 g in 10 ml of water, add 2 ml of *dilute sulphuric acid*, allow to stand for thirty minutes, and filter; to the filtrate add an excess of *potassium ferrocyanide solution*; no precipitate or colour is produced.

CHLORIDE. 1.0 g complies with the limit test for chlorides (350 parts per million).

WATER-INSOLUBLE MATTER. Dissolve 1 g in 10 ml of *carbon dioxide-free water*; the solution is not more than faintly opalescent and becomes clear on the addition of 0.05 ml of *acetic acid*.

CONTENT OF $C_4H_6O_4Pb,3H_2O$. Not less than 99.5 per cent and not more than the equivalent of 104.5 per cent, determined by the following method: Dissolve about 0.8 g, accurately weighed, in a mixture of 100 ml of water and 2 ml of *acetic acid*, add 5 g of *hexamine* and 0.2 ml of *xylenol orange solution* as indicator, and titrate with 0.05M disodium edetate until the solution becomes pale bright yellow; each ml of 0.05M disodium edetate is equivalent to 0.01897 g of $C_4H_6O_4Pb,3H_2O$.

Stability. It is efflorescent in warm air and absorbs carbon dioxide. It becomes anhydrous when dried at 40° and basic when heated.

Incompatibility. It is incompatible with carbonates, chlorides, iodides, sulphates, phosphates, and tannic acid.

Storage. It should be stored in airtight containers.

Uses. Preparations of lead salts are used empirically as lotions for the treatment of bruises and sprains. Lead salts should never be used internally.

POISONING. The common symptoms of acute lead poisoning are a burning pain in the stomach, vomiting, diarrhoea, intense thirst, and a metallic taste; these may be followed by giddiness or fainting, collapse, and coma. Immediate gastric lavage with a solution of magnesium sulphate, 25 grams in 5 litres of water, is the treatment of choice. Alternatively, the stomach may be emptied by administering an emetic, or demulcents such as milk or white of egg may be given. Shock should be treated by rest and warmth.

If sufficient lead has been absorbed to produce chronic poisoning, a diet high in calcium and vitamin D should be given to promote the deposition of lead in the bones in an insoluble form. Subsequent removal of the lead can be undertaken by the administration of sodium calciumedetate as an intravenous infusion, as described under Sodium Calciumedetate (page 445).

Preparations

LEAD LOTION, B.P.C. (page 728)

LEAD LOTION, EVAPORATING, B.P.C. (page 728)

LEAD SUBACETATE SOLUTION, DILUTE, B.P.C. (page 788)

LEAD SUBACETATE SOLUTION, STRONG, B.P.C. (page 788)

LEAD MONOXIDE

SYNONYMS: Litharge; Plumbi Monoxidum

$PbO = 223.2$

Solubility. Very slightly soluble in water; insoluble in alcohol; soluble in acetic acid, in dilute nitric acid, and in warm solutions of alkali hydroxides.

Standard

DESCRIPTION. Yellow, pale orange, or pale brick-red heavy scales or powder; odourless or almost odourless.

IDENTIFICATION TESTS. 1. When heated it darkens in colour and, on cooling, assumes a colour ranging from lemon-yellow to brick-red, according to the conditions of heating and cooling.

2. When heated with charcoal it is reduced to metallic lead.

3. When dissolved in *acetic acid* it gives the reactions characteristic of lead.

CARBONATE AND MOISTURE. Not more than 1.0 per cent, determined by igniting to constant weight.

CONTENT OF PbO. Not less than 99.0 per cent, calculated with reference to the substance ignited to constant weight, determined by the following method: Dissolve about 0.5 g, accurately weighed, in a mixture of 10 ml of water and 3 ml of *acetic acid* with the aid of gentle heat, cool, dilute to 100 ml with water, add 5 g of *hexamine* and 0.2 ml of *xylenol orange solution* as indicator, and titrate with 0.05M disodium edetate until the solution becomes pale bright yellow; each ml of 0.05M disodium edetate is equivalent to 0.01116 g of PbO.

Uses. Lead monoxide is used in the preparation of Strong Lead Subacetate Solution (page 788), and also in the preparation of diachylon plaster-masses.

LEMON OIL

SYNONYM: Oleum Limonis

Lemon Oil is expressed from the outer part of the fresh pericarp of the ripe or nearly ripe fruit of *Citrus limon* (L.) Burm. f. (Fam. Rutaceae).

Constituents. Lemon oil consists chiefly of (+)-limonene which, together with small quantities of other terpenes, constitutes about 90 per cent of the oil. The remaining 10 per cent consists of oxygenated compounds, of which citral is present in the largest amount. The quality of the oil is not determined solely by the citral content.

Solubility. Soluble, at 20°, in 12 parts of alcohol (90 per cent), the solution showing a slight opalescence; miscible with dehydrated alcohol.

Standard

DESCRIPTION. A pale yellow or greenish-yellow liquid; odour reminiscent of lemon.

OPTICAL ROTATION. At 20°, +57° to +65°.

REFRACTIVE INDEX. At 20°, 1·474 to 1·476.

WEIGHT PER ML. At 20°, 0·850 g to 0·856 g.

NON-VOLATILE MATTER. 2·0 to 3·0 per cent w/w, determined by the following method:
Evaporate about 5 g, accurately weighed, in a flat-bottomed dish of nickel or other suitable metal, 9 cm in diameter and 1·5 cm deep, by heating on a vigorously boiling water-bath for a total of 4 hours, and weigh the residue.

CONTENT OF ALDEHYDES. Not less than 3·5 per cent w/w, calculated as citral, $C_{10}H_{16}O$, determined by the following method:
Carry out the method for the determination of aldehydes given in Appendix 14, page 893, using about 10 g, accurately weighed, omitting the toluene, and using a volume, not less than 7 ml, of *hydroxylammonium chloride reagent in alcohol (60 per cent)* which exceeds by 1 to 2 ml the volume of 0·5N potassium hydroxide in alcohol (60 per cent) required; each ml of 0·5N potassium hydroxide in alcohol (60 per cent) is equivalent to 0·07673 g (*i.e.* 0·07612 × 1·008) of $C_{10}H_{16}O$.

Adulterants and substitutes. Lemon oil is sometimes adulterated with distilled lemon oil, with terpenes obtained as residues in the preparation of terpeneless oils, with low-grade orange oil, and with citral obtained from lemon grass oil.

Storage. It should be stored in well-filled airtight containers, protected from light, in a cool place.

Uses. The principal use of lemon oil is as a flavouring and perfumery agent. It is used to make Terpeneless Lemon Oil.

TERPENELESS LEMON OIL

SYNONYM: Oleum Limonis Deterpenatum

Terpeneless Lemon Oil may be prepared by concentrating Lemon Oil in vacuo until most of the terpenes have been removed, or by solvent partition.

Constituents. Terpeneless lemon oil consists chiefly of citral, with considerable quantities of esters, chiefly geranyl and linalyl acetates.

Solubility. Soluble, at 20°, in 1 part of alcohol (80 per cent).

Standard

DESCRIPTION. A colourless or pale yellow liquid; odour and taste of lemon.

OPTICAL ROTATION. At 20°, −4° to +1°.

REFRACTIVE INDEX. At 20°, 1·478 to 1·485.

WEIGHT PER ML. At 20°, 0·880 g to 0·890 g.

ESTER VALUE. 40 to 75, determined by the method of the British Pharmacopoeia for the determination of ester value, about 0·3 g, accurately weighed, being used, 10 ml of 0·1N alcoholic potassium hydroxide being substituted for 20 ml of 0·5N alcoholic potassium hydroxide, the refluxing being continued for 30 minutes, and the titration being made with 0·1N hydrochloric acid. The ester value is given by the formula: 5·60 m/w, where m = volume, in ml, of 0·1N

alcoholic potassium hydroxide required to saponify the esters, and w = weight, in g, of sample.

CONTENT OF ALDEHYDES. 40 to 50 per cent w/w, calculated as citral, $C_{10}H_{16}O$, determined by the method for Lemon Oil, about 1 g, accurately weighed, being used.

Storage. It should be stored in well-filled airtight containers, protected from light, in a cool place.

Uses. Terpeneless lemon oil is used almost exclusively as a flavouring agent; it has the advantages of being stronger in flavour and odour and more readily soluble in dilute alcoholic solution than the natural oil.

The terpeneless oil is equivalent in flavour to about twenty times its volume of lemon oil; a 1 per cent v/v solution in alcohol (70 per cent) is generally used for culinary purposes.

Preparations

LEMON SPIRIT, B.P.C. (page 793)

ORANGE SPIRIT, COMPOUND, B.P.C. (page 793)

DRIED LEMON PEEL

SYNONYM: Limonis Cortex Siccatus

Dried Lemon Peel consists of the dried outer part of the pericarp of the ripe, or nearly ripe, fruit of *Citrus limon* (L.) Burm. f. (Fam. Rutaceae), obtained principally from Spain, Italy, and Sicily.

Constituents. Dried lemon peel contains volatile oil, hesperidin, and pectin.

Standard
It complies with the requirements of the British Pharmacopoeia.
It contains not less than 2·5 per cent v/w of volatile oil.

Macroscopical characters: strips or pieces, outer surface yellow and somewhat rough from the presence of numerous minute pits, each corresponding to an oil gland; inner surface with only a small amount of white spongy pericarp; fracture short; some pieces with nipple-shaped apex attached.
Odour aromatic; taste aromatic and bitter.

Microscopical characters: the diagnostic characters are:

epidermis of small, polyhedral cells; tissue subjacent to the epidermis parenchymatous, many cells containing prismatic *crystals* of calcium oxalate, 15 to 25 μm long; numerous large lysigenous *oil glands* about 0·3 to 0·6 mm in diameter and small *vascular strands* embedded in the parenchyma.

Adulterants and substitutes. Peel which has been scarified by machines is dried and offered as dried lemon peel; it contains very little oil and can be distinguished by the fine lines of scarification or cuts on the outer surface.

Storage. It should be stored in airtight containers.

Actions and uses. Dried lemon peel is used as a flavouring agent.

LEVALLORPHAN TARTRATE

$C_{23}H_{31}NO_7 = 433.5$

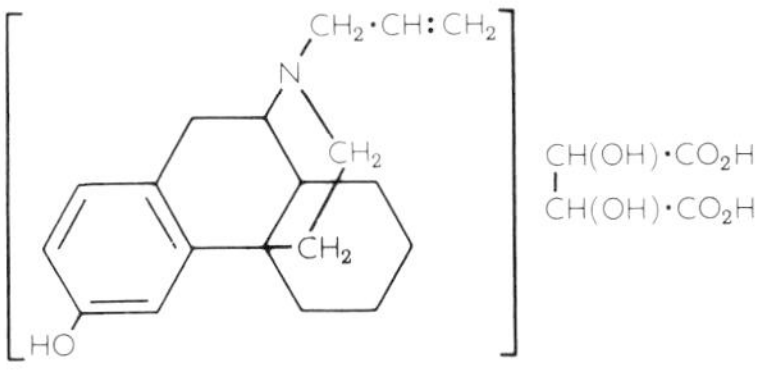

Levallorphan Tartrate is (−)-*N*-allyl-3-hydroxy-morphinan hydrogen tartrate.

Solubility. Soluble, at 20°, in 20 parts of water and in 100 parts of alcohol; very slightly soluble in ether.

Standard
It complies with the requirements of the British Pharmacopoeia.
It is a white, crystalline, odourless powder and contains not less than 98·5 and not more than the equivalent of 101·0 per cent of $C_{23}H_{31}NO_7$, calculated with reference to the dried substance. The loss on drying under the prescribed conditions is not more than 0·5 per cent. A 0·2 per cent solution in water has a pH of 3·2 to 4·0. It has a melting-point of about 176°.

Sterilisation. Solutions for injection are sterilised by heating in an autoclave or by filtration.

Storage. It should be stored in airtight containers, protected from light.

Actions and uses. Levallorphan is an antagonist of morphine and similar drugs. Its action resembles that of nalorphine (page 318),

but it is more potent. It is usually administered by intravenous injection as a 0·1 per cent solution.
Levallorphan is sometimes used in obstetrics in conjunction with a morphine-like agent such as pethidine with the object of reducing the respiratory depression for a given level of analgesia but there is no convincing evidence that this objective is achieved.

Dose. 0·2 to 2 milligrams by intravenous injection.

Preparation
LEVALLORPHAN INJECTION, B.P. A sterile solution of levallorphan tartrate in Water for Injections, the pH of the solution being adjusted to 4·5. Unless otherwise specified, a solution containing 1 mg in 1 ml is supplied. It should be protected from light.

OTHER NAME: *Lorfan®*

LEVODOPA

SYNONYM: L-Dopa

$C_9H_{11}NO_4 = 197.2$

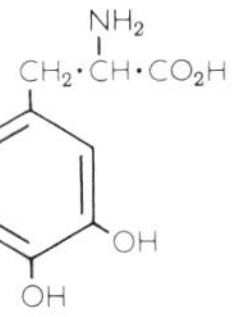

Levodopa is (−)-3-(3,4-dihydroxyphenyl)-L-alanine.

Solubility. Soluble, at 20°, in 300 parts of water; very slightly soluble in alcohol, in ether, and in chloroform; soluble in aqueous solutions of mineral acids and alkali carbonates.

Standard
It complies with the requirements of the British Pharmacopoeia.
It is a white or almost white, crystalline, odourless

powder and contains not less than 98·5 and not more than the equivalent of 101·0 per cent of $C_9H_{11}NO_4$, calculated with reference to the dried substance. The loss on drying under the prescribed conditions is not more than 0·5 per cent.

Storage. It should be stored in airtight containers, protected from light.

Actions and uses. Levodopa is a precursor of dopamine, which is depleted from the brain in Parkinson's disease. In the treatment of Parkinson's disease, levodopa is most effective in relieving hypokinesia, and may also decrease rigidity, oculogyric crises, and tremor.

Treatment may be commenced with a dosage of 125 milligrams or 250 milligrams four or five times daily, according to the weight of the patient, and in the absence of adverse effects the dosage may be increased by 250 milligrams per day every second or third day up to a maximum of 8 grams daily. Elderly patients may require a lower initial dosage such as 125 milligrams daily.

UNDESIRABLE EFFECTS. Anorexia and nausea are not uncommon. Giddiness due to postural hypotension may occur and palpitations and cardiac arrhythmias have been recorded. The commonest dose-limiting reaction, apart from nausea, is the appearance of involuntary movements, particularly affecting the tongue, jaw, and neck.

A wide variety of psychotic responses to levodopa has been described including confusion, depression, and hypomania.

PRECAUTIONS. It should not be given to patients who are being treated with pyridoxine or a monoamine-oxidase inhibitor, such as isocarboxazid, nialamide, phenelzine, or tranylcypromine, or within about ten days of the discontinuation of such treatment.

Dose. See above under **Actions and uses.**

Preparations

LEVODOPA CAPSULES, B.P. (*Syn.* L-Dopa Capsules). The quantity of levodopa in each capsule should be specified by the prescriber. Capsules containing 125, 250, and 500 mg are available.

LEVODOPA TABLETS, B.P. (*Syn.* L-Dopa Tablets). The quantity of levodopa in each tablet should be specified by the prescriber. Tablets containing 500 mg are available.

OTHER NAMES: *Berkdopa®*; *Brocadopa®*; *Larodopa®*; *Levopa®*; *Veldopa®*

LEVORPHANOL TARTRATE

$C_{21}H_{29}NO_7,2H_2O = 443·5$

Levorphanol Tartrate is the dihydrate of $(-)$-3-hydroxy-N-methylmorphinan hydrogen tartrate.

Solubility. Soluble in 45 parts of water, in 110 parts of alcohol, and in 50 parts of ether.

Standard
It complies with the requirements of the British Pharmacopoeia.
It is a white, crystalline, odourless powder and contains not less than 98·5 and not more than the equivalent of 101·0 per cent of $C_{21}H_{29}NO_7$, calculated with reference to the dried substance. The loss on drying under the prescribed conditions is 7·0 to 9·0 per cent. It has a melting-point of about 116°. A 0·2 per cent solution in water has a pH of 3·4 to 4·0.

Sterilisation. Solutions for injection are sterilised by heating in an autoclave or by filtration.

Storage. It should be stored in airtight containers.

Actions and uses. Levorphanol is an analgesic which has actions, uses, and undesirable effects similar to those described under Morphine Hydrochloride (page 314), but it differs from morphine in being almost as effective when given by mouth as by injection. Levorphanol tartrate is given by mouth in doses of 1·5 to 4·5 milligrams, by subcutaneous or intramuscular injection in doses of 2 to 4 milligrams, and by intravenous injection in doses of 1 to 1·5 milligrams; these doses may be repeated in accordance with the needs of the patient. In an emergency, 2 to 4 milligrams may be administered by slow intravenous injection.

DEPENDENCE. Prolonged administration of therapeutic doses may lead to the development of dependence of the morphine type, as described under Morphine Hydrochloride (page 314).

POISONING. The procedure described under Morphine Hydrochloride (page 314) should be adopted.

Dose. See above under **Actions and uses.**

Preparations

LEVORPHANOL INJECTION, B.P. It consists of a sterile solution of levorphanol tartrate in Water for Injections, the pH of the solution being adjusted to 5·5. It should be protected from light. The strength of the solution should be specified by the prescriber. Ampoules containing 2 mg in 1 ml are available.

LEVORPHANOL TABLETS, B.P. The quantity of levorphanol tartrate in each tablet should be specified by the prescriber. Tablets containing 1·5 mg are available.

OTHER NAME: *Dromoran®*

LIGNOCAINE HYDROCHLORIDE

SYNONYMS: Lidocaine Hydrochloride;
Lidocaini Hydrochloridum; Lignoc. Hydrochlor.

$C_{14}H_{23}ClN_2O,H_2O = 288 \cdot 8$

Lignocaine Hydrochloride is diethylaminoacet-2,6-xylidide hydrochloride monohydrate.

Solubility. Soluble, at 20°, in less than 1 part of water and in 1·5 parts of alcohol; soluble in chloroform; insoluble in ether.

Standard
It complies with the requirements of the European Pharmacopoeia.
It is a white, crystalline, odourless powder and contains not less than 99·0 per cent of $C_{14}H_{23}ClN_2O$, calculated with reference to the anhydrous substance. It contains 5·0 to 7·5 per cent w/w of water. It has a melting-point, without previous drying, of 76° to 79°. A 0·5 per cent solution in water has a pH of 4·0 to 5·5.

Sterilisation. Solutions for injection are sterilised by heating in an autoclave or by filtration.

Actions and uses. Lignocaine is a local anaesthetic, widely used by injection and for local application to mucous membranes. In equal concentration, it is more effective than procaine and gives a greater area of anaesthesia, but may be more toxic.
Solutions containing 0·5 to 2 per cent of lignocaine hydrochloride, with adrenaline 1 in 100,000 to 1 in 50,000, may be used for infiltration; except under special circumstances the concentration of lignocaine used should not exceed 1 per cent and the total quantity of lignocaine administered should not exceed 200 milligrams unless adrenaline is present, when up to 500 milligrams may be given. Solutions containing adrenaline should not be used for inducing anaesthesia in digits

because the profound ischaemia produced may lead to gangrene.
Preparations containing 1 to 4 per cent of lignocaine hydrochloride may be used to anaesthetise the pharynx, larynx, and trachea before endoscopic examination.
A 1 or 2 per cent solution is used for epidural anaesthesia.
In the treatment of cardiac arrhythmias, lignocaine hydrochloride has been given by intravenous injection in doses of 50 to 100 milligrams, administered as 5 to 10 millilitres of a 1 per cent solution over a period of two minutes, followed by intravenous infusion at a rate of 1 to 2 milligrams per minute in accordance with the needs of the patient.

POISONING. The procedure as described under Procaine Hydrochloride (page 404) should be adopted.

Preparations
LIGNOCAINE GEL, B.P.C. (page 701)
LIGNOCAINE AND ADRENALINE INJECTION, B.P. It consists of a sterile solution of lignocaine hydrochloride and adrenaline acid tartrate in Water for Injections containing 0·1 per cent of sodium metabisulphite. The strength of the solution should be specified by the prescriber. It should be protected from light.
LIGNOCAINE HYDROCHLORIDE INJECTION, B.P. It consists of a sterile solution of lignocaine hydrochloride in Water for Injections. The strength of the solution should be specified by the prescriber.

OTHER NAMES: *Xylocaine®*; *Xylotox®*

LINCOMYCIN HYDROCHLORIDE

$C_{18}H_{34}N_2O_6S,HCl,H_2O = 461 \cdot 0$

Lincomycin Hydrochloride is methyl 6,8-dideoxy-6-(1-methyl-4-propyl-2-pyrrolidinecarboxamido)-1-thio-D-*erythro*-D-*galacto*-octopyranoside hydrochloride monohydrate, an antimicrobial substance produced by *Streptomyces lincolnensis* var. *lincolnensis* or by any other means.

Solubility. Soluble, at 20°, in 1 part of water, in 40 parts of alcohol, and in 20 parts of dimethylformamide; insoluble in ether and in chloroform; very slightly soluble in acetone.

Standard
It complies with the requirements of the British Pharmacopoeia.
It is a white or almost white crystalline powder with a slight characteristic odour and contains not less than 82·5 per cent of lincomycin, $C_{18}H_{34}N_2O_6S$, calculated with reference to the anhydrous substance. It contains 3·0 to 6·0 per cent w/w of water. A 10 per cent solution in water has a pH of 3·0 to 5·5.

Labelling. If the material is not intended for parenteral administration, the label on the container states that the contents are not to be injected.

Storage. It should be stored in airtight containers at a temperature not exceeding 30°. If it is intended for parenteral administration, the containers should be sterile and sealed to exclude micro-organisms.

Actions and uses. Lincomycin is an antibiotic which is active against a narrow range of bacteria, mainly the pyogenic Gram-positive cocci and species of *Bacteroides*; it is ineffective against species of *Neisseria* and *Haemophilus*. It is bacteriostatic in low concentrations and bactericidal in high concentrations, and acts by interfering with the synthesis of deoxyribonucleic acid.

The hydrochloride is moderately well absorbed when given by mouth on an empty stomach but some reaches the large intestine where it is partly broken down. Lincomycin is weakly bound to plasma protein and readily diffuses into all tissues except the brain and cerebrospinal fluid. It is partly degraded in the body and partly excreted in the urine; it also crosses the placenta and is excreted in the bile and the breast milk. The biological half-life is five to seven hours.

Lincomycin is used chiefly for the treatment of susceptible infections in patients allergic to penicillins and for the treatment of infections that are not susceptible to penicillins. As it penetrates bone, it is also used for the treatment of osteomyelitis. Resistance is induced relatively easily, but cross-resistance is rare, except with erythromycin.

The usual dosage for adults is the equivalent of 1·5 grams of lincomycin daily in divided doses thirty minutes before food, or of 0·6 to 1·2 grams of lincomycin by intramuscular injection daily in two doses, or of 300 to 600 milligrams in Dextrose Injection (5 per cent) or Sodium Chloride Injection every eight to twelve hours by intravenous infusion.

Children may be given the equivalent of 8 to 16 milligrams of lincomycin per kilogram body-weight every eight hours by mouth or 5 to 10 milligrams per kilogram body-weight by intramuscular injection twice a day, or of 10 to 20 milligrams per kilogram body-weight by intravenous infusion daily in divided doses.

1·15 grams of lincomycin hydrochloride is approximately equivalent to 1 gram of lincomycin.

UNDESIRABLE EFFECTS. Diarrhoea, allergic reactions, and suprainfection with yeasts may occur, and, rarely, liver damage.

PRECAUTIONS AND CONTRA-INDICATIONS. Lincomycin should be administered with caution to patients with renal failure as accumulation may occur and the substance cannot be removed by dialysis. It should not be administered in pregnancy or to nursing mothers. Special precautions are required in prolonged treatment.

Dose. See above under **Actions and uses.**

Preparations

LINCOMYCIN CAPSULES, B.P. Unless otherwise specified, capsules each containing the equivalent of 500 mg of lincomycin are supplied.

LINCOMYCIN INJECTION, B.P. It consists of a sterile solution of lincomycin hydrochloride in Water for Injections. It should be protected from light and stored at a temperature not exceeding 20°. Under these conditions it may be expected to retain its potency for at least three years from the date of manufacture. Vials containing the equivalent of 600 mg of lincomycin in 2 ml are available.

OTHER NAMES: *Lincocin®*; *Mycivin®*

LIOTHYRONINE SODIUM

SYNONYM: L-Tri-iodothyronine Sodium

$C_{15}H_{11}I_3NNaO_4 = 673·0$

Liothyronine Sodium is sodium L-α-amino-β-[4-(4-hydroxy-3-iodophenoxy)-3,5-di-iodophenyl]propionate.

Solubility. Very slightly soluble in water, in ether, and in chloroform; soluble, at 20°, in 500 parts of alcohol; soluble in solutions of alkali hydroxides.

Standard

It complies with the requirements of the British Pharmacopoeia.

It is a white or buff-coloured odourless solid and contains organically combined iodine equivalent to not less than 95·0 and not more than the equivalent of 101·0 per cent of $C_{15}H_{11}I_3NNaO_4$, calculated with reference to the dried substance. The loss on drying under the prescribed conditions is not more than 4·0 per cent.

Storage. It should be stored in airtight containers, protected from light.

Actions and uses. Liothyronine has the actions and uses described under Thyroxine Sodium (page 510). It is an active principle of the thyroid gland and is believed to be the activated form of the thyroid hormone which has a stimulant effect on cellular metabolism. It is effective in smaller doses than thyroid or thyroxine and its action is quicker in onset but of shorter duration. It has the advantage over thyroid that it is of constant composition and biological assay is not necessary.

Liothyronine sodium is used in the treatment of severe hypothyroidism when a rapid therapeutic action is required, but it is less suitable than thyroxine for maintenance therapy, because of its shorter duration of action. It is given by mouth in an initial dosage of 10 to 20 micrograms daily, which is gradually increased by 10-microgram increments every three to seven days up to a total of 80 to 100 micrograms daily. A child may be given 10 to 40 micrograms daily according to age.

Liothyronine is used in a tri-iodothyronine

suppression test for the diagnosis of thyrotoxicosis; for this purpose it is given in a daily dosage of 120 micrograms for seven days.

UNDESIRABLE EFFECTS. Effects similar to those described under Thyroxine Sodium (page 510) may occur, but rapidly disappear if treatment is stopped or the dosage reduced.

CONTRA-INDICATIONS. Liothyronine is contra-indicated in patients with angina pectoris or cardiovascular disorders.

Dose. See above under **Actions and uses.**

Preparation
LIOTHYRONINE TABLETS, B.P. (*Syn.* L-Tri-iodothyronine Sodium Tablets). Unless otherwise specified, tablets each containing 20 μg of liothyronine sodium are supplied. They should be protected from light.

OTHER NAME: *Tertroxin*®

LIQUORICE

SYNONYMS: Glycyrrhiza; Liquiritiae Radix; Liquorice Root

Liquorice consists of the dried peeled or unpeeled root and stolon of various species of *Glycyrrhiza* (Fam. Leguminosae), yielding a drug having a sweet taste and almost free from bitterness.

The more important species of *Glycyrrhiza* are *G. glabra* L. and *G. glabra* var. *glandulifera* (Waldst. et Kit.) Boiss. *G. glabra* is a tall erect herbaceous perennial, widely distributed over southern Europe. It is imported chiefly from Russia, Turkey, Syria, and Iran.

Varieties. Russian liquorice is obtained from *G. glabra* var. *glandulifera*, which grows abundantly in southern Russia; it consists mainly of root and is usually imported in the unpeeled condition. The pieces are often much larger than those of *G. glabra* and are usually split longitudinally. The cork, when present, is somewhat purplish in colour and frequently scaly. The taste is sweet but has a slight bitterness; unpeeled Russian liquorice yields about 25 to 30 per cent of water-soluble extractive.
Persian liquorice, from Iran, is obtained from *G. glabra* var. *glandulifera* and is usually imported unpeeled; it resembles unpeeled Russian root in appearance.
Anatolian liquorice, from Turkey, and Syrian liquorice are derived from *G. glabra*; the pieces, which may be peeled or unpeeled, are sometimes of a very large size, up to 8 cm in diameter.

Constituents. Liquorice contains about 7 per cent of glycyrrhizin, a sweet white crystalline powder consisting of the calcium and potassium salts of glycyrrhizinic acid. The acid, which forms colourless crystals melting at 222°, is the diglucopyanosiduronic acid of the triterpenoid glycyrrhetic acid (glycyrrhetinic acid) (3β-hydroxy-11-oxo-18β-olean-12-en-30-oic acid).
Liquorice also contains glucose, sucrose, starch (about 30 per cent), other triterpenoid acids, and numerous flavonoid glycosides.

Standard
It complies with the requirements of the European Pharmacopoeia which describes only the unpeeled drug.
It contains not less than 25·0 per cent of water-soluble extractive.

UNGROUND DRUG. *Macroscopical characters:* pieces nearly cylindrical, about 0·5 to 3 cm in diameter and up to about 1 m in length, sometimes cut into lengths of about 10 to 15 cm. Unpeeled external surface longitudinally wrinkled, covered with a reddish-brown or purplish-brown corky layer, bearing small circular root scars and, on pieces of stolon, occasional small dark buds. Peeled drug: external surface smooth, yellow, and fibrous. Fracture fibrous in the bark and splintery in the wood. Smoothed, transversely cut surface showing a distinct cambium line at a depth of about one-third of the radius, separating the yellowish-grey bark from the finely radiate yellow wood; central pith only in the stolon. Xylem wedges narrow, finely porous, each with a phloem strand opposite, with groups of included fibres visible as a radial row of dark points.
When moistened with *sulphuric acid (80 per cent v/v)* the drug develops a deep yellow colour.
Odour faint and characteristic; taste sweet and almost free from bitterness.

Microscopical characters: the diagnostic characters are: *fibres* with thick, lignified or partially lignified walls present in groups of 10 to 50 in both phloem and xylem, often accompanied by rows of small rectangular cells each containing a prismatic *crystal* of calcium oxalate about 10 to 15 to 25 to 35 μm long; *vessels* large, walls with closely arranged bordered pits, frequently associated with lignified parenchyma; *starch* granules simple, oval, and rounded, 2 to 4 to 10 to 20 μm in diameter.
In the unpeeled drug, *cork cells* brownish, polyhedral, tabular.

POWDERED DRUG: Powdered Liquorice. A brownish-yellow powder possessing the diagnostic characters, odour, and taste of the unground drug. It is prepared from the unpeeled drug unless the peeled drug is specified.

Adulterants and substitutes. Manchurian liquorice, possibly from *G. uralensis* Fisch. ex DC., has a pale chocolate-brown, readily exfoliated cork, a lacunar xylem, and conspicuously wavy medullary rays. It contains glycyrrhizin but is practically free from sugars.
Liquorice derived from *G. glabra* has been imported from India: it varies considerably in thickness and is usually cut into short lengths.

Actions and uses. Liquorice is a demulcent and mild expectorant. Extracts of liquorice with sedatives and other expectorants are used in cough lozenges and cough pastilles; the liquid extract is used in cough mixtures.
Liquorice is used as a flavouring agent in the compound powder, and the liquid extract will disguise the taste of nauseous medicines, especially the alkali iodides, ammonium chloride, quinine, creosote, and Cascara Liquid Extract.

Powdered liquorice is used as an absorbent pill excipient.

Preparations
LIQUORICE EXTRACT, B.P.C. (page 683)

LIQUORICE LIQUID EXTRACT, B.P. Prepared from unpeeled liquorice by percolation with chloroform water, evaporation to a specified weight per ml, and addition of alcohol (90 per cent). Dose: 2 to 5 ml.
LIQUORICE LOZENGES, B.P.C. (page 733)
LIQUORICE POWDER, COMPOUND, B.P.C. (page 777)

LITHIUM CARBONATE

$Li_2CO_3 = 73·89$

Solubility. Soluble, at 20°, in 100 parts of water; less soluble in boiling water; insoluble in alcohol.

Standard
It complies with the requirements of the British Pharmacopoeia.
It is a white, crystalline, odourless powder and contains not less than 99·5 per cent of Li_2CO_3, calculated with reference to the dried substance. The loss on drying under the prescribed conditions is not more than 0·5 per cent.

Actions and uses. Lithium carbonate is used as a source of lithium ions, which may act by competing with sodium at various sites. It causes changes in the composition of electrolytes in body fluids and increases the intracellular and total body water content.
Lithium carbonate is used in the prophylaxis and treatment of refractory acute maniacal states and in the prophylaxis of manic depressive disease, but there is doubt whether it is effective for prophylaxis.
The initial dose in affective disorders is 250 milligrams daily and this may be gradually increased to 750 milligrams daily in divided doses; in manic depressive disease these doses may be doubled. It is advisable to control treatment by measurement of the plasma lithium level, which should be maintained between 0·6 and 1·6 millimoles per litre, above which side-effects commonly occur.

UNDESIRABLE EFFECTS. Side-effects depend upon the dose and the degree of accumulation and usually develop slowly over a period of several days; they include sluggishness, drowsiness, coarse tremor, loss of appetite, diarrhoea, and vomiting. The electrocardiogram may show flattening of the T-wave.
Administration of lithium carbonate may precipitate goitre requiring treatment with thyroxine.

CONTRA-INDICATIONS. Lithium carbonate should not be administered to patients with renal or cardiac disease.

Dose. 0·25 to 1·6 grams daily in divided doses.

Preparations
LITHIUM CARBONATE TABLETS, B.P. The quantity of lithium carbonate in each tablet should be specified by the prescriber. Tablets containing 250 mg are available.
SLOW LITHIUM CARBONATE TABLETS, B.P. These tablets are formulated to release the medicament over a period of several hours. The quantity of lithium carbonate in each tablet should be specified by the prescriber. Tablets containing 400 mg are available.

OTHER NAMES: *Camcolit*®; *Priadel*®

LOBELIA

SYNONYM: Lobelia Herb

Lobelia consists of the dried aerial parts of *Lobelia inflata* L. (Fam. Lobeliaceae). The plant is an erect annual herb, indigenous to the eastern United States of America and cultivated there and in Holland. It is cut down when the lower fruits are nearly ripe, and dried.

Constituents. Lobelia contains about 0·25 to 0·4 per cent of alkaloids, consisting of lobeline, lobelanine, lobelanidine, and a number of other alkaloids; the most important is lobeline. The drug also contains a neutral crystalline substance, inflatin, and lobelic acid.

Standard for unground drug
DESCRIPTION. *Macroscopical:* Stems green, often with a purplish tint, terete, hairy and winged in the upper part, channelled, angled, and nearly glabrous below; trichomes up to about 1·2 mm in length; alternate leaves or leaf scars present, phyllotaxis of 1:3.
Leaves pale green, broadly ovate to ovate-lanceolate and varying from about 3 to 8 cm in length, margin irregularly toothed, lamina bearing scattered bristly trichomes, especially on the veins of the lower surface. Inflorescence of racemes of about 6 to 20 flowers arising in the axils of the upper leaves; bracts foliaceous; pedicels slender, about 3 to 5 mm long; flowers hermaphrodite and zygomorphic, about 7 mm long; calyx superior; sepals 5, subulate, about 2·5 mm long; corolla epignous, tubular, about 4 mm long, bilabiate, upper lip of 2 lanceolate segments between which the corolla tube is split down to the base, lower lip of 3 spreading triangular-ovate lobes, pale violet-blue; androecium of 5 epignous stamens with syngynesious anthers, each anther having an apical tuft of trichomes; gynoecium of 2 carpels, ovary inferior, bilocular, ovules numerous, placentation axile, stigma bifid and surrounded by the anther tube.
Fruit an inflated, ovoid or ellipsoidal bilocular capsule, dehiscing by apical pores, and containing when ripe numerous brown ovoid reticulate seeds, about 0·5 to 0·7 mm long and about 0·3 mm wide.
Odour slight and somewhat irritating; taste slight at first but becoming burning and acrid when the drug is chewed.

Microscopical: the diagnostic characters are: Leaf: *epidermal cells* of adaxial surface with straight walls, *papillose, cuticle* striated; cells of abaxial surface with

wavy and beaded anticlinal walls; *stomata* anomocytic, on abaxial surface only; *trichomes* conical, unicellular or rarely 2-celled, with thin, warty walls and usually about 300 μm but sometimes as much as 1·2 mm long; *palisade ratio* about 4 to **4·3** to 5·3; *mesophyll* with many cells containing abundant *fat crystals* in the form of slender prisms 10 to 15 μm long and 2 μm thick, often arranged in small fan-shaped groups of 5 or 6; on warming the crystals are replaced by droplets of oil; *laticiferous vessels* anastomosing.
Stem: *epidermis* and *trichomes* as in leaf; *cuticle* striated; anastomosing *laticiferous vessels* also present; *pith* with lignified and pitted parenchyma.
Pollen grains spherical, about 24 to 30 μm in diameter, *extine* smooth, with 3 pores.
Pericarp with irregular, *pitted sclereids*.
Seed: *epidermal cells* about 100 μm by 25 μm, elongated-polygonal, with highly refractive lignified anticlinal walls.

ACID-INSOLUBLE ASH. Not more than 5·0 per cent.

FOREIGN ORGANIC MATTER. Not more than 2·0 per cent.

STEMS. Not more than 60·0 per cent.

CONTENT OF TOTAL ALKALOIDS. Not less than 0·25 per cent, calculated as lobeline, $C_{22}H_{27}NO_2$, determined by the following method:
Weigh accurately about 10 g, in fine powder, add 10 g of ignited sand, transfer to a stoppered flask, and add 75 ml of a mixture of 4 volumes of *solvent ether* and 1 volume of *alcohol (95 per cent)*; shake well, allow to stand for 15 minutes, add 5 ml of *dilute ammonia solution*, and shake frequently during one hour.
Transfer the mixture to a small percolator plugged with cotton wool, allow the liquid to flow into a separating funnel and, when the liquid ceases to flow, pack firmly and continue the percolation first with 25 ml of the ether–alcohol mixture and then with *solvent ether* until extraction of the alkaloids is complete.
To the percolate add 30 ml of 1N sulphuric acid, shake well, allow to separate, and run off the lower layer into another separator; repeat the extraction with a mixture of 25 ml of 0·5N sulphuric acid and 5 ml of *alcohol (95 per cent)*, run off the lower layer, and repeat the extraction with three or more successive 20-ml portions of the acid–alcohol mixture until extraction is complete.
Wash the mixed acid solutions, first with 10 ml and then with two successive 5-ml portions of *chloroform*, washing each chloroform solution with the same 20 ml of 0·5N sulphuric acid contained in another separator, discard the chloroform, transfer the acid liquid from the

second separator to the first separator, neutralise to *litmus paper* with *dilute ammonia solution* and add a further 5 ml in excess, and extract with successive 10-ml portions of *chloroform* until extraction of the alkaloids is complete, washing each chloroform solution separately with the same 5 ml of water and filtering through a 7-cm filter paper into a flask; wash the filter thoroughly with *chloroform*, collect the washings in the flask, heat on a water-bath to remove the chloroform until about 2 ml remains, add 2 ml of *dehydrated alcohol*, and continue the evaporation on the water-bath, using a gentle air-blast to complete the process; repeat with two further portions of *dehydrated alcohol*, and dry the residue for one hour at 80°.
Add to the residue 2 ml of *alcohol (95 per cent)*, warm until dissolved, add 10 ml of 0·02N sulphuric acid, cool, and titrate the excess of acid with 0·02N sodium hydroxide, using *methyl red solution* as indicator; each ml of 0·02N sulphuric acid is equivalent to 0·006749 g of $C_{22}H_{27}NO_2$.

Standard for powdered drug: Powdered Lobelia
DESCRIPTION. A dull greenish-yellow powder possessing the diagnostic microscopical characters, odour, and taste of the unground drug.

ACID-INSOLUBLE ASH; FOREIGN ORGANIC MATTER; CONTENT OF TOTAL ALKALOIDS. It complies with the requirements for the unground drug.

Adulterants and substitutes. Indian lobelia is derived from *L. nicotianifolia* Heyne ex Roem. et Schult. and from *L. leschenaultiana* (Presl) Skottsb. These drugs can be distinguished by the characters of their trichomes and by the palisade ratios.

Actions and uses. Lobelia is employed, usually as the ethereal tincture, in the treatment of asthma and chronic bronchitis to relieve bronchial spasm.
Lobelia is an ingredient of powders intended to be burnt for the relief of asthma, but such a procedure often aggravates chronic bronchitis.

POISONING. The stomach should be evacuated and symptomatic treatment given.

Dose. 200 to 600 milligrams.

Preparations
LOBELIA AND STRAMONIUM MIXTURE, COMPOUND, B.P.C. (page 746)
LOBELIA TINCTURE, ETHEREAL, B.P.C. (page 822)

LYMECYCLINE

Lymecycline is a soluble tetracycline, incorporating lysine, formaldehyde, and tetracycline, and having a molecular weight of approximately 603.

Solubility. Soluble, at 20°, in less than 1 part of water; slightly soluble in alcohol; insoluble in ether, in chloroform, and in acetone.

Standard
It complies with the requirements of the British Pharmacopoeia.
It is a yellow very hygroscopic powder and contains not less than 900 Units per mg, calculated with reference to the anhydrous substance. It contains not more than 5·0 per cent w/w of water. A 1 per cent solution in water has a pH of 7·8 to 8·1.

Stability. It is inactivated in solutions with a pH of less than 2 and is slowly destroyed at pH 7 or above.

Storage. It should be stored in airtight containers, protected from light, at a temperature not exceeding 25°.

Actions and uses. Lymecycline is an antibiotic having the actions and uses described under Tetracycline Hydrochloride (page 498), but when taken by mouth it is more rapidly absorbed and with doses containing the same amount of tetracycline a substantially higher concentration is produced in the blood.
Salts of aluminium, calcium, iron, and magnesium, which may decrease the absorption of tetracyclines from the gut, should not be given with lymecycline.
The usual dosage by mouth is the equivalent of 150 milligrams of tetracycline base four times a day; 200 milligrams of lymecycline is

approximately equivalent to 150 milligrams of tetracycline base or 160 milligrams of tetracycline hydrochloride.

Lymecycline may also be given by intramuscular injection in a dosage equivalent to 100 milligrams of tetracycline base two or three times daily. For intramuscular injection it is preferred to tetracycline hydrochloride because it is readily soluble at the pH of body fluids and so does not precipitate at the injection site to the same degree as tetracycline.

UNDESIRABLE EFFECTS; PRECAUTIONS AND CONTRA-INDICATIONS. As for Tetracycline Hydrochloride (page 498).

Dose. See above under **Actions and uses.**

Preparations
LYMECYCLINE CAPSULES, B.P. Unless otherwise specified, capsules each containing 204 mg of lymecycline are supplied.

LYMECYCLINE AND PROCAINE INJECTION, B.P. It consists of a sterile solution of lymecycline and procaine hydrochloride, with tartaric acid and magnesium ascorbate, in Water for Injections. It is prepared by dissolving the contents of a sealed container of lymecycline, tartaric acid, and magnesium ascorbate, in a solution of procaine hydrochloride and tartaric acid. It should be used immediately after preparation. Vials each containing 135 mg of lymecycline, equivalent to 100 mg of tetracycline base, are available; they are supplied with 3-ml ampoules of solvent.

OTHER NAME: *Tetralysal®*

LYNOESTRENOL

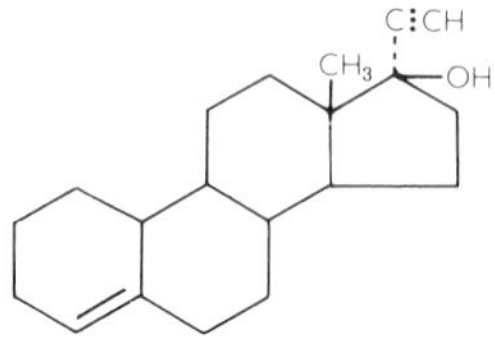

$C_{20}H_{28}O = 284.4$

Lynoestrenol is 19-nor-17α-pregn-4-en-20-yn-17-ol.

Solubility. Very slightly soluble in water; soluble, at 20°, in 15 parts of alcohol and of dehydrated alcohol, in 12 parts of ether and of acetone, and in 8 parts of chloroform.

Standard
It complies with the requirements of the British Pharmacopoeia.
It is a white or almost white, crystalline, odourless powder and contains not less than 97.0 and not more than the equivalent of 102.0 per cent of $C_{20}H_{28}O$, calculated with reference to the dried substance. The loss on drying under the prescribed conditions is not more than 0.5 per cent. It has a melting-point of 160° to 164°.

Storage. It should be stored in airtight containers, protected from light.

Actions and uses. Lynoestrenol is a synthetic progestational steroid which has actions similar to those described under Norethisterone (page 329). It is used, chiefly in conjunction with oestrogens, as an oral contraceptive to inhibit ovulation. For this purpose doses of 2.5 or 5 milligrams are given daily, usually with mestranol, from the fifth to the twenty-fourth day of each menstrual cycle. The course is repeated after an interval of one week. Regular administration is essential.

Lynoestrenol may also be used in doses of 5 milligrams daily for the treatment of dysfunctional uterine bleeding and in endometriosis; therapy in the latter condition must be continuous for nine to twelve months.

Lynoestrenol is available as tablets containing 2.5 milligrams together with ethinyloestradiol and as tablets containing 2.5 and 5 milligrams together with mestranol.

UNDESIRABLE EFFECTS. Lynoestrenol may give rise to headaches and tension, mental depression, nausea and vomiting, breast engorgement, fluid retention, and weight gain; a state of pseudopregnancy and premenstrual tension may be aggravated. It may give rise to break-through bleeding, and may cause hirsutism, acneiform skin rashes, and deepening of the voice. Prolonged use may lead to impairment of liver function. When taken without oestrogens it may not prevent conception.

Regular use of progestational oral contraceptives combined with oestrogens increases the risk of intravascular thrombosis and thromboembolic accidents.

PRECAUTIONS. These are as described under Norethisterone (page 329).

CONTRA-INDICATIONS. It is contra-indicated in patients with hepatic disturbances.

Dose. 5 to 15 milligrams daily in divided doses. As an oral contraceptive, 2.5 to 5 milligrams daily.

MACRISALB (^{131}I) INJECTION

SYNONYM: Macroaggregated Iodinated (^{131}I) Human Albumin Injection

This material is radioactive and any regulations in force must be complied with.

Macrisalb (^{131}I) Injection is a sterile suspension of human albumin which has been iodinated with iodine-131 and which has been denatured in such a way as to form insoluble aggregates. The aggregates are suspended in a saline solution isotonic with blood. The injection contains a suitable bactericide such as benzyl alcohol 0·9 per cent v/v.

Iodine-131 is a radioactive isotope of iodine, which emits β- and γ-radiation and has a half-life of 8 days; it may be prepared from the products of uranium fission or by the neutron irradiation of tellurium.

Standard
It complies with the requirements of the British Pharmacopoeia.
It is a dilute suspension of white or faintly yellow particles which may settle on standing and contains not less than 90·0 and not more than 110·0 per cent of the quantity of iodine-131 stated on the label at the date and hour stated on the label. The radioactivity is virtually all present in irregular particles with mean linear dimensions in the range 10 to 100 μm. It has a pH of 5·0 to 8·5.

Labelling. The label on the container states:
(1) the content of iodine-131 expressed in microcuries or millicuries at a given date and hour;
(2) the weight of human albumin in the container;
(3) that the injection is radioactive; and
(4) the date after which the injection is not intended to be used.

The label on the package also states:
(1) the total volume in the container;
(2) the conditions under which it should be stored; and
(3) the name of the bactericide.

Storage. It should be stored in an area assigned for the purpose at a temperature between 2° and 10°. The storage conditions should be such that the maximum radiation-dose-rate to which persons may be exposed is reduced to an acceptable level.
Glass containers may darken under the effects of radiation.

Actions and uses. Macrisalb (^{131}I) Injection is used mainly in the investigation of lung perfusion by external visualisation of the organ by scintiscanner or gamma-ray camera.

After intravenous injection, almost all the particles are trapped in the capillaries of the lung, the number in any region being dependent on the blood supply to that region. Only a very small percentage of the capillaries are occluded and within twenty-four hours all the particles have been cleared.

Pulmonary embolism is suggested by a silent area on the scan, indicating a reduced blood supply to the region. The emphysematous lung may show a patchy uptake. Tumours may produce large silent areas by pressure on the blood vessels.

Dose. 300 microcuries.

OTHER NAME: MAA (^{131}I) Injection

MACROGOL 300

SYNONYM: Polyethylene Glycol 300

Macrogol 300 is a mixture of the polycondensation products of ethylene oxide and water obtained under controlled conditions. It is represented by the formula $CH_2(OH)\cdot(CH_2\cdot O\cdot CH_2)_m\cdot CH_2OH$, where m may be 5 or 6. It has an average molecular weight of 285 to 325.

Solubility. Miscible with water, with alcohol, and with glycols; insoluble in ether.

Standard
It complies with the requirements of the British Pharmacopoeia.
It is a clear, colourless, viscous liquid with a faint characteristic odour. It has a weight per ml at 20° of 1·120 g to 1·130 g and contains not more than 1·0 per cent w/w of water. A 5·0 per cent solution in water has a pH of 4·0 to 7·0.
It has a viscosity at 25° of 59 to 73 centistokes.

Sterilisation. Aqueous solutions are sterilised by heating in an autoclave or by filtration.

Uses. The macrogols are strongly hydrophilic substances that are stable and non-irritant to the skin. They do not readily penetrate the skin, but as they are water-soluble and easily removed by washing, they are useful as ointment bases. An example is Macrogol Ointment which is a suitable mixture of macrogols 300 and 4000.

Macrogols 1540 and 4000 are used as water-soluble bases for pessaries and suppositories. The hardness, melting-point, and dissolution rate of the product can be modified by varying the proportions of the macrogols used. Since suppositories made with macrogols dissolve in water drawn from the rectal mucosa by osmosis, irritation may occur where the tissues are sensitive; to minimise irritant effects, about 20 per cent of water is often included in the basis.

Macrogol 4000 is employed as a binding agent and lubricant for tablets and, in alcoholic solution, for the film-coating of tablets.

Mixtures of the various liquid and solid grades of macrogol are used in the preparation of water-soluble bases for gauze dressings.

Macrogol 300 is used in preparations for

external application as a solvent for drugs such as hydrocortisone and undecenoic acid which are relatively insoluble in water. It has also been used as a vehicle for injections.

OTHER NAME: Liquid Macrogol

Preparations containing macrogols 300 and 1500 are hygroscopic.

Preparation
MACROGOL OINTMENT, B.P.C. (page 762)

MACROGOL 1540

SYNONYM: Polyethylene Glycol 1540

Macrogol 1540 is a mixture of the polycondensation products of ethylene oxide and water obtained under controlled conditions. It is represented by the formula $CH_2(OH) \cdot (CH_2 \cdot O \cdot CH_2)_m \cdot CH_2OH$, where m may be 28 to 36. It has an average molecular weight of 1300 to 1600.

Solubility. Soluble in 1 part of water, in 3 parts of chloroform, and in 100 parts of dehydrated alcohol; insoluble in solvent ether.

Standard
It complies with the requirements of the British Pharmacopoeia.
It is a creamy-white, soft, wax-like solid with a faint

characteristic odour. It has a freezing-point of 42° to 46°. A 5·0 per cent solution in water has a pH of 4·0 to 7·0.
It has a viscosity at 100° of 25 to 32 centistokes.

Uses. These are described under Macrogol 300.

MACROGOL 4000

SYNONYM: Polyethylene Glycol 4000

Macrogol 4000 is a mixture of the polycondensation products of ethylene oxide and water obtained under controlled conditions. It is represented by the formula $CH_2(OH) \cdot (CH_2 \cdot O \cdot CH_2)_m \cdot CH_2OH$, where m may be 69 to 84. It has an average molecular weight of 3100 to 3700.

Solubility. Soluble in 3 parts of water, in 2 parts of alcohol, and in 2 parts of chloroform; insoluble in ether.

Standard
It complies with the requirements of the British Pharmacopoeia.
It is a creamy-white, hard, wax-like solid or flakes with a faint characteristic odour. It has a freezing-point of 53° to 56°. A 5·0 per cent solution in water has a pH of 4·5 to 7·5.

It has a viscosity at 100° of 75 to 85 centistokes.

Sterilisation. It is sterilised by dry heat.

Uses. These are described under Macrogol 300.

Preparation
MACROGOL OINTMENT, B.P.C. (page 762)

OTHER NAME: Hard Macrogol

MAGENTA

SYNONYMS: Fuchsine; Basic Fuchsine; Rosaniline Hydrochloride

Magenta (Colour Index No. 42510) is a mixture of the hydrochlorides of pararosaniline [anhydrotri(p-aminophenyl)methanol] and rosaniline (anhydrotri-p-aminodiphenyl-m-tolyl-methanol).

Magenta may be prepared by heating a mixture of aniline and o- and p-toluidine and their hydrochlorides with nitrobenzene, or with a mixture of nitrobenzene and o-nitrotoluene, in the presence of a suitable catalyst.

Solubility. Soluble in water and in alcohol; insoluble in ether.

Standard
DESCRIPTION. Iridescent green crystals or a dark green lustrous crystalline powder; odourless.

IDENTIFICATION TESTS. 1. Dissolve 0·1 g in 100 ml of water; a dark red solution is produced. To 5 ml add

0·5 ml of *hydrochloric acid*; the solution becomes yellow.
2. To 5 ml of the solution prepared in test 1 add 0·5 ml of *dilute ammonia solution* and allow to stand for one minute; a red precipitate is formed.
3. Pass *sulphur dioxide* for 2 minutes through 5 ml of the solution prepared in test 1; the solution becomes pale yellow. Add 3 ml of *dilute nitric acid* and 0·05 ml of *silver nitrate solution*; a white precipitate is formed.

ZINC. Moisten 0·50 g with *sulphuric acid*, ignite, dissolve the residue in 2 ml of hot *dilute hydrochloric acid* and 10 ml of water, boil, add 2 ml of *dilute ammonia solution*, boil, filter, neutralise the filtrate to *litmus paper* with *dilute hydrochloric acid*, and add a further 4 ml of acid and 1 ml of *potassium ferrocyanide solution*; no turbidity is produced.

LOSS ON DRYING. Not more than 10·0 per cent, determined by drying at 130° for one hour.

SULPHATED ASH. Not more than 1·0 per cent.

CONTENT OF DYESTUFF. Not less than 85·0 per cent, calculated as rosaniline hydrochloride, $C_{20}H_{20}ClN_3$, with reference to the substance dried under the prescribed conditions, determined by the following method:
Dissolve about 0·3 g, accurately weighed, in 75 ml of *alcohol* (95 *per cent*) and 50 ml of water, add 25 ml of a 30 per cent w/v solution of *sodium potassium tartrate*

in water, heat to boiling, maintain a current of carbon dioxide through the flask, and titrate the hot solution with 0·1N titanous chloride; each ml of 0·1N titanous chloride is equivalent to 0·01689 g of $C_{20}H_{20}ClN_3$.

Actions and uses. Magenta has antifungal and antibacterial actions, especially against Gram-positive bacteria. Magenta Paint (Castellani's paint) is used in the treatment of superficial dermatophytoses, especially when moist eczematous dermatitis is present.

Preparation
MAGENTA PAINT, B.P.C. (page 766)

MAGNESIUM ACETATE
$C_4H_6MgO_4,4H_2O = 214·5$

$(CH_3 \cdot CO_2)_2Mg,4H_2O$

Solubility. Soluble, at 20°, in 1·5 parts of water and in 4 parts of alcohol.

Standard
DESCRIPTION. Colourless crystals or a white crystalline powder; odourless or almost odourless.

IDENTIFICATION TESTS. It gives the reactions characteristic of magnesium and of acetates.

ALKALINITY. pH of a 5·0 per cent w/v solution in *carbon dioxide-free water*, 7·5 to 8·5.

ARSENIC. It complies with the test given in Appendix 6, page 878 (2 parts per million).

CALCIUM. Not more than 100 parts per million, determined by the following method:
Dissolve 5·0 g in sufficient water to produce 100 ml and determine by atomic absorption spectroscopy at a wavelength of 422·7 nm, using Method II of the British Pharmacopoeia, Appendix XIA; use *calcium solution FP*, diluted if necessary with water, for the standard solution.

LEAD. It complies with the test given in Appendix 7, page 883 (20 parts per million).

POTASSIUM. Not more than 0·1 per cent, determined by the following method:
Dissolve 1·25 g in sufficient water to produce 250 ml and determine by emission spectroscopy at a wavelength of 766·7 nm, using Method II of the British Pharmacopoeia, Appendix XIA; use *potassium solution FP*, diluted if necessary with water, for the standard solution.

SODIUM. Not more than 0·5 per cent, determined by the following method:
Dissolve 1·0 g in sufficient water to produce 100 ml

and determine by emission spectroscopy at a wavelength of 589·0 nm, using Method II of the British Pharmacopoeia, Appendix XIA; use *sodium solution FP*, diluted if necessary with water, for the standard solution.

CHLORIDE. 1·0 g complies with the limit test for chlorides (350 parts per million).

NITRATE. Dissolve 1·0 g in 10 ml of water, add 5 mg of *sodium chloride*, 0·05 ml of *indigo carmine solution* and, with stirring, 10 ml of *nitrogen-free sulphuric acid*; the blue colour remains for at least 10 minutes.

SULPHATE. 1·0 g complies with the limit test for sulphates (600 parts per million).

READILY OXIDISABLE SUBSTANCES. Dissolve 2·0 g in 100 ml of water, add 2 ml of *dilute sulphuric acid* and 0·3 ml of 0·1N potassium permanganate and boil for 5 minutes; the colour of the solution is not completely discharged.

CONTENT OF $C_4H_6MgO_4,4H_2O$. Not less than 98·0 per cent, determined by the following method:
Dissolve about 0·5 g, accurately weighed, in 50 ml of water, add 10 ml of *ammonia buffer solution*, and titrate with 0·05M disodium edetate using *mordant black 11 solution* as indicator; each ml of 0·05M disodium edetate is equivalent to 0·01072 g of $C_4H_6MgO_4,4H_2O$.

Storage. It should be stored in airtight containers.

Uses. Magnesium acetate is a source of magnesium ions and may be used to adjust the magnesium content of solutions for haemodialysis.

HEAVY MAGNESIUM CARBONATE

SYNONYMS: Heavy Mag. Carb.; Magnesii Subcarbonas Ponderosus

Heavy Magnesium Carbonate is a hydrated basic magnesium carbonate of varying composition corresponding approximately to the formula $3MgCO_3,Mg(OH)_2,4H_2O$.

Heavy Magnesium Carbonate may be prepared by mixing boiling concentrated aqueous solutions of magnesium sulphate and sodium carbonate, evaporating to dryness, and washing the product.

Solubility. Very slightly soluble in water; insoluble in alcohol; soluble with effervescence in dilute acids.

Standard
It complies with the requirements of the European Pharmacopoeia.

It contains the equivalent of not less than 40·0 per cent and not more than 45·0 per cent of MgO; 15 g occupies a volume of about 30 ml.

DESCRIPTION. *Macroscopical:* an odourless, white powder.

Microscopical: mounted in dilute *glycerol* it is seen to consist mainly of subspherical particles, about 10 to 20 μm in diameter, many being arranged in clumps of 4 to 20; small numbers of particles resembling light magnesium carbonate occur amongst the spherites.

Between crossed polars each particle shows a well-marked black Maltese cross.

Hygroscopicity. At relative humidities between about 15 and 65 per cent, the equilibrium moisture content at 25° is about 1 per cent, but at relative humidities above about 75 per cent, the powder absorbs small amounts of moisture.

Actions and uses. Heavy magnesium carbonate has the actions and uses described under Light Magnesium Carbonate, but its smaller bulk renders it more suitable as an ingredient of antacid powders.

Dose. As an antacid: 250 to 500 milligrams,

repeated in accordance with the needs of the patient. As a laxative: 2 to 5 grams.

Preparations
BISMUTH LOZENGES, COMPOUND, B.P.C. (page 732)
BISMUTH POWDER, COMPOUND, B.P.C. (page 775)
CALCIUM CARBONATE POWDER, COMPOUND, B.P.C. (page 775)
MAGNESIUM CARBONATE POWDER, COMPOUND, B.P.C. (page 778)
MAGNESIUM TRISILICATE POWDER, COMPOUND, B.P.C. (page 778)
RHUBARB POWDER, COMPOUND, B.P.C. (page 778)
MAGNESIUM CARBONATE TABLETS, COMPOUND, B.P.C. (page 812)

LIGHT MAGNESIUM CARBONATE

SYNONYMS: Light Mag. Carb.; Magnesii Subcarbonas Levis

Light Magnesium Carbonate is a hydrated basic magnesium carbonate of varying composition corresponding approximately to the formula $3MgCO_3,Mg(OH)_2,3H_2O$.

Light Magnesium Carbonate may be prepared by boiling a mixture of dilute aqueous solutions of magnesium sulphate and sodium carbonate.

Solubility. Very slightly soluble in water; insoluble in alcohol; soluble with effervescence in dilute acids.

Standard
It complies with the requirements of the European Pharmacopoeia.
It contains the equivalent of not less than 40·0 per cent and not more than 45·0 per cent of MgO; 15 g occupies a volume of about 200 ml.

DESCRIPTION. *Macroscopical:* a very light, white, odourless powder.

Microscopical: mounted in dilute *glycerol* it is seen to consist of small acicular crystals, about 7 μm long and 1 to 2 μm thick, partly in clumps of about 10 to 200 crystals.

Actions and uses. Light magnesium carbonate has antacid and laxative actions. It is less effective for neutralising gastric acidity than magnesium hydroxide, and has the disadvantage of liberating carbon dioxide.

Light magnesium carbonate is more suitable for use in mixtures and the heavy variety for powders. It is used for dispersing volatile oils in inhalations having an aqueous vehicle.

Dose. As an antacid: 250 to 500 milligrams, repeated in accordance with the needs of the patient. As a laxative: 2 to 5 grams.

Preparations
CALCIUM CARBONATE MIXTURE, COMPOUND, PAEDIATRIC, B.P.C. (page 738)
KAOLIN MIXTURE, B.P.C. (page 745)
MAGNESIUM CARBONATE MIXTURE, B.P.C. (page 746)
MAGNESIUM CARBONATE MIXTURE, AROMATIC, B.P.C. (page 746)
MAGNESIUM SULPHATE MIXTURE, B.P.C. (page 747)
MAGNESIUM TRISILICATE MIXTURE, B.P.C. (page 747)
MAGNESIUM TRISILICATE AND BELLADONNA MIXTURE, B.P.C. (page 747)
RHUBARB MIXTURE, COMPOUND, B.P.C. (page 752)
RHUBARB MIXTURE, COMPOUND, PAEDIATRIC, B.P.C. (page 752)
RHUBARB POWDER, COMPOUND, B.P.C. (page 778)

MAGNESIUM CHLORIDE

SYNONYM: Mag. Chlor.

$MgCl_2,6H_2O = 203·3$

Solubility. Soluble, at 20°, in 1 part of water and in 2 parts of alcohol.

Standard
It complies with the requirements of the British Pharmacopoeia.
It occurs as deliquescent, colourless, odourless crystals.

Stability. When heated at 100°, it loses two molecules

of water of crystallisation; at 110° it begins to lose hydrogen chloride, forming basic salts.

Storage. It should be stored in airtight containers.

Uses. Magnesium chloride is used to adjust the concentration of magnesium ions in preparing solutions for haemodialysis and peritoneal dialysis.

MAGNESIUM HYDROXIDE

SYNONYM: Mag. Hydrox.

$Mg(OH)_2 = 58·32$

Magnesium Hydroxide may be prepared by boiling magnesium oxide with 20 to 30 times its weight of water for about 20 minutes, draining, and drying in thin layers at a temperature not exceeding 100°.

Solubility. Very slightly soluble in water; readily soluble in dilute acids.

Standard

DESCRIPTION. A white amorphous powder; odourless or almost odourless.

IDENTIFICATION TEST. It gives the reactions characteristic of magnesium.

ARSENIC. It complies with the test given in Appendix 6, page 878 (2 parts per million).

CALCIUM. Not more than 1·0 per cent, calculated as Ca, determined by the following method:
Suspend 0·60 g in 20 ml of water, add 10 ml of *hydrochloric acid*, dilute to 100 ml with water, further dilute 10 ml of this solution to 100 ml with water, and determine by the method of the British Pharmacopoeia for flame photometry, using *calcium solution FP*, diluted if necessary with 0·1N hydrochloric acid, for the standard solutions.

COPPER. Dissolve 0·6 g in a mixture of 5 ml of *hydrochloric acid* and 25 ml of water, boil to remove carbon dioxide, and make alkaline with *dilute ammonia solution*; no blue colour is produced.

IRON. 0·06 g dissolved in a mixture of 5 ml of water and 0·5 ml of *hydrochloric acid FeT* complies with the limit test for iron (660 parts per million).

LEAD. It complies with the test given in Appendix 7, page 883 (20 parts per million).

CARBONATE. Suspend 0·50 g in 10 ml of water, heat to boiling, cool, and add 10 ml of *dilute hydrochloric acid*; not more than a slight effervescence is produced.

CHLORIDE. 0·30 g dissolved in water with the addition of 1·5 ml of *nitric acid* complies with the limit test for chlorides (0·1 per cent).

SULPHATE. 0·06 g, dissolved in water with the addition of 3 ml of *dilute hydrochloric acid*, complies with the limit test for sulphates (1·0 per cent).

SOLUBLE MATTER. Boil 0·60 g with 50 ml of water for 5 minutes, filter, and evaporate the filtrate to dryness; the residue, after drying at 105°, weighs not more than 10 mg.

CONTENT OF $Mg(OH)_2$. Not less than 95·0 per cent, determined by the following method:
Dissolve about 1 g, accurately weighed, in 50 ml of 1N sulphuric acid and titrate the excess of acid with 1N sodium hydroxide, using *methyl orange solution* as indicator; each ml of 1N sulphuric acid is equivalent to 0·02916 g of $Mg(OH)_2$.

Storage. It should be stored in airtight containers.

Actions and uses. Magnesium hydroxide is an antacid and, owing to the formation of magnesium chloride in the stomach, it also acts as a mild saline laxative. It does not produce alkalosis.

Dose. As an antacid: 500 to 750 milligrams, repeated in accordance with the needs of the patient. As a laxative: 2 to 4 grams.

Preparations

LIQUID PARAFFIN AND MAGNESIUM HYDROXIDE EMULSION, B.P.C. (page 679)

MAGNESIUM HYDROXIDE MIXTURE, B.P. (*Syn.* Cream of Magnesia). It contains the equivalent of 7·9 per cent w/w of $Mg(OH)_2$. It should not be stored in a cold place. Dose: as an antacid, 5 to 10 millilitres, repeated in accordance with the needs of the patient; as a laxative, 25 to 50 millilitres.

LIGHT MAGNESIUM OXIDE

SYNONYMS: Light Mag. Ox.; Light Magnesia; Magnesii Oxidum Leve

$MgO = 40·30$

Light Magnesium Oxide may be prepared by heating light magnesium carbonate to dull redness. It forms a gelatinous mass on standing for about 30 minutes with fifteen times its weight of water.

Solubility. Very slightly soluble in water; insoluble in alcohol; soluble in dilute acids.

Standard

It complies with the requirements of the European Pharmacopoeia.
It is a very light, white, fine, amorphous, odourless powder, and contains not less than 98·0 per cent of MgO, calculated with reference to the ignited substance. The loss on ignition under the prescribed conditions is not more than 5·0 per cent. 20 g occupies a volume of not less than 150 ml.

Hygroscopicity. On exposure to air it rapidly absorbs moisture and carbon dioxide.

Storage. It should be stored in airtight containers.

Actions and uses. Light magnesium oxide has the actions and uses described under Magnesium Hydroxide. Because of its lightness, light magnesium oxide is suitable for inclusion in mixtures.

Dose. As an antacid: 250 to 500 milligrams, repeated in accordance with the needs of the patient. As a laxative: 2 to 5 grams.

Preparation

MAGNESIUM HYDROXIDE MIXTURE, B.P. (*Syn.* Cream of Magnesia). It contains in 10 ml the equivalent of about 550 mg of magnesium oxide. It should not be stored in a cold place. Dose: as an antacid, 5 to 10 millilitres, repeated in accordance with the needs of the patient; as a laxative, 25 to 50 millilitres.

MAGNESIUM STEARATE

Magnesium Stearate is the magnesium salt of a commercial stearic acid which consists chiefly of a mixture of stearic and palmitic acids.

Solubility. Insoluble in water, in alcohol, and in ether.

Standard
It complies with the requirements of the British Pharmacopoeia.
It is a fine, white, impalpable powder with a faint characteristic odour; it is unctuous and readily adherent to the skin. It contains the equivalent of 6·5 to 8·5 per cent of MgO, calculated with reference to the dried substance. The loss on drying under the prescribed conditions is not more than 4·0 per cent.

Storage. It should be stored in airtight containers.

Actions and uses. Magnesium stearate is used as a dusting-powder in the treatment of skin diseases, and in creams as a barrier to chemical irritants. It is also used as a lubricant for granules in the manufacture of tablets.

MAGNESIUM SULPHATE

SYNONYMS: Epsom Salts; Mag. Sulph.; Magnesii Sulfas

$MgSO_4,7H_2O = 246·5$

Solubility. Soluble, at 20°, in 1·5 parts of water; soluble in less than 0·2 part of boiling water; slightly soluble in alcohol.

Standard
It complies with the requirements of the European Pharmacopoeia.
It occurs as odourless, brilliant, colourless crystals or white crystalline powder and contains not less than 99·0 per cent of $MgSO_4$, calculated with reference to the dried substance. The loss on drying under the prescribed conditions is 48·0 to 52·0 per cent.
It effloresces in warm dry air and when heated at 150° to 160° is converted into the monohydrate; the last molecule of water of crystallisation is expelled at about 280°. A solution in water is neutral to phenol red.

Incompatibility. It is incompatible with alkali carbonates and bicarbonates; strong solutions are incompatible with potassium and ammonium bromides, the double sulphates crystallising out.

Sterilisation. Solutions for injection are sterilised by heating in an autoclave or by filtration.

Storage. It should be stored in airtight containers, in a cool place.

Actions and uses. Magnesium sulphate is a saline purgative. Such purgatives are not readily absorbed from the intestine. When taken by mouth in dilute solution they reduce the normal absorption of water from the intestine, with the result that the bulky fluid contents distend the bowel, active reflex peristalsis is excited, and evacuation of the contents of the intestine occurs in one to two hours. If hypertonic solutions are given by mouth the osmotic pressure in the bowel is raised and water is withdrawn from the tissues to restore the balance; the purgative action is then delayed.

Saline purgatives are often given in habitual constipation due to deficient peristalsis, the best results being obtained by taking the dose in a half to one tumblerful of water, preferably before breakfast.

The usual dose of magnesium sulphate is 5 to 15 grams.

A 50 per cent solution in water, in a dose of 60 to 180 millilitres, has been given as an enema.

In the treatment of cholecystitis, 50 millilitres of a 25 per cent solution of magnesium sulphate, administered directly into the duodenum by means of a duodenal tube, or given by mouth on an empty stomach, has been used to promote evacuation of the gall-bladder. The intravenous injection of 10 to 25 millilitres of a 10 per cent solution has been used to lower intracranial pressure and to control the convulsions in acute uraemia and eclampsia.

Wet dressings of a 25 per cent solution of magnesium sulphate are sometimes used in the treatment of carbuncles and boils.

Magnesium sulphate is a common ingredient of aperient mineral waters.

Dose. See above under **Actions and uses.**

Preparation
MAGNESIUM SULPHATE MIXTURE, B.P.C. (page 747)

DRIED MAGNESIUM SULPHATE

SYNONYMS: Dried Epsom Salts; Dried Mag. Sulph.

Dried Magnesium Sulphate may be prepared by drying magnesium sulphate at 100° until it has lost approximately 25 per cent of its weight.

Solubility. Soluble, at 20°, in 2 parts of water; more rapidly soluble in hot water.

Standard
It complies with the requirements of the British Pharmacopoeia.

It is a white odourless powder and contains 62·0 to 70·0 per cent of $MgSO_4$. A solution in water is neutral to phenol red.

Storage. It should be stored in airtight containers.

Actions and uses. Dried magnesium sulphate has the actions and uses described under Magnesium Sulphate, but it is employed only when the use of the hydrated salt would be disadvantageous. It is one of the chief ingredients of effervescent and non-effervescent aperient powders or granules.

As Magnesium Sulphate Paste it is used as an application to carbuncles and boils, but prolonged or repeated use may damage the surrounding skin and predispose to further boils.

Dose. 2 to 12 grams, as a single dose.

Preparation
MAGNESIUM SULPHATE PASTE, B.P.C. (page 767)

OTHER NAME: Exsiccated Magnesium Sulphate

MAGNESIUM TRISILICATE

SYNONYM: Mag. Trisil.

Magnesium Trisilicate is a hydrated magnesium silicate corresponding approximately to the formula $2MgO,3SiO_2$, with water of crystallisation.

Magnesium Trisilicate may be prepared by mixing aqueous solutions of magnesium sulphate and sodium silicate.

Solubility. Insoluble in water.

Standard
It complies with the requirements of the British Pharmacopoeia.
It contains 29·5 to 32·0 per cent of MgO and 65·0 to 68·5 per cent of SiO_2, both calculated with reference to the ignited substance. The loss on ignition under the prescribed conditions is 20·0 to 30·0 per cent.
Its capacity to absorb acid is determined by stirring continuously at 37° with 0·05N hydrochloric acid for three hours; the equivalent of 1·0 g of ignited substance requires not less than 250 ml.

DESCRIPTION. *Macroscopical:* a white or almost white, slightly hygroscopic, odourless powder.

Microscopical: magnesium trisilicate consists of irregular rounded particles, from about 10 by 15 μm to 40 by 60 μm, and thin flat lamellae, 10 by 10 μm up to 25 by 80 μm, together with numerous smaller particles about 5 to 10 μm across. With *safranine solution*, it stains deep red, and with *alcoholic methylene blue solution* deep blue.

Hygroscopicity. At relative humidities between about 15 and 65 per cent, the equilibrium moisture content at 25° is between about 17 and 23 per cent; at relative humidities between about 75 and 95 per cent, the equilibrium moisture content is between about 24 and 30 per cent.

Storage. It should be stored in airtight containers.

Actions and uses. Magnesium trisilicate has adsorbent and antacid properties and is non-toxic even in very large doses. Its action is exerted slowly, so that it does not give such rapid symptomatic relief as the alkali carbonates, bicarbonates, and oxides. However, the action continues for some time, and the substance is therefore of value in the treatment of dyspepsia. It does not give rise to alkalosis.

During neutralisation, magnesium chloride and a hydrated silica gel are formed; the latter also possesses adsorbent properties, although inferior in this respect to the original substance. The formation of magnesium chloride sometimes causes diarrhoea, but this is seldom severe.

Dose. 0·5 to 2 grams, repeated in accordance with the needs of the patient.

Preparations
MAGNESIUM TRISILICATE MIXTURE, B.P.C. (page 747)
MAGNESIUM TRISILICATE AND BELLADONNA MIXTURE, B.P.C. (page 747)
MAGNESIUM TRISILICATE POWDER, COMPOUND, B.P.C. (page 778)
MAGNESIUM TRISILICATE TABLETS, COMPOUND, B.P.C. (page 812)

MAIZE OIL

SYNONYM: Corn Oil

Maize Oil is the fixed oil obtained from the embryos of maize, *Zea mays* L. (Fam. Gramineae), which are separated during the preparation of maize starch.

Constituents. Maize oil consists of glycerides, the fatty acid constituents of which are mainly oleic and linoleic acids, with smaller proportions of palmitic and stearic acids.

Solubility. Very slightly soluble in alcohol; miscible with ether, with chloroform, and with light petroleum.

Standard
It complies with the requirements of the British Pharmacopoeia.
It is a pale yellow to golden yellow oil with a faint characteristic odour. It has a weight per ml at 20° of 0·915 g to 0·923 g.

Sterilisation. Maize oil is sterilised by dry heat.

Storage. It should be stored in well-filled airtight containers, protected from light, in a cool place.

Actions and uses. Maize oil has properties similar to those of olive oil. It is used, because of its high content of glycerides of unsaturated acids, as a constituent of diets intended to reduce high blood-cholesterol levels.

STERILISABLE MAIZE STARCH

Sterilisable Maize Starch is prepared by treating maize starch by chemical and physical means so that it does not gelatinise on exposure to moisture or steam sterilisation.

Standard
It complies with the requirements of the British Pharmacopoeia.
It is a white, free-flowing, odourless powder and contains up to 2·2 per cent of magnesium oxide. The loss on drying at 105° is not more than 12·0 per cent. A 10 per cent suspension in water has a pH of 9·5 to 10·8.

Sterilisation. It may be sterilised by heating at 150° to 160° for sufficient time to ensure that the whole of the powder is maintained at this temperature for one hour or by autoclaving, in thin layers, at 115° to 116° for thirty minutes.

Labelling. The label on the container states that care should be taken to avoid the use of excessive amounts of the powder on surgeons' gloves. ·

Uses. Sterilisable maize starch is used as a lubricant for surgeons' gloves; the lubricant properties are not affected by autoclaving. Unlike talc and similar substances it is completely absorbed by body tissues. It should, however, be used sparingly to minimise the possibility of inflammatory tissue reactions.

OTHER NAMES: Absorbable Dusting-powder; Modified Starch Dusting-powder

MALE FERN

SYNONYM: Filix Mas

Male Fern consists of the rhizome, frond-bases, and apical bud of *Dryopteris filix-mas* agg., which includes *D. filix-mas* (L.) Schott. s. str., *D. borreri* Newm., and *D. abbreviata* (DC) Newm. (Fam. Polypodiaceae).

Male fern is indigenous to Great Britain, other temperate regions, and the Indian subcontinent. It is usually collected late in the autumn, divested of its roots and dead portions, and then carefully dried. Internally, the freshly collected rhizome is green in colour, but during storage the green colour of the interior gradually disappears, often after a lapse of six months, and such drug is unfit for medicinal use.

Varieties. European male fern yields about 6 to 10 per cent of ethereal extractive, of which about 25 per cent is filicin. Indian male fern yields about 8 to 9·5 per cent of ethereal extractive, of which about 30 per cent is filicin.

Constituents. The drug contains a number of ether-soluble derivatives of phloroglucinol, some of which contribute to the anthelmintic action.
The phloroglucides are substituted partly with methyl or methoxyl groups and always with an acyl side-chain, mainly butyryl but also acetyl or propionyl, and occur as polymers linked by methylene bridges.
The active polymers are readily broken down in alkaline conditions to inactive monomers; aspidinol (2,6-dihydroxy-4-methoxy-3-methylbutyrophenone), a monomer with a butyryl side-chain, may be found in large amounts in *D. filix-mas*, but is not always present in *D. borreri* or *D. abbreviata*.
The proportions of different compounds vary but filicic acid (a trimer) and flavaspidic acid (a dimer) are invariably present as the major components, the latter being mainly responsible for the pharmacological activity of the drug. Albaspidin is usually present and there may be small proportions of desaspidin, which, if present, contributes to the anthelmintic activity.
In addition to the phloroglucinol derivatives, tannin (filicitannic acid) and volatile and fixed oils are present.
Filicin is the name given to the mixture of ether-soluble substances obtained in the assay of the drug and the extract.

Standard
It complies with the requirements of the British Pharmacopoeia.
It contains not less than 1·50 per cent of filicin.

UNGROUND DRUG. *Macroscopical characters:* pieces, 7 to 15 cm or more in length and about 5 cm wide, oblique in direction and ending in a large bud, the fronds showing circinate vernation; rhizome proper, about 2 cm in diameter, entirely covered with hard, persistent, ascending, hemicylindrical, dark brown bases of the fronds, about 3 to 6 cm long and 6 to 8 mm thick; phyllotaxis 5:8; rhizome and frond bases densely covered with ramenta; frond bases green internally; rhizome yellowish-green; transversely cut surface of both rhizome and each frond base showing a circle of about 7 to 9 pale yellowish vascular strands of various sizes. Odour slight; taste at first sweetish and astringent, later becoming bitter and nauseous.

Microscopical characters: the diagnostic characters are: *ramenta*, with marginal teeth of 2 or occasionally more cells, *glands* present at base only, usually 2, small, unicellular; *hypodermis* composed of yellowish-brown, longitudinally elongated cells with thickened walls; *ground tissue* composed of cellulosic parenchyma, cells filled with small *starch* granules up to 25 μm in diameter; *trichomes* glandular, short-stalked, pear-shaped, projecting into some intercellular spaces in ground tissue; *vascular system* dictyostelic, xylem with large lignified prismatic scalariform *tracheids* with pointed ends; cells of *endodermis* with thin, sinuous walls, surrounding each vascular strand.

POWDERED DRUG: Powdered Male Fern. A brown powder possessing the diagnostic microscopical characters, odour, and taste of the unground drug.

Adulterants and substitutes. The rhizomes and frond bases of several other ferns may occur as substitutes.
Lady-fern, *Athyrium filix-femina* (L.) Roth. is distinguished by the presence of only two dumb-bell shaped vascular strands in each frond base and by the absence of internal glandular trichomes and active phloroglucides.
Several European buckler ferns, including *D. villarii* (Bell.) Woynar, *D. aemula* (Ait.) O. Kuntze and members of the "*Dryopteris spinulosa*" complex [*D. carthusiana* (Vill.) H. P. Fuchs, *D. dilatata* (Hoffm.) A. Gray, *D. assimilis* S. Walker, and *D. cristata* (L.) A. Gray], as well as various hybrids belonging to the genus *Dryopteris*, all yield rhizomes and frond bases resembling those of male fern although some are more slender and elongated, with narrower rhizomes. The shape of the

ramenta and the microscopical appearance of the ramental margins may distinguish some of these taxa. All contain characteristic mixtures of phloroglucides which vary both qualitatively and quantitatively. Flavaspidic acid is present, usually with smaller amounts of desaspidin, tridesaspidin, para-aspidin, albaspidin, aspidinol, and, sometimes, phloropyrone; aspidin (not present in male fern) is a major active component in most of these taxa except *D. villarii* and *D. cristata*.

Actions and uses. Male fern is used, as Male Fern Extract, for the expulsion of tapeworms. The patient should be given a low-residue diet on the day before the extract is administered and a saline purgative during the evening. Next morning the extract should be given to the fasting patient in one dose or in several equal portions at half-hourly intervals, followed two hours after the last portion by a saline purgative.

Male Fern Extract may be administered in capsules but is more effective as a draught.

UNDESIRABLE EFFECTS. Toxic effects, which are rare, include headache, nausea, vomiting, severe abdominal cramp, diarrhoea, albuminuria, and dyspnoea. In severe cases, convulsions, loss of reflexes, and optic neuritis, leading to temporary or permanent blindness, may occur. Death sometimes ensues from respiratory or cardiac failure. Since absorption of Male Fern Extract may be increased by the presence of fat in the intestine, fatty meals and purgatives such as castor oil should not be given.

CONTRA-INDICATIONS. It is contra-indicated in anaemia and pregnancy and in old people and infants.

Preparations
MALE FERN EXTRACT, B.P. It contains 22 per cent w/w of filicin. It should be stored in airtight containers, protected from light, and should be thoroughly stirred or shaken before use. Dose: 3 to 6 millilitres after 24 hours' fasting.

MALE FERN EXTRACT DRAUGHT, B.P.C. (page 662)

MALEIC ACID

$C_4H_4O_4 = 116 \cdot 1$

$$\begin{array}{l} CH \cdot CO_2H \\ \parallel \\ CH \cdot CO_2H \end{array}$$

Solubility. Soluble, at 20°, in 1·5 parts of water, in 2 parts of alcohol, and in 12 parts of ether.

Standard
It complies with the requirements of the British Pharmacopoeia.
It is a white, crystalline, odourless powder and contains not less than 99·0 per cent of $C_4H_4O_4$, calculated with reference to the dried substance. The loss on drying under the prescribed conditions is not more than 1·5 per cent. It has a melting-point of 132° to 140°.

Uses. Maleic acid is used in the preparation of Ergometrine Injection and Methylergometrine Injection.

MALT EXTRACT

Malt Extract is obtained from sound malted grain of barley, *Hordeum distichon* L. or *H. vulgare* L. (Fam. Gramineae), or a mixture of this with not more than 33·0 per cent of sound malted grain of wheat, *Triticum aestivum* L. or *T. turgidum* L. (Fam. Gramineae). It contains 50 per cent or more of maltose, together with dextrin, glucose, and small amounts of other carbohydrates, and protein.

Malt Extract may be prepared by digesting at a suitable temperature, for an hour or more, a mixture of crushed malt with two to three times its weight of hot water, allowing to settle, drawing off the strained liquid, and extracting the mass with more hot water.

In order to obtain a product devoid of enzymic activity, the mixed liquids are heated at a convenient stage and kept at about 90° for an hour before finally evaporating under reduced pressure until a viscous product is obtained. Care must be taken not to overheat and darken the product.

Solubility. Miscible with water, giving a translucent solution.

Standard
DESCRIPTION. An amber or yellowish-brown viscous liquid; odour agreeable and characteristic.

REFRACTIVE INDEX. At 20°, 1·489 to 1·498.

WEIGHT PER ML. At 20°, 1·39 g to 1·42 g, determined by the following method:
Dissolve about 25 g, accurately weighed, by warming gently with 15 ml of water, cool, dilute to 50 ml, at 20°, with water, and weigh; calculate the weight per ml, at 20°, from the expression: $0 \cdot 9972W/(49 \cdot 86 + W - w)$, where W is the weight of the sample and w is the weight of the solution.

ARSENIC. It complies with the test given in Appendix 6, page 879 (1 part per million).

LIPASE. Mix 6·5 ml of *triacetin* with 95 ml of water, add 0·2 ml of *bromocresol purple solution (0·1 per cent w/v)*, neutralise the solution by the addition of 0·05N sodium hydroxide, and add sufficient water to produce 110 ml.
Transfer 50 ml of this solution to each of two large tubes, 20 cm long by 3 cm in diameter, and insert in each tube a rubber stopper having two holes, one for the drawn-out tip of a burette and the other for a short glass tube through which passes a thread operating a glass stirring coil.
Warm the contents of the tubes to a temperature of 30° and maintain at this temperature.

Prepare a solution containing 5·0 g of the sample in 10 ml of water and to the first prepared tube add 1 ml of this solution and to the second prepared tube add 1 ml of this solution which has been previously boiled; adjust the acidity of the solution in both tubes to between pH 6·2 and pH 6·4 by the dropwise addition of 0·05N sodium hydroxide from a burette and maintain the acidity of each solution between these limits for 6 hours, stirring frequently; the difference between the amounts of 0·05N sodium hydroxide added to the tubes is not more than 1·0 ml.

CONTENT OF PROTEIN. Not less than the equivalent of 4·0 per cent w/w, determined by the following method: Carry out Method I of the British Pharmacopoeia for the determination of nitrogen, using about 2·5 g, accurately weighed, and 13·5 ml of *nitrogen-free sul-phuric acid*; each ml of 0·1N sulphuric acid is equivalent to 0·00875 g of protein.

Actions and uses. Malt Extract is used chiefly as a vehicle for cod-liver oil and halibut-liver oil. It also has nutritive properties. It is a useful flavouring agent for masking bitter tastes. A diastatic malt extract, which is usually administered undiluted to children, is easily digested.

Preparations
MALT EXTRACT WITH COD-LIVER OIL, B.P.C. (page 684)
MALT EXTRACT WITH HALIBUT-LIVER OIL, B.P.C. (page 684)

MANGANESE SULPHATE

SYNONYM: Mang. Sulph.

$MnSO_4,4H_2O = 223·1$

Manganese Sulphate may be prepared by dissolving manganese carbonate in dilute sulphuric acid and evaporating the solution at a temperature of about 30°. At other temperatures other hydrates are formed.

Solubility. Soluble, at 20°, in 1 part of water; insoluble in alcohol.

Standard
DESCRIPTION. Pale pink crystals or crystalline powder; odourless or almost odourless.

IDENTIFICATION TESTS. 1. Dissolve 0·5 g in 10 ml of water and add 1 ml of *sodium sulphide solution*; a pink precipitate is formed which is soluble in *acetic acid*.

2. To 0·1 g add 2 g of *lead dioxide* and 5 ml of *nitric acid*, boil gently for a few minutes, add 100 ml of water, and filter; a purple solution is produced.

3. It gives the reactions characteristic of sulphates.

ARSENIC. It complies with the test given in Appendix 6, page 879 (4 parts per million).

HEAVY METALS AND ZINC. Dissolve 1·0 g in 25 ml of water and add 1 ml of *acetic acid* and 1 g of *sodium acetate*. Prepare a second solution by passing *hydrogen sulphide* for a few seconds into 25 ml of water. Pour the two solutions simultaneously into a small beaker; no immediate colour, turbidity, or precipitate is produced.

IRON. Dissolve 1·0 g in 10 ml of water and add 2 ml of *dilute hydrochloric acid* and 0·1N potassium permanganate, dropwise, until a permanent pink colour is produced; add 5 ml of *ammonium thiocyanate solution* and 20 ml of a mixture of equal volumes of *amyl alcohol* and *amyl acetate*, shake well, and allow to separate; any colour in the upper layer is not deeper than that produced by 2 ml of *standard iron solution FeT* when similarly treated (40 parts per million).

LEAD. It complies with the test given in Appendix 7, page 883 (20 parts per million).

CHLORIDE. 1·0 g complies with the limit test for chlorides (350 parts per million).

RESIDUE ON IGNITION. 66·0 to 69·0 per cent, determined by igniting to constant weight at 450° to 500°.

CONTENT OF $MnSO_4$. Not less than 98·0 per cent, calculated with reference to the ignited material, determined by the following method:
Dissolve about 0·15 g, accurately weighed, in 40 ml of water and add 8 ml of freshly boiled and cooled *nitric acid*; cool, add 1·5 g of *sodium bismuthate*, and shake for 2 minutes; add 25 ml of a mixture of 3 volumes of the nitric acid and 97 volumes of water, filter, wash the residue with 40 ml of the mixture, collecting the filtrate and washings in 50 ml of 0·1N ferrous ammonium sulphate, and titrate the excess of ferrous ammonium sulphate immediately with 0·1N potassium permanganate.
Repeat the procedure omitting the sample.
The difference between the two titrations represents the amount of ferrous ammonium sulphate required by the sample; each ml of 0·1N ferrous ammonium sulphate is equivalent to 0·003020 g of $MnSO_4$.

Sterilisation. Solutions are sterilised by heating in an autoclave or by filtration.

Actions and uses. Manganese sulphate is given for its effect in increasing the haematinic action of iron in the treatment of microcytic anaemia.

Dose. 0·5 to 2·5 milligrams.

Preparation
FERROUS SULPHATE TABLETS, COMPOUND, B.P.C. (page 811)

MANNITOL

$C_6H_{14}O_6 = 182.2$

$$HO \cdot CH_2 \cdot \overset{\overset{\displaystyle H}{|}}{\underset{\underset{\displaystyle OH}{|}}{C}} \cdot \overset{\overset{\displaystyle H}{|}}{\underset{\underset{\displaystyle OH}{|}}{C}} \cdot \overset{\overset{\displaystyle OH}{|}}{\underset{\underset{\displaystyle H}{|}}{C}} \cdot \overset{\overset{\displaystyle OH}{|}}{\underset{\underset{\displaystyle H}{|}}{C}} \cdot CH_2OH$$

Mannitol is a hexahydric alcohol related to mannose and may be prepared by the reduction of fructose.

Solubility. Soluble, at 20°, in 6 parts of water; slightly soluble in alcohol; insoluble in ether.

Standard
It complies with the requirements of the British Pharmacopoeia.
It is a white, crystalline, odourless powder and contains not less than 98·0 and not more than the equivalent of 102·0 per cent of $C_6H_{14}O_6$, calculated with reference to the dried substance. The loss on drying under the prescribed conditions is not more than 0·5 per cent. It has a melting-point of 166° to 169°.

Sterilisation. Solutions for injection are sterilised by heating in an autoclave or by filtration.

Actions and uses. Mannitol, when given by intravenous injection, acts as an osmotic diuretic. It is administered as a 20 per cent solution in a dosage of 50 to 100 grams daily to supplement the action of more potent diuretics; it is of little value when given alone.

A 2·5 per cent solution is used for irrigation of the bladder during transurethral resection of the prostate.
A 20 or 25 per cent solution is given by slow intravenous injection, in volumes up to 500 millilitres, to produce decompression in concussion and cerebral injury.
The 20 and 25 per cent solutions are supersaturated and may require warming before use to redissolve any crystals that have formed.

Dose. See above under **Actions and uses.**

Preparation
MANNITOL INJECTION, B.P. It consists of a sterile solution of mannitol in Water for Injections. It should be stored at temperatures between 20° and 30°; exposure to lower temperatures may result in the deposition of crystals, which should be dissolved by warming before use.

MANNOMUSTINE HYDROCHLORIDE

$C_{10}H_{24}Cl_4N_2O_4 = 378.1$

$$\left[Cl \cdot [CH_2]_2 \cdot NH \cdot CH_2 \cdot \overset{\overset{\displaystyle H}{|}}{\underset{\underset{\displaystyle OH}{|}}{C}} \cdot \overset{\overset{\displaystyle H}{|}}{\underset{\underset{\displaystyle OH}{|}}{C}} \cdot \overset{\overset{\displaystyle OH}{|}}{\underset{\underset{\displaystyle H}{|}}{C}} \cdot \overset{\overset{\displaystyle OH}{|}}{\underset{\underset{\displaystyle H}{|}}{C}} \cdot CH_2 \cdot NH \cdot [CH_2]_2 \cdot Cl \right] 2HCl$$

Mannomustine Hydrochloride is 1,6-di(2-chloroethylamino)-1,6-dideoxy-D-mannitol dihydrochloride.

Solubility. Soluble, at 20°, in 2 parts of water; slightly soluble in alcohol; insoluble in dehydrated alcohol, in ether, and in chloroform.

Standard
DESCRIPTION. A white crystalline powder; odourless or almost odourless.

IDENTIFICATION TESTS. 1. Dissolve 0·02 g in 2 ml of a 2 per cent w/v solution of *periodic acid* in water, allow to stand for 30 seconds, and add 0·5 ml of *barium chloride solution*; a white precipitate is formed.
2. It melts with decomposition at about 241°.
3. It gives the reactions characteristic of chlorides.

ACIDITY. pH of a 2·5 per cent w/v solution in *carbon dioxide-free water*, 2·0 to 3·5.

CLARITY OF SOLUTION. A 2·5 per cent w/v solution in water is clear.

SPECIFIC ROTATION. $+17°$ to $+22°$, calculated with reference to the substance dried under the prescribed conditions, determined, at 20°, in a 2·0 per cent w/v solution in water.

IONISABLE CHLORINE. 9·1 to 9·8 per cent, determined by the following method:
Dissolve about 0·05 g, accurately weighed, in 30 ml of water and titrate by the method given in Appendix 11, page 891, using 0·01N silver nitrate instead of 0·1N silver nitrate; each ml of 0·01N silver nitrate is equivalent to 0·0003545 g of ionisable chlorine.

ETHER-SOLUBLE MATTER. Not more than 0·5 per cent, determined by the following method:
Dissolve about 0·5 g, accurately weighed, in 20 ml of water, extract with three successive 15-ml portions of *solvent ether*, dry the combined extracts with *anhydrous sodium sulphate*, filter, evaporate off the ether, and dry the residue to constant weight at 105°.

LOSS ON DRYING. Not more than 1·0 per cent, determined by drying to constant weight at 105°.

SULPHATED ASH. Not more than 0·2 per cent.

CONTENT OF $C_{10}H_{24}Cl_4N_2O_4$. Not less than 99·0 and not more than the equivalent of 102·0 per cent, calculated with reference to the substance dried under the prescribed conditions, determined by the following method:
Dissolve about 0·03 g, accurately weighed, in 10 ml of water, add 10 ml of 0·1M periodic acid, shake, add 2 g of *sodium bicarbonate*, 25 ml of 0·1N sodium arsenite, and 0·5 g of *potassium iodide*, allow to stand for 20 minutes, and titrate with 0·1N iodine, using *starch mucilage* as indicator.
Repeat the procedure omitting the sample.
The difference between the two titrations represents the amount of 0·1M periodic acid required by the sample; each ml of 0·1N iodine is equivalent to 0·03781 g of $C_{10}H_{24}Cl_4N_2O_4$.

Actions and uses. Mannomustine is a cytotoxic agent with the actions, uses, and undesirable effects described under Mustine Hydrochloride (page 316).
It is used for the treatment of neoplastic disease, particularly of the lymphoid and haemopoietic systems. It is used for the palliative symptomatic treatment of chronic lymphatic leukaemia, Hodgkin's disease, reticulosarcoma, multiple myeloma, polycythaemia, and Brill-Symmers disease. When given in generalised carcinomatosis, pain may be relieved

and metastases in lymph nodes may regress, but these effects may be accompanied by severe bone-marrow depression.

Mannomustine may be useful in the treatment of acute leukaemia, particularly of the monocytic type, if the white-cell count is considerably increased.

Mannomustine hydrochloride is given by intravenous injection or infusion, or orally in enteric-coated tablets. It may also be given directly into body cavities, such as the pleural space. The parenteral dose is 50 to 100 milligrams dissolved in Sodium Chloride Injection to form a 0·5 to 2 per cent solution. It may be given once a day or on alternate days until a total dose of 600 to 800 milligrams has been administered; total doses of twice this quantity have been given.

Mannomustine hydrochloride may be given orally in enteric-coated tablets in doses of 50 to 100 milligrams.

PRECAUTIONS. Dosage should be controlled by response to the treatment, by periodic white-cell and red-cell counts, and also by observations on the bone marrow during the treatment of leukaemia and polycythaemia. Bone-marrow depression, when it occurs, may be prolonged.

Dose. See above under **Actions and uses.**

Preparation
MANNOMUSTINE INJECTION, B.P.C. (page 714)

OTHER NAME: *Degranol*®

MASTIC

SYNONYM: Mastiche

Mastic is a resinous exudation from certain forms or varieties of *Pistacia lentiscus* L. (Fam. Anacardiaceae), a small tree indigenous to the Mediterranean countries.

Mastic is exported mainly from the island of Chios (Scio) in the Aegean Sea, where it is obtained by puncturing the bark of the trees and allowing the oleoresin to exude and harden. It melts between 105° and 120°.

Constituents. Mastic consists mainly of triterpenoid acids, including mastic-adienonic acid, triterpene alcohols such as tirucallol, and about 2 per cent of volatile oil.

Solubility. Insoluble in water; partly soluble in alcohol and in turpentine oil; soluble, at 20°, in less than 1 part of chloroform and of ether.

Standard
DESCRIPTION. Small hard globular or pyriform pieces, about 4 to 8 mm in diameter, or more rarely in ovoid or nearly cylindrical pieces, up to 2 cm long and 1 cm wide; when fresh, pale yellow, clear, and glassy, the surface becoming dull and dusty on keeping; brittle, and breaking with a conchoidal fracture; when chewed, breaking up into sandy fragments which agglomerate into a plastic mass; odour somewhat aromatic; taste agreeable.

ACID VALUE. Not more than 70.

BENZENE-INSOLUBLE MATTER. Not more than 2·0 per cent, determined by the following method:
Shake vigorously 1·0 g, in powder, with 20 ml of *benzene* for 2 hours, filter, wash the residue with 5 ml of *benzene*, and dry to constant weight at 105°.

Adulterants and substitutes. East Indian or Bombay mastic is obtained from *P. khinjuk* Stocks and possibly other *Pistacia* species; it somewhat resembles genuine mastic, but the tears are darker, less vitreous, and not so clean. It is also more soluble in alcohol, less soluble in turpentine oil, and less disposed to agglomerate when chewed; the acid value varies from 103 to 109.

Uses. A solution of mastic in alcohol, ether, or chloroform is applied on cotton wool as a temporary filling for carious teeth. The compound paint is used as a protective covering for wounds and to hold gauze and radium needles in position.

Preparation
MASTIC PAINT, COMPOUND, B.P.C. (page 766)

MECLOZINE HYDROCHLORIDE

$C_{25}H_{29}Cl_3N_2 = 463·9$

Meclozine Hydrochloride is 1-*p*-chlorodiphenylmethyl-4-*m*-methylbenzylpiperazine dihydrochloride.

Solubility. Soluble, at 20°, in 1000 parts of water, in 25 parts of alcohol, and in 5 parts of chloroform.

Standard
It complies with the requirements of the British Pharmacopoeia.
It is a white or almost white, crystalline, almost odourless powder and contains not less than 98·0 and not more than the equivalent of 101·0 per cent of

$C_{25}H_{29}Cl_3N_2$, calculated with reference to the anhydrous substance. It contains not more than 5·0 per cent w/w of water.

Storage. It should be stored in airtight containers.

Actions and uses. Meclozine has the actions, uses, and undesirable effects of the antihistamine drugs, as described under Promethazine

Hydrochloride (page 409). It is used in the treatment of motion-sickness, nausea, and vomiting, particularly that of pregnancy, and for the relief of allergic states. For these purposes 25 to 50 milligrams of meclozine hydrochloride is given by mouth; the effect of a single dose lasts for twenty-four hours. For motion-sickness the dose is taken one hour before a journey.

POISONING. As for Promethazine Hydrochloride (page 409).

Dose. 25 to 50 milligrams daily, as a single dose or in divided doses.

Preparation
MECLOZINE TABLETS, B.P. Unless otherwise specified, tablets each containing 25 mg of meclozine hydrochloride are supplied. Tablets containing 12·5 mg are also available.

OTHER NAMES: *Ancolan®*; Meclizine Hydrochloride; *Postafène®*; *Sea-legs®*

MEFENAMIC ACID

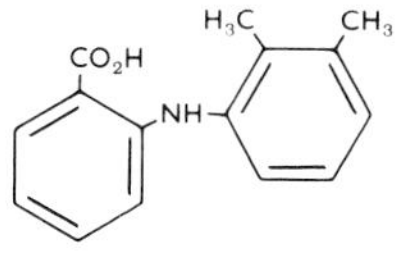

$C_{15}H_{15}NO_2 = 241·3$

Mefenamic Acid is *N*-2,3-xylylanthranilic acid.

Solubility. Very slightly soluble in water; soluble, at 20°, in 185 parts of alcohol, in 80 parts of ether, and in 150 parts of chloroform.

Standard
It complies with the requirements of the British Pharmacopoeia.
It is a white to greyish-white, microcrystalline, odourless powder and contains not less than 99·0 per cent of $C_{15}H_{15}NO_2$, calculated with reference to the dried substance. The loss on drying under the prescribed conditions is not more than 0·5 per cent.

Actions and uses. Mefenamic acid is an antipyretic and analgesic compound, similar in potency to aspirin, and it has a weak anti-inflammatory action. It is used to relieve the symptoms of rheumatic disorders and for minor pain.
It is available in capsules and as a paediatric

mixture containing 50 milligrams in 5 millilitres.

UNDESIRABLE EFFECTS. Mefenamic acid may give rise to gastro-intestinal irritation with changes in colonic function, producing constipation or diarrhoea necessitating discontinuation of treatment; more rarely, gastric ulceration and haematemesis may occur. Mefenamic acid may transiently lower the white-cell count and is a possible potentiator of coumarin anticoagulants. Skin rashes occur quite frequently.

Dose. 0·5 to 1 gram daily in divided doses.

Preparation
MEFENAMIC ACID CAPSULES, B.P. Unless otherwise specified, capsules each containing 250 mg of mefenamic acid are supplied.

OTHER NAME: *Ponstan®*

MEGESTROL ACETATE

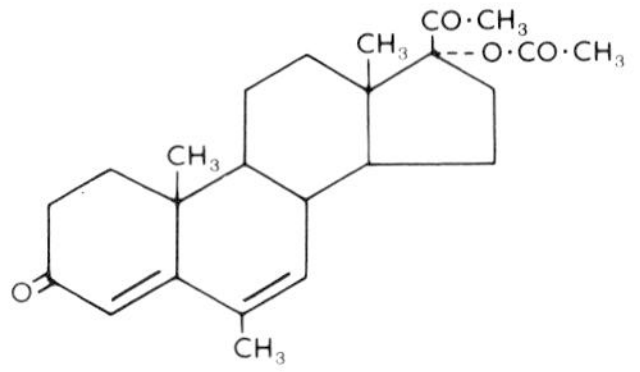

$C_{24}H_{32}O_4 = 384·5$

Megestrol Acetate is 17α-acetoxy-6-methylpregna-4,6-diene-3,20-dione.

Solubility. Very slightly soluble in water; soluble, at 20°, in 55 parts of alcohol, in 130 parts of ether, and in less than 1 part of chloroform; slightly soluble in fixed oils.

Standard
It complies with the requirements of the British Pharmacopoeia.
It is a white to creamy-white, crystalline, odourless powder and contains not less than 97·0 and not more than the equivalent of 103·0 per cent of $C_{24}H_{32}O_4$, calculated with reference to the dried substance. The loss on drying under the prescribed conditions is not more than 0·5 per cent. It has a melting-point of about 217°.

Storage. It should be protected from light.

Actions and uses. Megestrol acetate is a synthetic progestational steroid which has actions similar to those described under

Norethisterone (page 329) but is devoid of any significant oestrogenic or androgenic activity.
It is used, chiefly in conjunction with oestrogens, as an oral contraceptive to inhibit ovulation. For this purpose doses of 2 to 4 milligrams are given daily, usually with ethinyloestradiol, from the fifth to the twenty-fourth day of each menstrual cycle. It may also be given by the sequential method in which an oestrogen is given alone from the fifth to the nineteenth day of the menstrual cycle and then megestrol acetate in a dose of 1 milligram daily together with the oestrogen from the twentieth to the twenty-fourth day. The

regimen is repeated after an interval of one week. Regular administration is essential.

Megestrol acetate is available as tablets containing 1, 2, and 4 milligrams together with ethinyloestradiol.

UNDESIRABLE EFFECTS. Megestrol acetate may give rise to headaches and tension, mental depression, nausea and vomiting, breast engorgement, fluid retention, and weight gain. A state of pseudopregnancy and premenstrual tension may be aggravated; breakthrough bleeding is fairly common. Prolonged use may lead to impairment of liver function. When taken without oestrogens, megestrol acetate may not prevent conception.

Regular use of progestational oral contraceptives combined with oestrogens increases the risk of intravascular thrombosis and thromboembolic accidents.

PRECAUTIONS. These are described under Norethisterone (page 329).

Dose. As an oral contraceptive, 1 to 4 milligrams daily.

MEGLUMINE

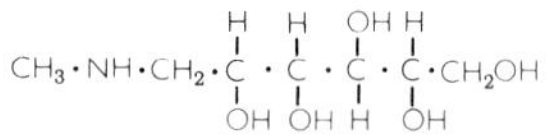

$C_7H_{17}NO_5 = 195·2$

Meglumine is *N*-methylglucamine.

$$CH_3 \cdot NH \cdot CH_2 \cdot \overset{H}{\underset{OH}{C}} \cdot \overset{H}{\underset{OH}{C}} \cdot \overset{OH}{\underset{H}{C}} \cdot \overset{H}{\underset{OH}{C}} \cdot CH_2OH$$

Solubility. Soluble, at 20°, in 1 part of water and in 100 parts of alcohol; insoluble in ether and in chloroform.

Standard
It complies with the requirements of the British Pharmacopoeia.
It is a white microcrystalline powder with a slight odour and contains not less than 99·0 per cent of $C_7H_{17}NO_5$, calculated with reference to the dried substance. The loss on drying under the prescribed conditions is not more than 1·0 per cent. It has a melting-point of 128° to 131°.

Uses. Meglumine is an organic base which is used for the preparation of salts of iodinated organic acids used as contrast media.

When the limited solubility of the sodium salt does not permit the preparation of the highly concentrated solutions that may be required for diagnostic procedures, the meglumine salts may be suitable for this purpose.

In the case of those contrast media which are available as highly soluble sodium salts, the meglumine salts may nevertheless be preferred for certain purposes on account of their lower toxicity to the heart, kidneys, and nerve tissues.

MEGLUMINE DIATRIZOATE INJECTION

SYNONYM: Meglumine Diatriz. Inj.

Meglumine Diatrizoate Injection is a sterile solution of the meglumine salt of 3,5-diacetamido-2,4,6-tri-iodobenzoic acid containing a suitable stabilising agent.

Standard
It complies with the requirements of the British Pharmacopoeia.
It is a clear, colourless to pale yellow, slightly viscous liquid and contains not less than 97·0 and not more than 103·0 per cent w/v of the content of meglumine diatrizoate stated on the label. A 65 per cent w/v solution has a pH of 6·0 to 7·0 and a weight per ml at 20° of 1·330 g to 1·360 g.

Storage. It should be protected from light.

Actions and uses. Meglumine diatrizoate injection is used as a contrast medium for angiography. The solution generally used for this purpose contains 65 per cent w/v of meglumine diatrizoate.

UNDESIRABLE EFFECTS. The effects described under Sodium Diatrizoate (page 450) may occur but are usually less marked.

PRECAUTIONS. As for Sodium Diatrizoate (page 450).

Dose. The strength of solution and the dose are determined by the physician in accordance with the diagnostic procedure.

OTHER NAME: *Angiografin*®

MELARSOPROL INJECTION

SYNONYM: Melarsoprol Inj.

Melarsoprol Injection is a sterile solution of melarsoprol, 2-[4-(4,6-diamino-1,3,5-triazin-2-ylamino)phenyl]-4-hydroxymethyl-1,3,2-dithiarsolan, in propylene glycol containing 5 per cent of water. It may be prepared by heating equimolar amounts of melarsen oxide and dimercaprol in propylene glycol and adding the water.

Standard
It complies with the requirements of the British Pharmacopoeia.
It is a clear solution with not more than a slightly alliaceous odour and contains not less than 3·4 and not more than 3·8 per cent w/v of melarsoprol, $C_{12}H_{15}AsN_6OS_2$. It has a weight per ml at 20° of 1·050 g to 1·060 g.

Sterilisation. It is sterilised by heating in an autoclave.

Actions and uses. Melarsoprol is a trypanocide. It is usually reserved for the treatment of advanced sleeping-sickness caused by *Trypanosoma rhodesiense* and *T. gambiense* in which the parasites have invaded the central nervous system.
The dosage is 3·6 milligrams per kilogram body-weight for an adult or 1·8 milligrams per kilogram body-weight for a child, given by intravenous injection daily for three days; this course of treatment should be repeated after an interval of ten days. During the administration of melarsoprol the patient should be kept in hospital.
If recrudescence occurs after adequate treatment with melarsoprol, the infection is usually resistant to all other organic arsenic derivatives.

UNDESIRABLE EFFECTS. Two kinds of undesirable effect may occur: Herxheimer reactions produced by the effect of the drug on the infection and toxic effects of arsenic such as encephalopathy. The toxic effects of arsenic may be alleviated by the injection of dimercaprol and the administration of sedatives.

Dose. See above under **Actions and uses.**

OTHER NAME: Mel B

MELPHALAN

$C_{13}H_{18}Cl_2N_2O_2 = 305·2$

Melphalan is *p*-di(2-chloroethyl)amino-L-phenylalanine.

Solubility. Very slightly soluble in water; soluble, at 20°, in 150 parts of methyl alcohol; insoluble in ether and in chloroform; soluble in dilute mineral acids.

Standard
It complies with the requirements of the British Pharmacopoeia.
It is a white or almost white odourless powder and contains not less than 93·0 per cent of $C_{13}H_{18}Cl_2N_2O_2$, calculated with reference to the dried substance. The loss on drying under the prescribed conditions is not more than 7·0 per cent. It melts with decomposition at about 177°.

Storage. It should be stored in airtight containers, protected from light, at a temperature not exceeding 25°.

Actions and uses. Melphalan, a cytotoxic drug, has the actions of mustine, from which it is derived. It acts mainly on dividing cells by causing cross linkage of deoxyribonucleic acid during the resting phase of mitosis. Like other cytotoxic drugs melphalan inhibits the growth of neoplastic cells but at the same time depresses bone-marrow activity, producing leucopenia and thrombocytosis. It is well absorbed orally and remains for about six hours in the bloodstream from which it is rapidly taken up by the tissues and organs, notably the kidneys.
Melphalan is used mainly for the treatment of myelomatosis and malignant melanoma. About a half to a third of cases of myelomatosis treated with melphalan show improvement for six months to two years and subjective remissions occur in 70 to 80 per cent of cases. In this disease melphalan produces a decrease in abnormal serum globulin, an increase in serum albumin, a reduction in proteinuria, and a rise in haemoglobin. Recurrence of melanomata can be prevented for several years.
Melphalan has also been used with variable results in the palliative treatment of Hodgkin's disease, Burkitt's lymphoma, reticulum cell sarcoma, and some other sarcomata (fibrosarcoma, neurofibrosarcoma, and Kaposi's sarcoma), seminoma, and carcinoma of the ovary.
For the treatment of myelomatosis the initial dose of melphalan is 6 to 10 milligrams daily by mouth for the first week. Dosage is then adjusted so that the white-cell and platelet counts do not fall below 2000 and 75,000 per cubic millimetre respectively. A course of treatment lasts from four to eight weeks. An alternative method is to give 2 to 4 milligrams daily for three to four months, keeping a care-

ful check on the white-cell and platelet counts. Provided these do not fall below the levels stated above, maintenance doses may be continued for nine months.

For the treatment of other conditions the dose of melphalan varies from 2 to 10 milligrams daily until a total dose of 100 to 200 milligrams is reached.

Melphalan has also been given intravenously in doses of 0·5 to 1 milligram per kilogram body-weight and by intra-arterial perfusion into an isolated limb in doses of 1 to 2 milligrams per kilogram body-weight.

UNDESIRABLE EFFECTS. Nausea, vomiting, diarrhoea, haemorrhage into the gastro-intestinal tract, temporary alopecia, and ulceration of the mouth and mucous membranes may occur, and may precede depression of the bone marrow, leucopenia, and thrombocytopenia. Regional perfusion of melphalan may cause oedema, neurotoxic effects, and blistering of the skin.

PRECAUTIONS. A haematological investigation, including white-cell and platelet counts,

should be made before and during treatment with melphalan. It should precede any change of dosage. The dosage for uraemic patients should be reduced.

CONTRA-INDICATIONS. Melphalan is contra-indicated in severe anaemia, leucopenia, or thrombocytopenia, and renal damage with azotaemia. It is also contra-indicated in the first trimester of pregnancy.

Dose. See above under **Actions and uses.**

Preparations

MELPHALAN INJECTION, B.P. It consists of a sterile solution prepared by dissolving the contents of a sealed container in alcohol (95 per cent) containing 2 per cent w/v of hydrogen chloride, and diluting the resulting solution with a 1·2 per cent w/v solution of dipotassium hydrogen phosphate in a 60 per cent v/v solution of propylene glycol in Water for Injections. It should be used immediately after preparation. Vials containing 100 mg are available.

MELPHALAN TABLETS, B.P. The quantity of melphalan in each tablet should be specified by the prescriber. They are compression coated or film coated. They should be stored at a temperature not exceeding 25°. Tablets containing 2 and 5 mg are available.

OTHER NAME: *Alkeran*®

MENTHOL

$C_{10}H_{20}O = 156·3$

Menthol, *p*-menthan-3-ol, is natural or synthetic $(-)$-menthol, or synthetic $(\pm)$-menthol.

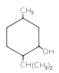

Natural $(-)$-menthol may be obtained from the volatile oils of various species of *Mentha* (Fam. Labiatae), chiefly from *M. arvensis* L. var. *piperascens* Holmes in Japan, var. *glabrata* Holmes in China, and *M. piperita* L. in America; it is separated from the oils by freezing.

Synthetic menthol may be obtained by the catalytic hydrogenation of thymol.

Solubility. Very slightly soluble in water and in glycerol; very soluble in alcohol and in essential oils; soluble, at 20°, in less than 1 part of ether, of chloroform, and of light petroleum, in 6 parts of liquid paraffin, and in 4 parts of olive oil.

Standard

It complies with the requirements of the British Pharmacopoeia.

It occurs as colourless acicular or prismatic crystals with a penetrating odour similar to that of peppermint oil. A 5 per cent solution in alcohol is neutral to litmus. $(-)$-Menthol, natural or synthetic, has a melting-point of 41° to 44° and a specific optical rotation of $-49°$ to $-50°$ when determined in a 10 per cent solution in alcohol.

$(\pm)$-Menthol has a freezing-point of 27° to 28°, rising on prolonged stirring to 30° to 32°.

Storage. It should be stored in airtight containers, in a cool place.

Actions and uses. Menthol is used to relieve the symptoms of bronchitis and sinusitis. For this purpose it is used, frequently mixed with camphor and eucalyptus oil, in pastilles, inhalations, and ointments.

Preparations

THYMOL GLYCERIN, COMPOUND, B.P.C. (page 702)
MENTHOL AND BENZOIN INHALATION, B.P.C. (page 705)
MENTHOL AND EUCALYPTUS INHALATION, B.P.C. (page 705)
BENZALKONIUM LOZENGES, B.P.C. (page 732)
BENZOCAINE LOZENGES, COMPOUND, B.P.C. (page 732)
FORMALDEHYDE LOZENGES, B.P.C. (page 732)
METHYL SALICYLATE OINTMENT, COMPOUND, B.P.C. (page 762)
MOUTH-WASH SOLUTION-TABLETS, B.P.C. (page 792)

MEPACRINE HYDROCHLORIDE

$C_{23}H_{32}Cl_3N_3O,2H_2O = 508\cdot9$

Mepacrine Hydrochloride is 3-chloro-9-(4-diethyl-amino-1-methylbutylamino)-7-methoxyacridine dihydrochloride dihydrate.

Solubility. Soluble, at 20°, in 40 parts of water, giving a clear yellow solution.

Standard
It complies with the requirements of the British Pharmacopoeia.
It is a bright yellow, crystalline, odourless powder and contains not less than 99·0 and not more than the equivalent of 101·0 per cent of $C_{23}H_{32}Cl_3N_3O$, calculated with reference to the dried substance. The loss on drying under the prescribed conditions is 5·0 to 8·0 per cent. A 2·0 per cent solution in water has a pH of 3·0 to 5·0.

Storage. It should be protected from light.

Actions and uses. Mepacrine has actions and uses similar to these described under Chloroquine Phosphate (page 101), but it has been largely replaced by chloroquine for the suppression and treatment of malaria.
A daily dosage of 100 milligrams of mepacrine hydrochloride by mouth in divided doses will suppress the symptoms of malaria and may be safely continued for long periods. Treatment should be continued until three weeks after leaving the endemic area.
For the curative treatment of malaria the dosage is 300 milligrams, three times on the first day and twice on the second day, followed by 100 milligrams three times a day for the next three to five days.
In the treatment of giardiasis, 100 milligrams of mepacrine hydrochloride three times a day for seven days is usually effective, although relapses may occur.
For the expulsion of tapeworms, doses of 100 milligrams are given at intervals of five minutes until a total of 1000 milligrams has been administered.

UNDESIRABLE EFFECTS. Mepacrine may occasionally cause gastric pain and headache; large doses may cause nausea, vomiting, diarrhoea and, rarely, transient mental disturbance. Yellow pigmentation of the skin usually accompanies its use and prolonged administration occasionally causes a condition of the skin resembling lichen planus.

Dose. See above under **Actions and uses.**

Preparation
MEPACRINE TABLETS, B.P. Unless otherwise specified, tablets each containing 100 mg of mepacrine hydrochloride are supplied. They should be protected from light.

OTHER NAMES: *Atabrine®*; *Quinacrine®*

MEPHENESIN

$C_{10}H_{14}O_3 = 182\cdot2$

Mephenesin is 3-(*o*-tolyloxy)propane-1,2-diol.

Solubility. Soluble, at 20°, in 100 parts of water, in 8 parts of alcohol, in 12 parts of chloroform, and in 7 parts of propylene glycol.

Standard
DESCRIPTION. White crystals or crystalline aggregates; odourless or almost odourless.

IDENTIFICATION TESTS. 1. To 1 g add 2 ml of *methyl carbonate* and 0·2 ml of a solution of 0·5 g of *sodium* in 10 ml of *dehydrated alcohol*, heat on a water-bath until a gelatinous precipitate remains, and remove the last traces of solvent by warming under reduced pressure; extract the residue by warming with 10 ml of *dehydrated alcohol*, filter, and evaporate the filtrate to dryness; the residue, after drying in a current of air, melts at about 95°.
2. The ultraviolet absorption spectrum exhibits the characteristics given in Appendix 3, page 855.

MELTING-POINT. 70° to 73°.

CHLORIDE. Shake 2·0 g with 40 ml of water and filter; the filtrate complies with the limit test for chlorides (175 parts per million).

CRESOL. To 0·10 g add 5·5 ml of water, 3 ml of a 4·0 per cent w/v solution of *sodium hexametaphosphate* in water, 1·5 ml of *lithium and sodium molybdophosphotungstate* solution, and 0·4 g of *anhydrous sodium carbonate*, heat on a water-bath for 5 minutes, and cool; any blue colour produced is not deeper than that produced when a mixture of 3 ml of a 0·001 per cent w/v solution of o-*cresol* in water and 2·5 ml of water is similarly treated (300 parts per million).

LOSS ON DRYING. Not more than 0·5 per cent, determined by drying for 24 hours over *phosphorus pentoxide* in vacuo.

SULPHATED ASH. Not more than 0·1 per cent.

CONTENT OF $C_{10}H_{14}O_3$. Not less than 99·0 per cent, calculated with reference to the substance dried under the prescribed conditions, determined by the method for Guaiphenesin (page 215); each ml of 1N sodium hydroxide is equivalent to 0·09111 g of $C_{10}H_{14}O_3$.

Sterilisation. Solutions for injection are sterilised by heating in an autoclave or by filtration.

Actions and uses. Mephenesin is a muscle relaxant which exerts a selective action on the spinal cord, probably through the anterior horn cells. Although it antagonises the action of strychnine on the spinal cord, it is ineffective in preventing leptazol convulsions. In small doses it relaxes hypertonic muscles without appreciably reducing motor power or producing respiratory depression. It lowers response to sensory stimuli and depresses superficial reflexes.

Mephenesin also has a central action, possibly on the basal ganglia and subcortical efferent pathways. Its effects are more prolonged when it is administered by mouth than when given by injection.

When given by mouth it is rapidly absorbed and broken down in the body and its break-down products can be detected in the urine after fifteen minutes, indicating that the effect of repeated administration is not normally cumulative. It may enhance the effects of narcotics and barbiturates.

Mephenesin has been given by mouth for the treatment of spastic, hypertonic, and hyper-kinetic conditions, such as parkinsonism, cere-bral palsy, choreoathetosis, and lesions of extrapyramidal origin. For the relief of spasms of tetanus a 10 per cent solution is admini-stered by intramuscular injection. It may also be given by intravenous injection, a 1 or 2 per cent solution being administered slowly or in a drip infusion.

Mephenesin is available as tablets containing 500 milligrams and as an elixir containing 1 gram in 15 millilitres.

UNDESIRABLE EFFECTS. When given by mouth mephenesin may cause drowsiness and, in some cases, nausea.

If a 10 per cent solution is given by intra-venous injection, it may give rise to intra-vascular haemolysis, haemoglobinuria, and local thrombosis at the site of injection; solu-tions containing more than 2 per cent may give rise to anuria if injected intravenously.

Overdosage with mephenesin may produce coarse nystagmus, blurred vision, and circum-oral numbness.

Dose. 0·5 to 1 gram by mouth once to six times daily; 0·1 to 1 gram by intramuscular or intravenous injection.

OTHER NAME: *Myanesin*®

MEPHENTERMINE SULPHATE

$C_{22}H_{36}N_2O_4S,2H_2O = 460·6$

$$\left[C_6H_5 \cdot CH_2 \cdot \overset{\overset{\displaystyle CH_3}{|}}{\underset{\underset{\displaystyle CH_3}{|}}{C}} \cdot NH \cdot CH_3 \right]_2 H_2SO_4, 2H_2O$$

Mephentermine Sulphate is $N\alpha\alpha$-trimethylphenethylamine sulphate dihydrate.

Solubility. Soluble, at 20°, in 20 parts of water and in 150 parts of alcohol; insoluble in chloroform.

Standard
It complies with the requirements of the British Pharmacopoeia.
It occurs as odourless colourless crystals or white crystalline powder and contains not less than 98·0 per cent of $C_{22}H_{36}N_2O_4S$, calculated with reference to the dried substance. The loss on drying under the pre-scribed conditions is 5·0 to 8·0 per cent. A 2 per cent solution in water has a pH of 4·0 to 6·5.

Sterilisation. Solutions for injection are sterilised by heating in an autoclave or by filtration.

Actions and uses. Mephentermine has the actions described under Methylamphetamine Hydrochloride (page 305); 1·4 milligrams of mephentermine sulphate is approximately equivalent to 1 milligram of the base.
It is used mainly for the treatment of hypo-tension due to trauma, anaesthesia, and sur-gery.

PRECAUTIONS. Mephentermine sulphate should not be given to patients who are being treated with a monoamine-oxidase inhibitor, such as isocarboxazid, nialamide, phenelzine, or tranyl-cypromine, or within about ten days of the discontinuation of such treatment. Its indis-criminate use is undesirable, as it may lead to dependence of the amphetamine type, as de-scribed under Amphetamine Sulphate (page 25).

Dose. The equivalent of 15 to 80 milligrams of mephentermine base by intramuscular or slow intravenous injection.

Preparation
MEPHENTERMINE INJECTION, B.P. It consists of a sterile solution of mephentermine sulphate in Water for In-jections. Unless otherwise specified, a solution con-taining the equivalent of 15 mg of the base in 1 ml is supplied.

MEPROBAMATE

$C_9H_{18}N_2O_4 = 218·3$

$$CH_3 \cdot \overset{\overset{\displaystyle CH_2 \cdot O \cdot CO \cdot NH_2}{|}}{\underset{\underset{\displaystyle CH_2 \cdot O \cdot CO \cdot NH_2}{|}}{C}} \cdot [CH_2]_2 \cdot CH_3$$

Meprobamate is 2,2-di(carbamoyloxymethyl)pentane.

Solubility. Soluble, at 20°, in 240 parts of water, in 7 parts of alcohol, and in 70 parts of ether.

Standard
It complies with the requirements of the British Pharmacopoeia.

It occurs as an almost odourless, white, crystalline powder or granular crystalline aggregates and contains not less than 98·0 per cent of $C_9H_{18}N_2O_4$, calculated with reference to the anhydrous substance. It contains not more than 0·5 per cent w/w of water. It has a melting-point of 104° to 107°.

Actions and uses. Meprobamate has tranquillising, anticonvulsant, and muscle relaxant properties. It is used in the treatment of psychoneurotic disorders when anxiety and nervous tension are present. The usual dosage is 400 milligrams three times a day.

UNDESIRABLE EFFECTS. Meprobamate sometimes provokes excitement instead of sedation. Idiosyncratic reactions may occur after a single dose and the drug should then be discontinued. It may cause hypotension, drowsiness, and blood dyscrasias and may enhance the effects of alcohol.

Meprobamate may give rise to dependence of the barbiturate-alcohol type as described under Phenobarbitone (page 366).

Dose. 0·4 to 1·2 grams daily in divided doses.

Preparation
MEPROBAMATE TABLETS, B.P. Unless otherwise specified, tablets each containing 400 mg of meprobamate are supplied. Tablets containing 200 mg are also available.

OTHER NAMES: *Equanil®*; *Mepavlon®*; *Meprate®*; *Miltown®*

MEPYRAMINE MALEATE

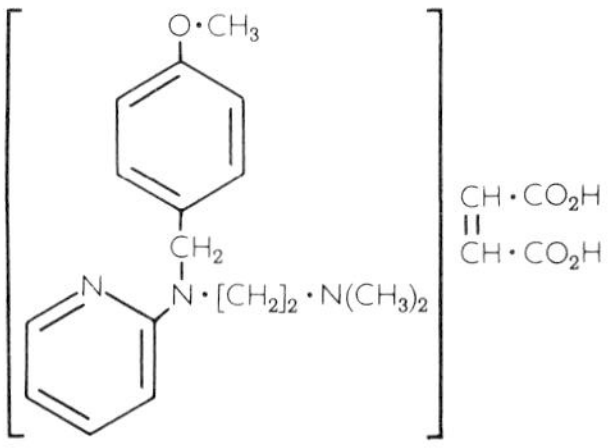

$C_{21}H_{27}N_3O_5 = 401·5$

Mepyramine Maleate is *N-p*-methoxybenzyl-*N'N'*-dimethyl-*N*-pyrid-2-ylethylenediamine hydrogen maleate.

Solubility. Soluble, at 20°, in less than 1 part of water, in 2·5 parts of alcohol, and in 1·5 parts of chloroform.

Standard
It complies with the requirements of the British Pharmacopoeia.
It is an odourless or almost odourless white or creamy-white powder and contains not less than 99·0 and not more than the equivalent of 101·0 per cent of $C_{21}H_{27}N_3O_5$, calculated with reference to the dried substance. The loss on drying under the prescribed conditions is not more than 0·5 per cent. It has a melting-point of 99° to 102°. A 1·0 per cent solution in water has a pH of 4·7 to 5·2.

Sterilisation. Solutions for injection are sterilised by heating in an autoclave.

Actions and uses. Mepyramine has the actions, uses, and undesirable effects of the antihistamine drugs, as described under Promethazine Hydrochloride (page 409), but it is less potent than promethazine and has a shorter duration of action. It is used mainly in the treatment of allergic and anaphylactic conditions, including hay fever, urticaria, and drug reactions.

Mepyramine maleate is usually given by mouth in a dosage of 50 milligrams every four to six hours; this may be increased gradually, according to the response and tolerance of the patient, but the daily dose should not exceed 1 gram. It may also be given by intramuscular or intravenous injection in a dose of 25 to 50 milligrams.

POISONING. As for Promethazine Hydrochloride (page 409).

Dose. See above under **Actions and uses.**

Preparations
MEPYRAMINE ELIXIR, B.P.C. (page 672)
MEPYRAMINE INJECTION, B.P. It consists of a sterile solution of mepyramine maleate in Water for Injections. Unless otherwise specified, a solution containing 25 mg in 1 ml is supplied.
MEPYRAMINE TABLETS, B.P. Unless otherwise specified, tablets each containing 50 mg of mepyramine maleate are supplied. They are sugar coated. Tablets containing 100 mg are also available.

OTHER NAME: *Anthisan®*

MERCAPTOPURINE

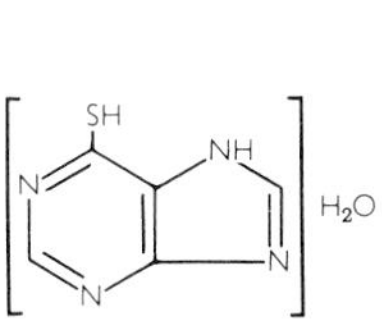

$C_5H_4N_4S,H_2O = 170·2$

Mercaptopurine is 6-mercaptopurine monohydrate.

Solubility. Very slightly soluble in water, in ether, and in acetone; soluble, at 20°, in 950 parts of alcohol; soluble in solutions of alkali hydroxides.

Standard
It complies with the requirements of the British Pharmacopoeia.
It is a yellow, crystalline, odourless powder and contains not less than 98·5 and not more than the equivalent of 101·0 per cent of $C_5H_4N_4S$, calculated with reference to the anhydrous substance. It contains 10·0 to 12·0 per cent w/w of water. It melts with decomposition at about 300°.

Storage. It should be stored in airtight containers, protected from light.

Actions and uses. Mercaptopurine is a cytotoxic agent. It is an analogue of adenine, a component of nucleic acid, and is believed to exert its effect in malignant disease by interfering with nucleic acid biosynthesis.

Although various natural purines protect micro-organisms from the inhibitory action of mercaptopurine, they do not interfere with its toxic or antitumour activity in animals or in man.

Mercaptopurine is used for the palliative treatment of acute leukaemia or chronic myeloid leukaemia; it has no value in other forms of cancer. In the treatment of acute leukaemia it produces remissions lasting from a few weeks to several months in a considerable proportion of children. Favourable results cannot be predicted and may be delayed. Patients with chronic myeloid leukaemia may also react favourably, but the administration of mercaptopurine is advisable only after other forms of treatment, such as irradiation or busulphan, have been fully utilised. However favourable the initial response may be, repeated courses of treatment invariably result in the development of a refractory state. Treatment with mercaptopurine is usually combined with other antineoplastic agents.

Mercaptopurine is also used as an immunosuppressive, for example in the treatment of the nephrotic syndrome and autoimmune haemolytic anaemia, and also with folic acid antagonists for the treatment of choriocarcinoma.

Mercaptopurine is administered by mouth, the usual dosage for a child or for an adult being 2·5 milligrams per kilogram body-weight daily in divided doses; this may have to be reduced or cautiously increased according to the response. Opinion varies about the advisability of maintenance therapy during remission periods.

UNDESIRABLE EFFECTS. The most serious toxic action of mercaptopurine is the production of hypoplasia of the bone marrow, and careful haematological control should be maintained. Other undesirable effects include oral ulceration and gastro-intestinal symptoms.

As with other cytotoxic agents the toxic effects may be delayed. They are usually quickly relieved by discontinuing treatment with the drug.

Dose. 100 to 200 milligrams daily in divided doses.

Preparation
MERCAPTOPURINE TABLETS, B.P. The quantity of mercaptopurine in each tablet should be specified by the prescriber. They should be stored in airtight containers, protected from light. Tablets containing 50 mg are available.

OTHER NAME: *Puri-Nethol*®

MERCURIC CHLORIDE

SYNONYMS: Corrosive Sublimate; Hydrargyri Perchloridum

$HgCl_2 = 271·5$

Mercuric Chloride, when heated, fuses to a colourless liquid at about 280°; above 300° it volatilises as a dense white cloud.

Solubility. Soluble, at 20°, in 15 parts of water and in 3 parts of alcohol; soluble in ether and in glycerol.

Standard
Material which complies with this standard meets the requirements of the European Pharmacopoeia.

DESCRIPTION. Heavy colourless or white crystals or crystalline masses, or a white crystalline powder.

IDENTIFICATION TESTS. It gives the reactions characteristic of mercuric salts and of chlorides.

APPEARANCE OF SOLUTION. A 5·0 per cent w/v solution in water complies with the following tests:
(i) The solution is clear or not more opalescent than a reference solution prepared by mixing 0·25 ml of *0·00002M sodium chloride*, 3·75 ml of water, 5·0 ml of *2M nitric acid*, and 1·0 ml of *dilute silver nitrate solution*, the comparison being made, 5 minutes after preparation of the reference solution, by viewing vertically 10 ml of the liquids in matched, colourless, transparent, neutral glass tubes, 16 mm internal diameter and with a flat base, against a black background in diffused light.
(ii) The solution has no colour when compared with water, the comparison being made by viewing horizontally 2 ml of the liquids in matched, colourless, transparent, neutral glass tubes, 12 mm internal diameter, against a white background in diffused daylight.

ACIDITY OR ALKALINITY. Dissolve 0·5 g in 10 ml of *carbon dioxide-free water* and add 0·1 ml of *methyl red solution*; the solution is red. Add 0·5 g of *sodium chloride*; the colour changes to yellow. Titrate with 0·01N hydrochloric acid; not more than 0·5 ml is required to change the colour of the solution to red.

MERCUROUS CHLORIDE. Dissolve 1 g in 30 ml of *solvent ether*; the solution is clear when compared with *solvent ether*, the comparison being made by viewing vertically 10 ml of the liquids in matched, colourless, transparent, neutral glass tubes, 16 mm internal diameter and with a flat base, against a black background in diffused light.

LOSS ON DRYING. Not more than 1·0 per cent, determined by drying 2·00 g for 24 hours over *anhydrous silica gel* in vacuo.

SULPHATED ASH. Not more than 0·1 per cent, determined on 2·0 g.

CONTENT OF $HgCl_2$. Not less than 99·5 per cent, calculated with reference to the substance dried under the prescribed conditions, determined by the following method:
Dissolve about 0·3 g, accurately weighed, in 100 ml of water, add about 40 ml of 0·05M disodium edetate, 5 ml of *ammonia buffer solution*, and, as indicator, *mordant black 11 solution*, and titrate with 0·05M zinc chloride until the blue colour changes to purple; add 3 g of *potassium iodide*, allow to stand for 2 minutes, and again titrate with 0·05M zinc chloride; each ml of 0·05M zinc chloride used in the second titration is equivalent to 0·01357 g of $HgCl_2$.

Incompatibility. It is incompatible with alkalis, lead acetate, silver nitrate, alkaloids (especially when iodides are present), and vegetable astringents.

Storage. It should be protected from light.

Actions and uses. The mercuric ion forms insoluble complexes with proteins and, by reason of this action on the proteins of bacterial cells, mercuric chloride is an antibacterial substance. To some extent its effect can be reversed by sulphydryl compounds.

Its use is limited by its toxicity, its precipitating action on proteins, its irritant action on raw surfaces, its corrosive action on metals, and by the fact that its activity is greatly reduced in the presence of excreta or body fluids.

Salicylic Acid and Mercuric Chloride Lotion is used for the treatment of follicular infections.

Solutions of mercuric chloride for external use should be coloured with indigo carmine as a warning of their toxic nature.

POISONING. In acute poisoning, death may ensue within a few hours from profound shock and circulatory collapse. Nephritis may sometimes develop if the patient survives, or symptoms resembling those of phosphorus poisoning may arise and may lead to death several weeks after the original poisoning occurred.

Acute mercurial poisoning should be treated as soon as possible by intramuscular injections of dimercaprol, 5 milligrams per kilogram body-weight being given, but this is an effective antidote only if given in the first hour or two after poisoning. It should be followed by two or three further injections of half this dose during the next twelve hours. Sodium Chloride Injection should be given by intravenous infusion for shock and the infusion should be continued, unless oedema occurs, to minimise kidney damage. If poisoning is mild, it usually responds readily to treatment with demulcents.

Preparation

SALICYLIC ACID AND MERCURIC CHLORIDE LOTION, B.P.C. (page 729)

YELLOW MERCURIC OXIDE

SYNONYM: Hydrargyri Oxidum Flavum

$HgO = 216·6$

Yellow Mercuric Oxide may be prepared by the interaction of aqueous solutions of mercuric chloride and sodium hydroxide.

Solubility. Insoluble in water and in alcohol; soluble in acids.

Standard

DESCRIPTION. An orange-yellow, amorphous powder; odourless.

IDENTIFICATION TESTS. 1. Heat gently; the colour changes to red. Heat strongly; decomposition to oxygen and mercury occurs.

2. A solution in *dilute hydrochloric acid* gives the reactions characteristic of mercuric salts.

ACIDITY OR ALKALINITY. Shake 1·0 g with 5 ml of *carbon dioxide-free water* and allow to settle; the supernatant liquid is neutral to *litmus paper*.

MERCUROUS SALTS. Dissolve 0·50 g in 25 ml of *dilute hydrochloric acid*; not more than a slight turbidity is produced.

CHLORIDE. To 0·20 g add 1 g of *zinc powder* and 10 ml of water, shake during 10 minutes, and filter; the filtrate complies with the limit test for chlorides (0·175 per cent).

LOSS ON DRYING. Not more than 1·0 per cent, determined by drying 1·0 g for one hour at 105°.

SULPHATED RESIDUE. Not more than 0·2 per cent, determined by moistening 1 g with *sulphuric acid* in a silica dish and heating strongly to constant weight.

CONTENT OF HgO. Not less than 99·3 per cent, calculated with reference to the substance dried under the prescribed conditions, determined by the following method:

Dissolve about 0·3 g, accurately weighed, in the minimum quantity of *dilute hydrochloric acid*, add 100 ml of water, about 40 ml of 0·05M disodium edetate, 5 ml of *ammonia buffer solution*, and, as indicator, *mordant black 11 solution*, and titrate with 0·05M zinc chloride to the first pink colour; add 3 g of *potassium iodide*, allow to stand for 2 minutes, and again titrate with 0·05M zinc chloride; each ml of 0·05M zinc chloride used in the second titration is equivalent to 0·01083 g of HgO.

Incompatibility. It is incompatible with cocaine hydrochloride, mercuric chloride being rapidly formed. Ointments containing yellow mercuric oxide should not be used while iodides are being given internally.

Storage. It should be protected from light.

Actions and uses. Yellow mercuric oxide has antibacterial properties and is used in eye ointments for the treatment of blepharitis and conjunctivitis, but such ointments should not be used for prolonged periods as there is a danger that mercury may be absorbed by the eye.

Preparation

MERCURIC OXIDE EYE OINTMENT, B.P.C. (page 699)

AMMONIATED MERCURY

SYNONYM: Hydrargyrum Ammoniatum

$NH_2 \cdot HgCl = 252 \cdot 1$

Ammoniated Mercury may be prepared by pouring a solution of mercuric chloride, with constant stirring, into a dilute solution of ammonia; the resulting precipitate is washed with cold water until the washings are nearly free from chloride, and dried at a low temperature.

Solubility. Insoluble in water, in alcohol, and in ether; soluble in warm hydrochloric, nitric, and acetic acids.

Standard
It complies with the requirements of the British Pharmacopoeia.
It is a white odourless powder and contains not less than 97·0 per cent of $NH_2 \cdot HgCl$.

Stability. It is decomposed slowly by warm water and rapidly by boiling water, a yellow basic salt of the composition $NH_2 \cdot HgCl, HgO$ being formed.

Storage. It should be protected from light.

Actions and uses. Ammoniated mercury is a mild antiseptic and is sometimes applied to the skin surrounding the perineum to destroy threadworms and to reduce reinfection. It was formerly used in the treatment of low-grade staphylococcal infections of the skin, and in psoriasis.

PRECAUTIONS. It should not be applied to raw surfaces because of the risk of absorption of mercury.

Preparations
AMMONIATED MERCURY OINTMENT, B.P. It contains 2·5 per cent of ammoniated mercury in Simple Ointment.

AMMONIATED MERCURY AND COAL TAR OINTMENT, B.P.C. (page 758)

AMMONIATED MERCURY, COAL TAR, AND SALICYLIC ACID OINTMENT, B.P.C. (page 758)

OTHER NAME: White Precipitate

MERSALYL ACID

$C_{13}H_{17}HgNO_6 = 483 \cdot 9$

Mersalyl Acid is a mixture of o-[(3-hydroxymercuri-2-methoxypropyl)carbamoyl]phenoxyacetic acid and its anhydrides.

Solubility. Slightly soluble in water and in dilute mineral acids; readily soluble in solutions of alkali hydroxides.

Standard
It complies with the requirements of the British Pharmacopoeia.
It is a white, slightly hygroscopic, odourless powder and contains not less than 98·0 and not more than the equivalent of 104·0 per cent of $C_{13}H_{17}HgNO_6$, calculated with reference to the dried substance. The loss on drying under the prescribed conditions is not more than 2·0 per cent.

Sterilisation. Solutions for injection are sterilised by heating with a bactericide, phenylmercuric nitrate being used, or by filtration. Contact with metal must be avoided.

Storage. It should be stored in airtight containers.

Actions and uses. Mersalyl acid, in the form of its salts, is a powerful diuretic which acts directly on the kidneys, increasing the excretion of water and sodium and thus decreasing the capacity of the body to retain fluid.
Mersalyl acid is used in the treatment of oedema and ascites in cardiac failure and is of value in relieving pulmonary oedema. It is also of value in ascites due to cirrhosis of the liver, in nephrotic oedema, and in carefully selected cases of subacute and chronic nephritis provided that there is no serious impairment of renal function. It has been largely superseded by oral diuretics.

Mersalyl acid is usually given, in the form of Mersalyl Injection, by deep intramuscular injection. Its diuretic action may be increased by producing a mild acidosis before administering the injection by giving three doses, each of 2 grams, of ammonium chloride on the previous day. The patient's tolerance to Mersalyl Injection may be tested by giving a preliminary intramuscular injection of 0·5 millilitre; in the absence of signs of intolerance, such as haematuria, diarrhoea, irritation of the skin, or prostration, 1 or 2 millilitres may be given on the following day. The intervals between injections are based on the therapeutic response; in the absence of a satisfactory diuretic response, repeated injections should not be given.
Overdosage may give rise to dehydration and consequently to uraemia. Some patients are intolerant of mercurial compounds; great care should be taken in the treatment of patients exhibiting numerous extrasystoles, those who have suffered recent myocardial infarction, and those receiving massive digitalis therapy. Intravenous injection is dangerous and may be followed by sudden death.

UNDESIRABLE EFFECTS. The most frequently occurring toxic effects following the administration of mersalyl acid are stomatitis, gastric disturbance, vertigo, febrile reactions, and skin irritation. To prevent the accumulation of excreted mercury in the intestine, constipation should be avoided. Some patients may be sensitive to mersalyl acid but tolerant to other mercurial compounds.

CONTRA-INDICATIONS. It should not be given in acute nephritis.

Dose. See above under **Actions and uses.**

Preparation
MERSALYL INJECTION, B.P. (*Syn.* Mersalyl and Theophylline Injection). It consists of a sterile solution containing 10 per cent of the sodium salt of mersalyl acid and 5 per cent of theophylline in Water for Injections, the pH of the solution being adjusted to 8.0. It should be protected from light. Dose: 0.5 to 2 millilitres by intramuscular injection on alternate days.

MESTRANOL

$C_{21}H_{26}O_2 = 310.4$

Mestranol is 3-methoxy-19-nor-17α-pregna-1,3,5(10)-trien-20-yn-17-ol.

Solubility. Very slightly soluble in water; soluble, at 20°, in 44 parts of alcohol, in 23 parts of ether, in 4.5 parts of chloroform, in 23 parts of acetone, and in 12 parts of dioxan.

Standard
It complies with the requirements of the British Pharmacopoeia.
It is a white or almost white, crystalline, odourless powder and contains not less than 97.0 and not more than the equivalent of 102.0 per cent of $C_{21}H_{26}O_2$, calculated with reference to the dried substance. The loss on drying under the prescribed conditions is not more than 0.5 per cent. It has a melting-point of 150° to 154°.

Storage. It should be protected from light.

Actions and uses. Mestranol has the actions of the oestrogens, as described under Oestradiol Benzoate (page 335). It is often included for these actions in amounts of 50 to 150 micrograms in oral contraceptive tablets.

UNDESIRABLE EFFECTS. Headache, dizziness, nausea, and vomiting may occur, but usually disappear if cyclic contraception is continued.

OTHER NAME: *Ovastol*®

METARAMINOL TARTRATE

$C_{13}H_{19}NO_8 = 317.3$

Metaraminol Tartrate is (−)-2-amino-1-(*m*-hydroxyphenyl)propan-1-ol hydrogen tartrate.

Solubility. Soluble, at 20°, in 3 parts of water and in 100 parts of alcohol; very slightly soluble in ether and in chloroform.

Standard
It complies with the requirements of the British Pharmacopoeia.
It is a white, crystalline, almost odourless powder and contains not less than 99.0 and not more than the equivalent of 101.0 per cent of $C_{13}H_{19}NO_8$, calculated with reference to the dried substance. The loss on drying under the prescribed conditions is not more than 0.5 per cent. It has a melting-point of 174° to 178°. A 5 per cent solution in water has a pH of 3.2 to 3.5.

Sterilisation. Solutions are sterilised by filtration.

Storage. It should be stored in airtight containers.

Actions and uses. Metaraminol is a long-acting vasopressor agent which is given by injection to raise the blood pressure in hypotensive emergencies. Its duration of action varies from twenty to ninety minutes according to the route of administration; when given by subcutaneous or intramuscular injection, metaraminol exerts a pressor effect in five to twelve minutes, and the peak effect is observed in about thirty minutes; a pressor effect

begins in one to two minutes after intravenous administration, and the peak occurs in about five minutes. Metaraminol may be given by intravenous infusion for the continuous maintenance of the blood pressure. 1.9 mg of metaraminol tartrate is approximately equivalent to 1 mg of metaraminol.

Dose. The equivalent of 2 to 10 milligrams of metaraminol by subcutaneous or intramuscular injection; the equivalent of 0.5 to 5 milligrams of metaraminol by intravenous injection; the equivalent of up to 100 milligrams of metaraminol, dissolved in not less than 500 millilitres of Sodium Chloride Injection or Dextrose Injection, by intravenous infusion.

Preparation
METARAMINOL INJECTION, B.P. It consists of a sterile solution of metaraminol tartrate in Water for Injections containing a suitable stabilising agent. Unless otherwise specified, a solution containing the equivalent of 10 mg of metaraminol in 1 ml is supplied. It should be protected from light.

OTHER NAME: *Aramine*®

METFORMIN HYDROCHLORIDE

$$\left[\begin{array}{c}(CH_3)_2N \cdot C \cdot NH \cdot C \cdot NH_2 \\ \underset{NH}{\parallel} \quad \underset{NH}{\parallel} \end{array}\right] HCl$$

$C_4H_{12}ClN_5 = 165 \cdot 6$

Metformin Hydrochloride is N^1,N^1-dimethylbiguanide hydrochloride.

Solubility. Soluble, at 20°, in 2 parts of water and in 100 parts of alcohol; insoluble in ether and in chloroform.

Standard
It complies with the requirements of the British Pharmacopoeia.
It is a white, crystalline, hygroscopic, almost odourless powder and contains not less than 98·5 and not more than the equivalent of 101·0 per cent of $C_4H_{12}ClN_5$, calculated with reference to the dried substance. The loss on drying under the prescribed conditions is not more than 0·5 per cent. It has a melting-point of about 225°.

Storage. It should be stored in airtight containers.

Actions and uses. Metformin is an oral hypoglycaemic agent with actions and uses similar to those of phenformin (page 363).
The initial dose is 500 milligrams two or three times a day with meals, gradually increased if necessary to 3 grams daily over a period of ten to fourteen days. Once control of the blood glucose has been achieved, it may be possible to reduce the dose without loss of control. The usual maintenance dosage is 1·0 to 1·5 grams daily, although more may be required.
Metformin may be given in conjunction with a sulphonylurea.
If the patient is already receiving insulin, the dosage of insulin should be given in full for two days and then gradually reduced while the dose of metformin is increased.

Metformin alone is unsuitable for the treatment of young diabetics.

UNDESIRABLE EFFECTS. Anorexia, nausea, and vomiting may occur and are usually dose-related. Urticarial reactions, weakness, and loss of weight occur rarely. Acidosis is less marked than with phenformin.

PRECAUTIONS AND CONTRA-INDICATIONS. Metformin should not be given to patients in diabetic coma or with severe acidosis or infection or after operations or trauma. It should be given with caution to patients with hepatic and renal disease and it should not be used during pregnancy.

POISONING. The procedure for the treatment of hypoglycaemia as described under Phenformin Hydrochloride (page 363) should be followed.

Dose. Initial dose, 1 to 1·5 grams daily in divided doses; subsequent doses up to 3 grams daily in divided doses.

Preparation
METFORMIN TABLETS, B.P. Unless otherwise specified, tablets each containing 500 mg of metformin hydrochloride are supplied. They may be film coated. Tablets containing 850 mg are also available.

OTHER NAMES: *Diguanil®*; *Glucophage®*; *Metiguanide®*

METHACHOLINE CHLORIDE

$C_8H_{18}ClNO_2 = 195 \cdot 7$

$$[CH_3 \cdot CO \cdot O \cdot CH(CH_3) \cdot CH_2 \cdot N(CH_3)_3]^+ \ Cl^-$$

Methacholine Chloride is 2-acetoxypropyltrimethylammonium chloride and may be prepared by acetylating β-methylcholine chloride.

Solubility. Soluble, at 20°, in less than 1 part of water and in 1·2 parts of alcohol; soluble in chloroform.

Standard
DESCRIPTION. Deliquescent colourless or white crystals or white crystalline powder; odourless or almost odourless.

IDENTIFICATION TESTS. 1. To 1 ml of a 10 per cent w/v solution in water add 1 ml of *alcohol (95 per cent)* and 1 ml of *sulphuric acid*; ethyl acetate, recognisable by its odour, is produced.
2. Heat gently 5 ml of a 10 per cent w/v solution in water with 2 g of *potassium hydroxide*; trimethylamine, recognisable by its odour, is produced.
3. To 1 ml of a 10 per cent w/v solution in water add a slight excess of a 10 per cent w/v solution of *gold chloride* in water; a precipitate is formed which, after recrystallising from hot water and drying at 105°, melts at about 127°.
4. It gives the reactions characteristic of chlorides.

ACIDITY. pH of a 2·0 per cent w/v solution in *carbon dioxide-free water*, 4·5 to 5·5.

MELTING-POINT. 170° to 173°.

ACETYLCHOLINE CHLORIDE. Dissolve 0·20 g in 10 ml of water, shake with 3 ml of *sodium perchlorate solution*, and cool in ice for 5 minutes; no precipitate is formed.

LOSS ON DRYING. Not more than 1·5 per cent, determined by drying to constant weight at 105°.

SULPHATED ASH. Not more than 0·1 per cent.

CONTENT OF $C_8H_{18}ClNO_2$. Not less than 98·0 and not more than the equivalent of 101·5 per cent, calculated with reference to the substance dried under the prescribed conditions, determined by the following method:
Dissolve about 0·5 g, accurately weighed, in 15 ml of water, add 50 ml of 0·1N sodium hydroxide, and heat on a water-bath for 45 minutes; cool, preventing the access of carbon dioxide, and titrate the excess of alkali with 0·1N sulphuric acid, using *phenolphthalein solution* as indicator.
Repeat the procedure omitting the sample.
The difference between the two titrations represents the amount of sodium hydroxide required by the sample; each ml of 0·1N sodium hydroxide is equivalent to 0·01957 g of $C_8H_{18}ClNO_2$.

Sterilisation. Solutions for injection are sterilised by filtration.

Storage. It should be stored in airtight containers.

Actions and uses. Methacholine chloride has the muscarinic actions of acetylcholine, but is more stable. It slows the heart, increases peristalsis, dilates peripheral blood vessels, and increases salivary, sweat, and bronchial secretions.

Methacholine chloride has been used to terminate attacks of auricular paroxysmal tachycardia when simpler methods have failed. It has also been used in the treatment of postoperative abdominal distension and retention of urine. The usual dose is 20 milligrams given by subcutaneous injection; this may be repeated in half an hour.

Eye-drops containing 2·5 per cent of methacholine chloride are used for the diagnosis of Adie's pupil; the affected pupil contracts within fifteen to thirty minutes of the instillation of the drops whereas the normal pupil does not respond. The eye-drops should be freshly prepared.

Methacholine chloride is available for injection as a solution in propylene glycol containing 25 milligrams per millilitre.

UNDESIRABLE EFFECTS. When given by injection, methacholine chloride may cause a terrifying sensation of choking; this may be stopped immediately by giving 600 micrograms of atropine sulphate by intravenous injection.

CONTRA-INDICATIONS. Methacholine chloride is contra-indicated in patients suffering from allergic conditions, especially asthma, as it may cause bronchial spasm and excessive bronchial secretion.

Dose. 10 to 25 milligrams by subcutaneous injection.

METHACYCLINE HYDROCHLORIDE

$C_{22}H_{23}ClN_2O_8 = 478·9$

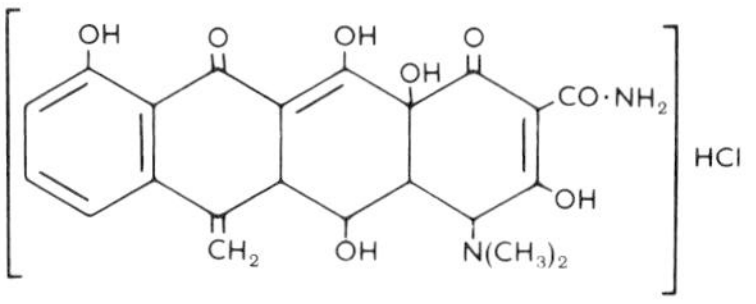

Methacycline Hydrochloride is 4-dimethylamino-1,4,4a,5,5a,6,11,12a-octahydro-3,5,10,12,12a-pentahydroxy-6-methylene-1,11-dioxonaphthacene-2-carboxyamide hydrochloride, an antimicrobial substance produced by chemical synthesis from oxytetracycline.

Solubility. Soluble, at 20°, in 65 parts of water and in 30 parts of methyl alcohol; insoluble in chloroform.

Standard
It complies with the requirements of the British Pharmacopoeia.
It is a yellow, crystalline, odourless powder and contains not less than 877 Units per mg, calculated with reference to the dried substance. The loss on drying under the prescribed conditions is not more than 2·0 per cent. A 1 per cent solution in water has a pH of 2·0 to 3·0.

Storage. It should be stored in airtight containers, protected from light.

Actions and uses. Methacycline has the actions described under Tetracycline Hydrochloride (page 498).

Salts of aluminium, calcium, iron, and magnesium, which may decrease the absorption of tetracyclines from the gut, should not be given with methacycline.

PRECAUTIONS AND CONTRA-INDICATIONS. As for Tetracycline Hydrochloride (page 498).

Dose. For an adult, 150 to 300 milligrams every six hours; for a child, 7 to 14 milligrams per kilogram body-weight daily in divided doses.

Preparation
METHACYCLINE CAPSULES, B.P. Unless otherwise specified, capsules each containing 150 mg of methacycline hydrochloride are supplied.

OTHER NAME: *Rondomycin®*

METHADONE HYDROCHLORIDE

SYNONYM: Amidone Hydrochloride

$C_{21}H_{28}ClNO = 345·9$

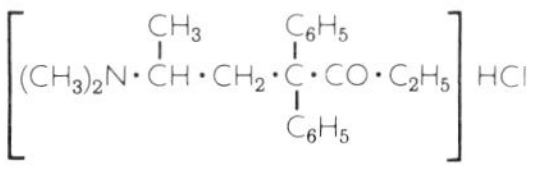

Methadone Hydrochloride is (±)-6-dimethylamino-4,4-diphenylheptan-3-one hydrochloride.

Solubility. Soluble, at 20°, in 12 parts of water and in 7 parts of alcohol; soluble in chloroform; insoluble in ether.

Standard
It complies with the requirements of the British Pharmacopoeia.
It occurs as odourless colourless crystals or white crystalline powder and contains not less than 99·0 and not more than the equivalent of 101·0 per cent of $C_{21}H_{28}ClNO$, calculated with reference to the dried substance. The loss on drying under the prescribed conditions is not more than 0·5 per cent. It has a melting-point of 233° to 236°. A 1 per cent solution in water has a pH of 4·5 to 6·5.

Incompatibility. It is incompatible with some dyes.

Sterilisation. Solutions for injection are sterilised by heating in an autoclave or by filtration. Chlorocresol should not be included as a bactericide.

Actions and uses. Methadone has actions and uses similar to those described under Morphine Hydrochloride (page 314).

It is a potent analgesic; this effect begins about fifteen minutes after subcutaneous injection and about forty-five minutes after oral administration and lasts from two to four hours. Its sedative action is much less marked than that of morphine and it is therefore not used as a pre-anaesthetic agent. Methadone depresses the cough centre. It also depresses the respiratory centre and is therefore undesirable as an obstetric analgesic. Its action on the gastro-intestinal tract is weaker than that of morphine and constipation seldom occurs.

Methadone is used extensively for the relief of pain where sedation is not necessary. For moderately severe pain, 5 to 10 milligrams of methadone hydrochloride by mouth every four hours is usually adequate; for a rapid effect it may be given by subcutaneous or intramuscular injection.

To suppress useless coughing, 1 to 2 milligrams of methadone hydrochloride is usually given by mouth in the form of a linctus.

Morphine addicts may be given methadone orally as substitution therapy; methadone effectively controls the symptoms of morphine withdrawal and dependence on methadone is easier to treat than dependence on morphine.

UNDESIRABLE EFFECTS. Nausea, vomiting, dizziness, faintness, and constriction of the pupil may occur. As with morphine, many of these effects occur more often in ambulant than in recumbent patients.

DEPENDENCE. When administered in therapeutic doses for prolonged periods, methadone may lead to the development of dependence of the morphine type, as described under Morphine Hydrochloride (page 314).

POISONING. The procedure described under Morphine Hydrochloride (page 314) should be adopted.

Dose. See above under **Actions and uses.**

Preparations
METHADONE INJECTION, B.P. It consists of a sterile solution of methadone hydrochloride in Water for Injections. The strength of the solution should be specified by the prescriber. Ampoules containing 10 mg in 1 ml are available.
METHADONE LINCTUS, B.P.C. (page 723)
METHADONE TABLETS, B.P. The quantity of methadone hydrochloride in each tablet should be specified by the prescriber. Tablets containing 5 mg are available.

OTHER NAME: *Physeptone*®

METHALLENOESTRIL

$C_{18}H_{22}O_3 = 286.4$

Methallenoestril is β-(6-methoxynaphth-2-yl)-$\alpha\alpha$-dimethylvaleric acid.

Solubility. Very slightly soluble in water; soluble, at 20°, in 10 parts of alcohol, in 8 parts of ether, and in 2 parts of chloroform; soluble in solutions of alkali hydroxides.

Standard
DESCRIPTION. A white or almost white crystalline powder; odourless or almost odourless.

IDENTIFICATION TESTS. 1. The ultraviolet absorption spectrum exhibits the characteristics given in Appendix 3, page 855.

2. It melts at about 138°.

LOSS ON DRYING. Not more than 0.5 per cent, determined by drying to constant weight at 105°.

SULPHATED ASH. Not more than 0.1 per cent.

CONTENT OF $C_{18}H_{22}O_3$. Not less than 97.5 and not more than the equivalent of 102.0 per cent, calculated with reference to the substance dried under the prescribed conditions, determined by the following method:
Dissolve about 0.25 g, accurately weighed, in 50 ml of *pyridine* and titrate with 0.1N tetrabutylammonium hydroxide to the maximum value of dE/dV (where E is the electromotive force and V is the volume of titrant) in a potentiometric titration; each ml of 0.1N tetrabutylammonium hydroxide is equivalent to 0.02864 g of $C_{18}H_{22}O_3$.

Actions and uses. Methallenoestril is a synthetic oestrogenic hormone which has actions and uses similar to those described under Oestradiol Benzoate (page 335).

For replacement therapy, it is generally given by mouth in a dosage of 3 milligrams two or three times a day for two to three weeks. In post-menopausal osteoporosis, this may be followed by a maintenance dosage of 3 milligrams daily.

For the suppression of lactation, 12 milligrams may be given three times a day for five days.

It may also be useful, when stilboestrol therapy is badly tolerated, for the symptomatic treatment of prostatic carcinoma, for which it may be given in a dosage of 3 to 6 milligrams three times a day.

UNDESIRABLE EFFECTS. These are as described under Oestradiol Benzoate (page 335). Methallenoestril seldom causes nausea, except when given in large doses, and gives rise to less withdrawal bleeding and gynaecomastia than oestradiol.

Dose. See above under **Actions and uses.**

Preparation
METHALLENOESTRIL TABLETS, B.P.C. (page 813)

OTHER NAME: *Vallestril*®

METHANDIENONE

$C_{20}H_{28}O_2 = 300.4$

Methandienone is 17-hydroxy-17α-methylandrosta-1,4-dien-3-one.

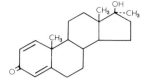

Solubility. Insoluble in water; soluble in alcohol, in chloroform, and in glacial acetic acid; slightly soluble in ether.

Standard
It complies with the requirements of the British Pharmacopoeia.
It is a white or faintly yellowish-white, crystalline, odourless powder and contains not less than 97·0 and not more than the equivalent of 103·0 per cent of $C_{20}H_{28}O_2$, calculated with reference to the dried substance. The loss on drying under the prescribed conditions is not more than 0·5 per cent. It has a melting-point of 163° to 167°.

Storage. It should be stored in airtight containers, protected from light.

Actions and uses. Methandienone has actions and uses similar to those described under Testosterone (page 494); its anabolic properties are more pronounced than its androgenic effects. It causes nitrogen and calcium retention and promotes protein synthesis, leading to an increase in skeletal weight and growth in bone. It has little progestational action.
Methandienone is used as an anabolic agent in the treatment of osteoporosis, and for the alleviation of low backache after the menopause. It is also given during post-operative recovery and during convalescence after chronic debilitating disease. It may be used in the palliative treatment of inoperable mammary carcinoma, especially where bone metastases have developed.
When combined with a high-calorie low-protein diet and with or without peritoneal dialysis or haemodialysis, methandienone may be of

value in the treatment of acute renal failure by reducing the speed at which the blood urea rises. In patients on chronic dialysis, methandienone may be helpful in preventing anaemia, although testosterone is more often used for this purpose in men.
Methandienone is also used to prevent extensive nitrogen loss after severe burns.
The initial dosage is 15 to 20 milligrams daily by mouth and this is reduced to 5 to 10 milligrams daily for maintenance. For long-term treatment, intermittent therapy is usually adequate, courses of four to six weeks' duration being given with intervals of two to four weeks. A child usually requires 0·1 milligram per kilogram body-weight daily; courses should be limited to four weeks and followed by an interval of one to two months before further treatment is given.

UNDESIRABLE EFFECTS. When given for prolonged periods, methandienone may give rise to androgenic effects and there may be some water retention and hypercalcaemia. Jaundice may develop occasionally.

CONTRA-INDICATIONS. Methandienone is contra-indicated in patients with prostatic carcinoma or hepatic dysfunction.

Dose. See above under **Actions and uses.**

Preparation
METHANDIENONE TABLETS, B.P. Unless otherwise specified, tablets each containing 5 mg of methandienone are supplied. They should be protected from light.

OTHER NAMES: *Dianabol®;* Methandrostenolone

METHAQUALONE

$C_{16}H_{14}N_2O = 250.3$

Methaqualone is 3,4-dihydro-2-methyl-3-*o*-tolylquinazolin-4-one.

Solubility. Insoluble in water; soluble, at 20°, in 12 parts of alcohol, in 50 parts of ether, and in 1 part of chloroform.

Standard
It complies with the requirements of the British Pharmacopoeia.
It is a white or almost white, crystalline, odourless powder and contains not less than 99·0 and not more than the equivalent of 101·0 per cent of $C_{16}H_{14}N_2O$, calculated with reference to the dried substance. The loss on drying under the prescribed conditions is not more than 0·5 per cent. It has a melting-point of 114° to 117°.

Storage. It should be stored in airtight containers, protected from light.

Actions and uses. Methaqualone has a hypnotic action resembling that of an intermediate-acting barbiturate, the actions and uses of which are described under Phenobarbitone (page 366).
Sleep lasting six to eight hours is produced within about fifteen minutes by an oral dose of 150 to 300 milligrams. The onset of sleep is rapid and may occur abruptly, particularly

when methaqualone is given in conjunction with an antihistamine such as diphenhydramine.

UNDESIRABLE EFFECTS. When sleep is delayed, a transient paraesthesia of the limbs and face may occur, but this does not appear to be associated with peripheral neuropathy. Headache, drowsiness, dizziness, and skin rashes may occur.

Methaqualone may reduce the ability of patients to drive motor cars or work with moving machinery, and may produce dependence of the barbiturate-alcohol type, as described under Phenobarbitone (page 366).

PRECAUTIONS AND CONTRA-INDICATIONS. Methaqualone should not be given to patients with hepatic dysfunction, eclampsia, or epilepsy. It may potentiate the action of neuroleptics, tranquillisers, barbiturates, and alcohol.

Particular care is necessary when methaqualone is prescribed in conjunction with an antihistamine as both stupor and convulsions may occur within the dose-range of both drugs.

POISONING. Conservative treatment as described under Phenobarbitone (page 366) should be adopted, but forced diuresis is ineffective and dialysis is rarely required.

Storage. It should be stored in airtight containers, protected from light.

Dose. As a hypnotic, 150 to 300 milligrams; as a sedative, 75 milligrams two or three times a day.

OTHER NAMES: *Melsed®*; *Quaalude®*; *Revonal®*

METHICILLIN SODIUM

$C_{17}H_{19}N_2NaO_6S,H_2O = 420.4$

Methicillin Sodium is sodium 6-(2,6-dimethoxybenzamido)penicillanate monohydrate.

Solubility. Soluble, at 20°, in 0·6 part of water and in 35 parts of alcohol; insoluble in fixed oils and in liquid paraffin.

Standard
It complies with the requirements of the British Pharmacopoeia.
It is a white microcrystalline powder and contains not less than 97·0 per cent of $C_{17}H_{19}N_2NaO_6S,H_2O$, and not less than 14·0 per cent of methoxyl, CH_3O. It contains not more than 4·8 per cent w/w of water. A 10 per cent solution in water has a pH of 5·5 to 7·5.

Hygroscopicity. It absorbs insignificant amounts of moisture at 25° at relative humidities up to about 65 per cent, but under damper conditions it absorbs significant amounts.

Labelling. If the material is not intended for parenteral administration, the label on the container states that the contents are not to be injected.

Storage. It should be stored in airtight containers at a temperature not exceeding 25°. If it is intended for parenteral administration, the containers should be sterile and sealed to exclude micro-organisms.

Actions and uses. Methicillin is a semi-synthetic penicillin which is not decomposed by staphylococcal penicillinase but which has a reduced antibiotic potency compared with benzylpenicillin. Unlike cloxacillin, it is not well absorbed when taken by mouth and should be given by injection. A smaller proportion of the drug in the tissues is protein bound compared with cloxacillin.

Its only use is in the treatment of severe penicillinase-producing staphylococcal infections when it should be given in a dose of 1 gram every four to six hours by intramuscular injection. In serious infections, the dose can be increased to 2 grams every four hours.

Strains of methicillin-resistant staphylococci have been reported.

PRECAUTIONS. The same precautions against allergy should be taken as for benzylpenicillin (page 51). It should not be used topically or in the treatment of non-penicillinase-producing staphylococcal infections.

Dose. See above under **Actions and uses.**

Preparation
METHICILLIN INJECTION, B.P. It consists of a sterile solution prepared by dissolving the sterile contents of a sealed container in Water for Injections. The quantity of methicillin sodium in each container should be specified by the prescriber. It should be used within two days of preparation and should be stored during this period at 2° to 10°. Vials containing 1 g are available.

OTHER NAME: *Celbenin®*

METHOHEXITONE INJECTION

Methohexitone Injection is a sterile solution of a mixture of one hundred parts by weight of sodium α-($\pm$)-5-allyl-1-methyl-5-(1-methylpent-2-ynyl)barbiturate and six parts by weight of dried sodium carbonate in Water for Injections free from carbon dioxide. It is prepared by dissolving the contents of a sealed container in the requisite amount of Water for Injections free from carbon dioxide.

Standard
It complies with the requirements of the British Pharmacopoeia.
The contents of the sealed container is a white or almost white, odourless powder and contains 90·0 to 95·0 per cent of $C_{14}H_{17}N_2NaO_3$ and 9·5 to 10·5 per cent of Na, both calculated with reference to the dried substance. The loss on drying under the prescribed conditions is not more than 3·0 per cent. A 5 per cent solution in water is clear and has a pH of 11·1 to 11·4.

Storage. It should be freshly prepared and used within twenty-four hours.

Actions and uses. Methohexitone is an anaesthetic for intravenous administration, with actions and uses similar to those described under Thiopentone Sodium (page 506), but it is more potent, acts for a shorter time, and is more rapidly eliminated from the tissues.
The usual dose for induction is 70 to 120 milligrams, administered in the form of a 1 per cent solution over a period of about thirty seconds. A 0·1 per cent solution may be used for continuous drip anaesthesia.

CONTRA-INDICATIONS. The only contra-indications are those common to all present-day general anaesthetics.

Dose. The equivalent of 30 to 120 milligrams of methohexitone sodium by slow intravenous injection.

OTHER NAMES: *Brietal Sodium*®; Sodium Methohexital

METHOIN

$C_{12}H_{14}N_2O_2 = 218\cdot3$

Methoin is 5-ethyl-3-methyl-5-phenylhydantoin.

Solubility. Slightly soluble in water; soluble, at 20°, in 13 parts of alcohol, in 85 parts of ether, and in 2·3 parts of chloroform; soluble in solutions of alkali hydroxides.

Standard
It complies with the requirements of the British Pharmacopoeia.
It occurs as colourless, lustrous, odourless plates and contains not less than 99·0 per cent of $C_{12}H_{14}N_2O_2$, calculated with reference to the dried substance. The loss on drying under the prescribed conditions is not more than 0·5 per cent. It has a melting-point of 136° to 139°.

Actions and uses. Methoin is an anti-convulsant which has actions similar to those described under Phenytoin Sodium (page 378), but it has a less hypnotic effect.
Methoin is used in the treatment of grand mal. It has also produced satisfactory results in some patients with psychomotor seizures, Jacksonian epilepsy, and behaviour disorders. In some cases the simultaneous administration of methoin and phenobarbitone has given the best results. Methoin is less effective in controlling petit mal attacks.
The initial daily dosage is 50 to 100 milligrams by mouth, given in divided doses; this may be increased by 50 milligrams at weekly intervals until a daily dosage of 600 milligrams is reached. The maximum daily dosage for a child is 400 milligrams.

UNDESIRABLE EFFECTS. Methoin gives rise to undesirable effects more frequently than phenytoin sodium, the commonest reactions being drowsiness, dizziness, muscular inco-ordination, and ataxia. The appearance of a rash indicates the need to reduce the dose or to discontinue the drug, but in some cases treatment can be maintained by reducing the dose of methoin and giving phenobarbitone in addition.
The most serious toxic effect of methoin is on the haemopoietic system, and cases of pancytopenia and aplastic anaemia have been reported.

PRECAUTIONS. Patients should be told to report immediately the occurrence of a sore throat or fever and to stop taking the drug pending further advice.

Dose. See above under **Actions and uses.**

Preparation
METHOIN TABLETS, B.P. Unless otherwise specified, tablets each containing 100 mg of methoin are supplied.

OTHER NAMES: Mephenytoin; *Mesantoin*®; *Mesontoin*®

METHOSERPIDINE

SYNONYM: Methoserp.

$C_{33}H_{40}N_2O_9 = 608.7$

Methoserpidine is methyl 11-demethoxy-10-methoxy-18-(3,4,5-trimethoxybenzoyl)-reserpate.

Solubility. Very slightly soluble in water; soluble, at $20°$, in 60 parts of alcohol, in 5 parts of chloroform, and in 8 parts of dioxan.

Standard
It complies with the requirements of the British Pharmacopoeia.
It is a cream-coloured, microcrystalline, hygroscopic, odourless powder and contains not less than 98·5 and not more than the equivalent of 101·5 per cent of $C_{33}H_{40}N_2O_9$, calculated with reference to the dried substance. The loss on drying under the prescribed conditions is not more than 2·0 per cent. It melts with decomposition at about $171°$.

Storage. It should be stored in airtight containers, protected from light. It darkens on exposure to light.

Actions and uses. Methoserpidine has actions and uses similar to those described under Reserpine (page 428).
When methoserpidine is used as a hypotensive agent for the treatment of mild to moderate hypertension, response to treatment is slow in onset, the full effect being observed about the second or third week after treatment is begun.
The initial dosage is up to 30 milligrams daily in divided doses for one week. The daily dosage is then adjusted by 5 or 10 milligrams at intervals of a week until a suitable maintenance dose is established; this should be between 15 and 60 milligrams daily in divided doses.

UNDESIRABLE EFFECTS. Nasal congestion, mild sedation, and gastro-intestinal disturbances may occur.

CONTRA-INDICATIONS. Methoserpidine should not be administered to patients with endogenous depression.

Dose. See above under **Actions and uses.**

Preparation
METHOSERPIDINE TABLETS, B.P. Unless otherwise specified, tablets each containing 5 mg of methoserpidine are supplied. They should be protected from light. Tablets containing 10 mg are also available.

OTHER NAME: *Decaserpyl*®

METHOTREXATE

Methotrexate is a mixture of N-{p-[(2,4-diaminopteridin-6-ylmethyl)methylamino]benzoyl}-L-glutamic acid and related substances.

Solubility. Very slightly soluble in water, in alcohol, in ether, and in chloroform; soluble in dilute solutions of alkali hydroxides and carbonates.

Standard
It complies with the requirements of the British Pharmacopoeia.
It is a yellow to orange crystalline powder and contains not less than 85·0 per cent of $C_{20}H_{22}N_8O_5$, calculated with reference to the anhydrous substance. It contains not more than 8·0 per cent w/w of water.

Storage. It should be stored in airtight containers, protected from light.

Actions and uses. Methotrexate is a cytotoxic antimetabolite that inhibits the hydrogenation of folic acid and prevents its participation in purine and nucleic acid synthesis. Although this interferes with the reproduction of malignant cells, normal cells are also affected, but to a lesser extent. Those most affected are neutrophil leucocytes, platelets, bone-marrow cells, and the epithelial cells of the mouth and gastro-intestinal tract. In addition, methotrexate is a powerful inhibitor of antibody synthesis and a teratogen in early pregnancy.

Methotrexate is used mainly for producing remissions in acute lymphoblastic leukaemia in children and for the treatment of choriocarcinoma. It is of limited value for the treatment of leukaemia in adults.
The dose, given orally for producing a remission in leukaemia in children, is 3 milligrams per square metre of body surface per day, or 0·07 to 0·14 milligram per kilogram body-weight. Alternatively, 20 to 40 milligrams per square metre of body surface may be administered intravenously or intramuscularly twice weekly. This dose is continued until signs of toxicity, such as ulceration of the mouth and diarrhoea, appear. The next dose is then omitted and subsequent dosage adjusted to 15 milligrams per square metre of body surface twice weekly.
For the treatment of leukaemic meningitis, methotrexate is given in a dose of 5 to 10 milligrams daily intrathecally until the blast-cell count is less than 10 per cubic millimetre in the cerebrospinal fluid.

The dose for the treatment of leukaemia in adults is 2·5 to 5 milligrams daily by mouth. In the treatment of leukaemia, methotrexate is usually given with other antileukaemic drugs such as mercaptopurine, a corticosteroid, and vincristine sulphate.

For choriocarcinoma, 15 to 25 milligrams of methotrexate is given intramuscularly once daily for five days, further courses being given after recovery of bone-marrow function. From five to twelve such courses are given.

Methotrexate has also been used for the palliative treatment of solid inoperable tumours in daily doses of 5 to 25 milligrams orally, or 25 to 50 milligrams parenterally, at weekly intervals. Doses of 30 to 50 milligrams daily have also been given by regional perfusion, and 25 milligrams dissolved in Sodium Chloride Injection instilled into body cavities. Improvement in selected cases of psoriasis has resulted from the administration of methotrexate given in two or three courses of 2·5 milligrams orally daily for six to twelve days, with six to twelve days between courses.

The immunosuppressive action of methotrexate has been used in the palliative treatment of dermatomyositis.

UNDESIRABLE EFFECTS. These include nausea, vomiting, ulceration and haemorrhage of the mouth and bowel, liver and kidney damage, bone-marrow depression, a fall in the white-cell and platelet counts, and alopecia.

In cases of overdosage 6 milligrams of calcium folinate may be given intramuscularly every four hours until the white-cell and platelet counts have recovered. The same dosage of calcium folinate may be given to protect against the systemic toxicity of methotrexate given by regional perfusion.

PRECAUTIONS. Periodic blood counts during treatment with methotrexate are essential; ulceration of the mouth, diarrhoea, and haemorrhagic enteritis are early signs of toxicity. A severe fall in the white-cell or platelet count necessitates stopping treatment for at least ten days. The simultaneous administration of salicylates or sulphonamides may increase the toxic effects of methotrexate.

CONTRA-INDICATIONS. Methotrexate should not be given to patients with depressed bone marrow or in early pregnancy.

Dose. See above under **Actions and uses.**

Preparations
METHOTREXATE INJECTION, B.P. It consists of a sterile solution of methotrexate with sodium chloride, sodium hydroxide, and suitable preservatives, prepared immediately before use by dissolving the sterile contents of a sealed container in Water for Injections. If a precipitate forms, the solution should be discarded. The quantity of methotrexate in each container should be specified by the prescriber. Vials containing 5 and 50 mg are available.

METHOTREXATE TABLETS, B.P. The quantity of methotrexate in each tablet should be specified by the prescriber. They should be protected from light. Tablets containing 2·5 mg are available.

METHOXAMINE HYDROCHLORIDE

$C_{11}H_{18}ClNO_3 = 247·7$

Methoxamine Hydrochloride is 2-amino-1-(2,5-dimethoxyphenyl)-propan-1-ol hydrochloride.

Solubility. Soluble, at 20°, in 2·5 parts of water and in 12 parts of alcohol; very slightly soluble in ether and in chloroform.

Standard
DESCRIPTION. Colourless or white plate-like crystals or white crystalline powder; odourless or with a faint odour.

IDENTIFICATION TESTS. 1. Dissolve 0·02 g in 2 ml of water, add 5 ml of *diazotised nitroaniline solution* and 1 ml of *sodium carbonate solution*, allow to stand for 2 minutes, and add 1 ml of 1N sodium hydroxide; a deep red colour is produced which is extractable with *butyl alcohol.*

2. The ultraviolet absorption spectrum exhibits the characteristics given in Appendix 3, page 855.

3. It gives the reactions characteristic of chlorides.

ACIDITY. pH of a 2·0 per cent w/v solution in *carbon dioxide-free water,* 4·0 to 6·0.

MELTING-POINT. 212° to 216°.

RELATED SUBSTANCES. Extinction at 345 nm of a 1-cm layer of a 0·50 per cent w/v solution in 0·01N hydrochloric acid, not more than 0·2.

LOSS ON DRYING. Not more than 0·5 per cent, determined by drying for 2 hours at 105°.

SULPHATED ASH. Not more than 0·1 per cent.

CONTENT OF $C_{11}H_{18}ClNO_3$. Not less than 99·0 per cent, calculated with reference to the substance dried under the prescribed conditions, determined by the following method:
Titrate about 0·5 g, accurately weighed, by Method I of the British Pharmacopoeia for non-aqueous titration; each ml of 0·1N perchloric acid is equivalent to 0·02477 g of $C_{11}H_{18}ClNO_3$.

Sterilisation. Solutions for injection are sterilised by heating in an autoclave or by filtration.

Actions and uses. Methoxamine is a synthetic sympathomimetic amine which causes prolonged peripheral vasoconstriction and consequently a rise in arterial blood pressure. It has little effect on the heart, although reflex bradycardia may occur. It has a marked pilomotor effect, but does not stimulate the central nervous system or cause bronchodilatation.

Methoxamine hydrochloride is administered by intramuscular injection in doses of 5 to 20 milligrams to maintain or restore the blood pressure during surgical operations and in hypotensive states such as post-operative shock or after ganglion blockade.

In emergencies, or when the systolic blood pressure has fallen to less than 60 mm of mercury, 5 to 10 milligrams may be given by intravenous injection at a rate of about 1 milligram per minute.

Its effect begins almost immediately after intravenous injection and lasts for about one hour; after intramuscular injection it begins within about fifteen minutes and lasts for about one and a half hours. A second intramuscular injection should not be given within fifteen minutes of the first dose, and the total daily dosage should not normally exceed 60 milligrams; a single intravenous dose should not exceed 10 milligrams. There is no diminution of effect with repeated doses. To prolong the effect of an intravenous dose, it may be supplemented by an intramuscular injection of 10 to 15 milligrams.

Methoxamine is especially suitable for maintaining blood pressure during spinal anaesthesia; a dose of 10 milligrams by intramuscular injection is usually sufficient for operations below the umbilical level and 15 to 20 milligrams for operations above this.

Methoxamine is applied locally for the relief of nasal congestion. It is suitable for infants and children. Applied intranasally as drops or spray it does not produce systemic side-effects, but occasionally may cause rebound congestion.

In addition to the injection, methoxamine hydrochloride is available as nasal drops and nasal spray containing 0·25 per cent.

UNDESIRABLE EFFECTS. Methoxamine may produce an undesirably high blood pressure with headache and vomiting. Bradycardia may occur, but this may be prevented or abolished by atropine. Methoxamine frequently induces the desire to urinate. After intravenous injection there may be a feeling of coldness.

PRECAUTIONS AND CONTRA-INDICATIONS. It is contra-indicated in coronary disease, severe hypertension or cardiovascular disease, and should be used with caution in patients with hyperthyroidism. It should not be given to patients who are being treated with a monoamine-oxidase inhibitor, such as iso-carboxazid, nialamide, phenelzine, or tranyl-cypromine, or within about ten days of the discontinuation of such treatment.

Dose. See above under **Actions and uses.**

Preparation
METHOXAMINE INJECTION, B.P.C. (page 714)

OTHER NAMES: *Vasoxine*®; *Vasylox*®

METHOXYFLURANE

$C_3H_4Cl_2F_2O = 165·0$

$CHCl_2 \cdot CF_2 \cdot O \cdot CH_3$

Methoxyflurane is 2,2-dichloro-1,1-difluoro-1-methoxyethane. It contains 0·01 per cent w/w of butylated hydroxytoluene as an antioxidant.

Solubility. Insoluble in water; miscible with alcohol, with ether, and with chloroform.

Standard
It complies with the requirements of the British Pharmacopoeia.
It is a clear, almost colourless, mobile liquid with a characteristic odour. It has a weight per ml at 20° of 1·423 g to 1·427 g. On heating it distils completely between 103·5° and 107·5°.

Storage. It should be stored in airtight containers, protected from light, in a cool place.

Actions and uses. Methoxyflurane is a volatile anaesthetic with actions similar to those described under Halothane (page 217), but induction is relatively slow. At operating theatre temperatures it is not inflammable or explosive and it may be used in conjunction with a cautery.

Methoxyflurane may be administered by any of the usual methods, alone or in combination with thiopentone, muscle relaxants, and other drugs used as aids to anaesthesia. For induction, a concentration of 2 to 2·8 per cent v/v may be given and the anaesthesia maintained with 0·5 per cent v/v in oxygen.

Good muscular relaxation can be obtained. There is some depression of respiration and blood pressure, but vomiting is unusual. The hypnotic effect of methoxyflurane is such that administration may be discontinued half an hour before the completion of operation.

For obstetric use a concentration of 0·5 per cent v/v in a mixture of nitrous oxide and oxygen may be used for anaesthesia and a concentration of 0·35 per cent v/v in air may be administered intermittently for analgesia; no depression of uterine contractions occurs. Methoxyflurane may cause the skin to look pale although the circulation remains stable.

PRECAUTIONS AND CONTRA-INDICATIONS. Methoxyflurane is contra-indicated in the presence of liver damage. It enhances the effects of muscle relaxants of the tubo-curarine type and of narcotics, which should therefore be used with caution, as also should adrenaline.

OTHER NAME: *Penthrane*®

METHYL HYDROXYBENZOATE

SYNONYM: Methylparaben

$C_8H_8O_3 = 152 \cdot 1$

Methyl Hydroxybenzoate is methyl p-hydroxybenzoate.

Solubility. Soluble, at 20°, in 500 parts of water, in 3·5 parts of alcohol, and in 3 parts of acetone; soluble in 20 parts of boiling water; readily soluble in ether and in solutions of alkali hydroxides; soluble in 60 parts of warm glycerol and in 40 parts of warm vegetable oils, the solutions remaining clear on cooling.

Standard
It complies with the requirements of the British Pharmacopoeia.
It is a fine, white, crystalline, almost odourless powder and contains not less than 99·0 and not more than the equivalent of 101·0 per cent of $C_8H_8O_3$. It has a melting-point of 125° to 128°.

Uses. Methyl hydroxybenzoate is employed, usually in conjunction with other hydroxybenzoate esters, as a preservative. For aqueous preparations, 0·1 to 0·2 per cent is usually sufficient.
Methyl hydroxybenzoate may be incorporated in preparations as a solution in alcohol or dissolved with the aid of heat.

OTHER NAMES: *Methyl Butex®*; *Nipagin M®*

METHYL SALICYLATE

SYNONYMS: Methyl Sal.; Methylis Salicylas

$C_8H_8O_3 = 152 \cdot 1$

Methyl Salicylate is methyl o-hydroxybenzoate.

Solubility. Slightly soluble in water; soluble, at 20°, in 10 parts of alcohol (70 per cent); miscible with alcohol (90 per cent), with ether, with chloroform, with carbon disulphide, with glacial acetic acid, and with fixed and volatile oils.

Standard
It complies with the requirements of the European Pharmacopoeia.
It is a colourless or slightly yellow liquid with a strong, persistent, characteristic, aromatic odour and contains not less than 99·0 per cent of $C_8H_8O_3$. It has a specific gravity at 20° of 1·182 to 1·187, equivalent to a weight per ml at 20° of about 1·179 g to 1·184 g.

Storage. It should be protected from light.

Actions and uses. Methyl salicylate has the actions of salicylates, as described under Sodium Salicylate (page 461), but is seldom given by mouth. It is readily absorbed through the skin and is applied in liniments and ointments for the relief of pain in lumbago, sciatica, and rheumatic conditions.

POISONING. The procedure as described under Aspirin (page 35) should be adopted.

NOTE. When Oil of Wintergreen, Wintergreen, or Wintergreen Oil is prescribed or demanded, Methyl Salicylate is dispensed or supplied.

Preparations
METHYL SALICYLATE LINIMENT, B.P.C. (page 726)
METHYL SALICYLATE OINTMENT, B.P.C. (page 762)
METHYL SALICYLATE OINTMENT, COMPOUND, B.P.C. (page 762)

METHYLAMPHETAMINE HYDROCHLORIDE

SYNONYMS: Methamphetamine Hydrochloride; Methylamphet. Hydrochlor.

$C_6H_5 \cdot CH_2 \cdot CH(CH_3) \cdot NHCH_3, HCl$

$C_{10}H_{16}ClN = 185 \cdot 7$

Methylamphetamine Hydrochloride is (+)-Nα-dimethylphenethylamine hydrochloride.

Solubility. Soluble, at 20°, in 2 parts of water and in 4 parts of alcohol; insoluble in ether and in acetone.

Standard
It complies with the requirements of the British Pharmacopoeia.
It occurs as odourless white crystals or crystalline powder and contains not less than 99·0 per cent of $C_{10}H_{16}ClN$, calculated with reference to the dried substance. The loss on drying under the prescribed conditions is not more than 1·0 per cent. It has a melting-point of 172° to 174°.

Sterilisation. Solutions for injection are sterilised by heating in an autoclave or by filtration.

Actions and uses. Methylamphetamine has actions, uses, and contra-indications similar to those described under Amphetamine Sulphate (page 25), but it takes effect more rapidly than amphetamine and its actions are more prolonged. Excessive doses produce restlessness, palpitations, and anxiety.
It has been given by mouth in the treatment of narcolepsy, parkinsonism, alcoholism, and certain depressive states, especially those which are associated with apathy and psychomotor retardation.
In Great Britain, the use of methylamphetamine is discouraged and supplies are restricted to hospitals.

UNDESIRABLE EFFECTS. Methylamphetamine may give rise to dependence of the amphetamine type as described under Amphetamine Sulphate (page 25) and it has a high dependence liability.

PRECAUTIONS. Methylamphetamine should not be given to patients who are being treated with a monoamine-oxidase inhibitor, such as isocarboxazid, nialamide, phenelzine, or tranylcypromine, or within about ten days of the discontinuation of such treatment.

POISONING. A very short-acting barbiturate should be administered by intravenous injection.

Dose. 2·5 to 10 milligrams by mouth; 10 to 30 milligrams by intramuscular or intravenous injection.

Preparations
METHYLAMPHETAMINE INJECTION, B.P. It consists of a sterile solution of methylamphetamine hydrochloride in Water for Injections. Unless otherwise specified, a solution containing 20 mg in 1 ml is supplied.
METHYLAMPHETAMINE TABLETS, B.P. Unless otherwise specified, tablets each containing 5 mg of methylamphetamine hydrochloride are supplied.

OTHER NAME: d-Deoxyephedrine Hydrochloride

INDUSTRIAL METHYLATED SPIRIT

SYNONYMS: I.M.S.; Industrial Methylated Spirits

Industrial Methylated Spirit is a mixture, made by a legally authorised methylator, of 19 volumes of alcohol (95 per cent) with 1 volume of approved wood naphtha, and is of the quality known as "66 O.P. Industrial Methylated Spirits".

Other strengths of industrial methylated spirit are available, such as "Absolute Industrial Methylated Spirits", which is 74 O.P. and contains less than 1 per cent of water, and "64 O.P. Industrial Methylated Spirits".

Standard
It complies with the requirements of the British Pharmacopoeia.
It is a clear, colourless, mobile, volatile liquid with an odour of alcohol and wood naphtha. It is highly inflammable, burning with a blue smokeless flame. The specific gravity at 20°/20° is not greater than 0·814.

Actions and uses. Industrial methylated spirit is applied externally for its astringent action, but mucous membranes and excoriated skin surfaces must be protected from such application. It is usually applied externally as Surgical Spirit.
The Board of Customs and Excise permit, subject to the observance of the conditions laid down in their regulations, the use of industrial duty-free spirit in the preparation of a range of specified preparations intended for external use only. These scheduled preparations include certain inhalations, liniments, lotions, sprays, spirits, and solutions of the British Pharmacopoeia and the British Pharmaceutical Codex, in addition to a formulary of medicinal, surgical, toilet, and other preparations.
Industrial methylated spirit may also be used in the preparation of certain extracts, resins, and surgical dressings, provided that in each case no alcohol remains in the finished product.
Provisions governing the dispensing, on the prescriptions of medical practitioners, dentists, and veterinary surgeons and practitioners, of industrial methylated spirit or of preparations of which it is an ingredient, and its use in ways other than those mentioned, are also contained in the regulations issued by the Board of Customs and Excise.
Industrial methylated spirit, as usually supplied, may contain small amounts of acetone and should not be used for the preparation of iodine solutions, as an irritating compound is formed by reaction between the iodine and acetone; for such preparations industrial methylated spirit (acetone-free) is used.

UNDESIRABLE EFFECTS. Industrial methylated spirit must not be taken by mouth, as its methyl alcohol content renders it poisonous. Symptoms include visual disturbances which often proceed to blindness, severe acidosis, and prolonged coma which may terminate in death from respiratory failure.

POISONING. Gastric lavage should be employed and the usual means adopted for the treatment of shock and respiratory failure. Acidosis should be treated by the administration of Compound Sodium Lactate Injection, and delirium, if it occurs, by hyoscine.

Preparation
SURGICAL SPIRIT, B.P.C. (page 794)

INDUSTRIAL METHYLATED SPIRIT (ACETONE-FREE)

Industrial Methylated Spirit (Acetone-free) is a mixture, made by a legally authorised methylator, of 19 volumes of alcohol (95 per cent) with 1 volume of approved wood naphtha or other denaturant approved by the Board of Customs and Excise, and is of the quality known as "66 O.P. Industrial Methylated Spirits" but free from acetone.

Other strengths of industrial methylated spirit (acetone-free) are available, such as "Absolute Industrial Methylated Spirits (Acetone-free)", which is 74 O.P., and "64 O.P., Industrial Methylated Spirits (Acetone-free)".

Standard

DESCRIPTION. A colourless, transparent, mobile, volatile liquid; odour of alcohol modified by the odour of the denaturant.

IDENTIFICATION TEST. Dilute 0·5 ml to 5 ml with water, add 2 ml of *potassium permanganate and phosphoric acid solution*, allow to stand for 10 minutes, and add 2 ml of *oxalic acid and sulphuric acid solution*; to the colourless solution add 5 ml of *decolorised magenta solution* and allow to stand at 15° to 30° for 30 minutes; a deep violet colour is produced.

ACIDITY OR ALKALINITY. 25 ml requires not more than 0·2 ml of 0·1N sodium hydroxide to give a pink colour with *phenolphthalein solution*, or not more than 1·0 ml of 0·1N hydrochloric acid to give a red colour with *methyl red solution*.

SPECIFIC GRAVITY (20°/20°). Not higher than 0·814.

ACETONE. Dilute 5 ml to 10 ml with water, add 1 ml of *2-nitrobenzaldehyde solution* followed by 1 ml of a 15 per cent w/v solution of *sodium hydroxide* in water, and allow to stand for 15 minutes; any colour which develops is not deeper than that produced by 10 ml of a 0·025 per cent v/v solution of *acetone* in *alcohol (50 per cent)* when similarly treated (500 parts per million).

OILY AND RESINOUS SUBSTANCES. Mix 5 ml with 95 ml of water; the solution remains clear.

NON-VOLATILE MATTER. Not more than 0·01 per cent w/v, determined by evaporating to dryness and drying the residue to constant weight at 105°.

Uses. Industrial methylated spirit (acetone-free) is used in the preparation of alcoholic solutions of iodine intended for external use.

UNDESIRABLE EFFECTS; POISONING. As for Industrial Methylated Spirit (above).

METHYLCELLULOSE

Methylcellulose is a methyl ether of cellulose. It may be prepared by methylating alkali cellulose with methyl chloride. The name "methylcellulose" is followed by a number indicating the approximate viscosity of a 2·0 per cent solution. The gel-point of a 2 per cent solution in water of Methylcellulose 4500 is about 50°.

Solubility. Soluble in cold water, forming a viscous colloidal solution; insoluble in hot water, in alcohol, in ether, and in chloroform.

Standard

METHYLCELLULOSE 20

DESCRIPTION. A white or creamy-white powder; odourless.

IDENTIFICATION TESTS. 1. Add 1 g to 100 ml of water; the powder swells and disperses, forming a viscous colloidal solution. Boil; a white precipitate is formed which redissolves on cooling.

2. Pour 2 ml of the cold solution prepared in test 1 onto a glass plate and allow the water to evaporate; a thin self-sustaining film is produced.

3. To 10 ml of the cold solution prepared in test 1 add 0·5 ml of a 0·05 per cent w/v solution of *brilliant yellow* in water, 0·05 ml of 0·1N sodium hydroxide, and 10 ml of a saturated solution of *sodium sulphate* in water; a voluminous, flocculent, red precipitate is formed. Filter; the filtrate is colourless.

4. Soak in *iodine water* for a few minutes and remove the excess of reagent; the powder is stained yellow. Add one or two drops of *sulphuric acid (66 per cent v/v)*; it is stained dark brown (distinction from microcrystalline cellulose).

ACIDITY OR ALKALINITY. pH of a 1·0 per cent w/v solution in *carbon dioxide-free water*, 6·0 to 8·0.

VISCOSITY. At 20°, 17·0 to 23·0 centistokes, determined by the following method:
Transfer 2·0 g, calculated with reference to the substance dried under the prescribed conditions, to a wide-mouthed bottle, add 100 ml of water previously heated to 85° to 90°, close the bottle with a stopper fitted with a stirrer, and stir for 10 minutes; place the bottle in an ice-bath, continue stirring until the solution is of uniform consistence, remove the bottle from the ice-bath, and allow the solution to attain room temperature.
Determine the viscosity of this solution by the method of the British Pharmacopoeia, Appendix IVH, for the determination of the viscosity of Methylcellulose, using a suspended-level viscometer with capillary diameter of 0·84 ± 0·02 mm.

ARSENIC. It complies with the test given in Appendix 6, page 879 (1 part per million).

LEAD. It complies with the test given in Appendix 7, page 883 (5 parts per million).

LOSS ON DRYING. Not more than 10·0 per cent, determined by drying to constant weight at 105°.

SULPHATED ASH. Not more than 1·0 per cent.

CONTENT OF METHOXYL. 27·0 to 29·0 per cent, calculated as CH_3O, with reference to the substance dried under the prescribed conditions, determined by the following method:
Carry out the method of the British Pharmacopoeia, Appendix X(I), for the determination of methoxyl, using about 0·05 g, accurately weighed, and a 25 per cent w/v solution of *sodium acetate* in the scrubber; each ml of 0·1N sodium thiosulphate is equivalent to 0·0005172 g of CH_3O.

METHYLCELLULOSE 450

It complies with the requirements of the British Pharmacopoeia.
It has a viscosity at 20° of 400 to 500 centistokes.

METHYLCELLULOSE 2500

DESCRIPTION; IDENTIFICATION TESTS; ACIDITY OR ALKALINITY; ARSENIC; LEAD; LOSS ON DRYING; SULPHATED ASH; CONTENT OF METHOXYL. It complies with the tests described under Methylcellulose 20.

VISCOSITY. At 20°, 2200 to 2800 centistokes, determined by the method given above for Methylcellulose 20, a suspended-level viscometer with capillary diameter of 3·70 ± 0·04 mm being used.

METHYLCELLULOSE 4500

DESCRIPTION; IDENTIFICATION TESTS; ACIDITY OR ALKALINITY; ARSENIC; LEAD; LOSS ON DRYING; SULPHATED ASH; CONTENT OF METHOXYL. It complies with the tests described under Methylcellulose 20.

VISCOSITY. At 20°, 4000 to 5000 centistokes, determined by the method given above for Methylcellulose 20, a suspended-level viscometer with capillary diameter of 3·70 ± 0·04 mm being used.

Storage. Methylcellulose should be stored in airtight containers, in a cool place.

Actions and uses. Methylcellulose disperses in cold water to form a viscous colloidal solution. A mucilage may be prepared by adding the methylcellulose to about one-third the required amount of boiling water and, when the powder is thoroughly hydrated, adding the remainder of the water, preferably in the form of ice, and stirring until homogeneous.

Various viscosity grades of methylcellulose are available. High-viscosity grades, such as methylcellulose 2500 and 4500, are used as thickening agents for medicated jellies and creams, as dispersing agents in suspensions, and as binding and disintegrating agents in tablets. A 0·5 to 1 per cent solution of a high-viscosity grade of methylcellulose is sometimes used to increase the viscosity of ophthalmic solutions, but for this purpose hypromellose (page 232) is usually preferred; an antimicrobial agent such as benzalkonium chloride should be incorporated.

Special grades with a high content of methoxyl, or having hydroxypropyl groups in place of some of the methyl groups (hypromellose, page 232) are used as adhesives in Plaster of Paris Bandage.

A low-viscosity grade, such as methylcellulose 20, is used as an emulsifying agent for liquid paraffin and other mineral oils and also for arachis and olive oils; it is less efficient for emulsifying cod-liver oil. Emulsions are prepared by mixing the oil with a methylcellulose mucilage, preferably using a mechanical stirrer.

Medium- and high-viscosity grades, such as methylcellulose 450, 2500, and 4500, are used as bulk laxatives, usually in the form of granules or tablets.

Dose. As a laxative: 1 to 4 grams daily in divided doses.

Preparation
METHYLCELLULOSE GRANULES, B.P.C. (page 703)

OTHER NAMES: *Celacol M®*; *Methocel MC®*

METHYLDOPA

$C_{10}H_{13}NO_4, 1\frac{1}{2}H_2O = 238·2$

Methyldopa is the sesquihydrate of $(-)$-β-(3,4-dihydroxyphenyl)-α-methyl-L-alanine.

Solubility. Soluble, at 20°, in 100 parts of water, in 400 parts of alcohol, and in less than 1 part of dilute hydrochloric acid; very slightly soluble in ether.

Standard
It complies with the requirements of the British Pharmacopoeia.
It is a white to yellowish-white, odourless, fine powder which may contain friable lumps and contains not less than 98·5 and not more than the equivalent of 101·0 per cent of $C_{10}H_{13}NO_4$, calculated with reference to the anhydrous substance. It contains 10·0 to 13·0 per cent w/w of water.

Storage. It should be stored in airtight containers, protected from light.

Actions and uses. Methyldopa inhibits the conversion of dopa to dopamine by competing for the enzyme dopa decarboxylase. In consequence, after the administration of methyldopa there is a reduction in the amount of noradrenaline formed from dopamine, but it has not been proved that this is entirely responsible for its hypotensive effect. Postural hypotension, although it occurs after administration of methyldopa, is never severe, nor does the blood pressure fall much on exercise.

Methyldopa is used in the treatment of moderate to severe hypertension. A thiazide diuretic may be given concurrently to potentiate the hypotensive effect.

The daily dosage of methyldopa is usually the equivalent of 0·5 to 2 grams of anhydrous methyldopa in divided doses; 1·13 grams of methyldopa is approximately equivalent to 1 gram of anhydrous methyldopa. Occasionally, the daily dosage may be increased to the equivalent of 4 grams.

UNDESIRABLE EFFECTS. Tolerance to methyldopa is rarely progressive and can usually be overcome by increasing the dose.

Undesirable effects include drowsiness, depression, dryness of the mouth, diarrhoea, and hyperpyrexia; liver damage, thrombocytopenia, and granulocytopenia have been reported.

Cases of acquired haemolytic anaemia have

rarely occurred, but some patients have developed a positive direct Coombs test without evidence of haemolysis, anaemia, or related clinical effects.

Drowsiness is particularly liable to occur following a rapid increase in dosage.

Oedema resulting from sodium retention may occur; this requires the administration of a diuretic.

CONTRA-INDICATIONS. Methyldopa is contra-indicated in patients with liver damage or dysfunction or with phaeochromocytoma.

Dose. See above under **Actions and uses.**

Preparation
METHYLDOPA TABLETS, B.P. Unless otherwise specified, tablets each containing the equivalent of 250 mg of anhydrous methyldopa are supplied. They are film coated. They should be protected from light. Tablets containing 125 and 500 mg are also available.

OTHER NAMES: *Aldomet®*; *Dopamet®*; *Medomet®*

METHYLENE BLUE

SYNONYM: Methylthionine Chloride

$C_{16}H_{18}ClN_3S,2H_2O = 355.9$

Methylene Blue (Colour Index No. 52015) is tetramethylthionine chloride dihydrate.

Solubility. Soluble, at 20°, in 40 parts of water, in 110 parts of alcohol, and in 450 parts of chloroform.

Standard
It complies with the requirements of the British Pharmacopoeia.

It is a hygroscopic, almost odourless, dark greenish, crystalline powder with a metallic lustre or dull, dark green or brown powder and contains not less than 96.0 and not more than the equivalent of 101.0 per cent of $C_{16}H_{18}ClN_3S$, calculated with reference to the dried substance. The loss on drying under the prescribed conditions is 8.0 to 15.0 per cent.

NOTE. Commercial methylene blue is the double chloride of tetramethylthionine and zinc and is not suitable for medicinal use.

Sterilisation. Solutions for injection are sterilised by heating in an autoclave or by filtration.

Storage. It should be stored in airtight containers.

Actions and uses. Methylene blue is used in the treatment of drug-induced methaemoglobinaemia, for which purpose it is administered by intravenous injection as a 1 per cent solution in doses of 1 to 4 milligrams per kilogram body-weight. It has also been used in the treatment of idiopathic methaemoglobinaemia in a daily dose of 300 milligrams, by mouth, with large doses of ascorbic acid.

Methylene blue is used in a renal function test, especially to compare the function of the two kidneys, but is inferior to indigo carmine for this purpose. For the test, 2 millilitres of a 2.5 per cent solution of methylene blue is injected intramuscularly and the ureteric orifices are examined by cystoscopy. Urine excreted by the normal kidney assumes a greenish colour in about half an hour; a delay in excretion is an indication of impairment of renal function.

Methylene blue has been used as a urinary antibacterial agent but it is of no value for this purpose.

Stains on the skin caused by methylene blue can be removed with a hypochlorite solution.

Dose. 50 to 300 milligrams by mouth; 1 to 4 milligrams per kilogram body-weight by intravenous injection.

METHYLERGOMETRINE MALEATE

$C_{24}H_{29}N_3O_6 = 455.5$

Methylergometrine Maleate is the hydrogen maleate of $(+)$-N-[1-(hydroxymethyl)propyl]-lysergamide, a partially synthetic homologue of ergometrine.

Solubility. Soluble, at 20°, in 200 parts of water, giving a solution with a blue fluorescence, and in 140 parts of alcohol.

Standard
It complies with the requirements of the British Pharmacopoeia.

It is a white or faintly yellow, crystalline powder and contains not less than 95.0 and not more than the equivalent of 105.0 per cent of $C_{24}H_{29}N_3O_6$, calculated with reference to the dried substance. The loss on drying under the prescribed conditions is not more than 2.0 per cent.

Sterilisation. Solutions for injection are sterilised by filtration or by heating in an autoclave in an atmosphere of nitrogen or other suitable gas.

Storage. It should be stored in hermetically sealed containers, protected from light, in an atmosphere of nitrogen.

Actions and uses. Methylergometrine has actions and uses similar to those described under Ergometrine Maleate (page 180), but it is effective in smaller doses. It must not be given in the first and second stages of labour and, because of its powerful oxytocic action, it is not usually administered before the expulsion of the placenta.

Methylergometrine maleate may be administered by mouth in a dose of 250 to 500 micrograms, or by intramuscular injection in a dose of 200 micrograms. It may also be given intravenously in a dose of 50 to 100 micrograms. If the patient is anaesthetised, 200 micrograms may be given intravenously, or 200 to 400 micrograms intramuscularly. If uterine inertia or haemorrhage persists, the dose may be repeated at intervals of two to four hours.

For the treatment of subinvolution or during post-partum convalescence, 250 micrograms may be given by mouth three or four times a day.

Dose. 250 to 500 micrograms by mouth; 100 to 200 micrograms by subcutaneous, intramuscular, or intravenous injection.

Preparations

METHYLERGOMETRINE INJECTION, B.P. It consists of a sterile solution of methylergometrine maleate in Water for Injections, the pH of the solution being adjusted to 3·2. Unless otherwise specified, a solution containing 200 μg in 1 ml is supplied. It should be protected from light.

METHYLERGOMETRINE TABLETS, B.P. Unless otherwise specified, tablets each containing 125 μg of methylergometrine maleate are supplied. They are sugar coated.

OTHER NAME: *Methergin*®

METHYLPREDNISOLONE

$C_{22}H_{30}O_5 = 374·5$

Methylprednisolone is 11β,17α,21-trihydroxy-6α-methylpregna-1,4-diene-3,20-dione.

Solubility. Very slightly soluble in water; soluble, at 20°, in 100 parts of dehydrated alcohol and in 530 parts of chloroform.

Standard
It complies with the requirements of the British Pharmacopoeia.
It is a white or almost white, crystalline, odourless powder and contains not less than 96·0 and not more than the equivalent of 104·0 per cent of $C_{22}H_{30}O_5$, calculated with reference to the dried substance. The loss on drying under the prescribed conditions is not more than 0·5 per cent. It melts with decomposition at about 243°.

Storage. It should be protected from light.

Actions and uses. Methylprednisolone has the actions, uses, and undesirable effects described under Prednisolone (page 399); it is effective in a slightly lower dosage than prednisolone.

PRECAUTIONS AND CONTRA-INDICATIONS. These are as described under Cortisone Acetate (page 132).

Dose. 8 to 80 milligrams daily in divided doses.

Preparation
METHYLPREDNISOLONE TABLETS, B.P. Unless otherwise specified, tablets each containing 4 mg of methylprednisolone are supplied. They should be protected from light. Tablets containing 2 mg are also available.

OTHER NAME: *Medrone*®

METHYLTESTOSTERONE

SYNONYM: Methyltestosteronum

$C_{20}H_{30}O_2 = 302·5$

Methyltestosterone is 17β-hydroxy-17α-methylandrost-4-en-3-one.

Solubility. Very slightly soluble in water; soluble, at 20°, in 5 parts of alcohol, in 10 parts of acetone, and in 160 parts of arachis oil; slightly soluble in ether.

Standard
It complies with the requirements of the European Pharmacopoeia.
It is a white or slightly yellowish-white, crystalline, odourless powder and contains not less than 97·0 and not more than the equivalent of 103·0 per cent of $C_{20}H_{30}O_2$, calculated with reference to the dried substance. The loss on drying under the prescribed conditions is not more than 1·0 per cent. It has a melting-point of 163° to 168°.

Storage. It should be stored in airtight containers, protected from light.

Actions and uses. Methyltestosterone has the actions and uses described under Testosterone (page 494). It has the advantage of being absorbed when given orally or sublingually. When given by mouth it has one-third to one-quarter of the androgenic activity of the same weight of testosterone propionate administered intramuscularly.

In the male, methyltestosterone is generally used for maintenance therapy after the full androgenic effect has been produced by parenteral administration of testosterone propionate. The dosage required varies considerably; it is usual to begin with 30 to 50 milligrams of methyltestosterone daily, in divided doses.

UNDESIRABLE EFFECTS. Jaundice may occur when the drug is given for long periods. Prolonged administration to women may give rise to excessive libido and, with large dosage, virilism may be produced.

PRECAUTIONS AND CONTRA-INDICATIONS. The precautions described under Testosterone (page 494) should be observed. Methyltesto-

sterone is contra-indicated in patients with impaired liver function and in pregnancy.

Dose. 25 to 50 milligrams daily for a man; 5 to 20 milligrams daily for a woman. For mammary carcinoma, 50 to 100 milligrams daily.

Preparation
METHYLTESTOSTERONE TABLETS, B.P. Unless otherwise specified, tablets each containing 5 mg of methyltestosterone are supplied. They should be protected from light. Tablets containing 10, 25, and 50 mg are also available.

OTHER NAMES: *Perandren®*; *Virormone-Oral®*

METHYLTHIOURACIL

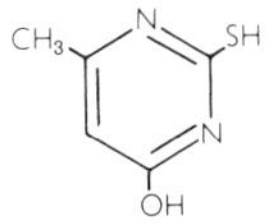

$C_5H_6N_2OS = 142.2$

Methylthiouracil is 4-hydroxy-2-mercapto-6-methylpyrimidine.

Solubility. Very slightly soluble in water, in alcohol, and in dilute mineral acids; soluble in dilute solutions of sodium hydroxide.

Standard
It complies with the requirements of the British Pharmacopoeia.
It is a white or pale cream-coloured odourless powder and contains not less than 98.0 per cent of $C_5H_6N_2OS$, calculated with reference to the dried substance. The loss on drying under the prescribed conditions is not more than 0.5 per cent. It melts with decomposition at about 330°.

Actions and uses. Methylthiouracil has actions and uses similar to those described under Carbimazole (page 77) by which it has been largely replaced.
In thyrotoxicosis, methylthiouracil is given in an initial dosage of 100 to 200 milligrams by mouth twice daily, reduced according to the

therapeutic response to a maintenance dose of 50 to 150 milligrams daily. Even after prolonged administration, relapse occurs in some patients within three months of withdrawal of the drug.

UNDESIRABLE EFFECTS. Toxic effects include granulocytopenia, sore throat, and rashes; less commonly lymphatic glandular enlargement, drug fever, purpura, and dermatitis occur.

Dose. See above under **Actions and uses.**

Preparation
METHYLTHIOURACIL TABLETS, B.P. Unless otherwise specified, tablets each containing 50 mg of methylthiouracil are supplied. Tablets containing 100 mg are also available.

METHYPRYLONE

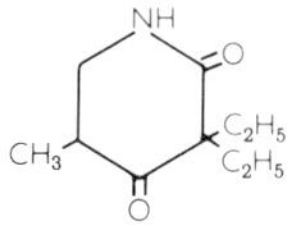

$C_{10}H_{17}NO_2 = 183.2$

Methyprylone is 3,3-diethyl-5-methylpiperidine-2,4-dione.

Solubility. Soluble, at 20°, in 14 parts of water, in less than 1 part of alcohol and of chloroform, and in 3.5 parts of ether.

Standard
It complies with the requirements of the British Pharmacopoeia.
It is a white or almost white, crystalline powder with a slight characteristic odour and contains not less than 98.5 and not more than the equivalent of 101.0 per cent of $C_{10}H_{17}NO_2$, calculated with reference to the dried substance. The loss on drying under the prescribed conditions is not more than 0.5 per cent. It has a melting-point of 74° to 77°.

Storage. It should be stored in airtight containers, protected from light.

Actions and uses. Methyprylone is used as a hypnotic and, less often, as a sedative.
The usual hypnotic dose is 200 to 400 milli-

grams; the effect develops in half to one hour and persists for about six hours. The sedative dose is 50 to 100 milligrams, repeated as required.

UNDESIRABLE EFFECTS. It may give rise to dependence of the barbiturate-alcohol type as described under Phenobarbitone (page 366), enhance the effects of alcohol, and reduce the ability to drive motor cars and operate moving machinery.
The higher hypnotic dose, when given at night, may result in giddiness or drowsiness the next morning.

POISONING. In severe poisoning, treatment should follow that recommended for barbiturate poisoning, as described under Pheno-barbitone (page 366), and may need to be supplemented by vasopressor drugs.

Dose. See above under **Actions and uses.**

Preparation
METHYPRYLONE TABLETS, B.P. Unless otherwise specified, tablets each containing 200 mg of methy-prylone are supplied. They should be stored in airtight containers. Tablets which are not sugar coated should be protected from light.

OTHER NAME: *Noludar*®

METRONIDAZOLE

$C_6H_9N_3O_3 = 171.2$

Metronidazole is 1-(2-hydroxyethyl)-2-methyl-5-nitroimidazole.

Solubility. Soluble, at 20°, in 100 parts of water, in 200 parts of alcohol, and in 250 parts of chloroform; slightly soluble in ether.

Standard
It complies with the requirements of the British Pharmacopoeia.
It is a white or creamy-white crystalline powder with a slight odour and contains not less than 99·0 and not more than the equivalent of 101·0 per cent of $C_6H_9N_3O_3$, calculated with reference to the dried substance. The loss on drying under the prescribed conditions is not more than 0·5 per cent. It has a melting-point of 159° to 162°.

Actions and uses. Metronidazole is a trichomonacide and amoebicide which is active by mouth. When given by mouth an effective concentration of the drug appears in the blood and urine; about half the dose is excreted by the kidneys. Its presence in the vagina does not interfere with the normal acidophilic flora and it has no effect on *Candida* species.
In the treatment of infections due to *Trichomonas vaginalis*, metronidazole is given by mouth, usually in a dosage of 200 milligrams three times a day for seven days; a micro-scopical examination of the vaginal secretion should be made to confirm the diagnosis and cure and to eliminate the possibility of a gonorrhoeal infection. Many relapses may be due to reinfection by the male partner, who may show no clinical signs of infection and may also need treatment. In elderly patients hormone therapy may be necessary in order to clear up any concomitant vaginitis.
Vincent's disease may also be treated with a similar course of metronidazole.
For intestinal and hepatic infections with *Entamoeba histolytica* it is given in dosages varying from 400 milligrams three times a day for five days to 800 milligrams three times a day for ten days.

UNDESIRABLE EFFECTS. Metronidazole may cause headache, malaise, transient rashes, anorexia, nausea, and gastro-intestinal upset. Consumption of alcohol increases the nausea, producing an effect which may then be severe. The urine of patients taking large doses of the drug is stained brown.

Dose. See above under **Actions and uses.**

Preparation
METRONIDAZOLE TABLETS, B.P. Unless otherwise specified, tablets each containing 200 mg of metro-nidazole are supplied.

OTHER NAME: *Flagyl*®

METYRAPONE

$C_{14}H_{14}N_2O = 226.3$

Metyrapone is 2-methyl-1,2-di(3-pyridyl)propan-1-one.

Solubility. Soluble, at 20°, in 100 parts of water, in 3 parts of alcohol, and in 3 parts of chloroform; soluble in dilute mineral acids.

Standard
It complies with the requirements of the British Pharmacopoeia.
It is a white to light amber crystalline powder with a characteristic odour and contains not less than 97·0 and not more than the equivalent of 103·0 per cent of $C_{14}H_{14}N_2O$, calculated with reference to the dried substance. The loss on drying under the prescribed conditions is not more than 0·5 per cent. It has a melting-point of 50° to 53°.
Storage. It should be protected from light.

Actions and uses. Metyrapone is a diag-nostic agent used to investigate the function of the anterior lobe of the pituitary gland. It inhibits 11β-hydroxylase, an enzyme neces-sary for the formation of cortisone and hydrocortisone from their precursors, and the resultant fall in the glucocorticoid blood level stimulates the anterior pituitary gland to secrete corticotrophin. This in turn stimulates production of further glucocorticoid pre-cursors by the adrenal cortex and since metyrapone blocks conversion of these to cortisone and hydrocortisone they are excreted in the urine. Estimation of urinary 17-hydroxycorticosteroids over the period of the test indicates whether or not the anterior pituitary is functioning effectively with regard to corticotrophin secretion.

Metyrapone also interferes with the formation of aldosterone but to a much lesser extent.

Metyrapone is used for the assessment of anterior pituitary lobe function and in the diagnosis of hypopituitarism. It is usually administered by mouth in doses of 250 to 750 milligrams every four hours for six doses; children may be given up to 15 milligrams per kilogram body-weight every four hours.

UNDESIRABLE EFFECTS. Nausea and vomiting may occur, with or without epigastric pain.

Giddiness and hypotension may be experienced if adrenal function is impaired.

PRECAUTIONS. Metyrapone may precipitate acute adrenal failure and should be used with great caution in patients with gross hypopituitarism.

Dose. 250 to 750 milligrams every four hours for six doses.

Preparation
METYRAPONE CAPSULES, B.P. The quantity of metyrapone in each capsule should be specified by the prescriber. They should be protected from light. Capsules containing 250 mg are available.

OTHER NAME: *Metopirone®*

MEXENONE

$C_{15}H_{14}O_3 = 242.3$

Mexenone is 2-hydroxy-4-methoxy-4'-methylbenzophenone.

$$H_3C-\bigcirc-CO-\bigcirc-O\cdot CH_3$$

Solubility. Insoluble in water; soluble, at 20°, in 70 parts of alcohol and in 7 parts of acetone.

Standard
DESCRIPTION. A pale yellow crystalline powder; odourless or almost odourless.

IDENTIFICATION TESTS. 1. It complies with the thin-layer chromatographic test given in Appendix 5, page 865.
2. The ultraviolet absorption spectrum exhibits the characteristics given in Appendix 3, page 855.
3. The infra-red absorption spectrum exhibits maxima which are only at the same wavelengths as, and have similar relative intensities to, those in the spectrum of *mexenone A.S.*

MELTING-POINT. 99° to 102°.

IRON. Ignite 1·0 g with 1 g of *anhydrous sodium carbonate*, cool, dissolve the residue in 5 ml of *hydrochloric acid FeT*, and dilute to 35 ml with water; the solution complies with the limit test for iron (40 parts per million).

RELATED COMPOUNDS. It complies with the test given in Appendix 5, page 865 (0·5 per cent).

LOSS ON DRYING. Not more than 0·5 per cent, determined by drying to constant weight at 60° in vacuo.

SULPHATED ASH. Not more than 0·1 per cent.

CONTENT OF $C_{15}H_{14}O_3$. Not less than 97·0 and not more than the equivalent of 103·0 per cent, calculated

with reference to the substance dried under the prescribed conditions, determined by the following method:
Dissolve about 0·06 g, accurately weighed, in *methyl alcohol* and dilute to 100 ml with *methyl alcohol*; dilute 10 ml of this solution to 100 ml with *methyl alcohol*, further dilute 10 ml of this solution to 100 ml with the same solvent, and measure the extinction of a 1-cm layer at the maximum at about 287 nm.
For purposes of calculation, use a value of 640 for the E(1 per cent, 1 cm) of $C_{15}H_{14}O_3$. Calculate the percentage of $C_{15}H_{14}O_3$ in the sample.

Actions and uses. Mexenone is characterised by its ability to absorb ultraviolet radiation over a wide range of wavelengths and even in low concentrations shows a sharp cut-off at about 350 nanometres, as the wavelength approaches that of visible light. It is used as a sun-screening compound in preparations designed to reduce the risk of sunburn and other light-induced dermatoses. It is applied in a concentration of 4 per cent in an aqueous cream basis.

Preparation
MEXENONE CREAM, B.P.C. (page 659)

OTHER NAME: *Uvistat 2211®*

SELF-EMULSIFYING MONOSTEARIN

SYNONYM: Glyceryl Monostearate Self-emulsifying

Self-emulsifying Monostearin is a mixture consisting principally of mono-, di-, and tri-glyceryl esters of stearic and palmitic acids, with small quantities of the corresponding esters of oleic and other fatty acids; it also contains free fatty acids, free glycerol, and a small percentage of potassium, sodium, or triethanolamine oleate or stearate.

Solubility. Dispersible in hot water; soluble in hot dehydrated alcohol, in hot liquid paraffin, and, subject to turbidity at concentrations below 20 per cent, in hot vegetable oils.

Standard
DESCRIPTION. A white to cream-coloured hard fat of waxy appearance; odour faint and fatty.

ACID VALUE. Not more than 18.

IODINE VALUE. Not more than 8, determined by the iodine monochloride method.

MELTING-POINT. 54° to 57°, determined by Method IV of the British Pharmacopoeia, Appendix IVA.

ALKALINITY. Shake 1·0 g with 20 ml of hot *carbon dioxide-free water* and allow to cool, with continuous shaking; the aqueous liquid has a pH of 8·0 to 10·0.

FREE GLYCEROL. Not more than 7·0 per cent, calculated as $C_3H_8O_3$, determined by the following method:
Dilute the aqueous extracts obtained in the determination of α-monoglyceride to 100 ml with water; add 50 ml of this solution to 25 ml of *periodic–acetic acid solution* and 25 ml of *glacial acetic acid* in an iodine flask and continue as for the determination of α-monoglyceride beginning with the words "and allow to stand for 30 minutes . . .".
The difference between the two titrations represents the amount or periodic–acetic acid required to oxidise the free glycerol; each ml of 0·1N sodium thiosulphate is equivalent to 0·002303 g of $C_3H_8O_3$.

SOAP. 2·5 to 7·0 per cent, calculated as sodium oleate, $C_{18}H_{33}NaO_2$, determined by the following method:
Add about 10 g, accurately weighed, to a mixture of 60 ml of *acetone* and 0·15 ml of *bromophenol blue solution (0·5 per cent)*, previously neutralised with 0·1N hydrochloric acid or 0·1N sodium hydroxide, warm gently on a water-bath until solution is completed, and titrate with 0·1N hydrochloric acid until the blue colour is discharged; allow to stand for 20 minutes, warm until any solidified matter has redissolved, and, if the blue colour reappears, continue the titration; each ml of 0·1N hydrochloric acid is equivalent to 0·03045 g of $C_{18}H_{33}NaO_2$.

CONTENT OF α-MONOGLYCERIDE. 30·0 to 40·0 per cent, calculated as $C_{21}H_{42}O_4$, determined by the following method:
Dissolve, by warming gently, about 0·8 g, accurately weighed, in 20 ml of *chloroform*, extract by shaking for one minute with 2 ml of *glacial acetic acid* diluted with 25 ml of water, followed by three successive 2-ml portions of *glacial acetic acid* diluted with 20 ml of water.
Wash the combined aqueous extracts with 5 ml of *chloroform*, reserve the aqueous extracts, and dilute the combined chloroformic solution and washings to 100 ml with *chloroform*; heat 25 ml of this solution in an iodine flask on a water-bath to remove the chloroform, dissolve the residue in 1 ml of *chloroform*, add 10 ml of *glacial acetic acid* and 20 ml of *periodic–acetic acid solution*, warm on a water-bath at a temperature not exceeding 45° until the mixture is just molten, shake for one minute, rinse the stopper and flask walls with *glacial acetic acid*, and allow to stand for 30 minutes at 20° to 30°; add 5 ml of a freshly prepared 20 per cent w/v solution of *potassium iodide* in water, and titrate the liberated iodine with 0·1N sodium thiosulphate, using *starch mucilage* as indicator.
Repeat the procedure omitting the sample.
The difference between the two titrations represents the amount of periodic–acetic acid required to oxidise the α-monoglyceride; each ml of 0·1N sodium thiosulphate is equivalent to 0·01793 g of $C_{21}H_{42}O_4$.

Incompatibility. Owing to the presence of soap, it is incompatible with acids and high concentrations of ionisable salts and with zinc oxide and oxides of heavy metals.

Uses. Self-emulsifying monostearin is used as an emulsifying agent for oils, fats, solvents, and waxes in the preparation of bases of the non-emulsified, emulsified, and vanishing-cream types. It produces stable, fine-grained creams, which are reasonably resistant to extremes of temperature. For ointments and more viscous creams, 5 to 20 per cent of self-emulsifying monostearin may be used. It is not intended for inclusion in preparations for internal use.
Aqueous preparations containing self-emulsifying monostearin should contain a preservative to prevent fungous or bacterial growth.

MORPHINE HYDROCHLORIDE

SYNONYMS: Morph. Hydrochlor.; Morphinii Chloridum

$C_{17}H_{20}ClNO_3,3H_2O = 375·8$

Morphine Hydrochloride may be prepared by treating morphine, the principal alkaloid of opium, with diluted hydrochloric acid.

Solubility. Soluble, at 20°, in 24 parts of water, in 100 parts of alcohol, and in 10 parts of glycerol; insoluble in ether and in chloroform.

Standard
It complies with the requirements of the European Pharmacopoeia.
It occurs as odourless, colourless, silky crystals, crystalline powder, or cubical white masses and contains not less than 98·0 per cent of $C_{17}H_{20}ClNO_3$, calculated with reference to the dried substance. The loss on drying under the prescribed conditions is 12·0 to 15·0 per cent.

Incompatibility. It is incompatible with solutions of ammonia and with vegetable astringents.

Sterilisation. Solutions for injection are sterilised by heating with a bactericide or by filtration.

Storage. It should be stored in airtight containers, protected from light.

Actions and uses. Morphine is a powerful analgesic and narcotic, but it also has central stimulant actions. It especially depresses the thalamus, sensory cortex, and respiratory and cough centres; it stimulates the spinal cord, the vagus and vomiting centres, and the third-nerve nucleus. Occasionally the stimulant actions are seen before or without the usual narcotic effects. Morphine increases tone in involuntary muscle, especially the sphincters of the gastro-intestinal tract. It reduces secretions, except those of the skin glands. It dilates skin vessels, but, in therapeutic doses, it has little effect on the circulation as a whole.
Morphine is used to relieve pain, anxiety, and sleeplessness due to pain. It reduces all disagreeable sensations apart from skin irritation. Where sleeplessness is not due to pain, dyspnoea, or cough, morphine usually fails to induce sleep when used in ordinary doses. Its analgesic action reaches a maximum in about an hour and persists for three or four hours. It is more effective when injected than when taken by mouth.
Morphine is invaluable in such emergencies as cardiac asthma and acute abdominal conditions such as perforation, and in the

treatment of severe trauma, for which it should be given in doses of 15 to 20 milligrams. Since it masks warning symptoms and physical signs, it is not given until a diagnosis has been made.

As a sedative and for pre-operative medication morphine is usually administered with atropine or hyoscine.

A dose of 5 to 10 milligrams of morphine hydrochloride often checks coughing, but for this action codeine is more commonly used. When the constipating effect of morphine is desired, it is often prescribed in a mixture containing kaolin.

Morphine has no local analgesic action and its use in local applications has no sound basis.

UNDESIRABLE EFFECTS. Tolerance is rapidly acquired and morphine produces marked euphoria and dependence (see below). Very young children are particularly susceptible to opiates; atypical and alarming effects sometimes occur in the elderly.

PRECAUTIONS. Morphine should not be given to patients who are being treated with a monoamine-oxidase inhibitor, such as isocarboxazid, nialamide, phenelzine, or tranylcypromine, or within about ten days of the discontinuation of such treatment.

DEPENDENCE. Dependence of the morphine type is characterised by (i) strong psychic dependence, (ii) an early development of physical dependence, which increases in intensity as the dosage is increased, and (iii) development of tolerance, necessitating increased dosage to obtain the initial effects.

POISONING. If the drug has been taken by mouth, the stomach should be washed out; a 0·2 per cent solution of potassium permanganate is commonly used for this purpose. A saline purgative may then be administered to reduce absorption from the gastrointestinal tract.

The most important aspect of treatment is to guard the patient from respiratory failure; for this purpose nalorphine or levallorphan should be used only when respiration is dangerously depressed. Artificial respiration may be required.

Dose. See above under **Actions and uses.**

Preparations
AMMONIUM CHLORIDE AND MORPHINE MIXTURE, B.P.C. (page 736)
IPECACUANHA AND MORPHINE MIXTURE, B.P.C. (page 745)
KAOLIN AND MORPHINE MIXTURE, B.P.C. (page 746)
MORPHINE HYDROCHLORIDE SOLUTION, B.P.C. (page 788)
MORPHINE SUPPOSITORIES, B.P.C. (page 798)
CHLOROFORM AND MORPHINE TINCTURE, B.P.C. (page 821)

MORPHINE SULPHATE

SYNONYM: Morph. Sulph.

$(C_{17}H_{19}NO_3)_2,H_2SO_4,5H_2O = 758·8$

Morphine Sulphate may be prepared by treating morphine, the principal alkaloid of opium, with diluted sulphuric acid.

Solubility. Soluble, at 20°, in 21 parts of water and in 1000 parts of alcohol; insoluble in ether and in chloroform.

Standard
It complies with the requirements of the British Pharmacopoeia.
It occurs as odourless, white, acicular crystals, cubical masses, or crystalline powder and contains not less than 98·0 and not more than the equivalent of 101·0 per cent of $(C_{17}H_{19}NO_3)_2,H_2SO_4$, calculated with reference to the dried substance. The loss on drying under the prescribed conditions is 9·0 to 12·0 per cent.

Incompatibility. It is incompatible with solutions of ammonia and with vegetable astringents.

Sterilisation. Solutions for injection are sterilised by heating with a bactericide or by filtration.

Storage. It should be stored in airtight containers, protected from light.

Actions and uses. Morphine sulphate has the actions, uses, and undesirable effects described under Morphine Hydrochloride.

PRECAUTIONS; DEPENDENCE. See under Morphine Hydrochloride.

POISONING. The procedure as described under Morphine Hydrochloride should be adopted.

Dose. 10 to 20 milligrams by mouth or by subcutaneous or intramuscular injection.

Preparations
MORPHINE AND ATROPINE INJECTION, B.P.C. (page 715)
MORPHINE SULPHATE INJECTION, B.P. (*Syn.* Morphine Injection). It consists of a sterile solution of morphine sulphate in Water for Injections containing 0·1 per cent of sodium metabisulphite. The strength of the solution should be specified by the prescriber. It should be protected from light. Ampoules containing 10, 15, 20, and 30 mg in 1 ml are available.
MORPHINE SUPPOSITORIES, B.P.C. (page 798)
MORPHINE SULPHATE TABLETS, B.P. The quantity of morphine sulphate in each tablet should be specified by the prescriber. They should be protected from light. Tablets containing 10, 15, 30, and 60 mg are available.

MUSTINE HYDROCHLORIDE

SYNONYMS: Mechlorethamine Hydrochloride; Nitrogen Mustard $[CH_3 \cdot N(CH_2 \cdot CH_2Cl)_2]HCl$

$C_5H_{12}Cl_3N = 192.5$

Mustine Hydrochloride is di(2-chloroethyl)methylamine hydrochloride.

CAUTION. *Mustine Hydrochloride is highly toxic; it is a powerful vesicant and a strong nasal irritant.*

Solubility. Very soluble in water.

Standard
It complies with the requirements of the British Pharmacopoeia.
It is white or almost white, crystalline, vesicant, hygroscopic powder or mass and contains not less than 98·0 and not more than the equivalent of 101·0 per cent of $C_5H_{12}Cl_3N$. It has a melting-point of about 108°.

Storage. It should be stored in airtight containers, in a cool place.

Actions and uses. Mustine is a cytotoxic agent which acts mainly on proliferating cells by alkylating the nucleic acids of the chromosomes. When administered by intravenous injection it causes a fall in the number of circulating lymphocytes and depresses the activity of the bone marrow, resulting in granulocytopenia, thrombocytopenia, and anaemia. Mustine hydrochloride is rapidly hydrolysed in the body.

Mustine is used in the treatment of Hodgkin's disease which has become resistant to irradiation treatment; it brings about a temporary remission of symptoms, but relapse occurs after a period of several months. Subsequent courses of treatment are usually less effective than the first. In the treatment of leukaemias and polycythaemia vera, mustine has been used as an alternative to irradiation.

The recommended dosage is 0·1 milligram of mustine hydrochloride per kilogram body-weight by intravenous injection daily on four consecutive days, after which there should be a rest period of at least six weeks. Regardless of body-weight, a single dose should not exceed 10 milligrams. The response should be assessed by examination of bone-marrow smears and blood counts. Necrosis may occur if the solution is not sufficiently diluted and not carefully administered directly into the vein.

A solution containing 1 milligram per millilitre in Sodium Chloride Injection is suitable for intravenous injection and a solution containing 1 milligram in 50 millilitres of Sodium Chloride Injection may be given by slow intravenous infusion.

Solutions for injection are prepared by an aseptic technique.

UNDESIRABLE EFFECTS. Mustine commonly causes nausea and vomiting; 0·5 to 1 milligram of hyoscine hydrobromide by subcutaneous injection or 4 to 8 milligrams of perphenazine by mouth may relieve these symptoms.

Other possible undesirable effects of mustine include liver damage, skin reactions, transient anorexia, light-headedness, drowsiness, and temporary amenorrhoea in women. Diarrhoea and gastric erosions may occur in some patients. Thrombophlebitis is a potential hazard if mustine is insufficiently diluted.

Mustine has a vesicant action on skin and mucous membrane, and care must be taken to avoid extravasation during injection. Should this occur, isotonic sodium thiosulphate solution (3 per cent) should be infiltrated into the affected area, and ice compresses then applied.

Overdosage with mustine causes severe haemopoietic depression, leading to severe anaemia, lymphocytopenia, granulocytopenia, and thrombocytopenic purpura. The last mentioned may cause bleeding from mucous membranes, and the granulocytopenia may be severe enough to be fatal.

PRECAUTIONS AND CONTRA-INDICATIONS. Mustine hydrochloride should not be given to patients with acute leukaemia, or with severe bone-marrow depression. Dosage should be controlled by blood counts. It should not be used in pregnancy.

Dose. See above under **Actions and uses.**

Preparation
MUSTINE INJECTION, B.P. It consists of a sterile solution of mustine hydrochloride prepared immediately before use by dissolving the sterile contents of a sealed container in Water for Injections. The quantity of mustine hydrochloride in each container should be specified by the prescriber. Vials containing 10 mg are available.

MYRRH

Myrrh is an oleo-gum-resin obtained from the stem of *Commiphora molmol* (Engl.) Engl. and possibly other species of *Commiphora* (Fam. Burseraceae), shrubs or small trees growing in north-eastern Africa and southern Arabia.

Constituents. Myrrh contains 25 to 40 per cent of resin, 57 to 61 per cent of gum, 7 to 17 per cent of volatile oil, a bitter principle, and 3 to 4 per cent of impurities. The resin consists principally of free resin acids. Both volatile oil and resin yield the same characteristic violet reaction with bromine vapour.

Standard

DESCRIPTION. Rounded or irregular tears, about 1·5 to 2·5 cm in diameter, or masses of agglutinated tears, up to about 10 cm across. Externally it is reddish-brown or reddish-yellow in colour, dry, and often covered with a fine dust. It breaks with a brittle fracture, exhibiting a granular, somewhat translucent surface, which is oily and of a rich brown colour and frequently exhibits whitish spots or veins.

Myrrh has an agreeably aromatic odour and an aromatic bitter acrid taste. When triturated with water, a yellowish emulsion is produced.

IDENTIFICATION TEST. Triturate 0·1 g with 0·5 g of sand, shake with 3 ml of *solvent ether*, filter, allow the filtrate to evaporate to a thin film, and pass the vapour of *bromine* over the film; a violet colour is produced.

ALCOHOL (90 PER CENT)-INSOLUBLE MATTER. Not more than 70·0 per cent, determined by the following method:

Macerate and wash about 2 g, accurately weighed, in a sintered-glass crucible with hot *alcohol (90 per cent)* until all soluble matter has been extracted; dry the residue to constant weight at 100°.

FOREIGN ORGANIC MATTER. Not more than 4·0 per cent.

VOLATILE OIL. Not less than 7·0 per cent v/w, determined by the method of Appendix 13, page 893.

ASH. Not more than 9·0 per cent.

Adulterants and substitutes. Fahdli or Arabian myrrh occurs in small masses of agglutinated tears with a less dusty surface and free from whitish marking

on the fractured surface. It is less bitter in taste and also less fragrant than genuine Somali myrrh.

Yemen myrrh occurs in large dusty pieces. It does not exhibit whitish streaks, does not exude oil when pressed with the finger-nail, and is less aromatic than myrrh.

Perfumed bdellium or bissabol closely resembles myrrh. It breaks with a waxy fracture and gives an oily exudate when pressed with the finger-nail. The whitish markings on the fractured surface are traversed by brown resin patches. It differs from myrrh both in odour and taste and does not respond to the colour test; it is probably obtained from *C. erythraea* (Ehrenb.) Engl. var. *glabrescens* Engl.

Opaque bdellium is a very hard, yellowish-brown, opaque gum-resin with a slight odour and a bitter taste.

African bdellium occurs in hard pieces, translucent in thin layers and breaking with a dull slaty fracture; it has a bitter taste and an odour recalling that of pepper.

Indian bdellium occurs in irregular, reddish-brown masses. The fractured surface is hard and, like the outer surface, covered with minute, shiny points of resin. It has a slight cedar-like odour, which develops on keeping, and an acrid but not bitter taste.

Gum hotai occurs in liver-coloured opaque masses. It contains an acid resin and a saponin.

Finely powdered myrrh is deficient in volatile oil and may yield as much as 13 per cent of ash.

Storage. It should be stored in a cool dry place.

Actions and uses. Myrrh is astringent to the mucous membrane; the tincture is used in mouth-washes and gargles for application to ulcers in the mouth and pharynx.

Preparation

MYRRH TINCTURE, B.P.C. (page 822)

NALIDIXIC ACID

$C_{12}H_{12}N_2O_3 = 232\cdot2$

Nalidixic Acid is 1-ethyl-7-methyl-4-oxo-1,8-naphthyridine-3-carboxylic acid.

Solubility. Insoluble in water; slightly soluble in alcohol; soluble, at 20°, in 25 parts of chloroform and in 350 parts of acetone; slightly soluble in solutions of alkali hydroxides.

Standard

DESCRIPTION. An almost white or very pale yellow crystalline powder; odourless or almost odourless.

IDENTIFICATION TESTS. 1. The ultraviolet absorption spectrum exhibits the characteristics given in Appendix 3, page 855.

2. The infra-red absorption spectrum exhibits maxima which are only at the same wavelengths as, and have the same relative intensities to, those in the spectrum of *nalidixic acid A.S.*

MELTING-POINT. 225° to 231°.

LOSS ON DRYING. Not more than 0·5 per cent, determined by drying to constant weight at 105°.

SULPHATED ASH. Not more than 0·2 per cent.

CONTENT OF $C_{12}H_{12}N_2O_3$. Not less than 98·0 and not more than the equivalent of 102·0 per cent, calculated with reference to the substance dried under the

prescribed conditions, determined by the following method:

Dissolve about 0·15 g, accurately weighed, in 25 ml of *dimethylformamide* and titrate with 0·1N tetrabutyl-ammonium hydroxide, using a 0·2 per cent w/v solution of *thymolphthalein* in *methyl alcohol* as indicator; each ml of 0·1N tetrabutylammonium hydroxide is equivalent to 0·02322 g of $C_{12}H_{12}N_2O_3$.

Storage. It should be stored in airtight containers, protected from light.

Actions and uses. Nalidixic acid is an antibacterial agent which is effective against infections by Gram-negative organisms, including *Escherichia coli*, *Aerobacter aerogenes*, *Klebsiella pneumoniae*, *Salmonella typhimurium*, *Shigella flexneri*, and species of *Proteus*. After oral administration it is rapidly absorbed and excreted by the kidneys, so that antibacterial concentrations are not reached in the tissues. Nalidixic acid is used for the treatment of infections of the urinary tract and gastro-intestinal tract when these are due to susceptible organisms. The usual dose for adults is 1 gram four times a day; children may be given 60 milligrams per kilogram body-weight daily in divided doses. When treatment is prolonged in chronic conditions these doses should be halved.

Nalidixic acid has also been used for the treatment of brucellosis.

UNDESIRABLE EFFECTS. Nausea, vomiting, dizziness, drowsiness, weakness, pruritus, and rashes may occur.

Disturbances of the central nervous system, including visual disturbances, excitement, depression, confusion, and hallucinations may occur, but these reactions are transient and reversible.

Patients should avoid unnecessary exposure to sunlight during treatment with nalidixic acid, as photosensitivity reactions may occur.

Dose. See above under **Actions and uses.**

Preparations
NALIDIXIC ACID MIXTURE, B.P.C. (page 747)
NALIDIXIC ACID TABLETS, B.P.C. (page 813)

OTHER NAME: *Negram*®

NALORPHINE HYDROBROMIDE

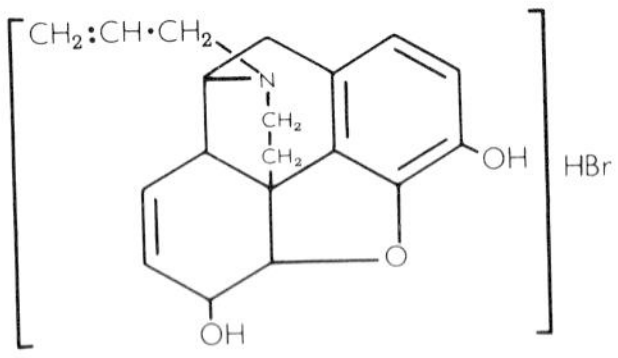

$C_{19}H_{22}BrNO_3 = 392\cdot3$

Nalorphine Hydrobromide is *N*-allylnormorphine hydrobromide.

Solubility. Soluble, at 20°, in 24 parts of water and in 35 parts of alcohol.

Standard
It complies with the requirements of the British Pharmacopoeia.
It is a white to creamy-white, crystalline, odourless powder and contains not less than 98·0 per cent of $C_{19}H_{22}BrNO_3$, calculated with reference to the dried substance. The loss on drying under the prescribed conditions is not more than 1·0 per cent. It melts with decomposition at about 260°.
Crystals of the dihydrate may be deposited from aqueous solutions; the anhydrous salt separates from solutions of the dihydrate in dehydrated alcohol.

Sterilisation. Solutions for injection are sterilised by heating in an autoclave or by filtration.

Storage. It should be stored in airtight containers, protected from light.

Actions and uses. Nalorphine reduces or abolishes most of the characteristic actions of morphine, other opiates, and many related synthetic substances, such as pethidine and methadone, and thus substantially lessens the toxicity of such drugs. It has no comparable action against the toxic effects of ether, cyclopropane, and barbiturates.

Nalorphine has analgesic properties similar to those described under Morphine Hydrochloride (page 314), but it is unsuitable for use as an analgesic, because of its unpleasant side-effects.

Nalorphine hydrobromide is given by intravenous injection in doses of 5 to 10 milligrams in the treatment of poisoning by mor-phine or its substitutes. It acts within twenty seconds, and the dose may have to be repeated, depending on the severity of the intoxication, up to a total of 40 milligrams. It is also used in the treatment of respiratory depression due to opiates and in opiate-induced respiratory depression in the newborn. Ten minutes or so before the expected time of delivery, nalorphine hydrobromide may be given to the mother in a dose of 10 milligrams, intravenously, or it may be injected into the umbilical vein of the newborn infant in a dose of 0·25 to 1 milligram.

Nalorphine is used in the diagnosis of drug dependence, as it provokes prompt and possibly severe withdrawal symptoms in the addict.

UNDESIRABLE EFFECTS. These include sweating, restlessness, pallor, nausea, bradycardia, and hypotension. Although it antagonises respiratory depression due to morphine and similar drugs, nalorphine is itself a potent respiratory depressant.

Dose. See above under **Actions and uses.**

Preparation
NALORPHINE INJECTION, B.P. It consists of a sterile solution of nalorphine hydrobromide in Water for Injections, the pH of the solution being adjusted to 3. Unless otherwise specified, a solution containing 10 mg in 1 ml is supplied. Ampoules containing 1 mg in 1 ml are also available. It should be protected from light.

OTHER NAME: *Lethidrone*®

NANDROLONE DECANOATE

$C_{28}H_{44}O_3 = 428 \cdot 7$

Nandrolone Decanoate is 17β-decanoyloxyoestr-4-en-3-one.

Solubility. Very slightly soluble in water; soluble, at 20°, in 1 part of alcohol; readily soluble in ether, in chloroform, in fixed oils, and in esters.

Standard
It complies with the requirements of the British Pharmacopoeia.
It is a white to creamy-white, crystalline powder with a faint characteristic odour and contains not less than 97·0 and not more than the equivalent of 103·0 per cent of $C_{28}H_{44}O_3$, calculated with reference to the dried substance. The loss on drying under the prescribed conditions is not more than 0·5 per cent. It has a melting-point of about 35°.

Sterilisation. Oily solutions for injection are sterilised by dry heat.

Storage. It should be stored under nitrogen at a temperature between 2° and 10° and protected from light.

Actions and uses. Nandrolone decanoate has the actions, uses, undesirable effects, and contra-indications described under Methandienone (page 299), but it is not active when given by mouth.
It is usually given by intramuscular injection in doses of 50 to 100 milligrams, and its action lasts for three or four weeks. For infants the dose is 10 to 25 milligrams. Jaundice has not been reported after its use.

Dose. See above under **Actions and uses.**

Preparation
NANDROLONE DECANOATE INJECTION, B.P. It consists of a sterile solution of nandrolone decanoate in ethyl oleate or other suitable ester, in a suitable fixed oil, or in any mixture of these. Unless otherwise specified, a solution containing 25 mg in 1 ml is supplied. A solution containing 50 mg in 1ml is also available. It should be protected from light.

OTHER NAME: *Deca-Durabolin®*

NANDROLONE PHENYLPROPIONATE

$C_{27}H_{34}O_3 = 406 \cdot 6$

Nandrolone Phenylpropionate is 17β-(β-phenylpropionyloxy)oestr-4-en-3-one.

Solubility. Very slightly soluble in water; soluble, at 20°, in 20 parts of alcohol.

Standard
It complies with the requirements of the British Pharmacopoeia.
It is a white to creamy-white crystalline powder with a characteristic odour and contains not less than 97·0 and not more than the equivalent of 103·0 per cent of $C_{27}H_{34}O_3$, calculated with reference to the dried substance. The loss on drying under the prescribed conditions is not more than 0·5 per cent. It has a melting-point of 95° to 99°

Sterilisation. Oily solutions for injection are sterilised by dry heat.

Storage. It should be protected from light.

Actions and uses. Nandrolone phenylpropionate has the actions, uses, and undesirable effects described under Methandienone (page 299), but it is not active when given by mouth.
It is usually given by intramuscular injection in a dosage of 25 to 50 milligrams weekly. Jaundice has not been reported after its use.

Dose. See above under **Actions and uses.**

Preparation
NANDROLONE PHENYLPROPIONATE INJECTION, B.P. It consists of a sterile solution of nandrolone phenylpropionate in ethyl oleate or other suitable ester, in a suitable fixed oil, or in any mixture of these. Unless otherwise specified, a solution containing 25 mg in 1 ml is supplied. It should be protected from light.

OTHER NAMES: *Durabolin®*; Nandrolone Phenpropionate

NAPHAZOLINE NITRATE

$C_{14}H_{15}N_3O_3 = 273 \cdot 3$

Naphazoline Nitrate is 2-(naphth-1-ylmethyl)-2-imidazoline nitrate.

Solubility. Soluble, at 20°, in 36 parts of water and in 16 parts of alcohol; very slightly soluble in ether and in chloroform.

Standard
It complies with the requirements of the British Pharmacopoeia.

It is a white or almost white, crystalline, odourless powder and contains not less than 99·0 and not more than the equivalent of 101·0 per cent of $C_{14}H_{15}N_3O_3$, calculated with reference to the dried substance. The loss on drying under the prescribed conditions is not more than 0·5 per cent. It has a melting-point of about 168°. A 1 per cent solution in water has a pH of 5·0 to 6·5.

Sterilisation. Solutions are sterilised by heating with a bactericide or by filtration.

Storage. It should be stored in airtight containers, protected from light.

Actions and uses. Naphazoline has a potent vasoconstrictor action comparable with that of adrenaline, but it does not produce prolonged vasoconstriction at the site of subcutaneous or intramuscular injection.

Naphazoline nitrate is applied in the form of nasal drops containing 0·05 or 0·1 per cent to reduce local swelling and congestion in cases of acute or chronic rhinitis of allergic or inflammatory origin, vasomotor rhinitis, and rhinosinusitis. It is also used as eye-drops containing 0·05 per cent to relieve inflammation of the cornea.

UNDESIRABLE EFFECTS. Naphazoline differs from the sympathomimetic amines in producing some central nervous depression after overdosage or accidental oral ingestion; drowsiness or even coma may result.

PRECAUTIONS. Frequent or prolonged use of naphazoline is undesirable as it usually gives rise to congestion of the mucosa and a return of symptoms; for this reason the smallest effective concentration should be used at intervals of not less than four to six hours.

OTHER NAME: *Privine®*

NEOMYCIN SULPHATE

SYNONYM: Neomycini Sulfas

Neomycin Sulphate is a mixture of the sulphates of the antimicrobial substances produced by the growth of certain selected strains of *Streptomyces fradiae*.

Solubility. Readily soluble in 3 parts of water; slowly soluble in 1 part of water; very slightly soluble in alcohol; insoluble in ether, in chloroform, and in acetone.

Standard
It complies with the requirements of the European Pharmacopoeia.
It is a white or yellowish-white, hygroscopic, almost odourless powder and contains not less than 650 Units per mg and 27·0 to 31·0 per cent of SO_4, calculated with reference to the dried substance. The loss on drying under the prescribed conditions is not more than 6·0 per cent. A 10 per cent solution in water has a pH of 5·0 to 7·5.

Storage. It should be stored in airtight containers, protected from light, at a temperature not exceeding 30°.

Actions and uses. Neomycin is an antibiotic belonging to the same group as kanamycin and having the same wide antibacterial spectrum as described under Kanamycin Sulphate (page 257). Kanamycin is preferred for systemic therapy as it has a slightly greater margin of safety.

Neomycin is used topically for the control of staphylococcal infections and staphylococcal carriage. It is also administered by mouth for the suppression of bacterial growth in the large bowel. However, because of the increasing prevalence of resistant staphylococci and large bowel flora these uses are being abandoned.

In the treatment of hepatic coma 1 gram may be given by mouth every four hours to reduce the absorption of protein breakdown products, but continued use may cause serious malabsorption.

UNDESIRABLE EFFECTS. Neomycin may give rise to hypersensitivity. It enhances the action of gallamine, suxamethonium, and tubocurarine, and may give rise to neuromuscular blockade.

Neomycin also enhances the effect of hypotensive drugs and the antihypertensive effect of thiazide diuretics.

PRECAUTIONS. Neomycin should not be used in the systemic treatment of infections because of its toxic effect on the kidneys and the eighth cranial nerve. Application to extensive raw areas, wounds, and cavities, and oral administration for long periods especially in the presence of ulceration should be avoided as it may give rise to symptoms of ototoxicity. Local application should be limited to the treatment of neomycin-sensitive staphylococcal infections and prolonged topical use should be avoided as it leads to skin sensitisation which may be obscured but not prevented by the concomitant use of corticosteroids.

Dose. As an intestinal antiseptic: 2 to 8 grams by mouth daily in divided doses.

Preparations
HYDROCORTISONE AND NEOMYCIN CREAM, B.P.C. (page 659)
NEOMYCIN CREAM, B.P.C. (page 660)
HYDROCORTISONE AND NEOMYCIN EAR-DROPS, B.P.C. (page 665)
NEOMYCIN ELIXIR, B.P.C. (page 673)

HYDROCORTISONE AND NEOMYCIN EYE-DROPS, B.P.C. (page 691)

NEOMYCIN EYE-DROPS, B.P.C. (page 693)

HYDROCORTISONE AND NEOMYCIN EYE OINTMENT, B.P.C. (page 699)

NEOMYCIN EYE OINTMENT, B.P.C. (page 700)

NEOMYCIN AND BACITRACIN OINTMENT, B.P.C. (page 762)

NEOMYCIN TABLETS, B.P. Unless otherwise specified, tablets each containing 350,000 Units of neomycin sulphate are supplied. They should be stored in airtight containers, protected from light, at a temperature not exceeding 30°.

OTHER NAMES: *Mycifradin*®; *Neolate*®; *Neomin*®; *Nivemycin*®

NEOSTIGMINE BROMIDE

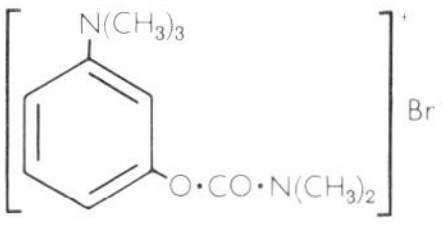

SYNONYMS: Neostig. Brom.; Neostigminii Bromidum

$C_{12}H_{19}BrN_2O_2$ = 303·2

Neostigmine Bromide is (*m*-dimethylcarbamoyloxyphenyl)trimethylammonium bromide.

Solubility. Soluble, at 20°, in less than 1 part of water and in 8 parts of alcohol; soluble in chloroform; almost insoluble in ether.

Standard
It complies with the requirements of the European Pharmacopoeia.
It occurs as odourless colourless crystals or white crystalline powder and contains not less than 98·5 per cent of $C_{12}H_{19}BrN_2O_2$, calculated with reference to the dried substance. The loss on drying under the prescribed conditions is not more than 1·0 per cent.

Storage. It should be stored in airtight containers, protected from light.

Actions and uses. Neostigmine bromide has the actions described under Neostigmine Methylsulphate. It is given by mouth in the treatment of myasthenia gravis.

UNDESIRABLE EFFECTS. As for Physostigmine Salicylate (page 380). In addition, neostigmine bromide, by increasing intestinal motility, may cause disruption of intestinal suture lines.

POISONING. As for Neostigmine Methylsulphate.

Dose. 15 to 30 milligrams by mouth, the frequency of the dose being determined in accordance with the needs of the patient.

Preparation
NEOSTIGMINE TABLETS, B.P. Unless otherwise specified, tablets each containing 15 mg of neostigmine bromide are supplied. They should be stored in airtight containers, protected from light.

OTHER NAME: *Prostigmin*®

NEOSTIGMINE METHYLSULPHATE

SYNONYM: Neostig. Methylsulph.

$C_{12}H_{18}N_2O_2,CH_4O_4S$ = 334·4

Neostigmine Methylsulphate is (*m*-dimethylcarbamoyloxyphenyl)trimethylammonium methyl sulphate.

Solubility. Soluble, at 20°, in less than 1 part of water and in 6 parts of alcohol.

Standard
It complies with the requirements of the British Pharmacopoeia.
It occurs as odourless colourless crystals or white crystalline powder and contains not less than 98·5 per cent of $C_{12}H_{18}N_2O_2,CH_4O_4S$, calculated with reference to the dried substance. The loss on drying under the prescribed conditions is not more than 1·0 per cent. It has a melting-point of 142° to 145°.

Sterilisation. Solutions are sterilised by heating in an autoclave or by filtration.

Storage. It should be stored in airtight containers, protected from light.

Actions and uses. Neostigmine inhibits cholinesterase activity and has actions similar to those described under Physostigmine Salicylate (page 380) but it does not act on the central nervous system. Its nicotinic action is more pronounced and its muscarinic action less pronounced than that of physostigmine. It is used mainly for its action on voluntary muscle and less frequently to increase the activity of involuntary muscle.

Neostigmine methylsulphate is used in the diagnosis and treatment of myasthenia gravis. For diagnosis 1 to 1·5 milligrams is given by intramuscular or intravenous injection; relief of signs and symptoms usually occurs within fifteen minutes in true cases of myasthenia. In the treatment of myasthenia gravis doses of 1 to 2·5 milligrams are given by subcutaneous, intramuscular or intravenous injection several times a day, according to the severity of the condition. Oral administration of neostigmine bromide or of pyridostigmine bromide are other methods of treatment. If the muscarinic effect of neostigmine is troublesome, it can be controlled by prior administration of atropine by mouth or by injection.

Neostigmine methylsulphate is also used to curtail the muscular relaxation produced by non-depolarising neuromuscular-blocking drugs such as tubocurarine and gallamine triethiodide; 2·5 to 5 milligrams is given intravenously after an injection of 0·5 to 1 milligram of atropine sulphate.

In the treatment of paralytic ileus and postoperative urinary retention, neostigmine methylsulphate is given by subcutaneous or intramuscular injection in doses of 0·5 to 1 milligram. A dose of 0·5 milligram is sometimes used to promote the expulsion of intestinal flatus before radiography of the gall-bladder, kidneys, or ureters.

Eye-drops containing 3 per cent are used in the treatment of glaucoma.

UNDESIRABLE EFFECTS. As for Physostigmine Salicylate (page 380). In addition, neostigmine methylsulphate, by increasing intestinal motility, may cause disruption of intestinal suture lines.

POISONING. Atropine sulphate should be given subcutaneously in doses of 1 to 2 milligrams.

Dose. See above under **Actions and uses.**

Preparation
NEOSTIGMINE INJECTION, B.P. It consists of a sterile solution of neostigmine methylsulphate in Water for Injections. Unless otherwise specified, a solution containing 500 μg in 1 ml is supplied. It should be protected from light. Ampoules containing 2·5 mg in 1 ml are also available.

OTHER NAME: *Prostigmin*®

NIALAMIDE

$C_{16}H_{18}N_4O_2 = 298·3$

Nialamide is *N*-benzyl-β-pyridine-4-carboxyhydrazidopropionamide.

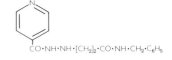

$CO·NH·NH·[CH_2]_2·CO·NH·CH_2·C_6H_5$

Solubility. Soluble, at 20°, in 400 parts of water, in 40 parts of alcohol, in 10 parts of methyl alcohol, and in 150 parts of chloroform.

Standard
It complies with the requirements of the British Pharmacopoeia.
It is a white, crystalline, almost odourless powder and contains not less than 97·0 and not more than the equivalent of 103·0 per cent of $C_{16}H_{18}N_4O_2$, calculated with reference to the dried substance. The loss on drying under the prescribed conditions is not more than 0·5 per cent. It has a melting-point of 151° to 153°.

Actions and uses. Nialamide is a monoamine-oxidase inhibitor and is used for the treatment of depression of neurotic or psychotic origin.

As an antidepressant the usual initial dosage is 150 milligrams daily by mouth in divided doses, and this may need to be increased to 300 milligrams daily in some cases. When a satisfactory response has been obtained the dose should be gradually reduced to the minimum which provides relief from symptoms; this may be as little as 75 milligrams daily.

UNDESIRABLE EFFECTS. The most frequently occurring reactions are headache, nausea, vertigo, dryness of the mouth, and excessive perspiration.

PRECAUTIONS. These are described under Phenelzine Sulphate (page 361).
Although nialamide appears to be free from hepatotoxicity, the fact that analogous compounds have given rise to hepatic reactions should be borne in mind when giving nialamide to patients with a history of liver damage or impaired liver function.

Dose. See above under **Actions and uses.**

Preparation
NIALAMIDE TABLETS, B.P. Unless otherwise specified, tablets each containing 25 mg of nialamide are supplied. Tablets containing 100 mg are also available.

OTHER NAME: *Niamid*®

NICLOSAMIDE

$C_{13}H_8Cl_2N_2O_4 = 327·1$

Niclosamide is 5-chloro-*N*-(2-chloro-4-nitrophenyl)-2-hydroxybenzamide.

Solubility. Slightly soluble in water; soluble, at 20°, in 150 parts of alcohol, in 350 parts of ether, and in 400 parts of chloroform.

Standard
It complies with the requirements of the British Pharmacopoeia.
It is a cream-coloured odourless powder and contains not less than 98·0 per cent of $C_{13}H_8Cl_2N_2O_4$, calculated with reference to the dried substance. The loss on drying under the prescribed conditions is not more than 0·5 per cent. It has a melting-point of about 228°.

Actions and uses. Niclosamide is a taenicide; it is effective against all the species of tapeworm that infect man. As with dichlorophen, the worms are partially digested before they are expelled, and the scolices cannot be found in the stools. A stool examination should be made after eight weeks to ensure that the worm has been killed.

The use of niclosamide against *Taenia solium*

may predispose to cysticercosis, as there is a possibility of ova from a partially digested worm migrating into the stomach.

The usual dose is 2 grams given on an empty stomach or after a light breakfast, either as a single dose or as two doses of 1 gram separated by an interval of one hour. Children under eight years of age are given half the adult dose. The tablets must be crushed or thoroughly chewed and washed down with water. A saline purge should be given two hours after treatment; if the patient is constipated it is advisable to purge on the day before treatment. Niclosamide is not appreciably absorbed from the intestine and therefore has no effect in

cysticercosis. *Hymenolepis nana* completes its life-cycle in man without passing through an intermediate host, and cysticerci of this tapeworm embedded in the intestinal mucosa escape the action of the drug and later develop into adults; they should be removed by a second treatment given one week after the first.

Dose. See above under **Actions and uses.**

Preparation
NICLOSAMIDE TABLETS, B.P. Unless otherwise specified, tablets each containing 500 mg of niclosamide are supplied. They should be chewed before being swallowed.

OTHER NAME: *Yomesan*®

NICOTINAMIDE

SYNONYMS: Niacinamide; Nicotinamidum

$C_6H_6N_2O = 122.1$

Nicotinamide is pyridine-3-carboxyamide.

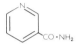

Solubility. Soluble, at 20°, in 1 part of water, in 1·5 parts of alcohol, and in 10 parts of glycerol; slightly soluble in ether.

Standard
It complies with the requirements of the European Pharmacopoeia.
It occurs as colourless crystals or white crystalline powder with a faint characteristic odour and contains not less than 99·0 per cent of $C_6H_6N_2O$, calculated with reference to the dried substance. The loss on drying under the prescribed conditions is not more than 0·5 per cent. It has a melting-point of 128° to 131°. A 5 per cent solution in water has a pH of 6·0 to 8·0.

Hygroscopicity. It absorbs insignificant amounts of moisture at 25° at relative humidities up to about 90 per cent.

Sterilisation. Solutions for injection are sterilised by heating in an autoclave or by filtration.

Storage. It should be stored in airtight containers.

Actions and uses. Nicotinamide has the actions of a vitamin as described under

Nicotinic Acid; it has no vasodilator action. It is used as an alternative to nicotinic acid for the treatment and prevention of pellagra; dosage and methods of administration are described under Nicotinic Acid.

Dose. Prophylactic, 15 to 30 milligrams by mouth, daily; therapeutic, 50 to 250 milligrams by mouth or by intravenous injection, daily.

Preparations
VITAMINS CAPSULES, B.P.C. (page 654)
VITAMINS B AND C INJECTION, B.P.C. (page 720)
NICOTINAMIDE TABLETS, B.P.C. (page 813)
VITAMIN B TABLETS, COMPOUND, B.P.C. (page 819)
VITAMIN B TABLETS, COMPOUND, STRONG, B.P.C. (page 819)

NICOTINIC ACID

SYNONYM: Niacin

$C_6H_5NO_2 = 123.1$

Nicotinic Acid is pyridine-3-carboxylic acid.

Solubility. Soluble, at 20°, in 55 parts of water; soluble in boiling water and in boiling alcohol; very slightly soluble in ether; soluble in solutions of alkalis.

Standard
It complies with the requirements of the British Pharmacopoeia.
It occurs as white or creamy-white odourless or almost odourless crystals or crystalline powder and contains not less than 99·0 per cent of $C_6H_5NO_2$, calculated with reference to the dried substance. The loss on drying under the prescribed conditions is not more than 0·5 per cent. It has a melting-point of 234° to 237°. A 1·3 per cent solution in water has a pH of 3·0 to 3·5.

Sterilisation. Solutions of the sodium salt for injection are sterilised by heating in an autoclave or by filtration.

Actions and uses. Nicotinic acid is essential for human nutrition, the normal daily requirement being probably about 6·6 to 8·8 milligrams per 1000 Calories or approximately 17 to 22 milligrams, depending on the protein intake. Its amide is a constituent of diphosphopyridine nucleotide (DPN) and triphosphopyridine nucleotide (TPN), two coenzymes associated with hydrogen transport in many biological oxidation-reduction processes. A deficiency of nicotinic acid is one factor in the etiology of pellagra, and the acid or its amide is used in the prophylaxis and treatment of this condition.

For the treatment of acute exacerbations of pellagra, up to 500 milligrams is given daily in divided doses by mouth. The amide, which is devoid of vasodilator action, may be given instead. The prophylactic or maintenance dose is 50 milligrams daily. If the patient is unable to swallow or absorb the nicotinic acid, it may be injected as a solution of the sodium salt in a dose not exceeding 50 milligrams, which may be repeated hourly; if nicotinamide is used, much larger doses may be given.

Nicotinic acid and its amide produce improvement in the mental, cutaneous, and alimentary manifestations of pellagra, but they have little influence on the neuropathy or the lesions of the lips and face that are frequently seen in pellagrins; foods or concentrates rich in the vitamin-B group should therefore be administered as well as nicotinic acid or its amide in the treatment of pellagra. It has a transient fibrinolytic action.

In addition to its action as a vitamin, nicotinic acid has a vasodilator action. When given by mouth or by injection in therapeutic doses, it may cause flushing of the face, a sensation of heat, and a pounding in the head; these symptoms are transient and harmless and may be avoided by substituting nicotinamide. Tolerance to the vasodilator effect develops rapidly when large doses are taken. Nicotinic acid has been employed for its vasodilator action in the treatment of peripheral vascular disease.

UNDESIRABLE EFFECTS. Nicotinic acid may cause dryness of the skin, anorexia, nausea, vomiting, diarrhoea, activation of peptic ulcer, hepatic disease, and hyperuricaemia.

Dose. See above under **Actions and uses.**

Preparation
NICOTINIC ACID TABLETS, B.P. Unless otherwise specified, tablets each containing 50 mg of nicotinic acid are supplied. Tablets containing 25 and 100 mg are also available.

NICOUMALONE

$C_{19}H_{15}NO_6 = 353.3$

Nicoumalone is 3-(α-acetonyl-p-nitrobenzyl)-4-hydroxycoumarin.

Solubility. Very slightly soluble in water and in ether; soluble, at 20°, in 400 parts of alcohol and in 200 parts of chloroform; soluble in solutions of alkali hydroxides.

Standard
It complies with the requirements of the British Pharmacopoeia.
It is an almost white to buff, odourless or almost odourless powder and contains not less than 98·5 per cent of $C_{19}H_{15}NO_6$, calculated with reference to the dried substance. The loss on drying under the prescribed conditions is not more than 0·5 per cent. It has a melting-point of about 198°.

Actions and uses. Nicoumalone has the actions and uses described under Phenindione (page 364). A therapeutic effect is obtained twenty-four to forty-eight hours after the initial dose has been given and ceases within thirty-six to forty-eight hours of the last dose. The initial dose is 8 to 16 milligrams by mouth on the first day, followed on the second day by 4 to 12 milligrams; thereafter the dose is carefully controlled by daily determinations of the prothrombin time.

Nicoumalone is sometimes tolerated by patients intolerant of other oral anticoagulants. Interactions with other drugs are similar to those described under Phenindione (page 364).

UNDESIRABLE EFFECTS. Nausea, loss of appetite, headache, and giddiness rarely occur; the usual safeguards during anticoagulant therapy should be observed.

Dose. See above under **Actions and uses.**

Preparation
NICOUMALONE TABLETS, B.P. The quantity of nicoumalone in each tablet should be specified by the prescriber. Tablets containing 1 and 4 mg are available.

OTHER NAMES: Acenocoumarol; *Sinthrome*®

NIKETHAMIDE

SYNONYM: Nicethamidum

$C_{10}H_{14}N_2O = 178.2$

Nikethamide is pyridine-3-carboxydiethylamide.

Solubility. Miscible with water, with alcohol, with ether, and with chloroform.

Standard

It complies with the requirements of the European Pharmacopoeia.

It is a colourless or slightly yellow oily liquid or crystalline mass with a slight characteristic odour and contains not less than 98·5 per cent of $C_{10}H_{14}N_2O$. It has a specific gravity at 20° of 1·060 to 1·066, corresponding to a weight per ml at 20° of about 1·057 g to 1·062 g. It has a freezing-point of 23° to 25°. A 25 per cent solution in water has a pH of 6·5 to 7·8.

Sterilisation. Solutions for injection are sterilised by heating in an autoclave or by filtration.

Actions and uses. Nikethamide is a respiratory stimulant, its site of action being the medullary centres of the brain. It increases the rate and depth of respiration and produces slight peripheral vasoconstriction, although in man it has very little effect on blood pressure. Any beneficial effect it has on the circulation is probably due to an improvement in the respiration. An increasing coronary flow has been demonstrated in animals, but there is no clinical evidence of the value of nikethamide in coronary and myocardial diseases, and there appears to be little justification for its use in cardiac conditions unless these are due to respiratory distress.

Because of its action on the peripheral vessels, it is used in circulatory failure occurring, for example, during acute infections and in surgical or traumatic shock, but in this condition it is being replaced by more effective vasoconstrictor drugs.

In emergencies, nikethamide is given by slow intravenous injection; doses as high as 2·5 grams may be necessary. Convulsive movements occur before the toxic dose is reached.

Dose. 0·5 to 2 grams by intravenous injection, repeated as necessary.

Preparation

NIKETHAMIDE INJECTION, B.P. It consists of a sterile solution containing 25 per cent of nikethamide in Water for Injections. Dose: 2 to 8 ml by intravenous injection, repeated as necessary.

NITRAZEPAM

$C_{15}H_{11}N_3O_3 = 281.3$

Nitrazepam is 2,3-dihydro-7-nitro-5-phenyl-1H-1,4-benzodiazepin-2-one.

Solubility. Very slightly soluble in water; soluble, at 20°, in 120 parts of alcohol, in 900 parts of ether, and in 45 parts of chloroform.

Standard

It complies with the requirements of the British Pharmacopoeia.

It is a yellow, crystalline, odourless powder and contains not less than 99·0 and not more than the equivalent of 101·0 per cent of $C_{15}H_{11}N_3O_3$, calculated with reference to the dried substance. The loss on drying under the prescribed conditions is not more than 0·5 per cent. It has a melting-point of 226° to 229°.

Storage. It should be stored in airtight containers, protected from light.

Actions and uses. Nitrazepam has properties similar to those described under Chlordiazepoxide Hydrochloride (page 96). It possesses marked sedative properties and is used principally as a hypnotic agent.

Sleep lasting six to eight hours is produced within thirty to sixty minutes of an oral dose of 5 to 10 milligrams. The dose should be reduced in elderly patients to 2·5 to 5 milligrams.

In addition to the tablets, it is also available as capsules containing 5 milligrams.

UNDESIRABLE EFFECTS. Nitrazepam may cause hang-over and light-headedness. In elderly patients it may cause confusion. There may be a danger of dependence of the barbiturate-alcohol type, as described under Phenobarbitone (page 366) and it may reduce the patient's ability to drive motor cars or operate moving machinery.

PRECAUTIONS. Caution should be exercised in using nitrazepam in conjunction with other drugs that act on the central nervous system.

Dose. See above under **Actions and uses.**

Preparation

NITRAZEPAM TABLETS, B.P. Unless otherwise specified, tablets each containing 5 mg are supplied. They should be protected from light.

OTHER NAME: *Mogadon*®

NITRIC ACID

$HNO_3 = 63.01$

Standard

DESCRIPTION. A clear colourless or almost colourless fuming liquid.

IDENTIFICATION TESTS. 1. Strongly acid, even when freely diluted.

2. Dilute 1 ml to 10 ml with water; the solution gives the reactions characteristic of nitrates.

WEIGHT PER ML. At 20°, about 1·41 g.

ARSENIC. It complies with the test given in Appendix 6, page 879 (1 part per million).

COPPER AND ZINC. To 1 ml add 20 ml of water and a slight excess of *dilute ammonia solution*; no blue colour is produced. Pass *hydrogen sulphide* through the solution; no precipitate is formed.

IRON. 0·5 ml complies with the limit test for iron (80 parts per million).

LEAD. It complies with the test given in Appendix 7, page 883 (2 parts per million).

CHLORIDE. 5 ml neutralised to *litmus paper* with *dilute ammonia solution* complies with the limit test for chlorides (70 parts per million).

SULPHATE. To 2·5 ml add 0·01 g of *sodium bicarbonate*, evaporate to dryness on a water-bath, and dissolve the residue in water; the solution complies with the limit test for sulphates (240 parts per million).

SULPHATED ASH. Not more than 0·01 per cent w/w.

CONTENT OF HNO_3. 69·0 to 71·0 per cent w/w, determined by the following method:
To about 4 g, accurately weighed, add 40 ml of water and titrate with 1N sodium hydroxide, using *methyl orange solution* as indicator; each ml of 1N sodium hydroxide is equivalent to 0·06301 g of HNO_3.

Actions and uses. Nitric acid is a powerful corrosive and stains the skin yellow. It is used in the preparation of Strong Ferric Chloride Solution (page 783).

POISONING. A stomach tube or emetics should not be used. The acid must be neutralised as quickly as possible; calcium hydroxide in water and Magnesium Hydroxide Mixture are good antidotes; carbonates should be avoided if possible, as they lead to the liberation of carbon dioxide and the consequent risk of perforation.

After neutralisation of the acid, demulcents, such as milk, raw eggs, or a vegetable oil such as olive oil should be given and shock should be treated by warmth and intravenous infusions if required. Morphine should be given for the relief of pain.

Nitric acid burns should be treated by immediately flooding with water, followed by the application of sodium bicarbonate or chalk in powder, or by the application of sodium bicarbonate or saline packs.

NITROFURANTOIN

$C_8H_6N_4O_5 = 238·2$

Nitrofurantoin is 1-(5-nitrofurfurylideneamino)hydantoin.

Solubility. Very slightly soluble in water; slightly soluble in alcohol and in glycerol; soluble, at 20°, in 200 parts of acetone, in 16 parts of dimethylformamide, and in 70 parts of macrogol 300.

Standard
It complies with the requirements of the British Pharmacopoeia.
It occurs as odourless or almost odourless yellow crystals or fine powder and contains not less than 98·0 and not more than the equivalent of 102·0 per cent of $C_8H_6N_4O_5$, calculated with reference to the dried substance. The loss on drying under the prescribed conditions is not more than 1·0 per cent.

Storage. It should be stored in airtight containers, protected from light, at a temperature not exceeding 25°.

Actions and uses. Nitrofurantoin is a broad-spectrum antibacterial agent whose mode of action on bacteria is unknown. It is well absorbed after oral administration but it is not possible to achieve effective levels in the tissues without intolerable side-effects. It is excreted in high concentration in the urine and its sole use is in the control of urinary infections.

Nitrofurantoin is not as effective in the eradication of urinary infections as agents that can be used to produce high tissue concentrations but it is useful as a long-term suppressive agent in chronic infections that cannot be treated by other means. Bacterial resistance does not develop readily but many strains of coliform organisms and *Pseudomonas* are now resistant. Doses of 5 to 8 milligrams per kilogram body-weight daily in divided doses are usually suitable but 10 milligrams per kilogram body-weight may be given for the treatment of severe infections. Treatment is usually continued for seven to fourteen days.

UNDESIRABLE EFFECTS. Nausea, abdominal discomfort, dizziness, and drowsiness may occur on full dosage but the symptoms usually subside when the dose is reduced. Serious complications are uncommon but include rashes and an alarming acute pulmonary syndrome that resembles pulmonary oedema. Polyneuritis may occur after prolonged administration, especially in patients with impaired renal function.

Undesirable effects may be minimised by adjusting the dose according to body-weight and administering the dose after meals.

PRECAUTIONS AND CONTRA-INDICATIONS. Nitrofurantoin should not be used in patients with a history of allergy to it or of the pulmonary syndrome or in those with glucose-6-phosphate-dehydrogenase deficiency in whom it may cause haemolytic anaemia. It should be used with caution in patients with renal impairment.

Dose. 50 to 150 milligrams four times daily.

OTHER NAMES: *Berkfurin*®; *Furadantin*®; *Furan*®; *Nitoin*®

Preparations
NITROFURANTOIN MIXTURE, B.P.C. (page 748)
NITROFURANTOIN TABLETS, B.P. Unless otherwise specified, tablets each containing 50 mg of nitrofurantoin are supplied. They should be stored in airtight containers, protected from light, at a temperature not exceeding 25°. Tablets containing 100 mg are also available.

NITROUS OXIDE

SYNONYM: Nitrogenii Oxidum

$N_2O = 44 \cdot 01$

Solubility. One volume, measured at normal temperature and pressure, dissolves, at 20°, in 2 volumes of water.

Standard
It complies with the requirements of the European Pharmacopoeia.
It is a colourless odourless gas and contains not less than 97·0 per cent v/v of N_2O in the gaseous phase. It is heavier than air and supports combustion; a glowing splinter of wood placed in it bursts into flame. When mixed with nitric oxide, no red fumes are produced (distinction from oxygen). It is supplied compressed in metal cylinders.

Storage, labelling, and colour-markings. It should be stored in metal cylinders in a special storage room, which should be cool and free from materials of an inflammable nature. The whole of the cylinder should be painted blue and the name of the gas or chemical symbol "N_2O" should be stencilled in paint on the shoulder of the cylinder. The name or chemical symbol of the gas should be clearly and indelibly stamped on the cylinder valve.

Actions and uses. Nitrous oxide is the oldest of the anaesthetics and is still the safest anaesthetic known.
When given alone, it produces anaesthesia lasting only for about forty-five seconds, recovery occurring within one to two minutes. When administered without air or oxygen, it produces complete anaesthesia in about one minute, with cyanosis, slow snoring respiration, dilated pupils, and raised blood pressure. These symptoms of anoxia disappear when air is breathed; they do not occur if mixtures containing 10 per cent of oxygen are used. Almost the only complications following the use of nitrous oxide are those due to varying degrees of oxygen lack.
Nitrous oxide is used extensively in dental and obstetric practice for producing both analgesia and light anaesthesia. In the production of full surgical anaesthesia nitrous oxide is usually used only for induction and as a vehicle for, or an adjuvant to, other anaesthetics. It is often used in conjunction with local anaesthetics and muscle relaxants.

POISONING. In the event of poisoning by nitrous oxide resulting in collapse and asphyxia, the procedure described under Chloroform (page 100) should be adopted.

NORADRENALINE ACID TARTRATE

SYNONYMS: Levarterenol Bitartrate; Noradren. Tart.; Noradrenaline Tartrate; Noradrenalini Tartras

$C_{12}H_{17}NO_9,H_2O = 337 \cdot 3$

Noradrenaline Acid Tartrate is (−)-2-amino-1-(3,4-dihydroxyphenyl)ethanol hydrogen tartrate monohydrate.

Solubility. Soluble, at 20°, in 2·5 parts of water; slightly soluble in alcohol; very slightly soluble in ether and in chloroform.

Standard
It complies with the requirements of the European Pharmacopoeia.
It is a white or almost white, crystalline, odourless powder and contains not less than 98·5 and not more than the equivalent of 101·0 per cent of $C_{12}H_{17}NO_9$, calculated with reference to the anhydrous substance. It contains 4·5 to 5·8 per cent w/w of water. A 1 per cent solution in water has a pH of 3·0 to 5·0.

Sterilisation. The strong solution containing 0·1 per cent of sodium metabisulphite and 0·8 per cent of sodium chloride is sterilised by heating in an autoclave or by filtration.

Storage. It should be stored in airtight containers, protected from light. It darkens on exposure to air and light.

Actions and uses. Noradrenaline is the neurohormone released at the terminations of post-ganglionic adrenergic nerve fibres when they are stimulated; it is also present in the adrenal medulla, from which it is liberated together with adrenaline.
In its effect it differs from adrenaline in

having little or no bronchodilator or vasodilator action (beta-effect). Its alpha-receptor actions are vasoconstriction, dilatation of the pupil, inhibition of the movements of the stomach, intestine, and bladder, and liberation of glucose from the liver.

The vasoconstrictor action of noradrenaline may be used to diminish the absorption and localise the effects of local anaesthetics, and to reduce haemorrhage during the subsequent operation; it should not, however, be used with cocaine. For these purposes it is given in solutions containing concentrations of noradrenaline of 1 in 100,000 to 1 in 50,000. When applied to mucous membranes it produces ischaemia by constricting the vessels. For the control of capillary bleeding, local application of a 1 in 5000 solution is usually effective.

Noradrenaline is preferred to adrenaline in the treatment of peripheral vasomotor collapse in which the blood volume is adequate, such as after the removal of phaeochromocytomata, sometimes following the use of ganglion-blocking drugs, in surgical shock, and in acute myocardial infarction.

In man, noradrenaline produces the desired pressor response mainly by peripheral vasoconstriction and with little myocardial stimulation; coronary flow is usually increased, and the diastolic interval is lengthened because of the compensatory vagal slowing which follows the increased arterial pressure.

Noradrenaline acid tartrate is usually administered by intravenous infusion as a solution containing 8 micrograms, equivalent to 4 micrograms of the base, per millilitre in Dextrose Injection (5 per cent w/v) or Sodium Chloride and Dextrose Injection; this solution is usually given initially at a rate of 1 millilitre per minute and subsequently at a rate sufficient to maintain the desired blood pressure, up to a maximum of 2·5 millilitres per minute. The infusion may be continued for days, if necessary, although there is a risk of gangrenous changes, especially at the site of infusion, and for this reason metaraminol is often preferred. Administration must not be stopped suddenly, but should be withdrawn gradually to guard against a disastrous fall in blood pressure.

PRECAUTIONS. Noradrenaline should not be used in the presence of ventricular hyperexcitability produced by chloroform, trichloroethylene, cyclopropane, mercurial diuretics, quinidine, or large dosage of digitalis.

Dose. 2 to 20 micrograms per minute by intravenous infusion, according to the blood pressure of the patient.

Preparations
NORADRENALINE INJECTION, B.P.C. (page 715)
NORADRENALINE SOLUTION, STRONG, STERILE, B.P.C. (page 789)

OTHER NAME: *Levophed*®

NORETHANDROLONE

$C_{20}H_{30}O_2 = 302·5$

Norethandrolone is 17-hydroxy-19-nor-17α-pregn-4-en-3-one.

Solubility. Insoluble in water; soluble, at 20°, in 8 parts of alcohol, in 5 parts of chloroform, and in 3 parts of methyl alcohol.

Standard
It complies with the requirements of the British Pharmacopoeia.
It is a white crystalline powder and contains not less than 95·0 per cent of $C_{20}H_{30}O_2$, calculated with reference to the dried substance. The loss on drying under the prescribed conditions is not more than 0·5 per cent. It has a melting-point of about 135°.

Storage. It should be protected from light.

Actions and uses. Norethandrolone has actions and uses similar to those described under Methandienone (page 299).
It is given by mouth or by intramuscular injection in a dosage of 25 to 50 milligrams daily. A child usually requires a daily dosage of 0·5 milligram per kilogram body-weight.

UNDESIRABLE EFFECTS. Because of its progestational activity, amenorrhoea and uterine bleeding may result from its withdrawal. It may also give rise to water retention and to jaundice.

CONTRA-INDICATIONS. It should not be given to patients with impaired liver function or during the first trimester of pregnancy.
Norethandrolone may give rise to androgenic effects and should not be used in patients with prostatic carcinoma.

Dose. 25 to 50 milligrams daily.

Preparation
NORETHANDROLONE TABLETS, B.P. Unless otherwise specified, tablets each containing 10 mg of norethandrolone are supplied. They should be protected from light.

OTHER NAME: *Nilevar*®

NORETHISTERONE

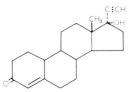

$C_{20}H_{26}O_2 = 298.4$

Norethisterone is 17-hydroxy-19-nor-17α-pregn-4-en-20-yn-3-one.

Solubility. Insoluble in water; soluble, at 20°, in 150 parts of alcohol, in 30 parts of chloroform, in 80 parts of acetone, and in 5 parts of pyridine; very slightly soluble in vegetable oils.

Standard
It complies with the requirements of the British Pharmacopoeia.
It is a white or creamy-white, crystalline, odourless powder and contains not less than 97.0 and not more than the equivalent of 102.0 per cent of $C_{20}H_{26}O_2$, calculated with reference to the dried substance. The loss on drying under the prescribed conditions is not more than 0.5 per cent. It has a melting-point of 201° to 206°.

Storage. It should be protected from light.

Actions and uses. Norethisterone is a synthetic progestational steroid which converts the proliferative uterine endometrium to the secretory phase. It has slight oestrogenic and androgenic activities. Norethisterone is active when taken by mouth and is generally used in conjunction with oestrogens.
In the treatment of primary and secondary amenorrhoea 10 to 20 milligrams is given daily, in divided doses, from the fifth day to the twenty-fourth day of each menstrual cycle; withdrawal bleeding usually occurs one to three days after discontinuing treatment. Norethisterone is also used for the treatment of menorrhagia, metrorrhagia, and endometriosis; in endometriosis, therapy must be continuous for nine to twelve months. It has also been used to reduce premenstrual tension and relieve dysmenorrhoea. To delay or prevent menstruation, it is given in a dosage of 20 to 30 milligrams daily.
Norethisterone is used in conjunction with oestrogens as an oral contraceptive to inhibit ovulation. For this purpose doses of 1 to 2 milligrams are given daily, usually with ethinyloestradiol or mestranol, from the fifth to the twenty-fourth day of each menstrual

cycle. The course is repeated after an interval of one week. Regular administration is essential.
Norethisterone is available as tablets containing 5 milligrams, and as tablets containing 1 and 2 milligrams together with mestranol.

UNDESIRABLE EFFECTS. Norethisterone may give rise to headache and tension, mental depression, nausea and vomiting, breast engorgement, fluid retention, and weight gain; a state of pseudopregnancy and premenstrual tension may be aggravated.
It may give rise to break-through bleeding and may cause hirsutism, acneiform skin rashes, and deepening of the voice. Virilisation of the female foetus may occur when doses of more than 15 milligrams daily of norethisterone are given. Prolonged use may lead to impairment of liver function. When taken without oestrogens it may not prevent conception.
Regular use of progestational oral contraceptives combined with oestrogens increases the risk of intravascular thrombosis and thromboembolic accidents.

PRECAUTIONS. Care is necessary when liver function is impaired and in patients with a previous medical history of venous thrombosis. Like other oral contraceptives, it is not reliable as a suppressant of ovulation in the first 10 to 12 days of the first regular course.

Dose. 10 to 20 milligrams daily in divided doses. As an oral contraceptive, 1 to 2 milligrams daily.

Preparation
NORETHISTERONE TABLETS, B.P. Unless otherwise specified, tablets each containing 5 mg of norethisterone are supplied. They should be protected from light.

OTHER NAMES: Norethindrone; *Primolut N*®

NORETHISTERONE ACETATE

$C_{22}H_{28}O_3 = 340.5$

Norethisterone Acetate is 17-acetoxy-19-nor-17α-pregn-4-en-20-yn-3-one.

Solubility. Very slightly soluble in water; soluble, at 20°, in 12.5 parts of alcohol and in 4 parts of acetone; slightly soluble in ether; soluble in chloroform.

Standard
It complies with the requirements of the British Pharmacopoeia.

It is a white or creamy-white, crystalline, odourless powder and contains not less than 97.0 and not more than the equivalent of 102.0 per cent of $C_{22}H_{28}O_3$, calculated with reference to the dried substance. The loss on drying under the prescribed conditions is not more than 0.5 per cent. It has a melting-point of about 163°.

Storage. It should be protected from light.

Actions and uses. Norethisterone acetate has the actions, uses, and undesirable effects described under Norethisterone, but it is effective in about half the dosage.

It is available as tablets containing 2·5 and 10 milligrams and as tablets containing 1, 2·5, 3, and 4 milligrams together with ethinyloestradiol.

PRECAUTIONS. These are as described under Norethisterone.

Dose. 2·5 to 20 milligrams daily in divided doses. As an oral contraceptive, 1 to 4 milligrams daily.

OTHER NAMES: Norethindrone Acetate; *Norlutin-A*®; *SH 420*®

NORETHYNODREL

$C_{20}H_{26}O_2 = 298·4$

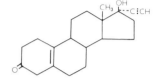

Norethynodrel is 17-hydroxy-19-nor-17α-pregn-5(10)-en-20-yn-3-one.

Solubility. Insoluble in water; soluble, at 20°, in 30 parts of alcohol, in 60 parts of ether, and in 7 parts of chloroform.

Standard
It complies with the requirements of the British Pharmacopoeia.
It is a white or almost white, crystalline, odourless powder and contains not less than 97·0 and not more than the equivalent of 102·0 per cent of $C_{20}H_{26}O_2$, calculated with reference to the dried substance. The loss on drying under the prescribed conditions is not more than 0·5 per cent. It has a melting-point of about 175°.
It contains not more than 1·0 per cent of mestranol.

Labelling. The label on the container states the percentage of mestranol present.

Storage. It should be protected from light.

Actions and uses. Norethynodrel is a synthetic progestational steroid which has actions similar to those described under Norethisterone (page 329). It is active when taken by mouth and is generally used in conjunction with oestrogens.

In the treatment of primary and secondary amenorrhoea it is given daily in a dosage of 5 to 10 milligrams from the fifth day to the twenty-fourth day of each menstrual cycle; withdrawal bleeding usually occurs one to three days after discontinuing treatment.

Norethynodrel is also used for the treatment of other dysfunctional uterine bleeding. For the treatment of endometriosis, doses of 20 to 30 milligrams daily are usually given continuously for nine to twelve months.

Norethynodrel is used in conjunction with oestrogens as an oral contraceptive to inhibit ovulation. For this purpose doses of 2·5 or 5 milligrams are given daily, usually with mestranol, from the fifth to the twenty-fourth day of each menstrual cycle. The course is repeated after an interval of one week. Regular administration is essential.

Norethynodrel is available as tablets containing 2·5, 3, and 5 milligrams together with mestranol.

UNDESIRABLE EFFECTS. Norethynodrel may give rise to headache and tension, mental depression, nausea and vomiting, breast engorgement, fluid retention, and weight gain; a state of pseudopregnancy and premenstrual tension may be aggravated.

It may give rise to break-through bleeding, and may cause hirsutism, acneiform skin rashes, and deepening of the voice. Prolonged use may lead to impairment of liver function. When taken without oestrogens it may not prevent conception.

Regular use of progestational oral contraceptives combined with oestrogens increases the risk of intravascular thrombosis and thromboembolic accidents.

PRECAUTIONS. These are described under Norethisterone (page 329).

Dose. 5 to 30 milligrams daily in divided doses. As an oral contraceptive, 2·5 to 10 milligrams daily.

NORTRIPTYLINE HYDROCHLORIDE

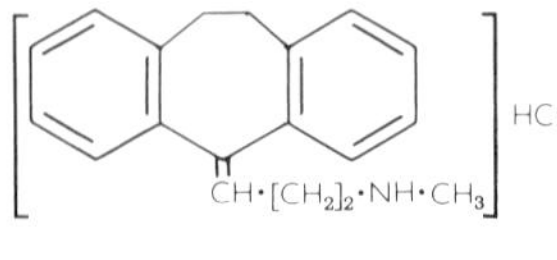

$C_{19}H_{22}ClN = 299·8$

Nortriptyline Hydrochloride is 10,11-dihydro-5-(3-methylaminopropylidene)-5*H*-dibenzo-[*a,d*]cycloheptene hydrochloride.

Solubility. Soluble, at 20°, in 50 parts of water, in 10 parts of alcohol, and in 5 parts of chloroform; insoluble in ether.

Standard
It complies with the requirements of the British Pharmacopoeia.

It is a white or almost white powder with a slight characteristic odour and contains not less than 98·0 and not more than the equivalent of 101·0 per cent of $C_{19}H_{22}ClN$, calculated with reference to the dried substance. The loss on drying under the prescribed conditions is not more than 0·5 per cent. It has a melting-point of about 218°.

Storage. It should be protected from light.

Actions and uses. Nortriptyline has the actions, uses, and undesirable effects described under Amitriptyline Hydrochloride (page 22) and is effective in similar dosage; 1·15 grams of nortriptyline hydrochloride is approximately equivalent to 1 gram of nortriptyline.

PRECAUTIONS AND CONTRA-INDICATIONS. Because of its anticholinergic activity, nortriptyline should not be given to patients with glaucoma or to those who might develop urinary retention.

Caution should be exercised when giving nortriptyline to patients who are being treated with a monoamine-oxidase inhibitor, such as isocarboxazid, nialamide, phenelzine, or tranylcypromine, or who have been so treated within the previous ten days.

Nortriptyline should be avoided in patients with ischaemic heart disease, especially when there is evidence of rhythm disturbance.

Dose. The equivalent of 20 to 100 milligrams of nortriptyline daily in divided doses.

Preparations
NORTRIPTYLINE CAPSULES, B.P. Unless otherwise specified, capsules each containing the equivalent of 10 mg of nortriptyline are supplied. Capsules containing the equivalent of 25 mg are also available.

NORTRIPTYLINE TABLETS, B.P. Unless otherwise specified, tablets each containing the equivalent of 10 mg of nortriptyline are supplied. Tablets containing the equivalent of 25 mg are also available.

OTHER NAMES: *Allegron*®; *Aventyl*®

NOSCAPINE

SYNONYM: Narcotine

$C_{22}H_{23}NO_7 = 413·4$

Noscapine is 5-(6,7-dimethoxy-1-oxophthalan-3-yl)-4-methoxy-6-methyl-1,3-dioxolo[4,5-g]isoquinoline, an alkaloid obtained from opium.

Solubility. Insoluble in water; slightly soluble in alcohol and in ether; soluble in chloroform.

Standard
It complies with the requirements of the British Pharmacopoeia.
It is an almost white, fine, crystalline, odourless powder and contains not less than 98·5 and not more than the equivalent of 101·0 per cent of $C_{22}H_{23}NO_7$, calculated with reference to the dried substance. The loss on drying under the prescribed conditions is not more than 1·0 per cent. It has a melting-point of 174° to 176°.

Storage. It should be stored in airtight containers.

Actions and uses. Noscapine has an antitussive action similar to that described under

Codeine Phosphate (page 123). It has no analgesic or narcotic action, it does not produce euphoria or drowsiness, and its use is unlikely to lead to dependence.

Noscapine is given by mouth to suppress irritant dry cough. It may also be used to suppress the cough of bronchitis and for the relief of whooping-cough in children.

Dose. 15 to 30 milligrams.

Preparation
NOSCAPINE LINCTUS, B.P.C. (page 723)

OTHER NAME: *Coscopin*®

NOVOBIOCIN CALCIUM

$(C_{31}H_{35}N_2O_{11})_2Ca = 1263·3$

Novobiocin Calcium is the calcium salt of an antimicrobial substance produced by the growth of *Streptomyces niveus* or related organisms or by any other means.

Solubility. Soluble, at 20°, in 300 parts of water, in 8 parts of alcohol, in 60 parts of acetone, in 100 parts of butyl acetate, and in 8 parts of methyl alcohol.

Standard
It complies with the requirements of the British Pharmacopoeia.
It is a white or yellowish-white, crystalline, odourless powder and contains not less than 850 Units per mg, calculated with reference to the anhydrous substance. It contains not more than 5·0 per cent w/w of water.

A 2·5 per cent suspension in water has a pH of 7·0 to 8·5.

Storage. It should be stored in airtight containers, protected from light.

Actions and uses. Novobiocin calcium has the antibacterial actions, uses, and undesirable effects of novobiocin, as described under Novobiocin Sodium. It is more stable in the presence of water than the sodium compound and can be used in the form of liquid suspensions for administration by mouth; 265 milligrams of novobiocin calcium is approximately equivalent to 250 milligrams of novobiocin.

PRECAUTIONS AND CONTRA-INDICATIONS. As for Novobiocin Sodium.

Dose. The equivalent of 1 to 2 grams of novobiocin daily in divided doses.

Preparations
NOVOBIOCIN MIXTURE, B.P.C. (page 748)
NOVOBIOCIN TABLETS, B.P. Unless otherwise specified, tablets each containing novobiocin calcium or novobiocin sodium equivalent to 250 mg of novobiocin are supplied. They may be sugar coated or compression coated.

OTHER NAME: *Albamycin*®

NOVOBIOCIN SODIUM

$C_{31}H_{35}N_2NaO_{11} = 634 \cdot 6$

Novobiocin Sodium is the monosodium salt of an antimicrobial substance produced by the growth of *Streptomyces niveus* or related organisms or by any other means.

Solubility. Soluble, at 20°, in 5 parts of water, in 7 parts of alcohol, and in 3 parts of methyl alcohol; slightly soluble in butyl acetate.

Standard
It complies with the requirements of the British Pharmacopoeia.
It is a white or yellowish-white, crystalline, odourless powder and contains not less than 850 Units per mg, calculated with reference to the anhydrous substance. It contains not more than 5·0 per cent w/w of water. A 2·5 per cent solution in water has a pH of 7·0 to 8·5.

Labelling. If the material is not intended for parenteral administration, the label on the container states that the contents are not to be injected.

Storage. It should be stored in airtight containers, protected from light. If it is intended for parenteral administration, the containers should be sterile and sealed to exclude micro-organisms.

Actions and uses. Novobiocin is an antibiotic which is active against a number of Gram-positive organisms, especially *Staphylococcus aureus*; in general, it has no significant action against Gram-negative bacteria, except some strains of *Proteus* species.

When given by mouth in therapeutic doses it is rapidly absorbed from the gastro-intestinal tract, producing a maximum concentration in the blood within two or three hours and effective levels for eight to twelve hours. It is excreted mainly in the bile.

Novobiocin is used in the treatment of staphylococcal infections, but its value is limited by the frequent occurrence of undesirable effects and the readiness with which bacterial resistance is acquired. Its use should be restricted to the treatment of staphylococcal infections in which the organisms are resistant to other antibiotics but have been proved to be sensitive to novobiocin, to the treatment of biliary tract infections by sensitive bacteria, and to the treatment of *Proteus* infections not suitable for treatment with other drugs.

Novobiocin is usually given by mouth, as either the sodium or calcium salt, the dosage for an adult being 250 milligrams every six hours or 500 milligrams every twelve hours; if tolerated, these doses may be doubled in severe or resistant infections; 260 milligrams of novobiocin sodium is approximately equivalent to 250 milligrams of novobiocin. A child may be given a total daily dosage of 20 to 45 milligrams per kilogram body-weight. Treatment should be continued for two or three days after the temperature has returned to normal.

When oral administration is impracticable, novobiocin, in the form of the sodium salt, may be given by the slow intravenous injection of a solution containing the equivalent of 500 milligrams of novobiocin in 30 millilitres of Sodium Chloride Injection over a period of five to ten minutes, or a more dilute solution may be given by intravenous infusion; solutions containing dextrose are incompatible with novobiocin sodium and should not be used as diluents. For a child the intravenous dosage is 15 milligrams per kilogram body-weight every twelve hours. Intramuscular injection is painful.

A yellow pigment which may appear in the serum of patients treated with novobiocin is a metabolite of the drug and does not indicate liver damage.

Solutions for injection are prepared by an aseptic technique.

UNDESIRABLE EFFECTS. Nausea and vomiting may occur during treatment and skin rashes and fever are relatively common. Leucopenia sometimes occurs when treatment is prolonged.

PRECAUTIONS AND CONTRA-INDICATIONS. The administration of novobiocin should be discontinued if jaundice develops. Novobiocin should not be given to children under six months, as it may interfere with the conjugation of bilirubin.

Dose. See above under **Actions and uses.**

Preparation

NOVOBIOCIN TABLETS, B.P. Unless otherwise specified, tablets each containing novobiocin calcium or novo- biocin sodium equivalent to 250 mg of novobiocin are supplied. They may be sugar coated or compression coated.

OTHER NAME: *Albamycin®*

NUTMEG

SYNONYM: Myristica

Nutmeg consists of the dried kernels of the seeds of *Myristica fragrans* Houtt. (Fam. Myristica- ceae), a tree indigenous to the Moluccas and cultivated in Indonesia and the West Indies (Grenada). The seed is divested of the arillus (mace) and slowly dried, an operation which takes from eight to ten weeks; the testa is then broken and the kernel removed.

Constituents. Nutmeg contains about 5 to 15 per cent of volatile oil and about 35 per cent of solid fat, the chief fatty acid constituents of which are myristic acid (about 60 per cent) and smaller amounts of palmitic, oleic, linoleic, and lauric acids. It also contains small amounts of myristicin, elemicin, and safrole.

Standard for unground drug

DESCRIPTION. *Macroscopical:* kernels ovoid, about 2 to 3 cm long and 1·5 to 2 cm broad; surface light brown, showing network of shallow reticulate grooves and marked with numerous small, dark brown points and lines; slight circular elevation about 5 mm in diameter, somewhat eccentrically placed at wider end, indicating tip of radicle, connected by a broad shallow groove to the chalaza showing as a slight circular depression at the opposite end; kernel consisting of a pale brown endosperm covered by a thin darker brown perisperm penetrating the endosperm by numerous infoldings, producing the characteristic ruminate appearance of the cut surface; embryo small, embedded in the endo- sperm near the micropyle; when pressed by the finger- nail the cut surface exudes oil.
Odour aromatic and characteristic; taste aromatic and somewhat bitter.

Microscopical: the diagnostic characters are: peripheral *perisperm* composed of strongly flattened polyhedral cells with brown contents and occasional prismatic *crystals*; inner ruminate portion of perisperm consist- ing of parenchyma containing isolated groups of yellow *oil cells*; endosperm of polyhedral cells each containing a single *aleurone grain* with a large crystal- loid, about 12 by 20 μm, and *starch* granules, 2- to 10- compound or simple, the latter up to about 20 μm in width, all frequently embedded in a dark brown, *fatty mass*; the fat forms radiating groups of feathery crystals when a preparation in hot *chloral hydrate solution* is allowed to cool.

ASH. Not more than 3·0 per cent.

VOLATILE OIL. Not less than 5·0 per cent v/w, deter- mined by the method of Appendix 13, page 893.

Standard for powdered drug: Powdered Nutmeg

DESCRIPTION. A reddish-brown powder possessing the diagnostic microscopical characters, odour, and taste of the unground drug.

ASH. It complies with the requirement for the un- ground drug.

VOLATILE OIL. Not less than 4·0 per cent v/w, deter- mined by the method of Appendix 13, page 893.

Adulterants and substitutes. Bombay nutmegs, from *M. malabarica* Lam., are longer, narrower and almost devoid of odour. Macassar or Papua nutmegs, from *M. argentea* Warb., are also longer and narrower and have a uniform scurfy surface, a safrole-like odour, and an acrid taste.
Limed nutmegs are nutmegs which have been dipped in milk of lime and subsequently dried, a process which is intended to protect them from the attacks of insects.

Storage. It should be stored in airtight containers, in a cool place.

Actions and uses. Nutmeg is a carminative and a flavouring agent.

UNDESIRABLE EFFECTS. In large doses, it excites the motor cortex and produces epileptiform convulsions.

Preparation

CHALK POWDER, AROMATIC, B.P.C. (page 776)

NUTMEG OIL

SYNONYMS: Myristica Oil; Oleum Myristicae

Nutmeg Oil is obtained by distillation from nutmeg.

Constituents. Nutmeg oil consists chiefly of terpenes, including α- and β-pinene. It also contains small amounts of myristicin.

Standard

DESCRIPTION. A colourless, pale yellow, or pale green liquid; odour that of nutmeg.

OPTICAL ROTATION. At 20°, East Indian oil, +10° to +25°; West Indian oil, +25° to +45°.

REFRACTIVE INDEX. At 20°, East Indian oil, 1·475 to 1·488; West Indian oil, 1·472 to 1·477.

SOLUBILITY IN ALCOHOL. Soluble, at 20°, East Indian oil, in 3 volumes of *alcohol (90 per cent)*; West Indian oil, in 4 volumes of *alcohol (90 per cent)*.

WEIGHT PER ML. At 20°, East Indian oil, 0·885 g to 0·915 g; West Indian oil, 0·860 g to 0·880 g.

NON-VOLATILE MATTER. Not more than 3·0 per cent w/w, determined by the following method:
Evaporate about 2 g, accurately weighed, in a flat- bottomed dish of nickel or other suitable metal, 9 cm in diameter and 1·5 cm deep, by heating on a vigorously boiling water-bath for a total of 4 hours, and weigh the residue.

Storage. It should be stored in well-filled airtight containers, protected from light, in a cool place.

Actions and uses. Nutmeg oil has carmina- tive properties and is used as a flavouring agent. When absorbed, large doses stimulate the cerebral cortex and may induce epilepti- form convulsions.

Dose. 0·05 to 0·2 millilitre.

NUX VOMICA

Nux Vomica consists of the dried ripe seeds of *Strychnos nux-vomica* L. (Fam. Loganiaceae), a small tree widely distributed over the Indian subcontinent and south-east Asia. The ripe fruit, which externally resembles an orange, contains a whitish bitter pulp, in which are embedded three to five seeds; the seeds are removed when ripe, washed free from pulp, and dried in the sun.

Constituents. Nux vomica contains the alkaloids strychnine and brucine, together with traces of strychnicine and vomicine and of a glycoside loganin (meliatin). It also contains fatty matter (about 3 per cent) and chlorogenic acid. The total alkaloidal content varies from 1·8 to 5·3 per cent, about half of which is strychnine, although the proportion is subject to some variation.

Standard
It complies with the requirements of the British Pharmacopoeia.
It contains not less than 1·20 per cent of strychnine.

UNGROUND DRUG. *Macroscopical characters:* seeds grey to greenish-grey, disk-shaped, nearly flat, umbonate, sometimes irregularly curved, 10 to 30 mm in diameter and 4 to 6 mm thick, edge rounded or subacute; umbo connected to micropyle by a radial ridge; trichomes crowded, radiating from centre of both flat faces, and appressed, giving seed a silky surface; endosperm abundant, translucent, horny, with a central disk-shaped cavity; embryo situated in central cavity next to micropyle, having 2 small, thin, cordate cotyledons and a cylindrical radicle.
Odourless; taste extremely bitter.

Microscopical characters: the diagnostic characters are: *trichomes* with strongly thickened, pitted, lignified bases and cylindrical limbs, up to about 1 mm long; limbs with several lignified *ribs* and breaking up in powder to form rod-like fragments; *endosperm* consisting of thick-walled unlignified polyhedral cells with well-marked plasmodesmata and containing *oil-plasma* and *aleurone grains*, the grains up to about 30 μm in diameter; *starch* and *crystals* of calcium oxalate absent; length of lignified rib per mg of seed: 167 to **184** to 206 cm.

POWDERED DRUG: Powdered Nux Vomica. A yellowish-grey powder possessing the diagnostic microscopical characters and taste of the unground drug; odourless.

Adulterants and substitutes. The following have been imported as nux vomica.
Seeds of *S. nux-blanda* Hill which may be distinguished by their regular shape, paler colour, and the presence of a distinct ridge on the edge of the seeds; they contain about 0·1 per cent of alkaloids, comprising diaboline, strychnine, and brucine.
Seeds of *S. potatorum* L.f., known as clearing nuts, are smaller and thicker; they contain about 0·1 per cent of alkaloids, consisting mainly of diaboline with small amounts of strychnine, brucine, and other bases.
Seeds of *S. wallichiana* Steud ex D.C. (*S. cinnamomifolia* Thwaites) are similar to nux vomica but are fawn rather than grey in colour; the alkaloidal content and composition is very similar to that of *S. nux-vomica*.

Actions and uses. Nux vomica has the actions, uses, and undesirable effects described under Strychnine Hydrochloride (page 474).

POISONING. The procedure as described under Strychnine Hydrochloride (page 474) should be adopted.

Preparations
NUX VOMICA ELIXIR, B.P.C. (page 673)
NUX VOMICA LIQUID EXTRACT, B.P. It contains 1·5 per cent of strychnine. Dose: 0·05 to 0·2 millilitre.
GENTIAN MIXTURE, ACID, WITH NUX VOMICA, B.P.C. (page 743)
GENTIAN MIXTURE, ALKALINE, WITH NUX VOMICA, B.P.C. (page 744)
NUX VOMICA MIXTURE, ACID, B.P.C. (page 748)
NUX VOMICA MIXTURE, ALKALINE, B.P.C. (page 749)
NUX VOMICA TINCTURE, B.P. It contains 0·125 per cent of strychnine. Dose: 0·5 to 2 millilitres.

NYSTATIN

Nystatin is an antifungal substance produced by the growth of *Streptomyces noursei* or by any other means.

Solubility. Very slightly soluble in water; slightly soluble in alcohol and in methyl alcohol; insoluble in ether and in chloroform.

Standard
It complies with the requirements of the British Pharmacopoeia.
It is a yellow to light brown, hygroscopic powder with a characteristic odour and contains not less than 3000 Units per mg, calculated with reference to the dried substance. The loss on drying under the prescribed conditions is not more than 5·0 per cent. A 3 per cent suspension in water has a pH of 6·5 to 8·0.

Storage. It should be stored in airtight containers, protected from light, at a temperature not exceeding 5°. Under these conditions, the potency may fall at the rate of about 1 per cent per month.

Actions and uses. Nystatin is an antibiotic which is active against a wide range of fungi and yeasts. When given by mouth, little is absorbed.
The chief use of nystatin is in the local treatment of monilial infections of the mucous membrane and of the skin and nails. In the treatment of monilial infections of the mouth, nystatin is used in the form of tablets which are allowed to dissolve slowly in the mouth or it is applied topically as a suspension. For intestinal moniliasis it is given by mouth in the form of tablets in a dosage of 500,000 to 1,000,000 Units three times a day. Vaginal moniliasis may be treated by means of soluble tablets or pessaries containing 100,000 Units; local treatment may be supplemented by oral administration of nystatin with a view to reducing the risk of reinfection from the intestinal tract. In monilial infections of the skin, nystatin is applied several times daily as an ointment or dusting-powder.
Although it is poorly absorbed from the

gastro-intestinal tract, nystatin has occasionally seemed to be of value when given by mouth
in systemic moniliasis.

UNDESIRABLE EFFECTS. Oral administration
of nystatin may give rise to diarrhoea,
nausea, and vomiting, but these effects are
rare and usually transient.

Dose. See above under **Actions and uses.**

OTHER NAMES: *Nitacin®*; *Nystan®*

Preparations
NYSTATIN MIXTURE, B.P.C. (page 749)
NYSTATIN OINTMENT, B.P.C. (page 763)
NYSTATIN PESSARIES, B.P.C. (page 773)
NYSTATIN TABLETS, B.P. Unless otherwise specified,
tablets each containing 500,000 Units of nystatin are
supplied. They are sugar coated. They should be
stored in airtight containers, at a temperature not
exceeding 25°; under these conditions they may be
expected to retain their potency for at least three
years.

OCTYL GALLATE

$C_{15}H_{22}O_5 = 282.3$

Octyl Gallate is octyl 3,4,5-trihydroxybenzoate.

Solubility. Insoluble in water; soluble, at 20°, in
2·5 parts of alcohol, in 3 parts of ether, in 30 parts of
chloroform, in 1 part of acetone, in 33 parts of arachis
oil, in 0·7 part of methyl alcohol, and in 7 parts of
propylene glycol.

Standard
It complies with the requirements of the British
Pharmacopoeia.
It is a white or creamy-white, odourless powder. The

loss on drying at 70° is not more than 0·5 per cent. It
has a melting-point of 100° to 102°.

Storage. It should be stored in airtight containers,
protected from light, contact with metals being
avoided.

Uses. Octyl gallate is used as an antoxidant
for preserving oils and fats, as described
under Propyl Gallate (page 413).

OESTRADIOL BENZOATE

SYNONYMS: Oestradiol Monobenzoate;
Oestradioli Benzoas

$C_{25}H_{28}O_3 = 376.5$

Oestradiol Benzoate is 3-benzoyloxyoestra-1,3,5(10)-trien-17β-ol.

Solubility. Insoluble in water and in solutions of
alkali hydroxides; soluble, at 20°, in 150 parts of
alcohol, in 50 parts of acetone, in 500 parts of arachis
oil, and in 200 parts of ethyl oleate.

Standard
It complies with the requirements of the European
Pharmacopoeia.
It occurs as odourless colourless crystals or white or
almost white crystalline powder and contains not less
than 97·0 and not more than the equivalent of 103·0
per cent of $C_{25}H_{28}O_3$, calculated with reference to the
dried substance. The loss on drying under the prescribed conditions is not more than 0·5 per cent. It has
a melting-point of 191° to 198°.

Sterilisation. Oily solutions for injection are
sterilised by dry heat.

Storage. It should be protected from light.

Actions and uses. Oestradiol is the most
active of the naturally occurring oestrogens.
These substances are concerned in producing
the oestrous changes in animals and in
controlling certain functions of the human
uterus and accessory organs, particularly
the proliferation of the endometrium, the
development of the decidua, and the cyclic
changes in the cervix and vagina. They
also influence the development of the
secondary sex characters and mammary

glands and affect the contractility of the
uterus and its response to oxytocin drugs.
Large doses of oestrogens depress the activities
of the anterior lobe of the pituitary gland.
The main therapeutic uses of the oestrogens
are: for replacement therapy in conditions
in which there is a deficiency of them; for the
treatment of conditions associated with hypoplasia of the genital tract, such as primary
amenorrhoea and delayed onset of puberty;
for the treatment of the menopausal syndrome,
particularly the vasomotor disturbances and
psychological upsets; for the treatment of
conditions such as senile vaginitis, vulvitis,
and kraurosis vulvae; and for the treatment,
in conjunction with progesterone, of some
disturbances of menstruation, including
secondary amenorrhoea due to ovarian deficiency, some types of dysmenorrhoea, and
functional uterine bleeding.
Oestrogens are also used to inhibit lactation;
for this purpose large doses are required,
which act by inhibiting the luteotropic
hormone of the anterior lobe of the pituitary
gland. They are also used for the palliative
treatment of carcinoma of the prostate and
breast, to diminish pain and to produce

temporary subjective improvement, particularly in bone metastases.

Oestrogens are administered orally, intramuscularly, and topically by inunction and in pessaries, tampons, and suppositories. The oral dose of the naturally occurring oestrogens is five to ten times that required by intramuscular injection.

Oestradiol benzoate is given by intramuscular injection to provide a depot from which the drug is slowly liberated during two to five days. The dosage is 1 to 5 milligrams at intervals of one to fourteen days; smaller doses may be used for maintenance therapy.

UNDESIRABLE EFFECTS. Oestrogens may sometimes cause undesirable uterine growth and proliferation and withdrawal bleeding in the menopause. If bleeding occurs following the use of oestrogens in the menopause, action should be taken to exclude its being due to cancer. The effects of the oestrogens on the uterus are enhanced by alternating courses of treatment with oestrogens and progesterone.

Dose. 1 to 5 milligrams daily by intramuscular injection.

Preparation
OESTRADIOL BENZOATE INJECTION, B.P. It is a sterile solution of oestradiol benzoate in ethyl oleate or other suitable ester, in a suitable fixed oil, or in any mixture of these; it may contain suitable alcohols. Unless otherwise specified, a solution containing 1 mg in 1 ml is supplied. It should be protected from light. Solid matter may separate on standing and should be redissolved by heating before use. Ampoules containing 2, 5, and 10 mg are also available.

OTHER NAME: *Benztrone®*

OLEIC ACID

$C_{18}H_{34}O_2 = 282.5$

$$CH_3 \cdot [CH_2]_7 \cdot CH : CH \cdot [CH_2]_7 \cdot CO_2H$$

Oleic Acid consists chiefly of octadec-9-enoic acid and may be prepared by the hydrolysis of fats or fixed oils or by treating commercial oleins with superheated steam. It also contains some stearic and palmitic acids and usually traces of iron, probably derived from the vessels in which it is stored.

Solubility. Insoluble in water; readily soluble in alcohol, in ether, in chloroform, and in light petroleum.

Standard
It complies with the requirements of the British Pharmacopoeia.
It is a yellowish to pale brown, oily liquid with a characteristic tallow-like odour. It has a weight per ml at 20° of 0.889 g to 0.895 g.

Storage. It should be stored in well-filled airtight containers, protected from light, contact with iron being avoided.

Uses. Oleic acid forms soaps with alkaline substances and is used in the preparation of injections, liniments, and lotions.

OLIVE OIL

SYNONYM: Oleum Olivae

Olive Oil is the fixed oil obtained by expression from the ripe fruits of *Olea europaea* L. (Fam. Oleaceae), a small tree cultivated in Portugal, countries bordering on the Mediterranean Sea, California, and South Australia; the oil may be refined.

Constituents. Olive oil consists of glycerides, the chief fatty acid of which is oleic acid, with smaller amounts of palmitic, linoleic, stearic, and myristic acids.

Solubility. Very slightly soluble in alcohol; miscible with ether, with chloroform, and with light petroleum.

Standard
It complies with the requirements of the British Pharmacopoeia.
It is a pale yellow or greenish-yellow oil with a slight but not rancid odour; at low temperatures it may be solid or partly solid. It has a weight per ml at 20° of 0.910 g to 0.913 g.

Adulterants and substitutes. Common adulterants of olive oil include cottonseed oil, arachis oil, tea-seed oil, obtained from *Camellia sasanqua* Thunb. and sometimes other species of *Camellia* (Fam. Theaceae), and sesame oil.
Tea-seed oil may be detected by the following test:
Add 0.2 ml to a cooled mixture of 0.8 ml of *acetic anhydride*, 1.5 ml of *chloroform*, and 0.2 ml of *sulphuric acid*, mix, and cool to room temperature; add *acetic anhydride*, dropwise, if necessary, to produce a clear solution and allow to stand for five minutes; the solution is green by reflected light, but no brown colour is seen by transmitted light. Add 10 ml of *anaesthetic ether* and mix immediately by inverting the tube; a transient faint pink colour may appear, but no red colour is produced.
Olive oil is sometimes prepared by refining oil obtained by solvent-extraction processes and such oil is often sold for edible or technical purposes.

Sterilisation. It is sterilised by dry heat.

Storage. It should be stored in well-filled airtight containers. If it has solidified, it should be completely melted and mixed before use.

Actions and uses. Olive oil is nutritious, demulcent, and mildly laxative. In the form of an emulsion, it may be given as a nitrogen-free diet during the treatment of renal failure.

Olive oil (100 to 500 millilitres) warmed to body temperature is injected per rectum to facilitate removal of impacted faeces.

Externally, olive oil is emollient and soothing to inflamed surfaces. It is applied to the skin to remove incrustations in eczema and psoriasis and is used as a lubricant in massage. Olive oil is employed in the preparation of liniments, ointments, plasters, and soaps and as a vehicle in oily suspensions for injection.

OPIUM

SYNONYM: Raw Opium

Opium consists of the dried or partly dried latex obtained from the unripe capsules of *Papaver somniferum* L. (Fam. Papaveraceae).

Opium is collected principally in the Indian subcontinent. It has also been collected in Asiatic Turkey, Yugoslavia, Greece, and Bulgaria. The exuded latex is partially dried by spontaneous evaporation together with artificial heat, and is manipulated to form cakes of uniform composition, variously shaped according to the country of origin, and known in commerce as Turkish, Indian, or European opium.

Varieties. Natural European and natural Turkish opiums are manipulated to form commercial products. Manipulated Turkish opium: brick-shaped masses, about 13 to 15 cm long, 10 to 12 cm wide, and 10 to 12 cm thick, usually bearing on one surface an indented monogram consisting of the letters T and M inside an O, covered with roughly powdered poppy leaves, weighing usually about 2 kg; outer surface firm, plastic, or very rarely brittle; internally softer, chocolate-brown or dark brown, and somewhat granular.

Manipulated European opium: elongated masses with rounded ends, weighing up to about 600 g, with or without a covering of broken poppy leaves; internally dark brown, soft when fresh, becoming plastic or brittle.

Indian opium: cubical or rectangular blocks or masses, weighing from 1 to 10 kg, wrapped in greaseproof paper or plastic material, varying in consistence from hard and brittle to plastic; internally dark brown to almost black, smooth and homogeneous.

Constituents. Opium contains about 25 alkaloids; morphine, which occurs in commercial varieties in proportions varying from about 9 to 17 per cent, exists in combination with meconic and sulphuric acids in the form of salts readily soluble in water. Turkish opium contains about 10 to 16 per cent of morphine, Yugoslavian about 15 to 17 per cent, and Indian about 9 to 12 per cent.

The proportion of noscapine [(−)-narcotine], which exists partly in the free state and partly as a salt, is usually about 2 to 9 per cent.

Codeine is present to the extent of about 0·3 to 4 per cent in combination with acids, Indian opium containing the highest proportion and Turkish opium the lowest.

The remaining alkaloids constitute about 2·5 to 6 per cent of the drug; they include thebaine, narceine, papaverine, (±)-reticuline, meconidine, codamine, (±)-laudanine, laudanosine, neopine, lanthopine, protopine, cryptopine, oxynarcotine, gnoscopine [(±)-narcotine], xanthaline (papaveraldine), tritopine [(−)-laudanine], hydrocotarnine, porphyroxine (in Indian opium), narcotoline, papaveramine, and possibly others. They exist partly in the free state and partly combined with meconic and sulphuric acids. Meconin, meconoidin, and opionin are neutral substances, present in small proportions only.

Other constituents are mucilage, sugar, wax, and caoutchouc, together with salts of calcium, magnesium, and potassium. Starch, tannin, calcium oxalate, and fat do not normally occur, and their presence therefore indicates sophistication.

When exhausted with water, undried opium gives an infusion which is acid and yields from 40 to 55 per cent of dry aqueous extract which contains most of the morphine present in the drug (constituting about 25 per cent of the extract).

Standard
It complies with the requirements of the British Pharmacopoeia.
It contains not less than 9·5 per cent of morphine, calculated as anhydrous morphine.

Macroscopical characters: characters of different varieties differ widely and are described under Varieties (above).
Odour strong, characteristic; taste bitter.

Microscopical characters: the diagnostic characters are: *latex* in abundant brown, granular, amorphous masses amongst which occur small quantities of structures insoluble in water:
Outer epidermis of capsule of poppy plant in fragments composed of polyhedral tabular cells in surface view, about 20 to 50 μm in either direction with strongly thickened unlignified walls sometimes strongly pitted, giving the lumen a stellate form; outer wall thick as seen in transverse section; *stomata* anomocytic, oval, about 17 μm wide and 25 μm long or sometimes circular and about 20 μm in diameter; *epidermis of leaf* of poppy plant present as rare fragments composed of thin-walled polyhedral cells; *stomata* anomocytic, confined to abaxial surface; *starch* almost absent, but a few small granules present measuring about 4 to 8 μm in diameter; *pollen grains* occasional, subspherical, with 3 pores, 16 to **20** to **30** to 40 μm in diameter.

Adulterants and substitutes. Smoking opium, produced by processes of maceration and digestion of opium in water, evaporation of the extract, and roasting, contains only about 5 per cent of morphine.

Powdered poppy capsule sometimes occurs as an adulterant and can be identified by the characters of the inner epidermis of the pericarp, which is composed of subrectangular and often slightly sinuous cells, as seen in surface view, about 85 to 245 μm long and 18 to 50 μm wide, with lignified and pitted anticlinal walls, about 7 μm thick; fairly numerous stomata, usually 5- or 6-sided and about 25 to 35 μm in diameter.

Actions and uses. The actions, uses, and undesirable effects of opium are substantially those of the morphine it contains and are described under Morphine Hydrochloride (page 314). The other alkaloids have little, if any, of the effects of morphine on pain and anxiety, and the claims that they enhance the actions of morphine, other than its constipating action, are not convincing.

The action of opium is exerted less rapidly than that of morphine, as absorption appears to take place less readily. Noscapine and papaverine relax intestinal muscle, in contrast to morphine and codeine which increase its tone; this action contributes to the greater constipating effect of opium as compared with that of morphine. Preparations of opium are therefore preferred in the treatment of diarrhoea and intestinal disorders, but their use in these conditions is diminishing.

Opium is given as a diaphoretic in the form of Ipecacuanha and Opium Powder or Tablets in the early stages of colds. For the action of opium on the intestine, Aromatic Chalk Powder with Opium is employed. Camphorated Opium Tincture is used to relieve coughing.

Although preparations containing opium have been used in a variety of local applications, the opium alkaloids have no action on motor or sensory nerve endings and there is no evidence that they are absorbed after local application in sufficient amount to produce any characteristic effect.

PRECAUTIONS. As for Morphine Hydrochloride (page 314).

DEPENDENCE. Opium may give rise to dependence of the morphine type, as described under Morphine Hydrochloride (page 314).

POISONING. The procedure as described under Morphine Hydrochloride (page 314) should be adopted.

NOTE. When Opium is prescribed, Powdered Opium is dispensed.

Preparations
OPIUM, POWDERED, B.P. (see below)
SQUILL LINCTUS, OPIATE, B.P.C. (page 725)
SQUILL LINCTUS, OPIATE, PAEDIATRIC, B.P.C. (page 725)
CHALK WITH OPIUM MIXTURE, AROMATIC, B.P.C. (page 739)
IPECACUANHA MIXTURE, OPIATE, PAEDIATRIC, B.P.C. (page 744)
OPIUM MIXTURE, CAMPHORATED, COMPOUND, B.P.C. (page 749)
SQUILL PASTILLES, OPIATE, B.P.C. (page 770)
OPIUM TINCTURE, B.P. It contains 1 per cent of anhydrous morphine. Dose: 0·25 to 2 millilitres.
OPIUM TINCTURE, CAMPHORATED, B.P. (*Syn.* Paregoric). It contains 5 per cent of Opium Tincture, 0·5 per cent of benzoic acid, 0·3 per cent of camphor, and 0·3 per cent of anise oil in alcohol (60 per cent). It contains 0·05 per cent of anhydrous morphine. Dose: 2 to 10 millilitres.
OPIUM TINCTURE, CAMPHORATED, CONCENTRATED, B.P.C. (page 822)

POWDERED OPIUM

SYNONYM: Opium Pulveratum

Powdered Opium is obtained by reducing Opium, dried at a moderate temperature, to a fine or moderately fine powder and adjusting, if necessary, to the required strength. When adjustment is necessary, powdered Lactose, coloured with burnt sugar, or powdered cocoa husk is added.

Standard
It complies with the requirements of the British Pharmacopoeia.
It is a light brown powder consisting of yellowish-brown or brownish-red particles and contains 10·0 per cent of morphine, calculated as anhydrous morphine (limits, 9·5 to 10·5 per cent).
It possesses the diagnostic microscopical characters, odour, and taste described under Opium; if powdered cocoa husk is present the structures which it exhibits are those described for the substance in the British Pharmacopoeia under Powdered Opium.

Storage. It should be stored in airtight containers.

Actions and uses. Powdered opium has the actions, uses, and undesirable effects described under Opium.

PRECAUTIONS. As for Morphine Hydrochloride (page 314).

DEPENDENCE. Powdered opium may give rise to dependence of the morphine type, as described under Morphine Hydrochloride (page 314).

POISONING. The procedure as described under Morphine Hydrochloride (page 314) should be adopted.

Dose. 25 to 200 milligrams.

Preparations
CHALK WITH OPIUM POWDER, AROMATIC, B.P.C. (page 776)
IPECACUANHA AND OPIUM POWDER, B.P.C. (page 777)
IPECACUANHA AND OPIUM TABLETS, B.P.C. (page 811)

ORANGE OIL

SYNONYMS: Sweet Orange Oil; Oleum Aurantii

Orange Oil is obtained by mechanical means from the fresh peel of the sweet orange, *Citrus sinensis* (L.) Osbeck (Fam. Rutaceae). It is produced in many tropical and subtropical countries.

Constituents. Orange oil contains at least 90 per cent of (+)-limonene. It also contains up to 3 per cent of aldehydes, calculated as decanal.

Solubility. Soluble, at 20°, in 7 parts of alcohol (90 per cent), but rarely with formation of bright solutions on account of the presence of waxy non-volatile substances.

Standard

DESCRIPTION. A yellow to yellowish-brown liquid; odour characteristic.

OPTICAL ROTATION. At 20°, +94° to +99°. When distilled, the first 10 per cent of the distillate has an optical rotation the same as, or only slightly lower than, the original oil.

REFRACTIVE INDEX. At 20°, 1·472 to 1·476.

WEIGHT PER ML. At 20°, 0·842 g to 0·848 g.

NON-VOLATILE MATTER. 1·0 to 5·0 per cent w/w, determined by the following method:
Evaporate about 2 g, accurately weighed, in a flat-bottomed dish of nickel or other suitable metal, 9 cm in diameter and 1·5 cm deep, by heating on a vigorously boiling water-bath for a total of 4 hours and weigh the residue.

CONTENT OF ALDEHYDES. Not less than 1·0 per cent w/w, calculated as decanal, $C_{10}H_{20}O$, determined by the method for Lemon Oil, page 264; each ml of 0·5N potassium hydroxide in alcohol (60 per cent) is equivalent to 0·07876 g (*i.e.* 0·07813 × 1·008) of $C_{10}H_{20}O$.

Adulterants and substitutes. Distilled orange oil is an inferior article, the effect of heat and steaming being detrimental to the oxygenated compounds. Bitter orange oil, from *C. aurantium* L., is chemically almost identical with sweet orange oil, but can be distinguished by its odour and bitter taste. The optical rotation at 20° varies from +92° to +97°, the weight per ml at 20° from 0·845 g to 0·851 g, and the aldehyde content from 0·3 to 1 per cent, calculated as decanal.

Stability. Orange oil deteriorates on keeping, acquiring a disagreeable terebinthinate taste.

Storage. It should be stored in well-filled airtight containers, protected from light, in a cool place.

Uses. Orange oil is employed as a flavouring agent, in perfumery, and for the preparation of the terpeneless oil.

TERPENELESS ORANGE OIL

SYNONYM: Oleum Aurantii Deterpenatum

Terpeneless Orange Oil may be prepared by concentrating Orange Oil in vacuo until most of the terpenes have been removed, or by solvent partition.

Constituents. Terpeneless orange oil consists chiefly of the free alcohols, (+)-linalol and (+)-terpineol, with considerable quantities of aldehydes, chiefly decanal, and smaller amounts of esters.

Solubility. Soluble, at 20°, in 1 part of alcohol (90 per cent).

Standard

DESCRIPTION. A yellow or orange-yellow liquid; odour that of orange.

OPTICAL ROTATION. At 20°, not more than +55°.

REFRACTIVE INDEX. At 20°, 1·461 to 1·473.

WEIGHT PER ML. At 20°, 0·860 g to 0·880 g.

CONTENT OF ALDEHYDES. 24 to 30 per cent w/w, calculated as decanal, $C_{10}H_{20}O$, determined by the method for Lemon Oil (page 264), about 1·5 g, accurately weighed, being used.

Storage. It should be stored in well-filled airtight containers, protected from light, in a cool place.

Uses. Terpeneless orange oil is used as a flavouring agent. It has a stronger flavour and odour and is more readily soluble than orange oil; 1 millilitre of terpeneless oil is equivalent in flavour to about 25 millilitres of the natural oil.

Preparation

ORANGE SPIRIT, COMPOUND, B.P.C. (page 793)

DRIED BITTER-ORANGE PEEL

SYNONYM: Aurantii Cortex Siccatus

Dried Bitter-Orange Peel is the dried outer part of the pericarp of the ripe or nearly ripe fruit of *Citrus aurantium* L. (Fam. Rutaceae). It is imported chiefly from Spain and other Mediterranean countries and from the West Indies.

Constituents. Dried bitter-orange peel contains volatile oil, the bitter glycoside aurantiamarin, the glycosides hesperidin and isohesperidin, hesperic acid, aurantiamaric acid, and an eriodictyol glycoside.
The peel also contains the carotenoid pigments kryptoxanthin, zeaxanthin, xanthophyll, citraurin, and violaxanthin. Pectin and a little fixed oil are also present, as well as small quantities of vitamins A, B₁,

and C. The bitter constituents occur chiefly in the white "zest" of the peel.
It yields to alcohol (60 per cent) about 30 to 40 per cent of extractive.

Standard
It complies with the requirements of the British Pharmacopoeia.

It contains not less than 2·5 per cent v/w of volatile oil.

Macroscopical characters: strips, ribbons, or quarters; outer surface red to dark orange-red and somewhat rough from the presence of numerous minute pits each corresponding to an oil gland; inner surface with only a small amount of white spongy pericarp; fracture short.

Odour aromatic; taste aromatic and bitter.

Microscopical characters: the diagnostic characters are: *epidermis,* small polyhedral cells about 5 to 13 μm wide with numerous circular *stomata* about 25 to 28 μm in diameter; tissues subjacent to epidermis parenchymatous, many cells containing prismatic *crystals* of calcium oxalate; numerous large *oil glands* and some small *vascular strands* embedded in the parenchyma.

Adulterants and substitutes. Owing to excessive rupturing of the oil glands, peel in narrow machine-cut strips (gelatin-cut) is not equal in aroma to hand-cut

dried peel and the volatile oil content is usually only about 1 per cent.

Dried sweet-orange peel may be distinguished by its paler, more yellowish colour and by being much less bitter in taste.

Indian orange peel is the fresh or the dried outer part of the pericarp of varieties of *C. aurantium* L. grown in the Indian sub-continent and Ceylon.

Storage. It should be stored in airtight containers.

Actions and uses. Dried bitter-orange peel is used as a flavouring agent.

Preparations
GENTIAN TINCTURE, COMPOUND, B.P.C. (page 822)
ORANGE PEEL INFUSION, CONCENTRATED, B.P.C. (page 704)
ORANGE SYRUP, B.P.C. (page 800)
ORANGE TINCTURE, B.P.C. (page 823)

ORCIPRENALINE SULPHATE

$C_{22}H_{36}N_2O_{10}S = 520·6$

Orciprenaline Sulphate is (±)-1-(3,5-dihydroxyphenyl)-2-isopropylaminoethanol sulphate. It contains variable amounts of water and methyl alcohol of crystallisation.

Solubility. Soluble, at 20°, in 2 parts of water and in 1 part of alcohol; very slightly soluble in chloroform and in ether.

Standard
It complies with the requirements of the British Pharmacopoeia.
It is a white odourless crystalline powder and contains not less than 98·0 and not more than the equivalent of 102·0 per cent of $C_{22}H_{36}N_2O_{10}S$, calculated with reference to the anhydrous and methyl-alcohol-free substance. The total content of water and methyl alcohol is not more than 6 per cent w/w of which not more than 2 per cent w/w is water. It has a melting-point of about 205°. A 10 per cent solution in water has a pH of 4·0 to 5·5.

Stability. It is more stable than adrenaline and other 3,4-substituted phenylalkanolamines but it is oxidised by atmospheric oxygen, especially in neutral or alkaline solution, in the presence of light and of heavy metal ions.

Sterilisation. Solutions are sterilised by heating in an autoclave or by filtration.

Storage. It should be protected from light.

Actions and uses. Orciprenaline is a sympathomimetic amine with actions similar to those described under Isoprenaline Sulphate (page 255). It differs in having a longer duration of action and in being effective when taken by mouth and swallowed.

In the treatment of bronchial asthma a dose of 20 milligrams may be given by mouth four times a day. A more rapid effect is obtained by the use of a spray solution or by the subcutaneous or deep intramuscular injection of 500 micrograms.

UNDESIRABLE EFFECTS. Tachycardia, headache, and dizziness are usually associated with overdosage, but are transient and seldom so severe as to necessitate withdrawal of the drug. Nausea may occur and, occasionally, difficulty in urination.

PRECAUTIONS AND CONTRA-INDICATIONS. Orciprenaline should not be given to patients who are being treated with a monoamine-oxidase inhibitor, such as isocarboxazid, nialamide, phenelzine, or tranylcypromine, or within about ten days of the discontinuation of such treatment. Orciprenaline should not be given to patients with thyrotoxicosis.

The excessive use of sprays containing orciprenaline should be avoided as it may lead to fatal results.

Dose. See above under **Actions and uses.**

Preparations
ORCIPRENALINE AEROSOL INHALATION, B.P.C. (page 646)
ORCIPRENALINE ELIXIR, B.P.C. (page 673)
ORCIPRENALINE INJECTION, B.P. It consists of a sterile solution of orciprenaline sulphate in Water for Injections containing suitable stabilising agents. Unless otherwise specified, a solution containing 500 μg in 1 ml is supplied. It should be protected from light.
ORCIPRENALINE TABLETS, B.P. Unless otherwise specified, tablets each containing 20 mg of orciprenaline sulphate are supplied. They should be protected from light.

OTHER NAME: *Alupent*®

ORPHENADRINE CITRATE

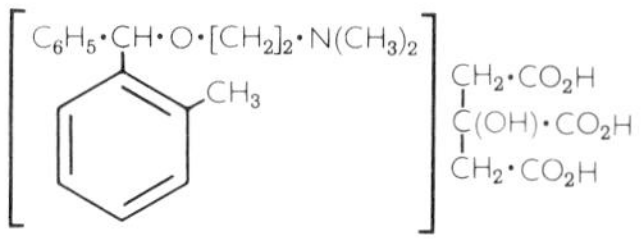

$C_{24}H_{31}NO_8 = 461 \cdot 5$

Orphenadrine Citrate is dimethyl[2-(α-o-tolylbenzyloxy)-ethyl]amine dihydrogen citrate.

$$\left[\begin{array}{c} C_6H_5 \cdot CH \cdot O \cdot [CH_2]_2 \cdot N(CH_3)_2 \\ \\ CH_3 \end{array} \right] \begin{array}{c} CH_2 \cdot CO_2H \\ C(OH) \cdot CO_2H \\ CH_2 \cdot CO_2H \end{array}$$

Solubility. Soluble, at 20°, in 70 parts of water; slightly soluble in alcohol; insoluble in ether and in chloroform.

Standard
It complies with the requirements of the British Pharmacopoeia.
It is a white or almost white, crystalline, almost odourless powder and contains not less than 98·5 and not more than the equivalent of 101·0 per cent of $C_{24}H_{31}NO_8$, calculated with reference to the dried substance. The loss on drying under the prescribed conditions is not more than 0·5 per cent. It has a melting-point of 135° to 138°.

Storage. It should be protected from light.

Actions and uses. Orphenadrine has a chemical structure closely related to that of diphenhydramine, but has only a weak antihistamine action and produces euphoria without sedation. By its action on the central nervous system it reduces spasm of voluntary muscle, and it is used, usually in conjunction with other drugs, in the treatment of parkinsonism; it relieves mental depression and reduces excessive salivation and perspiration. It is also used to reduce spasm and associated pain resulting from injury to voluntary muscle. The daily dosage is 200 milligrams of orphenadrine citrate by mouth, gradually increased to up to 400 milligrams according to the response of the patient.

There is some evidence that, with continued use, treatment with orphenadrine may become less effective.

In addition to the tablets, orphenadrine citrate is available as a solution for injection containing 60 milligrams in 2 millilitres; the usual dosage by intramuscular or intravenous injection is 60 milligrams once or twice daily.

UNDESIRABLE EFFECTS. Insomnia, mental excitement, increased tremor, and nausea may occur, but these usually disappear if the dosage is reduced.

PRECAUTIONS. Orphenadrine should be used with caution in patients with urinary retention or glaucoma.

Dose. See above under **Actions and uses.**

Preparation
SLOW ORPHENADRINE CITRATE TABLETS, B.P. Unless otherwise specified, tablets each containing 100 mg of orphenadrine citrate, formulated to release the medicament over several hours, are supplied. They should be protected from light.

OTHER NAME: *Norflex®*

ORPHENADRINE HYDROCHLORIDE

$C_{18}H_{23}NO,HCl = 305 \cdot 8$

Orphenadrine Hydrochloride is dimethyl[2-(α-o-tolylbenzyloxy)ethyl]amine hydrochloride.

Solubility. Soluble, at 20°, in 1 part of water, in 1 part of alcohol, and in 2 parts of chloroform; insoluble in ether.

Standard
It complies with the requirements of the British Pharmacopoeia.
It is a white or almost white, crystalline, odourless powder and contains not less than 98·5 and not more than the equivalent of 101·0 per cent of $C_{18}H_{23}NO,HCl$, calculated with reference to the dried substance. The loss on drying under the prescribed conditions is not more than 0·5 per cent. It has a melting-point of 159° to 162°.

Storage. It should be stored in airtight containers, protected from light.

Actions and uses. Orphenadrine hydrochloride has the actions, uses, and undesirable effects described under Orphenadrine Citrate (above).

PRECAUTIONS. As for Orphenadrine Citrate (above).

Dose. By mouth, 200 to 400 milligrams daily in divided doses; by intramuscular injection, up to 40 milligrams three times a day.

Preparation
ORPHENADRINE HYDROCHLORIDE TABLETS, B.P. Unless otherwise specified, tablets each containing 50 mg of orphenadrine hydrochloride are supplied. They are sugar coated.

OTHER NAME: *Disipal®*

OXIDISED CELLULOSE

Oxidised Cellulose is a sterilised polyanhydroglucuronic acid and may be prepared by oxidation of cotton, usually in the form of surgical gauze or lint, with nitrogen dioxide.

Solubility. Insoluble in water and in mineral acids; soluble in solutions of alkali hydroxides.

Standard
It complies with the requirements of the British Pharmacopoeia.
It is a white or creamy-white gauze, lint, or knitted material with a faint odour and contains 16·0 to 22·0 per cent of carboxyl, calculated with reference to the dried substance. The loss on drying under the prescribed conditions is not more than 15·0 per cent.

Storage. It should be stored in containers sealed to exclude micro-organisms, protected from light, in a cool place. It cannot be satisfactorily resterilised and if a portion only of the contents of a container is used on any one occasion, strict aseptic precautions should be taken to avoid contamination.

Actions and uses. Oxidised cellulose is an absorbable haemostatic, the action of which depends on the formation of a coagulum consisting of salts of polyanhydroglucuronic acid and haemoglobin.

When oxidised cellulose is applied to a bleeding surface it swells and forms a brown gelatinous mass which is gradually absorbed, usually within two to seven days of application. The rate of absorption depends on the size of the piece used and the vascularity of the area. Complete absorption of large amounts of blood-soaked material may take six weeks or longer. The haemostatic effect of oxidised cellulose is greater when dry material is used, hence moistening with water or saline is undesirable. If used with thrombin solution, however, it should first be neutralised by moistening with a solution of sodium bicarbonate in order to prevent inactivation of the thrombin.

Oxidised cellulose is used as a haemostatic in many types of surgery, including brain surgery. It is useful for packing cavities after surgical excisions and as a haemostatic uterine packing. Since it is non-irritant and completely absorbable, oxidised cellulose may be left in a wound. In dental surgery it is used to pack bleeding tooth sockets.

Except when used as a haemostatic, oxidised cellulose has no advantage as a surface dressing for open wounds, and since it delays the formation of callus, it is contra-indicated in clean bone surgery. It inactivates penicillin.

OTHER NAMES: *Oxycel®*; *Surgicel®*

OXYGEN

SYNONYM: Oxygenium

$O_2 = 32·00$

Oxygen may be obtained by the fractional distillation of liquid air, when it will contain a small proportion of argon and a trace of nitrogen, or by the electrolysis of water, when it will contain a small proportion of hydrogen. When mixed with nitric oxide, red fumes are produced (distinction from nitrous oxide).

Solubility. One volume, measured at normal temperature and pressure, dissolves, at 20°, in 32 volumes of water and in 3·6 volumes of alcohol.

Standard
It complies with the requirements of the European Pharmacopoeia.
It is a colourless odourless gas and contains not less than 99·0 per cent v/v of O_2.

Storage, labelling, and colour-markings. It should be stored compressed in metal cylinders in a special storage room which should be cool and free from materials of an inflammable nature. The valve end of the cylinder should be painted white down to the shoulder, and the remainder of the cylinder black; the name of the gas or chemical symbol "O_2" should be stencilled in paint on the shoulder of the cylinder. The name or chemical symbol of the gas should be clearly and indelibly stamped on the cylinder valve.

Oxygen and carbon dioxide mixtures should be stored in a similar manner. The valve end of the cylinder should be painted white and grey in four segments, two of each colour, down to the shoulder, and the remainder of the cylinder black; the names or chemical symbols of the gases should be stencilled in paint on the shoulder of the cylinder. The names or chemical symbols of the gases should be clearly and indelibly stamped on the cylinder valve.

Oxygen and helium mixtures should be stored in a similar manner. The valve end of the cylinder should be painted white and brown in four segments, two of each colour, down to the shoulder, and the remainder of the cylinder black; the names or chemical symbols of the gases should be stencilled in paint on the shoulder of the cylinder. The names or chemical symbols of the gases should be clearly and indelibly stamped on the cylinder valve.

Actions and uses. Oxygen inhalation is indicated in anoxia in such conditions as pneumonia, post-operative pulmonary complications, pulmonary oedema, shock, asphyxia neonatorum, congestive heart failure, and in poisoning due to coal gas, barbiturates, and other depressants. The addition of 5 or 7 per cent of carbon dioxide to inhaled oxygen stimulates the respiratory centre and causes deeper breathing, and such a mixture is often used in the treatment of carbon monoxide poisoning.

The concentration of oxygen for inhalation over long periods should be about 50 per cent at sea level; it should not as a rule exceed 60 per cent, except at high altitudes when as much as 80 per cent may be necessary, or when the administration is for short periods only. The continued inhalation of oxygen at concentrations above 70 per cent may be dangerous. The administration of concentrations above 50 per cent to premature infants may interfere with the development of a normal retinal blood supply.

The withdrawal of oxygen treatment should be gradual, especially in cases of chronic cyanosis.

Oxygen is administered by means of an oxygen tent, face mask, or nasal catheter. If a catheter is used the oxygen should be passed through a humidifier before inhalation. A flow rate of 5 to 8 litres per minute through a nasal catheter gives an oxygen concentration of 40 to 60 per cent; increasing the rate of flow beyond this does not result in an increased oxygen concentration in the lungs. To obtain concentrations above 60 per cent a mask must be used. A mask is not suitable for prolonged administration, as the percentage of oxygen in the inspired air depends on the depth of respiration and at low flow rates resistance to

breathing increases. An oxygen tent is used for children and those unable to tolerate catheters or masks; a flow rate up to 7 litres per minute will maintain an oxygen concentration of 60 per cent; it is impracticable to maintain concentrations higher than this.

Oxygen under pressure is used in the treatment of carbon monoxide poisoning, in some types of vascular injury, and to increase the effectiveness of irradiation in the treatment of malignant disease. For such purposes the patient is enclosed in a special high-pressure chamber.

Metal cylinders containing oxygen should be fitted with a reducing valve by which the rate of flow can be controlled. It is important that the reducing valve should be free from all traces of oil, as otherwise a violent explosion may occur. Also, if the reducing valve is of the rubber-bellows type, the tap of the reducer should always be opened before opening the main oxygen tap on the cylinder; opening the main tap with the reducing valve tap closed has been known to cause spontaneous fire.

OXYPHENBUTAZONE

$C_{19}H_{20}N_2O_3,H_2O = 342.4$

Oxyphenbutazone is 4-butyl-1-*p*-hydroxyphenyl-3,5-dioxo-2-phenylpyrazolidine monohydrate.

Solubility. Very slightly soluble in water; soluble, at 20°, in 3 parts of alcohol, in 20 parts of chloroform, in 20 parts of ether, and in 6 parts of acetone; soluble in solutions of alkali hydroxides.

Standard
It complies with the requirements of the British Pharmacopoeia.
It is a white, crystalline, odourless or almost odourless powder and contains not less than 99·0 per cent of $C_{19}H_{20}N_2O_3$, calculated with reference to the anhydrous substance. It contains 5·0 to 6·0 per cent w/w of water.

Actions and uses. Oxyphenbutazone has the actions, uses, and undesirable effects described under Phenylbutazone (page 374), of which it is a metabolite. It may be used in acute gout, active rheumatoid arthritis, and related diseases, when they do not respond to

safer medication. Oxyphenbutazone is even more slowly excreted than phenylbutazone and does not appear to have any advantage over it.

The usual initial dosage is 400 to 600 milligrams daily in divided doses after meals, reducing to a maintenance dose of 200 to 300 milligrams daily.

PRECAUTIONS. These are as described under Phenylbutazone (page 374).

Dose. See above under **Actions and uses.**

Preparation
OXYPHENBUTAZONE TABLETS, B.P. Unless otherwise specified, tablets each containing 100 mg of oxyphenbutazone are supplied. They are sugar coated.

OTHER NAME: *Tanderil*®

OXYPHENCYCLIMINE HYDROCHLORIDE

$C_{20}H_{29}ClN_2O_3 = 380.9$

Oxyphencyclimine Hydrochloride is 1,4,5,6-tetrahydro-1-methylpyrimidin-2-ylmethyl α-cyclohexyl-α-phenylglycollate hydrochloride.

Solubility. Soluble, at 20°, in 100 parts of water, in 60 parts of alcohol, in 20 parts of methyl alcohol, and in 200 parts of chloroform; very slightly soluble in ether.

Standard
It complies with the requirements of the British Pharmacopoeia.
It is a white, crystalline, odourless powder and contains

not less than 99·0 and not more than the equivalent of 101·0 per cent of $C_{20}H_{29}ClN_2O_3$, calculated with reference to the dried substance. The loss on drying under the prescribed conditions is not more than 0·5 per cent.

Actions and uses. Oxyphencyclimine is an anticholinergic drug with actions, uses, and undesirable effects similar to those described under Propantheline Bromide (page 411), but it has a prolonged action so that its effects may be obtained throughout the day with only two doses. Treatment should commence with 10 to 20 milligrams of oxyphencyclimine hydrochloride daily in divided doses; this should be reduced to a maintenance dose of 10 milligrams daily.

Dose. See above under **Actions and uses.**

Preparation
OXYPHENCYCLIMINE TABLETS, B.P. Unless otherwise specified, tablets each containing 5 mg of oxyphencyclimine hydrochloride are supplied.

OTHER NAME: *Daricon®*

OXYTETRACYCLINE DIHYDRATE

SYNONYM: Oxytetracyclini Dihydras

$C_{22}H_{24}N_2O_9,2H_2O = 496·5$

Oxytetracycline Dihydrate is the dihydrate of 4-dimethylamino-1,4,4a,5,5a,6,11,12a-octa-hydro-3,5,6,10,12,12a-hexahydroxy-6-methyl-1,11-dioxonaphthacene-2-carboxyamide, an antimicrobial substance produced by the growth of certain strains of *Streptomyces rimosus* or by any other means.

Solubility. Slightly soluble in water; readily soluble in dilute acids and in alkalis.

Standard
It complies with the requirements of the European Pharmacopoeia.
It is a yellow, crystalline, odourless powder and contains not less than 950 Units per mg, calculated with reference to the anhydrous substance. It contains 4·0 to 7·5 per cent w/w of water. A 1 per cent suspension in water has a pH of 5·0 to 7·5.

Storage. It should be stored in airtight containers, protected from light.

Actions and uses. Oxytetracycline dihydrate has the actions and uses described under Tetracycline Hydrochloride (page 498) and is given in similar dosage.
Salts of aluminium, calcium, iron, and magnesium, which may decrease the absorption of tetracyclines from the gut, should not be given with oxytetracycline.

UNDESIRABLE EFFECTS; PRECAUTIONS AND CONTRA-INDICATIONS. As for Tetracycline Hydrochloride (page 498).

Dose. For an adult, 1 to 3 grams daily in divided doses; for a child, 10 to 30 milligrams per kilogram body-weight daily in divided doses.

Preparation
OXYTETRACYCLINE TABLETS, B.P. Unless otherwise specified, tablets each containing 250 mg of oxytetracycline dihydrate are supplied. They are film coated or sugar coated. Tablets containing 50 and 100 mg are also available.

OTHER NAMES: *Abbocin®*; *Berkmycen®*; *Clinimycin®*; *Galenomycin®*; *Imperacin®*; *Oxydon®*; *Oxymycin®*; *Oxytetrin®*; *Stecsolin®*; *Terramycin®*; *Unimycin®*

OXYTETRACYCLINE HYDROCHLORIDE

SYNONYM: Oxytetracyclini Hydrochloridum

$C_{22}H_{24}N_2O_9,HCl = 496·9$

Oxytetracycline Hydrochloride is the hydrochloride of 4-dimethylamino-1,4,4a,5,5a,6,11,12a-octahydro-3,5,6,10,12,12a-hexahydroxy-6-methyl-1,11-dioxonaphthacene-2-carboxyamide, an antimicrobial substance produced by the growth of certain strains of *Streptomyces rimosus* or by any other means.

Solubility. Soluble, at 20°, in 2 parts of water, giving a clear solution which becomes turbid on standing, and in 45 parts of alcohol; soluble in propylene glycol.

Standard
It complies with the requirements of the European Pharmacopoeia.
It is a yellow, crystalline, hygroscopic, odourless powder and contains not less than 880 Units per mg, calculated with reference to the anhydrous substance. It contains not more than 2·0 per cent w/w of water. A 1 per cent solution in water has a pH of 2·3 to 2·9.

Sterilisation. Solutions for injection should be prepared by an aseptic technique.

Labelling. If the material is not intended for parenteral administration, the label on the container states that the contents are not be injected.

Storage. It should be stored in airtight containers, protected from light.

Actions and uses. Oxytetracycline hydrochloride has the actions and uses described under Tetracycline Hydrochloride (page 498) and is given in similar dosage.
Salts of aluminium, calcium, iron, and magnesium, which may decrease the absorption of tetracyclines from the gut, should not be given with oxytetracycline.

UNDESIRABLE EFFECTS; PRECAUTIONS AND CONTRA-INDICATIONS. As for Tetracycline Hydrochloride (page 498).

Dose. By mouth: for an adult, 1 to 3 grams daily in divided doses; for a child, 10 to 30 milligrams per kilogram body-weight daily in divided doses.
By intravenous infusion, in a concentration not exceeding 0·1 per cent w/v: for an adult, 1 to 2 grams daily; for a child, 10 to 20 milligrams per kilogram body-weight daily.

Preparations
OXYTETRACYCLINE CAPSULES, B.P. Unless otherwise specified, capsules each containing 250 mg of oxytetracycline hydrochloride are supplied.
OXYTETRACYCLINE INJECTION, B.P. It consists of a sterile solution prepared by dissolving the sterile contents of a sealed container in Water for Injections. The quantity of oxytetracycline hydrochloride in each container should be specified by the prescriber. It should be used within seventy-two hours of preparation and should be stored during this period at a temperature not exceeding 4°. For intravenous infusion. Vials containing 250 and 500 mg are available.

OTHER NAMES: *Berkmycen*®; *Imperacin*®; *Oxytetrin*®; *Terramycin*®; *Unimycin*®

OXYTOCIN INJECTION

Oxytocin Injection is a sterile aqueous solution containing the oxytocic principle of the posterior lobe of the pituitary body, which may be prepared by a process of fractionation from mammalian pituitary glands or by synthesis.

Standard
It complies with the requirements of the British Pharmacopoeia.
It is a clear colourless liquid with a pH of 3·0 to 4·5. Its potency is determined by a biological method. It contains not more than 1 Unit of vasopressin activity per 20 Units (oxytocic).

Sterilisation. It is sterilised by filtration.

Storage. It should be stored between 2° and 10°. Under these conditions it may be expected to retain its potency for at least three years from the date of manufacture. When stored at a temperature not exceeding 25° it may be expected to retain its potency for at least two years from the date of manufacture.

Actions and uses. Oxytocin Injection has the oxytocic action described under Powdered Pituitary (Posterior Lobe), but has little pressor or antidiuretic action. It is used principally for the induction of labour and to overcome uterine inertia.
For the induction of labour, 2 to 5 Units in 1000 millilitres of Dextrose Injection (5 per cent) may be given by slow intravenous infusion, and to overcome uterine inertia in labour, 1 to 5 Units similarly diluted may be given by intravenous infusion at a rate of thirty drops per minute until the inertia is overcome.
Oxytocin Injection is also used to control post-partum haemorrhage, a dose of 2 to 5 Units being given by subcutaneous or intramuscular injection or slow intravenous infusion; it may also be used in conjunction with ergometrine.
Oxytocin is also administered in buccal tablets and as a nasal spray, but it is then less effective and its action is more difficult to control.

PRECAUTIONS. The dosage must be carefully controlled in accordance with the requirements of the patient, as excessive doses give rise to violent contractions, with the danger of rupture of the uterus; the same care is required whether the drug is given transbuccally or by injection.

Dose. See above under **Actions and uses.**

OTHER NAMES: *Pitocin*®; *Syntocinon*®

OXYTOCIN TABLETS

Oxytocin Tablets contain synthetic oxytocin.

Standard
They comply with the requirements of the British Pharmacopoeia.

Storage. They should be stored in airtight containers at a temperature not exceeding 25°. Under these conditions, they may be expected to retain their potency for at least three years after the date of preparation.

Actions and uses. The actions and uses of oxytocin are described under Oxytocin Injection. The tablets are intended to be dissolved slowly in the mouth; absorption of oxytocin is incomplete and the effect is less reliable than when oxytocin is injected.
The usual dose by buccal administration for the induction of labour is 100 Units every thirty minutes.

Dose. See above under **Actions and uses.**

NOTE. Unless otherwise specified, tablets each containing 200 Units of oxytocin are supplied.

FRACTIONATED PALM KERNEL OIL

Fractionated Palm Kernel Oil is obtained by expression of the natural oil from the kernels of *Elaeis guineensis* (Fam. Palmae) followed by selective solvent fractionation and hydrogenation.

Solubility. Insoluble in water; very slightly soluble in alcohol; miscible with ether, with chloroform, and with light petroleum.

Standard
It complies with the requirements of the British Pharmacopoeia.

It is a white, solid, brittle, odourless fat. It has a melting-point of 31° to 36°.

Storage. It should be stored in a cool place.

Uses. Fractionated palm kernel oil is used instead of theobroma oil as a fatty basis for the preparation of suppositories.

OTHER NAMES: *Extracoa®*; *Supercoa®*

PANCREATIN

Pancreatin is a preparation of pancreas containing enzymes having protease, lipase, and amylase activity.

Pancreatin is usually obtained from the fresh or frozen pancreas of certain animals by extracting one part of pancreas with four parts of alcohol (25 per cent).
The dried product is assayed for enzymic activity in respect of protease, lipase, and amylase, and, if each activity is in excess of that required, the product may be diluted with Lactose, Sodium Chloride, or pancreatin of a lower digestive power, provided that the mixture still complies with the minimum requirements of the assay in respect of all three activities.

Solubility. Soluble or partly soluble in water, forming a slightly turbid solution; insoluble in alcohol and in ether.

Standard
It complies with the requirements of the British Pharmacopoeia.
It is a white or buff-coloured amorphous powder, free from unpleasant odour, and contains in 1 mg not less than 1 Unit of protease activity, not less than 15 Units of lipase activity, and not less than 12 Units of amylase activity. The loss on drying at 105° is not more than 5·0 per cent.

Stability. Its proteolytic activity is destroyed by treatment with more than traces of mineral acids and it is thereby distinguished from pepsin, which is active only in acid solution; all enzymic activity of pancreatin is destroyed by strong alkalis and by heat. When dissolved in water, it is precipitated by heat, acids, metallic salts, strong alcohol, and tannic acid, but not by a saturated solution of sodium chloride, differing in this last respect from pepsin.

Storage. It should be stored in airtight containers, in a cool place.

Actions and uses. Pancreatin may be administered by mouth, in the form of powder, tablets, or enteric-coated tablets or granules, to assist the digestion of starch and protein in patients with pancreatic deficiency.
In the treatment of fibrocystic disease, pancreatin is frequently used in the form of a powder having five times the minimum protease activity required by the British Pharmacopoeia; this enables the very high doses (equivalent to up to 40 grams daily of pancreatin conforming to the minimum requirements of the British Pharmacopoeia) to be given in reasonably small bulk.
Pancreatin is also used for the preparation of "predigested" protein foods. For peptonising milk, pancreatin is added to tepid water, and milk, previously heated to 38°, is then added; the mixture is stirred and maintained at 38° for fifteen minutes, or longer if complete peptonisation is desired, and then raised to boiling-point, after which it should be transferred to a cool place. The peptonised milk should be used within twenty-four hours of preparation. Gruel, arrowroot, and other farinaceous foods may be similarly predigested.

Dose. 0·5 to 6 grams with meals.

PAPAVERETUM

Papaveretum consists of the hydrochlorides of alkaloids of opium.

Papaveretum may be prepared from opium by converting the total alkaloids into their hydrochlorides and adjusting the mixture to contain the required proportions of alkaloids, or by mixing suitable proportions of the hydrochlorides of morphine, codeine, noscapine (narcotine), and papaverine.

Solubility. Soluble, at 20°, in 15 parts of water; less soluble in alcohol.

Standard
DESCRIPTION. A white, light brown, or brownish-grey powder.

IDENTIFICATION TESTS. 1. To 0·01 g add 0·2 ml of *sulphomolybdic acid solution*; a purple colour is produced.

2. To 0·01 g, dissolved in 1 ml of water, add 0·05 ml of *ferric chloride test solution*; a blue or greenish-blue colour is produced.

3. Heat 0·01 g with *sulphuric acid* containing a trace of *ferric chloride*; a violet to purple colour is produced.

CONTENT OF ANHYDROUS MORPHINE. 47·5 to 52·5 per cent, determined by the following method:
Transfer about 1 g, accurately weighed, to a separator with 20 ml of water, add 5 ml of 1N sodium hydroxide and 50 ml of *solvent ether*, shake thoroughly, allow to separate, run the lower layer into a second separator containing 25 ml of *solvent ether*, again shake well, allow to separate, and filter the lower layer, if necessary, through a tightly packed plug of cotton wool into a 50-ml graduated flask; wash the solvent ether in the two separators with a mixture of 2·5 ml of 1N sodium hydroxide and 5 ml of water, and then with successive 5-ml portions of water, filtering if necessary, until 50 ml of liquid has been collected.
Transfer the liquid to a small conical flask, add 5 ml of *alcohol (90 per cent)* and 25 ml of *solvent ether*, stopper the flask, shake, add 2·0 g of *ammonium chloride*, shake for 5 minutes and then occasionally during about 30 minutes, so that the total time of shaking is about 15 minutes, and allow to stand overnight.
Decant the ethereal layer as completely as possible into a funnel fitted with a small filter paper, rinse the flask and its contents with a further 10 ml of *solvent ether*, and again decant through the filter; wash the filter with 5 ml of *solvent ether*, added slowly and in portions, then pour the aqueous liquid from the flask into the filter without attempting to remove all the crystals, and, when all the liquid has passed through the filter, wash the flask and filter with *morphinated water* until the filtrate is free from chloride.
Wash the crystals on the filter back into the flask, add 30 ml of 0·1N sulphuric acid, boil, cool, and titrate the excess of acid with 0·1N sodium hydroxide, using *methyl red solution* as indicator; each ml of 0·1N sulphuric acid is equivalent to 0·2853 g of anhydrous morphine; to the amount indicated by the titration add 0·025 g in order to correct for the loss of morphine due to its solubility.

CONTENT OF ANHYDROUS CODEINE. 2·5 to 5·0 per cent, determined by the following method, the operations being carried out in subdued light:
Dissolve about 1 g, accurately weighed, in water and rinse into a separator containing 40 ml of *chloroform*, using a total of 20 ml of water; add 0·05 ml of *dilute hydrochloric acid*, shake vigorously for 30 to 40 seconds, and allow to separate; draw off the lower chloroform layer into a second separator containing 10 ml of 1N sodium hydroxide, shake, and allow to separate; run off the lower chloroform layer into a third separator containing 10 ml of water, shake, and allow to separate; repeat the extraction with four successive 20-ml portions of *chloroform*, washing each extract in turn with the same 10 ml of 1N sodium hydroxide and the same 10 ml of water.
Reserve the washed chloroform extracts for the determination of noscapine.
Transfer the aqueous layer remaining after the extraction with chloroform to a 100-ml beaker, rinsing in with the aqueous washing in the third separator, followed by 5 ml of water, passed in turn through the two separators; add the alkaline washings in the second separator, rinsing in with 5 ml of water.
Warm the contents of the beaker to remove dissolved chloroform, cool, add 3 ml of *dilute sodium hydroxide solution*, stir, and allow to stand for 30 minutes.
Filter through a small filter paper into a 100-ml separator, washing the beaker and filter with two successive 5-ml portions of water.
Extract the combined filtrate and washings with three successive 20-ml portions of *benzene*, washing each extract in turn with the same 10 ml of water; filter the benzene extracts into a clean separator, washing the filter with two successive 5-ml portions of *benzene*, and extract the combined filtrate and washings with 25 ml of *dilute sulphuric acid*, shaking vigorously for 5 minutes

and allowing to separate, and transfer the acid extract to a 100-ml beaker; wash the benzene layer once with 20 ml of water and add the washings to the acid extract; make the combined extract and washings alkaline with *strong ammonia solution* and boil until the volume has been reduced to 20 to 30 ml.
Determine the pH of the solution and adjust if necessary to 3·6 to 4·0 (yellowish-green to *bromocresol green paper*); filter into a 100-ml separator, wash the filter with two successive 5-ml portions of water, and extract the combined filtrate and washings with three successive 20-ml portions of *chloroform*, washing each extract in turn with the same 10 ml of water. Discard the chloroform extracts.
Combine the aqueous solution and washings, make alkaline with 2 ml of *dilute ammonia solution*, and extract with three successive 20-ml portions of *chloroform*, washing each extract in turn with the same 10 ml of water. Filter the chloroform extracts through a filter paper moistened with *chloroform* into a tared flask, evaporate off the chloroform, add 2 ml of *dehydrated alcohol*, evaporate on a water-bath in a current of air, with constant rotation of the flask to avoid undue heating, dry the residue for 10 minutes at 105°, cool, and weigh the residue of anhydrous codeine.

CONTENT OF NOSCAPINE. 16·0 to 22·0 per cent, determined by the following method:
Filter the washed chloroform extracts reserved in the determination of anhydrous codeine through a filter paper moistened with *chloroform* into a dry flask; evaporate off the chloroform, add 2 ml of *dehydrated alcohol*, and evaporate on a water-bath in a current of air, with constant rotation of the flask to avoid undue heating.
Dissolve the residue in 6 ml of *benzene*, add 3 ml of a 10 per cent w/v solution of *potassium hydroxide* in *dehydrated alcohol*, and place in a water-bath at 20° for 40 minutes.
Transfer the solution to a separator, rinsing in with three successive 5-ml portions of *benzene* and then with 10 ml of 1N sodium hydroxide, shake well, and allow to separate; transfer the aqueous layer to a second separator containing 10 ml of *benzene*, shake well, allow to separate, and transfer the aqueous layer to a small conical flask.
Wash the benzene layers in turn with two successive 5-ml portions of 1N sodium hydroxide and then with two successive 5-ml portions of water, adding all the washings to the aqueous solution in the flask.
Reserve the benzene layers for the determination of papaverine.
To the combined aqueous solution and washings add 6·5 ml of *hydrochloric acid* and heat in a water-bath until the temperature of the solution reaches 95°; cool, and transfer to a separator, rinsing in with three successive 5-ml portions of water; add about 7·5 ml of *strong ammonia solution* and extract with successive 20-, 10-, 10-, and 10-ml portions of *chloroform*, washing each extract in turn with the same 10 ml of water in a second separator.
Filter the chloroform extracts through a filter paper moistened with *chloroform* into a tared flask, evaporate off the chloroform, add 2 ml of *dehydrated alcohol*, evaporate on a water-bath in a current of air, with constant rotation of the flask to avoid undue heating, dry the residue for 10 minutes at 105°, cool, and weigh the residue of noscapine.

CONTENT OF PAPAVERINE. 2·5 to 7·0 per cent, determined by the following method:
Filter the benzene layer in the first separator reserved in the determination of noscapine into a dry flask, wash the separator and the filter first with the benzene washings in the second separator and then with 5 ml of *benzene*, evaporate off the benzene, add 2 ml of *dehydrated alcohol*, and evaporate on a water-bath in a current of air, with constant rotation of the flask to avoid undue heating.
Moisten the residue with 1 ml of *hydrochloric acid*, stir frequently with a glass rod during 15 minutes so that the whole of residue is thoroughly moistened with

the acid, wash into a separator through a small plug of cotton wool with a total of 20 ml of water used in small portions, and extract with successive 20-, 10-, 10-, and 10-ml portions of *chloroform*, washing each extract in turn, first with the same 10 ml of 1N sodium hydroxide and then with the same 10 ml of water.

Filter the chloroform extracts into a tared flask, evaporate off the chloroform, and dry, as described in the determination of noscapine; cool, and weigh the residue of papaverine.

Actions and uses. Papaveretum has the sedative and soporific actions described under Morphine Hydrochloride (page 314) but it produces milder secondary effects.

It is used as a means of administering the total alkaloids of opium by parenteral injection; it is given with hyoscine as a sedative before the administration of a general anaes-

thetic. It has also been given with hyoscine and atropine to produce light anaesthesia and "twilight sleep". Papaveretum is also given by mouth.

UNDESIRABLE EFFECTS; DEPENDENCE. These are as described under Morphine Hydrochloride (page 314).

POISONING. The procedure as described under Morphine Hydrochloride (page 314) should be adopted.

Dose. 10 to 20 milligrams by mouth or by injection.

Preparations
PAPAVERETUM INJECTION, B.P.C. (page 715)
PAPAVERETUM TABLETS, B.P.C. (page 814)

OTHER NAMES: *Omnopon®*; Opium Concentratum

PAPAVERINE HYDROCHLORIDE

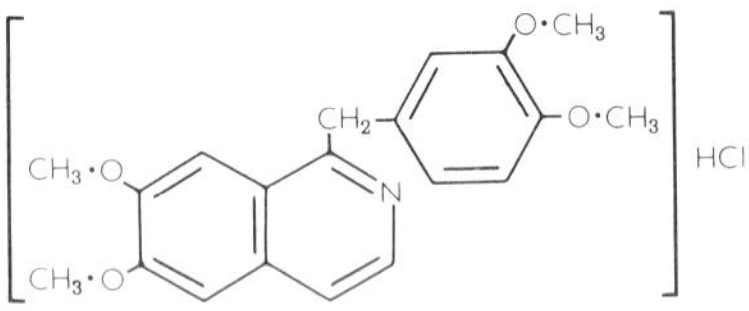

SYNONYMS: Papaver. Hydrochlor.; Papaverinii Chloridum

$C_{20}H_{22}ClNO_4 = 375.9$

Papaverine Hydrochloride is 6,7-dimethoxy-1-(3,4-dimethoxybenzyl)isoquinoline hydrochloride.

Papaverine is one of the alkaloids of opium and may be obtained, after the separation of morphine and codeine, from the mother liquors of opium extract, final purification being made through the acid oxalate (melting-point, 196° to 199°), which, unlike that of the accompanying narcotine, is sparingly soluble in alcohol. Papaverine may also be prepared synthetically.

Solubility. Soluble, at 20°, in 40 parts of water and in 120 parts of alcohol; soluble in chloroform; insoluble in ether.

Standard
It complies with the requirements of the European Pharmacopoeia.
It occurs as odourless white or almost white crystals or white crystalline powder and contains not less than 99.0 per cent of $C_{20}H_{22}ClNO_4$, calculated with reference to the dried substance. The loss on drying under the prescribed conditions is not more than 1.0 per cent. A 2 per cent solution in water has a pH of 3.0 to 4.5.

Sterilisation. Solutions for injection are sterilised by heating in an autoclave or by filtration.

Storage. It should be stored in airtight containers, protected from light.

Actions and uses. Papaverine has little, if any, hypnotic or analgesic action. It is used occasionally to produce relaxation of involuntary muscle in the treatment of peripheral vascular disease and in the treatment of coronary spasm, of intestinal, ureteric, and biliary colic, and of dysmenorrhoea.

It may be administered by mouth or by subcutaneous or intravenous injection, or may be applied to arteries during operations.

It is also used in bronchodilator sprays.

UNDESIRABLE EFFECTS. The intravenous administration of papaverine may give rise to cardiac arrhythmias.

Dose. 150 to 300 milligrams by mouth; 30 to 100 milligrams by injection.

Preparation
ADRENALINE AND ATROPINE SPRAY, COMPOUND, B.P.C. (page 794)

PARACETAMOL

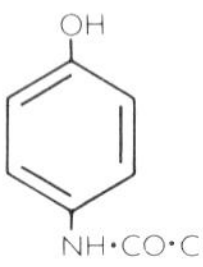

SYNONYM: Acetaminophen

$C_8H_9NO_2 = 151.2$

Paracetamol is *p*-acetamidophenol.

Solubility. Soluble, at 20°, in 70 parts of water, in 7 parts of alcohol, in 13 parts of acetone, in 40 parts of glycerol, and in 9 parts of propylene glycol; soluble in solutions of alkali hydroxides.

Standard
It complies with the requirements of the British Pharmacopoeia.
It occurs as odourless white crystals or crystalline

powder and contains not less than 98·0 and not more than the equivalent of 101·0 per cent of $C_8H_9NO_2$, calculated with reference to the dried substance. The loss on drying under the prescribed conditions is not more than 0·5 per cent. It has a melting-point of 169° to 172°.

Hygroscopicity. It absorbs insignificant amounts of moisture at 25° at relative humidities up to about 90 per cent.

Storage. It should be stored in airtight containers, protected from light.

Actions and uses. Paracetamol has analgesic and antipyretic actions similar to, but weaker than, those described under Aspirin (page 35), it has no anti-inflammatory properties. In the treatment of pain, such as headache, toothache, rheumatism, and neuralgia, paracetamol is given by mouth in a dosage of 0·5 to 1 gram every three or four hours, with a maximum of 4 grams in 24 hours. The usual dose for a child under one year is 120 milligrams, and for a child of one to five years 250 milligrams.

UNDESIRABLE EFFECTS. Purpura may occur. Doses exceeding 7 grams may cause hepatic damage and larger amounts cause irreversible hepatic necrosis. Paracetamol is therefore more hazardous, weight for weight, in suicide attempts than aspirin. Prolonged administration of large doses may give rise to renal damage.

Dose. See above under **Actions and uses.**

Preparations
PARACETAMOL ELIXIR, PAEDIATRIC, B.P.C. (page 674)

PARACETAMOL TABLETS, B.P. Unless otherwise specified, tablets each containing 500 mg are supplied. They should be stored in airtight containers, protected from light.

HARD PARAFFIN

SYNONYM: Paraffinum Durum

Hard Paraffin is a mixture of solid hydrocarbons consisting mainly of n-paraffins and, to a lesser extent, of their isomers.

Hard Paraffin may be obtained by distillation from petroleum, the hard paraffin being separated from the appropriate fractions by pressing or solvent processes, sweated and refined by clay or acid. It may also be obtained, in a similar manner, from the oil produced in the destructive distillation of shale.

Solubility. Insoluble in water and in alcohol; soluble in ether and in chloroform.

Standard
It complies with the requirements of the British Pharmacopoeia.
It is a colourless or white, somewhat translucent, wax-like, odourless solid, frequently showing a crystalline structure; it is slightly unctuous to the touch and burns with a luminous flame. It has a solidifying-point of 50° to 57° and is characterised by its stability to most chemical reagents. When melted, the liquid is free from fluorescence by daylight.

Sterilisation. It is sterilised by dry heat.

Uses. Hard paraffin is used to stiffen ointment bases.
A similar wax, melting at 43° to 46°, is used in the preparation of wax baths in physiotherapy. The wax is melted, applied to the affected part at a temperature as high as is comfortable for the patient and left in position until it has cooled and can be stripped off. The heat retained by the wax dilates the peripheral blood vessels and improves the blood supply to the affected part.

LIQUID PARAFFIN

Liquid Paraffin is a mixture of liquid hydrocarbons obtained from petroleum. It may contain up to 10 parts per million of tocopherol or butylated hydroxytoluene.

Liquid paraffin may be obtained from petroleum by distillation, a suitable fraction of the distillate being purified by washing with acid, neutralising with alkali, filtering while hot through activated charcoal, cooling to remove solid hydrocarbons, and redistilling. Liquid paraffin varies in composition according to the source of the petroleum.

Solubility. Insoluble in water and in alcohol; soluble in ether and in chloroform.

Standard
It complies with the requirements of the British Pharmacopoeia.
It is a transparent, colourless, oily, almost odourless liquid which is free from fluorescence by daylight. It has a weight per ml at 20° of 0·830 g to 0·890 g and a kinematic viscosity at 37·8° of not less than 64 centistokes.

Sterilisation. It is sterilised by dry heat.

Storage. It should be protected from light.

Actions and uses. Liquid paraffin, when taken by mouth, keeps the stools soft and is therefore particularly useful in the treatment of chronic constipation and in painful conditions of the anus and rectum, such as haemorrhoids and anal fissure, although excessive doses may result in seepage and anal irritation. Intestinal absorption of small amounts of liquid paraffin may occur, especially if it is emulsified, and if this absorption is long continued paraffinomata may develop; continued use of liquid paraffin may interfere with the absorption of the fat-soluble vitamins.

Liquid paraffin is not irritant when applied to mucous surfaces; it is used as an emollient in irritant skin conditions and for the removal of desquamative crusts. Sterile liquid paraffin is used as an aseptic surgical dressing and as a lubricant for surgical instruments.

Liquid paraffin is administered either alone or as an emulsion.

Dose. 10 to 30 millilitres.

Preparations

LIQUID PARAFFIN EMULSION, B.P.C. (page 678)

LIQUID PARAFFIN AND MAGNESIUM HYDROXIDE EMULSION, B.P.C. (page 679)

LIQUID PARAFFIN AND PHENOLPHTHALEIN EMULSION, B.P.C. (page 679)

LIQUID PARAFFIN EMULSION WITH CASCARA, B.P.C. (page 680)

WHITE SOFT PARAFFIN

SYNONYMS: Paraffinum Molle Album; White Petroleum Jelly

White Soft Paraffin is obtained by bleaching Yellow Soft Paraffin.

Solubility. Insoluble in water and in alcohol; soluble in ether, in chloroform, in light petroleum, the solutions sometimes showing a slight opalescence, and in fixed and volatile oils.

Standard
It complies with the requirements of the British Pharmacopoeia.
It is a white, translucent, soft, unctuous, odourless mass and is not more than slightly fluorescent by daylight, even when melted. It has a melting-point of 38° to 56°.

Sterilisation. It is sterilised by dry heat.

Uses. White soft paraffin has the uses described under Yellow Soft Paraffin.

Preparations
AQUEOUS CREAM, B.P. (*Syn.* Hydrous Emulsifying Ointment). It contains 30 per cent of Emulsifying Ointment and 0·1 per cent of chlorocresol, in water.
It should be stored in airtight containers, in a cool place.

EMULSIFYING OINTMENT, B.P. It contains 50 per cent of white soft paraffin, 30 per cent of Emulsifying Wax, and 20 per cent of liquid paraffin.

PARAFFIN OINTMENT, B.P.C. (page 763)

SIMPLE OINTMENT, B.P. It contains 85 per cent of white soft paraffin (or yellow soft paraffin), with wool fat, hard paraffin, and cetostearyl alcohol.

YELLOW SOFT PARAFFIN

SYNONYMS: Paraffinum Molle Flavum; Yellow Petroleum Jelly

Yellow Soft Paraffin is a purified mixture of semi-solid hydrocarbons obtained from petroleum.

Yellow Soft Paraffin is separated from certain crude residual fractions of petroleum or heavy lubricating oil fractions by chilling and it is purified by hot filtration through fuller's earth or activated charcoal.

Solubility. Insoluble in water and in alcohol; soluble in ether, in chloroform, in light petroleum, the solutions sometimes showing a slight opalescence, and in fixed and volatile oils.

Standard
It complies with the requirements of the British Pharmacopoeia.
It is a pale yellow to yellow, translucent, soft, unctuous mass, free or almost free from odour and is not more than slightly fluorescent by daylight, even when melted. It has a melting-point of 38° to 56°.

Sterilisation. It is sterilised by dry heat.

Uses. Yellow soft paraffin is bland, neutral, and non-irritant to the skin, but is poorly absorbed. It is used as a basis for ointments which are not intended to be absorbed. Sterile dressings containing yellow soft paraffin or its preparations are often used as wound dressings because they are easily removed.

Samples of yellow soft paraffin vary in rheological and other physical properties; in some samples hard waxy lumps are produced and there may be an excessive separation of liquid components. Differences in physical properties depend upon the chemical composition which varies according to the source, the type and degree of refining, and the blending processes.

Preparation
SIMPLE OINTMENT, B.P. It contains 85 per cent of yellow soft paraffin (or white soft paraffin), with wool fat, hard paraffin, and cetostearyl alcohol.

PARAFORMALDEHYDE

Paraformaldehyde is a solid polymer of formaldehyde. It volatilises at 100° and is readily converted into formaldehyde when heated to this temperature in the presence of water. A solution of paraformaldehyde in hot water exhibits the chemical properties of formaldehyde.

Paraformaldehyde may be prepared by evaporating a concentrated aqueous solution of formaldehyde or by adding to Formaldehyde Solution about one-fourth of its weight of sulphuric acid.

Solubility. Insoluble in water; soluble in solutions of alkali hydroxides.

Standard

DESCRIPTION. A white amorphous powder or friable amorphous mass; odour pungent.

IDENTIFICATION TEST. Warm 0·04 g with 10 ml of *sulphuric acid* containing 0·2 g of *salicyclic acid*; a deep red colour is produced.

ACIDITY OR ALKALINITY. Shake 1·0 g with 20 ml of *carbon dioxide-free water*, and filter; the filtrate is neutral to *litmus solution*.

MATTER INSOLUBLE IN WATER. Not more than 0·1 per cent, determined by the following method:
To about 5 g, accurately weighed, add 100 ml of water and 0·05 ml of *sodium hydroxide solution*, boil gently for 30 minutes, replacing any water lost by evaporation, filter through a sintered-glass crucible (British Standard grade No. 4), wash the residue with water, dry for 30 minutes at 105°, and weigh.

SULPHATED ASH. Not more than 0·1 per cent.

CONTENT OF PARAFORMALDEHYDE. Not less than 95·0 per cent, calculated as CH_2O, determined by the following method:
To about 0·8 g, accurately weighed, add 40 ml of

hydrogen peroxide solution and 50 ml of 1N sodium hydroxide, warm on a water-bath until effervescence ceases, and titrate with 1N hydrochloric acid, using *phenolphthalein solution* as indicator.
Repeat the procedure omitting the sample.
The difference between the two titrations represents the sodium hydroxide required by the formic acid produced by the oxidation; each ml of 1N sodium hydroxide is equivalent to 0·03003 g of CH_2O.

Storage. It should be stored in airtight containers.

Uses. Paraformaldehyde is used as a source of formaldehyde. For disinfecting rooms it is vaporised by heating on an electric hot-plate or by interaction with potassium permanganate, as described under Formaldehyde Solution (page 203), but as it produces a dry gas it is less satisfactory for this purpose than Formaldehyde Solution. Tablets prepared for disinfecting rooms by vaporisation should be coloured by the addition of a suitable blue dye.
In dentistry, it has been used as an obtundent for sensitive dentine and as an antiseptic in mummifying pastes and for root canals.
Paraformaldehyde is also used in lozenges.

Preparation
FORMALDEHYDE LOZENGES, B.P.C. (page 732)

PARALDEHYDE

SYNONYM: Paraldehydum

$(CH_3 \cdot CHO)_3 = 132·2$

Paraldehyde is the trimer of acetaldehyde containing a suitable amount of an antoxidant.

Solubility. Soluble, at 20°, in 9 parts of water; miscible with alcohol, with ether, with chloroform, and with volatile oils.

Standard
It complies with the requirements of the European Pharmacopoeia.
It occurs as a clear, colourless or slightly yellow liquid with a strong characteristic odour. On heating, not more than 10 per cent v/v distils below 123° and not less than 95 per cent distils below 126°. It has a freezing-point of 10° to 12° and a specific gravity at 20° of 0·993 to 0·996, corresponding to a weight per ml at 20° of about 0·990 g to 0·993 g.

Sterilisation. It is sterilised by filtration; contact with rubber should be avoided.

Storage. It should be stored in small, well-filled, airtight bottles, in complete darkness, in a cool place, avoiding contact with cork. If it has solidified, the whole contents of the bottle should be liquefied by warming and well mixed before use.

Actions and uses. Paraldehyde is a powerful and quick-acting hypnotic and anticonvulsant. Because of its objectionable odour and taste and slow part-excretion by the lungs, it is now rarely used as a hypnotic except in hospitals.

It is irritant to mucous membranes unless it has been diluted.
In the treatment of convulsions, paraldehyde is usually given by intramuscular injection in doses of 2 to 10 millilitres; not more than 5 millilitres should be injected into any one site. The injection is painful, and care should be taken to avoid the neighbourhood of nerve trunks. It has also been given by intravenous injection as a 10 per cent solution in water, but this is not recommended. Plastic syringes should not be used.
Paraldehyde is sometimes used as a basal anaesthetic, especially in children. The dose is 0·5 millilitre per kilogram body-weight, with an upper limit of 30 millilitres, as the enema; 1 millilitre of benzyl alcohol may be added to the enema to reduce local irritation. Children under one year may be given 0·5 to 1·5 millilitres and children from one to five years 2 to 4 millilitres of paraldehyde.

UNDESIRABLE EFFECTS. In spite of the unpleasantness of paraldehyde, dependence of the barbiturate-alcohol type, as described under Phenobarbitone (page 366), has occurred, especially among alcoholics.

POISONING. In cases of poisoning by paraldehyde, which may cause death by respiratory failure, oxygen with carbon dioxide and a respiratory stimulant should be administered.

Dose. 5 to 10 millilitres by mouth or by intramuscular injection. As a basal anaesthetic: 15 to 30 millilitres, suitably diluted, by rectal injection.

Preparations
PARALDEHYDE DRAUGHT, B.P.C. (page 662)
PARALDEHYDE ENEMA, B.P.C. (page 680)
PARALDEHYDE INJECTION, B.P.C. (page 716)

PARAMETHADIONE

$C_7H_{11}NO_3 = 157.2$

Paramethadione is 5-ethyl-3,5-dimethyloxazolidine-2,4-dione.

Solubility. Soluble in water, in alcohol, in ether, and in chloroform.

Standard
It complies with the requirements of the British Pharmacopoeia.
It is a clear colourless liquid with a characteristic odour and contains not less than 98.0 per cent w/w of $C_7H_{11}NO_3$. A 2.5 per cent solution in water has a pH of 4.0 to 7.5.

Actions and uses. Paramethadione has an anticonvulsant action similar to that described under Troxidone (page 523). It is used to control attacks of petit mal epilepsy, but is less effective than troxidone and less liable to produce severe toxic effects.

PRECAUTIONS AND CONTRA-INDICATIONS. Precautions are as described under Troxidone

(page 523). Paramethadione may produce renal damage and thrombocytopenic purpura and should not be administered to patients with renal or hepatic disease.

Dose. For an adult: initial dose, 900 milligrams daily in divided doses; subsequent doses, increasing to 1.8 grams in accordance with the needs of the patient.
For a child: initial dose, 300 milligrams daily in divided doses; subsequent doses, increasing to 900 milligrams, in accordance with the needs of the patient.

Preparation
PARAMETHADIONE CAPSULES, B.P. Unless otherwise specified, capsules each containing 300 mg of paramethadione are supplied.

OTHER NAME: *Paradione*®

PAROMOMYCIN SULPHATE

Paromomycin Sulphate is a mixture of the sulphates of the antimicrobial substances produced by the growth of certain strains of *Streptomyces rimosus* forma *paromomycinus*.

Solubility. Soluble, at 20°, in 1 part of water; insoluble in alcohol, in ether, and in chloroform; soluble in dilute acids and in solutions of alkali hydroxides.

Standard
DESCRIPTION. A creamy-white to light yellow hygroscopic powder; odourless or almost odourless.

IDENTIFICATION TESTS. 1. It complies with the thin-layer chromatographic test given in Appendix 5, page 866 (distinction from neomycin sulphate).
2. It gives the reactions characteristic of sulphates.

ACIDITY OR ALKALINITY. pH of a 3.0 per cent w/v solution in *carbon dioxide-free water*, 5.0 to 7.5.

CLARITY OF SOLUTION. A 3.0 per cent w/v solution in water is clear.

SPECIFIC ROTATION. +50° to +55°, calculated with reference to the substance dried under the prescribed conditions, determined, at 20°, in a 5.0 per cent w/v solution in water.

SULPHATE. 23.0 to 26.0 per cent, calculated with reference to the substance dried under the prescribed conditions, determined by the following method:
Dissolve about 1 g, accurately weighed, in 200 ml of water, add 3 ml of *hydrochloric acid*, heat to boiling, add 15 ml of hot *barium chloride solution*, heat on a water-bath for 4 hours with occasional stirring, filter, wash the filter with water, ignite the residue to constant weight, and weigh; each g of residue is equivalent to 0.4116 g of sulphate.

UNDUE TOXICITY. Inject subcutaneously into each of 10 male albino rats, each weighing between 100 and 135 g, a quantity equivalent to 100,000 Units per kg body-weight, dissolved in 3 ml of *water for injections*, twice a day for 5 consecutive days, preparing the solution daily and allowing an interval of 6 to 7 hours between the daily injections; none of the rats dies within 10 days of the last injection.
If one of the rats dies within 10 days, repeat the test; none of the second group of rats dies within 10 days of the last injection.

LOSS ON DRYING. Not more than 5.0 per cent, determined by drying to constant weight at 50° in vacuo.

SULPHATED ASH. Not more than 2.0 per cent.

MINIMUM POTENCY. Carry out an assay for paromomycin. A suggested method is given in Appendix 18, page 897.
The precision of any assay must be such that the fiducial limits of error (P = 0.95) are not less than 95 per cent and not more than 105 per cent of the estimated potency.
The upper fiducial limit of error is not less than 675 Units per mg, calculated with reference to the substance dried under the prescribed conditions.

Labelling. The label on the container states the number of Units per mg.

Storage. It should be stored in airtight containers.

Actions and uses. Paromomycin is active against a wide range of pathogenic intestinal bacteria and also against *Entamoeba histolytica*. As it is poorly absorbed from the gastro-intestinal tract, it is used in the treatment of intestinal infections.

The usual dosage in the treatment of bacterial dysentery is 35,000 to 60,000 Units per kilogram body-weight daily in divided doses for at least six days, and of intestinal amoebiasis, 25,000 Units per kilogram body-weight for at least five days. The daily dosage may be increased to 100,000 Units per kilogram body-weight in resistant infections.

For the suppression of the intestinal flora before surgery, 35,000 Units per kilogram body-weight may be given daily in divided doses for four days. Up to 6 mega Units daily may be given in the management of hepatic coma.

In addition to the capsules, paromomycin sulphate is available as a syrup containing 125,000 Units of paromomycin in 5 ml.

Paromomycin should not be given by injection on account of its toxicity.

UNDESIRABLE EFFECTS. These include diarrhoea and overgrowth of non-susceptible organisms.

Dose. See above under **Actions and uses.**

Preparation
PAROMOMYCIN CAPSULES, B.P.C. (page 653)

OTHER NAME: *Humatin®*

PENICILLAMINE

SYNONYM: D-Penicillamine

$C_5H_{11}NO_2S = 149.2$

Penicillamine is $(-)$-$\beta\beta$-dimethylcysteine.

$$HS \cdot \overset{\overset{\displaystyle CH_3}{|}}{\underset{\underset{\displaystyle CH_3}{|}}{C}} \cdot \overset{}{\underset{\underset{\displaystyle NH_2}{|}}{CH}} \cdot CO_2H$$

Solubility. Soluble, at 20°, in 9 parts of water and in 530 parts of alcohol; insoluble in ether and in chloroform.

Standard
It complies with the requirements of the British Pharmacopoeia.
It is a white or almost white, finely crystalline powder with a characteristic odour and contains not less than 95.0 per cent of $C_5H_{11}NO_2S$, calculated with reference to the dried substance. The loss on drying under the prescribed conditions is not more than 0.5 per cent. A 1 per cent solution in water has a pH of 4.5 to 5.5.

Storage. It should be stored in airtight containers.

Actions and uses. Penicillamine is an orally administered chelating agent which aids the elimination of certain toxic metal ions. It is used mainly in the treatment of hepato-lenticular degeneration (Wilson's disease). When it is given by mouth in a dosage of 0.5 to 1.5 grams daily, it increases the urinary output of copper from five to twenty times compared with that of untreated cases. The condition of some patients treated with penicillamine improves dramatically, but other patients, although their copper output increases considerably, show no improvement; improvement probably depends upon the amount of permanent and irreversible structural damage.

Penicillamine is also of value in the treatment of lead poisoning and poisoning by iron salts and of haemosiderosis. It is occasionally used empirically in the treatment of scleroderma and rheumatoid arthritis.

Penicillamine will chelate *in vitro* with silver, zinc, chromium, cadmium, cobalt, antimony, and bismuth ions.

UNDESIRABLE EFFECTS. It may give rise to proteinuria. Allergic reactions, gastro-intestinal symptoms, leucopenia, and thrombocytopenia rarely occur.

Dose. 0.5 to 1.5 grams daily in divided doses.

Preparations
PENICILLAMINE CAPSULES, B.P. Each capsule contains penicillamine or penicillamine hydrochloride. The quantity of penicillamine or penicillamine hydrochloride in each capsule should be specified by the prescriber. Capsules containing 250 mg of penicillamine and capsules containing 150 mg of penicillamine hydrochloride, equivalent to 120 mg of penicillamine, are available. They should be stored in airtight containers at a temperature not exceeding 25°

PENICILLAMINE TABLETS, B.P. The quantity in each tablet should be specified by the prescriber. They are film coated and should be stored at a temperature not exceeding 25°. Tablets containing 250 mg are available.

OTHER NAMES: *Distamine®*; *Cuprimine®*

PENICILLAMINE HYDROCHLORIDE

SYNONYM: D-Penicillamine Hydrochloride

$C_5H_{11}NO_2S,HCl = 185.7$

Penicillamine Hydrochloride is $(-)$-$\beta\beta$-dimethylcysteine hydrochloride.

Solubility. Soluble, at 20°, in 1 part of water, in 1.5 parts of alcohol, and in 230 parts of chloroform; insoluble in ether.

Standard
It complies with the requirements of the British Pharmacopoeia.

It is a white or almost white, finely crystalline, hygroscopic powder with a characteristic odour and contains not less than 95·0 per cent of $C_5H_{11}NO_2S,HCl$, calculated with reference to the dried substance. The loss on drying under the prescribed conditions is not more than 3·0 per cent. A 1 per cent solution in water has a pH of 1·6 to 2·2.

Storage. It should be stored in airtight containers at a temperature not exceeding 25°.

Actions and uses. Penicillamine hydrochloride has the actions, uses, and undesirable effects described under Penicillamine; 1·25 grams of penicillamine hydrochloride is

approximately equivalent to 1 gram of penicillamine.

Dose. The equivalent of 0·5 to 1·5 grams of penicillamine daily in divided doses.

Preparation
PENICILLAMINE CAPSULES, B.P. Each capsule contains penicillamine or penicillamine hydrochloride. The quantity of penicillamine or penicillamine hydrochloride in each capsule should be specified by the prescriber. Capsules containing 250 mg of penicillamine and capsules containing 150 mg of penicillamine hydrochloride equivalent to 120 mg of penicillamine, are available. They should be stored in airtight containers at a temperature not exceeding 25°.

OTHER NAME: *Distamine*®

DILUTED PENTAERYTHRITOL TETRANITRATE

SYNONYMS: Dil. Pentaerythr. Tetranit.; Diluted Pentaerythrityl Tetranitrate; Pentaerythritol Tetranitrate (20 per cent)

Diluted Pentaerythritol Tetranitrate is a mixture of pentaerythritol tetranitrate with lactose, or with a mixture of three parts of Lactose and one part of Starch.

Pentaerythritol tetranitrate is the 2,2-di(hydroxymethyl)propane-1,3-diol ester of nitric acid ($C_5H_8N_4O_{12} = 316·1$).

Standard
DESCRIPTION. A white crystalline powder; odourless or almost odourless.

IDENTIFICATION TESTS. 1. Suspend 0·01 g of the residue obtained in the determination of $C_5H_8N_4O_{12}$ in a mixture of 2 ml of *sulphuric acid* and 1 ml of water, cool, and carefully overlay with 3 ml of *ferrous sulphate solution*; a reddish-brown colour is produced at the interface.
2. The residue obtained in the determination of $C_5H_8N_4O_{12}$ melts at about 141°.
(The operator should be protected by a safety screen when making this determination.)

CONTENT OF $C_5H_8N_4O_{12}$. 18·5 to 21·5 per cent, determined by the following method:
Mix about 0·5 g, accurately weighed, with 25 ml of warm *dry acetone*, filter, and wash the residue with three successive 10-ml portions of *dry acetone*; combine the filtrate and washings, cautiously evaporate off the acetone in a current of warm air, dry the residue of $C_5H_8N_4O_{12}$ for 3 hours at 60°, and weigh. (The residue, which is explosive, should then be used for the identification tests and any remaining destroyed by dissolving in acetone and burning the solution in a large dish.)

Storage. It should be stored in airtight containers, protected from light, in a cool place.

Actions and uses. Pentaerythritol tetranitrate has the actions and uses described under Glyceryl Trinitrate Solution (page 212). When given by mouth, it is slowly absorbed from the gastro-intestinal tract; its effect commences about one hour after administration and lasts for about five hours.

POISONING. As for Glyceryl Trinitrate Solution (page 212).

Dose. 50 to 150 milligrams, equivalent to 10 to 30 milligrams of pentaerythritol tetranitrate.

Preparation
PENTAERYTHRITOL TABLETS, B.P. Unless otherwise specified, tablets each containing 10 mg of pentaerythritol tetranitrate are supplied. They should be stored in airtight containers, protected from light, in a cool place. Tablets containing 30 mg are also available.

OTHER NAMES: *Mycardol*®; *Peritrate*®

PENTAGASTRIN

$C_{37}H_{49}N_7O_9S = 767·9$

Pentagastrin is *N*-t-butoxycarbonyl-β-alanyl-L-tryptophyl-L-methionyl-L-aspartyl-L-phenylalanine amide.

Solubility. Insoluble in water; slightly soluble in alcohol; soluble in dilute ammonia solution and in dimethylformamide.

Standard
It complies with the requirements of the British Pharmacopoeia.
It is a white or almost white odourless powder and

NH·CO·[CH_2]_2·NH·CO·O·C(CH_3)_3
CH_2·CH·CO·NH
CH_3·S·[CH_2]_2·CH·CO·NH
HO_2C·CH_2·CH·CO·NH
C_6H_5·CH_2·CH·CO·NH_2

contains not less than 97·0 and not more than the equivalent of 103·0 per cent of $C_{37}H_{49}N_7O_9S$, calculated with reference to the dried substance. The loss on drying under the prescribed conditions is not more than 0·5 per cent.

Sterilisation. Solutions for injection are sterilised by filtration.

Storage. It should be protected from light.

Actions and uses. Pentagastrin stimulates the secretion of gastric acid, pepsin with intrinsic factor, pancreatic juice, and bile, and the segmenting activity of the bowel and sodium diuresis. It is not absorbed from the gut. When it is administered by intramuscular injection the peak effect occurs in ten to thirty minutes.

Pentagastrin is used to test gastric function as described under Histamine Acid Phosphate (page 221). For this purpose pentagastrin is administered by subcutaneous or intravenous injection, and as it does not give rise to the undesirable effects of histamine, it is preferred for this purpose. It is possible to determine the maximum acid secretion by recovering gastric juice while successively higher doses of pentagastrin are given by intravenous infusion.

UNDESIRABLE EFFECTS. Mild abdominal discomfort commonly occurs. Occasionally cramps, nausea, palpitation, and tachycardia occur about ten minutes after injection and these effects are more marked when the drug is administered intravenously.

Dose. By subcutaneous or intramuscular injection, 6 micrograms per kilogram body-weight.

By intravenous infusion, 0·6 to 6 micrograms per kilogram body-weight per hour.

Preparation
PENTAGASTRIN INJECTION, B.P. It consists of a sterile solution of pentagastrin in Water for Injections containing ammonium hydroxide. Vials containing 500 μg in 2 ml are available.

OTHER NAME: *Peptavlon®*

PENTAMIDINE ISETHIONATE

$C_{23}H_{36}N_4O_{10}S_2 = 592·7$

Pentamidine Isethionate is 1,5-di(*p*-amidinophenoxy)pentane di(2-hydroxyethanesulphonate).

Solubility. Soluble, at 20°, in 10 parts of water; soluble in glycerol; slightly soluble in alcohol; insoluble in ether, in chloroform, and in liquid paraffin.

Standard
It complies with the requirements of the British Pharmacopoeia.

It occurs as white or almost white, odourless, hygroscopic crystals or powder and contains not less than 98·5 and not more than the equivalent of 102·5 per cent of $C_{23}H_{36}N_4O_{10}S_2$, calculated with reference to the dried substance. The loss on drying under the prescribed conditions is not more than 4·0 per cent. It has a melting-point of 188° to 192°. A 5 per cent solution in water has a pH of 4·5 to 6·5.

Storage. It should be stored in airtight containers.

Actions and uses. Pentamidine is used in the prophylaxis and treatment of African trypanosomiasis. It does not attain a trypanocidal concentration in the cerebrospinal fluid after intramuscular injection and is therefore of little value in the treatment of advanced cases in which the central nervous system is involved.

For the treatment of early trypanosomiasis, 300 milligrams of pentamidine isethionate is given daily as a 10 per cent solution by intramuscular or intravenous injection on seven to fifteen successive days; this treatment is frequently supplemented with melarsoprol.

For prophylaxis, a dose of 300 milligrams is given every three to six months. Before pentamidine is used for prophylaxis in a community, a careful examination should be made to detect patients in whom the disease has advanced beyond the early stages and these must be given a full course of treatment with a drug such as melarsoprol.

Pentamidine is also used in the treatment of leishmaniasis; it is especially valuable in patients who do not respond to treatment with antimony. A dosage of 300 milligrams is given daily or on alternate days until twelve to fifteen doses have been given; a second course of treatment may be given one or two weeks later.

UNDESIRABLE EFFECTS. The intramuscular injection of pentamidine isethionate often causes pain and swelling at the site of injection. Intravenous injection, if made too rapidly, may produce a profound fall in blood pressure; this hypotensive effect may be prevented by giving the injection very slowly, or it may be relieved by the injection of a vasopressor drug such as adrenaline, noradrenaline, or metaraminol.

Pentamidine sometimes causes hypoglycaemia.

Dose. See above under **Actions and uses.**

Preparation
PENTAMIDINE INJECTION, B.P. It consists of a sterile solution of pentamidine isethionate prepared immediately before use by dissolving the sterile contents of a sealed container in Water for Injections. The quantity of pentamidine isethionate in each container should be specified by the prescriber. Vials containing 200 mg, 2 g, and 25 g are available.

PENTOBARBITONE SODIUM

SYNONYMS: Pentobarbital Sodium; Soluble
Pentobarbitone

$C_{11}H_{17}N_2NaO_3 = 248 \cdot 3$

Pentobarbitone Sodium is sodium 5-ethyl-5-(1-methylbutyl)barbiturate.

Solubility. Very soluble in water and in alcohol; very slightly soluble in ether.

Standard
It complies with the requirements of the British Pharmacopoeia.
It occurs as hygroscopic, odourless, white granules or crystalline powder and contains not less than 98·5 per cent of $C_{11}H_{17}N_2NaO_3$, calculated with reference to the dried substance. The loss on drying under the prescribed conditions is not more than 5·0 per cent. A 10 per cent solution in water has a pH of not more than 11.

Incompatibility. It is incompatible with acids, acidic salts such as ammonium bromide, acidic syrups such as lemon syrup, and chloral hydrate.

Storage. It should be stored in airtight containers.

Actions and uses. Pentobarbitone is an intermediate-acting barbiturate, the actions and uses of which are described under Phenobarbitone (page 366). The usual hypnotic dose is 100 to 200 milligrams.
Pentobarbitone sodium has been used as a basal anaesthetic before surgical operations, its sedative effect on the patient reducing the amount of general anaesthetic required. For this purpose 100 to 200 milligrams may be given by mouth in the evening preceding the operation, and the dose repeated two hours before the operation; this may be repeated again one hour before the operation if the sedative effect is inadequate.

Pentobarbitone sodium may be given slowly by intravenous injection as an anticonvulsant in the treatment of tetanus or of strychnine poisoning, the dose being 500 milligrams dissolved in 10 millilitres of Water for Injections. It is also given by mouth or by rectum.
Solutions for injection are prepared by an aseptic technique.

UNDESIRABLE EFFECTS; PRECAUTIONS; CONTRA-INDICATIONS; DEPENDENCE. These are as described under Phenobarbitone (page 366).

POISONING. The procedure as described under Phenobarbitone (page 366) should be adopted, but haemodialysis is not effective.

Dose. See above under **Actions and uses.**

Preparations
PENTOBARBITONE CAPSULES, B.P. (*Syn.* Soluble Pentobarbitone Capsules; Pentobarbital Sodium Capsules). The quantity of pentobarbitone sodium in each capsule should be specified by the prescriber. Capsules containing 30, 50, and 100 mg are available.
PENTOBARBITONE TABLETS, B.P. (*Syn.* Soluble Pentobarbitone Tablets; Pentobarbitone Sodium Tablets; Pentobarbital Sodium Tablets). The quantity of pentobarbitone sodium in each tablet should be specified by the prescriber. They should be stored in airtight containers. Tablets containing 100 mg are available.

OTHER NAME: *Nembutal*®

PENTOLINIUM TARTRATE

$C_{23}H_{42}N_2O_{12} = 538 \cdot 6$

Pentolinium Tartrate is pentamethylenebis(1-methylpyrrolidinium hydrogen tartrate).

Solubility. Soluble, at 20°, in less than 1 part of water and in 800 parts of alcohol; insoluble in ether and in chloroform.

Standard
It complies with the requirements of the British Pharmacopoeia.
It is a white or almost white, odourless powder and contains not less than 99·0 and not more than the equivalent of 101·0 per cent of $C_{23}H_{42}N_2O_{12}$, calculated with reference to the dried substance. The loss on drying under the prescribed conditions is not more than 2·0 per cent. It melts with decomposition at about 206°. A solution in water is acid to litmus.

Sterilisation. Solutions for injection are sterilised by heating in an autoclave or by filtration.

Storage. It should be stored in airtight containers, in a cool place.

Actions and uses. Pentolinium tartrate is a ganglion-blocking agent which inhibits the transmission of nerve impulses in both sym-pathetic and parasympathetic ganglia by raising the threshold of the ganglion cell to the acetylcholine released at preganglionic nerve endings. The sympathetic block produces peripheral dilatation, which causes increased blood flow, raised skin temperature, and reduced blood pressure. The parasympathetic block diminishes movement of the gastro-intestinal tract and bladder, reduces gastric and salivary secretion, and produces disturbances of visual accommodation.
Pentolinium is used to control severe or malignant hypertension but it has been largely replaced by drugs that selectively block sympathetic nerve transmission and do not produce the effects of parasympathetic blockade. As it is poorly and erratically absorbed from the gastro-intestinal tract it should not be

given by mouth. It may be administered by subcutaneous injection; the usual initial dose is 2·5 milligrams, and this may be increased by amounts of 0·5 to 1 milligram until the dose is effective.

To reduce side-effects, a smaller dose may be given in conjunction with reserpine (100 micrograms) or chlorothiazide (500 milligrams).

Pentolinum tartrate is given in the emergency treatment of hypertensive encephalopathy and eclampsia in a dose of 2 milligrams by subcutaneous injection; this dose may be repeated after fifteen minutes if the response is not satisfactory.

UNDESIRABLE EFFECTS. Constipation, dryness of the mouth, and blurring of vision may occur, but disappear when the drug is withdrawn.

CONTRA-INDICATIONS. Pentolinium is contra-indicated in patients with pyloric stenosis. As with all potent hypotensives it may enhance severe renal or cerebral vascular insufficiency.

POISONING. Patients with severe hypotension should be placed in the supine position with the feet raised; the blood pressure should be increased by an infusion of Noradrenaline Injection or by intramuscular injection of metaraminol.

Dose. See above under **Actions and uses.**

Preparation
PENTOLINIUM INJECTION, B.P. It consists of a sterile solution of pentolinium tartrate in Water for Injections, the pH of the solution being 6·0 to 7·0; when the injection is issued in multiple-dose containers containing chlorbutol as a preservative, the pH should be not less than 4·0. Unless otherwise specified, a solution containing 5 mg in 1 ml is supplied.

OTHER NAME: *Ansolysen®*

PEPPERMINT OIL

SYNONYM: Oleum Menthae Piperitae

Peppermint Oil is obtained by distillation from the fresh flowering tops of *Mentha* × *piperita* L. (Fam. Labiatae), a herb growing wild throughout Europe and cultivated in England, France, Italy, Bulgaria, Morocco, and America.

There are two varieties of peppermint, black peppermint and white peppermint, the former yielding more oil than the latter, but of a less delicate aroma. The oil is rectified if necessary. The odour and taste afford the best indication of the quality of the oil and by this means it is possible to distinguish between English, American, and other types of oils.

Constituents. Peppermint oil contains chiefly menthol, menthone, menthyl acetate, and terpenes. Menthofuran and other minor constituents contribute to the quality of the odour and flavour. Dimethyl sulphide is present in unrectified oil.

Solubility. Soluble, at 20°, in 4 parts of alcohol (70 per cent), with a slight opalescence, and in 0·5 part of alcohol (90 per cent), the solution sometimes becoming turbid on adding more of the solvent; miscible with dehydrated alcohol.

Standard
It complies with the requirements of the British Pharmacopoeia.
It is a colourless, pale yellow, or greenish-yellow liquid having the odour of peppermint and contains 4·0 to 9·0 per cent w/w of esters, calculated as menthyl acetate, $C_{12}H_{22}O_2$, and not less than 45·0 per cent w/w of free menthol, $C_{10}H_{20}O$. It has a weight per ml at 20° of 0·897 g to 0·910 g.

Stability. It darkens in colour and becomes viscous on keeping. On cooling to a low temperature, separation of menthol occurs, especially when a few crystals of this substance are added to start crystallisation.

Adulterants and substitutes. Japanese, Chinese, Formosan (Taiwan), and Brazilian mint oils obtained from varietal forms of *M. arvensis* L. are the richest of all in menthol, sometimes containing 85 per cent. Oils of these varieties are commonly partially dementholised; they still contain about 50 per cent of menthol and may occur as adulterants.

Storage. It should be stored in well-filled airtight containers, protected from light, in a cool place.

Actions and uses. Peppermint oil is a carminative. It may be administered on sugar or in tablets or lozenges.
Peppermint oil has mildly antiseptic properties; it is used to flavour dental preparations.

Dose. 0·05 to 0·2 millilitre.

Preparations
PEPPERMINT EMULSION, CONCENTRATED, B.P.C. (page 680)
PEPPERMINT SPIRIT, B.P.C. (page 793)
MAGNESIUM CARBONATE TABLETS, COMPOUND, B.P.C. (page 812)
MAGNESIUM TRISILICATE TABLETS, COMPOUND, B.P.C. (page 812)
SODIUM BICARBONATE TABLETS, COMPOUND, B.P. (*Syn.* Soda Mint Tablets). Each tablet contains 300 mg of sodium bicarbonate and 0·003 ml of peppermint oil. They should be stored in airtight containers, in a cool place. Dose: 2 to 6 tablets, which should be allowed to dissolve slowly in the mouth.
PEPPERMINT WATER, CONCENTRATED, B.P. It contains peppermint oil, 1 in 50. Dose: 0·25 to 1 millilitre.

PERPHENAZINE

$C_{21}H_{26}ClN_3OS = 404{\cdot}0$

Perphenazine is 2-chloro-10-{3-[4-(2-hydroxyethyl)pipe-razin-1-yl]propyl}phenothiazine.

Solubility. Very slightly soluble in water; soluble, at 20°, in 20 parts of alcohol, in 80 parts of ether, and in 1 part of chloroform; soluble in dilute hydrochloric acid.

Standard
It complies with the requirements of the British Pharmacopoeia.
It is a white or creamy-white, almost odourless powder and contains not less than 99·0 and not more than the equivalent of 101·0 per cent of $C_{21}H_{26}ClN_3OS$, calculated with reference to the dried substance. The loss on drying under the prescribed conditions is not more than 0·5 per cent. It has a melting-point of 96° to 100°.

Sterilisation. Solutions for injection are sterilised by heating in an autoclave or by filtration.

Storage. It should be protected from light.

Actions and uses. Perphenazine has the actions and uses described under Chlorpromazine Hydrochloride (page 107) but it is effective in much smaller doses, produces less sedation, and has a greater tendency to produce parkinsonism.

In psychotic patients the usual effective daily dosage by mouth is 12 to 24 milligrams and 5 to 15 milligrams daily by intramuscular injection. In the treatment of psychoneurosis, nausea, and vomiting, the daily dosage by mouth is usually 2 to 12 milligrams and should not exceed 24 milligrams. For the immediate relief of acute symptoms doses of 5 to 10 milligrams may be given by intramuscular injection at six-hourly intervals, the route being changed as soon as possible to oral administration.

For the prevention of post-operative vomiting 8 milligrams is given by mouth as a single dose prior to induction of anaesthesia. Vomiting arising from radiation therapy or occurring during pregnancy may be controlled by a dosage of 4 milligrams by mouth three times a day.

To control acute alcoholic mania 5 to 10 milligrams is given by intramuscular injection and to allay withdrawal symptoms during the treatment of addiction to drugs or alcohol 5 milligrams is given by intramuscular injection at six-hourly intervals for twenty-four hours, followed by 8 milligrams by mouth three times a day.

UNDESIRABLE EFFECTS. At therapeutic dosage levels, perphenazine rarely produces undesirable effects. However, extrapyramidal dysfunction, exhibited as pseudo-parkinsonism, may occur. At higher dosage levels, it may provoke extrapyramidal symptoms, such as dystonia and parkinsonism; these symptoms can be relieved or controlled by reducing the dosage or by using an antiparkinsonism drug.

POISONING. The procedure as described under Chlorpromazine Hydrochloride (page 107) should be adopted.

Dose. See above under **Actions and uses.**

Preparation
PERPHENAZINE TABLETS, B.P. The quantity of perphenazine in each tablet should be specified by the prescriber. They are sugar coated. Tablets containing 2, 4, and 8 mg are available.

OTHER NAME: *Fentazin*®

PERU BALSAM

SYNONYM: Peruvian Balsam

Peru Balsam is a viscous balsam exuded from the scorched and wounded trunk of *Myroxylon balsamum* (L.) Harms. var. *pereirae* (Royle) Harms. (Fam. Leguminosae), a tree growing in the forests of San Salvador in central America.

Constituents. Peru balsam contains 53 to 66 per cent of a colourless aromatic oily liquid and 20 to 28 per cent of a dark resin.
The liquid portion, sometimes called "cinnamein", consists of a mixture of benzyl benzoate and benzyl cinnamate in varying proportions, the former usually predominating.
The resin consists mainly of one or more resin alcohols esterified with cinnamic acid and to a small extent with benzoic acid.
Peru balsam also contains 10 to 22 per cent of free cinnamic acid and a small amount of vanillin.

Solubility. Soluble in chloroform; partly soluble in ether, in glacial acetic acid, and in light petroleum.
Water shaken with the balsam removes only traces of cinnamic acid.

Standard
DESCRIPTION. A dark brown viscous liquid which is transparent and reddish-brown when viewed in thin layers; it is free from stringiness or stickiness. It has an agreeable balsamic odour recalling that of vanillin.

SOLUBILITY IN ALCOHOL (90 PER CENT). Mix 1 volume with 1 volume of *alcohol (90 per cent)*; a clear solution is produced which becomes turbid on the addition of a further 2 volumes of *alcohol (90 per cent)*.

WEIGHT PER ML. At 20°, 1·140 g to 1·170 g.

BENZALDEHYDE AND TURPENTINE. Shake thoroughly 2 g with 10 ml of *light petroleum (boiling-range, 40° to 60°)*, filter, and evaporate 4 ml of the filtrate to dryness on a water-bath; the residue has no odour of benzaldehyde or turpentine.

COLOPHONY. Shake the remainder of the filtrate obtained in the test for benzaldehyde and turpentine with twice its volume of *dilute copper acetate solution*; the light-petroleum layer is not coloured green.

FATTY OILS. Shake 1·0 g with a solution of 3 g of *chloral hydrate* in 2 ml of water; a clear solution is produced.

SAPONIFICATION VALUE OF BALSAMIC ESTERS. Not less than 230, determined by the following method:
To the residue obtained in the determination of balsamic esters add 20 ml of 0·5N alcoholic potassium hydroxide and 20 ml of *alcohol (90 per cent)* and boil under a reflux condenser for 30 minutes; cool, and titrate the excess of alkali with 0·5N hydrochloric acid, using *phenolphthalein solution* as indicator.

CONTENT OF BALSAMIC ESTERS. 49·0 to 60·0 per cent, determined by the following method:
Dissolve about 1 g, accurately weighed, in 30 ml of *solvent ether*, extract with 20 ml, followed by 10 ml, of 0·5N sodium hydroxide, wash the combined extracts with 10 ml of *solvent ether*, and discard the alkaline extracts; wash the combined ethereal solutions with two successive 5-ml portions of water, shake with *anhydrous sodium sulphate*, filter through cotton wool, and wash the residue with *solvent ether*; evaporate off the ether at a temperature not exceeding 40° and dry the residue of balsamic esters to constant weight over *phosphorus pentoxide* at a pressure between 10 and 20 mm of mercury.

Adulterants and substitutes. Alcohol, benzaldehyde, colophony, copaiba, kerosene, fixed oil, and turpentine have been used as adulterants. They may be detected by a lowering in the weight per ml.
Peru balsam is also frequently adulterated with synthetic esters such as benzyl benzoate; samples containing added benzyl benzoate usually have a high proportion of balsamic esters and a high saponification value.

Actions and uses. Peru balsam has been used as an ointment (12·5 per cent v/v) for the treatment of scabies, but for this purpose it has been superseded by Benzyl Benzoate Application. Diluted with an equal part of castor oil, the balsam has been used as an application to bed-sores and chronic ulcers. Continued application of the balsam to the skin may cause sensitisation.

PETHIDINE HYDROCHLORIDE

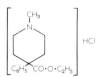

SYNONYM: Meperidine Hydrochloride

$C_{15}H_{22}ClNO_2 = 283·8$

Pethidine Hydrochloride is ethyl 1-methyl-4-phenylpiperidine-4-carboxylate hydrochloride.

Solubility. Very soluble in water; soluble, at 20°, in 20 parts of alcohol; soluble in chloroform; slightly soluble in ether and in acetone.

Standard
It complies with the requirements of the British Pharmacopoeia.
It occurs as odourless or almost odourless colourless crystals or white crystalline powder and contains not less than 99·0 and not more than the equivalent of 101·0 per cent of $C_{15}H_{22}ClNO_2$, calculated with reference to the dried substance. The loss on drying under the prescribed conditions is not more than 0·5 per cent. It has a melting-point of 187° to 189°. A 5 per cent solution in water has a pH of 4·0 to 6·0.

Sterilisation. Solutions for injection are sterilised by heating in an autoclave or by filtration.

Actions and uses. Pethidine has analgesic, sedative, spasmolytic, and local anaesthetic actions. Its spasmolytic action is less important than was originally claimed and may be largely dependent on its local effect on nerve fibres and nerve endings.
Pethidine is used to relieve the more severe types of pain which were previously controllable only by opiates; 100 milligrams of pethidine hydrochloride by mouth or by intramuscular or slow intermittent intravenous injection produces relief from pain in most medical or surgical conditions. Intravenous injection often produces undesirable effects. Intramuscular injection is more reliable than oral administration and produces an effect in ten to fifteen minutes which lasts for two to five hours.
Pethidine has been substituted for morphine in pre- and post-operative medication, but its action is not as powerful or prolonged as that of morphine for the control of severe post-operative pain. It is sometimes used in association with intravenous anaesthetics.
As it reduces the severity of labour pains without seriously diminishing the force of uterine contractions, pethidine is used as an obstetric analgesic; 100 milligrams is given by intramuscular injection as soon as regular contractions begin; the injection may be repeated one to three hours later if necessary, but more than four doses should not be given within twenty-four hours. Barbiturates or hyoscine may be given concurrently to enhance sedation and depress memory.

UNDESIRABLE EFFECTS. Pethidine produces mild euphoria in some patients and may lead to dependence of the morphine type, as described under Morphine Hydrochloride (page 314). It rarely produces toxic effects, although dizziness, nausea and dryness of the mouth may occur. Intravenous injection of pethidine may cause a fall in blood pressure.
The administration of pethidine as an analgesic during labour may give rise to respiratory depression in the infant at birth; this risk may be reduced by the simultaneous administration of levallorphan, 2 milligrams for every 100 milligrams of pethidine hydrochloride.

PRECAUTIONS. Pethidine should not be given to patients who are being treated with a monoamine-oxidase inhibitor, such as iso-carboxazid, nialamide, phenelzine, or tranyl-cypromine, or within about ten days of the discontinuation of such treatment. It should not be given in conjunction with meprobamate as the treatment may cause the development of hypotension.

POISONING. The procedure as described under Morphine Hydrochloride (page 314) should be adopted.

Dose. 50 to 100 milligrams by mouth; 25 to 100 milligrams by subcutaneous or intra-muscular injection; 25 to 50 milligrams by intravenous injection.

Preparations
PETHIDINE INJECTION, B.P. It consists of a sterile solution of pethidine hydrochloride in Water for Injections. The strength of the solution should be specified by the prescriber. Solutions containing 50 mg in 1 ml and 100 mg in 2 ml are available.

PETHIDINE TABLETS, B.P. The quantity of pethidine hydrochloride in each tablet should be specified by the prescriber. Tablets containing 25 and 50 mg are available.

PHENACETIN

SYNONYM: Phenacetinum

$C_{10}H_{13}NO_2 = 179.2$

Phenacetin is *p*-ethoxyphenylacetamide.

Solubility. Very slightly soluble in water; soluble, at 20°, in 20 parts of alcohol and in 20 parts of chloro-form; slightly soluble in glycerol.

Standard
It complies with the requirements of the European Pharmacopoeia.
It occurs as odourless, white, glistening, crystalline scales or fine, white, crystalline powder. It has a melting-point of 134° to 137°.

Hygroscopicity. At relative humidities between about 15 and 90 per cent the equilibrium moisture content at 25° is about 2 per cent.

Actions and uses. Phenacetin is metabolised to paracetamol and has analgesic and anti-pyretic actions similar to those described under Aspirin (page 35), but it has no anti-inflammatory properties. It is used to relieve headache, toothache, and rheumatic and neuralgic pains, but is of little value for the relief of severe pain.
It is sometimes prescribed in admixture with caffeine, aspirin, or codeine, and such mix-tures, in addition to causing the undesirable

effects described below, may give rise to dependence.

UNDESIRABLE EFFECTS. Phenacetin may cause sweating. Prolonged use may cause methae-moglobinaemia, sulphaemoglobinaemia, or haemolytic anaemia. Toxic effects on the kidney, both acute and chronic, have been described. The administration of very large doses may cause hepatic necrosis.

Dose. 300 to 600 milligrams as a single dose.

Preparations
ASPIRIN TABLETS, COMPOUND, B.P.C. (page 806)
ASPIRIN, PHENACETIN, AND CODEINE TABLETS, B.P. (*Syn*. Compound Codeine Tablets). Each tablet con-tains 250 mg each of aspirin and phenacetin and 8 mg of codeine phosphate. They should be stored in air-tight containers, protected from light. Dose: 1 or 2 tablets.
ASPIRIN, PHENACETIN, AND CODEINE TABLETS, SOLUBLE, B.P. (*Syn*. Soluble Compound Codeine Tablets). Each tablet contains 250 mg each of aspirin and phenacetin and 8 mg of codeine phosphate, with calcium carbonate, anhydrous citric acid, and saccharin sodium. They should be stored in airtight containers, protected from light. Dose: 1 or 2 tablets.

OTHER NAMES: Aceto-*p*-phenetidide; Acetophenetidin

PHENAZOCINE HYDROBROMIDE

$C_{22}H_{28}BrNO,\frac{1}{2}H_2O = 411.4$

Phenazocine Hydrobromide is 1,2,3,4,5,6-hexa-hydro-8-hydroxy-6,11-dimethyl-3-phenethyl-2,6-methano-3-benzazocine hydrobromide hemihydrate.

Solubility. Soluble, at 20°, in 350 parts of water, in 45 parts of alcohol, and in 140 parts of chloroform; insoluble in ether.

Standard
It complies with the requirements of the British Pharmacopoeia.
It is a white, microcrystalline, odourless powder and contains not less than 99·0 and not more than the equivalent of 101·0 per cent of $C_{22}H_{28}BrNO$, calcu-

lated with reference to the anhydrous substance. It contains 2·0 to 2·5 per cent w/w of water. A 0·2 per cent solution in water has a pH of 5·0 to 7·0

Sterilisation. Solutions for injection are sterilised by heating in an autoclave.

Storage. It should be protected from light.

Actions and uses. Phenazocine is a synthetic analgesic which has many of the actions and uses described under Morphine Hydrochloride (page 314). Its analgesic action is greater than that of morphine, quicker in onset, and longer in duration. It is less likely to cause constipation than morphine and in equipotent analgesic doses causes less respiratory depression; tolerance develops more slowly and less completely.

Phenazocine, like morphine, is used for preoperative medication, 1 to 2 milligrams of phenazocine hydrobromide being given by intramuscular injection forty-five to sixty minutes before the operation.

For post-operative pain, 1 to 2 milligrams may be given by intramuscular injection.

The dose as a general analgesic is 1 to 3 milligrams by intramuscular injection; the total dose should not exceed 12 milligrams during twenty-four hours.

The usual dose by mouth is 5 milligrams.

UNDESIRABLE EFFECTS. Phenazocine, like morphine, is addictive, inducing euphoria and relieving the withdrawal syndrome in morphine addicts. Undesirable effects include nausea, vomiting, dizziness, and constriction of the pupils.

CONTRA-INDICATIONS. Phenazocine is contra-indicated in coma, convulsive disorders, delirium tremens, hepatic insufficiency, myxoedema, and alcoholism.

POISONING. Phenazocine is a potent respiratory depressant. This action may be antagonised by the intravenous injection of nalorphine or levallorphan. The procedure as described under Morphine Hydrochloride (page 314) should be adopted.

Dose. See above under **Actions and uses.**

Preparations

PHENAZOCINE INJECTION, B.P. It consists of a sterile solution of phenazocine hydrobromide in Water for Injections containing 1·5 per cent v/v of propylene glycol and suitable buffering agents. It should be protected from light. The strength of the solution should be specified by the prescriber. Ampoules containing 2 mg of phenazocine hydrobromide in 1 ml are available.

PHENAZOCINE TABLETS, B.P. The quantity of phenazocine hydrobromide in each tablet should be specified by the prescriber. They should be protected from light. Tablets containing 5 mg of phenazocine hydrobromide are available.

OTHER NAME: *Narphen*®

PHENAZONE

SYNONYM: Antipyrin

$C_{11}H_{12}N_2O = 188·2$

Phenazone is 2,3-dimethyl-1-phenylpyrazol-5-one.

Solubility. Soluble, at 20°, in 1 part of water, of alcohol, and of chloroform, and in 50 parts of ether.

Standard

DESCRIPTION. Small colourless crystals or white, crystalline powder; odourless or almost odourless.

IDENTIFICATION TESTS. 1. Dissolve 0·1 g in 10 ml of water and add 2 ml of *tannic acid solution*; a white precipitate is formed.

2. Dissolve 0·1 g in 10 ml of water containing 0·1 g of *sodium nitrite* and add 1 ml of *dilute sulphuric acid*; a green colour is produced.

3. Dissolve 2 mg in 2 ml of water and add 0·05 ml of *ferric chloride test-solution*; a deep red colour is produced. Add 0·5 ml of *sulphuric acid*; the colour changes to light yellow.

4. A solution in water is neutral to *litmus solution*.

MELTING-POINT. 111° to 113°.

SULPHATED ASH. Not more than 0·1 per cent.

CONTENT OF $C_{11}H_{12}N_2O$. Not less than 99·0 per cent, determined by the following method:
Dissolve about 0·2 g, accurately weighed, in 20 ml of a 10 per cent w/v solution of *sodium acetate* in water, add 30 ml of 0·1N iodine, and allow to stand for 20 minutes with occasional shaking; add 10 ml of *chloroform*, shake until the precipitate has dissolved, and titrate the excess of iodine with 0·1N sodium thiosulphate.
Repeat the procedure omitting the sample.
The difference between the two titrations represents the amount of iodine required by the sample; each ml of 0·1N iodine is equivalent to 0·009412 g of $C_{11}H_{12}N_2O$.

Incompatibility. It is incompatible with nitrites in acid solution and with tannic acid in aqueous solution. With sodium salicylate in the dry state it forms an oily liquid on exposure to air; it acts similarly with butylchloral hydrate and betanaphthol.

Actions and uses. Phenazone has actions and uses similar to those described under Phenacetin (page 360).

After rapid and complete absorption, phenazone is distributed throughout the body water and is very slowly metabolised. It has therefore been used to estimate the body fluid volume.

UNDESIRABLE EFFECTS. Nausea and rashes may occur.

Dose. 300 to 600 milligrams.

PHENELZINE SULPHATE

$C_8H_{14}N_2O_4S = 234·3$

$C_6H_5·[CH_2]_2·NH·NH_2,H_2SO_4$

Phenelzine Sulphate is phenethylhydrazine hydrogen sulphate.

Solubility. Soluble, at 20°, in 7 parts of water; very slightly soluble in alcohol; insoluble in ether and in chloroform.

Standard

It complies with the requirements of the British Pharmacopoeia.

It occurs as a white powder or pearly platelets with a pungent odour and contains not less than 98·0 per cent of $C_8H_{14}N_2O_4S$, calculated with reference to the dried substance. The loss on drying under the prescribed conditions is not more than 1·0 per cent. It has a melting-point of 164° to 168°.

Storage. It should be stored in airtight containers, protected from light.

Actions and uses. Phenelzine is an antidepressant drug which inhibits monoamine oxidase and probably acts by influencing the metabolism of transmitter substances, such as noradrenaline and 5-hydroxytryptamine, in the brain.

Phenelzine appears to be of more value in the treatment of patients suffering from neurotic or reactive depressive illness than in the treatment of true endogenous depression. After three or four days of treatment with phenelzine, patients have considerable relief of fatigue and tension, sleeping habits are improved and emotional control is regained.

The usual dosage is the equivalent of 15 milligrams of the base by mouth three or four times a day, but for some patients only 15 milligrams a day may be required; 25 milligrams of phenelzine sulphate is approximately equivalent to 15 milligrams of phenelzine base. Such treatment is usually continued for one month; maintenance doses may be necessary for much longer periods. The drug should not be withdrawn abruptly because relapse may occur within a day or two. In refractory cases, treatment with phenelzine may be combined initially with electroconvulsive therapy.

UNDESIRABLE EFFECTS. The most frequently occurring undesirable effects are postural hypotension and attacks of giddiness, which usually disappear after suitable reduction in dosage. Dryness of the mouth, constipation, blurring of vision, rashes, headache, and liver damage may occur occasionally.

PRECAUTIONS. As monoamine-oxidase inhibitors may potentiate the action of other drugs, caution should be exercised in giving phenelzine in conjunction with any other drug. Amphetamine, atropine, carbamazepine, chloroquine, cocaine, dexamphetamine, ephedrine, ethamivan, fenfluramine, guanethidine, mephentermine, methoxamine, methylamphetamine, morphine, orciprenaline, pethidine, phenmetrazine, phenylephrine, phenylpropanolamine, and pseudoephedrine, should not be given at the same time as phenelzine. There is a danger if reserpine is given to patients who are already undergoing treatment with a monoamine-oxidase inhibitor.

Certain foodstuffs contain pressor agents, such as tyramine, which may be formed by microbial decomposition from amino-acids and may precipitate paroxysmal attacks in patients taking monoamine-oxidase inhibitors; the diet of such persons should therefore not include cheese, pickled herrings, broad bean pods, and certain protein extracts prepared from meat or yeast.

After the administration of phenelzine, an interval of about ten days should be allowed to elapse before any of the drugs or foods listed above are given so as to ensure that the monoamine-oxidase inhibitor has been eliminated and that tissue levels of monoamine oxidase have returned to normal.

Dose. See above under **Actions and uses.**

Preparation
PHENELZINE TABLETS, B.P. Unless otherwise specified, tablets each containing phenelzine sulphate equivalent to 15 mg of phenelzine are supplied. They are sugar coated.

OTHER NAME: *Nardil*®

PHENETHICILLIN POTASSIUM

$C_{17}H_{19}KN_2O_5S = 402.5$

Phenethicillin Potassium is a mixture of the potassium salts of 6-D(+)- and 6-L(−)-(α-phenoxypropionamido)penicillanic acid.

Solubility. Soluble, at 20°, in 1·5 parts of water, in 85 parts of alcohol, and in 800 parts of dehydrated alcohol; slightly soluble in chloroform; insoluble in ether.

Standard
It complies with the requirements of the British Pharmacopoeia.
It is a white or almost white, fine, crystalline powder with a slight sulphurous odour and contains not more than 97·0 per cent of $C_{17}H_{19}KN_2O_5S$, calculated with reference to the anhydrous substance. It contains not more than 1·5 per cent w/w of water. A 10 per cent solution in water has a pH of 5·5 to 7·5.

Hygroscopicity. It absorbs insignificant amounts of moisture at 25° at relative humidities up to about 65 per cent, but under damper conditions it absorbs significant amounts.

Storage. It should be stored in airtight containers.

Actions and uses. Phenethicillin has the actions and uses described under Phenoxymethylpenicillin (page 371).

Although phenethicillin gives rise to higher blood levels than phenoxymethylpenicillin it is less potent as an antibiotic and the effect of the two substances is therefore similar.

PRECAUTIONS AND CONTRA-INDICATIONS. As for Phenoxymethylpenicillin (page 371).

Dose. The equivalent of 0·5 to 1·5 grams of phenethicillin daily, in divided doses.

Preparations
PHENETHICILLIN CAPSULES, B.P. Unless otherwise specified, capsules each containing the equivalent of 250 mg of phenethicillin are supplied.

PHENETHICILLIN ELIXIR, B.P.C. (page 674).

PHENETHICILLIN TABLETS, B.P. Unless otherwise specified, tablets each containing the equivalent of 250 mg of phenethicillin are supplied. They should be stored in airtight containers. Tablets each containing the equivalent of 125 mg of phenethicillin are also available.

OTHER NAME: *Broxil*®

PHENFORMIN HYDROCHLORIDE

$C_{10}H_{16}ClN_5 = 241·7$

$$\left[C_6H_5 \cdot [CH_2]_2 \cdot NH \cdot \underset{\|}{C} \cdot NH \cdot \underset{\|}{C} \cdot NH_2 \right] HCl$$
$$ NH \quad\; NH$$

Phenformin Hydrochloride is N^1-phenethylbiguanide hydrochloride.

Solubility. Soluble, at 20°, in 8 parts of water and in 15 parts of alcohol; insoluble in ether and in chloroform.

Standard
It complies with the requirements of the British Pharmacopoeia.
It is a white or almost white, crystalline, odourless powder and contains not less than 99·0 and not more than the equivalent of 101·0 per cent of $C_{10}H_{16}ClN_5$, calculated with reference to the dried substance. The loss on drying under the prescribed conditions is not more than 1·0 per cent. It has a melting-point of 176° to 179°. A 2·5 per cent solution has a pH of 6·0 to 7·0.

Actions and uses. Phenformin is an oral hypoglycaemic agent which, unlike the sulphonylureas, as described under Chlorpropamide (page 109), has an action that is independent of the pancreatic beta-cells. Although the precise mode of action of phenformin is not known, it is thought that its main activities are to control the glucose level of the blood by increasing its peripheral utilisation and to inhibit gluconeogenesis in the diabetic.
Unlike insulin, phenformin does not encourage lipogenesis. It reduces the blood-glucose level in diabetes and in cortisone-induced hyperglycaemia in pre-diabetes, but it has no effect on the blood-sugar level of normal persons except in the fasting state. It reduces the insulin requirements of young diabetics. In a daily dosage of 50 to 100 milligrams, phenformin causes loss of weight in obese diabetics, whereas sulphonylureas usually give rise to a gain of weight.
Phenformin enhances fibrinolysis, particularly when it is given with oestrogens or anabolic steroids. It reduces the blood cholesterol in maturity-onset diabetes. In some diabetics it may cause ketosis.
Phenformin hydrochloride is absorbed after oral administration and its hypoglycaemic action lasts six to eight hours; this period may be extended to fourteen hours by the use of slow-release tablets or capsules. The drug is excreted largely unchanged by the kidneys within about twenty-four hours.
As the mode of action of phenformin is different from that of the sulphonylureas, it is sometimes used in conjunction with one of them when neither drug is fully effective alone. Phenformin used by itself is not suitable for unstable or juvenile diabetics or for diabetic patients requiring large doses of insulin, but it is sometimes used in conjunction with insulin; it should never completely replace insulin in brittle cases.
Phenformin hydrochloride is given initially in doses of 25 milligrams in the morning or morning and evening and the dose increased by 25 milligrams at intervals of two or three days until the blood-glucose level is controlled. Up to 300 milligrams may be given daily, divided into two, three, or four doses. A daily dosage of 100 to 150 milligrams is required by the average diabetic suitable for treatment with phenformin. A slow-release capsule of 50 milligrams may be given once or twice a day; higher doses may be required.

UNDESIRABLE EFFECTS. Phenformin may give rise to a metallic or bitter taste, anorexia, nausea, vomiting, and diarrhoea, particularly in patients on high dosage; these side-effects rarely necessitate withdrawal of the drug. Acute lactic acidosis is a rare but serious complication.

PRECAUTIONS AND CONTRA-INDICATIONS. During stabilisation the urine should be tested frequently for glucose and ketones. Phenformin should not be used in severe renal disease, congestive heart failure, diabetic coma, or the acute complications of diabetes, in pregnancy, before or after surgery, or during acute infections.
Juvenile diabetics should never be treated with phenformin alone.

POISONING. Hypoglycaemia should be treated by giving dextrose by mouth or, in serious cases, by the intravenous injection of a 20 to 50 per cent solution of dextrose.
Acidosis should be treated by the intravenous infusion of sodium bicarbonate solution.
When phenformin has been taken with a sulphonylurea the effects may be intensified, persist longer, and require treatment for a longer time.

Dose. See above under **Actions and uses.**

Preparation
PHENFORMIN TABLETS, B.P. Unless otherwise specified, tablets each containing 25 mg of phenformin hydrochloride are supplied.

OTHER NAME: *Dibotin*®

PHENINDAMINE TARTRATE

$C_{23}H_{25}NO_6 = 411.5$

Phenindamine Tartrate is 1,2,3,4-tetrahydro-2-methyl-9-phenyl-2-azafluorene hydrogen tartrate.

Solubility. Soluble, at 20°, in 70 parts of water and in 300 parts of alcohol; very slightly soluble in ether and in chloroform.

Standard
It complies with the requirements of the British Pharmacopoeia.
It is a white or almost white, almost odourless, voluminous powder and contains not less than 98·5 and not more than the equivalent of 101·0 per cent of $C_{23}H_{25}NO_6$, calculated with reference to the dried substance. The loss on drying under the prescribed conditions is not more than 1·0 per cent. It has a melting-point of 160° to 162°, resolidifies at about 163°, and remelts with decomposition at about 168°. A 1 per cent solution in water has a pH of 3·4 to 3·9.

Storage. It should be stored in airtight containers, protected from light.

Actions and uses. Phenindamine has the actions and uses of the antihistamine drugs, as described under Promethazine Hydrochloride (page 409) but it has no marked anti-emetic effect. Unlike some other antihistamines, it does not produce drowsiness and may even be mildly stimulating.

Phenindamine tartrate is given by mouth in a dosage of 25 to 50 milligrams once to four times a day. It is applied locally as a cream for the treatment of itching and other skin disorders, but the incidence of skin sensitisation is higher than with other antihistamine drugs. It has been used in the treatment of parkinsonism.

UNDESIRABLE EFFECTS. These occur frequently and may include dryness of the mouth, dizziness, and gastro-intestinal disturbances. Insomnia and convulsions may occur.

POISONING. See under Promethazine Hydrochloride (page 409).

Dose. See above under **Actions and uses.**

Preparation
PHENINDAMINE TABLETS, B.P. Unless otherwise specified, tablets each containing 25 mg of phenindamine tartrate are supplied. They are sugar coated.

OTHER NAME: *Thephorin®*

PHENINDIONE

$C_{15}H_{10}O_2 = 222.2$

Phenindione is 2-phenylindane-1,3-dione.

Solubility. Very slightly soluble in water; soluble, at 20°, in 125 parts of alcohol, in 110 parts of ether, and in 6·5 parts of chloroform. Solutions are yellow to red in colour.

Standard
It complies with the requirements of the British Pharmacopoeia.
It occurs as soft, white or creamy-white, almost odourless crystals and contains not less than 98·0 per cent of $C_{15}H_{10}O_2$, calculated with reference to the dried substance. The loss on drying under the prescribed conditions is not more than 1·0 per cent. It has a melting-point of 148° to 151°.

Storage. It should be stored in airtight containers.

Actions and uses. Phenindione is a synthetic anticoagulant which prolongs the prothrombin time by inhibiting the formation of "factor VII" and of prothrombin. A therapeutic effect is obtained twenty-four to thirty hours after the initial oral dose has been given and ceases within thirty-six hours of the last dose. To obtain an immediate effect on blood coagulation, heparin must be given intravenously for the first twenty-four to thirty hours of phenindione therapy. During treatment the plasma-prothrombin level should be determined frequently so that the daily dosage may be adjusted to the desired therapeutic level.

Phenindione is used in those conditions in which it is desirable to lower the coagulability of the blood. It is used in the prophylaxis and treatment of thrombosis in veins or arteries of the extremities. It prevents further thrombosis where this has already occurred, thereby markedly reducing the risk of embolism. Because of the risk of haemorrhage, its use in the treatment of such conditions as cerebral thrombosis may be dangerous, but it is sometimes used in the treatment of thrombosis of the central retinal vein. In the treatment of post-operative venous thrombosis, therapy is continued until the patient is fully ambulant.

Phenindione is given by mouth, usually in an initial dose of 200 to 300 milligrams which is repeated after twelve hours; the daily maintenance dosage is 25 to 100 milligrams according to the prothrombin activity of the blood.

The effect of phenindione may be modified by the concurrent administration of other drugs. Methandienone and other 17-alkylated steroids, clofibrate, phenylbutazone, and similar drugs, by plasma protein displacement, may increase the anticoagulant effect of phenindione, while barbiturates, chloral hydrate, glutethimide, and meprobamate, by promoting its metabolism, may reduce this effect. Aspirin and other salicylates may increase the danger of haemorrhage during anticoagulant therapy.

PRECAUTIONS AND CONTRA-INDICATIONS. Phenindione should be used with great caution in the presence of hepatic or severe renal disease and also in any condition where there is a real risk of serious haemorrhage, such as unhealed peptic ulceration. It should not be used within three days of parturition or of surgical operation, nor in the later months of pregnancy.

UNDESIRABLE EFFECTS. Rashes, pyrexia, diarrhoea, and sore throat may occur. Kidney damage may occur in patients sensitive to phenindione; serious toxic effects are rare, but may include liver damage, agranulocytosis, granulocytopenia, and eosinophilia.

Early clinical signs of overdosage are mild bleeding from the gums or elsewhere and the presence of erythrocytes in the urinary deposit.

Phytomenadione is the most effective antidote to overdosage; administration of water-soluble vitamin-K analogues and transfusion of whole blood are less effective. The usual dose of phytomenadione that is required is 2 to 20 milligrams by mouth. In severe hypoprothrombinaemia 10 to 50 milligrams of phytomenadione may be administered by slow intravenous injection in the form of Phytomenadione Injection, the dose depending on the degree of prothrombin time prolongation and the clinical urgency; overdosage may encourage thrombosis.

During treatment with phenindione the urine is sometimes coloured red, but this is of no clinical significance. Sensitivity to phenindione may develop during prolonged treatment and an alternative anticoagulant may have to be given.

Dose. See above under **Actions and uses**.

Preparation
PHENINDIONE TABLETS, B.P. The quantity of phenindione in each tablet should be specified by the prescriber. They should be stored in airtight containers. Tablets containing 10, 25, and 50 mg are available.

OTHER NAMES: *Dindevan*®; Phenylindanedione; *Theradione*®

PHENMETRAZINE HYDROCHLORIDE

$C_{11}H_{16}ClNO = 213\cdot7$

Phenmetrazine Hydrochloride is $(\pm)$-*trans*-3-methyl-2-phenylmorpholine hydrochloride.

Solubility. Soluble, at $20°$, in less than 1 part of water, in 2 parts of alcohol, and in 2 parts of chloroform; slightly soluble in ether.

Standard
It complies with the requirements of the British Pharmacopoeia.
It is a white, crystalline, odourless powder and contains not less than 98·5 and not more than the equivalent of 101·0 per cent of $C_{11}H_{16}ClNO$, calculated with reference to the dried substance. The loss on drying under the prescribed conditions is not more than 0·5 per cent. It has a melting-point of about 174°.

Stability. In alkaline preparations, phenmetrazine base is liberated and loss may occur by volatilisation of the base, particularly at high temperatures.

Actions and uses. Phenmetrazine is an anorectic agent which has little effect on the metabolic rate. In large doses it has a stimulant action on the central nervous system similar to that of amphetamine (page 25), but it has little action on the cardiovascular system. Phenmetrazine hydrochloride is used in the treatment of obesity to make a restricted diet more tolerable, a dosage of 12·5 to 25 milli-grams by mouth two or three times a day half an hour to one hour before meals being usually adequate. It is advisable not to administer the drug later than the late afternoon as it may cause insomnia. A course of treatment should not be continued for more than a month.

UNDESIRABLE EFFECTS. Large doses and prolonged treatment may lead to severe mental depression and dependence of the amphetamine type (see under Amphetamine Sulphate, page 25).

PRECAUTIONS. Phenmetrazine should not be given to patients who are being treated with a monoamine-oxidase inhibitor, such as isocarboxazid, nialamide, phenelzine, or tranylcypromine, or within about ten days of the discontinuation of such treatment.

Dose. See above under **Actions and uses**.

Preparation
PHENMETRAZINE TABLETS, B.P. Unless otherwise specified, tablets each containing 25 mg of phenmetrazine hydrochloride are supplied.

OTHER NAME: *Preludin*®

PHENOBARBITONE

SYNONYMS: Phenobarb.; Phenobarbital; Phenobarbitalum

$C_{12}H_{12}N_2O_3 = 232.2$

Phenobarbitone is 5-ethyl-5-phenylbarbituric acid.

Solubility. Soluble, at $20°$, in 1000 parts of water and in 10 parts of alcohol; soluble in ether, in chloroform, and in solutions of alkali hydroxides and carbonates.

Standard

It complies with the requirements of the European Pharmacopoeia.

It occurs as an odourless, white, crystalline powder or colourless crystals and contains not less than 99·0 and not more than the equivalent of 101·0 per cent of $C_{12}H_{12}N_2O_3$, calculated with reference to the dried substance. The loss on drying under the prescribed conditions is not more than 0·5 per cent. It has a melting-point of $174°$ to $178°$.

Actions and uses. Phenobarbitone is a member of the group of drugs known as the barbiturates. These drugs have a hypnotic action, but in therapeutic doses they have little or no effect on the medullary centres, so that blood pressure and respiration are not influenced. Barbiturates are used chiefly as hypnotics and sedatives.

There is considerable variation in the duration of action of the barbiturates and they may be roughly classified in the following groups, each of which has its special therapeutic indications:

Long-acting barbiturates: these include barbitone and phenobarbitone. Because of its depressant effect on the motor cortex phenobarbitone is used alone or with other anticonvulsants in the treatment of epilepsy. It is also used as a sedative in the treatment of disorders when anxiety and stress are present.

Intermediate-acting barbiturates: these include amylobarbitone, butobarbitone, cyclobarbitone, nealbarbitone, pentobarbitone, and quinalbarbitone. They are used as soporifics, their action ending not more than eight hours after administration. They may also be used for pre-operative medication to induce a quiet and restful condition in the patient.

Very short-acting barbiturates: these include methohexitone and thiopentone. They are used mainly as rapid-acting intravenous anaesthetics, either alone or, more usually, as a preliminary to inhalation anaesthesia.

Phenobarbitone has been used as a sedative in nervous and anxiety states, chorea, neurasthenia, climacteric disorders, dysmenorrhoea, and thyrotoxicosis, but it has been largely replaced by other sedatives. It is also used in the treatment of migraine, and in epilepsy to diminish the frequency and severity of attacks. In anticonvulsant dosage, phenobarbitone does not act as a hypnotic, but should it become necessary, in order to control the fits, to increase the dosage to a level at which the patient would become drowsy, phenytoin or primidone may be used to supplement the action of the barbiturate instead of increasing its dosage.

UNDESIRABLE EFFECTS. Patients vary in their response to the barbiturates, and the hypnotic state is occasionally preceded by excitement and delirium and by confusion in the elderly. Prolonged administration may lead to tolerance and the dosage may need to be increased to obtain the desired soporific effect. Increased dosage is liable to produce toxic effects, which may be either acute or chronic. The acute symptoms depend on the nature and dose of the barbiturate used; short-acting barbiturates give rise to respiratory and circulatory failure and the long-acting group to deep unconsciousness, which is followed by congestion of the lungs and "barbiturate pneumonia".

Symptoms of chronic poisoning include mild changes in the patient's mental condition, such as loss of memory, inability to concentrate, giddiness, depression, and dullness of mental perception, and also skin rashes of various types. Haemorrhagic bullae frequently accompany poisoning by long-acting barbiturates.

PRECAUTIONS. Phenobarbitone may increase the rate of metabolism of other drugs such as folic acid, griseofulvin, phenylbutazone, phenytoin, and anticoagulants of the coumarin type, and caution should therefore be exercised in giving phenobarbitone with other drugs. Sudden withdrawal of phenobarbitone from an epileptic should be avoided, as it may precipitate status epilepticus.

CONTRA-INDICATIONS. The majority of the barbiturates are detoxicated by the liver and are therefore contra-indicated where there is liver damage; phenobarbitone is, however, mainly excreted unchanged in the urine.

DEPENDENCE. Dependence of the barbiturate-alcohol type is characterized by a strong psychic dependence; intoxication manifested by sedation, sleep, coma, stupor, impaired cognition and judgement, and ataxia; development of tolerance; partial crossed tolerance between members of the group; a dangerous type of physical dependence manifested by anxiety, insomnia, weakness, tremors, abnormalities in the electro-encephalogram, convulsions, and delirium on withdrawal.

POISONING. The aims in treating barbiturate poisoning are to maintain respiration and to eliminate the drug. If the drug has been taken by mouth, the stomach should be washed out with warm water and filled with a dilute sodium sulphate solution to promote peristalsis.

Fluid may also be given by intravenous infusion, usually as Sodium Chloride and Dextrose Injection, but care must be taken not to give too much as it may increase the risk of bronchopneumonia due to oedema of the lungs.

The most important aspects of the treatment of barbiturate poisoning are careful nursing and the administration of oxygen if necessary.

In cases which do not respond to these measures, haemodialysis may be used in addition.

Dose. 30 to 125 milligrams three times daily.

Preparations
PHENOBARBITONE ELIXIR, B.P.C. (page 675)
BELLADONNA AND PHENOBARBITONE TABLETS, B.P.C. (page 807)
PHENOBARBITONE TABLETS, B.P. (*Syn.* Phenobarbital Tablets). The quantity of phenobarbitone in each tablet should be specified by the prescriber. Tablets containing 7·5, 10, 15, 30, 50, 60, 100, and 125 mg are available.
PHENOBARBITONE AND THEOBROMINE TABLETS, B.P.C. (page 814)

OTHER NAMES: *Gardenal®*; *Luminal®*

PHENOBARBITONE SODIUM

SYNONYMS: Phenobarb. Sod.; Phenobarbital Sodium; Soluble Phenobarbitone

$C_{12}H_{11}N_2NaO_3 = 254·2$

Phenobarbitone Sodium is sodium 5-ethyl-5-phenylbarbiturate.

Solubility. Soluble, at 20°, in 3 parts of water and in 25 parts of alcohol; insoluble in ether and in chloroform.

Standard
It complies with the requirements of the British Pharmacopoeia.
It is a white, hygroscopic, odourless powder and contains not less than 98·0 per cent of $C_{12}H_{11}N_2NaO_3$, calculated with reference to the dried substance. The loss on drying under the prescribed conditions is not more than 7·0 per cent. A 10 per cent solution in water has a pH of not more than 11.

Stability. In moist air it absorbs carbon dioxide, liberating phenobarbitone.

Incompatibility. It is incompatible with acids, acidic salts such as ammonium bromide, acidic syrups such as lemon syrup, and chloral hydrate. Phenobarbitone may be precipitated from mixtures containing the sodium derivative, depending on the concentration and the pH: in a mixture containing 30 mg of phenobarbitone sodium in 10 ml, precipitation of phenobarbitone occurs at pH 7·5 and below. The corresponding figures for other concentrations are: 60 mg, pH 7·9; 100 mg, pH 8·3; and 200 mg, pH 8·6.

Storage. It should be stored in airtight containers.

Actions and uses. Phenobarbitone sodium has the actions and uses described under Phenobarbitone. It may be given by injection to produce a more rapid effect.

Solutions for injection are prepared by an aseptic technique.

UNDESIRABLE EFFECTS; PRECAUTIONS; CONTRA-INDICATIONS; DEPENDENCE. These are as described under Phenobarbitone.

POISONING. The procedure as described under Phenobarbitone should be adopted.

Dose. 30 to 125 milligrams by mouth three times daily; 50 to 200 milligrams, as a single dose, by intravenous, intramuscular, or subcutaneous injection.

Preparations
PHENOBARBITONE INJECTION, B.P. It consists of a sterile solution of phenobarbitone sodium in a mixture of 9 volumes of propylene glycol and 1 volume of Water for Injections; it may contain not more than 0·02 per cent of disodium edetate. The quantity of phenobarbitone sodium in each container should be specified by the prescriber. Ampoules containing 200 mg in 1 ml are available.
GENTIAN MIXTURE, ALKALINE, WITH PHENOBARBITONE, B.P.C. (page 744)
PHENOBARBITONE SODIUM TABLETS, B.P. (*Syn.* Soluble Phenobarbitone Tablets; Phenobarbital Sodium Tablets). The quantity of phenobarbitone sodium in each tablet should be specified by the prescriber. They should be stored in airtight containers. Tablets containing 15, 30, and 60 mg are available.

OTHER NAME: *Gardenal Sodium®*

PHENOL

$C_6H_5 \cdot OH = 94·11$

Phenol is hydroxybenzene. It may be obtained from coal tar or prepared synthetically.

Solubility. Soluble, at 20°, in 12 parts of water; soluble in alcohol, in ether, in chloroform, in glycerol, in liquid paraffin, and in fixed and volatile oils; readily soluble in alkalis, forming solutions of alkali phenoxides.

At 20°, 100 parts of phenol is liquefied by the addition of 10 parts of water; this solution will dissolve about a further 30 parts of water, the solution remaining clear; on the further addition of water the liquid separates into two layers, one a solution of phenol in water and the other a solution of water in phenol, until about 1200 parts of water have been added, when a solution of phenol in water is formed.

Standard
It complies with the requirements of the British Pharmacopoeia.
It occurs as deliquescent, colourless or faintly pink, needle-shaped crystals or crystalline masses, with a characteristic and not tarry odour and contains not less than 99·0 per cent of C_6H_6O. It has a freezing-point not lower than 40·5° and a boiling-point of about 181°. A 1 in 12 solution in water at 20° is clear and alkaline to methyl orange.

Sterilisation. Oily solutions for injection are sterilised in hermetically sealed containers by dry heat.

Storage. It should be stored in airtight containers, protected from light, in a cool place.

Preparation and storage of solutions. See statement on aqueous solutions of antiseptics, under Solutions (page 779).

Actions and uses. Phenol is a bactericide, which, in concentrated solution, is destructive to tissues. Its use as a germicide has largely declined in favour of more active and less toxic compounds, but it is effective against certain viruses.
When strong solutions of phenol are applied to the skin the area becomes white through precipitation of proteins, and a slough is formed. With continued application, phenol penetrates into the deeper tissues causing paralysis of sensory nerve endings and painless gangrene. If preparations containing phenol are applied to large wounds, phenol may be absorbed in amounts sufficient to produce toxic effects.
The antiseptic properties of phenol are greatly reduced, and the caustic action delayed, if it is dissolved in alcohol, glycerol, or fixed oils.
An aqueous solution containing 0·5 per cent of phenol is used as a vehicle in some injections. A concentration of 1 per cent of phenol in water will kill most vegetative bacteria within a few minutes.
Liquefied Phenol has been used in dentistry as an analgesic for sensitive dentine and 5 per cent solutions have been used to devitalise the pulp in deciduous teeth. Diluted solutions containing 0·2 to 0·5 per cent of phenol, sometimes in the form of alkaline phenates, are used as astringent gargles and mouth-washes, but in these concentrations phenol can have little antibacterial action.
Phenol and Glycerol Injection is administered

intrathecally for the relief of severe intractable pain and spasticity.
Phenol Ear-drops are used in the treatment of otitis media and of boils in the ear.
Oily Phenol Injection is injected into the tissues around internal haemorrhoids as an analgesic thrombotic agent.
Phenol is rapidly absorbed from the surface of the body and from the gastro-intestinal tract. It is conjugated in the body and is excreted in the urine as benzenesulphonates and glycuronates which, upon oxidation, give the urine a green tint, and this may happen even when phenol preparations are applied locally to the skin.
Aqueous solutions of phenol should be coloured with amaranth or other suitable red dye, unless otherwise ordered.

POISONING. The stomach should be washed out repeatedly with a solution of magnesium or sodium sulphate, 30 g per gallon, or 30 g of magnesium or sodium sulphate in $\frac{1}{2}$ pint of water given by mouth. The patient should be kept warm to prevent circulatory collapse. Inhalation of oxygen with carbon dioxide or artificial respiration may be necessary.
Intravenous fluids must be given as the patient will be unable to take food or fluids by mouth, and an adequate flow of urine will hasten the excretion of phenol and its breakdown products. Care must be taken to adjust the fluid and electrolyte intake as there may be severe renal damage.
Burns caused by phenol on the skin or mucous surfaces should be swabbed with glycerol, alcohol, or oil to dissolve the phenol.

Preparations
LIQUEFIED PHENOL, B.P. It contains 80 per cent w/w of phenol in Purified Water. When phenol is to be mixed with collodion, fixed oils or paraffins, melted phenol should be used and not Liquefied Phenol. It should be stored in airtight containers, protected from light. If stored below 4°, it may congeal or deposit crystals; such material should be completely melted and well mixed before use.
PHENOL AND GLYCEROL INJECTION, B.P. (*Syn.* Phenol and Glycerin Injection). It consists of a sterile 5 per cent w/w solution of phenol in glycerol. It should be protected from light. Dose: 0·5 to 2 millilitres by intrathecal injection.
PHENOL EAR-DROPS, B.P.C. (page 665)
PHENOL GARGLE, B.P.C. (page 700)
POTASSIUM CHLORATE AND PHENOL GARGLE, B.P.C. (page 700)
PHENOL GLYCERIN, B.P.C. (page 701)
PHENOL INJECTION, OILY, B.P.C. (page 716)

OTHER NAME: Carbolic Acid

PHENOLPHTHALEIN

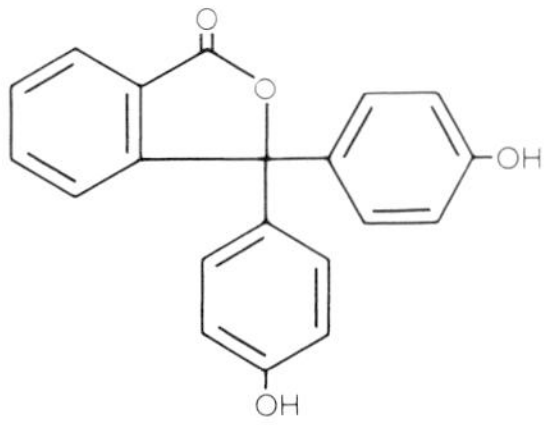

$C_{20}H_{14}O_4 = 318 \cdot 3$

Phenolphthalein is $\alpha\alpha$-di(p-hydroxyphenyl)phthalide.

Solubility. Very slightly soluble in water; soluble in alcohol and in ether.

Standard

It complies with the requirements of the British Pharmacopoeia.

It is a white or yellowish-white, crystalline or amorphous, odourless powder and contains not less than 98·0 and not more than the equivalent of 102·0 per cent of $C_{20}H_{14}O_4$, calculated with reference to the dried substance. The loss on drying under the prescribed conditions is not more than 1·0 per cent. It has a melting-point of 258° to 263°.

Hygroscopicity. It absorbs insignificant amounts of moisture at 25° at relative humidities up to about 90 per cent.

Actions and uses. Phenolphthalein is an irritant purgative which is usually taken at night to act in the morning. Some of it may be absorbed and excreted partly in the bile, so that purgative effects may continue for several days. It is excreted chiefly in the faeces, but some may be excreted by the kidneys, imparting a red colour to alkaline urine.

It is administered in pills or tablets, either alone or with aloin and other purgatives, and in Liquid Paraffin Emulsion.

UNDESIRABLE EFFECTS. Phenolphthalein may produce rashes and it has occasionally caused albuminuria and haemoglobinuria.

Dose. 50 to 300 milligrams.

Preparations

LIQUID PARAFFIN AND PHENOLPHTHALEIN EMULSION, B.P.C. (page 679)

PHENOLPHTHALEIN PILLS, COMPOUND, B.P.C. (page 774)

PHENOLPHTHALEIN TABLETS, B.P. Unless otherwise specified, tablets each containing 125 mg of phenolphthalein are supplied. They should be chewed before being swallowed. Tablets containing 60 mg are also available.

PHENOLSULPHONPHTHALEIN

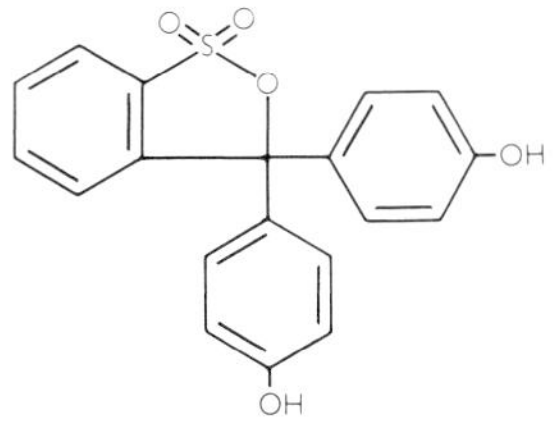

SYNONYM: Phenol Red

$C_{19}H_{14}O_5S = 354 \cdot 4$

Phenolsulphonphthalein is the sultone of di(p-hydroxyphenyl)-2-sulphophenylmethanol.

Solubility. Slightly soluble in water; soluble, at 20°, in 350 parts of alcohol; soluble in solutions of alkali hydroxides and of alkali carbonates.

Standard

DESCRIPTION. A bright to dark red crystalline powder; odourless or almost odourless.

IDENTIFICATION TESTS. 1. Dissolve 5 mg in 0·3 ml of 1N sodium hydroxide, add 2 ml of 0·1N bromine and 1 ml of *dilute hydrochloric acid*, shake well, allow to stand for 5 minutes, and make alkaline with 1N sodium hydroxide; an intense bluish-violet colour is produced. 2. When dissolved in solutions of alkali hydroxides or alkali carbonates, a violet-red to deep red colour is produced; the colour is changed to orange or yellow on the addition of a slight excess of acid and destroyed by warming with *zinc powder*.

ALKALI-INSOLUBLE MATTER. Not more than 0·5 per cent, determined by the following method:

To 1·0 g add 20 ml of a filtered 2·5 per cent w/v solution of *sodium bicarbonate* in water, rotate the container frequently during one hour, dilute to 100 ml with water, and allow to stand for 16 hours; centrifuge the solution, decant the supernatant liquid, and wash the residue by centrifuging and decantation successively with 25 ml of a filtered 1·0 per cent w/v solution of *sodium bicarbonate* in water and 25 ml of water; dry the residue at 105° and weigh.

UNDUE TOXICITY. Dissolve 0·50 g in a mixture of 40 ml of *water for injections* and 2·0 ml of 1N sodium hydroxide prepared with *water for injections*; adjust the pH to 6·0 to 7·5 by the addition of 1N hydrochloric acid prepared with *water for injections*, dilute to 50 ml with *water for injections*, and filter through a sintered-glass filter; 0·5 ml of this solution, when injected intravenously into each of 5 normal mice, each weighing approximately 20 g, does not cause the death of any of them within 24 hours.

If one of the mice dies, repeat the test; the sample complies if none of the second group dies within 24 hours.

PYROGENS. The filtered solution, prepared as described above in the test for undue toxicity, complies with the test for pyrogens, 1 ml being used for each kg of the rabbit's body-weight.

SULPHATED ASH. Not more than 0·5 per cent.

CONTENT OF $C_{19}H_{14}O_5S$. Not less than 94·0 per cent, determined by the following method:

Dissolve 0·87 to 0·90 g, accurately weighed, in 15 ml of 1N sodium hydroxide, dilute to 250 ml with water, and mix. To 50 ml of this solution in a glass-stoppered flask add 150 ml of water, 50 ml of 0·1N bromine, and 5 ml of *hydrochloric acid*, shake, allow to stand in the dark for 20 minutes, add 1 g of *potassium iodide*, and titrate the liberated iodine with 0·1N sodium thiosulphate, using *starch mucilage* as indicator; each ml of 0·1N bromine is equivalent to 0·004430 g of $C_{19}H_{14}O_5S$.

Sterilisation. Solutions for injection are sterilised by heating in an autoclave or by filtration.

Uses. Phenolsulphonphthalein has been used

as a test of renal function by estimating the rate of excretion in the urine after the intravenous injection of 6 milligrams, with 1·43 milligrams of sodium bicarbonate, in 1 millilitre of Sodium Chloride Injection. With normal renal function, at least 50 per cent is excreted in the urine in the first hour or 75 per cent in the first and second hours. The con-

centration in the urine can be determined colorimetrically after making alkaline with sodium hydroxide solution.

A neutralised solution of phenolsulphonphthalein is used in the diagnosis of hydrocephalus.

Dose. 6 milligrams by intravenous injection.

PHENOXYBENZAMINE HYDROCHLORIDE

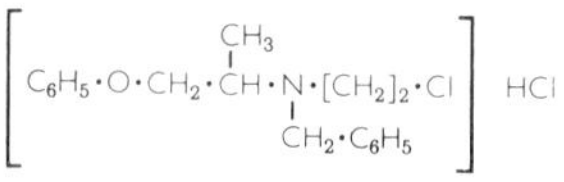

$C_{18}H_{23}Cl_2NO = 340·3$

$$\left[C_6H_5 \cdot O \cdot CH_2 \cdot \underset{\underset{CH_2 \cdot C_6H_5}{|}}{\overset{\overset{CH_3}{|}}{CH}} \cdot N \cdot [CH_2]_2 \cdot Cl \right] HCl$$

Phenoxybenzamine Hydrochloride is benzyl(2-chloroethyl)-(1-methyl-2-phenoxyethyl)amine hydrochloride.

CAUTION. *Phenoxybenzamine hydrochloride in powder should not be allowed to come into contact with the eyes and skin as it may cause irritation.*

Solubility. Slightly soluble in water; soluble, at 20°, in 9 parts of alcohol and in 9 parts of chloroform; soluble in propylene glycol.

Standard
It complies with the requirements of the British Pharmacopoeia.
It is a white or almost white, crystalline, odourless or almost odourless powder and contains not less than 98·5 and not more than the equivalent of 101·0 per cent of $C_{18}H_{23}Cl_2NO$, calculated with reference to the dried substance. The loss on drying under the prescribed conditions is not more than 0·5 per cent. It has a melting-point of 137·5° to 140°.

Stability of solutions. Neutral and alkaline solutions are unstable.

Actions and uses. Phenoxybenzamine has actions and uses similar to those described under Phentolamine Mesylate (page 373) but its effect lasts longer than that of phentolamine, a substantial dose being capable of causing postural hypotension for up to two days.

Phenoxybenzamine is used to control hypertension caused by phaeochromocytoma and occasionally in the treatment of peripheral vascular disease. Its effect cannot be reversed by noradrenaline.

Phenoxybenzamine hydrochloride is given by mouth, usually commencing with 10 milligrams daily and increasing the dosage according to the response of the patient up to a total of 240 milligrams daily in divided doses. It may also be given by slow intravenous injection in a daily dosage of 0·5 to 1 milligram per kilogram body-weight.

Dose. See above under **Actions and uses.**

Preparation
PHENOXYBENZAMINE CAPSULES, B.P. Unless otherwise specified, capsules each containing 10 mg of phenoxybenzamine hydrochloride are supplied.

OTHER NAME: *Dibenyline*®

PHENOXYETHANOL

SYNONYM: β-Phenoxyethyl Alcohol

$C_8H_{10}O_2 = 138·2$

$C_6H_5 \cdot O \cdot CH_2 \cdot CH_2OH$

Phenoxyethanol is 2-phenoxyethanol.

Solubility. Soluble, at 20°, in 43 parts of water and in 50 parts of arachis oil and of olive oil; miscible with alcohol, with acetone, and with glycerol.

Standard
DESCRIPTION. A colourless, slighty viscous liquid; odour faint and pleasant.

IDENTIFICATION TEST. Shake, until completely oxidised, 2 ml with a mixture of 4 g of *potassium permanganate*, 5·4 g of *sodium carbonate*, and 75 ml of water, and filter; saturate the filtrate with *sodium chloride* and acidify to *litmus paper* with *hydrochloric acid*; phenoxyacetic acid separates as soft crystals which, after recrystallising from water and drying, melt at about 99°.

WEIGHT PER ML. At 20°, 1·105 g to 1·110 g.

PHENOL. Not more than 0·1 per cent, determined by the following method:

Dilute 10·0 g to 100 ml with *methyl alcohol*; further dilute 10 ml of this solution to 100 ml with water and measure the extinction of a 1-cm layer at the maximum at about 287 nm. Repeat the procedure with a further 10 ml of the solution but adding 2 ml of 1N sodium hydroxide before diluting to 100 ml with water; the difference between the two extinctions is not greater than 0·25.

CONTENT OF $C_8H_{10}O_2$. Not less than 99·0 per cent w/w, determined by the following method:
To about 2 g, accurately weighed, add 10 ml of a freshly prepared 25 per cent w/w solution of *acetic anhydride* in *dehydrated pyridine*, heat on a water-bath for 45 minutes, add 10 ml of water, heat for a further 2 minutes, cool, add 10 ml of *butyl alcohol*, shake vigorously, and titrate the excess of acid with 1N sodium hydroxide, using *phenolphthalein solution* as indicator.

Repeat the procedure omitting the sample.
The difference between the two titrations represents the amount of acetic anhydride required by the sample; each ml of 1N sodium hydroxide is equivalent to 0·1382 g of $C_8H_{10}O_2$.

Preparation and storage of solutions. See statement on aqueous solutions of antiseptics, under Solutions (page 779).

Actions and uses. Phenoxyethanol has an antibacterial action against *Pseudomonas aeruginosa* and to a lesser extent against *Proteus vulgaris* and other Gram-negative organisms. Its action *in vitro* against *Ps. aeruginosa* is unaffected by the presence of 20 per cent of serum.

Phenoxyethanol has been used, as a 2·2 per cent solution or a 2 per cent cream, in the local treatment of *Ps. aeruginosa* infections of superficial wounds, burns, and abscesses. The solution may be applied by irrigation or instillation, or as a wet dressing; it is best prepared by shaking the phenoxyethanol with hot water until dissolved, cooling, and adjusting to volume.

Phenoxyethanol has been used, in conjunction with penicillin, sulphonamides, acridine derivatives, or quaternary ammonium compounds, in the local treatment of mixed infections.

PHENOXYMETHYLPENICILLIN

SYNONYMS: Penicillin V;
Phenoxymethylpenicillinum

$C_{16}H_{18}N_2O_5S = 350·4$

Phenoxymethylpenicillin is 6-phenoxyacetamidopenicillanic acid, an antimicrobial substance produced by the growth of certain strains of *Penicillium notatum* or related organisms on a culture medium containing an appropriate precursor or obtained by any other means.

Solubility. Slightly soluble in water; soluble, at 20°, in 7 parts of alcohol; insoluble in fixed oils and liquid paraffin.

Standard
It complies with the requirements of the European Pharmacopoeia.
It is a white finely crystalline powder and contains not less than 95·0 per cent of total penicillins and not less than 92·0 per cent of phenoxymethylpenicillin, both calculated as $C_{16}H_{18}N_2O_5S$ with reference to the anhydrous substance. It contains not more than 0·5 per cent w/w of water. A 0·5 per cent suspension in water has a pH of 2·4 to 4·0.

Storage. It should be stored in airtight containers.

Actions and uses. Phenoxymethylpenicillin is one of a group of penicillins that are stable in the acid of the stomach; therefore when they are given by mouth less is destroyed before absorption than with benzylpenicillin and the same blood level can be achieved with a smaller dose. In other respects these penicillins do not differ significantly in clinical effect from benzylpenicillin given orally (page 52); minor differences in protein binding, excretion rate, etc. are not of material importance in ordinary use.
Being relatively insoluble, phenoxymethylpenicillin cannot be used parenterally and it should not be used topically.
Because absorption in patients who are acutely ill may be unreliable, phenoxymethylpenicillin should only be used in those who are taking food readily by mouth.

Phenoxymethylpenicillin is administered either as the free acid or as its calcium or potassium salt. Treatment started with an initial dose of benzylpenicillin by injection may be maintained with doses of 250 milligrams of phenoxymethylpenicillin every four to six hours for an adult and proportionately smaller doses for a child. Larger doses may cause diarrhoea.

PRECAUTIONS AND CONTRA-INDICATIONS. Phenoxymethylpenicillin should be used with caution in patients with an allergic diathesis. Its use should be avoided when there is a definite history of penicillin allergy as serious reactions have been reported.

Dose. 0·5 to 1·5 grams daily in divided doses.

Preparations
PHENOXYMETHYLPENICILLIN CAPSULES, B.P. (*Syn.* Penicillin V Capsules). Unless otherwise specified, capsules each containing 250 mg of phenoxymethylpenicillin, or an equivalent quantity of the calcium or potassium salt, are supplied. Capsules containing 125 mg are also available.
PHENOXYMETHYLPENICILLIN MIXTURE, B.P.C. (page 749)
PHENOXYMETHYLPENICILLIN TABLETS, B.P. (*Syn.* Penicillin V Tablets). Unless otherwise specified, tablets each containing 250 mg of phenoxymethylpenicillin, or an equivalent quantity of the calcium or potassium salt, are supplied. They may be film coated. They should be stored in airtight containers, in a cool place. Tablets containing 125 and 300 mg are also available.

OTHER NAME: *Distaquaine V*®

PHENOXYMETHYLPENICILLIN CALCIUM

SYNONYM: Penicillin V Calcium

$(C_{16}H_{17}N_2O_5S)_2Ca,2H_2O = 774\cdot9$

Phenoxymethylpenicillin Calcium is the dihydrate of the calcium salt of phenoxymethyl-penicillin.

Solubility. Slowly soluble, at 20 , in 120 parts of water; insoluble in fixed oils and in liquid paraffin.

Standard
It complies with the requirements of the British Pharmacopoeia.
It is a white finely crystalline powder, which is odourless or has a slight characteristic odour and contains not less than 87·0 per cent of total penicillins and not less than 85·0 per cent of phenoxymethylpenicillin, both calculated as $C_{16}H_{18}N_2O_5S$ with reference to the dried substance. The loss on drying under the prescribed conditions is not more than 1·5 per cent. A 0·5 per cent solution in water has a pH of 5·0 to 7·5.

Storage. It should be stored in airtight containers.

Actions and uses. Phenoxymethylpenicillin calcium has the actions and uses described under Phenoxymethylpenicillin, but when given by mouth in equivalent doses it is absorbed more readily from the gastro-intestinal tract than the free acid and gives somewhat higher blood levels.

PRECAUTIONS AND CONTRA-INDICATIONS. As for Phenoxymethylpenicillin.

Dose. The equivalent of 0·5 to 1·5 grams of phenoxymethylpenicillin daily in divided doses.

Preparations
PHENOXYMETHYLPENICILLIN CAPSULES, B.P. (*Syn.* Penicillin V Capsules). Unless otherwise specified, capsules each containing 250 mg of phenoxymethylpenicillin, or an equivalent quantity of the calcium or potassium salt, are supplied. Capsules containing 125 mg are also available.

PHENOXYMETHYLPENICILLIN MIXTURE, B.P.C. (page 749)

PHENOXYMETHYLPENICILLIN TABLETS, B.P. (*Syn.* Penicillin V Tablets). Unless otherwise specified, tablets each containing 250 mg of phenoxymethylpenicillin, or an equivalent quantity of the calcium or potassium salt, are supplied. They may be film coated. They should be stored in airtight containers, in a cool place. Tablets containing 125 and 300 mg are also available.

OTHER NAMES: *Crystapen V*®; *Penicals*®

PHENOXYMETHYLPENICILLIN POTASSIUM

SYNONYM: Penicillin V Potassium

$C_{16}H_{17}KN_2O_5S = 388\cdot5$

Phenoxymethylpenicillin Potassium is the potassium salt of phenoxymethylpenicillin.

Solubility. Soluble, at 20 , in 1·5 parts of water; insoluble in ether, in fixed oils, and in liquid paraffin.

Standard
It complies with the requirements of the British Pharmacopoeia.
It is a white finely crystalline powder, which is odourless or has a slight characteristic odour and contains not less than 87·0 per cent of total penicillins and not less than 85·0 per cent of phenoxymethylpenicillin, both calculated as $C_{16}H_{18}N_2O_5S$ with reference to the dried substance. The loss on drying under the prescribed conditions is not more than 1·5 per cent. A 0·5 per cent solution in water has a pH of 5·0 to 7·5.

Storage. It should be stored in airtight containers.

Actions and uses. Phenoxymethylpenicillin potassium has the actions and uses described under Phenoxymethylpenicillin, but when given by mouth in equivalent doses it is absorbed more readily from the gastro-intestinal tract than the free acid and gives somewhat higher blood levels.

PRECAUTIONS AND CONTRA-INDICATIONS. As for Phenoxymethylpenicillin.

Dose. The equivalent of 0·5 to 1·5 grams of phenoxymethylpenicillin daily in divided doses.

Preparations
PHENOXYMETHYLPENICILLIN CAPSULES, B.P. (*Syn.* Penicillin V Capsules). Unless otherwise specified, capsules each containing 250 mg of phenoxymethylpenicillin, or an equivalent quantity of the calcium or potassium salt, are supplied. Capsules containing 125 mg are also available.

PHENOXYMETHYLPENICILLIN ELIXIR, B.P.C. (page 675)

PHENOXYMETHYLPENICILLIN MIXTURE, B.P.C. (page 749)

PHENOXYMETHYLPENICILLIN TABLETS, B.P. (*Syn.* Penicillin V Tablets). Unless otherwise specified, tablets each containing 250 mg of phenoxymethyl-penicillin, or an equivalent quantity of the calcium or potassium salt, are supplied. They may be film coated. They should be stored in airtight containers, in a cool place. Tablets containing 125 and 300 mg are also available.

OTHER NAMES: *CVK*®; *Crystapen V*®; *Distaquaine V-K*®; *Econopen V*®; *Icipen*®; *Ospeneff*®; *Penoxyl VK*®; *Stabillin V-K*®; *V-Cil-K*®

PHENSUXIMIDE

$C_{11}H_{11}NO_2 = 189.2$

Phensuximide is N-methyl-α-phenylsuccinimide.

Solubility. Soluble, at $20°$, in 250 parts of water, in 20 parts of alcohol, and in 35 parts of ether.

Standard

DESCRIPTION. A white crystalline powder; odourless or almost odourless.

IDENTIFICATION TESTS. 1. Heat 0.1 g with 5 ml of *sodium hydroxide solution*; the odour of methylamine slowly develops.

2. The ultraviolet absorption spectrum exhibits the characteristics given in Appendix 3, page 856.

3. The infra-red absorption spectrum exhibits maxima which are only at the same wavelengths as, and have similar relative intensities to, those in the spectrum of *phensuximide A.S.*

ACIDITY. Dissolve 5 g in 100 ml of *alcohol (95 per cent)*, previously neutralised to *phenolphthalein solution*, and titrate with $0.1N$ sodium hydroxide, using *phenolphthalein solution* as indicator; not more than 1.5 ml is required.

MELTING-POINT. $69°$ to $72°$.

CYANIDE. To 1.0 g add 1 ml of $0.1N$ sodium hydroxide, warm on a water-bath for 2 minutes, cool, add 1 ml of $1N$ hydrochloric acid, 25 ml of water, and 1 ml of *bromine solution*, and allow to stand for 2 minutes; add 2 ml of *arsenic trioxide solution*, remove the bromine vapour with a current of air, add 10 ml of *barbituric acid and pyridine solution*, warm on a water-bath at $40°$ for 45 minutes, cool, and dilute to 50 ml with water. The extinction of a 1-cm layer of this solution at the maximum at about 586 nm is not more than 0.55.

LOSS ON DRYING. Not more than 0.5 per cent, determined by drying to constant weight at $50°$ over *phosphorus pentoxide* in vacuo.

SULPHATED ASH. Not more than 0.1 per cent.

CONTENT OF $C_{11}H_{11}NO_2$. Not less than 99.0 per cent, calculated with reference to the substance dried under the prescribed conditions, determined by the following method:
To about 0.6 g, accurately weighed, add 30 ml of a 50 per cent w/v solution of *sodium hydroxide* in water, boil for $1\frac{1}{2}$ hours under a reflux condenser, allowing any vapours issuing from the top of the condenser to pass through a distillation apparatus and into 50 ml of $0.1N$ hydrochloric acid. Carefully add 50 ml of

water through the top of the reflux condenser, re-attach the distillation apparatus, turn off the water flowing through the reflux condenser, and distil until crystals appear in the distillation flask, collecting the distillate in the same 50 ml of $0.1N$ hydrochloric acid. Carefully add two further quantities, each of 50 ml, of water, distilling as before after each addition, and titrate the combined distillates with $0.1N$ sodium hydroxide, using *methyl red solution* as indicator.
Repeat the procedure omitting the sample.
The difference between the two titrations represents the amount of acid required to neutralise the ammonia formed; each ml of $0.1N$ hydrochloric acid is equivalent to 0.01892 g of $C_{11}H_{11}NO_2$.

Actions and uses. Phensuximide is an anticonvulsant used in the treatment of petit mal. In the majority of cases it reduces the severity, frequency, and duration of the attacks, even if complete control cannot be obtained.

The usual dosage for an adult is 1 to 3 grams daily in divided doses, but the initial dosage should not exceed 1 gram daily. For a child up to 5 years, the usual initial dosage is 250 milligrams daily; the subsequent dosage is increased by 250 milligrams at intervals of two to three weeks to 1.5 grams daily. For a child of six to twelve years, the usual initial dosage is 500 milligrams daily; the subsequent dosage is increased by 500 milligrams at intervals of two to three weeks to 3 grams daily.

UNDESIRABLE EFFECTS. Drowsiness, nausea, and dizziness may occur, but they are usually transient. Blood dyscrasias and renal damage may rarely occur.

PRECAUTIONS. It is advisable that blood counts and examination of the urine should be carried out periodically.

Dose. See above under **Actions and uses.**

Preparation
PHENSUXIMIDE CAPSULES, B.P.C. (page 653)

OTHER NAME: *Milontin®*

PHENTOLAMINE MESYLATE

$C_{18}H_{23}N_3O_4S = 377.5$

Phentolamine Mesylate is 2-(N-m-hydroxyphenyl-p-toluidinomethyl)imidazoline methanesulphonate.

Solubility. Soluble, at $20°$, in 1 part of water, in 5 parts of alcohol, and in 700 parts of chloroform.

Standard
It complies with the requirements of the British Pharmacopoeia.
It is a white, crystalline, slightly hygroscopic, odourless powder and contains not less than 99.0 per cent of $C_{18}H_{23}N_3O_4S$, calculated with reference to the dried substance. The loss on drying under the prescribed conditions is not more than 0.5 per cent. It has a melting-point of $177°$ to $181°$.

Incompatibility. It is incompatible with iron.

Sterilisation. Solutions for injection are sterilised by filtration.

Storage. It should be stored in airtight containers, protected from light.

Actions and uses. Phentolamine antagonises the vasoconstrictor effects of adrenaline and noradrenaline.
It has been used in the diagnosis of phaeochro-

mocytomata, but the test is not considered satisfactory on account of the high incidence of false positives and it has been largely replaced by the direct estimation of circulating and excreted catecholamines. The diagnostic dose for an adult is 5 to 10 milligrams of phentolamine mesylate by intravenous injection; for a child it is 1 milligram. In patients with phaeochromocytomata, the blood pressure immediately falls, by at least 35/25 mm of mercury, into the normal range and remains depressed for several minutes. The maximum effect occurs within two minutes of the injection. The test may be vitiated by the simultaneous administration of other hypotensive agents.

Phentolamine may also be used, pre-operatively and during operations for the removal of phaeochromocytomata, to prevent a paroxysm caused by the anaesthetic or by

handling the tumour. The dose is the same as the diagnostic dose and is given one to two hours before the operation; it may be repeated if necessary during the operation.

UNDESIRABLE EFFECTS. Moderate or light tachycardia may follow intramuscular injection, and intravenous injection may cause tachycardia with angina and, rarely, weakness, vertigo, and flushing.

Dose. 5 to 10 milligrams by intravenous injection.

Preparation
PHENTOLAMINE INJECTION, B.P. It consists of a sterile solution of phentolamine mesylate in Water for Injections containing anhydrous dextrose and sodium metabisulphite. Unless otherwise specified, a solution containing 10 mg in 1 ml is supplied. It should be stored protected from light, in an atmosphere of nitrogen or other suitable gas.

OTHER NAMES: Phentolamine Methanesulphonate; *Rogitine*®

PHENYLBUTAZONE

SYNONYM: Phenylbutazonum

$C_{19}H_{20}N_2O_2 = 308.4$

Phenylbutazone is 4-butyl-1,2-diphenylpyrazolidine-3,5-dione.

Solubility. Very slightly soluble in water; soluble, at 20°, in 28 parts of alcohol, in 15 parts of ether, and in 1.25 parts of chloroform; soluble in solutions of alkali hydroxides.

Standard
It complies with the requirements of the European Pharmacopoeia.
It is a white or almost white, crystalline, almost odourless powder and contains not less than 99.0 and not more than the equivalent of 101.0 per cent of $C_{19}H_{20}N_2O_2$, calculated with reference to the dried substance. The loss on drying under the prescribed conditions is not more than 0.2 per cent. It has a melting-point of 104° to 107°.

Stability of solutions. Aqueous solutions prepared by dissolving phenylbutazone in water with the addition of alkali hydroxide are slowly hydrolysed and oxidised by atmospheric oxygen.

Actions and uses. Phenylbutazone is a non-steroidal anti-inflammatory agent that is more potent than aspirin. It exhibits uricosuric and sodium-retaining effects and it blocks iodine uptake by the thyroid and a variety of other intracellular enzymatic processes including mucopolysaccharide production. It is metabolised and excreted slowly and its therapeutic effect is therefore prolonged. It is used mainly to relieve symptoms of rheumatic disorders and acute thrombophlebitis.

Phenylbutazone is given by mouth with meals in a dosage of 200 to 400 or, rarely, 600 milligrams daily in divided doses. When prolonged administration is necessary it is advisable, because of the increased incidence of undesirable effects at higher dosage levels, to keep the dosage below 400 milligrams daily.

Phenylbutazone may also be administered by rectum in suppositories in a dosage of 250 milligrams once or twice daily.

UNDESIRABLE EFFECTS. Toxic effects occur frequently, even when the dosage does not exceed 400 milligrams daily, and may include oedema, rashes, gastric upset, and mucosal ulceration of the mouth, oesophagus, stomach, or duodenum, with haematemesis and melaena.
Granulocytopenia is common and is an indication to withdraw the drug as otherwise the condition may become irreversible.

PRECAUTIONS. Because of its salt-retaining and antidiuretic action, patients with mild cardiac congestive failure may be precipitated into complete decompensation; it is therefore advisable to restrict salt in the diet of such patients.
Changes in the leucocyte count may be delayed for several days after the onset of febrile symptoms; frequent counts are therefore no safeguard against the development of agranulocytosis and the patient should be advised by his medical practitioner to discontinue the drug and report to him at the first sign of any of the toxic effects noted above. These toxic effects may occur with regular daily therapy or on resuming the drug after a lapse of two weeks or more, which suggests a sensitisation effect.
In many patients, toxic effects occur within a few days of starting treatment and phenyl-

butazone should not be used, particularly in rheumatoid arthritis, without close day-to-day observation.

The use of phenylbutazone in conjunction with anticoagulants of the coumarin type should be avoided as it may displace them from protein binding sites with a consequent risk of haemorrhage.

Dose. See above under **Actions and uses.**

Preparations

PHENYLBUTAZONE SUPPOSITORIES, B.P. Unless otherwise specified, suppositories each containing 250 mg are supplied.

PHENYLBUTAZONE TABLETS, B.P. Unless otherwise specified, tablets each containing 100 mg of phenylbutazone are supplied. They are sugar coated or film coated. Tablets containing 200 mg are also available.

OTHER NAME: *Butazolidin®*

PHENYLEPHRINE HYDROCHLORIDE

$C_9H_{14}ClNO_2 = 203\cdot7$

Phenylephrine Hydrochloride is $(-)$-1-*m*-hydroxyphenyl-2-methylaminoethanol hydrochloride.

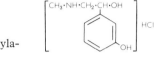

Solubility. Soluble, at 20°, in 2 parts of water, in 4 parts of alcohol, and in 2 parts of glycerol; insoluble in fixed oils.

Standard

It complies with the requirements of the British Pharmacopoeia.

It is a white or almost white, odourless, crystalline powder and contains not less than 98·5 and not more than the equivalent of 101·0 per cent of $C_9H_{14}ClNO_2$, calculated with reference to the dried substance. The loss on drying under the prescribed conditions is not more than 1·0 per cent. It has a melting-point of 141° to 144°.

Sterilisation. Solutions for injection are sterilised by filtration.

Storage. It should be stored in airtight containers, protected from light.

Actions and uses. Phenylephrine is a sympathomimetic drug which has actions similar to those described under Noradrenaline Acid Tartrate (page 327) but it has weaker pressor activity and a longer duration of action than noradrenaline and lacks the cardiac and central adverse effects of adrenaline. After injection it produces peripheral vasoconstriction and increased arterial pressure; it also causes reflex bradycardia.

Phenylephrine is probably the safest vasoconstrictor to use with cyclopropane and other anaesthetics liable to cause cardiac irregularities, and is used to combat hypotension during spinal anaesthesia. It is also a satisfactory vasoconstrictor for use with local anaesthetics. The initial dose is 5 milligrams of phenylephrine hydrochloride by subcutaneous or intramuscular injection, followed by supplementary doses of 1 to 10 milligrams if necessary. Alternatively, 5 to 20 milligrams may be given in 500 millilitres of Sodium Chloride Injection or Dextrose Injection by slow intravenous infusion.

In the treatment of peripheral vascular collapse, 500 micrograms may be given slowly by intravenous injection as a 0·02 per cent solution, or 5 milligrams by intramuscular injection.

Solutions containing 0·25 to 0·5 per cent of phenylephrine hydrochloride may be applied locally as vasoconstrictors in nasal congestion. For use in ophthalmology as a mydriatic and vasoconstrictor, solutions containing 0·5 to 2 per cent are employed. Stronger solutions may be used, but are liable to cause irritation, although this can be prevented by the addition of a local anaesthetic.

Phenylephrine hydrochloride is occasionally used as an inhalation in bronchial asthma, in conjunction with a bronchodilator such as isoprenaline sulphate.

PRECAUTIONS. Phenylephrine should not be given to patients who are being treated with a monoamine-oxidase inhibitor, such as isocarboxazid, nialamide, phenelzine, or tranylcypromine, or within about ten days of the discontinuation of such treatment.

Dose. See above under **Actions and uses.**

Preparations

PHENYLEPHRINE EYE-DROPS, B.P.C. (page 693)

PHENYLEPHRINE INJECTION, B.P. It consists of a sterile solution of phenylephrine hydrochloride in Water for Injections. Unless otherwise specified, a solution containing 10 mg in 1 ml is supplied. When intended for intravenous injection, a solution of this strength should be diluted before use. It should be protected from light.

OTHER NAMES: *Fenox®*; *Neophryn®*

PHENYLMERCURIC ACETATE

SYNONYM: Phenylhydrargyri Acetas

$C_6H_5 \cdot Hg \cdot O \cdot CO \cdot CH_3$

$C_8H_8HgO_2 = 336 \cdot 7$

Phenylmercuric Acetate may be prepared by boiling together benzene and a solution of mercuric acetate in glacial acetic acid and recrystallising the product from alcohol.

Solubility. Soluble, at 20°, in 600 parts of water, in 24 parts of alcohol, and in 19 parts of acetone.

Standard

DESCRIPTION. A white or creamy-white crystalline powder or small white prisms or leaflets; odourless or almost odourless.

IDENTIFICATION TESTS. 1. To 5 ml of a saturated solution in water add 0·2 ml of *sodium sulphide solution*; a white precipitate is formed which turns black on boiling the mixture and allowing it to stand.

2. To 0·1 g add 0·5 ml of *nitric acid*, warm gently until a dark brown colour is produced, and dilute with 10 ml of water; the odour of nitrobenzene is produced.

3. To 0·1 g add 0·5 ml of *sulphuric acid* and 1 ml of *alcohol (95 per cent)* and warm; the odour of ethyl acetate is produced.

MELTING-POINT. 149° to 153°.

MERCURIC SALTS AND HEAVY METALS. Shake 1·0 g with a mixture of 10 ml of *dilute hydrochloric acid* and 40 ml of water for 5 minutes and filter, rejecting the first 10 ml of the filtrate; to 25 ml of the clear filtrate add 5 ml of *alcohol (95 per cent)* and pass *hydrogen sulphide* through the solution.
Any colour that develops is not deeper than that produced by passing *hydrogen sulphide* through a mixture of 25 ml of a 0·002 per cent w/v solution of *mercuric chloride* in water and 5 ml of *alcohol (95 per cent)* (0·1 per cent calculated as $HgCl_2$).

POLYMERCURATED BENZENE COMPOUNDS. Not more than 1·5 per cent, determined by the following method: Shake about 2 g, accurately weighed, with 100 ml of *toluene* at 20°, filter, and wash the residue with succes-

sive portions of *toluene*, using a total of 50 ml; dry the residue at 105° for one hour and weigh.

SULPHATED ASH. Not more than 0·2 per cent.

CONTENT OF $C_8H_8HgO_2$. Not less than 98·0 per cent determined by the following method:
Boil about 0·3 g, accurately weighed, with 5 ml of an 85 per cent w/v solution of *formic acid* in water, 15 ml of water, and 1 g of *zinc powder* under a reflux condenser for half an hour; wash the condenser with 10 ml of water and filter the combined solution and washings, retaining as much as possible of the precipitate in the flask, and washing with water until the washings are neutral to *litmus paper*.
Re-attach the condenser to the flask, add 20 ml of *nitric acid* and 10 ml of water, boil for 10 minutes, wash the condenser with 10 ml of water, cool the flask, and use the solution in the flask to dissolve the precipitate retained on the filter; heat the solution on a water-bath for 3 minutes, add 0·5 g of *urea*, and sufficient 0·1N potassium permanganate to produce a permanent pink colour, cool, add sufficient *hydrogen peroxide solution* to decolorise the solution, and titrate with 0·1N ammonium thiocyanate, using *ferric ammonium sulphate solution* as indicator; each ml of 0·1N ammonium thiocyanate is equivalent to 0·01684 g of $C_8H_8HgO_2$.

Storage. It should be protected from light.

Preparation and storage of solutions. See statement on aqueous solutions of antiseptics, under Solutions (page 779).

Actions and uses. Phenylmercuric acetate has antibacterial, antifungal, and spermicidal properties similar to those described under Phenylmercuric Nitrate.

PHENYLMERCURIC NITRATE

SYNONYM: Phenylhydrargyri Nitras

$C_6H_5 \cdot Hg \cdot OH, C_6H_5 \cdot Hg \cdot NO_3$

$C_{12}H_{11}Hg_2NO_4 = 634 \cdot 4$

Phenylmercuric Nitrate is a basic phenylmercuric nitrate.

Solubility. Soluble, at 20°, in 1500 parts of water and in 1000 parts of alcohol; more soluble in glycerol and in fixed oils; soluble in 160 parts of boiling water.

Standard

It complies with the requirements of the British Pharmacopoeia.
It occurs as white, odourless, lustrous plates or crystalline powder and contains not less than 98·0 and not more than the equivalent of 102·0 per cent of $C_{12}H_{11}Hg_2NO_4$, calculated with reference to the dried substance. The loss on drying under the prescribed conditions is not more than 1·0 per cent. It melts with decomposition at about 188°. A 0·02 per cent solution in water is neutral to bromocresol green.

Incompatibility. It is incompatible with chlorides, bromides, and iodides, with which it forms the less soluble halogen compounds.

Storage. It should be protected from light.

Preparation and storage of solutions. See statement on aqueous solutions of antiseptics, under Solutions (page 779).

Actions and uses. Phenylmercuric nitrate has antibacterial and antifungal properties. It is used as a bactericide in a concentration of 0·001 per cent in preparations for parenteral administration and in a concentration of 0·002 per cent in some eye-drops, but its inclusion in eye-drops intended for use over long periods is not recommended.
Phenylmercuric nitrate may be used in the process of sterilisation by heating with a bactericide, in which a solution or suspension of the medicament in a 0·002 per cent solution of phenylmercuric nitrate in Water for Injections is heated in the final sealed containers at 98° to 100° for 30 minutes. It should not be used in solutions intended for intrathecal, intracisternal, or peridural injection, or in solutions intended for intra-

venous injection where the dose exceeds 15 millilitres.

Preparations of phenylmercuric nitrate are used as chemical contraceptives. The spermicidal activity is much reduced in vaginal secretions of pH greater than 7·2.

PHENYLPROPANOLAMINE HYDROCHLORIDE

$C_9H_{14}ClNO = 187·7$ $C_6H_5 \cdot CH(OH) \cdot CH(NH_2) \cdot CH_3, HCl$

Phenylpropanolamine Hydrochloride is the hydrochloride of ($\pm$)-2-amino-1-phenylpropan-1-ol.

Solubility. Soluble, at 20°, in 2·5 parts of water and in 9 parts of alcohol; insoluble in ether and in chloroform.

Standard
It complies with the requirements of the British Pharmacopoeia.
It is a white to creamy-white, crystalline, odourless or almost odourless powder and contains not less than 99·0 and not more than the equivalent of 102·0 per cent of $C_9H_{14}ClNO$, calculated with reference to the dried substance. The loss on drying under the prescribed conditions is not more than 0·5 per cent. It has a melting-point of 193° to 196°. A 3 per cent solution in water has a pH of 4·5 to 6·0.

Sterilisation. Solutions are sterilised by heating in an autoclave or by filtration.

Actions and uses. Phenylpropanolamine is a sympathomimetic amine with actions similar to those of ephedrine (page 178) but it is somewhat more active as a vasoconstrictor and less active as a central stimulant and bronchodilator.

Phenylpropanolamine hydrochloride is given by mouth in doses of 25 to 50 milligrams for the symptomatic treatment of allergic conditions such as bronchial asthma or hay fever. It is applied as a 1 to 3 per cent solution or jelly for the relief of nasal congestion.

PRECAUTIONS AND CONTRA-INDICATIONS. Phenylpropanolamine should be given with caution to hypertensive patients.
It should not be given to patients who are being treated with a monoamine-oxidase inhibitor, such as isocarboxazid, nialamide, phenelzine, or tranylcypromine, or within about ten days of the discontinuation of such treatment.

Dose. 25 to 50 milligrams.

PHENYTOIN

$C_{15}H_{12}N_2O_2 = 252·3$

Phenytoin is 5,5-diphenylhydantoin.

Solubility. Very slightly soluble in water; soluble, at 20°, in 70 parts of alcohol, in 600 parts of ether, and in 500 parts of chloroform; soluble in solutions of alkali hydroxides.

Standard
DESCRIPTION. A white or almost white crystalline powder; odourless or almost odourless.
IDENTIFICATION TESTS. 1. Dissolve 0·1 g in a mixture of 0·5 ml of 1N sodium hydroxide and 2 ml of a 10 per cent w/v solution of *pyridine* in water, add a further 8 ml of the pyridine solution, shake, add 1 ml of *copper sulphate with pyridine solution*, and allow to stand for 10 minutes; a blue precipitate is produced.
2. The infra-red absorption spectrum exhibits maxima which are only at the same wavelengths as, and have similar relative intensities to, those in the spectrum of *phenytoin A.S.*
SOLUBILITY IN SODIUM HYDROXIDE. A solution prepared by dissolving 1 g in a mixture of 5 ml of 1N sodium hydroxide and 20 ml of water is clear and not darker than pale yellow.
BENZILIC ACID. Dissolve 0·1 g in 5 ml of *sulphuric acid*; a yellow colour is produced. If a red colour is produced it is less intense than that produced when 100 µg of *benzilic acid* is dissolved in 5 ml of *sulphuric acid*.

LOSS ON DRYING. Not more than 0·5 per cent, determined by drying to constant weight at 105°.
SULPHATED ASH. Not more than 0·1 per cent.
CONTENT OF $C_{15}H_{12}N_2O_2$. Not less than 99·0 and not more than the equivalent of 101·0 per cent, calculated with reference to the substance dried under the prescribed conditions, determined by the following method:
Dissolve about 0·5 g, accurately weighed, in 25 ml of *dimethylformamide* and titrate with 0·1N sodium methoxide, using *quinaldine red solution* as indicator.
Repeat the procedure omitting the sample.
The difference between the two titrations represents the amount of sodium methoxide required by the sample; each ml of 0·1N sodium methoxide is equivalent to 0·02523 g of $C_{15}H_{12}N_2O_2$.

Actions and uses. Phenytoin has the actions, uses, and undesirable effects described under Phenytoin Sodium; 0·9 gram of phenytoin is approximately equivalent to 1 gram of phenytoin sodium.

Preparation
PHENYTOIN MIXTURE, B.P.C. (page 750)

OTHER NAME: Diphenylhydantoin; *Epanutin*®

PHENYTOIN SODIUM

SYNONYM: Soluble Phenytoin

$C_{15}H_{11}N_2NaO_2 = 274.3$

Phenytoin Sodium is the sodium derivative of 5,5-diphenylhydantoin.

Solubility. Soluble in water and in alcohol; insoluble in ether and in chloroform; solutions in water are sometimes turbid owing to partial hydrolysis.

Standard
It complies with the requirements of the British Pharmacopoeia.
It is a white, somewhat hygroscopic, odourless powder and contains not less than 98·5 and not more than the equivalent of 101·0 per cent of $C_{15}H_{11}N_2NaO_2$, calculated with reference to the dried substance. The loss on drying under the prescribed conditions is not more than 3·0 per cent.

Stability. It absorbs carbon dioxide from the atmosphere with liberation of diphenylhydantoin.

Sterilisation. Solutions are sterilised by heating in an autoclave or by filtration.

Storage. It should be stored in airtight containers.

Actions and uses. Phenytoin has an anticonvulsant action but relatively little hypnotic effect. It is used in the treatment of epilepsy and for this purpose has the advantage over phenobarbitone of being less likely to produce drowsiness and mental dullness. It is frequently effective in conjunction with phenobarbitone in patients in whom phenobarbitone alone causes too much depression. In changing from phenobarbitone or other sedatives to phenytoin, the transition should be made gradually with some overlapping of the use of the two drugs; too rapid withdrawal of phenobarbitone may lead to an increase in the frequency of seizures. Phenytoin is more effective in controlling seizures of the grand mal type than of the petit mal type.
The dosage for an adult is 50 to 100 milligrams of phenytoin sodium by mouth three times a day, increased if necessary to a maximum of 200 milligrams three times a day. A child over six years of age may be given 100 milligrams three or four times a day; younger children may be given 30 to 60 milligrams of phenytoin sodium three times a day.

Because phenytoin sodium is strongly alkaline, it may irritate the gastric mucosa; this may be avoided by giving the dose with a copious draught of water after meals, although it is more effective if given before meals.
Phenytoin sodium may be given by intramuscular or intravenous injection at a rate not exceeding 50 milligrams per minute.
It is administered by slow intravenous infusion in the treatment of cardiac arrhythmias, the usual dose being 5 milligrams per kilogram body-weight.

UNDESIRABLE EFFECTS. Minor toxic effects such as dizziness, nausea, and rashes occur frequently, but may usually be overcome by reducing the dosage for a few days, after which they do not usually return on increasing the dosage to the original amount. Tenderness and hyperplasia of the gums may also occur. Other toxic symptoms sometimes observed are fever, ataxia, diplopia, muscular tremors, hallucinations, and mental confusion. Leucopenia, exfoliative dermatitis, and purpura are more serious reactions which may be severe enough to necessitate the withdrawal of the drug.
Phenytoin lowers the plasma folate concentration and may induce megaloblastic anaemia. Hirsutism may also occur.

Dose. See above under **Actions and uses.**

Preparations
PHENYTOIN CAPSULES, B.P.C. (page 653)
PHENYTOIN INJECTION, B.P.C. (page 716)
PHENYTOIN TABLETS, B.P. (*Syn.* Phenytoin Sodium Tablets; Soluble Phenytoin Tablets). Unless otherwise specified, tablets each containing 100 mg of phenytoin sodium are supplied. They are sugar coated. Tablets containing 30 mg and 50 mg are also available.

OTHER NAMES: Diphenylhydantoin Sodium; *Epanutin*®; *Epiphen*®

PHOLCODINE

$C_{23}H_{30}N_2O_4,H_2O = 416.5$

Pholcodine is the monohydrate of the 3-(2-morpholinoethyl) ether of morphine.

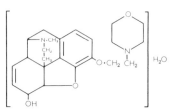

Solubility. Soluble, at 20°, in 50 parts of water and in 3 parts of dehydrated alcohol; slightly soluble in ether; very soluble in chloroform and in acetone; soluble in dilute hydrochloric acid.

Standard
It complies with the requirements of the British Pharmacopoeia.
It is a white or almost white, crystalline, odourless

powder and contains not less than 98·0 and not more than the equivalent of 101·0 per cent of $C_{23}H_{30}N_2O_4$, calculated with reference to the dried substance. The loss on drying under the prescribed conditions is 3·9 to 4·5 per cent. It has a melting-point of about 99°, after sintering at about 95°.

Storage. It should be stored in airtight containers.

Actions and uses. Pholcodine resembles codeine in suppressing cough and is used for the relief of unproductive cough. It has less depressant effect on the respiratory centre than morphine and does not cause constipation.

Dose. Up to 60 milligrams daily in divided doses.

Preparations
PHOLCODINE LINCTUS, B.P.C. (page 724)
PHOLCODINE LINCTUS, STRONG, B.P.C. (page 724)

PHOSPHORIC ACID

SYNONYMS: Acidum Phosphoricum Concentratum; Concentrated Phosphoric Acid

$H_3PO_4 = 98·0$

Phosphoric Acid is orthophosphoric acid.

When phosphoric acid is heated, it loses water and is converted finally into metaphosphoric acid, HPO_3, which on cooling forms a transparent glassy mass.

Solubility. Miscible with water and with alcohol.

Standard
It complies with the requirements of the European Pharmacopoeia.
It is a clear, colourless, corrosive, syrupy, odourless liquid and contains 85·0 to 90·0 per cent w/w of H_3PO_4. It may solidify at low temperatures, forming colourless crystals which do not melt until the temperature reaches 28°. It has a weight per ml at 20° of about 1·7 g.

Storage. It should be stored in glass containers.

Actions and uses. Dilute phosphoric acid is occasionally prescribed in mixtures containing vegetable bitters to stimulate appetite.

PHTHALYLSULPHATHIAZOLE

$C_{17}H_{13}N_3O_5S_2 = 403·4$

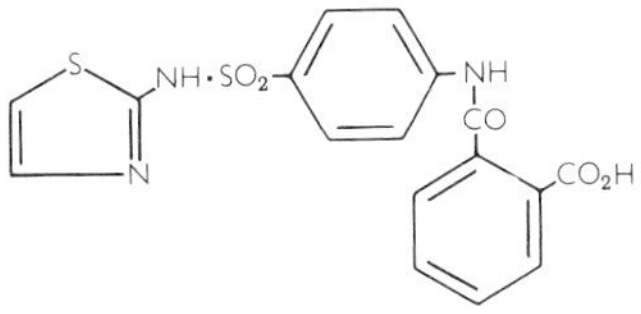

Phthalylsulphathiazole is 4'-[N-(thiazol-2-yl)sulphamoyl]-phthalanilic acid.

Solubility. Very slightly soluble in water and in chloroform; soluble, at 20°, in 600 parts of alcohol; readily soluble in aqueous solutions of alkali hydroxides and carbonates and in hydrochloric acid.

Standard
It complies with the requirements of the British Pharmacopoeia.
It occurs as odourless or almost odourless white or yellowish-white crystals or powder and contains not less than 98·5 and not more than the equivalent of 102·5 per cent of $C_{17}H_{13}N_3O_5S_2$, calculated with reference to the dried substance. The loss on drying under the prescribed conditions is not more than 2·0 per cent.

Storage. It should be protected from light.

Actions and uses. Phthalylsulphathiazole is a relatively insoluble compound which is only slowly broken down in the gastro-intestinal tract so that when it is given by mouth the bulk of the dose reaches the large intestine and is excreted in the faeces. A proportion of the dose is absorbed as sulphathiazole and in certain conditions, particularly where there is extensive ulceration of the intestinal mucosa, sufficient can be absorbed to cause systemic effects and renal tubular obstruction.
Phthalylsulphathiazole has the antibacterial actions of the sulphonamides, as described under Sulphadimidine (page 478), and is still sometimes used to treat bacterial dysentery and to reduce the incidence of postoperative infection after large bowel surgery.

Dose. 5 to 10 grams daily in divided doses.

Preparation
PHTHALYLSULPHATHIAZOLE TABLETS, B.P. Unless otherwise specified, tablets each containing 500 mg of phthalylsulphathiazole are supplied. They should be protected from light.

OTHER NAME: *Thalazole®*

PHYSOSTIGMINE

SYNONYM: Eserine

$C_{15}H_{21}N_3O_2 = 275\cdot3$

Physostigmine is an alkaloid obtained from the calabar bean,
the seed of *Physostigma venenosum* Balfour (Fam. Leguminosae), a woody climbing plant indi
genous to the west coast of Africa.

Solubility. Soluble, at 20°, in 75 parts of water, in 10 parts of alcohol, in 30 parts of ether, and in 1 part of chloroform; soluble, on warming, in 100 parts of castor oil.

Standard
DESCRIPTION. Colourless or almost colourless crystals; odourless or almost odourless. It becomes pink on exposure to light and air.

IDENTIFICATION TESTS. 1. Warm 5 mg with 0·3 ml of *dilute ammonia solution*; a yellowish-red solution is produced. Evaporate the solution; a bluish residue remains which complies with the following tests:
(i) it is soluble in *alcohol (95 per cent)*, producing a blue solution which, on the addition of *acetic acid*, appears blue by transmitted light and shows a red fluorescence which is intensified by dilution with water;
(ii) it is soluble in *sulphuric acid*, producing a green solution which, on the gradual addition of *alcohol (95 per cent)*, changes to red but reverts to green when the alcohol is evaporated.
2. Dissolve 0·1 g in 2 ml of *alcohol (95 per cent)*, add 10 ml of *trinitrophenol solution*, and cool in ice; a precipitate is formed which, after recrystallising from water and drying, melts at about 114°.
3. It melts at about 106°.

SPECIFIC ROTATION. $-76°$ to $-80°$, determined, at 20°, in a 2·0 per cent w/v solution in *chloroform*.

SULPHATED ASH. Not more than 0·1 per cent.

CONTENT OF $C_{15}H_{21}N_3O_2$. Not less than 97·0 and no more than the equivalent of 102·0 per cent, determined by the following method:
Dissolve about 0·17 g, accurately weighed, in 25 ml of *chloroform* and 25 ml of *glacial acetic acid* and titrate the solution by Method I of the British Pharmacopoeia for non-aqueous titration, using 0·02N perchloric acid in dioxan as the titrant and determining the end-point potentiometrically; each ml of 0·02N perchloric acid in dioxan is equivalent to 0·005507 g of $C_{15}H_{21}N_3O_2$.

Sterilisation. Sterile oily solutions are prepared by an aseptic technique.

Storage. It should be stored in airtight containers protected from light.

Actions and uses. Physostigmine has the actions described under Physostigmine Sali
cylate. It has been used for the preparation of eye-drops containing up to 1 per cent w/v in sterile castor oil.

PHYSOSTIGMINE SALICYLATE

SYNONYMS: Eserine Salicylate; Eserinii Salicylas; Physostig. Sal.; Physostigminii Salicylas

$C_{15}H_{21}N_3O_2,C_7H_6O_3 = 413\cdot5$

Solubility. Soluble, at 20°, in 90 parts of water and in 25 parts of alcohol.

Standard
It complies with the requirements of the European Pharmacopoeia.
It occurs as colourless or faintly yellow odourless crystals and contains not less than 98·5 per cent of $C_{15}H_{21}N_3O_2,C_7H_6O_3$, calculated with reference to the dried substance. The loss on drying under the prescribed conditions is not more than 1·0 per cent. It has a melting-point of 184° to 187°. A solution in water is acid to methyl red and alkaline to bromophenol blue.

Stability. The salt and its aqueous solution become red on exposure to light and air, owing to formation of rubreserine; the change is less rapid in faintly acid solution.

Sterilisation. Solutions are sterilised by heating with a bactericide or by filtration. The pH of the solution should be kept below 4 and an antioxidant should be included.

Storage. It should be stored in airtight containers, protected from light. Solutions should be freshly prepared or, if kept, should be stored in hermetically sealed containers.

Actions and uses. Physostigmine inhibits cholinesterase activity and prevents the rapid destruction of acetylcholine, thereby enhancing its action. It increases salivary, gastric, and bronchial secretions and intestinal move
ments, slows the heart, and dilates peripheral blood vessels; these effects are antagonised by atropine. When applied to the eye, physostig
mine constricts the pupil, reduces intra
ocular pressure if this is raised, and contracts the ciliary muscles. It may cause nausea, vomiting, and diarrhoea. With large doses muscular twitchings followed by muscular weakness and respiratory paralysis may occur. Physostigmine salicylate is used chiefly as a miotic. The pupils begin to constrict within ten minutes of its application and its effect lasts for about twelve hours. It is also used to counteract the dilatation of the pupil caused by atropine, homatropine, or cocaine; in these circumstances it may, however, produce considerable irritation and pain due to spasm. Physostigmine salicylate is also used to decrease intra-ocular pressure in glaucoma.

POISONING. The stomach should be washed out with a 0·2 per cent solution of potassium permanganate. A short-acting barbiturate should be given, if necessary by intravenous injection, to control muscular twitching, and atropine may be given to relieve the muscarinic actions.

PHYSOSTIGMINE SULPHATE

SYNONYMS: Eserine Sulphate; Physostig. Sulph.

$(C_{15}H_{21}N_3O_2)_2,H_2SO_4 = 648\cdot8$

Solubility. Soluble, at 20°, in less than 1 part of water and of alcohol; slightly soluble in ether.

Standard

DESCRIPTION. A white, microcrystalline, deliquescent powder; odourless or almost odourless.

IDENTIFICATION TESTS. 1. Dissolve 0·05 g in 5 ml of water and add 1N sodium hydroxide, dropwise; a white precipitate is produced which dissolves in excess of the reagent to give a red solution.

2. It complies with test 1 given under Physostigmine, page 380.

3. It gives the reactions characteristic of sulphates.

ACIDITY OR ALKALINITY. A 1·0 per cent w/v solution in carbon dioxide-free water is neutral to methyl orange solution.

MELTING-POINT. 144° to 148°, determined after drying at 105°.

SPECIFIC ROTATION. −116° to −120°, calculated with reference to the substance dried under the prescribed conditions, determined, at 20°, on a 2·0 per cent w/v solution in water.

LOSS ON DRYING. Not more than 1·0 per cent, determined by drying to constant weight at 105°.

SULPHATED ASH. Not more than 0·1 per cent.

CONTENT OF $(C_{15}H_{21}N_3O_2)_2,H_2SO_4$. Not less than 7·0 and not more than the equivalent of 102·0 per cent, calculated with reference to the substance dried under the prescribed conditions, determined by the following method:

Dissolve about 0·17 g, accurately weighed, in 25 ml of water, make alkaline by the addition of 1 g of sodium bicarbonate, and extract with three successive 25-ml portions of chloroform, filtering each extract through a dry filter paper; combine the extracts, add 25 ml of glacial acetic acid, and continue the determination by Method I of the British Pharmacopoeia for non-aqueous titration, 0·02N perchloric acid being used; each ml of 0·02N perchloric acid is equivalent to 0·006488 g of $(C_{15}H_{21}N_3O_2)_2,H_2SO_4$.

Stability. Physostigmine sulphate and its aqueous solution become red on exposure to light and air, owing to formation of rubreserine; the change is less rapid in acid solution.

Sterilisation. Solutions are sterilised by heating with a bactericide or by filtration.

Storage. It should be stored in airtight containers, protected from light.

Actions and uses. Physostigmine sulphate has the actions and uses described under Physostigmine Salicylate.

As the sulphate is more soluble than the salicylate and is compatible with a wider range of preservatives, it is now preferred for the preparation of eye-drops. Eye-drops containing up to 4 per cent of physostigmine sulphate may be used in the treatment of glaucoma.

Preparations

PHYSOSTIGMINE AND PILOCARPINE EYE-DROPS, B.P.C. (page 693)

PHYSOSTIGMINE EYE-DROPS, B.P.C. (page 693)

PHYTOMENADIONE

SYNONYM: Vitamin K_1

$C_{31}H_{46}O_2 = 450\cdot7$

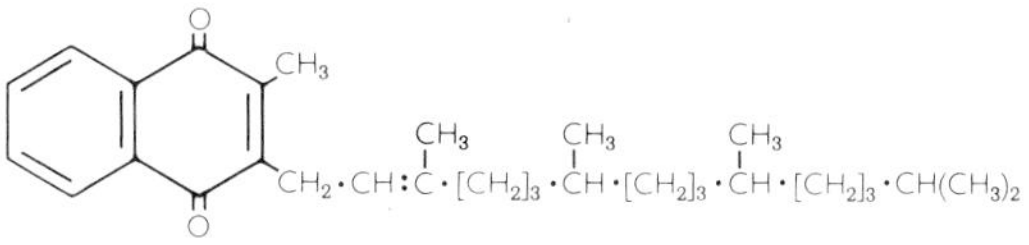

Phytomenadione is 2-methyl-3-phytyl-1,4-naphthaquinone.

Solubility. Insoluble in water; soluble, at 20°, in 70 parts of alcohol; soluble in ether, in chloroform, and in fixed oils.

Standard

It complies with the requirements of the British Pharmacopoeia.

It is a clear, deep yellow, almost odourless oil and contains not less than 97·0 and not more than the equivalent of 102·0 per cent w/w of $C_{31}H_{46}O_2$.

Stability. It decomposes on exposure to sunlight.

Sterilisation. Dispersions for injection are sterilised by heating in an autoclave.

Storage. It should be stored in airtight containers, protected from light.

Actions and uses. Phytomenadione is a naturally occurring vitamin K. It maintains a normal level of prothrombin in the blood plasma.

In hypoprothrombinaemia the intravenous administration of phytomenadione causes a rise in the plasma-prothrombin level within fifteen minutes and a reduction in the clotting-time. It acts more rapidly than the synthetic vitamin-K analogues and its effect is more prolonged.

Phytomenadione is used in the treatment of severe haemorrhage due to a low prothrombin level caused by anticoagulant therapy with phenindione or the coumarin derivatives. It is administered by slow intravenous infusion in doses of 5 to 20 milligrams, usually as a dispersion; the dose may be repeated in a few hours. For less severe hypoprothrombin-aemia, it may be given by mouth, initially in doses of 5 to 10 milligrams and subsequently in doses increased, if necessary, to 15 to 20 milligrams. For haemorrhagic disease of the newborn, 0·5 to 1 milligram is given by intra-muscular or intravenous injection.

UNDESIRABLE EFFECTS. Excessive doses of phytomenadione may produce haemolytic anaemia, hyperbilirubinaemia, and kernicterus in the newborn, particularly in premature infants.

The administration of large doses of phytomenadione in an attempt to correct the hypothrombinaemia associated with severe liver disease may further depress the prothrombin level.

The intravenous administration of phytomenadione injection may produce flushing, sweating, a sense of suffocation, and peripheral vascular failure. Intravenous injections should therefore be given very slowly.

Dose. See above under **Actions and uses.**

Preparations

PHYTOMENADIONE INJECTION, B.P. (*Syn.* Vitamin K Injection). It consists of a sterile dispersion of phyto menadione in Water for Injections. The strength c the dispersion should be specified by the prescriber. **I** deteriorates on exposure to light and should be store in the dark; it should not be allowed to freeze. If o droplets have appeared or separation has occurred, **i** should not be used. Ampoules containing 1 and 10 m are available.

PHYTOMENADIONE TABLETS, B.P. (*Syn.* Vitamin K Tablets). The quantity of phytomenadione in eac tablet should be specified by the prescriber. They ar sugar coated. They should be chewed or allowed t dissolve slowly in the mouth.

OTHER NAME: *Konakion®*; Phytonadione

PILOCARPINE HYDROCHLORIDE

SYNONYM: Pilocarp. Hydrochlor.

$C_{11}H_{17}ClN_2O_2 = 244\cdot7$

Pilocarpine Hydrochloride is the hydrochloride of pilocarpine, an alkaloid obtained from th leaves of *Pilocarpus microphyllus* Stapf (jaborandi) and other species of *Pilocarpus* (Fam Rutaceae).

Solubility. Soluble, at 20°, in less than 1 part of water, in 3 parts of alcohol, and in 360 parts of chloroform; insoluble in ether.

Standard

DESCRIPTION. Colourless crystals or a white crystalline powder; hygroscopic; odourless or almost odourless.

IDENTIFICATION TESTS. 1. Dissolve 10 mg in 5 ml of water, add 0·1 ml of *dilute sulphuric acid*, 1 ml of *hydrogen peroxide solution*, 1 ml of *benzene*, and 0·05 ml of *potassium chromate solution*, shake well, and allow to separate; the benzene layer is coloured bluish-violet and the aqueous layer remains yellow.

2. It gives the reactions characteristic of chlorides.

ACIDITY. pH of a 0·5 per cent w/v solution in *carbon dioxide-free water*, 3·8 to 5·2.

MELTING-POINT. 200° to 205°.

SPECIFIC ROTATION. +89·0° to +93·0°, calculated with reference to the substance dried under the prescribed conditions, determined, at 20°, in a 2·0 per cent w/v solution in water.

NITRATE. Dissolve 0·05 g in 5 ml of water and carefully add the solution to 5 ml of *diphenylamine solution*, ensuring that the liquids do not mix; no blue colour is produced at the liquid interface.

CERTAIN OTHER ALKALOIDS. It complies with the test given in Appendix 5, page 866.

LOSS ON DRYING. Not more than 3·0 per cent, determined by drying for 2 hours at 105°.

SULPHATED ASH. Not more than 0·1 per cent.

CONTENT OF $C_{11}H_{17}ClN_2O_2$. Not less than 99·0 pe cent, calculated with reference to the substance drie under the prescribed conditions, determined by th following method:
Titrate about 0·5 g, accurately weighed, by Method of the British Pharmacopoeia for non-aqueous titration each ml of 0·1N perchloric acid is equivalent t 0·02447 g of $C_{11}H_{17}ClN_2O_2$.

Incompatibility. It is incompatible with chlor hexidine acetate and phenylmercuric salts.

Sterilisation. Solutions are sterilised by heating in a autoclave or by filtration.

Storage. It should be stored in airtight containers protected from light.

Actions and uses. Pilocarpine hydrochlorid has the actions and uses of pilocarpine, a described under Pilocarpine Nitrate. Th hydrochloride is now preferred to the nitrat for the preparation of eye-drops because it i compatible with a more useful range o preservatives.

POISONING. Gastric lavage should be em ployed and atropine given subcutaneously.

Preparations

PHYSOSTIGMINE AND PILOCARPINE EYE-DROPS, B.P.C (page 693)

PILOCARPINE EYE-DROPS, B.P.C. (page 694)

PILOCARPINE NITRATE

SYNONYMS: Pilocarp. Nit.; Pilocarpinii Nitras

$C_{11}H_{16}N_2O_2,HNO_3 = 271\cdot3$

Pilocarpine Nitrate is the nitrate of pilocarpine, an alkaloid obtained from the leaves o *Pilocarpus microphyllus* Stapf (jaborandi) and other species of *Pilocarpus* (Fam. Rutaceae).

Solubility. Soluble, at 20°, in 8 parts of water and in 160 parts of alcohol; very slightly soluble in ether and in chloroform.

Standard

It complies with the requirements of the Europea Pharmacopoeia.

t occurs as odourless colourless crystals or white crystalline powder and contains not less than 99·0 and not more than the equivalent of 101·0 per cent of $C_{11}H_{16}N_2O_2,HNO_3$, calculated with reference to the dried substance. The loss on drying under the prescribed conditions is not more than 0·5 per cent. It melts with decomposition at 174° to 179°. A 5 per cent solution in water is acid to methyl red and alkaline to bromophenol blue.

Incompatibility. It is incompatible with chlorhexidine acetate and solutions containing more than 1 per cent are incompatible with benzalkonium chloride.

Sterilisation. Solutions are sterilised by heating in an autoclave or by filtration.

Storage. It should be protected from light.

Actions and uses. Pilocarpine has the muscarinic actions of acetylcholine, as described under Physostigmine Salicylate (page 380). Like physostigmine, it has been used to constrict the pupil and decrease the intra-ocular pressure in glaucoma and detachment of the retina, but it is only about half as active; for this purpose, a 1 per cent solution may be used.

Its action on the eye is less complete and of shorter duration than that of physostigmine and a slight increase of intra-ocular pressure may occur at first.

It is used to antagonise the effects of atropine on the eye and has been used to counteract some of the common side-effects of ganglion-blocking agents, such as dryness of the mouth, constipation, and impaired vision.

POISONING. Gastric lavage should be employed and atropine given subcutaneously.

PIPERAZINE ADIPATE

$C_4H_{10}N_2,C_6H_{10}O_4 = 232·3$

Solubility. Soluble, at 20°, in 18 parts of water; insoluble in alcohol.

Standard
It complies with the requirements of the British Pharmacopoeia.
It is a white, crystalline, odourless powder and contains not less than 98·5 per cent of $C_4H_{10}N_2,C_6H_{10}O_4$, calculated with reference to the dried substance. The loss on drying under the prescribed conditions is not more than 0·5 per cent. It melts with decomposition at about 250°. A 5 per cent solution in water has a pH of 5·0 to 6·0.

Actions and uses. Piperazine adipate has the actions, uses, and undesirable effects described under Piperazine Hydrate; 120 milligrams of piperazine adipate is approximately equivalent to 100 milligrams of piperazine hydrate.

Dose. See under **Actions and uses** of Piperazine Hydrate.

Preparation
PIPERAZINE ADIPATE TABLETS, B.P. Unless otherwise specified, tablets each containing 300 mg of piperazine adipate are supplied.

OTHER NAME: *Entacyl®*

PIPERAZINE CITRATE

$(C_4H_{10}N_2)_3,2C_6H_8O_7 = 642·7$

Piperazine Citrate is a hydrated piperazine citrate containing a variable amount of water of hydration, corresponding to five or six molecules of water.

Solubility. Soluble, at 20°, in 1·5 parts of water; very slightly soluble in alcohol and in ether.

Standard
It complies with the requirements of the British Pharmacopoeia.
It is a fine, white, granular, almost odourless powder and contains not less than 98·5 per cent of $(C_4H_{10}N_2)_3$, $2C_6H_8O_7$, calculated with reference to the anhydrous substance. It contains 10·0 to 14·0 per cent w/w of water. It has a melting-point, after drying at 105°, of about 190°. A 5 per cent solution in water has a pH of 5·0 to 6·0.

Storage. It should be protected from light.

Actions and uses. Piperazine citrate has the actions, uses, and undesirable effects described under Piperazine Hydrate; 125 milligrams of piperazine citrate is approximately equivalent to 100 milligrams of piperazine hydrate.

Dose. See under **Actions and uses** of Piperazine Hydrate.

Preparation
PIPERAZINE CITRATE ELIXIR, B.P.C. (page 675)

OTHER NAMES: *Antepar®*; *Helmezine®*; *Minox®*

PIPERAZINE HYDRATE

$C_4H_{10}N_2,6H_2O = 194.2$

Piperazine Hydrate is the hexahydrate of piperazine.

Solubility. Soluble, at 20°, in 3 parts of water and in 1 part of alcohol.

Standard

DESCRIPTION. Colourless, glassy, deliquescent crystals; odour faint and characteristic.

IDENTIFICATION TESTS. 1. Dissolve 0·1 g in 5 ml of water, add 0·5 g of *sodium bicarbonate*, 2·5 ml of *potassium ferricyanide solution*, and 0·1 ml of *mercury*, shake vigorously for one minute, and allow to stand for 20 minutes; a reddish colour slowly develops.

2. Dissolve 0·3 g in 5 ml of *alcohol (95 per cent)* and add 3 ml of a 20 per cent w/v solution of *trichloroacetic acid* in *alcohol (95 per cent)*; a precipitate is formed which, after washing with *alcohol (95 per cent)*, recrystallising from *alcohol (95 per cent)*, and drying for 4 hours over *phosphorus pentoxide* in vacuo, melts at about 122°.

3. Dissolve 0·2 g in 3 ml of water, add 2 ml of *sodium hydroxide solution* and 0·5 ml of *benzoyl chloride*, and shake vigorously for 15 minutes, cooling the tube in running water; a precipitate is formed which, after washing with *sodium carbonate solution*, recrystallising from *alcohol (95 per cent)*, and drying for 4 hours over *phosphorus pentoxide* in vacuo, melts at about 190°.

4. A 1 per cent w/v solution in water is alkaline to *litmus paper*.

MELTING-POINT. 43° to 45°.

LEAD. It complies with the test given in Appendix 7, page 883 (10 parts per million).

SULPHATED ASH. Not more than 0·1 per cent.

CONTENT OF $C_4H_{10}N_2,6H_2O$. Not less than 98·0 per cent, determined by the following method:
Dissolve about 0·2 g, accurately weighed, in a mixture of 3·5 ml of 1N sulphuric acid and 10 ml of water, add 100 ml of *trinitrophenol solution*, heat on a water-bath for 15 minutes, allow to stand for 1 hour, and filter through a sintered glass crucible (British Standard Grade No. 4).
Wash the residue with successive 10-ml portions of a mixture of equal volumes of water and a saturated solution of *trinitrophenol* in water until the washings are free from sulphate, continue washing the residue with 5 successive 10-ml portions of *dehydrated alcohol*, and dry the residue to constant weight at 105°; each g of residue is equivalent to 0·3567 g of $C_4H_{10}N_2,6H_2O$.

Storage. It should be stored in airtight containers, protected from light.

Actions and uses. Piperazine is an anthelmintic which is effective against threadworms and roundworms. Roundworms are narcotised and unable to maintain their position in the gut of the host; they are expelled with the stools. Narcosis of roundworms takes at least five hours to develop; worms at all stages of maturity in the gut are affected, but larval forms in the tissues are not. The fact that piperazine does not stimulate the worms to muscular activity makes it the safest drug available for the treatment of heavy infections.

Little is known about the mode of action of piperazine on threadworms. It has no significant action upon hookworms, whipworms, or tapeworms.

For the treatment of threadworm infections in an adult and in a child aged over twelve years, a daily dose equivalent to 2 grams of piperazine hydrate is given by mouth for one week. For a child aged from seven to twelve years, the daily dose is 1·5 grams; for a child aged from four to six years, 1 gram; for a child aged from two to three years, 750 milligrams; and for a child aged from nine to twenty-four months, 375 milligrams. The doses should preferably be divided and administered in two or three portions during the day.

For the treatment of roundworm infections, a single dose with the evening meal is usually sufficient to narcotise the worms, which are passed with the next stool. The dose for an adult is the equivalent of 4 grams of piperazine hydrate, and for a child weighing less than 20 kilograms, 3 grams. If the patient has normal bowel movement, a purgative is not necessary; if the patient is constipated, a purgative should be given on the morning after the dose of the anthelmintic so that the worms are expelled before the effect of the drug wears off. In very sick children with heavy roundworm infections, piperazine should be given in divided doses as described for the treatment of threadworm infections. It is also necessary to correct fluid balance and electrolyte balance, and this is usually best achieved by intravenous drip.

Piperazine is usually administered as the adipate, citrate, or phosphate; the equivalent of 100 milligrams of piperazine hydrate is contained in about 120 milligrams of adipate, 125 milligrams of citrate, and 104 milligrams of phosphate.

UNDESIRABLE EFFECTS. Piperazine salts rarely produce toxic effects unless prolonged treatment with large doses is given so that the drug accumulates in the tissues of the host; dizziness, paraesthesia, muscular incoordination, vomiting and blurred vision have been reported under these conditions. Toxic effects cease when treatment is discontinued.

Dose. See above under **Actions and uses.**

OTHER NAME: *Antepar*®

PIPERAZINE PHOSPHATE

$C_4H_{10}N_2,H_3PO_4,H_2O = 202.1$

Solubility. Soluble, at 20°, in 60 parts of water; insoluble in alcohol.

Standard
It complies with the requirements of the British Pharmacopoeia.
It is a white, crystalline, odourless powder and contains not less than 98.5 per cent of $C_4H_{10}N_2,H_3PO_4$, calculated with reference to the anhydrous substance. It contains 8.0 to 9.5 per cent w/w of water. A 1 per cent solution in water has a pH of 6.0 to 6.5.

Actions and uses. Piperazine phosphate has the actions, uses, and undesirable effects described under Piperazine Hydrate; 104 milligrams of piperazine phosphate is approximately equivalent to 100 milligrams of piperazine hydrate.

Dose. See under **Actions and uses** of Piperazine Hydrate.

Preparation
PIPERAZINE PHOSPHATE TABLETS, B.P. Unless otherwise specified, tablets each containing 260 mg of piperazine phosphate are supplied. Tablets containing 500 mg are also available.

OTHER NAMES: *Antepar®*; *Helmezine®*

POWDERED PITUITARY (POSTERIOR LOBE)

Powdered Pituitary (Posterior Lobe) is a powder prepared from the posterior lobe of mammalian pituitary bodies.

When the powder is issued for use as an antidiuretic it is assayed by the method given in Appendix 18 (page 900); the strength is expressed as Units per g.

The active principles in the lobes of the pituitary bodies are rapidly destroyed after death by autolytic enzymes, but the process may be slowed by freezing and almost stopped by defatting and dehydrating. The pituitary bodies are accordingly removed from the animals and frozen as soon as possible after death. The posterior lobes are dissected, defatted, and dehydrated by immersion in acetone, dried, and powdered.

Solubility. Partly soluble in water.

Standard
DESCRIPTION. A yellowish-white or grey amorphous powder; odour characteristic.

IDENTIFICATION TESTS. Extract with a 0.25 per cent w/v solution of *acetic acid* in water sufficiently warm to coagulate the proteins and destroy the autolytic enzymes, filter, and adjust the filtrate to pH 3 to 4; the solution complies with the following tests:

1. It causes contraction of the muscle of the mammalian uterus, suspended in a bath as described in the biological assay of Oxytocin Injection given in the British Pharmacopoeia, Appendix XIVC7.
2. It causes a rise in blood pressure when injected into the vein of a mammal anaesthetised by a general anaesthetic or by destruction of the brain.
3. When injected under the skin of a mammal, at the same time as a volume of water is administered by mouth, it causes a delay in the excretion of the water.
4. When mixed with an equal volume of 2N sodium hydroxide and allowed to stand for one hour at room temperature and then neutralised, the actions on the blood pressure and on the excretion of water disappear and the activity on the muscle of the mammalian uterus is reduced to not more than 5 per cent of that originally present.

ACETONE. Transfer 1.0 g to a small distillation flask, add 20 ml of water and 1 drop of a suitable anti-foaming agent, and attach the flask to a condenser which has its outlet dipping below the surface of 5 ml of water contained in a test-tube; gently distil until the volume of liquid in the receiver is about 14 ml and dilute the distillate to 15 ml with water.

To 2 small test tubes add, respectively, 0.5 ml of the diluted distillate and 0.5 ml of water; to each tube add 0.1 ml of a 15 per cent w/v solution of *sodium nitroprusside* in water and 0.05 ml of *strong sodium hydroxide solution*, allow to stand for 2 minutes, add 0.1 ml of *glacial acetic acid*, and immediately compare the colour of the two solutions by viewing them vertically against a white background.
The solution prepared from the sample shows no greater pink or brownish-pink colour than the solution prepared from water.

MICROBIAL CONTAMINATION. 25 g is free from salmonellae and 1 g is free from *E. coli*, the method given in the British Pharmacopoeia, Appendix XVIB, being used.

SPECIFIC OXYTOCIC ACTIVITY. The estimated potency is not less than 800 Units per g, determined by the following method:
Carry out the method of the British Pharmacopoeia, Appendix XIVC7 for the biological assay of Oxytocin Injection, an extract being prepared by the method described for the Extract of the Standard Preparation or of the Laboratory Standard Preparation. The precision of the assay must be such that the fiducial limits of error (P = 0.95) are between 80 and 125 per cent of the estimated potency.
For the purpose of the assay and calculations the stated potency is taken to be 889 Units per g. The estimated potency is not less than 90 per cent of the stated potency.

Labelling. The label on the container states:
(1) the number of Units of oxytocic activity per g and, when issued for use as an antidiuretic, the number of Units of antidiuretic activity per g.

The label or wrapper on the package or the label on the container states:
(1) the date of manufacture; and
(2) the date after which the preparation is not intended to be used.

Storage. It should be stored in a cool place.

Actions and uses. Powdered pituitary (posterior lobe) has oxytocic, pressor, antidiuretic, and hyperglycaemic actions. It causes contraction of the uterus by a direct stimulation of the uterine muscle, the effect varying with the period in the menstrual cycle in which it is given and depending on whether or not the uterus is pregnant and on the stage of pregnancy. The response is greatest in the first two weeks of the menstrual cycle and in the later stages of pregnancy. Small doses increase the tone and amplitude of the uterine contractions; large or repeated doses result in tetany lasting for five to ten minutes; oestrogens intensify and progesterone diminishes the effect.

In the normal person, pituitary (posterior lobe) delays the excretion of urine for one to two hours, but the exact mode of action is unknown.

In the control of the polyuria of diabetes insipidus, a sterile aqueous solution containing 5 to 10 Units is given subcutaneously morning and evening or it may be applied on a pledget or tampon to the nasal mucous membrane; Pituitary (Posterior Lobe) Insufflation is used for the same purpose.

CONTRA-INDICATIONS. It should not be used in obstetrics, as preparations of oxytocin free from pressor action are available for this purpose.

Dose. The dose is determined by the physician in accordance with the needs of the patient.

Preparation
PITUITARY (POSTERIOR LOBE) INSUFFLATION, B.P.C. (page 721)

PODOPHYLLUM

SYNONYMS: American Mandrake; Podoph.; Podophyllum Rhizome

Podophyllum consists of the dried rhizome and roots of *Podophyllum peltatum* L. (Fam. Berberidaceae), a small herb with a long perennial rhizome, common in the eastern United States of America and eastern Canada. The rhizome is collected in the late summer, cut into pieces, and dried.

Constituents. Podophyllum contains the three closely related lignans, podophyllotoxin (up to about 1 per cent) and α- and β-peltatins, all derivatives of naphthofuran which differ only in the number and position of the hydroxyl and methyl groups, and their glycosides. It also contains another lignan (a deoxypodophyllin-1β-D-glucosopyranosyl ester), the flavonoids quercetin and astragalin (kaempferol 3-glucoside), starch, and resinous matter.

Podophyllotoxin is converted by alkalis into a salt of podophyllic acid, which readily loses water to form a crystalline lactone, picropodophyllin.

Podophyllum yields 2 to 8 per cent or more of resin. The acid-insoluble ash is about 1 to 2·5 per cent and the total ash about 4 to 7 per cent. It yields to alcohol (90 per cent) 11 to 16 per cent of extractive.

Standard for unground drug
DESCRIPTION. *Macroscopical:* rhizome occurring in subcylindrical pieces about 5 to 10 cm or more long and about 5 mm thick; externally reddish-brown, smooth or slightly wrinkled longitudinally; at intervals of about 5 to 10 cm, rhizome enlarged for about 1 to 2 cm to a thickness of about 1·5 cm; upper surface of enlargement bearing a concave scar, left by the fall of the flowering stem, surrounded by several circular leaf scars; under surface of enlargement bearing up to 12 roots or root scars; roots, when present, cylindrical or flattened, about 1·5 mm thick, brown and brittle; fracture of rhizome short; smoothed, transversely cut surface white and starchy, unless rhizome has been dried at a temperature sufficient to gelatinise starch, when yellowish and horny; showing a thin cork and a circle of about 20 to 30 small oval vascular bundles situated about half-way between centre and circumference of rhizome.

Odour slight, characteristic; taste somewhat bitter and acrid.

Microscopical: the diagnostic characters are: Rhizome: *epidermis* of longitudinally elongated tabular cells with dark *tannin* contents and brown suberised walls; *cork* in 1 to 3 layers, cells rectangular, about two and a half times as long as wide, those from enlarged regions more nearly isodiametric; *cortex* with outer collenchyma and wide zone of parenchyma; *pith* similar to cortical parenchyma, cells of both containing abundant *starch* granules, mostly compound with 2 to **4** to 15 components, some simple, 2 to **15** to 30 μm in diameter, and also cluster *crystals* of calcium oxalate often 60 to 100 μm in diameter, in idioblasts; vascular bundles with *vessels* with spirally thickened and pitted walls, pits elongated and bordered; bundles often accompanied by perimedullary *sclereids*, up to 630 μm long and with thick, pitted walls.

Root: *epidermis* slightly papillose and having somewhat thickened outer walls; *exodermis* with thin suberised walls; *cortical cells* parenchymatous, with pitted walls, containing *starch* granules and calcium oxalate *crystals* as in the rhizome; primary *xylem* strands 4 to 9; *pith* of thin-walled parenchyma and a central core of *sclereids*, each about 30 to 230 μm long with thick, pitted walls.

IDENTIFICATION TEST. Macerate 0·5 g for 10 minutes with 10 ml of *alcohol (95 per cent)*, filter, and to the filtrate add 0·6 ml of *strong copper acetate solution*; a bright green colour, but no brown precipitate, is produced.

FOREIGN ORGANIC MATTER. Not more than 2·0 per cent.

CONTENT OF RESIN. Not less than 4·0 per cent, determined by the following method:
Extract about 10 g, accurately weighed, in moderately coarse powder, with *alcohol (90 per cent)* for 4 hours in an apparatus for the continuous extraction of drugs, remove most of the alcohol from the extract, transfer the residue to a small beaker, evaporate the extract to a syrupy consistence (about 3 g), and pour, stirring continuously, into a mixture of 20 ml of water and 0·2 ml of *hydrochloric acid*, cooled below 5°, contained in a second beaker.
Allow to settle, pour a little of the clear supernatant liquid back into the first beaker, mix well with the syrupy liquid remaining in it, and again pour into the second beaker, repeating the operation until all the syrup is well mixed with the precipitation liquid.
Allow to stand for 2 hours below 5°, stir well to break any coagulated resin, and filter, transferring the bulk of the precipitate from the beaker to the filter with the aid of a small portion of the filtrate and then with **three**

successive 5-ml portions of a mixture of 20 ml of water and 0·1 ml of *hydrochloric acid*, cooled below 5°. Wash the residue with a further 5 ml of the acidified water and dissolve the residue on the filter and any residue remaining in the beaker in hot *alcohol (90 per cent)*; evaporate off the alcohol and dry the residue to constant weight at 105°.

Standard for powdered drug: Powdered Podophyllum

DESCRIPTION. A light brown powder possessing the diagnostic microscopical characters, odour, and taste of the unground drug.

IDENTIFICATION TEST; FOREIGN ORGANIC MATTER; CONTENT OF RESIN. It complies with the requirements for the unground drug.

Uses. Podophyllum is used almost entirely for the preparation of podophyllum resin.

INDIAN PODOPHYLLUM

SYNONYMS: Ind. Podoph.; Indian Podophyllum Rhizome; Podophyllum Emodi

Indian Podophyllum consists of the dried rhizome and roots of *Podophyllum emodi* Wall. ex Hook. f. et Thoms. (*P. hexandrum* Royle) (Fam. Berberidaceae), a plant growing in the temperate forests on the lower slopes of the Himalayas. The roots form a large proportion of the drug and are mainly detached from the rhizome.

Constituents. Indian podophyllum contains the lignans, podophyllotoxin (1 to 4 per cent) and its β-D-glucoside (0·5 to 1 per cent), 4'-demethylpodophyllotoxin and its glucoside and a deoxypodophyllin-1β-D-glucosopyranosyl ester, and the flavonoid astragalin (kaempferol 3-glucoside), but peltatins are absent.

Indian podophyllum yields 6 to 12 per cent of resin, the composition of which is not identical with that from podophyllum.

Standard for unground drug

DESCRIPTION. *Macroscopical:* rhizome occurring in irregularly cylindrical or dorsiventrally flattened, contorted knotty pieces, yellowish-brown to earthy-brown; pieces about 2 to 4 cm long and 1 to 2 cm thick; upper surface with about 3 to 4 cup-shaped scars of aerial stems, under surface with numerous stout roots or circular root scars; fracture of rhizome short; smoothed, transversely cut surface pale brown and starchy, unless rhizome has been dried at a temperature sufficient to gelatinise starch, when horny; showing large central pith and a circle of about 20 radially elongated vascular bundles.

Odour slight, characteristic; taste somewhat bitter and acrid.

Microscopical: the diagnostic characters are: Rhizome: *epidermis* absent; *cork* in up to 6 layers, cells polyhedral, not more than twice as long as wide; *cortex, medullary rays,* and *pith* parenchymatous, cells moderately thick-walled, with simple pits, and containing abundant *starch* granules, compound, usually 2 to **4** to 20 components, 2 to **7** to 34 μm in diameter, and cluster *crystals* of calcium oxalate, 20 to **30** to 60 μm in diameter; xylem *vessels* usually with elongated bor-

dered pits; perimedullary groups of *sclereids*, up to 320 μm long with thick, pitted walls.

Root: *epidermis* slightly papillose and having very much thickened outer and anticlinal walls; *exodermis* suberised, with wavy walls; cortex very wide, parenchymatous, with *starch* granules but no calcium oxalate *crystals; xylem* in 4 to 9 primary strands; *pith* with large central core of *sclereids*, axially elongated or nearly isodiametric, walls very thick and pitted.

IDENTIFICATION TEST. Macerate 0·5 g for 10 minutes in 10 ml of *alcohol (95 per cent)*, filter, and to the filtrate add 0·6 ml of *strong copper acetate solution*; a brown precipitate, but no green colour, is formed.

FOREIGN ORGANIC MATTER. Not more than 2·0 per cent.

CONTENT OF RESIN. Not less than 8·0 per cent, determined by the method for Podophyllum (page 386), the extract being evaporated to about 5 g and poured into a mixture of 40 ml of water and 0·4 ml of *hydrochloric acid*.

Standard for powdered drug: Powdered Indian Podophyllum

DESCRIPTION. A light brown powder possessing the diagnostic microscopical characters, odour, and taste of the unground drug.

IDENTIFICATION TEST; FOREIGN ORGANIC MATTER; CONTENT OF RESIN. It complies with the requirements for the unground drug.

Uses. Indian podophyllum is used almost entirely for the preparation of podophyllum resin.

PODOPHYLLUM RESIN

SYNONYMS: Podoph. Resin; Podophyllin

Podophyllum Resin is the resin obtained from Indian Podophyllum or more rarely from Podophyllum. It may be extracted by percolating with alcohol and pouring the concentrated percolate into water acidified with hydrochloric acid. The precipitated resin is well washed and dried at a low temperature.

Constituents. Podophyllum resin contains podophyllotoxin, at least 40 per cent in resin from Indian Podophyllum and about 10 per cent in resin from Podophyllum, picropodophyllin and its glucoside, the flavonoids quercetin and astragalin (kaempferol 3-glucoside), and resinous substances.

Resin from Indian Podophyllum contains in addition

4'-demethylpodophyllotoxin and its glucoside; that from Podophyllum contains α- and β-peltatins.

Solubility. Very slightly soluble in cold water, but partly soluble in hot water, from which it is precipitated on cooling; soluble completely, or almost completely, in alcohol; partly soluble in ether, in chloroform, and in dilute ammonia solution.

Standard
It complies with the requirements of the British Pharmacopoeia.

It occurs as a light brown to greenish-yellow amorphous powder or brownish-grey masses with a characteristic odour and a bitter acrid taste; it darkens in colour on exposure to light or when heated above 25°. The resin from Podophyllum may be distinguished from that from Indian Podophyllum by gently shaking 3 ml of a 13 per cent w/v solution of the finely powdered resin in *alcohol (60 per cent)* with 0·5 ml of 1N potassium hydroxide; the resin from Podophyllum does not gelatinise, whereas that from Indian Podophyllum forms a jelly on standing.

Labelling. The label on the container states the botanical source.

Storage. It should be stored in airtight containers, protected from light.

Actions and uses. Because of its cytotoxic action, podophyllum resin is used as a paint in the treatment of soft venereal and other warts. It has also been used as a purgative, but its use for this purpose constitutes an unnecessarily unpleasant treatment.

CONTRA-INDICATIONS. It should not be used in pregnancy.

UNDESIRABLE EFFECTS. Powdered podophyllum resin is strongly irritant to the skin and mucous membrane.

Dose. 15 to 60 milligrams.

Preparation
PODOPHYLLIN PAINT, COMPOUND, B.P.C. (page 766)

POLDINE METHYLSULPHATE

$C_{22}H_{29}NO_7S = 451\cdot5$

Poldine Methylsulphate is 2-benziloyloxymethyl-1,1-dimethylpyrrolidinium methyl sulphate.

Solubility. Soluble, at 20°, in 1 part of water and in 20 parts of alcohol; slightly soluble in chloroform.

Standard
It complies with the requirements of the British Pharmacopoeia.

It is a white, crystalline, odourless powder and contains not less than 98·5 per cent of $C_{22}H_{29}NO_7S$, calculated with reference to the dried substance. The loss on drying under the prescribed conditions is not more than 0·5 per cent. It has a melting-point of 137° to 142°. A 1 per cent solution in water has a pH of 5·0 to 7·0.

Stability. Aqueous solutions at a pH of less than 4·0 are stable for long periods when stored at a temperature not exceeding 30°. The rate of hydrolysis at the ester linkage increases with rise in pH and temperature and hydrolysis is rapid in solutions of pH greater than 7·0.

Actions and uses. Poldine is an anticholinergic drug with actions and uses similar to those described under Propantheline Bromide (page 411). Its effects are longer lasting than those of atropine (page 36).

A dosage of 2 to 6 milligrams every six hours may be required to reduce gastric secretion and spasm in ulcer patients; treatment should begin with the lower dose, which should be gradually increased until the symptoms are controlled.

UNDESIRABLE EFFECTS. Blurring of vision, constipation, hesitancy over micturition, and tachycardia may occur. If necessary the dose should be reduced progressively by 1 milligram until the undesirable effect is relieved.

Dose. See above under **Actions and uses.**

Preparation
POLDINE TABLETS, B.P. Unless otherwise specified tablets each containing 2 mg of poldine methylsulphate are supplied. Tablets containing 4 mg are also available.

OTHER NAME: *Nacton*®

POLYMYXIN B SULPHATE

SYNONYMS: Polymyx. B Sulph.; Polymyxini B Sulfas

Polymyxin B Sulphate is a mixture of the sulphates of certain antimicrobial polypeptides produced by the growth of certain strains of *Bacillus polymyxa* or obtained by any other means.

Solubility. Soluble in water; slightly soluble in alcohol.

Standard
It complies with the requirements of the European Pharmacopoeia.

It is a white or creamy-white, hygroscopic, odourless or almost odourless powder and contains not less than 6500 Units per mg, calculated with reference to the dried substance. The loss on drying under the prescribed conditions is not more than 6·0 per cent. A 2 per cent solution in water has a pH of 5·0 to 7·0.

Sterilisation. Solutions for injection are sterilised by filtration.

Labelling. If the material is intended for the preparation of injections the label states "Polymyxin B Sulphate for Injection".

Storage. It should be stored in airtight containers, protected from light. If it is intended for parenteral administration the containers are sealed to exclude micro-organisms.

Actions and uses. Polymyxin B is an antibiotic which is active against a wide variety of Gram-negative bacteria, including *Escherichia coli*, *Aerobacter aerogenes*, and *Pseudomonas aeruginosa*.

Polymyxin B sulphate is administered by mouth or applied topically. For intestinal infections by sensitive bacteria it may be given in a dose of 1,000,000 Units every four hours for adults or 40,000 Units per kilogram body-weight for children. Very little is absorbed unless there is extensive ulceration.

Specific bacterial skin infections, especially of burns, may be treated topically with solutions containing 0·1 to 1·0 per cent, applied as a wet dressing or a spray. Systemic toxicity may result from the treatment of large raw areas.

Polymyxin B sulphate is irritant to the tissues and sulphomyxin sodium (page 486) should preferably be used if it is essential to give polymyxin by injection.

UNDESIRABLE EFFECTS. Systemic toxicity may give rise to dizziness and paraesthesia, especially of the face. More serious but apparently reversible damage may occur to the renal tubules.

Dose. See above under **Actions and uses.**

Preparation
POLYMYXIN INJECTION, B.P.C. (page 717)

OTHER NAME: *Aerosporin®*

POLYSORBATE 20

SYNONYM: Polyoxyethylene (20) Sorbitan Monolaurate

Polysorbate 20 is a complex mixture of partial lauric esters of sorbitol and its mono- and di-anhydrides condensed with approximately 20 moles of ethylene oxide for each mole of sorbitol and its anhydrides. It has a weight per ml at 20° of about 1·10 g; the viscosity at 20° is about 500 centipoises.

Solubility. Miscible with water, with alcohol, with ethyl acetate, and with methyl alcohol; soluble, at 20°, in 125 parts of cottonseed oil and in 200 parts of toluene; slightly soluble in liquid paraffin.

Standard
DESCRIPTION. A clear yellow oily liquid with a characteristic odour.

IDENTIFICATION TESTS. 1. To 2 ml of a 5 per cent w/v solution in water add 10 ml of *ammonium cobalto-thiocyanate solution* and 5 ml of *chloroform*, shake well, and allow to separate; a blue colour is produced in the chloroform layer.

2. To 5 ml of a 5 per cent w/v solution in water add 5 ml of 1N sodium hydroxide, boil, cool, and acidify with *dilute hydrochloric acid*; the solution is strongly opalescent.

3. On saponification it yields a mixture of fatty acid and polyols; the fatty acid produced has an acid value of about 260.

ACIDITY OR ALKALINITY. pH of a 5·0 per cent w/v solution in *carbon dioxide-free water*, 5·0 to 7·0.

ACID VALUE. Not more than 2·0.

HYDROXYL VALUE. 96·0 to 108·0, determined by the method given in Appendix 21, page 902, about 3 g, accurately weighed, being used.

SAPONIFICATION VALUE. 40·0 to 50·0.

ARSENIC. It complies with the test given in Appendix 6, page 879 (3 parts per million).

LEAD. It complies with the test given in Appendix 8 page 887 (10 parts per million).

WATER. Not more than 3·0 per cent w/w, determined by the method given in Appendix 16, page 895.

SULPHATED ASH. Not more than 0·25 per cent.

Uses. Polysorbate 20 has the uses of the polysorbates, as described under Polysorbate 80. It is more hydrophilic than polysorbate 60 and polysorbate 80.

It is used alone or in conjunction with polysorbate 80 for the solubilisation of oils. It has also been used for the dispersion of coal tar in ointment bases.

OTHER NAMES: *Crillet 1®*; *Sorbester Q12®*; *Tween 20®*

POLYSORBATE 60

SYNONYM: Polyoxyethylene (20) Sorbitan Monostearate

Polysorbate 60 is a complex mixture of partial stearic esters of sorbitol and its mono- and di-anhydrides condensed with approximately 20 moles of ethylene oxide for each mole of sorbitol and its anhydrides. It usually contains a very small amount of added water in order to obtain a product which is liquid at room temperature. It has a weight per ml at 20° of about 1·10 g.

Solubility. Soluble, at 20°, in 30 parts of cottonseed oil; soluble in water; miscible with acetone and with dioxan; insoluble in mineral oils.

Standard
DESCRIPTION. An opaque yellow semi-gel which becomes a clear oily liquid at temperatures above 24°; odour faintly sweet or oily.

IDENTIFICATION TESTS. 1. It complies with tests 1 and 2 described under Polysorbate 20.

2. On saponification it yields a mixture of fatty acid and polyols; the fatty acid produced has an acid value of about 205 and a solidifying-point not lower than 50°.

ACID VALUE. Not more than 2·0.

HYDROXYL VALUE. 81·0 to 96·0, determined by the method given in Appendix 21, page 902, about 3 g, accurately weighed, being used.

SAPONIFICATION VALUE. 45·0 to 55·0.

ARSENIC. It complies with the test given in Appendix 6, page 879 (3 parts per million).

LEAD. It complies with the test given in Appendix 8, page 887 (10 parts per million).

WATER. Not more than 3·0 per cent w/w, determined by the method given in Appendix 16, page 895.

SULPHATED ASH. Not more than 0·25 per cent.

Uses. Polysorbate 60 has the uses of the polysorbates, as described under Polysorbate 80, from which it differs in solubility.

OTHER NAMES: *Crillet 3®*; *Sorbester Q18®*; *Tween 60®*

POLYSORBATE 80

SYNONYM: Polyoxyethylene (20) Sorbitan Mono-oleate

Polysorbate 80 is a complex mixture of partial oleic esters of sorbitol and its mono- and di-anhydrides condensed with approximately 20 moles of ethylene oxide for each mole of sorbitol and its anhydrides. It has a weight per ml at 20° of about 1·08 g; the viscosity at 20° is about 600 centipoises.

Solubility. Miscible with water, with alcohol, with ethyl acetate, and with methyl alcohol; soluble, at 20°, in 125 parts of cottonseed oil; slightly soluble in liquid paraffin.

Standard

DESCRIPTION. A clear yellow oily liquid; odour characteristic of fatty acids.

IDENTIFICATION TESTS. 1. It complies with tests 1 and 2 described under Polysorbate 20.
2. To a 5 per cent solution in water add *bromine solution*, dropwise; the bromine solution is de-colorised.

ACIDITY OR ALKALINITY. pH of a 5·0 per cent w/v solution in water, 6·0 to 8·0.

ACID VALUE. Not more than 2·0.

HYDROXYL VALUE. 65·0 to 80·0, determined by the method given in Appendix 21, page 902, about 3 g, accurately weighed, being used.

SAPONIFICATION VALUE. 45·0 to 55·0.

ARSENIC. It complies with the test given in Appendix 6, page 879 (3 parts per million).

LEAD. It complies with the test given in Appendix 8, page 887 (10 parts per million).

WATER. Not more than 3·0 per cent w/w, determined by the method given in Appendix 16, page 895.

SULPHATED ASH. Not more than 0·25 per cent.

Uses. Polysorbates are non-ionic surface-active agents. They are used in the preparation of emulsions, creams, ointments, and suppository bases.

When used alone, the polysorbates, being hydrophilic, yield oil-in-water emulsions, but emulsions and creams of varying character, including both oil-in-water and water-in-oil types, may be produced by incorporating varying proportions of sorbitan ether–esters. The emulsions are stable, being little affected by high concentrations of electrolytes or changes in pH.

Polysorbates are also used as solubilising agents for essential oils, oil-soluble vitamins, and phenobarbitone, and as wetting agents in suspensions for administration by mouth or injection.

OTHER NAMES: *Crillet 4®*; *Sorbester Q17®*; *Tween 80®*

POTASSIUM ACETATE

$CH_3 \cdot CO_2 K = 98·14$

Solubility. Soluble, at 20°, in less than 1 part of water and in 2 parts of alcohol.

Standard

DESCRIPTION. Colourless crystals or a white crystalline powder; odourless or almost odourless.

IDENTIFICATION TESTS. It gives the reactions characteristic of potassium and of acetates.

ALKALINITY. pH of a 5·0 per cent w/v solution in *carbon dioxide-free water*, 7·5 to 9·5.

ARSENIC. It complies with the test given in Appendix 6, page 879 (2 parts per million).

CALCIUM. Not more than 100 parts per million, determined by the method given under Magnesium Acetate (page 275).

LEAD. It complies with the test given in Appendix 7, page 883 (2 parts per million).

MAGNESIUM. Not more than 100 parts per million, determined by the method given under Calcium Acetate (page 66), 1·0 g dissolved in sufficient water to produce 100 ml being used.

SODIUM. Not more than 0·5 per cent determined by the method given under Magnesium Acetate (page 275).

CHLORIDE. 1·0 g complies with the limit test for chlorides (350 parts per million).

NITRATE. It complies with the test given under Magnesium Acetate (page 275).

SULPHATE. 1·0 g complies with the limit test for sulphates (600 parts per million).

READILY OXIDISABLE SUBSTANCES. It complies with the test given under Magnesium Acetate (page 275).

LOSS ON DRYING. Not more than 5·0 per cent, determined by drying to constant weight at 105°.

CONTENT OF $C_2H_3KO_2$. Not less than 99·0 per cent, calculated with reference to the substance dried under the prescribed conditions, determined by the following method:

Titrate about 0·2 g, accurately weighed, by Method I of the British Pharmacopoeia, Appendix XIB, for non-aqueous titration; each ml of 0·1N perchloric acid is equivalent to 0·009814 g of $C_2H_3KO_2$.

Storage. It should be stored in airtight containers.

Uses. Potassium acetate is a source of potassium ions and may be used to adjust the potassium content of solutions for haemodialysis.

POTASSIUM ACID TARTRATE

SYNONYMS: Pot. Acid Tart.; Potassium Hydrogen Tartrate; Purified Cream of Tartar

$C_4H_5KO_6 = 188.2$

Potassium Acid Tartrate may be obtained by purification of crude cream of tartar, or argol, which is deposited from grape juice during fermentation and is also found in the lees of wine.

Solubility. Soluble, at 20°, in 190 parts of water; soluble in 16 parts of boiling water; insoluble in alcohol.

Standard

DESCRIPTION. Colourless crystals or white crystalline powder; odourless or almost odourless.

IDENTIFICATION TESTS. 1. Ignite, neutralise the residue with *dilute hydrochloric acid*, and filter; the solution gives the reactions characteristic of potassium.

2. It gives the reactions characteristic of tartrates. Neutralise a solution in water with *sodium hydroxide solution*; it gives the reactions characteristic of solutions of tartrates.

ACIDITY. A solution in *carbon dioxide-free water* is neutral to *bromophenol blue solution*.

ARSENIC. It complies with the test given in Appendix 6, page 879 (1 part per million).

COPPER AND IRON. Dissolve 2·0 g in a mixture of 5 ml of *dilute ammonia solution* and 40 ml of water and add 0·3 ml of *sodium sulphide solution PbT*; any colour which develops is not more than slightly deeper than that produced when a similar solution to which 1 ml of *potassium cyanide solution PbT* has been added is similarly treated.

LEAD. It complies with the test given in Appendix 7, page 883 (10 parts per million).

CHLORIDE. 1·0 g, dissolved by warming, complies with the limit test for chlorides (350 parts per million).

SULPHATE. 0·50 g dissolved in hot water with the addition of 3 ml of *dilute hydrochloric acid* complies with the limit test for sulphates (0·12 per cent).

FREE TARTARIC ACID. Not more than 0·2 per cent, determined by the following method:
Shake about 1 g, in fine powder, accurately weighed, with 20 ml of *alcohol (90 per cent)*, filter, evaporate 10 ml of the filtrate to dryness, and dry the residue to constant weight at 105°.

LOSS ON DRYING. Not more than 0·5 per cent, determined by drying to constant weight at 105°.

CONTENT OF $C_4H_5KO_6$. Not less than 99·5 per cent, calculated with reference to the substance dried under the prescribed conditions, determined by the following method:
Dissolve about 1·5 g, accurately weighed, in 100 ml of boiling water and titrate the hot solution with 0·2N sodium hydroxide, using *phenolphthalein solution* as indicator; each ml of 0·2N sodium hydroxide is equivalent to 0·03764 g of $C_4H_5KO_6$.

Hygroscopicity. It absorbs insignificant amounts of moisture at 25° at relative humidities up to about 90 per cent.

Uses. Potassium acid tartrate has been used as a saline purgative.

Dose. 1 to 4 grams.

POTASSIUM BICARBONATE

SYNONYMS: Pot. Bicarb.; Potassium Hydrogen Carbonate

$KHCO_3 = 100.1$

Potassium Bicarbonate may be prepared by saturating a concentrated aqueous solution of potassium carbonate with carbon dioxide.

Solubility. Soluble, at 20°, in 3 parts of water; very slightly soluble in alcohol.

Standard

DESCRIPTION. Colourless, monoclinic prisms or white, granular powder; odourless or almost odourless.

IDENTIFICATION TESTS. 1. It gives the reaction characteristic of potassium. Neutralise a solution in water with *dilute hydrochloric acid*; it gives the reactions characteristic of solutions of potassium salts.

2. It gives the reactions characteristic of bicarbonates.

ALKALINITY. pH of a 1·0 per cent w/v solution in *carbon dioxide-free water*, not more than 8·6.

ALUMINIUM, CALCIUM, AND INSOLUBLE MATTER. Boil 5·0 g with 50 ml of water and 10 ml of *dilute ammonia solution*, filter, wash the residue with water, and ignite to constant weight; the residue weighs not more than 5 mg.

ARSENIC. It complies with the test given in Appendix 6, page 879 (2 parts per million).

IRON. 2·0 g dissolved in a mixture of 2 ml of *hydrochloric acid FeT* and 10 ml of water and diluted to 40 ml with water complies with the limit test for iron (20 parts per million).

LEAD. It complies with the test given in Appendix 7, page 883 (5 parts per million).

SODIUM. Dissolve 0·30 g in 3·5 ml of water, add 2 ml of *alcohol (95 per cent)* and 3 ml of *potassium antimonate solution*, and allow to stand for 15 minutes; no white crystalline precipitate or sediment, visible to the naked eye, is formed.

CHLORIDE. 0·50 g dissolved in water with the addition of 1·5 ml of *nitric acid* complies with the limit test for chlorides (700 parts per million).

SULPHATE. 0·50 g dissolved in water with the addition of 3·5 ml of *dilute hydrochloric acid* complies with the limit test for sulphates (0·12 per cent).

CONTENT OF $KHCO_3$. Not less than 99·0 per cent, determined by the following method:
Dissolve about 1·5 g, accurately weighed, in 20 ml of water, and titrate with 0·5N hydrochloric acid, using *methyl orange solution* as indicator; each ml of 0·5N hydrochloric acid is equivalent to 0·05006 g of $KHCO_3$.

Use. Potassium bicarbonate is an ingredient of Colchicum and Sodium Salicylate Mixture (page 740).

POTASSIUM BROMIDE

SYNONYMS: Kalii Bromidum; Pot. Brom.

KBr = 119·0

Solubility. Soluble, at 20°, in 1·6 parts of water and in 200 parts of alcohol; soluble in glycerol.

Standard
It complies with the requirements of the European Pharmacopoeia.
It occurs as odourless colourless crystals or white crystalline powder and contains not less than 98·0 per cent of KBr, calculated with reference to the dried substance. The loss on drying under the prescribed conditions is not more than 1·0 per cent.

Incompatibility. It is incompatible with oxidising agents and with salts of mercury and silver.

Actions and uses. Bromides are depressants of the central nervous system and are more effective as sedatives than as hypnotics.
Mixtures containing bromides have been widely used as sedatives and anticonvulsants, but in view of their undesirable effects they have been largely replaced by more effective substances such as chloral hydrate and barbiturates.

UNDESIRABLE EFFECTS. During prolonged administration accumulation of bromide may occur, giving rise to symptoms of poisoning (bromism) which may consist of skin eruptions of various types, nausea and vomiting, mental dullness, lapses of memory, and even mental derangement. The symptoms usually subside when bromides are withheld and chlorides are administered.

PRECAUTIONS. Special care should be taken in prescribing bromides for the aged or for patients suffering from impaired renal function or on a salt-restricted diet.

Dose. 1 to 6 grams daily in divided doses.

Preparation
GELSEMIUM AND HYOSCYAMUS MIXTURE, COMPOUND, B.P.C. (page 743)

POTASSIUM CHLORATE

KClO$_3$ = 122·6

Potassium Chlorate may be prepared by electrolysis of a hot solution of potassium chloride.

CAUTION. *Potassium chlorate is liable to explode under certain conditions, and, when mixing it with any dry substance, friction and percussion should be avoided.*

Solubility. Soluble, at 20°, in 14 parts of water and of glycerol; soluble in 2 parts of boiling water; very slightly soluble in alcohol.

Standard
DESCRIPTION. Colourless crystals or white powder; odourless or almost odourless.

IDENTIFICATION TESTS. 1. Add 0·2 g to 1 ml of *hydrochloric acid*; the liquid becomes yellow and chlorine and oxides of chlorine are evolved.
2. Heat; it melts and evolves oxygen. The residue gives the reactions characteristic of potassium and of chlorides.

ACIDITY OR ALKALINITY. A 5·0 per cent w/v solution in *carbon dioxide-free water* is neutral to *bromothymol blue solution*.

ARSENIC. It complies with the test given in Appendix 6, page 879 (2 parts per million).

LEAD. It complies with the test given in Appendix 7, page 883 (10 parts per million).

CHLORIDE. 0·50 g complies with the limit test for chlorides (700 parts per million).

SULPHATE. 0·50 g dissolved in water with the addition of 3 ml of *dilute hydrochloric acid* complies with the limit test for sulphates (0·12 per cent).

CONTENT OF KClO$_3$. Not less than 99·0 per cent, determined by the following method:
Dissolve about 0·3 g, accurately weighed, in 10 ml of water contained in a glass-stoppered flask, add 10 ml of *sodium nitrite solution*, followed by 20 ml of *nitric acid*, stopper the flask, and allow to stand for 10 minutes; add 100 ml of water and sufficient *potassium permanganate solution* to produce a permanent pink colour and decolorise by the addition of a trace of

ferrous sulphate; add 0·1 g of *urea*, shake vigorously with 30 ml of 0·1N silver nitrate, filter, wash the residue with water, and titrate the excess of silver nitrate in the combined filtrate and washings with 0·1N ammonium thiocyanate, using *ferric ammonium sulphate solution* as indicator; each ml of 0·1N silver nitrate is equivalent to 0·01226 g of KClO$_3$.

Stability. Potassium chlorate is unstable and liable to explode when in contact with organic compounds or readily oxidisable substances such as charcoal, phosphorus, or sulphur, especially if heated or subjected to friction or percussion.

Storage and handling of tablets. Potassium chlorate tablets should not be allowed to come into contact with matches or surfaces containing phosphorus compounds and should be dispensed in bottles or boxes.

Actions and uses. Potassium chlorate is a sialogogue and mild astringent. It is used in the form of a gargle or in lozenges or tablets. The assumption that it has an antiseptic action is without rational basis.

UNDESIRABLE EFFECTS. The internal administration of potassium chlorate may cause kidney damage or methaemoglobinaemia. In a susceptible person, it may produce acute haemolytic anaemia, giving rise to methaemoglobinuria.

POISONING. The symptoms of acute poisoning by potassium chlorate are nausea, vomiting, abdominal pain, albuminuria, and haematuria. Treatment consists in gastric lavage, the use of alkalis to prevent anuria, and, if necessary, transfusion of blood to combat the anaemia.

POTASSIUM CHLORIDE

SYNONYM: Kalii Chloridum

KCl = 74·55

Solubility. Soluble, at 20°, in 3 parts of water; insoluble in dehydrated alcohol and in ether.

Standard
It complies with the requirements of the European Pharmacopoeia.
It occurs as odourless colourless crystals or white crystalline powder and contains not less than 99·0 per cent of KCl, calculated with reference to the dried substance. The loss on drying under the prescribed conditions is not more than 1·0 per cent.

Sterilisation. Solutions for injection are sterilised by heating in an autoclave or by filtration.

Actions and uses. Potassium ions play an important part in cellular metabolism. Their concentration is much higher in the cells than in the extracellular fluid, and there is an uptake of potassium during glycogen storage. When administered by mouth, potassium salts are rapidly excreted in the urine and toxic concentrations are not usually achieved by this route even with large doses, but an excess of potassium ions, when injected intravenously, produces depression of the heart and may cause cardiac arrest. Electrocardiographic tracings show typical changes, but owing to the migration of potassium from the intracellular fluid to the serum during excretion, such changes are not always parallel with directly determined potassium concentrations.

Deficiency of potassium ions causes acute muscular weakness, paraesthesia, and cardiac arrhythmias. It is important to maintain the body-potassium in patients with diabetic acidosis, persistent diarrhoea and vomiting, following the abuse of purgatives, and during treatment with chlorothiazide and related substances. When potassium supplements are given in conjunction with diuretic therapy, they should be given on the day following that on which the diuretic is administered.

In acute potassium deficiency, a solution of potassium chloride may be administered intravenously; administration should be slow in order to avoid toxic effects on the heart. The total amount of potassium chloride administered intravenously should not exceed 6 grams (80 millimoles) daily and the concentration of the solution should not exceed 3·2 grams (43 millimoles) per litre.

Compound Sodium Lactate Injection is used in the treatment of acidosis.

UNDESIRABLE EFFECTS. Potassium salts by mouth are more irritant than the corresponding sodium salts; their low renal threshold excretion promotes diuresis.

Tablets containing potassium salts may cause ulceration of the gastro-intestinal tract with bleeding and intestinal obstruction. Potassium chloride should therefore be given as a well-diluted solution or in the form of slow-release tablets. Potassium Chloride Tablets should be crushed and dissolved in water before administration.

Colonic irritation may occur during treatment with tablets containing potassium chloride together with a diuretic of the thiazide group.

POISONING. Overdosage with potassium salts should be treated with calcium, dextrose, and insulin, and fluids should be given intravenously, if necessary.

Dose. The dose is determined by the physician in accordance with the needs of the patient.

Preparations
POTASSIUM CHLORIDE AND DEXTROSE INJECTION, B.P. It consists of a sterile solution of potassium chloride and anhydrous dextrose in Water for Injections. Unless otherwise specified, a solution containing 0·3 per cent of potassium chloride (40 millimoles, or milliequivalents, each of K^+ and Cl^- per litre) and 5 per cent of anhydrous dextrose is supplied. On storage, this solution may cause separation of small solid particles from glass containers; solutions containing such particles must not be used. It should be stored at a temperature not exceeding 25°.

POTASSIUM CHLORIDE AND SODIUM CHLORIDE INJECTION, B.P. It consists of a sterile solution of potassium chloride and sodium chloride in Water for Injections. Unless otherwise specified, a solution containing 0·3 per cent of potassium chloride and 0·9 per cent of sodium chloride is supplied (approximately 40 millimoles, or milliequivalents, of K^+, 150 millimoles, or milliequivalents, of Na^+, and 190 millimoles, or milliequivalents, of Cl^- per litre).

SODIUM LACTATE INJECTION, COMPOUND, B.P. (Syn. Hartmann's Solution for Injection; Ringer-Lactate Solution for Injection). It consists of a sterile solution containing sodium lactate, prepared from 2·4 ml of lactic acid and 1·15 g of sodium hydroxide, with sodium chloride, potassium chloride, and calcium chloride, in Water for Injections to 1000 ml. This solution provides approximately 2 millimoles, or 4 milliequivalents, of Ca^{2+}, 131 millimoles, or milliequivalents, of Na^+, 5 millimoles, or milliequivalents, of K^+, 111 millimoles, or milliequivalents, of Cl^-, and the equivalent of 29 millimoles, or milliequivalents, of HCO_3^- per litre. On storage, this solution may cause separation of small solid particles from glass containers; solutions containing such particles must not be used.

STRONG POTASSIUM CHLORIDE SOLUTION, B.P. It consists of a sterile 15 per cent solution of potassium chloride in Water for Injections. Each 10 ml of the

Dose. 300 to 600 milligrams.

Preparation
POTASSIUM CHLORATE AND PHENOL GARGLE, B.P.C. (page 700)

solution contains approximately 20 millimoles, or milliequivalents, each of K^+ and of Cl^-. The solution must be diluted before use with not less than 50 times its volume of Sodium Chloride Injection or other suitable diluent.

POTASSIUM CHLORIDE TABLETS, B.P. Unless otherwise specified, tablets each containing 500 mg of potassium chloride are supplied. They should be dissolved in water before administration. They should be stored in airtight containers.

POTASSIUM CITRATE

SYNONYM: Pot. Cit.

$C_6H_5K_3O_7,H_2O = 324\cdot4$

Solubility. Soluble, at 20°, in 1 part of water and in 2 parts of glycerol; very slightly soluble in alcohol.

Standard
It complies with the requirements of the British Pharmacopoeia.
It occurs as a slightly hygroscopic, white, odourless, crystalline powder or granular crystals and contains not less than 99·0 and not more than the equivalent of 101·0 per cent of $C_6H_5K_3O_7,H_2O$.

Storage. It should be stored in airtight containers.

Actions and uses. Potassium citrate has the actions of the alkali citrates and is used principally to make the urine alkaline, as described under Sodium Citrate (page 449).

Dose. Up to 10 grams daily in divided doses.

Preparations
POTASSIUM CITRATE AND HYOSCYAMUS MIXTURE, B.P.C. (page 751)
POTASSIUM CITRATE MIXTURE, B.P.C. (page 750)

POTASSIUM GLUCONATE

$C_6H_{11}KO_7 = 234\cdot2$

$$HO\cdot CH_2\cdot[CH(OH)]_4\cdot CO_2K$$

Potassium Gluconate is the potassium salt of gluconic acid and may be prepared by neutralising gluconic acid with potassium carbonate and evaporating the solution.

Solubility. Soluble, at 20°, in 3 parts of water; very slightly soluble in alcohol; insoluble in chloroform and in ether.

Standard
DESCRIPTION. A white crystalline powder; odourless or almost odourless.

IDENTIFICATION TESTS. 1. Dissolve 0·05 g in 1 ml of water and add 0·05 ml of *ferric chloride test-solution*; an intense yellow colour is produced.
2. Dissolve 0·5 g in 5 ml of warm water, add 0·65 ml of *glacial acetic acid* and 1 ml of *phenylhydrazine*, heat on a water-bath for 30 minutes, cool, and induce crystallisation; white crystals are formed which, after recrystallising from water, with the addition of *decolorising charcoal*, and drying at 105°, melt at about 200°, with decomposition.
3. Ignite 0·5 g; dissolve the residue in 2 ml of *dilute hydrochloric acid* and filter; the filtrate gives the reactions characteristic of solutions of potassium salts.

ACIDITY OR ALKALINITY. 1·0 g dissolved in 25 ml of *carbon dioxide-free water* requires for neutralisation not more than 0·5 ml of 0·1N sodium hydroxide or of 0·1N hydrochloric acid, *phenolphthalein solution* being used as indicator.

ARSENIC. It complies with the test given in Appendix 6, page 879 (2 parts per million).

LEAD. It complies with the test given in Appendix 7, page 883 (10 parts per million).

CHLORIDE. 0·5 g complies with the limit test for chlorides (700 parts per million).

SULPHATE. 1·0 g complies with the limit test for sulphates (600 parts per million).

DEXTROSE AND SUCROSE. Dissolve 0·50 g in 10 ml of hot water, add 2 ml of *dilute hydrochloric acid*, boil for 2 minutes, cool, and add 15 ml of *sodium carbonate solution*; add 5 ml of this solution to 2 ml of *potassium cupri-tartrate solution* and boil for one minute; no red precipitate is formed.

LOSS ON DRYING. Not more than 2·0 per cent, determined by drying to constant weight at 105°.

CONTENT OF $C_6H_{11}KO_7$. Not less than 99·0 per cent, calculated with reference to the substance dried under the prescribed conditions, determined by the following method:
Titrate about 0·5 g, accurately weighed, by Method I of the British Pharmacopoeia, Appendix XIB, for non-aqueous titration; each ml of 0·1N perchloric acid is equivalent to 0·02342 g of $C_6H_{11}KO_7$.

Actions and uses. Potassium gluconate is almost tasteless and is therefore convenient for the oral administration of potassium supplements to patients undergoing diuretic therapy when there is danger of potassium depletion.

Dose. 5 to 10 grams (20 to 40 millimoles, or milliequivalents, of K^+).

OTHER NAME: *Katorin*®

POTASSIUM HYDROXIDE

SYNONYM: Caustic Potash

KOH = 56·11

Potassium Hydroxide may be obtained by the electrolysis of an aqueous solution of potassium chloride.

Solubility. Soluble or almost completely soluble, at 20°, in 1 part of water and in 3 parts of alcohol; very soluble in boiling dehydrated alcohol.

Standard
It complies with the requirements of the British Pharmacopoeia.
It occurs as white sticks, pellets, or fused masses, which are dry, hard, and brittle, very deliquescent, and break with a crystalline fracture. It contains not less than 85·0 per cent of total alkali, calculated as KOH, and not more than 4·0 per cent of K_2CO_3.
It is strongly alkaline and corrosive and rapidly destroys organic tissues.
It may be freed from carbonate by solution in alcohol, filtration, and evaporation.

Hygroscopicity. When exposed to the air, it absorbs moisture and carbon dioxide.

Storage. It should be stored in airtight containers; if the containers are made of glass they should be closed by waxed corks or plastic-lined screw caps.

Actions and uses. Potassium hydroxide is a powerful caustic. A 2·5 per cent solution in glycerol is used as a cuticle solvent.

POISONING. Large draughts of water containing vinegar, acetic acid, citric acid, or lemon juice should be given, followed by demulcent drinks and olive oil or arachis oil.
Burns due to potassium hydroxide should be flooded with water and then with dilute acetic acid.

Preparation
POTASSIUM HYDROXIDE SOLUTION, B.P. (*Syn.* Potash Solution). It contains 5 per cent w/v of total alkali, calculated as KOH. It should be stored in airtight bottles of lead-free glass or of a suitable plastic.

POTASSIUM HYDROXYQUINOLINE SULPHATE

SYNONYM: Potassium Oxyquinoline Sulphate

Potassium Hydroxyquinoline Sulphate consists of an equimolecular mixture of 8-hydroxyquinoline sulphate, $(C_9H_7NO)_2,H_2SO_4$, and potassium sulphate, and may be prepared by mixing intimately the two substances.

Potassium Hydroxyquinoline Sulphate partly liquefies between 172° and 184°. A 5 per cent solution in carbon dioxide-free water has a pH of about 3. On extraction with hot alcohol, a residue of potassium sulphate and a solution of 8-hydroxyquinoline sulphate are obtained.

Solubility. Soluble, at 20°, in 2 parts of water; insoluble in ether.

Standard
DESCRIPTION. A pale yellow microcrystalline powder; odour slight.

IDENTIFICATION TESTS. 1. To 5 ml of a 5 per cent w/v solution in water add 0·5 ml of *ferric chloride test-solution*; a bright green colour is produced.
2. To 5 ml of a 5 per cent w/v solution in water add 1 ml of *dilute hydrochloric acid* and 1 ml of *barium chloride solution*; a white precipitate is formed.
3. To 5 ml of a 5 per cent w/v solution in water add 2 ml of *bromine solution*; a precipitate is formed, which, after washing with water and drying at 105°, melts at about 190°.
4. To 5 ml of a 5 per cent w/v solution in water add 0·5 ml of *sodium hydroxide solution*; a precipitate of 8-hydroxyquinoline, melting at about 75°, is formed, which redissolves in excess of alkali.
5. Ignite; the residue gives the reactions characteristic of potassium.

WATER. Not more than 5·0 per cent w/w, determined by the method given in Appendix 16, page 895.

SULPHATED ASH. 31·0 to 34·0 per cent, calculated with reference to the anhydrous substance.

CONTENT OF 8-HYDROXYQUINOLINE. 49·0 to 51·0 per cent, calculated as C_9H_7NO, with reference to the anhydrous substance, determined by the following method:
Dissolve about 0·35 g, accurately weighed, in 50 ml of water and 20 ml of *hydrochloric acid* in a glass-stoppered flask; add 50 ml of 0·1N bromine, shake repeatedly during 15 minutes, allow to stand for 15 minutes, and dilute to 200 ml with water; add 10 ml of *potassium iodide solution* and titrate the liberated iodine with 0·1N sodium thiosulphate, using *starch mucilage* as indicator.
Repeat the procedure omitting the sample.
The difference between the two titrations represents the amount of bromine required by the sample; each ml of 0·1N bromine is equivalent to 0·003629 g of C_9H_7NO.

Incompatibility. A solution of potassium hydroxyquinoline sulphate gives with many metallic salts precipitates of co-ordination complexes of 8-hydroxyquinoline (oxine).

Actions and uses. Potassium hydroxyquinoline sulphate has antibacterial and deodorant properties.
For mycosis and secondarily infected eczema it is applied to the skin as a lotion or application containing 0·05 to 0·2 per cent.

POTASSIUM IODIDE

SYNONYMS: Kalii Iodidum; Pot. Iod.

KI = 166·0

Solubility. Soluble, at 20°, in less than 1 part of water, in 23 parts of alcohol, and in 2 parts of glycerol.

AQUEOUS SOLUTIONS. A marked fall in the temperature of the solution occurs when potassium iodide dissolves in water to form a strong solution; when sodium iodide dissolves a considerable rise in temperature occurs. Iodine readily dissolves in an aqueous solution of potassium iodide, forming a dark-brown solution containing potassium tri-iodide. Certain iodides, such as mercuric iodide, which are insoluble in water, also dissolve in an aqueous solution, double iodides being formed.

Standard

It complies with the requirements of the European Pharmacopoeia.

It occurs as odourless, colourless crystals or white powder and contains not less than 99·0 per cent of KI, calculated with reference to the dried substance. The loss on drying under the prescribed conditions is not more than 1·0 per cent. A solution in water may be slightly alkaline.

Incompatibility. It is incompatible with salts of iron, bismuth, and mercury, with potassium chlorate and other oxidising agents, and with strychnine hydrochloride, quinine sulphate, and other alkaloidal salts.

Storage. It should be stored in airtight containers, protected from light.

Actions and uses. Potassium iodide is rapidly absorbed when given by mouth and is rapidly excreted, mainly by the kidneys and partly by the salivary, mucous, and other glands. Its secretion by the salivary glands is the cause of the persistent unpleasant taste.

It may be used for the prophylaxis and treatment of simple goitre, which is endemic in districts where the diet is deficient in iodides. Potassium iodide, or Aqueous Iodine Solution, is administered by mouth for ten to fourteen days prior to surgical operation on the thyroid gland in order to produce a firm texture suitable for operation. This treatment should not be continued for more than three weeks after the operation.

Potassium iodide is also used as an expectorant.

Potassium iodide is usually administered in mixtures or in solution, freely diluted, since concentrated solutions have an irritant action on the gastric mucosa.

UNDESIRABLE EFFECTS. Intolerance to iodides sometimes occurs, the symptoms being nasal catarrh, lachrymation, rashes of variable character, headache, and depression. Some patients showing idiosyncrasy to small doses appear to tolerate larger doses.

Dose. As an expectorant: 250 to 500 milligrams.

In the pre-operative treatment of thyrotoxicosis: 150 milligrams daily in divided doses.

Preparations

BELLADONNA AND EPHEDRINE MIXTURE, PAEDIATRIC, B.P.C. (page 737)

LOBELIA AND STRAMONIUM MIXTURE, COMPOUND, B.P.C. (page 746)

POTASSIUM IODIDE MIXTURE, AMMONIATED, B.P.C. (page 751)

STRAMONIUM AND POTASSIUM IODIDE MIXTURE, B.P.C. (page 753)

POTASSIUM NITRATE

KNO$_3$ = 101·1

Potassium Nitrate may be obtained by the interaction of sodium nitrate and potassium chloride.

Solubility. Soluble, at 20°, in 3·3 parts of water; slightly soluble in alcohol.

Standard

It complies with the requirements of the British Pharmacopoeia.

It occurs as an odourless, white, crystalline powder or colourless crystals and contains not less than 99·0 per cent of KNO$_3$.

Stability. When heated above 350°, potassium nitrate decomposes, giving off oxygen and leaving a residue of potassium nitrate and nitrite. In contact with red-hot carbon it deflagrates.

Use. Potassium nitrate is an ingredient of Toughened Silver Nitrate.

POTASSIUM PERMANGANATE

SYNONYMS: Kalii Permanganas; Pot. Permang.

KMnO$_4$ = 158·0

Solubility. Soluble, at 20°, in 16 parts of water; freely soluble in boiling water.

Standard

It complies with the requirements of the European Pharmacopoeia.

It occurs as dark purple or almost black crystals, often with a metallic lustre, and contains not less than 99·0 per cent of KMnO$_4$.

Incompatibility. It is incompatible with iodides, reducing agents, and most organic matter.

An acidified solution in water is readily reduced by hydrogen peroxide, by easily oxidisable substances, and by organic matter.

Storage. It should be stored so as to avoid contact with organic substances.

Actions and uses. Potassium permanganate, because of its oxidising action, possesses disinfectant and deodorant properties. It is used as a 1 in 1000 solution in water as a cleansing application to ulcers or abscesses, 1 in 4000 as a gargle, mouth-wash, or vaginal irrigation, and 1 in 10,000 to 1 in 5000 for application to weeping skin lesions and for urethral irrigation.

Potassium permanganate has been widely used as a first-aid treatment in snake bite but it is of no value for this purpose although a solution will destroy any venom on the surface of the skin.

Solutions of potassium permanganate rapidly stain the skin brown; the stain can be removed by means of oxalic or sulphurous acid.

POTASSIUM SORBATE

$C_6H_7KO_2 = 150 \cdot 2$

$$CH_3 \cdot CH:CH \cdot CH:CH \cdot CO_2K$$

Potassium Sorbate is the potassium salt of 2,4-hexadienoic acid.

Solubility. Soluble, at 20°, in less than 1 part of water and in 70 parts of alcohol; very slightly soluble in acetone.

Standard
DESCRIPTION. A white or creamy-white powder; odour faint and characteristic.

IDENTIFICATION TESTS. 1. To a solution in water add *bromine solution*, dropwise; the bromine solution is decolorised.

2. The ultraviolet absorption spectrum exhibits the characteristics given in Appendix 3, page 856.

3. The infra-red absorption spectrum exhibits maxima which are only at the same wavelengths as, and have similar relative intensities to, those in the spectrum of *potassium sorbate A.S.*

4. Ignite; the residue gives the reactions characteristic of potassium.

ACIDITY OR ALKALINITY. A solution in water is neutral to *litmus solution*.

ARSENIC. It complies with the test given in Appendix 6, page 879 (2 parts per million).

LEAD. It complies with the test given in Appendix 7, page 883 (10 parts per million).

WATER. Not more than 1·0 per cent w/w, determined by the method given in Appendix 16, page 895.

CONTENT OF $C_6H_7KO_2$. Not less than 99·0 and not more than the equivalent of 101·0 per cent, calculated with reference to the anhydrous substance, determined by the following method:
Titrate about 0·5 g, accurately weighed, by Method I of the British Pharmacopoeia, Appendix XIB, for non-aqueous titration; each ml of 0·1N perchloric acid is equivalent to 0·01502 g of $C_6H_7KO_2$.

Storage. It should be stored in airtight containers, protected from light, in a cool place.

Uses. Potassium sorbate has the uses described under Sorbic Acid (page 465) but it is more soluble in water.

POVIDONE

SYNONYM: Polyvinylpyrrolidone

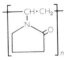

Povidone is the pharmaceutical grade of polyvinylpyrrolidone. There are two types, one suitable for oral ingestion and topical application and the other for parenteral administration. The standard in this monograph applies only to the former type used as a pharmaceutical adjuvant in oral preparations; additional requirements are necessary for the injectable material. Povidone is sometimes commercially designated with a "K number", which is a figure derived from the viscosity. Materials of different "K numbers" have slightly differing properties.

Polyvinylpyrrolidone consists of essentially linear polymers of 1-vinylpyrrolid-2-one. Variation in the degree of polymerisation results in the production of polymers with different chain lengths and consequently various molecular weights.
Polyvinylpyrrolidone is available commercially as a number of mixtures of polymers, each product having a particular mean molecular weight, which is in the range 10,000 to 700,000. Some of the physical properties of polyvinylpyrrolidone depend upon the mean molecular weight; for example, solubilities decrease with increasing molecular weight and viscosities of solutions increase. The viscosities of aqueous solutions containing up to 10 per cent of povidone do not differ significantly from that of water.

Solubility. Readily soluble in water, in alcohol, and in chloroform, the solubility depending on the mean molecular weight; insoluble in ether.

Standard
DESCRIPTION. A white or creamy-white powder; odourless or almost odourless.

IDENTIFICATION TESTS. 1. To 10 ml of a 2 per cent w/v solution in water add 20 ml of 1N hydrochloric acid and 5 ml of *potassium dichromate solution*; an orange-yellow precipitate is formed.

2. Add 5 ml of a 2 per cent w/v solution in water to 2 ml of *ammonium cobaltothiocyanate solution* which has been acidified with 5N hydrochloric acid; a pale blue precipitate is formed.

3. To 5 ml of a 0·5 per cent w/v solution in water add 0·2 ml of 0·1N iodine; a deep red colour is produced.

ARSENIC. It complies with the test given in Appendix 6, page 879 (2 parts per million).

LEAD. It complies with the test given in Appendix 7, page 883 (10 parts per million).

ALDEHYDES. Not more than 0·5 per cent, calculated as CH₃·CHO, determined by the following method: Add 10 g to 180 ml of *sulphuric acid (25 per cent v/v)* contained in a round-bottom flask, and attach the flask to a reflux condenser, the top of which is connected by means of an inverted U-shaped adaptor to the top of another vertical condenser at the lower end of which is attached a receiver, cooled in ice and containing 20 ml of 1N hydroxyammonium chloride.
Heat the solution in the flask under reflux for 45 minutes, discontinue the water supply to the reflux condenser, distil until about 100 ml of distillate is collected in the receiver, and titrate the contents of the receiver with 0·1N sodium hydroxide, using *bromophenol blue solution* as indicator.
Repeat the procedure omitting the sample.
The difference between the two titrations represents the amount of 0·1N sodium hydroxide equivalent to the aldehydes present; each ml of 0·1N sodium hydroxide is equivalent to 0·004405 g of CH₃·CHO.

VINYLPYRROLIDONE. Not more than 1·0 per cent, calculated as C₆H₉NO, determined by the following method:
Dissolve about 4 g, accurately weighed, in 30 ml of water, add 0·50 g of *sodium acetate*, and titrate the solution with 0·1N iodine until the colour due to iodine no longer fades; add a further 3 ml of 0·1N iodine, allow to stand for 10 minutes, and titrate the excess iodine with 0·1N sodium thiosulphate, using *starch mucilage* as indicator; each ml of 0·1N iodine is equivalent to 0·005557 g of C₆H₉NO.

WATER. Not more than 5·0 per cent w/w, determined by the method given in Appendix 16, page 895.

SULPHATED ASH. Not more than 0·1 per cent.

TOTAL NITROGEN. 12·0 to 13·0 per cent, calculated as N, with reference to the anhydrous substance, determined by Method I of the British Pharmacopoeia, Appendix X(L), for the determination of nitrogen, about 0·3 g, accurately weighed, and 11 ml of *nitrogen-free sulphuric acid* being used.

Hygroscopicity. Povidone is hygroscopic, significant amounts of moisture being absorbed even at low relative humidities; its equilibrium moisture content at 30, 50, and 70 per cent relative humidity is 10, 20, and 40 per cent, respectively.

Labelling. The label on the container states that the contents are not suitable for the preparation of injections.

Storage. It should be stored in airtight containers.

Uses. The type of povidone covered by the above standard is used in concentrations up to 10 per cent as a suspending and dispersing agent in aqueous oral preparations. As a tablet binder it is used in concentrations of 0·5 to 5 per cent; it is particularly useful in effervescent tablets and for other granulation processes in which a non-aqueous liquid excipient is used. It is also used in conjunction with acetylated monoglycerides or polyvinyl alcohol in the film coating of tablets. An injectable type of povidone, which is not covered by the above standard, has been used as a plasma extender.
Non-pharmaceutical grades of polyvinyl-pyrrolidone are used in a number of cosmetic preparations such as skin sprays and hair lacquers.

OTHER NAME: *Plasdone K®*

PRACTOLOL

C₁₄H₂₂N₂O₃ = 266·3

Practolol is (±)-4-(2-hydroxy-3-isopropylaminopropoxy)acetanilide.

Solubility. Soluble in 400 parts of water, in 40 parts of alcohol, and in 200 parts of chloroform.

Standard
It complies with the requirements of the British Pharmacopoeia.
It is a fine, white or almost white, odourless powder and contains not less than 99·0 and not more than the equivalent of 101·0 per cent of C₁₄H₂₂N₂O₃, calculated with reference to the dried substance. The loss on drying under the prescribed conditions is not more than 0·5 per cent. It has a melting-point of 141° to 144°.

Stability of solutions. Aqueous solutions are most stable at pH6, and such solutions may be sterilised by heating in an autoclave and stored at room temperature, protected from light.

Hygroscopicity. It absorbs insignificant amounts of moisture at 25° at relative humidities up to about 80 per cent.

Storage. It should be protected from light.

Actions and uses. Practolol has actions and uses similar to those described under Propranolol Hydrochloride (page 412) but it is more specific in its inhibiting effect on sympathetic stimulation of the heart and has less effect on respiratory function.

UNDESIRABLE EFFECTS. These are as described under Propranolol Hydrochloride (page 412).

Dose. 200 to 900 milligrams daily in divided doses by mouth; 5 to 20 milligrams by slow intravenous injection.

Preparations
PRACTOLOL INJECTION, B.P. It consists of a sterile solution of practolol in Water for Injections containing citric acid. Unless otherwise specified, a solution containing 2 mg in 1 ml is supplied.

PRACTOLOL TABLETS, B.P. Unless otherwise specified, tablets each containing 100 mg of practolol are supplied.

OTHER NAME: *Eraldin®*

PREDNISOLONE

SYNONYM: Prednisolonum

$C_{21}H_{28}O_5 = 360.4$

Prednisolone is $11\beta,17\alpha,21$-trihydroxypregna-1,4-diene-3,20-dione.

Solubility. Slightly soluble in water; soluble, at 20°, in 27 parts of dehydrated alcohol; soluble in dioxan and in methyl alcohol.

Standard
It complies with the requirements of the European Pharmacopoeia.
It is a white or almost white, crystalline, hygroscopic, odourless powder and contains not less than 96.0 and not more than the equivalent of 104.0 per cent of $C_{21}H_{28}O_5$, calculated with reference to the dried substance. The loss on drying under the prescribed conditions is not more than 1.0 per cent. It melts with decomposition at about 230°.

Preparation of solid dosage forms. In order to achieve a satisfactory rate of dissolution, prednisolone in the form of an ultra-fine powder should be used.

Storage. It should be stored in airtight containers, protected from light.

Actions and uses. Prednisolone has the actions and uses described under Cortisone Acetate (page 132) but it is effective in about one-fifth to one-quarter of the dosage; in such dosage it has a weaker sodium-retaining effect than cortisone.

It is used especially for its anti-inflammatory action in the treatment of conditions where a cortisone-like action is required and, because of its weaker sodium-retaining action, it is usually to be preferred to cortisone in such conditions as rheumatoid arthritis, rheumatic fever, status asthmaticus, and ulcerative colitis. It is useful in the treatment of nephrotic oedema, as it produces diuresis. It is not used alone in the treatment of adrenal-deficiency states because of its weak salt-retaining effect.

Prednisolone is given by mouth, the dosage being adjusted to the needs of the patient and varying widely according to the disorder being treated.

In rheumatoid arthritis a single dose of 5 milligrams given by mouth at night will often ease night and early morning symptoms. For long-term suppressive treatment of rheumatoid arthritis the minimum dosage giving a satisfactory response should be used; not more than 7 milligrams daily should be given as otherwise the usual undesirable effects of long-term corticosteroid therapy will inevitably occur.

A somewhat higher regular maintenance dosage is usually necessary in the treatment of asthma, and prednisolone is also used in large daily doses such as 100 to 200 milligrams as an immunosuppressive agent for organ transplantation. In addition, single large doses such as 1 gram have been given intravenously in the form of soluble prednisolone compounds to prevent organ rejection after renal transplantation.

In conditions dangerous to life, such as pemphigus vulgaris, systemic lupus erythematosus, leukaemia, and acute haemolytic crises, high dosage, if necessary up to 100 milligrams daily, is permissible. In conditions such as status asthmaticus up to 60 milligrams daily may be given, although in severe crises intravenous administration of hydrocortisone or corticotrophin may be preferred.

UNDESIRABLE EFFECTS. These are the same as those described under Cortisone Acetate (page 132), the features of Cushing's syndrome becoming apparent on full dosage. Dyspepsia is common and peptic ulceration may occur.

PRECAUTIONS AND CONTRA-INDICATIONS. As for Cortisone Acetate (page 132).

Dose. See above under **Actions and uses.**

Preparation
PREDNISOLONE TABLETS, B.P. Unless otherwise specified, tablets each containing 5 mg of prednisolone are supplied. They should be stored in airtight containers, protected from light. Tablets containing 1 mg are also available.

OTHER NAMES: *Codelcortone®*; *Delta-cortef®*; *Deltacortril®*; *Delta-genacort®*; *Deltalone®*; *Deltastab®*; *Di-Adreson-F®*; *Marsolone®*; *PreCortisyl®*; *Prednelan®*

PREDNISOLONE PIVALATE

SYNONYM: Prednisolone Trimethylacetate

$C_{26}H_{36}O_6 = 444.6$

Prednisolone Pivalate is $11\beta,17\alpha$-dihydroxy-21-pivaloyl-oxypregna-1,4-diene-3,20-dione.

Solubility. Very slightly soluble in water; soluble, at 20°, in 150 parts of alcohol and in 16 parts of chloroform.

Standard
It complies with the requirements of the British Pharmacopoeia.

It is a white or almost white, crystalline, odourless powder and contains not less than 96·0 and not more than the equivalent of 104·0 per cent of $C_{26}H_{36}O_6$, calculated with reference to the dried substance. The loss on drying under the prescribed conditions is not more than 0·5 per cent. It has a melting-point of about 229°.

Storage. It should be stored in airtight containers, protected from light.

Actions and uses. Prednisolone pivalate may be given as a microcrystalline suspension by intra-articular injection in rheumatoid and other forms of arthritis to reduce swelling and facilitate movement.

Suspensions for injection are prepared by an aseptic technique.

PRECAUTIONS AND CONTRA-INDICATIONS. As for Cortisone Acetate (page 132).

Dose. 5 to 20 milligrams by intra-articular injection or local infiltration.

Preparation
PREDNISOLONE PIVALATE INJECTION, B.P. It consists of a sterile suspension of prednisolone pivalate, in very fine particles, in Water for Injections containing suitable dispersing, stabilising, and buffering agents. Unless otherwise specified, a suspension containing 10 mg in 1 ml is supplied. It should be stored at room temperature and protected from light. A suspension containing 50 mg in 1 ml is also available.

OTHER NAME: *Ultracortenol*®

PREDNISOLONE SODIUM PHOSPHATE

SYNONYM: Prednisolone Sod. Phos.

$C_{21}H_{27}Na_2O_8P = 484·4$

Prednisolone Sodium Phosphate is the disodium salt of the 21-phosphate ester of $11\beta,17\alpha,21$-trihydroxypregna-1,4-diene-3,20-dione.

Solubility. Soluble, at 20°, in 3 parts of water and in 1000 parts of alcohol; insoluble in chloroform.

Standard
It complies with the requirements of the British Pharmacopoeia.
It is a white or almost white, hygroscopic, odourless powder and contains not less than 96·0 and not more than the equivalent of 103·0 per cent of $C_{21}H_{27}Na_2O_8P$, calculated with reference to the anhydrous substance. It contains not more than 8·0 per cent w/w of water. A 0·5 per cent solution in water has a pH of 7·5 to 9·0.

Stability. Aqueous solutions having a pH of about 8·0 are stable if protected from light. Particular care must be taken to prevent microbial contamination of the solutions so as to avoid hydrolysis of the ester by phosphatase which is a common product of microbial metabolism.

Sterilisation. Solutions for injection are sterilised by filtration.

Storage. It should be stored in airtight containers, protected from light.

Actions and uses. Prednisolone sodium phosphate has the actions, uses, and undesirable effects described under Prednisolone (page 399).
It is soluble in water and is used in eye-drops and other preparations for topical therapy in inflammatory or allergic conditions of the eye or skin.
It may be given by intravenous injection, in a dose equivalent to 20 to 100 milligrams of prednisolone, when a more rapid effect is required; 135 milligrams of prednisolone sodium phosphate is approximately equivalent to 100 milligrams of prednisolone.
It is also given by intra-articular injection in rheumatoid arthritis to relieve local pain and swelling in affected joints.

PRECAUTIONS AND CONTRA-INDICATIONS. As for Cortisone Acetate (page 132).

Dose. See above under **Actions and uses.**

Preparations
PREDNISOLONE ENEMA, B.P.C. (page 681)
PREDNISOLONE EYE-DROPS, B.P.C. (page 694)
PREDNISOLONE SODIUM PHOSPHATE INJECTION, B.P. It consists of prednisolone sodium phosphate in Water for Injections; it contains suitable stabilising agents and may contain a suitable buffering agent. Unless otherwise specified, a solution containing the equivalent of 20 mg of prednisolone in 1 ml is supplied. It should be stored protected from light at a temperature not exceeding 25°.

OTHER NAMES: *Codelsol*®; *Prednesol*®; *Predsol*®

PREDNISONE

SYNONYM: Prednisonum

$C_{21}H_{26}O_5 = 358·4$

Prednisone is $17\alpha,21$-dihydroxypregna-1,4-diene-3,11,20-trione.

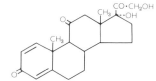

Solubility. Very slightly soluble in water; soluble, at 20°, in 190 parts of alcohol, in 300 parts of dehydrated alcohol, and in 200 parts of chloroform.

Standard
It complies with the requirements of the European Pharmacopoeia.

It is a white or almost white, crystalline, odourless powder and contains not less than 96·0 and not more than the equivalent of 104·0 per cent of $C_{21}H_{26}O_5$, calculated with reference to the dried substance. The loss on drying under the prescribed conditions is not more than 1·0 per cent. It melts with decomposition at about 230°.

Preparation of solid dosage forms. In order to achieve a satisfactory rate of dissolution, prednisone in the form of an ultra-fine powder should be used.

Storage. It should be protected from light.

Actions and uses. Prednisone is readily converted in the liver to prednisolone (page 399)

and there is no significant difference between the effects of the two substances.

UNDESIRABLE EFFECTS. As for Prednisolone (page 399).

PRECAUTIONS AND CONTRA-INDICATIONS. As for Cortisone Acetate (page 132).

Dose. As for Prednisolone (page 399).

Preparation
PREDNISONE TABLETS, B.P. Unless otherwise specified, tablets each containing 5 mg of prednisone are supplied. They should be protected from light. Tablets containing 1 mg are also available.

OTHER NAMES: *Anpisone®*; Deltadehydrocortisone; *DeCortisyl®*; *Delta-Cortelan®*; *Deltacortone®*; *Di-Adreson®*; *Marsone®*

PRILOCAINE HYDROCHLORIDE

$C_{13}H_{21}ClN_2O = 256·8$

Prilocaine Hydrochloride is α-propylaminopropio-*o*-toluidide hydrochloride.

Solubility. Soluble, at 20°, in 5 parts of water and in 6 parts of alcohol; insoluble in ether.

Standard
It complies with the requirements of the British Pharmacopoeia.
It is a white, crystalline, odourless powder and contains not less than 99·0 and not more than the equivalent of 101·0 per cent of $C_{13}H_{21}ClN_2O$, calculated with reference to the dried substance. The loss on drying under the prescribed conditions is not more than 0·5 per cent. It has a melting-point of 167° to 169°.

Sterilisation. Solutions for injection are sterilised by heating in an autoclave or by filtration.

Storage. It should be stored in airtight containers.

Actions and uses. Prilocaine is a local anaesthetic with properties similar to lignocaine but it is less toxic and less liable to cause vasodilatation. It is used in dentistry and to produce infiltration and spinal anaesthesia. The total quantity of prilocaine hydrochloride should not exceed 400 milligrams unless adrenaline is present, when up to 600 milligrams may be given.
Solutions containing 0·5, 1·0, 1·5, and 4·0 per

cent of prilocaine hydrochloride, and 0·5 per cent of prilocaine hydrochloride with adrenaline 1 in 250,000, and 1·0 per cent of prilocaine hydrochloride with adrenaline 1 in 200,000 are available; solutions containing 3·0 per cent of prilocaine hydrochloride with adrenaline 1 in 300,000 or felypressin 0·03 unit per millilitre are available for dental purposes.

UNDESIRABLE EFFECTS. Like other local anaesthetics, prilocaine may stimulate the central nervous system.

PRECAUTIONS AND CONTRA-INDICATIONS. Overdosage may give rise to methaemoglobinaemia, and hence the use of prilocaine should be avoided in patients with anaemia. It should be used with caution in pregnancy as it may give rise to foetal methaemoglobinaemia.
Solutions containing adrenaline should not be used for inducing anaesthesia in digits because the profound ischaemia produced may lead to gangrene.

OTHER NAME: *Citanest®*

PRIMAQUINE PHOSPHATE

$C_{15}H_{27}N_3O_9P_2 = 455·3$

Primaquine Phosphate is 8-(4-amino-1-methylbutylamino)-6-methoxyquinoline di(dihydrogen phosphate).

Solubility. Soluble, at 20°, in 16 parts of water; insoluble in alcohol, in ether, and in chloroform.

Standard
It complies with the requirements of the British Pharmacopoeia.
It is an orange-red, crystalline, odourless or almost odourless powder and contains not less than 97·5 per cent of $C_{15}H_{27}N_3O_9P_2$, calculated with reference to the dried substance. The loss on drying under the prescribed conditions is not more than 0·5 per cent. It has

a melting-point of about 200°. A 1 per cent solution in water has a pH of 2·5 to 3·5.

Stability. It is affected by light. Aqueous solutions are thermolabile; approximately half their activity is lost in 24 hours at 100°.

Hygroscopicity. It absorbs insignificant amounts of moisture at temperatures up to 37° at relative humidities up to about 80 per cent.

Storage. It should be protected from light.

Actions and uses. Primaquine is an anti-malarial drug which kills the exoerythrocytic stages of *Plasmodium vivax*, *P. ovale*, and *P. malariae* and the early pre-erythrocytic form of *P. falciparum*. It also kills gametocytes, or renders them incapable of development in the mosquito, but has little action on other erythrocytic stages and therefore should not be used alone in the treatment of a malarial attack.

Its chief use is for the radical cure of *P. vivax* infections in people returning from malarious areas. For this purpose, a short intensive course of treatment with a schizonticide such as chloroquine is given to kill any erythrocytic parasites, and this is followed by a course of fourteen daily doses of primaquine phosphate, each equivalent to 15 milligrams of the base, by mouth, to kill the tissue forms; 15 mg of primaquine base is approximately equivalent to 26·34 mg of primaquine phosphate.

Primaquine phosphate may also be given once a week for the prophylaxis of malaria in a dose equivalent to 30 to 60 milligrams of the base, together with the equivalent of 300 milligrams of chloroquine or amodiaquine.

UNDESIRABLE EFFECTS. The most common symptoms of overdosage are abdominal pain, methaemoglobinaemia, and, less frequently, haemolytic anaemia and methaemoglobinuria. Toxic effects occur most commonly in genetic groups with glucose-6-phosphate-dehydrogenase deficiency, a condition which is prevalent mostly among dark-skinned people.

Dose. See above under **Actions and uses.**

Preparation
PRIMAQUINE TABLETS, B.P. Unless otherwise specified, tablets each containing primaquinine phosphate equivalent to 7·5 mg of primaquine base are supplied. They are sugar coated.

PRIMIDONE

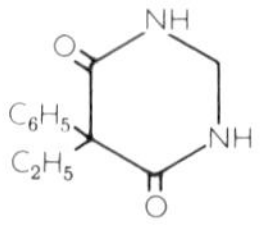

$C_{12}H_{14}N_2O_2 = 218·3$

Primidone is 5-ethylhexahydro-5-phenylpyrimidine-4,6-dione.

Solubility. Slightly soluble in water; soluble, at 20°, in 170 parts of alcohol; very slightly soluble in most organic solvents.

Standard
It complies with the requirements of the British Pharmacopoeia.
It is a white, crystalline, odourless powder and contains not less than 99·0 per cent of $C_{12}H_{14}N_2O_2$, calculated with reference to the dried substance. The loss on drying under the prescribed conditions is not more than 0·5 per cent. It has a melting-point of about 280°.

Actions and uses. Primidone is an effective anticonvulsant, particularly in grand mal and psychomotor attacks. It is used when adequate control is not obtainable with phenobarbitone and phenytoin. Any change-over of treatment should be gradual, both in introducing primidone and in withdrawing the previous treatment.
The initial dosage for adults and children over

nine years is 500 milligrams by mouth daily in divided doses, increased by 250 milligrams at intervals of three days up to a total daily dosage of 1 to 2 grams; for children under nine years these doses should be halved.

UNDESIRABLE EFFECTS. Toxic effects such as drowsiness, nausea, and rashes may occur, particularly during the first week of treatment, but are usually transient and the treatment may be continued, possibly with reduced dosage. Megaloblastic anaemia may occur.

Dose. See above under **Actions and uses.**

Preparations
PRIMIDONE MIXTURE, B.P.C. (page 751)
PRIMIDONE TABLETS, B.P. Unless otherwise specified, tablets each containing 250 mg of primidone are supplied.

OTHER NAME: *Mysoline*®

PROBENECID

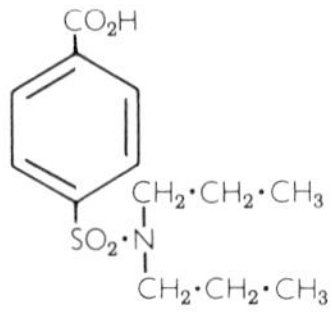

$C_{13}H_{19}NO_4S = 285·4$

Probenecid is *p*-(dipropylsulphamoyl)benzoic acid.

Solubility. Insoluble in water and in dilute mineral acids; soluble, at 20°, in 25 parts of alcohol and in 12 parts of acetone; soluble in dilute solutions of alkali hydroxides and of sodium bicarbonate.

Standard
It complies with the requirements of the British Pharmacopoeia.
It is a white or almost white, odourless, crystalline

powder and contains not less than 99·0 per cent of $C_{13}H_{19}NO_4S$, calculated with reference to the dried substance. The loss on drying under the prescribed conditions is not more than 0·5 per cent. It has a melting-point of about 199°.

Actions and uses. Probenecid is a uricosuric agent which is rapidly absorbed when given by mouth. In the treatment of gout it promotes excretion of urates by inhibiting tubular resorption, which results in a lowering of the elevated plasma–uric-acid levels and a slow depletion of urate deposits (tophi) in the tissues.

Probenecid reduces tubular excretion of penicillins, thereby increasing the plasma levels up to tenfold, and is therefore used as an adjunct to therapy in conditions such as subacute bacterial endocarditis, where very high levels of penicillins may be required. It may be used to reduce the rate of excretion of various penicillins, including ampicillin, benzylpenicillin, cloxacillin, methicillin, and phenoxymethylpenicillin, and it is also effective with cephalexin and cephalothin.

Probenecid has no analgesic action and no part to play in the treatment of acute gout, although acute attacks usually diminish some weeks after beginning treatment with the drug.

Probenecid is used to reduce the frequency of acute attacks of gout and to prevent the formation of new tophi and reduce those already present. Acute attacks of gout may be precipitated in the first few weeks or months of treatment with probenecid, particularly with high dosage; it is therefore usual to start treatment with a dosage of 250 milligrams twice daily by mouth and to increase it gradually, usually to 1·5 to 2 grams daily. Colchicine, in a dosage of 500 micrograms once or twice daily, may be given concurrently with the aim of reducing the incidence of such attacks. The dosage should be uninterrupted, as any irregularity of dosage leads to reduced urate output and increased plasma–uric-acid levels. Treatment must usually be continued for life.

Aspirin, citrates, and salicylates should not be given with probenecid as they antagonise its uricosuric effect.

UNDESIRABLE EFFECTS. These are rare with a daily dosage of up to 1 gram, but with dosage above this level, gastro-intestinal upsets, rashes and, occasionally, drug fever and hypersensitivity reactions may occur.

Dose. See above under **Actions and uses.**

Preparation
PROBENECID TABLETS, B.P. Unless otherwise specified, tablets each containing 500 mg of probenecid are supplied.

OTHER NAME: *Benemid*®

PROCAINAMIDE HYDROCHLORIDE

$C_{13}H_{22}ClN_3O = 271·8$

Procainamide Hydrochloride is *p*-amino-*N*-(2-diethylaminoethyl)-benzamide hydrochloride.

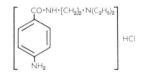

Solubility. Soluble, at 20°, in less than 1 part of water, in 2 parts of alcohol, and in 140 parts of chloroform; very slightly soluble in ether.

Standard
It complies with the requirements of the British Pharmacopoeia.
It is a white to yellowish-white, crystalline, hygroscopic, odourless powder and contains not less than 98·0 and not more than the equivalent of 101·0 per cent of $C_{13}H_{22}ClN_3O$, calculated with reference to the dried substance. The loss on drying under the prescribed conditions is not more than 1·0 per cent. It has a melting-point of 165° to 169°. A 10 per cent solution in water has a pH of 5·0 to 6·5.

Sterilisation. Solutions for injection are sterilised by heating in an autoclave.

Storage. It should be stored in airtight containers.

Actions and uses. Procainamide has actions similar to those described under Procaine Hydrochloride, but its effects, particularly on the heart, are more sustained than those of procaine. Like quinidine, it diminishes the excitability, conductivity, and contractility of both atrium and ventricle, and increases the refractory period of the atrium.

Procainamide is used to reduce the risk of fibrillation during thoracic surgery and in the treatment of arrhythmias and extrasystoles, especially those provoked by anaesthetics. It is given by slow intravenous infusion as a 2·5 per cent solution of procainamide hydrochloride in doses of up to 1 gram. It may also be given by mouth; the dosage should rarely exceed 1 gram every three hours.

UNDESIRABLE EFFECTS. Intravenous administration of procainamide may precipitate a grave fall in blood pressure. Large oral doses may cause such nausea that treatment has to be discontinued. A condition resembling lupus erythematosus may develop, especially when the procainamide is given orally over a long period.

Dose. See above under **Actions and uses.**

Preparations
PROCAINAMIDE INJECTION, B.P. It consists of a sterile

solution of procainamide hydrochloride with benzyl alcohol and 0·1 per cent of sodium metabisulphite in Water for Injections. Unless otherwise specified, a solution containing 100 mg in 1 ml is supplied.

PROCAINAMIDE TABLETS, B.P. Unless otherwise specified, tablets each containing 250 mg of procainamide hydrochloride are supplied. They should be stored in airtight containers.

OTHER NAME: *Pronestyl*®

PROCAINE HYDROCHLORIDE

SYNONYM: Procainii Chloridum

$C_{13}H_{21}ClN_2O_2 = 272\cdot8$

Procaine Hydrochloride is 2-diethylaminoethyl *p*-aminobenzoate hydrochloride.

Solubility. Soluble, at 20°, in 1 part of water and in 25 parts of alcohol; slightly soluble in chloroform; insoluble in ether.

Standard
It complies with the requirements of the European Pharmacopoeia.
It occurs as odourless colourless crystals or white crystalline powder and contains not less than 99·0 per cent of $C_{13}H_{21}ClN_2O_2$, calculated with reference to the dried substance. The loss on drying under the prescribed conditions is not more than 0·5 per cent. It has a melting-point of 154° to 157°. A 2 per cent solution in water has a pH of 5·0 to 6·5.

Sterilisation. Solutions for injection are sterilised by heating in an autoclave or by filtration.

Storage. It should be protected from light.

Actions and uses. Procaine is a short-acting local anaesthetic. It is less toxic than cocaine, but because of its poor penetration of intact mucous membranes, it is useless for surface application. To prolong its effect, adrenaline, in a concentration of 1 in 400,000 to 1 in 50,000, is added to constrict the blood vessels at the site of injection.
Procaine and Adrenaline Injection is used for infiltration anaesthesia. Solutions containing adrenaline should not, however, be used for inducing anaesthesia in digits, because the profound ischaemia produced may lead to gangrene.
Procaine hydrochloride may be given intrathecally as a 2 to 10 per cent aqueous solution or as a 5 to 10 per cent solution in cerebrospinal fluid. A 5 per cent aqueous solution is

isotonic with blood serum; to increase its specific gravity for intrathecal injection, 5 per cent of dextrose may be added. A 1 per cent solution is used in caudal anaesthesia. For epidural anaesthesia the strength of the solution should not be more than 5 per cent.
In dental practice, procaine has been largely replaced by lignocaine for the production of local anaesthesia. It was formerly used as Procaine and Adrenaline Injection; the effect of 1 to 2 millilitres appears in about five minutes and lasts for half an hour to two hours.

UNDESIRABLE EFFECTS. Constant wetting of the skin with solutions of procaine hydrochloride may cause a dermatitis characterised by dryness and cracking of the skin.

POISONING. Artificial respiration should be applied and a barbiturate administered intravenously to control the convulsions. The toxic action of procaine may be reduced by a preliminary dose of phenobarbitone or other barbiturate.

Preparations
PROCAINE AND ADRENALINE INJECTION, B.P. (*Syn.* Strong Procaine and Adrenaline Injection). It consists of a sterile solution containing 2 per cent of procaine hydrochloride and adrenaline 1 in 50,000. It should be protected from light.

TETRACYCLINE AND PROCAINE INJECTION, B.P.C. (page 719)

PROCAINE PENICILLIN

SYNONYMS: Procaine Benzylpenicillin; Procaine Penicillin G

$C_{13}H_{20}N_2O_2,C_{16}H_{18}N_2O_4S,H_2O = 588\cdot7$

Procaine Penicillin is the monohydrate of the procaine salt of benzylpenicillin.

Solubility. Soluble, at 20°, in 200 parts of water.

Standard
It complies with the requirements of the British Pharmacopoeia.
It is a white crystalline powder and contains not less than 96·0 per cent of total penicillins and 37·5 to 40·5 per cent of procaine, $C_{13}H_{20}N_2O_2$. It contains not more than 4·2 per cent w/w of water. A 30 per cent suspension in water has a pH of 5·0 to 7·5.

Labelling. If the material is not intended for parenteral administration, the label on the container states that the contents are not to be injected.

Storage. It should be stored in airtight containers at a temperature not exceeding 30°. If it is intended for parenteral administration, the containers should be sterile and sealed to exclude micro-organisms.

Actions and uses. Procaine penicillin is a sparingly soluble salt of benzylpenicillin. It is administered intramuscularly to create a depot from which benzylpenicillin is slowly released into the blood stream. A dose of 300 to 900 milligrams may be expected to maintain an effective concentration in the blood for about twenty-four hours, so that injections need not be given more frequently than once a day; 300 milligrams of procaine penicillin is approximately equivalent to 200 milligrams of benzylpenicillin.

Procaine penicillin has the uses described under Benzylpenicillin (page 51); it is frequently mixed with benzylpenicillin, as in the fortified injection, the mixture being particularly useful at the beginning of treatment.

Procaine penicillin is usually administered by injection as an aqueous suspension. Injections prepared with an oily medium are also available, sometimes with the addition of aluminium stearate, but they appear to have no advantage over an adequate dose of one of the aqueous suspensions.

UNDESIRABLE EFFECTS. Large doses given more frequently than once daily may give rise to undesirable effects due to the absorption of procaine and leave painful lumps at the injection site.

PRECAUTIONS. The precautions against allergy described under Benzylpenicillin (page 51) should be observed.

Dose. See above under **Actions and uses.**

Preparations
BENETHAMINE PENICILLIN INJECTION, FORTIFIED, B.P.C. (page 709)

BENZATHINE PENICILLIN INJECTION, FORTIFIED, B.P.C. (page 710)

PROCAINE PENICILLIN INJECTION, B.P. (*Syn.* Procaine Benzylpenicillin Injection). It consists of a sterile suspension of procaine penicillin in Water for Injections containing suitable buffering and dispersing agents. Unless otherwise specified, a suspension containing 300 mg in 1 ml is supplied. It should be stored at a temperature not exceeding 20° and protected from light; under these conditions it may be expected to retain its potency for at least eighteen months.

PROCAINE PENICILLIN INJECTION, FORTIFIED, B.P. It consists of a sterile suspension of 5 parts of procaine penicillin in Water for Injections containing 1 part of benzylpenicillin in solution. It is prepared by adding Water for Injections to the contents of a sealed container, which contain suitable dispersing agents and may also contain a suitable buffering agent. Unless otherwise specified, an injection containing 300 mg of procaine penicillin and 60 mg of benzylpenicillin in a suitable dose-volume is supplied. It should be used within seven days of preparation, the date of which is stated on the label, or within fourteen days if a buffering agent is present, provided that it is stored during this period at 2° to 10°; at temperatures approaching 20° it should be used within twenty-four hours of preparation or within four days if a buffering agent is present.

OTHER NAME: *Distaquaine G®*

PROCHLORPERAZINE MALEATE
$C_{28}H_{32}ClN_3O_8S = 606\cdot1$

Prochlorperazine Maleate is 2-chloro-10-[3-(4-methylpiperazin-1-yl)propyl]phenothiazine di(hydrogen maleate).

Solubility. Very slightly soluble in water and in alcohol; insoluble in ether.

Standard
It complies with the requirements of the British Pharmacopoeia.
It is a white or pale yellow, crystalline, almost odourless powder and contains not less than 98·0 and not more than the equivalent of 101·0 per cent of $C_{28}H_{32}ClN_3O_8S$, calculated with reference to the dried substance. The loss on drying under the prescribed conditions is not more than 1·0 per cent. It has a melting-point of 198° to 203°.

Storage. It should be protected from light.

Actions and uses. Prochlorperazine has the actions and uses described under Chlorpromazine Hydrochloride (page 107) but it is less sedating, more effective as an anti-emetic, and more liable to give rise to extrapyramidal side-effects. It is particularly effective for the prevention and relief of vomiting, for which it is given three times daily as a suppository or by mouth in a dose of 25 milligrams; it may be given by injection. It may also be effective in the treatment of Ménière's disease and other forms of vestibular disorder. In the treatment of psychiatric states it is given in a dosage of 15 to 100 milligrams daily in divided doses.

UNDESIRABLE EFFECTS. Prochlorperazine may give rise to parkinsonism, particularly in children, in whom severe dystonic reactions may occur. Drowsiness may occur in the early stages of treatment.

Dose. See above under **Actions and uses.**

Preparation
PROCHLORPERAZINE TABLETS, B.P. The quantity of prochlorperazine maleate in each tablet should be specified by the prescriber. They should be protected from light. Tablets containing 5 and 25 mg are available.

OTHER NAME: *Stemetil®*

PROCHLORPERAZINE MESYLATE

$C_{20}H_{24}ClN_3S,(CH_3SO_3H)_2 = 566 \cdot 1$

Prochlorperazine Mesylate is 2-chloro-10-[3-(4-methylpiperazin-1-yl)propyl]phenothiazine dimethanesulphonate.

Solubility. Soluble, at $20°$, in less than $0 \cdot 5$ part of water and in 40 parts of alcohol; slightly soluble in chloroform; insoluble in ether.

Standard
It complies with the requirements of the British Pharmacopoeia.
It is a white or almost white, odourless powder and contains not less than $98 \cdot 0$ and not more than the equivalent of $101 \cdot 0$ per cent of $C_{20}H_{24}ClN_3S$, $(CH_3SO_3H)_2$, calculated with reference to the dried substance. The loss on drying under the prescribed conditions is not more than $1 \cdot 0$ per cent. A 2 per cent solution in water has a pH of $2 \cdot 0$ to $3 \cdot 0$.

Sterilisation. Solutions for injection are sterilised by heating in an autoclave in an atmosphere of nitrogen or other suitable gas.

Storage. It should be protected from light.

Actions and uses. Prochlorperazine mesylate has the actions, uses, and undesirable effects described under Prochlorperazine Maleate.

It is administered by deep intramuscular injection in a dosage of $12 \cdot 5$ to 25 milligrams twice or thrice daily in the treatment of psychiatric disorders.
As an anti-emetic, $12 \cdot 5$ milligrams is given by intramuscular injection.
For the treatment of acute alcoholism, it is given by intravenous injection in a dose of 100 milligrams.

Dose. See above under **Actions and uses.**

Preparation
PROCHLORPERAZINE INJECTION, B.P. It consists of a sterile solution of prochlorperazine mesylate in Water for Injections free from dissolved air and containing suitable buffering and stabilising agents. The strength of the solution should be specified by the prescriber. It should be protected from light. A solution containing $12 \cdot 5$ mg in 1 ml is available.

OTHER NAMES: Prochlorperazine Methanesulphonate; *Stemetil*®

PROCYCLIDINE HYDROCHLORIDE

$C_{19}H_{30}ClNO = 323 \cdot 9$

Procyclidine Hydrochloride is 1-cyclohexyl-1-phenyl-3-(pyrrolidin-1-yl)propan-1-ol hydrochloride.

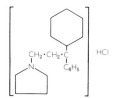

Solubility. Soluble, at $20°$, in 40 parts of water and in 15 parts of alcohol; insoluble in ether and in acetone.

Standard
It complies with the requirements of the British Pharmacopoeia.
It is a white crystalline powder with a faint odour and contains not less than $99 \cdot 0$ and not more than the equivalent of $101 \cdot 0$ per cent of $C_{19}H_{30}ClNO$, calculated with reference to the dried substance. The loss on drying under the prescribed conditions is not more than $0 \cdot 5$ per cent. It has a melting-point of $225°$ to $227°$. A 1 per cent solution in water has a pH of $4 \cdot 5$ to $6 \cdot 5$.

Actions and uses. Procyclidine is used for the symptomatic treatment of parkinsonism. It decreases rigidity more than tremor and improves muscular co-ordination and mobility of the patient, but it has little effect on salivation. The initial dosage by mouth is usually $2 \cdot 5$ milligrams of procyclidine hydrochloride three times a day and this is gradually increased by $2 \cdot 5$ milligrams a day until the optimum effect is obtained; 20 milligrams a day is often required and doses of up to 60 milligrams have

occasionally been necessary. Post-encephalitic patients usually require larger doses than arteriosclerotic patients.
Procyclidine hydrochloride is usually administered by mouth but when necessary it may be given by intramuscular or intravenous injection in doses of 5 to 10 milligrams.
Solanaceous alkaloids and other drugs used for the relief of parkinsonism are sometimes given in conjunction with procyclidine.

UNDESIRABLE EFFECTS. Drowsiness, ataxia, giddiness, blurred vision, confusion, nausea and vomiting may occur; they usually disappear when the dose is reduced.

Dose. See above under **Actions and uses.**

Preparations
PROCYCLIDINE INJECTION, B.P.C. (page 717)
PROCYCLIDINE TABLETS, B.P. Unless otherwise specified, tablets each containing 5 mg of procyclidine hydrochloride are supplied.

OTHER NAME: *Kemadrin*®

PROFLAVINE HEMISULPHATE

SYNONYMS: Neutral Proflavine Sulphate; Proflavine

$C_{26}H_{24}N_6O_4S,2H_2O = 552\cdot6$

Proflavine Hemisulphate is 3,6-diaminoacridine sulphate dihydrate.

Solubility. Soluble, at 20°, in 300 parts of water and in 35 parts of glycerol; soluble in 1 part of boiling water; very slightly soluble in alcohol; insoluble in ether and in chloroform.

Standard

DESCRIPTION. An orange to red, crystalline, hygroscopic powder; odourless or almost odourless.

IDENTIFICATION TESTS. Dissolve 0·1 g in 30 ml of water. This solution complies with the following tests:
(i) Add 0·2 ml to a large volume of water; a greenish fluorescence is produced.
(ii) To 1 ml add 0·1 ml of *sulphuric acid*; an immediate precipitate of bright reddish-orange needles is produced.
(iii) To 2 ml add *sodium hydroxide solution*; a lemon-yellow precipitate is produced.
(iv) To 5 ml add 1 ml of 1N hydrochloric acid and 5 ml of a 10 per cent w/v solution of *sodium nitrite* in water and boil for 1 minute; a brown precipitate is produced. Filter the solution; the filtrate is yellow (distinction from certain other flavines).
(v) It gives the reactions characteristic of sulphates.

ACIDITY OR ALKALINITY. pH of a saturated solution in *carbon dioxide-free water*, 6·0 to 8·0.

CERTAIN OTHER ACRIDINE DERIVATIVES. Dissolve 0·10 g in 100 ml of a 0·9 per cent w/v solution of *sodium chloride* at 35°; the solution is clear, or almost clear, and does not visibly deteriorate when allowed to stand in the dark at 15° to 20° for 24 hours.

WATER. 3·0 to 7·0 per cent w/w, determined by the method given in Appendix 16, page 895, 20 ml of a mixture of equal parts of *dehydrated pyridine* and *glacial acetic acid* being used in place of methyl alcohol.

SULPHATED ASH. Not more than 0·5 per cent.

CONTENT OF $C_{26}H_{24}N_6O_4S$. Not less than 98·0 per cent, calculated with reference to the anhydrous substance, determined by the following method:
Dissolve about 2 g, accurately weighed, in 750 ml of water, make the solution faintly acid to *congo red paper* by the addition of 1N hydrochloric acid, add 5 g of *sodium acetate* and, with stirring, 50 ml of 0·1M potassium ferricyanide, and allow to stand for 10 minutes.
Filter the solution, wash the filter with three successive 50-ml portions of water, and to the combined filtrate and washings add, successively and with mixing after each addition, 10 ml of *hydrochloric acid*, 10 g of *sodium chloride*, 1 g of *potassium iodide*, and a solution containing 3 g of *zinc sulphate* in 10 ml of water, and allow to stand for 3 minutes.
Titrate the liberated iodine with 0·1N sodium thiosulphate, using *starch mucilage* as indicator, and, when the titration is nearly complete, allow to stand for a further 3 minutes before completing the titration. Repeat the procedure omitting the sample.
The difference between the two titrations represents the amount of potassium ferricyanide required to precipitate the proflavine; each ml of 0·1M potassium ferricyanide is equivalent to 0·07749 g of $C_{26}H_{24}N_6O_4S$.

Storage. It should be stored in airtight containers, protected from light.

Preparation and storage of solutions. See statement on aqueous solutions of antiseptics, under Solutions (page 779).

Actions and uses. Proflavine and other acridine derivatives are slow-acting antiseptics which are effective against many Gram-positive and Gram-negative bacteria; they are used in the treatment of infected wounds. In the concentrations usually employed, they are not effective against *Proteus vulgaris, Pseudomonas aeruginosa,* and some strains of *Escherichia coli.* Their activity is not reduced by tissue fluids and serum, and, in concentrations of 0·01 per cent or less, they do not interfere with the action of phagocytic cells.

For the dressing of wounds or burns, a 0·1 per cent solution is used, but, if treatment is prolonged, weaker solutions or another antiseptic should be used, as the acridine derivatives tend to delay healing.

For the treatment of certain local infections of the external ear, mouth, throat, and skin, 0·1 to 1 per cent w/v alcoholic or aqueous solutions are used.

Stains on the skin caused by acridine derivatives may be removed by washing with a dilute solution of sulphurous acid or of hydrochloric acid.

Preparation

PROFLAVINE CREAM, B.P.C. (page 660)

PROGESTERONE

SYNONYM: Progesteronum

$C_{21}H_{30}O_2 = 314\cdot5$

Progesterone is pregn-4-ene-3,20-dione.

Solubility. Insoluble in water; soluble, at 20°, in 8 parts of alcohol, in 16 parts of ether, in less than 1 part of chloroform, in 60 parts of arachis oil, in 60 parts of ethyl oleate, and in 100 parts of light petroleum.

Standard

It complies with the requirements of the European Pharmacopoeia.
It occurs as odourless colourless crystals or white or at most slightly yellowish-white crystalline powder and

contains not less than 97·0 and not more than the equivalent of 103·0 per cent of $C_{21}H_{30}O_2$, calculated with reference to the dried substance. The loss on drying under the prescribed conditions is not more than 0·5 per cent. It has a melting-point of 128° to 133° but it may also occur in a form which melts at about 121°, due to polymorphism.

Sterilisation. Oily solutions for injection are sterilised by dry heat.

Storage. It should be protected from light.

Actions and uses. Progesterone, which is secreted by the corpus luteum, converts the proliferative endometrium to a secretory phase and, if pregnancy ensues, helps to maintain the decidua. It has been largely replaced by progestational compounds which are active when given by mouth and which have a less marked virilising action.

Progesterone is administered intramuscularly or by implantation.

In addition to the oily injection, progesterone is available as aqueous suspensions for injection containing 5, 10, 25, and 50 milligrams per millilitre, and as implants containing 100 and 200 milligrams.

PRECAUTIONS AND CONTRA-INDICATIONS. It should not be used in pregnancy because of the virilising effect on a female foetus.

Dose. 20 to 60 milligrams daily by intramuscular injection.

Preparation
PROGESTERONE INJECTION, B.P. It consists of a sterile solution of progesterone in ethyl oleate or other suitable ester, in a suitable fixed oil, or in any mixture of these; it may contain suitable alcohols. Unless otherwise specified, a solution containing 10 mg in 1 ml is supplied. Solutions containing 25 and 50 mg in 1 ml are also available. It should be protected from light. Solid matter may separate on standing and should be redissolved by heating before use.

OTHER NAME: *Gestone*®

PROGUANIL HYDROCHLORIDE

$C_{11}H_{17}Cl_2N_5 = 290·2$

Proguanil Hydrochloride is N^1-*p*-chlorophenyl-N^5-isopropyldiguanide hydrochloride.

Solubility. Soluble, at 20°, in 110 parts of water and in 40 parts of alcohol; very slightly soluble in ether and in chloroform.

Standard
It complies with the requirements of the British Pharmacopoeia.
It is a white, crystalline, odourless powder and contains not less than 99·0 and not more than the equivalent of 101·0 per cent of $C_{11}H_{17}Cl_2N_5$, calculated with reference to the dried substance. The loss on drying under the prescribed conditions is not more than 0·5 per cent. It has a melting-point of about 245°.

Hygroscopicity. It absorbs insignificant amounts of moisture at temperatures up to 37° at relative humidities up to about 80 per cent.

Actions and uses. Proguanil is used for the prevention and treatment of malaria. When given by mouth it is rapidly absorbed and is excreted mainly in the urine; its action is dependent upon the formation of an active metabolite, 2,4-diamino-5-*p*-chlorophenyl-5,6-dihydro-6,6-dimethyl-1,3,5-triazine.

When used in the treatment of malaria caused by *Plasmodium falciparum*, proguanil kills parasites undergoing schizogony in the red blood cells and also the tissue forms. It thus acts as a causal prophylactic and effects a radical cure, so that attacks do not recur when treatment is stopped. In the treatment of malaria caused by *P. vivax*, proguanil kills the asexual parasites in the red blood cells, but will not always eradicate latent tissue infection, so that attacks may sometimes recur after

treatment is stopped. Proguanil does not kill the gametocytes, but renders them non-infective for the mosquito while the drug is present in the blood. Malaria parasites in the red blood cells are killed more rapidly by quinine, chloroquine, or mepacrine than by proguanil, which is therefore not the best drug to use for the treatment of acute malaria.

To suppress the symptoms of malaria, a dosage of 100 to 300 milligrams is given by mouth twice a week during exposure to infection, but in some areas it is necessary to give 100 milligrams every day.

Strains of *Plasmodium* sometimes become resistant to proguanil; in such circumstances, chloroquine or mepacrine should be used for a time to prevent the transmission of resistant strains.

A dosage of 100 milligrams twice a week for six months following exposure to infection greatly reduces the chance of relapse in malaria caused by *P. vivax*.

UNDESIRABLE EFFECTS. These very rarely occur during the administration of therapeutic doses.

Dose. See above under **Actions and uses.**

Preparation
PROGUANIL TABLETS, B.P. Unless otherwise specified, tablets each containing 100 mg of proguanil hydrochloride are supplied. Tablets containing 25 mg are also available.

OTHER NAME: *Paludrine*®

PROMAZINE HYDROCHLORIDE

$C_{17}H_{21}ClN_2S = 320.9$

Promazine Hydrochloride is 10-(3-dimethylaminopropyl)phenothiazine hydrochloride.

Solubility. Soluble, at 20°, in 1 part of water and in 2 parts of alcohol and of chloroform.

Standard
It complies with the requirements of the British Pharmacopoeia.
It is a white or almost white, crystalline, slightly hygroscopic, odourless or almost odourless powder and contains not less than 99·0 and not more than the equivalent of 101·0 per cent of $C_{17}H_{21}ClN_2S$, calculated with reference to the dried substance. The loss on drying under the prescribed conditions is not more than 0·5 per cent. It has a melting-point of 177° to 181°. A 5 per cent solution in water has a pH of 4·2 to 5·4.

Stability. It is affected by air and light and by traces of heavy metals. On decomposition, solutions may be coloured pink or red.

Sterilisation. Solutions for injection are sterilised by heating in an autoclave in an atmosphere of nitrogen or other suitable gas.

Storage. It should be stored in airtight containers, protected from light.

Actions and uses. Promazine has actions, uses, and undesirable effects similar to those described under Chlorpromazine Hydrochloride (page 107).

POISONING. The procedure as described under Chlorpromazine Hydrochloride (page 107) should be followed.

Dose. 50 to 800 milligrams by mouth or by intramuscular or intravenous injection daily in divided doses.

Preparations
PROMAZINE INJECTION, B.P. It consists of a sterile solution of promazine hydrochloride in Water for Injections free from dissolved air and containing suitable buffering and stabilising agents. Unless otherwise specified, a solution containing 50 mg in 1 ml is supplied. It should be protected from light.

PROMAZINE TABLETS, B.P. Unless otherwise specified, tablets each containing 25 mg of promazine hydrochloride are supplied. These tablets are sugar coated. Tablets containing 50 and 100 mg are also available.

OTHER NAME: *Sparine*®

PROMETHAZINE HYDROCHLORIDE

$C_{17}H_{21}ClN_2S = 320.9$

Promethazine Hydrochloride is 10-(2-dimethylaminopropyl)-phenothiazine hydrochloride.

Solubility. Soluble, at 20°, in less than 1 part of water, in 9 parts of alcohol, and in 2 parts of chloroform.

Standard
It complies with the requirements of the British Pharmacopoeia.
It is a white or slightly cream-coloured odourless or almost odourless powder and contains not less than 99·0 and not more than the equivalent of 101·0 per cent of $C_{17}H_{21}ClN_2S$, calculated with reference to the dried substance. The loss on drying under the prescribed conditions is not more than 0·5 per cent. A 10 per cent solution in water has a pH of 3·5 to 5·0.

Sterilisation. Solutions for injection are sterilised by heating in an autoclave in an atmosphere of nitrogen or other suitable gas.

Storage. It should be protected from light.

Actions and uses. Promethazine is a powerful and long-acting antagonist of histamine.
The antihistamine drugs resemble each other in their effects of diminishing or abolishing most of the actions of histamine; they do not, however, affect its stimulant action on gastric secretion. The action of histamine most readily affected is that on the involuntary muscle of the intestine, bladder, uterus and bronchioles; the vasodilator and vasoconstrictor actions of histamine are also antagonised. The dilatation and increased permeability of capillaries produced by histamine are prevented and the weals caused by intradermal injections of histamine are reduced by these drugs.

Anaphylactic reactions produced in animals and certain allergic reactions in man are modified by the antihistamine drugs, although larger doses are necessary for this purpose than are required to antagonise the effects of injected histamine. The histamine antagonists are not entirely specific, for when used in higher concentrations they may also antagonise the actions of acetylcholine and of adrenaline. Most of the histamine antagonists depress the central nervous system and cause drowsiness; they also produce local anaesthesia when applied locally or injected subcutaneously, but their administration by the latter route is not recommended, as irritation often results.

The antihistamine drugs are active when given by mouth. When assessing their activity, attention must be paid not only to the time taken for the drug to produce its maximum effect, but also to the duration of its action. The action of promethazine lasts for about twenty hours, and it may therefore be given less frequently than most other antihistamines. The daily dosage of promethazine hydrochloride required to maintain an effect against an intradermal injection of histamine in man is about one-fourteenth of that of mepyramine maleate.

The antihistamine drugs have been used in the treatment of allergic reactions of the skin and mucous membranes, such as acute urticaria, atopic dermatitis, allergic rhinitis, and hay fever. They are also used in treating allergic reactions caused by such drugs as the antibiotics and sulphonamides. Itching skin affections, such as atopic dermatitis, contact dermatitis, pruritus ani and vulvae, generalised pruritus, and insect bites, are often temporarily relieved either by giving antihistamines internally or by applying them externally in the form of an ointment or cream. Topical application is not without risk, as skin sensitisation and dermatitis may result. Since the cause of the reaction is not removed, symptoms may reappear when the drug is stopped. In the treatment of chronic conditions, the general condition of the skin and mucous membrane remains unaltered, although symptoms such as itching and sneezing may be relieved.

Certain types of bronchial asthma respond to treatment with the antihistamine drugs, but such treatment is unlikely to be effective during an acute attack unless supplemented by bronchodilators.

Some of the antihistamines have powerful anti-emetic properties and are used for the prevention and treatment of vomiting from various causes, including post-operative vomiting, irradiation sickness, drug-induced nausea, motion-sickness, vomiting of pregnancy, and Ménière's disease and other labyrinthine disturbances. There is evidence that infection with the common cold is in no way influenced by these compounds.

Promethazine hydrochloride is administered by mouth, the usual daily dosage for an adult being 25 to 50 milligrams and for a child up to 30 milligrams. It may also be given by deep intramuscular injection in a dose not exceeding 50 milligrams.

UNDESIRABLE EFFECTS. Toxic effects commonly encountered with most of the antihistamine drugs are dryness of the mouth, throat, and nose, and abdominal pain with vomiting or diarrhoea.

Because the antihistamines may cause drowsiness in some persons their use constitutes a danger to patients who drive vehicles or work with moving machinery. The danger is increased if alcohol is also taken.

POISONING. Large doses of the antihistamines may cause convulsions and may precipitate fits in epileptics; if this stage is reached a short-acting barbiturate, such as thiopentone sodium, should be administered intravenously. Gastric lavage should be employed if the drug has recently been taken by mouth.

Dose. See above under **Actions and uses.**

Preparations
PROMETHAZINE ELIXIR, B.P.C. (page 676)

PROMETHAZINE HYDROCHLORIDE INJECTION, B.P. It consists of a sterile solution of promethazine hydrochloride in Water for Injections free from dissolved air and containing suitable stabilising agents. Unless otherwise specified, a solution containing 25 mg in 1 ml is supplied. It should be protected from light.

PROMETHAZINE HYDROCHLORIDE TABLETS, B.P. Unless otherwise specified, tablets each containing 10 mg of promethazine hydrochloride are supplied. They are sugar coated. Tablets containing 25 mg are also available.

OTHER NAME: *Phenergan*®

PROMETHAZINE THEOCLATE

$C_{24}H_{27}ClN_6O_2S = 499{\cdot}0$

Promethazine Theoclate is the 10-(2-dimethylaminopropyl)phenothiazine salt of 8-chlorotheophylline (theoclic acid).

Solubility. Very slightly soluble in water; soluble, at 20°, in 70 parts of alcohol and in 2·5 parts of chloroform; insoluble in ether.

Standard
It complies with the requirements of the British Pharmacopoeia.
It is a white or almost white odourless powder and contains not less than 98·0 and not more than the equivalent of 101·0 per cent of $C_{24}H_{27}ClN_6O_2S$, calculated with reference to the dried substance. The loss on drying under the prescribed conditions is not more than 0·5 per cent.

Storage. It should be stored in airtight containers, protected from light.

Actions and uses. Promethazine theoclate has the actions, uses, and undesirable effects of the antihistamine drugs, as described under Promethazine Hydrochloride; 1·5 grams of promethazine theoclate is approximately equivalent to 1 gram of promethazine hydrochloride.

Promethazine theoclate is given by mouth for the prevention and relief of motion-sickness.

POISONING. As for Promethazine Hydrochloride.

Dose. 25 to 50 milligrams daily.

Preparation
PROMETHAZINE THEOCLATE TABLETS, B.P. Unless otherwise specified, tablets each containing 25 mg of promethazine theoclate are supplied. They should be stored in airtight containers, protected from light.

OTHER NAMES: *Avomine®*; Promethazine Chlorotheophyllinate

PROPANIDID

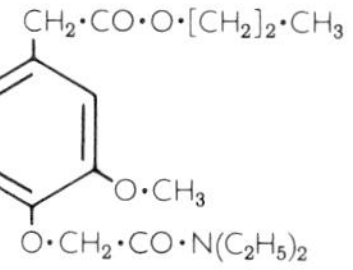

$C_{18}H_{27}NO_5 = 337.4$

Propanidid is propyl 4-diethylcarbamoylmethoxy-3-methoxyphenylacetate.

Solubility. Very slightly soluble in water; miscible with alcohol, with ether, and with chloroform.

Standard
It complies with the requirements of the British Pharmacopoeia.
It is a pale, greenish-yellow, viscous, hygroscopic liquid with a slight odour and contains not less than 98.0 per cent of $C_{18}H_{27}NO_5$.

Actions and uses. Propanidid is a short-acting anaesthetic for intravenous administration. It also has local anaesthetic activity. It is metabolised by esterases in the plasma and the liver.
The usual dose for the induction of anaesthesia is 100 to 750 milligrams by intravenous injection as a 5 per cent solution and the resulting anaesthesia usually lasts for three to six minutes. Hyperventilation commonly occurs during induction and this may be followed by hypoventilation or apnoea. The action of suxamethonium may be enhanced and doses of the order of 8 to 10 milligrams per kilogram body-weight may depress the circulation.
Propanidid has been used to produce ultra-light anaesthesia during conservative dental treatment but its use for this purpose has been questioned.

Dose. See above under **Actions and uses.**

OTHER NAME: *Epontol®*

PROPANTHELINE BROMIDE

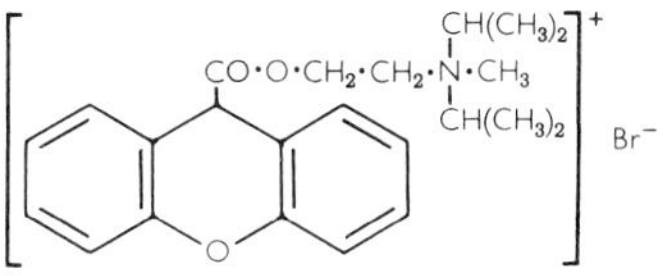

$C_{23}H_{30}BrNO_3 = 448.4$

Propantheline Bromide is 2-di-isopropylaminoethyl xanthen-9-carboxylate methobromide.

Solubility. Very soluble in water, in alcohol, and in chloroform; insoluble in ether.

Standard
It complies with the requirements of the British Pharmacopoeia.
It is a white or yellowish-white, slightly hygroscopic, odourless powder and contains not less than 98.0 and not more than the equivalent of 102.0 per cent of $C_{23}H_{30}BrNO_3$, calculated with reference to the dried substance. The loss on drying under the prescribed conditions is not more than 1.5 per cent. It has a melting-point of 157° to 162°.

Storage. It should be stored in airtight containers.

Actions and uses. Propantheline has the peripheral but not the central actions of atropine (page 36). It is administered, chiefly to reduce gastric secretion and intestinal mobility, in a dosage of 15 milligrams three times daily, with double the dose at bedtime. It has also been used to diminish biliary and ureteric spasm and to control excessive salivation, sweating, and nocturnal enuresis.

UNDESIRABLE EFFECTS. Hypotension, urinary retention, and constipation may occur. Propantheline has ganglion-blocking effects, but these are not important in therapeutic dosage. It is less liable than atropine to produce dryness of the mouth, tachycardia, and disturbances of vision.

PRECAUTIONS. It should be used with caution in patients with glaucoma, because of its liability to increase intra-ocular pressure, and in those with prostatic enlargement.

Dose. See above under **Actions and uses.**

Preparation
PROPANTHELINE TABLETS, B.P. Unless otherwise specified, tablets each containing 15 mg of propantheline bromide are supplied. They are sugar coated. They should be stored in airtight containers.

OTHER NAMES: *Aclobrom®*; *Pro-banthine®*

PROPICILLIN POTASSIUM

$C_{18}H_{21}KN_2O_5S = 416.5$

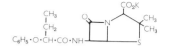

Propicillin Potassium is a mixture of the potassium salts of 6-D(+)- and 6-L(−)-(α-phenoxybutyramido)penicillanic acid.

Solubility. Soluble, at 20°, in 1·2 parts of water, in 25 parts of alcohol, and in 65 parts of dehydrated alcohol; very slightly soluble in ether and in chloroform.

Standard
It complies with the requirements of the British Pharmacopoeia.
It is a white or almost white finely crystalline powder and contains not less than 97·0 per cent of $C_{18}H_{21}KN_2O_5S$, calculated with reference to the anhydrous substance. It contains not more than 1·0 per cent w/w of water. A 10 per cent solution in water has a pH of 5·0 to 7·0.

Storage. It should be stored in airtight containers at a temperature not exceeding 25°.

Actions and uses. Propicillin has the actions and uses described under Phenoxymethyl-penicillin (page 371).
Although propicillin potassium gives rise to higher blood levels than phenoxymethyl-penicillin it is less potent as an antibiotic and

the effect of the two substances is therefore similar. Although it is more resistant to staphylococcal penicillinase than phenoxy-methylpenicillin, the difference is not suffi-ciently great to be of value in the treatment of penicillinase-producing staphylococcal infec-tions.

PRECAUTIONS AND CONTRA-INDICATIONS. As for Phenoxymethylpenicillin (page 371).

Dose. The equivalent of 0·5 to 1·5 grams of propicillin daily in divided doses.

Preparations
PROPICILLIN ELIXIR, B.P.C. (page 676)
PROPICILLIN TABLETS, B.P. Unless otherwise specified, tablets each containing the equivalent of 250 mg of propicillin are supplied. They may contain peppermint oil as a flavouring agent. Tablets containing the equivalent of 125 mg of propicillin are also available.

OTHER NAMES: *Brocillin*®; *Ultrapen*®

PROPRANOLOL HYDROCHLORIDE

$C_{16}H_{22}ClNO_2 = 295.8$

Propranolol Hydrochloride is (±)-1-isopropylamino-3-naphth-1′-yloxypropan-2-ol hydrochloride.

Solubility. Soluble, at 20°, in 20 parts of water and in 20 parts of alcohol; slightly soluble in chloroform.

Standard
It complies with the requirements of the British Pharmacopoeia.
It is a white or almost white, odourless powder and contains not less than 99·0 and not more than the equivalent of 101·0 per cent of $C_{16}H_{22}ClNO_2$, calcu-lated with reference to the dried substance. The loss on drying under the prescribed conditions is not more than 0·5 per cent. A 1 per cent solution in water has a pH of 5·0 to 6·0.

Stability. It is affected by light. In aqueous solutions, it decomposes with oxidation of the isopropylamine side-chain, accompanied by reduction in the pH and discoloration of the solution. Solutions are most stable at pH 3 and decompose rapidly when alkaline.

Hygroscopicity. It absorbs less than 1 per cent of water at 25° at relative humidities up to 80 per cent.

Storage. It should be protected from light.

Actions and uses. Propranolol has a specific blocking action on the adrenergic beta-receptors and inhibits the sympathetic stimu-lation of the heart. It is used in the treatment of cardiac arrhythmias associated with heart disease, digitalis intoxication, or anaesthesia.
In urgent cases propranolol may be given in-travenously in a dose of 1 milligram, dissolved in 1 millilitre of water, over a period of one

minute, the injection being preceded, if the heart rate is already slow, by the intravenous administration of 1 to 2 milligrams of atro-pine; this dose may be repeated every two minutes until a response is observed or until 10 milligrams has been given to con-scious patients or 5 milligrams to patients under anaesthesia.
In the treatment of arrhythmias, 10 to 30 milli-grams may be given by mouth three or four times a day. In angina pectoris the usual initial dosage is 80 milligrams daily in divided doses; this is increased by 40 milligrams daily at intervals of three days up to 160 milli-grams daily, which may be further increased to 600 milligrams daily if necessary.
In patients with poor myocardial function it may be necessary to give digitalis at the same time. Propranolol may also be used in con-junction with digitalis in the treatment of auricular fibrillation.

UNDESIRABLE EFFECTS. Propranolol may pre-cipitate cardiac failure in some patients and, if the failure persists after full digitalisation, pro-pranolol must be withdrawn. It may also give rise to bronchospasm.

Nausea, vomiting, insomnia, lassitude, and mild diarrhoea may occur, but can usually be avoided by increasing the dose gradually during the first week of treatment.

Non-thrombocytopenic purpura, erythematous rash, and paraesthesia of the hands may occur, but these reactions are rare.

CONTRA-INDICATIONS. It should not be given to patients with a history of bronchial asthma.

Dose. See above under **Actions and uses.**

Preparations

PROPRANOLOL INJECTION, B.P. It consists of a sterile solution of propranolol hydrochloride in Water for Injections containing citric acid. Unless otherwise specified, a solution containing 1 mg in 1 ml is supplied.

PROPRANOLOL TABLETS, B.P. Unless otherwise specified, tablets each containing 10 mg of propranolol hydrochloride are supplied. Tablets containing 40 and 80 mg are also available.

OTHER NAME: *Inderal®*

PROPYL GALLATE

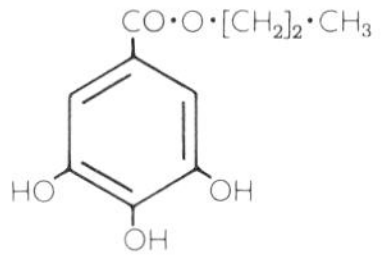

$C_{10}H_{12}O_5 = 212 \cdot 2$

Propyl Gallate is propyl 3,4,5-trihydroxybenzoate.

Solubility. Soluble, at 20°, in 1000 parts of water, in 3 parts of alcohol, in 3 parts of ether, and in 2000 parts of arachis oil.

Standard

It complies with the requirements of the British Pharmacopoeia.
It is a white to creamy-white, crystalline, odourless powder. The loss on drying at 105° is not more than 1·0 per cent. It has a melting-point of 146° to 148°.

Storage. It should be stored in airtight containers, protected from light, contact with metals being avoided.

Uses. Propyl gallate is used as an antoxidant for preserving oils and fats; it is also used to inhibit autoxidation of ether, paraldehyde, and similar substances which develop peroxides in the presence of oxygen.

Anhydrous oils and fats may contain up to 0·01 per cent of propyl gallate and volatile oils up to 0·1 per cent; propyl gallate is dissolved in fixed oils by warming the mixture to 70° to 80° and in solid fats by warming until the fat is just melted.

The formation of peroxides in ether is inhibited by 0·01 per cent of propyl gallate and the oxidation of paraldehyde is retarded by 0·05 per cent.

PROPYL HYDROXYBENZOATE

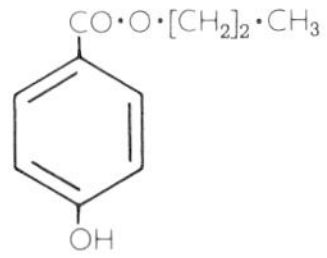

SYNONYM: Propylparaben

$C_{10}H_{12}O_3 = 180 \cdot 2$

Propyl Hydroxybenzoate is propyl *p*-hydroxybenzoate.

Solubility. Very slightly soluble in water; soluble, at 20°, in 3·5 parts of alcohol, in 3 parts of acetone, in 40 parts of fixed oils, and in 140 parts of glycerol; readily soluble in solutions of alkali hydroxides.

Standard

It complies with the requirements of the British Pharmacopoeia.
It is a white, crystalline, odourless powder and contains not less than 99·0 and not more than the equivalent of 101·0 per cent of $C_{10}H_{12}O_3$. It has a melting-point of 95° to 98°.

Uses. Propyl hydroxybenzoate is employed, usually in conjunction with other hydroxybenzoate esters, as a preservative in a concentration of 0·05 per cent for aqueous preparations and 0·1 per cent for emulsions and creams. It may be dissolved with the aid of heat or incorporated as a solution in alcohol.

OTHER NAMES: *Nipasol M®*; *Propyl Butex®*

PROPYLENE GLYCOL

$C_3H_8O_2 = 76 \cdot 10$

$CH_3 \cdot CH(OH) \cdot CH_2OH$

Propylene Glycol is (±)-propane-1,2-diol.

Solubility. Miscible with water, with alcohol, with chloroform, and with acetone; soluble, at 20°, in 6 parts of ether; immiscible with light petroleum and with fixed oils.

Standard

It complies with the requirements of the British Pharmacopoeia.

It is a clear, colourless, viscous, hygroscopic, odourless liquid. It has a weight per ml at 20° of 1·035 g to 1·037 g and a boiling-point of about 187°, not less than 95·0 per cent v/v distilling between 185° and 189°.

Sterilisation. It is sterilised by heating in sealed ampoules in an autoclave or by filtration.

Storage. It should be stored in airtight containers.

Uses. Propylene glycol is a useful solvent of low toxicity for some vitamins, barbiturates, and other substances which are insufficiently soluble in water or are unstable in aqueous solution.

It may be used, suitably diluted, in the preparation of injections and oral solutions and may be included in spray solutions to stabilise the droplet size. Examples of preparations in which propylene glycol is used are Chloramphenicol Ear-drops, Digoxin Injection, Phenobarbitone Injection, and Benzoic Acid Solution.

Propylene glycol is also used as a solvent for topical corticosteroids in the formulation of ointments.

PROPYLHEXEDRINE

$C_{10}H_{21}N = 155 \cdot 3$

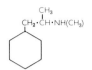

Propylhexedrine is (2-cyclohexyl-1-methylethyl)methylamine.

Solubility. Miscible with alcohol, with ether, and with chloroform; soluble in dilute acids.

Standard
DESCRIPTION. A clear colourless liquid; odour characteristic and amine-like.

IDENTIFICATION TESTS. 1. Dissolve 0·1 g in a mixture of 3 ml of water and 0·2 ml of *dilute hydrochloric acid*. To 1 ml add 3 ml of *mercuric chloride test-solution*; a bulky white granular precipitate is formed (distinction from adrenaline, ephedrine, and phenylephrine).

2. To the remainder of the solution prepared in test 1 add 20 ml of *trinitrophenol solution* and cool in ice; a precipitate is formed which, after washing with water, recrystallising from *alcohol (20 per cent)* and drying for 2 hours at 80°, melts at about 107°.

3. It boils at about 204°, determined by the method given in Appendix 9B, page 888.

4. The infra-red absorption spectrum exhibits maxima which are only at the same wavelengths as, and have similar relative intensities to, those in the spectrum of *propylhexedrine A.S.*

WEIGHT PER ML. At 20°, 0·853 g to 0·861 g.

RELATED COMPOUNDS. It complies with the test given in Appendix 5A, page 867.

SULPHATED ASH. Not more than 0·1 per cent w/w.

CONTENT OF $C_{10}H_{21}N$. Not less than 98·0 and not more than the equivalent of 101·0 per cent w/w, determined by the following method:

Dissolve about 0·3 g, accurately weighed, in 30 ml of 0·1N sulphuric acid, add 50 ml of water, and titrate the excess of acid with 0·1N sodium hydroxide, using *methyl red solution* as indicator; each ml of 0·1N sulphuric acid is equivalent to 0·01553 g of $C_{10}H_{21}N$.

Storage. It should be stored in airtight containers.

Actions and uses. Propylhexedrine is a volatile sympathomimetic amine with a local vasoconstrictor action, but when inhaled it has little stimulating effect on the central nervous system.

It is used in inhalers, containing 250 milligrams, for the relief of congested nasal mucous membranes in hay fever, asthma, coryza, and vasomotor rhinitis and to relieve blockage of the eustachian tubes.

OTHER NAME: *Benzedrex®*

PROPYLIODONE

$C_{10}H_{11}I_2NO_3 = 447 \cdot 0$

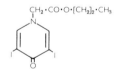

Propyliodone is propyl 1,4-dihydro-3,5-di-iodo-4-oxopyrid-1-ylacetate.

Solubility. Very slightly soluble in water and in ether; soluble, at 20°, in 500 parts of alcohol and in 150 parts of chloroform.

Standard
It complies with the requirements of the British Pharmacopoeia.

It is a white or almost white, crystalline, odourless or almost odourless powder and contains not less than 99·0 and not more than the equivalent of 101·0 per cent of $C_{10}H_{11}I_2NO_3$, calculated with reference to the dried substance. The loss on drying under the prescribed conditions is not more than 0·5 per cent. It has a melting-point of 187° to 190°.

Sterilisation. It is sterilised by dry heat.

Storage. It should be protected from light.

Actions and uses. Propyliodone is a contrast medium used in bronchography. It is a slightly soluble compound related to diodone and is rapidly eliminated from the lungs. It gives well-defined bronchograms, however, for at least thirty minutes.

It is used in either oily or aqueous suspension and is introduced either by a cannula through the cricothyroid membrane or by a catheter through the nose, the trachea and larynx having been previously anaesthetised by means of a local anaesthetic.

A dose of 300 milligrams for each year of age, up to a maximum of 9 grams for an adult, is usually adequate.

UNDESIRABLE EFFECTS. The toxicity of propyliodone is low, but it causes frequent coughing and for this reason adequate local anaesthesia of the trachea is essential.

Dose. See above under **Actions and uses.**

Preparations

PROPYLIODONE INJECTION, B.P. It consists of a sterile suspension containing 50 per cent of propyliodone in Water for Injections. It contains suitable dispersing and suspending agents; it may contain a suitable

buffering agent and bactericide. It should be stored protected from light at a temperature between 10° and 30°.

PROPYLIODONE INJECTION, OILY, B.P. It consists of a sterile suspension containing 60 per cent of propyliodone in arachis oil. It should be stored protected from light at a temperature below 30°.

OTHER NAME: *Dionosil*®

PROPYLTHIOURACIL

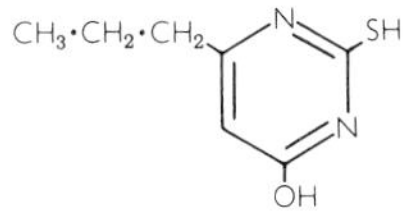

$C_7H_{10}N_2OS = 170.2$

Propylthiouracil is 4-hydroxy-2-mercapto-6-propylpyrimidine.

Solubility. Very slightly soluble in water; slightly soluble in alcohol, in ether, and in chloroform; soluble in solutions of alkali hydroxides.

Standard

It complies with the requirements of the British Pharmacopoeia.

It occurs as odourless white or pale cream-coloured crystals or crystalline powder and contains not less than 98.0 per cent of $C_7H_{10}N_2OS$, calculated with reference to the dried substance. The loss on drying under the prescribed conditions is not more than 0.5 per cent. It has a melting-point of about 220°.

Actions and uses. Propylthiouracil is an antithyroid substance which has the actions,

uses, and undesirable effects described under Carbimazole (page 77).

PRECAUTIONS. As for Carbimazole (page 77).

Dose. Controlling dosage, 200 to 600 milligrams daily; maintenance dosage, 50 to 200 milligrams daily.

Preparation

PROPYLTHIOURACIL TABLETS, B.P. Unless otherwise specified, tablets each containing 50 mg of propylthiouracil are supplied.

PROTAMINE SULPHATE INJECTION

SYNONYM: Protamine Sulph. Inj.

Protamine Sulphate Injection is a sterile solution in Sodium Chloride Injection of protamine sulphate prepared from the sperm or mature testes of fish belonging to the family Clupeidae or Salmonidae.

Standard

It complies with the requirements of the British Pharmacopoeia.

It is a clear colourless solution and contains not less than 80.0 per cent of the prescribed or stated amount of protamine sulphate. It has a pH of 2.5 to 3.5.

Sterilisation. It is sterilised by filtration.

Storage. It should be stored at room temperature.

Actions and uses. Protamine sulphate neutralises the anticoagulant property of heparin and is used in the treatment of heparin overdosage. It is administered by slow intravenous injection, 5 millilitres of a 1 per cent solution being injected over a period of ten minutes. Not more than 50

milligrams of protamine sulphate should be given at any one time.

If administered within fifteen minutes of the injection of heparin, the amount of protamine sulphate required is 1 milligram for each 100 Units of heparin injected; proportionately less is required if more time has elapsed, especially as protamine sulphate itself possesses an anticoagulant action. A 5 per cent solution is used to neutralise the action of heparin in regional heparinisation.

Dose. The dose is determined by the physician in accordance with the needs of the patient.

Unless otherwise specified, a solution containing 10 mg of protamine sulphate in 1 ml is supplied.

PROTHIONAMIDE

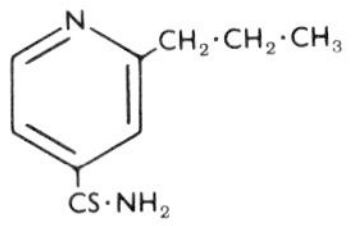

$C_9H_{12}N_2S = 180.3$

Prothionamide is 2-propylisonicotinthioamide.

Solubility. Insoluble in water; soluble, at 20°, in 30 parts of alcohol, in 300 parts of ether, in 200 parts of chloroform, and in 16 parts of methyl alcohol.

Standard

DESCRIPTION. Yellow crystals or yellow crystalline powder; odourless or almost odourless.

IDENTIFICATION TESTS. 1. Heat 0·1 g with 5 ml of *sodium hydroxide solution*; vapours are evolved which turn *red litmus paper* blue.

2. Heat 0·1 g with 5 ml of 1N hydrochloric acid; vapours are evolved which blacken *lead paper*.

3. Dissolve 0·01 g in 5 ml of *methyl alcohol* and add 5 ml of 0·1N silver nitrate; a brownish-black precipitate is produced.

4. The ultraviolet absorption spectrum exhibits the characteristics given in Appendix 3, page 856.

5. The infra-red absorption spectrum exhibits maxima which are only at the same wavelengths as, and have similar relative intensities to, those in the spectrum of *prothionamide A.S.*

ACIDITY. Dissolve 2·0 g in 20 ml of warm *methyl alcohol*, add 20 ml of water, cool, shake until crystallisation occurs, and titrate with 0·1N sodium hydroxide, using *cresol red solution* as indicator; not more than 0·2 ml is required.

MELTING-POINT. 140° to 143°.

LEAD. It complies with the test given in Appendix 7, page 883 (10 parts per million).

RELATED COMPOUNDS. It complies with the test given in Appendix 5A, page 867 (0·5 per cent).

LOSS ON DRYING. Not more than 1·0 per cent, determined by drying to constant weight at 105°.

SULPHATED ASH. Not more than 0·1 per cent.

CONTENT OF $C_9H_{12}N_2S$. Not less than 99·0 per cent, calculated with reference to the substance dried under the prescribed conditions, determined by the following method:
Titrate about 0·45 g, accurately weighed, by Method I of the British Pharmacopoeia, Appendix XIB, for non-aqueous titration; each ml of 0·1N perchloric acid is equivalent to 0·01803 g of $C_9H_{12}N_2S$.

Storage. It should be protected from light.

Actions and uses. Prothionamide is a tuberculostatic agent with actions and uses similar to those of ethionamide (page 188) but it causes a lower incidence of gastro-intestinal side-effects. Bacterial resistance develops simultaneously to both ethionamide and prothionamide and there is also some cross-resistance between them and thiacetazone.

The use of prothionamide is normally restricted to patients with infections that are resistant to other drugs. It should always be given simultaneously with other tuberculostatic agents to delay the development of resistance.

The usual dose for an adult is 0·75 to 1 gram daily in single or divided doses. For children under ten years of age the usual initial dose is 10 milligrams per kilogram body-weight daily, gradually increased, if tolerated, up to a maximum of 20 milligrams per kilogram body-weight daily.

UNDESIRABLE EFFECTS. These are as described under Ethionamide (page 188).

PRECAUTIONS AND CONTRA-INDICATIONS. Treatment should be discontinued if signs of liver damage occur. Prothionamide may cause damage to the foetus and should not be used in pregnancy unless no safer drug is available.

Dose. See above under **Actions and uses.**

Preparation
PROTHIONAMIDE TABLETS, B.P.C. (page 814)

OTHER NAME: *Trevintix*®

PROTRIPTYLINE HYDROCHLORIDE

$C_{19}H_{22}ClN = 299·8$

Protriptyline Hydrochloride is 5-(3-methylaminopropyl)-5*H*-dibenzo[*a,d*]cycloheptene hydrochloride.

Solubility. Soluble, at 20°, in 2 parts of water, in 4·5 parts of alcohol, and in 3 parts of chloroform; insoluble in ether.

Standard
It complies with the requirements of the British Pharmacopoeia.
It is a white to yellowish-white, odourless or almost odourless powder and contains not less than 99·0 and not more than the equivalent of 101·0 per cent of $C_{19}H_{22}ClN$, calculated with reference to the dried substance. The loss on drying under the prescribed conditions is not more than 0·5 per cent. It has a melting-point of about 168°. A 1 per cent solution in water has a pH of 5·0 to 6·5.

Actions and uses. Protriptyline has the actions and uses described under Amitriptyline Hydrochloride (page 22) but it has a more rapid onset of action, varying from four to eight days after inception of treatment. Although it lacks the sedative action of amitriptyline, it may reduce alertness and ability to perform complex tasks.

UNDESIRABLE EFFECTS. These are as described under Amitriptyline Hydrochloride (page 22) but dystonias and photosensitivity may also occur.

PRECAUTIONS AND CONTRA-INDICATIONS. These are as described under Amitriptyline Hydrochloride (page 22).
Caution should be exercised when giving protriptyline to patients who are being treated with a monoamine-oxidase inhibitor, such as isocarboxazid, nialamide, phenelzine, or tranylcypromine, or who have been so treated within the previous ten days.

Dose. 15 to 60 milligrams daily in divided doses, reducing as depression becomes controlled.

Preparation
PROTRIPTYLINE TABLETS, B.P. Unless otherwise specified, tablets each containing 5 mg of protriptyline hydrochloride are supplied. They are film coated. Tablets containing 10 mg are also available.

OTHER NAME: *Concordin*®

PROXYMETACAINE HYDROCHLORIDE

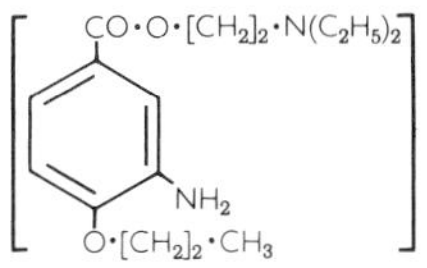

SYNONYM: Proparacaine Hydrochloride

$C_{16}H_{27}ClN_2O_3 = 330.9$

Proxymetacaine Hydrochloride is 2-diethylaminoethyl 3-amino-4-propoxybenzoate hydrochloride.

Solubility. Soluble, at 20°, in 30 parts of water and in 50 parts of alcohol.

Standard
DESCRIPTION. A white or almost white crystalline powder; odourless or almost odourless.

IDENTIFICATION TESTS. 1. Dissolve about 0·1 g in 10 ml of water, heat to boiling, add, with stirring, 1 ml of a saturated solution of *trinitrophenol* in *alcohol (20 per cent)*, and allow to cool slowly; a precipitate is formed which, after washing with water and drying in vacuo, melts at about 119°.
2. The ultraviolet absorption spectrum exhibits the characteristics given in Appendix 3, page 856.
3. It gives the reaction characteristic of primary aromatic amines, forming a bright orange-red precipitate.
4. It gives the reactions characteristic of chlorides.

ACIDITY. pH of a 1·0 per cent w/v solution in *carbon dioxide-free water*, 5·5 to 6·1.

MELTING-POINT. 178° to 185°.

LOSS ON DRYING. Not more than 0·5 per cent, determined by drying at 105° for 3 hours.

SULPHATED ASH. Not more than 0·15 per cent.

CONTENT OF $C_{16}H_{27}ClN_2O_3$. Not less than 98·0 and not more than the equivalent of 102·0 per cent, calculated with reference to the substance dried under the prescribed conditions, determined by the following method:
Titrate about 0·25 g, accurately weighed, by Method I of the British Pharmacopoeia, Appendix XIB, for non-aqueous titration; each ml of 0·1N perchloric acid is equivalent to 0·01654 g of $C_{16}H_{27}ClN_2O_3$.

Sterilisation. Solutions are sterilised by filtration in an atmosphere of nitrogen or other inert gas.

Storage. It should be stored in airtight containers.

Actions and uses. Proxymetacaine is a local anaesthetic which is suitable for use in the eye. It has a potency somewhat greater than that of amethocaine.
The instillation of one drop of a 0·5 per cent solution of proxymetacaine hydrochloride produces anaesthesia lasting about fifteen minutes; deep anaesthesia, as required for cataract extraction, may be obtained by instilling one drop every five to ten minutes until five to seven drops have been administered.

UNDESIRABLE EFFECTS. Sensitivity reactions occur rarely.

Preparation
PROXYMETACAINE EYE-DROPS, B.P.C. (page 694)

OTHER NAME: *Ophthaine®*

PSEUDOEPHEDRINE HYDROCHLORIDE

$C_{10}H_{16}ClNO = 201.7$

$[C_6H_5 \cdot CH(OH) \cdot CH(NHCH_3) \cdot CH_3]HCl$

Pseudoephedrine Hydrochloride is the hydrochloride of (+)-2-methylamino-1-phenylpropan-1-ol, an alkaloid obtained from species of *Ephedra*.

Solubility. Soluble, at 20°, in 1·6 parts of water, in 4 parts of alcohol, and in 60 parts of chloroform.

Standard
It complies with the requirements of the British Pharmacopoeia.
It is a white, crystalline, almost odourless powder and contains not less than 99·0 and not more than the equivalent of 101·0 per cent of $C_{10}H_{16}ClNO$, calculated with reference to the dried substance. The loss on drying under the prescribed conditions is not more than 0·5 per cent. It has a melting-point of 183° to 186°.

Actions and uses. Pseudoephedrine is a sympathomimetic amine with actions resembling those of ephedrine (page 178).
It is used as a bronchodilator and peripheral vasoconstrictor in preparations for the relief of nasal and bronchial congestion, particularly in bronchial asthma.

PRECAUTIONS AND CONTRA-INDICATIONS. Pseudoephedrine should be given with caution to hypertensive patients and those with prostatic enlargement. It should not be given to patients who are being treated with a monoamine-oxidase inhibitor, such as isocarboxazid, nialamide, phenelzine, or tranylcypromine, or within about ten days of the discontinuation of such treatment.

Dose. 60 to 180 milligrams daily in divided doses.

OTHER NAME: *d-Isoephedrine Hydrochloride*

PSYLLIUM

SYNONYM: Flea Seed

Psyllium consists of the dried ripe seed of *Plantago afra* L. (*P. psyllium*) or of *P. indica* L. (*P. arenaria* Waldst. et Kit.) (Fam. Plantaginaceae). The plants are annual herbs which are indigenous to the Mediterranean region (*P. afra*) and parts of Europe, Asia, and North Africa (*P. indica*).

Psyllium is produced mainly in southern France.

Constituents. Psyllium contains mucilage as its principal constituent, together with fixed oil and proteins. It yields about 2·5 to 4 per cent of ash.

Standard for unground drug
DESCRIPTION. *Macroscopical: P. afra* seeds about 2 to 3 mm long and 0·8 to 1·2 mm wide, rounded-oblong in outline, dark reddish-brown, surface shining and glossy, very transparent and showing the embryo as a paler longitudinal area about one-third width of seed as seen through the outer layers; hilum pale coloured, in centre of concave surface, a slight transverse constriction across the centre of the convex surface; endosperm hard; embryo straight, almost as long as the seed, lying near the convex surface, and having two cotyledons and their contiguous flattened upper surfaces in the median plane; seeds becoming surrounded by a layer of colourless translucent mucilage when soaked in water.
P. indica seeds similar to those of *P. afra* but more elliptical in outline; blackish-brown in colour and not very transparent; surface rather dull; from 2 to 2·5 mm long and 1 to 1·5 mm wide at the centre; the furrow of the concave surface frequently extending to the extreme end of the seed.
Odour not marked; taste mucilaginous.

Microscopical: the diagnostic characters are: *epidermis* with polyhedral cells, transparent and full of mucilage; *endosperm* composed of cells with thick, cellulose walls with numerous pits, cell contents granular; *embryo* of thin-walled polyhedral cells containing *fixed oil* and *aleurone grains*.

FOREIGN ORGANIC MATTER. Not more than 3·0 per cent.

ABSORBENCY. Transfer 1·0 g to a 25-ml stoppered cylinder, fill to the 20-ml mark with water, shake gently and occasionally during 24 hours, and allow to stand for one hour; the swollen seeds occupy a volume of not less than 14 ml.

WEIGHT. 100 seeds weigh 0·09 g to 0·14 g.

Standard for powdered drug: Powdered Psyllium
DESCRIPTION. A light brown to brown powder possessing the diagnostic microscopical characters of the unground drug.

FOREIGN ORGANIC MATTER; ABSORBENCY. It complies with the requirements for the unground drug.

Adulterants and substitutes. The seeds of *P. lanceolata* L. are distinguished by their yellowish-brown colour, the dark furrow with a black central hilum, and the failure to produce any appreciable layer of mucilage when soaked in water; 100 seeds weigh about 0·16 g.

Actions and uses. Psyllium has the property of absorbing and retaining water and has therefore been used as a bulk-providing medium in the treatment of chronic constipation. It is taken with a draught of water. Preparations of psyllium are also used to assist the production of a smooth solid faecal mass after colostomy.

Psyllium, on account of its content of mucilage, has been used as a demulcent.

Dose. 5 to 15 grams.

PUMILIO PINE OIL

Pumilio Pine Oil is obtained by distillation from the fresh leaves of *Pinus mugo* Turra var. *pumilio* (Haenke) Zenari (Fam. Pinaceae), a tree growing chiefly in the Austrian Alps, more especially in the Tyrol.

Constituents. Pumilio pine oil consists largely of terpenes and sesquiterpenes, with up to 10 per cent of bornyl acetate.

Solubility. Soluble, at 20°, in 10 parts of alcohol, with opalescence.

Standard
DESCRIPTION. A colourless or faintly yellow liquid; odour pleasant and aromatic.

OPTICAL ROTATION. At 20°, −4° to −15°.

REFRACTIVE INDEX. At 20°, 1·470 to 1·480.

WEIGHT PER ML. At 20°, 0·858 g to 0·870 g.

CONTENT OF ESTERS. 4·0 to 10·0 per cent w/w, calculated as bornyl acetate, $C_{12}H_{20}O_2$, determined by the method of the British Pharmacopoeia, Appendix IXA, for the determination of esters; each ml of 0·5N alcoholic potassium hydroxide is equivalent to 0·09814 g of $C_{12}H_{20}O_2$.

Adulterants and substitutes. Other commercially available oils are Oil of Siberian Fir from *Abies sibirica* Ledeb., which has a weight per ml at 20° of 0·900 g to 0·920 g and contains 33 to 45 per cent of esters, calculated as bornyl acetate, and Oil of Scots Pine, formerly from *P. sylvestris* L. but now distilled from the leaves and twigs of various conifers, which has a weight per ml at 20° of 0·860 g to 0·870 g and contains 1·0 to 2·5 per cent of esters, calculated as bornyl acetate.
Aromatic Oil of Pine, which is obtained as a by-product in the manufacture of steam-distilled wood turpentine in America, differs considerably in odour from the above oils, and consists largely of terpineol. It has a weight per ml at 20° of 0·927 g to 0·942 g.

Storage. It should be stored in well-filled airtight containers, protected from light, in a cool place.

Actions and uses. Pumilio pine oil is pleasantly aromatic and is inhaled with steam, sometimes with the addition of menthol, eucalyptus oil, and Compound Benzoin Tincture, to relieve cough and nasal congestion.

PYRAZINAMIDE

$C_5H_5N_3O = 123·1$

Pyrazinamide is pyrazinecarboxyamide.

Solubility. Soluble, at 20°, in 60 parts of water and in 110 parts of alcohol; soluble in ether and in chloroform.

Standard
It complies with the requirements of the British Pharmacopoeia.
It is a white or almost white, crystalline, odourless or almost odourless powder and contains not less than 99·0 per cent of $C_5H_5N_3O$, calculated with reference to the anhydrous substance. It contains not more than 0·5 per cent w/w of water. It has a melting-point of 188° to 191°.

Storage. It should be stored in airtight containers.

Actions and uses. Pyrazinamide is a tuberculostatic drug with uses similar to those described under Sodium Aminosalicylate (page 442), but it is used only in infections that are resistant to other tuberculostatic drugs. Bacterial resistance to pyrazinamide may develop in six to eight weeks and therefore it should always be used in conjunction with another drug to which the organism is sensitive.
The usual daily dosage for an adult is 20 to 35 milligrams per kilogram body-weight up to a maximum of 3 grams, given in three or four doses at equally spaced intervals.

UNDESIRABLE EFFECTS. Signs of liver damage occur in a small proportion of patients taking 3 grams of pyrazinamide daily and jaundice occurs less frequently. Anorexia, malaise, nausea, vomiting, fever, arthralgia, difficulty in micturition, rashes, and photosensitivity may also occur.

PRECAUTIONS AND CONTRA-INDICATIONS. Pyrazinamide should not be given to patients with liver damage and tests for liver function should be made before commencing treatment and at frequent intervals during treatment. Care should be taken if the drug is given to patients with renal disease or a history of gout. If it is given to patients with diabetes mellitus it may cause difficulty in controlling the diabetes.

Dose. See above under **Actions and uses.**

Preparation
PYRAZINAMIDE TABLETS, B.P. Unless otherwise specified, tablets each containing 500 mg of pyrazinamide are supplied.

OTHER NAME: *Zinamide®*

PYRIDOSTIGMINE BROMIDE

SYNONYM: Pyridostig. Brom.

$C_9H_{13}BrN_2O_2 = 261·1$

Pyridostigmine Bromide is 3-dimethylcarbamoyloxy-1-methylpyridinium bromide.

Solubility. Soluble, at 20°, in less than 1 part of water and of alcohol and in 1 part of chloroform; very slightly soluble in ether; slightly soluble in light petroleum.

Standard
It complies with the requirements of the British Pharmacopoeia.
It is a white or almost white, deliquescent, crystalline powder with an agreeable characteristic odour and contains not less than 98·5 and not more than the equivalent of 101·0 per cent of $C_9H_{13}BrN_2O_2$, calculated with reference to the dried substance. The loss on drying under the prescribed conditions is not more than 2·0 per cent. It has a melting-point of 153° to 156°.

Sterilisation. Solutions for injection are sterilised by heating in an autoclave or by filtration.

Storage. It should be stored in airtight containers, protected from light.

Actions and uses. Pyridostigmine has actions similar to those described under Neostigmine Methylsulphate (page 321) but is only about one-fourth as active as neostigmine.
Pyridostigmine is used in the treatment of myasthenia gravis; when given by mouth in doses of 60 to 240 milligrams of pyridostigmine bromide, it acts within thirty to forty-five minutes and the effect lasts for four to six hours. It may also be given by subcutaneous or intramuscular injection in a dose of 1 to 5 milligrams.
Pyridostigmine does not always relieve the symptoms of myasthenia gravis as completely as neostigmine, but its prolonged effect often provides more sustained relief and it is therefore particularly suitable for treatment at night.

UNDESIRABLE EFFECTS. As for Physostigmine Salicylate (page 380).
Pyridostigmine is less liable to cause nausea, vomiting, abdominal pain, and diarrhoea than neostigmine, but by increasing intestinal mobility it may cause disruption of intestinal suture lines.

Dose. See above under **Actions and uses.**

Preparations
PYRIDOSTIGMINE INJECTION, B.P. It consists of a sterile solution of pyridostigmine bromide in Water for

Injections. Unless otherwise specified, a solution containing 1 mg in 1 ml is supplied. It should be protected from light. A solution containing 5 mg in 1 ml is also available.

PYRIDOSTIGMINE TABLETS, B.P. Unless otherwise specified, tablets each containing 60 mg of pyridostigmine bromide are supplied. They should be stored in airtight containers, protected from light.

OTHER NAME: *Mestinon®*

PYRIDOXINE HYDROCHLORIDE

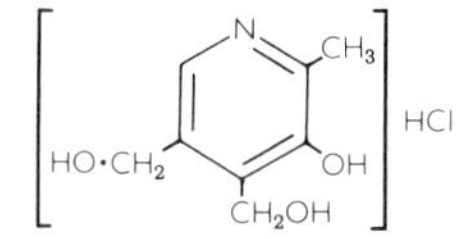

SYNONYMS: Pyridox. Hydrochlor.; Pyridoxinii Chloridum; Vitamin B_6

$C_8H_{12}ClNO_3 = 205.6$

Pyridoxine Hydrochloride is 3-hydroxy-4,5-di(hydroxymethyl)-2-methylpyridine hydrochloride.

Solubility. Soluble, at 20°, in 5 parts of water and in 100 parts of alcohol; very slightly soluble in ether and in chloroform.

Standard
It complies with the requirements of the European Pharmacopoeia.
It is a white or whitish, crystalline, odourless powder and contains not less than 98.0 and not more than the equivalent of 101.0 per cent of $C_8H_{12}ClNO_3$, calculated with reference to the dried substance. The loss on drying under the prescribed conditions is not more than 0.5 per cent. It melts with decomposition at about 205°. A 5 per cent solution in water has a pH of 2.3 to 3.5.

Sterilisation. Solutions for injection are sterilised by heating in an autoclave or by filtration.

Storage. It should be protected from light.

Actions and uses. Pyridoxine, pyridoxal, and pyridoxamine, which occur in foodstuffs, particularly in yeast, liver, cereals, and meat, are collectively known as vitamin B_6. In the body they are converted to pyridoxal phosphate, which is a coenzyme for a wide variety of metabolic transformations, including decarboxylation, transamination, racemization, and the metabolism of tryptophan, sulphur-containing amino-acids, and hydroxyamino-acids.

Pyridoxine plays a part in protein metabolism, the synthesis of fat from protein, haemopoiesis, and the nutrition of the skin. Convulsions and hypochromic anaemia have occurred in infants deficient in pyridoxine and in adults deprived of the vitamin. Lesions of the skin and mouth resembling those of ariboflavinosis and nicotinic acid deficiency have been observed in adults deprived of pyridoxine.

The daily requirement of pyridoxine in man is probably about 2 milligrams.

Pyridoxine has been used in the treatment of the nausea and vomiting of pregnancy and irradiation sickness, but the evidence of its value in these conditions is not impressive. The dosage of pyridoxine hydrochloride employed for this purpose has been purely empirical, quantities ranging from 20 to 100 milligrams daily having been given.

For convulsions in infants caused by pyridoxine deficiency, the dosage is 4 milligrams per kilogram body-weight daily for short periods. For the treatment of anaemia induced by pyridoxine deficiency in an adult, the dosage is 50 to 150 milligrams daily in divided doses.

Some types of megaloblastic anaemia, possibly due to pyridoxine deficiency, have responded to treatment with 100 to 200 milligrams of pyridoxine hydrochloride daily.

To prevent the possible occurrence of peripheral neuritis and anaemia in patients receiving isoniazid, pyridoxine is given in doses of 20 to 150 milligrams daily.

Pyridoxine, even in small doses, blocks the action of levodopa.

Dose. See above under **Actions and uses.**

Preparations
PYRIDOXINE INJECTION, B.P.C. (page 718)
VITAMINS B AND C INJECTION, B.P.C. (page 720)
PYRIDOXINE TABLETS, B.P.C. (page 815)
VITAMIN B TABLETS, COMPOUND, STRONG, B.P.C. (page 819)

OTHER NAME: *Benadon®*

PYRIMETHAMINE

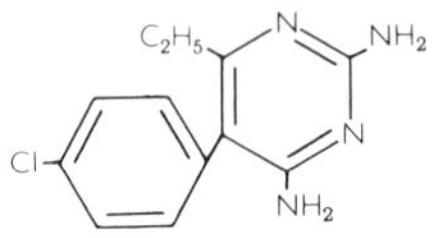

$C_{12}H_{13}ClN_4 = 248.7$

Pyrimethamine is 2,4-diamino-5-*p*-chlorophenyl-6-ethylpyrimidine.

Solubility. Insoluble in water; soluble, at 20°, in 200 parts of alcohol and in 125 parts of chloroform; soluble in warm, dilute, mineral acids.

Standard
It complies with the requirements of the British Pharmacopoeia.

It is a white, crystalline, odourless powder and contains not less than 99·0 and not more than the equivalent of 101·0 per cent of $C_{12}H_{13}ClN_4$, calculated with reference to the dried substance. The loss on drying under the prescribed conditions is not more than 0·5 per cent. It has a melting-point of 239° to 242°.

Actions and uses. Pyrimethamine is an antimalarial drug which has actions and uses similar to those described under Proguanil Hydrochloride (page 408). It affects the nucleoprotein metabolism of the parasite by interference in the folic-folinic acid systems, and this action is exerted mainly at the time when the nucleus divides. It has little effect upon immature schizonts in the red corpuscles and is therefore slow to control a malarial attack; for this purpose it is better to use a rapidly acting drug such as chloroquine.

The chief value of pyrimethamine is as a suppressant. It usually kills the primary exoerythrocytic parasites of *Plasmodium vivax* and, if used regularly, will therefore prevent relapses of most strains of benign tertian malaria. Pyrimethamine also affects gametocytes, rendering them incapable of complete development in the mosquito.

Strains of *Plasmodium* occur which are resistant to pyrimethamine, and there is evidence that some strains of proguanil-resistant malaria in man are cross-resistant to pyrimethamine. This is a further reason for using a drug of a different type for the treatment of acute infections.

A dosage of 25 milligrams of pyrimethamine by mouth once weekly is usually adequate for the prophylaxis of all forms of malaria in an adult. For a child under five years a dosage of 6·25 milligrams, and for a child from five to fifteen years 12·5 milligrams, is given once weekly. The drug is acceptable to children because it is tasteless.

Mass-treatment with pyrimethamine, given during the malaria season, is effective in maintaining a very low incidence of infection in populations in areas where seasonal epidemics of malaria occur.

Pyrimethamine is given together with chloroquine for the treatment of malarial fever during eradication campaigns; the chloroquine rapidly eliminates asexual parasites and the pyrimethamine helps to prevent transmission by the mosquito.

Sulphonamides and sulphones enhance the action of pyrimethamine, and combined courses of treatment may be used against chloroquine-resistant strains of malaria parasite.

In the treatment of toxoplasmosis 25 milligrams of pyrimethamine may be given daily, together with 500 milligrams of sulphadiazine thrice daily, for fourteen days. The dose of pyrimethamine may be increased if the patient can tolerate it.

UNDESIRABLE EFFECTS. No toxic effects have been observed during the administration of 25 milligrams of pyrimethamine once weekly. When 25 milligrams is given every day for long periods, depression of haemopoiesis is observed in some persons because of the antagonistic effect of the drug to folic acid. When treatment ceases, haemopoiesis is restored. Very large doses of pyrimethamine cause vomiting and convulsions.

POISONING. The stomach should be washed out and an injection of calcium folinate given to counteract the effect of the drug upon the processes mediated by folic acid. Convulsions should be controlled by the injection of a suitable barbiturate.

Dose. See above under **Actions and uses.**

Preparation
PYRIMETHAMINE TABLETS, B.P. Unless otherwise specified, tablets each containing 25 mg of pyrimethamine are supplied.

OTHER NAME: *Daraprim®*

PYROXYLIN

Pyroxylin is a nitrated cellulose prepared by treating defatted cotton wool with a mixture of nitric and sulphuric acids, under carefully controlled conditions, and purifying the product.

Pyroxylin is a mixture of nitrates of a polysaccharide of high molecular weight, $(C_6H_{10}O_5)_n$, consisting of at least two hundred glycopyranose units. On this basis pyroxylin has a composition corresponding to the introduction of two to two and a half nitrate groups per sugar unit.

The properties of nitrated cellulose, such as its solubility and the viscosity of its solutions, depend largely upon the number of nitrate groups introduced into the cellulose molecule, and this number depends upon the conditions of nitration, including the composition of the acid mixture and the temperature and length of time of nitration.

Nitrated celluloses which contain an average of more or less nitrate groups than pyroxylin are insoluble in a mixture of alcohol and ether; by this test gun-cotton, which contains an average of three nitrate groups per sugar unit, may be distinguished from pyroxylin.

Solubility. Readily soluble, at 20°, in a mixture of 1 volume of alcohol (90 per cent) and 3 volumes of ether, yielding an almost clear and colourless solution; soluble in acetone.

Standard
It complies with the requirements of the British Pharmacopoeia.
It occurs as a white felted mass of filaments similar in appearance to cotton wool but harsher to the touch. It is highly inflammable. A 3 per cent w/v solution in acetone (95 per cent) has a kinematic viscosity at 20° of 1100 to 2450 centistokes.

Storage. It should be stored, loosely packed, in air-tight containers, protected from light, in a cool place. It should be kept moist with industrial methylated spirit.

Uses. Pyroxylin is used in the preparation of collodions, which are convenient applications for the protection of small cuts and abrasions and for use as vehicles for drugs when prolonged local action is required.

Preparations
FLEXIBLE COLLODION, B.P. (*Syn.* Collodion). It contains 1·6 per cent of pyroxylin, with colophony, castor oil and alcohol (90 per cent), in solvent ether.

SALICYLIC ACID COLLODION, B.P.C. (page 654)

QUASSIA

SYNONYM: Quassia Wood

Quassia is the dried stem-wood of *Picrasma excelsa* (Sw.) Planch. (Fam. Simarubaceae), a tree of moderate size indigenous to the West Indies and northern Venezuela but exported only from Jamaica. The trunks and larger branches are freed from the bark, cut into thin transverse slices or chips, and dried.

Constituents. Quassia contains about 0·2 per cent of the bitter principles quassin (a lactone) and neoquassin (the hemiacetal of quassin) and a minute quantity of a yellow crystalline substance which exhibits a blue fluorescence in an acidified alcoholic solution. Quassia yields to water about 4 to 8 per cent of extractive.

Standard for unground drug
DESCRIPTION. *Macroscopical:* transverse slices or chips; density about 0·54 to 0·56, pale yellow or sometimes bright yellow; diffuse porous, with false annual rings; tough, but easily split longitudinally; tangential surface ripple-marked.
Odourless; taste intensely bitter.

Microscopical: the diagnostic characters are: *vessels* in groups of 2 to 11; walls with very numerous, minute bordered pits; vessel elements up to 200 μm wide and about 250 to 325 μm long, with transverse ends; *xylem fibres* about 750 to 900 μm long and 18 μm wide, with moderately thick walls having simple, oblique, slit-like pits; *xylem parenchyma* chiefly in interrupted tangential bands about 2 to 4 to occasionally 15 rows wide, some paratracheal parenchyma in 1 to several layers around parts of the vessels not adjacent to medullary rays; axial parenchyma in files about 4 cells long or up to 12 small cells each containing a prismatic *crystal* of calcium oxalate, 12 to **18** to **24** to 40 μm long; *medullary rays* storied, about 6 to 8 per mm of arc, mostly 2 to 4 cells wide, about 10 to 20 per cent being uniseriate, some cells containing prisms of calcium oxalate and some cells of both parenchyma and rays containing small *starch* granules, about 4 to 12 μm in diameter, mostly simple and spherical or occasionally compound with 2 components.

BITTERNESS. Macerate 5·0 g, in moderately fine powder, with 100 ml of *alcohol (70 per cent)*, with occasional shaking, for 24 hours, filter, and dilute 1 ml of the filtrate to 500 ml with water; at least 2 of 3 persons agree that 3 ml of this solution retained in the mouth for 20 seconds is not less bitter than 3 ml of a 0·00002 per cent w/v solution of *quassin* in water.
Between tests, 10 ml of a 0·1 per cent w/v solution of *citric acid* in a 5 per cent w/v solution of *sucrose* in water should be used as a mouth-wash.

WATER-SOLUBLE EXTRACTIVE. Not less than 4·0 per cent.

ASH. Not more than 5·0 per cent.

FOREIGN ORGANIC MATTER. Not more than 2·0 per cent.

Standard for powdered drug: Powdered Quassia
DESCRIPTION. A yellow to pale buff powder possessing the diagnostic microscopical characters and taste of the unground drug; odourless.

BITTERNESS; WATER-SOLUBLE EXTRACTIVE; ASH; FOREIGN ORGANIC MATTER. It complies with the requirements for the unground drug.

Adulterants and substitutes. Surinam quassia, from *Quassia amara* L. (Fam. Simarubaceae), is distinguished by the medullary rays, which are mostly one cell wide, and by the absence of crystals of calcium oxalate; it contains quassin and neoquassin.
Exhausted quassia may be differentiated by the lower yield of aqueous extractive and by the less bitter taste.
Quassia showing greyish patches is wood which has been attacked by fungus.

Actions and uses. Quassia is a bitter and, on account of its freedom from tannin, an infusion prepared from quassia, 1 to 100, may be given with salts of iron.

QUILLAIA

SYNONYMS: Quillaia Bark; Quillaiae Cortex

Quillaia consists of the dried inner part of the bark of *Quillaja saponaria* Molina, a tree indigenous to Chile and Peru, and cultivated in the Indian subcontinent, and of other species of *Quillaja* (Fam. Rosaceae).

Quillaia is exported only from Chile under the commercial designation of Valparaiso or San Antonio quillaia.

Constituents. Quillaia contains two colourless amorphous saponin glycosides, quillaic acid and quillaia-sapotoxin; they both impart to water the property of frothing, but the acrid taste and sternutatory effect are due to quillaiasapotoxin alone. Quillaia also contains sucrose and yields to alcohol (45 per cent) 28 to 40 per cent of extractive.

Standard
It complies with the requirements of the British Pharmacopoeia.

UNGROUND DRUG. *Macroscopical characters:* pieces hard, tough, flat, up to about 1 m long, 10 to 20 cm broad and 3 to **6** to 10 mm thick; outer surface brownish-white bearing pale reddish-brown or blackish-brown streaks or patches of adherent outer bark; inner surface yellowish-white, smooth, and very hard; fracture splintery and laminated, the broken surface showing numerous large prisms of calcium oxalate as glistening points; smoothed, transversely cut surface appearing chequered, with delicate radial lines representing medullary rays and tangential lines formed by alternating tangential bands of phloem containing fibres.
Taste acrid and astringent; sternutatory.

Microscopical characters: the diagnostic characters are: *outer bark,* when present, consisting of reddish-brown *cork cells* alternating with bands of brown parenchyma interspersed with numerous groups of *phloem fibres* and containing large prismatic *crystals* of calcium oxalate; *inner bark* composed of bands of tortuous *fibres* irregularly enlarged at intervals, about 500 to 1000 µm long and 20 to 50 µm wide, alternating with mixed *sieve tissue* and parenchyma; *medullary rays* mostly 3 to 4 but sometimes up to 6 cells wide with occasional subrectangular *sclereids* adjacent to the bundles of *phloem fibres; starch* grains 5 to **10** to 20 µm in diameter, and prismatic *crystals* of calcium oxalate, usually 50 to 170 µm long and up to 30 µm wide, present in the parenchymatous cells.

POWDERED DRUG: Powdered Quillaia. A pale buff powder with a pink tinge, possessing the diagnostic microscopical characters and taste of the unground drug; strongly sternutatory; forms a copious persistent froth when shaken with water.

Actions and uses. The saponins of quillaia in aqueous solution lower surface tension and the extract and tincture are used as emulsifying agents, especially for tar preparations and for volatile oils. Powdered quillaia has a powerful sternutatory action.

Preparations
QUILLAIA LIQUID EXTRACT, B.P.C. (page 684)
QUILLAIA TINCTURE, B.P.C. (page 823)

OTHER NAMES: Panama Wood; Soap Bark

QUINALBARBITONE SODIUM

SYNONYMS: Quinalbarb. Sod.; Secobarbitalum Natricum; Secobarbitone Sodium

$C_{12}H_{17}N_2NaO_3 = 260.3$

Quinalbarbitone Sodium is sodium 5-allyl-5-(1-methylbutyl)barbiturate.

Solubility. Soluble, at 20°, in 3 parts of water and in 5 parts of alcohol; very slightly soluble in ether.

Standard
It complies with the requirements of the European Pharmacopoeia.
It is a white, hygroscopic, odourless powder and contains not less than 98·5 and not more than the equivalent of 102·0 per cent of $C_{12}H_{17}N_2NaO_3$, calculated with reference to the dried substance. The loss on drying under the prescribed conditions is not more than 5·0 per cent. A 10 per cent solution in water has a pH of not more than 11.

Incompatibility. It is incompatible with acids, acidic salts such as ammonium bromide, acidic syrups such as lemon syrup, and chloral hydrate.

Storage. It should be stored in airtight containers.

Actions and uses. Quinalbarbitone sodium is an intermediate-acting barbiturate, the actions and uses of which are described under Phenobarbitone (page 366). The usual hypnotic dose is 100 to 200 milligrams.

UNDESIRABLE EFFECTS; CONTRA-INDICATIONS; PRECAUTIONS. These are as described under Phenobarbitone (page 366).

POISONING. The procedure as described under Phenobarbitone (page 366) should be adopted.

Dose. See above under **Actions and uses.**

Preparations
QUINALBARBITONE CAPSULES, B.P. The quantity of quinalbarbitone sodium in each capsule should be specified by the prescriber. Capsules containing 50 and 100 mg are available.
QUINALBARBITONE TABLETS, B.P. The quantity of quinalbarbitone sodium in each tablet should be specified by the prescriber. They are sugar coated. Tablets containing 50 and 100 mg are available.

OTHER NAMES: Secobarbital Sodium; *Seconal Sodium*®

QUINIDINE SULPHATE

$C_{40}H_{50}N_4O_8S,2H_2O = 782.9$

Quinidine Sulphate is the sulphate dihydrate of quinidine, an alkaloid obtained from the bark of various species of *Cinchona*; the base is an optical isomer of quinine.

Solubility. Soluble, at 20°, in 80 parts of water and in 10 parts of alcohol.

Standard
It complies with the requirements of the British Pharmacopoeia.

It occurs as white, needle-like, odourless crystals and contains not less than 99·0 and not more than the equivalent of 101·0 per cent of $C_{40}H_{50}N_4O_8S$, calculated with reference to the dried substance. The loss on drying under the prescribed conditions is 3·0 to 5·0 per cent. A 1 per cent solution in water has a pH of 6·0 to 6·8.

Stability. It darkens in colour on exposure to light. When heated, one molecule of water of crystallisation is lost at 100° and the second at 120°.

Sterilisation. Solutions for injection are sterilised by heating in an autoclave or by filtration.

Storage. It should be stored in airtight containers, protected from light.

Actions and uses. Quinidine prolongs the refractory period of cardiac muscle and therefore reduces the rate at which successive contractions can take place.

Quinidine is used in the treatment of paroxysmal ventricular tachycardia, and of auricular fibrillation of recent origin in the absence of congestive heart failure; it is valuable in cases of thyrotoxicosis in which fibrillation persists after thyroidectomy.

A preliminary dose of 200 milligrams of quinidine sulphate is given by mouth in the morning and, if there are no signs of idiosyncrasy, 400 milligrams is given four hours later, followed by 600 milligrams after a further four hours. This treatment is continued as long as toxic symptoms do not occur, the maximum dosage being usually 3 grams a day. If there is no improvement after treatment

for ten days, the quinidine should be discontinued, as it is unlikely to be of any benefit. In successful cases, the change from auricular fibrillation to normal rhythm occurs suddenly and the dose should then be reduced gradually. It may be necessary to continue treatment with a dosage of 300 milligrams once or twice a day for a considerable time in order to maintain normal rhythm.

For the prophylaxis of cardiac arrhythmias, 200 milligrams may be given three or four times a day.

Rarely in an emergency, quinidine may be given by intravenous injection, but extreme care must be taken.

UNDESIRABLE EFFECTS. Occasionally, quinidine produces such effects as palpitation, headache, nausea, vomiting, dizziness, dimness of vision, scarlatiniform eruptions, and precordial pain.

Dose. See above under **Actions and uses.**

Preparation
QUINIDINE SULPHATE TABLETS, B.P. Unless otherwise specified, tablets each containing 200 mg of quinidine sulphate are supplied. They should be stored in airtight containers, protected from light.

OTHER NAMES: *Auriquin®*; *Quinicardine®*

QUININE BISULPHATE

SYNONYM: Quinine Acid Sulphate

$C_{20}H_{24}N_2O_2,H_2SO_4,7H_2O = 548\cdot6$

Quinine Bisulphate is the hydrogen sulphate heptahydrate of quinine, an alkaloid obtained from the bark of various species of *Cinchona*.

Solubility. Soluble, at 20°, in 8 parts of water, giving a solution with a blue fluorescence, and in 50 parts of alcohol.

Standard
It complies with the requirements of the British Pharmacopoeia.
It occurs as odourless colourless crystals or white crystalline powder and contains not less than 99·0 and not more than the equivalent of 101·0 per cent of $C_{20}H_{24}N_2O_2,H_2SO_4$, calculated with reference to the dried substance. The loss on drying under the prescribed conditions is 19·0 to 24·0 per cent. A 1 per cent solution in water has a pH of 2·8 to 3·8.

Hygroscopicity. It is efflorescent in dry air.

Storage. It should be stored in airtight containers, protected from light.

Actions and uses. Quinine bisulphate has the actions, uses, and undesirable effects of

quinine, as described under Quinine Dihydrochloride. It is used for the preparation of tablets.

Dose. In the suppression of malaria, 300 to 600 milligrams daily.
In the treatment of malaria, 1·2 to 2 grams daily in divided doses.

Preparation
QUININE BISULPHATE TABLETS, B.P. (*Syn.* Quinine Acid Sulphate Tablets). These tablets may be sugar coated or film coated. Unless otherwise specified, sugar-coated tablets each containing 300 mg of quinine bisulphate are supplied. They should be stored in airtight containers and, unless sugar coated, should be protected from light.

QUININE DIHYDROCHLORIDE

SYNONYM: Quinine Acid Hydrochloride

$C_{20}H_{24}N_2O_2,2HCl = 397.3$

Quinine Dihydrochloride is the dihydrochloride of quinine, an alkaloid obtained from the bark of various species of *Cinchona*.

Solubility. Soluble, at 20°, in less than 1 part of water, in 14 parts of alcohol, and in 7 parts of chloroform; insoluble in ether.

Standard
It complies with the requirements of the British Pharmacopoeia.
It is a white or almost white, odourless powder and contains not less than 99·0 and not more than the equivalent of 101·0 per cent of $C_{20}H_{26}Cl_2N_2O_2$, calculated with reference to the dried substance. The loss on drying under the prescribed conditions is not more than 3·0 per cent. A 3 per cent solution in water has a pH of 2·0 to 3·0.

Sterilisation. Solutions for injection are sterilised by heating in an autoclave or by filtration.

Storage. It should be stored in airtight containers, protected from light.

Actions and uses. Quinine suppresses the asexual cycle of development of malaria parasites in the erythrocytes. It has no action on the tissue forms of the malaria parasite and therefore will not prevent relapse of *Plasmodium vivax* infection; it also has no action on *P. falciparum* gametocytes and therefore does not prevent transmission of the infection by the mosquito.

Quinine has been used to prevent and control overt attacks of malaria, but has now been largely superseded by less toxic and more effective antimalarial drugs. A dosage of 300 to 600 milligrams daily has been used as a suppressant. For the treatment of an attack, 600 milligrams has been given by mouth three times a day for four days or until the symptoms are relieved; for this purpose, tablets containing the bisulphate are usually preferred. If vomiting prevents the retention of oral doses, a soluble salt of quinine may be given by intravenous injection or by slow intravenous infusion in 200 millilitres of Sodium Chloride Injection. Intramuscular injections are slower in action than intravenous injections; they are painful and may cause tissue necrosis.

Quinine dihydrochloride is the salt usually employed for the preparation of injections. It is given by injection to patients with cerebral malaria, or when vomiting prevents the retention of the orally administered drug; 20 millilitres of a 3 per cent solution may be given by slow intravenous injection or 200 millilitres of a 0·3 per cent solution in warm saline may be given by slow intravenous infusion.

UNDESIRABLE EFFECTS. Therapeutic doses of quinine frequently produce mild toxic symptoms such as deafness, ringing in the ears, visual disturbances, and slight giddiness and tremors. Excessive doses may cause permanent deafness or blindness, and may also cause abortion in pregnant women.

The administration of quinine to a patient who has previously been suffering from a chronic and inadequately controlled malarial infection may precipitate an attack of blackwater fever.

Dose. See above under **Actions and uses.**

Preparations
QUININE DIHYDROCHLORIDE INJECTION, B.P. It consists of a sterile solution of quinine dihydrochloride in Water for Injections. Unless otherwise specified, a solution containing 300 mg in 1 ml is supplied. A solution of this strength must be diluted with at least ten times its volume of Water for Injections before administration, and injected slowly. It should be protected from light.
QUININE DIHYDROCHLORIDE TABLETS, B.P.C. (page 815)

QUININE HYDROCHLORIDE

SYNONYM: Chininii Chloridum

$C_{20}H_{24}N_2O_2,HCl,2H_2O = 396.9$

Quinine Hydrochloride is the hydrochloride dihydrate of quinine, an alkaloid obtained from the bark of various species of *Cinchona*.

Solubility. Soluble, at 20°, in 23 parts of water and in less than 1 part of alcohol.

Standard
It complies with the requirements of the European Pharmacopoeia.
It occurs as colourless, fine, silky, acicular, odourless crystals, often grouped in clusters, and contains not less than 98·0 and not more than the equivalent of 101·0 per cent of $C_{20}H_{24}N_2O_2,HCl$, calculated with reference to the dried substance. The loss on drying under the prescribed conditions is 6·0 to 10·0 per cent.
On exposure to light it gradually becomes yellowish in colour. It is efflorescent in dry air.

Sterilisation. Solutions for injection are sterilised by heating in an autoclave or by filtration.

Storage. It should be stored in airtight containers, protected from light.

Actions and uses. Quinine hydrochloride has the actions, uses, and undesirable effects of quinine, as described under Quinine Dihydrochloride.

It has been used in conjunction with urethane as a sclerosing agent in the treatment of varicose veins.

Dose. In the suppression of malaria, 300 to 600 milligrams daily.

In the treatment of malaria, 1·2 to 2 grams daily in divided doses.

QUININE SULPHATE

$(C_{20}H_{24}N_2O_2)_2,H_2SO_4,2H_2O = 782·9$

Quinine Sulphate is the sulphate dihydrate of quinine, an alkaloid obtained from the bark of various species of *Cinchona*.

Solubility. Soluble, at 20°, in 810 parts of water and in 95 parts of alcohol; slightly soluble in ether and in chloroform; readily soluble in a mixture of 2 parts of chloroform and 1 part of dehydrated alcohol.

Standard

It complies with the requirements of the British Pharmacopoeia.

It occurs as white, usually lustreless, acicular, odourless crystals and contains not less than 99·0 and not more than the equivalent of 101·0 per cent of $(C_{20}H_{24}N_2O_2)_2$, H_2SO_4, calculated with reference to the dried substance. The loss on drying under the prescribed conditions is 3·0 to 5·0 per cent. A 1 per cent suspension in water has a pH of 5·7 to 6·6.

On exposure to light it becomes brown in colour.

Incompatibility. It is incompatible with alkalis and their carbonates, iodides, tannic acid, and mercuric chloride.

Storage. It should be stored in airtight containers, protected from light.

Actions and uses. Quinine sulphate has the actions, uses, and undesirable effects of quinine, as described under Quinine Dihydro-chloride. It may be given in tablets, but the bisulphate is usually preferred for this purpose. It is not sufficiently soluble for the preparation of injections, the dihydrochloride being more generally used.

The chief use of quinine sulphate is as a bitter.

Dose. In the suppression of malaria, 300 to 600 milligrams daily.

In the treatment of malaria, 1·2 to 2 grams daily in divided doses.

Preparations

FERROUS PHOSPHATE, QUININE, AND STRYCHNINE TABLETS, B.P.C. (page 810)

QUININE SULPHATE TABLETS, B.P. These tablets may be sugar coated or film coated. Unless otherwise specified, sugar-coated tablets each containing 300 mg of quinine sulphate are supplied. Tablets containing 125 and 200 mg are also available. They should be stored in airtight containers and, unless sugar coated, should be protected from light.

RAUWOLFIA SERPENTINA

SYNONYM: Rauwolfia

Rauwolfia Serpentina consists of the dried roots of *Rauwolfia serpentina* Benth. (Fam. Apocynaceae), an erect shrub growing in the Indian subcontinent, Burma, Thailand, and Java.

Constituents. Rauwolfia serpentina contains numerous alkaloids, the most active as hypotensive agents being the ester alkaloids, which consist of methyl reserpate, with an indole structure, esterified with trimethoxybenzoic acid (reserpine) or with trimethoxycinnamic acid (rescinnamine).

Other alkaloids present have structures related to reserpic acid but are not esterified and include ajmaline (rauwolfine), ajmalinine, ajmalicine, isoajmaline (isorauwolfine), serpentine, rauwolfinine, and sarpagine.

Standard for unground drug

DESCRIPTION. *Macroscopical:* pieces about 8 to 15 cm long and 0·5 to 1 cm thick, some pieces as long as 40 cm and attaining a diameter of 2 cm; subcylindrical or slightly tapering, rather tortuous, rarely branched; rootlets usually absent; outer surface greyish to yellowish-brown, dull, with faint longitudinal ridges and a few small, circular root scars in a tetrastichous arrangement, somewhat scaly in the older pieces with small patches of exfoliating bark exposing the pale yellowish-white wood; fracture short; smoothed, transversely cut surface showing a large whitish, finely radiate, dense, and very finely porous xylem, occupying about three-quarters of the diameter, and a narrow yellowish-brown bark; starchy throughout. Odourless; taste bitter.

Microscopical: the diagnostic characters are: *cork* stratified with about 2 to 7 alternating bands of smaller cells, in 3 to 7 rows, and larger cells in 1 to 3 rows; cells isodiametric in surface view, about 20 to 70 μm, the smaller, flattened cells about 5 to 20 μm and the larger cells about 40 to 75 μm in the radial direction; *phelloderm* of a few rows of parenchyma; *phloem* narrow, parenchymatous, with small scattered groups of sieve tissue; parenchyma filled with small *starch* granules, mostly rounded but a few muller-shaped or irregular, 5 to 8 to 12 to 20 occasionally 40 μm in diameter, some showing a hilum as a simple or radiate split; numerous cells of the phloem parenchyma starch-free but containing prismatic and conglomerate *crystals* of calcium oxalate; *xylem* with well-marked growth rings and a denser core about 0·5 mm wide and containing numerous small *vessels*, remaining secondary xylem very parenchymatous and with numerous *medullary rays*; parenchyma of xylem and medullary rays lignified, with numerous rounded simple pits and filled with small starch granules; *tracheids* and *vessels* in narrow interrupted radial rows, about 35 to 54 μm in diameter, with numerous bordered pits; *xylem fibres* few with small, slanting, slit-like pits; *latex cells* occasional, in medullary rays of phloem and in cortex of rhizome; *sclereids* and *phloem fibres* absent.

FOREIGN ORGANIC MATTER. Not more than 2·0 per cent.

CONTENT OF RESERPINE-LIKE ALKALOIDS. Not less than 0·15 per cent, determined by the following method, all operations being carried out in subdued light: Triturate about 2·5 g, in fine powder, accurately weighed, with 10 ml of a 5 per cent w/v solution of *glacial acetic acid* in *alcohol (95 per cent)*, allow to stand for 2 hours, stirring occasionally, transfer to an apparatus for the continuous extraction of drugs, extract for 4 hours with 90 ml of *alcohol (95 per cent)*, and dilute the extract to 100 ml with *alcohol (95 per cent)*.
To 20 ml of this solution add 200 ml of 0·5N sulphuric acid, extract with three successive 25-ml portions of *trichloroethane*, washing each extract with the same 50 ml of 0·5N sulphuric acid, retain the washings and discard the extracts; extract the aqueous solution with 20 ml of *chloroform*, followed by five successive 15-ml portions of *chloroform*, and extract the washings retained from the first extraction, successively, with each chloroform extract; wash each extract with two successive 10-ml portions of a 2 per cent w/v solution of *sodium bicarbonate* in water, filter the extracts through a cotton-wool plug, and dilute the combined extracts to 100 ml with *chloroform*.
Evaporate 20 ml of this solution to dryness in a boiling-tube, add 10 ml of *alcohol (95 per cent)* and 2 ml of 0·5N sulphuric acid, warm to dissolve the residue, cool, and add 2 ml of a 0·3 per cent w/v solution of *sodium nitrite* in water; maintain at 55° for 30 minutes, cool, add 1 ml of a 5 per cent w/v solution of *sulphamic acid* in water, dilute to 20 ml with *alcohol (95 per cent)*, and

measure the extinction of a 1-cm layer at 390 nm, using as a blank a solution prepared by evaporating a further 20 ml to dryness and following the above procedure, but omitting the addition of the sodium nitrite solution. Calculate the proportion of reserpine-like alkaloids present by comparing the values obtained with a calibration curve prepared using a solution of *reserpine* in *alcohol (95 per cent)*.

Standard for powdered drug: Powdered Rauwolfia Serpentina

DESCRIPTION. A brownish-grey powder possessing the diagnostic microscopical characters and taste of the unground drug; odourless.

FOREIGN ORGANIC MATTER; CONTENT OF RESERPINE-LIKE ALKALOIDS. It complies with the requirements for the unground drug.

Adulterants and substitutes. Roots from other species of *Rauwolfia* resemble those of *R. serpentina* in external characters; they are most readily distinguished by the microscopical characters of transverse sections. The root of *R. tetraphylla* L. has a uniform cork and abundant sclereids and fibres in the bark; its vessels are quite numerous, averaging about 75 μm in diameter; it contains reserpine, but no rescinnamine.

Actions and uses. Rauwolfia serpentina has the actions, uses, and undesirable effects described under Reserpine (page 428). It is given by mouth as tablets of the powdered root or as an extract containing the constituent alkaloids.

PRECAUTIONS. As for Reserpine (page 428).

Dose. 1 to 2 grams.

RAUWOLFIA VOMITORIA

SYNONYM: African Rauwolfia

Rauwolfia Vomitoria consists of the dried roots of *Rauwolfia vomitoria* Afz. (Fam. Apocynaceae), a bush or tree indigenous to tropical Africa from the Guinea coast to Mozambique.

Constituents. Rauwolfia vomitoria contains numerous alkaloids, the most active as hypotensive agents being the ester alkaloids reserpine (about 0·2 per cent) and rescinnamine.
Other alkaloids present include reserpoxidine and seredine of the reserpine type, and ajmaline, alstonine, isoajmaline, isoreserpiline, raumitorine, rauvomitine, reserpiline, sarpagine, vomalidine, yohimbine, and α-yohimbine.

Standard for unground drug
DESCRIPTION. *Macroscopical:* roots occasionally branched, subcylindrical, very slightly tapering, up to about 30 cm long and 0·15 to 1·5 cm, rarely up to 9 cm, thick; outer surface greyish-brown, deeply longitudinally cracked or rubbed smooth, with a few oblique rootlet stumps; cork, if present, easily removed as flakes; fracture difficult, splintery in the wood, short in the bark; smoothed, transversely cut surface showing a narrow, pale brown bark, up to about 3 mm thick, and a buff or yellowish, finely radiate porous wood forming the majority of the drug.
Odourless; taste bitter.

Microscopical: the diagnostic characters are: *cork* stratified with zones of flattened suberised cells, each 3 to 4 layers in radial width, alternating with zones of larger lignified cells, each from 1 to about 120 layers in radial width; cells isodiametric in surface view, about 10 to 55 μm, the flattened cells about 5 to 15 μm and the larger cells about 14 to 200 μm in the radial direction; *phelloderm* of about 5 to 16 layers of parenchyma and *sclereids* about 12 to 180 μm in width or length, singly

or in small groups, occasionally containing prismatic *crystals* of calcium oxalate; *phloem* having scattered secretion cells with granular contents and isolated groups of *sclereids* forming in larger roots several discontinuous bands alternating in the outer phloem with collapsed sieve tissue, *sieve elements* clearly defined in the inner region; phloem parenchyma with several cells containing prismatic or conglomerate *crystals* of calcium oxalate; *xylem* with numerous *vessels*, about 36 to 180 μm in diameter, solitary or paired, subcylindrical, walls with small bordered pits; vessel elements about 75 to 1200 μm long, lignified *tyloses* occasionally present in the older vessels; *fibres* numerous, about 200 to 1500 μm long and up to 32 μm wide, with oblique, slit-like pits; *medullary rays* up to 3 cells wide, heterogeneous, with isolated groups of sclereids; *starch* granules in all parenchymatous tissues, rounded, 1 to 10 to 20 μm in diameter, with central hila or stellate clefts, also some 2- to 4-compound granules with muller-shaped components.

ACID-INSOLUBLE ASH. Not more than 2·0 per cent.

FOREIGN ORGANIC MATTER. Not more than 2·0 per cent.

CONTENT OF RESERPINE-LIKE ALKALOIDS. Not less than 0·2 per cent, determined by the method for Rauwolfia Serpentina.

Standard for powdered drug: Powdered Rauwolfia Vomitoria

DESCRIPTION. A brownish-grey powder possessing the diagnostic microscopical characters and taste of the unground drug; odourless.

ACID-INSOLUBLE ASH; FOREIGN ORGANIC MATTER; CONTENT OF RESERPINE-LIKE ALKALOIDS. It complies with the requirements for the unground drug.

Adulterants and substitutes. The stems of *R. vomitoria* contain negligible quantities of reserpine and can be distinguished from the roots by the smoother cork, the presence of unlignified pericyclic fibres, a dense wood with marked growth rings and a central pith; xylem vessels, about 18 to 70 μm in diameter; latex canals occur in the pith and bark.

R. caffra Sond., which occurs in districts extending from the Cameroons to the Cape; the roots are similar, but the cork is unstratified and entirely lignified. Roots of other common African *Rauwolfia* species have smaller xylem vessels, their diameters not exceeding 125 μm.

Uses. Rauwolfia vomitoria is used almost entirely for the production of reserpine.

RESERPINE

$C_{33}H_{40}N_2O_9 = 608.7$

Reserpine is an alkaloid obtained from the roots of species of *Rauwolfia* (Fam. Apocynaceae), mainly *R. serpentina* Benth. and *R. vomitoria* Afz., or prepared synthetically. The material obtained from natural sources may contain closely related alkaloids.

Solubility. Very slightly soluble in water and in ether; slightly soluble in alcohol and in methyl alcohol; soluble, at 20°, in 6 parts of chloroform and in 90 parts of acetone.

Standard
It complies with the requirements of the British Pharmacopoeia.
It occurs as white to pale fawn, odourless, small crystals or crystalline powder and contains not less than 98·0 and not more than the equivalent of 101·0 per cent of total alkaloids and not less than 98·0 and not more than the equivalent of 102·0 per cent of $C_{33}H_{40}N_2O_9$, both calculated with reference to the dried substance. The loss on drying under the prescribed conditions is not more than 1·0 per cent. It melts with decomposition at about 270°.

Sterilisation. Solutions for injection are sterilised by filtration.

Storage. It should be stored in airtight containers, protected from light.

Actions and uses. Reserpine has a central depressant action and produces sedation and a lowering of blood pressure accompanied by bradycardia. Its antihypertensive effect is due to the depletion of stores of catecholamines.
When given by mouth its effects are slow in onset, seldom appearing within three to six days of administration, and continue for some time after its withdrawal; it has a cumulative effect. Reserpine is of most value in younger patients with mild labile hypertension associated with tachycardia. In long-established hypertension it is best used in conjunction with more potent hypotensive drugs.
Patients vary in their response to reserpine and dosage must be adjusted to individual requirements. To control mild or moderate cases of hypertension, the dosage for an adult is in the range 100 to 500 micrograms, usually about 250 micrograms, daily by mouth. A thiazide diuretic may be given concurrently to potentiate the antihypertensive effect.
Reserpine is used for its sedative action in mild anxiety states and chronic psychoses. It has a tranquillising rather than hypnotic

action and produces less somnolence than the barbiturates. Patients with chronic mental illness treated with reserpine often become relaxed, sociable, and cooperative.
In mild anxiety states, doses of 0·5 to 2 milligrams by mouth are usually adequate. In severe psychosis a daily dosage of 2 to 3 milligrams by mouth, in conjunction with 5 to 10 milligrams daily by intramuscular injection, may be given initially, the dosage being subsequently reduced according to the patient's response; the optimum dosage may vary widely between patients. Treatment may have to be continued over a long period and the drug should not be abruptly withdrawn.

UNDESIRABLE EFFECTS. Reserpine, even in the minimum therapeutic doses, may give rise to a number of toxic effects. Of these, the most common are nasal congestion, lethargy, drowsiness, peculiar dreams, vertigo, and gastro-intestinal upsets.
Dyspnoea and urticarial rash sometimes occur, and a few patients increase in weight.
Higher doses may cause flushing, injection of conjunctivae, insomnia, bradycardia, and occasionally parkinsonism and severe mental depression which may lead to suicide. Cases of oedema have also been reported.
Intramuscular or intravenous injection of reserpine may cause postural hypotension.
Toxic effects are usually transient and quickly disappear on reducing the dosage or discontinuing treatment.
Tolerance to reserpine does not develop and it does not appear to be habit-forming.

PRECAUTIONS. Reserpine should be used with caution in anxiety depressive states. If used in conjunction with electroconvulsive therapy an interval of at least seven days should be allowed to elapse between the last dose of reserpine and the commencement of the shock treatment.

Reserpine should also be given with caution to patients with cardiac arrhythmias, myocardial infarction or severe cardiac damage, bronchitis, asthma, or gastric ulcer. It may give rise to hypotension in patients undergoing anaesthesia.

Dose. See above under **Actions and uses.**

Preparation

RESERPINE TABLETS, B.P. The quantity of reserpine in each tablet should be specified by the prescriber. They should be protected from light. Tablets containing 0·1, 0·25, and 1 mg are available.

OTHER NAME: *Serpasil®*

RESORCINOL

SYNONYM: Resorcin

$C_6H_6O_2 = 110·1$

Resorcinol is *m*-dihydroxybenzene.

Solubility. Soluble, at 20°, in less than 1 part of water and in 1 part of alcohol; soluble in ether, in glycerol, and in fixed oils; very slightly soluble in chloroform and in carbon disulphide.

Standard

It complies with the requirements of the British Pharmacopoeia.
It occurs as colourless or almost colourless acicular crystals or powder with a slight but characteristic odour; when exposed to light and air it becomes pinkish in colour. It contains not less than 99·0 per cent of $C_6H_6O_2$. It has a melting-point of 109° to 111° and sublimes on further heating. A 5 per cent solution in water is not acid to methyl orange.

Storage. It should be stored in airtight containers, protected from light.

Actions and uses. Resorcinol causes peeling of the skin, which may help in the treatment of acne. A 2·5 per cent alcoholic solution has been used to remove dandruff, but may slightly discolour fair hair unless all traces of soap or alkali are removed before application.

UNDESIRABLE EFFECTS. Myxoedema has been reported as a result of prolonged application of resorcinol preparations to raw surfaces.

Preparations

RESORCINOL OINTMENT, COMPOUND, B.P.C. (page 763)
MAGENTA PAINT, B.P.C. (page 766)
RESORCINOL AND SULPHUR PASTE, B.P.C. (page 768)
BISMUTH SUBGALLATE SUPPOSITORIES, COMPOUND, B.P.C. (page 796)

RHUBARB

SYNONYMS: Rhei Rhizoma; Rheum

Rhubarb consists of the rhizome of *Rheum palmatum* L. and possibly of other species and hybrids of *Rheum* (Fam. Polygonaceae), excepting *R. rhaponticum* L., cultivated in China and Tibet, deprived of most of its bark, and dried.

Varieties. High-grade rhubarb, corresponding to that formerly known as Shensi rhubarb and now sometimes marketed as Chinghai rhubarb, has a bright yellow surface and shows distinct whitish reticulations which give rise to the characteristic "nutmeg" fracture, which exhibits a bright pink tint. Much of this material shows a single hole through which passed the cord by which the rhubarb was suspended during drying.
Another quality, similar to that formerly known as Canton rhubarb, may be poorly trimmed with greyish patches on the outer surface, is of a less agreeable odour and taste, and the whitish reticulations are much less distinct. The fracture of this rhubarb is more or less uniformly granular, shows no obvious marbling and can be of a paler pink colour than Chinghai. Inferior consignments will only contain a small proportion of rhubarb giving a pink fracture, the bulk of the pieces exhibiting a grey, mauve, or brown fracture.
All Chinese rhubarb is exported from Shanghai or Tientsin in wooden cases, lined with tin-plate, and containing 280 lb or 50 kg respectively, with the inferior grades sometimes packed in hessian bags. Such commercial designations as "East Indian", "Turkey", or "Muscovy" rhubarb are now rarely used, and referred to the route by which the drug once reached the European markets.

Constituents. Rhubarb contains a number of anthraquinone derivatives based on emodin, 6-methoxy-chrysophanol (physcione), chrysophanol, aloe-emodin (9,10-dihydro-1,8-dihydroxy-3-hydroxymethyl-9,10-dioxoanthracene), and rhein. These occur free and as the glycosides of their quinone, anthrone, or dianthrone forms.
The chief purgative constituent is said to be an amorphous resin which, on hydrolysis, yields rhein, chrysophanol, and other substances.
Rhubarb also contains cinnamic acid, gallic acid and tannins, rheinolic acid, volatile oil, starch and calcium oxalate.
Chinese Rhubarb yields to alcohol about 35 to 45 per cent of extractive.

Standard

It complies with the requirements of the British Pharmacopoeia.
It contains not less than 35·0 per cent of alcohol (45 per cent)-soluble extractive.

UNGROUND DRUG. *Macroscopical characters:* pieces varying from subcylindrical and barrel-shaped to conical and plano-convex, or somewhat prismatic; often perforated with a hole; about 5 to 15 cm long and 3 to 10 cm wide; pieces usually covered with a bright brownish-yellow powder which on removal exposes the surface showing numerous longitudinal, dark reddish-brown lines or spots embedded in a whitish matrix; fracture granular and uneven; smoothed, transversely cut surface pinkish-brown or greyish; cambium line darker, near periphery (sometimes removed with external tissues on peeling); secondary phloem, when present, consisting of dark reddish-brown medullary rays containing colouring matter alternating with white lines of phloem parenchyma containing starch and calcium oxalate. Normal secondary xylem narrow, situated immediately to inner side of cambium, with an internal ring of more or less united star-like vascular strands consisting of dark red medullary rays radiating through central white phloem and peripheral xylem; these strands are known as star spots.

Odour characteristic, somewhat aromatic; taste bitter, slightly astringent.

Tests. Rhubarb complies with the following tests:

(1) Shake 0·1 g, in powder or small pieces, with 10 ml of *ferric chloride solution* mixed with 5 ml of *hydrochloric acid*, and immerse in a water-bath for about 10 minutes; filter immediately, cool the filtrate, and extract with 10 ml of *carbon tetrachloride*; separate the carbon tetrachloride layer, wash with 5 ml of water, and shake with 5 ml of *dilute ammonia solution*; a rose-pink to cherry-red colour is produced in the ammoniacal layer (presence of anthraquinone derivatives).

(2) Macerate 0·5 g of rhubarb in coarse powder or of material peeled from the outside of the drug with 10 ml of *alcohol (45 per cent)* for 15 to 20 minutes, shaking occasionally, and filter. Place one drop of the filtrate on a filter paper and examine under ultraviolet radiation, including radiation of wavelength 366 nm; no distinct blue fluorescence is produced (absence of rhapontic rhubarb).

Microscopical characters: the diagnostic characters are: *starch* granules, abundant in parenchyma, either simple or compound, with up to 5 components and showing a hilum usually in the form of a radiate split, individual granules about 4 to 18 μm, compound granules about 20 to 30 μm in diameter; large cluster *crystals* of calcium oxalate about 20 to 200 μm in diameter and frequently more than 100 μm; amorphous *yellow substance* insoluble in *alcohol (90 per cent)* but soluble in water and in *chloral hydrate solution*, and becoming reddish-pink on treatment with *dilute ammonia solution* and deep red with solutions of caustic alkalis; *vessels* mostly with reticulately pitted walls giving no reaction for lignin; *cork* and *sclerenchyma* absent.

POWDERED DRUG: Powdered Rhubarb. An orange-yellow to yellowish-brown powder possessing the diagnostic microscopical characters, odour, and taste of the unground drug.

Adulterants and substitutes. Rhapontic rhubarb, the rhizome of *R. rhaponticum*, is imported from China and is known commercially as "Chinese rhapontica", although it may be offered by exporters as "Tai-Hwang" or "Tze-Hwang" rhubarb without indicating that it is of a rhapontic nature. The rhizome occurs as untrimmed pieces, sometimes split longitudinally, and has a distinctive, slightly sweet odour, which readily distinguishes it from the official drug.

Chinese rhapontica may be hollow in the centre and the radiate transverse section shows alternate paler and darker concentric circles and a diffuse ring of isolated star-spots. When examined by the tests given above under *Tests*, it complies with test (1) for anthraquinone derivatives, but in test (2) for absence of rhapontic rhubarb it gives a distinct blue fluorescence which is intensified in colour by exposure to ammonia vapour.

Indian rhubarb, obtained from *R. emodi* Wall., occurs in cylindrical or irregular pieces, much shrunken, light in weight, and easily cut; sometimes with adherent bark, rather dark in colour, almost odourless, and taste bitter. It contains anthraquinone derivatives and yields about 25 to 30 per cent of alcohol-soluble extractive.

Storage. It should be stored in airtight containers, protected from light.

Actions and uses. Rhubarb is a mild anthraquinone purgative which has actions and uses similar to those described under Senna Fruit (page 437). Its action differs from that of other anthraquinone-containing drugs in that the tannin present may exert an astringent action after purgation.

Dose. 0·2 to 1 gram.

Preparations
GENTIAN AND RHUBARB MIXTURE, B.P.C. (page 744)
RHUBARB MIXTURE, COMPOUND, B.P.C. (page 752)
RHUBARB MIXTURE, COMPOUND, PAEDIATRIC, B.P.C. (page 752)
RHUBARB AND SODA MIXTURE, AMMONIATED, B.P.C. (page 752)
RHUBARB POWDER, COMPOUND, B.P.C. (page 778)
FIGS SYRUP, COMPOUND, B.P.C. (page 800)
RHUBARB TINCTURE, COMPOUND, B.P. It is prepared from rhubarb, 1 in 10, cardamom seed, coriander, glycerol, and alcohol (60 per cent). Dose: up to 15 millilitres daily in divided doses.

RIBOFLAVINE

SYNONYM: Riboflavinum

$C_{17}H_{20}N_4O_6 = 376·4$

Riboflavine is 7,8-dimethyl-10-(D-ribit-1-yl)isoalloxazine.

Solubility. Slightly soluble in water and in alcohol; more soluble in saline solution and in a 10 per cent w/v solution of urea in water; insoluble in ether and in chloroform; soluble in dilute solutions of alkali hydroxides.

Standard
It complies with the requirements of the European Pharmacopoeia.
It is a yellow to orange-yellow crystalline powder with a slight odour and contains not less than 98·0 and not more than the equivalent of 102·0 per cent of $C_{17}H_{20}N_4O_6$, calculated with reference to the dried substance. The loss on drying under the prescribed conditions is not more than 1·5 per cent. A saturated solution in water has a pH of 5·5 to 7·2.

Stability. When dry it is not appreciably affected by diffused light, but in solution, especially in the presence of alkali, it deteriorates rapidly, the decomposition being accelerated by light.

Sterilisation. Solutions for injection are sterilised by filtration.

Storage. It should be stored in airtight containers, protected from light.

Actions and uses. Riboflavine, a member of the vitamin-B group, is a component of the flavoprotein enzymes which form part of an enzyme system for the transference of hydrogen. The flavoproteins are necessary for the oxidation of carbohydrates, amino-acids, aldehydes, and other products of metabolism. Before it can be utilised, riboflavine must be phosphorylated, the process occurring in the intestinal wall, liver, and red blood cells.

The rôle of riboflavine in human nutrition is unknown, but it probably plays a part in the nutrition of mucous membranes, formation of red blood cells and protein metabolism. Riboflavine is absorbed from the intestinal mucosa, stored chiefly in the liver and kidneys, and excreted in the urine.

Riboflavine deficiency in man is characterised by a well-defined syndrome, the features of which are angular stomatitis, glossitis (magenta tongue), reddened, shiny, and denuded lips, seborrhoeic follicular keratosis of the nasolabial folds, nose, and forehead, and dermatitis of the ano-genital region. For normal health, an adult requires about 1·5 to 3 milli-grams of riboflavine daily, and a child 0·6 to 1·8 milligrams. Requirements are increased in pregnancy and lactation.

There is little evidence that riboflavine is of therapeutic value except in the treatment of ariboflavinosis, for which a dosage of 2 to 10 milligrams daily is given according to the severity of the condition.

Riboflavine is normally administered by mouth, but, if for any reason it cannot be absorbed or utilised by this route, it may be injected.

Dose. See above under **Actions and uses.**

Preparations
VITAMINS CAPSULES, B.P.C. (page 654)
VITAMINS B AND C INJECTION, B.P.C. (page 720)
RIBOFLAVINE TABLETS, B.P.C. (page 815)
VITAMIN B TABLETS, COMPOUND, B.P.C. (page 819)
VITAMIN B TABLETS, COMPOUND, STRONG, B.P.C. (page 819)

OTHER NAMES: *Beflavit*®; Lactoflavin; Vitamin B₂

RIBOFLAVINE PHOSPHATE (SODIUM SALT)

$C_{17}H_{20}N_4O_9NaP,2H_2O = 514·4$

Riboflavine Phosphate (Sodium Salt) is sodium 7,8-dimethyl-10-(D-ribit-1-yl)isoalloxazine 5'-phosphate dihydrate.

Solubility. Soluble, at 20°, in 20 parts of water; very slightly soluble in alcohol; insoluble in ether and in chloroform.

Standard
DESCRIPTION. A yellow to orange-yellow, hygroscopic, crystalline powder; odourless or almost odourless.

IDENTIFICATION TESTS. 1. To 1 ml of a 0·01 per cent w/v solution in water add 1 ml of 1N sodium hydroxide, expose the solution to ultraviolet radiation for 30 minutes, add sufficient *acetic acid* to make the solution acid to *blue litmus paper*, and shake the mixture with 2 ml of *chloroform*; the chloroform layer exhibits a yellow fluorescence.

2. Dissolve, with the aid of heat, 0·1 g in 1 ml of 5N hydrochloric acid, add 10 ml of *alcohol (95 per cent)*, cool in an ice-bath, induce crystallisation, and filter through a sintered-glass crucible (British Standard Grade No. 4); the residue, after washing with *solvent ether* and drying, has a melting-point of about 200°.

3. The ultraviolet absorption spectrum exhibits the characteristics given in Appendix 3, page 856.

4. To 0·5 g add 10 ml of *nitric acid*, evaporate the mixture to dryness on a water-bath, ignite the residue until the carbon is removed, dissolve the final residue in 5 ml of water, and filter; the filtrate gives the reactions characteristic of sodium and of phosphates.

ACIDITY. pH of a 2·0 per cent w/v solution in water, 4·0 to 6·3.

SPECIFIC ROTATION. +38° to +42°, calculated with reference to the substance dried under the prescribed conditions and determined, at 20°, in a 1·5 per cent w/v solution in 5N hydrochloric acid.

FREE PHOSPHATE. Not more than 0·5 per cent, calculated as H_3PO_4 and with reference to the substance dried under the prescribed conditions, determined by the following method:
Dissolve about 0·02 g, accurately weighed, in 15 ml of water, add 2·5 ml of *ammonium molybdate with sulphuric acid solution* and 1 ml of *1-amino-2-naphthol-4-sulphonic acid solution*, dilute to 25 ml with water, mix, allow to stand for 50 minutes, filter through a sintered-glass crucible (British Standard Grade No. 4), if necessary, and compare the extinction of a 1-cm layer at 740 nm with that of a similarly prepared solution using 5 ml of *standard phosphoric acid solution* in place of the sample solution, and using as the blank a solution prepared by treating 5 ml of water in the same manner. Calculate the content of free phosphate, as H_3PO_4, in the sample.

LUMIFLAVIN. To 0·035 g add 10 ml of *alcohol-free chloroform*, shake for 5 minutes, and filter; the colour of the filtrate is not deeper than that of a solution prepared by diluting 3·0 ml of 0·1N potassium dichromate to 1000 ml with water.

LOSS ON DRYING. 4·0 to 10·0 per cent, determined by drying for 5 hours at 100° over *phosphorus pentoxide* in vacuo.

CONTENT OF RIBOFLAVINE. Not less than 73·0 and not more than 79·0 per cent, calculated with reference to the substance dried under the prescribed conditions, determined by the following method:
The procedure should be carried out in subdued light or in low-actinic glassware. Dissolve about 0·1 g, accurately weighed, in sufficient *dilute acetic acid* to produce 1000 ml; dilute 10 ml of this solution to 50 ml with *dilute acetic acid* and measure the extinction of a 1-cm layer at the maximum at about 444 nm. Immediately after measuring the extinction, decolorise the solution by the addition of 0·02 g of *sodium dithionite* and immediately measure the extinction again; repeat the procedure using, in place of the sample, about 0·075 g, accurately weighed, of *riboflavine A.S.* From the differences in the two extinctions found for the sample and for the riboflavine A.S., calculate the content of riboflavine in the sample.

Storage. It should be stored in airtight containers, protected from light.

Actions and uses. Riboflavine phosphate (sodium salt) is a soluble compound of riboflavine which is used for the preparation of injections. It has the actions described under

Riboflavine; 1·4 grams of riboflavine phosphate (sodium salt) is approximately equivalent to 1 gram of riboflavine.

Preparation
VITAMINS B AND C INJECTION, B.P.C. (page 720)

ROSEMARY OIL

SYNONYM: Oleum Rosmarini

Rosemary Oil is obtained by distillation from flowering tops or leafy twigs of *Rosmarinus officinalis* L. (Fam. Labiatae), an evergreen shrub indigenous to southern Europe, and growing abundantly on dry rocky hills in the Mediterranean regions.

Most rosemary oil is imported from Spain, the south of France, and other western Mediterranean countries, but that distilled in Great Britain is superior to the imported oil.

Constituents. Rosemary oil contains 2 to 5 per cent of esters, notably bornyl acetate, and from 10 to 18 per cent of free alcohols, including borneol and linalol. It also contains camphor, pinene, camphene, and cineole.

Standard
DESCRIPTION. A colourless or pale yellow liquid; odour that of rosemary.

OPTICAL ROTATION. At 20°, −5° to +10°.

REFRACTIVE INDEX. At 20°, 1·466 to 1·474.

SOLUBILITY IN ALCOHOL. Soluble, at 20°, in 1 part of *alcohol (90 per cent)* with not more than a slight opalescence.

WEIGHT PER ML. At 20°, 0·893 g to 0·910 g.

ESTER VALUE. Not less than 5·5.

ESTER VALUE AFTER ACETYLATION. 37·0 to 65·0, determined by the method given in Appendix 14, page 893.

FREEZING-POINT OF *o*-CRESOL COMPLEX. Into a stout-walled test-tube, about 15 mm in diameter and 80 mm in length, place 1·05 g, accurately weighed, of melted *o*-cresol and 2·55 g, accurately weighed, of *cineole*-*o*-*cresol compound* and add 1·5 g, accurately weighed, of the oil, previously dried by shaking with *anhydrous magnesium sulphate*. Warm the mixture gently until melted and complete the determination as described in Appendix IXD of the British Pharmacopoeia, beginning with the words "Insert a thermometer graduated in fifths of a degree . . .", and ending at the words ". . . lower than the true freezing-point". The freezing-point is not higher than 39·8°.

Adulterants and substitutes. Camphor oil and eucalyptus oil have been used as adulterants, and the presence of either of these oils will raise the freezing-point of the complex of the oil with *o*-cresol above 39·8°.

Storage. It should be stored in well-filled airtight containers, protected from light, in a cool place.

Actions and uses. Rosemary oil is used as a perfumery agent and is an ingredient of Soap Liniment (page 726).

SACCHARIN

$C_7H_5NO_3S = 183·2$

Saccharin is *o*-benzoicsulphimide.

Solubility. Soluble, at 20°, in 290 parts of water, in 30 parts of alcohol, in 12 parts of acetone, and in 50 parts of glycerol; soluble in about 25 parts of boiling water; slightly soluble in ether and in chloroform; readily soluble in dilute ammonia solution, in solutions of alkali hydroxides, and, with evolution of carbon dioxide, in solutions of alkali bicarbonates.

Standard
It complies with the requirements of the British Pharmacopoeia.
It occurs as white crystals or crystalline powder; it is odourless or has a faint aromatic odour and contains not less than 98·0 per cent of $C_7H_5NO_3S$, calculated with reference to the dried substance. The loss on drying under the prescribed conditions is not more than 1·0 per cent. It has a melting-point of 226° to 230°. A saturated solution in water is acid to litmus.

Actions and uses. Saccharin is a sweetening agent. It is usually accepted as being about 550 times sweeter than sugar.
Saccharin is used as a substitute for sugar, especially in diabetes mellitus and obesity, as it has no food value. It is excreted unchanged in the urine. It is preferably used as saccharin sodium, which is more soluble and comparatively free from the unpleasant after-taste of saccharin.

Preparation
SACCHARIN TABLETS, B.P.C. (page 816)

SACCHARIN SODIUM

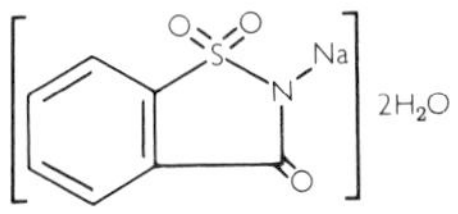

SYNONYM: Soluble Saccharin

$C_7H_4NNaO_3S,2H_2O = 241·2$

Saccharin Sodium is the dihydrate of the sodium derivative of *o*-benzoicsulphimide.

Solubility. Soluble, at 20°, in 1·5 parts of water and in 50 parts of alcohol.

Standard
It complies with the requirements of the British Pharmacopoeia.
It is a white, efflorescent, crystalline powder; it is odourless or has a faint aromatic odour and contains not less than 98·0 per cent of $C_7H_4NNaO_3S$, calculated with reference to the dried substance. The loss on drying under the prescribed conditions is 12·0 to 16·0 per cent.

Sterilisation. Solutions for injection are sterilised by heating in an autoclave.

Storage. It should be stored in airtight containers.

Actions and uses. Saccharin sodium is used for the same purposes as saccharin. The addition of about 1 per cent of a solution containing 10 per cent of saccharin sodium is suitable for sweetening most liquid preparations. Saccharin sodium is injected intravenously for the determination of circulation time; a suitable dose is 2·5 grams in 5 millilitres of Water for Injections.

Preparation
SACCHARIN TABLETS, B.P.C. (page 816)

SALBUTAMOL

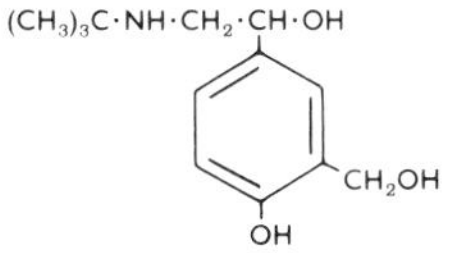

$C_{13}H_{21}NO_3 = 239·3$

Salbutamol is 1-(4-hydroxy-3-hydroxymethylphenyl)-2-t-butylaminoethanol.

Solubility. Soluble, at 20°, in 70 parts of water and in 25 parts of alcohol; slightly soluble in ether.

Standard
It complies with the requirements of the British Pharmacopoeia.
It is a white or almost white, crystalline, odourless powder and contains not less than 98·0 and not more than the equivalent of 101·0 per cent of $C_{13}H_{21}NO_3$, calculated with reference to the dried substance. The loss on drying under the prescribed conditions is not more than 0·5 per cent. It has a melting-point of about 156°.

Storage. It should be protected from light.

Actions and uses. Salbutamol is a sympathomimetic amine with actions similar to those described under Isoprenaline Sulphate (page 255). Its main action, however, is on the adrenergic receptors in the bronchi and the respiratory tract rather than on the cardiac receptors. For this reason it induces broncho-

dilatation and inhibits bronchospasm in doses which do not produce marked cardiac acceleration.
Salbutamol is administered as an aerosol spray in doses of up to 200 micrograms.

UNDESIRABLE EFFECTS. Palpitations and tachycardia may occur in some cases when salbutamol is given by inhalation.

PRECAUTIONS AND CONTRA-INDICATIONS. It is contra-indicated in patients with hypertension, myocardial insufficiency, and hyperthyroidism. The excessive use of sprays containing salbutamol should be avoided as it may lead to fatal results.

Dose. See above under **Actions and uses.**

Preparation
SALBUTAMOL AEROSOL INHALATION, B.P.C. (page 647)

OTHER NAME: *Ventolin®*

SALBUTAMOL SULPHATE

$C_{13}H_{21}NO_3,\frac{1}{2}H_2SO_4 = 288·4$

Salbutamol Sulphate is 1-(4-hydroxy-3-hydroxymethylphenyl)-2-t-butylaminoethanol hemisulphate.

Solubility. Soluble, at 20°, in 4 parts of water; soluble in alcohol, in ether, and in chloroform.

Standard
It complies with the requirements of the British Pharmacopoeia.
It is a white or almost white odourless powder and contains not less than 98·0 and not more than the equivalent of 101·0 per cent of $C_{13}H_{21}NO_3,\frac{1}{2}H_2SO_4$, calculated with reference to the dried substance. The loss on drying under the prescribed conditions is not more than 0·5 per cent.

Storage. It should be protected from light.

Actions and uses. Salbutamol sulphate has the actions described under Salbutamol. It is administered by mouth as tablets or as an elixir. It may also be used as a respirator solution containing the equivalent of 0·5 per cent of salbutamol.
In addition to the tablets described below, **an**

elixir containing the equivalent of 2 milligrams of salbutamol in 5 millilitres and sustained-release tablets each containing the equivalent of 8 milligrams of salbutamol are available.

UNDESIRABLE EFFECTS. Palpitations and tachycardia may occur in some patients when salbutamol sulphate is given by inhalation or by mouth. Oral administration may give rise to muscle tremors.

PRECAUTIONS AND CONTRA-INDICATIONS. As for Salbutamol.

Dose. The equivalent of 6 to 16 milligrams of salbutamol daily in divided doses.

Preparation
SALBUTAMOL TABLETS, B.P. These tablets contain salbutamol sulphate. Unless otherwise specified, tablets each containing the equivalent of 2 mg of salbutamol are supplied. Tablets containing the equivalent of 4 mg are also available.

OTHER NAME: *Ventolin*®

SALICYLIC ACID

$C_7H_6O_3 = 138 \cdot 1$

Salicylic Acid is *o*-hydroxybenzoic acid.

Solubility. Soluble, at 20°, in 550 parts of water and in 4 parts of alcohol; soluble in ether, in chloroform, and in solutions of ammonium acetate, sodium phosphate, potassium citrate, and sodium citrate.

Standard
It complies with the requirements of the British Pharmacopoeia.
It occurs as almost odourless, colourless, feathery crystals or white powder and contains not less than 99·5 per cent of $C_7H_6O_3$. It has a melting-point of 158·5° to 161°. A solution in water is acid to methyl red.

Incompatibility. It is incompatible with iron salts and with oxidising substances.

Actions and uses. Salicylic acid is a keratolytic substance with bacteriostatic and fungicidal properties.
It is used externally in dusting-powders, lotions, and ointments for the treatment of chronic ulcers, dandruff, and fungous infections of the skin. In the form of a paint in a collodion basis or as a plaster, it is employed to destroy warts or corns.

Preparations
SALICYLIC ACID COLLODION, B.P.C. (page 654)
SALICYLIC ACID AND SULPHUR CREAM, B.P.C. (page 660)
SALICYLIC ACID LOTION, B.P.C. (page 728)
SALICYLIC ACID AND MERCURIC CHLORIDE LOTION, B.P.C. (page 729)
AMMONIATED MERCURY, COAL TAR, AND SALICYLIC ACID OINTMENT, B.P.C. (page 758)
BENZOIC ACID OINTMENT, COMPOUND, B.P.C. (page 758)
COAL TAR AND SALICYLIC ACID OINTMENT, B.P.C. (page 760)
SALICYLIC ACID OINTMENT, B.P. It contains 2 per cent of salicylic acid in wool alcohols ointment.
SALICYLIC ACID AND SULPHUR OINTMENT, B.P.C. (page 763)
ZINC AND SALICYLIC ACID PASTE, B.P. (*Syn.* Lassar's Paste). It contains 24 per cent each of zinc oxide and starch and 2 per cent of salicylic acid, in white soft paraffin.

SECBUTOBARBITONE

$C_{10}H_{16}N_2O_3 = 212 \cdot 2$

Secbutobarbitone is 5-ethyl-5-s-butylbarbituric acid.

Solubility. Soluble, at 20°, in 1400 parts of water, in 12 parts of alcohol, in 30 parts of chloroform, and in 30 parts of ether; also soluble in aqueous solutions of alkali hydroxides and carbonates.

Standard
It complies with the requirements of the British Pharmacopoeia.
It is a fine, white, microcrystalline, odourless powder. The loss on drying at 80° is not more than 0·5 per cent. It has a melting-point of 165° to 168°. A saturated solution is acid to litmus.

Actions and uses. Secbutobarbitone is an intermediate-acting barbiturate, the actions and uses of which are described under Phenobarbitone (page 366).

UNDESIRABLE EFFECTS; CONTRA-INDICATIONS; PRECAUTIONS; DEPENDENCE; POISONING. As for Phenobarbitone (page 366).

Dose. 100 to 200 milligrams.

SELENIUM SULPHIDE

$SeS_2 = 143 \cdot 1$

Solubility. Insoluble in water and in organic solvents.

Standard
DESCRIPTION. A bright orange to reddish-brown powder with a faint odour of hydrogen sulphide.

IDENTIFICATION TESTS. 1. Boil gently about 0·05 g with 5 ml of *nitric acid* for 30 minutes, dilute to 50 ml with water, and filter; to 5 ml of the filtrate add 10 ml of water and 5 g of *urea*, boil, cool, and add 2 ml of *potassium iodide solution*; a yellow to orange colour is produced which darkens rapidly on standing.

2. Allow the coloured solution obtained in test 1 to

stand for 10 minutes and then filter through a bed of *kieselguhr*; the filtrate gives the reactions characteristic of sulphates.

SOLUBLE SELENIUM COMPOUNDS. Not more than 5 parts per million, calculated as Se, determined by the following method:
To 10·0 g add 100 ml of water at 20°, mix well, allow to stand for 1 hour with frequent shaking, and filter; to 10 ml of the filtrate add 2 ml of *2·5M formic acid*, dilute to 50 ml with water, adjust the pH to between 2·0 and 3·0 with *2·5M formic acid*, add 2 ml of a 0·5 per cent w/v solution of *3,3′-diaminobenzidine tetrahydrochloride* in water, allow to stand for 45 minutes, adjust the pH to between 6·0 and 7·0 by the addition of *dilute ammonia solution*, and extract the solution by shaking for 1 minute with 10 ml of *toluene* and allowing to separate; measure the extinction of a 1-cm layer of the toluene solution at 420 nm.
The extinction is less than that of a solution prepared by treating 5 ml of *standard selenium solution* in the same manner.
Caution. 3,3′-Diaminobenzidine tetrahydrochloride is potentially carcinogenic and should be handled with appropriate precautions.

CONTENT OF Se. 52·0 to 55·0 per cent, determined by the following method:
To about 0·1 g, accurately weighed, add 25 ml of *fuming nitric acid*, heat on a water-bath for 1 hour, cool, and dilute to 100 ml with water; to 25 ml of this solution add 10 g of *urea* and 25 ml of water, boil, cool, add 10 ml of *potassium iodide solution* and 10 ml of *chloroform*, and titrate immediately with 0·02N sodium thiosulphate until the aqueous layer is a pale straw colour; stopper the flask, shake vigorously for 30 seconds, add 0·1 ml of *starch mucilage*, and continue the titration to the complete absence of blue colour in the aqueous layer; each ml of 0·02N sodium thiosulphate is equivalent to 0·0003948 g of Se.

Actions and uses. Selenium sulphide, although highly toxic if taken by mouth, is only absorbed in traces when applied to the skin and is used as an application, containing 2·5 per cent in suspension, in the control of dandruff and seborrhoeic dermatitis of the scalp.
After the hair has been washed and rinsed, 5 to 10 millilitres of the application should be applied to the scalp together with a small volume of warm water to produced a lather. After rinsing, a second treatment should be made so that the time of exposure of the scalp to the action of the selenium sulphide is at least five minutes. The hair should then be thoroughly rinsed and all traces of the suspension removed from the hands and the finger nails. The application should be used twice a week, later once a week, and then less often as the condition is controlled.

PRECAUTIONS. Selenium sulphide should not be applied to inflamed or weeping areas because of the risk of cutaneous absorption. Care should be taken that it does not enter the conjunctival sac as it may cause keratitis and conjunctivitis.

POISONING. Vomiting, anorexia, anaemia, and fatty degeneration of the liver may follow the ingestion of selenium sulphide.
The stomach should be emptied and symptomatic treatment may be given as appropriate, but dimercaprol and sodium edetate should not be used.

Preparation
SELENIUM SULPHIDE SCALP APPLICATION, B.P.C. (page 649)

L-SELENOMETHIONINE (^{75}Se) INJECTION

This material is radioactive and any regulations in force must be complied with.

L-Selenomethionine (^{75}Se) Injection is a sterile solution of L-selenomethionine (^{75}Se).

Selenium-75 is a radioactive isotope of selenium which emits γ-radiation and has a half-life of 120 days; it is prepared by neutron irradiation of natural selenium or of selenium enriched in selenium-74.
L-Selenomethionine (^{75}Se) may be prepared either by chemical synthesis or by the growth of certain micro-organisms in a medium containing selenite ion (^{75}Se).

Standard
It complies with the requirements of the British Pharmacopoeia.
It is a clear colourless or faintly yellow liquid and contains not less than 90·0 and not more than 110·0 per cent of the quantity of selenium-75 stated on the label at the date stated on the label. Not less than 90 per cent of the selenium-75 is in the form of selenomethionine at the date stated on the label. It has a pH of 6·0 to 8·0.

Sterilisation. It is sterilised by heating in an autoclave.

Labelling. The label on the container states:
(1) the content of selenium-75 expressed in microcuries or millicuries at a given date;
(2) the volume of the injection;
(3) that the injection is radioactive; and
(4) either that the injection does not contain a bactericide or the name and proportion of any added bactericide.

Storage. It should be stored in an area assigned for the purpose. The storage conditions should be such that the maximum radiation-dose-rate to which persons may be exposed is reduced to an acceptable level.
Glass containers may darken under the effects of radiation.

Actions and uses. Selenomethionine (^{75}Se) is an amino-acid in which a selenium-75 atom replaces a sulphur atom. Although it does not occur in nature it is metabolised similarly to methionine and after injection its uptake and distribution in the body may be determined by scintiscanning or the use of the gamma-ray camera.
Pancreas scanning may be used in the detection of space-occupying lesions of the organ and in the investigation of pancreatitis. The uptake of selenomethionine by the pancreas may be increased in various ways although none of them is outstandingly successful. The

interpretation of gamma-scans of the pancreas is difficult because of the much larger amount of material taken up by the liver, and sometimes by the spleen.

Localisation of the parathyroid glands has been attempted with only very limited success.

Dose. 250 microcuries.

SENEGA

SYNONYM: Senega Root

Senega is the dried rootstock and root of *Polygala senega* L. or *P. senega* var. *latifolia* Torr. et Gray (Fam. Polygalaceae), a perennial herbaceous plant indigenous to southern Canada and the United States of America; it is also cultivated in Japan. Commercial supplies come mainly from Canada or Japan.

Varieties. Canadian senega usually consists of a rootstock, 1 to 4 cm wide, from which arises a tapering tap root, 3 to 6 mm in diameter, which frequently divides into two or more branches.

Japanese senega is obtained from young plants and is much smaller and more slender than the Canadian variety; it is paler in colour and the branched root bears numerous fine fibrous rootlets which form a tangled mass.

Constituents. Senega contains two saponins, senegin and polygalic acid, but it is probable that neither is a pure compound. The crude saponin on hydrolysis yields glucose, arabinose, a methylpentose, and a mixture of sapogenins, one of which has been named senegenin, a chlorine-containing triterpenoid.

Senega also contains α-spinasterol, polygalitol (1,5-anhydrosorbitol), sucrose, free fatty acids, and a small amount of volatile oil consisting largely of methyl salicylate. It yields about 5 per cent of ash.

Standard for unground drug

DESCRIPTION. *Macroscopical:* rootstock knotty, up to about 4 cm wide, bearing the remains of slender aerial stems and buds with purplish scale leaves, and a descending tap root, about 4 to 20 cm long and 2 to 6 mm wide just below the rootstock; tap root yellowish-brown, longitudinally or transversely wrinkled, usually tortuous with rather angular bends, on the concave side of which may occasionally be seen a distinct keel following a rapidly descending spiral; root bearing one or more spreading lateral roots and, in the Japanese variety, numerous fibrous rootlets about 0·5 to 2 mm thick and 4 to 10 cm long; fracture short and splintery in the wood, smooth in the bark; smoothed, transversely cut surface showing a thin layer of cork, a light brown bark, and a central whitish xylem traversed by almost imperceptible medullary rays; anomalous secondary thickening occurring, resulting in increased development of phloem in the keel region (where present) and in formation in the xylem of one or sometimes two wedge-shaped parenchymatous medullary rays with their apices adjacent to the primary xylem. Odour characteristic, recalling that of wintergreen; taste sweetish at first, but afterwards acrid; drug imparting to water the property of frothing.

Microscopical: the diagnostic characters are: Root: *cork* of about 2 to 6 layers of yellowish-brown tabular cells; parenchyma containing droplets of *oil* but no *starch*; *xylem* consisting of numerous *tracheids* with pitted walls and fewer small *vessels*, with reticulately thickened or pitted walls, up to 65 μm in diameter and often with lateral perforations; primary xylem diarch; *fibres*, *sclereids*, and *crystals* absent.

Stem: *epidermis* of elongated subrectangular cells; *cortex* parenchymatous; *pericyclic fibres* unlignified, in a band; *phloem* of slender elements; *xylem* containing *tracheids* with pitted walls and *vessels* with pitted or reticulately or spirally thickened walls; *pith* parenchymatous.

Scale leaves: ovate, blunt, about 2 to 3 mm long, shortly ciliate with blunt unicellular *trichomes*, up to 115 μm long, often curved at the tip, walls striated, tip filled with a refractive deposit; *epidermal cells* with sinuous anticlinal walls; *stomata* anomocytic.

ACID-INSOLUBLE ASH. Not more than 3·0 per cent.

SULPHATED ASH. Not more than 8·0 per cent.

ALCOHOL (60 PER CENT)-SOLUBLE EXTRACTIVE. Not less than 29·0 per cent.

FOREIGN ORGANIC MATTER. Not more than 2·0 per cent.

STEMS. Not more than 2·0 per cent.

Standard for powdered drug: Powdered Senega

DESCRIPTION. A grey powder possessing the diagnostic microscopical characters, odour, and taste of the unground drug. The powder is very irritating to mucous membranes of the nose and throat.

ACID-INSOLUBLE ASH; SULPHATED ASH; ALCOHOL (60 PER CENT)-SOLUBLE EXTRACTIVE; FOREIGN ORGANIC MATTER; STEMS. It complies with the requirements for the unground drug.

Adulterants and substitutes. Indian or Pakistan senega consists of the roots of *Andrachne aspera* (L.) Spreng. (Fam. Euphorbiaceae), which are contorted, with two or three longitudinal ridges but no keel, a reddish-brown bark, and a normal whitish wood with up to three or four growth rings; fragments of the bark warmed with water acquire a reddish tint, whereas similar fragments of senega acquire a yellowish tint, similar delicate tints being imparted to the water; odourless.

Another Indian senega consists of the roots of *Glinus oppositifolius* (L.) A.DC. (Fam. Aizoaceae), the transversely cut surface of which shows a series of concentric rings of vascular tissue.

Actions and uses. The actions of senega are attributed to its saponin constituents, which, although not absorbed, are irritant to the gastric mucosa and give rise to a reflex secretion of mucus in the bronchioles.

Senega has been employed, usually with other expectorants, in the treatment of chronic bronchitis.

Preparations

SENEGA LIQUID EXTRACT, B.P.C. (page 685)
SENEGA INFUSION, CONCENTRATED, B.P.C. (page 704)
SENEGA TINCTURE, B.P.C. (page 823)

SENNA FRUIT

SYNONYMS: Senna Pod; Sennae Fructus

Senna Fruit consists of the dried fruits of *Cassia senna* L. (*C. acutifolia* Delile; *C. angustifolia* Vahl.) (Fam. Leguminosae), known in commerce as Alexandrian or Khartoum senna, which is indigenous to and cultivated in the Sudan, or Tinnevelly senna, which is cultivated largely in Southern India. Small quantities of the fruits of both varieties are also exported from Eritrea.

Varieties. Alexandrian senna pods are pale to greenish-brown, with a brown central zone where the positions of the seeds are indicated by slight swellings. The width of the pod varies from 2 to 2·5 cm.
Tinnevelly senna pods are usually darker, slightly narrower (not more than 1·8 cm wide), and somewhat straighter than the Alexandrian, and the remains of the base of the style are usually more pronounced.
The testa of the seeds of Alexandrian senna is reticulately wrinkled and that of Tinnevelly seeds has transverse ridges.

Constituents. Senna fruit contains active constituents similar to those of the leaf. Commercial samples of Alexandrian pods contain about 2·5 to 4·5 per cent of sennosides A and B [glucosides of stereoisomers of rhein dianthrone, 10,10'-bis(9,10-dihydro-1,8-dihydroxy-9-oxoanthracene-3-carboxylic acid)]; Tinnevelly pods contain about 1·2 to 2·5 per cent.
Smaller quantities of the following anthraquinone glycosides are also present: sennosides C and D, based on the heterodianthrones of rhein and aloe-emodin [9,10 - dihydro - 10 - (9,10 - dihydro - 1,8 - dihydroxy - 3 - hydroxymethyl - 9 - oxoanthr - 10 - yl) - 1,8 - dihydroxy-9-oxoanthracene-3-carboxylic acid], rhein anthrone 8-glucoside, rhein 8-glucoside, rhein 8-diglucoside, aloe-emodin 8-glucoside, and aloe-emodin anthrone diglucoside.
Alexandrian senna pods yield to water about 35 to 40 per cent of extractive, and Tinnevelly pods about 18 to 35 per cent.

Standard
It complies with the requirements of the European Pharmacopoeia, as specified in the monographs for Sennae Fructus Acutifoliae and Sennae Fructus Angustifoliae.
Fruits derived from Alexandrian senna contain not less than 4·0 per cent of hydroxyanthracene derivatives, calculated as sennoside B, and those derived from Tinnevelly senna contain not less than 2·5 per cent of hydroxyanthracene derivatives, calculated as sennoside B.

Macroscopical characters: Fruit rounded-oblong to slightly reniform in shape, pale green to greenish-brown, texture parchment-like, laterally flattened, about 4 to 5 cm long and up to 2·5 cm wide; apex rounded, with a slightly projecting point formed by the base of the style; base cuspidate or shortly stalked; each pod containing about 6 to 7 flat obovate-cuneate hard seeds, about 5 to 6 mm long, having a wrinkled whitish-green surface and a short raised ridge on each side at the pointed end.
Average weight of a single senna pod is about 0·16 g. Odour and taste slight.

Microscopical characters: the diagnostic characters are: *Pericarp: epidermal cells* isodiametric, with thick outer walls; *stomata* occasional, paracytic or anomocytic; *trichomes* unicellular, warty; *endocarp* fibrous, *fibres* 5 to 7 μm wide and 0·5 to 1·4 mm long, in 2 to 4 layers crossing one another obliquely; walls thick, lignified; *mesocarp* parenchymatous, innermost layer, in contact with endocarp, with many cells containing a single prismatic *crystal* of calcium oxalate about 7 to 10 μm long; *vascular strands* of sutures each surrounded by a *crystal sheath* with prisms of calcium oxalate.
Seed coat: *epidermis* of small cells, *cuticle* thick, mucilaginous; *hypodermis* of palisade cellulosic *sclereids* followed to inner side by a layer of cells shaped like inverted mushrooms, anticlinal walls of cells thickened, giving a horseshoe-shaped outline to intercellular spaces as seen in transverse section; these cells followed to inner side by parenchyma and then a similar layer of upright mushroom-shaped cells; *endosperm* composed of polyhedral cells with thick mucilaginous walls; *embryo* consisting of thin-walled tissue.

Adulterants and substitutes. Italian or dog senna pods, derived from *Cassia italica* (Mill.) Lam. ex F. W. Andr. (*Cassia obovata* Collad.), are about 3·5 to 5·5 cm long and 1·5 cm broad; they are reniform and strongly curved with rounded ends and contain about 8 to 10 seeds, the pericarp having a small crescent-shaped ridge over each seed.

Storage. Senna fruit should be protected from light.

Actions and uses. Senna fruit is an anthraquinone purgative. The glycosides are absorbed from the intestinal tract and the active anthraquinones liberated in the course of their breakdown are excreted into the colon, which they then stimulate; the stomach and small intestine are not normally affected. As purgation occurs eight to ten hours after administration, senna preparations should preferably be given at bedtime.
Senna fruit is usually administered in the form of an infusion, four to twelve pods being soaked in about 5 fluid ounces of warm water for about twelve hours.
Some of the anthraquinones are excreted by the kidneys, and the urine of patients taking senna preparations may acquire a marked yellow colour, which changes to red on the addition of an alkali. These compounds may also appear in other secretions, notably in the milk.

Dose. 0·5 to 2 grams.

Preparations
SENNA LIQUID EXTRACT, B.P.C. (page 685)
FIGS SYRUP, COMPOUND, B.P.C. (page 800)
SENNA TABLETS, B.P. They contain the powdered pericarp of senna fruit. Unless otherwise specified, tablets each containing the equivalent of 7·5 mg of total sennosides are supplied. Dose: the equivalent of up to 30 milligrams of total sennosides.

SENNA LEAF

SYNONYM: Sennae Folium

Senna Leaf consists of the dried leaflets of the paripinnate leaves of *Cassia senna* L. (*C. acutifolia* Delile; *C. angustifolia* Vahl.) (Fam. Leguminosae), known in commerce as Alexandrian or Khartoum senna, which is indigenous to and cultivated in the Sudan, or Tinnevelly senna, which is cultivated largely in Southern India. Small quantities of the leaflets of both varieties are also exported from Eritrea.

Varieties. Alexandrian senna leaflets are pale greyish-green, ovate-lanceolate and usually slightly curved and twisted; they are brittle and often broken.

Tinnevelly senna leaflets are yellowish-green, lanceolate, flat and mostly unbroken. They are less pubescent than Alexandrian senna and are marked by occasional oblique and transverse lines produced by the hydraulic pressure used in packing the bales.

The vein islet number of Alexandrian senna is 25 to 30 and that of Tinnevelly senna is 20 to 23. The stomatal index of Alexandrian senna is 10 to **12·5** to 15 and that of Tinnevelly senna is 14 to **17·5** to 20.

Constituents. Senna leaf contains sennosides A and B [glucosides of stereoisomers of rhein dianthrone, 10,10′-bis(9,10-dihydro-1,8-dihydroxy-9-oxoanthracene-3-carboxylic acid)]; the aglycone of sennoside A is dextrorotatory, while that of sennoside B is the *meso*-form. Commercial samples of the leaf contain about 2 to 3 per cent of the sennosides.

Smaller quantities of the following anthraquinone glycosides are also present: sennosides C and D, based on the heterodianthrones of rhein and aloe-emodin [9,10-dihydro-10-(9,10-dihydro-1,8-dihydroxy-3-hydroxymethyl-9-oxoanthr-10-yl)-1,8-dihydroxy-9-oxoanthracene-3-carboxylic acid], rhein anthrone 8-glucoside, rhein 8-glucoside, rhein 8-diglucoside, aloe-emodin 8-glucoside, and aloe-emodin anthrone diglucoside.

Senna leaf also contains rhein, aloe-emodin, kaempferol, and isorhamnetin in the free state and combined as glycosides. Myricyl alcohol, salicylic acid, a phytosterolin, mucilage, resin, and calcium oxalate are also present.

Senna leaf yields to water about 30 to 40 per cent of extractive.

Standard for unground drug

Material which complies with this standard meets the requirements of the European Pharmacopoeia.

DESCRIPTION. *Macroscopical:* Leaflets lanceolate to ovate-lanceolate, about 2 to 5 cm long and 0·5 to 1·6 cm wide, pale greyish-green or yellowish-green, texture thin and brittle; asymmetrical and occasionally unequal at the base, covered with a very short fine pubescence, visible under a lens; margin entire and slightly revolute, apex acute and mucronate, petiole about 1 mm long, veins more distinct on under surface; rachis, when present, slender, about 7 to 10 cm long, with 4 to 6 pairs of leaflet scars and a longitudinal groove on the upper surface; young stem thicker and somewhat angled, bearing alternate leaf scars.

Odour slight and characteristic; taste mucilaginous at first, then slightly bitter and unpleasant.

Microscopical: the diagnostic characters are: *epidermis,* both surfaces with straight-walled polyhedral cells, many containing *mucilage* in the inner half, staining with *ruthenium red solution*; *stomata* paracytic, present on both surfaces; *trichomes* conical, unicellular, up to 250 μm long, frequently curved near the base, with thick warty walls; *mesophyll* isobilateral, with 1 layer of palisade cells below each epidermis, those beneath lower epidermis with wavy anticlinal walls; *veins* with upper and lower *bundle caps* composed of fibres, caps with outer sheath of parenchymatous cells, some of which containing a single prismatic *crystal* of calcium oxalate; cluster *crystals* of calcium oxalate present in some cells of the intercostal mesophyll.

IDENTIFICATION TEST. Heat about 25 mg, in fine powder, with 50 ml of water and 2 ml of *hydrochloric acid* in a water-bath for 15 minutes; allow the mixture to cool, add 40 ml of *solvent ether,* shake, allow to separate, and dry the ethereal layer with *anhydrous sodium sulphate*; evaporate 5 ml of the ethereal solution to dryness, allow the residue to cool, and add 5 ml of *dilute ammonia solution*; a yellow or, at most, orange colour is produced. Heat the solution on a water-bath for 2 minutes; a reddish-violet colour is produced.

CHROMATOGRAPHIC TEST. It complies with the test given in Appendix 5A, page 867.

FOREIGN ORGANIC MATTER. 1. Not more than 1 per cent. 2. Absence of *C. auriculata,* determined by the following tests: (i) Moisten about 5 mg, in fragments, with 1 drop of *sulphuric acid (80 per cent v/v)*; no crimson colour is produced. (ii) Shake 0·20 g, in powder, with 3 ml of *alcohol (95 per cent)* for 3 minutes and filter; shake the filtrate with about 0·2 g of *decolorising charcoal* and filter; mix the filtrate with an equal volume of *sulphuric acid (33 per cent w/v)*; no red colour is produced in the cold or on heating for 1 minute on a water-bath.

STALKS. Not more than 2 per cent.

SULPHATED ASH. Not more than 12·0 per cent, determined on 2 g of the powdered drug.

ACID-INSOLUBLE ASH. Not more than 2·0 per cent.

CONTENT OF TOTAL ANTHRAQUINONE GLYCOSIDES. Not less than 2·5 per cent, calculated as sennoside B, determined by the following method:

The procedure should be carried out in subdued light, or low-actinic glassware should be used.

To about 0·15 g, in fine powder, accurately weighed, in a 100-ml flask add 30 ml of water, swirl to mix, weigh, attach a reflux condenser, and immerse the flask in a water-bath, with the water level in the bath just above that of the liquid in the flask, for 15 minutes.

Allow the mixture to cool, and adjust the weight of the flask and its contents to the original weight with water. Centrifuge the mixture, transfer 20·0 ml of the clear supernatant liquid to a separating funnel, add 0·05 ml of *hydrochloric acid,* and extract with two successive 15-ml portions of *chloroform*; discard the extracts.

Centrifuge the aqueous liquid, transfer 10·0 ml of the clear supernatant liquid to a 100-ml round-bottomed flask, adjust to pH 7 to 8 with a 5 per cent w/v solution of *sodium carbonate* in water, add 20 ml of a 6·3 per cent w/v solution of *ferric chloride* in water, mix, attach a reflux condenser to the flask, and heat on a water-bath for 20 minutes. Without cooling the liquid, add 1 ml of *hydrochloric acid.* Continue the heating for a further 20 minutes, swirling the liquid in the flask frequently, to dissolve the precipitate, and allow to cool.

Transfer the liquid to a separating funnel and extract with three 25-ml portions of *solvent ether,* having used each portion to rinse the flask first. Wash the combined ethereal extracts with two 15-ml portions of water and dilute to 100·0 ml with *solvent ether.*

Evaporate 10·0 ml of the ethereal solution just to dryness on a water-bath, dissolve the residue in 10·0 ml of 1N *potassium hydroxide,* and filter the solution, if necessary, through a sintered-glass filter. Immediately measure the extinction of a 1-cm layer at 500 nm using water as the blank.

For purposes of calculation, use a value of 210 for the $E(1 \text{ per cent, } 1 \text{ cm})$ of sennoside B under these conditions.

Calculate the percentage of total anthraquinone glycosides in the sample.

Standard for powdered drug: Powdered Senna Leaf

DESCRIPTION. A green to yellowish-green powder possessing the diagnostic microscopical characters, odour, and taste of the unground drug.

IDENTIFICATION TEST; CHROMATOGRAPHIC TEST; FOREIGN ORGANIC MATTER; SULPHATED ASH; ACID-INSOLUBLE ASH; CONTENT OF ANTHRAQUINONE GLYCO-SIDES. It complies with the requirements for the unground drug.

Adulterants and substitutes. Leaflets of *Cassia italica* (Mill.) Lam. ex F. W. Andr. (*Cassia obovata* Collad.), known as "dog senna", are distinguished by their obovate shape and, microscopically, by the papillose cells of the lower epidermis.

Leaflets of *C. montana* Hayne, which are darker in colour, have a rounded apex and a dark network of veins.

Leaflets of *C. angustifolia*, growing wild in Arabia, known as Arabian or Mecca senna, are narrow, lanceolate, and usually discoloured.

Palthé senna, from *C. auriculata* L., consists of small oblong to obovate leaflets, which are coloured crimson by *sulphuric acid (80 per cent v/v)*.

Leaflets of *C. holosericea* Fresen. are small and hairy. Argel leaves, derived from *Solenostemma argel* Hayne (Fam. Apocynaceae), have been found admixed with Alexandrian senna, and occasionally the dehisced follicles and plumed seeds are also present; the texture of the leaves is thick and rigid; they are peculiarly curled, curved, or twisted; the surface is finely rugose and the veins are not evident; the leaf is equal at the base, the trichomes are three-celled, and the taste is distinctly bitter.

Storage. Senna leaf should be protected from light.

Actions and uses. Senna leaf has the actions and uses described under Senna Fruit.

Dose. 0·5 to 2 grams.

Preparation

LIQUORICE POWDER, COMPOUND, B.P.C. (page 777)

SILVER NITRATE

SYNONYM: Argenti Nitras

$AgNO_3 = 169·9$

Solubility. Soluble, at 20°, in less than 1 part of water and in 27 parts of alcohol; slightly soluble in ether and in glycerol.

Standard

It complies with the requirements of the European Pharmacopoeia.

It occurs as odourless, transparent, colourless crystals or white crystalline powder and contains not less than 99·5 per cent of $AgNO_3$. A 4 per cent solution in water has a pH of 5·4 to 6·4.

Incompatibility. It is incompatible with alkalis, halogen acids and their salts, phosphates, tannin, and astringent preparations.

Sterilisation. Solutions are sterilised by heating in an autoclave or by filtration.

Storage. It should be protected from light. Solutions should be freshly prepared and supplied in amber-coloured bottles.

Actions and uses. Silver nitrate is caustic, astringent, and bactericidal. It has been used as a caustic to destroy warts and other small skin growths.

Compresses soaked in a 0·5 per cent solution of silver nitrate have been applied to severe burns to reduce infection.

Silver nitrate stains the skin black and prolonged use of solutions may cause permanent staining of the tissues.

POISONING. A solution of common salt should be given and, after vomiting has been induced, copious draughts of milk, demulcent drinks and, finally, a dose of castor oil administered.

Preparation

SILVER NITRATE, TOUGHENED, B.P. It contains 95 per cent of silver nitrate and 5 per cent of potassium nitrate. It should be protected from light.

SOFT SOAP

SYNONYM: Sapo Mollis

Soft Soap is soap made by the interaction of aqueous solutions of either potassium hydroxide or sodium hydroxide with a suitable vegetable oil or oils, or with fatty acids derived therefrom. The soap, if prepared from oil, contains the glycerol formed during saponification.

Solubility. Soluble, at 20°, in 4 parts of water and in 1 part of alcohol; soluble in 1 part of boiling water. Some varieties of soft soap tend to separate as a gel from concentrated alcoholic solutions.

Standard

It complies with the requirements of the British Pharmacopoeia.

It is a yellowish-white to green or brown unctuous substance, yielding not less than 44·0 per cent of fatty acids.

It may be coloured with chlorophyll or not more than 0·015 per cent of an innocuous green soap dye.

Uses. Soft soap is used to remove incrustations in chronic scaly skin diseases such as psoriasis, and to cleanse the scalp before the application of antiseptic lotions. A solution in industrial methylated spirit, with the addition of solvent ether, is used to cleanse the skin. A solution of 1 part of soft soap in 20 parts of warm water is used as an enema.

Preparations

TURPENTINE LINIMENT, B.P. It contains 65 per cent of turpentine oil, 7·5 per cent of soft soap, and 5 per cent of camphor.

SOAP SPIRIT, B.P.C. (page 794)

SODA LIME

Soda Lime is a mixture of sodium hydroxide, or sodium hydroxide and potassium hydroxide, with calcium hydroxide.

Soda lime may be prepared by fusion and subsequent granulation of the fused mass.

Solubility. Partly soluble in water; almost completely soluble in dilute acetic acid.

Standard
It complies with the requirements of the British Pharmacopoeia.
It occurs as hard granules, which may be white or greyish-white or coloured with an indicator to show their capacity for absorbing carbon dioxide; suitable indicators include phenolphthalein, potassium permanganate, and methyl violet.
It absorbs not less than 20·0 per cent of its weight of carbon dioxide. The loss on drying at 105° is 15·0 to 19·0 per cent.

Storage. It should be stored in airtight containers.

Uses. Soda lime is used to absorb carbon dioxide in closed-circuit anaesthetic apparatus. Limits are specified for particle size to eliminate small granules, which cause excessive resistance to respiration, and large granules, which give inefficient absorption. The granules should be free from dust, which otherwise would be inhaled and cause irritation.
The containers for soda lime attached to the machines usually hold about 500 grams; if used continuously, this amount of soda lime will absorb carbon dioxide for two to three hours, in which time the granules will become coated with carbonate and further absorption prevented. After an interval of an hour, the soda lime will partially recover its absorptive capacity and may be used again. By using it intermittently in this way 500 grams of soda lime will provide efficient absorption for a total period of about seven to eight hours. The condition of the soda lime may be judged from the colour of the indicator which is usually incorporated.
Absorption of carbon dioxide by soda lime is accompanied by the evolution of heat, the temperature of the container usually reaching about 40°; if it becomes much hotter than this the soda lime should be discarded. It is preferable to change the soda lime container after each patient, as this allows the soda lime to cool and to recover. It is also advisable to moisten the soda lime with a few millilitres of water when filling the containers, as this increases the rate of absorption. Further moisture will be supplied by the water vapour exhaled by the patient.
Soda lime is similarly used to absorb carbon dioxide during determination of the basal metabolic rate.

PRECAUTIONS. Soda lime must not be used with trichloroethylene, as this is decomposed by warm alkali into toxic products which give rise to lesions of the nervous system.

SODIUM ACETATE

SYNONYM: Sod. Acet.

$CH_3 \cdot CO_2Na, 3H_2O = 136 \cdot 1$

Solubility. Soluble, at 20°, in less than 1 part of water and in 19 parts of alcohol.

Standard
It complies with the requirements of the British Pharmacopoeia.
It occurs as colourless crystals or a white crystalline powder which is efflorescent in warm air. It is odourless or has a very faint odour of acetic acid and contains not less than 99·5 and not more than the equivalent of 101·0 per cent of $CH_3 \cdot CO_2Na$, calculated with reference to the dried substance. The loss on drying under the prescribed conditions is 39·0 to 40·5 per cent.

Uses. Sodium acetate is used as a source of sodium ions in preparing solutions for haemodialysis and intraperitoneal dialysis. It is preferred to sodium bicarbonate on account of its greater solubility.

SODIUM ACID CITRATE

SYNONYMS: Disodium Hydrogen Citrate; Sod. Acid Cit.

$C_6H_6Na_2O_7, 1\frac{1}{2}H_2O = 263 \cdot 1$

Solubility. Soluble, at 20°, in less than 2 parts of water; insoluble in alcohol.

Standard
It complies with the requirements of the British Pharmacopoeia.
It is a white odourless powder and contains not less than 98·0 and not more than the equivalent of 104·0 per cent of $C_6H_6Na_2O_7, 1\frac{1}{2}H_2O$. A 3 per cent solution in water has a pH of 4·9 to 5·2.

Sterilisation. Solutions for injection are sterilised by heating in an autoclave or by filtration.

Actions and uses. Sodium acid citrate is an anticoagulant. It is used, generally in solution with dextrose, to prevent the clotting of blood intended for transfusion. For this purpose it is preferable to sodium citrate, as the dextrose–

sodium acid citrate solution may be sterilised by heating in an autoclave with little danger of caramelisation. Sodium acid citrate solutions are less likely to damage the surface of glass containers with the production of glass spicules than sodium citrate solutions.

A suitable solution contains 1·7 to 2 per cent of sodium acid citrate and 2·5 per cent of dextrose in Water for Injections; 120 millilitres is sufficient to prevent the clotting of about 420 millilitres of blood.

When very large transfusions are given, sufficient sodium acid citrate to affect the patient's coagulation mechanism may be inadvertently administered; in these circumstances heparinised blood should be used.

SODIUM ACID PHOSPHATE

SYNONYMS: Sod. Acid Phos.; Sodium Dihydrogen Phosphate

$NaH_2PO_4,2H_2O = 156·0$

Sodium Acid Phosphate may be prepared by the interaction of sodium phosphate and phosphoric acid.

Solubility. Soluble, at 20°, in 1 part of water; very slightly soluble in alcohol.

Standard
It complies with the requirements of the British Pharmacopoeia.
It occurs as odourless colourless crystals or white crystalline powder and contains not less than 98·0 per cent of $NaH_2PO_4,2H_2O$.
When heated, it loses its water of crystallisation at 100°, melts with decomposition at 205° forming sodium hydrogen pyrophosphate, $Na_2H_2P_2O_7$, and at 250° leaves a final residue of sodium metaphosphate, $NaPO_3$.

Actions and uses. Sodium acid phosphate is a saline purgative, the actions and uses of which are described under Magnesium Sulphate (page 278). It is also given to render the urine acid. It is administered by mouth in dilute aqueous solution.

Dose. 2 to 4 grams.

Preparation
PHOSPHATES ENEMA, B.P.C. (page 680)

SODIUM ALGINATE

Sodium Alginate consists chiefly of the sodium salt of alginic acid.

Various grades of sodium alginate are available which yield aqueous solutions having various viscosities covering the range 20 to 400 centipoises in 1 per cent solution at 20°.

The apparent viscosity at 20° of a solution of sodium alginate containing 1 g of the material in 100 ml of water is not less than 70 per cent and not more than 130 per cent of that stated on the label for viscosity grades of 100 centipoises or less and not less than 80 per cent and not more than 120 per cent of that stated on the label for viscosity grades higher than 100 centipoises.

The solution for the determination of viscosity is prepared by stirring 95 ml of water with a high-speed stirrer, slowly adding 1·0 g of the sample by sprinkling it into the vortex formed in the water, diluting to 100 ml with water, and allowing to stand for 16 hours.

Solubility. Slowly soluble in water, forming a viscous solution; insoluble in alcohol, in ether, and in chloroform.

Standard
DESCRIPTION. A white or buff powder; odourless or almost odourless.

IDENTIFICATION TESTS. 1. To 5 ml of a 1 per cent w/v solution in water add 1 ml of *calcium chloride solution*; a voluminous gelatinous precipitate is formed.
2. To 10 ml of a 1 per cent solution in water add 1 ml of *dilute sulphuric acid*; a heavy gelatinous precipitate is formed.

3. It complies with test 1 given for Alginic Acid, page 11.

ARSENIC. It complies with the test given in Appendix 6, page 879 (3 parts per million).

IRON. Ignite 1·0 g, cool, dissolve the residue in 3 ml of *hydrochloric acid FeT*, and dilute to 50 ml with water; 5 ml of this solution complies with the limit test for iron (400 parts per million).

LEAD. It complies with the test given in Appendix 7, page 883 (10 parts per million).

LOSS ON DRYING. Not more than 22·0 per cent, determined by drying to constant weight at 105°.

SULPHATED ASH. 30·0 to 35·0 per cent, calculated with reference to the substance dried under the prescribed conditions.

Incompatibilities. It is incompatible with acridine derivatives, crystal violet, calcium salts, phenylmercuric salts, alcohol in concentrations above 5 per cent, and heavy metals.
Solutions are most stable between pH 4 and 10; alginic acid is precipitated below pH 3. Solutions should not be stored in metal containers.

Sterilisation. It is sterilised by heating in an autoclave. Solutions may be similarly sterilised, but some loss of viscosity occurs to an extent which varies according to the nature of the other substances present.

Labelling. The viscosity grade should be stated on the label.

Uses. High and medium viscosity grades of sodium alginate are used for the preparation of gels, pastes, and creams and for thickening and stabilising emulsions. Medium viscosity sodium alginate is also used for its haemostatic properties as a surgical dressing. Low viscosity sodium alginate is used as a pharmaceutical adjuvant. A 1 per cent solution has suspending properties similar to those of Tragacanth Mucilage and is a useful stabiliser of oil-in-water emulsions.

For the preparation of pastes and creams, 1 to 10 per cent of sodium alginate is used according to the viscosity required; the addition of a trace of a soluble calcium salt increases the viscosity.

In preparing a solution, dispersion of the alginate may be aided by first mixing it with a suitable dispersing agent such as sugar, alcohol, glycerol, or propylene glycol. The solution should be prepared with a high-speed stirrer.

SODIUM AMINOSALICYLATE

SYNONYMS: Natrii Aminosalicylas; Sod. Aminosal.; Sodium Para-aminosalicylate

$C_7H_6NNaO_3,2H_2O = 211 \cdot 1$

Sodium Aminosalicylate is sodium 4-amino-2-hydroxybenzoate dihydrate.

Solubility. Soluble, at 20°, in 2 parts of water; soluble in alcohol; very slightly soluble in ether and in chloroform.

Standard
It complies with the requirements of the European Pharmacopoeia.
It occurs as odourless, white or almost white crystals or crystalline powder and contains not less than 99·0 and not more than the equivalent of 101·0 per cent of $C_7H_6NNaO_3$, calculated with reference to the dried substance. The loss on drying under the prescribed conditions is 16·0 to 17·5 per cent. A 2 per cent solution in water has a pH of 6·5 to 8·5.

Stability. Aqueous solutions are unstable and should be freshly prepared; oxidation and darkening in colour are retarded by adding 0·1 per cent of sodium metabisulphite.

Storage. It should be stored in airtight containers, protected from light.

Actions and uses. Sodium aminosalicylate is used in the treatment of tuberculosis, but only in conjunction with streptomycin or isoniazid or both, as the development of resistance by the infecting organisms is thereby delayed.

When taken by mouth it is rapidly absorbed, the maximum concentration in the blood being attained in about one hour, and is rapidly excreted, mainly by the kidneys. The greater proportion of a single dose is eliminated within six hours, and frequent doses are therefore necessary to maintain an adequate concentration in the blood. High concentrations are found in the lungs, liver, and kidneys; it also diffuses into the cerebrospinal fluid, pleural cavity, and aqueous humour.

The daily dosage of sodium aminosalicylate for an adult is usually 10 to 20 grams by mouth in divided doses; ideally, each dose is given at four-hourly intervals, but for convenience it is usually given twice daily.

UNDESIRABLE EFFECTS. Sodium aminosalicylate is liable to cause the usual undesirable effects of salicylates, such as drug fever, cutaneous eruptions, nausea, vomiting, diarrhoea, hypokalaemia with paralysis and cardiac arrhythmia, and jaundice; lymphadenopathy may sometimes occur.

Hypoprothrombinaemia may occur, but is of no clinical significance unless surgical procedures are to be undertaken.

Albuminuria, haematuria, and anuria have been reported.

PRECAUTIONS. The urine of patients taking sodium aminosalicylate reduces Benedict's solution; this should be borne in mind when treating diabetic patients with the drug.

Patients hypersensitive to sodium aminosalicylate may also be hypersensitive to other compounds with a *p*-aminophenyl group, including sulphonamides and certain hair dyes. Desensitisation may be attempted by reducing the dose of sodium aminosalicylate to that which avoids toxic symptoms and then increasing the dose each day within the limits of toleration until the desired daily quantity is again being given.

Dose. See above under **Actions and uses.**

Preparations
SODIUM AMINOSALICYLATE CACHETS, B.P.C. (page 650)
SODIUM AMINOSALICYLATE AND ISONIAZID CACHETS, B.P.C. (page 650)
SODIUM AMINOSALICYLATE AND ISONIAZID GRANULES, B.P.C. (page 703)
SODIUM AMINOSALICYLATE TABLETS, B.P. Unless otherwise specified, tablets each containing 500 mg of sodium aminosalicylate are supplied. They are sugar coated. Tablets containing 750 mg are also available.

OTHER NAMES: *Aminacyl Sodium*®; *Paramisan Sodium*®; Sodium PAS

SODIUM AUROTHIOMALATE

Sodium Aurothiomalate consists chiefly of the sodium salt of aurothiomalic acid,
$CO_2H \cdot CH(S \cdot Au) \cdot CH_2 \cdot CO_2H$.

Sodium Aurothiomalate may be prepared by the interaction of solutions of sodium thiomalate and gold iodide, precipitation of the sodium aurothiomalate formed by the addition of sodium chloride, and purification of the product.

Solubility. Soluble, at 20°, in less than 1 part of water; very slightly soluble in alcohol and in fixed oils.

Standard
It complies with the requirements of the British Pharmacopoeia.
It is a fine, pale yellow, hygroscopic powder with a faint odour and contains 44·5 to 46·0 per cent of Au and 10·8 to 11·5 per cent of Na, both calculated with reference to the dried substance. The loss on drying under the prescribed conditions is not more than 2·0 per cent. A 10 per cent solution in water has a pH of 6·0 to 7·0 and, when heated in a sealed ampoule at 100° for one hour and cooled, remains bright and is not more deeply coloured than a 0·05 per cent solution of potassium dichromate.

Sterilisation. Solutions for injection are sterilised by heating with a bactericide or by filtration.

Storage. It should be stored in airtight containers, protected from light.

Actions and uses. Compounds of gold, when given intramuscularly, are absorbed slowly and stored in the reticulo-endothelial cells. They are excreted slowly, mainly in the urine. No satisfactory explanation of their action has yet been found.
Sodium aurothiomalate is used chiefly in the treatment of rheumatoid arthritis. It is given by deep intramuscular injection, usually as an aqueous solution. It may be given in an initial dose of 10 milligrams, followed by gradually increasing doses, given at weekly intervals, up to a dose of 50 milligrams. Treatment may also be given in one course of weekly injections of 50 milligrams up to a total of 1 gram unless toxic effects occur, but after an initial improvement, which is usually maintained for several months after the last injection, the therapeutic effects gradually diminish. For this reason it is preferable to give sodium aurothiomalate over a much longer period, injections being either reduced in amount or given less frequently, such as every two to four weeks, or both, in order to maintain an effective deposit of the drug in the tissues.
Treatment should not be given to patients with skin reactions, stomatitis, unexplained fevers or malaise, sore throats, or haemorrhagic manifestations, and enquiries should therefore be made of patients and the urine examined for protein before each injection.
An injection may produce a transient exacerbation of rheumatoid symptoms; this occasionally necessitates a reduction in dosage.

UNDESIRABLE EFFECTS. Toxic effects are relatively common, especially skin reactions such as pruritus, purpura, erythema, papular eruptions, and urticaria. More serious reactions such as exfoliative dermatitis, toxic hepatitis, nephrosis, agranulocytosis, thrombocytopenia, and aplastic anaemia may occur, and if there are any signs of intolerance, treatment should be stopped immediately and dimercaprol or penicillamine given.
Blood dyscrasias may occur suddenly and sometimes fatally; red and white cell and platelet counts should therefore be carried out every three to four weeks and the patients should be asked to report untoward symptoms such as fever, sore throat, skin reactions, pyrexia, or marked unexplained malaise, as soon as they occur.
Undesirable effects are more likely to occur when the erythrocyte sedimentation rate has fallen below 25 millimetres per hour and the patient's condition has improved considerably.

Dose. See above under **Actions and uses.**

Preparation
SODIUM AUROTHIOMALATE INJECTION, B.P. It consists of a sterile solution of sodium aurothiomalate in Water for Injections. Unless otherwise specified, a solution containing 10 mg in 1 ml is supplied. It should be protected from light. Solutions containing 1, 5, 20, and 50 mg of sodium aurothiomalate are also available.

OTHER NAMES: *Myocrisin®*; Sodium Aurothiosuccinate

SODIUM BENZOATE

SYNONYM: Sod. Benz.

$C_7H_5NaO_2 = 144 \cdot 1$

Solubility. Soluble, at 20°, in 2 parts of water and in 90 parts of alcohol.

Standard
It complies with the requirements of the British Pharmacopoeia.
It is a white, amorphous, granular, flaky, or crystalline powder which is odourless or has a faint odour of benzoin and contains not less than 99·0 per cent of $C_7H_5NaO_2$, calculated with reference to the dried substance. The loss on drying under the prescribed conditions is not more than 1·5 per cent.

Incompatibility. It is incompatible with acids and with ferric salts.

Sterilisation. Solutions for injection are sterilised by heating in an autoclave or by filtration.

Actions and uses. Sodium benzoate, when given internally, is conjugated with glycine in the liver to form hippuric acid. This is the basis of a liver-function test. For the test, 6 grams dissolved in 200 millilitres of water is administered by mouth and the hippuric acid content of the urine is determined in specimens collected at suitable intervals. The test may also be carried out by the intravenous injection

of 1·8 grams of sodium benzoate dissolved in 20 millilitres of Water for Injections.

Sodium benzoate has also been used as a urinary antiseptic in a dosage of 0·3 to 2 grams given by mouth.

Sodium benzoate is sometimes used as a preservative instead of benzoic acid because of its greater solubility in water, but it is effective only in acidic preparations.

SODIUM BICARBONATE

SYNONYMS: Natrii Hydrogenocarbonas; Sod. Bicarb.; Sodium Hydrogen Carbonate

$NaHCO_3 = 84·01$

Solubility. Soluble, at 20°, in 11 parts of water; insoluble in alcohol.

Standard
It complies with the requirements of the European Pharmacopoeia.
It is a white, crystalline, odourless powder and contains not less than 99·0 and not more than the equivalent of 101·0 per cent of $NaHCO_3$. A 5 per cent solution in water is slightly alkaline.

Stability. When heated it decomposes and, at 250° to 300°, is converted into anhydrous sodium carbonate. Solutions in water slowly decompose at ordinary temperatures with partial conversion into the normal carbonate; the decomposition is accelerated by agitation or warming.

Hygroscopicity. At relative humidities up to about 80 per cent, the equilibrium moisture content at 25° is less than 1 per cent, but at relative humidities above about 85 per cent, it rapidly absorbs excessive amounts of moisture and this may be associated with decomposition by loss of carbon dioxide.

Sterilisation. Solutions are sterilised by heating in an autoclave or by filtration. When a solution is sterilised by heating in an autoclave, carbon dioxide is first passed through the solution in the final container, which is then hermetically sealed and not opened until at least two hours after the solution has cooled to room temperature.

Actions and uses. Sodium bicarbonate, and similar alkaline compounds, neutralise the acid secretion in the stomach. After absorption, the alkali carbonates increase the alkali reserve of the plasma and there is an increased excretion of urine, which is rendered less acid.

Sodium bicarbonate is given by mouth in the treatment of hyperchlorhydria to relieve the pain and distension; it is given with bitters, such as gentian, thirty minutes before meals to neutralise excessive secretion in the stomach. It is also of value as an antacid in the

treatment of dyspepsia and flatulence and of vomiting in children.

Solutions containing 1 to 4 per cent of sodium bicarbonate are administered intravenously to correct sodium depletion; solutions containing up to 8·4 per cent are used for the correction of metabolic acidosis caused by cardiac arrest. For its action in rendering mucus less viscid, sodium bicarbonate is added to spray solutions and washes for the throat and nose.

Sodium bicarbonate is an ingredient of Compound Sodium Chloride Mixture, which is taken as an expectorant. A weak solution (1 in 150) applied to the skin relieves itching, urticaria, and eczema.

Sodium Bicarbonate Eye Lotion is used as a first-aid treatment for irrigating burns and injuries in the eye.

Dose. 1 to 5 grams.

Preparations
SODIUM BICARBONATE EAR-DROPS, B.P.C. (page 665)
SODIUM BICARBONATE INJECTION, B.P. It consists of a sterile solution of sodium bicarbonate in Water for Injections. Unless otherwise specified, a solution containing 1·4 per cent of sodium bicarbonate is supplied.
GENTIAN MIXTURE, ALKALINE, B.P.C. (page 743)
NUX VOMICA MIXTURE, ALKALINE, B.P.C. (page 749)
RHUBARB AND SODA MIXTURE, AMMONIATED, B.P.C. (page 752)
SODIUM BICARBONATE MIXTURE, PAEDIATRIC, B.P.C. (page 752)
SODIUM CHLORIDE MIXTURE, COMPOUND, B.P.C. (page 753)
SODIUM BICARBONATE TABLETS, COMPOUND, B.P. (*Syn.* Soda Mint Tablets). Each tablet contains 300 mg of sodium bicarbonate, with peppermint oil. They should be stored in airtight containers, in a cool place. Dose: 2 to 6 tablets, which should be allowed to dissolve slowly in the mouth.

SODIUM BROMIDE

SYNONYM: Sod. Brom.

$NaBr = 102·9$

Solubility. Soluble, at 20°, in 1·5 parts of water and in 17 parts of alcohol.

Standard
It complies with the requirements of the British Pharmacopoeia.

It occurs as small, odourless, colourless, transparent, or opaque, cubical crystals or, more generally, white granular powder and contains not less than 99·0 per cent of NaBr, calculated with reference to the dried substance. The loss on drying under the prescribed conditions is not more than 5·0 per cent.

Hygroscopicity. It is deliquescent, but, owing to the formation of $NaBr,2H_2O$, does not appear moist until over 20 per cent of water has been absorbed.

Incompatibilities. It is incompatible with oxidising agents and with salts of mercury and silver.

Storage. It should be stored in airtight containers.

Actions and uses. Sodium bromide has the actions, uses, and undesirable effects of the bromides, as described under Potassium Bromide (page 392).

PRECAUTIONS. These are as described under Potassium Bromide (page 392).

Dose. 1 to 6 grams daily in divided doses.

SODIUM CALCIUMEDETATE

$C_{10}H_{12}CaN_2Na_2O_8,2H_2O = 410\cdot3$

Sodium Calciumedetate is the dihydrate of the calcium chelate of the disodium salt of ethylenediamine-$NNN'N'$-tetra-acetic acid, and may be prepared from a calcium salt and disodium dihydrogen ethylenediamine-$NNN'N'$-tetra-acetate.

Solubility. Soluble, at $20°$, in 2 parts of water; very slightly soluble in alcohol; insoluble in ether and in chloroform.

Standard
It complies with the requirements of the British Pharmacopoeia.
It is a white or creamy-white powder with a slight odour and contains not less than $97\cdot0$ and not more than the equivalent of $103\cdot0$ per cent of $C_{10}H_{12}CaN_2Na_2O_8$, calculated with reference to the dried substance. The loss on drying under the prescribed conditions is $8\cdot0$ to $11\cdot0$ per cent. A $2\cdot0$ per cent solution in water has a pH of $6\cdot5$ to $8\cdot0$.

Sterilisation. Solutions for injection are sterilised by heating in an autoclave or by filtration. Containers are made from lead-free glass.

Actions and uses. The pharmacological action of sodium calciumedetate is due to its ability to exchange its calcium atom for lead ions in the blood, thereby forming a stable non-ionisable lead compound which is water-soluble and readily excreted unchanged by the kidneys. The exchange between the lead and calcium is preferential because other metals, such as iron, copper, and cobalt, are more strongly bound to tissue proteins. Sodium calciumedetate is therefore useful in the treatment of lead poisoning and lead encephalopathy.

Sodium calciumedetate is usually given by intravenous infusion as a $0\cdot5$ to 3 per cent solution in Sodium Chloride Injection or Dextrose Injection. The infusion fluid is usually administered over a period of one hour, to a maximum of 40 milligrams of the anhydrous salt per kilogram body-weight, twice daily for up to five days. The treatment may be repeated, if necessary, after an interval of two or three days.

Sodium calciumedetate given by mouth also produces a rapid excretion of lead in the urine, which continues for some days after the cessation of treatment; the usual dosage is the equivalent of 4 grams of the anhydrous salt daily in divided doses.

UNDESIRABLE EFFECTS. Although the toxicity of sodium calciumedetate is very low, there is evidence that the repeated administration of moderate doses may produce a toxic nephrosis which, however, clears up in a few days after the drug is withdrawn.

Dose. See above under **Actions and uses.**

Preparations
SODIUM CALCIUMEDETATE INJECTION, B.P. It consists of a sterile solution of sodium calciumedetate in Water for Injections. It contains in $0\cdot2$ ml the equivalent of 40 mg of anhydrous sodium calciumedetate. It should be diluted before administration to 6 to 40 times its volume with Sodium Chloride Injection or Dextrose Injection. Dose: a maximum of $0\cdot2$ millilitre per kg body-weight by intravenous infusion over a period of one hour, twice daily for up to 5 days, in accordance with the needs of the patient.

SODIUM CALCIUMEDETATE TABLETS, B.P. Each tablet contains the equivalent of 500 mg of anhydrous sodium calciumedetate. Dose: a maximum of 8 tablets daily in divided doses.

OTHER NAME: *Calcium Disodium Versenate*®

SODIUM CARBONATE

SYNONYMS: Natrii Carbonas Decahydricus; Sodium Carbonate Decahydrate

$Na_2CO_3,10H_2O = 286\cdot1$

Sodium Carbonate may be prepared by heating sodium bicarbonate and crystallising the product from water.

Solubility. Soluble, at $20°$, in 2 parts of water; insoluble in alcohol.

Standard
Material which complies with this standard meets the requirements of the European Pharmacopoeia.

DESCRIPTION. Colourless, transparent, efflorescent crystals or a white crystalline powder; odourless.

IDENTIFICATION TESTS. A 10 per cent solution in water has a pH greater than 10 and gives the reactions characteristic of sodium and of carbonates.

APPEARANCE OF SOLUTION. A 40 per cent w/v solution in water complies with the following tests:
(i) The solution is clear or not more opalescent than a reference solution prepared by mixing, without vigorous shaking, 3·75 ml of *0·00002M sodium chloride*, 0·25 ml of water, 5·0 ml of *2M nitric acid*, and 1·0 ml of *dilute silver nitrate solution*, the comparison being made, 5 minutes after preparation of the reference solution, by viewing vertically 10 ml of the liquids in matched, colourless, transparent, neutral glass tubes, 16 mm internal diameter and with a flat base, against a black background in diffused light.
(ii) The solution is not more intensely coloured than a reference solution prepared by mixing 0·1 ml of *yellow standard solution* with 1·9 ml of *diluted hydrochloric acid* (*1 per cent w/v*), the comparison being made by viewing horizontally 2 ml of the liquids in matched, colourless, transparent, neutral glass tubes, 12 mm internal diameter, against a white background in diffused daylight.

ARSENIC. It complies with the test given in Appendix 6, page 879 (2 parts per million).

HEAVY METALS. It complies with the test given in Appendix 8, page 887 (20 parts per million as Pb).

IRON. Dissolve 0·5 g, in portions, in a mixture of 2·5 ml of water and 0·5 ml of *hydrochloric acid FeT*, boil, cool, neutralise to *litmus paper* with *dilute sodium hydroxide solution*, and dilute to 10 ml with water. This solution complies with the following test:
Add 2 ml of a 20 per cent w/v solution of *citric acid FeT* in water and 0·1 ml of *thioglycollic acid*, mix, make alkaline with *strong ammonia solution*, dilute to 20 ml with water, and allow to stand for 5 minutes; any pink colour produced is not more intense than that produced when 10 ml of *weak iron standard solution* is treated in the same manner (20 parts per million).

ALKALI HYDROXIDES AND CARBONATES. Dissolve 1·0 g in 20 ml of water, add 20 ml of *0·25M barium chloride*, filter, and to 10 ml of the filtrate add 0·1 ml of *phenolphthalein solution*; the solution does not become red. Boil the remainder of the filtrate for 2 minutes; the solution remains clear.

CHLORIDE. Dissolve 1·0 g in a mixture of 5 ml of water and 2 ml of *nitric acid* and dilute to 15 ml with water. This solution complies with the following test:
Add the prepared solution to a mixture of 0·3 ml of *dilute silver nitrate solution* and 0·15 ml of *2M nitric acid* and allow to stand for 2 minutes protected from light; any opalescence produced is not more intense than that produced when a mixture of 10 ml of *chloride standard solution* and 5 ml of water are treated in the same manner (50 parts per million).

SULPHATE. Dissolve 1·5 g, in portions, in a mixture of 7·5 ml of water and 1·5 ml of *hydrochloric acid*, boil, cool, neutralise to *litmus paper* with *dilute sodium hydroxide solution*, dilute to 15 ml with water, and add 0·3 ml of *acetic acid*. This solution complies with the following test:
To 1·5 ml of *sulphate standard solution* add successively and with continuous shaking 0·75 ml of *alcohol* (*95 per cent*), 0·5 ml of *0·25M barium chloride*, and 0·25 ml of *acetic acid*, shake for a further 30 seconds, add the prepared solution, and allow to stand for 5 minutes; any opalescence produced is not more intense than that produced when 15 ml of *standard sulphate solution*, acidified with 0·3 ml of *acetic acid*, is used in place of the prepared solution (100 parts per million).

CONTENT OF Na₂CO₃. Not less than 36·7 and not more than 39·0 per cent, determined by the following method:
Dissolve about 3 g, accurately weighed, in 25 ml of water and titrate with 1N hydrochloric acid using *methyl orange solution* as indicator; each ml of 1N hydrochloric acid is equivalent to 0·05300 g of Na₂CO₃.

Storage. It should be stored in airtight containers.

Uses. Sodium carbonate is employed in the preparation of alkaline baths (250 g in 150 litres) and of Surgical Chlorinated Soda Solution.

Preparation
CHLORINATED SODA SOLUTION, SURGICAL, B.P.C. (page 782)

SODIUM CARBOXYMETHYLCELLULOSE

SYNONYM: Sodium Cellulose Glycollate

Sodium Carboxymethylcellulose is the sodium salt of carboxymethylcellulose, and is prepared from chloroacetic acid, cellulose, and sodium hydroxide. Sodium carboxymethylcellulose may be represented by the formula $[C_6H_{10-x}O_5(CH_2 \cdot CO_2Na)_x]_n$, where x represents the degree of substitution and n the number of anhydroglucose units in the molecule. The degree of polymerisation, n, affects the viscosity of solution.

Different grades of sodium carboxymethylcellulose are available which yield aqueous solutions having various viscosities covering the range 6 to 4000 centipoises in 1 per cent solution.

The apparent viscosity of a solution of sodium carboxymethylcellulose at 20° containing 1 g of the material in 100 millilitres of water is not less than 60 per cent and not more than 140 per cent of that stated on the label for viscosity grades of 100 centipoises or less and not less than 70 per cent and not more than 130 per cent of that stated on the label for viscosity grades higher than 100 centipoises.

Solubility. Soluble in water at all temperatures, giving a clear solution; insoluble in most organic solvents.

Standard
DESCRIPTION. A white to cream-coloured hygroscopic powder; odourless or almost odourless.

IDENTIFICATION TESTS. 1. Adjust 10 ml of the 1 per cent solution prepared in the test for acidity or alkalinity to pH 0·5 with *dilute hydrochloric acid*; a fine white precipitate is formed (distinction from methylcellulose).

2. Boil 10 ml of the 1 per cent solution for 5 minutes; no precipitate is formed (distinction from methylcellulose and ethylcellulose).

3. To 5 ml of the 1 per cent solution add 5 ml of *hydrochloric acid*, boil under a reflux condenser for 30 minutes, cool, and neutralise to *litmus paper* with *sodium hydroxide solution*; add 0·1 ml of this solution to 5 ml of hot *potassium cupri-tartrate solution*; a red precipitate is formed (presence of reducing sugar).

4. It complies with Identification Test 4 given for Methylcellulose, page 307 (distinction from microcrystalline cellulose).

5. To 10 ml of the 1 per cent solution add 10 ml of a 1 per cent w/v solution of *calcium chloride* in water; no gelatinous precipitate is formed (distinction from sodium alginate).

6. Ignite; the residue gives the reactions characteristic of sodium.

ACIDITY OR ALKALINITY. pH of a 1 per cent w/v solution in *carbon dioxide-free water*, 6·0 to 8·0, the solution being prepared by the following method:
Weigh accurately an amount equivalent to 2·0 g of the dry substance in a beaker, place a mechanical stirrer 1 in. above the powder, add 160 ml of *carbon dioxide-free water*, and stir for 30 minutes, avoiding undue aeration of the solution and preventing access of carbon dioxide. Dilute to 200 ml with *carbon dioxide-free water* and allow to stand for 16 hours.

ARSENIC. It complies with the test given in Appendix 6, page 879 (1 part per million).

IRON. 0·25 g complies with the limit test for iron (160 parts per million).

LEAD. It complies with the test given in Appendix 7, page 883 (10 parts per million).

WATER-INSOLUBLE MATTER. Not more than 1·0 per cent, calculated with reference to the substance dried under the prescribed conditions, determined by the following method:
Centrifuge 100 g of the solution prepared in the test for acidity or alkalinity at 3000 r.p.m. for 15 minutes or until all the fibre has settled, decant the supernatant liquid, replace it with an equal volume of water, shake, and again centrifuge; repeat the procedure until all the gelatinous material has been dispersed.
Replace the supernatant liquid with an equal volume of 0·01N hydrochloric acid, stir, and centrifuge; finally replace the acid with an equal volume of *acetone* and centrifuge; filter through a tared sintered-glass crucible (British Standard Grade No. 3), wash the residue with *acetone*, dry for 2 hours at 105°, cool, and weigh.

ALCOHOL-SOLUBLE MATTER. Not more than 2·0 per cent, calculated with reference to the substance dried under the prescribed conditions, determined by the following method:
To about 2 g, accurately weighed, add 150 ml of *alcohol (80 per cent)* and stir for 30 minutes; transfer the residue to a tared sintered-glass crucible (British Standard Grade No. 3) with the aid of about 150 ml of *alcohol (80 per cent)*, followed by about 150 ml of *alcohol (95 per cent)*, wash with *solvent ether* until the alcohol is removed, draw air through the crucible until the ether is removed, and dry the residue to constant weight at 105°.

LOSS ON DRYING. Not more than 10·0 per cent, determined by drying to constant weight at 105°.

DEGREE OF SUBSTITUTION. Not less than 0·4, determined by the following method:
Transfer about 1 g, accurately weighed, of the dried residue obtained in the determination of alcohol-soluble matter to a platinum or silica crucible, ignite gently until charring is complete, and ignite at 700°

until all the carbon is removed; dissolve the residue in water and titrate with 0·1N sulphuric acid, using *methyl red solution* as indicator, adding about 1·0 ml of the acid in excess; boil to remove carbon dioxide, cool, and titrate the excess of acid with 0·1N sodium hydroxide. Calculate the degree of substitution from the formula:

$$\text{degree of substitution} = \frac{0 \cdot 162\,(0 \cdot 1b/g)}{1 - 0 \cdot 08\,(0 \cdot 1b/g)}$$

where g = weight of dry alcohol-insoluble matter taken, and
b = volume, in millilitres, of 0·1N sulphuric acid required to neutralise the ash.

Incompatibility. It is incompatible with strongly acid solutions and with soluble salts of iron and some other metals.

Sterilisation. Sodium carboxymethylcellulose can be sterilised in the dry state by maintaining at 160° for 1 hour, but this leads to a substantial decrease in viscosity and some deterioration in the properties of solutions prepared from the sterilised material.
Sterilisation of solutions by heating also causes some lowering of viscosity, but this is much less marked. When a solution is heated in an autoclave at 125° for 15 minutes and allowed to cool, the viscosity may be expected to decrease by about 25 per cent; allowance should therefore be made for this when calculating the amount of sodium carboxymethylcellulose to be included in a preparation which is to be sterilised.

Uses. Sodium carboxymethylcellulose is used for suspending powders in aqueous preparations intended for external application or for oral or parenteral administration. It can also be used for stabilising emulsions and for dispersing the precipitate formed when resinous tinctures are added to water. For these purposes 0·25 to 1 per cent of the medium-viscosity grades is usually adequate.
Higher concentrations, such as 4 to 6 per cent, of the medium-viscosity grades produce gels which can be used as the basis for applications and pastes; glycerol is usually included in such preparations to prevent drying-out.
Aqueous preparations of sodium carboxymethylcellulose which are likely to be stored for long periods should contain a preservative. Medium- and high-viscosity grades of sodium carboxymethylcellulose, like those of methylcellulose, are used as bulk laxatives; for this purpose 4 to 10 grams is given daily in divided doses, each dose being taken with plenty of water.

Dose. As a bulk laxative, 4 to 10 grams daily in divided doses.

OTHER NAMES: *Cekol®*; *Courlose®*; *Edifas B®*

SODIUM CHLORIDE

SYNONYMS: Natrii Chloridum; Sod. Chlor.

NaCl = 58·44

Solubility. Soluble, at 20°, in 3 parts of water, in 250 parts of alcohol, and in 10 parts of glycerol.

Standard
It complies with the requirements of the European Pharmacopoeia.
It occurs as odourless, colourless, cubical crystals or white crystalline powder and contains not less than 99·5 per cent of NaCl, calculated with reference to the dried substance. The loss on drying under the pre-

scribed conditions is not more than 1·0 per cent. It contains no added substances.

Sterilisation. Solutions for injection are sterilised by heating in an autoclave or by filtration.

Storage. It should be stored in airtight containers. Solutions, on keeping, may cause the separation of small solid particles from glass containers; solutions containing such particles must not be used.

Actions and uses. Sodium chloride is the most important salt for maintaining the osmotic tension of the blood and tissues; changes in osmotic tension influence the movement of fluids and diffusion of salts in the cellular tissues. Normal tissue fluid contains about 140 millimoles of sodium ions and about 100 millimoles of chloride ions per litre. About 5 to 12 grams of sodium chloride is taken daily in the food and a corresponding amount is excreted in the urine.

Excess of sodium chloride will act as a saline diuretic; when sodium chloride is absorbed from the intestine, or injected, the osmotic equilibrium of the blood is maintained by the excretion of the surplus salt and water by the kidneys. Sodium chloride in a dosage of 10 to 12 grams a day, by aiding excretion, is of value in the treatment of poisoning by bromides or iodides.

Solutions of sodium chloride, usually with the addition of dextrose, are given intravenously and sometimes by rectum to patients who are unable to take fluids by mouth. It may be necessary to give saline intravenously for four or five days until the patient can take fluids orally; if no fluid is taken by mouth, 3·5 litres is required daily in temperate climates and rather more in the tropics. This is best given as Sodium Chloride and Dextrose Injection. If the patient is not excreting chloride in his urine, his salt intake is insufficient. Sodium Chloride Injection has been used to combat dehydration, but it is found that the administration of large quantities may produce oedema, owing to accumulation of salt in the tissues.

Severe sweating, such as occurs when heavy work is done in a hot atmosphere, may cause a marked loss of sodium chloride, producing muscle cramps and involuntary tremors. This can be prevented or relieved by taking sufficient saline drink (a 0·5 per cent salt solution is suitable) to compensate for the loss of sodium chloride in the sweat.

In Addison's disease the patient loses large quantities of sodium chloride in the urine owing to deficiency of adrenocortical hormones; such hormones, for example cortisone, may be given in replacement therapy. Additional salt is necessary to maintain the electrolyte balance, and as much as 10 to 15 grams of sodium chloride by mouth daily in enteric-coated capsules or tablets, or a mixture of sodium citrate, chloride, and bicarbonate may

be given. During replacement therapy with corticosteroids, care must be taken to ensure that abnormal retention of sodium chloride, with resultant oedema, does not occur.

Sodium Chloride Injection is often given parenterally in the treatment of poisoning by mercurial salts, phenol, and other substances eliminated by the kidneys, except where there is pulmonary oedema. A strong salt solution given by mouth is a useful emetic in an emergency.

Sodium chloride injections may be given intraperitoneally to infants; for rectal administration half-strength saline is usually used, as it is more readily absorbed than normal saline.

Preparations

SODIUM CHLORIDE EYE LOTION, B.P.C. (page 697)

POTASSIUM CHLORIDE AND SODIUM CHLORIDE INJECTION, B.P. It consists of a sterile solution of sodium chloride and potassium chloride in Water for Injections. Unless otherwise specified, a solution containing 0·9 per cent of sodium chloride and 0·3 per cent of potassium chloride is supplied (approximately 40 millimoles, or milliequivalents, of K^+, 150 millimoles, or milliequivalents, of Na^+, and 190 millimoles, or milliequivalents, of Cl^- per litre).

SODIUM CHLORIDE INJECTION, B.P. It consists of a sterile solution of sodium chloride in Water for Injections. The strength is stated on the label as the percentage w/v of sodium chloride; the label also states the approximate concentration, in millimoles per litre, of the sodium ions and the chloride ions. Unless otherwise specified, a solution containing 0·9 per cent of sodium chloride is supplied. This solution contains approximately 150 millimoles, or milliequivalents, of Na^+ and of Cl^- per litre.

When Normal Saline Solution for Injection is prescribed, Sodium Chloride Injection (0·9 per cent) is dispensed.

On storage, this solution may cause separation of small solid particles from glass containers; solutions containing such particles must not be used.

SODIUM CHLORIDE AND DEXTROSE INJECTION, B.P. It consists of a sterile solution of sodium chloride and anhydrous dextrose in Water for Injections. Unless otherwise specified, a solution containing 0·18 per cent of sodium chloride (approximately 30 millimoles, or milliequivalents, per litre) and 4·0 per cent of anhydrous dextrose is supplied. It should be stored at a temperature not exceeding 25°.

On storage, this solution may cause separation of small solid particles from glass containers; solutions containing such particles must not be used.

SODIUM CHLORIDE MIXTURE, COMPOUND, B.P.C. (page 753)

SODIUM CHLORIDE MOUTH-WASH, COMPOUND, B.P.C. (page 755)

SODIUM CHLORIDE SOLUTION, B.P.C. (page 789)

SODIUM CHLORIDE TABLETS, B.P. Unless otherwise specified, tablets each containing 300 mg of sodium chloride are supplied. They should be dissolved in water before administration.

SODIUM CHROMATE (^{51}Cr) SOLUTION

This material is radioactive and any regulations in force must be complied with.

Sodium Chromate (^{51}Cr) Solution is a sterile solution of sodium chromate (^{51}Cr), made isotonic with blood by the addition of sodium chloride.

Chromium-51 is a radioactive isotope of chromium, having a half-life of 28 days; it may be prepared by the neutron irradiation of chromium, either of natural isotopic composition or enriched in chromium-50.

Standard
It complies with the requirements of the British Pharmacopoeia.
It is a clear colourless or faintly yellow solution and contains not less than 90·0 and not more than 110·0 per cent of the quantity of chromium-51 stated on the label at the date and hour stated on the label. The specific activity is not less than 20 millicuries per milligram of chromium at the date and hour stated on the label. It has a pH of 5·0 to 8·0.

Sterilisation. It is sterilised by heating in an autoclave.

Labelling. The label on the container states:
(1) the content of chromium-51 expressed in microcuries or millicuries at a given date and hour;
(2) that the solution is radioactive; and
(3) that it does not contain a bactericide.

The label on the package also states:
(1) the total volume in the container; and
(2) the content of total chromium.

Storage. It should be stored in an area assigned for the purpose. The storage conditions should be such that the maximum radiation-dose-rate to which persons may be exposed is reduced to an acceptable level.
Glass containers may darken under the effects of radiation.

Actions and uses. Sodium chromate (^{51}Cr) is used for labelling red blood cells. It crosses the red-cell membrane and becomes attached to the β-polypeptide chains of the haemoglobin molecules, from which it is only slowly eluted. Doses of about 100 microcuries are used to determine the life span of red cells in the investigation of haemolytic anaemias. The γ-emission of sodium chromate (^{51}Cr) is of sufficiently high energy to permit the estimation of radioactivity at the body surface, thus enabling the sites of isotope accumulation due to red-cell destruction or pooling to be determined.
Sodium chromate (^{51}Cr) may also be used for the detection of red-cell loss due to haemorrhage into the gastro-intestinal tract and for the determination of the circulating red-cell volume; smaller doses of about 50 microcuries may be used for these purposes.

Dose. For labelling red blood cells in the investigation of haematological disorders: up to 200 microcuries.

SODIUM CITRATE

SYNONYM: Sod. Cit.

$C_6H_5Na_3O_7,2H_2O = 294·1$

Solubility. Soluble, at 20°, in less than 2 parts of water; insoluble in alcohol.

Standard
It complies with the requirements of the British Pharmacopoeia.
It occurs as white, odourless, granular crystals or crystalline powder and contains not less than 99·0 and not more than the equivalent of 101·0 per cent of $C_6H_5Na_3O_7,2H_2O$.
In moist air it is slightly deliquescent and in warm dry air it is efflorescent.

Sterilisation. Solutions for injection are sterilised by heating in an autoclave or by filtration.

Storage. It should be stored in airtight containers. Solutions, on keeping, may cause the separation of small solid particles from glass containers; solutions containing such particles must not be used.

Actions and uses. Sodium citrate is oxidised in the tissues and is partly excreted as carbon dioxide; it increases the alkali reserve and renders the urine less acid, having the ultimate effect of bicarbonates without their neutralising action upon gastric secretion. As the alkali citrates are absorbed more readily than the tartrates, their laxative action is less marked.
Sodium citrate has been used to allay symptoms in urinary infections, to make the urine alkaline in the treatment of inflammatory conditions of the bladder and in some types of antibiotic therapy, and to prevent crystalluria during treatment with certain sulphonamides.
Sodium citrate is added to milk in the feeding of infants and invalids to prevent the formation of large curds; for invalids, from 60 to 180 milligrams of sodium citrate is added to each 40 millilitres of milk, and for infant feeding a solution containing 125 milligrams in 5 millilitres is added to each feed.
Sodium citrate prevents the clotting of blood *in vitro*, a 2·5 to 3·8 per cent solution being employed; a 3 per cent solution is also used for washing out syringes and apparatus before collection of blood. Its use as an anticoagulant for whole human blood is described under Whole Human Blood (page 582), but it has been largely replaced for this purpose by sodium acid citrate.

Dose. Up to 10 grams daily in divided doses.

Preparations
SODIUM CITRATE MIXTURE, B.P.C. (page 753)
SODIUM CITRATE SOLUTION FOR BLADDER IRRIGATION, STERILE, B.P.C. (page 789)
SODIUM CITRATE TABLETS, B.P. Unless otherwise

specified, tablets each containing 125 mg of sodium citrate are supplied. They should be stored in airtight containers. They are intended for use in infant feeding; they should be dissolved in water and the solution added to the feed. Tablets containing 60 and 300 mg are also available.

SODIUM CROMOGLYCATE

$C_{23}H_{14}Na_2O_{11} = 512 \cdot 3$

Sodium Cromoglycate is sodium 5,5'-(2-hydroxytri-methylenedioxy)bis(4-oxo-4H-chromene-2-carboxy-late).

Solubility. Soluble, at 20°, in 20 parts of water; insoluble in alcohol and in chloroform.

Standard
It complies with the requirements of the British Pharmacopoeia.
It is a white, crystalline, odourless, hygroscopic powder and contains not less than 98·0 and not more than the equivalent of 101·0 per cent of $C_{23}H_{14}Na_2O_{11}$, calculated with reference to the dried substance. The loss on drying under the prescribed conditions is not more than 10·0 per cent.

Storage. It should be stored in airtight containers.

Actions and uses. Sodium cromoglycate is used in the prophylactic treatment of asthma. It appears to block intermediate steps in the immediate allergic reaction. It is administered only by inhalation, either alone or in admixture with a small quantity of isoprenaline to prevent bronchospasm due to inhalation of the powder. Other drugs may be required to

treat inflammatory and other non-allergic aspects of the disease.

UNDESIRABLE EFFECTS. Slight irritation of the throat and bronchi commonly occurs, especially during infective illnesses.
Sudden withdrawal may precipitate asthma, particularly in cases where the use of sodium cromoglycate has permitted a reduction in corticosteroid dose.

Dose. By inhalation, 20 milligrams every three to twelve hours.

Preparation
SODIUM CROMOGLYCATE CARTRIDGES, B.P. They consist of hard gelatin capsules each containing 20 mg of sodium cromoglycate and an equal quantity of lactose. They should be protected from moisture and stored at a temperature not exceeding 30°. They are intended for use by inhalation and are not to be swallowed.

OTHER NAMES: *Intal*®; *Rynacrom*®

SODIUM DIATRIZOATE

$C_{11}H_8I_3N_2NaO_4 = 635 \cdot 9$

Sodium Diatrizoate is sodium 3,5-diacetamido-2,4,6-tri-iodobenzoate.

Solubility. Soluble, at 20°, in 2 parts of water; slightly soluble in alcohol; insoluble in ether and in acetone.

Standard
It complies with the requirements of the British Pharmacopoeia.
It is a white odourless powder and contains not less than 98·0 and not more than the equivalent of 101·0 per cent of $C_{11}H_8I_3N_2NaO_4$, calculated with reference to the anhydrous substance. It contains 4·5 to 9·0 per cent w/w of water. A 50 per cent solution in water has a pH of 7·0 to 9·0.

Sterilisation. Solutions for injection are sterilised by heating in a autoclave or by filtration.

Storage. It should be protected from light.

Actions and uses. Sodium diatrizoate is used as a contrast medium in diagnostic radiology for the examination of a wide range of systems of the body. For many purposes it has replaced diodone; in common with other tri-iodo-compounds it gives a higher degree of radio-opacity and is less toxic than diodone in similar concentration. It is available in solutions containing 25 and 45 per cent. Stronger

solutions are available; these solutions consist of mixtures of the sodium and meglumine salts of diatrizoic acid and contain the equivalent of 65, 76, and 85 per cent of sodium diatrizoate.
For intravenous pyelography, 20 millilitres of the 45 per cent solution is usually sufficient, but if inadequate contrast is obtained larger volumes may be used. Usually, X-ray photographs can be obtained without preliminary preparation of the patient, but better results will be obtained if the patient avoids taking fluids for twelve hours prior to the examination and if a laxative is given on the night before to eliminate gas and faeces from the bowel. The total volume of medium should be injected in one to three minutes. Its excretion by the kidneys is almost immediately detectable by serial films. For retrograde pyelography the 25 per cent solution is usually adequate.

For operative and post-operative cholangiography three successive injections of 4 millilitres of the 25 per cent solution directly into the biliary system is usually sufficient for visualisation of the bile duct.

For translumbar aortography in adults where the injection is to be made immediately above the renal arteries, a single injection of between 20 and 30 millilitres of the 65 or 76 per cent solution is used. The reason for this limitation of dosage is the nephrotoxic effect of larger doses. If, however, the injection is to be given some distance below the renal arteries, a quantity greater than 30 millilitres can be used with safety.

For angiocardiography, 1 millilitre of the 76 or 85 per cent solution per kilogram body-weight is used. In calculating the volume, account must be taken of the dead space in the apparatus and pump which is used for the administration.

For peripheral arteriography and cerebral angiography a suitable concentration is 45 per cent. In cerebral angiography an average of 8 millilitres should be used for each injection and a maximum of 80 millilitres should not be exceeded in any one complete investigation, because of the possibility of causing cerebral oedema. The injections are made into the common carotid artery or, for the study of the intracerebral structure, into the internal carotid artery.

UNDESIRABLE EFFECTS. The occasional undesirable reactions which may occur include nausea, vomiting, sensations of heat, weakness, headache, thirst, coughing, sneezing, itching, pallor, tachycardia, and hypotension. Urticarial rashes may occur and these can usually be relieved by the immediate intravenous injection of an antihistamine. In rare cases, profound shock leading to cardiac arrest may occur and supplies of adrenaline, oxygen, and a suitable corticosteroid for injection should be available.

PRECAUTIONS. There is no wholly satisfactory test which will enable the radiologist to predict a severe reaction, but some workers make a preliminary sensitivity test by injecting intravenously 1 millilitre of medium and observing the patient for a period prior to the administration of the full injection.

CONTRA-INDICATIONS. An idiosyncrasy to inorganic iodine does not necessarily contra-indicate the use of an organic compound of iodine. Sodium diatrizoate should not be used for pyelography in patients with multiple myeloma because renal failure may occur.

Dose. The strength of solution and the dose are determined by the physician in accordance with the diagnostic procedure.

Preparation
SODIUM DIATRIZOATE INJECTION, B.P. It consists of a sterile solution of sodium diatrizoate in Water for Injections containing suitable buffering and stabilising agents. The strength of the solution should be specified by the prescriber. It should be protected from light.

SODIUM FLUORIDE

NaF = 41·99

Solubility. Soluble, at 20°, in 25 parts of water; insoluble in alcohol.

Standard
It complies with the requirements of the British Pharmacopoeia.
It is a white odourless powder and contains not less than 98·0 per cent of NaF, calculated with reference to the dried substance. The loss on drying under the prescribed conditions is not more than 0·5 per cent.

Storage. It should be stored in airtight containers.

Actions and uses. Sodium fluoride is used for the prophylaxis of dental caries in communities where the intake of fluoride from drinking water and food is low. It may be added to water supplies to give a final concentration of 1 part of fluoride ion per million. A 2 per cent solution of sodium fluoride in water may be applied to children's teeth, after preliminary cleansing, three times at intervals of one week at three, seven, ten, and thirteen years of age to correspond with tooth eruption. Alternatively, a paste containing 75 per cent of sodium fluoride and 25 per cent of glycerol is applied to the teeth, rubbed in for one minute, and removed by a mouth-wash.

The continued ingestion of excessive amounts of fluoride in food or drinking water during the period of tooth development leads to mottling of the tooth enamel.

Sodium fluoride is a constituent of some insecticides and rodenticides.

UNDESIRABLE EFFECTS. Sodium fluoride taken by mouth in quantities in excess of 250 milligrams causes nausea and vomiting, epigastric pain, and diarrhoea; large doses cause muscular weakness and clonic convulsions, followed by respiratory and cardiac failure, collapse, and death.

POISONING. When sodium fluoride has been swallowed, the stomach should be washed out with a 1 per cent solution of calcium chloride or with lime water; a purgative dose of castor oil and demulcents should be given.

If considerable absorption of fluoride has taken place, a 10 per cent solution of calcium gluconate may be administered intravenously and, if necessary, morphine given by subcutaneous injection.

SODIUM FUSIDATE

$C_{31}H_{47}NaO_6 = 538.7$

Sodium Fusidate is the sodium salt of fusidic acid, an antimicrobial substance produced by the growth of certain strains of *Fusidium coccineum* (K. Tubaki).

Solubility. Soluble, at 20°, in 1 part of water and of alcohol and in 350 parts of chloroform; very slightly soluble in ether and in acetone.

Standard
It complies with the requirements of the British Pharmacopoeia.
It is a white or almost white, crystalline, slightly hygroscopic, odourless or almost odourless powder and contains not less than 97.5 per cent of $C_{31}H_{47}NaO_6$, calculated with reference to the anhydrous substance. It contains not more than 1.0 per cent w/w of water. A 1.25 per cent solution in water has a pH of 7.5 to 9.0.

Storage. It should be stored in airtight containers, protected from light.

Actions and uses. Sodium fusidate has an antibacterial action against Gram-positive organisms, including penicillin-resistant strains of *Staphylococcus aureus*, and also against some Gram-negative organisms. Used alone or in conjunction with other antibiotics, it may be effective in the treatment of infections due to penicillin-resistant staphylococci.

UNDESIRABLE EFFECTS. Mild gastro-intestinal disturbances may occur, but these may be minimised if the dose is given with food.

Dose. 1 to 2 grams daily in divided doses.

Preparation
SODIUM FUSIDATE CAPSULES, B.P. Unless otherwise specified, capsules each containing 250 mg of sodium fusidate are supplied.

OTHER NAME: *Fucidin*®

SODIUM HYDROXIDE

SYNONYMS: Caustic Soda; Sod. Hydrox.

$NaOH = 40.00$

Sodium Hydroxide may be obtained by the electrolysis of an aqueous solution of sodium chloride.

Solubility. Soluble, or almost completely soluble, at 20°, in 1 part of water; very soluble in alcohol.
A solution free from carbonate may be prepared by dissolving sodium hydroxide in alcohol or in an equal weight of water, followed by filtration or decantation.

Standard
It complies with the requirements of the British Pharmacopoeia.
It occurs as white sticks, scales, pellets, or fused masses, which are dry, hard, and brittle, breaking with a crystalline fracture, and contains not less than 97.5 per cent of total alkali, calculated as NaOH, and not more than 2.5 per cent of Na_2CO_3.

Hygroscopicity. When exposed to the air it rapidly absorbs moisture and liquefies, but subsequently becomes solid again, due to absorption of carbon dioxide and formation of sodium carbonate, and effloresces.

Storage. It should be stored in airtight containers; if the containers are made of glass they should be closed by waxed corks or plastic-lined screw caps.

Actions and uses. Sodium hydroxide is a powerful caustic. A 2.5 per cent solution in glycerol is used as a cuticle solvent.
Sodium hydroxide is also used in a variety of pharmaceutical preparations.

POISONING. Large draughts of water containing vinegar, acetic acid, citric acid, or lemon juice should be given, followed by demulcent drinks and olive oil or arachis oil.
Burns due to sodium hydroxide should be flooded with water and then with dilute acetic acid.

SODIUM IODIDE

SYNONYMS: Natrii Iodidum; Sod. Iod.

$NaI = 149.9$

Solubility. Soluble, at 20°, in less than 1 part of water, in 2 parts of alcohol, and in 1 part of glycerol.

AQUEOUS SOLUTIONS. A marked rise in the temperature of the solution occurs when sodium iodide dissolves in water to form a strong solution; when potassium iodide dissolves, a considerable fall in temperature occurs.

Standard
It complies with the requirements of the European Pharmacopoeia.
It occurs as odourless colourless crystals or white crystalline powder and contains not less than 99.0 per cent of NaI, calculated with reference to the dried substance. The loss on drying under the prescribed conditions is not more than 5.0 per cent.

Stability. Sodium iodide is deliquescent in moist air and decomposes, becoming yellow in colour owing to the liberation of iodine. It melts at a dull red heat with some loss of iodine; at high temperatures it slowly volatilises.
A solution of sodium iodide in water gradually becomes

coloured on exposure to light and air due to liberation of iodine.

Incompatibility. It is incompatible with salts of iron, bismuth, and mercury, with potassium chlorate and other oxidising agents, and with strychnine hydrochloride, quinine sulphate, and other alkaloidal salts.

Sterilisation. Solutions for injection are sterilised by heating in an autoclave or by filtration.

Storage. It should be stored in airtight containers, protected from light.

Actions and uses. Sodium iodide has actions, uses, and undesirable effects similar to those described under Potassium Iodide (page 396).

It is used for the prophylaxis of simple goitre, 0·01 per cent of sodium iodide being added to table salt (iodised salt). Alternatively, for this purpose it may be given by mouth in a dosage of not more than 0·5 to 1 milligram daily, 5 to 10 milligrams once a week, or 200 milligrams daily for ten days twice a year.

It is also used, similarly to potassium iodide, in the pre-operative treatment of patients with thyrotoxicosis.

Dose. As an expectorant, 250 to 500 milligrams.

In the pre-operative treatment of thyrotoxicosis, 150 milligrams daily in divided doses.

Preparation

CAFFEINE IODIDE ELIXIR, B.P.C. (page 667)

SODIUM IODIDE (^{125}I) SOLUTION

This material is radioactive and any regulations in force must be complied with.

Sodium Iodide (^{125}I) Solution is a solution suitable for oral administration containing sodium iodide (^{125}I); it also contains sodium thiosulphate or other suitable reducing agent.

Iodine-125 is a radioactive isotope of iodine which emits γ- and X-radiation and has a half-life of 60 days; it may be prepared by the neutron irradiation of xenon.

Standard
It complies with the requirements of the British Pharmacopoeia.
It is a clear colourless solution and contains not less than 85·0 and not more than 115·0 per cent of the quantity of iodine-125 stated on the label at the date stated on the label. The specific activity is not less than 2 millicuries per microgram of iodine at the date stated on the label. Not more than 1·0 per cent of the total activity, expressed as disintegrations per second, is due to iodine-126 at the date stated on the label. It has a pH of 7·0 to 10·0.

Labelling. The label on the container states:
(1) the content of iodine-125 expressed in microcuries or millicuries at a given date;
(2) that the solution is radioactive; and
(3) that the solution is not to be used for parenteral injection.

The label on the package also states the total volume in the container.

Storage. It should be stored in an area assigned for the purpose. The storage conditions should be such that the maximum radiation-dose-rate to which persons may be exposed is reduced to an acceptable level.

Actions and uses. Sodium iodide (^{125}I) solution may be administered by mouth to study the uptake of iodine by the thyroid gland, but owing to the low energy of the radiation emitted by iodine-125 it is rarely used for this purpose.

Sodium iodide (^{125}I) solution, or a similar solution free from thiosulphate or other reducing agent, may be used for the radioactive labelling of albumin, fibrinogen, protein hormones, and other proteins which are to be administered to patients or used for assay procedures *in vitro*. Iodine-125 is preferred for this purpose to iodine-131 because of the reduced risk to workers carrying out diagnostic procedures and the reduced radiation dose to the patient. The dose of iodine-125 as sodium iodide solution or in the form of iodinated proteins is up to 100 microcuries.

PRECAUTIONS AND CONTRA-INDICATIONS. See under Sodium Iodide (^{131}I) Solution (page 454) and Iodinated (^{125}I) Human Albumin Injection (page 244).

SODIUM IODIDE (^{131}I) INJECTION

This material is radioactive and any regulations in force must be complied with.

Sodium Iodide (^{131}I) Injection is a sterile solution containing sodium iodide (^{131}I); it also contains sodium thiosulphate or other suitable reducing agent.

Iodine-131 is a radioactive isotope of iodine which emits β- and γ-radiation and has a half-life of 8 days; it may be prepared from the products of uranium fission or by the neutron irradiation of tellurium.

Standard
It complies with the requirements of the British Pharmacopoeia.

It is a clear colourless solution and contains not less than 90·0 and not more than 110·0 per cent of the quantity of iodine-131 stated on the label at the date and hour stated on the label. The specific activity is not less than 5 millicuries per microgram of iodine at the date and hour stated on the label. It has a pH of 7·0 to 8·0.

Sterilisation. It is sterilised by heating in an autoclave.

Labelling. The label on the container states:
(1) the content of iodine-131 expressed in microcuries or millicuries at a given date and hour;
(2) that the injection is radioactive; and
(3) either that it does not contain a bactericide or the name and proportion of any added bactericide.

The label on the package also states the total volume in the container.

Storage. It should be stored in an area assigned for the purpose. The storage conditions should be such that the maximum radiation-dose-rate to which

persons may be exposed is reduced to an acceptable level.
Glass containers may darken under the effects of radiation.

Actions and uses. Sodium Iodide (^{131}I) Injection has the actions and uses described under Sodium Iodide (^{131}I) Solution and is administered by intravenous injection in similar dosage.

PRECAUTIONS AND CONTRA-INDICATIONS. As for Sodium Iodide (^{131}I) Solution.

SODIUM IODIDE (^{131}I) SOLUTION

This material is radioactive and any regulations in force must be complied with.

Sodium Iodide (^{131}I) Solution is a solution suitable for oral administration containing sodium iodide (^{131}I); it also contains sodium thiosulphate or other suitable reducing agent.

Iodine-131 is a radioactive isotope of iodine which emits β- and γ-radiation and has a half-life of 8 days; it may be prepared from the products of uranium fission or by the neutron irradiation of tellurium.

Standard
It complies with the requirements of the British Pharmacopoeia.
It is a clear colourless solution and contains not less than 90·0 and not more than 110·0 per cent of the quantity of iodine-131 stated on the label at the date and hour stated on the label. The specific activity is not less than 5 millicuries per microgram of iodine at the date and hour stated on the label. It has a pH of 7·0 to 10·0.

Labelling. The label on the container states:
(1) the content of iodine-131 expressed in microcuries or millicuries at a given date and hour;
(2) that the solution is radioactive; and
(3) that the solution is not to be used for parenteral injection.

The label on the package also states the total volume in the container.

Storage. It should be stored in an area assigned for the purpose. The storage conditions should be such that the maximum radiation-dose-rate to which persons may be exposed is reduced to an acceptable level.
Glass containers may darken under the effects of radiation.

Actions and uses. Sodium Iodide (^{131}I) Solution is used for the oral administration of radioactive iodine-131. The volume containing the requisite dose is calculated from the content of radioactivity at a given time and date, as stated on the label, and from the rate of radioactive decay.
Doses of 2 to 10 microcuries, but occasionally up to 50 microcuries, are used to study the iodine uptake of the thyroid gland, the iodine-binding activity of the plasma, and the iodine-excretion rate in the diagnosis of hypo-thyroidism or hyperthyroidism. Recent administration of any preparation containing iodine or thyroid hormone will, however, interfere with the iodine uptake of the gland. Doses of 100 to 200 microcuries are used to locate aberrant thyroid tissue, and to detect nodules in the thyroid gland which will take

up iodine in greater or lesser amounts than the rest of the gland.
Similar or smaller doses are sometimes used to determine the rate of iodine uptake of the thyroid in hyperthyroidism or of secondary deposits from a carcinoma of the thyroid, and to calculate the dose of Sodium Iodide (^{131}I) Solution required for the treatment of hyper-thyroidism.
Doses of 1 to 15 millicuries, repeated if necessary, are given for the treatment of hyper-thyroidism, but it is not normally regarded as the treatment of choice in patients less than forty-five years old. This treatment carries a risk that permanent hypothyroidism may develop, perhaps months or even years after the treatment has ceased.
Doses of 10 to 40 millicuries may be used in some patients with angina pectoris and heart failure to reduce the activity of the thyroid gland.
Doses of 60 to 150 millicuries are used for the treatment of carcinoma of the thyroid with secondary deposits, if these have been shown to take up significant amounts of iodine.

PRECAUTIONS AND CONTRA-INDICATIONS. The patient's urine must be monitored, because, when doses greater than 1 millicurie are administered, significant amounts of iodine-131 may be excreted; it may be necessary to store the urine until its radioactivity is low enough for it to be disposed of in accordance with any regulations of the appropriate authorities.
The use of Sodium Iodide (^{131}I) Solution is contra-indicated, even in diagnostic doses, during pregnancy and lactation. Foetal thyroid tissue takes up significant amounts of iodine-131 by the twelfth week of gestation and is highly susceptible to irradiation. Infants may receive dangerous amounts of radioactivity in the mother's milk.
Children, too, are very sensitive to thyroid irradiation and should not be given radioactive iodine-131.

Dose. See above under **Actions and uses.**

SODIUM IODOHIPPURATE (^{131}I) INJECTION

This material is radioactive and any regulations in force must be complied with.

Sodium Iodohippurate (^{131}I) Injection is a sterile solution containing sodium *o*-iodohippurate (^{131}I).

Iodine-131 is a radioactive isotope of iodine which emits β- and γ-radiation and has a half-life of 8 days; it may be prepared from the products of uranium fission or by the neutron irradiation of tellurium.

Standard
It complies with the requirements of the British Pharmacopoeia.
It is a clear colourless solution which may become brown on storage and contains not less than 90·0 and not more than 110·0 per cent of the content of iodine-131 stated on the label at the date and hour stated on the label. Not less than 95·0 per cent of the iodine-131 is in the form of sodium *o*-iodohippurate at the date and hour stated on the label. It has a pH of 7·0 to 8·5.

Stability. Sodium Iodohippurate (^{131}I) Injection decomposes with an accompanying decrease in radiochemical purity. It should be issued in such a form that when stored under the prescribed conditions the rate of decomposition, measured in terms of radiochemical purity, does not exceed 2 per cent during a period of ten days from the date stated on the label.

Sterilisation. It is sterilised by heating in an autoclave; benzyl alcohol 0·9 per cent v/v is a suitable bactericide.

Labelling. The label on the container states:
(1) the content of iodine-131 expressed in microcuries or millicuries at a given date and hour; and
(2) that the injection is radioactive.

The label on the package also states:
(1) the total volume of the injection;
(2) the total content of sodium *o*-iodohippurate; and
(3) the name and proportion of any added bactericide.

Storage. It should be stored protected from light at a temperature not exceeding 25° in an area assigned for the purpose. The storage conditions should be such that the maximum radiation-dose-rate to which persons may be exposed is reduced to an acceptable level.
Glass containers may darken under the effects of radiation.

Actions and uses. Sodium iodohippurate (^{131}I) is used in a test of renal function.
The material is selectively and rapidly excreted by the kidneys, and no tubular reabsorption takes place. Its passage through the kidneys is detected by a pair of collimated scintillation counters, one located accurately over each kidney; sometimes a third similar counter is located over the bladder, so that the rise of radioactivity in the urine can be recorded graphically at the same time as records are made from each kidney, and in addition a fourth detector is sometimes placed over the head to enable a record of blood radioactivity to be made simultaneously.
A suitable dose for this diagnostic procedure is about 20 microcuries administered intravenously in 1 to 2 millilitres of isotonic solution. The test is completed in 20 to 30 minutes.

Dose. In the investigation of renal function, by intravenous injection, 20 microcuries.

SODIUM LAURYL SULPHATE

SYNONYM: Sod. Lauryl Sulph.

Sodium Lauryl Sulphate is a mixture of the sodium salts of sulphated normal primary alcohols; these sulphated alcohols are sometimes incorrectly referred to as "sulphonated fatty alcohols". It consists chiefly of sodium lauryl sulphate, $C_{12}H_{25}O \cdot SO_2 \cdot ONa$.

Sodium Lauryl Sulphate may be prepared by treating with sulphuric acid the mixture of alcohols obtained by hydrogenation of coconut oil and neutralising the product with sodium hydroxide.

Solubility. Very soluble in water, forming a turbid solution; partly soluble in alcohol.

Standard
It complies with the requirements of the British Pharmacopoeia.
It occurs as white or pale yellow crystals or powder with a slight characteristic odour and contains the equivalent of not less than 85·0 per cent w/w of sodium alkyl sulphates, calculated as $C_{12}H_{25}O \cdot SO_2 \cdot ONa$.

Uses. Sodium lauryl sulphate is an anionic emulsifying agent. It is used in the preparation of Emulsifying Wax, which is used as an emulsifying agent for producing oil-in-water creams. Such creams are stable over a wide pH range and suitable for the incorporation of anionic and non-ionic medicaments. For cationic medicaments, Cetrimide Emulsifying Wax and Cetomacrogol Emulsifying Wax are more suitable emulsifying agents.
Sodium lauryl sulphate reduces surface tension and is used as a wetting agent and detergent. It is not affected by hard water on account of the solubility of the corresponding calcium and magnesium salts, and the addition of sodium lauryl sulphate to soap retards the formation of insoluble calcium soaps.
Aqueous solutions which are sufficiently concentrated to contain micelles will solubilise many water-insoluble materials.

Preparation
EMULSIFYING WAX, B.P. (*Syn.* Anionic Emulsifying Wax). It contains cetostearyl alcohol and sodium lauryl sulphate or similar sodium salts of sulphated higher primary aliphatic alcohols. A suitable preparation may be prepared from 90 g of cetostearyl alcohol, 10 g of sodium lauryl sulphate, and 4 ml of water.

SODIUM METABISULPHITE

SYNONYM: Sodium Pyrosulphite

$Na_2S_2O_5 = 190 \cdot 1$

Sodium Metabisulphite may be prepared by saturating a hot concentrated solution of sodium hydroxide or sodium carbonate with sulphur dioxide and allowing to cool, whereupon sodium metabisulphite crystallises out.

Solubility. Soluble, at 20°, in 2 parts of water; less soluble in alcohol.

Standard
It complies with the requirements of the British Pharmacopoeia.
It occurs as colourless prismatic crystals or white or creamy-white crystalline powder with a sulphurous odour and contains not less than 95·0 per cent of $Na_2S_2O_5$. A solution in water is acid to phenol red and has the odour of sulphur dioxide.
It usually contains small amounts of sodium sulphite and sodium sulphate.

Stability. It is a powerful reducing agent, and on exposure to air and moisture it is slowly oxidised to sulphate, with disintegration of the crystals.

Storage. It should be stored in airtight containers.

Uses. Sodium metabisulphite is an antoxidant and reducing agent and is widely employed in pharmaceutical preparations, especially in those containing substances which are readily oxidised to form coloured decomposition products. It is often used in a concentration of 0·1 per cent, but concentrations of 0·01 to 1 per cent have been employed.
In the formulation of a pharmaceutical preparation, the minimum concentration should be chosen which will give the desired antoxidant effect. A chelating agent such as sodium edetate is sometimes used in conjunction with sodium metabisulphite to remove heavy metallic ions which often catalyse oxidation reactions.
Sodium metabisulphite is usually employed as an antoxidant in acidic preparations; for alkaline preparations, sodium sulphite is usually preferred.
Sodium metabisulphite decomposes in air, especially on heating, and an appreciable amount may be lost during sterilisation before the substance has had time to exert its antoxidant effect; decomposition in solutions is accompanied by a fall in pH. Injections containing sodium metabisulphite should preferably be filled into containers in which the air has been replaced by an inert gas such as nitrogen.
Rubber caps used to close multidose containers should be pretreated with sodium metabisulphite solution if sodium metabisulphite is included in the contents of the containers.
Under certain conditions, sodium metabisulphite may react with adrenaline and other drugs which are derivatives of o- or p-hydroxybenzyl alcohol, and with some dyes and flavouring agents.
Preparations containing sodium metabisulphite should be thoroughly tested to determine its effect on the active constituents and other ingredients.
Sodium metabisulphite is used as a preservative in acidic solutions and syrups, its antimicrobial action being due to the presence of sulphur dioxide liberated by the reaction between the metabisulphite and the acid.

SODIUM METHYL HYDROXYBENZOATE

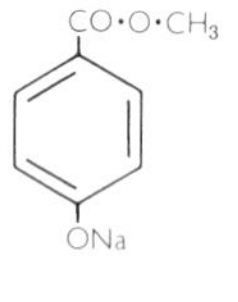

SYNONYM: Sodium Methylparaben

$C_8H_7NaO_3 = 174 \cdot 1$

Sodium Methyl Hydroxybenzoate is the sodium derivative of methyl p-hydroxybenzoate.

Solubility. Soluble in 2 parts of water and in 50 parts of alcohol; almost insoluble in fixed oils.

Standard
It complies with the requirements of the British Pharmacopoeia.
It is a white, crystalline, hygroscopic, almost odourless powder and contains not less than 99·0 and not more than the equivalent of 102·0 per cent of $C_8H_7NaO_3$, calculated with reference to the anhydrous substance.

It contains not more than 5·0 per cent w/w of water. A 0·1 per cent solution in water has a pH of 9·5 to 10·5.

Storage. It should be stored in airtight containers.

Uses. Sodium methyl hydroxybenzoate is used in place of methyl hydroxybenzoate (page 305) when it is desirable to have a material which is more soluble in water.

OTHER NAMES: *Nipagin M Sodium*®; Soluble Methyl Hydroxybenzoate

SODIUM NITRITE

$NaNO_2 = 69.00$

Solubility. Soluble, at 20°, in 1·5 parts of water and in 160 parts of alcohol.

Standard

DESCRIPTION. Deliquescent colourless or slightly yellow crystals or a white or slightly yellow crystalline powder; odourless or almost odourless.

IDENTIFICATION TESTS. 1. For nitrite: (a) heat with *dilute sulphuric acid*—red fumes are evolved; (b) dissolve 0·01 g in 1 ml of water and add to a mixture of 0·5 ml of *aniline* and 5 ml of *glacial acetic acid*—a deep orange-red colour is produced; (c) to 5 ml of a 1 per cent w/v solution in water add 5 ml of *ferrous sulphate solution*—a deep-brown colour is produced.

2. It gives the reactions characteristic of sodium.

ARSENIC. It complies with the test given in Appendix 6, page 879 (2 parts per million).

LEAD. It complies with the test given in Appendix 7, page 883 (10 parts per million).

CHLORIDE. 0·50 g complies with the limit test for chlorides (700 parts per million).

SULPHATE. 0·25 g dissolved in water with the addition of 3 ml of *dilute hydrochloric acid* complies with the limit test for sulphates (0·24 per cent).

CONTENT OF $NaNO_2$. Not less than 95·0 per cent, determined by the following method:
Dissolve about 0·5 g, accurately weighed, in water, dilute to 100 ml with water, and determine by slow titration the volume of the solution required to decolorise a mixture of 50·0 ml of 0·1N potassium permanganate, 5 ml of *sulphuric acid* and 100 ml of water, warmed to about 40°; 50·0 ml of 0·1N potassium permanganate is equivalent to 0·1725 g of $NaNO_2$.

Incompatibility. It is incompatible with oxidising agents, phenazone, and caffeine citrate.

Sterilisation. Solutions for injection are sterilised by heating in an autoclave or by filtration.

Storage. It should be stored in airtight containers.

Actions and uses. The actions and uses of sodium nitrite are similar to but less marked than those described under Glyceryl Trini-

trate Solution (page 212). The onset of its effect is delayed for about fifteen minutes and its actions last for about one hour.

Sodium nitrite occupies a special place in the treatment of cyanide poisoning; 10 millilitres of Sodium Nitrite Injection is given intravenously during three minutes, followed after five minutes by 50 millilitres of Sodium Thiosulphate Injection given intravenously during ten minutes. The injections may be repeated in two hours if necessary. The sodium nitrite produces methaemoglobinaemia and the cyanide ions combine with the methaemoglobin to produce cyanmethaemoglobin, thus protecting essential enzymes from the cyanide ion. The cyanmethaemoglobin dissociates, setting free cyanide, which is converted to thiocyanate by the sodium thiosulphate.

Sodium nitrite is added to aqueous antiseptic solutions to give a concentration of 1 per cent in order to prevent rusting of surgical instruments.

POISONING. The procedure as described under Glyceryl Trinitrate Solution (page 212) should be adopted.

Methaemoglobinaemia, severe enough to cause asphyxia, may be reversed by the administration of methylene blue, 2 milligrams per kilogram body-weight, by mouth or by intravenous injection.

Dose. 30 to 120 milligrams by mouth.

In cyanide poisoning: 300 milligrams by intravenous injection.

Preparation

SODIUM NITRITE INJECTION, B.P.C. (page 718)

SODIUM PERBORATE

$NaBO_2,H_2O_2,3H_2O = 153.9$

Solubility. Soluble, at 20°, in 40 parts of water, with some decomposition.

Standard

DESCRIPTION. Colourless, prismatic crystals or a white powder, stable in crystalline form; odourless or almost odourless.

IDENTIFICATION TESTS. 1. Mix 1 ml of a saturated solution in water with 1 ml of *dilute sulphuric acid* and 0·2 ml of *potassium dichromate solution*, shake with 2 ml of *solvent ether*, and allow to stand; a blue colour is produced in the ether layer.

2. The mixture obtained on the addition of *sulphuric acid* and *methyl alcohol* burns, when ignited, with a flame tinged with green.

3. A solution in water is alkaline to *litmus solution*.

4. It gives the reactions characteristic of sodium.

ARSENIC. It complies with the test given in Appendix 6, page 879 (8 parts per million).

IRON. Dissolve 0·50 g in 5 ml of water and 2·5 ml of *dilute hydrochloric acid*, and evaporate to dryness on a water-bath with frequent stirring; the residue dissolved

in 40 ml of water complies with the limit test for iron (80 parts per million).

LEAD. It complies with the test given in Appendix 7, page 883 (10 parts per million).

CHLORIDE. 1·0 g complies with the limit test for chlorides (350 parts per million).

SULPHATE. 0·05 g complies with the limit test for sulphates (1·2 per cent).

CONTENT OF $NaBO_2,H_2O_2,3H_2O$. Not less than 96·0 and not more than the equivalent of 103·0 per cent, determined by the following method:
Dissolve about 0·3 g, accurately weighed, in 50 ml of water, add 10 ml of *dilute sulphuric acid*, and titrate with 0·1N potassium permanganate; each ml of 0·1N potassium permanganate is equivalent to 0·007693 g of $NaBO_2,H_2O_2,3H_2O$.

Storage. It should be stored in airtight containers.

Actions and uses. Sodium perborate readily releases oxygen in contact with oxidisable matter and has been used in aqueous solution for purposes similar to those described under Hydrogen Peroxide Solution (page 227). Mixed with two to four parts of calcium carbonate it has been employed also as a dentifrice, but frequent use may cause blistering and oedema.

SODIUM PERTECHNETATE (^{99m}Tc) INJECTION

This material is radioactive and any regulations in force must be complied with.

Sodium Pertechnetate (^{99m}Tc) Injection is a sterile solution containing technetium-99m in the form of pertechnetate ion and sufficient sodium chloride to make the solution isotonic with blood.

Technetium-99m is a radioactive nuclide which emits γ-radiation and has a half-life of 6 hours; it is formed by the radioactive decay of molybdenum-99, a radioactive isotope of molybdenum produced by the neutron irradiation of natural molybdenum or molybdenum enriched in molybdenum-98.

The injection is prepared by the elution of a column containing molybdenum-99 adsorbed on a suitable material such as alumina.

Standard
It complies with the requirements of the British Pharmacopoeia.
It is a clear colourless solution and contains not less than 90 and not more than 110 per cent of the content of technetium-99m stated on the label at the date and hour stated on the label. Up to the date and hour after which the injection is not intended to be used, not more than 0·01 per cent of the total radioactivity is due to radionuclides other than technetium-99m, except that technetium-99 resulting from the decay of technetium-99m may be present, and except that molybdenum-99m may be present to the extent of 0·1 per cent of the total radioactivity, all calculated at the time of administration. It has a pH of 4·5 to 7·5.

Sterilisation. It is either prepared aseptically using a sterile preparation of molybdenum-99 or sterilised by heating in an autoclave or by filtration.

Labelling. The label on the container and the label on the package state:
(1) the content of technetium-99m at a given date and hour;
(2) the volume;
(3) that the injection is radioactive; and
(4) the date and hour after which the injection is not intended to be used.

Storage. It should be stored in an area assigned for the purpose. The storage conditions should be such that the maximum radiation-dose-rate to which persons may be exposed is reduced to an acceptable level.

Actions and uses. Technetium-99m is the radionuclide that is most widely used for diagnostic procedures. Its monoenergetic 140 keV gamma-rays, which are easily and efficiently collimated, and the absence of any β-radiation make it an almost ideal radiation source for external gamma-scintigraphy with either rectilinear scanners or gamma-ray cameras.

Sodium pertechnetate, which is the form in which technetium-99m is obtained from a radionuclide generator, is selectively concentrated in various organs, including the brain, thyroid gland, and salivary glands, and in the choroid plexuses.

Sodium pertechnetate crosses the blood-brain barrier and is gradually taken up in many brain tumours. This property is utilised in the detection of both primary and secondary brain tumours. A short time after an injection, gamma-scanning of the suspected area is begun. To avoid confusion, uptake in the choroid plexuses and glands is blocked by administering potassium perchlorate about an hour before the injection.

Other organs are visualised by technetium-99m scintigraphy with extemporaneously prepared injections in which sodium pertechnetate (^{99m}Tc) has been converted to a physical or chemical form which will localise in the organ concerned.

For external gamma-scanning of the liver the ^{99m}Tc-radioactivity is required in the form of a colloid. A sulphur colloid or an antimony sulphide colloid is commonly used.

A suspension of particles having a diameter of 20 to 50 μm is used for lung scanning. It is prepared as a suspension of human albumin particles or of iron hydroxide particles carrying ^{99m}Tc activity.

An intravenous injection prepared by the addition of a chelating agent such as diethylenetriaminepenta-acetic acid to sodium pertechnetate solution in the presence of a suitable buffer is used for scanning the kidneys and as an alternative to sodium pertechnetate injection for brain scanning.

Sodium pertechnetate (^{99m}Tc) has been used to prepare an injection of technetium-99m in the form of a polyphosphate for bone scanning.

Sodium pertechnetate (^{99m}Tc) has also been used to prepare labelled human albumin for blood pool studies, and particularly for placenta location.

SODIUM PHOSPHATE

SYNONYMS: Disodium Hydrogen Phosphate; Natrii Phosphas; Sod. Phos.

$Na_2HPO_4,12H_2O = 358.1$

Sodium Phosphate may be prepared by the interaction of sodium carbonate and acid calcium phosphate.

Solubility. Soluble, at 20°, in 5 parts of water; very slightly soluble in alcohol.

Standard
It complies with the requirements of the European Pharmacopoeia.
It occurs as colourless, transparent, strongly efflorescent, odourless crystals and contains not less than 98.5 and not more than the equivalent of 101.0 per cent of Na_2HPO_4, calculated with reference to the dried substance. The loss on drying under the prescribed conditions is 57.0 to 61.0 per cent.

Stability. When heated to 40° it fuses; at 100° it loses its water of crystallisation, and at a dull-red heat it is converted into the pyrophosphate, $Na_4P_2O_7$.

Storage. It should be stored in airtight containers.

Actions and uses. Sodium phosphate is a saline purgative, the actions and uses of which are described under Magnesium Sulphate (page 278). When given by mouth a small proportion of the salt, however, is absorbed and it therefore also exerts a mild diuretic action. It is usually administered in solution.

Dose. 2 to 16 grams.

SODIUM PHOSPHATE (^{32}P) INJECTION

This material is radioactive and any regulations in force must be complied with.

Sodium Phosphate (^{32}P) Injection is a sterile isotonic solution containing sodium phosphate (^{32}P) and added phosphate.

Phosphorus-32 is a radioactive isotope of phosphorus having a half-life of 14.3 days; it may be prepared by the neutron irradiation of sulphur.

Standard
It complies with the requirements of the British Pharmacopoeia.
It is a clear colourless solution and contains not less than 90.0 and not more than 110.0 per cent of the quantity of phosphorus-32 stated on the label at the date and hour stated on the label. The specific activity is not less than 0.3 millicurie per milligram of phosphate ion. It has a pH of 6.0 to 7.0.

Sterilisation. It is sterilised by heating in an autoclave.

Labelling. The label on the container states:
(1) the content of phosphorus-32 expressed in microcuries or millicuries at a given date and hour;
(2) that the injection is radioactive; and
(3) either that it does not contain a bactericide or the name and proportion of any added bactericide.

The label on the package also states:
(1) the total volume in the container; and
(2) the content of total phosphate.

Storage. It should be stored in an area assigned for the purpose. The storage conditions should be such that the maximum radiation-dose-rate to which persons may be exposed is reduced to an acceptable level.
Glass containers may darken under the effects of radiation.

Actions and uses. Sodium Phosphate (^{32}P) Injection is a solution suitable for the intravenous administration of radioactive phosphorus-32.
Phosphorus-32 has a half-life of just over fourteen days, but because it is metabolised and excreted, its effective half-life in the human body is estimated to be only eight days. Phosphorus-32 is deposited in bone and nucleoprotein and rapidly dividing cells have a particular affinity for the element.
Sodium Phosphate (^{32}P) Injection is used for irradiating the body with β-rays. It is used as a palliative agent in the treatment of polycythaemia vera and its use may be preceded, if required, by phlebotomy. Initially, a single dose of 5 millicuries may be injected intravenously, followed, if necessary, by doses of not more than 3 or 4 millicuries at intervals of not less than two months.
The full effect of treatment with radioactive phosphorus-32 may not be seen for three or four months but, if the platelet count falls below 50,000 per cubic millimetre, a remission, usually lasting for four months to two years, is likely to occur. Relapses may be treated with further courses of radioactive phosphorus-32 but an interval of at least three months should elapse between any two courses of the treatment.
In the treatment of chronic myeloid leukaemia, Sodium Phosphate (^{32}P) Injection produces results resembling those obtained with X-ray treatment. An intravenous dose of 1 to 2 millicuries once a week may be required for four to eight weeks to reduce the leucocyte count to about 10,000 to 20,000 per cubic millimetre. After a course of treatment, remissions last from three to ten months in about half of the patients. Chronic lymphatic leukaemia does not respond so readily, and local irradiation of lymph nodes is sometimes more beneficial.
Radioactive phosphorus-32 has little effect during exacerbations in the course of chronic

leukaemias and is of little value in the treatment of the acute leukaemias, Hodgkin's disease, and lymphosarcoma. In those reticuloses, however, in which the tumour is highly sensitive to irradiation, satisfactory results may be obtained by treatment with radioactive phosphorus-32.

Sodium Phosphate (^{32}P) Injection is of no value for the treatment of multiple myeloma or of most forms of carcinoma or sarcoma.

Radioactive phosphorus-32 has also been used for the diagnosis and localisation of intraocular tumours and skin tumours.

PRECAUTIONS AND CONTRA-INDICATIONS. Significant amounts of radioactive phosphorus-32 are excreted in the urine and, after oral administration, in the faeces. The excreta must therefore always be monitored and, if necessary, stored until the radioactivity is low enough for it to be disposed of in accordance with any regulations of the appropriate authorities.

Because of its depressant effect on the red bone marrow, Sodium Phosphate (^{32}P) Injection, even in therapeutic doses, may produce aplastic anaemia, leucopenia, and thrombocytopenic purpura. Paradoxically, it has been reported that radioactive phosphorus-32, used for the treatment of polycythaemia vera, has induced leukaemia. Frequent examination of the blood during and after radioactive phosphorus-32 therapy is essential. Symptoms of radiation sickness have followed its use.

Special caution should be exercised when giving Sodium Phosphate (^{32}P) Injection to leukaemic patients with an erythrocyte count of less than 2,500,000 per cubic millimetre. It is contra-indicated if the reticulocyte count, in the presence of significant anaemia, is less than 0·2 per cent and also if the leucocyte count is less than 3000 per cubic millimetre or the platelet count is less than 150,000 per cubic millimetre.

Dose. See above under **Actions and uses.**

SODIUM POLYMETAPHOSPHATE

Sodium Polymetaphosphate may be prepared by heating anhydrous sodium dihydrogen phosphate to a temperature above its melting-point, sufficient disodium hydrogen phosphate having been added to yield a product containing about 10 per cent of tetrasodium pyrophosphate, $Na_4P_2O_7$, and cooling the melt rapidly. The presence of the pyrophosphate increases the pH of solutions to approximately 7.

Although this substance has been called sodium hexametaphosphate, it exists, in fact, in much higher degrees of polymerisation.

Solubility. Slowly soluble in water; insoluble in alcohol.

Standard

DESCRIPTION. Colourless, translucent, vitreous, deliquescent plates or powder; odourless or almost odourless.

IDENTIFICATION TESTS. 1. Dissolve 0·4 g in 20 ml of water and add the solution, in portions, to 10 ml of a 1 per cent w/v solution of *anhydrous calcium chloride* in water; a white precipitate is first formed which subsequently dissolves. Make slightly alkaline to *litmus paper* with *dilute ammonia solution* and add *ammonium oxalate solution*; no precipitate is formed.

2. Moisten a small portion with *hydrochloric acid* and introduce into the flame of a Bunsen burner on a platinum wire loop; the flame becomes yellow.

3. To a solution in water add *potassium antimonate solution*; a white crystalline precipitate is slowly produced.

4. A solution prepared by boiling a sample with *2M nitric acid* for 30 minutes gives the reactions characteristic of phosphates.

ALKALINITY. pH of a 0·25 per cent w/v solution in *carbon dioxide-free water*, 7·0 to 7·5.

ARSENIC. It complies with the test given in Appendix 6, page 879 (2 parts per million).

LEAD. It complies with the test given in Appendix 7, page 884 (25 parts per million).

IRON, ALUMINIUM, CALCIUM, AND MAGNESIUM. Boil 0·50 g for 30 minutes with 20 ml of water and 2 ml of *hydrochloric acid*, cool, dilute to 25 ml with water, make alkaline to *litmus paper* with *dilute ammonia solution*, and allow to stand for 5 minutes; not more than an opalescence is produced.

CHLORIDE. 0·50 g complies with the limit test for chlorides (700 parts per million).

SULPHATE. 0·25 g boiled for 30 minutes with 20 ml of water and 3 ml of *dilute hydrochloric acid* complies with the limit test for sulphates (0·24 per cent).

CONTENT OF $Na_4P_2O_7$. 8·0 to 15·0 per cent, determined by the following method:
Dissolve about 10 g, accurately weighed, in 100 ml of water and titrate with 1N hydrochloric acid, using *methyl orange solution* as indicator; each ml of 1N hydrochloric acid is equivalent to 0·1330 g of $Na_4P_2O_7$.

CONTENT OF $(NaPO_3)_x$. Not less than 85·0 per cent, determined by the following method:
Dissolve about 3 g, accurately weighed, in 50 ml of 1N hydrochloric acid, boil gently under a reflux condenser for 30 minutes, cool, add 12 g of *sodium chloride* and *phenolphthalein solution* as indicator, and titrate with 1N sodium hydroxide to a definite pink colour; each ml of 1N sodium hydroxide in excess of 50 ml is equivalent to 0·1020 g of $(NaPO_3)_x$.

Stability. Aqueous solutions of sodium polymetaphosphate slowly revert to orthophosphate; the rate of hydration is considerably increased by high temperatures and by the addition of sufficient acid or alkali.

Storage. It should be stored in airtight containers.

Uses. Sodium polymetaphosphate combines with calcium and magnesium ions to form complex soluble compounds and it is therefore used, in a concentration of 1 in 600 to 1 in

300, to prevent the precipitation of calcium and magnesium compounds from water. Sodium polymetaphosphate may also be used as a dusting-powder (5 per cent) in hyperhidrosis and bromidrosis and as a prophylactic against mycotic infection of the toes.

OTHER NAME: *Calgon®*

SODIUM POTASSIUM TARTRATE

SYNONYMS: Rochelle Salt; Sod. Pot. Tart.

$C_4H_4KNaO_6,4H_2O = 282.2$

Solubility. Soluble, at 20°, in 1·5 parts of water; very slightly soluble in alcohol.

Standard
DESCRIPTION. Colourless crystals or white crystalline powder; odourless or almost odourless.

IDENTIFICATION TESTS. It gives the reactions characteristic of sodium, of potassium, and of tartrates.

ACIDITY OR ALKALINITY. Dissolve 1·0 g in 10 ml of *carbon dioxide-free water* and titrate with 0·1N sodium hydroxide or with 0·1N hydrochloric acid, using *phenolphthalein solution* as indicator; not more than 0·1 ml is required.

ARSENIC. It complies with the test given in Appendix 6, page 879 (2 parts per million).

IRON. 0·50 g complies with the limit test for iron (80 parts per million).

LEAD. It complies with the test given in Appendix 7, page 884 (10 parts per million).

CHLORIDE. 1·0 g complies with the limit test for chlorides (350 parts per million).

SULPHATE. 0·25 g dissolved in water with the addition of 3 ml of *dilute hydrochloric acid* complies with the limit test for sulphates (0·24 per cent).

CONTENT OF $C_4H_4KNaO_6,4H_2O$. Not less than 99·0 and not more than the equivalent of 102·0 per cent, determined by the following method:

Ignite gently about 2 g, accurately weighed, cool, boil the residue with 50 ml of water and 50 ml of 0·5N hydrochloric acid, and filter; wash the residue with water and titrate the excess of acid in the combined filtrate and washings with 0·5N sodium hydroxide, using *methyl orange solution* as indicator; each ml of 0·5N hydrochloric acid is equivalent to 0·07056 g of $C_4H_4KNaO_6,4H_2O$.

Actions and uses. Sodium potassium tartrate is a saline purgative, the actions and uses of which are described under Magnesium Sulphate (page 278). It causes a watery evacuation of the bowel without producing irritation.

The tartrates of the alkali metals are less readily absorbed than the citrates; their purgative action is therefore greater, while their diuretic action and effect in reducing the acidity of the urine are less pronounced.

Dose. 8 to 16 grams.

Preparations
EFFERVESCENT POWDER, COMPOUND, B.P.C. (page 776)
EFFERVESCENT POWDER, COMPOUND, DOUBLE-STRENGTH, B.P.C. (page 777)

SODIUM PROPYL HYDROXYBENZOATE

SYNONYM: Sodium Propylparaben

$C_{10}H_{11}NaO_3 = 202.2$

Sodium Propyl Hydroxybenzoate is the sodium derivative of propyl *p*-hydroxybenzoate.

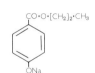

Solubility. Soluble in 1 part of water, in 50 parts of alcohol, and in 2 parts of alcohol (50 per cent); almost insoluble in fixed oils.

Standard
It complies with the requirements of the British Pharmacopoeia.
It is a white, crystalline, hygroscopic, odourless powder and contains not less than 99·0 and not more than the equivalent of 102·0 per cent of $C_{10}H_{11}NaO_3$, calculated with reference to the anhydrous substance. It

contains not more than 5·0 per cent w/w of water. A 0·1 per cent solution in water has a pH of 9·5 to 10·5.

Storage. It should be stored in airtight containers.

Uses. Sodium propyl hydroxybenzoate is used in place of propyl hydroxybenzoate (page 413) when it is desirable to have a material which is more soluble in water.

OTHER NAMES: *Nipasol M Sodium®*; Soluble Propyl Hydroxybenzoate

SODIUM SALICYLATE

SYNONYM: Sod. Sal.

$C_7H_5NaO_3 = 160.1$

Sodium Salicylate is sodium *o*-hydroxybenzoate.

Solubility. Soluble, at 20°, in 1 part of water and in 11 parts of alcohol.
A saturated aqueous solution is liable to deposit crystals of a less-soluble hydrated salt, $C_7H_5NaO_3,6H_2O$.

Standard
It complies with the requirements of the British Pharmacopoeia.
It occurs as colourless small crystals or crystalline

flakes or as a white powder; it is odourless or has a faint characteristic odour. It contains not less than 99·5 per cent of $C_7H_5NaO_3$, calculated with reference to the dried substance. The loss on drying under the prescribed conditions is not more than 0·5 per cent.

Incompatibility. It is incompatible with most acids and with solutions of some alkaloids. With alkali bicarbonates, a sodium salicylate solution gradually acquires a reddish-brown colour; if the prescriber will authorise the addition, sodium metabisulphite (0·1 per cent) will retard this change. Sodium salicylate forms a deep purple solution with iron salts.

Actions and uses. Sodium salicylate has antipyretic and analgesic actions. When given by mouth, it is absorbed mainly through the intestine and is rapidly excreted; frequent doses are therefore required to maintain a satisfactory concentration in the blood. The usual dose is 0·6 to 2 grams.

Sodium salicylate is a gastric irritant and sodium bicarbonate is often given with it to reduce this effect; however, the bicarbonate also increases the rate of excretion and thus lowers the concentration of salicylate in the blood to less effective levels.

Sodium salicylate causes dilatation of the skin vessels and some perspiration and the increased loss of heat results in a fall in body temperature.

The principal use of sodium salicylate is in the treatment of acute rheumatic fever; a dosage of 1·3 grams may be given by mouth every two hours, or 2 grams every three hours, until the temperature is reduced. For acute rheumatism, it is given in a daily dosage of 5 to 10 grams in divided doses. For the control of rheumatoid arthritis, aspirin is preferred because it is a more effective analgesic.

The unpleasant taste of sodium salicylate may be disguised with Orange Peel Infusion.

UNDESIRABLE EFFECTS. Some patients exhibit an idiosyncrasy to salicylates, as described under Aspirin (page 35). After large doses, most patients are liable to experience certain undesirable effects, which include headache, tinnitus, confusion, dimness of vision, excessive sweating, skin eruptions, and dyspnoea. Salicylates must be used with care in patients with acute renal disease. The prothrombin time may be prolonged after repeated large doses.

POISONING. The procedure as described under Aspirin (page 35) should be adopted.

Dose. See above under **Actions and uses**.

Preparations
COLCHICUM AND SODIUM SALICYLATE MIXTURE, B.P.C. (page 740)
SODIUM SALICYLATE MIXTURE, B.P.C. (page 753)
SODIUM SALICYLATE MIXTURE, STRONG, B.P.C. (page 753)

SODIUM STIBOGLUCONATE

Sodium Stibogluconate is a pentavalent antimony compound of indefinite composition. It has been represented by the formula $C_6H_9Na_2O_9Sb$, but it usually contains less than two atoms of sodium for each atom of antimony.

Sodium Stibogluconate may be prepared by the interaction of antimonic acid, gluconic acid, and sodium hydroxide, or by adding antimony pentachloride to a solution of gluconic acid and treating the reaction mixture with sodium hydroxide. The product is purified by dissolving in water and precipitating with methyl alcohol.

Solubility. Very soluble in water; insoluble in alcohol and in ether.

Standard
It complies with the requirements of the British Pharmacopoeia.
It is a colourless odourless powder consisting mainly of amorphous particles and contains 30·0 to 34·0 per cent of total antimony, calculated with reference to the dried substance. The loss on drying under the prescribed conditions is 10·0 to 15·0 per cent. A 10 per cent solution in water has a pH of 5·0 to 5·6.

Storage. It should be stored in airtight containers.

Actions and uses. Sodium stibogluconate is used in the treatment of leishmaniasis. It is much less toxic than antimony sodium tartrate (page 32), and it forms a stable aqueous solution which is non-irritant. After parenteral administration a large proportion of the drug is excreted rapidly by the kidneys.

Sodium stibogluconate is administered by intramuscular or intravenous injection; a course of treatment usually consists of six to ten daily injections, each of 6 millilitres of Sodium Stibogluconate Injection. More than one course is usually necessary for the treatment of *Leishmania donovani* infections in East Africa, Ethiopia, and the Sudan.

For the treatment of oriental sore the injection may be infiltrated around the edges of the lesions, a total of not more than 2 millilitres being injected at one time, but intravenous or intramuscular injections combined with bland local dressings are generally more satisfactory.

UNDESIRABLE EFFECTS. Toxic effects, such as nausea, vomiting, or rigors, are rare.

POISONING. As for Antimony Sodium Tartrate (page 32).

Dose. See above under **Actions and uses**.

Preparation
SODIUM STIBOGLUCONATE INJECTION, B.P. It consists of a sterile solution containing sodium stibogluconate, equivalent to 10 per cent of total antimony, in Water for Injections; 6 ml contains 2 g of sodium stibogluconate. It should be protected from light.

OTHER NAME: *Pentostam®*

SODIUM SULPHATE

SYNONYMS: Glauber's Salt; Natrii Sulfas Decahydricus; Sod. Sulph.

$Na_2SO_4,10H_2O = 322 \cdot 2$

Solubility. Soluble, at 20°, in 2·5 parts of water, at 33°, in 0·3 part, and then decreasing with increase in temperature to 0·5 part at 100°; insoluble in alcohol. Sodium sulphate readily forms a supersaturated solution when a saturated solution prepared at a temperature above 33° is cooled.

Standard
It complies with the requirements of the European Pharmacopoeia.
It occurs as odourless, colourless, transparent crystals or white crystalline powder and contains not less than 99·0 per cent of Na_2SO_4, calculated with reference to the dried substance. The loss on drying under the prescribed conditions is 52·0 to 57·0 per cent. It rapidly effloresces in dry air.
When heated to a temperature of 33°, the crystals liquefy. The anhydrous salt fuses at red heat without decomposition.

Sterilisation. Solutions for injection are sterilised by heating in an autoclave or by filtration.

Storage. It should be stored in airtight containers.

Actions and uses. Sodium sulphate is a saline purgative, the actions and uses of which are described under Magnesium Sulphate (page 278).
A 4·3 per cent solution of sodium sulphate given by intravenous infusion has been used as a diuretic in the treatment of anuria due to deposition of calculi in the renal pelvis during sulphonamide treatment.
A 12 to 25 per cent solution is of value as a lymphagogue when applied to infected wounds.

Dose. 5 to 15 grams.

ANHYDROUS SODIUM SULPHATE

SYNONYMS: Anhyd. Sod. Sulph.; Dried Glauber's Salt; Dried Sodium Sulphate; Natrii Sulfas Anhydricus

$Na_2SO_4 = 142 \cdot 0$

Anhydrous Sodium Sulphate may be prepared by drying Sodium Sulphate to constant weight at 100°.

Solubility. Soluble, at 20°, in 5 parts of water; insoluble in alcohol.

Standard
Material which complies with this standard meets the requirements of the European Pharmacopoeia.

DESCRIPTION. A white hygroscopic powder; odourless.

IDENTIFICATION TESTS. It gives the reactions characteristic of sodium and of sulphates.

APPEARANCE OF SOLUTION. A 2·2 per cent w/v solution in water complies with the following tests:
(i) The solution is clear when compared with water, the comparison being made by viewing vertically 10 ml of the liquids in matched, colourless, transparent, neutral glass tubes, 16 mm internal diameter and with a flat base, against a black background in diffused light.
(ii) The solution has no colour when compared with water, the comparison being made by viewing vertically 10 ml of the liquids in matched, colourless, transparent, neutral glass tubes, 16 mm internal diameter and with a flat base, against a white background in diffused daylight.

ACIDITY OR ALKALINITY. 0·22 g dissolved in 10 ml of *carbon dioxide-free water* requires for neutralisation not more than 0·5 ml of either 0·01N hydrochloric acid or 0·01N sodium hydroxide, *bromothymol blue solution* being used as indicator.

ARSENIC. It complies with the test given in Appendix 6, page 879 (3·3 parts per million).

CALCIUM. Mix 0·25 ml of *calcium standard solution* with 2 ml of *ammonium oxalate solution* and allow to stand for 1 minute; add 10 ml of a 2·2 per cent w/v solution of the sample in water, 1 ml of *acetic acid*, and 5 ml of *alcohol (95 per cent)*, shake, and allow to stand for 15 minutes; any opalescence produced is not more intense than that produced when 10 ml of *calcium standard solution* is used in place of 0·25 ml (450 parts per million).

HEAVY METALS. It complies with the test given in Appendix 8, page 887 (45 parts per million).

IRON. 0·11 g dissolved in 10 ml of water complies with the test for the prepared solution in the test for Iron given under Sodium Carbonate, page 445 (90 parts per million).

MAGNESIUM. To 10 ml of a 2·2 per cent w/v solution in water add 1 ml of *glycerin*, 0·15 ml of *titan yellow solution*, 0·5 ml of *ammonium oxalate solution*, and 5 ml of 2N sodium hydroxide, and shake; any pink colour produced is not more intense than that produced when 5 ml of *magnesium standard solution* and 5 ml of water are used in place of the test solution (200 parts per million).

ZINC. To 10 ml of a 2·2 per cent w/v solution in water add 0·1 ml of *potassium ferrocyanide solution* and allow to stand for 30 minutes; any opalescence produced is not more intense than that produced when a mixture of 10 ml of *zinc standard solution*, 0·1 ml of *potassium ferrocyanide solution*, and 0·05 ml of *acetic acid* is allowed to stand for 30 minutes (450 parts per million).

CHLORIDE. 0·11 g dissolved in 15 ml of water complies with the test for the prepared solution in the test for Chloride given under Sodium Carbonate, page 445 (450 parts per million).

LOSS ON DRYING. Not more than 5·0 per cent, determined by drying to constant weight at 130°.

CONTENT OF Na_2SO_4. Not less than 99·0 per cent, calculated with reference to the substance dried under the prescribed conditions, determined by the following method:
Dissolve about 0·1 g, accurately weighed, in 250 ml of *dilute hydrochloric acid*, heat to boiling, add slowly a slight excess of *0·25M barium chloride*, heat for 30 minutes on a water-bath, shaking occasionally, and filter; wash the residue with water, dry, and ignite to constant weight; each g of residue is equivalent to 0·6084 g of Na_2SO_4.

Storage. It should be stored in airtight containers.

Actions and uses. Anhydrous sodium sulphate has the actions described under Sodium Sulphate. It is used for preparing effervescent granules and powders and in preparations for which the powdered crystals of sodium sulphate are not suitable.

Dose. 1 to 8 grams.

OTHER NAMES: Exsiccated Glauber's Salt; Exsiccated Sodium Sulphate

SODIUM SULPHITE

$Na_2SO_3,7H_2O = 252.1$

Solubility. Soluble, at 20°, in 2 parts of water and in 28 parts of glycerol; insoluble in alcohol.

Standard

DESCRIPTION. Colourless monoclinic prisms; odourless or almost odourless.

IDENTIFICATION TESTS. 1. For sulphite: (a) heat with *hydrochloric acid*—sulphur dioxide is evolved; (b) add a 5 per cent w/v solution in water to *iodine solution*—the reagent is decolorised and the solution gives the reactions characteristic of sulphates; (c) add a 5 per cent w/v solution in water to *potassium permanganate solution* acidified to *litmus paper* with *dilute sulphuric acid*—the reagent is decolorised; (d) to a 5 per cent w/v solution in water add *lead acetate solution*—a white precipitate, soluble in cold *dilute nitric acid*, is formed; boil—a white precipitate is formed.

2. It gives the reactions characteristic of sodium.

ARSENIC. It complies with the test given in Appendix 6, page 879 (2 parts per million).

COPPER. Dissolve 10.0 g in 30 ml of water, add 1 ml of a 20 per cent w/v solution of *copper-free citric acid* in water and 1 ml of *acacia solution*, adjust the alkalinity of the solution to pH 9.0 by the addition of *dilute ammonia solution*, dilute to 50 ml with water, add 2 ml of *sodium diethyldithiocarbamate solution*, mix, and allow to stand for 2 minutes; any colour which develops is not deeper than that produced by 5 ml of *dilute copper sulphate solution* when similarly treated (5 parts per million).

IRON. Dissolve 4.0 g in 25 ml of water, add 15 ml of *hydrochloric acid FeT*, and evaporate to dryness; dissolve the residue in a mixture of 1 ml of *hydrochloric acid FeT* and 2 ml of water and dilute to 50 ml with water; 20 ml of this solution complies with the limit test for iron (25 parts per million).

LEAD. It complies with the test given in Appendix 7, page 884 (10 parts per million).

THIOSULPHATE. Dissolve 1.0 g in 10 ml of water, add 3 ml of *hydrochloric acid*, and heat on a water-bath for 10 minutes; no turbidity is produced.

CONTENT OF $Na_2SO_3,7H_2O$. Not less than 96.0 per cent, determined by the following method: Dissolve about 0.5 g, accurately weighed, in 50 ml of 0.1N iodine, add 1 ml of *hydrochloric acid*, and titrate the excess of iodine with 0.1N sodium thiosulphate, using *starch mucilage* as indicator; each ml of 0.1N iodine is equivalent to 0.01261 g of $Na_2SO_3,7H_2O$.

Stability. Sodium sulphite is efflorescent in air, becoming opaque and slowly oxidised to sulphate.
A solution in water is alkaline to litmus and is more rapidly oxidised than the solid salt. On boiling a saturated aqueous solution, the anhydrous salt separates out as a crystalline powder which redissolves on cooling.
On gently heating the salt, it softens but does not fuse; above 100° the crystals lose their water of crystallisation without melting or losing their shape; at a red heat the salt fuses, yielding an orange-red mixture of sodium sulphide and sodium sulphate.

Storage. It should be stored in airtight containers.

Uses. Sodium sulphite is used as a preservative in alkaline solutions and syrups.

SODIUM THIOSULPHATE

SYNONYM: Sodium Hyposulphite

$Na_2S_2O_3,5H_2O = 248.2$

Solubility. Soluble, at 20°, in less than 1 part of water; insoluble in alcohol.

Standard

DESCRIPTION. Colourless monoclinic prisms; odourless or almost odourless. Efflorescent in warm dry air and slightly hygroscopic in moist air.

IDENTIFICATION TESTS. 1. Dissolve 0.25 g in 5 ml of water and add 1 ml of *hydrochloric acid*; a white precipitate, which quickly changes to yellow, is formed and sulphur dioxide is evolved.

2. Dissolve 0.25 g in 5 ml of water and add *iodine solution* dropwise; the reagent is decolorised and the mixture does not give the reactions characteristic of sulphates.

3. It gives the reactions characteristic of sodium.

ACIDITY OR ALKALINITY. 10.0 g dissolved in 100 ml of *carbon dioxide-free water* requires for neutralisation not more than 0.1 ml of 0.1N sodium hydroxide or 0.1N hydrochloric acid, *bromothymol blue solution* being used as indicator.

CALCIUM. Dissolve 0.25 g in 5 ml of water, add 5 ml of *ammonium oxalate solution*, and allow to stand for 5 minutes; no turbidity is produced.

CONTENT OF $Na_2S_2O_3,5H_2O$. Not less than 99.0 and not more than the equivalent of 101.0 per cent, determined by the following method: Dissolve about 1 g, accurately weighed, in 20 ml of water and titrate with 0.1N iodine; each ml of 0.1N iodine is equivalent to 0.02482 g of $Na_2S_2O_3,5H_2O$.

Stability. When rapidly heated it melts in its water of crystallisation at 50°; at 100° it loses all its water of crystallisation and at a red heat it is decomposed. It is slowly decomposed when boiled in aqueous solution.

Sterilisation. Solutions for injection are sterilised by heating in an autoclave in an atmosphere of nitrogen.

Storage. It should be stored in airtight containers.

Actions and uses. Sodium thiosulphate is used, in conjunction with sodium nitrite, in the treatment of cyanide poisoning; 10 millilitres of Sodium Nitrite Injection is given intravenously during three minutes, followed after five minutes by 50 millilitres of Sodium Thiosulphate Injection given intravenously during ten minutes. The injections may be repeated in two hours if necessary.

The sodium nitrite produces methaemoglobinaemia and the cyanide ions combine with the methaemoglobin to produce cyanmethaemoglobin, thus protecting essential enzymes from the cyanide ions. The cyanmethaemoglobin dissociates, setting free cyanide, which is converted to thiocyanate by the sodium thiosulphate.

Dose. In the treatment of cyanide poisoning, 25 grams by intravenous injection.

Preparation
SODIUM THIOSULPHATE INJECTION, B.P.C. (page 718)

SORBIC ACID

$C_6H_8O_2 = 112\cdot1$

$$CH_3\cdot CH:CH\cdot CH:CH\cdot CO_2H$$

Sorbic Acid is 2,4-hexadienoic acid.

Solubility. Soluble, at 20°, in 700 parts of water, in 10 parts of alcohol, in 20 parts of ether, and in about 150 parts of fats and of fatty oils.

Standard
DESCRIPTION. A white or creamy-white powder; odour faint and characteristic.

IDENTIFICATION TESTS. 1. To a saturated solution in water add *bromine solution*, dropwise; the bromine solution is decolorised.

2. The ultraviolet absorption spectrum exhibits the characteristics given in Appendix 3, page 856.

3. The infra-red absorption spectrum exhibits maxima which are only at the same wavelengths as, and have similar relative intensities to, those in the spectrum of *sorbic acid A.S.*

MELTING-POINT. 133° to 137°.

ARSENIC. It complies with the test given in Appendix 6, page 879 (2 parts per million).

LEAD. It complies with the test given in Appendix 7, page 884 (10 parts per million).

WATER. Not more than 0·5 per cent w/w, determined by the method given in Appendix 16, page 895.

SULPHATED ASH. Not more than 0·2 per cent.

CONTENT OF $C_6H_8O_2$. Not less than 99·0 per cent, calculated with reference to the anhydrous substance, determined by the following method:
Dissolve about 1·5 g, accurately weighed, in 25 ml of *alcohol (95 per cent)*, previously neutralised to *phenolphthalein solution*, and titrate with 1N sodium hydroxide, using *phenolphthalein solution* as indicator; each ml of 1N sodium hydroxide is equivalent to 0·1121 g of $C_6H_8O_2$.

Storage. It should be stored in airtight containers, protected from light, in a cool place.

Uses. Sorbic acid has antifungal and antibacterial properties. In concentrations of 0·1 to 0·2 per cent it is an efficient preservative for acidic preparations but is much less effective in neutral or alkaline media.

It is sometimes preferred to the hydroxybenzoate esters as a preservative in preparations containing non-ionic emulsifying agents but its use may give rise to skin irritation.

SORBITAN MONOLAURATE

Sorbitan Monolaurate is a mixture of the partial esters of sorbitol and its mono- and dianhydrides with lauric acid. It has a weight per ml at 20° of about 1·00 g; the viscosity at 25° is about 4500 centipoises.

Solubility. Insoluble but dispersible in water; soluble, at 20°, in 100 parts of cottonseed oil; slightly soluble in ethyl acetate; miscible with alcohol.

Standard
DESCRIPTION. An amber-coloured viscous liquid; odour characteristic.

IDENTIFICATION TESTS. It complies with tests 2 and 3 described under Polysorbate 20 (page 389).

ACID VALUE. 4·0 to 7·0.

HYDROXYL VALUE. 330 to 358, determined by the method given in Appendix 21, page 902, about 1 g, accurately weighed, being used.

SAPONIFICATION VALUE. 158 to 170.

ARSENIC. It complies with the test given in Appendix 6, page 879 (3 parts per million).

LEAD. It complies with the test given in Appendix 8, page 887 (10 parts per million).

SULPHATED ASH. Not more than 0·25 per cent.

Uses. Sorbitan esters are non-ionic surface-active agents which are used in the preparation of emulsions, creams, and ointments. They are lipophilic in character and, when used alone, produce water-in-oil emulsions. They are also used in conjunction with suitable polysorbates, when, by appropriate choice of ester and concentration, the character of the emulsion can be varied and either water-in-oil or oil-in-water types may be obtained.

Sorbitan monolaurate is less lipophilic in character than the mono-oleate or the mono-stearate.

OTHER NAMES: *Crill 1*® ; *Sorbester P12*® ; *Span 20*®

SORBITAN MONO-OLEATE

Sorbitan Mono-oleate is a mixture of the partial esters of sorbitol and its mono- and di-anhydrides with oleic acid. It has a weight per ml at 20° of about 1·00 g; the viscosity at 25° is about 1000 centipoises.

Solubility. Insoluble but dispersible in water; miscible with alcohol; insoluble in propylene glycol.

Standard
DESCRIPTION. An amber-coloured viscous liquid; odour characteristic of fatty acids.

IDENTIFICATION TESTS. It complies with test 2 described under Polysorbate 20 (page 389) and with test 2 described under Polysorbate 80 (page 390).

ACID VALUE. 5·0 to 8·0.

HYDROXYL VALUE. 193 to 209, determined by the method given in Appendix 21, page 902, about 2 g, accurately weighed, being used.

SAPONIFICATION VALUE. 149 to 160.

ARSENIC. It complies with the test given in Appendix 6, page 879 (3 parts per million).

LEAD. It complies with the test given in Appendix 8, page 887 (10 parts per million).

SULPHATED ASH. Not more than 0·25 per cent.

Uses. Sorbitan mono-oleate has the uses of the sorbitan esters, as described under Sorbitan Monolaurate. It is more lipophilic in character than the monolaurate, and is useful for the preparation of creams of the water-in-oil type; a small proportion of polysorbate 60 or polysorbate 80 may be added to reduce viscosity and to aid the formation of an emulsion, thus avoiding the necessity for passing the cream through a homogeniser or mill.

Up to 10 per cent of sorbitan mono-oleate may be incorporated in paraffin-type bases to form anhydrous bases capable of absorbing large amounts of water.

OTHER NAMES: *Crill 4*®; *Sorbester P17*®; *Span 80*®

SORBITAN MONOSTEARATE

Sorbitan Monostearate is a mixture of the partial esters of sorbitol and its mono- and di-anhydrides with stearic acid.

Solubility. Insoluble but dispersible in water; soluble, at 20°, in 120 parts of alcohol.

Standard
DESCRIPTION. A pale yellow solid; odour faint and oily.

IDENTIFICATION TESTS. 1. It complies with test 2 described under Polysorbate 20 (page 389) and with test 2 described under Polysorbate 60 (page 389).
2. It has a setting-point of about 50°.

ACID VALUE. 5·0 to 10·0.

HYDROXYL VALUE. 235 to 260, determined by the method given in Appendix 21, page 902, about 1 g, accurately weighed, being used.

SAPONIFICATION VALUE. 147 to 157.

ARSENIC. It complies with the test given in Appendix 6, page 880 (3 parts per million).

LEAD. It complies with the test given in Appendix 8 page 887 (10 parts per million).

SULPHATED ASH. Not more than 0·25 per cent.

Uses. Sorbitan monostearate has the uses of the sorbitan esters, as described under Sorbitan Monolaurate. It has lipophilic properties similar to those of sorbitan mono-oleate.

OTHER NAMES: *Crill 3*®; *Sorbester P18*®; *Span 60*®

SORBITOL

$C_6H_{14}O_6 = 182·2$

$$HO·CH_2·\overset{\overset{\displaystyle H}{|}}{C}·\overset{\overset{\displaystyle H}{|}}{\underset{\underset{\displaystyle OH}{|}}{C}}·\overset{\overset{\displaystyle OH}{|}}{\underset{\underset{\displaystyle H}{|}}{C}}·\overset{\overset{\displaystyle H}{|}}{\underset{\underset{\displaystyle OH}{|}}{C}}·CH_2OH$$

Solubility. Soluble, at 20°, in less than 1 part of water and in 25 parts of alcohol; insoluble in ether and in chloroform.

Standard
It complies with the requirements of the British Pharmacopoeia.
It is a white, microcrystalline, odourless, slightly hygroscopic powder and contains not less than 98·0 per cent of $C_6H_{14}O_6$, calculated with reference to the anhydrous substance. It contains not more than 1·5 per cent w/w of water. It has a melting-point of about 95°.

Sterilisation. Solutions are sterilised by heating in an autoclave.

Storage. It should be stored in airtight containers.

Actions and uses. Sorbitol is used for the intravenous administration of carbohydrate in parenteral feeding. It is usually given as a 30 per cent w/v solution at a rate not exceeding 2 millilitres per minute. According to the United Kingdom Labelling of Food Regulations 1970, 1 gram of sorbitol contributes 3·75 Calories, and a 30 per cent solution therefore provides 1125 Calories per litre.

Sorbitol has also been used as an ingredient of some solutions for peritoneal dialysis.

The pharmaceutical uses of sorbitol are described under Sorbitol Solution (page 790).

Preparation
SORBITOL INJECTION, B.P. It consists of a sterile solution of sorbitol in Water for Injections. Unless otherwise specified, a solution containing 30 per cent w/v is supplied.

SPEARMINT OIL

SYNONYMS: Oleum Menthae Crispae; Oleum Menthae Viridis

Spearmint Oil is obtained by distillation from fresh flowering plants of *Mentha spicata* L. and *Mentha × cardiaca* (Gray) Bak. (Fam. Labiatae), grown in Europe and America, most of the oil of commerce being imported from north America.

Constituents. Spearmint oil contains about 55 to 70 per cent of (−)-carvone.

Solubility. Soluble, at 20°, in 1 part of alcohol (80 per cent). The solution may become opalescent on further dilution with alcohol (80 per cent).

Standard
DESCRIPTION. A colourless pale yellow or greenish-yellow liquid when recently distilled, but becoming darker and viscous on keeping; odour that of spearmint.

OPTICAL ROTATION. At 20°, −45° to −60°.

REFRACTIVE INDEX. At 20°, 1·484 to 1·491.

WEIGHT PER ML. At 20°, 0·917 g to 0·934 g.

CONTENT OF CARVONE. Not less than 55·0 per cent w/w, determined by the method given in Appendix 14, page 893.

Storage. It should be stored in well-filled airtight containers, protected from light, in a cool place.

Actions and uses. The properties of spearmint oil resemble those of peppermint oil. It is used as a flavouring agent and carminative.

Dose. 0·05 to 0·2 millilitre.

SPIRONOLACTONE

$C_{24}H_{32}O_4S = 416·6$

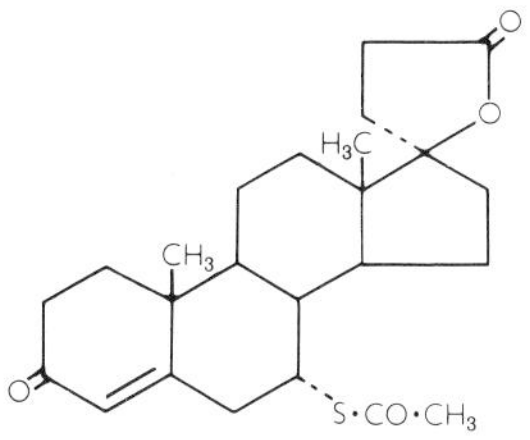

Spironolactone is 7α-acetylthio-17β-hydroxy-3-oxo-17α-pregn-4-ene-21-carboxylic acid γ-lactone.

Solubility. Very slightly soluble in water; soluble, at 20°, in 80 parts of alcohol, in 100 parts of ether, and in 3 parts of chloroform.

Standard
It complies with the requirements of the British Pharmacopoeia.
It is a buff-coloured powder which is odourless or has a slight odour of thioacetic acid and contains not less than 96·0 and not more than the equivalent of 102·0 per cent of $C_{24}H_{32}O_4S$, calculated with reference to the dried substance. The loss on drying under the prescribed conditions is not more than 0·5 per cent. It has a melting-point of about 205°.

Storage. It should be protected from light.

Actions and uses. Spironolactone is a competitive inhibitor of the natural corticosteroid hormone aldosterone, which promotes retention of sodium and excretion of potassium by the distal renal tubules. It thus increases sodium and reduces potassium excretion and so differs from chlorothiazide and similar diuretics, which act on the proximal tubules and increase sodium excretion but do not prevent excretion of potassium by the distal tubules.
Provided that production of aldosterone is

sufficiently high, spironolactone is active when given by mouth to patients on a low-salt diet. It is ineffective if aldosterone output is low.
The use of spironolactone is justified in the treatment of oedema when the condition is associated with excessive secretion of aldosterone. It is administered in conjunction with chlorothiazide and similar diuretics to reduce potassium loss while enhancing the excretion of sodium. It is usually given by mouth in a dosage of 25 milligrams four times a day.

UNDESIRABLE EFFECTS. Spironolactone may give rise to headache and, when taken in large doses, to drowsiness; skin rashes may occasionally occur, but usually clear when the drug is discontinued.

Dose. See above under **Actions and uses.**

Preparation
SPIRONOLACTONE TABLETS, B.P. Unless otherwise specified, tablets each containing 25 mg of spironolactone are supplied. They should be protected from light.

OTHER NAME: *Aldactone-A*®

SQUILL

SYNONYM: Scilla

Squill consists of the bulb of *Urginea maritima* (L.) Baker (Fam. Liliaceae). The plant is indigenous to the Mediterranean region. The bulbs are collected soon after the plant has flowered, divested of their dry outer membranous coats, and usually cut into transverse slices and dried. It is known in commerce as white squill.

Constituents. Squill contains the glycosides scillarin A and scillarin B. The former is a pure crystalline glycoside, which gives on hydrolysis scillaridin A (bufa-3,5,20,22-tetraenolide) and a sugar, scillabiose (a glucosidorhamnoside). Scillarin B is a mixture of glycosides.

Squill also contains a small amount of glucoscillarin A, about 4 to 11 per cent of mucilage, and a polyfructosan, sinistrin.

It yields to alcohol (60 per cent) about 65 to 80 per cent of extractive.

Standard for unground drug

DESCRIPTION. *Macroscopical:* slices transverse, about 5 to 8 mm thick, occurring as straight or curved triangular pieces about 0·5 to 5 cm long and 3 to 8 mm wide at mid-point, tapering towards each end, yellowish-white, texture horny, somewhat translucent, breaking with an almost glassy fracture when quite dry, but readily absorbing moisture when exposed to the air and becoming tough and flexible; transversely cut surface showing a single row of prominent vascular bundles near the concave edge and numerous smaller bundles scattered throughout the mesophyll.

Almost odourless; taste mucilaginous, disagreeably bitter, and acrid.

Microscopical: the diagnostic characters are: *epidermis,* cells polygonal and axially elongated, 1 to 2 times longer than wide, outer wall thick, stratified; *stomata* very rare, anomocytic, and nearly circular in outline, about 50 to 60 μm in diameter; *mesophyll* of colourless, thin-walled parenchyma containing very occasional *starch* granules, many cells containing bundles of acicular *crystals* of calcium oxalate embedded in *mucilage,* crystals up to about 1 mm long and about 1 to 15 μm wide; other cells containing *sinistrin; vascular bundles* collateral, scattered throughout the mesophyll; *xylem vessels* with spiral and annular wall thickening; *trichomes* absent.

IDENTIFICATION TEST. The mucilage contained in the cells of the mesophyll stains red with *alkaline corallin solution* but gives no red colour with *ruthenium red solution* and no purple colour with *iodine water.*

ACID-INSOLUBLE ASH. Not more than 1·5 per cent.

ALCOHOL (60 PER CENT)-SOLUBLE EXTRACTIVE. Not less than 68·0 per cent, determined on the material dried for one hour at 105° and powdered.

Standard for powdered drug: Powdered Squill

DESCRIPTION. A very hygroscopic white or yellowish-white powder possessing the diagnostic microscopical characters, odour, and taste of the unground drug.

IDENTIFICATION; ACID-INSOLUBLE ASH; ALCOHOL (60 PER CENT)-SOLUBLE EXTRACTIVE. It complies with the requirements for the unground drug.

Adulterants and substitutes. A red variety of *U. maritima* is used in French pharmacy in addition to the white variety; it has a more intensely bitter taste. This red variety is also used for the manufacture of rat poison. It contains the toxic principle scilliroside, a glycoside similar to scillarin A.

Urginea is the sliced bulb of *U. indica* Kunth (Fam. Liliaceae), indigenous to the Indian subcontinent and known in commerce as Indian squill. It is usually cut into longitudinal slices and may be distinguished by the somewhat darker colour of the pieces, which are ridged in the direction of their length and are occasionally grouped three or four together and attached to a portion of the axis. The epidermal cells are three to five times longer than they are broad; mucilage, which stains red with *alkaline corallin solution* and reddish-purple with *iodine water,* occurs in the cells of the mesophyll and also in association with the acicular crystals of calcium oxalate.

Urginea contains bitter principles similar to the glycosidal substances found in European squill; the drug contains about 35 to 40 per cent of mucilage and yields to *alcohol (60 per cent)* 20 to 50 per cent of extractive.

Storage. It should be stored in a cool dry place. Powdered Squill should be kept in a desiccated atmosphere.

Actions and uses. The glycosides of squill have an action upon the heart resembling that of digitalis, but are poorly absorbed from the gastro-intestinal tract and are less potent.

Squill irritates the gastric mucosa, and in large doses produces nausea and vomiting. In smaller doses it has a reflex expectorant action and its preparations are common constituents of cough mixtures.

Dose. 60 to 200 milligrams.

Preparations

STARCH

SYNONYM: Amylum

Starch consists of polysaccharide granules obtained from the grains of maize, *Zea mays* L., of rice, *Oryza sativa* L., or of wheat, *Triticum aestivum* L. (*T. vulgare* Vill.) and other species of *Triticum* (Fam. Gramineae), or from the tubers of the potato, *Solanum tuberosum* L. (Fam. Solanaceae). Maize starch is also known as corn starch.

SOLUBLE STARCH, which is used as a reagent, is prepared from the starch of potato or of maize by a process involving treatment with dilute hydrochloric acid, carefully adjusted so as to destroy the gelatinising power of the starch. Soluble starch shows the microscopical appearance almost unchanged of potato starch or maize starch, but has the property of being readily soluble in hot water to form a transparent mobile liquid.

Varieties. The diagnostic microscopical characters are: Maize starch: polyhedral, subspherical or, occasionally, muller-shaped granules, about 5 to **10** to **20** to 30 μm in diameter; the hilum is represented by a central triangular or 2- to 5-rayed fissure, and striations are not visible; it shows a well-marked cross when viewed between crossed polars.

Rice starch: simple and compound granules; single granules are polyhedral and are usually 2 to **5** to **8** to 12 μm in diameter; the hilum is sometimes evident as a minute central point; spindle-shaped and lemon-shaped granules are absent (distinction from oat starch); the compound grains are ovate, usually about 12 to 30 μm long and 7 to 20 μm wide; they contain about 2 to 150 components.

Wheat starch: principally simple lenticular granules, which are circular, oval, or subreniform in outline; the hilum appears as a central point or, if the granule is on its edge, as a line; the granules are mostly simple, the smaller ones being usually 5 to 10 μm and the larger ones 20 to 25 or up to 50 μm in greatest width. A few compound granules of 2 to 4 components are present; there are always more than 400 granules per milligram having a maximum diameter exceeding 40 μm (distinction from barley starch). When viewed between crossed polars, a dull cross of the maltese shape is seen.

Potato starch (sometimes known as English arrowroot): ovoid, irregularly ovoid, or subspherical, and often somewhat flattened; the hilum is a point towards the narrower end of the granule, and has an eccentricity of $\frac{1}{3}$ to $\frac{1}{4}$; the striations are well-marked and concentric; some rings appear darker than others. The granules are mostly simple, the subspherical ones measuring about 10 to 35 μm and the ovoid ones 30 to 100 μm. A few compound granules of 2 to 3 components are always present. The granules show a well-marked cross when viewed between crossed polars. Potato starch is easily distinguished from arrowroot and from other official starches by its rapid gelatinisation when mounted in a 0·9 per cent w/v solution of potassium hydroxide in water.

Constituents. Starch contains amylose and amylopectin, both polysaccharides based on α-glucose; the proportions vary somewhat in different starches, but the ratio of amylose (β-amylose) to amylopectin (α-amylose) is usually about 1 to 4.

Amylose consists of linear chains of 250 to 300 1,4-linked α-glucose residues arranged in the form of a helix; amylopectin is also a polymer of α-glucose but the macromolecule is built up of branched chains of glucose units linked in both the 1,4 and 1,6 positions. Amylopectin yields a gelatinous solution with water, whereas amylose yields a limpid solution which is coloured blue with iodine solution.

Solubility. Insoluble in cold water and in alcohol.

Standard

It complies with the appropriate requirements of the European Pharmacopoeia for Amylum Maydis (maize starch), Amylum Oryzae (rich starch), Amylum Solani (potato starch), or Amylum Tritici (wheat starch). It occurs as an odourless fine white powder or irregular

angular masses readily reducible to powder. The loss on drying at 100° to 105° is not more than 15 per cent for maize, rice, and wheat starch, and not more than 20 per cent for potato starch.

When 1 g of starch is boiled with 50 ml of water and the mixture cooled, a mucilage is formed, which is coloured deep blue by *iodine solution*; the colour disappears on warming and reappears on cooling.

Adulterants and substitutes. Manihot (Manioc) starch, often known as cassava or tapioca starch, obtained from *Manihot esculenta* Crantz (Fam. Euphorbiaceae), occurs as a substitute and is described under Arrowroot (page 34); this cassava starch may be used as Starch in tropical and subtropical parts of the world where official starches are not available.

Hygroscopicity. At relative humidities between about 25 and 55 per cent, the equilibrium moisture content of maize, rice, and wheat starches at 25° is between about 10 and 14 per cent and that for potato starch between about 10 and 18 per cent. At relative humidities above about 75 per cent, all starches absorb substantial amounts of moisture.

Labelling. The label states the botanical source.

Storage. It should be stored in airtight containers, in a cool dry place.

Actions and uses. Starch acts as an absorbent and is used as a dusting-powder for application to chafed or excoriated skin, either alone or mixed with zinc oxide or other similar substances.

Starch Mucilage may be employed as an emollient for the skin and is the basis of some enemas; it may also be used as an antidote in the treatment of poisoning by iodine.

A poultice may be prepared by boiling one part of starch with ten parts of water.

Starch is incorporated in some tablets as a disintegrating agent.

Preparations

CHLORPHENESIN DUSTING-POWDER, B.P.C. (page 663)

TALC DUSTING-POWDER, B.P.C. (page 663)

ZINC, STARCH, AND TALC DUSTING-POWDER, B.P.C. (page 664)

ZINC UNDECENOATE DUSTING-POWDER, B.P.C. (page 664)

STARCH MUCILAGE, B.P.C. (page 756)

RESORCINOL OINTMENT, COMPOUND, B.P.C. (page 763)

ZINC PASTE, COMPOUND, B.P. (*Syn.* Zinc Paste). It contains 25 per cent each of starch and zinc oxide in white soft paraffin.

ZINC AND SALICYLIC ACID PASTE, B.P. (*Syn.* Lassar's Paste). It contains 24 per cent each of starch and zinc oxide and 2 per cent of salicylic acid in white soft paraffin.

STEARIC ACID

Stearic Acid is a mixture of fatty acids, chiefly stearic and palmitic acids. It may contain a suitable antioxidant, such as 0·005 per cent of butylated hydroxytoluene.

Stearic Acid may be obtained by hydrolysis of various fats and subsequent removal of the liquid acids by cooling and filtration.
It may be powdered by sprinkling it with alcohol during trituration.

NOTE. Pure stearic acid, $C_{17}H_{35}·CO_2H = 284·5$, is obtained from an alcoholic solution of commercial stearic acid by fractional crystallisation, followed by conversion to magnesium stearate and subsequent acidification; it occurs in white shining flaky crystals or as a hard, somewhat glossy solid, melting at 69·3°.

Solubility. Insoluble in water; soluble, at 20°, in 15 parts of alcohol; soluble in ether and in chloroform.

Standard
DESCRIPTION. White greasy flaky crystals or hard masses showing signs of crystallisation; odourless or almost odourless.

ACID VALUE. 200 to 210.

IODINE VALUE. Not more than 4, determined by the iodine monochloride method.

MELTING-POINT. Not lower than 54°, determined by Method IV of the British Pharmacopoeia, Appendix IVA.

MINERAL ACID. Melt 5·0 g, shake with 5 ml of hot carbon dioxide-free water for 2 minutes, cool, and filter; the filtrate is not acid to methyl orange solution.

NEUTRAL FAT AND PARAFFIN. Boil 1·0 g with a solution of 1 g of sodium carbonate in 30 ml of water; the solution is not more than opalescent.

SULPHATED ASH. Not more than 0·1 per cent.

Labelling. The label on the container states the name and proportion of any added antioxidant.

Uses. Stearic acid, partly neutralised with alkalis or triethanolamine, is used in the preparation of creams. In the form of a powder it has been used as a lubricant in making compressed tablets.
When partly neutralised, stearic acid forms a creamy basis with five to fifteen times its weight of aqueous liquid and in this form it is sometimes used as the basis of vanishing creams; the proportion of alkali used largely determines the appearance and plasticity of the cream. After being neutralised and dissolved by heat in glycerol or alcohol, it will solidify when cold with at least ten times its weight of liquid.

STERCULIA

SYNONYMS: Sterculia Gum; Indian Tragacanth; Karaya Gum

Sterculia is the gum obtained from *Sterculia urens* Roxb. and other species of *Sterculia* (Fam. Sterculiaceae). It is produced in India, Pakistan, and Africa.

Constituents. Sterculia yields on hydrolysis, among other products, galacturonic acid (about 43 per cent), D-galactopyranose, L-rhamnopyranose, and acetic acid. Unlike tragacanth, sterculia does not contain methoxyl groups. When hydrolysed with phosphoric acid, the volatile acidity is about 14 to 16 per cent, calculated as acetic acid. The drug contains no oxidase and yields 5 to 7 per cent of ash.

Solubility. Partly soluble in water, in which it swells to a homogeneous, adhesive, gelatinous mass; insoluble in alcohol.

Standard for unground drug
DESCRIPTION. *Macroscopical:* irregular or vermiform pieces, about 0·5 to 2 cm thick; greyish or pinkish in colour; surface striated.
Odour of acetic acid.

Microscopical: when powdered and mounted in alcohol, it appears as small, transparent, angular particles of various sizes and shapes; the particles lose their sharp edges when water is added and each gradually swells until a large, indefinite, almost structureless mass results; when mounted in *ruthenium red solution*, the particles are stained red; no starch granules visible when mounted in *iodine water*.

IDENTIFICATION TESTS. 1. Shake 1 g with 80 ml of water during 24 hours; a tacky and viscous granular mucilage is produced.
2. Boil 4 ml of the mucilage obtained in test 1 with 0·5 ml of *hydrochloric acid*, add 1 ml of *sodium hydroxide solution*, filter, to the filtrate add 3 ml of *potassium cupri-tartrate solution*, and heat; a red precipitate is formed.
3. Warm 0·5 g with 2 ml of *sodium hydroxide solution*; a brown colour is produced.

ACID-INSOLUBLE ASH. Not more than 1·0 per cent.

ASH. Not more than 7·0 per cent.

VOLATILE ACID. Not less than 14·0 per cent, calculated as acetic acid, $C_2H_4O_2$, determined by the following method:
To about 1 g, accurately weighed, contained in a 700-ml long-necked flask, add 100 ml of water and 5 ml of *phosphoric acid*, allow to stand for several hours, or until the gum is completely swollen, and boil gently for 2 hours under a reflux condenser; steam-distil until 800 ml of distillate is obtained and the acid residue measures about 20 ml, and titrate the distillate with 0·1N sodium hydroxide, using *phenolphthalein solution* as indicator.
Repeat the procedure omitting the sample.
The difference between the two titrations represents the amount of alkali required to neutralise the volatile acid; each ml of 0·1N sodium hydroxide is equivalent to 0·006005 g of $C_2H_4O_2$.

Standard for powdered drug: Powdered Sterculia
DESCRIPTION. A white or buff-coloured powder possessing the diagnostic microscopical characters and odour of the unground drug.

IDENTIFICATION; ACID-INSOLUBLE ASH; ASH. It complies with the requirements for the unground drug.

VOLATILE ACID. Not less than 10·0 per cent, calculated as acetic acid, $C_2H_4O_2$, determined by the method for the unground drug.

Storage. It should be stored in a cool dry place. Powdered Sterculia should be stored in airtight containers.

Uses. Sterculia is used as a substitute for tragacanth in lozenges, pastes, and denture-fixative powders.

STILBOESTROL

SYNONYM: Diethylstilbestrol

$C_{18}H_{20}O_2 = 268\cdot4$

Stilboestrol is 3,4-di-p-hydroxyphenylhex-3-ene.

CAUTION. *Stilboestrol is a powerful oestrogen. Contact with the skin or inhalation of the dust should be avoided. Rubber gloves should be worn when handling the powder and, if the powder is dry, a face mask should also be worn.*

Solubility. Very slightly soluble in water; soluble, at 20°, in 5 parts of alcohol, in 3 parts of ether, and in 40 parts of arachis oil; soluble in solutions of alkali hydroxides.

Standard
It complies with the requirements of the British Pharmacopoeia.
It is a white or almost white, crystalline, odourless powder and contains not less than 98·0 and not more than the equivalent of 101·0 per cent of $C_{18}H_{20}O_2$, calculated with reference to the dried substance. The loss on drying under the prescribed conditions is not more than 0·5 per cent. It has a melting-point of about 172°.

Hygroscopicity. It absorbs insignificant amounts of moisture at 25° at relative humidities up to about 90 per cent.

Sterilisation. Oily solutions for injection are sterilised by dry heat.

Storage. It should be protected from light.

Actions and uses. Stilboestrol has the actions, uses, and undesirable effects of the oestrogens, as described under Oestradiol Benzoate (page 335). Like the other synthetic oestrogens it is readily absorbed from the gastro-intestinal tract.
For the treatment of menopausal symptoms it is advisable to start with a low dosage, such as 0·1 milligram by mouth two or three times a day, and subsequently to adjust the dosage to the minimum necessary to control the symptoms.

In the treatment of amenorrhoea due to ovarian insufficiency, 0·25 to 1 milligram is given daily during the proliferative phase of the menstrual cycle. Larger doses may be needed for such conditions as senile vaginitis and kraurosis vulvae.

For the suppression of lactation, 5 milligrams is given two or three times a day for three days and subsequently the dosage is gradually reduced.

For the palliative treatment of carcinoma of the prostate and mammary carcinoma, 10 to 20 milligrams or more is given daily.

UNDESIRABLE EFFECTS. In excessive dosage, stilboestrol may give rise to nausea and vomiting.

Dose. See above under **Actions and uses.**

Preparations
STILBOESTROL PESSARIES, B.P.C. (page 773)

STILBOESTROL TABLETS, B.P. (*Syn.* Diethylstilbestrol Tablets). Unless otherwise specified, tablets each containing 500 μg of stilboestrol are supplied. They should be protected from light. Tablets containing 100 μg and 1, 5, 25, and 100 mg are also available.

OTHER NAME: *Pabestrol®*

PREPARED STORAX

SYNONYM: Styrax Praeparatus

Prepared Storax is the purified balsam obtained from the trunk of *Liquidambar orientalis* Mill. (Fam. Hamamelidaceae), a tree indigenous to the south-west of Asiatic Turkey.

The secretion of the crude balsam, which is not a normal product of the tree, is induced by wounding the bark. The crude balsam forms an opaque greyish viscous liquid, which on standing separates into a supernatant aqueous liquid and a dark brown oleoresinous layer. It contains about 20 to 30 per cent of water, together with fragments of bark and other extraneous material; from these it is purified by solution in alcohol, filtration, and evaporation.

Constituents. Prepared storax consists of a resin mixed with an oily liquid. The resin consists of compounds of unknown structure, including one or more resin alcohols which are partly free and partly esterified with cinnamic acid. The oily liquid contains styrene, vanillin, and free cinnamic acid, together with the ethyl, phenylpropyl, and cinnamyl esters of cinnamic acid.

Solubility. Soluble in alcohol (90 per cent), in carbon disulphide, in chloroform, and in glacial acetic acid; partly soluble in ether.

Standard
DESCRIPTION. A brown viscous liquid which is transparent in thin layers; odour agreeable and balsamic.

IDENTIFICATION TEST. Mix 1 g with 3 g of sand, add 5 ml of *potassium permanganate solution*, and warm gently; a distinct odour of benzaldehyde is produced.

ACID VALUE. 55 to 80, calculated with reference to the substance dried under the prescribed conditions.

SAPONIFICATION VALUE. 170 to 200, calculated with reference to the substance dried under the prescribed conditions.

LOSS ON DRYING. Not more than 5·0 per cent, determined by drying in a thin layer on a water-bath for one hour.

CONTENT OF TOTAL BALSAMIC ACIDS. Not less than 30·0 per cent, calculated with reference to the substance dried under the prescribed conditions, determined by the method for Benzoin (page 49).

Adulterants and substitutes. American storax, or sweet gum, is a transparent viscous yellowish fluid obtained from *L. styraciflua* L.

Partly exhausted storax is a balsam which has been partially deprived of its cinnamyl alcohol and cinnamic acid.
Factitious storax is also available.

Uses. Prepared storax is an ingredient of Benzoin Inhalation (page 705) and of Compound Benzoin Tincture (page 820).

STRAMONIUM

SYNONYMS: Stramonii Folium; Stramonium Leaf

Stramonium consists of the dried leaves or dried leaves and flowering tops of *Datura stramonium* L. (Fam. Solanaceae) and its varieties. The plants are annuals cultivated in the Balkans and the United States of America. The leaves and young shoots are collected while the plant is in flower, from about June to September.

Varieties. The leaves and stems of *D. stramonium* are green in colour and the corollas of the flowers are white when fresh and a pale buff colour when dry.
The stems and petioles and the main veins of the leaves of *D. stramonium* L. var. *tatula* (L.) Torr. vary in colour from a red tint to purple-black; the corollas are purplish blue when fresh and brown, sometimes with a purplish tint, when dry; the leaves are a somewhat darker green than those of *D. stramonium*.
D. stramonium L. var. *inermis* (Jacq.) Timm. and *D. stramonium* L. var. *godronii* Danert bear fruits devoid of spines.
Stramonium is sometimes imported in a broken (laminated) condition and is then frequently found to be adulterated.

Constituents. Stramonium contains 0·25 to 0·5 per cent of alkaloids, which consist chiefly of (−)-hyoscyamine and (−)-hyoscine with a small amount of atropine [(±)-hyoscyamine]; about 30 per cent of the alkaloids consist of (−)-hyoscine.

Standard
It complies with the requirements of the European Pharmacopoeia.
It contains not less than 0·25 per cent of alkaloids, calculated as hyoscyamine, $C_{17}H_{23}NO_3$, with reference to the drug dried at 100° to 105°.

UNGROUND DRUG. *Macroscopical characters:* leaves dark greyish-green and much shrivelled and twisted as a result of drying; when expanded, outline ovate or triangular-ovate, dentately lobed with an irregularly serrated margin, mostly 8 to 25 cm long and 7 to 15 cm broad; apex acuminate, base usually unequal; petiole often short and twisted; trichomes numerous on young leaves, older leaves almost glabrous; stems dichasially branched, slender with transverse and longitudinal wrinkles; flowers occurring solitarily at the forks, being about 7·5 cm long, erect and shortly pedicellate; corolla buff-coloured or brown, sometimes with a purplish tint, plicate and trumpet-shaped, but much twisted when dry; ovary superior, conical, spuriously tetralocular in the lower part, covered with short emergences, ovules numerous and campylotropous; immature fruit may be covered with numerous spinous emergences; seeds brown to black, flattened, subreniform, about 3 mm long, testa minutely pitted and vaguely reticulate, embryo curved in an oily endosperm.
Odour disagreeable and characteristic; taste bitter and unpleasant.

Microscopical characters: the diagnostic characters are: Leaf: *epidermis,* cells with a smooth *cuticle,* those of adaxial surface with straight or somewhat curved anticlinal walls and those of abaxial surface with sinuous anticlinal walls; *stomata* anisocytic, more numerous on abaxial epidermis; *trichomes* (a) *non-glandular,* straight or slightly curved, uniseriate, 3- to 5-celled, conical,

with thin warty walls, the basal cell being largest and usually exceeding 50 μm in length and 35 μm in breadth, (b) *glandular,* usually curved and composed of short 1- or 2-celled stalk and 2- to 7-celled pyriform glandular head; *palisade cells* in 1 layer beneath the epidermis; *crystal layer* composed of cells most of which containing a single cluster crystal of calcium oxalate or occasional prisms or microsphenoidal crystals; *phloem* intraxylary in midrib.
Stem: *trichomes* as in leaf, but up to 800 μm long; *pericyclic fibres* occasional; *xylem fibres* and *vessels* numerous; *crystals* of calcium oxalate represented by cluster crystals in cells of phloem and pith and occasional microsphenoidal crystals.
Pollen grains: 60 to 80 μm in diameter, with 3 large pores and coarsely warty *extine.*

POWDERED DRUG: Powdered Stramonium. A greyish-green powder possessing the diagnostic microscopical characters, odour, and taste of the unground drug.

Adulterants and substitutes. Datura leaf, which contains about 0·5 per cent alkaloids, the majority (−)-hyoscyamine, consists of the dried leaves and flowering tops of *D. innoxia* Miller and *D. metel* L., annual plants growing in the Indian subcontinent, although *D. innoxia* is indigenous to Mexico.
Datura leaves are about the same size as those of stramonium, those of *D. innoxia* are ovate to somewhat cordate, the margin entire, undulate or sometimes with two or three low teeth; both surfaces are densely pubescent; the trichomes are of three types, the most numerous being slender with a 2- or 4-celled uniseriate stalk and usually a unicellular glandular head, their length varying from 175 to 600 μm.
Leaves of *D. metel* are ovate to cordate and usually have three to four coarse teeth, but there are no small teeth in the sinuses; although glabrous to the unaided eye they have trichomes similar to those of stramonium, but the non-glandular trichomes are usually less than 35 μm in width at the base and the basal cell is rarely as long as 50 μm.
The leaves of *Xanthium strumarium* L. (Fam. Compositae), *Carthamus helenoides* Desf. (Fam. Compositae) and *Chenopodium hybridum* L. (Fam. Chenopodiaceae) have been recorded as adulterants.

Storage. It should be stored in a cool dry place, protected from light.

Actions and uses. The actions of stramonium are similar to those described under Belladonna Herb (page 42) and Hyoscyamus (page 231). It has been used to control the salivation, muscular rigidity, and tremor of parkinsonism.
Stramonium is an ingredient of powders intended to be burnt and the fumes inhaled for

the relief of asthma, but such a procedure often aggravates chronic bronchitis.

PRECAUTIONS. The dose should not be increased too rapidly as this may lead to paralysis of accommodation.

POISONING. As for Atropine (page 36).

OTHER NAME: Thornapple Leaf

Preparations

LOBELIA AND STRAMONIUM MIXTURE, COMPOUND, B.P.C. (page 746)

STRAMONIUM AND POTASSIUM IODIDE MIXTURE, B.P.C. (page 753)

STRAMONIUM TINCTURE, B.P. It contains 0·025 per cent of alkaloids. Dose: up to 6 millilitres daily in divided doses.

STREPTOMYCIN SULPHATE

SYNONYM: Streptomycini Sulfas

$C_{42}H_{84}N_{14}O_{36}S_3 = 1457·4$

Streptomycin Sulphate is the sulphate of an antimicrobial base produced by the growth of certain strains of *Streptomyces griseus* or obtained by any other means.

CAUTION. *Streptomycin may cause severe dermatitis in sensitised persons, and pharmacists, nurses, and others who handle the drug frequently should wear masks and rubber gloves.*

Solubility. Very soluble in water; very slightly soluble in alcohol, in ether, and in chloroform.

Standard

It complies with the requirements of the European Pharmacopoeia.

It is a white or almost white hygroscopic powder which is odourless or has a slight odour and contains not less than 720 Units per mg, calculated with reference to the dried substance. The loss on drying under the prescribed conditions is not more than 7·0 per cent. A 25 per cent solution in water has a pH of 4·5 to 7·0.

Labelling. If the material is not intended for parenteral administration, the label on the container states that the contents are not to be injected.

Storage. It should be stored in airtight containers at a temperature not exceeding 30°. If it is intended for parenteral administration, the containers should be sterile and sealed to exclude micro-organisms.

Actions and uses. Streptomycin is an antibiotic which is active against a wide range of bacteria, both Gram-positive and Gram-negative, but its clinical use depends on its action against *Mycobacterium tuberculosis*, *Escherichia coli*, *Klebsiella pneumoniae*, and some species of *Proteus* and of *Salmonella*.

When streptomycin is given by mouth it is poorly absorbed except in newborn infants and in patients with extensive ulceration, as in ulcerative colitis, and it normally appears unchanged in the faeces. When streptomycin is administered by intramuscular injection to normal adults, blood levels reach a peak after one hour and from 30 to 90 per cent of a dose is excreted unchanged in the urine within twenty-four hours. Excretion is delayed when renal function is impaired. Streptomycin does not readily pass the blood-brain barrier.

Streptomycin is used in the treatment of all forms of tuberculosis. Because relatively rapid induction of bacterial resistance may occur, streptomycin must always be used in conjunction with at least one other effective antituberculous drug.

The usual dose for an adult is 750 milligrams daily by intramuscular injection, but other dosage schemes such as 1 gram two or three times a week are also effective. Patients over sixty years should receive a reduced dosage, such as 500 milligrams daily in divided doses, and the drug should preferably not be given to patients over seventy years. Doses for children should be based on those for young adults, reduced in proportion to body-weight. This treatment is suitable for the treatment of tuberculous meningitis provided that streptomycin is used in conjunction with drugs such as isoniazid which enter the cerebrospinal fluid; it is no longer considered to be generally essential to give streptomycin by intrathecal injection for this purpose. When the clinical situation demands it, streptomycin may be given by intrathecal injection in a daily dose of up to 100 milligrams, dissolved in 10 millilitres of Sodium Chloride Injection, provided that meningeal irritation, as shown by increasing numbers of polymorphs in the cerebrospinal fluid, is absent.

Streptomycin is of value in the treatment of severe pulmonary infections due to *Haemophilus influenzae* and *Klebsiella pneumoniae*. It has also been used for the treatment of other non-tuberculous infections, particularly infections of the large bowel, cholecystitis, and peritonitis, but because of the rapid development of resistance and the prevalence of strains of bacteria that are already resistant it should only be used when the causative organisms are known to be sensitive to its action.

UNDESIRABLE EFFECTS. Allergic reactions are relatively common, the usual symptoms being fever and rash occurring during the second week of treatment in patients who have not previously been treated with streptomycin or immediately after starting treatment in those patients who have previously been sensitised to the drug; desensitisation is possible but is rarely necessary because alternative drugs are available.

Damage to the auditory and vestibular divisions of the eighth cranial nerve occurs if the concentration of the drug in the tissues is allowed to rise slightly above the minimum that is necessary for effective therapy; vertigo, nausea, tinnitus, deafness, and nystagmus may come on suddenly and regress when the drug is withdrawn, but permanent damage to hearing and balance may also develop insidiously during treatment or even some weeks afterwards.

Damage to the renal tubules, bone marrow, and liver rarely occurs at the usual therapeutic tissue levels.

Streptomycin impairs neuromuscular transmission and while this action is too weak to cause symptoms in normal subjects it may give rise to severe muscular weakness in patients with myasthenia gravis and also prolong the effect of neuromuscular blocking agents.

It may occasionally give rise to lupus erythematosus.

PRECAUTIONS AND CONTRA-INDICATIONS. The doses recommended for the treatment of tuberculosis are close to the toxic level and should be reduced if the blood urea is raised. The serum level of streptomycin should not be allowed to exceed 15 micrograms per millilitre even transiently, and for this reason intravenous administration should be avoided. Since streptomycin crosses the placenta and may cause damage to the eighth cranial nerve of the foetus, it should not be used in pregnancy.

NOTE. When Streptomycin is prescribed the quantity is interpreted as referring to streptomycin base and the equivalent amount of Streptomycin Sulphate is dispensed; 1·25 grams of the sulphate is approximately equivalent to 1·0 gram of the base.

Dose. The equivalent of 0·5 to 1 gram of streptomycin base by intramuscular injection daily or at longer intervals.

As an intestinal antiseptic: the equivalent of 500 milligrams of streptomycin base by mouth every eight hours.

Preparations

STREPTOMYCIN ELIXIR, PAEDIATRIC, B.P.C. (page 677)

STREPTOMYCIN SULPHATE INJECTION, B.P. (*Syn.* Streptomycin Injection). It consists of a sterile solution of streptomycin sulphate in Water for Injections containing suitable stabilising agents. It may contain a suitable buffering agent.

Unless otherwise specified, a solution containing the equivalent of 330 mg of streptomycin base in 1 ml is supplied. It should be stored at a temperature not exceeding 20°, protected from light; under these conditions it may be expected to retain its potency for at least eighteen months from the date of manufacture.

OTHER NAME: *Streptaquaine*®

STRYCHNINE HYDROCHLORIDE

SYNONYM: Strych. Hydrochlor.

$C_{21}H_{23}ClN_2O_2,2H_2O = 406·9$

Strychnine Hydrochloride is the hydrochloride of the alkaloid strychnine, which is obtained from the seeds of *Strychnos nux-vomica* L. and other species of *Strychnos* (Fam. Loganiaceae).

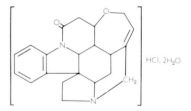

Solubility. Soluble, at 20°, in 40 parts of water and in 85 parts of alcohol; insoluble in ether.

Standard

DESCRIPTION. Colourless prismatic crystals or a white crystalline powder.

IDENTIFICATION TESTS. 1. Dissolve 0·1 mg in 0·2 ml of *sulphuric acid* and slowly move a small crystal of *potassium dichromate* through the solution; an intense violet colour is produced, which changes through red to yellow.

2. To 0·5 mg add 0·2 ml of *sulphuric acid*, followed by 0·05 g of *ammonium vanadate*, and stir; a deep violet colour is produced, which changes to red. Add 1 ml of water; the colour changes to cherry-red.

3. It gives the reactions characteristic of chlorides.

ACIDITY. Dissolve 0·20 g in 10 ml of *carbon dioxide-free water* and titrate with 0·02N sodium hydroxide, using

methyl red solution as indicator; not more than 0·2 ml is required.

SULPHATE. 0·25 g complies with the limit test for sulphates (0·24 per cent).

BRUCINE. To 0·1 g add 1 ml of a mixture of equal volumes of *nitric acid* and water; no red or reddish colour is produced.

LOSS ON DRYING. 7·0 to 9·0 per cent, determined by drying to constant weight at 130°.

SULPHATED ASH. Not more than 0·1 per cent.

CONTENT OF $C_{21}H_{23}ClN_2O_2$. Not less than 97·5 per cent, calculated with reference to the substance dried under the prescribed conditions, determined by the following method:

Titrate about 0·5 g, accurately weighed, by Method I of the British Pharmacopoeia, Appendix XIB, for non-aqueous titration; each ml of 0·1N perchloric acid is equivalent to 0·03709 g of $C_{21}H_{23}ClN_2O_2$.

Incompatibility. It is incompatible with alkali hydroxides and carbonates, Aromatic Ammonia Spirit, bromides, and iodides.

Sterilisation. Solutions for injection are sterilised by heating in an autoclave or by filtration.

Actions and uses. Strychnine stimulates all parts of the nervous system. It is rapidly absorbed from the gastro-intestinal tract and is slowly excreted, so that its action may be cumulative. Its use as a therapeutic agent has now been largely abandoned.

Because of its bitter taste strychnine has been used as a stomachic and tonic, but there is no evidence to show that it is of special value for these purposes. It has also been used with cathartics, but its incorporation in purgative pills and tablets is without therapeutic justification and may cause fatal accidental poisoning, especially in young children.

Small doses of strychnine delay the onset of fatigue, but this delay is followed by a phase of depression of muscular activity. It has been used as an analeptic, but it stimulates the respiratory and cardiovascular centres only in convulsant doses.

Liquid medicines containing strychnine should be made slightly acid.

UNDESIRABLE EFFECTS. Toxic doses of strychnine produce convulsions of all voluntary muscle. Since extensor muscles are generally the stronger, the body is arched backwards and assumes a position of generalised extension, the head is retracted, the feet are turned inwards, and the arms are extended. All forms of sensation are rendered more acute. Death results from spasm of the respiratory muscles.

POISONING. The stomach should be emptied and washed out with 1 in 5000 potassium permanganate solution or 2 per cent tannic acid solution. An emetic should not be given owing to the danger of aspirating vomitus.

Convulsions may be controlled by the intravenous injection of a 5 or 10 per cent solution of thiopentone sodium and by the intravenous injection of muscle relaxants such as tubocurarine chloride or gallamine triethiodide.

The patient should be sheltered from external stimuli in a quiet darkened room.

Artificial respiration or controlled respiration using oxygen is necessary if the respiratory muscles are fixed in spasm.

Dose. 2 to 8 milligrams.

Preparation

FERROUS PHOSPHATE, QUININE, AND STRYCHNINE TABLETS, B.P.C. (page 810)

SUCCINYLSULPHATHIAZOLE

SYNONYM: Succinylsulfathiazolum

$C_{13}H_{13}N_3O_5S_2,H_2O = 373·4$

Succinylsulphathiazole is 4'-(thiazol-2-ylsulphamoyl)succinanilic acid monohydrate.

Solubility. Very slightly soluble in water; soluble, at 20°, in 200 parts of alcohol; slightly soluble in acetone; insoluble in ether and chloroform; soluble in solutions of alkali hydroxides, and, with evolution of carbon dioxide, in solutions of alkali bicarbonates.

Standard

It complies with the requirements of the European Pharmacopoeia.

It occurs as odourless white or yellowish-white crystals or powder and contains not less than 99·0 per cent of $C_{13}H_{13}N_3O_5S_2$, calculated with reference to the dried substance. The loss on drying under the prescribed conditions is 4·0 to 5·5 per cent. It melts with decomposition at about 190°.

Stability. It slowly darkens on exposure to light.

Storage. It should be stored in airtight containers, protected from light.

OTHER NAME: *Sulfasuxidine*®

Actions and uses. Succinylsulphathiazole has the actions and uses described under Phthalylsulphathiazole (page 379).

UNDESIRABLE EFFECTS. The toxicity of succinylsulphathiazole is very low. Because of its effect on intestinal bacteria, prolonged use may lead to overgrowth of *Candida* species.

Dose. 10 to 20 grams daily in divided doses.

Preparations

SUCCINYLSULPHATHIAZOLE MIXTURE, PAEDIATRIC, B.P.C. (page 754)

SUCCINYLSULPHATHIAZOLE TABLETS, B.P. Unless otherwise specified, tablets each containing 500 mg of succinylsulphathiazole are supplied. They should be stored in airtight containers, protected from light.

SUCROSE

SYNONYMS: Refined Sugar; Sucrosum

$C_{12}H_{22}O_{11} = 342.3$

Sucrose is β-D-fructofuranosyl-α-D-glucopyranoside and may be obtained from the juice of the sugar-cane, *Saccharum officinarum* L. (Fam. Gramineae), or of white-rooted varieties of the sugar-beet, *Beta vulgaris* (Fam. Chenopodiaceae).

Sugar is extracted from sugar-cane by boiling the neutralised expressed juice with milk of lime and evaporating the filtered liquid under reduced pressure. The solution is decolorised with charcoal, the lime precipitated by means of carbon dioxide, and the sucrose recrystallised.

Sucrose is obtained from sugar-beet by allowing the non-colloidal materials to diffuse from the cells into hot water, the resulting solution being treated as described above.

The mother liquors from both processes contain a considerable quantity of sugar and are marketed as syrups in various forms or used in the manufacture of alcohol.

Solubility. Soluble, at 20°, in less than 1 part of water and in 370 parts of alcohol.

Standard

It complies with the requirements of the European Pharmacopoeia.

It occurs as odourless, lustrous, dry, colourless crystals or white crystalline powder.

Hygroscopicity. It absorbs insignificant amounts of moisture at 25° at relative humidities up to about 85 per cent, but under damper conditions it absorbs substantial amounts.

Sterilisation. Solutions for injection are sterilised by heating in an autoclave or by filtration.

Actions and uses. Sucrose is used as a sweetening agent and as a demulcent. Solutions of sucrose in concentrations of less than 65 per cent w/w ferment, but more concentrated solutions, such as syrups, have an osmotic pressure sufficiently great to inhibit the growth of most bacteria and fungi. The syrups may be used as flavouring agents.

Preparation

SYRUP, B.P. It contains 66·7 per cent w/w of sucrose. A suitable preservative or mixture of preservatives may be added. The label on the container states the names and proportions of any added preservatives.

Syrup should not be exposed to any undue fluctuations of temperature.

SULPHACETAMIDE SODIUM

SYNONYM: Soluble Sulphacetamide

$C_8H_9N_2NaO_3S,H_2O = 254.2$

Sulphacetamide Sodium is the monohydrate of the sodium derivative of *N*-*p*-aminobenzenesulphonylacetamide.

Solubility. Soluble, at 20°, in 1·5 parts of water; slightly soluble in alcohol and in acetone.

Standard

It complies with the requirements of the British Pharmacopoeia.

It occurs as odourless white or yellowish-white crystals or microcrystalline powder and contains not less than 99·0 and not more than the equivalent of 101·0 per cent of $C_8H_9N_2NaO_3S$, calculated with reference to the dried substance. The loss on drying under the prescribed conditions is 6·0 to 8·0 per cent. A 5 per cent solution in water has a pH of 8·0 to 9·5.

A mixture of Sulphacetamide Sodium and 1 per cent of sulphacetamide gives a solution in water which has a pH of about 7·4.

Stability. The discoloration of solutions can be retarded by the addition of sodium metabisulphite and protection from light.

Sterilisation. Solutions are sterilised by heating in an autoclave, by heating with a bactericide, or by filtration; powders for local application are sterilised by the method described under Sulphadimidine (page 478). When sulphacetamide solutions are sterilised by heat, some hydrolysis occurs with the formation of sulphanilamide, which may be deposited as crystals, especially in concentrated solutions and under cold storage conditions.

Storage. It should be protected from light.

Actions and uses. Sulphacetamide sodium has the actions of the sulphonamides, as described under Sulphadimidine (page 478). It is used chiefly for local application in infections and injuries of the conjunctiva.

In the treatment of acute conjunctivitis and in the prophylaxis of ocular infections after injuries or burns, a 10 per cent solution is applied every two hours, or a 30 per cent solution twice a day; alternatively, an ointment may be used.

Preparations

SULPHACETAMIDE EYE-DROPS, B.P.C. (page 695)

SULPHACETAMIDE EYE OINTMENT, B.P. Unless otherwise specified, an eye ointment containing 6 per cent of sulphacetamide sodium is supplied. Eye ointments containing 2·5 and 10 per cent are also available.

OTHER NAME: *Albucid*®

SULPHADIAZINE

$C_{10}H_{10}N_4O_2S = 250.3$

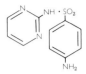

Sulphadiazine is 2-(p-aminobenzenesulphonamido)pyrimidine.

Solubility. Very slightly soluble in water; slightly soluble in alcohol and in acetone; insoluble in ether and in chloroform; readily soluble in dilute mineral acids and in solutions of alkali hydroxides and carbonates.

Standard
It complies with the requirements of the British Pharmacopoeia.
It occurs as almost odourless, white, yellowish-white, or pinkish-white crystals or powder and contains not less than 99.0 per cent of $C_{10}H_{10}N_4O_2S$, calculated with reference to the dried substance. The loss on drying under the prescribed conditions is not more than 0.5 per cent. It melts with decomposition at about 255°.

Stability. It slowly darkens on exposure to light.

Sterilisation. Powders for local application are sterilised by the method described under Sulphadimidine (page 478).

Storage. It should be protected from light.

Actions and uses. Sulphadiazine has the actions of the sulphonamides, as described under Sulphadimidine (page 478). It is absorbed from the gastro-intestinal tract and distributed approximately equally in the joints, pleura, peritoneum, and cavities; diffusion into the cerebrospinal system takes place more slowly. It is excreted less rapidly than sulphathiazole.

Sulphadiazine is effective in the treatment of infections due to haemolytic streptococci, pneumococci, meningococci, gonococci, *Escherichia coli*, and, to a lesser extent, staphylococci and the organisms of gas-gangrene. It is important to give sulphadiazine during the acute phase of the infection.

For systemic infections, sulphadiazine is usually given by mouth in an initial dose of 3 grams; the subsequent dosage should be 1 gram every six hours until the fever subsides or for a maximum of seven days. This dosage is usually sufficient to produce a satisfactory blood level.

For urinary tract infections, the initial dose is usually 2 grams; the subsequent dosage should be 0.5 to 1 gram every six to eight hours.

In severe meningitis, sulphadiazine is administered intravenously as Sulphadiazine Injection. Because orally administered sulphadiazine is not absorbed from the gastro-intestinal tract sufficiently quickly in patients with toxaemia and low blood pressure, conditions often found in patients with severe meningitis, intravenous administration is necessary during the first few days of treatment. It is necessary to maintain a blood concentration of 10 to 15 milligrams per 100 millilitres in this infection; for an adult a dosage of 1 to 1.5 grams every four hours is required. Sulphadiazine Injection should therefore be given, preferably diluted with Sodium Chloride Injection or Dextrose Injection to give a concentration not exceeding 5 per cent of sulphadiazine, by intravenous infusion during the first two days of the infection. If this method is impracticable, the drug may be given by intravenous injection, but it should never be given intrathecally. When it is given by intravenous injection, leakage into the subcutaneous tissue should be avoided, as the injection is strongly alkaline. Subsequently sulphadiazine should be given by mouth, the treatment being continued for two or three days after clinical recovery.

UNDESIRABLE EFFECTS. The undesirable effects of the sulphonamides are described under Sulphadimidine (page 478).

Sulphadiazine rarely causes toxic effects and is generally well tolerated, but anuria and haematuria must be guarded against and sufficient fluid should be given to maintain a large urinary output. The urine should be kept alkaline to prevent crystallisation of the acetyl derivative during excretion.

Frequent leucocyte counts should be made.

CONTRA-INDICATIONS. As for Sulphadimidine (page 478).

Dose. See above under **Actions and uses.**

Preparations
SULPHADIAZINE INJECTION, B.P. It consists of a sterile solution of the sodium salt of sulphadiazine in Water for Injections free from dissolved air; it contains not more than 0.1 per cent of sodium thiosulphate. Unless otherwise specified, a solution containing the equivalent of 1 g of sulphadiazine in 4 ml is supplied.
It should be protected from light.

SULPHADIAZINE TABLETS, B.P. Unless otherwise specified, tablets each containing 500 mg of sulphadiazine are supplied. They should be stored in airtight containers, protected from light.

SULPHADIMETHOXINE

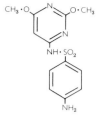

$C_{12}H_{14}N_4O_4S = 310.3$

Sulphadimethoxine is 4-*p*-aminobenzenesulphonamido-2,6-dimethoxypyrimidine.

Solubility. Very slightly soluble in water; slightly soluble in alcohol; soluble in dilute mineral acids and in solutions of alkali hydroxides and carbonates.

Standard

It complies with the requirements of the British Pharmacopoeia.

It is a white or creamy-white, crystalline, almost odourless powder and contains not less than 99.0 per cent of $C_{12}H_{14}N_4O_4S$, calculated with reference to the dried substance. The loss on drying under the prescribed conditions is not more than 0.5 per cent. It has a melting-point of 198° to 204°.

Storage. It should be protected from light.

Actions and uses. Sulphadimethoxine is a long-acting compound which has the actions of the sulphonamides, as described under Sulphadimidine. When given by mouth it is rapidly absorbed and blood levels are maintained for at least twenty-four hours. It is extensively bound to blood protein; the protein-adsorbed fraction is not active against infecting organisms, the antibacterial action being due to the free sulphonamide which is slowly released.

There is no evidence that the long-acting sulphonamides are more effective than short-acting ones, such as sulphadimidine, and some of them may be less safe.

UNDESIRABLE EFFECTS. Headache and nausea may occur and, more rarely, skin eruptions, the most serious of which is the Stevens-Johnson syndrome, a life-threatening variety of erythema multiforme.

CONTRA-INDICATIONS. As for Sulphadimidine.

Dose. Initial dose, 1 to 2 grams; subsequent doses, 500 milligrams every twenty-four hours.

Preparation

SULPHADIMETHOXINE TABLETS, B.P. Unless otherwise specified, tablets each containing 500 mg of sulphadimethoxine are supplied. They should be stored in airtight containers, protected from light.

OTHER NAME: *Madribon®*

SULPHADIMIDINE

SYNONYM: Sulfadimidinum

$C_{12}H_{14}N_4O_2S = 278.3$

Sulphadimidine is 2-*p*-aminobenzenesulphonamido-4,6-dimethylpyrimidine.

Solubility. Very slightly soluble in water; soluble, at 20°, in 120 parts of alcohol; soluble in dilute mineral acids and in solutions of alkali hydroxides and carbonates.

Standard

It complies with the requirements of the European Pharmacopoeia.

It occurs as odourless or almost odourless white or creamy-white crystals or powder and contains not less than 99.0 per cent of $C_{12}H_{14}N_4O_2S$, calculated with reference to the dried substance. The loss on drying under the prescribed conditions is not more than 0.5 per cent. It has a melting-point of 197° to 200°.

Stability. Exposure to light gives rise to discoloration and decomposition.

Sterilisation. Sulphadimidine for local application is first reduced to a fine powder and dried at 100° and then sterilised by dry heat in the final sealed containers; the sterilised powder should show not more than a slight discoloration.

Storage. It should be protected from light.

Actions and uses. The actions of the sulphonamides, of which sulphadimidine may be taken as a typical example, is bacteriostatic rather than bactericidal and is considered to be due to the similarity of their chemical structure to that of *p*-aminobenzoic acid, which is essential to the normal development of bacteria. Hence, if a sulphonamide is present in a concentration greater than that of *p*-aminobenzoic acid, it is taken up by the bacterial enzyme system, which thus becomes blocked and incapable of its normal function. The relative potencies of the sulphonamides used systemically appear to depend mainly on differences in solubility, absorption, and excretion rather than on any specificity. Infections due to the less susceptible organisms, such as pneumococci, respond best to those sulphonamides with which it is possible to maintain a high blood concentration. Virus infections in general are unaffected, although those accompanying secondary infections by haemolytic streptococci may be favourably influenced.

When sulphonamides are used for the treatment of systemic infections, it is important to obtain rapidly an optimal concentration of the drug in the blood and to maintain this in order to prevent the development of resistant strains of the infecting organism.

Sulphadimidine is rapidly absorbed from the gastro-intestinal tract, so that with regular dosage by mouth the blood concentration can be readily maintained at 5 to 10 milligrams per 100 millilitres. Sulphadimidine crosses the blood–brain barrier less easily than sulphadiazine; thus, while sulphadimidine is often the sulphonamide of choice in pneumococcal or streptococcal infections and in *Escherichia coli* infections of the urinary tract, sulphadiazine is usually preferred in meningeal infections.

Sulphonamides are concentrated in the urine. In the treatment of non-gonococcal genito-urinary infections, especially those due to *Esch. coli*, they are effective in relatively small doses.

For systemic infections, sulphadimidine should be given by mouth in an initial dose of up to 3 grams; the subsequent dosage should be 1 gram every four hours or 1·5 grams every six hours. For urinary tract infections, the initial dose is 2 grams; subsequent dosage should be up to 4 grams daily in divided doses. Infants and children usually tolerate sulphonamides better than adults; for a child of average weight the recommended dosage is one-sixth the adult dose from six months to one year of age, one-third the adult dose from one to five years of age, one-half the adult dose from six to twelve years of age, and two-thirds the adult dose from thirteen to fifteen years of age.

UNDESIRABLE EFFECTS. A variety of toxic symptoms may follow the administration of sulphonamides. Nausea and vomiting are relatively common, but may be avoided by giving the drug in divided doses.

Cyanosis, which may be due to methaemoglobinaemia, to sulphaemoglobinaemia, or to the action of an oxidation product, is occasionally seen; usually, however, it is not sufficiently severe to necessitate the suspension of treatment.

Skin rashes occur occasionally, and in such cases it is advisable to stop treatment and give abundant fluids; in general, patients undergoing sulphonamide therapy should avoid exposure to direct sunlight.

There is a danger of haematuria, due to the insolubility of the acetyl derivatives; it may occur whenever the fluid intake is restricted or the urine is acid. Granulocytopenia is rare, especially if the duration of a course of treatment does not exceed a week or ten days and if an interval of several weeks is allowed between courses.

Sulphonamides applied to the skin are liable to give rise to sensitisation.

Sulphadimidine itself is well tolerated and serious toxic effects are infrequent. Nausea and vomiting seldom occur and the nausea is so slight as not to interfere with the continuation of treatment. Owing to the relatively high solubility of its acetyl derivative, even in acid urine, sulphadimidine is less likely to cause anuria and haematuria than sulphathiazole.

CONTRA-INDICATIONS. Sulphonamides are contra-indicated in the presence of renal disease or jaundice and in hypersensitive patients.

Dose. See above under **Actions and uses.**

Preparations

SULPHADIMIDINE MIXTURE, PAEDIATRIC, B.P.C. (page 754)

SULPHADIMIDINE TABLETS, B.P. Unless otherwise specified, tablets each containing 500 mg of sulphadimidine are supplied. They should be stored in airtight containers, protected from light.

OTHER NAME: *Sulphamezathine®*

SULPHADIMIDINE SODIUM

$C_{12}H_{13}N_4NaO_2S = 300·3$

Sulphadimidine Sodium is the sodium derivative of sulphadimidine.

Solubility. Soluble, at 20°, in 2·5 parts of water and in 60 parts of alcohol.

Standard
It complies with the requirements of the British Pharmacopoeia.
It occurs as hygroscopic, odourless or almost odourless, white or creamy-white crystals or powder and contains not less than 98·0 and not more than the equivalent of 101·0 per cent of $C_{12}H_{13}N_4NaO_2S$, calculated with reference to the dried substance. The loss on drying under the prescribed conditions is not more than 2·0 per cent. A 10 per cent solution in water has a pH of 10·0 to 11·0.

Stability. Exposure to light gives rise to discoloration and decomposition. Exposure to air results in absorption of carbon dioxide and decrease in solubility.
Aqueous solutions are most stable at pH 10 to 11 and are decomposed by light and by the presence of salts of heavy metals. Precipitation of sulphadimidine occurs below pH 10 or in the presence of carbon dioxide.

Sterilisation. Solutions for injection are sterilised by heating in an autoclave in an atmosphere of nitrogen or other suitable gas.

Storage. It should be protected from light.

Actions and uses. Sulphadimidine sodium has the actions, uses, undesirable effects, and contra-indications described under Sulpha-dimidine.

The dose may be given in a 33·3 per cent solution by intravenous injection to patients in whom a satisfactory concentration of sulpha-dimidine cannot be obtained by oral administration. It should not be given intrathecally.

Dose. 1 to 2 grams by intravenous or intra-muscular injection.

Preparation

SULPHADIMIDINE INJECTION, B.P. It consists of a sterile solution of sulphadimidine sodium in Water for Injections free from dissolved air. Unless otherwise specified, a solution containing 1 g in 3 ml is supplied. It should be protected from light.

OTHER NAMES: Soluble Sulphadimidine; *Sulphamezathine Sodium*®

SULPHAFURAZOLE

SYNONYM: Sulfisoxazole

$C_{11}H_{13}N_3O_3S = 267·3$

Sulphafurazole is 5-*p*-aminobenzenesulphonamido-3,4-dimethyli-soxazole.

Solubility. Very slightly soluble in water; soluble, at 20°, in 50 parts of alcohol, in 800 parts of ether, in 1000 parts of chloroform, and in 30 parts of a 5 per cent aqueous solution of sodium bicarbonate.

Standard
It complies with the requirements of the British Pharmacopoeia.
It is a white or yellowish-white, crystalline, odourless powder and contains not less than 99·0 per cent of $C_{11}H_{13}N_3O_3S$, calculated with reference to the dried substance. The loss on drying under the prescribed conditions is not more than 0·5 per cent. It has a melting-point of 195° to 198°.

Storage. It should be protected from light.

Actions and uses. Sulphafurazole has the actions and uses of the sulphonamides, as described under Sulphadimidine. A daily dosage of 6 grams by mouth is usually sufficient to maintain a satisfactory blood level. Because of its relatively high solubility in urine (about 300 milligrams in 100 millilitres of urine at

pH 6), it is especially useful in urinary tract infections.

UNDESIRABLE EFFECTS. The undesirable effects of the sulphonamides are described under Sulphadimidine. Sulphafurazole is relatively free from toxic effects.

CONTRA-INDICATIONS. These are described under Sulphadimidine.

Dose. For systemic infections: initial dose, 3 grams; subsequent doses, up to 6 grams daily in divided doses.
For urinary tract infections: initial dose, 2 grams; subsequent doses, up to 4 grams daily in divided doses.

Preparation
SULPHAFURAZOLE TABLETS, B.P. Unless otherwise specified, tablets each containing 500 mg of sulpha-furazole are supplied. They should be stored in airtight containers, protected from light.

OTHER NAME: *Gantrisin*®

SULPHAGUANIDINE

$C_7H_{10}N_4O_2S,H_2O = 232·3$

Sulphaguanidine is *N-p*-aminobenzenesulphonylguanidine monohydrate.

Solubility. Soluble, at 20°, in 1000 parts of water and in 250 parts of alcohol; soluble in 10 parts of boiling water; readily soluble in dilute mineral acids; slightly soluble in acetone; insoluble in solutions of alkali hydroxides.

Standard
DESCRIPTION. White or almost white crystals or powder, darkening slowly on exposure to light; odourless or almost odourless.

IDENTIFICATION TESTS. 1. To 0·2 g add 5 ml of *sodium hydroxide solution*; the powder does not dissolve. Boil; the powder dissolves and the odour of ammonia is produced.

2. Dissolve 0·05 g in 2 ml of warm *dilute hydrochloric acid*, cool in ice, add 2 ml of *sodium nitrite solution*, mix, and add 2 ml of water and 1 ml of *β-naphthol solution*; a scarlet gelatinous precipitate is formed.

3. The infra-red absorption spectrum exhibits maxima which are only at the same wavelengths as, and have

similar relative intensities to, those in the spectrum of *sulphaguanidine*.

ACIDITY. Heat 1·0 g for 5 minutes at 70° with 50 ml of *carbon dioxide-free water*, cool quickly to 20°, filter, and titrate 25 ml of the filtrate with 0·1N sodium hydroxide, using *phenolphthalein solution* as indicator; not more than 0·1 ml is required.

MELTING-POINT. 190° to 192·5°.

LEAD. It complies with the test given in Appendix 7, page 884 (10 parts per million).

RELATED COMPOUNDS. It complies with the test given in Appendix 5A, page 868 (0·5 per cent).

LOSS ON DRYING. 6·0 to 8·0 per cent, determined by drying to constant weight at 105°.

SULPHATED ASH. Not more than 0·1 per cent.

CONTENT OF $C_7H_{10}N_4O_2S$. Not less than 99·0 per cent, calculated with reference to the substance dried under

the prescribed conditions, determined by the following method:
Dissolve about 0·5 g, accurately weighed, in 75 ml of water and 10 ml of *hydrochloric acid* and titrate with 0·1M sodium nitrite, determining the end-point electrometrically; each ml of 0·1M sodium nitrite is equivalent to 0·02142 g of $C_7H_{10}N_4O_2S$.

Storage. It should be protected from light.

Actions and uses. Sulphaguanidine has the actions of the sulphonamides, as described under Sulphadimidine (page 478). It is not readily absorbed from the gastro-intestinal tract and is therefore used in the treatment of local intestinal infections, such as bacillary dysentery, although phthalylsulphathiazole and succinylsulphathiazole are now considered to be more effective, as the amounts of these drugs absorbed into the blood stream are much smaller.

In the treatment of dysentery, 3 grams of sulphaguanidine is given by mouth three or four times a day for three days, followed by 3 grams twice a day for four days, or 5 grams twice a day in severe cases. The earlier the treatment is begun, the more rapid is the clinical cure; if improvement does not occur within three to four days it is unlikely that the drug will be effective on further administration. For prophylaxis, succinylsulphathiazole is to be preferred.

Sulphaguanidine may be of value in refractory cases of amoebic dysentery by controlling secondary bacterial infections, although some antibiotics are more effective in this respect.

In cases of ulcerative colitis, sulphaguanidine may be absorbed into the blood stream in dangerous amounts; in this condition, therefore, the use of phthalylsulphathiazole is to be preferred.

UNDESIRABLE EFFECTS. Toxic effects, in conditions other than ulcerative colitis, are slight, although rashes and haematuria have been reported.

During prolonged treatment with sulphaguanidine, vitamins of the B group should be administered to replace a possible loss of these vitamins through the action of the drug on the organisms normally present in the gastro-intestinal tract.

Because of its effect on intestinal bacteria, prolonged use may lead to proliferation of *Candida* species.

CONTRA-INDICATIONS. As for Sulphadimidine (page 478).

Dose. See above under **Actions and uses.**

Preparation
SULPHAGUANIDINE TABLETS, B.P.C. (page 816)

SULPHAMETHIZOLE

$C_9H_{10}N_4O_2S_2 = 270·3$

Sulphamethizole is 2-*p*-aminobenzenesulphonamido-5-methyl-1,3,4-thiadiazole.

Solubility. Slightly soluble in water, in ether, and in chloroform; soluble, at 20°, in 25 parts of alcohol and in 15 parts of acetone; soluble in 60 parts of boiling water, in solutions of alkali hydroxides, and in dilute mineral acids.

Standard
It complies with the requirements of the British Pharmacopoeia.
It occurs as odourless or almost odourless colourless crystals or white or creamy-white crystalline powder and contains not less than 99·0 and not more than the equivalent of 101·0 per cent of $C_9H_{10}N_4O_2S_2$, calculated with reference to the dried substance. The loss on drying under the prescribed conditions is not more than 0·5 per cent. It has a melting-point of 208° to 211°.

Storage. It should be protected from light.

Actions and uses. Sulphamethizole has the actions, uses, undesirable effects, and contra-indications of the sulphonamides, as described under Sulphadimidine (page 478).

When given by mouth it is rapidly absorbed from the gastro-intestinal tract and rapidly excreted. It is used chiefly for the treatment of coliform infections of the urinary tract in a dosage of 100 to 200 milligrams by mouth five times a day for five to seven days.

The risk of crystalluria is less than with sulphathiazole, and in temperate climates the fluid intake may be reduced to maintain the urinary concentration of the drug.

Dose. See above under **Actions and uses.**

Preparation
SULPHAMETHIZOLE TABLETS, B.P. Unless otherwise specified, tablets each containing 100 mg of sulphamethizole are supplied. They should be stored in air-tight containers, protected from light.

OTHER NAMES: *Methisul*®; *Mizol*®; *Urolucosil*®

SULPHAMETHOXAZOLE

$C_{10}H_{11}N_3O_3S = 253.3$

Sulphamethoxazole is 3-*p*-aminobenzenesulphonamido-5-methylisoxazole.

Solubility. Very slightly soluble in water; soluble, at 20°, in 50 parts of alcohol and in 3 parts of acetone; soluble in solutions of alkali hydroxides.

Standard
It complies with the requirements of the British Pharmacopoeia.
It is a white or yellowish-white, crystalline, odourless powder and contains not less than 99·0 per cent of $C_{10}H_{11}N_3O_3S$, calculated with reference to the dried substance. The loss on drying under the prescribed conditions is not more than 0·5 per cent. It has a melting-point of 169° to 172°. A 10 per cent suspension in water has a pH of 4·0 to 6·0.

Storage. It should be protected from light.

Actions and uses. Sulphamethoxazole is an antibacterial agent with the actions of the sulphonamides, as described under Sulphadimidine (page 478). Therapeutic blood levels are reached within two hours of administration of the drug and may be maintained by doses at intervals of eight to twelve hours; peak levels are reached within four hours of administration.

Because of its pharmacokinetic similarity to trimethoprim, sulphamethoxazole is the sulphonamide most commonly used in conjunction with it. The two components act on two successive reactions in the bacterial synthesis of folic acid, and while either component alone has bacteriostatic properties, if an organism is sensitive to both drugs, the mixture is bactericidal; the mixture may be of value even when some degree of resistance to sulphonamides is evident. The mixture is used in the treatment of Gram-positive and Gram-negative infections of the respiratory, alimentary, and urinary tracts; gonococci, pneumococci, staphylococci, haemolytic streptococci, *Escherichia coli, Haemophilus influenzae*, and species

of *Klebsiella, Proteus, Salmonella*, and *Shigella* are usually sensitive to it; *Pseudomonas aeruginosa* and *Streptococcus faecalis* are generally resistant.

UNDESIRABLE EFFECTS. These are as described under Sulphadimidine (page 478).

PRECAUTIONS AND CONTRA-INDICATIONS. The contra-indications are as described under Sulphadimidine (page 478).
Preparations of trimethoprim and sulphamethoxazole should not be given to patients hypersensitive to sulphonamides. Repeated haematological investigations are required during prolonged therapy because of possible interference with the patient's folic acid metabolism. The use of preparations of trimethoprim and sulphamethoxazole during pregnancy is not recommended.

Dose. Sulphamethoxazole: initial dose, 2 grams, followed by 1 gram every twelve hours, unless used with trimethoprim.
In conjunction with trimethoprim: 160 to 480 milligrams of trimethoprim with 0·8 to 2·4 grams of sulphamethoxazole daily, divided into two or three doses.

Preparations
Co-TRIMOXAZOLE MIXTURE, B.P.C. (page 740)
Co-TRIMOXAZOLE MIXTURE, PAEDIATRIC, B.P.C. (page 741)
Co-TRIMOXAZOLE TABLETS, B.P. (*Syn.* Trimethoprim and Sulphamethoxazole Tablets). These tablets contain sulphamethoxazole and trimethoprim in the proportion of five parts to one. Unless otherwise specified, tablets each containing 400 mg of sulphamethoxazole and 80 mg of trimethoprim are supplied. They should be stored in airtight containers, protected from light.
Co-TRIMOXAZOLE TABLETS, PAEDIATRIC, B.P.C. (page 810)

OTHER NAMES: *Gantanol*®. In conjunction with trimethoprim: *Bactrim*®; *Septrin*®

SULPHAMETHOXYDIAZINE

$C_{11}H_{12}N_4O_3S = 280.3$

Sulphamethoxydiazine is 2-*p*-aminobenzenesulphonamido-5-methoxy-pyrimidine.

Solubility. Very slightly soluble in water; slightly soluble in alcohol and in dilute hydrochloric acid; soluble in solutions of alkali hydroxides and carbonates.

Standard
It complies with the requirements of the British Pharmacopoeia.
It is a white or yellowish-white, crystalline, odourless or almost odourless powder and contains not less than 99·0 per cent of $C_{11}H_{12}N_4O_3S$, calculated with re-

ference to the dried substance. The loss on drying under the prescribed conditions is not more than 0·5 per cent. It has a melting-point of 209° to 213.°

Storage. It should be protected from light.

Actions and uses. Sulphamethoxydiazine has the actions, uses, and undesirable effects of the long-acting sulphonamides, as described under Sulphadimethoxine (page 478).

When given by mouth, it is rapidly absorbed from the gastro-intestinal tract and slowly excreted; the peak concentration in the blood is attained about four hours after administration and therapeutic blood levels may be maintained for up to forty-eight hours. An initial dose of 1 to 2 grams by mouth followed by 500 milligrams daily is usually sufficient to maintain a satisfactory blood level.

In addition to the tablets, sulphamethoxydiazine is available as a suspension containing 500 milligrams in 5 millilitres.

CONTRA-INDICATIONS. As for Sulphadimidine (page 478).

Dose. See above under **Actions and uses.**

Preparation
SULPHAMETHOXYDIAZINE TABLETS, B.P. Unless otherwise specified, tablets each containing 500 mg are supplied. They should be stored in airtight containers, protected from light.

OTHER NAME: *Durenate®*

SULPHAMETHOXYPYRIDAZINE

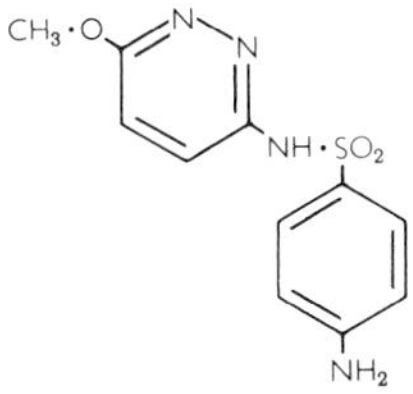

$C_{11}H_{12}N_4O_3S = 280·3$

Sulphamethoxypyridazine is 3-*p*-aminobenzenesulphonamido-6-methoxypyridazine.

Solubility. Very slightly soluble in water; slightly soluble in alcohol; soluble, at 20°, in 25 parts of acetone; soluble in dilute mineral acids and in solutions of alkali hydroxides.

Standard
It complies with the requirements of the British Pharmacopoeia.
It is a white or yellowish-white, crystalline, odourless or almost odourless powder and contains not less than 99·0 per cent of $C_{11}H_{12}N_4O_3S$, calculated with reference to the dried substance. The loss on drying under the prescribed conditions is not more than 0·5 per cent. It has a melting-point of 180° to 183°.

Storage. It should be protected from light.

Actions and uses. Sulphamethoxypyridazine has the actions, uses, and undesirable effects of the long-acting sulphonamides, as described under Sulphadimethoxine (page 478). As it is very soluble in neutral or acid urine, it is given by mouth in the treatment of urinary tract infections.

The initial dose is 1 to 2 grams, with a subsequent dosage of 500 milligrams daily.

CONTRA-INDICATIONS. As for Sulphadimidine (page 478).

Dose. See above under **Actions and uses.**

Preparation
SULPHAMETHOXYPYRIDAZINE TABLETS, B.P. Unless otherwise specified, tablets each containing 500 mg of sulphamethoxypyridazine are supplied. They should be stored in airtight containers, protected from light.

OTHER NAMES: *Lederkyn®*; *Midicel®*

SULPHAPYRIDINE

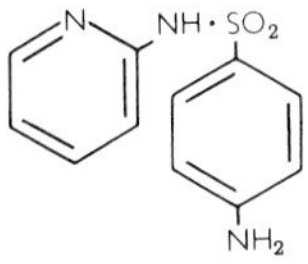

$C_{11}H_{11}N_3O_2S = 249·3$

Sulphapyridine is 2-(*p*-aminobenzenesulphonamido)pyridine.

Solubility. Very slightly soluble in water; soluble, at 20°, in 400 parts of alcohol and in 65 parts of acetone; soluble in dilute mineral acids, in aqueous solutions of alkali hydroxides, and in 100 parts of boiling water.

Standard
It complies with the requirements of the British Pharmacopoeia.
It is a white or yellowish-white, crystalline, odourless or almost odourless powder and contains not less than 99·0 and not more than the equivalent of 101·0 per cent of $C_{11}H_{11}N_3O_2S$, calculated with reference to the dried substance. The loss on drying under the prescribed conditions is not more than 0·5 per cent. It has a melting-point of 191° to 193°.

Storage. It should be protected from light.

Actions and uses. Sulphapyridine is now rarely used in medicine, except in the treatment of patients with dermatitis herpetiformis which does not respond to dapsone. It is given by mouth in a dosage of 3 to 4 grams daily until no further blisters develop and then in a dosage of 0·5 to 1 gram daily.

UNDESIRABLE EFFECTS. The undesirable effects are similar to those described under Sulphathiazole; an adequate output of urine must be ensured.

CONTRA-INDICATIONS. As for Sulphadimidine (page 478).

Dose. See above under **Actions and uses.**

Preparation
SULPHAPYRIDINE TABLETS, B.P. Unless otherwise specified, tablets each containing 500 mg of sulphapyridine are supplied. They should be stored in airtight containers, protected from light.

OTHER NAME: *M. & B. 693®*

SULPHATHIAZOLE

$C_9H_9N_3O_2S_2 = 255\cdot3$

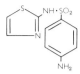

Sulphathiazole is 2-(*p*-aminobenzenesulphonamido)thiazole.

Solubility. Very slightly soluble in water; slightly soluble in alcohol; soluble in dilute mineral acids and in solutions of alkali hydroxides and carbonates.

Standard
DESCRIPTION. A white or almost white crystalline powder; odourless or almost odourless.

IDENTIFICATION TESTS. 1. Heat 0·05 g in a dry tube; a brown to red colour is produced; on further heating, the odours of ammonia, aniline, and hydrogen sulphide are produced.

2. Dissolve 0·01 g in 10 ml of water and 2 ml of 0·1N sodium hydroxide, and add 0·5 ml of *copper sulphate solution*; a greyish-purple precipitate is formed.

3. Diazotise 0·05 g and treat with *β-naphthol solution*, as described under Sulphaguanidine (page 480); a bright orange-red precipitate is formed.

4. The infra-red absorption spectrum exhibits maxima which are at the same wavelengths as, and have similar relative intensities to, those in the spectrum of *sulphathiazole A.S.*

ACIDITY. Heat 1·0 g for 5 minutes at 70° with 50 ml of *carbon dioxide-free water*, cool quickly to 20°, filter, and titrate 25 ml of the filtrate with 0·1N sodium hydroxide, using *bromothymol blue solution* as indicator; not more than 0·1 ml is required.

MELTING-POINT. 200° to 203°.

LEAD. It complies with the test given in Appendix 7, page 884 (10 parts per million).

RELATED COMPOUNDS. It complies with the test given in Appendix 5A, page 868 (0·5 per cent).

LOSS ON DRYING. Not more than 0·5 per cent, determined by drying to constant weight at 105°.

SULPHATED ASH. Not more than 0·1 per cent.

CONTENT OF $C_9H_9N_3O_2S_2$. Not less than 99·0 and not more than the equivalent of 101·0 per cent, calculated with reference to the substance dried under the prescribed conditions, determined by the method for Sulphaguanidine (page 480); each ml of 0·1M sodium nitrite is equivalent to 0·02553 g of $C_9H_9N_3O_2S_2$.

Sterilisation. Powders for local application are sterilised by the method described under Sulphadimidine (page 478).

Storage. It should be protected from light.

Actions and uses. Sulphathiazole has the actions and uses of the sulphonamides, as described under Sulphadimidine (page 478). It is the only sulphonamide which has any effect in staphylococcal infections; it is also effective in the treatment of infections due to *β*-haemolytic streptococci, pneumococci, and gonococci.

When given by mouth, sulphathiazole is rapidly absorbed, and the maximum concentration in the blood, 5 to 10 milligrams per 100 millilitres, is attained in about four to six hours. It does not readily cross the blood–brain barrier into the cerebrospinal fluid and is therefore unsuitable for the treatment of meningeal infections. It is more rapidly excreted than sulphadimidine or sulphadiazine, a single dose being almost completely excreted in twenty-four hours.

In the treatment of pneumococcal pneumonia and other respiratory tract infections, as well as of localised staphylococcal infections such as otitis media and tonsillitis, it is usual to give an initial dose of 3 grams, followed by 1 gram every four hours until the temperature has remained normal for three days. The dosage for a child should be based on the scheme outlined under Sulphadimidine (page 478).

UNDESIRABLE EFFECTS. Toxic symptoms are common; the most usual undesirable effect is drug fever, and rashes are more frequent than with the other sulphonamides. Agranulocytosis occasionally occurs.

Sulphathiazole is excreted partly as the insoluble crystalline acetyl derivative and this occasionally causes blocking of the renal tubules and anuria, while milder degrees of renal damage may be indicated by haematuria. These risks, which are greater with sulphathiazole than with other sulphonamides, may be reduced to a minimum by maintaining a high fluid intake during treatment with the drug and by the administration of alkalis.

PRECAUTIONS AND CONTRA-INDICATIONS. Sulphathiazole should not be given to patients with renal disease and great care should be taken in its administration in hot climates; if haematuria develops the drug must be discontinued.

Dose. See above under **Actions and uses.**

Preparation
SULPHATHIAZOLE TABLETS, B.P.C. (page 816)

OTHER NAME: *Thiazamide*®

SULPHINPYRAZONE

$C_{23}H_{20}N_2O_3S = 404\cdot5$

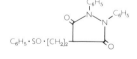

Sulphinpyrazone is 1,2-diphenyl-4-(2-phenylsulphinylethyl)pyrazolidine-3,5-dione.

Solubility. Slightly soluble in water; soluble, at 20°, in 40 parts of alcohol, in 750 parts of ether, and in 2 parts of chloroform; very slightly soluble in light petroleum; soluble in aqueous solutions of alkali hydroxides.

Standard
It complies with the requirements of the British Pharmacopoeia.
It is a white or almost white, odourless powder and contains not less than 99·0 per cent of $C_{23}H_{20}N_2O_3S$,

calculated with reference to the dried substance. The loss on drying under the prescribed conditions is not more than 0·5 per cent. It has a melting-point of 131° to 135°.

Actions and uses. Sulphinpyrazone is a uricosuric agent which is used in the treatment of gout to deplete the tissues of urates, to reduce the plasma–uric-acid level by increasing urinary urate excretion, and to diminish the incidence of acute attacks. Its effectiveness is reduced in the presence of citrates and salicylates.

Sulphinpyrazone may be given in conjunction with other uricosuric agents such as probenecid or with allopurinol when one drug alone has proved inadequate.

The usual dosage is 300 to 600 milligrams daily, given in divided doses every six to twelve hours, but at the beginning of treatment acute episodes may be precipitated and it is safer to begin with a reduced dosage. Colchicine, in a dosage of 500 micrograms once or twice daily, may be given concurrently with the aim of reducing the incidence of such attacks.

Treatment must be continued for many months or years before the tophaceous deposits are very much reduced, and regular dosage is essential. In such prolonged treatment, the possibility that blood dyscrasias may occur should be borne in mind.

CONTRA-INDICATIONS. It is contra-indicated in patients with impaired renal function.

Dose. See above under **Actions and uses.**

Preparation
SULPHINPYRAZONE TABLETS, B.P. Unless otherwise specified, tablets each containing 100 mg of sulphinpyrazone are supplied.

OTHER NAME: *Anturan*®

SULPHOBROMOPHTHALEIN SODIUM

$C_{20}H_8Br_4Na_2O_{10}S_2 = 838·0$

Sulphobromophthalein Sodium is the disodium salt of 3,4,5,6-tetrabromo-$\alpha\alpha$-di(4-hydroxy-3-sulphophenyl)phthalide.

Solubility. Soluble, at 20°, in 12 parts of water; insoluble in alcohol and in acetone.

Standard
It complies with the requirements of the British Pharmacopoeia.
It is a white, crystalline, hygroscopic, odourless, powder and contains 36·0 to 39·0 per cent of Br and 7·4 to 8·2 per cent of S, both calculated with reference to the dried substance. The loss on drying under the prescribed conditions is not more than 5·0 per cent.

Sterilisation. Solutions for injection are sterilised by filtration.

Storage. It should be stored in airtight containers.

Actions and uses. Sulphobromophthalein sodium is used for testing the functional capacity of the liver, particularly of its reticuloendothelial cells. After intravenous injection the dye combines with plasma proteins, but it is normally rapidly removed from the blood and excreted in the bile.

The test is usually performed in the morning after the patient has had a fat-free breakfast; no food must be given during the test. A dose of sulphobromophthalein sodium, usually 5 milligrams per kilogram body-weight, is given very slowly as a 5 per cent solution by intravenous injection over a period of about three minutes. When fluid retention is present, the dose to be given should be calculated from the patient's ideal weight obtained from tables. Forty-five minutes after the injection, 10 millilitres of blood is collected from another vein and allowed to clot, special care being taken to avoid haemolysis, and the amount of dye remaining in the serum is determined colorimetrically. In patients with normal liver function not more than 7 per cent of the dye is present in the blood forty-five minutes after the injection.

The test should not be performed on patients with a history of drug sensitivity, because of the risk of severe allergic reactions.

The 5 per cent solution may yield, on standing, a deposit which may not be readily observed. Immediately before use, therefore, the ampoules containing the solution must be immersed in boiling water for twenty minutes, well shaken, and cooled to body temperature.

Dose. See above under **Actions and uses.**

OTHER NAMES: B.S.P.; *Bromsulphalein*®; S.B.P.

SULPHOMYXIN SODIUM

Sulphomyxin Sodium is a mixture of sulphomethylated polymyxin B and sodium bisulphite.

Sulphomyxin Sodium may be prepared from polymyxin B by the action of formaldehyde and sodium bisuphite, whereby amino-groups of the polymyxin B are sulphomethylated.

Solubility. Soluble, at 20°, in less than 1 part of water and in 750 parts of alcohol.

Standard
It complies with the requirements of the British Pharmacopoeia.
It is a white almost odourless powder and contains not less than 5000 Units per mg, calculated with reference to the dried substance. The loss on drying under the prescribed conditions is not more than 3·0 per cent. A 2 per cent solution in water has a pH of 6·0 to 8·0.

Storage. It should be stored in airtight containers, protected from light. If it is intended for parenteral administration, the containers should be sterile and sealed to exclude micro-organisms.

Actions and uses. Sulphomyxin sodium has the antibacterial activity described under Polymyxin B Sulphate (page 388). It should be used only in the treatment of life-threatening systemic and urinary infections due to strains of such organisms as *Pseudomonas aeruginosa* which are not susceptible to or fail to respond to less toxic preparations.

It is given by intramuscular injection, the usual dose being 2,000,000 Units daily in divided doses. The dose must be reduced in patients with impaired renal function.

UNDESIRABLE EFFECTS. Paraesthesiae of the face and hands are common and proteinuria with impairment of renal function may follow. If sulphomyxin is allowed to accumulate in the body, neurological complications due to neuromuscular blockage may occur, leading to respiratory failure.

Dose. Up to 2 mega Units daily in divided doses, by intramuscular injection.

Preparation
SULPHOMYXIN INJECTION, B.P. It consists of a sterile solution prepared by dissolving the sterile contents of a sealed container in Water for Injections. It should be used within forty-eight hours of its date of preparation, which is stated on the label, and should be stored during this period at 2° to 10°. The quantity of sulphomyxin sodium in each container should be specified by the prescriber. Vials containing 500,000 Units are available.

OTHER NAME: *Thiosporin*®

PRECIPITATED SULPHUR

S = 32·06

Precipitated Sulphur may be prepared by boiling sublimed sulphur with calcium hydroxide and water for about an hour, filtering, and decomposing the resulting solution of calcium poly-sulphides and thiosulphate by means of hydrochloric acid diluted with an equal volume of water and added in a thin stream with constant stirring until only a slight alkalinity remains. The precipitate is washed and dried rapidly at a moderate temperature.

Precipitated Sulphur melts at about 115°, forming a yellow mobile liquid which becomes dark and viscous on heating at about 160°. At higher temperatures it burns with a blue flame, producing sulphur dioxide. It dissolves in hot aqueous solutions of alkali hydroxides, with the formation of polysulphides and thiosulphates.

Solubility. Very slightly soluble in water and in alcohol; almost completely soluble in carbon disulphide, the solution depositing the insoluble variety of sulphur on exposure to light.

Standard
It complies with the requirements of the British Pharmacopoeia.

DESCRIPTION. *Macroscopical:* a soft, pale greyish-yellow or greenish-yellow, odourless powder, free from grittiness.

Microscopical: minute, colourless *spherules*, about 1·5 to 11 μm in diameter, a few occurring singly or in small groups of 2 to 20, but the majority in large irregular clumps of about 100 or more, each clump consisting of spherules of different sizes, the larger ones being less numerous; *crystalline particles* absent.
When mounted in *cresol* and examined in polarised light on a dark field precipitated sulphur assumes a brilliant golden tint with numerous bright green and red points.

Actions and uses. Precipitated sulphur is a mild antiseptic and parasiticide.
Preparations of sulphur are applied externally in the treatment of acne.
It has also been used as a mild laxative.

Dose. 1 to 4 grams.

Preparations
SALICYLIC ACID AND SULPHUR CREAM, B.P.C. (page 660)
SULPHUR LOTION, COMPOUND, B.P.C. (page 729)
SALICYLIC ACID AND SULPHUR OINTMENT, B.P.C. (page 763)
SULPHUR OINTMENT, B.P. It contains 10 per cent of precipitated sulphur in Simple Ointment.
RESORCINOL AND SULPHUR PASTE, B.P.C. (page 768)

SUBLIMED SULPHUR

SYNONYM: Flowers of Sulphur

S = 32·06

Sublimed Sulphur may be obtained by sublimation of native sulphur or from sulphides or as a by-product of the refining of crude petroleum. It is only partially soluble in carbon disulphide and is thereby distinguished from crushed lump sulphur which is completely soluble.

Solubility. Very slightly soluble in water and in alcohol.

Standard
DESCRIPTION. *Macroscopical:* a fine yellow slightly gritty powder; odour faint and not unpleasant.

Microscopical: yellowish *spherules*, about 5 to 40 μm in diameter, a very few isolated, but mostly in fairly large clumps of about 50 to 100 or more; occasional *semi-crystalline lumps*, about 150 μm in diameter, occur and result from a somewhat higher temperature in the cooling chamber.
When mounted in *cresol* and examined in polarised light on a dark field, sublimed sulphur shines brightly with a dull golden-yellow colour.

IDENTIFICATION TESTS. 1. It melts at about 115° to a yellow mobile liquid, which becomes dark and viscid on heating at about 160°.
2. It burns with a blue flame, forming sulphur dioxide.
3. Dissolve 1 mg in 2 ml of hot *pyridine*, add 0·2 ml of *sodium bicarbonate solution*, and boil; a blue or green colour is produced.

ACIDITY. Shake 2·0 g vigorously with 50 ml of *carbon dioxide-free water* and titrate with 0·1N sodium hydroxide, using *phenolphthalein solution* as indicator; not more than 1·0 ml is required.

ARSENIC. It complies with the test given in Appendix 6, page 880 (2 parts per million).

MATTER INSOLUBLE IN CARBON DISULPHIDE. Shake 1·0 g with 20 ml of *carbon disulphide*, allow to stand for 10 minutes, filter, wash the residue with *carbon disulphide*, and dry; the residue weighs not less than 0·2 g.

ASH. Not more than 0·2 per cent.

Actions and uses. Sublimed sulphur has actions and uses similar to those described under Precipitated Sulphur.

Dose. 1 to 4 grams.

Preparation
LIQUORICE POWDER, COMPOUND, B.P.C. (page 777)

SULPHURATED POTASH

SYNONYMS: Liver of Sulphur; Potassa Sulphurata

Sulphurated Potash is a mixture of potassium polysulphides and other potassium compounds, including sulphite and thiosulphate, and may be prepared by fusing 2 parts of potassium carbonate with 1 part of sublimed sulphur.

Solubility. Almost completely soluble, at 20°, in 2 parts of water.

Standard
DESCRIPTION. Solid fragments, externally greenish-yellow, internally pale liver-brown rapidly changing to greenish-yellow on exposure to air; odour that of hydrogen sulphide.

IDENTIFICATION TEST. Dissolve 0·1 g in 2 ml of water and add 1 ml of *hydrochloric acid*; hydrogen sulphide is evolved and sulphur precipitated. Boil, filter and to the filtrate add 2 ml of *platinic chloride solution*; a yellow precipitate is formed.

WATER-INSOLUBLE MATTER. Not more than 0·5 per cent, determined by the following method:
Shake about 5 g, accurately weighed, with 50 ml of water, filter, wash the residue with water, and dry to constant weight at 105°.

CONTENT OF S. 42·0 to 45·0 per cent determined by the following method:
Dissolve about 0·2 g, accurately weighed, in 10 ml of water, add 5 ml of *sodium hydroxide solution*, heat to

boiling, and add slowly, with stirring, *bromine solution AsT* until a clear solution is obtained and bromine is present in excess; acidify to *litmus paper* with *hydrochloric acid*, boil until the excess of bromine is removed, and dilute to 100 ml with water; whilst still hot add slowly a slight excess of hot *barium chloride solution*, heat for 30 minutes on a water-bath, and filter; wash the residue with water, dry, and ignite to constant weight; each g of residue is equivalent to 0·1373 g of S.

Stability. It readily absorbs moisture and carbon dioxide from the air and undergoes oxidation.

Incompatibility. It is incompatible with acids.

Storage. It should be stored in airtight containers.

Actions and uses. Sulphurated potash is used as a peeling agent in acne, sometimes in the form of a lotion containing also zinc sulphate and Camphor Water.

Preparation
ZINC SULPHIDE LOTION, B.P.C. (page 730)

SULPHURIC ACID

H₂SO₄ = 98·07

Sulphuric Acid may be prepared by dissolving the product of the oxidation of sulphur dioxide in water.

Impure sulphuric acid of commerce, known as concentrated oil of vitriol, "C.O.V.", contains about 95 to 98 per cent w/w of H₂SO₄;

brown oil of vitriol, "B.O.V.", contains 75 to 85 per cent w/w of H₂SO₄.
Battery or accumulator acid is pure sulphuric

acid diluted with distilled water to a specific gravity ranging from 1·20 to 1·26.

Nordhausen or fuming sulphuric acid, known commercially as "oleum", is prepared by the addition of sulphur trioxide to sulphuric acid and is available containing various proportions of SO_3.

When diluting sulphuric acid, the acid should be added slowly, with constant stirring, to the water.

Standard

DESCRIPTION. A colourless corrosive liquid of oily consistence, evolving much heat when added to water.

IDENTIFICATION TESTS. 1. Strongly acid, even when freely diluted.

2. Carefully add 1 ml to 10 ml of water; the solution gives the reactions characteristic of sulphates.

WEIGHT PER ML. At 20°, about 1·84 g.

ARSENIC. It complies with the test given in Appendix 6, page 880 (2 parts per million).

IRON. 1 ml complies with the limit test for iron (40 parts per million).

LEAD. It complies with the test given in Appendix 7, page 884 (10 parts per million).

CHLORIDE. 5 ml carefully added to water and neutralised to *litmus paper* with *dilute ammonia solution* complies with the limit test for chlorides (70 parts per million).

NITRATE. Add 5 ml carefully to a mixture of 5 ml of water and 0·5 ml of *indigo carmine solution* and allow to stand for one minute; the colour is not discharged.

OXIDISABLE SUBSTANCES. Add 5 ml carefully to 20 ml of water, cool, add 0·1 ml of 0·1N potassium permanganate, and allow to stand for 5 minutes; the colour is not discharged.

RESIDUE ON EVAPORATION. Not more than 0·01 per cent w/w, determined by the following method:
Evaporate about 10 g, accurately weighed, by heating gently, and ignite the residue to constant weight.

CONTENT OF H_2SO_4. Not less than 95·0 per cent w/w, determined by the following method:
To 40 ml of water add carefully about 2 g, accurately weighed, and titrate with 1N sodium hydroxide, using *methyl orange solution* as indicator; each ml of 1N sodium hydroxide is equivalent to 0·04904 g of H_2SO_4.

Storage. It should be stored in airtight containers.

Actions and uses. Sulphuric acid is a powerful corrosive which chars organic substances. In contact with the skin or mucous membrane it causes intense pain and rapid destruction of tissue.

POISONING. A stomach tube or emetics should not be used. The acid must be neutralised as quickly as possible. Calcium hydroxide in water and Magnesium Hydroxide Mixture are good antidotes; carbonates should be avoided if possible, as they lead to the liberation of carbon dioxide and the consequent risk of perforation.

After neutralisation of the acid, demulcents such as milk, raw eggs, or a vegetable oil such as olive oil should be given and shock should be treated by warmth and intravenous infusions if required. Morphine should be given for the relief of pain.

Sulphuric acid burns should be treated by immediately flooding with water, followed by the application of sodium bicarbonate or chalk in powder, or by the application of sodium bicarbonate or saline packs.

DILUTE SULPHURIC ACID

Dilute Sulphuric Acid may be prepared by adding 104 g of Sulphuric Acid gradually, with constant stirring and cooling, to 896 g of Purified Water.

Standard

WEIGHT PER ML. At 20°, 1·062 g to 1·072 g.

CONTENT OF H_2SO_4. 9·5 to 10·5 per cent w/w, determined by the following method:
Dilute about 10 g, accurately weighed, with 40 ml of water and titrate with 1N sodium hydroxide, using

methyl orange solution as indicator; each ml of 1N sodium hydroxide is equivalent to 0·04904 g of H_2SO_4.

Actions and uses. Dilute sulphuric acid has actions similar to those of other dilute mineral acids. It is occasionally prescribed in mixtures containing vegetable bitters to stimulate appetite.

POISONING. The procedure as described under Sulphuric Acid should be adopted.

Dose. 0·3 to 5 millilitres, well diluted.

SULTHIAME

$C_{10}H_{14}N_2O_4S_2 = 290·4$

Sulthiame is tetrahydro-2-*p*-sulphamoylphenyl-1,2-thiazine 1,1-dioxide.

Solubility. Slightly soluble in water; soluble, at 20°, in 350 parts of alcohol, in 500 parts of ether, and in 700 parts of chloroform.

Standard

It complies with the requirements of the British Pharmacopoeia.

It is a white, crystalline, odourless powder and contains

not less than 98·0 per cent of $C_{10}H_{14}N_2O_4S_2$, calculated with reference to the dried substance. The loss on drying under the prescribed conditions is not more than 0·5 per cent. It has a melting-point of 185° to 187°.

Actions and uses. Sulthiame is an anticonvulsant of low toxicity which is more effective in controlling myoclonic seizures, focal epilepsy, and hyperkinetic behaviour than in influencing grand mal; it is not recommended for the treatment of petit mal. In changing from other anticonvulsants to sulthiame, the transition should be gradual.

The usual adult dose is 200 milligrams three times daily, but, when other therapy has already been instituted, 100 milligrams may be given twice daily as the initial dosage. For children the usual dosage is 10 to 15 milligrams per kilogram body-weight daily in divided doses, but one-third of this dosage should be given initially when other drugs are already being given.

Crystalluria occurs with overdosage but can be prevented by making the urine alkaline.

UNDESIRABLE EFFECTS. The most usual undesirable effects are anorexia, ataxia, and paraesthesia which often disappear in a few days.

Dose. See above under **Actions and uses.**

Preparation
SULTHIAME TABLETS, B.P. Unless otherwise specified, tablets each containing 50 mg of sulthiame are supplied. They are film coated. Tablets containing 200 mg are also available.

OTHER NAMES: *Ospolot®*; Sultiame

SURAMIN

SYNONYM: Suramin Sodium

$C_{51}H_{34}N_6Na_6O_{23}S_6 = 1429.2$

Suramin is the symmetrical 3″-urea of the sodium salt of 8-(3-benzamido-4-methylbenzamido)-naphthalene-1,3,5-trisulphonic acid.

Solubility. Soluble, at 20°, in less than 1 part of water; very slightly soluble in alcohol; insoluble in ether and in chloroform.

Standard
DESCRIPTION. A white, pinkish-white, or faintly cream-coloured, hygroscopic powder; odourless or almost odourless.

IDENTIFICATION TESTS. 1. Boil 0·05 g for 5 minutes with 2 ml of a mixture containing equal volumes of *sulphuric acid* and water, cool, add 20 ml of water and 0·02 g of *sodium nitrite*, allow to stand for 1 minute, add 0·2 g of *urea*, shake, and allow to stand for 2 minutes. Add 0·2 ml of this solution to a solution of 10 mg of N-(1-*naphthyl*)*ethylenediamine hydrochloride* and 0·5 g of *sodium acetate* in 5 ml of *acetic acid*; a magenta colour rapidly develops.
2. The residue after ignition gives the reactions characteristic of sodium.

CLARITY OF SOLUTION. Dissolve 1·0 g in 100 ml of *carbon dioxide-free water*; not more than a minute trace is left undissolved and the solution is clear.

ACIDITY. 5·0 g dissolved in 50 ml of water, previously neutralised to *methyl red and methylene blue solution*, requires for neutralisation not more than 0·5 ml of either 0·02N hydrochloric acid or 0·02N sodium hydroxide, using *methyl red and methylene blue solution* as indicator.

LEAD. It complies with the test given in Appendix 7, page 884 (10 parts per million).

CHLORIDE. Dissolve 0·50 g in 10 ml of water, add 5 ml of *dilute nitric acid* and 5 ml of 0·1N silver nitrate, filter, wash the filter with water, and titrate the combined filtrate and washings with 0·1N ammonium thiocyanate, using *ferric ammonium sulphate solution* as indicator; not less than 3·3 ml of 0·1N ammonium thiocyanate is required.

SULPHATE. 1·0 g complies with the limit test for sulphates (600 parts per million).

FREE AMINE. Dissolve 5·0 g in 50 ml of water, add 2·5 ml of *hydrochloric acid* and 1 g of *potassium bromide*, and titrate with 0·1M sodium nitrite, determining the dead-stop end-point by the method of the British Pharmacopoeia, Appendix XID.
Repeat the procedure omitting the sample.
The difference between the two titrations is not more than 0·4 ml.

ABSENCE OF UNDUE TOXICITY. It is tested on at least 10 mice by the intravenous injection of doses of 0·32 mg per g of body-weight. It passes the test if the total number of mice which die within 3 days does not exceed 50 per cent of the total number of mice injected.
A suggested method of test is given in Appendix 18, page 901.

THERAPEUTIC POTENCY. It is tested on mice infected with a strain of *Trypanosoma equiperdum*, or other suitable species of trypanosome sensitive to suramin, so that the blood contains between 1000 and 20,000 trypanosomes per ml.
The sample is tested on at least 10 mice by intravenous injection of doses of 0·8 μg per g of body-weight. On the third day after the injection, the blood of each mouse is examined microscopically in 20 fields using a microscope with a 4-mm objective.
The sample passes the test if 50 per cent or more of the total number of mice injected show absence of visible trypanosomes in the blood.
A suggested method of test is given in Appendix 18, page 901.

WATER. Not more than 10·0 per cent w/w, determined by the method given in Appendix 16, page 895.

CONTENT OF $C_{51}H_{34}N_6Na_6O_{23}S_6$. Not less than 97·5 per cent, calculated with reference to the anhydrous substance, determined by the following method:
To about 1 g, accurately weighed, add 20 ml of *sulphuric acid* (50 per cent v/v), boil under a reflux condenser for 1 hour, cool, dilute to 100 ml with water, add 1 g of *potassium bromide*, and titrate with 0·1M sodium nitrite, determining the dead-stop end-point by

the method given in the British Pharmacopoeia, Appendix XID.

Repeat the procedure omitting the sample.

The difference between the two titrations represents the amount of sodium nitrite required by the sample; each ml of 0.1 M sodium nitrite is equivalent to 0.02382 g of $C_{51}H_{34}N_6Na_6O_{23}S_6$.

Storage. It should be stored in airtight containers, protected from light, in a cool place.

Actions and uses. Suramin is effective against the early stages of trypanosomiasis, particularly in patients infected with *Trypanosoma rhodesiense*. It does not cross the blood–brain barrier and is valueless in more advanced stages of trypanosomiasis in which the central nervous system is involved.

Suramin is also of value in the treatment of onchocerciasis.

Before starting a course of treatment, the patient's tolerance to suramin should be tested by a dose of 200 milligrams given intravenously. If no untoward reactions occur within twenty-four to forty-eight hours, a dose of 1 gram is given; this is repeated weekly, usually until 5 grams has been given. The urine should be tested before each dose is given and if protein is present the dosage should be reduced or administration delayed. The interval between doses may be shortened if no proteinuria develops.

Suramin is also used prophylactically against trypanosomiasis, a dose of 2 grams conferring protection for at least three months.

In onchocerciasis, suramin is effective against the adult parasites but it has no direct action on the microfilariae of *Onchocerca volvulus*.

Solutions for injection are prepared by an aseptic technique.

UNDESIRABLE EFFECTS. Suramin may produce toxic effects, the chief of which is damage to the kidneys; the occurrence of proteinuria indicates the need for caution in further treatment. Other toxic reactions include vomiting, rashes, peripheral neuritis, and amblyopia.

PRECAUTIONS. As with pentamidine, it is important to detect more advanced infections and to treat these with a drug such as melarsoprol.

Dose. See above under **Actions and uses.**

Preparation

SURAMIN INJECTION, B.P.C. (page 718)

OTHER NAME: *Antrypol*®

SUXAMETHONIUM BROMIDE

SYNONYM: Succinylcholine Bromide

$$[(CH_3)_3N \cdot [CH_2]_2 \cdot O \cdot CO \cdot [CH_2]_2 \cdot CO \cdot O \cdot [CH_2]_2 \cdot N(CH_3)_3]^{2+} \ 2Br^-, 2H_2O$$

$C_{14}H_{30}Br_2N_2O_4, 2H_2O = 486.2$

Suxamethonium Bromide is 2-dimethylaminoethyl succinate dimethobromide dihydrate.

Solubility. Soluble, at $20°$, in less than 1 part of water and in 5 parts of alcohol; insoluble in ether and in chloroform.

Standard

It complies with the requirements of the British Pharmacopoeia.

It is a white or creamy-white, almost odourless powder and contains not less than 99.0 and not more than the equivalent of 101.0 per cent of $C_{14}H_{30}Br_2N_2O_4$, calculated with reference to the dried substance. The loss on drying under the prescribed conditions is 6.0 to 8.0 per cent. It has a melting-point of about $225°$. A 1 per cent solution in water has a pH of 4.0 to 5.0.

Incompatibility. In solution, suxamethonium bromide is rapidly destroyed by alkalis and therefore should not be mixed with thiopentone sodium.

Storage. It should be protected from light.

Actions and uses. Suxamethonium bromide has the actions, uses, and undesirable effects described under Suxamethonium Chloride.

The intravenous dose for an adult is 0.5 to 1 milligram of the base per kilogram body-weight; 1.67 milligrams of suxamethonium bromide is approximately equivalent to 1 milligram of the base.

Dose. The dose is determined by the physician in accordance with the needs of the patient.

Preparation

SUXAMETHONIUM BROMIDE INJECTION, B.P. (*Syn.* Succinylcholine Bromide Injection). It consists of a sterile solution of suxamethonium bromide prepared immediately before use by dissolving the sterile contents of a sealed container in Water for Injections. The quantity of suxamethonium bromide in each container should be specified by the prescriber. Ampoules containing 67 and 335 mg of suxamethonium bromide, equivalent to 40 and 200 mg respectively of suxamethonium, are available.

OTHER NAME: *Brevidil M*®

SUXAMETHONIUM CHLORIDE

SYNONYMS: Succinylcholine Chloride; Suxamethonii Chloridum

$$[(CH_3)_3N \cdot [CH_2]_2 \cdot O \cdot CO \cdot [CH_2]_2 \cdot CO \cdot O \cdot [CH_2]_2 \cdot N(CH_3)_3]^{2+} \ 2Cl^-, 2H_2O$$

$C_{14}H_{30}Cl_2N_2O_4, 2H_2O = 397 \cdot 3$

Suxamethonium Chloride is 2-dimethylaminoethyl succinate dimethochloride dihydrate.

Solubility. Soluble, at 20°, in 1 part of water; less soluble in alcohol; insoluble in ether.

Standard
It complies with the requirements of the European Pharmacopoeia.
It is a white or almost white, crystalline, almost odourless powder and contains not less than 98·0 and not more than the equivalent of 101·0 per cent of $C_{14}H_{30}Cl_2N_2O_4$, calculated with reference to the anhydrous substance. It contains 8·0 to 10·0 per cent w/w of water. It has a melting-point, without previous drying, of about 160°. A 1 per cent solution in water has a pH of 4·0 to 5·0.

Incompatibility. In solution, suxamethonium chloride is rapidly destroyed by alkalis and therefore should not be mixed with thiopentone sodium.

Sterilisation. Solutions for injection are sterilised by heating with a bactericide or by filtration.

Storage. It should be protected from light.

Actions and uses. Suxamethonium chloride is a short-acting relaxant of voluntary muscle. It produces muscular paralysis by a depolarisation of the neuromuscular end-plate. This effect is increased rather than antagonised by the anticholinesterase drugs, such as neostigmine.

Suxamethonium chloride given intravenously in a dose of 30 to 60 milligrams to an adult will produce an immediate but short-lasting muscular relaxation with respiratory paralysis. The onset of relaxation is preceded by diffuse incoordinated muscular contractions which are painful; pain may also be experienced during recovery. The administration of suxamethonium chloride should therefore always be preceded by an intravenous anaesthetic such as thiopentone sodium.

The contractions occur in about fifteen seconds after administration of the suxamethonium and last for about twenty seconds, their disappearance indicating the onset of paralysis. In the majority of patients, paralysis lasts for two to six minutes, after which time muscle power returns and becomes normal in a further three or four minutes.

Suxamethonium chloride is given intravenously, in single doses, for short operative manipulative procedures, such as endotracheal intubation, for the prevention of traumatic complications in electro-convulsion therapy, and in the symptomatic treatment of convulsions of tetanus. For long operations, repeated intravenous doses may be given; no cumulative effect or tachyphylaxis occurs. Alternatively, it may be given as a 1 in 1000 solution by continuous intravenous infusion, by which means the degree of relaxation can easily be controlled.

The dose of suxamethonium is often given in terms of the base; 1·37 milligrams of suxamethonium chloride is approximately equivalent to 1 milligram of the base.

Suxamethonium chloride may be used with any of the commonly employed anaesthetics.

UNDESIRABLE EFFECTS. Bradycardia and hypertension may occur, but these are of no significance except during electroconvulsive therapy or after severe burns when cardiac arrest has been attributed to them.

In normal persons, suxamethonium chloride is rapidly inactivated by cholinesterase enzymes, but occasionally paralysis may be prolonged and this is usually associated with low serum-cholinesterase activity which may occur in carcinoma of the bronchus, liver disease, malnutrition, and poisoning due to organophosphorus compounds, or as a result of genetic factors.

Pain in the muscles of the chest, shoulder, and neck sometimes follows the administration of suxamethonium chloride, particularly in patients who are ambulant shortly after its use.

PRECAUTIONS. Respiratory paralysis will occur with adequate muscular relaxation and facilities for controlled respiration should be available when the drug is used.

In therapeutic doses, suxamethonium chloride does not cause liberation of histamine and it has no significant effect on the cardiovascular or any other system.

With high doses, especially when given by intravenous infusion, there may be a rise in blood pressure due to the stimulatory action of suxamethonium chloride on the sympathetic ganglia (nicotinic action); this may be counteracted by the administration of ganglion-blocking drugs, such as pentolinium tartrate.

POISONING. Respiratory depression should be combated by controlled respiration, an insufflator or closed-circuit anaesthetic machine being used.

Dose. The dose is determined by the physician in accordance with the needs of the patient.

Preparation
SUXAMETHONIUM CHLORIDE INJECTION, B.P. (*Syn.* Succinylcholine Chloride Injection). It consists of a sterile solution of suxamethonium chloride in Water for Injections. Unless otherwise specified, a solution containing 50 mg in 1 ml is supplied. It should be stored at as low a temperature as possible above its freezing-point and not exceeding 4°; under these conditions it may be expected to retain its potency for at least two years from the date of preparation, which is stated on the label.

OTHER NAMES: *Anectine*®; *Scoline*®

PURIFIED TALC

SYNONYM: Talc

Purified Talc is a purified native magnesium silicate, corresponding approximately to the formula $Mg_6(Si_2O_5)_4(OH)_4$.

Solubility. Insoluble in water, in dilute mineral acids, and in dilute solutions of alkali hydroxides.

Standard
It complies with the requirements of the British Pharmacopoeia.
It is a very fine, white, unctuous, impalpable, odourless powder. The loss on drying at 105° is not more than 1·0 per cent and the loss on ignition under the prescribed conditions is not more than 6·0 per cent.

Microscopical characters: irregular, sharply angled particles, either as small flakes or as pieces with jagged and laminated ends, up to 135 μm in length or width, the smaller ones about 3 to 5 μm; it does not stain with *safranine solution* or *alcoholic methylene blue solution*; mounted in *cresol* or *chloral hydrate*, it shines brightly on a dark field between crossed polars (distinction from magnesium trisilicate).

Hygroscopicity. It absorbs insignificant amounts of moisture at 25° at relative humidities up to about 90 per cent.

Sterilisation. It is sterilised by heating at a temperature not lower than 160° for sufficient time to ensure

that the whole of the powder is maintained at this temperature for one hour or it may be sterilised by exposure to ethylene oxide under suitable conditions.

Actions and uses. Purified talc is used in massage and as a dusting-powder to allay irritation and prevent chafing; it is usually mixed with starch and zinc oxide. Purified talc used in dusting-powders should be sterilised. It is unsuitable for dusting surgical gloves, since it may cause foreign-body granulomata.

Purified talc is also used to clarify liquids and as a lubricant in making tablets.

Preparations
CHLORPHENESIN DUSTING-POWDER, B.P.C. (page 663)
TALC DUSTING-POWDER, B.P.C. (page 663)
ZINC, STARCH, AND TALC DUSTING-POWDER, B.P.C. (page 664)

OTHER NAMES: Powdered Talc; Purified French Chalk

TANNIC ACID

SYNONYM: Tannin

Tannic Acid may be obtained from oak galls by subjecting them to a process of fermentation and extracting with water-saturated ether.

Tannic Acid is not a carboxylic acid; on hydrolysis with dilute sulphuric acid it yields gallic acid and glucose, and this decomposition indicates that its minimum complexity is represented by a pentadigalloylglucose, $C_{76}H_{52}O_{46}$, a formula which is in accordance with its slightly acid reaction and dextrorotation.

Many commercial samples of tannic acid contain gallic acid, the presence of which reduces the solubility and may be detected by the production of a pink colour on the addition of a 5 per cent w/v solution of potassium cyanide in water. These varieties of tannic acid are used in dyeing and in the manufacture of ink and are not suitable for medicinal use; they occur in coarse powder or lumps, darker in colour than the official substance.

Solubility. Soluble, at 20°, in less than 1 part of water and of alcohol; very slightly soluble in ether, in chloroform, and in light petroleum; very soluble in acetone; slowly soluble in 1 part of glycerol.

Standard
It complies with the requirements of the British Pharmacopoeia.
It occurs as yellowish-white or light-brown glistening scales, light masses, or impalpable powder with a characteristic odour. The loss on drying at 105° is not more than 9·0 per cent. A solution in water is dextrorotatory and acid to methyl red.

Stability. Aqueous solutions decompose on keeping.

Incompatibility. It is incompatible with salts of iron, lead, antimony, and silver, and with alkaloids, albumin, and gelatin.

Actions and uses. Tannic acid precipitates proteins and forms insoluble complexes with many heavy metals, alkaloids, and glycosides. It is therefore useful as an antidote in poisoning by these substances, as it delays their absorption.

Tannic acid has little action on intact skin, but on abraded surfaces it forms a hard coagulum and on this account has been employed in the treatment of burns; it is now seldom used for this purpose because the coagulum causes contractures and, moreover, sufficient tannic acid may be absorbed from large areas to cause damage to the liver.

The astringent action on the mucous membrane of the gastro-intestinal tract exerted by the combined tannic acids in catechu and in similar drugs has been used for the symptomatic management of diarrhoea.

In lozenges, gargles, or sprays, tannic acid is used as an astringent for the mucous membrane of the mouth and throat.

UNDESIRABLE EFFECTS. Fatal hepatotoxic manifestations have followed the administration of barium sulphate enemas containing tannic acid, which has been added to improve the clarity of X-ray photographs.

Preparation
TANNIC ACID GLYCERIN, B.P.C. (page 702)

TAR

SYNONYM: Pix Liquida

Tar is the bituminous liquid obtained by the destructive distillation of the wood of the Scots pine, *Pinus sylvestris* L., and other trees of the family Pinaceae, and is known in commerce as Stockholm tar.

Constituents. Tar contains many substances, including hydrocarbons, which are chiefly terpenoid in character, and phenols, most of which are high-boiling dihydric phenols and their methyl ethers.

Solubility. Very slightly soluble in water; soluble, at 20°, in 10 parts of alcohol (90 per cent); soluble in ether, in chloroform, and in fixed and volatile oils.

Standard
It complies with the requirements of the British Pharmacopoeia.
It is a dark brown or almost black semi-liquid substance with a strong, characteristic, empyreumatic odour.
It is transparent in thin layers if free from water.

When stored for some time it separates into a layer which is granular in character due to minute crystallisation of catechol, resin acids, etc., and a surface layer of a syrupy consistence. Tar has an acid reaction which is imparted to water when shaken with it, and it may thereby be distinguished from coal tar, which has an alkaline reaction.

Actions and uses. Tar has antipruritic properties, but its action is less marked than that of coal tar. It has been applied as an ointment in the treatment of chronic skin diseases, especially psoriasis and eczema.

COAL TAR

SYNONYM: Pix Carbonis

Coal Tar is a product obtained by the destructive distillation of bituminous coal at about 1000°. It has a weight per ml at 20° of about 1·15 g.

Constituents. The chief constituents are benzene, phenols, naphthalene, and pitch, together with small quantities of basic compounds such as pyridine and quinoline.

Solubility. Slightly soluble in water; partly soluble in alcohol, in ether, in chloroform, and in volatile oils.

Standard
DESCRIPTION. A thick, nearly black, viscous liquid; odour strong, penetrating, and characteristic. On exposure to air, it gradually becomes more viscous. It burns with a luminous sooty flame.

IDENTIFICATION TESTS. 1. A saturated solution in water is alkaline to *litmus solution* (distinction from tar obtained from wood or lignite, or by the destructive distillation of bituminous coal at temperatures below 600°).

2. Shake 0·5 g with 10 ml of *light petroleum (boiling-range, 40° to 60°)* and allow to stand; a greenish-blue colour is produced in the light-petroleum layer.

ASH. Not more than 2·0 per cent.

Actions and uses. Coal tar has actions and uses similar to those described under Prepared Coal Tar. It is sometimes preferred to Prepared Coal Tar but it is liable to be more irritating to the skin.

Preparations
COAL TAR, PREPARED, B.P. (see below)
COAL TAR PAINT, B.P.C. (page 765)
ZINC AND COAL TAR PASTE, B.P.C. (page 769)

PREPARED COAL TAR

SYNONYM: Pix Carbonis Praeparata

Prepared Coal Tar is obtained by heating commercial coal tar in a shallow vessel for one hour at 50° with frequent stirring.

Constituents. The constituents are those of coal tar, with a smaller proportion of the more volatile constituents.

Solubility. Very slightly soluble in water; partly soluble in alcohol (90 per cent) and in ether; almost completely soluble in chloroform.

Standard
It complies with the requirements of the British Pharmacopoeia.
It is a nearly black viscous liquid with a strongly empyreumatic odour; in very thin layers it is brown.

Actions and uses. Prepared Coal Tar has antipruritic properties. It is used in the form of lotions and ointments in the treatment of

pruritus, psoriasis, eczema, and other skin affections.

Preparations
AMMONIATED MERCURY AND COAL TAR OINTMENT, B.P.C. (page 758)
CALAMINE AND COAL TAR OINTMENT, B.P.C. (page 760)
COAL TAR AND SALICYLIC ACID OINTMENT, B.P.C. (page 760)
COAL TAR AND ZINC OINTMENT, B.P.C. (page 760)
COAL TAR PASTE, B.P.C. (page 767)
COAL TAR SOLUTION, B.P. It consists of an alcoholic extract of Prepared Coal Tar (1 in 5) and quillaia.
COAL TAR SOLUTION, STRONG, B.P.C. (page 783)

TARTARIC ACID

$C_4H_6O_6 = 150 \cdot 1$ $CO_2H \cdot CH(OH) \cdot CH(OH) \cdot CO_2H$

Tartaric Acid is (+)-tartaric acid and may be obtained from argol, the crude potassium hydrogen tartrate deposited during the fermentation of grape juice.

Solubility. Soluble, at 20°, in less than 1 part of water and in 2·5 parts of alcohol; slightly soluble in ether.

Standard
It complies with the requirements of the British Pharmacopoeia.
It occurs as odourless colourless crystals or white powder and contains not less than 99·5 per cent of $C_4H_6O_6$, calculated with reference to the dried substance. The loss on drying under the prescribed conditions is not more than 1·0 per cent.

Hygroscopicity. It absorbs insignificant amounts of moisture at relative humidities up to about 65 per cent, but at relative humidities above about 75 per cent, it is deliquescent.

Storage. It should be stored in airtight containers.

Actions and uses. Tartaric acid is a saline purgative which has actions similar to those

described under Sodium Potassium Tartrate (page 461). It is a constituent of effervescent powders and granules and of cooling drinks and should be taken well diluted with water. Approximately neutral solutions are formed when 10 parts of tartaric acid are mixed in solution with 11 parts of ammonium bicarbonate, $6\frac{1}{2}$ parts of magnesium carbonate, $13\frac{1}{4}$ parts of potassium bicarbonate, or $11\frac{1}{4}$ parts of sodium bicarbonate.

Dose. 0·3 to 2 grams.

Preparations
EFFERVESCENT POWDER, COMPOUND, B.P.C. (page 776)
EFFERVESCENT POWDER, COMPOUND, DOUBLE-STRENGTH, B.P.C. (page 777)

TERPINEOL

$C_{10}H_{18}O = 154 \cdot 3$

Terpineol is a mixture of isomers in which (±)-α-terpineol largely predominates. It may be prepared by treating terpin hydrate with dilute mineral acid and fractionating the crude product by distillation.

Solubility. Very slightly soluble in water; soluble, at 20°, in 2 parts of alcohol (70 per cent); soluble in ether.

Standard
DESCRIPTION. A colourless, slightly viscous, optically inactive liquid, which may deposit crystals; odour pleasant.

REFRACTIVE INDEX. At 20°, 1·4825 to 1·4855.

WEIGHT PER ML. At 20°, 0·931 g to 0·935 g.

LOW-BOILING SUBSTANCES. Not more than 4·0 per cent v/v distils below 214°, determined by the method

described in Appendix 9A, page 887, for the determination of distillation range, 50 ml of sample being used and the distillate being collected in a 10-ml graduated cylinder.

Actions and uses. Terpineol has antibacterial properties and is a useful solvent. It prevents the crystallisation of chloroxylenol from Chloroxylenol Solution; solvents such as alcohol do not have this effect.

TESTOSTERONE

$C_{19}H_{28}O_2 = 288 \cdot 4$

Testosterone is 17β-hydroxyandrost-4-en-3-one.

Solubility. Very slightly soluble in water; soluble, at 20°, in 5 parts of alcohol and in 150 parts of ethyl oleate.

Standard
It complies with the requirements of the British Pharmacopoeia.
It is a white, crystalline, odourless powder and contains not less than 97·0 and not more than the equivalent of 103·0 per cent of $C_{19}H_{28}O_2$, calculated with reference to the dried substance. The loss on drying under the prescribed conditions is not more than 0·5 per cent. It has a melting-point of 152° to 156°.

Storage. It should be protected from light.

Actions and uses. Testosterone is the androgenic hormone formed in the interstitial (Leydig) cells of the testes under the control

of the anterior lobe of the pituitary gland. It controls the development and maintenance of the male sex organs and the male secondary sex characteristics. In small doses it increases the number of spermatozoa produced, but in large doses it inhibits the activity of the anterior lobe of the pituitary gland and suppresses the formation of spermatozoa. In underdeveloped or adolescent males, testosterone increases the size of the scrotum, phallus, seminal vesicles, and the prostate; libido and sexual activity may also be increased.

Testosterone is essential for the development

of the secondary sex characteristics of the male—deep voice, facial and body hair, flat chest and pelvis, and aggressive drive. Testosterone also produces systemic effects such as increased nitrogen retention which leads to an increase in skeletal weight, water retention, increased vascularity of the skin, and increased growth of bone. Large and repeated doses given in early puberty may cause closure of the epiphyses and stop growth.

Testosterone inhibits the gonadotrophic activity of the anterior lobe of the pituitary gland, thereby suppressing ovarian activity and menstruation. Continued administration of large doses, in excess of about 300 milligrams monthly, to women produces symptoms of virilism, such as male-like hirsutism, deepening of the voice, atrophy of breast tissue and the uterine endometrium, and hypertrophy of the clitoris; libido is increased and lactation suppressed.

Testosterone and its derivatives are used in the male when the testes are absent or maldeveloped, when the sex organs are imperfectly developed as in eunuchoidism, and when the secondary sex characteristics are absent or their development is delayed. They are also used in the treatment of gynaecomastia. They are of no value in the treatment of sterility, unless this is due to sexual underdevelopment, or of undescended testicles, of impotence, or of prostatic hypertrophy.

Testosterone and its derivatives are used in the female in selected cases for the treatment of dysmenorrhoea, functional uterine bleeding (menorrhagia, metrorrhagia) and chronic mastitis, for suppression of lactation, for relief of after-pains in labour, and for the palliative treatment of carcinoma of the breast in those patients beyond the scope of surgery or irradiation therapy. Small doses are used with oestrogens in the treatment of the climacteric.

Testosterone has been used in both the male and the female to increase weight in patients suffering from emaciation or wasting diseases, such as Simmonds's disease, but less-virilising anabolic agents such as norethandrolone are now preferred for this purpose.

To achieve a prolonged action, testosterone is implanted subcutaneously. For parenteral administration, testosterone propionate is generally used, and for oral use, methyltestosterone or fluoxymesterone.

PRECAUTIONS. Patients under treatment with testosterone or its derivatives should be carefully watched for signs of hypercalcaemia, oedema, and virilism.

Dose. 100 to 600 milligrams, as total implantation dose.

Preparation
TESTOSTERONE IMPLANTS, B.P. Unless otherwise specified, sterile implants each consisting of 100 mg of testosterone are supplied. They should be protected from light. Implants consisting of 200 mg are also available.

TESTOSTERONE PHENYLPROPIONATE

$C_{28}H_{36}O_3 = 420.6$

Testosterone Phenylpropionate is 17β-(β-phenylpropionyloxy)androst-4-en-3-one.

Solubility. Very slightly soluble in water; soluble, at 20°, in 40 parts of alcohol.

Standard
It complies with the requirements of the British Pharmacopoeia.
It is a white to almost white crystalline powder with a characteristic odour and contains not less than 97·0 and not more than the equivalent of 103·0 per cent of $C_{28}H_{36}O_3$, calculated with reference to the dried substance. The loss on drying under the prescribed conditions is not more than 0·5 per cent. It has a melting-point of 114° to 117°.

Sterilisation. Oily solutions for injection are sterilised by dry heat.

Storage. It should be protected from light.

Actions and uses. Testosterone phenylpropionate has the actions and uses described under Testosterone, but is more potent than testosterone and has a longer duration of action. It is given by subcutaneous or intramuscular injection in a dosage of 10 to 50 milligrams every four to fourteen days, according to the condition under treatment.

PRECAUTIONS. These are described under Testosterone.

Dose. See above under **Actions and uses.**

Preparation
TESTOSTERONE PHENYLPROPIONATE INJECTION, B.P. It consists of a sterile solution of testosterone phenylpropionate in ethyl oleate or other suitable ester, in a suitable fixed oil, or in any mixture of these. Unless otherwise specified, a solution containing 10 mg in 1 ml is supplied. It should be protected from light.

TESTOSTERONE PROPIONATE

SYNONYM: Testosteroni Propionas

$C_{22}H_{32}O_3 = 344 \cdot 5$

Testosterone Propionate is 17β-propionyloxyandrost-4-en-3-one.

Solubility. Very slightly soluble in water; soluble, at 20°, in 6 parts of alcohol, in 4 parts of acetone, in 35 parts of arachis oil, and in 20 parts of ethyl oleate.

Standard
It complies with the requirements of the European Pharmacopoeia.
It occurs as odourless, colourless or at most slightly yellowish-white crystals or white, crystalline powder and contains not less than 97·0 and not more than the equivalent of 103·0 per cent of $C_{22}H_{32}O_3$, calculated with reference to the dried substance. The loss on drying under the prescribed conditions is not more than 0·5 per cent. It has a melting-point of 119° to 122°.

Sterilisation. Oily solutions for injection are sterilised by dry heat.

Storage. It should be protected from light.

Actions and uses. Testosterone propionate has actions similar to those described under Testosterone. It is an effective androgen for parenteral use, but is inactive when given by mouth. It is given by intramuscular injection in a dosage of 10 to 50 milligrams two or three times a week for replacement therapy in the male; persistent priapism is a sign of overdosage.

For the palliative treatment of carcinoma of the breast beyond the aid of surgery, 100 to 300 milligrams a week is given in divided doses. A dosage in excess of 300 milligrams monthly may produce virilism in the female.

Dose. See above under **Actions and uses.**

Preparation
TESTOSTERONE PROPIONATE INJECTION, B.P. It consists of a sterile solution of testosterone propionate in ethyl oleate or other suitable ester, in a suitable fixed oil, or in any mixture of these. Unless otherwise specified, a solution containing 10 mg in 1 ml is supplied. It should be protected from light. Solutions containing 5, 25, and 50 mg in 1 ml are also available.

OTHER NAME: *Virormone*®

TETRACHLOROETHYLENE

SYNONYM: Perchloroethylene

$CCl_2{:}CCl_2 = 165 \cdot 8$

Solubility. Insoluble in water; soluble in alcohol; miscible with ether and with oils.

Standard
It complies with the requirements of the British Pharmacopoeia.
It is a colourless mobile liquid with a characteristic odour. It has a weight per ml at 20° of 1·620 g to 1·626 g, and a boiling-point of 119° to 122°, not less than 95 per cent v/v distilling within a range of 1·5°. Thymol, 0·01 per cent w/w, is added as a preservative.

Storage. It should be stored in airtight containers, protected from light.

Actions and uses. Tetrachloroethylene is given by mouth for the expulsion of hookworms; it is of little value against threadworms and is ineffective against liver flukes.

The usual dose for an adult is 3 millilitres, and for a child 0·2 millilitre for each year of age up to fifteen years. The patient is given a saline purgative on an empty stomach, followed two hours later by the dose of tetrachloroethylene and then by a further dose of a saline purgative. If possible, the patient should be kept in bed during treatment; food or alcohol should not be given. When large numbers of people are treated under field conditions, the dose of tetrachloroethylene is usually given at the same time as the saline purgative.

Tetrachloroethylene may be given without purgation and this is of advantage in anaemic patients, because the disturbance of the fluid balance brought about by saline purgatives is avoided; for such patients, however, bephenium hydroxynaphthoate is to be preferred.

UNDESIRABLE EFFECTS. Toxic effects are rare; liver damage may occur occasionally, and a few patients may experience a transitory sensation of unsteadiness and vertigo after administration of the drug.

Tetrachloroethylene is used as a solvent in industry. Prolonged inhalation of its vapour in concentrations of over 200 parts per million produces toxic effects on the central nervous system, kidneys and liver, initial symptoms including dizziness, excessive perspiration, nausea and vomiting, and stupor. Some deaths have occurred.

DEPENDENCE. Dependence of the barbiturate–alcohol type, as described under Phenobarbitone (page 366), may occur in persons who habitually inhale small quantities of tetrachloroethylene vapour.

POISONING. Industrial poisoning by tetrachloroethylene is treated by removal of the patient from the source of the vapour, by artificial respiration, and by the administration of oxygen containing 5 per cent of carbon dioxide.

Dose. See above under **Actions and uses.**

Preparation
TETRACHLOROETHYLENE CAPSULES, B.P. Unless otherwise specified, capsules each containing 1 ml of tetrachloroethylene are supplied. They should be stored in a cool place and protected from light.

TETRACOSACTRIN ACETATE

Tetracosactrin Acetate is the hexa-acetate of L-seryl-L-tyrosyl-L-seryl-L-methionyl-L-glutamyl-L-histidyl-L-phenylalanyl-L-arginyl-L-tryptophylglycyl-L-lysyl-L-prolyl-L-valylglycyl-L-lysyl-L-lysyl-L-arginyl-L-arginyl-L-prolyl-L-valyl-L-lysyl-L-valyl-L-tyrosyl-L-proline.

Solubility. Soluble in 70 parts of water.

Standard
It complies with the requirements of the British Pharmacopoeia.
It is a white to yellow amorphous powder and contains not less than 76·0 per cent of peptide and 5 to 16 per cent w/w of water.

Storage. It should be stored in airtight containers.

Actions and uses. Tetracosactrin is a synthetic analogue of corticotrophin; it contains the first 24 of the 39 amino-acids and has the complete therapeutic activity of the natural substance corticotrophin. It is used for the same purposes as corticotrophin (page 129).
It may be administered as lyophilised powder containing mannitol, dissolved in Dextrose Injection (5 per cent), as a test for adrenocortical function, or in long-acting form in a zinc phosphate or hydroxide complex for subcutaneous or intramuscular injection every one to four days. As a rough guide to dosage

1 milligram of tetracosactrin is equivalent to 100 to 150 Units of corticotrophin zinc injection.

UNDESIRABLE EFFECTS. The undesirable effects described under Corticotrophin (page 129) may occur. Occasionally, a local tissue reaction may occur following the use of the long-acting preparation.

PRECAUTIONS AND CONTRA-INDICATIONS. As for Corticotrophin (page 129).

Preparation
TETRACOSACTRIN ZINC INJECTION, B.P. It consists of a sterile aqueous suspension of tetracosactrin acetate with zinc hydroxide and suitable stabilising agents. It should be stored at 2° to 15° and should not be allowed to freeze; under these conditions it may be expected to retain its potency for at least three years after the date of manufacture.
The strength of the suspension should be specified by the prescriber. Suspensions containing the equivalent of 0·5 and 1 mg of tetracosactrin in 1 ml are available in vials of 2 ml.

OTHER NAMES: *Cortrosyn®*; *Synacthen®*

TETRACYCLINE

$C_{22}H_{24}N_2O_8 = 444·4$

Tetracycline is a hydrated form of 4-dimethylamino-1,4,4a,5,5a,6,11,12a-octahydro-3,6,10,12,12a-pentahydroxy-6-methyl-1,11-dioxonaphthacene-2-carboxyamide, an antimicrobial substance which may be prepared by dechlorinating chlortetracycline, by reducing oxytetracycline, or by fermentation.

Solubility. Very slightly soluble in water; soluble, at 20°, in 50 parts of alcohol; insoluble in ether and in chloroform; soluble in dilute acids and, with decomposition, in solutions of alkali hydroxides.

Standard
DESCRIPTION. A yellow crystalline powder; odourless or almost odourless.

IDENTIFICATION TESTS. 1. To 0·5 mg add 2 ml of *sulphuric acid*; an intense violet colour is produced. Add 1 drop of *ferric chloride solution*; the colour changes to brown or reddish-brown.
2. It complies with the thin-layer chromatographic test given in Appendix 5A, page 869.

ACIDITY. pH of a suspension prepared by shaking 0·1 g with 10 ml of water, 3·5 to 6·0.

LIGHT ABSORPTION. To 10 ml of a 0·01 per cent w/v solution in 0·01N hydrochloric acid add 75 ml of water and 5 ml of *sodium hydroxide solution*, dilute to 100 ml with water, mix immediately, and measure the extinction of a 1-cm layer at 380 nm exactly 6 minutes after the addition of the sodium hydroxide solution;

the extinction is not less than 0·40 and not more than 0·42, calculated with reference to the substance dried under the prescribed conditions.

LIGHT ABSORBING IMPURITIES. Extinction, at 430 nm, of a 1-cm layer of a 0·2 per cent w/v solution in 0·01N hydrochloric acid, measured within 1 hour of preparing the solution, not more than 0·50.

SPECIFIC ROTATION. −260° to −280°, calculated with reference to the substance dried under the prescribed conditions, determined, at 20°, in a 1·0 per cent w/v solution in 0·1N hydrochloric acid.

LOSS ON DRYING. Not more than 13·0 per cent, determined by drying for 2 hours at 105°.

MINIMUM POTENCY. Carry out an assay for tetracycline. A suggested method is given in Appendix 18, page 897. The precision of any assay must be such that the fiducial limits of error (P = 0·95) are not less than 95 per cent and not more than 105 per cent of the estimated potency.
The upper fiducial limit of error is not less than 1000

Units per mg, calculated with reference to the substance dried under the prescribed conditions.

Stability. It is inactivated in solutions of pH less than 2 and is slowly destroyed at pH 7 or above. It darkens in strong sunlight in a moist atmosphere.

Labelling. The label on the container states that the contents are not to be injected.

Storage. It should be stored in airtight containers, protected from light.

Actions and uses. Tetracycline has the actions, uses, and undesirable effects described under Tetracycline Hydrochloride. It is used in the preparation of oral liquid pre-

parations of the antibiotic; 1 gram of tetracycline (trihydrate) is approximately equivalent to 1 gram of tetracycline hydrochloride. Salts of aluminium, calcium, iron, and magnesium, which may decrease the absorption of tetracyclines from the gut, should not be given with tetracycline.

PRECAUTIONS AND CONTRA-INDICATIONS. As for Tetracycline Hydrochloride.

Preparation
TETRACYCLINE MIXTURE, B.P.C. (page 754)

OTHER NAMES: *Achromycin®*; *Clinitetrin®*; *Steclin®*; *Telotrex®*; *Tetrachel®*; *Tetracyn®*; *Totomycin®*

TETRACYCLINE HYDROCHLORIDE

$C_{22}H_{24}N_2O_8,HCl = 480.9$

Tetracycline Hydrochloride is 4-dimethylamino-1,4,4a,5,5a,6,11,12a-octahydro-3,6,10,12,12a-pentahydroxy-6-methyl-1,11-dioxonaphthacene-2-carboxyamide hydrochloride, an antimicrobial substance which may be prepared by dechlorinating chlortetracycline or reducing oxytetracycline.

Solubility. Soluble, at 20°, in 10 parts of water, giving a clear solution which becomes turbid on standing, and in 100 parts of alcohol; very slightly soluble in ether, in chloroform, and in acetone; soluble in solutions of alkali hydroxides and carbonates.

Standard
It complies with the requirements of the British Pharmacopoeia.
It is a yellow, crystalline, odourless powder and contains not less than 950 Units per mg, calculated with reference to the dried substance. The loss on drying under the prescribed conditions is not more than 2·0 per cent. A 1 per cent solution in water has a pH of 1·8 to 2·8.

Stability. It darkens in strong sunlight in a moist atmosphere; it is inactivated in solutions of pH less than 2 and is slowly destroyed at pH 7 or above.

Labelling. If the material is not intended for parenteral administration, the label on the container states that the contents are not to be injected.

Storage. It should be stored in airtight containers, protected from light.

Actions and uses. Tetracycline and its analogues are antibiotics which are effective against a wide range of pathogenic bacteria, both Gram-positive and Gram-negative, including some which are resistant to penicillin.

The organisms which are sensitive to the tetracyclines in the concentrations usually achieved in the body during treatment are *Brucella abortus*, *Escherichia coli*, *Haemophilus* species, *Klebsiella* species, *Actinomyces* species, *Entamoeba histolytica*, *Trichomonas vaginalis*, staphylococci, streptococci, treponemata, and certain rickettsiae and viruses. *Proteus vulgaris*, *Pseudomonas aeruginosa*, and *Salmonella* species are less susceptible, and tubercle bacilli, yeasts, and fungi are resistant. Resistance to the tetracyclines develops relatively slowly in susceptible organisms, but when it occurs it is often a complete cross-resistance amongst all members of the group.

In such cases treatment should be continued with another class of antibiotic or with a suitable sulphonamide.

When given by mouth, the tetracyclines are only partly absorbed from the gastro-intestinal tract; therapeutic blood levels are achieved more readily by increasing the frequency of administration than by increasing the dose. After absorption, the tetracyclines readily diffuse into the body fluids, although chlortetracycline does not pass the blood–brain barrier unless the meninges are damaged or inflamed. The tetracyclines are slowly excreted in the urine and bile.

Salts of aluminium, calcium, iron, and magnesium, which may decrease the absorption of tetracyclines from the gut, should not be given with tetracycline hydrochloride.

The tetracyclines are used in the treatment of infections caused by susceptible organisms, especially those that are resistant to penicillin and the sulphonamides; these infections include anthrax, brucellosis, Friedländer and viral pneumonias, whooping-cough, rickettsial fevers such as scrub typhus, Q fever, and Rocky Mountain spotted fever, and some diseases, such as psittacosis and lymphogranuloma inguinale, caused by the large viruses.

The tetracyclines are used, in conjunction with other amoebicides, in the treatment of amoebic dysentery. They are also of value in the treatment of staphylococcal and streptococcal infections in penicillin-sensitive patients and in chronic bronchitis to prevent infection of the respiratory tract by sensitive organisms.

All the tetracyclines are effective against the susceptible organisms named above, but tetracycline is the drug of choice in infections of the central nervous system and, like oxytetracycline, is preferred to chlortetracycline in the treatment of urinary tract infections, especially when these are caused by *Klebsiella* species and *Esch. coli*.

The usual dosage of tetracycline hydrochloride for an adult is 250 to 500 milligrams by mouth every six hours, but up to 4 grams daily may be given in more severe infections. The usual dosage for a child is 2·5 to 7·5 milligrams per kilogram body-weight every six hours. Treatment should be continued for at least forty-eight hours after the patient's temperature has returned to normal and acute symptoms have subsided. In severe acute infections, 0·5 to 1 gram may be given every twelve hours by slow intravenous infusion of a solution containing not more than 0·1 per cent; oral treatment should be substituted as soon as practicable, because the injection may cause phlebitis.

The tetracyclines may be given by intramuscular injection, in a solution containing not more than 5 per cent, in a dosage of 200 to 400 milligrams for an adult and 5 milligrams per kilogram body-weight for a child daily, in divided doses; as the injection is painful, procaine is usually included in the solution.

The tetracyclines are also applied topically in the treatment of some localised infections.

Solutions for injection are prepared by an aseptic technique.

UNDESIRABLE EFFECTS. Treatment with tetracyclines may cause gastro-intestinal disturbances, with flatulence, nausea, vomiting, and diarrhoea.

Overgrowth of resistant organisms, such as *Candida* and other fungi, may occur in the mouth and intestines, producing angular stomatitis, glossitis, and rectal and vaginal irritation; marked changes in the intestinal flora result from the destruction of susceptible organisms, which facilitates the multiplication of resistant organisms such as *Candida*, some strains of staphylococci, and yeasts, and may also result in a deficiency of vitamins of the B group.

The most serious toxic effect is the occurrence of staphylococcal enterocolitis, caused by organisms which have developed resistance; the onset of this condition is often sudden and it may end fatally. If it occurs, the tetracycline should be withdrawn and methicillin or cloxacillin given by injection in conjunction with benzylpenicillin, pending the results of sensitivity tests on the causative organism.

Drug fever and allergic skin rashes occur on rare occasions, but can usually be controlled by the administration of antihistamines.

PRECAUTIONS AND CONTRA-INDICATIONS. Tetracyclines readily cross the placental barrier and should not be given to pregnant women or to infants, unless no other drug will control the infection, because they interfere with the growth and development of the teeth; the permanent front teeth may also be affected if tetracyclines are given to children up to six years and the permanent back teeth if tetracyclines are given to children up to twelve years.

The antibiotics of this group readily decompose on storage, especially in the presence of warmth and moisture, giving toxic decomposition products which cause nausea, glycosuria, proteinuria, and aminoaciduria.

Dose. See above under **Actions and uses.**

Preparations
TETRACYCLINE CAPSULES, B.P. Unless otherwise specified, capsules each containing 250 mg of tetracycline hydrochloride are supplied. Capsules containing 50 mg are also available.

TETRACYCLINE INJECTION, B.P. It consists of a sterile solution prepared by dissolving the sterile contents of a sealed container in Water for Injections. The quantity of tetracycline hydrochloride in each container should be specified by the prescriber. It should be used within seventy-two hours of preparation and it should be stored during this period at a temperature not exceeding 4°. For intravenous infusion. Vials containing 250 and 500 mg are available.

TETRACYCLINE AND PROCAINE INJECTION, B.P.C. (page 719)

TETRACYCLINE TABLETS, B.P. Unless otherwise specified, tablets each containing 250 mg of tetracycline hydrochloride are supplied. These tablets are film coated or sugar coated. Tablets containing 50, 100, and 500 mg are also available.

OTHER NAMES: *Achromycin*®; *Clinitetrin*®; *Economycin*®; *Steclin*®; *Telotrex*®; *Tetrachel*®; *Tetracyn*®; *Totomycin*®

PREPARED THEOBROMA

SYNONYMS: Non-alkalised Cocoa Powder; Prep. Theobrom.; Theobroma Praeparata

Prepared Theobroma is roasted theobroma seed deprived of most of its shell, pressed to remove a portion of its fat, and finely ground. Theobroma seed consists of the fermented and dried seeds of *Theobroma cacao* L. (Fam. Sterculiaceae), a tree cultivated in West Africa and other tropical countries.

Prepared Theobroma should not have undergone any process of "alkalisation" during its manufacture. It is often flavoured by the addition of vanillin or cinnamon.

Constituents. Prepared Theobroma contains about 15 to 30 per cent of fat (cocoa butter) and 0·5 to 2 per cent of theobromine; it yields about 6 per cent of ash.

Standard
DESCRIPTION. *Macroscopical:* A light-brown to dark reddish-brown powder; odour and taste similar to

those of theobroma seed but generally more aromatic.

Microscopical: The diagnostic characters are: polyhedral parenchymatous cells of the cotyledons, some containing a reddish-brown pigment (cocoa red), starch granules, simple or 2- or 3-compound, up to 15 μm in diameter, fat, and aleurone grains; traces only of shell tissue are present.

ALKALI. pH, determined electrometrically, of a suspension of 10 g in 30 ml of *carbon dioxide-free water*, not more than 6·0.

FOREIGN STARCHES. Absent.

CONTENT OF FAT. Not less than 15·0 per cent, determined by extraction with *light petroleum (boiling-range, 40° to 60°)* in an apparatus for the continuous extraction of drugs.

Adulterants and substitutes. Cocoa shell, the seed coat of the cocoa seed, has a layer, one cell thick, of sclereids, each about 5 to 10 μm wide and 10 to 30 μm long, a subepidermal layer of mucilage cells which stain with *ruthenium red solution*, and a few slender spiral vessels, about 10 to 20 μm wide, singly or in groups of up to about 6, traversing a spongy parenchyma with subcircular intercellular spaces enclosed by the arm-like projections of the cells.

Storage. It should be stored in airtight containers.

Uses. Prepared Theobroma is used as a basis in the preparation of some tablets. The "chocolate basis" for tablets consists of a mixture of Prepared Theobroma 15 parts, sucrose 15 parts, and lactose 70 parts.

THEOBROMA OIL

SYNONYMS: Cocoa Butter; Oleum Theobromatis

Theobroma Oil is the solid fat obtained from the crushed and roasted seeds of *Theobroma cacao* L. (Fam. Sterculiaceae), a tree cultivated in West Africa and other tropical countries, and is obtained as a by-product in the manufacture of cocoa.

Constituents. Theobroma oil contains about 55 per cent of oleopalmitostearin with small quantities of the glycerides of linoleic and other fatty acids.

Solubility. Slightly soluble in alcohol; soluble in ether, in chloroform, in boiling dehydrated alcohol, and in light petroleum.

Standard
It complies with the requirements of the British Pharmacopoeia.
It is a yellowish-white solid, becoming white on keeping. It has a faint agreeable odour resembling that of

cocoa; it is sometimes deodorised. It is usually supplied in oblong cakes; it is brittle when cold and breaks with a smooth fracture which shows indications of crystalline structure; it becomes soft at 25° and has a melting-point of 31° to 34°.

Adulterants and substitutes. Paraffin, stearin, tallow, Borneo tallow, and other fats have been reported as adulterants.

Uses. Theobroma oil is used for the preparation of suppositories, pessaries, and bougies.

THEOBROMINE

SYNONYM: Theobrominum

$C_7H_8N_4O_2 = 180·2$

Theobromine is 3,7-dimethylxanthine, an alkaloid contained in the seeds of *Theobroma cacao* L. (Fam. Sterculiaceae).

With alkali hydroxides, theobromine forms salts and is not extracted from alkaline solution by shaking with immiscible solvents. Theobromine sublimes at about 290° without decomposition.

Solubility. Very slightly soluble in water, in alcohol, and in chloroform; insoluble in ether; soluble in solutions of alkali hydroxides and in dilute mineral acids.

Standard
Material which complies with this standard meets the requirements of the European Pharmacopoeia.

DESCRIPTION. A white crystalline powder or rhombic needles; odourless.

IDENTIFICATION TESTS. 1. Mix 5 mg with 0·25 ml of *strong hydrogen peroxide solution*, add 0·25 ml of *dilute hydrochloric acid*, and evaporate to dryness on a waterbath; the residue is yellowish-red. Add 0·05 ml of *dilute ammonia solution*; the colour changes to reddish-violet.

2. Dissolve, with the aid of gentle heat, 0·02 g in 2 ml of *dilute ammonia solution*, cool, and add 2 ml of *dilute*

silver nitrate solution; the solution remains clear. Boil the solution gently for a few minutes; a white crystalline precipitate is produced.

ACIDITY. pH of a solution prepared by boiling 1·0 g in 50 ml of water, cooling, and filtering, 5·5 to 7·0.

FOREIGN CARBONISABLE SUBSTANCES. Dissolve 0·10 g in 2 ml of *sulphuric acid*. This solution complies with the following tests:

(i) The solution is clear when compared with *sulphuric acid*, the comparison being made by viewing 2 ml of the liquids in matched, colourless, transparent, neutral glass tubes, 12 mm internal diameter, in darkness and with a beam of light being passed laterally through the liquids from an electric lamp giving a luminosity of 1000 lux at a distance of 1 m.

(ii) The solution is not more intensely coloured than a reference solution prepared by mixing 0·1 ml of *yellow standard solution* with 1·9 ml of *diluted hydrochloric acid (1 per cent w/v)*, the comparison being made by viewing horizontally 2 ml of the liquids in matched, colourless, transparent, neutral glass tubes, 12 mm internal diameter, against a white background in diffused daylight.

ALKALOIDS. To 0·50 g add 5 ml of water and 1 ml of *dilute sulphuric acid*, shake vigorously, filter, and to the filtrate add 0·25 ml of *potassium mercuri-iodide solution*.
Compare the solution with *dilute sulphuric acid* in the manner described in test (i), given above under Foreign Carbonisable Substances; the solution remains clear for not less than 5 minutes.

THEOPHYLLINE. Dissolve 0·50 g in 10 ml of 4N sodium hydroxide. This solution complies with the following tests:
(i) The solution is clear or not more opalescent than a reference solution prepared by mixing 0·05 ml of 0·00002M sodium chloride, 0·75 ml of water, 1·0 ml of 2M nitric acid, and 0·2 ml of *dilute silver nitrate solution*, the comparison being made, 5 minutes after preparation of the reference solution, in the manner described in test (i), given above under Foreign Carbonisable Substances.
(ii) It complies with test (ii), given above under Foreign Carbonisable Substances.

CAFFEINE. Not more than 0·8 per cent, determined by the following method:
Transfer the solution prepared in the test for Theophylline to a separating funnel, add 30 ml of water and 50 ml of *chloroform*, shake, and allow to separate; dry the chloroform layer over *anhydrous sodium sulphate*, filter, evaporate 25 ml of the filtrate to dryness, dry the residue in a desiccator, and weigh.

LOSS ON DRYING. Not more than 0·5 per cent, determined by drying to constant weight at 105°.

SULPHATED ASH. Not more than 0·1 per cent.

CONTENT OF $C_7H_8N_4O_2$. Not less than 99·0 per cent, calculated with reference to the substance dried under the prescribed conditions, determined by the following method:
Dissolve, by boiling gently, about 0·3 g, accurately weighed, in 125 ml of water, cool to about 50° to 60°, add 25 ml of 0·1N silver nitrate, and titrate with 0·1N sodium hydroxide, using *bromothymol blue solution* as indicator; each ml of 0·1N sodium hydroxide is equivalent to 0·01802 g of $C_7H_8N_4O_2$.

Actions and uses. Theobromine has an action on the kidney similar to that described under Caffeine (page 63) but has no stimulant effect upon the central nervous system. In the form of Phenobarbitone and Theobromine Tablets, it has been employed to allay the nervous excitement and insomnia associated with hypertension, but this preparation has no advantage over phenobarbitone alone.

UNDESIRABLE EFFECTS. In large doses, theobromine may cause nausea and loss of appetite.

Dose. 300 to 600 milligrams.

Preparation
PHENOBARBITONE AND THEOBROMINE TABLETS, B.P.C. (page 814)

THEOPHYLLINE

SYNONYMS: Anhydrous Theophylline; Theophyllinum

$C_7H_8N_4O_2 = 180·2$

Theophylline is 1,3-dimethylxanthine, an alkaloid isomeric with theobromine.

Theophylline is a weak base, forming salts with acids and soluble derivatives with alkali metals. It may be extracted from slightly acid solution by a mixture of isopropyl alcohol and chloroform.

Solubility. Soluble, at 25°, in 120 parts of water and in 80 parts of alcohol; slightly soluble in ether; soluble in solutions of alkali hydroxides.

Standard
It complies with the requirements of the European Pharmacopoeia.
It is a white, crystalline, odourless powder and contains not less than 99·0 and not more than the equivalent of 101·0 per cent of $C_7H_8N_4O_2$, calculated with reference to the dried substance. The loss on drying under the prescribed conditions is not more than 0·5 per cent. It has a melting-point of 270° to 274° after drying at 100° to 105°.

Actions and uses. Theophylline has actions resembling those of the other xanthine derivatives, caffeine and theobromine. Its diuretic action, although stronger than that of caffeine, is of short duration. It is a more powerful relaxant of involuntary muscle than theobromine or caffeine. It has only a slight stimulant action on the cerebrum. Because of its low solubility, theophylline itself is seldom used, its more soluble derivatives, such as aminophylline and choline theophyllinate, being preferred.

UNDESIRABLE EFFECTS. Theophylline may cause gastric irritation, nausea, and vomiting.

Dose. 60 to 200 milligrams.

Preparations
AMINOPHYLLINE INJECTION, B.P. (*Syn.* Theophylline and Ethylenediamine Injection). It consists of a sterile solution of aminophylline in Water for Injections free from carbon dioxide. For intravenous injection, unless otherwise specified, a solution containing 250 mg in 10 ml is supplied.
MERSALYL INJECTION, B.P. (*Syn.* Mersalyl and Theophylline Injection). It consists of a sterile solution containing 10 per cent of the sodium salt of mersalyl acid and 5 per cent of theophylline in Water for Injections, the pH of the solution being adjusted to 8·0. It should be protected from light. Dose: 0·5 to 2 millilitres by intramuscular injection, on alternate days.

THEOPHYLLINE HYDRATE

SYNONYM: Theophyllinum Monohydricum

$C_7H_8N_4O_2,H_2O = 198.2$

Theophylline hydrate is 1,3-dimethylxanthine monohydrate.

Solubility. Soluble, at $25°$, in 120 parts of water and in 80 parts of alcohol; slightly soluble in ether; soluble in solutions of alkali hydroxides.

Standard
It complies with the requirements of the European Pharmacopoeia.
It is a white, crystalline, odourless powder and contains not less than 99.0 and not more than the equivalent of

101.0 per cent of $C_7H_8N_4O_2$, calculated with reference to the dried substance. The loss on drying under the prescribed conditions is 8.0 to 9.5 per cent. It has a melting-point of $270°$ to $274°$ after drying at $100°$ to $105°$.

Actions and uses. Theophylline hydrate has the actions, uses, and undesirable effects described under Theophylline.

THIABENDAZOLE

$C_{10}H_7N_3S = 201.2$

Thiabendazole is 2-(4-thiazolyl)benzimidazole.

Solubility. Very slightly soluble in water; soluble, at $20°$, in 150 parts of alcohol and in 300 parts of chloroform; slightly soluble in ether; soluble in dilute mineral acids.

Standard
DESCRIPTION. A white or almost white powder; odourless or almost odourless.

IDENTIFICATION TESTS. 1. Dissolve 5 mg in 5 ml of 0.1N hydrochloric acid, add 3 mg of p-*phenylene-diamine dihydrochloride*, shake until dissolved, add 0.1 g of *zinc powder*, mix, and allow to stand for 2 minutes; the odour of hydrogen sulphide is produced. Add 10 ml of *ferric ammonium sulphate solution*; a deep blue or blue-violet colour is produced.
Caution. p-Phenylenediamine dihydrochloride may cause dermatitis. It should be handled with care and contact with the skin should be avoided.

2. It melts at about $300°$.

3. The ultraviolet absorption spectrum exhibits the characteristics given in Appendix 3, page 856.

4. The infra-red absorption spectrum exhibits maxima which are only at the same wavelengths as, and have similar relative intensities to, those in the spectrum of *thiabendazole A.S.*

LOSS ON DRYING. Not more than 0.5 per cent, determined by drying to constant weight at $105°$.

SULPHATED ASH. Not more than 0.1 per cent.

CONTENT OF $C_{10}H_7N_3S$. Not less than 98.0 and not more than the equivalent of 101.0 per cent, calculated with reference to the substance dried under the prescribed conditions, determined by the following method:
Titrate about 0.16 g, accurately weighed, by Method I of the British Pharmacopoeia, Appendix XIB, for non-aqueous titration; each ml of 0.1N perchloric acid is equivalent to 0.02013 g of $C_{10}H_7N_3S$.

Actions and uses. Thiabendazole is an anthelmintic which is administered orally and absorbed from the gastro-intestinal tract, reaching maximal concentration in the blood three hours after ingestion. Excretion is mainly in the urine and a single dose is almost completely eliminated in five days.
Its principal use in human medicine is against *Strongyloides stercoralis* and *Trichuris*

trichiura, and in creeping eruption (infection with larval forms of *Ancyclostoma caninum* or *A. braziliense*). For infections with round-worm, threadworm, and hookworm in man other less toxic drugs are available.
It has been used against *Trichinella spiralis* but its action against the larval forms of this parasite in human tissue is uncertain.

UNDESIRABLE EFFECTS. Anorexia, nausea, vomiting, and epigastric discomfort may occur, and less commonly xanthopsia (yellow vision), pruritus, rashes, diarrhoea, headache, and drowsiness. Fever, chills, and lymphadeno-pathy have been reported but may represent allergic response to dead parasites. A decrease in blood pressure and pulse rate may be noted. Crystalluria without haematuria has been reported but promptly disappears on discontinuing ingestion of the drug.
Some persons during treatment may excrete a metabolite that imparts to the urine an odour similar to that which may occur after ingestion of asparagus. The odour usually disappears not more than twenty-four hours after taking the last dose.

PRECAUTIONS AND CONTRA-INDICATIONS. No teratogenic effect has been observed, but in the case of pregnant women, unless the symptoms produced by a helminthic infection are severe, it is in general best to postpone anthelmintic therapy until after parturition.

Dose. 25 milligrams per kilogram body-weight twice daily for two to three days, or for mass therapy 50 milligrams per kilogram body-weight as a single dose.

Preparation
THIABENDAZOLE TABLETS, B.P.C. (page 817)

OTHER NAME: *Mintezol®*

THIACETAZONE

$C_{10}H_{12}N_4OS = 236·3$

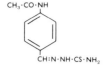

Thiacetazone is *p*-formylacetanilide thiosemicarbazone.

Solubility. Very slightly soluble in water; soluble, at 20°, in 500 parts of alcohol and in 100 parts of propylene glycol.

Standard

DESCRIPTION. Pale yellow crystals or crystalline powder; odourless or almost odourless.

IDENTIFICATION TESTS. 1. Boil 0·01 g with 5 ml of 1N hydrochloric acid for 3 minutes, cool, and add sufficient water to produce 200 ml. Mix 5 ml of this solution with 0·25 ml of *sodium nitrite solution* and add the mixture to 0·5 ml of *β-naphthol solution*; a red colour is produced.
2. Dissolve, with the aid of heat, 0·01 g in 1 ml of 6N sodium hydroxide, add 0·25 ml of *lead acetate solution*, and boil for 1 minute; a black precipitate is produced.
3. It complies with the thin-layer chromatographic test given in Appendix 5A, page 869.
4. The ultraviolet absorption spectrum exhibits the characteristics given in Appendix 3, page 856.
5. The infra-red absorption spectrum exhibits maxima which are only at the same wavelengths as, and have similar relative intensities to, those in the spectrum of *thiacetazone A.S.*

LEAD. It complies with the test given in Appendix 7, page 884 (10 parts per million).

p-ACETAMIDOBENZALAZINE. It complies with the test given in Appendix 5A, page 869 (0·2 per cent).

THIOSEMICARBAZIDE. Not more than 0·1 per cent, determined by the following method:
To 2·0 g, finely powdered, add sufficient water to produce 50 ml, shake, allow to stand for 1 hour with occasional shaking, and filter, discarding the first portion of the filtrate; acidify 25 ml of the clear filtrate with *dilute sulphuric acid*, add 0·1 ml of *ferroin sulphate solution*, and titrate with 0·1N ceric ammonium sulphate to a blue end-point which persists for 1 minute; not more than 0·8 ml is required.

LOSS ON DRYING. Not more than 0·5 per cent, determined by drying to constant weight at 105°.

SULPHATED ASH. Not more than 0·2 per cent.

CONTENT OF $C_{10}H_{12}N_4OS$. Not less than 98·0 and not more than the equivalent of 102·0 per cent, calculated with reference to the substance dried under the prescribed conditions, determined by the following method:
Dissolve about 0·1 g, accurately weighed, in 60 ml of *methyl alcohol* by heating to 60° on a water-bath, slowly add 20 ml of hot *methanolic silver nitrate solution*, maintain the solution at 60° until the precipitate coagulates and leaves a clear supernatant liquid, cool, filter through a sintered-glass crucible (British Standard Grade No. 4), wash the residue with *methyl alcohol* until the washings are free from silver nitrate, and dry to constant weight at 105°; each g of residue is equivalent to 0·4606 g of $C_{10}H_{12}N_4OS$.

Storage. It should be stored in airtight containers, protected from light.

Actions and uses. Thiacetazone inhibits the growth of *Mycobacterium tuberculosis* and of *M. leprae* and is used in the treatment of tuberculosis and leprosy. Peak tissue levels are achieved three to five hours after administration by mouth and excretion is complete in about forty-eight hours. There are marked regional differences in the incidence of undesirable effects which seem to depend on the state of nutrition and presence of other endemic diseases in the populations concerned. In tolerant populations thiacetazone may be used in conjunction with streptomycin and isoniazid as a first choice in the treatment of susceptible infections. In most countries, however, its use is limited to the treatment of infections that are resistant to other drugs. Cross-resistance between thiacetazone and ethionamide or prothionamide may occur.

The usual adult dose in the treatment of tuberculosis is 150 milligrams, or 2 milligrams per kilogram body-weight, given daily in a single dose, but it is preferable to commence treatment with approximately one-tenth of the quantity and gradually increase the dose over a period of a week or ten days to establish the maximum that the patient will tolerate.

Thiacetazone should always be given simultaneously with other drugs to delay the development of resistance.

In the treatment of leprosy, the usual initial dose is 50 milligrams daily, gradually increasing over a period of four to eight weeks to a total daily dose of 150 milligrams.

UNDESIRABLE EFFECTS. Allergic reactions commonly occur but are usually mild and subside rapidly when treatment is discontinued, but rashes and fever may be followed by the Stevens-Johnson syndrome, agranulocytosis, and similar serious or fatal responses if treatment is continued.

Dizziness, deafness, nausea, vomiting, and hepatitis may occur in patients being treated with thiacetazone in conjunction with other drugs. Displacement of streptomycin from protein binding sites or interference with renal excretion may be responsible for increased eighth-nerve damage when thiacetazone is used in treatment schemes that include streptomycin.

Dose. See above under **Actions and uses.**

Preparation

THIACETAZONE TABLETS, B.P.C. (page 817)

OTHER NAME: *Thioparamizone*®

THIAMBUTOSINE

$C_{19}H_{25}N_3OS = 343.5$

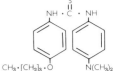

Thiambutosine is *N-p*-butoxyphenyl-*N'-p*-dimethylaminophenyl-thiourea.

Solubility. Very slightly soluble in water; soluble, at 20°, in 300 parts of ether and in 1.5 parts of chloroform; soluble in acetone.

Standard
It complies with the requirements of the British Pharmacopoeia.
It is a white or creamy-white, crystalline, odourless powder and contains not less than 99.0 and not more than the equivalent of 101.0 per cent of $C_{19}H_{25}N_3OS$. It has a melting-point of 123° to 127°.

Storage. It should be stored in airtight containers, protected from light.

Actions and uses. Thiambutosine, like dapsone, is given by mouth in the treatment of leprosy, but it causes less reaction than dapsone. It is particularly valuable in dimorphous cases with considerable tissue exacerbation and in tuberculoid cases.

It is used in a dosage of 500 milligrams daily, which is increased when necessary up to a maximum of 2 grams. Treatment may be continued for up to two years, after which time resistance may occur; thereafter dapsone can usually be given.

Thiambutosine has been used in conjunction with sulphones or with isoniazid, but it is more valuable when used alone in patients who react badly to dapsone. It has also proved useful in patients with severe neuritis who are sometimes intolerant of sulphones.

UNDESIRABLE EFFECTS. Antithyroid actions may occur with high dosage, but this is very rare. Occasional skin eruptions may occur, but usually it is not necessary to discontinue treatment.

Dose. See above under **Actions and uses.**

Preparation
THIAMBUTOSINE TABLETS, B.P. Unless otherwise specified, tablets each containing 500 mg of thiambutosine are supplied. They should be stored in airtight containers, protected from light.

OTHER NAME: *Ciba-1906®*

THIAMINE HYDROCHLORIDE

SYNONYMS: Aneurine Hydrochloride; Thiaminii Chloridum; Vitamin B_1

$C_{12}H_{18}Cl_2N_4OS = 337.3$

Thiamine Hydrochloride is 3-(4-amino-2-methylpyrimidin-5-ylmethyl)-5-(2-hydroxyethyl)-4-methylthiazolium chloride hydrochloride.

Solubility. Soluble, at 20°, in 1 part of water, in 100 parts of alcohol, and in 20 parts of glycerol; soluble in methyl alcohol; very slightly soluble in dehydrated alcohol, in ether, and in acetone.

Standard
It complies with the requirements of the European Pharmacopoeia.
It occurs as colourless crystals or white or almost white crystalline powder with a characteristic odour and contains not less than 98.5 cent of $C_{12}H_{18}Cl_2N_4OS$, not less than 20.6 and not more than 21.2 per cent of total Cl, and not less than 10.4 and not more than 10.7 per cent of Cl present as monohydrochloride, calculated with reference to the dried substance. The loss on drying under the prescribed conditions is not more than 5.0 per cent. A 2.5 per cent solution in water has a pH of 2.7 to 3.3.

Stability. Solutions of pH 4.0 or less deteriorate only slowly, but neutral or alkaline solutions deteriorate rapidly, especially on exposure to air.

Sterilisation. Solutions for injection are sterilised by filtration.

Storage. It should be stored in airtight containers, protected from light, contact with metal being avoided.

Actions and uses. Thiamine, in the form of its pyrophosphate (co-carboxylase), is the prosthetic group for the enzymes involved in the decarboxylation of pyruvic and α-ketoglutaric acids. It therefore plays an important part in the intermediary metabolism of carbohydrate. In thiamine deficiency the oxidation of α-ketoacids is impaired and the blood pyruvate rises.

Thiamine is widely distributed in foods, the richest sources being whole grains, pulses, yeast, and pork. It is absorbed mainly from the small intestine, although there is some evidence that bacterial synthesis and absorption occur in the large intestine. Before utilisation, thiamine must be phosphorylated, a process which occurs in all nucleated cells, particularly in the liver, kidney, and white blood cells. The optimum intake is believed to be about 1 milligram daily.

Requirements are directly related to the carbohydrate intake and metabolic rate and are increased in pregnancy, lactation, hyperthyroidism, pyrexia, exercise, and conditions causing increased metabolism or diuresis.

Thiamine has no therapeutic value apart from the treatment of thiamine deficiency. In beriberi there is a severe deficiency, not only of thiamine but of other factors of the vitamin-B group. Thiamine has been administered for the treatment of neuritis of varying etiology, but evidence of its value is lacking, unless the neuritis is due to thiamine deficiency.

There are a number of diseases in which thiamine deficiency may be caused by interference with its ingestion, absorption, and utilisation or by increasing its destruction or excretion. This is likely to occur, for example, in patients on restricted diets and in those suffering from gastro-intestinal diseases, some forms of mental disease, or alcoholism. Some cases of pregnancy neuritis may be due to thiamine deficiency. It is rational to supplement the diet in such cases not only with thiamine but also with other vitamins.

Thiamine is usually given by mouth; parenteral administration is unnecessary, except for patients with impaired absorption or acute cardiac beriberi.

UNDESIRABLE EFFECTS. Toxic effects have been produced by injections of 50 milligrams of thiamine hydrochloride. Large doses may also interfere with the metabolism of other vitamins of the vitamin-B group and may precipitate the symptoms of other deficiency states in poorly nourished patients. Except in the initial treatment of acute cardiac beriberi, there is no justification for the administration of single doses in excess of 10 milligrams.

Dose. Prophylactic, 2 to 5 milligrams by mouth daily; therapeutic, 25 to 100 milligrams by mouth or by subcutaneous or intramuscular injection daily.

Preparations
VITAMINS CAPSULES, B.P.C. (page 654)
THIAMINE HYDROCHLORIDE INJECTION, B.P. (*Syn.* Vitamin B$_1$ Injection). It consists of a sterile solution of thiamine hydrochloride in Water for Injections. Unless otherwise specified, a solution containing 25 mg in 1 ml is supplied. It should be protected from light. A solution containing 100 mg in 2 ml is also available.
VITAMINS B AND C INJECTION, B.P.C. (page 720)
THIAMINE HYDROCHLORIDE TABLETS, B.P. (*Syn.* Vitamin B$_1$ Tablets). Unless otherwise specified, tablets each containing 3 mg of thiamine hydrochloride are supplied. They should be stored in airtight containers, contact with metal being avoided, and protected from light. Tablets containing 5, 10, 25, 50, 100, and 300 mg are also available.
VITAMIN B TABLETS, COMPOUND, B.P.C. (page 819)
VITAMIN B TABLETS, COMPOUND, STRONG, B.P.C. (page 819)

OTHER NAME: *Benerva*®

THIOMERSAL

SYNONYM: Thimerosal

$C_9H_9HgNaO_2S = 404.8$

Thiomersal is sodium *o*-(ethylmercurithio)benzoate

Solubility. Soluble, at 20°, in 1 part of water and in 8 parts of alcohol; very slightly soluble in ether.

Standard
It complies with the requirements of the British Pharmacopoeia.
It is a light, cream-coloured, crystalline powder with a slight characteristic odour and contains not less than 98.0 per cent of $C_9H_9HgNaO_2S$, calculated with reference to the dried substance. The loss on drying under the prescribed conditions is not more than 0.5 per cent. A 1 per cent solution in water has a pH of 6.8 to 8.0.

Incompatibility. It is incompatible with acids, salts of heavy metals, and iodine, and it forms precipitates with many alkaloids.
The rate of oxidation of thiomersal in solution is greatly increased when traces of copper ions are present. In slightly acid solutions thiomersal is converted to *o*-(ethylmercurithio)benzoic acid which is soluble in about 3500 parts of water and so may be precipitated; solutions of the free acid undergo slow decomposition with the formation of insoluble products.

Sterilisation. Solutions are sterilised by heating in an autoclave or by filtration.

Storage. It should be protected from light.

Preparation and storage of solutions. See statement on aqueous solutions of antiseptics, under Solutions (page 779).

Actions and uses. Thiomersal has an antibacterial action on some non-sporing organisms; it is also a fungicide. A 0.1 per cent solution is used for the pre-operative sterilisation of the skin. A cream containing 0.1 per cent is applied in mycotic infections of the skin.

Thiomersal is also used as a preservative in biological products, usually in a concentration of 0.01 to 0.02 per cent.

OTHER NAMES: *Merthiolate*®; Thiomersalate

THIOPENTONE SODIUM

SYNONYMS: Soluble Thiopentone; Thiopent. Sod.;
Thiopentalum Natricum

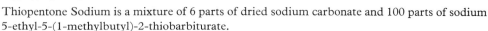

$C_{11}H_{17}N_2NaO_2S = 264·3$

Thiopentone Sodium is a mixture of 6 parts of dried sodium carbonate and 100 parts of sodium 5-ethyl-5-(1-methylbutyl)-2-thiobarbiturate.

Solubility. Soluble, at 20°, in 1·5 parts of water; partly soluble in alcohol; insoluble in ether.

Standard
It complies with the requirements of the European Pharmacopoeia.
It is a yellowish-white hygroscopic powder with a characteristic alliaceous odour and contains the equivalent of not less than 84·0 and not more than 87·0 per cent of $C_{11}H_{18}N_2O_2S$ and not less than 10·0 and not more than 11·0 per cent of Na, both calculated with reference to the dried substance. The loss on drying under the prescribed conditions is not more than 2·5 per cent.

Storage. It should be stored in airtight containers.

Actions and uses. Thiopentone is a very short-acting barbiturate, the actions and uses of which are described under Phenobarbitone (page 366). It is administered intravenously for the induction of general anaesthesia or for the production of complete anaesthesia of short duration. It is most useful for short operations, especially when inhalation anaesthetics are not available or are contra-indicated. In dental practice, it may be used for short easy extractions. For inducing anaesthesia, 100 to 150 milligrams, as a 2·5 or, occasionally, 5 per cent solution, is injected over ten to fifteen seconds; if relaxation has not occurred in about thirty seconds, a further 100 to 150 milligrams may be given. Injections should be given with the patient in the recumbent position and care should be taken to see that none of the solution is injected outside the vein, as it may cause tissue necrosis.

For longer procedures, repeated or continuous administration may be used. It may be administered by rectum as a basal anaesthetic in a dose of 40 milligrams per kilogram body-weight, with a maximum of 2 grams, dissolved in about 30 millilitres of Purified Water.

Solutions for injection are prepared by an aseptic technique.

PRECAUTIONS AND CONTRA-INDICATIONS. Thiopentone should not be used in patients with impaired liver function or low blood pressure. The chief danger arising during anaesthesia with thiopentone is respiratory depression and means for treating respiratory failure should be at hand.

POISONING. As for Phenobarbitone (page 366).

Dose. See above under **Actions and uses.**

Preparation
THIOPENTONE INJECTION, B.P. It consists of a sterile solution prepared immediately before use by dissolving the sterile contents of a sealed container in Water for Injections. The quantity of thiopentone sodium in each container should be specified by the prescriber. Vials containing 0·25, 0·5, 1, 2·5, and 5 g are available.

OTHER NAMES: *Intraval Sodium*®; *Pentothal*®

THIOPROPAZATE HYDROCHLORIDE

$C_{23}H_{30}Cl_3N_3O_2S = 518·9$

Thiopropazate Hydrochloride is 10-{3-[4-(2-acetoxyethyl)piperazin-1-yl]propyl}-2-chloro-phenothiazine dihydrochloride.

CAUTION. *Thiopropazate may cause severe dermatitis in sensitised persons, and pharmacists, nurses, and others who handle the drug frequently should wear masks and rubber gloves.*

Solubility. Soluble, at 20°, in 4 parts of water, in 126 parts of alcohol, and in 65 parts of chloroform; insoluble in ether.

Standard
DESCRIPTION. An almost white crystalline powder; odour faint.

IDENTIFICATION TESTS. 1. Dissolve 5 mg in 1 ml of *sulphuric acid*; a red colour is produced. Warm; the colour changes to brown.
2. It complies with the thin-layer chromatographic test given in Appendix 5C, page 873.
3. The ultraviolet absorption spectrum exhibits the characteristics given in Appendix 3, page 856.
4. The infra-red absorption spectrum exhibits maxima which are only at the same wavelengths as, and have similar relative intensities to, those in the spectrum of *thiopropazate hydrochloride A.S.*
5. It gives the reactions characteristic of chlorides.

ACIDITY. pH of a 10·0 per cent w/v solution in water, 1·4 to 1·7.

MELTING-POINT. 228° to 232°.

LOSS ON DRYING. Not more than 1·0 per cent, determined by drying to constant weight at 105°.

SULPHATED ASH. Not more than 0·1 per cent.

CONTENT OF $C_{23}H_{30}Cl_3N_3O_2S$. Not less than 98·0 and not more than the equivalent of 101·0 per cent, calculated with reference to the substance dried under the prescribed conditions, determined by the following method:
Dissolve about 0·6 g, accurately weighed, in a mixture

of 30 ml of *glacial acetic acid* and 20 ml of *acetone* and titrate by Method I of the British Pharmacopoeia, Appendix XIB, for non-aqueous titration, using 0·1N perchloric acid in dioxan as the titrant; each ml of 0·1N perchloric acid in dioxan is equivalent to 0·02595 g of $C_{23}H_{30}Cl_3N_3O_2S$.

Actions and uses. Thiopropazate has the actions and uses described under Chlorpromazine Hydrochloride (page 107), but it is effective in much smaller doses and has relatively little sedative effect. It is valuable as an antisialagogue before induction of anaesthesia and in the control of Huntingdon's chorea and cerebellar ataxia.

UNDESIRABLE EFFECTS. Although thiopropazate does not produce the jaundice which may occur during treatment with chlorpromazine, it occasionally produces hypotension, blurring of vision, and an erythematous rash.

Coating of the tablets reduces the risk of sensitisation amongst persons who handle the drug frequently.

In high doses, extrapyramidal effects may occur; in these circumstances the dosage should be reduced, or an antiparkinsonism drug may be given at the same time.

PRECAUTIONS. Thiopropazate may enhance the sedative effect of barbiturates, alcohol, and narcotic drugs. When it is used in epileptic states the dosage of anticonvulsant drugs should not be reduced.

POISONING. As for Chlorpromazine Hydrochloride (page 107).

Dose. 5 to 10 milligrams three times daily.

Preparation
THIOPROPAZATE TABLETS, B.P.C. (page 817)

OTHER NAME: *Dartalan*®

THIORIDAZINE HYDROCHLORIDE

$C_{21}H_{27}ClN_2S_2 = 407·0$

Thioridazine Hydrochloride is 10-[2-(1-methylpiperid-2-yl)ethyl]-2-methylthiophenothiazine hydrochloride.

Solubility. Soluble, at 20°, in 9 parts of water, in 10 parts of alcohol, and in 1·5 parts of chloroform; very slightly soluble in ether.

Standard
It complies with the requirements of the British Pharmacopoeia.
It is a white or cream-coloured, crystalline powder with a slight odour and contains not less than 99·0 and not more than the equivalent of 101·0 per cent of $C_{21}H_{27}ClN_2S_2$, calculated with reference to the dried substance. The loss on drying under the prescribed conditions is not more than 0·5 per cent. It has a melting-point of 159° to 163°. A 10 per cent solution in water has a pH of 3·5 to 4·5.

Storage. It should be stored in airtight containers, protected from light.

Actions and uses. Thioridazine has a tranquillising action similar to that described under Chlorpromazine Hydrochloride (page 107) but it has no therapeutically significant anti-emetic or hypothermic action and does not potentiate the action of anaesthetics.
Thioridazine is used mainly for the treatment of schizophrenia and for the control of mania and agitation. It may be used in the management of anxiety states and in children with behaviour problems. It is contra-indicated in severely depressed patients.
In severe mental illness the usual initial daily

dosage for an adult is up to 600 milligrams of thioridazine hydrochloride by mouth; this is later reduced to a maintenance dosage of 100 to 200 milligrams daily.
In treating children with behaviour problems, the basic dosage is 1 milligram per kilogram body-weight daily in divided doses.

UNDESIRABLE EFFECTS. The incidence of extrapyramidal side-effects is low. Amenorrhoea, galactorrhoea, hypotension, ventricular arrhythmias and, rarely, oedema, weight gain, blood dyscrasias, and photo-allergic and phototoxic reactions may occur. Pigmentary retinopathy may occur within four to eight weeks of treatment with a dose of 1 gram or more daily.

POISONING. The procedure described under Chlorpromazine Hydrochloride (page 107) should be adopted.

Dose. See above under **Actions and uses.**

Preparation
THIORIDAZINE TABLETS, B.P. The quantity of thioridazine hydrochloride in each tablet should be specified by the prescriber. They are sugar coated. Tablets containing 10, 25, 50, and 100 mg are available.

OTHER NAME: *Melleril*®

THIOTEPA

$C_6H_{12}N_3PS = 189·2$

Thiotepa is triaziridin-1-ylphosphine sulphide.

Solubility. Soluble, at 20°, in 8 parts of water, in 2 parts of alcohol, and in 2 parts of chloroform.

Standard
It complies with the requirements of the British Pharmacopoeia.
It occurs as fine, white, crystalline flakes with a faint odour and contains not less than 97·0 and not more than the equivalent of 102·0 per cent of $C_6H_{12}N_3PS$, calculated with reference to the anhydrous substance. It contains not more than 2·0 per cent w/w of water. It has a melting-point of 52° to 57°.

Storage. It should be stored in airtight containers at a temperature between 2° and 10°. At higher temperatures it polymerises and becomes inactive.

Actions and uses. Thiotepa, a cytotoxic alkylating agent with actions similar to those of mustine, is believed to act by releasing ethyleneimine radicals which have a marked cytotoxic effect on rapidly dividing cells by inhibiting nucleic acid synthesis. Like other drugs of this type, thiotepa prevents mitosis and damages the chromosomes.

Thiotepa is one of the less toxic alkylating agents and, although it produces destruction of tissues composed of rapidly dividing cells such as the bone marrow, the gastro-intestinal mucosa, and the gonads, cells with a low rate of mitosis are less affected. There is no selective uptake of thiotepa by any organ or tissue and it is rapidly broken down and excreted.

Thiotepa is used for the palliative treatment of widespread malignant disease, particularly carcinoma of the breast and ovary, chronic leukaemia, lymphosarcoma, reticulosarcoma, and Hodgkin's disease. It has also been used for the treatment of advanced malignant disease of the lung, gastro-intestinal tract, and genito-urinary and central nervous systems, although with less benefit. Remissions have been obtained in some cases of malignant melanoma.

Local instillation is sometimes employed to prevent the reaccumulation of fluid in patients with malignant pleural effusions and ascites. For the latter purpose thiotepa is preferred to mustine as it is not vesicant.

Thiotepa has been used in combination with the surgical ablation of malignant tumours to prevent the spread of tumour cells.

Thiotepa may be administered by intramuscular, intravenous, intra-arterial, intrapleural, or intraperitoneal injection, as well as by direct injection into the tumour mass. It can also be introduced directly into body cavities such as the bladder and pericardium. The dose must be adjusted according to the severity of the condition, the size and accessibility of the tumour, and the condition of the patient, and must be carefully controlled by repeated observations of the white-cell count.

As thiotepa can be given by a number of different routes according to the site, type, and grade of tumour, there is a wide range of dosage. For all routes of administration, except intravenous, the initial dose is 200 micrograms per kilogram body-weight daily, continued for three to five days. The maximum maintenance dose is 200 micrograms per kilogram body-weight every one to three weeks. It should be controlled by frequent white-cell counts; if the white-cell count is less than 3000 per cubic millimetre or the platelet count under 150,000 per cubic millimetre, treatment should be stopped or the dose should be reduced. Half these doses should be employed if thiotepa is given intravenously.

As an adjunct to the surgery of malignant disease, 1 milligram per kilogram body-weight, divided into three equal doses, is given on the day of operation and on the first and second post-operative days. A dose of 10 to 60 milligrams may be injected into a tumour mass or, dissolved in 20 to 60 millilitres of fluid, it may be instilled into cavities at weekly intervals.

UNDESIRABLE EFFECTS. Vomiting, headache, and anorexia may occur. The main toxic effect is depression of the haemopoietic system, particularly of the white cells. Thrombocytopenia with haemorrhagic manifestations may occur.

These toxic effects are not related to the size of the dose.

PRECAUTIONS. Thiotepa should only be given to patients under close supervision. The blood of all patients receiving thiotepa should be examined weekly or more frequently if necessary.

Dose. See above under **Actions and uses.**

Preparation
THIOTEPA INJECTION, B.P. It consists of a sterile solution prepared by dissolving the sterile contents of a sealed container in Water for Injections containing sodium chloride and sodium bicarbonate.
It should be stored at a temperature of 2° to 10° and used within 5 days. Vials containing 15 mg are available.

THYMOL

$C_{10}H_{14}O = 150·2$

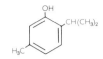

Thymol is 2-isopropyl-5-methylphenol.

Thymol may be prepared synthetically from piperitone, menthone, or *p*-cymene, or extracted from the volatile oils of *Thymus vulgaris* L., *Monarda punctata* L. (Fam. Labiatae), or *Trachyspermum ammi* (L.) Sprague (Fam. Umbelliferae). Thyme oil yields about 20 to 30 per cent of thymol; the other two oils yield respectively about 60 per cent and about 45 to 55 per cent.

Thymol is obtained from the oils by distilling off the hydrocarbons and extracting the residue with aqueous sodium hydroxide solution, which forms with thymol a soluble sodium derivative; the extract is acidified, and the liberated thymol is recrystallised from alcohol or light petroleum.

Solubility. Soluble, at 20°, in 1000 parts of water and in less than 1 part of alcohol, of ether, and of chloroform.

Standard
It complies with the requirements of the British Pharmacopoeia.
It occurs as colourless crystals with a pungent, aromatic, thyme-like odour. It sinks in cold water, but on heating to about 45° it melts and rises to the surface. It has a freezing-point not lower than 49·3°. A 4 per cent solution in alcohol (50 per cent) is neutral to litmus.

Storage. It should be stored in airtight containers, protected from light.

Preparation and storage of solutions. See statement on aqueous solutions of antiseptics, under Solutions (page 779).

Actions and uses. Thymol is a bactericide of higher potency than phenol but its use is limited by its low solubility in water.

It is an ingredient of deodorant mouth-washes, toothpastes, and gargles. Compound Thymol Glycerin and similar preparations are used as deodorant mouth-washes and gargles, but they are not effective as antiseptics.

Mixed with phenol and camphor, thymol is used in dentistry to prepare cavities and, mixed with zinc oxide, as a protective cap to the dentine prior to filling.

Thymol is added as an antoxidant to trichloroethylene and tetrachloroethylene in a concentration of 0·01 per cent.

Preparations
THYMOL GLYCERIN, COMPOUND, B.P.C. (page 702)
MOUTH-WASH SOLUTION-TABLETS, B.P.C. (page 792)

THYROID

SYNONYMS: Dry Thyroid; Thyroid Extract; Thyroid Gland; Thyroideum Siccum

Thyroid is dried, powdered, defatted thyroid gland of the ox, sheep, or pig; the powder is diluted with Lactose to the required strength.

The organic iodine compounds present in thyroid occur in combination with protein as thyroglobulins, which are soluble in water. On drying the thyroid gland at a temperature of 40° or below, as much as 70 per cent of the thyroglobulins remains unaltered and is therefore extractable by water.

If drying has been carried out at 100°, or by treatment with alcohol followed by drying at 60°, the thyroglobulins are almost completely denatured and made insoluble, and the product will not comply with the requirements of the British Pharmacopoeia.

Solubility. Partly soluble in water, the solution containing the inorganic iodine and the thyroglobulins not denatured during drying.

Standard
It complies with the requirements of the British Pharmacopoeia.
It contains 0·23 to 0·27 per cent of iodine in thyroid combination. The loss on drying at 105° is not more than 7·5 per cent.

DESCRIPTION. *Macroscopical:* a cream-coloured, amorphous powder; odour and taste, faint and meat-like.

Microscopical: numerous highly refractive, smooth, vitreous, angular fragments of the colloid contents of the vesicles, having striated conchoidal surfaces and varying in size from about 10 µm by 15 µm to 95 µm by 140 µm; less conspicuous fragments of connective tissue, subcyclindrical in shape, slightly undulate and having frayed fibrous ends; occasional irregularly ovoid particles composed of small vesicles adhering together and filled with their colloid contents; a few isolated epithelial cells, often with conspicuous nuclei and sparsely scattered fragments of striated muscle fibre.

The colloid particles stain readily with *eosin solution* and with *iodine solution*.

Storage. It should be stored in airtight containers, in a cool place.

Actions and uses. Thyroid has the actions, uses, and undesirable effects described under Thyroxine Sodium. Approximately 60 milligrams of thyroid is equivalent in therapeutic activity to 0·1 milligram of thyroxine sodium.

Dose. 30 to 250 milligrams daily.

Preparation
THYROID TABLETS, B.P. Unless otherwise specified, tablets each containing 30 mg of thyroid are supplied. They should be stored in airtight containers, in a cool place. Tablets containing 15, 60, 125, 200, and 300 mg are also available.

THYROXINE SODIUM

SYNONYM: L-Thyroxine Sodium

$C_{15}H_{10}I_4NNaO_4,5H_2O = 888.9$

Thyroxine Sodium is sodium L-α-amino-β-[4-(4-hydroxy-3,5-di-iodophenoxy)-3,5-di-iodophenyl]propionate pentahydrate.

Solubility. Soluble, at 20°, in 600 parts of water and in 250 parts of alcohol; very slightly soluble in ether and in chloroform; soluble in solutions of alkali hydroxides.

Standard
It complies with the requirements of the British Pharmacopoeia.
It is an odourless, white or pale buff, amorphous or crystalline powder and contains not less than 97.0 and not more than the equivalent of 101.0 per cent of $C_{15}H_{10}I_4NNaO_4$, calculated with reference to the dried substance. The loss on drying under the prescribed conditions is 6.0 to 12.0 per cent.

Storage. It should be stored in airtight containers, protected from light.

Actions and uses. Thyroxine sodium produces an increase in oxygen consumption and an increase in general metabolism, with which are associated an increased excretion of nitrogen, calcium, and water in the urine and a decrease of body-weight.
Thyroxine sodium is indicated only in the treatment of thyroid-deficiency states; it should never be given to a patient with a normally functioning intact gland, as such administration diminishes the intrinsic secretion. A dosage of 150 to 300 micrograms daily by mouth will restore patients with myxoedema to normality and maintain them in the euthyroid state.
After prolonged hypothyroidism, it is wise to restore a myxoedematous subject to normality only gradually, as some weeks are needed for mental and physical adaptation to the normal state.

Thyroxine sodium is used in the treatment of cretinism, the average dosage for a child of six months being 10 micrograms daily, increased to 100 to 200 micrograms daily at puberty. The only other indication for thyroid therapy, apart from primary and post-operative myxoedema, is hypothyroidism secondary to anterior pituitary destruction (Simmonds's disease). In these cases, however, thyroxine sodium is never administered alone, but only in conjunction with other hormones such as cortisone.
Obesity is not an indication for thyroxine administration, unless accompanied by clear evidence of hypothyroidism.

UNDESIRABLE EFFECTS. Attempts to restore the patient to a normal state too rapidly may result in sweating, tachycardia, diarrhoea, restlessness, excitability, and cardiac arrhythmias, possibly with signs of cardiac strain or decompensation, particularly in the aged.
Even slight overdosage may induce angina pectoris in certain patients, with or without electrocardiographic abnormalities; pain in a limb and aggravation of symptoms due to pre-existing osteo-arthritis may also occur.

Dose. See above under **Actions and uses.**

Preparation
THYROXINE TABLETS, B.P. (*Syn.* L-Thyroxine Sodium Tablets). Unless otherwise specified, tablets each containing 50 μg of thyroxine sodium are supplied. They should be protected from light. Tablets containing 100 μg are also available.

OTHER NAMES: *Eltroxin®*; Levothyroxine Sodium

TITANIUM DIOXIDE

SYNONYM: Titanium Oxide

$TiO_2 = 79.90$

Titanium Dioxide may be prepared from ilmenite or other titanium ores by processes which generally involve roasting and subsequent separation of the purified dioxide from iron and other impurities. It has a density of about 4.0. It forms titanates when fused with alkali hydroxides or carbonates.

Solubility. Insoluble in water, in hydrochloric acid, and in nitric acid; soluble in hydrofluoric acid and in hot sulphuric acid.

Standard
DESCRIPTION. A white amorphous powder; odourless or almost odourless.

IDENTIFICATION TESTS. 1. Fuse 0.5 g with 2.5 g of *potassium carbonate*, ignite in a furnace at about 950° for 30 minutes, cool, extract with 20 ml of *dilute sulphuric acid*, and filter. To 5 ml of the filtrate add *sodium hydroxide solution* or *dilute ammonia solution*; a white gelatinous precipitate is formed.

2. To 5 ml of the filtrate obtained in test 1 add a piece of *granulated zinc* and allow to stand; a violet colour is produced.

3. To 5 ml of the filtrate obtained in test 1 add 0.2 ml of *hydrogen peroxide solution*; a yellow to orange-red colour is produced.

ACIDITY OR ALKALINITY. Shake 5.0 g with 50 ml of *carbon dioxide-free water*; the suspension is not acid to *bromothymol blue solution*, and requires for neutralisation not more than 0.5 ml of 0.1N hydrochloric acid.

TOTAL ANTIMONY. Not more than 100 parts per million, determined by the following method:

To 5 ml of the solution reserved in the determination of the content of TiO_2, add 7 ml of *hydrochloric acid* and 5 ml of water, cool, if necessary, to 20°, and add successively, mixing well after each addition, 0·25 ml of *sodium nitrite solution*, 25 ml of *sodium hexametaphosphate solution* and 5 ml of *brilliant green solution*; extract with 5·0 ml of *toluene*, shaking vigorously for 30 seconds, filter the toluene extract through a dry filter paper, and measure the extinction of a 1-cm layer at the maximum at about 640 nm, using *toluene* as the blank.

Calculate the amount of antimony, Sb, present by reference to a calibration curve prepared in the following manner:

To suitable aliquots of *standard antimony solution* add 7 ml of *hydrochloric acid*, dilute to 15 ml with water, and treat each solution by the method described above, beginning with the words "cool, if necessary, to 20° . . .".

ACID-SOLUBLE ANTIMONY. Not more than 2 parts per million, determined by the following method:

Boil about 10 g, accurately weighed, with 50 ml of 0·5N hydrochloric acid for 15 minutes, with occasional stirring, allow to settle, decant and filter the supernatant liquid through a filter previously washed with 0·5N hydrochloric acid, and extract the residue with four successive 10-ml portions of 0·5N hydrochloric acid, decanting and filtering each extract through the same filter; allow the combined filtrate and washings to cool, and dilute to 100 ml with water; reserve a portion of the solution for the test for acid-soluble lead.

To 5 ml add 7 ml of *hydrochloric acid* and 5 ml of water and continue by the method for total antimony, beginning with the words "cool, if necessary, to 20°. . .".

ARSENIC. It complies with the test given in Appendix 6, page 880 (5 parts per million).

BARIUM COMPOUNDS. To 10 ml of the solution reserved in the determination of the content of TiO_2 add 1 ml of *dilute sulphuric acid* and allow to stand; no precipitate or turbidity is produced.

IRON. Mix intimately 0·2 g with 0·4 g of *potassium carbonate* and ignite in a furnace at about 950° for 30 minutes; allow to cool, transfer the mass to a flask with the aid of 4 ml of water and 6 ml of *hydrochloric acid*, heat gently until a clear solution is obtained, cool, and dilute to 100 ml with water; 20 ml of this solution complies with the limit test for iron, 0·08 g of *potassium carbonate* dissolved in 1 ml of *hydrochloric acid* being included in the standard colour (0·1 per cent).

ACID-SOLUBLE LEAD. Not more than 10 parts per million, determined by the method given in Appendix 7, page 884, the solution reserved in the determination of acid-soluble antimony being used.

SOLUBLE MATTER. Not more than 0·5 per cent, determined by the following method:

Boil about 4 g, accurately weighed, with 150 ml of water containing 0·5 g of *ammonium sulphate*, cool, dilute to 200 ml with water, and filter; evaporate 100 ml of the filtrate to dryness and ignite the residue to constant weight.

CONTENT OF TiO_2. Not less than 98·0 per cent, determined by the following method:

Mix intimately about 1 g, accurately weighed, with 2 g of *potassium carbonate* and ignite in a furnace at about 950° for 30 minutes; allow to cool, tranfer the mass to a flask with the aid of 20 ml of water and, in small portions, 30 ml of *hydrochloric acid*, heat gently until a clear solution is obtained, cool, and dilute to 100 ml with water.

Reserve a portion of this solution for the test for total antimony and for barium compounds; the solution should be used soon after preparation and should be discarded if a precipitate forms.

Dilute 10 ml to 200 ml with water, add 4 ml of *strong hydrogen peroxide solution*, mix well, cool, add 50 ml of 0·05M disodium edetate, and allow to stand for 5 minutes; adjust the solution to pH 5·0 by the addition of *sodium hydroxide solution*, add 5g of *hexamine*, and titrate the excess of disodium edetate with 0·05M zinc chloride, using *xylenol orange solution* as indicator; each ml of 0·05M disodium edetate is equivalent to 0·003995 g of TiO_2.

Actions and uses. Titanium dioxide has an action on the skin similar to that described under Zinc Oxide (page 539). It is used in the treatment of dermatoses with exudation and to relieve pruritus. It is an ingredient of face powders and other cosmetics and is used to prevent sunburn.

Titanium dioxide is also used to pigment and opacify hard gelatin capsules and also as a delustring agent for regenerated cellulose and other man-made fibres.

Preparation

TITANIUM DIOXIDE PASTE, B.P.C. (page 768)

TOLAZOLINE HYDROCHLORIDE

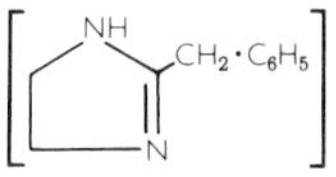

$C_{10}H_{13}ClN_2 = 196·7$

Tolazoline Hydrochloride is 2-benzyl-2-imidazoline hydrochloride.

Solubility. Soluble, at 20°, in less than 1 part of water, in 2 parts of alcohol, and in 2·5 parts of chloroform; insoluble in ether.

Standard

It complies with the requirements of the British Pharmacopoeia.

It is a white or creamy-white, crystalline, odourless or almost odourless powder and contains not less than 99·0 and not more than the equivalent of 101·0 per cent of $C_{10}H_{13}ClN_2$, calculated with reference to the dried substance. The loss on drying under the prescribed conditions is not more than 0·5 per cent. It has a melting-point of 172° to 176°. A 1 per cent solution in water has a pH of 5·0 to 7·0.

Sterilisation. Solutions for injection are sterilised by heating in an autoclave or by filtration.

Storage. It should be stored in airtight containers, protected from light.

Actions and uses. Tolazoline causes marked dilatation of arterioles and capillaries, and increases the skin temperature to a greater extent and for a longer period than most other vasodilator drugs. It also stimulates gastric secretion.

Tolazoline also antagonises those effects of noradrenaline and adrenaline that are attributed to alpha-receptor stimulation, but it has poor adrenergic-blocking activity and hence is of no value in the treatment of hypertension.

Tolazoline is used mainly for the treatment of peripheral vascular disorders due to arterial spasm or occlusion. In the treatment of Raynaud's disease, 25 to 50 milligrams of tolazoline hydrochloride may be given by mouth. It has been given by intramuscular or intravenous injection in doses of 10 to 20 milligrams and has also been applied topically in the treatment of local vascular disorders.

UNDESIRABLE EFFECTS. Tolazoline may produce nausea, vomiting, diarrhoea, and postural hypotension.

CONTRA-INDICATIONS. It is contra-indicated in patients with coronary insufficiency or other severe heart disease and in cases of peptic ulceration.

Dose. 25 to 50 milligrams four times a day by mouth.

Preparation
TOLAZOLINE TABLETS, B.P. Unless otherwise specified, tablets each containing 25 mg of tolazoline hydrochloride are supplied. They should be stored in airtight containers, protected from light.

OTHER NAMES: *Priscol®*; *Zoline®*

TOLBUTAMIDE

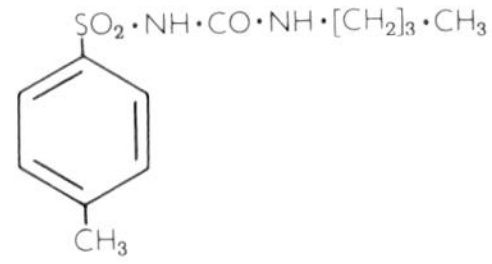

SYNONYM: Tolbutamidum

$C_{12}H_{18}N_2O_3S = 270.3$

Tolbutamide is *N*-butyl-*N'*-toluene-*p*-sulphonylurea.

Solubility. Insoluble in water; soluble, at 20°, in 10 parts of alcohol and in 3 parts of acetone; soluble in sodium hydroxide solution and in dilute mineral acids.

Standard
It complies with the requirements of the European Pharmacopoeia.
It is a white, crystalline, almost odourless powder and contains not less than 99.0 per cent of $C_{12}H_{18}N_2O_3S$, calculated with reference to the dried substance. The loss on drying under the prescribed conditions is not more than 0.5 per cent. It has a melting-point of 128° to 130°.

Actions and uses. Tolbutamide has the actions and uses described under Chlorpropamide (page 109).
It is active when taken by mouth but, as it is excreted more rapidly than chlorpropamide, it has a shorter duration of action. After a single dose, the blood-sugar level falls within two to four hours and the reduced level is maintained for eight to ten hours.
The usual initial daily dosage is 1 to 4 grams by mouth in divided doses. The dose and frequency of administration is subsequently adjusted to achieve a suitable balance adequate for controlling the blood-sugar level and preventing glycosuria; the maintenance dose is usually 0.5 to 1.5 grams daily in divided doses.
Tolbutamide may also be given, in the form of its sodium derivative, by intravenous injection in a dose of 1 gram for the diagnosis of insulinomas, but this is not without risk.

UNDESIRABLE EFFECTS. Rashes, gastro-intestinal disturbances, and intolerance to alcohol may occur and, rarely, blood dyscrasies and jaundice.

Dose. See above under **Actions and uses.**

Preparation
TOLBUTAMIDE TABLETS, B.P. Unless otherwise specified, tablets each containing 500 mg of tolbutamide are supplied.

OTHER NAME: *Rastinon®*

TOLNAFTATE

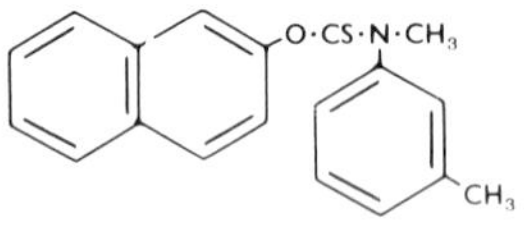

$C_{19}H_{17}NOS = 307.4$

Tolnaftate is *O*-naphth-2-yl methyl-*m*-tolylthiocarbamate.

Solubility. Very slightly soluble in water and in alcohol; soluble, at 20°, in 55 parts of ether, in 3 parts of chloroform, and in 9 parts of acetone.

Standard
It complies with the requirements of the British Pharmacopoeia.
It is a white to creamy-white odourless powder. The loss on drying at 60° at a pressure not exceeding 5 mmHg for three hours is not more than 0.5 per cent. It has a melting-point of 109° to 112°.

Actions and uses. Tolnaftate is an antifungal agent used for the topical treatment of ringworm and other skin infections due to *Epidermophyton floccosum*, *Microsporum au-* *douinii*, *M. canis*, *Trichophyton mentagrophytes*, and *T. verrucosum*; infections due to *T. rubrum*, *T. tonsurans*, and *Malassezia furfur* may also respond. It is not active against species of *Candida* or bacteria.
Tolnaftate, like other topical agents, is not suitable for the treatment of tinea of the nails and scalp, but it may be used as an adjunct to systemic treatment with griseofulvin.
Since tolnaftate is not keratolytic, skin tolerance is very good; primary irritation and allergic sensitisation occasionally occur.
Tolnaftate is applied in the form of cream or dusting-powder containing 1 per cent.

OTHER NAME: *Tinaderm®*

TOLU BALSAM

Tolu Balsam is a solid or semi-solid balsam obtained by incision from the trunk of *Myroxylon balsamum* (L.) Harms (Fam. Leguminosae), a tree indigenous to Colombia and adjoining regions in South America.

Constituents. Tolu balsam contains 12 to 15 per cent of free cinnamic acid, about 8 per cent of free benzoic acid, a trace of vanillin, and about 7·5 per cent of an oily liquid consisting of benzyl benzoate with a little benzyl cinnamate. The resin, of which the balsam contains about 80 per cent, yields, on saponification, one or more resin alcohols, cinnamic acid, and a little benzoic acid.

Good fresh tolu balsam yields, when distilled with water, 1·5 to 3 per cent of a very fragrant volatile oil.

Solubility. Soluble in alcohol (90 per cent), in ether, in chloroform, and in glacial acetic acid; partly soluble in carbon disulphide, the soluble portion consisting chiefly of cinnamic acid; very slightly soluble in light petroleum; partly soluble in solutions of caustic alkalis.

Standard

DESCRIPTION. A soft, tenacious, brownish-yellow or brown, resinous solid when first imported, subsequently becoming harder and finally brittle; transparent in thin films; odour aromatic and vanilla-like; taste aromatic. When warmed and pressed between pieces of glass and examined with a lens, it exhibits crystals of cinnamic acid.

IDENTIFICATION TESTS. 1. Warm gently about 1 g, in powder, with 5 ml of *potassium permanganate solution*; the odour of benzaldehyde is produced.

2. To a solution in *alcohol (90 per cent)* add *ferric chloride test-solution*; a green colour is produced.

ACIDITY. A solution in *alcohol (90 per cent)* is acid to *litmus solution*.

ACID VALUE. 100 to 160, calculated with reference to the dry alcohol-soluble matter, determined by the following method:
Dissolve about 2·5 g, accurately weighed, in 50 ml of boiling *alcohol (90 per cent)*, add 5 ml of *phenolphthalein solution*, and titrate the hot solution with 0·5N alcoholic potassium hydroxide prepared with *alcohol (90 per cent)*.

ALCOHOL (90 PER CENT)-INSOLUBLE MATTER. Not more than 5·0 per cent, determined by the following method: Warm about 2 g, in coarse powder, accurately weighed, with 25 ml of *alcohol (90 per cent)*, filter, wash the residue with hot *alcohol (90 per cent)* until extraction is complete, and dry to constant weight at 105°.

COLOPHONY. Warm 5·0 g with 25 ml of *carbon disulphide* under a reflux condenser, with shaking, filter, and evaporate the filtrate to dryness.
Triturate the residue with 6 ml of *light petroleum (boiling-range, 40° to 60°)*, filter, wash the filter with sufficient of the same solvent to adjust the filtrate to 6 ml, shake the filtrate with 10 ml of *dilute copper acetate solution*, and allow to separate; the light petroleum layer is not coloured green.

ESTER VALUE. 40 to 85, calculated with reference to the dry alcohol-soluble matter.

SAPONIFICATION VALUE. 170 to 230, calculated with reference to the dry alcohol-soluble matter.

LOSS ON DRYING. Not more than 4·0 per cent, determined by the following method:
Spread evenly about 2 g, in coarse powder, accurately weighed, in a flat-bottomed dish, 9 cm in diameter and 1·5 cm deep, and dry over *phosphorus pentoxide* for 4 hours in vacuo.

CONTENT OF TOTAL BALSAMIC ACIDS. Not less than 35·0 and not more than 50·0 per cent, calculated as cinnamic acid with reference to the dry alcohol-soluble matter, determined by the method for Benzoin, page 49.
Subtract from the weight of the sample taken the proportion of alcohol (90 per cent)-insoluble matter and the loss on drying and calculate the content of total balsamic acids.

Adulterants and substitutes. Exhausted balsam may be detected by the deficiency of balsamic acids. Factitious tolu balsam made by adding synthetic balsamic acids to the exhausted balsam lacks the fragrance associated with the volatile oil.

Uses. Tolu balsam, in the form of Tolu Syrup, is frequently used to flavour cough mixtures.

Preparations

TOLU LINCTUS, COMPOUND, PAEDIATRIC, B.P.C. (page 725)

TOLU SOLUTION, B.P.C. (page 791)

TOLU SYRUP, B.P.C. (page 801)

BENZOIN TINCTURE, COMPOUND, B.P.C. (page 820)

TRAGACANTH

SYNONYM: Trag.

Tragacanth is the dried gummy exudation obtained by incision from *Astragalus gummifer* Labill. and some other species of *Astragalus* (Fam. Leguminosae), shrubs indigenous to Iran, Greece, Turkey, Iraq, and Syria; it is known in commerce as Persian tragacanth.

Some indication of its suspending properties may be obtained from the apparent viscosity of its mucilage; commercial samples vary considerably in this property.

Constituents. Tragacanth can be separated into two fractions, one termed tragacanthin, which is soluble in water, and the other termed bassorin, which contains about 5 per cent of methoxyl and is insoluble, but swells, in water. The gum also contains about 15 per cent of moisture, traces of starch and of altered cell-walls. It yields on hydrolysis, among other products, galacturonic acid, D-galactopyranose, L-arabinofuranose, and D-xylopyranose. Tragacanth has a volatile acidity of about 2 to 3 per cent, calculated as acetic acid.

Solubility. Partly soluble in water, in which it swells to a homogeneous, adhesive, gelatinous mass; insoluble in alcohol.

Standard
It complies with the requirements of the British Pharmacopoeia.

UNGROUND DRUG. *Macroscopical characters:* thin, flattened, more or less curved, ribbon-like flakes, about 25 mm long and 12 mm broad; white or pale yellowish-

white, horny, translucent, marked on flat sides with concentric ridges; fracture short.
Odourless; almost tasteless.
When warmed with *sodium hydroxide solution*, a canary-yellow colour slowly develops.

Microscopical characters: the diagnostic characters are: when powdered and mounted in alcohol, it appears as small, transparent, angular particles of various sizes and shapes; the particles lose their sharp edges when water is added, each gradually swelling until large indefinite masses containing a few groups of small rounded starch granules result.

POWDERED DRUG: Powdered Tragacanth. A white powder possessing the diagnostic microscopical characters and taste of the unground drug; odourless.

Adulterants and substitutes. "Vermicelli" tragacanth is composed of tears and vermiform pieces.
Smyrna tragacanth occurs in flakes, but is more opaque and less ribbon-like than the official drug; it contains appreciable quantities of starch.
Hog gum, or Caramania gum, occurs in yellowish or yellowish-brown, opaque tears or vermiform pieces; it is said to be obtained from a species of *Prunus* (Fam. Rosaceae).
Indian tragacanth (karaya gum) is described under Sterculia (page 470).
Ceratonia, or Carob gum, consisting of the endosperms of the seeds of *Ceratonia siliqua* L. (Fam. Leguminosae), occurs as translucent white oval concavo-convex disks containing about 58 per cent of mannan and about 29 per cent of galactan.

Storage. It should be stored in airtight containers. Powdered Tragacanth should be similarly stored.

Uses. Tragacanth forms viscous solutions or gels with water, depending on the concentration. Being almost tasteless and non-toxic it is used as a suspending agent in mixtures containing resinous tinctures and heavy insoluble powders, and to stabilise emulsions prepared with acacia. Compound Tragacanth Powder combines the suspending powers of tragacanth and acacia.

Tragacanth is also used in medicated and toilet creams and jellies containing glycerol. A thick mucilage is used as a drying application to the skin, for example as a basis for medicaments such as ichthammol, salicylic acid, resorcinol, and sulphur.
In dispensing lotions, creams, and jellies the tragacanth is first dispersed in a distributing agent, such as alcohol, essential oil, or glycerol, to prevent agglomeration on the addition of water.
Tragacanth is used in the preparation of lozenges and as an excipient for pills and tablets. It is also used in obstetric creams and as the basis of lubricants for catheters and surgical instruments. The powder is used as an adhesive for dentures.
Aqueous tragacanth preparations which do not contain a drug with an antimicrobial action should include a preservative if an appreciable storage life is required.

Preparations
TRAGACANTH MUCILAGE, B.P.C. (page 756)
TRAGACANTH POWDER, COMPOUND, B.P. It contains 15 per cent of tragacanth, 20 per cent each of acacia and starch, and 45 per cent of sucrose. It should be stored in airtight containers.

TRANYLCYPROMINE SULPHATE

$C_{18}H_{24}N_2O_4S = 364 \cdot 5$

Tranylcypromine Sulphate is (±)-*trans*-2-phenylcyclopropylamine sulphate.

Solubility. Soluble, at 20°, in 20 parts of water; very slightly soluble in alcohol; slightly soluble in ether; insoluble in chloroform.

Standard
It complies with the requirements of the British Pharmacopoeia.
It is a white or almost white crystalline powder, which is odourless or has a faint odour of cinnamaldehyde and contains not less than 98·0 and not more than the equivalent of 102·0 per cent of $C_{18}H_{24}N_2O_4S$, calculated with reference to the dried substance. The loss on drying under the prescribed conditions is not more than 0·5 per cent.

Actions and uses. Tranylcypromine is a monoamine-oxidase inhibitor. It is used in the treatment of depressive states, including endogenous, reactive, and psychoneurotic depression. It usually produces a response in susceptible patients within three days.
The usual dosage is 20 milligrams daily in two doses by mouth, increased if necessary to 30 milligrams daily. For the intensive treatment of severe depression, a commencing dose of 40 milligrams daily may be given, increased at weekly intervals to a maximum of 60 milligrams daily; when a satisfactory response has been achieved, dosage may be reduced to a maintenance level of 20 milligrams daily.
Unlike other monoamine-oxidase inhibitors, the effects of tranylcypromine persist for only forty-eight to seventy-two hours after the withdrawal of the drug.

UNDESIRABLE EFFECTS. The most frequently occurring reactions are insomnia, dizziness, muscular weakness, dryness of the mouth, and hypotension. In some patients, hypertension accompanied by severe headache may occur, requiring discontinuation of treatment with tranylcypromine and treatment with antihypertensive drugs such as phentolamine or pentolinium.

PRECAUTIONS. These are as described under Phenelzine Sulphate (page 361).

Dose. See above under **Actions and uses.**

Preparation
TRANYLCYPROMINE TABLETS, B.P. Unless otherwise specified, tablets each containing tranylcypromine sulphate equivalent to 10 mg of tranylcypromine are supplied. They are sugar coated.

OTHER NAME: *Parnate*®

TRIAMCINOLONE

$C_{21}H_{27}FO_6 = 394.4$

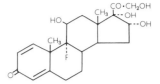

Triamcinolone is 9α-fluoro-11β,16α,17α,21-tetrahydroxypregna-1,4-diene-3,20-dione.

Solubility. Soluble, at 20°, in 500 parts of water and in 240 parts of alcohol; very slightly soluble in ether and in chloroform.

Standard

DESCRIPTION. A white or almost white crystalline powder; odourless or almost odourless.

IDENTIFICATION TESTS. 1. Dissolve 1 mg in 6 ml of *alcohol (95 per cent)*, add 5 ml of a 1 per cent w/v solution of *di-t-butyl-p-cresol* in *alcohol (95 per cent)* and 5 ml of *dilute sodium hydroxide solution*, and heat on a water-bath under a reflux condenser for 20 minutes; a pinkish-lavender colour is produced.

2. Heat 0·5 ml of *chromic-sulphuric acid mixture* in a test-tube 2 in long and ¼ in in diameter in a water-bath for 5 minutes; the solution wets the sides of the tube readily and there is no greasiness.
Add 3 mg of the sample and again heat in a water-bath for 5 minutes; the solution does not wet the sides of the tube and does not pour easily from the tube.

3. It complies with the thin-layer chromatographic test given in Appendix 5A, page 869.

4. The ultraviolet absorption spectrum exhibits the characteristics given in Appendix 3, page 856.

5. The infra-red absorption spectrum exhibits maxima which are only at the same wavelengths as, and have similar relative intensities to, those in the spectrum of *triamcinolone A.S.*

SPECIFIC ROTATION. $+65°$ to $+71°$, calculated with reference to the substance dried under the prescribed conditions, determined, at 20°, in a 1·0 per cent w/v solution in *dimethylformamide*.

RELATED FOREIGN STEROIDS. It complies with the test given in Appendix 5A, page 869 (2·0 per cent).

LOSS ON DRYING. Not more than 2·0 per cent, determined by drying for 3 hours at 60° in vacuo.

SULPHATED ASH. Not more than 0·2 per cent.

CONTENT OF $C_{21}H_{27}FO_6$. Not less than 96·0 per cent and not more than the equivalent of 104·0 per cent, calculated with reference to the substance dried under the prescribed conditions, determined by the following method:
Dissolve about 0·025 g, accurately weighed, in sufficient *alcohol (95 per cent)* to produce 100 ml, dilute 2 ml of this solution to 50 ml with *alcohol (95 per cent)*, and

measure the extinction of a 2-cm layer at the maximum at about 238 nm.
For purposes of calculation use a value of 380 for the E(1 per cent, 1 cm) of $C_{21}H_{27}FO_6$.
Calculate the percentage of $C_{21}H_{27}FO_6$ in the sample.

Actions and uses. Triamcinolone has the actions and uses described under Cortisone Acetate (page 132) but has virtually no sodium-retaining effect. During the first days of administration it may even cause a loss of sodium from the body, and an initial mild diuretic action is sometimes observed. It is used, therefore, in all conditions for which cortisone is indicated, except in adrenocortical deficiency states, where some salt-retaining action is desirable.

It is given by mouth in a dosage slightly lower than that of prednisone or prednisolone; the dosage is usually 4 to 48 milligrams daily in divided doses, but for extended use as an anti-inflammatory agent it should not exceed 6 milligrams daily.

UNDESIRABLE EFFECTS. These are described under Cortisone Acetate (page 132) but salt retention and oedema are unlikely to occur. The voracious appetite which occurs occasionally in patients during treatment with other cortisone analogues does not occur with triamcinolone.

Dizziness, anorexia, somnolence, muscle weakness, and post-prandial flushing may occur.

PRECAUTIONS AND CONTRA-INDICATIONS. As for Cortisone Acetate (page 132).

Dose. See above under **Actions and uses.**

Preparation
TRIAMCINOLONE TABLETS, B.P.C. (page 817)

OTHER NAMES: *Adcortyl®*; *Ledercort®*

TRIAMCINOLONE ACETONIDE

$C_{24}H_{31}FO_6 = 434.5$

Triamcinolone Acetonide is 9α-fluoro-11β,21-dihydroxy-16α,17α-isopropylidenedioxypregna-1,4-diene-3,20-dione.

Solubility. Very slightly soluble in water; soluble, at 20°, in 150 parts of alcohol, in 40 parts of chloroform, and in 11 parts of acetone.

Standard
It complies with the requirements of the British Pharmacopoeia.

It is a white or almost white, crystalline, odourless or almost odourless powder and contains not less than 97·0 and not more than the equivalent of 103·0 per cent of $C_{24}H_{31}FO_6$, calculated with reference to the dried substance. The loss on drying under the prescribed conditions is not more than 1·5 per cent.

Storage. It should be protected from light.

Actions and uses. Triamcinolone acetonide has the actions and uses of topically applied hydrocortisone (page 224) but, being more potent, it is used in lower concentrations, usually 0·1 per cent.

Preparations
TRIAMCINOLONE CREAM, B.P.C. (page 660)
TRIAMCINOLONE LOTION, B.P.C. (page 729)
TRIAMCINOLONE OINTMENT, B.P.C. (page 764)
TRIAMCINOLONE DENTAL PASTE, B.P.C. (page 769)

OTHER NAMES: *Adcortyl®*; *Kenalog®*; *Ledercort®*

TRIAMTERENE

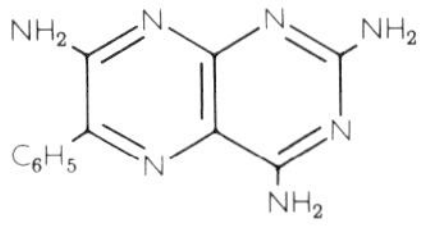

$C_{12}H_{11}N_7 = 253·3$

Triamterene is 2,4,7-triamino-6-phenylpteridine.

Solubility. Slightly soluble in water; very slightly soluble in alcohol and in chloroform; insoluble in ether.

Standard
It complies with the requirements of the British Pharmacopoeia.
It is a yellow, crystalline, odourless powder and contains not less than 98·5 and not more than the equivalent of 101·0 per cent of $C_{12}H_{11}N_7$, calculated with reference to the dried substance. The loss on drying under the prescribed conditions is not more than 0·5 per cent.

Actions and uses. Triamterene is a diuretic which exerts its effect directly on the tubule. It increases sodium, chloride, and, to a lesser extent, bicarbonate excretion and thereby increases water diuresis. It is a weaker diuretic than the thiazides and it causes potassium retention rather than loss.

It is active when given by mouth, diuresis beginning after about two hours and reaching a peak level after about four to eight hours; occasionally the maximum effect is not obtained until after two or three days' treatment. Triamterene is used for the treatment of oedema, especially if due to corticosteroid treatment or secondary hyperaldosteronism. In conjunction with other diuretics it may be useful in patients who have become refractory to treatment. It does not activate latent diabetes mellitus and may be used in place of thiazide diuretics for diabetic patients.

Triamterene may be administered in doses of 100 milligrams, once or twice daily after meals. Maintenance doses may be administered on alternate days, with a thiazide diuretic on the days when triamterene is omitted, to prevent a rise in blood urea which may occur with prolonged daily dosage.

UNDESIRABLE EFFECTS. Triamterene may give rise to nausea, vomiting, mild diarrhoea, dryness of the mouth, headache, and muscle weakness; rashes may rarely occur.

PRECAUTIONS. Triamterene may cause electrolyte imbalance and nitrogen retention. Periodic estimations of potassium and urea-nitrogen blood levels should be undertaken.

Dose. See above under **Actions and uses.**

Preparation
TRIAMTERENE CAPSULES, B.P. Unless otherwise specified, capsules each containing 50 mg of triamterene are supplied.

OTHER NAME: *Dytac®*

TRICHLOROACETIC ACID

SYNONYM: Trichloracetic Acid

$C_2HCl_3O_2 = 163·4$

$CCl_3 \cdot CO_2H$

Trichloroacetic Acid may be prepared by the oxidation of chloral with nitric acid.

Solubility. Soluble, at 20°, in about 0·1 part of water; soluble in alcohol and in ether.

Standard
It complies with the requirements of the British Pharmacopoeia.
It occurs as colourless very deliquescent crystals or crystalline masses with a slight characteristic pungent odour and contains not less than 98·0 per cent of $C_2HCl_3O_2$. It has a melting-point of 55° to 57°.

Storage. It should be stored in airtight containers.

Actions and uses. Liquefied trichloroacetic acid, prepared by the addition of 10 per cent by weight of water, is applied externally in the treatment of warts. A 10 per cent aqueous solution has been used for application to corneal warts.

TRICHLOROETHYLENE

$CHCl:CCl_2 = 131\cdot4$

Trichloroethylene may be prepared by chlorinating acetylene, boiling the tetrachloroethane produced with milk of lime, and purifying the product by distillation; thymol, $0\cdot01$ per cent w/w, is added as a preservative.

It may contain not more than $0\cdot001$ per cent w/w of a suitable blue colouring matter to distinguish it, when used for anaesthetic purposes, from chloroform, which it closely resembles in physical characteristics.

Solubility. Very slightly soluble in water; miscible with dehydrated alcohol, with ether, with chloroform, and with fixed and volatile oils.

Standard
It complies with the requirements of the British Pharmacopoeia.
It is a colourless or pale blue, transparent, mobile liquid with a characteristic odour resembling that of chloroform. It has a weight per ml at 20° of $1\cdot460$ g to $1\cdot466$ g and a boiling-point of 86° to 88°, not less than 95 per cent v/v distilling within a range of 1°.

Stability. It is stable in the presence of moisture but undergoes decomposition on exposure to bright light in the presence of air.

Storage. It should be stored in airtight containers, protected from light, in a cool place.

Actions and uses. Trichloroethylene is the least volatile of the liquid anaesthetics and is less potent than either chloroform or ether. It is non-irritant to mucous membranes and is non-inflammable when used with air or oxygen. It induces anaesthesia smoothly and rapidly.

Its main disadvantage is that it does not produce full muscular relaxation or deep anaesthesia and is therefore unsuitable for long operations and for those requiring complete relaxation. It may also increase the respiratory rate, inducing short jerky inspirations, and, like chloroform, may produce cardiac irregularities, such as auricular or ventricular extrasystoles.

Trichloroethylene is used by inhalation for analgesia in obstetrics, a concentration of $0\cdot5$ per cent in air being recommended for this purpose. It is also used by inhalation to alleviate the pain of trigeminal neuralgia.

Trichloroethylene is used to produce light anaesthesia, the vapour being mixed with air or nitrous oxide and oxygen. Owing to its low volatility it is difficult to administer on an open mask. For the induction of anaesthesia it may be given by means of suitable inhalers, some of which are for self-administration in obstetrics, by drawing air over the liquid in a bottle, or by means of a semi-closed apparatus.

In less pure form, trichloroethylene is used commercially in the dry-cleaning industry, for the degreasing of metals, and for oil and fat extraction. Improper working conditions may give rise to acute poisoning or narcosis which may be fatal, although temporary unconsciousness is a more common manifestation.

PRECAUTIONS. Trichloroethylene must never be used in a closed-circuit apparatus, because the heat produced by the action of carbon dioxide and water vapour on the soda lime causes it to react with the soda lime to form dichloroacetylene, which may cause cranial palsies and may even be lethal. Adrenaline should never be administered at the same time as trichloroethylene owing to the danger of ventricular fibrillation.

Prolonged exposure to trichloroethylene vapour may cause cardiac irregularities and degenerative changes in the nervous system, particularly in the sensory fibres of the first and fifth cranial nerves. The maximum allowable concentration for an eight-hour daily exposure is 100 parts per million by volume.

DEPENDENCE. Dependence of the barbiturate–alcohol type, as described under Phenobarbitone (page 366), may occur in persons who habitually inhale small quantities of trichloroethylene vapour.

POISONING. Industrial poisoning by trichloroethylene is treated by removal of the patient from the source of the vapour, by artificial respiration, and by the administration of oxygen containing 5 per cent of carbon dioxide.

Dose. 1 millilitre by inhalation.

OTHER NAME: *Trilene*®

TRICHLOROFLUOROMETHANE

SYNONYMS: Propellent 11; Refrigerant 11; Fluorotrichloromethane

$CCl_3F = 137\cdot4$

Trichlorofluoromethane is liquid at ordinary temperatures, but because of its low boiling-point it is supplied as a liquefied gas under pressure in suitable metal containers. It has a weight per ml of about $1\cdot61$ g at $-35°$ and of about $1\cdot50$ g at $15°$.

Solubility. In the liquid state: immiscible with water; miscible with dehydrated alcohol.

Standard
DESCRIPTION. A clear colourless non-inflammable volatile liquid; odour faint and ethereal.

IDENTIFICATION TEST. It boils at about $23\cdot7°$.

DISTILLATION RANGE. When determined by the method given in Appendix 17A, page 896, the specified fraction distils within a range of $0\cdot3°$.

HIGH-BOILING IMPURITIES. Not more than $0\cdot01$ per cent v/v, determined by the following method:
Allow the boiling-tube containing the remaining 15 ml of sample from the determination of distillation range

to stand in a water-bath at $54°$ for 30 minutes and measure the volume of the residue.

FREE ACIDITY; CHLORIDE. It complies with the tests described under Dichlorodifluoromethane, page 155.

WATER. Not more than $0\cdot0010$ per cent w/w, determined by the method given in Appendix 17B, page 896.

Storage. It should be stored in suitable metal containers, in a cool place, away from any fire risk.

Uses. Trichlorofluoromethane is used as a refrigerant and aerosol propellent, as described under Dichlorodifluoromethane (page 155).

TRICLOFOS SODIUM

$C_2H_3Cl_3NaO_4P = 251\cdot4$

$$Cl_3C \cdot CH_2 \cdot O \cdot \underset{\underset{OH}{|}}{\overset{\overset{O}{\|}}{P}} \cdot ONa$$

Triclofos Sodium is sodium hydrogen 2,2,2-trichloroethyl phosphate.

Solubility. Soluble, at $20°$, in 2 parts of water and in 250 parts of alcohol; very slightly soluble in ether.

Standard
It complies with the requirements of the British Pharmacopoeia.
It is a white or almost white, hygroscopic, odourless powder and contains not less than $41\cdot3$ and not more than $43\cdot2$ per cent of Cl and not less than $97\cdot0$ and not more than the equivalent of $102\cdot0$ per cent of $C_2H_3Cl_3NaO_4P$, both calculated with reference to the dried substance. The loss on drying under the prescribed conditions is not more than $5\cdot0$ per cent. A 2 per cent solution in water is clear and has a pH of $3\cdot0$ to $4\cdot5$.

Incompatibility. Aqueous solutions are incompatible with salts of heavy metals, calcium, magnesium, and alkaloids.

Storage. It should be stored in airtight containers.

Actions and uses. Triclofos sodium has sedative and hypnotic actions similar to those of dichloralphenazone (page 155) and other

chloral compounds. It is suitable for use as a sedative in domiciliary midwifery.
The sedative dose is 500 milligrams once or twice daily and the hypnotic dose is 1 to 2 grams thirty minutes before bedtime.

UNDESIRABLE EFFECTS. Rashes may occur. Prolonged use may lead to dependence of the barbiturate-alcohol type as described under Phenobarbitone (page 366) and it may enhance the effects of alcohol.

Dose. See above under **Actions and uses.**

Preparations
TRICLOFOS ELIXIR, B.P.C. (page 677)

TRICLOFOS TABLETS, B.P. Unless otherwise specified, tablets each containing 500 mg of triclofos sodium are supplied. They are film coated. They should be stored in airtight containers.

OTHER NAME: *Tricloryl®*

TRIETHANOLAMINE

Triethanolamine is a variable mixture of bases consisting mainly of tri(2-hydroxyethyl)amine, $(CH_2OH \cdot CH_2)_3N$, together with di(2-hydroxyethyl)amine and smaller amounts of 2-hydroxyethylamine.

Triethanolamine forms crystalline salts with mineral acids, the hydrochloride and the hydriodide being sparingly soluble in alcohol. With the higher fatty or olefinic acids, it forms salts which are soluble in water and have the general characters of soaps.
Triethanolamine volatilises slowly at $100°$.

Solubility. Miscible with water and with alcohol; slightly soluble in ether.

Standard
DESCRIPTION. A clear colourless or slightly yellow hygroscopic liquid; odourless or almost odourless.

IDENTIFICATION TESTS. 1. A 10 per cent w/v solution in *dilute hydrochloric acid* gives with *phosphotungstic acid solution* a copious precipitate, with *iodine solution* a slight precipitate, and with *potassium mercuri-iodide solution* or *platinic chloride solution* no precipitate.

2. Mix 1 ml with 1 ml of water and neutralise to *litmus paper* with *hydrochloric acid*; a crystalline precipitate is formed which, after washing with *alcohol (95 per cent)* and drying, melts at about 178°.

3. A 10 per cent w/v solution in water is strongly alkaline to *litmus solution*.

REFRACTIVE INDEX. At 20°, 1·482 to 1·485.

WEIGHT PER ML. At 20°, 1·120 g to 1·130 g.

SULPHATED ASH. Not more than 0·1 per cent.

CONTENT OF TOTAL BASES. Not less than 99·0 and not more than the equivalent of 110·0 per cent w/w, calculated as $C_6H_{15}NO_3$, determined by the following method:
Mix about 3 g, accurately weighed, with 20 ml of water, and titrate with 1N hydrochloric acid, using *methyl red solution* as indicator; each ml of 1N hydrochloric acid is equivalent to 0·1492 g of $C_6H_{15}NO_3$.

CONTENT OF TRI(2-HYDROXYETHYL)AMINE. Not less than 80·0 per cent w/w, calculated as $C_6H_{15}NO_3$, determined by the following method:
Mix about 0·5 g, accurately weighed, with 5 ml of *dilute hydrochloric acid* and evaporate to dryness on a water-bath; stir the residue with 5 ml of *isopropyl alcohol*, transfer to a tared sintered-glass crucible, and wash the dish and residue with three successive 5-ml portions of *isopropyl alcohol*, thoroughly drying the residue in the crucible by suction after each washing, and dry the residue to constant weight at 105°; add to the weight so obtained a correction of 0·2 mg for each ml of isopropyl alcohol used; each g is equivalent to 0·8035 g of $C_6H_{15}NO_3$.

Storage. It should be stored in airtight containers.

Uses. Triethanolamine is used chiefly combined with fatty acids such as stearic and oleic acids; equimolecular proportions of base and fatty acid form a soap which may be used as an emulsifying agent to produce fine-grained stable emulsions of the oil-in-water type with a pH of about 8. The emulsion is conveniently formed by adding, with constant stirring, a warm solution of the acid in the oil, together with other oil-soluble ingredients, to an aqueous solution of the triethanolamine and other water-soluble ingredients warmed to the same temperature; violent stirring should be avoided, as it may produce a persistent froth. Although emulsions made with triethanolamine soaps are slightly more stable than those prepared with alkali soaps, they too break down in the presence of acids and high concentrations of ionisable salts.

For the emulsification of fixed oils, triethanolamine equal to 2 to 4 per cent of the weight of oil, with two to five times as much fatty acid, is adequate; for liquid paraffin, the amount of triethanolamine should be increased to about 5 per cent of the weight of liquid paraffin, with a proportionate increase in the weight of fatty acid.

Triethanolamine can also be used to neutralise carboxyvinylpolymers in the formation of aqueous gels containing glycerol or propylene glycol.

Preparations made with triethanolamine soaps are liable to darken on exposure to light.

TRIFLUOPERAZINE HYDROCHLORIDE

$C_{21}H_{26}Cl_2F_3N_3S = 480·4$

Trifluoperazine Hydrochloride is 10-[3-(4-methyl-piperazin-1-yl)propyl]-2-trifluoromethylphenothiazine dihydrochloride.

Solubility. Soluble, at 20°, in 2 parts of water; slightly soluble in alcohol and in isopropyl alcohol; insoluble in ether.

Standard
It complies with the requirements of the British Pharmacopoeia.
It is a white to pale yellow, crystalline, odourless or almost odourless, hygroscopic powder and contains not less than 99·0 and not more than the equivalent of 101·0 per cent of $C_{21}H_{26}Cl_2F_3N_3S$, calculated with reference to the dried substance. The loss on drying under the prescribed conditions is not more than 1·0 per cent. A 5 per cent solution in water has a pH of 1·7 to 2·6.

Stability. In aqueous solution it is readily oxidised by atmospheric oxygen.

Sterilisation. Solutions for injection are sterilised by heating in an autoclave in an atmosphere of nitrogen or other suitable gas or by filtration.

Storage. It should be stored in airtight containers, protected from light.

Actions and uses. Trifluoperazine has the actions and uses described under Chlorpromazine Hydrochloride (page 107) but it is effective in much smaller doses than chlorpromazine and may be effective in patients who do not respond to chlorpromazine. It acts rapidly in blocking conditioned responses and as an anti-emetic.

In psychotic patients, trifluoperazine may be stimulating rather than sedating, and the usual effective daily dosage by mouth is the equivalent of 15 to 30 milligrams of trifluoperazine, although higher dosage may be necessary. The equivalent of up to 5 milligrams daily may be given by intramuscular injection. In the treatment of psychoneurosis and nausea and vomiting, the equivalent of 2 to 4 milligrams daily is usually sufficient; 6 milligrams daily by mouth or 3 milligrams daily by intramuscular injection should not be exceeded.

Trifluoperazine is unlikely to produce hypotension or hypothermia or to enhance the actions of narcotics and analgesics and is not used for these purposes.

In addition to the tablets, trifluoperazine hydrochloride is available as sustained-release capsules containing the equivalent of

2, 10, and 15 mg of trifluoperazine, as an elixir containing the equivalent of 1 mg of trifluoperazine in 5 ml, and as an injection containing the equivalent of 1 mg of trifluoperazine in 1 ml.

UNDESIRABLE EFFECTS. It may cause drowsiness, dizziness and, occasionally, stimulation; it rarely gives rise to jaundice, blood dyscrasias, and galactorrhoea. High dosage may cause extrapyramidal symptoms, dystonias, and akathisia, particularly in children.

POISONING. The procedure as described under Fluphenazine Hydrochloride (page 202) should be followed. If necessary, hypotension may be treated by the intravenous infusion of noradrenaline.

Dose. See above under **Actions and uses.**

Preparation
TRIFLUOPERAZINE TABLETS, B.P. The equivalent quantity of trifluoperazine base in each tablet should be stated by the prescriber. They are sugar coated. Tablets containing 1 and 5 mg are available.

OTHER NAME: *Stelazine*®

TRIMEPRAZINE TARTRATE

$C_{40}H_{50}N_4O_6S_2 = 747\cdot0$

Trimeprazine Tartrate is 10-(3-dimethylamino-2-methylpropyl)phenothiazine tartrate.

Solubility. Soluble, at 20°, in 4 parts of water, in 30 parts of alcohol, and in 75 parts of chloroform; very slightly soluble in ether.

Standard
DESCRIPTION. A white or slightly cream-coloured powder; odourless or almost odourless. It darkens in colour on exposure to light.

IDENTIFICATION TESTS. 1. Dissolve 0·5 g in 10 ml of water and add 1 ml of *nitric acid*; a red colour is produced and a white precipitate is formed which rapidly redissolves. Warm; the colour changes suddenly to dark green.

2. Dissolve 0·5 g in 5 ml of water, add 1·5 ml of *sodium hydroxide solution*, extract with two successive 10-ml portions of *anaesthetic ether*, and reserve the aqueous liquid; shake the combined extracts with *anhydrous sodium sulphate*, filter, evaporate off the ether, and induce crystallisation; the residue, after drying for 16 hours over *phosphorus pentoxide* in vacuo, melts at about 67°.

3. Make 2 ml of the aqueous solution obtained in test 1 slightly acid to *litmus paper* with *acetic acid* and add 1 ml of *ammonium vanadate solution*; an orange-red colour is produced.

4. It complies with the thin-layer chromatographic test given in Appendix 5C, page 873.

5. The ultraviolet absorption spectrum exhibits the characteristics given in Appendix 3, page 856.

ACIDITY. pH of a 2·0 per cent w/v solution in *carbon dioxide-free water*, 5·0 to 6·5.

MELTING-POINT. 159° to 163°.

LOSS ON DRYING. Not more than 1·0 per cent, determined by drying to constant weight at 100° in vacuo.

SULPHATED ASH. Not more than 0·1 per cent.

CONTENT OF $C_{40}H_{50}N_4O_6S_2$. Not less than 99·0 and not more than the equivalent of 101·0 per cent, calculated with reference to the substance dried under the prescribed conditions, determined by the following method:
Titrate about 1 g, accurately weighed, by Method I of the British Pharmacopoeia, Appendix XIB, for non-aqueous titration; each ml of 0·1N perchloric acid is equivalent to 0·03735 g of $C_{40}H_{50}N_4O_6S_2$.

Storage. It should be protected from light.

Actions and uses. Trimeprazine has an antihistamine action resembling that of promethazine (page 409) and an action on the central nervous system resembling that of chlorpromazine (page 107). Its most marked effect, however, is an antipruritic action.

For the relief of pruritus, trimeprazine tartrate is given by mouth, the usual daily dosage for an adult being 10 to 40 milligrams and for a child 7·5 to 25 milligrams, divided into three or four doses.

It is also used for pre-operative medication of children, 2 to 5 milligrams per kilogram body-weight being given by mouth approximately one hour before operation. It may also be given for pre-operative medication by deep intramuscular injection in doses of 600 to 900 micrograms per kilogram body-weight about one to two hours before operation.

UNDESIRABLE EFFECTS. Trimeprazine frequently produces drowsiness; if this is pronounced, the dosage should be reduced or another antihistamine should be substituted. Other undesirable effects seen occasionally are dizziness, dryness of the mouth, allergic skin reactions and, rarely, agranulocytosis.

POISONING. In acute poisoning the procedure as described under Chlorpromazine Hydrochloride (page 107) should be adopted.

Dose. See above under **Actions and uses.**

Preparations
TRIMEPRAZINE ELIXIR, PAEDIATRIC, B.P.C. (page 677)
TRIMEPRAZINE ELIXIR, PAEDIATRIC, STRONG, B.P.C. (page 678)
TRIMEPRAZINE INJECTION, B.P.C. (page 719)
TRIMEPRAZINE TABLETS, B.P.C. (page 818)

OTHER NAME: *Vallergan*®

TRIMETHOPRIM

$C_{14}H_{18}N_4O_3 = 290\cdot3$

Trimethoprim is 2,4-diamino-5-(3,4,5-trimethoxybenzyl)pyrimidine.

Solubility. Very slightly soluble in water; soluble, at 20°, in 300 parts of alcohol, in 55 parts of chloroform, and in 80 parts of methyl alcohol; insoluble in ether.

Standard
It complies with the requirements of the British Pharmacopoeia.
It is a white odourless powder and contains not less than 98·5 and not more than the equivalent of 101·0 per cent of $C_{14}H_{18}N_4O_3$, calculated with reference to the dried substance. The loss on drying under the prescribed conditions is not more than 1·0 per cent. It has a melting-point of about 200°.

Actions and uses. Trimethoprim is an anti-bacterial agent which is active against approximately the same range of organisms as the antibacterial sulphonamides. It inhibits bacterial dihydrofolate reductases which utilise as substrate the product of a reaction sensitive to the sulphonamides.
It is well absorbed after oral administration and is slowly excreted by the kidney, the biological half-life being approximately fifteen hours; therapeutic blood levels may be maintained by doses at intervals of eight to twelve hours.
Trimethoprim is used mainly in admixture with sulphamethoxazole—see under Sulpha-methoxazole (page 482).
It is also used in conjunction with a sulphon-amide in the treatment of malaria due to susceptible strains of *Plasmodium falciparum* that are resistant to chloroquine. For this purpose doses of 0·5 to 1·5 grams of trimethoprim and 0·75 to 1·5 grams of sulfametopyrazine may be given over a period of twenty-four hours, or

10 milligrams of trimethoprim per kilogram and 20 milligrams of sulfametopyrazine per kilogram body-weight may be given as a single dose. When these doses are given, anti-microbial blood levels of sulfametopyrazine may be expected to persist for five to seven days.

UNDESIRABLE EFFECTS. Nausea may follow the administration of high doses of trimethoprim.

PRECAUTIONS AND CONTRA-INDICATIONS. Although the affinity of trimethoprim for mammalian dihydrofolate reductase is very low, repeated haematological investigations are required during prolonged therapy.
The use of trimethoprim in early pregnancy is not recommended.

Dose. Trimethoprim, for the treatment of malaria, see above under **Actions and uses.**
In conjunction with sulphamethoxazole, see under Sulphamethoxazole (page 482).

Preparations
Co-TRIMOXAZOLE MIXTURE, B.P.C. (page 740).

Co-TRIMOXAZOLE MIXTURE, PAEDIATRIC, B.P.C. (page 741)

Co-TRIMOXAZOLE TABLETS, B.P. (*Syn.* Trimethoprim and Sulphamethoxazole Tablets). These tablets contain sulphamethoxazole and trimethoprim in the proportion of five parts to one. Unless otherwise specified, tablets each containing 400 mg of sulphamethoxazole and 80 mg of trimethoprim are supplied. They should be stored in airtight containers, protected from light.

Co-TRIMOXAZOLE TABLETS, PAEDIATRIC, B.P.C. (page 810)

OTHER NAMES: In conjunction with sulphamethoxazole: *Bactrim®*; *Septrin®*

TRIMIPRAMINE MALEATE

$C_{24}H_{30}N_2O_4 = 410\cdot5$

Trimipramine Maleate is 5-(3-dimethylamino-2-methyl-propyl)-10,11-dihydro-5H-dibenz[b,f]azepine hydrogen maleate.

Solubility. Soluble in water, in alcohol, and in chloroform; very slightly soluble in ether.

Standard
It complies with the requirements of the British Pharmacopoeia.
It is a white, crystalline, odourless or almost odourless powder and contains not less than 99·0 and not more than the equivalent of 101·0 per cent of $C_{24}H_{30}N_2O_4$, calculated with reference to the dried substance. The loss on drying under the prescribed conditions is not more than 0·5 per cent. It has a melting-point of 141° to 145°.

Storage. It should be protected from light.

Actions and uses. Trimipramine has actions and uses similar to those of Imipramine Hydrochloride (page 234) but its sedative action is more pronounced. It is available as the tablets and as capsules, the latter containing 50 mg.

UNDESIRABLE EFFECTS. These are as described under Imipramine Hydrochloride (page 234);

extrapyramidal effects rarely occur. Changes in plasma transaminase may occur.

PRECAUTIONS. Caution should be exercised when giving trimipramine to patients who are being treated with a monoamine-oxidase inhibitor, such as isocarboxazid, nialamide, phenelzine, or tranylcypromine, or who have been so treated within the previous ten days.

OTHER NAME: *Surmontil*®

Dose. The equivalent of 25 to 125 milligrams of trimipramine daily in divided doses.

Preparation
TRIMIPRAMINE TABLETS, B.P. Unless otherwise specified, tablets each containing the equivalent of 10 mg of trimipramine are supplied. They are compression coated. Tablets containing the equivalent of 25 mg are also available.

TRIPROLIDINE HYDROCHLORIDE

$C_{19}H_{23}ClN_2,H_2O = 332.9$

Triprolidine Hydrochloride is *trans*-1-pyrid-2'-yl-3-pyrrolidin-1''-yl-1-*p*-tolylprop-1-ene hydrochloride monohydrate.

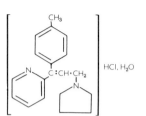

Solubility. Soluble, at 20°, in 2 parts of water, in 1·5 parts of alcohol, and in less than 1 part of chloroform; insoluble in ether.

Standard
It complies with the requirements of the British Pharmacopoeia.
It is a white, crystalline, odourless powder and contains not less than 98·5 and not more than the equivalent of 101·0 per cent of $C_{19}H_{23}ClN_2$, calculated with reference to the anhydrous substance. It contains 4·5 to 6·0 per cent w/w of water. It has a melting-point of 118° to 121°.

Actions and uses. Triprolidine has the actions, uses, and undesirable effects of the antihistamine drugs, as described under Promethazine Hydrochloride (page 409). It is

effective when given by mouth and its action lasts for about twelve hours.

In addition to the tablets, triprolidine hydrochloride is available as an elixir containing 2 mg in 5 ml.

POISONING. As for Promethazine Hydrochloride (page 409).

Dose. 5 to 7·5 milligrams daily in divided doses.

Preparation
TRIPROLIDINE TABLETS, B.P. Unless otherwise specified, tablets each containing 2·5 mg are supplied.

OTHER NAME: *Actidil*®

TROPICAMIDE

$C_{17}H_{20}N_2O_2 = 284.4$

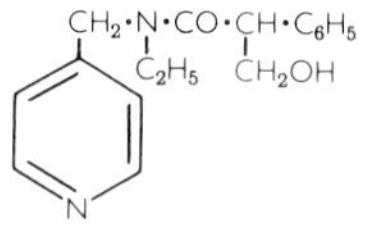

Tropicamide is *N*-ethyl-*N*-(4-pyridylmethyl)tropamide.

Solubility. Soluble, at 20°, in 160 parts of water, in 3·5 parts of alcohol, and in 2 parts of chloroform.

Standard
It complies with the requirements of the British Pharmacopoeia.
It is a white or almost white, crystalline, odourless or almost odourless powder and contains not less than 99·0 and not more than the equivalent of 101·0 per cent of $C_{17}H_{20}N_2O_2$, calculated with reference to the dried substance. The loss on drying under the prescribed conditions is not more than 0·5 per cent. It has a melting-point of 95° to 98°.

Actions and uses. Tropicamide has mydriatic and cycloplegic properties similar to those described under Atropine (page 36) but it acts more quickly and its effect lasts for a shorter time.

The usual quantity required for refraction procedures is two drops of a 1 per cent solution followed after five minutes by a further two drops; the duration of action may be extended by repeating the instillation of drops at intervals of thirty minutes.

For examination of the fundus 2 drops of a 0·5 per cent solution may be used.

PRECAUTIONS AND CONTRA-INDICATIONS. Tropicamide has little effect on intra-ocular tension in the normal eye, but it should be used with caution in cases where the intra-ocular pressure is high.

It is contra-indicated in narrow-angle glaucoma.

OTHER NAME: *Mydriacyl*®

TROXIDONE

$C_6H_9NO_3 = 143.1$

Troxidone is 3,5,5-trimethyloxazolidine-2,4-dione.

Solubility. Soluble, at 20°, in 13 parts of water and in 2 parts of alcohol; soluble in ether and in chloroform.

Standard
It complies with the requirements of the British Pharmacopoeia.
It occurs as colourless granular crystals with a slightly camphoraceous odour and contains not less than 98.0 per cent of $C_6H_9NO_3$. It has a melting-point, without previous drying, of 45° to 47°.

Storage. It should be stored in airtight containers, in a cool place.

Actions and uses. Troxidone prevents leptazol-induced convulsions in animals without causing general depression of the central nervous system, but does not control spon-'taneous convulsions in man.
Troxidone is used in the treatment of true petit mal epilepsy. The initial daily dosage for a child up to two years is 300 milligrams, from two to six years, 600 milligrams, and for an adult, 900 milligrams by mouth, in divided doses; if no toxic effects are observed, these doses may be increased, if necessary, at intervals of not less than a week up to a total daily dose of not more than twice these amounts.
The clinical improvement, usually observed within one to four weeks of beginning treatment, is accompanied by a marked reduction or disappearance of spike and wave formations in the electroencephalogram.

UNDESIRABLE EFFECTS. The most frequent undesirable effect is photophobia, which is usually experienced as a glare effect in brightly lit surroundings, and if this is severe and persistent the wearing of dark glasses may be necessary. Rashes, nausea, headache, fatigue, and muscular weakness occur occasionally.
Rarer but potentially fatal toxic effects are due to hypersensitivity reactions affecting the bone marrow, skin, kidney, and liver.

PRECAUTIONS   and   CONTRA-INDICATIONS.
Troxidone does not diminish the frequency or severity of convulsive seizures in patients with grand mal epilepsy and must not be used for the treatment of those patients, as it may precipitate status epilepticus. It does not relieve patients with psychomotor seizures, but in some of those patients it may augment the therapeutic action of phenytoin sodium.

Dose. See above under **Actions and uses.**

Preparations
TROXIDONE CAPSULES, B.P. Unless otherwise specified, capsules each containing 300 mg of troxidone are supplied.
TROXIDONE TABLETS, PAEDIATRIC, B.P.C. (page 818)

OTHER NAMES: *Tridione®*; Trimethadione

TUBOCURARINE CHLORIDE

SYNONYMS: Tubocurar. Chlor.; Tubocurarinii Chloridum

$C_{37}H_{42}Cl_2N_2O_6,5H_2O = 771.7$

Tubocurarine Chloride is the chloride of an alkaloid, (+)-tubocurarine, obtained from extracts of the stems of *Chondodendron tomentosum* Ruiz et Pav. (Fam. Menispermaceae) and possessing the specific biological activity of curare on neuromuscular transmission.

Solubility. Soluble, at 20°, in 20 parts of water and in 30 parts of alcohol; soluble in solutions of alkali hydroxides; very slightly soluble in ether, in chloroform, and in acetone.

Standard
It complies with the requirements of the European Pharmacopoeia.
It is a white or slightly yellowish-white, crystalline, odourless powder and contains not less than 98.0 and not more than the equivalent of 102.0 per cent of $C_{37}H_{42}Cl_2N_2O_6$, calculated with reference to the dried substance. The loss on drying under the prescribed conditions is 9.0 to 12.0 per cent. It melts with decomposition at about 270°. A 1 per cent solution in water has a pH of 4.0 to 6.0.

Sterilisation. Solutions for injection are sterilised by heating in an autoclave in an atmosphere of nitrogen or other suitable gas.

Actions and uses. Tubocurarine produces relaxation of voluntary muscle by reducing its response to acetylcholine.
When administered intravenously it produces first fatigue, then weakness, and, finally, paralysis of voluntary muscle, beginning in the eyes and spreading to the face, neck, limbs, abdomen, intercostal muscles, and diaphragm; recovery of muscle function occurs in the reverse order.

The effects of moderate doses are transient, owing to their rapid elimination and destruction. The peak effect is reached within three to five minutes of intravenous injection, and the effect begins to decline after about twenty minutes. When respiratory paralysis occurs, it will do so within seven to ten minutes of intravenous injection.

In the dosage used clinically, tubocurarine has no central stimulant, depressant, or analgesic action. Its action is antagonised by anticholinesterase drugs.

Tubocurarine chloride is used chiefly as an adjunct to anaesthesia to secure muscular relaxation in surgery and obstetrics. For this purpose, 10 to 20 milligrams of tubocurarine chloride is given by intravenous injection, followed, if necessary, as indicated by the degree of muscular relaxation, by further doses of 2 to 4 milligrams at intervals of about thirty minutes up to a total of 45 milligrams, provided that adequate methods for dealing with respiratory failure are at hand.

It can be used with the usual anaesthetic agents, barbiturates, and intravenous analgesic drugs. In the presence of ether, however, the action of tubocurarine is enhanced; when ether is used as the anaesthetic, it is important, therefore, to reduce the dose of tubocurarine chloride to one-half to one-third of that used with other anaesthetics.

The additional doses of tubocurarine are sometimes given alternately with small doses of a barbiturate during operation. Since precipitation may occur when a solution of tubocurarine chloride is mixed with certain barbiturates, admixture with these barbiturates must be avoided.

It is also used, usually by the intravenous route, to produce muscular relaxation before such procedures as bronchoscopy and laryngoscopy; 0·6 to 1·2 milligrams of atropine should be given to counteract the increased salivation caused by tubocurarine.

Tubocurarine is used in certain neurological conditions for the symptomatic relief of hypertonia, tremor, and incoordination. It is also used in tetanus and shock therapy to diminish the severity of the convulsions and to prevent fractures, and in the treatment of fractures and dislocations.

UNDESIRABLE EFFECTS. The chief dangers arising from the use of tubocurarine are respiratory failure and regurgitation of the stomach contents due to relaxation of the oesophageal muscle and sphincters.

CONTRA-INDICATIONS. Tubocurarine is contra-indicated in patients with myasthenia gravis and in asthmatics, because it causes the release of histamine.

POISONING. Neostigmine methylsulphate should be given intravenously in a dose of 5 milligrams after the intravenous injection of atropine sulphate 0·5 to 1 milligram; this dose of atropine may be repeated if necessary. Artificial respiration is essential until spontaneous breathing is resumed.

Dose. See above under **Actions and uses.**

Preparation
TUBOCURARINE INJECTION, B.P. It consists of a sterile solution containing 1 per cent of tubocurarine chloride in Water for Injections.

OTHER NAMES: *Tubarine*®; *d*-Tubocurarine Chloride

TURPENTINE OIL

SYNONYM: Oleum Terebinthinae

Turpentine Oil is the oil obtained by distillation and rectification from turpentine, an oleoresin obtained from various species of *Pinus* (Fam. Pinaceae), notably *P. palustris* Mill. and *P. elliottii* Engelm. (*P. caribaea* Mor.) in North America and *P. pinaster* Ait. in southern Europe. The unrectified oil is the turpentine of commerce.

French and Portuguese turpentine oils are always strongly laevorotatory, but American oils may be either laevo- or dextro-rotatory.

Constituents. Turpentine oil consists principally of pinenes, together with smaller amounts of other terpenes.

Solubility. Soluble, at 20°, in 7 parts of alcohol (90 per cent) and in 3 parts of alcohol (95 per cent); miscible with dehydrated alcohol, with ether, with chloroform, with carbon disulphide, and with glacial acetic acid.

Standard
It complies with the requirements of the British Pharmacopoeia.
It is a clear, bright, colourless liquid with a strong characteristic odour which becomes stronger and less pleasant on storage and on exposure to the air. It has a weight per ml at 20° of 0·855 g to 0·868 g.

Stability. On prolonged exposure to the air, turpentine oil undergoes rapid change, especially in the presence of moisture; it becomes viscous and yellow and acquires an acid reaction, the weight per ml increases, the boiling-point rises, and the solubility in alcohol increases.

Adulterants and substitutes. Petroleum, resin oil, and wood turpentine are common adulterants.
Petroleum may be detected by its effect in lowering the weight per ml, and also by the flash-point, which for pure turpentine oil is about 95°F. White spirit, which is commonly used as a turpentine substitute, consists of petroleum fractions and has a flash-point of about 82°F.
Resin oil, a product of the destructive distillation of

colophony, may be detected by the fatty stain which the adulterated oil leaves when evaporated from paper.

Wood turpentine, which is obtained by distilling the roots and stumps of various species of *Pinus*, has a higher weight per ml.

Sulphate turpentine, obtained during the manufacture of wood pulp by the sulphate process, resembles turpentine oil but contains sulphur compounds.

Storage. It should be stored in well-filled airtight containers, protected from light, in a cool place.

Actions and uses. Turpentine oil is applied externally in liniments as a counter-irritant and rubefacient.

POISONING. Emetics and demulcent drinks should be given, with magnesium sulphate to promote purgation and with morphine to relieve pain.

Preparations
TURPENTINE LINIMENT, B.P. It contains 65 per cent of turpentine oil, with soft soap and camphor.

WHITE LINIMENT, B.P.C. (page 726)

UNDECENOIC ACID

SYNONYM: Undecylenic Acid

$C_{11}H_{20}O_2 = 184.3$

$$CH_2:CH \cdot [CH_2]_8 \cdot CO_2H$$

Undecenoic Acid consists mainly of undec-10-enoic acid.

Solubility. Very slightly soluble in water; miscible with alcohol, with ether, with chloroform, and with fixed and volatile oils.

Standard
It complies with the requirements of the British Pharmacopoeia.
It is a colourless to pale yellowish-brown liquid or a white to cream-coloured crystalline mass with a characteristic odour and contains not less than 96.0 per cent of $C_{11}H_{20}O_2$. It has a freezing-point of 21° to 24°.

Storage. It should be stored in airtight containers, protected from light.

Actions and uses. Undecenoic acid is a fungicide used for the prophylaxis and treatment of superficial dermatophytoses of the head, ears, feet, axillae, and groin and of candidiasis and mycotic infections of the vulva and vagina.

For application to the skin, concentrations of 2 to 15 per cent are used, sometimes in conjunction with zinc undecenoate, in ointments, emulsions, and dusting-powders.

For application to mucous surfaces the concentration should not exceed 1 per cent, as stronger preparations may cause irritation.

Preparations
ZINC UNDECENOATE DUSTING-POWDER, B.P.C. (page 664)

ZINC UNDECENOATE OINTMENT, B.P. It contains 20 per cent of zinc undecenoate and 5 per cent of undecenoic acid in Emulsifying Ointment.

UREA

$CH_4N_2O = 60.06$

$$NH_2 \cdot CO \cdot NH_2$$

Urea is the diamide of carbonic acid.

Solubility. Soluble, at 20°, in 1 part of water and in 12 parts of alcohol; soluble in 1.5 parts of boiling alcohol; insoluble in ether and in chloroform.

Standard
It complies with the requirements of the British Pharmacopoeia.
It occurs as odourless or almost odourless, colourless, transparent, slightly hygroscopic, prismatic crystals and contains not less than 99.5 per cent of CH_4N_2O. It has a melting-point of 132° to 134°.

Sterilisation. Solutions for injection are sterilised by filtration.

Storage. It should be stored in airtight containers.

Actions and uses. Urea exerts a diuretic action. When given by mouth, it is rapidly excreted and its excretion is accompanied by an increase in urinary output; the rate of excretion of 15 grams of urea administered in 100 millilitres of water is used as a test for renal function. The usual dose as a diuretic is 5 to 15 grams.

To produce decompression in concussion and cerebral injury, urea is administered by slow intravenous injection in a 30 per cent w/v solution in Dextrose Injection (5 or 10 per cent). The dose is usually 40 to 90 grams of urea, but not exceeding 1.5 grams per kilogram body-weight, in twenty-four hours. The solution is irritant and care must be taken to avoid extravasation during injection.

Dose. See above under **Actions and uses.**

Preparation
UREA INJECTION, B.P. It consists of a sterile solution prepared immediately before use by dissolving the sterile contents of a sealed container in Dextrose Injection (5 or 10 per cent w/v). The sealed container also contains a small proportion of citric acid.

OTHER NAMES: Carbamide; *Ureaphil®*; *Urevert®*

VANCOMYCIN HYDROCHLORIDE

Vancomycin Hydrochloride is an antibiotic produced by the growth of certain strains of *Streptomyces orientalis* or by any other means.

Solubility. Soluble, at 20°, in 10 parts of water and in 700 parts of alcohol; slightly soluble in ether; very slightly soluble in chloroform.

Standard
It complies with the requirements of the British Pharmacopoeia.
It is a light brown odourless powder and contains not less than 900 Units per mg, calculated with reference to the anhydrous substance. It contains not more than 4·5 per cent w/w of water. The pH of a 5 per cent solution in water is 2·8 to 4·5.

Storage. It should be stored in sterile containers, sealed to exclude micro-organisms.

Actions and uses. Vancomycin is an antibiotic which is effective against Gram-positive cocci. It is given by intravenous injection, mainly in the treatment of systemic infections caused by staphylococci which are resistant to other antibiotics; it is also of value in the treatment of endocarditis and other infections caused by non-haemolytic streptococci resistant to penicillin.

The usual daily dosage for an adult is 2 grams of vancomycin hydrochloride given by slow intravenous infusion over a period of twenty-four hours, or 500 milligrams given by slow intravenous injection over a period of twenty to thirty minutes every six to eight hours; the daily dosage for a child is 45 milligrams per kilogram body-weight.

When given by slow intravenous injection the dose of vancomycin hydrochloride is dissolved in 100 to 200 millilitres of Sodium Chloride Injection or Dextrose Injection (5 per cent); when given by intravenous infusion, the dose is dissolved in a larger volume. The solution is irritant and care should be taken to avoid extravasation during injection. To guard against accumulation, regular blood-level determinations should be made; a blood concentration of 10 to 20 micrograms per millilitre should be maintained.

UNDESIRABLE EFFECTS. Nausea, shivering, and rashes may occur. Impaired hearing is a more serious hazard, but is unlikely to occur unless treatment is prolonged or there is impairment of kidney function resulting in a lowered excretion rate and higher blood concentration of the antibiotic.

Dose. See above under **Actions and uses.**

Preparation
VANCOMYCIN INJECTION, B.P. It consists of a sterile solution prepared immediately before use by dissolving the sterile contents of a sealed container in Water for Injections. The quantity of vancomycin hydrochloride in each container should be specified by the prescriber. Ampoules containing 500 mg are available.

OTHER NAME: *Vancocin®*

VANILLIN

$C_8H_8O_3 = 152·1$

Vanillin is 4-hydroxy-3-methoxybenzaldehyde and may be obtained from *Vanilla planifolia* Andrews or other species of *Vanilla* (Fam. Orchidaceae), or prepared synthetically.

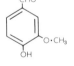

Solubility. Soluble, at 20°, in 100 parts of water and in 20 parts of glycerol; soluble in alcohol, in fixed and volatile oils, and in solutions of alkali hydroxides.

Standard
DESCRIPTION. White or cream-coloured crystalline needles or powder; odour characteristic of vanilla.

IDENTIFICATION TESTS. 1. To 1 ml of a saturated solution in water, add 1 ml of *lead acetate solution*; a white precipitate is formed which is soluble in hot water from which it separates in scales on cooling.

2. To 10 ml of a saturated solution in water, add 0·2 ml

of *ferric chloride test-solution*; a blue colour is produced. Heat at 80° for 3 minutes; the solution becomes brown. Cool; a white or almost white precipitate is formed.

MELTING-POINT. 81° to 83°.

SULPHATED ASH. Not more than 0·1 per cent.

Storage. It should be stored in airtight containers, protected from light.

Uses. Vanillin is used as a flavouring agent and in perfumery.

VASOPRESSIN INJECTION

SYNONYM: Vasopressin Inj.

Vasopressin Injection is a sterile aqueous solution containing the pressor and antidiuretic principles, prepared by a process of fractionation, of the posterior lobe of mammalian pituitary bodies.

Standard
It complies with the requirements of the British Pharmacopoeia.
It is a clear colourless liquid and contains 20 Units (pressor) and not more than 1·2 Units (oxytocic) per

ml; the activities are determined by biological methods. It has a pH of 3·0 to 4·0.

Sterilisation. It is sterilised by filtration.

Storage. It should be stored at temperatures between

2° and 10°. Under these conditions it may be expected to retain its potency for at least three years from the date of manufacture. If stored at temperatures not exceeding 25°, it may be expected to retain its potency for at least two years from the date of manufacture.

Actions and uses. Vasopressin Injection has the pressor and antidiuretic actions described under Powdered Pituitary (Posterior Lobe) (page 385) but has practically no oxytocic activity.

Vasopressin Injection is administered by subcutaneous or intramuscular injection in the treatment of diabetes insipidus to control the polyuria; it must be given at least twice a day and, if given by intravenous injection, it must be well diluted.

Vasopressin Injection has been used to stimulate the muscle of the intestinal tract, but it has been superseded by cholinergic drugs because they are safer. It should not be used to raise the blood pressure.

UNDESIRABLE EFFECTS. The administration of Vasopressin Injection may be followed by marked pallor, nausea, eructation, cramp, and a desire to defaecate.

CONTRA-INDICATIONS. It is contra-indicated in vascular disease, especially of the coronary arteries.

Dose. 0·1 to 1 millilitre, equivalent to 2 to 20 Units, by subcutaneous or intramuscular injection.

OTHER NAME: *Pitressin®*

VINBLASTINE SULPHATE

$C_{46}H_{60}N_4O_{13}S = 909.1$

Vinblastine Sulphate is the sulphate of an alkaloid occurring in *Catharanthus roseus* (L.) G. Don (*Vinca rosea* L.) (Fam. Apocynaceae).

Solubility. Soluble, at 20°, in 10 parts of water, in 1200 parts of alcohol, and in 50 parts of chloroform; insoluble in ether.

Standard
It complies with the requirements of the British Pharmacopoeia.
It is a white to slightly yellow, amorphous or crystalline, very hygroscopic, odourless powder and contains not less than 96·0 and not more than the equivalent of 101·0 per cent of $C_{46}H_{60}N_4O_{13}S$, calculated with reference to the dried substance. The loss on drying under the prescribed conditions is not more than 17·0 per cent. A 0·15 per cent solution in water has a pH of 3·5 to 5·0.

Storage. It should be stored in airtight containers, protected from light, at a temperature between 2° and 10°.

Actions and uses. Vinblastine sulphate is a cytotoxic drug that arrests cell growth at the metaphase. Its actions are more pronounced on the rapidly dividing cell than on the normal cell. In clinical dosage it depresses bone-marrow activity, affecting mainly the white cells, with relative sparing of the erythroid elements. The bone-marrow depression is reversible on stopping the drug.

Vinblastine sulphate suppresses the immune response and in high doses is neurotoxic. Like other cytotoxic drugs it is teratogenic. It is cleared from the blood after intravenous injection in about an hour, and is excreted mainly by the liver through the bile, less than 5 per cent of a given dose appearing in the urine.

Vinblastine sulphate is used mainly for the treatment of Hodgkin's disease and other lymphomas and choriocarcinoma. It is more likely to induce a remission in Hodgkin's disease than cyclophosphamide (page 138), although a combination of the two drugs with prednisolone is more effective than either

drug alone. Some response has been reported in the treatment of inoperable solid tumours, such as those of the breast, female genital tract, lung, testes, and gastro-intestinal tract. The results are stated to be better if vinblastine sulphate is used in conjunction with other cytotoxic drugs, such as cyclophosphamide and chlorambucil.

Vinblastine sulphate is administered by the intravenous injection of a solution of 1 milligram per millilitre in Water for Injections or Sodium Chloride Injection. It is given weekly, starting with a dose of 100 micrograms per kilogram body-weight, which is raised by weekly increments of 50 micrograms per kilogram body-weight. The dose should not be increased beyond that which reduces the white-cell count to 3000 per cubic millimetre. The maximum single dose in patients previously treated with cytotoxic agents or deep X-rays should not generally exceed 150 micrograms per kilogram body-weight; in previously untreated patients, higher doses may be tolerated. Higher doses are tolerated by children with leukaemia. The average weekly dose is 150 to 200 micrograms per kilogram body-weight.

Response to treatment may take one or two weeks, as in cases of Hodgkin's disease and choriocarcinoma, or may be delayed as long as twelve weeks in the case of solid tumours. Once response has occurred a maintenance dose may be given indefinitely every one or two weeks. This is the maximum dose that the patient will tolerate without the production of serious leucopenia. White-cell counts should therefore be done before each injection and the dose of vinblastine sulphate adjusted so that the count does not fall below 4000 per cubic millimetre.

Vinblastine sulphate may also be administered in Dextrose Injection (5 per cent w/v) by intravenous infusion, by continuous intra-arterial infusion, and into body cavities. Withdrawal of the drug usually results in relapse within three weeks.

UNDESIRABLE EFFECTS. In general, these are dose-related. Effects on the haemopoietic system include neutropenia, and rarely thrombocytopenia, which may occur if vinblastine sulphate is given after courses of other cytotoxic drugs or after irradiation. Recovery occurs within seven to fourteen days of stopping the drug.

Other side-effects are epilation, nausea, vomiting, anorexia, diarrhoea, stomatitis, and urticaria.

The neurological manifestations, apart from bone-marrow depression, are the most serious side-effects. They include peripheral neuropathy, neuromyopathy, paraesthesia, loss of deep tendon reflexes, psychoses, and mental depression.

Dysfunction of the autonomic nervous system may also occur, with urinary retention, severe constipation, leading to ileus, and parotid gland pain and tenderness.

PRECAUTIONS. Vinblastine sulphate should be used with care in cachectic patients. Its use in pregnancy is not advised as it is teratogenic. Care should be used when it is injected intravenously as perivenous infiltration may cause cellulitis, phlebitis, and venous thrombosis.

CONTRA-INDICATIONS. Vinblastine sulphate should not be given if the white-cell count is below 4000 per cubic millimetre, if bacterial infection is present, or if the bone marrow is infiltrated with neoplastic cells.

Dose. See above under **Actions and uses.**

Preparation

VINBLASTINE INJECTION, B.P. It consists of a sterile solution prepared by dissolving the sterile contents of a sealed container in Water for Injections. It should be stored at a temperature between 2° and 10° and used within four days of preparation, or within thirty days of preparation if a bactericide is present. Vials containing 10 mg of vinblastine sulphate are available.

OTHER NAME: *Velbe*®

VINCRISTINE SULPHATE

$C_{46}H_{58}N_4O_{14}S = 923·0$

Vincristine Sulphate is the sulphate of an alkaloid occurring in *Catharanthus roseus* (L.) G. Don (*Vinca rosea* L.) (Fam. Apocynaceae).

Solubility. Soluble, at 20°, in 2 parts of water, in 600 parts of alcohol, and in 30 parts of chloroform; insoluble in ether.

Standard

It complies with the requirements of the British Pharmacopoeia.

It is a white to slightly yellow, amorphous or crystalline, very hygroscopic, odourless powder and contains not less than 90·0 and not more than the equivalent of 105·0 per cent of $C_{46}H_{58}N_4O_{14}S$, calculated with reference to the dried substance. The loss on drying under the prescribed conditions is not more than 12·0 per cent. A 0·1 per cent solution in water has a pH of 3·5 to 4·5.

Storage. It should be stored in airtight containers, protected from light, at a temperature between 2° and 10°.

Actions and uses. Vincristine sulphate is a cytotoxic drug which, like vinblastine sulphate, arrests mitosis in the metaphase. Although the depressant action of vincristine sulphate on the bone marrow is less than that of vinblastine sulphate, it has a more pronounced neurotoxic effect. In clinical dosage it may cause peripheral neuropathy, neuromuscular disturbances, and effects on the autonomic nervous system. It is administered intravenously. It is rapidly cleared from the blood and is excreted mainly through the bile.

Although the range of clinical activity resembles that of vinblastine sulphate, there are some differences. There is no cross-resistance between the two and vincristine sulphate is less effective in the treatment of Hodgkin's disease. It is more effective in the treatment of the acute leukaemias, particularly in children, but as it does not readily penetrate the blood–brain barrier, it should always be used with other oncolytic agents if the leukaemic process involves the central nervous system.

Other conditions in which vincristine sulphate has produced remissions are lymphosarcoma, reticulum sarcoma, neuroblastoma, Wilm's tumour, and tumours of the brain, breast, and lung.

Vincristine sulphate is administered intravenously at weekly intervals, almost invariably in conjunction with other oncolytic drugs. For children with leukaemia the commencing weekly dose is 50 micrograms per kilogram body-weight with weekly increments of 25 micrograms per kilogram, until a maximum of 150 micrograms per kilogram is reached. After remission has occurred the dosage is reduced to a maintenance level of 50 to 75 micrograms per kilogram weekly. For adult leukaemia the weekly dose is from 25 to 75 micrograms per kilogram body-weight.

For other malignant conditions the dose is smaller, of the order of 25 micrograms per kilogram body-weight weekly until a remission occurs. The dose is then reduced to 5 to 10 micrograms per kilogram for as long as any anti-tumour effect can be observed.

UNDESIRABLE EFFECTS. These are dose-related and less likely to occur if the weekly dose is below 100 micrograms per kilogram body-weight.

The commonest adverse reactions are alopecia, neuromuscular and neurological disturbances, gastro-intestinal upsets, particularly abdominal colic, severe constipation, leucopenia, loss of weight, and dysuria. These effects may decrease or disappear on reducing the dose.

PRECAUTIONS AND CONTRA-INDICATIONS. Although neuromuscular rather than bone-

marrow toxicity limits dosage, white-cell counts should be carried out before giving each dose. Dosage should be reduced or temporarily omitted if infection is present.

Care should be taken against extravasation during intravenous injection as this may cause phlebitis or cellulitis.

The concentration of the solution for injection should be from 10 to 100 micrograms per millilitre.

Dose. See above under **Actions and uses.**

Preparation
VINCRISTINE INJECTION, B.P. It consists of a sterile solution of a mixture of 1 part by weight of vincristine sulphate and 10 parts by weight of lactose prepared by dissolving the sterile contents of a sealed container in Water for Injections. It should be stored at a temperature between 2° and 10° and used within 24 hours of preparation or within fourteen days if a bactericide is present. Vials containing 1 mg and 5 mg of vincristine sulphate are available.

OTHER NAME: *Oncovin*®

VINYL ETHER

$C_4H_6O = 70.09$ $(CH_2:CH)_2O$

Vinyl Ether is divinyl ether to which has been added about 4 per cent v/v of dehydrated alcohol and not more than 0.01 per cent w/v of phenyl-α-naphthylamine or other suitable stabiliser.

CAUTION. *Vinyl Ether is inflammable and mixtures with oxygen or air at certain concentrations are explosive; it should not be used in the presence of a naked flame or of an electrical apparatus liable to produce a spark. Precautions should be taken against the production of static electrical discharge.*

Divinyl ether has a flash-point below $-22°F$ (closed-cup test). On exposure to air and light, divinyl ether decomposes into formaldehyde and formic acid, ultimately polymerising to a jelly; the rate of decomposition is retarded by the presence of the stabiliser. The dehydrated alcohol is added to reduce the rate of evaporation of Vinyl Ether when used in anaesthesia and so reduce the possibility of ice formation on masks.

Solubility. Soluble, at 20°, in 100 parts of water; miscible with alcohol, with ether, and with chloroform.

Standard
It complies with the requirements of the British Pharmacopoeia.
It is a clear, colourless, liquid with a characteristic odour and often a slight purplish fluorescence due to the presence of the stabiliser. It has a weight per ml at 20° of 0·770 g to 0·778 g and a boiling-point of 28° to 31°. When shaken with water, the aqueous layer is neutral to litmus.

Storage. It should be stored in airtight containers of not more than 200-ml capacity, protected from light, in a cool place. It should be used within forty-eight hours of first opening the container.

Actions and uses. Vinyl ether is a very volatile anaesthetic which has a potency about four times that of ether. It is more toxic and

more rapid in action than ether and considerable care must therefore be exercised in its administration, as the stage of overdosage is very quickly reached. Recovery is very rapid. The degree of muscular relaxation induced by vinyl ether is more variable than that induced by ether and cannot be relied upon during surgical operations.

It is important to note that the eye signs which are usually depended upon in anaesthesia are entirely unreliable in the case of vinyl ether, and the extent of anaesthesia must be gauged by the rate, depth, and regularity of the respiration; overdosage is usually indicated by the development of cyanosis.

Other disadvantages of vinyl ether are the frequency with which excessive salivation occurs and the toxic effect on the liver.

Post-operative complications are rare, and nausea and vomiting relatively infrequent.

Vinyl ether is indicated for use in minor operative procedures of short duration. It has been used in dental surgery and in obstetrics. It is also useful as an induction anaesthetic and, in minimal doses, as an adjuvant to other anaesthetics; one part of vinyl ether with three parts of anaesthetic ether forms a mixture which gives a vapour of constant composition.

For short operations or as an induction anaesthetic, vinyl ether is commonly administered on an open mask or in an inhaler. For longer procedures the semi-closed or closed method is used, with admixture of nitrous oxide and oxygen.

POISONING. In the event of poisoning resulting in collapse, the procedure described under Chloroform (page 100) should be adopted.

OTHER NAME: *Vinesthene®*

VIOMYCIN SULPHATE

Viomycin Sulphate is the sulphate of an antimicrobial base produced by certain strains of *Streptomyces griseus* var. *purpureus* or by any other means.

Solubility. Very soluble in water; slightly soluble in alcohol; very slightly soluble in ether.

Standard
It complies with the requirements of the British Pharmacopoeia.
It is a white or almost white, somewhat hygroscopic, odourless or almost odourless powder and contains not less than 700 Units per mg, calculated with reference to the dried substance. The loss on drying under the prescribed conditions is not more than 5·0 per cent. A solution in water containing 100,000 Units per ml is clear and has a pH between 4·5 and 7·0.

Storage. It should be stored in airtight sterile containers, sealed to exclude micro-organisms, in a cool place.

Actions and uses. Viomycin is an antibiotic which is active against *Mycobacterium tuberculosis*, including strains which are resistant to streptomycin. It is readily absorbed when given by intramuscular injection and is excreted mainly by the kidneys.

The main use of viomycin is in the treatment of all forms of tuberculosis when an antibiotic of the streptomycin group cannot be used because the organism is resistant or the patient hypersensitive. Like other antituberculous drugs, it has little effect when extensive caseation or fibrosis is present. As with streptomycin, treatment with viomycin should be combined with the administration of isoniazid or an aminosalicylate in order to minimise the emergence of resistant strains.

The usual dosage is 1 mega Unit of viomycin sulphate, dissolved in not less than 2 millilitres of Water for Injections or Sodium Chloride Injection, twice a week in two equal doses, morning and evening. Treatment must be continued for six months or more.

UNDESIRABLE EFFECTS. Rashes, renal irritation, disturbances of electrolyte and fluid balances, abnormalities in the electrocardiogram, dizziness, and loss of hearing occur infrequently with normal dosage.

PRECAUTIONS AND CONTRA-INDICATIONS. Because of its potential toxicity, viomycin should not be used unless streptomycin is contra-indicated; it should not be used for patients with impaired kidney function.

If injections are given more frequently than recommended a check must be made on the electrolyte balance and kidney function.

Dose. See above under **Actions and uses.**

Preparation
VIOMYCIN SULPHATE INJECTION, B.P. It consists of a sterile solution prepared by dissolving the sterile contents of a sealed container in Water for Injections. The quantity of viomycin sulphate in each container should be specified by the prescriber. It should be used within one week of its date of preparation, which is stated on the label, when stored at room temperature, or within one month when stored at 2° to 10°.

OTHER NAME: *Viocin®*

VIPRYNIUM EMBONATE

$C_{75}H_{70}N_6O_6 = 1151·4$

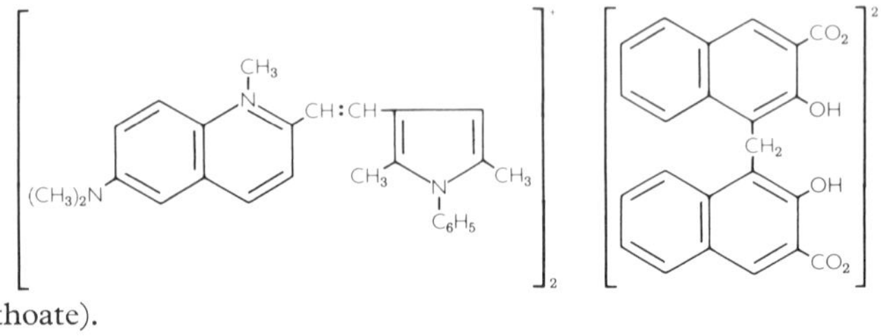

Viprynium Embonate is 6-dimethylamino-2-[2-(2,5-dimethyl-1-phenylpyrrol-3-yl)vinyl]-1-methylquinolinium 4,4'-methylenebis(3-hydroxy-2-naphthoate).

Solubility. Very slightly soluble in water, in alcohol, and in ether; slightly soluble in chloroform; soluble, at 20°, in 330 parts of methoxyethanol.

Standard
It complies with the requirements of the British Pharmacopoeia.

It is a bright orange-red to almost black, crystalline, almost odourless powder and contains not less than 96·0 and not more than the equivalent of 104·0 per cent of $C_{75}H_{70}N_6O_6$, calculated with reference to the dried substance. The loss on drying under the prescribed conditions is not more than 6·0 per cent. It melts with decomposition at about 206°.

Storage. It should be stored in airtight containers, protected from light.

Actions and uses. Viprynium embonate is a dye which is used as an anthelmintic against threadworms. It is poorly absorbed.

It is administered by mouth as a single dose equivalent to 5 milligrams of the base per kilogram body-weight; 75 milligrams of viprynium embonate is approximately equivalent to 50 milligrams of viprynium base. It may be

desirable to repeat the dose after one or two weeks.

Viprynium embonate stains the stools red and also stains any clothing with which it comes into contact. The tablets should be swallowed whole as otherwise the mouth is deeply stained.

UNDESIRABLE EFFECTS. Nausea and vomiting occasionally occur.

Dose. See above under **Actions and uses.**

Preparations
VIPRYNIUM MIXTURE, B.P.C. (page 755)
VIPRYNIUM TABLETS, B.P. Unless otherwise specified, tablets each containing the equivalent of 50 mg of viprynium are supplied. They are sugar coated.

OTHER NAMES: *Vanquin®*; Viprynium Pamoate

VITAMIN A ESTER CONCENTRATE

Vitamin A Ester Concentrate consists of an ester or a mixture of esters of retinol, or of a solution of the ester or mixture of esters in arachis oil or other suitable vegetable oil; esters of natural or synthetic origin or mixtures of such esters may be used. It may contain a suitable antoxidant or mixture of antoxidants.

Solubility. Insoluble in water; soluble or partly soluble in alcohol; miscible with ether, with chloroform, and with light petroleum.

Standard
It complies with the requirements of the British Pharmacopoeia.
It is a yellow oil or mixture of oil and crystalline material which when warmed yields a homogeneous, yellow oil; it has a faint odour.
It contains in 1 g not less than 485,000 Units of vitamin-A activity and not less than 97·0 per cent of the number of Units of vitamin-A activity stated on the label; it

may contain a suitable antoxidant or mixture of antoxidants.

Storage. It should be stored in hermetically sealed containers in an atmosphere of nitrogen or other suitable gas, protected from light, in a cool place.

Actions and uses. Vitamin A ester concentrate has the actions, uses, and undesirable effects described under Concentrated Vitamin A Solution (below).

CONCENTRATED VITAMIN A SOLUTION

Concentrated Vitamin A Solution may consist of a suitable fish-liver oil or blend of such oils, or it may be prepared by dissolving, at a temperature not exceeding 60°, a source of vitamin A in a vegetable oil such as arachis oil.

In preparing Concentrated Vitamin A Solution, any suitable source of vitamin A may be used, such as a fish-liver oil rich in the vitamin, a concentrate prepared therefrom, or synthetic vitamin A or its esters.

A concentrate may be prepared by molecular distillation from oils of suitable potency. It may also be prepared from fish-liver oils by saponifying with alcoholic potash, extracting the unsaponifiable matter with ether, evaporating off the ether, dissolving the residue in twice its weight of methyl alcohol, cooling to 0°, removing the cholesterol which crystallises out, and finally distilling off the methyl alcohol.

A concentrate so prepared from mammalian livers contains a very small amount of vitamin D, but may contain more vitamin A than a concentrate prepared in the same way from

cod-liver oil. It is mixed with a suitable vegetable oil to give a solution of the required strength.

Solubility. Slightly soluble in alcohol; miscible with ether, with chloroform, and with light petroleum.

Standard
DESCRIPTION. A pale yellow or yellow oily liquid; odour faint but not rancid.

ACID VALUE. Not more than 2·5.

ANTIRACHITIC ACTIVITY (VITAMIN D). The estimated potency is not more than 500 Units per g, determined by the following method:
Carry out the method of the British Pharmacopoeia, Appendix XIVG, for the biological assay of antirachitic vitamin (vitamin D).
The precision of the assay must be such that the fiducial limits of error (P = 0·95) are between 60 and 170 per cent of the estimated potency.

VITAMIN-A ACTIVITY. Not less than 45,000 and not more than 55,000 Units per g, determined by the method of the British Pharmacopoeia, Appendix XVIIA, for the assay of vitamin A.

Storage. It should be stored in well-filled airtight containers, protected from light, in a cool place.

Actions and uses. Vitamin A maintains the development and normal function of epithelial tissue. The human requirements of vitamin A cannot be accurately assessed, but are believed to be in the region of 5000 Units daily, with an additional 1000 Units during pregnancy and 3000 Units during lactation.

Deficiency of vitamin A leads to impaired dark-adaptation and atrophy of epithelial cells with differentiation into a stratified keratinising epithelium. In the eye, the conjunctiva is dry and wrinkled; there is also dryness of the cornea. This xerophthalmia may lead to secondary infection and panophthalmitis.

The earliest symptom indicating deficiency is night blindness, caused by failure of the retinal rods to resynthesise visual purple. Dryness and roughness of the skin may also occur. The epithelial changes may favour secondary infection, but the vitamin should not be called "anti-infective"; additional vitamin A given to persons who are not suffering from a deficiency of the vitamin does not increase their resistance to infection.

Deficient absorption of the precursors of vitamin A occurs in certain conditions, such as coeliac disease and sprue. Therapeutically, vitamin A may be administered in these conditions and when there is reason to suspect inadequate absorption of the fat-soluble vitamin due to defective absorption of fat.

Excessive use of liquid paraffin may inhibit absorption of appreciable amounts of vitamin A and its precursors from the small and large intestines.

A person suffering from vitamin A deficiency is prone to develop infections, particularly of the respiratory tract, and will benefit from the administration of vitamin A. But there is no evidence that vitamin A will influence the course of respiratory or other infections in a person receiving an adequate intake of vitamin A.

For the treatment of vitamin A deficiency, 25,000 to 50,000 Units should be given daily until a clinical response is obtained.

UNDESIRABLE EFFECTS. Signs of vitamin-A intoxication may occur in young children if the intake is grossly excessive, e.g. over 50,000 Units daily taken over long periods. The symptoms are a rough itching skin, dry coarse hair, tender firm deep swellings in the limbs, enlarged liver, a raised erythrocyte sedimentation rate, anaemia, and an increase in serum alkaline phosphatase.

Treatment consists in withdrawing the vitamin A, when most manifestations disappear within a week.

Dose. 0·06 to 1·2 millilitres, equivalent to approximately 2500 to 50,000 Units of vitamin-A activity, daily.

Preparations
VITAMINS A AND D CAPSULES, B.P.C. (page 653)
VITAMINS CAPSULES, B.P.C. (page 654)

CONCENTRATED VITAMIN D SOLUTION

Concentrated Vitamin D Solution may consist of a suitable fish-liver oil or blend of such oils, or it may be prepared by dissolving, at a temperature not exceeding 60°, a source of vitamin D in a vegetable oil such as arachis oil.

In preparing Concentrated Vitamin D Solution, any suitable source of vitamin D may be used, such as calciferol, a fish-liver oil rich in vitamin D, a concentrate prepared from such oils, or any other source of the antirachitic substance found in fish livers.

Solubility. Slightly soluble in alcohol; miscible with ether, with chloroform, and with light petroleum.

Standard
DESCRIPTION. A pale yellow or yellow oily liquid; odour faint but not rancid.

ACID VALUE. Not more than 2·5.

VITAMIN-A ACTIVITY. Not more than 5000 Units per g, determined by the method of the British Pharmacopoeia, Appendix XVIIA, for the assay of vitamin A.

ANTIRACHITIC ACTIVITY (VITAMIN D). The estimated potency is not less than 9000 and not more than 11,000 Units per g, determined by the following method:
Carry out the method of the British Pharmacopoeia, Appendix XIVG, for the biological assay of antirachitic vitamin (vitamin D).
The precision of the assay must be such that the fiducial limits of error (P = 0·95) are between 60 and 170 per cent of the estimated potency.

Storage. It should be stored in well-filled airtight containers, protected from light, in a cool place.

Actions and uses. Concentrated Vitamin D Solution has the actions, uses, and undesirable effects described under Calciferol (page 65).

PRECAUTIONS. These are as described under Calciferol (page 65).

Dose. For an infant or for an adult: prophylactic, 0·04 to 0·08 millilitre, equivalent to approximately 400 to 800 Units, daily; therapeutic, 0·1 to 2 millilitres, equivalent to approximately 1000 to 20,000 Units, daily.

For hypoparathyroidism: 5 to 20 millilitres, equivalent to approximately 50,000 to 200,000 Units, daily.

For lupus vulgaris: 5 to 10 millilitres, equivalent to approximately 50,000 to 100,000 Units, daily.

Preparations
VITAMINS A and D CAPSULES, B.P.C. (page 653)
VITAMINS CAPSULES, B.P.C. (page 654)

CONCENTRATED VITAMINS A AND D SOLUTION

Concentrated Vitamins A and D Solution may consist of a suitable fish-liver oil or blend of such oils, or it may be prepared by dissolving, at a temperature not exceeding 60°, a source of vitamin A and a source of vitamin D in a vegetable oil such as arachis oil.

In preparing Concentrated Vitamins A and D Solution, any source of vitamin A or D used in the preparation of Concentrated Vitamin A Solution or of Concentrated Vitamin D Solution, respectively, may be used.

Solubility. Slightly soluble in alcohol; miscible with ether, with chloroform, and with light petroleum.

Standard
DESCRIPTION. A pale yellow or yellow oily liquid; odour faint but not rancid; taste bland or slightly fishy.

ACID VALUE. Not more than 2·5.

VITAMIN-A ACTIVITY. Not less than 45,000 and not more than 55,000 Units per g, determined by the method of the British Pharmacopoeia, Appendix XVIIA, for the assay of vitamin A.

ANTIRACHITIC ACTIVITY (VITAMIN D). Not less than 4500 and not more than 5550 Units per g, determined by the following method:
Carry out the method of the British Pharmacopoeia,

Appendix XIVG, for the biological assay of antirachitic vitamin (vitamin D).
The precision of the assay must be such that the fiducial limits of error (P = 0·95) are between 60 and 170 per cent of the estimated potency.

Storage. It should be stored in well-filled airtight containers, protected from light, in a cool place.

Actions and uses. Concentrated Vitamins A and D Solution is used as a dietary supplement to correct or prevent symptoms arising from a deficiency of these two vitamins.

Dose. 0·06 to 0·6 millilitre, equivalent to approximately 2500 to 25,000 Units of vitamin-A activity and approximately 250 to 2500 Units of antirachitic activity (vitamin D), daily.

Preparation
VITAMINS A AND D CAPSULES, B.P.C. (page 653)

WARFARIN SODIUM

$C_{19}H_{15}NaO_4 = 330·3$

Warfarin Sodium is the sodium derivative of 4-hydroxy-3-(3-oxo-1-phenylbutyl)-*2H*-1-benzopyran-2-one or the clathrate of this substance with isopropyl alcohol.

Solubility. Soluble, at 20°, in less than 1 part of water and of alcohol; slightly soluble in ether and in chloroform.

Standard
It complies with the requirements of the British Pharmacopoeia.
It is a white, crystalline, odourless powder and contains not less than 98·0 and not more than the equivalent of 102·0 per cent of $C_{19}H_{15}NaO_4$, calculated with reference to the anhydrous isopropyl-alcohol-free substance. It contains not more than 2·0 per cent w/w of water and 4·3 to 8·3 per cent w/w of isopropyl alcohol in the clathrate. A 5 per cent solution in water is not more than faintly opalescent. A 1 per cent solution in water has a pH of 7·2 to 8·3.

Storage. It should be stored in airtight containers, protected from light.

Actions and uses. Warfarin sodium is an anticoagulant which has actions, uses, and undesirable effects similar to those described under Phenindione (page 364). Warfarin is usually preferred to phenindione, as it is less liable to give rise to toxic effects. The effect of a single oral dose appears in twelve to eighteen hours and lasts for five to six days.

The initial dose is usually 15 to 25 milligrams; in no circumstances should the initial dose exceed 50 milligrams. Subsequent doses of 3 to 10 milligrams should be given daily after the prothrombin time has begun to recede from its peak; the dosage must be adjusted in accordance with the prothrombin activity of the blood, which must be estimated periodically.
In addition to its use in medicine, warfarin is also used as a rodenticide.

PRECAUTIONS AND CONTRA-INDICATIONS. As for Phenindione (page 364).

Dose. See above under **Actions and uses.**

Preparation
WARFARIN TABLETS, B.P. The quantity of warfarin sodium in each tablet should be specified by the prescriber. They should be stored in airtight containers, protected from light. Tablets containing 1, 3, 5, 10, and 20 mg are available.

OTHER NAME: *Marevan*®

PURIFIED WATER

SYNONYM: Aqua Purificata

$H_2O = 18.02$

Purified Water is prepared from suitable potable water by distillation, by treatment with ion-exchange materials, or by any other suitable method.

The ion-exchange materials used in the preparation of Purified Water are known as "deionising resins" and consist of hard organic polymer particles, each containing ionised functional groups of a single type distributed throughout the mass of the material. The potable water is passed through two columns containing a cation-exchange resin and an anion-exchange resin respectively, or through a single column containing a mixture of the two resins.

Resins which may be used include a strong cation exchanger containing sulphonic acid functional groups ($RSO_3^- H^+$, where R stands for the resin structure) and a strong anion exchanger containing quaternary ammonium groups ($R \cdot NZ_3^+ OH^-$, where Z stands for an aliphatic group).

Micro-organisms may multiply in ion-exchange columns, but their growth can be minimised by using the column continuously and regenerating regularly after a thorough backwashing.

It is inadvisable to use the ion-exchange method for preparing Purified Water unless facilities are available for controlling the quality of the water.

Standard
It complies with the requirements of the European Pharmacopoeia.
It is a clear, colourless, odourless liquid.

Storage. It should be stored in airtight containers which do not alter the properties of the water.

Uses. Purified water is used as a solvent and vehicle. Aqueous preparations intended for parenteral injection should be prepared with Water for Injections.

NOTE. When Distilled Water is prescribed or demanded, Purified Water is dispensed or supplied.

WATER FOR INJECTIONS

SYNONYM: Aqua pro Injectionibus

Water for Injections is sterilised distilled water free from pyrogens.

Water for Injections may be prepared by distilling potable water from a neutral-glass or metal still fitted with an efficient device for preventing entrainment; the first portion of the distillate is rejected and the remainder is collected in suitable containers and immediately sterilised by heating in an autoclave or by filtration without the addition of a bactericide.

Water for Injections free from carbon dioxide is prepared by boiling the distillate for ten minutes, cooling, and transferring to the final containers with as little exposure to air as possible and immediately sterilising by heating in an autoclave.

Standard
It complies with the requirements of the British Pharmacopoeia.

Uses. Water for Injections is used in preparations intended for parenteral administration and in other sterile products. For these purposes it may be replaced by freshly distilled water, prepared by the process described for Water for Injections but omitting the sterilisation stage, provided that the final preparation is immediately sterilised.

When supplied in multidose containers, a suitable bactericide should be added, and the name and concentration of the bactericide given on the label. If it is to be used for the preparation of intrathecal injections, or of intravenous injections with doses of more than 15 millilitres, a bactericide must not be added and the water should be distributed in single-dose containers.

WILD CHERRY BARK

SYNONYMS: Prunus Serotina; Virginian Prune; Virginian Prune Bark

Wild Cherry Bark is the dried bark of the wild or black cherry, *Prunus serotina* Ehrh. (Fam. Rosaceae), a tree widely distributed over North America.

The bark is collected in the states of Virginia, North Carolina, and Tennessee during the months of July to October, dried, and exported under the commercial designation of Thin Natural Wild Cherry Bark. The most esteemed bark is that collected in the autumn, preferably from young stems and branches.

Constituents. Wild cherry bark contains (+)-mandelonitrile glucoside (prunasin) and an enzyme system, which interact in the presence of water yielding benzaldehyde, hydrocyanic acid, and glucose. Benzoic, trimethylgallic, and *p*-coumaric acids and a small amount of volatile oil are present.

Other constituents are tannin, fatty acids, and resinous substances which yield β-methylaesculetin (scopoletin) on hydrolysis with acid. Good specimens of the drug yield 0·075 to 0·16 per cent of hydrocyanic acid.

Wild cherry bark yields to alcohol (60 per cent) 17 to 23 per cent of extractive. The ash is about 3 to 4 per cent and the acid-insoluble ash 0·2 to 0·6 per cent.

Standard for unground drug

DESCRIPTION. *Macroscopical:* irregular fragments or curved or channelled pieces up to 12 cm long and 5 cm wide and not more than 4 mm thick; young bark covered externally with a thin, smooth, reddish-brown to brownish-black papery cork sometimes exfoliated and revealing the smooth greenish-brown cortex, both cork and underlying cortex showing numerous, transversely elongated lenticels about 0·5 to 1·5 cm long; older bark darker and rougher; inner surface cinnamon-brown, showing fine wavy longitudinal striations anastomosing to form a fine reticulation with raised pale areas in the meshes, patches of narrowly lanceolate fissures, about 1·0 to 5·0 mm long, frequently present, reticulation less pronounced in young bark; fracture short, granular; smoothed, transversely cut surface with outer, thin, brown cork covering a narrow green cortex followed internally by a narrow line of pericyclic sclerenchyma and reddish-brown secondary phloem containing small groups of sclereids and traversed by numerous paler medullary rays.

Odour slight; taste astringent, aromatic, bitter, recalling that of bitter almonds; when moistened, developing a strong odour of benzaldehyde.

Microscopical: the diagnostic characters are: *phelloderm* and *cortex* parenchymatous, containing chlorophyll; *pericycle* consisting of an almost continuous zone of *sclereids* with very occasional *fibres*; sclereids, some branched, in numerous groups; *starch* granules about 5 to 9 μm in diameter, in cells of the *medullary rays*; *secondary phloem* and medullary rays with large, irregular fissures between them; *crystals* of calcium oxalate prismatic, 10 to **30** to **40** to 80 μm long, and clusters, 10 to **18** to 30 μm wide, chiefly in cells of phloem bordering upon the fissures; typical *phloem fibres* absent.

HYDROCYANIC ACID. To 1 g, broken into small pieces or in powder, in a stoppered tube, add 1 ml of water.

Suspend a strip of filter-paper moistened with *trinitrophenol solution* above the liquid, stopper the tube, and allow to stand for 30 minutes; the paper becomes brick-red.

ASH. Not more than 4·0 per cent.

WATER-SOLUBLE EXTRACTIVE. Not less than 10·0 per cent.

FOREIGN ORGANIC MATTER. Not more than 2·0 per cent.

Standard for powdered drug. Powdered Wild Cherry Bark

DESCRIPTION. A light-brown powder possessing the diagnostic microscopical characters, odour, and taste of the unground drug.

HYDROCYANIC ACID; ASH; WATER-SOLUBLE EXTRACTIVE; FOREIGN ORGANIC MATTER. It complies with the requirements for the unground drug.

Adulterants and substitutes. A form of the bark, known as "rossed" bark, sometimes occurs in commerce; this consists of bark from which the cortex, in addition to the cork, has been removed; its uniformly dark cinnamon-brown outer surface has a rough or rasped appearance and exhibits under a lens pale longitudinal strands of sclerenchymatous cells alternating with darker medullary rays.

Thick bark from the trunk and larger branches is characterised by numerous depressions on the outer surface and the absence of lenticels.

Barks from other species of *Prunus* are occasionally substituted for the official drug and may be recognised by the presence of fibres or by the taste, which is astringent and deficient in the flavour of bitter almond.

Storage. It should be stored in a cool dry place. Powdered Wild Cherry Bark should be stored in airtight containers, in a cool place.

Actions and uses. In the form of the syrup, wild cherry bark has been used in the treatment of cough, but it has little therapeutic value.

The chief use of Wild Cherry Syrup is as a flavouring agent.

Preparation
WILD CHERRY SYRUP, B.P.C. (page 801)

WOOL ALCOHOLS

SYNONYM: Wool Wax Alcohols

Wool Alcohols may be obtained by treating wool fat with alkali and separating the fraction containing cholesterol and other alcohols.

Constituents. Wool alcohols is a crude mixture of steroid and triterpene alcohols, including 28 to 34 per cent of cholesterol and 10 to 13 per cent of isocholesterol.

Solubility. Insoluble in water; slightly soluble in alcohol; completely soluble in 25 parts of boiling dehydrated alcohol; soluble in ether, in chloroform, and in light petroleum.

Standard
It complies with the requirements of the British Pharmacopoeia.

It is a somewhat brittle golden-brown solid with a smooth and shiny fracture and with a faint odour resembling that of wool fat. It contains not less than 30·0 per cent of cholesterol and 500 to 1000 parts per million of butylated hydroxyanisole or of butylated hydroxytoluene. The loss on drying at 105° for one hour is not more than 0·5 per cent. When warmed, it becomes plastic and melts at a temperature not lower than 58°. It has an acid value of not more than 2·0.

Storage. It should be stored in airtight containers, protected from light, in a cool place.

Uses. Wool alcohols resembles wool fat in being a good emulsifying agent for water-in-oil emulsions. Emulsions made with it are usually preferred to those made with wool fat, since they do not darken on the surface or emit an objectionable odour in hot weather.

The proportion of water that can be incorporated in soft paraffin is increased threefold by the addition of 5 per cent of wool alcohols. Such emulsions are not "cracked" by the addition of weak acids such as citric, lactic, or tartaric acid, and they may be improved and made more stable by the addition of cetostearyl alcohol.

Proportions of wool alcohols up to 2·5 per cent may be added to oil-in-water emulsions in order to improve the texture, stability, and emollient properties.

Although wool alcohols may contain small amounts of phenolic antoxidants, higher concentrations of phenols may cause an incompatibility if included in emulsions containing wool alcohols.

UNDESIRABLE EFFECTS. Wool alcohols some-times has a slightly irritant action and in rare instances may give rise to a bullous eruption. Occasional cases of skin sensitivity have occurred.

Preparations

OILY CREAM, B.P. It contains equal parts of Wool Alcohols Ointment and water. It should be stored in airtight containers made from non-absorbent material, in a cool place.

WOOL ALCOHOLS OINTMENT, B.P. It contains 6 per cent of wool alcohols, with hard, soft, and liquid paraffins.

WOOL FAT

SYNONYMS: Adeps Lanae; Anhydrous Lanolin

Wool Fat is the purified anhydrous fat-like substance obtained from the wool of the sheep, *Ovis aries* L. (Fam. Bovidae).

In preparing wool fat, the natural grease is extracted from the wool by scouring with dilute alkali, with which it readily forms an emulsion; the emulsion is acidified and the wool fat separates as a distinct layer at the surface of the liquid. Purification may be effected by repeated treatment with water in a centrifuge.

Wool fat may be saponified by alcoholic potassium hydroxide solution.

Constituents. Wool fat consists mainly of fatty acid esters of cholesterol, lanosterol, and fatty alcohols, together with free alcohols, free fatty acids, and hydrocarbons.

Solubility. Insoluble in water; slightly soluble in cold alcohol; soluble in 75 parts of boiling alcohol, depositing most of the wool fat as a flocculent precipitate on cooling; also soluble in ether, in chloroform, in acetone, and in carbon disulphide.

Standard

It complies with the requirements of the British Pharmacopoeia.

It is a pale yellow, tenacious, unctuous substance with a slight but characteristic odour. It has a melting-point of 36° to 42°.

It may contain not more than 200 parts per million of butylated hydroxyanisole or of butylated hydroxytoluene.

Adulterants and substitutes. Paraffins and animal and vegetable fats and oils are possible adulterants.

Sterilisation. It is sterilised by dry heat.

Uses. Wool fat is used in the formulation of ointment bases. It can absorb about 30 per cent of water and may be of value in stabilising water-in-oil emulsions. On storage, such emulsions are liable to darken on the surface. Occasional cases of skin sensitivity to wool fat have occurred.

Preparations

HYDROUS WOOL FAT, B.P. (*Syn.* Adeps Lanae Hydrosus; Lanolin). It contains 70 per cent of wool fat, with water. It should be stored in airtight containers, in a cool place.

HYDROUS WOOL FAT OINTMENT, B.P.C. (page 761)

SIMPLE OINTMENT, B.P. It contains 5 per cent each of wool fat, hard paraffin, and cetostearyl alcohol in white or yellow soft paraffin.

XENON (^{133}Xe) INJECTION

This material is radioactive and any regulations in force must be complied with.

Xenon (^{133}Xe) Injection is a sterile solution of xenon-133 made isotonic with blood by the addition of sodium chloride.

Xenon-133 is a radioactive isotope of xenon which emits β- and γ-radiation and has a half-life of 5·3 days; it may be prepared from the products of uranium fission.

Standard

It complies with the requirements of the British Pharmacopoeia.

It is a clear colourless solution and contains not less than 80·0 and not more than 120·0 per cent of the quantity of xenon-133 stated on the label at the date and hour stated on the label. It has a pH of 5·0 to 8·0.

Sterilisation. It is sterilised by heating in an autoclave.

Labelling. The label on the container states:

(1) the content of xenon-133 expressed in microcuries or millicuries at a given date and hour;

(2) the volume of the injection;

(3) that the injection is radioactive; and

(4) either that the injection does not contain a bactericide, or the name and proportion of any added bactericide.

Storage. It should be stored in an area assigned for the purpose. The storage conditions should be such that the maximum radiation-dose-rate to which persons may be exposed is reduced to an acceptable level.

Glass containers may darken under the effects of radiation.

Actions and uses. Xenon has a low solubility in blood plasma and when xenon (^{133}Xe) injection is administered intravenously its radioactivity is removed on first passing through the lungs.

Xenon (^{133}Xe) injection is used for measurements of lung perfusion. The radioactivity is examined by means of detectors placed over various regions of the lungs or by the use of the gamma-ray camera.

Xenon (^{133}Xe) injection is also administered intra-arterially or intravenously for cerebral and other regional blood flow studies and for circulation measurements. Blood flow in muscle and skin is determined after intramuscular or subcutaneous injection by recording the rate of disappearance of ^{133}Xe radioactivity from the relevant area.

Dose. In studies of pulmonary function, 1 to 2 millicuries by intravenous injection.

In studies of the circulatory system, 300 microcuries by intra-arterial or intravenous injection.

XYLOSE

SYNONYM: D-Xylose

$C_5H_{10}O_5 = 150.1$

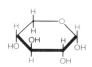

Solubility. Soluble in less than 1 part of water; soluble in hot alcohol.

Standard
It complies with the requirements of the British Pharmacopoeia.
It occurs as odourless colourless needles or white crystalline powder. The loss on drying at 100° at a pressure not exceeding 5 mmHg is not more than 0.5 per cent.

Actions and uses. Xylose is used orally in a dose of 25 grams to test the absorptive capacity of the intestinal mucosa. In normal subjects, at least 5 grams is excreted in the urine within five hours.

DRIED YEAST

Dried Yeast consists of unicellular fungi belonging to the family Saccharomycetaceae, a subdivision of the Ascomycetales, which have been dried by a process which avoids decomposition of the vitamins present.

The chief species of yeast used in the fermentation industries are *Saccharomyces cerevisiae* Meyen *emend.* Hansen, *S. carlsbergensis* Hansen, and *S. monacensis* Hansen, of which many different strains and races exist.

Constituents. Dried Yeast contains vitamins of the B group, the amount in each gram being about 100 to 200 μg of thiamine hydrochloride, 300 to 600 μg of nicotinic acid, and 40 to 60 μg of riboflavine; it also contains pyridoxine, pantothenic acid, biotin, folic acid, vitamin B_{12}, *p*-aminobenzoic acid, and inositol, and is one of the richest known sources of the vitamin-B group.

It contains about 46 per cent of proteins, some of which are combined with nucleic acid to form nucleins and nucleoproteins, and about 36 per cent of carbohydrates.

A number of enzymes are present, including zymase, invertase, maltase, emulsin, and a proteolytic endo-tryptase.

Among other constituents are fat, choline, ergosterol, zymosterol, glycogen, various other carbohydrates, and glutathione.

It yields about 8.5 per cent of ash.

Standard
DESCRIPTION. *Macroscopical:* a buff or brownish-buff, somewhat granular powder; odour characteristic.

Microscopical: the diagnostic characters are: somewhat angular masses of loosely agglutinated, rounded or ovoid cells, or short-branched filaments composed of united cells; cells colourless, about 3 to 8 μm in diameter, containing a somewhat granular protoplasm with one or two vacuoles; cells occasionally containing four small spores formed under conditions of low nutrition, scanty moisture, and free aeration. Occasional starch grains may be present, derived from the filtration process.

ARSENIC. It complies with the test given in Appendix 6, page 880 (2 parts per million).

COPPER. It complies with the test given in Appendix 8, page 886 (120 parts per million).

LEAD. It complies with the test given in Appendix 8, page 886 (7 parts per million).

STARCH. On the addition of *iodine solution,* no blue colour is produced.

VIABLE CELLS. Add 4.5 g of *yeast nutrient* to a 100-ml Pasteur flask containing 50 ml of tap water and sterilise by heating in an autoclave at 115° for 20 minutes; add, with aseptic precautions, 2 g of sample and incubate at 28°.

Collect the gas evolved in a graduated tube inverted over the outlet tube in a trough of water and measure the volume of gas at the end of 6 hours.

Repeat the procedure, omitting the sample, and subtract the volume of gas evolved from that obtained in the first determination; the difference is not more than 10 ml.

If the difference is more than 10 ml, add 0.05 ml of *methylene blue solution* to 0.05 ml of a 1.0 per cent w/v suspension in water and examine microscopically; not more than an occasional unstained cell is visible.

LOSS ON DRYING. Not more than 9.0 per cent, determined by drying to constant weight at 100°.

CONTENT OF NICOTINIC ACID. Not less than 0.3 mg per g, determined by the method given in Appendix 24, page 907.

CONTENT OF RIBOFLAVINE. Not less than 0.04 mg per g, determined by the method given in Appendix 24, page 908.

CONTENT OF THIAMINE. Not less than 0.1 mg per g, calculated as thiamine hydrochloride, determined by the method given in Appendix 24, page 909.

Storage. It should be stored in airtight containers.

Actions and uses. Dried yeast is a source of the vitamin-B group and has been used for the prevention and treatment of vitamin-B-deficiency diseases.

As a dietary supplement, infants may be given 1 to 2·5 grams daily, mixed with milk, children, 4 to 6 grams daily, and adults, 6 to 8 grams daily. In severe vitamin-B-deficiency diseases, such as beriberi, pellagra, or aribo-flavinosis, doses of up to 30 grams daily have been given.

UNDESIRABLE EFFECTS. Large doses may cause diarrhoea.

Dose. 1 to 8 grams.

Preparation
YEAST TABLETS, B.P.C. (page 820)

ZINC CHLORIDE

SYNONYM: Zinci Chloridum

$ZnCl_2 = 136·3$

Zinc Chloride may be prepared by dissolving zinc in hydrochloric acid, evaporating the resulting solution, and fusing the residue; it is usually poured into moulds to solidify.

When heated, zinc chloride melts to a clear liquid at about 260°, and at a higher temperature it is partly volatilised, forming dense white fumes and leaving a residue of zinc oxide.

Zinc chloride almost always contains some oxychloride and is therefore not completely soluble in water; when a solution in water is made neutral to methyl orange by adding a few drops of dilute hydrochloric acid, a clear solution is obtained./

When a strong aqueous solution is heated, hydrogen chloride is given off and a precipitate of zinc oxychloride is formed on dilution.

Solubility. Soluble, at 20°, in less than 1 part of water, in 1·5 parts of alcohol, and in 2 parts of glycerol.

Standard
Material which complies with this standard meets the requirements of the European Pharmacopoeia.

DESCRIPTION. A white crystalline powder or opaque white sticks; very deliquescent and caustic; odourless.

IDENTIFICATION TESTS. 1. A solution in water to which *dilute hydrochloric acid* is added dropwise, to give a clear solution, gives the reactions characteristic of zinc.

2. A solution in *dilute nitric acid* gives the reactions characteristic of chlorides.

ACIDITY. pH of a solution prepared by dissolving 1·0 g in 9 ml of *carbon dioxide-free water*, 4·6 to 6·0. Any slight turbidity in the solution should be ignored.

AMMONIUM. Dissolve 2·0 g in 38 ml of *carbon dioxide-free water* and add *dilute hydrochloric acid*, dropwise, until a clear solution is obtained. Reserve the unused portion of this solution for the test for Aluminium, Calcium, Magnesium, Heavy Metals, and Iron and for the test for Sulphate. 0·5 ml of this solution diluted to 14 ml with water complies with the test given for Aluminium Sulphate, page 18 (400 parts per million).

ALUMINIUM, CALCIUM, MAGNESIUM, HEAVY METALS, AND IRON. To 8 ml of the solution prepared in the test for Ammonium add 2 ml of *strong ammonia solution* and shake. This solution complies with the following tests:

(i) The solution is clear when compared with water, the comparison being made by viewing vertically 10 ml of the liquids in matched, colourless, transparent, neutral glass tubes, 16 mm internal diameter and with a flat base, against a black background in diffused light.

(ii) The solution has no colour when compared with water, the comparison being made by viewing horizontally 2 ml of the liquids in matched, colourless, transparent, neutral glass tubes, 12 mm internal diameter, against a white background in diffused daylight.

(iii) To the prepared solution add 1 ml of *sodium phosphate solution*; the solution remains clear for at least 5 minutes. Add 0·15 ml of *sodium sulphide and glycerin solution*; a white precipitate is produced and, on standing, the supernatant liquid remains colourless.

ARSENIC. It complies with the test given in Appendix 6, page 880 (10 parts per million).

OXYCHLORIDE. Dissolve 1·5 g in 1·5 ml of *carbon dioxide-free water*; the solution is clear or not more than slightly opalescent. Add 7·5 ml of *alcohol (95 per cent)*; a cloudiness is produced which disappears on the addition of 0·3 ml of *dilute hydrochloric acid*.

SULPHATE. 5 ml of the solution prepared in the test for Ammonium, diluted to 15 ml with water, complies with the test for the prepared solution in the test for Sulphate given under Sodium Carbonate, page 445, 5 ml of *sulphate standard solution* diluted to 15 ml with water being used in the preparation of the reference solution (200 parts per million).

CONTENT OF $ZnCl_2$. Not less than 95·0 per cent, determined by the following method:
Dissolve about 0·15 g, accurately weighed, in 10 ml of *dilute acetic acid*, add 45 ml of water and 0·05 g of *xylenol orange mixture* followed by sufficient *hexamine* to change the colour of the solution to red; add a further 2 g of *hexamine* and titrate with 0·05M disodium edetate; each ml of 0·05M disodium edetate is equivalent to 0·006815 g of $ZnCl_2$.

Storage. It should be stored in airtight containers.

Actions and uses. Zinc chloride is a powerful caustic and astringent. A solution containing zinc chloride and zinc sulphate is used as an astringent mouth-wash. A 10 per cent solution of zinc chloride is used as an obtundent.

POISONING. Poisoning by zinc chloride is characterised by corrosion and inflammation of the mucous membrane of the mouth and stomach, which is usually rendered white. Ulceration, often followed by perforation, may also occur.

Alkali carbonate, milk, or white of egg should be administered liberally.

Preparation
ZINC SULPHATE AND ZINC CHLORIDE MOUTH-WASH, B.P.C. (page 756)

ZINC OXIDE

SYNONYM: Zinci Oxidum

ZnO = 81·4

Zinc Oxide may be prepared by the combustion of metallic zinc in a current of air or by igniting zinc carbonate.

Commercial zinc oxide, manufactured for use as a pigment, is known as "zinc white".

Solubility. Insoluble in water and in alcohol; soluble in dilute mineral acids.

Standard
It complies with the requirements of the European Pharmacopoeia.
It is a soft, white or faintly yellowish-white, odourless powder free from grittiness and contains not less than 99·0 per cent of ZnO, calculated with reference to the substance ignited at 500°. The loss on ignition is not more than 1·0 per cent.

NOTE. Zinc oxide forms cement-like products when mixed with a strong solution of zinc chloride or with phosphoric acid, owing to the formation of oxy-salts.

Hygroscopicity. When exposed to the air it gradually absorbs moisture and carbon dioxide.

Sterilisation. It is sterilised by dry heat.

Actions and uses. Zinc oxide is applied externally, in dusting-powders, ointments, pastes, and lotions, as a mild astringent for the skin, as a soothing and protective application in eczema and as a protective for slight excoriations.

Preparations
CALAMINE APPLICATION, COMPOUND, B.P.C. (page 648)
CALAMINE CREAM, AQUEOUS, B.P.C. (page 656)
ZINC CREAM, B.P. It contains 32 per cent of zinc oxide, in a cream prepared from calcium hydroxide, oleic acid, arachis oil, wool fat, and purified water.
ZINC AND ICHTHAMMOL CREAM, B.P.C. (page 661)
CHLORPHENESIN DUSTING-POWDER, B.P.C. (page 663)

HEXACHLOROPHANE DUSTING-POWDER, B.P.C. (page 663)
ZINC, STARCH, AND TALC DUSTING-POWDER, B.P.C. (page 664)
CALAMINE LOTION, B.P. It contains 15 per cent of calamine and 5 per cent of zinc oxide, with bentonite, sodium citrate, glycerol, and liquefied phenol.
BENZOCAINE OINTMENT, COMPOUND, B.P.C. (page 758)
CALAMINE AND COAL TAR OINTMENT, B.P.C. (page 760)
COAL TAR AND ZINC OINTMENT, B.P.C. (page 760)
RESORCINOL OINTMENT, COMPOUND, B.P.C. (page 763)
ZINC OINTMENT, B.P. It contains 15 per cent of zinc oxide in Simple Ointment.
ZINC AND CASTOR OIL OINTMENT, B.P. (*Syn.* Zinc and Castor Oil Cream; Zinc and Castor Oil). It contains 7·5 per cent of zinc oxide and 50 per cent w/w of castor oil.
ALUMINIUM PASTE, COMPOUND, B.P.C. (page 767)
COAL TAR PASTE, B.P.C. (page 767)
RESORCINOL AND SULPHUR PASTE, B.P.C. (page 768)
TITANIUM DIOXIDE PASTE, B.P.C. (page 768)
ZINC PASTE, COMPOUND, B.P. (*Syn.* Zinc Paste). It contains 25 per cent each of starch and zinc oxide in white soft paraffin.
ZINC AND COAL TAR PASTE, B.P.C. (page 769)
ZINC AND SALICYLIC ACID PASTE, B.P. (*Syn.* Lassar's Paste). It contains 24 per cent each of starch and zinc oxide and 2 per cent of salicylic acid in white soft paraffin.
BISMUTH SUBGALLATE SUPPOSITORIES, COMPOUND, B.P.C. (page 796)
HAMAMELIS AND ZINC OXIDE SUPPOSITORIES, B.P.C. (page 797)

ZINC STEARATE

Zinc Stearate may be prepared by the interaction of a soluble zinc salt and a solution of the sodium salt of stearic acid. It consists chiefly of zinc stearate, $(C_{17}H_{35}\cdot CO_2)_2Zn$, but contains also a variable proportion of zinc palmitate, $(C_{15}H_{31}\cdot CO_2)_2Zn$, and usually a small amount of zinc oleate, $(C_{17}H_{33}\cdot CO_2)_2Zn$.

Solubility. Insoluble in water, in alcohol, and in ether.

Standard
DESCRIPTION. A light white amorphous powder, free from gritty particles; odour faint and characteristic.
IDENTIFICATION TEST. Boil 1 g with 25 ml of water and 5 ml of *hydrochloric acid*; an oily layer of fatty acids is produced which floats on the surface of the liquid; the aqueous layer, after neutralisation to *litmus paper*, gives the reactions characteristic of zinc.

ACIDITY OR ALKALINITY. Shake 1·0 g with 5 ml of *alcohol* (*95 per cent*), previously neutralised to *phenol red solution*, and 20 ml of *carbon dioxide-free water*; not more than 0·1 ml of 0·1N hydrochloric acid or 0·1N sodium hydroxide is required for neutralisation, *phenol red solution* being used as indicator.

SULPHATE. Heat 0·10 g with 25 ml of water containing 2·5 ml of *dilute hydrochloric acid* and filter; the filtrate complies with the limit test for sulphates (0·6 per cent).

ALKALIS AND ALKALINE EARTHS. Not more than 2·0 per cent, determined by the following method:
Boil about 1 g, accurately weighed, with 25 ml of water and 5 ml of *hydrochloric acid*, filter while hot, and wash with 25 ml of hot water; to the combined filtrate and washings add *dilute ammonia solution* until the solution is just alkaline to *litmus paper*, followed by an excess of *ammonium sulphide solution*, filter, evaporate the filtrate to dryness, and ignite the residue; extract with 10 ml of water, filter, evaporate the filtrate to dryness, and ignite to constant weight.

ETHER-SOLUBLE MATTER. Not more than 1·0 per cent, determined by the following method:
Mix about 5 g, accurately weighed, with 100 ml of *solvent ether*, shake for 30 minutes, filter, evaporate 50 ml of the filtrate to dryness, and dry the residue.

CONTENT OF ZINC. 10·45 to 12·45 per cent, determined by the following method:
Boil about 1 g, accurately weighed, with 50 ml of 0·1N hydrochloric acid for 10 minutes, cool, filter,

wash the residue with water, and titrate the combined filtrate and washings with 0·1N sodium hydroxide, using *methyl red solution* as indicator; each ml of 0·1N hydrochloric acid is equivalent to 0·003269 g of Zn.

Actions and uses. Zinc stearate is used as a soothing and protective application in the treatment of skin inflammation. It is used either alone or combined with other powders or in the form of a cream.

Preparation
CALAMINE APPLICATION, COMPOUND, B.P.C. (page 648)

ZINC SULPHATE

SYNONYM: Zinci Sulfas

$ZnSO_4,7H_2O = 287·5$

Zinc Sulphate may be prepared by dissolving zinc in dilute sulphuric acid or by roasting zinc blende, a native zinc sulphide, in air, extracting the product with water, and crystallising from the resulting solution.

Crude zinc sulphate is sometimes known as "white vitriol" or "white copperas".

Solubility. Soluble, at 20°, in less than 1 part of water; insoluble in alcohol.

Standard
It complies with the requirements of the European Pharmacopoeia.
It occurs as odourless, efflorescent, colourless, transparent crystals or a white crystalline powder and contains not less than 99·0 and not more than the equivalent of 105·0 per cent of $ZnSO_4,7H_2O$. A 5 per cent solution in water has a pH of 4·4 to 5·6.

Incompatibility. It is incompatible with alkali carbonates and hydroxides and with astringent infusions and decoctions.

Sterilisation. Solutions are sterilised by heating in an autoclave or by filtration.

Storage. It should be stored in airtight containers.

Actions and uses. Zinc sulphate is sometimes used to promote healing in granulating wounds in a dose of 220 milligrams three times a day with meals. Higher doses such as 2 grams, administered as a 1 per cent solution, produce emesis.

Zinc sulphate is used externally in the form of astringent lotions for indolent ulcers and to assist granulation. Dilute aqueous solutions may be applied locally to relieve chronic inflammation of the cornea in conjunctivitis.

POISONING. Alkali carbonate, milk, or white of egg should be administered liberally.

Dose. As an emetic: 0·6 to 2 grams.

Preparations
ZINC SULPHATE EYE-DROPS, B.P.C. (page 695)
ZINC SULPHATE AND ADRENALINE EYE-DROPS, B.P.C. (page 696)
COPPER AND ZINC SULPHATES LOTION, B.P.C. (page 727)
ZINC SULPHATE LOTION, B.P.C. (page 729)
ZINC SULPHATE AND ZINC CHLORIDE MOUTH-WASH, B.P.C. (page 756)
ZINC SULPHIDE LOTION, B.P.C. (page 730)

ZINC UNDECENOATE

SYNONYM: Zinc Undecylenate

$(C_{10}H_{19}·CO_2)_2Zn = 431·9$

Zinc Undecenoate is zinc undec-10-enoate.

Solubility. Very slightly soluble in water and in alcohol.

Standard
It complies with the requirements of the British Pharmacopoeia.
It is a fine white or creamy-white powder and contains not less than 98·0 and not more than the equivalent of 102·0 per cent of $C_{22}H_{38}O_4Zn$, calculated with reference to the dried substance. The loss on drying under the prescribed conditions is not more than 1·5 per cent. It has a melting-point of 117° to 121°.

Actions and uses. Zinc undecenoate has a fungicidal action similar to that of undecenoic acid (page 525) and is used for similar purposes. It is applied to the skin, usually in conjunction with undecenoic acid, in ointments and dusting-powders.

Preparations
ZINC UNDECENOATE DUSTING-POWDER, B.P.C. (page 664)
ZINC UNDECENOATE OINTMENT, B.P. It contains 20 per cent of zinc undecenoate and 5 per cent of undecenoic acid in Emulsifying Ointment.

PART 2

Immunological Products and Related Preparations

ANTISERA

Antisera are preparations from native sera containing substances that have a specific prophylactic or therapeutic action when injected into persons exposed to or suffering from a disease due to a specific micro-organism.

This general monograph applies to the following products:

ANTITOXIC SERA

Botulinum Antitoxin, page 553
Diphtheria Antitoxin, page 554
Gas-gangrene Antitoxin (Oedematiens), page 558
Gas-gangrene Antitoxin (Perfringens), page 559
Gas-gangrene Antitoxin (Septicum), page 559
Mixed Gas-gangrene Antitoxin, page 559
Scorpion Venom Antiserum, page 568
Snake Venom Antiserum, page 570
Tetanus Antitoxin, page 571

ANTIBACTERIAL SERUM

Leptospira Antiserum, page 560

ANTIVIRAL SERUM

Rabies Antiserum, page 564

In preparing antisera, preparations from cultures of the specific organisms or their products are injected into horses or other animals so as to produce immunity, a condition which is manifested by the formation of *antibodies* in the animals' blood. Antibodies are associated with the globulin fraction of serum.

The general term *antigen* is used to describe any substance which, when injected into the body, will elicit the formation of antibodies, substances which are antagonistic to or otherwise reactive with the antigen. The antigens in common use include toxins, toxoids, and bacterial and viral vaccines.

Antisera are usually concentrated; leptospira antiserum and snake venom antiserum are exceptions. In the case of antitoxic sera, the globulins or their derivatives are obtained by treatment with a proteolytic enzyme; pepsin-treated antitoxic sera are usually termed refined antitoxins. It is desirable to use purified products whenever possible so as to avoid the injection of excessive amounts of foreign proteins which may give rise to reactions.

ANTITOXIC SERA. In preparing antitoxic sera, the antigen used is either the specific toxin or, more usually, the toxoid. Toxins are poisonous substances which are excreted into the substrate when certain pathogenic bacteria are grown in artificial culture media and they can be demonstrated in the media after the organisms have been removed by filtration; they are sometimes referred to as soluble toxins or *exotoxins*. These exotoxins can be rendered non-toxic or harmless by adding formaldehyde solution and incubating for some days or weeks, usually at 37°; filtrates detoxicated in this way are known as *toxoids* or *formol toxoids*.

Non-lethal amounts of toxin, or the corresponding toxoid, are injected in gradually increasing doses into animals, usually horses. Specific antitoxins develop in the serum and the animals become actively immune. When the examination of small samples of blood shows that a satisfactory degree of immunity has been produced, larger volumes of blood are withdrawn from the jugular vein and the plasma or serum is processed.

ANTIBACTERIAL SERA are prepared against certain bacteria which do not produce exotoxins. When graded doses of suspensions of living or dead bacteria, or preparations from these suspensions, are injected into horses or other animals, antibodies develop that can combine with the antigens of the organisms and render them susceptible to phagocytosis or lysis by the action of complement. When the blood contains a sufficient amount of antibody it is collected and processed.

ANTIVIRAL SERA are not usually obtained from animals injected with specific viruses; rabies antiserum is an exception. The immune globulins are usually obtained from the plasma or serum of human patients who have recovered from certain virus diseases, of adults who have had the disease in the past, or of persons who have been artificially immunised. Human immunoglobulin, prepared from pools of adult human plasma and containing the antibodies of normal adults, is used in the prophylaxis of certain virus diseases.

Rabies antiserum is obtained from animals, usually horses, by injecting gradually increasing doses of a rabies vaccine. It is customary first to use a killed vaccine and then, when some immunity is established, to use living virus as an antigen. When a sufficient virus-neutralising titre is reached the blood is collected and may be processed.

ANTISERA issued in liquid form are distributed under aseptic conditions into sterile containers which are then sealed to exclude micro-organisms. A suitable antibacterial substance, in a concentration sufficient to prevent the growth of micro-organisms, is usually added; this is essential when antisera are issued in multiple-dose containers.

For native antisera, solutions of globulins, and liquid preparations obtained by simple fractionation with salts, the rate of deterioration during storage at 0° is negligible for five years and at 5° does not exceed in each year 5 per cent of the previous year's activity. At higher temperatures the annual rate of deterioration is greater; at 15° it may be about 10 per cent, at 20° it may approach 20 per cent, and at 37° preparations may lose 25 to 50 per cent of their activity in a year. With enzyme-treated antisera the rate of deterioration is usually less; they are most stable at pH 5·0 to 6·5, when the rate of deterioration at 0° to 5° is negligible; up to 15° it does not exceed 3 per cent, and at 20°, 5 per cent; at 37° preparations may lose 10 to 20 per cent of their activity in a year.

General Standard

DESCRIPTION. Liquid antisera are almost colourless or very faintly yellow liquids free from turbidity and almost odourless except for the odour of any antibacterial substance that may have been added. Freeze-dried antisera are white or pale yellow friable solids which dissolve in water to form colourless or pale yellow liquids.

POTENCY. The potency of each preparation, when the methods available permit, is determined in relation to the appropriate standard preparation by a biological method and expressed in Units per ml. The Unit is a specified amount of standard antiserum.

STERILITY. Antisera comply with the test for sterility of the European Pharmacopoeia.

ABNORMAL TOXICITY. Antisera comply with the tests for abnormal toxicity of the European Pharmacopoeia.

REACTION. pH 6·0 to 7·0.

TOTAL PROTEINS. Not more than 17·0 per cent w/v, determined by the method of the European Pharmacopoeia.

ALBUMINS. Unless otherwise specified, antisera show not more than a trace of albumins when examined electrophoretically.

FOREIGN PROTEINS. When examined by precipitation reactions with specific antisera, they are shown to consist exclusively of protein of the declared animal species.

PHENOL. Not more than 0·25 per cent w/v, determined by the method of the European Pharmacopoeia.

Storage. Antisera should be protected from light and stored at 2° to 10°; they should not be allowed to freeze. The amount of antiserum placed in each container must be sufficient to ensure that, when stored under these conditions, the number of Units stated on the label is still present at the end of the period during which the preparation is intended to be used.

Actions and uses. When antitoxins and other antibodies developed in the blood of one individual are transferred to a second individual by injecting a suitable quantity of the blood or serum containing the antibodies, passive immunity is conferred. This type of immunity is relatively quickly established, the rapidity depending upon the route of injection; antibodies do not remain in the blood of the second individual for longer than a few weeks, owing to the elimination of the foreign protein by the body. The rate of elimination is much slower, however, when homologous serum is used. Individuals who have received foreign protein in serum on a previous occasion may eliminate this protein subsequently with extreme rapidity. It is important, therefore, to follow the conferment of passive immunity, which is largely an emergency procedure, by the injection of suitable antigens to produce active immunity.

Antitoxic sera have the specific power of neutralising the toxins formed by micro-organisms and rendering them harmless to susceptible animals.

Antibacterial sera appear to act by rendering the micro-organisms susceptible to phagocytosis.

Antiviral sera are believed to act mainly by preventing the specific virus from entering the tissue cells and, as they cannot repair the harmful cell damage, their chief value is prophylactic rather than therapeutic.

SERUM REACTIONS. These are liable to occur after the injection of any serum of animal origin. The more serious general reactions are: (1) *Serum anaphylaxis*, a condition of severe shock appearing within a few minutes of the injection, or with less intensity up to two hours afterwards. (2) *Serum sickness*, a syndrome of rashes, pyrexia, and joint-pains occurring typically seven to twelve days, or less commonly three to four days, after the injection; the accelerated reaction is seen in persons who have previously received serum. (3) *Thermal reaction*, a sudden pyrexia accompanied by rigor occurring after the intravenous injection of certain batches of serum; it is not due to serum sensitivity, but is probably caused by pyrogenic substances produced during processing.

The use of enzyme-treated serum has considerably diminished the incidence of serum sickness and the symptoms are usually mild and transient. Serum anaphylaxis, although very rare, may still occur and may prove dangerous in susceptible subjects.

Intradermal, conjunctival, and scratch tests for the detection of serum sensitivity are unreliable and are not recommended.

Before injecting serum, information should be obtained as to whether previous injections of serum have been received and whether the patient is subject to allergic diseases, especially asthma and infantile eczema. If there is no history of previous serum injection or of allergic reaction, the dose of serum may be given intramuscularly; if there is time, however, or if injections of serum have been given previously, a trial dose of 0·2 ml of the serum should be given subcutaneously; if no *general* reaction develops within thirty minutes, the main dose of serum is given intramuscularly.

If the patient is subject to allergic diseases, the first trial dose should be 0·2 ml of a 1 in 10 dilution of the serum, given subcutaneously; if no *general* reaction develops during an interval of thirty minutes, a subcutaneous injection of 0·2 ml of undiluted serum is given and, if a further thirty minutes elapses without incident, the main dose is given intramuscularly.

Whenever serum is to be injected, by whatever route, the patient must be kept under observation for at least thirty minutes after the injection and adrenaline injection and corticosteroids kept in readiness for emergency use.

Serum should never be given by the intravenous route unless a preliminary intramuscular injection, given at least thirty minutes beforehand, has been tolerated. For intravenous use the serum should be at room temperature, the injection should be given very slowly, and the patient should be recumbent during the injection and for at least an hour afterwards.

VACCINES

Vaccines are preparations of antigenic materials that are administered with the object of inducing in the recipient a specific active immunity to infection or intoxication by the corresponding infecting agents. They may contain living or dead micro-organisms or bacterial toxins or toxoids or they may be purified products derived from bacteria. They may be simple vaccines prepared from one species only or mixed vaccines which are mixtures of two or more simple vaccines.

This general monograph applies to the following products:

SIMPLE BACTERIAL VACCINES

Sterile vaccines
Cholera Vaccine, page 554
Eltor Vaccine, page 558
Pertussis Vaccine, page 562
Plague Vaccine, page 562
Typhoid Vaccine, page 575

Living vaccines
Bacillus Calmette-Guérin Vaccine, page 552
Bacillus Calmette-Guérin Vaccine, Percutaneous, page 553

BACTERIAL TOXOIDS

Diphtheria Vaccine, page 555
Diphtheria Vaccine, Adsorbed, page 556
Tetanus Vaccine, page 572
Tetanus Vaccine, Adsorbed, page 572

VIRAL AND RICKETTSIAL VACCINES

Inactivated vaccines
Influenza Vaccine, page 560
Poliomyelitis Vaccine (Inactivated), page 563
Rabies Vaccine, page 565
Typhus Vaccine, page 577

Living vaccines
Measles Vaccine (Live Attenuated), page 561
Poliomyelitis Vaccine (Oral), page 563
Rubella Vaccine (Live Attenuated), page 566
Smallpox Vaccine, page 569
Smallpox Vaccine, Dried, page 570
Yellow Fever Vaccine, page 577

MIXED VACCINES

Diphtheria and Tetanus Vaccine, page 556
Diphtheria and Tetanus Vaccine, Adsorbed, page 556
Diphtheria, Tetanus, and Pertussis Vaccine, page 557
Diphtheria, Tetanus, and Pertussis Vaccine, Adsorbed, page 557

The methods of preparation are designed to ensure that the identity of the specific antigens is maintained and that no microbial contaminants are introduced. The final products are distributed under aseptic conditions into sterile containers which are then sealed to exclude extraneous micro-organisms. All forms, with the exception of certain living vaccines, comply with the test for sterility of the European Pharmacopoeia.

BACTERIAL VACCINES may be prepared from one species only or may contain two or more different species or varieties. Each culture used for the preparation of bacterial vaccines is first carefully examined for its identity, antigenic properties, and purity. The culture is grown on a solid medium under appropriate conditions and is then washed off the medium with Sodium Chloride Injection or other suitable solution; alternatively, it is grown in a fluid medium. The whole culture, or an extract or derivative of the culture, is used for preparing the vaccine.

In preparing sterile bacterial vaccines the bacteria are killed in such a manner that the antigenic potency of the product is not impaired. A suitable antibacterial substance, in a concentration sufficient to prevent the growth of micro-organisms, may be added to sterile bacterial vaccines and is invariably added to such vaccines when they are issued in multiple-dose containers.

Bacterial vaccines containing living bacteria are prepared from strains which are avirulent for man but which stimulate the production of antibodies active against pathogenic strains of the same species.

Bacterial vaccines are suspensions of varying opacity, usually white, in colourless or slightly coloured liquids. They may be standardised by determining the number of bacteria per ml, either by direct count in a counting chamber or by comparison of the opacity of the suspension with that of a preparation of standard opacity.

BACTERIAL TOXOIDS are toxins or material derived therefrom, the specific toxicity of which has been reduced to a low level or completely removed by chemical or physical means without destroying the immunising potency.

Toxoids produced by the action of formaldehyde, the most commonly used detoxicating agent, are sometimes called *formol toxoids* or *anatoxins*.

Adsorbed toxoids may be prepared by adsorbing formol toxoids on a suspension of aluminium hydroxide, hydrated aluminium phosphate, or other suitable substance;

the precipitate may be separated, washed, and suspended in a saline or other appropriate solution isotonic with blood.

Bacterial toxoids are clear colourless or yellow liquids, or suspensions of white or grey particles in colourless or yellow liquids. They comply with tests for minimum potency as immunising antigens.

MIXED VACCINES are mixtures of two or more simple bacterial vaccines or bacterial toxoids. They are clear liquids or suspensions of varying opacity, usually white, in colourless or slightly coloured liquids.

VIRAL AND RICKETTSIAL VACCINES are prepared from infected tissue or blood obtained from artificially infected animals, from cultures in fertile eggs, or from cell or tissue cultures. The material may be inactivated by exposure to formaldehyde or by other suitable chemical or physical means. Living vaccines are usually prepared with attenuated antigenic strains of the specific organisms. A suitable antibacterial substance may be added to inactivated or living viral or rickettsial vaccines, provided that it has no action against the specific organisms.

Viral and rickettsial vaccines vary in appearance from clear colourless liquids to suspensions of varying opacity and colour.

Storage. Bacterial vaccines, bacterial toxoids, and bacterial toxins should be protected from light and stored at 2° to 10°. They deteriorate at temperatures approaching 20°. Unless otherwise specified, liquid vaccines should not be allowed to freeze.

Viral and rickettsial vaccines should be stored under the conditions described in the individual monographs.

Immunisation of Children

It is now possible to provide protection against several infectious diseases in early life by active immunisation and the schedule on page 550 is based upon the recommendations of the Department of Health and Social Security (1972).

The basic course of immunisation against diphtheria, pertussis, tetanus, and poliomyelitis should be completed at as early an age as possible consistent with the likelihood of a good immunological response. Routine primary vaccination against smallpox is not now recommended in the United Kingdom, but in countries where smallpox is endemic, vaccination should be carried out as early as practicable. Reinforcement of immunisation against diphtheria, tetanus, and poliomyelitis, and revaccination against smallpox in endemic areas, should be carried out at the age of first entry to school. Further reinforcement of immunisation against tetanus and poliomyelitis and revaccination against smallpox in endemic areas should be given at school-leaving age.

Examples of timing of doses for the basic course of immunisation against diphtheria, tetanus, pertussis, and poliomyelitis are given below; in all examples there is an interval of six to eight weeks between the first and second doses and of four to six months between the second and third doses.

First dose	Second dose	Third dose
3 months	5 months	9 to 12 months
4 months	6 months	10 to 12 months
5 months	7 months	11 to 13 months
6 months	8 months	12 to 14 months

Age	Vaccine
During the first year of life NOTE: The earliest age at which the first dose should be given is three months.	diphtheria, tetanus, and pertussis ⎫ poliomyelitis (oral)　　　　　　⎭ Three doses, with an interval of 6 to 8 weeks between the first and second doses and 4 to 6 months between the second and third.
During the second year of life	measles (live)
Five years or school entry NOTE: These may be given, if desired, at nursery school entry at three years of age.	diphtheria and tetanus ⎫ poliomyelitis (oral)　　 ⎭ or diphtheria, tetanus, and poliomyelitis
Ten to thirteen years NOTE: For tuberculin-negative children. Normally at thirteen years but the local epidemiological situation may sometimes call for earlier vaccination. In some areas B.C.G. vaccine is given as a routine in infancy.	bacillus Calmette-Guérin
Fifteen to nineteen years or on leaving school	poliomyelitis (oral or inactivated) ⎫ tetanus　　　　　　　　　　　　 ⎭
Girls eleven to thirteen years	rubella

NOTE. Where an age range is specified in the above table it includes the following birthday, that is, eleven to thirteen years means from the eleventh to the fourteenth birthday.

If no immunisation or an incomplete basic course has been given before entry to nursery or primary school, measles vaccine should be given followed by full courses of diphtheria and tetanus vaccine and poliomyelitis (oral) vaccine.

Routine vaccination against smallpox is not now recommended in the United Kingdom. Vaccination is still recommended for those at special risk, such as doctors, nurses, and other health service staff, and for travellers to areas of the world where smallpox is still occurring or to countries where eradication programmes are in progress. When anyone is vaccinated against smallpox, the possibility of accidental infection of eczematous members of the family must be borne in mind.

While routine vaccination of women of childbearing age against rubella is not recommended, rubella vaccination may be given to women of childbearing age who request it and are found to be seronegative, to women in the post-partum period found during their pregnancy to have been seronegative, and to seronegative women at special risk either of acquiring rubella or of transmitting it to others. Women so vaccinated should be advised to avoid pregnancy for eight weeks after vaccination because of possible harm to the foetus if pregnancy occurs within that period.

An interval of three to four weeks should normally be allowed to elapse before the administration of any two live vaccines or between the administration of diphtheria, tetanus, and pertussis vaccine and any live vaccine other than poliomyelitis vaccine (oral), whichever is given first.

Immunisation of Travellers

Two schedules are given as a guide to the inoculation of travellers. They may be amended according to the immunological history of the traveller and the time available before departure. When sufficient time is not available to follow the suggested procedures, the responses to some antigens may be suboptimal and there is a risk of undesirable reactions of various kinds.

For travellers who have to go abroad from time to time, the following schedule is recommended, provided that there is sufficient time before departure:

Week	Vaccine
1	yellow fever
4	smallpox
5	*read result of smallpox*
7	typhoid-paratyphoid A and B and tetanus (*1*)
10	poliomyelitis (oral) (*1*)
13	typhoid-paratyphoid A and B and tetanus (*2*)
16	poliomyelitis (oral) (*2*)
22	poliomyelitis (oral) (*3*)
39	typhoid-paratyphoid A and B and tetanus (*3*)

When the schedule is completed, an occasional reinforcing dose may be all that is required before a subsequent journey. Reinforcing injections should be given as follows:

Vaccine	Frequency of reinforcing dose
yellow fever vaccine	every 10 years
smallpox vaccine	every 3 years
typhoid-paratyphoid A and B vaccine	every year as long as the individual is at special risk; every 3 years in other circumstances
tetanus vaccine	every 5 years

It should be noted that the International Certificate of Vaccination becomes valid, in respect of smallpox, eight days after the date of a successful primary vaccination, or on the date of revaccination, and, in respect of yellow fever, ten days after the first vaccination, or immediately on revaccination within six years.

Cholera vaccine is injected only in special circumstances. As the International Certificate is valid in respect of cholera for a period of six months only, this vaccine has been omitted from the recommended schedule; the Certificate becomes valid six days after the first cholera vaccination and immediately on revaccination within six months. The International Certificate does not recognise Eltor Vaccine as complying with requirements for international travel; for this purpose cholera vaccine must contain the classical serotypes of Inaba and Ogawa and may also contain the El Tor biotypes.

ALTERNATIVE SCHEDULE. For travellers who have little warning of their journey, the following alternative schedule may be adopted:

Day	Vaccine
1	cholera (1) typhoid-paratyphoid A and B and tetanus (1), and poliomyelitis (oral) (1)
5	yellow fever and smallpox (at separate sites)
13	cholera (2)
	read results of smallpox
28	typhoid-paratyphoid A and B and tetanus (2) and poliomyelitis (oral) (2)

When smallpox vaccine and yellow fever vaccine must be given to the same person at short notice, the two vaccines may be given at the same time but at different sites; this is preferable to shortening the interval between the two vaccinations, a practice which might lead to interference between the two vaccines.

The third doses of typhoid-paratyphoid A and B and tetanus vaccine and of poliomyelitis vaccine (oral) will be required some months later in order to complete the primary courses of immunisation.

This alternative schedule is unsatisfactory from the immunological standpoint and longer intervals are desirable when the time available permits.

BACILLUS CALMETTE-GUÉRIN VACCINE

SYNONYMS: BCG Vaccine; Freeze-dried BCG Vaccine; Vaccinum Tuberculosis (BCG) Cryodesiccatum

Bacillus Calmette-Guérin Vaccine is a freeze-dried preparation containing live bacteria obtained from a strain derived from the bacillus of Calmette and Guérin and known to protect man against tuberculosis.

The production of the vaccine is based on the seed lot system. The strain of bacillus used is maintained so as to preserve its power of sensitising man to tuberculin and its relative non-pathogenicity to man and laboratory animals. The seed lot is maintained at a temperature not exceeding 6°.

The bacilli are grown in or on a suitable

medium for not more than fourteen days and the harvested growth is diluted in a sterile liquid medium designed to preserve the antigenicity and viability of the vaccine, distributed into sterile glass containers, and dried from the frozen state. The containers are then sealed so as to exclude micro-organisms.

Standard
It complies with the requirements of the European Pharmacopoeia.
The dried product is a white solid which, when reconstituted by adding the appropriate quantity of a suitable reconstituting liquid indicated on the label, forms a suspension intended for intracutaneous injection.
The reconstituted vaccine complies with specific tests for virulent mycobacteria, contaminating micro-organisms, toxicity, excessive reactivity, and virulence.

Storage. It should be stored as described under Vaccines (page 549). Under these conditions it may be expected to retain its potency for two years from the date of completion of manufacture. The reconstituted vaccine should be used immediately after preparation.

Actions and uses. Bacillus Calmette-Guérin Vaccine is used for active immunisation against tuberculosis, principally for the vaccination of selected groups of the population and of persons likely to be exposed to infection. It is given only to persons who give a negative tuberculin reaction, as described under Old Tuberculin (page 573).

A suitable schedule for the immunisation of children is given under Vaccines (page 549). The vaccine is generally administered intracutaneously over the insertion of the deltoid muscle.

Dose. Prophylactic, as a single dose, 0·1 millilitre by intracutaneous injection.

ABBREVIATED NAME: Dried Tub/Vac/BCG

PERCUTANEOUS BACILLUS CALMETTE-GUÉRIN VACCINE

SYNONYM: Percut. BCG Vaccine

Percutaneous Bacillus Calmette-Guérin Vaccine is a suspension of living cells of an authentic strain of the bacillus of Calmette and Guérin with a higher viable bacterial count than Bacillus Calmette-Guérin Vaccine. It is prepared immediately before use by reconstituting the dried vaccine with an appropriate volume of a suitable sterile liquid.

The vaccine is produced in a similar manner to Bacillus Calmette-Guérin Vaccine. The strain of bacillus used is maintained so as to preserve its power of sensitising man to tuberculin and its relative non-pathogenicity to man and laboratory animals.

Standard
It complies with the requirements of the British Pharmacopoeia.
The dried product is a solid which, when reconstituted by adding the appropriate quantity of a suitable reconstituting liquid indicated on the label, forms an opalescent suspension intended for percutaneous injection.
The reconstituted vaccine complies with specific tests for skin-sensitising potency, freedom from extraneous micro-organisms, toxicity, and virulence.

Storage. It should be stored as described under Vaccines (page 549). Under these conditions it may be expected to retain its potency for two years from the date of completion of manufacture. The reconstituted vaccine should be used immediately after preparation.

Actions and uses. Percutaneous Bacillus Calmette-Guérin Vaccine has the actions and uses described under Bacillus Calmette-Guérin Vaccine, but it is administered by the percutaneous route with the aid of a suitable instrument. On account of its higher viable bacterial count, it is not suitable for intracutaneous administration.

ABBREVIATED NAME: Tub/Vac/BCG(Perc)

BOTULINUM ANTITOXIN

SYNONYM: Immunoserum Antibotulinum

Botulinum Antitoxin is a preparation from native serum containing the antitoxic globulins that have the specific power of neutralising the toxins formed by *Clostridium botulinum*, type A, type B, or type E, or any mixture of types A, B, and E.

Botulinum Antitoxin is prepared by the method for antitoxic sera described under Antisera (page 543). Horses are immunised separately against type A, type B, and type E toxins and the sera blended and standardised.

Standard
It complies with the requirements of the European Pharmacopoeia.
It contains not less than 500 Units per ml for each of types A and B and not less than 50 Units per ml for type E.

NOTE. When Mixed Botulinum Antitoxin or Botulinum Antitoxin is prescribed or demanded and the types to be present are not stated, Botulinum Antitoxin prepared from types A, B, and E is dispensed or supplied.

Storage. It should be stored as described under Antisera (page 545).

Actions and uses. Botulism is a condition of acute toxaemia characterised by paralysis of muscles caused by toxin present in infected food at the time it is consumed. Botulinum toxin is an extremely powerful poison acting peripherally by interfering with the release of acetylcholine at the neuromuscular junction. The earliest symptoms of its action are blurred or double vision, giddiness, ptosis, vomiting, diarrhoea, and difficulty in swallowing and speaking.

Botulinum Antitoxin has been successfully used in the treatment of intoxication due to type E, the antitoxin neutralising circulating toxin. Similar considerations apply to intoxications with type B but treatment with antitoxin is probably less effective against the more powerful and rapidly acting type A toxin. However, since no alternative treat-ment is known, it is advisable to give the antitoxin.

Antitoxin should be given as early as possible in the course of the disease, but since type B and type E toxins may persist for some time in the circulation, late administration may be of some help. Since the type of toxin is seldom known, the polyvalent antitoxin is usually given.

Dose. Prophylactic, not less than 10,000 Units each of type A and type B and not less than 1000 Units of type E by subcutaneous or intramuscular injection.

Therapeutic, not less than 50,000 Units each of type A and type B and not less than 5000 Units of type E by intramuscular or intravenous injection.

ABBREVIATED NAME: Bot/Ser

CHOLERA VACCINE

SYNONYM: Vaccinum Cholerae

Cholera Vaccine is a sterile suspension of suitable strains of the cholera vibrio, *Vibrio cholerae*.

Cholera Vaccine consists of a mixture of equal parts of vaccines, prepared separately by the method for sterile bacterial vaccines described under Vaccines (page 548), from the two main serotypes, Inaba and Ogawa. It may contain, in addition to not less than 8000 million vibrios per ml prepared from the classical biotype, vaccines prepared from the Inaba and Ogawa serotypes of the El Tor biotype.

Standard
It complies with the requirements of the European Pharmacopoeia.
It contains not less than 8000 million *V. cholerae* of the classical biotype in each human dose, which does not exceed 1 ml.

Storage. It should be stored as described under Vaccines (page 549).

Actions and uses. Cholera Vaccine is used only as an immunising agent and the immunity conferred is short-lived. A primary prophylactic course of two injections is recommended, preferably with an interval of four weeks between the injections, and this may confer immunity for five to six months. Further doses of 1 millilitre should therefore be given at intervals of six months. Reactions to this vaccine are usually mild.

Dose. Prophylactic, by subcutaneous or intramuscular injection: the volume stated on the label as the dose, usually initial dose 0·5 millilitre, second dose 1 millilitre after an interval of one to four weeks.

ABBREVIATED NAME: Cho/Vac

DIPHTHERIA ANTITOXIN

SYNONYM: Immunoserum Antidiphthericum

Diphtheria Antitoxin is a preparation from native serum containing the antitoxic globulins that have the specific power of neutralising the toxin formed by *Corynebacterium diphtheriae* and rendering it harmless to susceptible animals.

The antitoxin is prepared by the method for antitoxic sera described under Antisera (page 543).

Standard
It complies with the requirements of the European Pharmacopoeia.
It contains not less than 1000 Units per ml in the case of antitoxin obtained from horse serum and not less that 500 Units per ml for antitoxin obtained from the serum of other species.

Storage. It should be stored as described under Antisera (page 545).

Actions and uses. Diphtheria Antitoxin neutralises the toxin produced by *C. diphtheriae* locally at the site of infection, but does not affect the pathological changes already induced by the toxin. It can neutralise the toxin present in the circulation, but it is unlikely that it can neutralise that which is fixed to the tissues.

The dose of antitoxin varies according to the severity and stage of the disease, but not with the age of the patient; a child requires at least as large a dose as an adult. As mortality increases rapidly with delay in administering antitoxin, an adequate dose should be given as soon as the disease is diagnosed or suspected without waiting for the results of the culture.

When the attack is mild or of moderate severity, doses of 10,000 to 30,000 Units should be given intramuscularly; doses of 40,000 to 100,000 Units or even more should be given in severe cases.

Whenever a dose of more than 40,000 Units is thought to be necessary, the intravenous route should be used; first a portion of the dose is given intramuscularly, followed one-half to two hours later by the bulk of the dose intravenously.

It should be appreciated that twenty-four hours after the intramuscular injection of a dose, the antitoxin titre in the patient's circulation is only about half that attained after the intravenous injection of the same amount. If at any time the amount of antitoxin given is considered to be inadequate, an additional dose should be administered intravenously.

The prophylactic dose is 500 to 2000 Units, usually injected intramuscularly. The passive immunity thus conferred usually lasts about two weeks. Passive immunisation may be combined with active immunisation, as described under Diphtheria Vaccine.

Dose. Prophylactic, 500 to 2000 Units by subcutaneous or intramuscular injection.
Therapeutic, 10,000 to 100,000 Units by intramuscular or intravenous injection.

ABBREVIATED NAME: Dip/Ser

DIPHTHERIA VACCINE

SYNONYM: Diphtheria Prophylactic

Diphtheria Vaccine is prepared from diphtheria toxin produced by the growth of *Corynebacterium diphtheriae*. The toxin is converted to diphtheria formol toxoid by treatment with Formaldehyde Solution.

Standard
It complies with the requirements of the British Pharmacopoeia, which includes tests for potency and specific toxicity.
It contains not less than 25 *flocculation equivalents* (25 Lf) in the recommended dose.

Storage. It should be stored as described under Vaccines (page 549).

Actions and uses. Diphtheria vaccines are used for active immunisation against diphtheria. For primary immunisation of infants, the most commonly used preparation is Diphtheria, Tetanus, and Pertussis Vaccine. In this vaccine the pertussis component acts as an adjuvant for the diphtheria toxoid. Primary immunisation should consist of three injections, the second following the first after an interval of six to eight weeks, and the third following the second after an interval of four to six months; immunisation should be completed by the end of the first fourteen months of life.

For the primary immunisation of children to whom the administration of pertussis vaccine is considered undesirable, Adsorbed Diphtheria and Tetanus Vaccine should be used. If primary vaccination against diphtheria only is required, Adsorbed Diphtheria Vaccine must be used; Diphtheria Vaccine is no longer regarded as adequate for the primary immunisation of children.

At school entry a further reinforcing dose is recommended; for this purpose Diphtheria Vaccine, Adsorbed Diphtheria Vaccine, or Diphtheria, Tetanus, and Poliomyelitis Vaccine may be used.

Some guide to the liability of patients to suffer undue reactions during immunisation is provided by the response to the control in the Schick test.

Dose. Prophylactic, by intramuscular or by deep subcutaneous injection: the volume indicated on the label as the dose, repeated as directed under Actions and uses.

ABBREVIATED NAME: Dip/Vac/FT

ADSORBED DIPHTHERIA VACCINE

SYNONYM: Adsorbed Diphtheria Prophylactic

Adsorbed Diphtheria Vaccine is prepared from diphtheria formol toxoid containing not less than 1500 *flocculation equivalents* (1500 Lf) per mg of protein nitrogen and a mineral carrier which may be aluminium hydroxide or aluminium phosphate.

The antigenic properties of this vaccine are adversely affected by exposure to the action of phenol or cresol; bactericides of this type are not added to the vaccine.

Standard
It complies with the requirements of the British Pharmacopoeia, which includes tests for potency and specific toxicity.
It contains not more than 1·25 mg of Al in the recommended dose.

Storage. It should be stored as described under Vaccines (page 549).

Actions and uses. Adsorbed Diphtheria Vaccine is used for active immunisation against diphtheria. Primary immunisation should consist of three injections, the second following the first after an interval of six to eight weeks, and the third following the second after an interval of four to six months; immunisation should be completed by the end of the first fourteen months of life. When primary immunisation is required, Adsorbed Diphtheria Vaccine is used. For the reinforcement of primary immunisation, Diphtheria Vaccine or Adsorbed Diphtheria Vaccine is used.

Some guide to the liability of patients to suffer undue reactions during immunisation is provided by the response to the control in the Schick test.

Dose. Prophylactic, by intramuscular or by deep subcutaneous injection: the volume indicated on the label as the dose, repeated as directed under Actions and uses.

ABBREVIATED NAME: Dip/Vac/Adsorbed

DIPHTHERIA AND TETANUS VACCINE

SYNONYM: Diphtheria-Tetanus Prophylactic

Diphtheria and Tetanus Vaccine is a mixture of diphtheria formol toxoid and tetanus formol toxoid.

Standard
It complies with the requirements of the British Pharmacopoeia, which includes tests for potency of the constituent vaccines and a test for specific toxicity.

Storage. It should be stored as described under Vaccines (page 549).

Actions and uses. Diphtheria and Tetanus Vaccine is especially useful for reinforcing doses for children at about five years of age or at school entry who no longer require immunisation against pertussis. A suitable schedule for the immunisation of children is given under Vaccines (page 549).

Dose. Prophylactic, by intramuscular or by deep subcutaneous injection: 0·5 or 1 millilitre as indicated on the label as the dose.

ABBREVIATED NAME: DT/Vac/FT

ADSORBED DIPHTHERIA AND TETANUS VACCINE

SYNONYM: Adsorbed Diphtheria-Tetanus Prophylactic

Adsorbed Diphtheria and Tetanus Vaccine is prepared from diphtheria formol toxoid containing not less than 1500 *flocculation equivalents* (1500 Lf) per mg of protein nitrogen, tetanus formol toxoid, and a mineral carrier which may be aluminium hydroxide or aluminium phosphate.

Standard
It complies with the requirements of the British Pharmacopoeia, which includes tests for potency of the constituent vaccines and a test for specific toxicity.
It contains not more than 1·25 mg of Al in the recommended dose.

Storage. It should be stored as described under Vaccines (page 549).

Actions and uses. Adsorbed Diphtheria and Tetanus Vaccine is used for both the primary immunisation and reinforcing dose for children in the prophylaxis of diphtheria and tetanus. A suitable schedule for the immunisation of children is given under Vaccines (page 549).

Dose. Prophylactic, by intramuscular or by deep subcutaneous injection: 0·5 or 1 millilitre as indicated on the label as the dose.

ABBREVIATED NAME: DT/Vac/Adsorbed

DIPHTHERIA, TETANUS, AND PERTUSSIS VACCINE

SYNONYM: Diphtheria-Tetanus-Whooping-cough Prophylactic

Diphtheria, Tetanus, and Pertussis Vaccine is a mixture of diphtheria formol toxoid, tetanus formol toxoid, and a suspension of killed *Bordetella pertussis*.

Standard
It complies with the requirements of the British Pharmacopoeia, which includes tests for potency of the constituent vaccines, a limit of opacity, and a test for specific toxicity.

Storage. It should be stored as described under Vaccines (page 549).

Actions and uses. Diphtheria, Tetanus, and Pertussis Vaccine is used for primary immunisation against diphtheria, tetanus, and whooping-cough.
A suitable schedule for the immunisation of children is given under Vaccines (page 549). A reinforcing dose is desirable at school entry;

as it is considered that the risk of whooping-cough is over by then, Diphtheria and Tetanus Vaccine is generally used. Diphtheria and Tetanus Vaccine is also used in those rare cases where a reaction to pertussis vaccine contra-indicates the use of this constituent and in these cases, for primary immunisation, Adsorbed Diphtheria and Tetanus Vaccine is used.

Dose. Prophylactic, by intramuscular or by deep subcutaneous injection: three doses each of 0·5 or 1 millilitre as indicated on the label as the dose and as directed under Actions and uses.

ABBREVIATED NAME: DTPer/Vac

ADSORBED DIPHTHERIA, TETANUS, AND PERTUSSIS VACCINE

SYNONYM: Adsorbed Diphtheria-Tetanus-Whooping-cough Prophylactic

Adsorbed Diphtheria, Tetanus, and Pertussis Vaccine is prepared from diphtheria formol toxoid, tetanus formol toxoid, a suspension of killed *Bordetella pertussis*, and a mineral carrier which may be aluminium hydroxide or aluminium phosphate.

Standard
It complies with the requirements of the British Pharmacopoeia, which includes tests for potency of the constituent vaccines and a test for specific toxicity.
It contains not more than 1·25 mg of Al in the recommended dose.

Storage. It should be stored as described under Vaccines (page 549).

Actions and uses. Adsorbed Diphtheria, Tetanus, and Pertussis Vaccine is used for

primary immunisation against diphtheria, tetanus, and whooping-cough in the same manner as Diphtheria, Tetanus, and Pertussis Vaccine (above).

Dose. Prophylactic, by intramuscular or by deep subcutaneous injection: three doses each of 0·5 or 1 millilitre as indicated on the label as the dose.

ABBREVIATED NAME: DTPer/Vac/Adsorbed

DIPHTHERIA, TETANUS, AND POLIOMYELITIS VACCINE

Diphtheria, Tetanus, and Poliomyelitis Vaccine is a mixture of diphtheria formol toxoid, tetanus formol toxoid, and poliomyelitis vaccine (inactivated).

In preparing this vaccine, the poliomyelitis vaccine (inactivated) is tested for the absence of infective poliomyelitis virus before it is incorporated with the other ingredients because such a test is not applicable to the mixed vaccine.

Standard
It complies with the requirements of the British Pharmacopoeia, which includes tests for potency of the constituent vaccines and a test for specific toxicity.

Storage. It should be stored as described under Vaccines (page 549). Under these conditions it may be expected to retain its potency for at least one year from the date of manufacture.

Actions and uses. Diphtheria, Tetanus, and Poliomyelitis Vaccine is used to reinforce the immunity of children who have previously been immunised against diphtheria, tetanus, and poliomyelitis, particularly at the time of school entry.
A suitable schedule for the immunisation of children is given under Vaccines (page 549).

Dose. Prophylactic, by intramuscular or by deep subcutaneous injection, the volume stated on the label as the dose.

ABBREVIATED NAME: DTPol/Vac

DIPHTHERIA, TETANUS, PERTUSSIS, AND POLIOMYELITIS VACCINE

SYNONYM: Diphtheria-Tetanus-Whooping-cough-Poliomyelitis Prophylactic

Diphtheria, Tetanus, Pertussis, and Poliomyelitis Vaccine is a mixture of diphtheria formol toxoid, tetanus formol toxoid, a suspension of killed *Bordetella pertussis*, and poliomyelitis vaccine (inactivated).

In preparing this vaccine, the poliomyelitis vaccine (inactivated) is tested for the absence of infective poliomyelitis virus before it is incorporated with the other ingredients because such a test is not applicable to the mixed vaccine.

Standard
It complies with the requirements of the British Pharmacopoeia, which includes tests for potency of the constituent vaccines, a limit of opacity, and a test for specific toxicity.

Storage. It should be stored as described under Vaccines (page 549). Under these conditions it may be expected to retain its potency for at least one year from the date of manufacture.

Actions and uses. Diphtheria, Tetanus, Pertussis, and Poliomyelitis Vaccine is used for the active immunisation of infants against diphtheria, tetanus, whooping-cough, and poliomyelitis. Primary immunisation should consist of three injections, the second following the first after an interval of six to eight weeks, and the third following the second after an interval of four to six months; immunisation should be completed by the end of the first fourteen months of life.

Dose. Prophylactic, by intramuscular or by deep subcutaneous injection: three doses each of 0·5 or 1 millilitre as indicated on the label as the dose and as directed under Actions and uses.

ABBREVIATED NAME: DTPerPol/Vac

ELTOR VACCINE

Eltor Vaccine is a suspension of suitable killed strains of the El Tor biotype of *Vibrio cholerae*.

Eltor Vaccine consists of a mixture of equal parts of vaccines prepared separately by the method for sterile bacterial vaccines described under Vaccines (page 548) from smooth strains of the two main serotypes, Inaba and Ogawa.

Standard
It complies with the requirements of the British Pharmacopoeia.
It contains not less than 8000 million *V. cholerae* of the El Tor biotype in 1 ml.

Storage. It should be stored as described under Vaccines (page 549).

Actions and uses. Eltor Vaccine is used for the same purpose as Cholera Vaccine (page 554) but it is not recognised as complying with the requirements for vaccination certificates required for international travel—see under Immunisation of Travellers (page 551).

Dose. Prophylactic, by subcutaneous or intramuscular injection: the volume stated on the label as the dose, usually initial dose 0·5 millilitre, second dose 1 millilitre after an interval of one to four weeks.

ABBREVIATED NAME: Eltor/Vac

GAS-GANGRENE ANTITOXIN (OEDEMATIENS)

SYNONYM: Immunoserum Anticlostridium Oedematiens

Gas-gangrene Antitoxin (Oedematiens) is a preparation from native serum containing the antitoxic globulins that have the specific power of neutralising the alpha toxin formed by *Clostridium oedematiens* and rendering it harmless to susceptible animals.

The antitoxin is prepared by the method for antitoxic sera described under Antisera (page 543).

Standard
It complies with the requirements of the European Pharmacopoeia.
It contains not less than 3750 Units in 1 ml.

Storage. It should be stored as described under Antisera (page 5!5).

Actions and uses. Gas-gangrene Antitoxin (Oedematiens) is used mainly in conjunction with other gas-gangrene antitoxins, especially those of *Clostridium perfringens* and *Clostridium septicum*, as in Mixed Gas-gangrene Antitoxin.

The monovalent antitoxin is not much used in practice owing to the difficulty of rapidly identifying the infecting organism. The suggested initial therapeutic dose is not less than

30,000 Units by intravenous injection; further injections may be given every four to six hours, according to the response of the patient.

Dose. By intramuscular or intravenous injection: prophylactic, 10,000 Units; therapeutic, not less than 30,000 Units.

GAS-GANGRENE ANTITOXIN (PERFRINGENS)

SYNONYMS: Gas-gangrene Antitoxin (Welchii); Immunoserum Anticlostridium Perfringens

Gas-gangrene Antitoxin (Perfringens) is a preparation from native serum containing the antitoxic globulins that have the specific power of neutralising the alpha toxin formed by *Clostridium perfringens* (*Cl. welchii*, type A) and rendering it harmless to susceptible animals.

The antitoxin is prepared by the method for antitoxic sera described under Antisera (page 543).

Standard
It complies with the requirements of the European Pharmacopoeia.
It contains not less than 1500 Units in 1 ml.

Storage. It should be stored as described under Antisera (page 545).

Actions and uses. Gas-gangrene Antitoxin (Perfringens) is used mainly in conjunction with other gas-gangrene antitoxins, especially those of *Clostridium oedematiens* and *Clostridium septicum*, as in Mixed Gas-gangrene Antitoxin.

The monovalent antitoxin is not much used in practice owing to the difficulty of rapidly identifying the infecting organism. The suggested initial therapeutic dose is not less than 30,000 Units by intravenous injection; further injections may be given every four to six hours, according to the response of the patient.

For prophylactic treatment Gas-gangrene antitoxin (Perfringens) may be given together with Tetanus Antitoxin.

Dose. By intramuscular or intravenous injection: prophylactic, 10,000 Units; therapeutic, not less than 30,000 Units.

GAS-GANGRENE ANTITOXIN (SEPTICUM)

SYNONYM: Immunoserum Anticlostridium Septicum

Gas-gangrene Antitoxin (Septicum) is a preparation from native serum containing the antitoxic globulins that have the specific power of neutralising the alpha toxin formed by *Clostridium septicum*, also known as Vibrion septique, and rendering it harmless to susceptible animals.

The antitoxin is prepared by the method for antitoxic sera described under Antisera (page 543).

Standard
It complies with the requirements of the European Pharmacopoeia.
It contains not less than 1500 Units in 1 ml.

Storage. It should be stored as described under Antisera (page 545).

Actions and uses. Gas-gangrene Antitoxin (Septicum) is used mainly in conjunction with other gas-gangrene antitoxins, especially those of *Clostridium perfringens* and *Clostridium*

oedematiens, as in Mixed Gas-gangrene Antitoxin.

The monovalent antitoxin is not much used in practice owing to the difficulty of rapidly identifying the infecting organism. The suggested initial therapeutic dose is not less than 15,000 Units by intravenous injection; further injections may be given every four to six hours, according to the response of the patient.

Dose. By intramuscular or intravenous injection: prophylactic, 5000 Units; therapeutic, not less than 15,000 Units.

MIXED GAS-GANGRENE ANTITOXIN

SYNONYM: Immunoserum Anticlostridium Mixtum

Mixed Gas-gangrene Antitoxin is prepared by mixing Gas-gangrene Antitoxin (Perfringens), Gas-gangrene Antitoxin (Oedematiens), and Gas-gangrene Antitoxin (Septicum).

Standard
It complies with the requirements of the European Pharmacopoeia.
It contains in each ml not less than 1000 Units of

Gas-gangrene Antitoxin (Perfringens), not less than 1000 Units of Gas-gangrene Antitoxin (Oedematiens), and not less than 500 Units of Gas-gangrene Antitoxin (Septicum).

Storage. It should be stored as described under Antisera (page 545).

Actions and uses. Mixed Gas-gangrene Antitoxin should be given, as soon as possible after infliction of a wound, as a prophylactic measure against the development of gas-gangrene. Intravenous injection ensures rapid distribution of the antitoxin, but if this route is impracticable the injection may be given intramuscularly into healthy tissue. Mixed Gas-gangrene Antitoxin has been given with Tetanus Antitoxin. There is no hard and fast rule about dosage; the dose indicated may be doubled or repeated if the clinical condition of the patient deteriorates or if an operation is necessary.

The therapeutic dose is at least three times the prophylactic dose and is administered by intravenous injection in order to neutralise the toxaemia with a minimum of delay. Repeated administration may be required every four to six hours, according to the response of the patient.

As soon as the infecting micro-organism has been identified, monovalent antitoxin may be substituted for polyvalent antitoxin, although this course is seldom possible in practice.

Dose. Prophylactic, 25,000 Units by intramuscular or intravenous injection; therapeutic, not less than 75,000 Units by intravenous injection.

ABBREVIATED NAME: Gas/Ser

INFLUENZA VACCINE

SYNONYMS: Influenza Vaccine (Inactivated); Vaccinum Influenzae Inactivatum

Influenza Vaccine is an aqueous suspension of a suitable strain or strains of influenza virus, inactivated so that they are non-infective but retain their antigenic properties. Suitable strains of influenza virus are those currently recommended by the World Influenza Centre of the World Health Organisation.

The vaccine is prepared by the method for viral and rickettsial vaccines described under Vaccines (page 549). The virus of each strain is grown in the allantoic cavity of ten- to thirteen-day-old fertile chick embryos and the allantoic fluid harvested after incubation for two to three days at 33° to 37°. Bacteriologically sterile fluids are pooled and inactivated. If formaldehyde is used it is added to give a concentration of about 1 in 10,000 of HCHO and inactivation is allowed to proceed for two to three days at 0° to 4°.

The virus is then purified by centrifugation or other suitable means and suspended in a neutral buffered saline solution containing thiomersal or other suitable antibacterial substance.

Vaccine containing more than one strain of virus is made by mixing purified inactivated suspensions of each strain.

Standard
It complies with the requirements of the European Pharmacopoeia, which includes tests for abnormal toxicity, viral inactivation, antigenic content, and sterility.

It is a slightly opalescent liquid.

Storage. It should be stored protected from light at 2° to 10°. It should not be allowed to freeze. Under these conditions it may be expected to retain its potency for eighteen months.

Actions and uses. Influenza Vaccine is used for active immunisation against epidemic influenza. It is usually given by deep subcutaneous injection during the autumn, when it may be expected to give substantial protection against infection by the same antigenic variety of virus. Protection develops in two to three weeks, but is, however, short-lived.

As a rule, influenza vaccination is not prescribed annually, except for persons considered to be under special risk, for example, patients with chronic cardiac or pulmonary insufficiency. It may be given during an influenza epidemic, particularly to such people as medical and nursing staff who are required to remain at work during the epidemic.

Dose. Prophylactic, as a single dose, 1 millilitre by deep subcutaneous injection.

ABBREVIATED NAME: Flu/Vac

LEPTOSPIRA ANTISERUM

SYNONYM: Leptospira Icterohaemorrhagiae Antiserum

Leptospira Antiserum is native serum, or a preparation from native serum, containing the antibodies that give a specific protection against strains of *Leptospira icterohaemorrhagiae*.

Leptospira Antiserum is prepared by the method for antibacterial sera described under Antisera (page 544), successively increasing doses of killed whole cultures of *Leptospira* being injected intravenously into horses.

Standard

DESCRIPTION. A clear, almost colourless to yellow or yellowish-brown liquid which may become turbid with age.

IDENTIFICATION. It renders virulent strains of *L. icterohaemorrhagiae* harmless to susceptible animals.

STERILITY; ABNORMAL TOXICITY. It complies with the requirements of the General Standard for Antisera (page 545) for sterility and abnormal toxicity.

POTENCY. In laboratory tests, the antiserum protects groups of guinea-pigs against lethal infection induced by a method of scarification or by the subcutaneous or intraperitoneal injection of virulent passaged strains of *Leptospira*.

Storage. It should be stored as described under Antisera (page 545).

Actions and uses. Leptospira Antiserum is occasionally used in the treatment of spirochaetal jaundice (Weil's disease), mainly as an adjuvant to various forms of chemotherapy. Administration by the intravenous route is preferable in severe cases and by the intramuscular route in patients less severely affected.

Leptospira Antiserum is not used routinely in prophylaxis. It is not effective against infections due to *L. canicola*, for which no specific antiserum is available for therapeutic use.

Dose. Therapeutic, 20 to 40 millilitres by intravenous or intramuscular injection.

ABBREVIATED NAME: Lep/Ser

MEASLES VACCINE (LIVE ATTENUATED)

SYNONYMS: Measles Vaccine (Live); Vaccinum Morbillorum

Measles Vaccine (Live Attenuated) is an aqueous suspension of an approved strain of live attenuated measles virus grown in cultures of chick-embryo cells.

Production of the vaccine is based on a seed lot system, the final vaccine representing not more than ten subcultures from the culture on which the original laboratory and clinical tests were made showing the strain to be suitable.

The virus is grown under aseptic conditions in chick-embryo cell cultures in a suitable maintenance medium containing no penicillin and no extraneous protein capable of producing hypersensitivity when injected into human subjects. If animal serum is used, it must not be in a concentration of more than one part per million in the final vaccine. The chick-embryo cells are derived from embryonated chicken eggs from a healthy flock free from adventitious agents.

The virus is grown at a constant temperature and harvested not later than fourteen days after inoculation. The virus suspensions are tested for freedom from bacterial, mycoplasmal, and extraneous viral contamination, and the pooled harvest is clarified by a method which ensures the removal of all tissue cells. A suitable stabiliser is added to the pool, which is then distributed into the final sterile containers, freeze-dried, and the containers sealed.

The final batches of vaccine are tested for identity by a suitable serological test, for virus concentration by titration against a reference preparation, and for freedom from abnormal toxicity by animal inoculation.

The dry product is reconstituted immediately before use by dissolving the contents of a sealed container in the appropriate quantity of Water for Injections. The vaccine may have a reddish tinge if phenol red has been used as a pH indicator in the production.

Standard

It complies with the requirements of the European Pharmacopoeia, which includes tests for extraneous viruses, contaminating micro-organisms, abnormal toxicity, and virus titre.

Storage. It should be stored between 2° and 10°; under these conditions it may be expected to retain its potency for at least one year after the date of manufacture.

The reconstituted vaccine should be used immediately after preparation.

Actions and uses. Measles Vaccine (Live Attenuated) is used for active immunisation against measles. Susceptible subjects develop protective antibodies towards the end of the second week after vaccination.

Mild clinical effects, lasting a day or two and consisting mainly of pyrexia, general irritability, and a transient rash, may develop in a minority of patients from six to twelve days after vaccination. The clinical effects are not transmissible to other individuals.

The virus present in the vaccine is rendered ineffective by the presence of measles antibodies in the circulation, whether derived transplacentally from the mother or as a result of injection of measles immunoglobulin in prophylactic doses during the previous six weeks, or actively stimulated by previous infection with epidemic measles or vaccination previously with Measles Vaccine (Live Attenuated). The vaccine is therefore unlikely to be effective in the majority of children under six months of age and a substantial proportion of those aged six to twelve months.

A suitable schedule for the immunisation of children is given under Vaccines (page 549).

PRECAUTIONS AND CONTRA-INDICATIONS. The vaccine should be used with care in individuals having a history of febrile convulsions and in the presence of brain damage or egg-protein sensitivity.

It is contra-indicated in leukaemia, lymphoma, and other generalised malignant diseases, hypogammaglobulinaemia, acute febrile illness, and pregnancy.

It should not be given at the same time as therapy that depresses the immune response.

CAUTION. The vaccine is readily inactivated by traces of viricidal agents, including chemical disinfectants, antiseptics, spirits, bactericidal soaps, and heavy metals.

Disposable syringes sterilised by gamma-irradiation should preferably be used for reconstituting and administering the vaccine. Glass syringes and steel needles, if they are used, should be thoroughly cleansed in recently distilled water and sterilised by autoclaving or by dry heat.

Chlorinated or other chemically treated water must be avoided.

Dose. Prophylactic, as a single dose, by subcutaneous or intramuscular injection: 0·5 millilitre.

ABBREVIATED NAME: Meas/Vac (Live)

PERTUSSIS VACCINE

SYNONYMS: Vaccinum Pertussis; Whooping-cough Vaccine

Pertussis Vaccine is a sterile suspension of killed *Bordetella pertussis*.

The vaccine is prepared by the method for sterile bacterial vaccines described under Vaccines (page 548). The bacilli are killed by heat or by the action of a suitable chemical and a concentrated suspension, in a saline or other appropriate solution isotonic with blood, containing a suitable antibacterial substance, is prepared; if necessary it is stored in the cold for about three months to lower the toxicity. This suspension is then diluted to the final strength with a saline or other appropriate solution isotonic with blood which may contain a suitable antibacterial substance.

Standard
It complies with the requirements of the European Pharmacopoeia, which includes tests for potency sterility, abnormal toxicity, and a limit of opacity.
It contains not less than 4 Units in each single human dose, which must not exceed 1 ml.

Storage. It should be stored as described under Vaccines (page 549). Under these conditions it may be expected to retain its potency for two years from the date of manufacture.

Actions and uses. Pertussis Vaccine is used for active immunisation against whooping-cough, but it is best used in the form of the combined Diphtheria, Tetanus, and Pertussis Vaccine. Whooping-cough is most dangerous in early life, and the vaccine should be injected when the infant is three to six months old. A suitable schedule for the immunisation of children is given under Vaccines (page 549). Reactions to the vaccine in children are usually mild, but a few may be severe.

Dose. Prophylactic, by intramuscular or by deep subcutaneous injection: three doses each of 0·5 or 1 millilitre as indicated on the label as the dose and as directed under Actions and uses.

ABBREVIATED NAME: Per/Vac

PLAGUE VACCINE

Plague Vaccine is a suspension of suitable killed strains of *Pasteurella pestis*.

The vaccine is prepared by the method for sterile bacterial vaccines described under Vaccines (page 548) from cultures of the capsulated form of *P. pestis* in such a manner that it contains the greatest possible amount of capsular material. The bacteria are killed by Formaldehyde Solution.

The concentrated suspension is stored at 2° to 10° and is diluted as required with a saline or other appropriate solution isotonic with blood containing sufficient phenol to give a final concentration of 0·5 per cent w/v of phenol, not more than 0·025 per cent w/v of

formaldehyde, and 3000 million bacteria (*P. pestis*) in 1 ml.

Standard
It complies with the requirements of the British Pharmacopoeia.
It contains 3000 million bacteria (*P. pestis*) in 1 ml.

Storage. It should be stored as described under Vaccines (page 549).

Actions and uses. Plague Vaccine gives a useful degree of protection against attack. Persons exposed to infection should be given a reinforcing dose of 1 millilitre every year.

The vaccine sometimes causes moderately

severe local and general reactions which usually subside after one or two days.

Dose. Prophylactic, by subcutaneous or intra-muscular injection: initial dose, 0·5 millilitre; second dose, 1 millilitre after an interval of one to four weeks.

ABBREVIATED NAME: Plague/Vac

POLIOMYELITIS VACCINE (INACTIVATED)

SYNONYMS: Poliomyelitis Vaccine (Killed); Vaccinum Poliomyelitidis Inactivatum

Poliomyelitis Vaccine (Inactivated) is an aqueous suspension of suitable strains of poliomyelitis virus, types 1, 2, and 3, grown in cultures of monkey kidney tissue and inactivated by a suitable method. When injected into animals, it stimulates the production of neutralising antibodies to poliomyelitis virus, types 1, 2, and 3, in the circulating blood.

Poliomyelitis Vaccine (Inactivated) may be prepared by the following method.

The virus of each type is grown with aseptic precautions in cultures of monkey kidney cells that have not been propagated in series. If animal serum is used in the medium for initiating cell growth, its calculated concentration in the final vaccine does not exceed one part per million. The medium for maintaining cell growth, as distinct from that for initiating it, contains no protein, but may contain a non-toxic pH indicator such as phenol red and may also contain antibiotics, except penicillin, in the smallest effective concentration. The virus suspension is passed through a bacteria-proof filter.

After filtration and before inactivation, each monovalent virus suspension is titrated for infective virus and is not used unless it has a titre of at least 30 million TCID50 per ml for types 1 and 3 and at least 10 million TCID50 per ml for type 2; the TCID50 is the tissue-culture infective dose 50 per cent, which is the dose of virus that produces infection in 50 per cent of the monkey-kidney tissue-culture tubes.

Within seventy-two hours of filtration, inactivation is initiated by the addition of Formaldehyde Solution to give a concentration of about 1 in 10,000 of HCHO. Inactivation is allowed to proceed at 37°, usually for not less than twelve days. During this period its progress is followed by determining virus titres at suitably spaced intervals. Tests for effective inactivation are made on a sample of at least 500 ml from each monovalent suspension by inoculation into tissue cultures; the procedure is repeated after three days. The suspension is regarded as inactivated if neither sample is shown to contain infective virus, the second sample being taken at the end of the inactivation period.

The trivalent vaccine is made by mixing inactivated suspensions of each type of poliomyelitis virus in suitable proportions. Free formaldehyde is removed by the addition of sodium metabisulphite, and suitable antibacterial substances are then added. The trivalent vaccine is subjected to safety tests both in tissue culture and in monkeys.

Standard
It complies with the requirements of the European Pharmacopoeia, which includes tests for potency, infective virus, sterility, and abnormal toxicity.
It is a clear liquid which may have a reddish tinge if phenol red has been used as a pH indicator in its production.

Storage. It should be stored at 2° to 10°. Under these conditions it may be expected to retain its potency for eighteen months after the date of manufacture.

Actions and uses. Poliomyelitis Vaccine (Inactivated) is used for active immunisation against poliomyelitis, although the live oral vaccine is often preferred.
Reactions to the injection of the vaccine are negligible.

Dose. Prophylactic, by subcutaneous or intramuscular injection: three doses, each of 1 millilitre, with an interval of six to eight weeks between the first and second dose and six months between the second and third.

ABBREVIATED NAME: Pol/Vac (Inact)

POLIOMYELITIS VACCINE (ORAL)

SYNONYMS: Poliomyelitis Vaccine (Live); Vaccinum Poliomyelitidis Perorale

Poliomyelitis Vaccine (Oral) is an aqueous suspension of suitable live attenuated strains of poliomyelitis virus, types 1, 2, or 3, grown in suitable cell cultures; it may contain any one of the three virus types or combinations of them. It contains a stabilising agent.

The vaccine may be prepared by the following method.
Production is based on a seed lot system and the final vaccine represents not more than three subcultures of types 1 and 2 and not more than two subcultures of type 3 from the

vaccines on which were made the original laboratory and clinical tests which established the suitability of the strains.

The virus of each type is grown with aseptic precautions in suitable cell cultures that have been shown not to contain extraneous micro-organisms. The medium for maintaining cell growth, as distinct from that for initiating it, contains no serum but may contain a suitable pH indicator such as phenol red and may also contain antibiotics, except penicillin, in the smallest effective concentration.

The virus is grown at a temperature not exceeding 35° for not more than four days after inoculation. The virus suspension is then tested for identity, bacterial and mycotic sterility, and freedom from extraneous viruses, and those suspensions which pass these tests are pooled and filtered through a bacteria-proof filter.

The filtered vaccine is tested for identity and virus concentration. It is also compared with appropriate reference preparations for ability to replicate in tissue cultures at 36° to 38° and at 39° to 41° and for neurovirulence by intra-spinal and intrathalamic injection into *Macaca irus* (cynomolgus monkeys) or equally suscep-tible monkeys. The vaccine is issued if it is shown by these tests not to differ significantly from the reference preparations.

Standard
It complies with the requirements of the European Pharmacopoeia, which includes tests for extraneous viruses, contaminating micro-organisms, abnormal toxicity, and virus titre.
It is a clear liquid which, if phenol red has been used as a pH indicator in its production, has a reddish tinge, but may be colourless or coloured by a distinctive dye when diluted for human use.

Storage. It should be stored in the frozen state; in this condition it may be expected to retain its potency for at least two years. When thawed and kept at a tempera-ture between 2° and 10° it may be expected to retain its potency for twelve months. At higher temperatures it deteriorates rapidly and if kept at ambient temperatures not exceeding 20° it may be expected to lose its potency within seven days.

Actions and uses. Poliomyelitis Vaccine (Oral) is used for active immunisation against poliomyelitis. It is given by mouth either as three doses of a trivalent vaccine or as one dose each of three monovalent vaccines con-taining virus types 1, 2, and 3 respectively.
Suitable schedules for the immunisation of children and travellers are given under Vaccines (page 549).

Dose. Prophylactic, the quantity stated on the label, either as a single dose of each of the three virus types at suitable intervals or as three doses of a vaccine containing all three types (trivalent vaccine) at suitable inter-vals.

ABBREVIATED NAME: Pol/Vac (Oral)

RABIES ANTISERUM

SYNONYMS: Antirabies Serum; Immunoserum Antirabicum

Rabies Antiserum is a preparation of rabies immunoglobulins or their derivatives obtained by purification from native serum. Rabies Antiserum specifically neutralises rabies virus.

The antiserum is prepared by the method for antiviral sera described under Antisera (page 544), increasing doses of killed or living rabies virus being injected into horses or other animals. The vaccines used for immunising the animals must be prepared in a species different from that used for the preparation of human rabies vaccine. The globulins or their derivatives containing the specific immune substances may be obtained from the serum by fractional precipitation, by enzyme treat-ment, or by other chemical or physical methods; the refined product is in liquid form.

Standard
It complies with the requirements of the European Pharmacopoeia.
It contains not less than 80 Units in 1 ml.

Storage. It should be stored as described under Antisera (page 545).

Actions and uses. Rabies Antiserum is used for the prevention of rabies in patients who have received bites on areas of special danger,

such as the head and the neck, from rabid animals or animals suspected of being rabid. It is given in conjunction with Rabies Vaccine.

The antiserum must be given as soon as possible after exposure, preferably within twenty-four hours. The dose is approximately 40 Units per kilogram body-weight intra-muscularly on the first day, followed by daily injections of rabies vaccine. Up to 5 millilitres of antiserum should, when feasible, be in-filtrated around and under bites. The number of injections of vaccine will depend on the severity of the possible infection—see under Rabies Vaccine.

It is often useful to give the antiserum im-mediately and then start the vaccine treatment on the first sign of rabies in the biting animal. If signs suggestive of rabies are already present in the biting animal, then the antiserum must be given immediately, followed by the vaccine, which may be stopped on the fifth day after exposure if the animal is normal; the anti-serum must not be given after the second day of vaccine treatment as it will interfere with the production of active immunity by the vaccine.

Dose. *Local treatment:* a volume of not less than 5 millilitres should be infiltrated around the wound.
Systemic treatment: in patients who have been exposed to severe risk, by intramuscular injection, a single dose of 2000 to 3000 Units

given within forty-eight hours and preferably within twenty-four hours of infection and followed immediately by a dose of Rabies Vaccine and subsequently by not fewer than thirteen daily doses of the vaccine.
Two reinforcing doses of vaccine should be given on the tenth and twentieth days after completion of the primary course to overcome possible interference by passive antibody with active immune responses.

ABBREVIATED NAME: Rab/Ser

RABIES VACCINE

Rabies Vaccine consists of a suitable killed rabies fixed virus in an aqueous suspension of uncontaminated brain tissue derived from animals previously infected intracerebrally with fixed virus.

Rabies Vaccine protects susceptible animals against subsequent infection by an authentic strain of rabies virus. When first isolated from man or animal, rabies virus is known as "street virus"; after repeated passage through animals by intracerebral infection it becomes modified in its properties and is known as "fixed virus".
The vaccine may be prepared by infecting intracerebrally suitable animals, usually sheep or rabbits, with fixed virus. When the animals have shown typical symptoms of rabies for at least twenty-four hours and have developed complete paralysis, they are killed and the brains are harvested. The brains are homogenised in sodium chloride injection and the virus killed by treatment with a chemical agent such as chloroform, ether, phenol, or Formaldehyde Solution. The vaccine is then usually diluted to contain not more than 5 per cent w/v of brain material calculated on a wet weight.
The vaccine has also been prepared from embryonic chicken or duck tissue infected with fixed rabies virus. β-Propiolactone may be used for inactivation.

Standard
It complies with the requirements of the British Pharmacopoeia, which includes tests for abnormal toxicity and absence of infective virus and a limit of solids.
It occurs as a white flocculent suspension in a clear liquid or a slightly turbid liquid.

Storage. It should be protected from light and stored at 2° to 10°. Under these conditions it may be expected to retain its potency for at least six months from the date of manufacture.

Actions and uses. Rabies Vaccine is used for the prevention of rabies in patients who have been bitten by rabid animals or animals suspected of being rabid; in the latter case treatment is stopped if the animal is normal on the fifth day after exposure or attack or if acceptable laboratory findings are negative in the animal killed at the time of the attack. Infection cannot take place through unbroken skin, but it is possible through uninjured mucous membranes. Rabies antiserum may be administered before beginning treatment with the vaccine.
The vaccine should be given subcutaneously into the cellular tissue on the side of the abdomen well below the margin of the ribs. As the inoculations are given daily, it is advisable to vary the site of inoculation with each succeeding dose. Patients undergoing antirabies treatment should avoid fatigue but are ordinarily able to attend to their work.
Before initiating antirabies treatment the following factors should be considered:
(1) Whether enzootic rabies exists in the country where the bite occurred or whether the biting animal has been recently imported from an enzootic area. Animals more likely to be infected than others are bats and carnivores (especially dogs, cats, skunks, foxes, coyotes, raccoons). Although rodents (squirrels, rats, and mice) are rarely infective, in enzootic areas any wild animal that bites or scratches, particularly those that escape, must be suspect.
(2) The circumstances of the biting incident. *Unprovoked* attacks mean that the animal is more likely to be rabid. Bites suffered while attempting to handle or feed apparently healthy animals may be regarded as *provoked*. The biting animal should be captured and confined under veterinary observation for signs of rabies for at least ten days. Adult animals that have been adequately immunised with rabies vaccine are unlikely to develop rabies *or transmit virus*.
(3) The extent and location of bite wound. It is calculated that only 10 to 15 per cent of human exposures to known rabid animals result in infection. Infection is more likely to occur after severe multiple or deep penetrating wounds or bites on the head, neck, or

hands; it is less likely to occur after mild scratches, lacerations, or single bites on areas of the body other than the head, neck, or hands. Open wounds and abrasions suspected of being contaminated with saliva are also considered mild. Indirect contact or a lick on unabraded skin is not considered exposure.

PRECAUTIONS. The vaccine should be administered cautiously to subjects with a history of hypersensitivity and recourse made to antihistamine drugs or adrenaline in the event of an anaphylactoid reaction occurring. If serious allergic manifestations preclude continuation of prophylaxis, vaccine of avian origin should be substituted. If meningeal or neuroparalytic reactions develop, vaccine treatment should be stopped and corticosteroid therapy instituted.

Rabies Antiserum should be used as well as vaccine in all severe exposures and in unprovoked attacks by wild animals.

Dose. *Post-exposure prophylaxis.*
Primary immunisation: fourteen daily doses of not less than 2 millilitres of vaccine are injected subcutaneously as indicated above under Actions and uses; twenty-one doses may be given in *severe* exposures either daily for twenty-one days or fourteen doses in the first seven days (either as two separate injections or as a double dose) then seven daily doses.
Reinforcing doses: two reinforcing doses are given, one ten days and the other at least twenty days after completing the primary course. Reinforcing doses are particularly important if rabies antiserum was used in the initial therapy.

ABBREVIATED NAME: Rab/Vac

RUBELLA VACCINE (LIVE ATTENUATED)

SYNONYM: Rubella Vaccine (Live)

Rubella Vaccine (Live Attenuated) is an aqueous suspension of a suitable live attenuated strain of rubella virus grown in suitable cell cultures. It is prepared immediately before use by reconstituting the dried vaccine with Water for Injections; bactericides must not be added.

Production of the vaccine is based on a seed lot system and the final vaccine represents not more than five subcultures from the vaccine on which were made the original laboratory and clinical tests showing the strain to be suitable.

The virus is grown with aseptic precautions in suitable cell cultures. The cell cultures from mammals or birds are derived from a healthy group or flock known to be free from known adventitious agents and the cell cultures are shown not to contain extraneous micro-organisms. If human diploid cells are used they must be of an approved strain.

The medium added for maintaining cell growth, as distinct from that for initiating it, contains no serum but may contain a suitable pH indicator such as phenol red and also antibiotics (except penicillin and streptomycin) in the smallest effective concentration. The temperature of incubation is accurately controlled during the growth of the virus.

The virus suspension is harvested within twenty-eight days of inoculation and is tested for identity, bacterial and mycotic sterility, and freedom from extraneous viruses. Virus harvests which pass these tests are pooled and clarified to remove tissue cells. A suitable stabiliser is added to the clarified vaccine, which is then distributed into sterile containers of glass or other suitable material and dried from the frozen state before the containers are sealed.

The vaccine is tested for identity and virus concentration and is issued if it is shown by these tests to be satisfactory.

Standard
It complies with the requirements of the British Pharmacopoeia.
The dried product is a pellet which, when reconstituted by adding the appropriate quantity of Water for Injections indicated on the label, yields a suspension which may have a reddish tinge if phenol red has been used in the preparation. The reconstituted vaccine complies with tests for abnormal toxicity and virus titre.

Storage. It should be stored at a temperature between 2° and 10°. Under these conditions it may be expected to retain its potency for at least one year.
The reconstituted vaccine should be used immediately after preparation.

Actions and uses. Rubella Vaccine (Live Attenuated) is used for active immunisation against German measles. Susceptible subjects develop protective antibodies towards the end of the third week after vaccination.

Mild clinical effects lasting a day or two and consisting mainly of pyrexia, general irritability, and a transient rash develop in a minority of patients from six to fourteen days after vaccination. Arthralgia occasionally occurs and is more likely to occur after rubella vaccination in adults than in children.

Suitable schedules for the immunisation of children are given under Vaccines (page 549).

PRECAUTIONS AND CONTRA-INDICATIONS. The vaccine should be used with care in individuals having a history of brain damage because of the possibility of severe reactions occurring.

It is contra-indicated in leukaemia, lymphoma, and other generalised malignant diseases, hypogammaglobulinaemia, acute febrile illness, and especially pregnancy.

It is important that any woman vaccinated is not pregnant and does not become pregnant for eight weeks after vaccination.

Dose. Prophylactic, as a single dose by subcutaneous or intramuscular injection: 0·5 millilitre.

ABBREVIATED NAME: Rub/Vac (Live)

SCHICK TEST TOXIN

Schick Test Toxin is a sterile filtrate from a culture in nutrient broth of *Corynebacterium diphtheriae* which, after being allowed to mature, is diluted so that 0·2 millilitre contains the Test Dose.

The diluent used for Schick Test Toxin may be a sterile aqueous solution containing 1·5 per cent w/v of a mixture of 57 g of borax, 85 g of boric acid, and 99 g of sodium chloride, or some other solution which will equally well stabilise the hydrogen-ion concentration and render the mixture isotonic with blood.

Schick Test Toxin causes a local reaction when injected into the skin of a healthy white or light-coloured guinea-pig which has not previously been treated with any antigenic material, but fails to cause this reaction when mixed before injection with a sufficient quantity of Diphtheria Antitoxin.

Standard
It complies with the requirements of the British Pharmacopoeia.
It is a clear colourless liquid.
The Test Dose is measured by tests in guinea-pigs for combining power and for toxicity. In the test for combining power it gives a local reaction, known as a "positive Schick reaction", when one Test Dose, mixed with $\frac{1}{1250}$ Unit or more of Diphtheria Antitoxin, is injected intracutaneously and it gives no local reaction of any kind when one Test Dose is mixed with $\frac{1}{750}$ Unit or less of Diphtheria Antitoxin and injected intracutaneously. In the test for toxicity, a positive Schick reaction is produced by a 1 in 25 dilution but not by a 1 in 50 dilution.

Storage. Schick Test Toxin prepared with borate-boric acid buffer solution in saline and stored below 25° may be expected to retain its potency for at least two months; when stored at 2° to 10° it may be expected to retain its potency for six months.

Actions and uses. Schick Test Toxin is a reagent employed for the diagnosis of susceptibility to diphtheria. It is used in the Schick test, which consists in the intracutaneous injection of a specified amount of diphtheria toxin, known as the Schick dose; administration is followed by reactions which are readily recognised and can be used as a test for the presence or absence of a certain amount of diphtheria antitoxin.

The flexor surface of the forearms is a convenient site for the Schick test. The skin is first cleansed with alcohol, which is allowed to dry, or with soap and water, and 0·2 millilitre of Schick Test Toxin is then injected intracutaneously into the left arm, while 0·2 millilitre of Schick Control is injected intracutaneously into the right arm. The reactions to these injections may be read after an interval of twenty-four to forty-eight hours, although five to seven days are necessary to detect late reactors and to reconsider earlier doubtful readings.

If it is possible to take a reading on only one occasion, this should be done not earlier than the fourth day and not later than the seventh. In most cases any pseudo-reaction will have subsided by this time.

The reactions which can be distinguished in the test are as follows:

A *positive* Schick reaction, indicating that the patient is susceptible to diphtheria, is shown by a red flush about 10 to 15 millimetres in diameter in the skin at the site of administration on the test arm, but no reaction on the control arm. The reaction fades slowly during the second week after injection, showing superficial desquamation and brown pigmentation.

A *negative* Schick reaction, indicating that the patient is immune to diphtheria, is one in which there is no redness on either arm.

A *negative-and-pseudo* Schick reaction, or "pseudo-reaction", indicating that the patient is immune to diphtheria, is shown by a flush which develops rapidly in twenty-four hours, equally or nearly equally, on each arm. It is less circumscribed than the positive reaction, fades more rapidly, and may leave some pigmentation but little or no desquamation. It is produced in some immune patients, particularly children over ten years of age and adults, who are sensitive to constituents of the test material other than the specific toxin.

A *combined* or *positive-and-pseudo* Schick reaction, indicating that the patient is susceptible to diphtheria, is one in which a pseudo-reaction develops rapidly on both arms, but as this fades the positive reaction develops on the test arm. In this way, the test arm tends to acquire the characters of a true positive reaction, while the reaction on the control arm is fading.

All doubtful reactors should be regarded as positive, except well-marked pseudo-reactors, who are almost invariably immune. The latter are usually older children and adults who have been exposed to diphtheria infection; the exposures which have sensitised them have presumably led also to the development of specific antitoxin.

Infants born of immune mothers have an inherited immunity for the first few months of life; they do not respond very well to the vaccine on account of interference from the passive antitoxin.

Children between the ages of six months and ten years who have not been given diphtheria toxoid are mostly Schick-positive and the Schick test is not considered essential for children up to eight to ten years old.

Above ten years of age the state of immunity varies greatly and the test should always be performed.

Dose. Diagnostic, 0·2 millilitre by intracutaneous injection.

SCHICK CONTROL

Schick Control is Schick Test Toxin that has been heated at 70° to 85° for not less than five minutes in order to destroy the specific toxin.

Schick Control is prepared from the same batch of Schick Test Toxin as that with which it is issued for use.

Standard
It complies with the requirements of the British Pharmacopoeia.

Actions and uses. Schick Control is used in the Schick test to distinguish between the true Schick-positive reaction, due to the absence of diphtheria antitoxin in the blood, and a pseudo-reaction, due to susceptibility to non-specific substances.

Dose. Diagnostic, 0·2 millilitre by intracutaneous injection.

SCORPION VENOM ANTISERUM

SYNONYM: Antiscorpion Serum

Scorpion Venom Antiserum is a preparation containing the specific globulins or their derivatives which neutralise the activity of the venom of one or more types of scorpion.

The antiserum is prepared by the method for antitoxic sera described under Antisera (page 543), dried venom being used as an immunising agent.

Scorpions are widespread in tropical and subtropical areas and their venoms vary in potency and toxicity. *Buthus occitanus* occurs widely in North Africa, the Middle East, and some parts of Southern Europe, *B. maurus* occurs in the Sudan, *B. judaicus* in Syria, Turkey, and Iran, and *B. tamulus* in India; *Leiurus quinquestriatus* is common in Egypt, the Sudan, and the Middle East; *Androctonus australis* occurs in North West Africa and *A. crassicauda* in Turkey and Syria; various species of *Palamneus* are found in India.

The venom of Central and South American scorpions is much more potent and toxic and is frequently lethal. The most important are *Tityus* and *Centruroides* species.

Some of the venoms of scorpions are antigenically similar and antisera produced against these may neutralise the venoms of several different species of scorpions.

Standard
DESCRIPTION; STERILITY; ABNORMAL TOXICITY; REACTION; TOTAL PROTEINS; ALBUMINS; FOREIGN PROTEINS. It complies with the requirements of the General Standard for Antisera (page 545).

IDENTIFICATION. It renders the corresponding venom, or venoms, harmless to susceptible animals.

POTENCY. In view of the numerous toxic fractions and venoms and the varying requirements of different localities, no standard for potency is included. The antiserum should be assayed in animals against a dry standard venom or against a control antiserum of established potency.

The potency of the antiserum should be such that the dose stated on the label will completely neutralise the maximum amount of venom likely to be delivered by a single sting. This is determined by injecting appropriate mixtures of antiserum and venom into mice.

Storage. It should be stored as described under Antisera (page 545).

Actions and uses. The intensity of pain caused by a scorpion sting varies according to the site of sting, the species of scorpion, and the amount of venom injected. The pain may last for between six and forty-eight hours but is usually intense for the first six to ten hours and rigors, sweating, and symptoms of shock are very common. The sting is not usually fatal in the African and Middle East areas but children and debilitated people may die; death frequently results from the sting of South and Central American scorpions.

An antiserum suitable for the species of scorpion prevalent in the area can prevent the symptoms and reduce the pain in a short time.

The injection is often made in or near the site of the sting, but injection in a suitable proximal position is also effective.

Dose. The quantity stated on the label as the dose, injected intramuscularly or into and around the site of the sting.

SMALLPOX VACCINE

SYNONYMS: Liquid Smallpox Vaccine (Dermal); Vaccinum Variolae Fluidum Dermicum; Vaccinum Vacciniae

Smallpox Vaccine contains the living virus of vaccinia and produces the characteristic lesions of vaccinia virus when applied to a scarified area of the skin of man, calves, sheep, rabbits, or guinea-pigs.

Smallpox Vaccine obtained from the lesions produced on the skin of living animals may be called "Vaccine Lymph".

In preparing the vaccine, vaccinal dermal pulp or crude lymph is homogenised in buffer (0·003M phosphate, pH 7·3) and trichloro-trifluoroethane, separated by centrifuging, and the supernatant fluid treated with phenol. Glycerol and bacteriological peptone are added to give concentrations of 40 per cent v/v and 1 per cent w/v respectively.

The vaccine may also be prepared in chick chorio-allantoic membranes which are ground and tested for bacteriological sterility and suspended in a final concentration of 40 per cent v/v of glycerol.

The vaccine is distributed under aseptic conditions into sterile plastic tubing or glass capillary tubes which hold one human dose. Multiple-dose containers may also be used.

Standard
It complies with the requirements of the European Pharmacopoeia.
It is a viscid colourless or straw-coloured liquid and does not contain antibiotics. It contains not more than 500 extraneous living micro-organisms in 1 ml and complies with a test for the absence of pathogenic organisms.
Its potency is determined on the chorio-allantoic membrane of the chick embryo by comparison with a reference vaccine which has been calibrated against the International Reference Preparation of Smallpox Vaccine. The vaccine passes the test if it contains not less than 1×10^8 pock-forming units per ml.

Storage. It should be protected from light and stored below $-20°$ until required for use. Under these conditions it may be expected to retain its potency for twelve months. After removal from such storage it may be kept for three months at a temperature not exceeding $4°$, provided the total time from the date of passing the test does not exceed one year. When stored between $4°$ and $10°$, it may be expected to retain its potency for fourteen days.

Actions and uses. Smallpox Vaccine is inoculated by multiple pressure or by scarification; it is not intended to be administered

intradermally. The characteristic eruption of vaccinia is produced at the site of inoculation. As a result of this infection, immunity to smallpox develops. Generally all other preventive inoculations should be avoided within three weeks of primary vaccination. When a rapid programme of inoculations is necessary, vaccinations against yellow fever and smallpox may be done either simultaneously or within two days of each other at different sites. If this is not feasible an interval of at least two weeks should separate the respective vaccinations to minimise the likelihood of viral interference.

PRECAUTIONS AND CONTRA-INDICATIONS. Important contra-indications to vaccination are the presence of eczema or a history of eczema, septic skin infections, leukaemia or other reticulo-endothelial malignancies, hypogammaglobulinaemia, and corticosteroid or other immunosuppressive treatment.

The danger of death following the vaccination of those suffering from allergic eczema is so great that such patients should not be vaccinated unless they are directly exposed to infection with smallpox. Equally at risk of potentially lethal eczema vaccinatum are eczematous persons who come into contact with recently vaccinated subjects.

If persons suffering from the conditions cited are vaccinated they should be given human vaccinial immunoglobulin at the same time.

Additional contra-indications to vaccination include septic skin conditions and pregnancy.

In the presence of suspected smallpox there are no absolute contra-indications to the immediate vaccination of close contacts.

Dose. Prophylactic, about 0·02 millilitre applied to the skin by scarification or by pressure inoculation.

ABBREVIATED NAME: Var/Vac

DRIED SMALLPOX VACCINE

SYNONYMS: Freeze-dried Smallpox Vaccine (Dermal); Vaccinum Variolae Cryodesiccatum Dermicum

Dried Smallpox Vaccine has much greater heat resistance than the liquid vaccine and is therefore particularly suitable for storage and use in hot climates where refrigeration is inadequate.

The vaccine is prepared from a suitable strain of vaccinia virus propagated in the skin of healthy animals. The virus is extracted from the vaccinial dermal pulp in a buffer solution containing a fluorocarbon and treated with phenol to reduce the bacterial contamination. Bacteriological peptone is added to a final concentration of 5 per cent w/v.

The suspension is distributed aseptically into vials and dried by vacuum sublimation from the frozen state. The vials are stoppered under vacuum or at atmospheric pressure in the presence of oxygen-free nitrogen or other suitable inert gas.

The dried vaccine is supplied only in multiple-dose containers together with reconstituting fluid.

Standard
It complies with the requirements of the European Pharmacopoeia.

It is an almost white powder and does not contain antibiotics. The reconstituted vaccine complies with the bacteriological requirements for Smallpox Vaccine (page 569) and is assayed for potency in the chick chorioallantoic membrane as described under Smallpox Vaccine.

The dried vaccine also complies with a heat resistance test which requires that it should retain at least one-tenth of the initial viral infectivity after not less than four weeks' storage at a temperature not below 37°.

Storage. It should be protected from light and stored continuously at a constant temperature below 5°. Under these conditions it may be expected to retain its potency for three years. The reconstituted vaccine may be kept for seven days at a temperature between 2° and 10°.

Actions and uses. Dried Smallpox Vaccine has the actions and uses described under Smallpox Vaccine (page 569).

Dose. Prophylactic, about 0·02 millilitre of the reconstituted vaccine applied to the skin by scarification or by pressure inoculation.

ABBREVIATED NAME: Var/Vac

SNAKE VENOM ANTISERUM

SYNONYMS: Antivenene; Antivenin; Antivenom; Antivenom Serum; Venom Antitoxin; Anti-snakebite Serum

Snake Venom Antiserum is native serum, or a preparation from native serum, containing the antitoxic globulins, or their derivatives, that have the power of neutralising the venom of one or more kinds of snake.

The main toxic fractions of venom are neurotoxins, cytotoxins, including haemolysins, and coagulants. Neurotoxin predominates in the venom of elapine snakes (cobra, mamba, etc.) and cytotoxins and coagulants in viperine venoms (viper, adder, rattlesnake) but some viperine venoms, particularly those of certain rattlesnakes, are strongly neurotoxic. Snake Venom Antiserum may be prepared by the method for antitoxic sera as described under Antisera (page 543). The antigens and methods used vary from country to country.

No antiserum effective against all venoms is available because of the great immunological differences in the venoms of the snakes of different continents. The custom is for each country to prepare antisera able to neutralise the venoms of the indigenous snakes.

Specific monovalent antisera are prepared, but more commonly antivenin preparations are polyvalent, that is, they have a neutralising effect upon the venoms of more than one species. For example, in South Africa an antiserum is prepared primarily to neutralise the venoms of the Cape cobra, the ringhals, and the puff-adder and, in the Indian sub-continent, to neutralise those of the krait, cobra, Russell's viper, and the saw-scaled viper.

The only poisonous snake found in Great Britain is the adder, or common viper, *Vipera berus*.

Methods of immunising horses vary, some laboratories using formolised venom (anavenom) throughout, some using unmodified venom, and others anavenom followed, when the horses have developed some immunity, by unmodified venom. Several months may be required to produce a potent antiserum.

Standard
DESCRIPTION. If a native antiserum, it is a yellow or yellowish-brown liquid; if a preparation from native serum, it is usually almost colourless but may be yellowish-brown or greenish-yellow.

IDENTIFICATION. It renders the corresponding venom, or venoms, harmless to susceptible animals.

ACIDITY OR ALKALINITY. pH of native antiserum, 7·0 to 8·5 depending upon the concentration of plasma bicarbonate; pH of preparations of antitoxic globulins, 6·0 to 7·0.

STERILITY; ABNORMAL TOXICITY. It complies with the requirements of the General Standard for Antisera (page 545) for sterility and abnormal toxicity.

POTENCY. In view of the numerous toxic fractions and venoms and the varying requirements of different localities, no standard for potency is included. The antiserum should be assayed in animals against a dry standard venom or against a control antiserum of established potency. In view of certain special problems in the assay of venom antisera, such assays should be made against a standard preparation at two or more dose-levels.

An International Biological Standard for *Naja* antivenin is available.

Storage. It should be stored as described under Antisera (page 545).

Actions and uses. A bite by an elapine snake does not usually produce a severe local reaction, but death may ensue within a few minutes to several hours from the respiratory paralysis caused by the neurotoxin.

Viperine venom produces a severe local reaction, with pain, swelling, haemorrhage, and tissue damage, followed by generalised vascular injury, widespread internal haemorrhagic lesions, and blood loss, with resultant shock. Some viperine venoms, notably that of Russell's viper, contain powerful coagulants which may cause death by producing intravascular clotting.

Ideally, specific antiserum should be administered, but this requires that the reptile responsible for the bite is seen and identified accurately. If this is not possible it should always be assumed to be venomous and a large dose of polyvalent snake venom antiserum should be administered at the earliest possible moment, preferably intravenously; ideally, an intramuscular "trial dose" should be given half an hour before an intravenous injection, but in practice this is usually omitted owing to the urgency of the situation. In addition, as much antiserum as possible should be injected into and around the bitten area, the remaining antiserum being given subcutaneously or intramuscularly; the local injection of antiserum is particularly indicated in viperine bite. If improvement does not occur after an hour, a further dose should be given intravenously.

A scale of dosage cannot be laid down because the venoms of the snakes of different countries differ in toxicity and the antivenoms differ in potency; detailed instructions relating to dosage are issued with the antiserum.

It should be noted that the use of antisera entails the injection of large doses of globulins of animal origin, usually from horses, and that even when the globulins have been purified and pepsin-treated they will probably induce serum sickness. However, this is a transient disorder and preferable to the severe systemic disturbances, or death, caused by snake bite.

In Great Britain the effect of an adder bite is not usually fatal in a healthy person. The use of snake venom antiserum is no longer recommended by the Department of Health and Social Security because the efficacy of the available antiserum against *Vipera berus* is unproved.

Dose. Large doses, usually 20 to 50 millilitres, injected intravenously and into and around the bitten site as soon as possible, followed by further amounts as indicated.

TETANUS ANTITOXIN

SYNONYM: Immunoserum Antitetanicum

Tetanus Antitoxin is a preparation containing the specific antitoxic globulins or their derivatives that have the power of neutralising the toxin formed by *Clostridium tetani* and rendering it harmless to susceptible animals.

The antitoxin is prepared by the method for antitoxic sera described under Antisera (page 543).

Standard
It complies with the requirements of the European Pharmacopoeia.
It contains not less than 1000 Units in 1 ml when intended for prophylactic use and not less than 3000 Units in 1 ml when intended for therapeutic use.

Storage. It should be stored as described under Antisera (page 545).

Actions and uses. Tetanus toxin has such an affinity for nerve cells that once it is present in the cells, antitoxin is unlikely to influence it. In the treatment of the acute disease antitoxin can be expected to neutralise only toxin which is still circulating.

For prophylactic use antitoxin may be injected into all non-immune or partially immunised persons as soon as possible after a wound. A suitable dose is 1500 Units, or 3000 Units in heavily infected wounds. It is doubtful if repeated doses are either useful or advisable; sensitivity to horse serum is rapidly induced and second or later doses of antitoxin may be so rapidly removed from the circulation as to render them useless.

In patients who have received horse serum of any kind on a previous occasion the first dose of antitoxin after wounding may similarly be rapidly eliminated and fail to give any protection. In such patients and in those who are hypersensitive to horse serum, bovine or ovine serum or Human Tetanus Immunoglobulin (page 589) may be safer.

When tetanus antitoxin in any form is given,

the patient should also be given a dose of Adsorbed Tetanus Vaccine and arrangements should be made to complete his active immunisation later.

If antitoxin is used in the treatment of tetanus, it should be given as early as possible. The maximum dose need not be more than 100,000 Units and repeated doses are unnecessary. Before surgical procedures involving old injured tissues, a similar dose may be given.

PRECAUTIONS AND CONTRA-INDICATIONS. Reactions to equine tetanus antitoxin are unfortunately common and often severe and opinion is turning against its routine use. Such reac-

tions may be avoided by the use of Human Tetanus Immunoglobulin (page 589).

Thorough wound toilet and the administration of penicillin for several days afterwards is now accepted as sound practice, though many would still give antitoxin in wounds thought to carry a high risk of tetanus. Whatever treatment is given, the opportunity should be taken to immunise the patient actively against tetanus with tetanus toxoid.

Dose. Prophylactic, not less than 1500 Units by subcutaneous or intramuscular injection. Therapeutic, 50,000 to 100,000 Units by intramuscular injection.

ABBREVIATED NAME: Tet/Ser

TETANUS VACCINE

SYNONYM: Tetanus Toxoid

Tetanus Vaccine is prepared from tetanus toxin produced by the growth of *Clostridium tetani*. The toxin is converted to tetanus formol toxoid by treatment with Formaldehyde Solution.

When injected into animals the vaccine stimulates the production of tetanus antitoxin in the circulating blood or increases the amount of this antitoxin if it is already present.

Standard
It complies with the requirements of the British Pharmacopoeia, which includes tests for potency and specific toxicity.

Storage. It should be stored as described under Vaccines (page 549).

Actions and uses. Tetanus Vaccine is used for active immunisation against tetanus. The intramuscular injection of three well-spaced doses gives rise to the production of a considerable amount of tetanus antitoxin in the blood. The antitoxin present in the blood after injection of the vaccine can usually be expected to persist for at least five years. A booster dose many years after the primary immunisation will stimulate the production of antibodies rapidly.

Immunisation of patients following injury must depend upon assessment of the risk associated with the type of wound involved. If the patient's immune status is known, it

may already be adequate or require only the administration of a booster dose of vaccine. Non-immune subjects may require passive immunisation with tetanus antitoxin, but the opportunity should also be taken to initiate the active immunisation of the subject.

When tetanus vaccine and tetanus antitoxin are to be given at the same time, Adsorbed Tetanus Vaccine should be used, the vaccine must not be injected into the same limb as the antitoxin, and the same syringe must not be used.

As a prophylactic for the routine immunisation of children, tetanus vaccine is best used in the form of the combined Diphtheria, Tetanus, and Pertussis Vaccine, with a booster dose of Tetanus Vaccine at school-leaving age; a suitable schedule is described under Vaccines (page 549).

Dose. Prophylactic, by intramuscular or deep subcutaneous injection: 0·5 or 1 millilitre as indicated on the label as the dose, followed after six to twelve weeks by a second dose, followed after six to twelve months by a third dose.

ABBREVIATED NAME: Tet/Vac/FT

ADSORBED TETANUS VACCINE

SYNONYM: Adsorbed Tetanus Toxoid

Adsorbed Tetanus Vaccine is prepared from tetanus formol toxoid and a mineral carrier which may be aluminium hydroxide or aluminium phosphate.

Standard
It complies with the requirements of the British Pharmacopoeia, which includes tests for potency and specific toxicity.
It contains not more than 1·25 mg of Al in the recommended dose.

Storage. It should be stored as described under Vaccines (page 549).

Actions and uses. Adsorbed Tetanus Vaccine is used for the prophylaxis of tetanus as described under Tetanus Vaccine.

Dose. Prophylactic, by intramuscular or deep subcutaneous injection: 0·5 or 1 millilitre as indicated on the label as the dose, followed after six to twelve weeks by a second dose, followed after six to twelve months by a third dose.

ABBREVIATED NAME: Tet/Vac/Adsorbed

TETANUS AND PERTUSSIS VACCINE

SYNONYM: Tetanus-Whooping-cough Prophylactic

Tetanus and Pertussis Vaccine is a mixture of tetanus formol toxoid and a suspension of killed *Bordetella pertussis*.

Standard
It complies with the requirements of the British Pharmacopoeia, which includes tests for potency of the constituent vaccines, a limit of opacity, and a test for specific toxicity.

Storage. It should be stored as described under Vaccines (page 549).

Actions and uses. Tetanus and Pertussis Vaccine is used for active immunisation against tetanus and whooping-cough. Its use is limited to those cases where simultaneous immunisation with a diphtheria component is contra-indicated, as for instance when a child is known to be sensitive to diphtheria toxoid.

Dose. Prophylactic, by intramuscular or deep subcutaneous injection: three doses each of 0·5 or 1 millilitre as indicated on the label as the dose, the second following the first after an interval of six to eight weeks, and the third following the second after an interval of four to six months.

ABBREVIATED NAME: TPer/Vac

OLD TUBERCULIN

SYNONYM: Tuberculinum Crudum

Old Tuberculin is the heat-concentrated filtrate from a fluid medium on which the human or bovine strain of *Mycobacterium tuberculosis* has been grown.

The culture medium on which the organisms are grown may be glycerol broth or, more commonly, a synthetic medium in which the source of nitrogen for bacterial growth is usually asparagin and the sources of carbon are usually glycerol and dextrose.

The organisms are grown rapidly and abundantly for six weeks or more at 37°. The cultures are steamed for at least one hour and the culture fluid, from which the organisms may or may not have been removed previously by filtration, is concentrated by evaporation on a water-bath, usually to one-tenth of its original volume. It is clarified by filtration, commonly after the addition of 0·5 per cent of phenol, and assayed against a reference preparation by biological assay in guinea-pigs rendered specifically hypersensitive with the homologous organism.

Old Tuberculin is distributed under aseptic conditions into sterile containers which are then sealed to exclude micro-organisms.

Standard
It complies with the requirements of the European Pharmacopoeia, which includes tests for potency, freedom from living mycobacteria, sensitising effect, toxicity, and sterility.
It is a transparent, yellow to brown, viscous liquid and contains not less than 100,000 Units in 1 ml. It possesses a specific toxicity for animals infected with the tubercle bacillus.
The reference preparation used in determining the potency should have the same potency as the Standard Preparation for Old Tuberculin. The Unit is con-

tained in 0·000011111 ml of the Standard Preparation of Old Tuberculin at present in use (1973) and has the same activity as the International Unit.

Storage. Old Tuberculin should be protected from light and stored at 2° to 10°. Undiluted Old Tuberculin is stable for at least 8 years.
Diluted solutions of Old Tuberculin are much less stable, their stability depending upon their mode of preparation and the nature of the diluent. Diluted solutions should be kept in full containers and should be used as soon as possible after preparation. Once a container is opened any portion of the contents not used at once should be discarded.

Actions and uses. Old Tuberculin is used as a diagnostic agent for tuberculosis.
A person showing a specific sensitivity to tuberculin is considered to have been infected with the tubercle bacillus, although the infection may be inactive. There is no significant difference between the active principle in preparations of the human type of *M. tuberculosis* and that in preparations of the bovine type.
Sensitivity tests to tuberculin can be performed in different ways, the intracutaneous test of Mantoux giving the most precise results. The diagnostic dose varies with the circumstances because of the great variation in sensitivity to tuberculin. In a full-scale test, the initial dose injected is 1 Unit of either old tuberculin or tuberculin purified protein derivative in 0·1 millilitre. The test is read at seventy-two hours. A positive reaction is characterised by an area of palpable infiltra-

tion of not less than 5 or 6 millimetres in diameter which may or may not be surrounded by erythema. Necrosis may occur in hypersensitive persons. If the reaction is negative, the test is repeated with 10 Units of tuberculin in 0·1 millilitre. If the second test is negative a final test may be made with 100 Units in 0·1 millilitre before regarding the person as "Mantoux-negative". Frequently, where the sensitivity of the person is not expected to be unduly high, the initial test is with 5 or 10 Units followed, if negative, by the test with 100 Units. It is also common practice in epidemiological surveys to use a single test with 5 or 10 Units.

A multiple-puncture (Heaf) method may be employed using a concentrated solution of tuberculin containing 100,000 Units in 1 millilitre. Results are obtained similar to those with a two-stage Mantoux test. The test is read at three to seven days, preferably the latter.

In children aged less than three years, who have not been vaccinated with BCG vaccine, a positive tuberculin reaction indicates an infection which should be suspected as active; between the ages of three and five years this inference is doubtful; in children over five years the possibility of active lesions must still be considered; in adolescence and adult life the diagnostic value of a positive reading is less than in childhood as the disease is less likely to be active.

A strong positive reaction in a person recently known to be negative signifies a recent tuberculous infection.

A negative reaction to 100 Units in the Mantoux test, with some rare exceptions, excludes an active tuberculous infection. The test can be negative, however, when performed early in the infection before hypersensitivity to tuberculoprotein has developed, and also in certain very acute forms of the disease.

Temporary diminution of skin sensitivity to tuberculin may occur during an attack of measles, after ultraviolet light treatment, and during cortisone therapy.

CAUTION. As traces of tuberculin are apt to adhere to glassware, syringes used for tuberculin tests should not be used for other purposes.

Dose. Diagnostic, 1, 5, 10, or 100 Units, contained in 0·1 millilitre of the appropriate dilution, by intracutaneous injection.

TUBERCULIN PURIFIED PROTEIN DERIVATIVE

SYNONYMS: Tuberculin P.P.D.; Tuberculini Derivatum Proteinosum Purificatum

Tuberculin Purified Protein Derivative is the active principle of Old Tuberculin and is prepared from the fluid medium on which the tubercle bacilli have been grown.

In preparing the product, the filtrate of the culture, either with or without previous concentration, is submitted to a process of fractional precipitation with trichloroacetic acid, ammonium sulphate, or other suitable protein precipitant. It is more constant in composition and potency than Old Tuberculin.

The potency is compared with that of a reference preparation by biological assay in guinea-pigs rendered specifically hypersensitive to the homologous organism.

Tuberculin Purified Protein Derivative is distributed under aseptic conditions into sterile containers which are then sealed to exclude micro-organisms.

Standard
It complies with the requirements of the European Pharmacopoeia, which includes tests for potency, sensitising effect, toxicity, and sterility, and a limit of phenol (not more than 0·5 per cent).
It occurs as a colourless to pale straw-coloured liquid with a pH of 6·5 to 7·5 or as a sterile freeze-dried powder or pellets. The liquid contains 100,000 Units in 1 ml and the powder contains 30,000 Units in 1 mg. It produces no reactions when injected into normal guinea-pigs, but if the guinea-pigs have been infected with *M. tuberculosis*, small intracutaneous doses cause erythema and swelling while large doses may produce necrosis at the site of injection.
Mammalian Tuberculin Purified Protein Derivative is prepared from the human or bovine type of *M. tuberculosis* and the potency is compared with that of the Standard Preparation of Purified Protein Derivative of mammalian tuberculin.
Avian Tuberculin Purified Protein Derivative is prepared from the avian type of *M. tuberculosis* and the potency is compared with that of the Standard Preparation of Purified Protein Derivative of avian tuberculin.

Storage. It should be protected from light and stored at 2° to 10°. Undiluted Tuberculin Purified Protein Derivative in concentrated solution preserved with 0·5 per cent of phenol is stable for at least 8 years and in the dried form the Purified Protein Derivative will retain its potency indefinitely.
Diluted solutions are much less stable, their stability depending upon their mode of preparation and the nature of the diluent. Diluted solutions should be kept in full containers and should be used as soon as possible after preparation.
Once a container is opened any portion of the contents not used at once should be discarded.

Actions and uses. Tuberculin Purified Protein Derivative has the actions and uses described under Old Tuberculin.

CAUTION. As traces of tuberculin are apt to adhere to glassware, syringes used for tuberculin tests should not be used for other purposes.
Tuberculin Purified Protein Derivative may produce toxic effects when inhaled, and care must be taken when handling the powder.

Dose. Diagnostic, 1, 5, 10, or 100 Units, contained in 0·1 millilitre of the appropriate dilution, by intracutaneous injection.

TYPHOID VACCINE

SYNONYM: Vaccinum Typhoidi

Typhoid Vaccine is a suspension of killed *Salmonella typhi*.

The vaccine is prepared from one or more strains of *S. typhi* that are smooth and have the full complement of O, H, and Vi antigens. The bacteria are killed by heating the suspension or by treatment with formaldehyde or phenol.

Standard
It complies with the requirements of the European Pharmacopoeia, which includes tests for sterility and abnormal toxicity.
It contains not less than 1000 million *S. typhi* per human dose, which does not exceed 1 ml.

Storage. It should be stored as described under Vaccines (page 549).

Actions and uses. Typhoid Vaccine has been shown to be an effective prophylactic against typhoid fever, and as the value of paratyphoid vaccines has not been established, some practitioners prefer to prescribe simple Typhoid Vaccine and thus avoid injecting possibly inert bacteria which may contribute to the reaction rate with typhoid-paratyphoid vaccines.

The vaccine should be administered by subcutaneous injection in two doses separated by an interval of four to six weeks. Immunity usually lasts for at least two years.

Suitable schedules for the immunisation of travellers are given under Vaccines (page 551).

Local erythema, swelling, tenderness, pain, general malaise, nausea, and headache may sometimes occur after the subcutaneous injection of this vaccine.

Dose. The volume stated on the label as the first dose, followed after an interval of four to six weeks by a second dose, by subcutaneous injection.

ABBREVIATED NAME: Typhoid/Vac

TYPHOID AND TETANUS VACCINE

Typhoid and Tetanus Vaccine is a mixture of a suspension of killed *Salmonella typhi* and tetanus formol toxoid.

The suspension of bacteria is prepared from one or more strains of *S. typhi* that are smooth and have the full complement of O, H, and Vi antigens; the bacteria are killed either by heat or by treatment with formaldehyde or phenol.

Standard
It complies with the requirements of the British Pharmacopoeia, which includes tests for potency and specific toxicity.
It contains 1000 million or 2000 million typhoid bacilli (*S. typhi*) in 1 ml.

Storage. It should be stored as described under Vaccines (page 549).

Actions and uses. Typhoid and Tetanus Vaccine may be used for primary immunisation against typhoid fever and tetanus; three well-spaced intramuscular doses are required to immunise satisfactorily against tetanus.

The vaccine is used for reinforcing doses when it is advisable to boost the immunity against tetanus as well as typhoid.

The vaccine is usually administered by intramuscular injection in two doses separated by an interval of at least four to six weeks, the second dose being followed after an interval of preferably four to six months by a dose of Tetanus Vaccine or Adsorbed Tetanus Vaccine.

A single intramuscular dose is given as a reinforcing dose.

Dose. The volume stated on the label as the dose, followed after an interval of four to six weeks by a second dose, followed after an interval of preferably four to six months by a dose of Tetanus Vaccine or Adsorbed Tetanus Vaccine.

ABBREVIATED NAME: Typhoid/Tet/Vac

TYPHOID-PARATYPHOID VACCINES

Typhoid-paratyphoid Vaccines are mixed suspensions of killed *Salmonella typhi*, *S. paratyphi A*, and *S. paratyphi B*. They may also contain Cholera Vaccine or Tetanus Vaccine as described below.

TYPHOID-PARATYPHOID A AND B VACCINE (TAB/Vac). *Synonym:* T.A.B. Vaccine.
It contains 1000 million *S. typhi*, 500 or 750 million *S. paratyphi A*, and 500 or 750 million *S. paratyphi B* in 1 ml.

INTRACUTANEOUS TYPHOID-PARATYPHOID A AND B VACCINE [TAB/Vac (Intracutaneous)]. *Synonyms:* Intracut. T.A.B. Vaccine; Intradermal Typhoid-paratyphoid A and B Vaccine.
It contains either 2500 million *S. typhi*, 1250 million *S. paratyphi A*, and 1250 million *S. paratyphi B*, or 2000 million *S. typhi*, 1500 million *S. paratyphi A*, and 1500 million *S. paratyphi B* in 1 ml (dose, 0·1 ml).

TYPHOID-PARATYPHOID A AND B AND CHOLERA VACCINE (TABCho/Vac). *Synonym:* T.A.B. and Cholera Vaccine.
It contains 1000 million *S. typhi*, 500 or 750 million *S. paratyphi A*, 500 or 750 million *S. paratyphi B*, and 8000 million cholera vibrios in 1 ml. The cholera component consists of equal parts of the two main serotypes, Inaba and Ogawa, of the classical biotype of *Vibrio cholerae*. This vaccine is suitable for use when an international certificate in respect of cholera vaccination is required.

TYPHOID-PARATYPHOID A AND B AND TETANUS VACCINE (TABT/Vac). *Synonyms:* T.A.B. and Tetanus Vaccine; Typhoid-paratyphoid A and B Vaccine-Tetanus Toxoid.
It contains tetanus formol toxoid and 500 or 1000 million *S. typhi*, 250 or 500 million *S. paratyphi A*, and 250 or 500 million *S. paratyphi B* in 1 ml.

They consist of vaccines prepared from strains of *S. typhi*, *S. paratyphi A*, and *S. paratyphi B* that are smooth and have the full complement of O and H antigens and, in the case of *S. typhi*, contain also the Vi antigen. Either a single strain or several strains of each species may be included. The bacteria are killed by heat or by a bactericide.

Standard
They comply with the requirements of the British Pharmacopoeia.

Storage. They should be stored as described under Vaccines (page 549).

Actions and uses. Typhoid Vaccine has been shown to be an effective prophylactic against typhoid fever. It is widely used in the form of Typhoid-paratyphoid A and B Vaccine for the prevention of typhoid and paratyphoid fevers, although the value of the paratyphoid components has not been established.
Typhoid-paratyphoid A and B and Cholera Vaccine is used for primary immunisation against enteric fevers and cholera. Typhoid-paratyphoid A and B and Tetanus Vaccine is used for primary immunisation against enteric fevers and tetanus, for which three intramuscular doses are required to immunise satisfactorily against tetanus, there being an interval of at least four to six weeks between the first and second doses and preferably four to six months between the second and third doses. These vaccines are seldom used for reinforcing doses as the intervals before a reinforcing dose is required for the various components do not correspond; it is preferable therefore to use the simple typhoid-paratyphoid, cholera, or tetanus vaccines separately for this purpose.
Typhoid-paratyphoid vaccines are usually administered by subcutaneous injection in two doses, preferably separated by an interval of four to six weeks, and immunity usually lasts two to three years. When an epidemic or other major risk of infection arises it may be desirable to administer a reinforcing dose. Suitable schedules for the immunisation of travellers are given under Vaccines (page 551). Local erythema, swelling, tenderness, pain, general malaise, nausea, and headache may sometimes occur after subcutaneous or intramuscular injection of these vaccines.
Intracutaneous Typhoid-paratyphoid Vaccine is suitable for intracutaneous administration only. The dose is 0·1 millilitre and overdosage may give rise to an area of skin necrosis. The intracutaneous route is reliable only if the inoculation technique is satisfactory. Typhoid-paratyphoid vaccines prepared for subcutaneous injection are unsuitable for intracutaneous use.

Dose. The volume stated on the label as the dose, administered as described above under Actions and uses.

TYPHUS VACCINE

Typhus Vaccine is a suspension of killed epidemic (Breinl strain) typhus rickettsiae. It specifically protects susceptible animals against epidemic typhus.

The vaccine may be prepared by injecting virulent rickettsiae into the yolk-sacs of fertile eggs which have been incubated for seven days. Incubation is continued until heavy yolk-sac infection has been established. The yolk-sacs are then collected and suitably treated to liberate the maximum number of rickettsiae. The material is suspended in a saline or other appropriate solution isotonic with blood, containing 0·2 to 0·5 per cent of formaldehyde, so that the suspension contains 10 to 15 per cent w/w of yolk-sac tissue; it is purified by treatment with ether or trichlorotrifluoroethane.

It is distributed into sterile containers sealed to exclude micro-organisms; the bactericide may be thiomersal 1 in 10,000 with a trace of formaldehyde solution.

Standard
It complies with the requirements of the British Pharmacopoeia, which includes tests for potency and toxicity.
It is a slightly turbid liquid from which the rickettsiae settle out, on prolonged standing, as a delicate, powdery, white deposit which is readily redispersed on shaking.

Storage. It should be stored protected from light at 2° to 10°. It should not be allowed to freeze. Under these conditions it may be expected to retain its potency for at least one year after the date of manufacture.

Actions and uses. Typhus vaccine is of value in the prophylaxis of louse-borne typhus. The vaccine lessens the severity of the disease and the mortality rate, although it may not materially influence the attack rate.

The primary course is two doses, each of 1 millilitre, for persons over the age of nine years, given at intervals of seven to ten days. Children between the ages of six months and four years should have 0·2-millilitre doses and those between four and nine years 0·5-millilitre doses.

Reinforcing doses of 1 millilitre should be given annually, except during an epidemic when they should be given every three months. General reactions resulting from administration of the recommended doses are uncommon.

Dose. Prophylactic, 0·2 to 1 millilitre by subcutaneous injection.

ABBREVIATED NAME: Typhus/Vac

YELLOW FEVER VACCINE

Yellow Fever Vaccine is an aqueous suspension of chick-embryo tissue containing the attenuated yellow fever virus 17D strain which, although avirulent for man, is nevertheless highly immunogenic. When injected intracerebrally into susceptible mice, the vaccine produces encephalitis characteristic of infection by yellow fever virus, ending fatally within twenty-one days. When injected into susceptible rhesus monkeys, it stimulates the production of specific antibodies in the blood of most of the monkeys.

Yellow Fever Vaccine may be prepared by injecting the living attenuated virus into the embryos of fertile eggs which have been incubated for seven to eight days. Incubation is continued for a further three to four days and the embryos are then collected, pooled in batches, ground, and extracted with purified water.

The resultant suspension is centrifuged and the supernatant liquid is transferred to sterile ampoules and dried from the frozen state; the containers are filled with pure dry sterile nitrogen and then sealed by fusion of the glass.

The dry product is reconstituted immediately before use by dissolving the contents of a sealed container in saline or other appropriate solution isotonic with blood.

Standard
It complies with the requirements of the British Pharmacopoeia, which includes tests for potency, toxicity, and sterility.

It occurs as a dry cream-coloured to reddish-yellow powder, scales, or small lumps.
The potency of the vaccine is determined as the number of LD50 doses in 1 ml. The LD50 dose is that amount of vaccine which when injected intracerebrally into an adequate number of susceptible adult mice causes the death within twenty-one days, from specific yellow fever virus encephalitis, of one-half of the mice used.

Storage. The dried vaccine should be protected from light and stored at approximately 0°. Under these conditions, it may be expected to retain its potency for at least one year after the date of manufacture; at lower temperatures it retains its potency for longer periods. At 20° it loses its potency within a few days.

Actions and uses. Yellow Fever Vaccine produces an active immunity which is usually established within ten days of administration and persists for many years. Only one dose is required for immunisation, but reinoculation every ten years is desirable.

Suitable schedules for the immunisation of

travellers are given under Vaccines (page 551). Reactions to the vaccine seldom occur. Allergic symptoms, which can usually be effectively controlled by the administration of adrenaline or an antihistamine, have been observed in persons sensitive to egg protein. Mild encephalitis occasionally occurs in infants under the age of nine months and it is recommended that, when possible, vaccination against yellow fever should be postponed until an infant is at least nine months old.

The precautions to be taken when vaccinating simultaneously against yellow fever and smallpox are described under Smallpox Vaccine (page 569).

Dose. Prophylactic, not less than 1000 LD50 doses by subcutaneous injection.

ABBREVIATED NAME: Yel/Vac

PART 3
Preparations of Human Blood

PREPARATIONS OF HUMAN BLOOD

This section contains monographs on whole human blood and related products, arranged in the following order:

Whole Human Blood
Concentrated Human Red Blood Corpuscles
Human Albumin
Dried Human Albumin
Human Albumin Fraction (Saline)
Dried Human Albumin Fraction (Saline)
Dried Human Antihaemophilic Fraction
Human Fibrin Foam
Dried Human Fibrinogen
Dried Human Fibrinogen for Isotopic Labelling
Human Normal Immunoglobulin Injection
Human Tetanus Immunoglobulin
Human Vaccinia Immunoglobulin
Dried Human Plasma
Dried Human Serum
Dried Human Thrombin

It is essential that all the apparatus and materials brought into contact with preparations of human blood are free from pyrogens. Water for Injections should be used to prepare all aqueous solutions, and apparatus should be thoroughly rinsed with it before sterilisation. A suitable filter should be included in transfusion apparatus.

Preparations of human blood are not prepared commercially in the United Kingdom. In England and Wales, they are provided by the Department of Health and Social Security. Human immunoglobulin for the prevention of infectious diseases is available from the Public Health Laboratory Service, and for treating hypogammaglobulinaemia or immune deficiency states from the Division of Immunology, Clinical Research Centre, Harrow, Middlesex, or the Regional Immunology Laboratory, East Birmingham General Hospital, Bordesley, Birmingham. Human fibrin foam and human thrombin are available from the Blood Products Laboratory and the other preparations are available from Regional Transfusion Centres.

In Scotland, preparations of human blood are available from the centres of the Scottish National Blood Transfusion Association, and in Northern Ireland through the Regional Transfusion Centre.

Serum Hepatitis

Transfusion of blood containing Australia (hepatitis-associated) antigen is associated with the occurrence of hepatitis in recipients; hepatitis may however follow transfusion of blood in which the antigen cannot be detected by screening methods at present used to detect Australia antigen. Thus the exclusion of donors whose blood

contains the antigen diminishes but does not necessarily eliminate the risk of transmitting hepatitis. Donors whose blood has been shown to contain antibody to Australia
antigen are also excluded.

Whole human blood, concentrated red blood corpuscles, human antihaemophilic
fraction, dried human fibrinogen, dried human fibrinogen for isotopic labelling, dried
human plasma, dried human serum, and dried human thrombin therefore carry a risk
of transmitting serum hepatitis.

Preparations of albumin that have been heated for ten hours at 60° and preparations
of immunoglobulin, made by ethanol fractionation, do not transmit hepatitis.

WHOLE HUMAN BLOOD

Whole Human Blood is blood withdrawn from adult human beings and mixed with an anticoagulant solution.

Blood donors must be healthy adults, who
have not suffered or are not suffering from
syphilis, malaria, or jaundice and whose
blood has given a negative test for Australia
(hepatitis-associated) antigen and antibody;
who are, as far as can be ascertained by a
registered medical practitioner after inspection or simple clinical examination and
consideration of their medical history, free
from other diseases transmissible by blood
transfusion, and the haemoglobin content of
whose blood, estimated against the Cyanmethaemoglobin Solution for Photometric
Haemoglobinometry (British Standard 3985:
1966) is not less than 12·5 grams per 100
millilitres (female donors) or 13·3 grams per
100 millilitres (male donors). Not more than
420 millilitres of blood is drawn on one
occasion.

Preferably, a donor should not be called upon
to give blood more often than once every six
months.

The blood is withdrawn aseptically through a
closed system of sterile tubing which leads
into the sterile final container in which the
anticoagulant solution has been placed before
sterilisation. During collection the container
should be gently agitated to mix the blood and
anticoagulant solution.

The blood remaining in the tubing after
collection is used for grouping the blood and
for the tests for freedom from syphilis and
from Australia (hepatitis-associated) antigen;
the ABO group is determined by examination
of both cells and serum, and the Rh group by
examination of the cells.

Immediately after collection, the container is
sealed and cooled to 4° to 6° and thereafter is
opened only for administering the blood; a
separate sample of the blood mixed with anticoagulant should be provided for compatibility testing.

The anticoagulant solution most generally
used consists of Water for Injections containing 1·7 to 2·1 per cent of sodium acid
citrate and 2·5 per cent of anhydrous dextrose;
120 millilitres is sufficient to prevent clotting
in 420 millilitres of blood. The acidity of
the solution prevents caramelisation during
sterilisation and the dextrose delays haemolysis
of the red blood corpuscles. Whole Human
Blood prepared with this solution may be used
up to twenty-one days after collection.

Standard
It complies with the requirements of the British
Pharmacopoeia.
It is a dark red fluid which separates on standing into a
sediment of red blood corpuscles and a yellow supernatant plasma free from visible products of haemolysis;
the line of demarcation is sharp, but a continuous or
interrupted greyish layer of leucocytes may form on the
surface of the red blood corpuscles. The plasma may be
clear, or turbid due to the presence of fat, which may
form a white layer on the surface of the plasma.
It has a haemoglobin concentration of not less than
9·7 g per 100 ml in terms of the Cyanmethaemoglobin
Solution for Photometric Haemoglobinometry (British
Standard 3985:1966).

Labelling. The label on the container states:
(1) the ABO group;
(2) the Rh group and the nature of specific antisera
used in testing;
(3) the total volume of fluid, the proportion of blood,
and the nature and percentage of anticoagulant and of
any other material introduced;
(4) the date on which the blood was withdrawn;
(5) the date after which the preparation is not intended
to be used;
(6) the conditions to be observed for maintaining the
fitness for transfusion of the preparation;
(7) that the preparation should not be used if there is
any visible evidence of deterioration; and
(8) for blood of group O, that a test for haemolysins
has been carried out and, if a positive result has been
obtained, that the blood is unsafe for transfusion to
recipients of other groups.

Storage. It should be stored, in sterile containers
sealed to exclude micro-organisms, at 4° to 6° until
needed for use, except during any periods necessary
for its examination and transport at higher temperatures;
such periods should not exceed thirty minutes, after
which the blood should immediately be cooled again
to 4° to 6°.
During storage, certain elements in the blood diminish
in amount or disappear; leucocytes disintegrate in a

few hours, most of the platelets and certain clotting factors, particularly Factor VIII, disappear in a few days, and prothrombin and complement gradually decrease.

Stored Whole Human Blood is a potentially dangerous fluid, the maintenance of the sterility of which depends entirely upon meticulous attention to cleanliness, faultless asepsis, and accurate and constant refrigeration from collection until use.

The fitness of Whole Human Blood for transfusion can be judged only by its appearance. During storage, haemolysis of the red blood corpuscles occurs, and a red colour, which obscures the line of demarcation between the plasma and the sediment of corpuscles, may develop in the plasma immediately above the corpuscular layer. Whole Human Blood which shows these signs of haemolysis should not be used.

Haemolysis also results if blood is frozen or heated and if it becomes infected; infection usually causes rapid and total haemolysis, but certain Gram-negative organisms may flourish at 4° to 6° without causing any visible haemolysis.

Actions and uses. Whole human blood is used for transfusion, either to replace red blood corpuscles, clotting factors, or other normal constituents partly or completely missing from the patient's blood, or to restore blood volume.

The amount of whole human blood transfused and the rate at which it is given depend upon the patient's age and general condition, and on the state of his circulatory system, and upon the indication for transfusion. The haemoglobin concentration of the blood of the average adult is raised by about 1 gram per 100 millilitres by the transfusion of 540 millilitres of whole human blood.

Whole human blood should not be transfused, except in grave emergency, unless the ABO and Rh groups of the patient's and the donor's blood have been verified and a compatibility check made between the patient's serum and the donor's red cells.

The Rh group of a recipient should always be determined, as at least 50 per cent of Rh-negative recipients may develop Rh antibodies if transfused with Rh-positive blood. A proportion of Rh-negative mothers may become immunised to the Rh factor during pregnancy by bearing Rh-positive foetuses which have inherited the Rh factor from their fathers.

Any of these immunised persons, if subsequently transfused with Rh-positive blood, may suffer a haemolytic reaction which may be fatal. Moreover, a transfusion of Rh-positive blood may sensitise a Rh-negative female, so that subsequent Rh-positive children may be affected with haemolytic disease of the newborn. Ideally all patients should be transfused with blood of homologous Rh group.

In grave emergencies, group O Rh-negative blood, plasma, human albumin factor (saline), or plasma substitute, may be given while the patient's group is determined and a compatibility test is done; there are, however, few occasions on which there is not time to do these tests before transfusion.

SERUM HEPATITIS—*see note on page 581.*

CONCENTRATED HUMAN RED BLOOD CORPUSCLES

SYNONYM: Concentrate of Human Red Blood Cells

Concentrated Human Red Blood Corpuscles is Whole Human Blood from which part of the plasma and anticoagulant solution has been removed.

The product is prepared, not more than twelve hours before use, from Whole Human Blood which is not more than fourteen days old.

The blood is centrifuged or allowed to stand until the corpuscles have settled, and a quantity of the supernatant liquid equivalent to not less than 40 per cent of the volume of the Whole Human Blood is removed. The red blood corpuscles in the sediment are matched with the recipient's serum and, after matching, may be mixed with the sediment from other containers similarly prepared and matched.

The removal of the plasma and mixing of the sediments should be effected by siphoning through a closed system of sterile tubing; full aseptic precautions must be observed throughout the preparation.

Standard

It complies with the requirements of the British Pharmacopoeia.

It is a dark red fluid which may separate on standing into a sediment of red blood corpuscles and a supernatant layer of yellow plasma.

It has a haemoglobin concentration of not less than 15·5 g per 100 ml in terms of the Cyanmethaemoglobin Solution for Photometric Haemoglobinometry (British Standard 3985:1966).

Labelling. The label on the container states:

(1) the reference numbers of the containers of the whole human blood from which it was made;

(2) the ABO group of the whole human blood from which it was made;

(3) the Rh group of the whole human blood from which it was made and the nature of specific antisera used in testing;

(4) the time after which the preparation is not intended to be used;

(5) the conditions to be observed for maintaining the fitness for transfusion of the preparation; and

(6) that the preparation should not be used if there is any visible evidence of deterioration.

Storage. It should be stored, in sterile containers sealed to exclude micro-organisms, at 4° to 6°; it should be used within twelve hours of its preparation.

Actions and uses. Transfusions of concentrated human red blood corpuscles are given for the treatment of various forms of anaemia; the haemoglobin concentration of the blood of the average adult is raised by about 2 grams per 100 millilitres by the concentrated human red blood corpuscles obtained from 1080 millilitres of whole human blood.

SERUM HEPATITIS—*see note on page* 581.

HUMAN ALBUMIN

Human Albumin is a solution in water of human albumin containing a low proportion of salt.

Human Albumin is obtained from pooled human plasma and may be prepared by precipitation with organic solvents such as alcohol, under controlled conditions of pH, ionic strength, and temperature. No bactericide or antibiotic is added at any stage during preparation. Freeze-drying or other suitable treatment is used to remove residual solvent. The resultant protein is dissolved in water and sodium caprylate or other suitable substances are added to stabilise it to heat at pH 7·0.

The solution is sterilised by filtration and distributed aseptically into containers which are then sealed to exclude micro-organisms. The solution is then heated to and maintained at 59·5° to 60·5° for ten hours to prevent the transmission of serum hepatitis.

Finally, the containers are incubated for not less than fourteen days at 30° to 32° and examined visually for signs of microbial contamination.

Standard
It complies with the requirements of the British Pharmacopoeia.
It is a clear amber to deep orange-brown liquid and contains 15 to 25 per cent of protein and not more than 0·65 millimole of sodium ions, not more than 0·05 millimole of potassium ions, and not more than 0·1 millimole of citrate ions per g of protein. It has a pH of 6·7 to 7·3.

Labelling. The label on the container states:
(1) the volume;
(2) the total amount of protein;

(3) the concentration of sodium, potassium, and citrate ions;

(4) the names and concentrations of stabilising agents and any other added substances present in the final solution;

(5) that the contents should not be used if the solution is turbid or contains a deposit;

(6) the date after which the solution is not intended to be used; and

(7) the conditions under which it should be stored.

Storage. It should be protected from light and stored at 2° to 25°.

Actions and uses. Human albumin is used when it is desired to administer relatively large amounts of protein in a small volume and with minimal amounts of sodium and potassium.

It has been used in the treatment of certain liver disorders such as cirrhosis in which hypoalbuminaemia occurs; its value for this purpose is uncertain, but benefit to patients with predominantly peripheral oedema has been reported. It has also been used in nephrotic nephritis with the object of inducing diuresis, but its value has not been established. Human albumin is also used to restore a depleted blood volume. Additional fluid should be given by mouth if the patient is dehydrated. The amount of human albumin transfused and the rate at which it is given depend on the patient's age and general condition, the state of his circulatory system, and the indication for its use.

DRIED HUMAN ALBUMIN

Dried Human Albumin is prepared by freeze-drying human albumin of protein concentration not exceeding 10 per cent w/v. Before drying, the solution in the final containers is heated to and maintained at 59·5° to 60·5° for ten hours to prevent the transmission of serum hepatitis.

Standard
It complies with the requirements of the British Pharmacopoeia.
It is a cream-coloured powder. When dissolved in a volume of water equal to the volume of Water for Injections stated on the label the solution contains 24·0 to 26·0 per cent of protein and not more than 0·65 millimole of sodium ions, not more than 0·05 millimole of potassium ions, and not more than 0·1 millimole of citrate ions per g of protein.

Labelling. The label on the container states:
(1) the volume of Water for Injections necessary to reconstitute the solution to 25 per cent protein concentration;

(2) the concentration of sodium, potassium, and citrate ions;

(3) the names and concentrations of stabilising agents and any other added substances present;

(4) that the container should not be shaken to hasten solution of the solids;

(5) that the contents should not be used if, after adding water, a gel forms or solution is incomplete;

(6) that the solution should be discarded if not used within three hours;

(7) the date after which the contents are not intended to be used; and

(8) the conditions under which it should be stored.

Storage. It should be stored in an atmosphere of nitrogen, in sterile containers sealed to exclude micro-organisms and moisture, at 2° to 25°, and protected from light.

Actions and uses. Dried human albumin is used for the purposes described under Human Albumin.

HUMAN ALBUMIN FRACTION (SALINE)

SYNONYM: Human Plasma Protein Fraction

Human Albumin Fraction (Saline) is a solution of the proteins of liquid human plasma containing albumin and some globulins that retain their solubility on heating. It exerts a colloidal osmotic pressure equivalent to that of pooled liquid human plasma containing 5·2 per cent w/v of protein. It contains no fibrinogen and only traces of gamma globulin.

Human Albumin Fraction (Saline) is obtained from pooled liquid human plasma and may be prepared by precipitation with organic solvents such as alcohol under controlled conditions of pH, ionic strength, and temperature.

No bactericide or antibiotic is added at any stage during preparation. Freeze-drying or other suitable treatment is used to remove residual solvent. The resultant protein is dissolved in water and sodium caprylate or other suitable substances are added to stabilise it to heat and sodium chloride to adjust the concentration of sodium ions to about 150 millimoles per litre at pH 7·0.

The solution is sterilised by filtration and distributed aseptically into containers which are then sealed to exclude micro-organisms and heated to and maintained at 59·5° to 60·5° for ten hours to prevent the transmission of serum hepatitis.

Finally, the containers are incubated for not less than fourteen days at 30° to 32° and examined visually for signs of microbial contamination.

Standard
It complies with the requirements of the British Pharmacopoeia.
It is a clear amber-coloured liquid and contains not less than 4·3 per cent w/v of protein, 130 to 160 millimoles of sodium ions, not more than 15 millimoles of citrate ions, and not more than 2 millimoles of potassium ions per litre. It has a pH of 6·7 to 7·3.

Labelling. The label on the container states:
(1) the volume;
(2) the total amount of protein;
(3) the concentrations of sodium, potassium, and citrate ions;
(4) the names and concentrations of stabilising agents and any other added substances present in the final solution;
(5) that the contents must not be used if the solution is turbid or contains a deposit;
(6) the date after which the preparation is not intended to be used; and
(7) the conditions under which it should be stored.

Storage. It should be protected from light and stored at a temperature between 2° and 25°.

Actions and uses. Human albumin fraction (saline) is used in the same way as reconstituted plasma for the purposes described under Dried Human Plasma (page 590).

DRIED HUMAN ALBUMIN FRACTION (SALINE)

Dried Human Albumin Fraction (Saline) is prepared by freeze-drying Human Albumin Fraction (Saline) immediately after it has been heated at 59·5° to 60·5° for ten hours.

Standard
It complies with the requirements of the British Pharmacopoeia.
It is a cream-coloured powder which, when dissolved in a volume of water equal to the volume of Water for Injections stated on the label, yields a solution that contains not less than 4·3 per cent w/v of protein, 130 to 160 millimoles of sodium ions, not more than 15 millimoles of citrate ions, and not more than 2 millimoles of potassium ions per litre.

Labelling. The label on the container states:
(1) the volume of Water for Injections necessary to reconstitute the solution;
(2) the total amount of protein in the reconstituted solution;
(3) the concentrations of sodium, potassium, and citrate ions;
(4) the names and concentrations of stabilising agents and any other added substances;

(5) that the contents must not be used if, after adding water, a gel forms or solution is incomplete;
(6) that the reconstituted solution should be discarded if not used within three hours;
(7) the date after which the contents are not intended to be used; and
(8) the conditions under which it should be stored.

Storage. It should be stored in an atmosphere of nitrogen, in sterile containers sealed to exclude micro-organisms and moisture, at a temperature below 25°, and protected from light.

Actions and uses. Dried human albumin fraction (saline) is used for the purposes described under Dried Human Plasma (page 590).

DRIED HUMAN ANTIHAEMOPHILIC FRACTION

Dried Human Antihaemophilic Fraction is prepared from human plasma; it is rich in clotting factor VIII.

The human plasma is obtained from blood from human subjects who comply with the requirements for donors given under Whole Human Blood (page 582). The blood is withdrawn aseptically into a suitable anticoagulant solution. During withdrawal there should be no interruption in the flow from the donor and the container should be gently agitated.

Immediately after withdrawal is complete the blood is cooled to 4° and if the plasma is to be stored frozen it should be separated from cellular components by centrifugation and frozen to −30° or below within twelve hours of collection.

If the plasma is not to be frozen it should be separated from cellular components as soon as possible, and not later than eighteen hours after collection, and fractionation begun without delay.

Human antihaemophilic fraction may be prepared from human plasma so obtained by precipitation under controlled conditions of pH, ionic strength, and temperature, with organic solvents or by freezing and thawing. The precipitate may be washed by extraction with suitable solvents dissolved in sodium citrate solution adjusted to pH 6·8 to 7·2, which may also contain sodium chloride.

The solution is sterilised by filtration through a membrane filter and immediately frozen and dried. No preservative is added.

Standard
It complies with the requirements of the British Pharmacopoeia.
It is a white powder or friable solid which, when dissolved in a volume of water equal to the volume of Water for Injections stated on the label, yields a solution which contains not less than 3 Units per ml, not more than 2·5 per cent of fibrinogen, not more than 3·0 per cent of total protein, not more than 200 millimoles of sodium ions per litre, and not more than 55 millimoles of citrate ions per litre.

The reconstituted solution has a pH of 6·8 to 7·2.

Labelling. The label on the container states:
(1) the number of Units contained in it;
(2) that 1 Unit is approximately equivalent to the antihaemophilic activity of 1 ml of average normal plasma;
(3) that the reconstituted preparation contains not more than 2·5 per cent of fibrinogen and not more than 3·0 per cent of total protein;
(4) the amounts of total sodium and citrate ions and the amount of any other added substance contained in it;
(5) that the preparation should be allowed to warm to 20° to 25° before reconstitution;
(6) the volume of Water for Injections necessary to reconstitute the solution and that reconstitution may occupy up to thirty minutes;
(7) that only gentle mixing should be employed during reconstitution to avoid frothing;
(8) that if a gel forms on reconstitution the preparation should not be used;
(9) the number of donations in the pool from which the preparation was obtained;
(10) the date after which the preparation is not intended to be used;
(11) the conditions under which it should be stored; and
(12) that the reconstituted solution should be used immediately.

Storage. It should be stored in an atmosphere of nitrogen, in sterile containers sealed to exclude micro-organisms and moisture, at a temperature below 6°, and protected from light.

Actions and uses. Dried human antihaemophilic fraction is used specifically to control bleeding in haemophiliacs. The amount transfused depends upon the circumstances, particularly the immediate cause of the bleeding and the severity of the haemophilia. The object of treatment is to raise the concentration of plasma antihaemophilic globulin to at least thirty per cent of normal and to maintain it at this level until bleeding has ceased.

SERUM HEPATITIS—see note on page 581.

HUMAN FIBRIN FOAM

Human Fibrin Foam is a dry artificial sponge of human fibrin.

Human Fibrin Foam is prepared by clotting with human thrombin a foam of a solution of Human Fibrinogen. The clotted foam is dried from the frozen state, cut into strips, and sterilised by heating at 130° for three hours.

Solubility. Insoluble in water.

Standard
DESCRIPTION. A firm, light, white, spongy material.

LOSS ON DRYING. Not more than 0·5 per cent, determined by drying at a pressure not exceeding 0·02 mmHg over *phosphorus pentoxide* for twenty-four hours.

STERILITY. It complies with the test for sterility of the European Pharmacopoeia.

Labelling. The label on the container states:
(1) the date after which the preparation is not intended to be used; and
(2) the conditions under which it should be stored.

Storage. It should be stored in sterile containers sealed to exclude micro-organisms and moisture, at a temperature below 25°, and protected from light.

Actions and uses. Human fibrin foam is used, in conjunction with human thrombin, as a haemostatic agent in surgery in sites in which bleeding cannot easily be controlled by the commoner methods of haemostasis.

A piece of the foam is cut to the required size,

saturated with a solution of thrombin in Sodium Chloride Injection, and placed in contact with the bleeding-point. Blood coagulates in contact with the thrombin in the interstices of the foam, which acts as a scaffold for the clot thus formed. Since all the clotting materials are of human origin, they may be left in place when the wound is closed.

DRIED HUMAN FIBRINOGEN

Dried Human Fibrinogen is a sterile dried preparation of the soluble constituent of liquid human plasma which, on the addition of human thrombin, is transformed into fibrin.

Dried Human Fibrinogen may be prepared from human plasma separated from Whole Human Blood by precipitation with organic solvents such as alcohol under controlled conditions of pH, ionic strength, and temperature. The precipitate is dissolved in a solution of sodium chloride and sodium citrate and dried from the frozen state; no preservative is added.

Standard
It complies with the requirements of the British Pharmacopoeia.
It is a white powder or friable solid which, when reconstituted with a volume of water equal to the volume of Water for Injections stated on the label, forms an almost colourless, opalescent solution which clots on the addition of thrombin on standing.
When fibrinogen is so reconstituted the resultant solution contains: (a) 1·0 to 1·5 per cent w/v of fibrinogen, comprising not less than 70 per cent of the total protein present; (b) not more than 200 millimoles of sodium ions per litre; and (c) not more than 25 millimoles of citrate ions per litre.

Labelling. The label on the container states:
(1) the amounts of fibrinogen, sodium ions, and citrate ions and the name and amount of any other added substance contained in it;
(2) the quantity of Water for Injections necessary to reconstitute the original volume of the liquid human fibrinogen;
(3) the date after which the preparation is not intended to be used;
(4) the conditions under which it should be stored; and
(5) that the preparation should be used immediately after reconstitution.

Storage. It should be stored in an atmosphere of nitrogen, in sterile containers sealed to exclude micro-organisms and moisture, at a temperature below 25°, and protected from light.

Actions and uses. Dried human fibrinogen is used to control haemorrhage associated with the defibrination syndrome which may occur in the presence of certain obstetrical conditions such as premature separation of the placenta or death of the foetus *in utero* or in association with cardiac operations. Haemorrhage does not usually occur until the fibrinogen level, which should be determined before treatment, has fallen below 100 mg per 100 ml of plasma. The transfusion of a solution of 2 to 6 grams of dried fibrinogen will usually control haemorrhage in these conditions.
Fibrinogen is also used to raise the fibrinogen level during operations on patients with the very rare abnormality, congenital afibrinogenaemia.
Dried human fibrinogen is used in conjunction with human thrombin to fix nerve sutures and to improve the adhesion of skin and mucous membrane grafts.
Dried human fibrinogen is reconstituted by adding, using an aseptic technique, a volume of Water for Injections not greater than the original volume of the fibrinogen solution before drying. The fibrinogen dissolves slowly and the container may be rocked but should not be shaken to aid solution; if shaken, frothing will occur which will impede solution.
Dried human fibrinogen should be used immediately after reconstitution; it must not be used more than three hours after reconstitution.
SERUM HEPATITIS—*see note on page* 581.

DRIED HUMAN FIBRINOGEN FOR ISOTOPIC LABELLING

Dried Human Fibrinogen for Isotopic Labelling is a preparation of the soluble constituent of liquid human plasma which, on the addition of human thrombin, is transformed into fibrin.

The product is prepared from liquid human plasma obtained from selected donors by precipitating with organic solvents such as alcohol under controlled conditions of pH, ionic strength, and temperature, dissolving the precipitate in a solution of sodium chloride and sodium citrate, and drying from the frozen state.

Standard
It complies with the requirements of the British Pharmacopoeia.
It is a white powder or friable solid. When dissolved in a volume of water equal to the volume of Water for Injections stated on the label not less than 90 per cent of the total protein present is clottable.
Labelling. The label on the container states:
(1) the amounts of fibrinogen, sodium ions, and citrate ions contained in it;

(2) the volume of Water for Injections necessary to reconstitute the solution;

(3) the date after which the contents are not intended to be used;

(4) the conditions under which it should be stored; and

(5) that the reconstituted solution should be used immediately after preparation.

Storage. It should be stored in an atmosphere of nitrogen, in sterile containers sealed to exclude micro-organisms and moisture, at 2° to 10°, and protected from light.

Actions and uses. Dried human fibrinogen for isotopic labelling is used mainly in the form of iodine-125 or iodine-131 labelled preparations for the detection of deep venous thrombosis.

SERUM HEPATITIS—*see note on page* 581.

HUMAN NORMAL IMMUNOGLOBULIN INJECTION

SYNONYMS: Human Normal Immunoglobulin; Immunoglobulinum Humanum Normale

Human Normal Immunoglobulin Injection is a sterile preparation containing almost all the gamma-G globulins of human plasma together with smaller amounts of other plasma proteins. It contains the antibodies of normal adults.

Human Normal Immunoglobulin Injection is usually prepared from pooled human plasma by precipitation with organic solvents such as alcohol under controlled conditions of pH, ionic concentration, and temperature.

The separated globulins are dissolved in a 0·8 per cent w/v solution of sodium chloride or other suitable vehicle containing a suitable preservative such as 0·01 per cent w/v of thiomersal.

The solution is sterilised by filtration and distributed into single-dose containers; it may also be prepared as a freeze-dried product.

Human Normal Immunoglobulin Injection is also sometimes prepared from saline extracts of intact placentae from healthy women or from retroplacental blood obtained from such placentae.

Human Normal Immunoglobulin Injection is prepared from pools of not less than 1000 donations.

Standard

It complies with the requirements of the European Pharmacopoeia.

The liquid preparation is a clear pale yellow to light brown liquid, free from turbidity and particulate matter at the time of preparation; during storage, slight turbidity or a small amount of particulate matter may form.

The freeze-dried preparation is a white to slightly yellowish powder or friable solid which is completely soluble in water.

The liquid preparation and the reconstituted freeze-dried material contain 10·0 to 17·0 per cent w/v of protein and specific precipitation tests show that they contain proteins of human origin only.

Labelling. The label on the container states:

(1) the name and amount of any added substance;

(2) the date after which the preparation is not intended to be used;

(3) the conditions under which it should be stored;

(4) the volume containing a specified amount of protein;

(5) the amount of any specific antibody claimed by the manufacturer; and

(6) "for intramuscular use only".

The label on the container of the freeze-dried product also states:

(7) the volume of Water for Injections necessary to reconstitute the product; and

(8) that the reconstituted product should be used immediately after preparation.

Storage. The liquid preparation should be protected from light and stored at 2° to 10°; under these conditions it may be expected to retain its potency for three years from the date of manufacture.

The freeze-dried preparation should be stored in an atmosphere of nitrogen, at a temperature below 25°, and protected from light; under these conditions it may be expected to retain its potency for five years from the date of manufacture.

Actions and uses. Human normal immunoglobulin injection is used to protect susceptible contacts against infectious hepatitis and measles and to a lesser extent rubella and poliomyelitis. It is unlikely to be of value in the prevention of chicken pox, mumps, serum hepatitis, smallpox, or whooping-cough. It should be administered by intramuscular injection as soon as possible after exposure is thought to have occurred. Protection is achieved in a proportion of subjects and lasts for not more than four to six weeks.

Human normal immunoglobulin injection is also used for the treatment of congenital or acquired hypogammaglobulinaemia and other immune deficiency states in which immunoglobulin G is diminished or absent.

INFECTIOUS HEPATITIS. Human normal immunoglobulin injection is used to control outbreaks of the disease in institutions or to modify the disease in known contacts for whom an attack would be dangerous. It is also used to protect persons travelling to countries where infectious hepatitis is endemic. Protection lasts about three months.

Dose. By intramuscular injection: for prevention, children under one year, 250 milligrams; one to two years, 500 milligrams; three years or over, 750 milligrams; for attenuation, 250 milligrams.

MEASLES. Human normal immunoglobulin injection is used for controlling outbreaks of the disease in hospitals and institutions and for preventing or attenuating the disease in children under three years of age or in persons suffering from intercurrent illness or living in an unfavourable environment, for whom an attack of measles might be dangerous.

Dose. By intramuscular injection: for prevention, children under one year, 250 milligrams; one to two years, 500 milligrams; three years and over, 750 milligrams; for attenuation, 250 milligrams.

RUBELLA. Human normal immunoglobulin injection is given to pregnant women who have been exposed to rubella during the early months of pregnancy to prevent the disease and its effects on the foetus. It is not necessary to give immunoglobulin if anti-

bodies to rubella virus are already present, and about ninety per cent of adult women have such antibodies.

Dose. By intramuscular injection, 0·75 to 1·5 grams.

HYPOGAMMAGLOBULINAEMIA AND OTHER IMMUNE DEFICIENCY STATES:

Dose. Initially, 50 milligrams per kilogram body-weight for five successive days; maintenance dose 25 to 50 milligrams per kilogram body-weight per week depending upon the severity of the condition.

NOTE. When Human Gamma Globulin Injection or Human Gamma-G Immunoglobulin is prescribed or demanded, Human Normal Immunoglobulin Injection is supplied.

HUMAN TETANUS IMMUNOGLOBULIN

SYNONYM: Immunoglobulinum Humanum Antitetanicum

Human Tetanus Immunoglobulin contains specific antibodies against the toxin of *Clostridium tetani.*

The product is prepared from a pool of plasma from persons immunised against tetanus.

Standard
It complies with the requirements of the European Pharmacopoeia and with the requirements for Human Normal Immunoglobulin Injection with the exception of that concerning pool size.
It contains not less than 50 Units of tetanus antitoxin per ml.

Labelling; Storage. As for Human Normal Immunoglobulin Injection.

Actions and uses. Human tetanus immunoglobulin is used to protect unimmunised individuals at risk who are known to be sensitive to the animal preparation (Tetanus Antitoxin). When available in sufficient amounts it is the preparation of choice for the protection of unimmunised individuals at risk.

Dose. By intramuscular injection, for prevention, 250 Units.

HUMAN VACCINIA IMMUNOGLOBULIN

SYNONYM: Immunoglobulinum Humanum Antivaccinium

Human Vaccinia Immunoglobulin contains specific antibodies against the vaccinia virus.

The product is prepared from a pool of plasma from persons recently vaccinated against smallpox.

Standard
It complies with the requirements of the European Pharmacopoeia and with the requirements for Human Normal Immunoglobulin Injection with the exception of that concerning pool size.
It contains not less than 500 Units of vaccinia antibody per ml.

Labelling; Storage. As for Human Normal Immunoglobulin Injection.

Actions and uses. Human vaccinia immunoglobulin is used to treat patients with generalised vaccinia and also those in whom localised vaccinial infection endangers the eye. It is also given simultaneously with smallpox vaccination when this has to be done

under circumstances which increase the attendant risks. When the time since exposure is too long for vaccination alone to protect smallpox contacts, this form of immunoglobulin may be given as a prophylactic likely to be of value as a supplement to smallpox vaccine.

Dose. By intramuscular injection: for generalised vaccinia, vaccinial lesions of the eye, and smallpox vaccination in the presence of contra-indications, children under one year, 500 milligrams, one to six years, 1 gram, seven to fourteen years, 1·5 grams, and adults and children over fourteen years, 2 grams; for previously unvaccinated contacts of cases of smallpox, children under one year, 500 milligrams, one to six years, 1 gram, and adults and children over six years, 1·5 grams.

DRIED HUMAN PLASMA

Dried Human Plasma is prepared by drying a pool of the supernatant fluids which are separated, by centrifuging or by standing, from quantities of Whole Human Blood.

The supernatant fluid from each sample of whole human blood is siphoned through a closed system of sterile tubing by an aseptic technique and pooled with other supernatant fluids so that contributions from donors of A, O, and either B or AB groups are represented in approximately the ratio 9 : 9 : 2. In order to avoid untoward effects due to the products of bacterial growth, no individual contribution of plasma is used if there is any evidence of bacterial contamination and no pool is used unless it complies with the tests for sterility.

Not more than ten separate donations of plasma should be pooled, unless an effective method of destroying the causative agent of serum hepatitis can be applied. The pool is dried either from the frozen state or by any other method which will avoid denaturing the proteins and will yield a product readily soluble in a quantity of water equal to the volume of the liquid from which the substance was prepared.

Standard
It complies with the requirements of the British Pharmacopoeia.
It is a sterile pale to deep cream-coloured powder, which is completely soluble, at 15° to 20°, within ten minutes, in a volume of water equal to the volume of Water for Injections stated on the label. Such a solution contains not less than 4·5 per cent w/v of protein, and must be shown by specific precipitation tests to contain only human plasma proteins. Coagulation occurs when an aqueous solution of calcium chloride is added to the reconstituted plasma.

Labelling. The label on the container states:
(1) the nature and percentage of anticoagulant and of any other material introduced;
(2) that the contents are derived from not more than 10 donations of blood;
(3) the quantity of diluent necessary to reconstitute the original volume of liquid human plasma;
(4) the protein content of the reconstituted liquid human plasma;

(5) the date after which the preparation must not be used;
(6) the conditions under which it should be stored; and
(7) that the preparation should be used immediately after reconstitution.

Storage. It should be stored in an atmosphere of nitrogen, in sterile containers sealed to exclude micro-organisms and moisture, at a temperature below 25°, and protected from light.
It may be stored for several years in temperate and tropical climates if it is kept free from moisture. The only practical criterion of its fitness for use is complete solution within ten minutes when reconstituted. If solution is incomplete or if a gel forms, the plasma should not be used, even though the expiry date has not been reached.

Actions and uses. Dried human plasma dissolved in a volume of Water for Injections, Sodium Chloride Injection, or a solution containing 2·5 per cent of anhydrous dextrose and 0·45 per cent of sodium chloride, equivalent to the volume of the liquid plasma from which it was prepared, gives a reconstituted plasma which is mainly used for the restoration of plasma volume in patients suffering from burns, scalds or crush injuries. It is also used in emergencies when whole human blood is not available, or while awaiting the results of compatibility tests.

Because of its keeping properties and ease of storage, dried human plasma is valuable as a transfusion medium in small hospitals without a blood bank and in isolated communities, but it should not be used in place of whole human blood merely for convenience.

The amount of plasma transfused and the rate at which it is given depend upon the patient's age and general condition, on the state of his circulatory system, and on the indication for its use.

Reconstituted dried human plasma should be used immediately after reconstitution.

SERUM HEPATITIS—*see note on page* 581.

DRIED HUMAN SERUM

Dried Human Serum is prepared by drying a pool of the fluid which separates from human blood which has clotted in the absence of any anticoagulant.

For the preparation of Dried Human Serum, blood is collected by the method described under Whole Human Blood, except that the anticoagulant solution is omitted from the receiving vessel, from donors who fulfil the same requirements.

The blood is allowed to clot, and the serum is removed aseptically by siphoning through a closed system of sterile tubing. The serum is mixed with that from other samples of blood so that contributions from donors of A, O,

and either B or AB groups are represented in approximately the ratio 9 : 9 : 2. In order to avoid untoward effects due to the products of bacterial growth, no individual contribution of serum is used if there is any evidence of bacterial contamination and no pool is used unless it complies with the tests for sterility.

Not more than ten separate donations of serum are pooled. The pool is dried either from the frozen state or by any other method which will avoid denaturing the proteins and will yield a product readily soluble in a quantity of water equal to the volume of the liquid from which the substance was prepared.

Standard
It complies with the requirements of the British Pharmacopoeia.
It is a sterile pale to deep cream-coloured powder or friable solid, which is completely soluble, at 15° to 20°, within ten minutes, in a volume of water equal to the volume of Water for Injections stated on the label. Such a solution contains not less than 6·5 per cent w/v of protein, and must be shown by specific precipitation tests to contain only human serum proteins. No coagulation occurs when an aqueous solution of calcium chloride is added to the reconstituted serum.

Labelling. The label on the container states:
(1) that the contents are derived from not more than 10 donations of blood;
(2) the quantity of diluent necessary to reconstitute the original volume of liquid human serum;
(3) the protein content of the reconstituted liquid human serum;
(4) the date after which the preparation is not intended to be used;

(5) the conditions under which it should be stored; and
(6) that the preparation should be used immediately after reconstitution.

Storage. It should be stored, in an atmosphere of nitrogen, in sterile containers sealed to exclude micro-organisms and moisture, at a temperature below 25°, and protected from light.
It may be stored for several years in temperate and tropical climates if it is kept free from moisture. The only practical criterion of its fitness for use is complete solution within ten minutes when reconstituted. If solution is incomplete or if a gel forms, the serum should not be used, even though the expiry date has not been reached.

Actions and uses. Dried human serum is used for the same purposes as those described under Dried Human Plasma and is reconstituted in a similar manner.
Reconstituted serum should be used immediately after reconstitution.

SERUM HEPATITIS—*see note on page* 581.

DRIED HUMAN THROMBIN

Dried Human Thrombin is a preparation of the enzyme which converts human fibrinogen into fibrin.

The product is obtained from liquid human plasma and may be prepared by precipitation with suitable salts and organic solvents under controlled conditions of pH, ionic strength, and temperature. The prothrombin of the human plasma is converted into thrombin in solution by the addition of a minimum amount of calcium ions and human thromboplastin. The solution is clarified by filtration and dried from the frozen state.

Standard
It complies with the requirements of the British Pharmacopoeia.
It is a cream-coloured powder which is readily soluble in saline solution, forming a cloudy, pale yellow solution. It contains not less than 10 clotting doses per mg.

Labelling. The label on the container states:
(1) the number of clotting doses contained in it;
(2) the conditions under which it should be stored;
(3) that the reconstituted solution should be used immediately after reconstitution; and

(4) the date after which the preparation is not intended to be used.

Storage. It should be stored, in an atmosphere of nitrogen, in sterile containers sealed to exclude micro-organisms and moisture, at a temperature below 25°, and protected from light.

Actions and uses. A solution of human thrombin in Sodium Chloride Injection, prepared by means of an aseptic technique, is used in conjunction with human fibrinogen and human fibrin foam. When it is used with human fibrinogen, the strength of solution will depend upon the desired rapidity of clotting; when it is used with human fibrin foam, a solution containing 30 to 50 clotting doses per millilitre is employed. Solutions of human thrombin should never be injected.

SERUM HEPATITIS—*see note on page* 581.

PART 4

Surgical Ligatures and Sutures

SURGICAL LIGATURES AND SUTURES

This section contains monographs for a number of surgical ligatures and sutures, which are classified as absorbable or non-absorbable materials. Sterilised surgical catgut is the only suture in the first category.

STERILISED SURGICAL CATGUT

SYNONYMS: Chorda Resorbilis Aseptica; Sterile Catgut; Sterilised Surgical Ligature (Catgut); Sterilised Surgical Suture (Catgut)

Sterilised Surgical Catgut consists of sterile strands prepared from collagen derived from healthy mammals. They may be prepared from the washed intestines of sheep, *Ovis aries* L. (Fam. Bovidae), or other herbivorous animals. The intestines, on removal from the animal, are cleaned and either processed immediately or frozen, dried, or otherwise suitably preserved. They are prepared by splitting longitudinally into ribbons, scraping to remove the mucosa and muscular layers, and, according to the gauge required, twisting one, two, or more ribbons uniformly under tension to form a strand. The strands are air-dried under tension and their surface polished to produce an even gauge throughout their length. Strands may also be prepared from other collagen fibres, such as those obtained from beef serosa.

Surgical catgut is liable to bacterial contamination, particularly with the dried resistant spores of pathogenic anaerobes, such as those responsible for tetanus and gas-gangrene; the spores are deeply embedded in the material, which is itself not easily penetrated either by heat or bactericides. As it consists chiefly of collagen, which is readily converted into gelatin by heat in the presence of moisture, it must be thoroughly dehydrated by careful drying if it is to be subjected to heat.

Each strand, of a length not exceeding 350 cm, is placed in a glass tube or other suitable container. Ethyl alcohol with a water content of 3 to 5 per cent or another suitable hydrated fluid may be added to the container; such hydrated fluids keep the strand flexible. A bactericide, but not an antibiotic, may have been added to the fluid. The container is sealed and the contents are sterilised. Heat must not be used for this purpose, as at high temperatures the small amount of water in the strand or in a hydrated fluid causes swelling and a serious diminution in the tensile strength of the strand. Any suitable method, such as exposure to ionising radiation or prolonged exposure to bactericides, may be used for sterilisation, but the process chosen must not unduly increase the rate at which the suture is absorbed.

In order to sterilise the exterior of glass containers before they are opened, they should be washed in a cold detergent solution and immersed in a 1 per cent solution of formaldehyde in alcohol or some other equally effective bactericide; the period of immersion should be not less than twenty-four hours. For containers other than glass the bactericide used should be suitable for the material from which the container is made.

After removal from the container the strand should not be immersed before use in an aqueous fluid, such as sterile saline, as the strand may swell and lose tensile strength.

"Plain" or "non-hardened" sterilised surgical catgut is Sterilised Surgical Catgut which has not been processed to reduce the rate of absorption by the body tissues; it is generally effective in normal muscle for about 5 to 10 days.

"Hardened" sterilised surgical catgut is Sterilised Surgical Catgut which has been treated with a suitable hardening agent designed to prolong its resistance to digestion; catgut hardened by treatment with chromium compounds is known as "chromicised" catgut. The hardening process may be controlled to vary the rate of absorption.

Standard
It complies with the requirements of the European Pharmacopoeia.

Packaging. It is packed in sealed containers which maintain sterility and which, once opened, cannot be re-sealed.

Labelling. The label on or in the container states, by indelible marking or perforation:
(1) the name of the suture;
(2) the size number;
(3) the length of the strand(s) (in cm or m);
(4) whether the strand(s) are "plain", "hardened", or "chromicised";
(5) that the container should not be subjected to heat treatment; and
(6) a number or other indication by which the history of the suture may be traced.

The label on the package or the label on or in the container states:
(7) the name and percentage of any bactericide in the fluid in the container.

Storage. It should be stored in a cool place, protected from light.

NON-ABSORBABLE SURGICAL SUTURES

Non-absorbable Surgical Sutures consist of strands which, when introduced into a living organism, are not metabolised by the organism.

This general monograph applies to the following sutures:

Linen Suture
Sterile Linen Suture
Polyamide 6 Suture
Sterile Polyamide 6 Suture
Polyamide 6/6 Suture
Sterile Polyamide 6/6 Suture
Plaited Polyester Suture
Sterile Plaited Polyester Suture
Plaited Silk Suture
Sterile Plaited Silk Suture
Monofilament Stainless Steel Suture
Sterile Monofilament Stainless Steel Suture

Plaited Stainless Steel Suture
Sterile Plaited Stainless Steel Suture
Twisted Stainless Steel Suture
Sterile Twisted Stainless Steel Suture

Strands which have been treated to reduce capillarity are designated "non-capillary".

General Standard

Unless otherwise indicated, for batches of 500 strands or less, use 5 strands as the sample for each test; for batches of more than 500, use 1 per cent of the strands or 10, whichever is the fewer.

DESCRIPTION. A uniform strand of metal or of natural or synthetic material which effectively resists absorption by the body tissues and does not cause undue tissue reaction. The strand consists of a single filament or fibre, or of a thread prepared by spinning, twisting, or plaiting (braiding) single filaments or fibres; the threads may be sheathed. The strands may be dyed or pigmented with a suitable non-toxic non-irritant colouring matter to give a uniform colour which is fast to boiling in water, in alcohol, and in the fluid in which the strand is packed.

LENGTH. *Non-sterilised sutures and stainless steel sutures.* Not less than the length stated on the label, determined while the strand is subjected to just sufficient tension to keep it straight during the measurement.

Sterile sutures other than stainless steel sutures. The total length of strand(s) in each container does not exceed 350 cm. The length of each strand is not less than 95 per cent of the length stated on the label, determined while the strand is subjected to just sufficient tension to keep it straight during the measurement, after conditioning the strand by the following method:

If the strand is packed in the dry state, remove it from the container and then condition it by maintaining it in an atmosphere of 60 to 80 per cent relative humidity at 16° to 21° for not less than 2 hours before testing; if the strand is packed in a fluid, remove it from the container, dry it in a current of air, and then subject it to the same conditioning.

DIAMETER. *Sutures other than stainless steel sutures.* The average of the diameters recorded for all the strands in the sample is within the limits specified in Table 1 (page 599) for the average diameter of the size stated on the label, and none of the diameters recorded is less than the minimum diameter or greater than the maximum diameter specified. In addition, not less than two-thirds of the diameters recorded on each individual strand are within the limits specified for the average diameter.

Make the measurements in an atmosphere of 60 to 80 per cent relative humidity at 16° to 21° with a suitable mechanical measuring instrument of the dial-reading type with a dial graduated to read directly to 0·01 mm. The table of the instrument is about 5 cm in diameter and the pressor foot is circular with a diameter of about 1·25 cm. The pressor foot and the moving parts connected to it are weighted so as to apply a total load of 200 ± 10 g to the strand under test.

Remove a strand from its container and immediately, unless otherwise stated in the individual monograph, apply, as described below under Tensile Strength, a tension equal to half the minimum breaking force specified in column A of Table 3 (page 600) for the size stated on the label and the type of material in the strand. Without delay, measure diameters along the length of the strand: for a strand not greater than 90 cm in length, make the measurements at the three quarterly points; for a strand greater than 90 cm in length, make the measurements at points 30 cm apart over the whole length of the strand. At each point, measure the diameter, rotate the strand about its longitudinal axis through 90°, and again measure the diameter. Record the diameter at each point on the strand as the average of the two measurements.

Repeat the above procedure on each strand in the sample, and calculate the average of all the diameters recorded.

Stainless steel sutures. The diameter at each point at which a measurement is made on all the strands in the sample is within the limits specified in Table 2 for size stated on the label.

Make the measurements with a mechanical measuring instrument. A suitable instrument is described above under *Sutures other than stainless steel sutures.*

Apply, as described below under Tensile Strength, to each strand in the sample, a tension equal to a quarter of the minimum breaking force specified in Table 2 for the size and type of suture stated on the label; do not allow twisted strands to untwist. Measure the diameter at the points specified above under *Sutures other than stainless steel sutures*; for braided and twisted sutures, at each point make two measurements at right angles to each other, and record the average of the two measurements as the diameter.

TENSILE STRENGTH. *Sutures other than stainless steel sutures.* Not less than 80 per cent of the strands in the sample have a breaking force over a simple knot equal to or more than that specified in column A of Table 3 for the size stated on the label and the type of material in the strand, and no strand has a breaking load less than that specified in column B.

Carry out the determinations on a tensilometer in an atmosphere of 60 to 80 per cent relative humidity at 16° to 21°. If the strand is packed in fluid, complete the determination within 15 minutes of removing the strand from its container; if the strand is packed in the dry state, first condition it by immersion for 24 hours in *alcohol (95 per cent)* or *isopropyl alcohol (90 per cent)* and again complete the determination within 15 minutes of removing the strand from the fluid.

Carry out the determination on a hand- or electrically-operated machine of the dead-weight type having a fixed clamp and a mobile clamp with a constant rate of traverse of 30 cm per minute and having a capacity such that, when the strand breaks, the angle which the pendulum arm makes with the vertical is not less than 9° and not more than 45°. The clamps should be so designed that the strand can be attached without the possibility of slipping and that not more than a quarter of them break within 10 mm of the clamp.

Remove a strand from the fluid in which it is packed or conditioned. For strands longer than 25 m, discard the first 30 cm from one end and use a 2-m portion for the test. Immediately tie a simple knot in the strand by passing one end over the other and through the loop and pull both ends until the strand is taut. Attach the strand to the clamps in such a way that the knot is midway between them and the distance between the clamps is not less than 12·5 cm and not more than 20 cm. Apply a tension to the strand between the clamps equal to one quarter of the minimum breaking force specified in column A for the stated size and type of material and then set the mobile clamp in motion. Note the force indicated on the scale when the strand breaks. If the strand breaks in a clamp or within 10 mm of one, discard the result and repeat the determination on another portion of the strand. If the strand is longer than 50 cm, repeat the determination on another portion and take the lower result as the breaking force of the strand.

Stainless steel sutures. The average breaking force on a straight pull is within the range given in the appropriate column of Table 2 for the size stated on the label.

Determine the breaking load for each of the unknotted strands in the sample on the tensilometer described above under *Sutures other than stainless steel sutures*, making not less than two determinations on each strand and taking the lowest result as the breaking force. Calculate the average breaking force for the strands in the sample.

STRENGTH OF NEEDLE ATTACHMENT. If the strand is attached to an eyeless needle, the average force necessary to detach the strand from the needle when 5 sutures are tested is not less than the minimum force specified in column A of Table 4 for the size stated on the label and none of the individual forces is less than the minimum force specified in column B. If not more than one of the individual forces is less than the specified value, the determination may be repeated on a further 10 sutures; the needle attachment meets the requirements if none of the 10 values is less than the specified value.

Carry out the determinations on a tensilometer of the same type as that used for the determination of tensile strength above.

Fix an unknotted strand in the mobile clamp of the machine and the needle in the fixed clamp in such a manner that the whole of the swaged end of the needle is free of the clamp and in line with the direction of pull on the suture when the force is applied. Determine the force required to break the strand or detach it from the needle. Repeat the determination on 4 further sutures and calculate the average force required.

STERILITY. Sterile sutures comply with the test for sterility described in Appendix 28, page 917.

TABLE 1

Diameter of non-absorbable sutures other than stainless steel

Size No.	Diameter (mm)		
	Average	Minimum	Maximum
0·1	0·010 to 0·029	0·007	0·040
0·3	0·030 to 0·049	0·020	0·060
0·5	0·050 to 0·069	0·040	0·080
0·7	0·070 to 0·090	0·060	0·12
1	0·10 to 0·14	0·080	0·17
1·5	0·15 to 0·19	0·12	0·22
2	0·20 to 0·24	0·17	0·27
2·5	0·25 to 0·29	0·22	0·35
3	0·30 to 0·39	0·27	0·45
4	0·40 to 0·49	0·35	0·55
5	0·50 to 0·59	0·45	0·65
6	0·60 to 0·69	0·55	0·75
7	0·70 to 0·79	0·65	0·85
8	0·80 to 0·89	0·75	0·95

TABLE 2

Diameter and tensile strength of stainless steel sutures

Size No.	Diameter (mm)		Average breaking force over a simple knot (kgf)	
			Monofilament	Plaited and Twisted
0·5	0·05		0·10 to 0·15	0·08 to 0·12
1	0·10		0·45 to 0·66	0·36 to 0·53
1·2	0·125		0·72 to 0·99	0·58 to 0·79
1·5	0·16	±0·0064	1·0 to 1·6	0·8 to 1·3
2	0·20		1·7 to 2·5	1·4 to 2·0
2·5	0·25		2·7 to 4·1	2·2 to 3·3
3	0·315		4·3 to 6·4	3·4 to 5·1
3·5	0·35		5·5 to 8·2	4·4 to 6·6
4	0·40		7·1 to 10·5	5·7 to 8·4
4·5	0·45	±0·0127	9·0 to 13·3	7·2 to 10·6
5	0·50		11·3 to 16·6	9·0 to 13·3
6	0·63		16·1 to 23·7	12·9 to 19·0

TABLE 3

Tensile strength of non-absorbable sutures other than stainless steel

Size No.	Minimum breaking force over simple knot (kgf)									
	Linen		Mono-filament and sheathed polyamide		Plaited polyamide		Plaited polyester		Plaited silk	
	A	B	A	B	A	B	A	B	A	B
0·1	—	—	—	—	—	—	—	—	—	—
0·3	—	—	0·05	0·03	0·05	0·03	—	—	—	—
0·5	—	—	0·08	0·04	0·08	0·04	0·10	0·06	0·05	0·03
0·7	—	—	0·12	0·05	0·12	0·05	0·17	0·09	0·10	0·04
1	—	—	0·14	0·08	0·20	0·08	0·20	0·10	0·20	0·05
1·5	0·50	0·30	0·30	0·12	0·35	0·12	0·40	0·17	0·37	0·10
2	0·80	0·45	0·60	0·14	0·65	0·20	0·80	0·20	0·70	0·20
2·5	1·1	0·50	0·80	0·30	1·0	0·35	1·2	0·40	1·1	0·37
3	1·3	0·80	1·3	0·60	1·4	0·65	1·7	0·80	1·4	0·70
4	2·2	1·1	2·0	0·80	2·2	1·0	2·9	1·2	2·3	1·1
5	3·5	1·3	2·7	1·3	3·5	1·4	4	1·7	3·5	1·4
6	4·5	2·2	3·5	2·0	4·5	2·2	5	2·9	4	2·3
7	6	3·5	5	2·7	6	3·5	7	4	5	3·5
8	6·8	4·5	—	—	7	4·5	9	5	6·5	4

TABLE 4

Strength of needle attachment

Size No.	Minimum breaking or detaching force (kgf)	
	A	B
1	0·24	0·12
1·5	0·50	0·25
2	0·70	0·32
2·5	1·0	0·50
3 and 3·5	1·4	0·70
4 and larger	1·8	0·90

Sterilisation. Non-absorbable surgical sutures may be sterilised by autoclaving or by any other suitable method, such as exposure to ionising radiation, as described in Appendix 29, page 921, or by prolonged exposure to bactericides.

Some plastics may be adversely affected if heated above 116°, and if autoclaving at higher temperatures is used for sterilisation, care must be taken to ensure that any suture of a synthetic material withstands the selected combination of temperature and time.

Packaging. Sterile non-absorbable surgical sutures are supplied, either in the dry state or in a sterile preserving fluid, in glass tubes sealed by fusion of the glass or in other suitable containers which maintain sterility and which, once opened, cannot be resealed. A bactericide, but not an antibiotic, may have been added to the fluid. The total length of suture in a container does not exceed 350 cm.

Labelling. The label on or in the container states, by indelible marking or perforation:
(1) the name of the suture;
(2) the size number;
(3) the length of the strand(s) (in cm or m); and
(4) a number or other indication by which the history of the suture may be traced.

The label on the package or the label on or in the container states:
(5) that, for treated sutures, the suture is non-capillary;
(6) the name and percentage of any bactericide in the fluid; and
(7) that, for sterile sutures, unless otherwise indicated in the individual monograph, any portion of the suture not used on the occasion when the container is first opened should be discarded.

Linen Suture

Linen Suture consists of a twisted strand prepared from the pericyclic fibres of the stem of flax, *Linum usitatissimum* L. (Fam. Linaceae). On sterilisation by exposure to ionising radiation, the strand will lose some of its tensile strength.

Standard
DESCRIPTION. A three-cord satin-finished, uniformly and firmly twisted strand, free from fuzziness and undue irregularities, complying with the requirements described under Non-absorbable Surgical Sutures.

IDENTIFICATION TESTS. 1. Isolate a few individual fibres and examine them under a microscope. The fibres, 25 to 50 mm in length and 12 to 31 μm in width, have long finely pointed ends and, along the greater part of their length, a narrow lumen and thick walls occasionally marked with fine longitudinal striations. Sometimes there are unilateral swellings with transversal lines.

2. Impregnated with *iodinated zinc chloride solution*, the individual fibres are coloured violet-blue.

LENGTH; STRENGTH OF NEEDLE ATTACHMENT. It complies with the requirements described under Non-absorbable Surgical Sutures.

DIAMETER. It complies with the requirements described under Non-absorbable Surgical Sutures. Condition the strands in an atmosphere of 60 to 80 per cent relative humidity at 16° to 21° for 4 hours immediately before testing.

TENSILE STRENGTH. It complies with the requirements described under Non-absorbable Surgical Sutures. Immerse the strands in water at 16° to 21° for 30 minutes immediately before testing.

Labelling. The directions given under Non-absorbable Surgical Sutures should be followed.

Sterile Linen Suture

SYNONYMS: Sterile Linen Thread; Filum Lini Asepticum

Sterile Linen Suture is Linen Suture which has been subjected to a sterilisation process.

Standard
Strands which comply with this standard will meet the requirements of the European Pharmacopoeia.

DESCRIPTION; IDENTIFICATION TESTS; DIAMETER. It complies with the requirements described under Linen Suture, above.

LENGTH; STRENGTH OF NEEDLE ATTACHMENT; STERILITY. It complies with the requirements described under Non-absorbable Surgical Sutures.

TENSILE STRENGTH. It complies with the requirements described under Non-absorbable Surgical Sutures. If the suture is in the dry state or has been packed in an anhydrous fluid, immerse the strands in water at 16° to 21° for 30 minutes immediately before testing; if it is packed in an aqueous fluid, dry the strands in a current of air before subjecting to the same treatment.

Sterilisation. It may be sterilised as described under Non-absorbable Surgical Sutures.

Packaging; Labelling. The directions given under Non-absorbable Surgical Sutures should be followed.

Polyamide 6 Suture

SYNONYM: Nylon 6 Suture

The general use of the synonym "nylon" is limited and in any country in which the name "nylon" is a trade mark it may be used only when applied to the product made by the owners of the trade mark.

Polyamide 6 Suture consists of a strand (monofilament), plaited (braided) strands, or sheathed strands of the polyamide produced by the polymerisation of ε-caprolactam.

Standard
DESCRIPTION. A smooth uniform strand, circular in cross-section, or a uniformly plaited strand, or lightly twisted strands, sheathed with the same material, complying with the requirements described under Non-absorbable Surgical Sutures.

IDENTIFICATION TESTS. 1. Heat about 0·05 g with 0·5 ml of *hydrochloric acid* in a sealed glass tube at 110° for 18 hours and allow to stand for several hours; no crystals are formed.

2. To about 0·05 g add 10 ml of *hydrochloric acid*; the strand disintegrates and dissolves completely within a few minutes (distinction from polyester suture).

3. Place about 0·05 g in an ignition tube clamped in a vertical position and heat gently until heavy vapours are evolved; when the vapours fill the tube, remove it from the flame, and hold in the vapours a strip of unglazed white paper impregnated with a freshly prepared saturated solution of *2-nitrobenzaldehyde* in *sodium hydroxide solution*; a violet-brown colour, which fades slowly and is discharged on washing with *dilute sulphuric acid* and water, is slowly produced on the paper (distinction from polyester suture).

MONOMER AND OLIGOMER. Not more than 2·0 per cent, determined by the following method:
Extract about 1 g, accurately weighed, with 30 ml of *methyl alcohol* in an apparatus for the continuous extraction of drugs for 7 hours, ensuring 18 to 20 changes. Evaporate the extract to dryness on a water-bath, dry the residue for 10 minutes at 110°, allow to cool, and weigh the extracted monomer and oligomer.

LENGTH; DIAMETER; TENSILE STRENGTH; STRENGTH OF NEEDLE ATTACHMENT. It complies with the requirements described under Non-absorbable Surgical Sutures.

Incompatibility. It is incompatible with phenol and its homologues, and with other phenolic substances.

Labelling. The directions given under Non-absorbable Surgical Sutures should be followed; the name on the label indicates the type of suture, i.e. monofilament, plaited (braided), or sheathed, as appropriate.

Sterile Polyamide 6 Suture

SYNONYMS: Sterile Nylon 6 Suture; Filum Polyamidicum-6 Asepticum

The general use of the synonym "nylon" is limited and in any country in which the name "nylon" is a trade mark it may be used only when applied to the product made by the owners of the trade mark.

Sterile Polyamide 6 Suture is Polyamide 6 Suture which has been subjected to a sterilisation process.

Standard
Strands which comply with this standard will meet the requirements of the European Pharmacopoeia.

DESCRIPTION; IDENTIFICATION TESTS; MONOMER AND OLIGOMER. It complies with the requirements described under Polyamide 6 Suture, above.

LENGTH; DIAMETER; TENSILE STRENGTH; STRENGTH OF NEEDLE ATTACHMENT; STERILITY. It complies with the requirements described under Non-absorbable Surgical Sutures.

Incompatibility. It is incompatible with phenol and its homologues and with other phenolic substances.

Sterilisation. It may be sterilised as described under Non-absorbable Surgical Sutures.

Packaging. The directions given under Non-absorbable Surgical Sutures should be followed.

Labelling. The directions given under Non-absorbable Surgical Sutures should be followed; the name on the label indicates the type of suture, i.e. monofilament, plaited (braided), or sheathed, as appropriate.

Polyamide 6/6 Suture

SYNONYM: Nylon 6/6 Suture

The general use of the synonym "nylon" is limited and in any country in which the name "nylon" is a trade mark it may be used only when applied to the product made by the owners of the trade mark.

Polyamide 6/6 Suture consists of a strand (monofilament), plaited (braided) strands, or sheathed strands of the polyamide produced by the combination of hexamethylenediamine and adipic acid.

Standard

DESCRIPTION. A smooth uniform strand, circular in cross-section, or a uniformly plaited strand, or lightly twisted strands, sheathed with the same material, complying with the requirements described under Non-absorbable Surgical Sutures.

IDENTIFICATION TESTS. 1. Heated over a flame, it melts and burns, forming a hard globule of residue and giving off a characteristic odour resembling that of celery.

2. To about 0·05 g add 10 ml of *hydrochloric acid*; the strand disintegrates and dissolves completely within a few minutes (distinction from polyester suture).

3. Place about 0·05 g in an ignition tube clamped in a vertical position and heat gently until heavy vapours are evolved; when the vapours fill the tube, remove it from the flame, and hold in the vapours a strip of unglazed white paper impregnated with a freshly prepared saturated solution of *2-nitrobenzaldehyde* in *sodium hydroxide solution*; a violet-brown colour, which fades slowly and is discharged on washing with *dilute sulphuric acid* and water, is slowly produced on the paper (distinction from polyester suture).

LENGTH; DIAMETER; TENSILE STRENGTH; STRENGTH OF NEEDLE ATTACHMENT. It complies with the requirements described under Non-absorbable Surgical Sutures.

Incompatibility. It is incompatible with phenol and its homologues and with other phenolic substances.

Labelling. The directions given under Non-absorbable Surgical Sutures should be followed; the name on the label indicates the type of suture, i.e. monofilament, plaited (braided), or sheathed, as appropriate.

Sterile Polyamide 6/6 Suture

SYNONYMS: Sterile Nylon 6/6 Suture; Filum Polyamidicum 6/6 Asepticum

The general use of the synonym "nylon" is limited and in any country in which the name "nylon" is a trade mark it may be used only when applied to the product made by the owners of the trade mark.

Sterile Polyamide 6/6 Suture is Polyamide 6/6 Suture which has been subjected to a sterilisation process.

Standard

Strands which comply with this standard will meet the requirements of the European Pharmacopoeia.

DESCRIPTION; IDENTIFICATION TESTS. It complies with the requirements described under Polyamide 6/6 Suture, above.

LENGTH; DIAMETER; TENSILE STRENGTH; STRENGTH OF NEEDLE ATTACHMENT; STERILITY. It complies with the requirements described under Non-absorbable Surgical Sutures.

Incompatibility. It is incompatible with phenol and its homologues and with other phenolic substances.

Sterilisation. It may be sterilised as described under Non-absorbable Surgical Sutures.

Packaging. The directions given under Non-absorbable Surgical Sutures should be followed.

Labelling. The directions given under Non-absorbable Surgical Sutures should be followed; the name on the label indicates the type of suture, i.e. monofilament, plaited (braided), or sheathed, as appropriate.

Plaited Polyester Suture

SYNONYM: Braided Polyester Suture

Plaited Polyester Suture consists of a plaited strand of the polyester produced by the combination of ethylene glycol and terephthalic acid.

Standard

DESCRIPTION. A uniformly plaited strand, complying with the requirements described under Non-absorbable Surgical Sutures.

IDENTIFICATION TESTS. 1. The strand dissolves very slowly when heated in *dimethylformamide* or *dichlorobenzene*.

2. To about 0·05 g add 10 ml of *hydrochloric acid*; the strand remains intact even after prolonged immersion (distinction from polyamide suture).

3. Carry out test 3 described under Polyamide 6 Suture, page 602; a greenish-blue colour, which changes to blue on washing with *dilute sulphuric acid* and water, is produced on the paper (distinction from polyamide suture).

LENGTH; DIAMETER; TENSILE STRENGTH; STRENGTH OF NEEDLE ATTACHMENT. It complies with the requirements described under Non-absorbable Surgical Sutures.

Labelling. The directions given under Non-absorbable Surgical Sutures should be followed.

Sterile Plaited Polyester Suture

SYNONYMS: Sterile Braided Polyester Suture; Sterile Polyester Suture; Filum Polyestericum Asepticum

Sterile Plaited Polyester Suture is Plaited Polyester Suture which has been subjected to a sterilisation process.

Standard

Strands which comply with this standard will meet the requirements of the European Pharmacopoeia.

DESCRIPTION; IDENTIFICATION TESTS. It complies with the requirements described under Plaited Polyester Suture, above.

LENGTH; DIAMETER; TENSILE STRENGTH; STRENGTH OF NEEDLE ATTACHMENT; STERILITY. It complies with the requirements described under Non-absorbable Surgical Sutures.

Sterilisation. It may be sterilised as described under Non-absorbable Surgical Sutures.

Packaging; Labelling. The directions given under Non-absorbable Surgical Sutures should be followed.

Plaited Silk Suture

SYNONYM: Braided Silk Suture

Plaited Silk Suture consists of a plaited strand of silk prepared from the degummed cocoon filaments spun by the silkworm, *Bombyx mori* L. and other species of *Bombyx* (Fam. Bombycidae). On sterilisation, the strand may lose some of its tensile strength.

Standard

DESCRIPTION. A uniformly plaited unbleached discharged unloaded strand, complying with the requirements described under Non-absorbable Surgical Sutures.

IDENTIFICATION TESTS. 1. Isolate a few individual fibres and examine them under a microscope. The fibres are approximately triangular to semicircular in cross-section with rounded edges and without a lumen. They are sometimes marked with very fine longitudinal striations parallel to the axis of the strand.

2. Impregnated with *iodinated potassium iodide solution*, the individual fibres are coloured pale yellow.

3. Warm with *mercury nitrate solution*; a brick-red colour is produced.

SULPHATED ASH. Not more than 4·0 per cent.

LENGTH; DIAMETER; STRENGTH OF NEEDLE ATTACHMENT. It complies with the requirements described under Non-absorbable Surgical Sutures.

TENSILE STRENGTH. It complies with the requirements described under Non-absorbable Surgical Sutures. If the strand is packed in the dry state, omit the conditioning before testing.

Labelling. The directions given under Non-absorbable Surgical Sutures should be followed.

Sterile Plaited Silk Suture

SYNONYMS: Sterile Braided Silk Suture; Filum Bombycis Tortum Asepticum

Sterile Plaited Silk Suture is Plaited Silk Suture which has been subjected to a sterilisation process.

Standard
Strands which comply with this standard will meet the requirements of the European Pharmacopoeia.

DESCRIPTION; IDENTIFICATION TESTS; TENSILE STRENGTH. It complies with the requirements described under Plaited Silk Suture, above.

LENGTH; DIAMETER; STRENGTH OF NEEDLE ATTACHMENT; STERILITY. It complies with the requirements described under Non-absorbable Surgical Sutures.

Sterilisation. It may be sterilised as described under Non-absorbable Surgical Sutures.

Packaging; Labelling. The directions given under Non-absorbable Surgical Sutures should be followed.

Monofilament Stainless Steel Suture

SYNONYMS: Monofilament Surgical Steel; Surgical Stainless Steel Monofilament Wire

Monofilament Stainless Steel Suture consists of a strand of fully softened stainless steel wire.

Standard
DESCRIPTION. A smooth uniform single strand, circular in cross-section, and free from grease. The composition of the steel is in accordance with British Standard 4106:1967. The strand does not snap on bending.

DIAMETER; LENGTH; TENSILE STRENGTH; STRENGTH OF NEEDLE ATTACHMENT. It complies with the requirements described under Non-absorbable Surgical Sutures.

ELONGATION. In the determination of tensile strength, the elongation of each strand before it breaks is not less than 30 per cent.

Labelling. The directions given under Non-absorbable Surgical Sutures should be followed.

Sterile Monofilament Stainless Steel Suture

SYNONYM: Sterile Monofilament Surgical Steel

Sterile Monofilament Stainless Steel Suture is Monofilament Stainless Steel Suture which has been subjected to a sterilisation process.

Standard
DESCRIPTION; ELONGATION. It complies with the requirements described under Monofilament Stainless Steel Suture.

DIAMETER; LENGTH; TENSILE STRENGTH; STRENGTH OF NEEDLE ATTACHMENT; STERILITY. It complies with the requirements described under Non-absorbable Surgical Sutures.

Sterilisation. It may be sterilised by autoclaving or by any other suitable method. The bulk and arrangement of the wire must allow complete penetration of the sterilising agent.
The length of wire sterilised should be kept to a minimum in order to minimise the risk of contamination and avoid the need for resterilisation.
If sterilised repeatedly at high temperatures, it may be liable to stress corrosion.

Packaging. The directions given under Non-absorbable Surgical Sutures should be followed; once the container has been opened, any unused suture should be either discarded or resterilised.

Labelling. The directions given under Non-absorbable Surgical Sutures should be followed.

Plaited Stainless Steel Suture

SYNONYMS: Braided Stainless Steel Suture; Plaited Surgical Steel; Braided Surgical Steel

Plaited Stainless Steel Suture consists of a plaited strand of fully softened stainless steel wire.

Standard
DESCRIPTION. A uniformly plaited strand, free from grease. The composition of the steel is in accordance with British Standard 4106:1967. The strand does not snap on bending.

DIAMETER; LENGTH; TENSILE STRENGTH; STRENGTH OF NEEDLE ATTACHMENT. It complies with the requirements described under Non-absorbable Surgical Sutures.

ELONGATION. It complies with the requirements described under Monofilament Stainless Steel Suture.

Labelling. The directions given under Non-absorbable Surgical Sutures should be followed.

Sterile Plaited Stainless Steel Suture

SYNONYMS: Sterile Braided Stainless Steel Suture; Sterile Plaited Surgical Steel; Sterile Braided Surgical Steel

Sterile Plaited Stainless Steel Suture is Plaited Stainless Steel Suture which has been subjected to a sterilisation process.

Standard
DESCRIPTION. It complies with the requirements described under Plaited Stainless Steel Suture, above.

DIAMETER; LENGTH; TENSILE STRENGTH; STRENGTH OF NEEDLE ATTACHMENT; STERILITY. It complies with the requirements described under Non-absorbable Surgical Sutures.

ELONGATION. It complies with the requirements described under Monofilament Stainless Steel Suture.

Sterilisation. It may be sterilised as described under Sterile Monofilament Stainless Steel Suture.

Packaging. The directions given under Sterile Monofilament Stainless Steel Suture should be followed.

Labelling. The directions given under Non-absorbable Surgical Sutures should be followed.

Twisted Stainless Steel Suture

SYNONYM: Twisted Surgical Steel

Twisted Stainless Steel Suture consists of a twisted strand of fully softened stainless steel wire.

Standard
DESCRIPTION. A uniformly and firmly twisted strand, free from grease. The composition of the steel is in accordance with British Standard 4106:1967. The strand does not snap on bending.

DIAMETER; LENGTH; TENSILE STRENGTH; STRENGTH OF NEEDLE ATTACHMENT. It complies with the requirements described under Non-absorbable Surgical Sutures.

ELONGATION. It complies with the requirements described under Monofilament Stainless Steel Suture.

Labelling. The directions given under Non-absorbable Surgical Sutures should be followed.

Sterile Twisted Stainless Steel Suture

SYNONYM: Sterile Twisted Surgical Steel

Sterile Twisted Stainless Steel Suture is Twisted Stainless Steel Suture which has been subjected to a sterilisation process.

Standard
DESCRIPTION. It complies with the requirements described under Twisted Stainless Steel Suture.

DIAMETER; LENGTH; TENSILE STRENGTH; STRENGTH OF NEEDLE ATTACHMENT; STERILITY. It complies with the requirements described under Non-absorbable Surgical Sutures.

ELONGATION. It complies with the requirements described under Monofilament Stainless Steel Suture.

Sterilisation. It may be sterilised as described under Sterile Monofilament Stainless Steel Suture.

Packaging. The directions given under Sterile Monofilament Stainless Steel Suture should be followed.

Labelling. The directions given under Non-absorbable Surgical Sutures should be followed.

PART 5

Surgical Dressings

SURGICAL DRESSINGS

The monographs in this section provide standards for a number of surgical dressings and for fibres and fabrics used in their preparation. Information is given on their uses, packaging, labelling, and sterilisation. The monographs are arranged in the following groups:

Rayon. Where "rayon" is specified in the following monographs it means Regenerated Cellulose or Delustred Regenerated Cellulose.

Rubber. Where "rubber" is specified in the following monographs it means natural rubber.

Medicated dressings. Those surgical dressings that are permitted or required in a particular monograph to contain a suitable antiseptic shall be impregnated so as to contain about 0·1 per cent of either aminacrine hydrochloride or chlorhexidine hydrochloride (or an equivalent amount of the gluconate), or about 0·15 per cent of either domiphen bromide or euflavine.

Dyed dressings. Those surgical dressings that are permitted or required in a particular monograph to be dyed shall be impregnated with a suitable non-toxic dye; the choice of dye is not restricted to one that is permitted for colouring food.

Sterilisation. Methods suitable for the sterilisation of surgical dressings are given in Appendix 29 (page 926). Any other method of sterilisation may be used, provided that the sterilised dressing complies with the test for sterility of surgical dressings given in Appendix 28 (page 917) and with all the other requirements of the standard, except that a sterilised dressing may be slightly less white than an unsterilised dressing.

Standards and testing. In the absence of specific directions in the monographs, the methods described in Appendix 27 (page 912) are used in the examination of surgical dressings for adhesiveness, area per unit weight, sulphated ash, colour fastness, elasticity, extensibility, foreign matter, sterility, tensile strength, threads per stated length, water-soluble extractive, water-vapour permeability, waterproofness, weight per unit area, weight of fabric, weight of film, weight of adhesive mass, and content of antiseptic.

Unless otherwise stated, all weights, counts, and tensile strengths given in the standards refer to those obtained under standard atmospheric conditions of 63 to 67 per cent relative humidity and 18° to 22°.

Yarn Counts. Yarn counts are now specified in U.K. TEX Equivalents; English yarn counts given afterwards in parentheses are for information only. The TEX count is the weight, in grams, of 1 kilometre (1000 metres) of yarn. The U.K. TEX Equivalent is a rounded number, which involves the use of decimals in the medium and fine counts ranges, sufficiently close to the TEX number to satisfy normal commercial tolerances; these equivalents differ from the range of selected TEX numbers recommended by the International Organisation for Standardisation because there are insufficient ISO rounded numbers to accommodate all the counts available in the present range of English cotton counts.

Foreign matter and added foreign matter. Foreign matter is regarded as being made up of the natural impurities of a material, together with residues of any substances used in its processing. Added foreign matter includes any substances not specifically permitted in the monograph but excluding foreign matter as defined here.

The requirement in a number of monographs that the foreign matter does not exceed 1·0 per cent and that the dressing contains no added foreign matter is intended to allow the presence of traces of natural impurities and textile finishing materials, but to exclude the presence of unauthorised substances, for example, wetting agents, starches, filling materials, and antiseptics; in monographs where such additives are permissible the limit for foreign matter is higher.

Absorbency. The initial absorbency of surgical dressings is generally lost or much diminished after long storage or exposure to heat or damp. When stored under suitable conditions in temperate climates there is usually little loss of absorbency within two years of the date of manufacture, but occasionally the loss is more rapid. Repeated sterilisation by autoclaving is likely to impair the absorbency of some materials, particularly cotton.

Packaging. A *well-closed package* protects the contents from contamination with extraneous solids and does not allow the contents to be released unintentionally under normal conditions of handling, storage, and transport.

A *sealed package* is a well-closed package which is sealed in such a manner that the seal must be broken, and be seen to be broken, before the contents are used; the seal is not replaceable. In addition, if the product is labelled "sterile", the package must also exclude micro-organisms.

Unless otherwise specified in a particular monograph, all dressings must be packed in well-closed packages. Special considerations applicable to sterile surgical dressings are given in Appendix 29 (page 926).

Packaging materials must be sufficiently strong to withstand normal handling, storage, and transport.

Labelling. The label on the outer wrapper of a package of a sterile surgical dressing states: "Sterile. This package shall not be issued nor the contents used if the wrapper(s) or seal is broken". In addition, if the inner wrapper encloses more than one dressing which are all intended to be used only on the occasion when the package is first opened, the label on the outer wrapper also states: "Unused contents should be discarded as non-sterile".

Storage. Surgical dressings should be stored in a cool, dry, well-ventilated place. Special storage requirements are indicated in certain monographs.

BANDAGES

Calico Bandage, Triangular

Triangular Calico Bandage consists of a triangular-shaped piece of unbleached calico.

Standard
DESCRIPTION. A piece of unbleached calico, which complies with the standard for Unbleached Calico, page 635, in the shape of a right-angled isosceles triangle; the warp and weft threads of the cloth are parallel with the two equal sides of the triangle.

Uses. Triangular calico bandage is used as a sling. If the bandage is likely to be in contact with areas of broken skin, it should be sterilised before use.

Cotton and Rubber Elastic Bandage

SYNONYM: Cotton Elastic Bandage

Cotton and Rubber Elastic Bandage consists of characteristic fabric of plain weave, in which the warp threads are of cotton and combined cotton and rubber yarn and the weft threads are of cotton.

Standard
DESCRIPTION. Characteristic fabric of plain weave, in one continuous length containing no joins, clean, reasonably free from weaving defects, cotton leaf and shell, and having fast edges. It may be dyed flesh colour with a suitable non-toxic dye.

YARN. A uniform, good medium grade.

FABRIC. The warp threads consist of singles cotton threads and combined rubber and cotton threads:
Cotton threads consist of cotton yarn of a count not finer than 13·4 tex (44's).
Combined cotton and rubber threads consist of two threads spirally folded, each of these threads being composed of one rubber thread and two singles cotton threads. The unstretched threads have a finished resultant count, after final spiral folding, not finer than 98·4 tex (6's) and contain not less than 8 turns per cm in the final spirally folded yarn.

They are arranged as follows: one cotton and rubber thread, four singles cotton threads, repeated, ending with one cotton and rubber thread.

The fast edges may be formed of one cotton thread woven between two combined rubber and cotton threads; the cotton thread, which consists of twofold, threefold, or fourfold yarns with a resultant count of 39·4 tex (15's), has a weaving crimp of about 500 per cent, and the combined rubber and cotton threads are similar to those used in the body of the bandage. Other types of fast edge may be used.

The weft threads consist of singles cotton threads of a count not finer than 11·8 tex (50's).

THREADS PER STATED LENGTH. Warp: average not less than 17·5 singles threads and not less than 4·5 combined threads per cm, determined by counting the total numbers of each type of thread in the warp and dividing by the width, in cm, of the unstretched bandage.

Weft: average not less than 15 per cm, determined on the fully stretched bandage.

WEIGHT PER UNIT AREA. Not less than 70 g per m², calculated from the unstretched width and the fully stretched length.

ELASTICITY. The fully stretched length is not less than twice the unstretched length and the regain length is not more than three-fifths of the fully stretched length.

FOREIGN MATTER. Not more than 1·0 per cent; contains no added foreign matter.

Labelling. If the bandage is dyed, the colour is stated on the label.

Uses. Cotton and rubber elastic bandage has the uses described under Crêpe Bandage (page 613).

Cotton and Rubber Elastic Net Bandage

SYNONYM: Cotton and Elastic Net Bandage

Cotton and Rubber Elastic Net Bandage consists of characteristic fabric of lace construction, in which the warp threads are of combined cotton and rubber yarn and the bobbin threads are of cotton.

Standard

DESCRIPTION. Characteristic net fabric of lace construction, in one continuous length containing no joins, clean, and reasonably free from weaving defects, cotton leaf and shell. The construction is such that the bandage is elastic in both the width and the length. It may be dyed flesh colour with a suitable non-toxic dye.

YARN. A uniform high grade.

FABRIC. The warp threads consist of combined cotton and rubber yarn of two singles cotton yarns twisted together with a rubber thread; the diameter of the rubber thread is not less than 0·020 cm. The unstretched combined threads have a finished resultant count, after final spiral folding, not finer than 90·8 tex (6½'s) and contain not less than 23 turns per cm in the final spirally folded yarn.

The bobbin threads consist of normal twofold well-mercerised cotton yarn with a finished resultant count, after doubling, not finer than 19·6 tex (2/60's).

THREADS PER STATED LENGTH. Warp: average not less than 8·6 per cm, determined by counting the total number of threads in the warp and dividing by the width, in cm, of the unstretched bandage.

MESHES. Not less than 8 per cm along the length of the unstretched bandage.

WEIGHT PER UNIT AREA. Not less than 140 g per m², calculated on the unstretched bandage.

ELASTICITY. The fully stretched width and length are not less than twice the unstretched width and length, respectively. The regain width is not more than three-fifths of the fully stretched width and the regain length is not more than one-half of the fully stretched width.

FOREIGN MATTER. Not more than 1·0 per cent; contains no added foreign matter.

Labelling. If the bandage is dyed, the colour is stated on the label.

Uses. Cotton and rubber elastic net bandage has the uses described under Crêpe Bandage (page 613).

Cotton Conforming Bandage

Cotton Conforming Bandage consists of cotton cloth of plain weave, suitably treated in order to impart elasticity in both the weft and warp directions. Two types of cotton conforming bandage are available.

Standard for Type A

DESCRIPTION. Cotton cloth of plain weave, bleached to a good white, in one continuous length containing no joins, clean, and reasonably free from weaving defects, cotton leaf and shell. The edges are evenly cut parallel to the warp threads and folded over.

YARN. A uniform, good medium grade.

THREADS PER STATED LENGTH. Warp: not less than 11·5 per cm.
Weft: not less than 57 per 10 cm.
Both measurements are made on the bandage stretched in the warp direction by application of a force of 1 kgf per 2·5-cm width.

WEIGHT PER UNIT AREA. Not less than 24 g per m², calculated from the unstretched width and the length stretched by application of a force of 1 kgf per 2·5-cm width.

EXTENSIBILITY. The fully stretched width and length are not less than 1¼ times the unstretched width and length respectively, the extension being measured on application of a force of 1 kgf per 2·5-cm width.

FLUORESCENCE. Examine under ultraviolet radiation, including radiation of wavelength 365 nm; not more than an occasional point of fluorescence is visible (absence of fluorescent brightening agents).

Standard for Type B

DESCRIPTION; YARN; EXTENSIBILITY; FLUORESCENCE. It complies with the Standard for Type A given above.

THREADS PER STATED LENGTH. Warp: not less than 84 per 10 cm.
Weft: not less than 52 per 10 cm.
Both measurements are made on the bandage stretched in the warp direction by application of a force of 1 kgf per 2·5-cm width.

WEIGHT PER UNIT AREA. Not less than 30 g per m², calculated from the unstretched width and the length stretched by application of a force of 1 kgf per 2·5-cm width.

Labelling. The type of bandage is stated on the label.

Uses. Cotton conforming bandage is used to protect dressings and hold them in place.

Cotton Crêpe Bandage

Cotton Crêpe Bandage consists of characteristic fabric of plain weave, in which the warp threads are of cotton and the weft threads are of cotton or rayon or of combined cotton and rayon yarn.

Standard

DESCRIPTION. Characteristic fabric of plain weave, in one continuous length containing no joins, clean, reasonably free from weaving defects, cotton leaf and shell, and having fast edges. It may be dyed flesh colour with a suitable non-toxic dye.
The width is that portion between and including the fast edges of the unstretched bandage.

YARN. A uniform, good medium grade.

FABRIC. The warp threads consist of twofold cotton threads with a finished count, after crêpe-twisting, not finer than 45·4 tex (2/26's) and containing not less than 17 folding turns per cm; they are arranged as follows: two threads S-twist and two threads Z-twist, repeated.
The weft threads consist of cotton or rayon staple fibre, or cotton and rayon staple fibre spun together, with a count not finer than 69·4 tex (8·5's).

THREADS PER STATED LENGTH. Warp: average not less than 17 per cm, determined by counting the total number of threads in the warp and dividing by the width, in cm, of the unstretched bandage.
Weft: average not less than 78 per 10 cm, determined on the fully stretched bandage.

WEIGHT PER UNIT AREA. Not less than 140 g per m², calculated from the unstretched width and the fully stretched length.

ELASTICITY. The regain length is not more than four-fifths of the fully stretched length.

FOREIGN MATTER. Not more than 1·0 per cent; contains no added foreign matter.

Labelling. If the bandage is dyed, the colour is stated on the label.

Uses. Cotton crêpe bandage is used in the treatment of sprains and strains and in other conditions in which light support is required;

it may be used for this purpose in conjunction with other surgical appliances. It is also used for correctional purposes.

Much of the elasticity of the bandage is lost during use, but it can be largely restored by washing the bandage in hot soapy water.

Cotton Stretch Bandage

Cotton Stretch Bandage consists of characteristic fabric of plain weave, in which both the warp and weft threads are of cotton.

Standard

DESCRIPTION. Characteristic fabric of plain weave, in one continuous length containing no joins, clean, reasonably free from weaving defects, cotton leaf and shell, and having fast edges. It may be dyed flesh colour with a suitable non-toxic dye.

The width is that portion between and including the fast edges of the unstretched bandage.

YARN. A uniform, good medium grade.

FABRIC. The warp threads consist of singles cotton threads with a finished count not finer than 59·0 tex (10's) and twofold cotton threads with a finished count, after crêpe-twisting, not finer than 59·0 tex (2/20's), each containing not less than 21 folding turns per cm. They are arranged as follows: one twofold thread (S-twist), one singles thread, one twofold thread (Z-twist), one singles thread, repeated, together with two twofold binding threads at each cut edge.

The weft threads consist of singles cotton threads of a count not finer than 29·6 tex (20's).

THREADS PER STATED LENGTH. Warp: average not less than 6 singles threads and not less than 6 twofold threads per cm, determined by counting the total numbers of each type of thread in the warp and dividing by the width, in cm, of the unstretched bandage.

Weft: average not less than 80 per 10 cm, determined on the fully stretched bandage.

WEIGHT PER UNIT AREA. Not less than 105 g per m², calculated from the unstretched width and the fully stretched length.

ELASTICITY. The fully stretched length is not less than twice the unstretched length and the regain length not more than two-thirds of the fully stretched length.

FOREIGN MATTER. Not more than 1·0 per cent; contains no added foreign matter.

Labelling. If the bandage is dyed, the colour is stated on the label.

Uses. Cotton stretch bandage is used to protect dressings and hold them in place and to give support and, if necessary, immobilisation. In use, there is less likelihood of this bandage slipping than there is with open-wove bandage.

Crêpe Bandage

Crêpe Bandage consists of characteristic fabric of plain weave, in which the warp threads are of cotton and of wool and the weft threads are of cotton.

Standard

DESCRIPTION. Characteristic fabric of plain weave, in one continuous length containing no joins, clean, reasonably free from weaving defects, cotton leaf and shell, and having fast edges. It may be dyed flesh colour with a suitable non-toxic dye.

The width is that portion between and including the fast edges of the unstretched bandage.

YARN. A uniform, good medium grade.

FABRIC. The warp threads consist of twofold cotton threads with a finished count, after crêpe twisting, not finer than 59·0 tex (2/20's), each containing not less than 21 folding turns per cm, and wool threads with a count not coarser than 35·0 tex (25's worsted count) and not finer than 30·0 tex (30's worsted count), or equivalent twofold threads with the same resultant count. They are arranged as follows: one twofold cotton thread (S-twist), two wool threads, one twofold cotton thread (Z-twist), two wool threads, repeated, together with two twofold cotton binding threads at each cut edge.

The weft threads consist of singles cotton thread with a count not finer than 29·6 tex (20's).

THREADS PER STATED LENGTH. Warp: average not less than 6 cotton threads and not less than 12 wool threads per cm, determined by counting the total number of each type of thread in the warp and dividing by the width, in cm, of the unstretched bandage.

Weft: average not less than 10 per cm, determined on the fully stretched bandage.

WEIGHT PER UNIT AREA. Not less than 115 g per m², calculated from the unstretched width and the fully stretched length.

ELASTICITY. The fully stretched length is not less than twice the unstretched length and the regain length is not more than two-thirds of the fully stretched length.

FOREIGN MATTER. Not more than 1·0 per cent; contains no added foreign matter.

CONTENT OF WOOL. Not less than 33·3 per cent, all contained in the warp, determined by the following method:

Place an accurately weighed quantity of the dried extracted sample from the determination of foreign matter in a beaker containing 250 ml of boiling *dilute sodium hydroxide solution*, boil for 10 minutes, decant the liquid through a No. 150 sieve, and return any loose threads or fibres from the sieve to the beaker; add a further 250 ml of the sodium hydroxide solution, and repeat the process.

Wash the residue with water until free from alkali, passing all the washings through the sieve, combine any loose threads or fibres on the sieve with the residue, and dry to constant weight at 105°.

To the weight of residue add 4 per cent to allow for the loss of natural constituents of the cotton; the weight thus obtained is that of the dry cotton and the difference between this weight and that of the dried extracted sample taken is the weight of dry wool.

To the weights of dry cotton and dry wool add allowances for moisture regain of 8·5 and 16 per cent, respectively, and hence calculate the percentage of wool.

Labelling. If the bandage is dyed, the colour is stated on the label.

Uses. Crêpe bandage is used in the treatment of sprains and strains and in other conditions in which light support is required; it may be used for this purpose in conjunction with other surgical appliances. It is also used for correctional purposes and as a compression bandage.

Much of the elasticity of the bandage is lost during use, but it can be largely restored by washing the bandage in hot soapy water.

Domette Bandage

Domette Bandage consists of union fabric of plain weave, in which the warp threads are of cotton and the weft threads are of wool.

Standard

DESCRIPTION. Union fabric of plain weave, in one continuous length containing no joins, clean, and reasonably free from weaving defects, cotton leaf and shell; the edges are evenly cut, parallel with the warp threads, and are reasonably free from loose threads.

YARN. A uniform, good medium grade.

FABRIC. The warp threads are of cotton and the weft threads are of wool.

THREADS PER STATED LENGTH. Warp: average not less than 15 per cm.
Weft: average not less than 86 per 10 cm.

WEIGHT PER UNIT AREA. Not less than 100 g per m².

FOREIGN MATTER. Not more than 2·0 per cent.

CONTENT OF WOOL. Not less than 66·6 per cent, determined by the method for Crêpe Bandage, page 613.

Uses. Domette bandage is used for orthopaedic purposes, especially in cases where a high degree of warmth, protection, and support is required; these qualities are provided by the heavy wool weft.

Open-wove Bandage

SYNONYMS: White Open-wove Bandage; Cambric Bandage

Open-wove Bandage consists of cotton cloth of plain weave.

Standard

DESCRIPTION. Cotton cloth of plain weave, bleached to a good white, in one continuous length containing no joins, clean, and reasonably free from weaving defects, leaf, and shell; the edges are evenly cut, parallel with the warp threads, and are reasonably free from loose threads.

YARN. A uniform, good medium grade. The warp yarn has a bleached count not finer than 14·8 tex (40's) and not coarser than 17·8 tex (33's).

THREADS PER STATED LENGTH. Warp: average 17·1 per cm; standard deviation 0·55.
Weft: average 10·7 per cm; standard deviation 0·25.

WEIGHT PER UNIT AREA. Average 71 g per m²; standard deviation 2·5.

FOREIGN MATTER. Not more than 1·5 per cent.

FLUORESCENCE. Examine under ultraviolet radiation, including radiation of wavelength 365 nm; not more than an occasional point of fluorescence is visible (absence of fluorescent brightening agents).

Uses. Open-wove bandage is used to protect dressings and hold them in place and to give support and, if necessary, immobilisation; the heavy weft gives added protection in the form of bulk and better gripping between layers of the bandage. When applied wet, allowance should be made for possible shrinkage. It is also used to secure splints.

Plaster of Paris Bandage

SYNONYM: Plaster of Paris Dressing

Plaster of Paris Bandage consists of cotton cloth impregnated with dried calcium sulphate, consisting of a mixture of the amorphous and crystalline forms, and suitable adhesives so that the calcium sulphate is adherent to the fabric. The setting time of the bandage may be varied by the incorporation of various modifiers.

Standard

DESCRIPTION. Cotton cloth impregnated with dried calcium sulphate and suitable adhesives; the cotton cloth is of gauze (leno) weave, in one continuous length containing no joins, bleached to a good white, clean, and reasonably free from weaving defects, leaf, and shell. The bandage is reasonably free from loose powder.

THREADS PER STATED LENGTH. Warp: average not less than 15 per cm.
Weft: average not less than 75 per 10 cm.

WEIGHT PER UNIT AREA. Not less than 340 g per m².

WEIGHT OF FABRIC. Not less than 26 g per m², determined by the following method:
Take about 25 g of the bandage and measure its area.
Wash the sample thoroughly with cold water, wringing the material by hand after each washing and passing all the washings through a fine sieve.
Remove any remaining foreign matter from the combined extracted material and any loose threads or fibres from the sieve by treatment similar to that described for the determination of foreign matter in Appendix 27, page 914, and dry the extracted material at 105°.
To the weight of the dried material, add 8·5 per cent to allow for moisture regain, and hence, from the area of the original sample, calculate the weight of fabric in g per m².

TIME OF SETTING. Loosely roll a strip of the bandage about 5 cm wide and weighing about 20 g, and immerse it for 15 seconds in 100 ml of water at 30° in a cylindrical vessel about 5 cm in diameter.
Remove the sample from the water without squeezing, allow to drain for 10 seconds, and wind on a glass rod, or smooth mandrel of non-absorbent material, about 1 cm in diameter; the bandage sets within 8 minutes of removal from the water.
After setting, remove the glass rod or mandrel; the test specimen does not crumble under pressure of the fingers.

CONTENT OF CALCIUM SULPHATE. Not less than 85·0 per cent, calculated as $CaSO_4,\frac{1}{2}H_2O$, determined by the following methods:
(i) Weigh accurately about 5 g of the bandage, taking care to avoid loss of any loosely adherent material, ignite in a platinum or silica dish at 500° to 600° until the residue is white, cool, and weigh.
Weigh accurately about 0·5 g of the ash and dissolve in the minimum amount of *dilute hydrochloric acid*. Remove any silica, iron, and aluminium, and finally precipitate the calcium as oxalate by the usual gravimetric procedure.
Filter, and wash the residue with a 0·2 per cent w/v solution of *ammonium oxalate* in water until free from chloride; transfer the residue and paper to a tared platinum crucible, moisten thoroughly with *dilute sulphuric acid*, and heat carefully, finally burning the paper; cool, add sufficient *sulphuric acid* to saturate the residue thoroughly, and heat to remove the excess of acid; ignite at 800°, cool, and weigh; each g of residue is equivalent to 1·066 g of $CaSO_4,\frac{1}{2}H_2O$.
(ii) Weigh accurately about 0·25 g of the ash prepared in (i) above, dissolve in *dilute hydrochloric acid* containing a little *bromine*, boil, and filter to remove any insoluble matter; dilute the filtrate to 250 ml with water, boil, and add, dropwise, with stirring, 30 ml of a 4 per cent w/v solution of *barium chloride* in water.
Heat on a water-bath for at least 2 hours or until the precipitate has settled and filter through a prepared and ignited Gooch crucible; wash the residue with hot water until the washings are free from chloride, dry, and ignite at 900° to constant weight; each g of residue is equivalent to 0·6216 g of $CaSO_4,\frac{1}{2}H_2O$.

Packaging. It should be enclosed in containers which prevent access of moisture and damage by pressure.

Uses. Plaster of Paris bandage is used for the immobilisation and splinting of fractures and for the construction of rest splints and body supports. In orthopaedic surgery it is used for immobilisation, support, and correction splinting.

In order to reduce the possibility of infecting wounds under the bandage, care should be taken that only clean water is used to wet the bandage before its application. It should be realised that bacteria can pass through the applied bandage while it is still moist and, to a lesser extent, after it has dried.

Zinc Paste and Coal Tar Bandage

Zinc Paste and Coal Tar Bandage consists of open-wove cotton cloth impregnated with a paste containing zinc oxide and prepared coal tar.

Standard

DESCRIPTION. Cotton cloth impregnated evenly with a paste containing zinc oxide and 3·0 per cent w/w of Prepared Coal Tar. The paste may have the following composition:
Zinc Oxide 150 g, Prepared Coal Tar 30 g, Wool Fat 20 g, Emulsifying Wax 100 g, and water to 1000 g.

FABRIC; YARN; THREADS PER STATED LENGTH; WEIGHT OF FABRIC; WEIGHT OF PASTE. It complies with the requirements described under Zinc Paste Bandage.

CONTENT OF ZINC OXIDE IN THE PASTE. Not less than 6·0 per cent, calculated as ZnO, determined by the following method:
Ignite about 6 g of the bandage until all the carbon is removed, cool the residue, dissolve in 30 ml of *dilute nitric acid*, and dilute to 250 ml with water.
Neutralise 50 ml of this solution to *litmus paper* with *dilute ammonia solution*, add 5 ml of *ammonia buffer solution* and 100 ml of water, and titrate with 0·05M disodium edetate, using *mordant black 11 solution* as indicator; each ml of 0·05M disodium edetate is equivalent to 0·004068 g of ZnO.
The weight of paste taken in this determination is calculated as described in Appendix 27, page 916, under "Weight of adhesive mass" for weight of adhesive mass taken.

Packaging. It should be enclosed in sealed packages which prevent the passage of moisture.

Uses. Zinc paste and coal tar bandage is used in the treatment of skin disorders arising as a complication of leg ulcers and of other skin affections such as neurodermatitis, prurigo, verrucous lichen planus of the legs, and infantile, seborrhoeal, and chronic vesicular eczemas.

Zinc Paste and Ichthammol Bandage

Zinc Paste and Ichthammol Bandage consists of open-wove cotton cloth impregnated with a paste containing zinc oxide and ichthammol.

Standard

DESCRIPTION. Cotton cloth impregnated evenly with a paste containing zinc oxide and 2·0 per cent w/w of Ichthammol. The paste may have the following composition:
Zinc Oxide 62·5 g, Ichthammol 20 g, Gelatin 94 g, Glycerol 374 g, Sodium Propyl Hydroxybenzoate 0·6 g, and water to 1000 g.

FABRIC; YARN; THREADS PER STATED LENGTH; WEIGHT OF FABRIC; WEIGHT OF PASTE. It complies with the requirements described under Zinc Paste Bandage.

CONTENT OF ZINC OXIDE IN THE PASTE. Not less than 6·0 per cent, calculated as ZnO, determined by the method for Zinc Paste and Coal Tar Bandage.

Packaging. It should be enclosed in sealed packages which prevent the passage of moisture.

Uses. Zinc paste and ichthammol bandage is used in the treatment of leg ulcers, varicose eczemas, and chronic dermatitis.

Zinc Paste Bandage

Zinc Paste Bandage consists of open-wove cotton cloth impregnated with a paste containing zinc oxide.

Standard

DESCRIPTION. Cotton cloth impregnated evenly with a paste containing zinc oxide. The paste may have the following composition:
Zinc Oxide 180 g, Gelatin 160 g, Glycerol 255 g, Calcium Chloride (dihydrate) 115 g, Boric Acid 20 g, and water to 1000 g.

FABRIC. The cotton cloth is of plain weave, bleached to a good white, in one continuous length containing no joins, clean, and reasonably free from weaving defects, leaf, and shell; the edges are parallel to the warp threads, reasonably free from long loose threads, and may be serrated to prevent fraying.

YARN. A uniform, good medium grade. The warp and weft yarns have counts not finer than 14·8 tex (40's) and 24·6 tex (24's) respectively.

THREADS PER STATED LENGTH. Warp: average not less than 12 per cm.
Weft: average not less than 78 per 10 cm.

WEIGHT OF FABRIC. Not less than 42 g per m², determined by the following method:
Take about 10 g of the bandage, accurately weighed, and measure its area; boil the sample with water until the soluble ingredients of the mass have completely dissolved and the insoluble ingredients have become loosened, add sufficient *dilute hydrochloric acid* to remove any adhering zinc oxide, and decant the liquid through a No. 150 sieve; transfer the residual material to the sieve, wash thoroughly, and dry to constant weight at 105°.
To the weight of the dried material add 8·5 per cent to allow for moisture regain and hence, from the area of the original sample, calculate the weight of fabric in g per m².
In bandages with a serrated edge, allowance is made for the area of serration.

WEIGHT OF PASTE. Not less than 175 g per m², determined as described in Appendix 27, page 916, for weight of adhesive mass.
In bandages with a serrated edge, allowance is made for the area of serration.

CONTENT OF ZINC OXIDE IN THE PASTE. Not less than 6·0 per cent, calculated as ZnO, determined by the following method:
Boil about 6 g of the bandage, accurately weighed, with 150 ml of water for 5 minutes, add 30 ml of *dilute nitric acid*, decant the liquid on to a Buchner funnel, and wash the material and the filter with warm water until the washings are free from nitrate; evaporate the combined filtrate and washings to 200 ml, cool, and dilute to 250 ml with water.
To 50 ml of the solution add 1 g of *ammonium chloride*, 1 g of *ammonium oxalate*, and sufficient *dilute ammonia solution* until the solution is just alkaline to *litmus paper*; add a further 5 ml of *dilute ammonia solution*,

heat to boiling, allow to stand for 1 hour, filter, and wash the residue with hot water.

Dilute the cooled combined filtrate and washings to 150 ml with water, add 5 ml of *ammonia buffer solution*, and titrate with 0·05M disodium edetate, using *mordant black 11 solution* as indicator; each ml of 0·05M disodium edetate is equivalent to 0·004068 g of ZnO.

The weight of paste taken in this determination is calculated as described in Appendix 27, page 916, under "Weight of adhesive mass" for weight of adhesive mass taken.

Packaging. It should be enclosed in sealed packages which prevent the passage of moisture.

Uses. Zinc paste bandage is used to support and prevent the swelling of fractured limbs after the removal of plaster casts and to support varicose veins. It is also used in the treatment of ulcers, varicose eczemas, phlebitis, and oedema of the legs.

ADHESIVE BANDAGES

Adhesive bandages are of two types: self-adhesive bandages, which are normally sticky, and diachylon adhesive bandages, which need to be warmed before application.

This monograph applies to the following adhesive bandages:

> Diachylon Elastic Adhesive Bandage
> Diachylon Elastic Adhesive Bandage, Ventilated
> Zinc Oxide Elastic Self-adhesive Bandage
> Zinc Oxide Elastic Self-adhesive Bandage, Half-spread
> Zinc Oxide Elastic Self-adhesive Bandage, Ventilated

These bandages are unsuitable for extemporaneous preparation. For convenience during use of adhesive bandages, a narrow margin of supporting material may be left unspread along each edge.

Diachylon adhesive bandages are lead-base adhesive bandages and are prepared by spreading diachylon masses, which are plastic or resinous masses having as a basis the reaction products of lead monoxide and vegetable oils or their derivatives, on elastic cloth. In tropical or subtropical climates, the formulation may be varied to meet conditions of temperature, provided that the required proportion of the active ingredients is maintained.

Diachylon adhesive bandages require to be warmed before application to the skin to secure adequate adhesion; the skin should be rendered free from hair and thoroughly dry before the bandage is applied.

Self-adhesive bandages are prepared by spreading a self-adhesive mass upon a supporting material. The constituents of the mass other than specific medicaments should be innocuous to the skin.

Self-adhesive bandages adhere closely to the skin at body temperature and do not require warming before application; the skin should be rendered free from hair and thoroughly dry before the bandage is applied.

Storage. Adhesive bandages should be stored in a dry place below 20°, protected from light and from deleterious vapours or contaminants.

Diachylon Elastic Adhesive Bandage

SYNONYM: Elastic Diachylon Bandage

Diachylon Elastic Adhesive Bandage consists of elastic cloth spread evenly with a diachylon mass.

Standard

DESCRIPTION. Elastic cloth spread evenly with a diachylon mass. The elastic cloth is in one continuous length containing no joins, clean, and reasonably free from weaving defects, cotton leaf and shell; it may be dyed flesh colour with a suitable non-toxic dye.

The diachylon mass consists of lead soaps of the higher fatty acids to which suitable adhesives are added.

FABRIC; THREADS PER STATED LENGTH. It complies with the requirements described under Cotton Crêpe Bandage, page 612.

WEIGHT OF FABRIC. Not less than 140 g per m², calculated from the unstretched width and the fully stretched length.

WEIGHT OF ADHESIVE MASS. Not less than 135 g per m², calculated from the unstretched spread width and the fully stretched length.

ELASTICITY. The regain length is not more than nine-tenths of the fully stretched length.

CONTENT OF LEAD IN THE ADHESIVE MASS. Not less than 26·5 per cent, calculated as PbO, with reference to the mass dried for 3 hours at 105°, determined by the following method:
Extract about 2 g of the bandage with *trichloroethylene* in an apparatus for the continuous extraction of drugs, evaporate the extract to dryness, dry the residue at 105° for 3 hours, and weigh.
To the residue add 40 ml of *acetic acid*, boil until a clear oily layer is obtained, cool, add 40 ml of water, decant through a moistened filter paper, and wash the oily layer with 25 ml of *dilute acetic acid* and then with hot water until about 150 ml of filtrate has been collected.
Boil the filtrate, add, with constant stirring, 25 ml of a 10 per cent w/v solution of *potassium dichromate* in water, heat for 15 minutes on a water-bath, with constant stirring, and filter while hot.
Wash the residue with hot water, then with *alcohol (95 per cent)*, followed by *solvent ether*, and dry to constant weight at 105°; each g of residue is equivalent to 0·6906 g of PbO.

Labelling. If the cloth is dyed, the colour is stated on the label.

Storage. It should be stored as described under Adhesive Bandages (page 616).

Uses. Diachylon elastic adhesive bandage is used in the treatment of chronic leg ulcers in ambulant patients and for the support of varicose veins. It is occasionally used in chiropody for support bandaging when the patient is hypersensitive to extension plaster.

Diachylon Elastic Adhesive Bandage, Ventilated

SYNONYM: Ventilated Elastic Diachylon Bandage

Ventilated Diachylon Elastic Adhesive Bandage consists of elastic cloth spread evenly with a diachylon mass so as to leave strips of unspread fabric along its length.

Standard
DESCRIPTION. Elastic cloth spread evenly with a diachylon mass in a regular manner so that portions of the fabric running along its length are left unspread; the area of the unspread portions, excluding any margin, does not exceed 50 per cent of the total area.
The elastic cloth is in one continuous length containing no joins, clean, and reasonably free from weaving defects, cotton leaf and shell; it may be dyed flesh colour with a suitable non-toxic dye.
The diachylon mass consists of lead soaps of the higher fatty acids to which suitable adhesives are added.

FABRIC; THREADS PER STATED LENGTH. It complies with the requirements described under Cotton Crêpe Bandage, page 612.

WEIGHT OF FABRIC. Not less than 140 g per m², calculated from the unstretched width and the fully stretched length.

WEIGHT OF ADHESIVE MASS. Not less than 135 g per m² on the spread portions, calculated from the unstretched width, the fully stretched length, and the measured spread and unspread areas.

ELASTICITY. The regain length is not more than nine-tenths of the fully stretched length.

CONTENT OF LEAD IN THE ADHESIVE MASS. Not less than 26·5 per cent, calculated as PbO, with reference to the mass dried for 3 hours at 105°, determined by the method for Diachylon Elastic Adhesive Bandage, using about 3 g of the bandage.

Labelling. If the cloth is dyed, the colour is stated on the label.

Storage. It should be stored as described under Adhesive Bandages (page 616).

Uses. Ventilated diachylon elastic adhesive bandage has the uses described under Diachylon Elastic Adhesive Bandage.

Zinc Oxide Elastic Self-adhesive Bandage

SYNONYM: Elastic Adhesive Bandage

Zinc Oxide Elastic Self-adhesive Bandage consists of elastic cloth spread evenly with a self-adhesive plaster mass containing zinc oxide.

Standard
DESCRIPTION. Elastic cloth spread with a self-adhesive plaster mass containing zinc oxide; it must be spread evenly, except that the mass may be made porous or permeable to air.
The elastic cloth is in one continuous length containing no joins, clean, and reasonably free from weaving defects, cotton leaf and shell; it may be dyed flesh colour with a suitable non-toxic dye.

FABRIC; THREADS PER STATED LENGTH; ELASTICITY. It complies with the requirements described under Cotton Crêpe Bandage, page 612.

WEIGHT OF FABRIC. Not less than 140 g per m², calculated from the unstretched width and the fully stretched length.

WEIGHT OF ADHESIVE MASS. Not less than 120 g per m², calculated from the unstretched spread width and the fully stretched length.

CONTENT OF ZINC OXIDE IN THE ADHESIVE MASS. Not less than 10·0 per cent, calculated as ZnO, determined by the method for Zinc Oxide Self-adhesive Plaster, page 633.

Labelling. If the self-adhesive plaster mass is porous, this is stated on the label. If the cloth is dyed, the colour is also stated on the label.

Storage. It should be stored as described under Adhesive Bandages (page 616).

Uses. Zinc oxide elastic self-adhesive bandage is used in the treatment of conditions where support or compression is required, such as fractured ribs and clavicles, swollen or sprained joints, varicose veins, and leg ulcers. It is also used to secure dressings and appliances.

Zinc Oxide Elastic Self-adhesive Bandage, Half-spread

SYNONYMS: Semi-spread Elastic Adhesive Bandage; Half-spread Elastic Adhesive Bandage

Half-spread Zinc Oxide Elastic Self-adhesive Bandage is elastic adhesive bandage with half the width of fabric unspread.

Standard
DESCRIPTION. Elastic cloth spread evenly over half its width with a self-adhesive plaster mass containing zinc oxide; the area of the unspread portion, excluding any margin, does not exceed 50 per cent of the total area.
The elastic cloth is in one continuous length containing no joins, clean, and reasonably free from weaving defects, cotton leaf and shell; it may be dyed flesh colour with a suitable non-toxic dye.

FABRIC; THREADS PER STATED LENGTH; ELASTICITY. It complies with the requirements described under Cotton Crêpe Bandage, page 612.

WEIGHT OF FABRIC. Not less than 140 g per m², calculated from the unstretched width and the fully stretched length.

WEIGHT OF ADHESIVE MASS. Not less than 120 g per m² on the spread portion, calculated from the unstretched width, the fully stretched length, and the measured spread and unspread areas.

CONTENT OF ZINC OXIDE IN THE ADHESIVE MASS. Not less than 10·0 per cent, calculated as ZnO, determined by the method for Zinc Oxide Self-adhesive Plaster, page 633, using about 2 g of the bandage, accurately weighed.

Labelling. If the cloth is dyed, the colour is stated on the label.

Storage. It should be stored as described under Adhesive Bandages (page 616).

Uses. Half-spread zinc oxide self-adhesive bandage has the uses described under Zinc Oxide Elastic Self-adhesive Bandage (page 617).

Zinc Oxide Elastic Self-adhesive Bandage, Ventilated

SYNONYM: Ventilated Elastic Adhesive Bandage

Ventilated Zinc Oxide Elastic Self-adhesive Bandage is elastic adhesive bandage spread so as to leave strips of unspread fabric along its length.

Standard
DESCRIPTION. Elastic cloth spread evenly with a self-adhesive plaster mass containing zinc oxide in a regular manner so that portions of the fabric running along its length are left unspread; the area of the unspread portions, excluding any margins, does not exceed 50 per cent of the total area.
The elastic cloth is in one continuous length containing no joins, clean, and reasonably free from weaving defects, cotton leaf and shell; it may be dyed flesh colour with a suitable non-toxic dye.

FABRIC; THREADS PER STATED LENGTH; ELASTICITY. It complies with the requirements described under Cotton Crêpe Bandage, page 612.

WEIGHT OF FABRIC. Not less than 140 g per m², calculated from the unstretched width and the fully stretched length.

WEIGHT OF ADHESIVE MASS. Not less than 120 g per m² on the spread portions, calculated from the unstretched width, the fully stretched length, and the measured spread and unspread areas.

CONTENT OF ZINC OXIDE IN THE ADHESIVE MASS. Not less than 10·0 per cent, calculated as ZnO, determined by the method for Zinc Oxide Self-adhesive Plaster, page 633, using about 2 g of the bandage, accurately weighed.

Labelling. If the cloth is dyed, the colour is stated on the label.

Storage. It should be stored as described under Adhesive Bandages (page 616).

Uses. Ventilated zinc oxide elastic self-adhesive bandage has the uses described under Zinc Oxide Elastic Self-adhesive Bandage (page 617).

COTTON WOOLS

Absorbent Cotton Wool

SYNONYMS: Absorbent Cotton; Lanugo Gossypii Absorbens

Absorbent Cotton Wool is prepared from cotton, which consists of the epidermal trichomes of the seeds of *Gossypium herbaceum* L. and other cultivated species of *Gossypium* (Fam. Malvaceae).
The seeds are removed mechanically and the trichomes freed from fatty matter by treatment with alkali, bleached, washed, and mechanically loosened and separated to form a fleecy mass of soft white filaments which consist almost entirely of cellulose.
Absorbent Cotton Wool absorbs water readily but its absorbency may be reduced considerably by medication, by prolonged storage, or by exposure to heat. It may be attacked by moulds when stored under conditions where the moisture in the cotton wool exceeds about 9 per cent.

Solubility. Soluble, at 20°, in *sulphuric acid (66 per cent v/v)*. Swollen uniformly by *ammoniacal copper oxide solution* and ultimately dissolved with the exception of the contents of the lumen. Insoluble in *dilute sodium hydroxide solution*.

Standard
Material which complies with this standard will meet the requirements of the European Pharmacopoeia.

DESCRIPTION. *Macroscopical:* well-carded cotton fibres, of average length not less than 10 mm, bleached to a good white, free from pieces of thread and reasonably free from leaf, shell, and foreign matter. It offers appreciable resistance when pulled and does not shed any appreciable quantity of dust when gently shaken. The quality and material is the same throughout. It is odourless or almost odourless. It may be slightly off-white if it has been sterilised.
Microscopical: each trichome consists of a single cell, up to 4 cm in length and 15 to 40 μm in width,

forming a flattened tubular band with slightly thickened rounded edges and showing 50 to 120 twists per cm; the apex is rounded and often solid. It consists exclusively of typical cotton fibres.

IDENTIFICATION TEST. Treat with *iodinated zinc chloride solution*; a violet colour is produced.

NEPS. Spread 1 g evenly between two colourless glass plates, each 10 cm × 10 cm, and examine by transmitted light for neps.
The sample is not more neppy than the European Pharmacopoeia Standard Sample for Neps (obtainable from the Manchester Chamber of Commerce Testing House, 10 Barlow Moor Road, Didsbury, Manchester, M20 0TR, or from The Secretary, European Pharmacopoeia Commission, Strasbourg, France).

ABSORBENCY. Place about 5 g, accurately weighed, taken in approximately equal quantities from five different places in the sample, loosely in a dry cylindrical copper wire basket, 8·0 cm in height, 5·0 cm in diameter, and 2·7 ± 0·3 g in weight, constructed of wire 0·4 mm in diameter and with a mesh 1·5 to 2·0 cm.
Hold the packed basket with its long axis horizontal and drop it from a height of about 10 mm into water at 20° contained in a beaker, 11 to 12 cm in diameter and filled to a depth of 10 cm. Measure with a stopwatch the time taken by the basket to sink below the surface of the water.
Remove the basket from the water, hold it over the the beaker with its long axis horizontal, allow the water to drain for 30 seconds, and transfer the basket to a previously tared beaker and reweigh. Calculate the weight of water retained by each gram of the sample.
Repeat the entire test twice.
Calculate the sinking time and the water-holding capacity as the average of the three tests.
The sinking time is not more than 10 seconds and the water-holding capacity is not less than 23·0 g per gram of sample.

COLOUR OF AQUEOUS EXTRACT. To 10 g add 100 ml of water, allow to stand for 2 hours in a closed vessel, decant, pressing the sample with a glass rod to express the residual liquid, and mix. Reserve 10 ml of the liquid for the test for Surface-active Substances.
Filter the remainder of the liquid; the filtrate does not differ in colour from the water used to prepare the extract. Reserve the filtrate for the test for Acidity or Alkalinity.

ACIDITY OR ALKALINITY. To 25 ml of the filtrate reserved in the test for Colour of Aqueous Extract add 0·15 ml of *phenolphthalein solution*; the solution does not show a pink colour.
To another 25 ml of the filtrate add 0·05 ml of *methyl orange solution*; the solution is yellow.

SURFACE-ACTIVE SUBSTANCES. Shake vigorously in a clean test tube the decanted liquid reserved in the test for Colour of Aqueous Extract and allow to stand for 10 minutes. Not more than a ring of froth, in contact with the walls of the test tube, remains.

WATER-SOLUBLE SUBSTANCES. Not more than 0·50 per cent, determined by the following method:
Boil about 5 g, accurately weighed, with 500 ml of water for 30 minutes, stirring frequently, and replacing the water lost by evaporation. Decant the hot liquid, pressing the sample with a glass rod to express the residual liquid, mix, and filter the liquid while it is still hot.
Evaporate 400 ml of the filtrate (equivalent to four-fifths of the weight of sample taken) to dryness and dry the residue to constant weight at 105°.

ETHER-SOLUBLE SUBSTANCES. Not more than 0·50 per cent, determined by the following method:
Extract about 5 g, accurately weighed, with *solvent ether* for 4 hours in an apparatus for the continuous extraction of drugs or for intermittent extraction, with not less than four extractions per hour; evaporate the extract to dryness and dry the residue to constant weight at 105°.

COLOURING MATTER. Slowly extract 10 g, packed into a narrow percolator, with *alcohol* (*95 per cent*) until 50 ml of extract is obtained and examine a 20-cm layer of the extract against a white background.
The extract is not more than a very faint yellow and has no bluish or greenish tinge.

FLUORESCENCE. Examine a layer, about 5 mm in thickness, under ultraviolet radiation, including radiation of wavelength 365 nm. The sample shows only a slight brownish-violet fluorescence and not more than an occasional yellow particle. It shows no intense blue fluorescence except that which may be shown by a few isolated fibres (absence of fluorescent brightening agents).

LOSS ON DRYING. Not more than 8·0 per cent, determined on 5 g, by drying to constant weight at 105°.

SULPHATED ASH. Not more than 0·40 per cent, determined on 5 g.

STERILITY. If the label on the package states that the material is sterile, the contents comply with the test for sterility described in Appendix 28, page 917.

Sterilisation. It may be sterilised by one of the methods described for surgical dressings in Appendix 29 (page 926) or by any other suitable process.

Packaging. It should be enclosed in either well-closed packages or sealed packages, according to the requirements of the user. Waxed paper should not be used for any wrapping in contact with the cotton wool, as it reduces the absorbency of the material.
If the material is sterile, it should be enclosed in a sealed package and the directions given in Appendix 29, page 926 should be followed; the inner wrapper may enclose a number of pieces or "balls".

Labelling. If the material is supplied sterile, it is labelled as described in the general monograph, page 611.

Uses.
Absorbent cotton wool complying with the requirements in this monograph for staple length and neps is suitable for cleansing and swabbing wounds, for pre-operative skin preparation, and for the application of medicaments to wounds. It is sufficiently resilient to provide an effective pad for use over dressings to protect the wound and for the absorption of fluids. It may be available as small pieces or "balls".
For insertion into orifices such as the ear and nose, for application to the throat and eye, and for the preparation of swabs for taking specimens, it is advisable to use a cotton wool with a longer staple length than is specified in this monograph.
Grades with shorter staple lengths and more neps have less resilience and are more dusty.

Capsicum Cotton Wool

SYNONYM: Capsicum Cotton

Capsicum Cotton Wool consists of absorbent cotton wool impregnated with capsicum oleoresin and methyl salicylate.
It may be prepared by compressing the cotton wool and pouring over it an alcoholic solution of capsicum oleoresin, methyl salicylate, and a suitable dye. The alcoholic solution contains sufficient capsicum oleoresin to give

a product which, when dried, complies with the Standard.

Capsicum Cotton Wool contains, when freshly prepared, about 1 per cent of methyl salicylate.

In making this preparation, the alcohol may be replaced by Industrial Methylated Spirit, provided that the law and statutory regulations governing the use of industrial methylated spirit are observed.

Standard

DESCRIPTION. Cotton wool, which complies with the standard for Absorbent Cotton Wool, impregnated as uniformly as possible with Capsicum Oleoresin and Methyl Salicylate and dyed orange-brown; it has an odour of methyl salicylate.

DESCRIPTION; NEPS; SULPHATED ASH. It complies with the requirements described under Absorbent Cotton Wool.

CONTENT OF CAPSAICIN. 0·030 to 0·070 per cent, determined by the following method:

Transfer about 10 g, accurately weighed, to an apparatus for the continuous extraction of drugs and extract with *dehydrated methyl alcohol* for not less than 6 hours.

Evaporate the extract on a water-bath until the volume is reduced to about 20 ml, cool, dilute to 25 ml with *dehydrated methyl alcohol*, and continue by the method for Capsicum, page 72, beginning with the words "to 10 ml of this solution add 15 ml of *dehydrated methyl alcohol*, . . .".

Packaging. It should be enclosed in sealed packages, doubly wrapped to prevent loss of pungency.

Uses. Capsicum cotton wool is used as a counter-irritant and to produce heat on undamaged skin; it is used in the treatment of rheumatic conditions. The heating effect can be increased by slight moistening.

DRESSINGS

Elastic Adhesive Dressing

Elastic Adhesive Dressing consists of an absorbent pad fixed to extension plaster so as to leave a suitable margin of adhesive; the pad and the adhesive margin are covered by a protector. The dressing may be sterilised.

The pad is medicated with one of the permitted antiseptics specified in the general monograph (page 609) and dyed yellow if necessary with a suitable non-toxic dye; the antiseptic and the dye may be omitted if the dressing is sterile.

Standard

DESCRIPTION. The dressing is one of two types:

Wound dressing is circular, square, or rectangular. The pad is substantially the same shape as the dressing and is fixed as centrally as possible to a piece of plaster, which complies with the standard for Extension Plaster, page 631, except that it may be perforated or ventilated, so as to leave a margin of adhesive surface surrounding the pad.

The width of the adhesive margin is not less than 5 mm or not less than 15 per cent of the overall dimensions of the dressing, whichever is the greater, and the width of the margin on any one side is not less than half the width of the margin on the opposite side.

Rectangular dressings may have an adhesive margin of not less than 1·5 mm on each of one pair of opposite sides, provided that the adhesive margin on each of the other two sides is at least 25 per cent of the overall dimension of the dressing in that direction.

If, for convenience in use of the dressing, the corners of the plaster are cut to a radius, this is ignored in defining the shape and dimensions of the dressing.

The pad and the margin of the adhesive surface are covered by a suitable protector. The pad does not become detached from the plaster when the protector is removed.

Dressing strip is a square or rectangular piece of plaster, which complies with the standard for Extension Plaster, page 631, except that it may be perforated or ventilated, and to which has been fixed a pad of equal length in such a way as to leave adhesive margins on the two sides which are parallel with the warp.

Except in the case of special-purpose dressing strips, the pad is placed as centrally as possible and the width of each adhesive margin is not less than 8 mm or not less than 20 per cent of the overall dimension of

the dressing, whichever is the greater, and the width of the margin on either side is not less than half the width of the margin on the other side.

In the case of special-purpose dressing strips the pad is fixed off-centre, the width of the narrower adhesive margin being between 12 mm and 28 mm and not more than half the width of the wider margin.

The pad and the margins are covered by a suitable protector. The pad does not become detached from the plaster when the protector is removed.

PERFORATIONS. If the plaster is perforated, the perforations are not more than 3 mm in diameter, are regularly distributed, and do not exceed in area 10 per cent of the total area of the dressing.

SPREAD AREA. If the plaster is ventilated, the area of the unspread portion does not exceed 50 per cent of the total area. In calculating the weight of adhesive mass the actual spread area is used.

STERILITY. If the dressing is sterile, it complies with the test for sterility described in Appendix 28, page 917.

Standard for the pad

DESCRIPTION. A piece of suitable absorbent material medicated as uniformly as possible with one of the permitted antiseptics and dyed yellow if necessary with a suitable dye; the medicament and dye may be omitted if the dressing is sterile.

The dimensions of the pad are not less than 33 per cent of the overall dimensions of the dressing, except that in the case of special-purpose dressing strips the width of the pad is not less than 12 mm.

WEIGHT PER UNIT AREA. Not less than 34 g per m².

CONTENT OF ANTISEPTIC. If the pad is medicated, it complies with the requirements given in Appendix 27, page 916.

Sterilisation. It may be sterilised by exposure to ethylene oxide or ionising radiation as described for surgical dressings in Appendix 29 (page 926) or by any other suitable process.

Packaging. If the dressing is sterile, it should be enclosed in an individual sealed package and the directions given in Appendix 29 (page 926) should be followed.

Labelling. The label on the package states:

(1) "Apply to clean dry skin",

(2) "Store in a cool place",

(3) the name and proportion of the medicament, if present, and

(4) whether the dressing is porous, perforated, or ventilated.

If the plaster is dyed, the colour is also stated on the label.

In addition, if the dressing is sterile, it is labelled as described in the general monograph (page 611).

Storage. It should be stored in a dry place at a temperature between 15° and 20°, protected from light and from deleterious vapours and contaminants.

Uses. Elastic adhesive dressing is used as a protective covering for wounds.

Paraffin Gauze Dressing

SYNONYM: Tulle Gras Dressing

Paraffin Gauze Dressing consists of bleached cotton or rayon or combined cotton and rayon cloth impregnated with yellow soft paraffin.

It is prepared by cutting the cloth to the required size, packing into a suitable container, and completely impregnating with a sufficient quantity of yellow soft paraffin.

When the dressing is required for use in tropical or subtropical countries, the yellow soft paraffin may be replaced by a suitable mixture of yellow soft paraffin and hard paraffin.

The dressing may be supplied in single or multiple packs, in pieces or in strip form. It is supplied sterile and it is essential to use a method of sterilisation appropriate to the form of packaging. The material is liable to shrink during sterilisation by heating.

Standard

DESCRIPTION. Bleached cotton or rayon cloth, or combined cotton and rayon cloth, packed with or without interleaving paper and evenly impregnated with Yellow Soft Paraffin. The cloth is of gauze (leno) weave with two picks in each shed.

YARN. A uniform, good medium grade.

THREADS PER STATED LENGTH. Determined on the impregnated cloth: warp, average not less than 75 per 10 cm; weft, average not less than 82 per 10 cm.

WEIGHT OF FABRIC. Not less than 42 g per m², determined by the following method:
Dry the extracted cloth obtained in the test for ether-soluble extractive, condition the dried cloth by exposing it for not less than 12 hours to the standard atmospheric conditions for testing described in Appendix 27, page 913, and reweigh.
Determine the area of the conditioned cloth and hence calculate the weight of fabric in g per m².

ETHER-SOLUBLE EXTRACTIVE. Not less than 200 g per m², determined by the following method:
Condition the dressing in its container by maintaining it at 18° to 22° for not less than 6 hours immediately before testing. By means of forceps, remove the dressing from the container, and transfer it to an apparatus for the continuous extraction of drugs, leaving behind any soft paraffin adhering to the walls of the container.
Extract the dressing with *solvent ether* for 6 hours, or longer if necessary to remove all the ether-soluble extractive, remove the solvent from the extract, and dry the residue to constant weight at 105°.
Remove the extracted cloth from the apparatus, allow the solvent to evaporate, determine the area of the dry cloth, and hence calculate the weight of extractive per m².
If the pack contains two dressings, similarly treat both of them and calculate the average weight of extractive per m² of the two dressings.

If the dressing is in a multiple pack, similarly treat a dressing selected from the top, centre, and bottom of the pile, removing and discarding any interleaving paper, and calculate the average weight of extractive per m² of the three dressings.

STERILITY. It complies with the test for sterility given in Appendix 28, page 917.

Standard for the interleaving paper

When interleaving paper is used, it complies with the following requirements:

BURSTING STRENGTH. Average of 6 tests, not less than 14,060 kgf per m², determined on a Mullen-type Bursting Tester.

WEIGHT PER UNIT AREA. Not less than 70 g per m², determined by extracting a measured area of the paper with *solvent ether* for 6 hours in an apparatus for the continuous extraction of drugs, allowing the solvent to evaporate from the extracted paper, conditioning the dry paper by exposing it for not less than 6 hours to the standard atmospheric conditions for testing described in Appendix 27, page 913, weighing, and calculating the weight in g per m².

Packaging. Each piece is enclosed in a sealed container which will withstand the process of sterilisation and normal handling and prevent the access of microorganisms; alternatively, several dressings, preferably separated by interleaving paper, may be enclosed in the container.

If a metal container is used, it must be sufficiently strong not to distort during normal handling and transport and should preferably be pressed and free from soldered joints; if solder is used, care should be taken to ensure that it is capable of withstanding the temperature of sterilisation.

The edges of the lid of a metal container are covered by means of a continuous strip of suitable adhesive tape and the container is sealed by means of the label or a wrapper covering one or more sides of the container in such a manner that the seal is torn when the tape is removed. If the seal is broken, the package must not be issued.

Labelling. The label on the container states that the dressing is sterile provided that the seal is unbroken and that the package shall not be issued if the seal is broken.

Uses. Paraffin gauze dressing is used in the treatment of wounds, such as burns and scalds, and for skin grafts.

Preferably, the dressing should be taken from a freshly opened pack which contains only a sufficient number of dressings for use on a single occasion. If, however, any dressings in a multiple pack remain unused, they can be resterilised; if they are not resterilised, they must be discarded.

Plastic Wound Dressing, Perforated

SYNONYM: Porous Plastic Dressing

Perforated Plastic Wound Dressing consists of an absorbent pad fixed to perforated plastic self-adhesive plaster so as to leave a margin of adhesive surface surrounding the pad; the pad and adhesive margin are covered with a protector. The dressing may be sterilised.

The pad is medicated with one of the permitted antiseptics specified in the general monograph (page 609) and dyed yellow if necessary with a suitable non-toxic dye; the antiseptic and the dye may be omitted if the dressing is sterile.

Standard

DESCRIPTION. The dressing is circular, square, or rectangular.

The pad is substantially the same shape as the dressing and is fixed as centrally as possible to a piece of plaster, which complies with the standard for Perforated Plastic Self-adhesive Plaster, page 632, so as to leave a margin of adhesive surface surrounding the pad. The width of the adhesive margin is not less than 5 mm or not less than 15 per cent of the overall dimension of the dressing, whichever is the greater, and the width of the margin on any one side is not less than half the width of the margin on the opposite side.

Rectangular dressings may have an adhesive margin of not less than 1·5 mm on each of one pair of opposite sides, provided that the adhesive margin on each of the other two sides is at least 25 per cent of the overall dimension of the dressing in that direction.

If, for convenience in use of the dressing, the corners of the plaster are cut to a radius, this is ignored in defining the shape and dimensions of the dressing.

The pad and the margin of the adhesive surface are covered by a suitable protector. The pad does not become detached from the plaster when the protector is removed.

EXTENSIBILITY. It complies with the test described in Appendix 27, page 914.

STERILITY. If the dressing is sterile, it complies with the test for sterility described in Appendix 28, page 917.

Standard for the pad

DESCRIPTION. It complies with the requirements described under Elastic Adhesive Dressing, page 620, except that the statement relating to special-purpose dressing strips is not applicable.

WEIGHT PER UNIT AREA; CONTENT OF ANTISEPTIC. It complies with the requirements described under Elastic Adhesive Dressing, page 620.

Sterilisation. It may be sterilised by exposure to ethylene oxide or ionising radiation as described for surgical dressings in Appendix 29 (page 926) or by any other suitable process.

Packaging. It is packed as described under Elastic Adhesive Dressing (page 620).

Labelling. It is labelled as described under Elastic Adhesive Dressing (page 620).

Storage. It should be stored as described under Elastic Adhesive Dressing (page 620).

Uses. Perforated plastic wound dressing is used as a protective covering for wounds when complete permeability is required.

Plastic Wound Dressing, Waterproof

SYNONYM: Occlusive Plastic Dressing

Waterproof Plastic Wound Dressing consists of an absorbent pad fixed to waterproof plastic self-adhesive plaster so as to leave a margin of adhesive surface surrounding the pad; the pad and adhesive margin are covered with a protector. The dressing may be sterilised.

The pad is medicated with one of the permitted antiseptics specified in the general monograph (page 609) and dyed yellow if necessary with a suitable non-toxic dye; the antiseptic and the dye may be omitted if the dressing is sterile.

Standard

DESCRIPTION. The dressing is circular, square, or rectangular.

The pad is substantially the same shape as the dressing and is fixed as centrally as possible to a piece of plaster,

which complies with the standard for Waterproof Plastic Self-adhesive Plaster, page 633, so as to leave a margin of adhesive surface surrounding the pad.

The width of the adhesive margin is not less than 3 mm, or not less than 10 per cent of the overall dimension of the dressing, whichever is the greater, and the width of the margin on any one side is not less than half the width of the margin on the opposite side.

If, for convenience in use of the dressing, the corners of the plaster are cut to a radius, this is ignored in defining the shape and dimensions of the dressing.

The pad and the margin of adhesive surface are covered by a suitable protector. The pad does not become detached from the plaster when the protector is removed.

EXTENSIBILITY. It complies with the test described in Appendix 27, page 914.

STERILITY. If the dressing is sterile, it complies with the test for sterility described in Appendix 28, page 917.

Standard for the pad

DESCRIPTION. It complies with the requirements described under Elastic Adhesive Dressing, page 620, except that the statement relating to special-purpose dressing strips is not applicable.

WEIGHT PER UNIT AREA; CONTENT OF ANTISEPTIC. It complies with the requirements described under Elastic Adhesive Dressing, page 620.

Sterilisation. It may be sterilised by exposure to ethylene oxide or ionising radiation as described for surgical dressings in Appendix 29 (page 926) or by any other suitable process.

Packaging. It is packed as described under Elastic Adhesive Dressing (page 620).

Labelling. It is labelled as described under Elastic Adhesive Dressing (page 620).

Storage. It should be stored as described under Elastic Adhesive Dressing (page 620).

Uses. Waterproof plastic wound dressing is used as a protective covering for wounds when an occlusive dressing is required.

Plastic Wound Dressing, Waterproof Microporous

SYNONYMS: Microporous Plastic Dressing; Semipermeable Plastic Dressing

Waterproof Microporous Plastic Wound Dressing consists of an absorbent pad fixed to waterproof microporous plastic self-adhesive plaster so as to leave a margin of adhesive surface surrounding the pad; the pad and adhesive margin are covered with a protector. The dressing may be sterilised.

The pad is medicated with one of the permitted antiseptics specified in the general monograph (page 609) and dyed yellow if necessary with a suitable non-toxic dye; the antiseptic and the dye may be omitted if the dressing is sterile.

Standard

DESCRIPTION. The dressing is circular, square, or rectangular.

The pad is substantially the same shape as the dressing and is fixed as centrally as possible to a piece of plaster, which complies with the standard for Waterproof Microporous Plastic Self-adhesive Plaster, page 632, so as to leave a margin of adhesive surface surrounding the pad.

The width of the adhesive margin is not less than 3 mm,

or not less than 10 per cent of the overall dimension of the dressing, whichever is the greater, and the width of the margin on any one side is not less than half the width of the margin on the opposite side.

If, for convenience in use of the dressing, the corners of the plaster are cut to a radius, this is ignored in defining the shape and dimensions of the dressing.

The pad and the margin of adhesive surface are covered by a suitable protector. The pad does not become detached from the plaster when the protector is removed.

EXTENSIBILITY. It complies with the test described in Appendix 27, page 914.

STERILITY. If the dressing is sterile, it complies with the test for sterility described in Appendix 28, page 917.

Standard for the pad

DESCRIPTION. It complies with the requirements described under Elastic Adhesive Dressing, page 620, except that the statement relating to special-purpose dressing strips is not applicable.

WEIGHT PER UNIT AREA; CONTENT OF ANTISEPTIC. It complies with the requirements described under Elastic Adhesive Dressing, page 620.

Sterilisation. It may be sterilised by exposure to ethylene oxide or ionising radiation as described for surgical dressings in Appendix 29 (page 926) or by any other suitable process.

Packaging. It is packed as described under Elastic Adhesive Dressing (page 620).

Labelling. It is labelled as described under Elastic Adhesive Dressing (page 620).

Storage. It should be stored as described under Elastic Adhesive Dressing (page 620).

Uses. Waterproof microporous plastic wound dressing is used as a protective covering for wounds when a waterproof dressing which allows the passage of air and water vapour is required.

Standard Dressing No. 7

SYNONYM: Plain Lint Finger Dressing

Standard Dressing No. 7 consists of a sterile unmedicated open finger-stall formed by attaching an open tube of absorbent lint to an open-wove bandage.

Standard
Standard Dressing No. 7 is prepared from:

Absorbent Lint, two pieces, each	..	5 cm by 4·5 cm
or one piece	..	5 cm by 9 cm
Open-wove Bandage	.. ..	2·5 cm by 50 cm

DESCRIPTION. An open tube of absorbent lint, which complies with the standard for Absorbent Lint, page 630, attached obliquely by the continuous stitching of its seams across the outer surface of the rolled open-wove bandage, which complies with the standard for Open-wove Bandage, page 614, approximately 15 cm from one end.

The lint tube consists either of the two small pieces of absorbent lint sewn together down their longer sides with the raised surfaces facing outwards, one side being sewn completely and the other side along half its length, or of the single large piece of absorbent lint suitably folded to produce a tube of the same dimensions and sewn along half the length of the open longer side.

STERILITY. It complies with the test for sterility described in Appendix 28, page 917.

Sterilisation. It is sterilised by one of the methods described for surgical dressings in Appendix 29 (page 926) or by any other suitable process.

Packaging. The lint tube is folded so that the open ends are brought together and protected from contamination on opening, the rolled bandage is placed on the outside of the folded lint, and the loose end of the bandage is wound round the rolled bandage and the lint.

The dressing is enclosed in an inner sealed wrapper, which will withstand the process of sterilisation and prevent access of micro-organisms, and in an outer sealed wrapper or carton fitted with a quick-tearing or quick-opening device.

Labelling. It is labelled as described in the general monograph (page 611).

Uses. Standard dressing No. 7 is used as a sterile wound dressing for fingers and toes.

Standard Dressing No. 8

SYNONYM: Medium Plain Lint Dressing

Standard Dressing No. 8 consists of an unmedicated pad, of absorbent cotton wool faced with absorbent lint, attached to an open-wove bandage; the dressing is sterile.

Standard
Standard Dressing No. 8 is prepared from:

Absorbent Cotton Wool	..	approximately 1·5 g
Absorbent Lint	.. ..	.. 7·5 cm by 10 cm
Open-wove Bandage	..	.. 5 cm by 1·5 m

DESCRIPTION. A pad, measuring 7·5 cm by 10 cm, attached lengthwise, by continuous stitching across its narrow ends, to the outer surface of the rolled open-wove bandage, which complies with the standard for Open-wove Bandage, page 614, approximately 40 cm from one end.

The pad consists of the rectangular piece of absorbent lint, which complies with the standard for Absorbent Lint, page 630, superimposed, with the raised surface downwards, on to a pad of the absorbent cotton wool, which complies with the standard for Absorbent Cotton Wool, page 618.

STERILITY. It complies with the test for sterility described in Appendix 28, page 917.

Sterilisation. It is sterilised by one of the methods described for surgical dressings in Appendix 29 (page 926) or by any other suitable process.

Packaging. The pad is folded in half with the lint facing inwards, the rolled bandage is placed on the outside of the folded pad, and the loose end of the bandage is wound round the rolled bandage and the pad.

The dressing is enclosed in an inner sealed wrapper, which will withstand the process of sterilisation and prevent access of micro-organisms, and in an outer sealed wrapper or carton fitted with a quick-tearing or quick-opening device.

Labelling. It is labelled as described in the general monograph (page 611).

Uses. Standard dressing No. 8 is used as a sterile wound dressing for hands and feet.

Standard Dressing No. 9

SYNONYM: Large Plain Lint Dressing

Standard Dressing No. 9 consists of an unmedicated pad, of absorbent cotton wool faced with absorbent lint, attached to an open-wove bandage; the dressing is sterile.

Standard

Standard Dressing No. 9 is prepared from:

Absorbent Cotton Wool   ..   approximately 3 g
Absorbent Lint   ..   ..   ..   10 cm by 15 cm
Open-wove Bandage   ..   ..   7·5 cm by 2 m

DESCRIPTION. A pad, measuring 10 cm by 15 cm, attached lengthwise, by continuous stitching across its narrow ends, to the outer surface of the rolled open-wove bandage, which complies with the standard for Open-wove Bandage, page 614, approximately 40 cm from one end.

The pad consists of the rectangular piece of absorbent lint, which complies with the standard for Absorbent Lint, page 630, superimposed, with the raised surface downwards, on to a pad of the absorbent cotton wool, which complies with the standard for Absorbent Cotton Wool, page 618.

STERILITY. It complies with the test for sterility described in Appendix 28, page 917.

Sterilisation. It is sterilised by one of the methods described for surgical dressings in Appendix 29 (page 926) or by any other suitable process.

Packaging. It should be packed as described under Standard Dressing No. 8.

Labelling. It is labelled as described in the general monograph (page 611).

Uses. Standard dressing No. 9 is used as a sterile wound dressing for large areas.

Standard Dressing No. 10

SYNONYM: Medicated Lint Finger Dressing

Standard Dressing No. 10 consists of a sterile medicated open finger-stall formed by attaching an open tube of euflavine lint to an open-wove bandage.

Standard

Standard Dressing No. 10 is prepared from:

Euflavine Lint, two pieces, each ..   5 cm by 4·5 cm
        or one piece   ..   5 cm by 9 cm
Open-wove Bandage   ..   ..   2·5 cm by 50 cm

DESCRIPTION. An open tube of euflavine lint, which complies with the standard for Euflavine Lint, page 630, attached obliquely by the continuous stitching of its seams across the outer surface of the rolled open-wove bandage, which complies with the standard for Open-wove Bandage, page 614, approximately 15 cm from one end.

The lint tube consists either of the two small pieces of euflavine lint sewn together down their longer sides with the raised surfaces facing outwards, one side being sewn completely and the other side along half its length, or of the single large piece of euflavine lint suitably folded to produce a tube of the same dimensions and sewn along half the length of the open longer side.

STERILITY. It complies with the test for sterility described in Appendix 28, page 917.

Sterilisation. It is sterilised by one of the methods described for surgical dressings in Appendix 29 (page 926) or by any other suitable process.

Packaging. It should be packed as described under Standard Dressing No. 7.

Labelling. It is labelled as described in the general monograph (page 611).

Uses. Standard dressing No. 10 is used as a sterile dressing for the first-aid treatment of mild burns of the fingers and toes.

Standard Dressing No. 11

SYNONYM: Medium Medicated Lint Dressing

Standard Dressing No. 11 consists of a pad, of absorbent cotton wool faced with euflavine lint, attached to an open-wove bandage; the dressing is sterile.

Standard

Standard Dressing No. 11 is prepared from:

Absorbent Cotton Wool   ..   approximately 1·5 g
Euflavine Lint   ..   ..   7·5 cm by 10 cm
Open-wove Bandage   ..   ..   5 cm by 1·5 m

DESCRIPTION. A pad, measuring 7·5 cm by 10 cm, attached lengthwise, by continuous stitching across its narrow ends, to the outer surface of the rolled open-wove bandage, which complies with the standard for Open-wove Bandage, page 614, approximately 40 cm from one end.

The pad consists of the rectangular piece of euflavine lint, which complies with the standard for Euflavine Lint, page 630, superimposed, with the raised surface downwards, on to a pad of the absorbent cotton wool, which complies with the standard for Absorbent Cotton Wool, page 618.

STERILITY. It complies with the test for sterility described in Appendix 28, page 917.

Sterilisation. It is sterilised by one of the methods described for surgical dressings in Appendix 29 (page 926) or by any other suitable process.

Packaging. It is packed as described under Standard Dressing No. 8.

Labelling. It is labelled as described in the general monograph (page 611).

Uses. Standard dressing No. 11 is used as a sterile dressing for the first-aid treatment of mild burns of the hands and feet.

Standard Dressing No. 12

SYNONYM: Large Medicated Lint Dressing

Standard Dressing No. 12 consists of a pad, of absorbent cotton wool faced with euflavine lint, attached to an open-wove bandage; the dressing is sterile.

Standard

Standard Dressing No. 12 is prepared from:

Absorbent Cotton Wool   ..   approximately 3 g
Euflavine Lint   ..   ..   10 cm by 15 cm
Open-wove Bandage   ..   ..   7·5 cm by 2 m

DESCRIPTION. A pad, measuring 10 cm by 15 cm, attached lengthwise, by continuous stitching across its narrow ends, to the outer surface of the rolled open-wove bandage, which complies with the standard for Open-wove Bandage, page 614, approximately 40 cm from one end.

The pad consists of the rectangular piece of euflavine lint, which complies with the standard for Euflavine Lint, page 630, superimposed, with the raised surface downwards, on to a pad of absorbent cotton wool, which complies with the standard for Absorbent Cotton Wool, page 618.

STERILITY. It complies with the test for sterility described in Appendix 28, page 917.

Sterilisation. It is sterilised by one of the methods described for surgical dressings in Appendix 29 (page 926) or by any other suitable process.

Packaging. It is packed as described under Standard Dressing No. 8.

Labelling. It is labelled as described in the general monograph (page 611).

Uses. Standard dressing No. 12 is used as a sterile dressing for the first-aid treatment of mild burns.

Standard Dressing No. 13

SYNONYM: Small Plain Wound Dressing

Standard Dressing No. 13 consists of an unmedicated pad, of absorbent cotton wool enclosed in absorbent gauze, attached to an open-wove bandage; the dressing is sterile.

Standard
Standard Dressing No. 13 is prepared from:

Absorbent Cotton Wool ..	approximately 6 g
Absorbent gauze	20 cm by 10 cm

or

Tubular absorbent gauze	17 cm in circumference by 10 cm
Open-wove Bandage	5 cm by 2 m

DESCRIPTION. A pad, measuring 7·5 cm by 10 cm, attached lengthwise, by continuous stitching across its narrow ends, to the outer surface of the rolled open-wove bandage, which complies with the standard for Open-wove Bandage, page 614, approximately 25 cm from one end.
The pad consists of the absorbent cotton wool, which complies with the standard for Absorbent Cotton Wool, page 618, enclosed in a piece of absorbent gauze, woven tubular or single width, which complies with the standard for Absorbent Cotton Gauze (13 Light), page 626, with the exception that the weft has an average of not less than 45 threads per 10 cm and the weight per unit area has an average of 13 g per m².

STERILITY. It complies with the test for sterility described in Appendix 28, page 917.

Sterilisation. It is sterilised by one of the methods described for surgical dressings in Appendix 29 (page 926) or by any other suitable process.

Packaging. The pad is folded in half with the surface of the gauze facing inwards, the rolled bandage is placed on the outside of the folded pad, and the loose end of the bandage is wound round the rolled bandage and the pad.
The dressing is enclosed in an inner sealed wrapper, which will withstand the process of sterilisation and prevent access of micro-organisms, and in an outer sealed wrapper or carton fitted with a quick-tearing or quick-opening device.

Labelling. It is labelled as described in the general monograph (page 611).

Uses. Standard dressing No. 13 is used as a sterile, absorbent, and protective dressing for wounds of small area.

Standard Dressing No. 14

SYNONYM: Medium Plain Wound Dressing

Standard Dressing No. 14 consists of an unmedicated pad, of absorbent cotton wool enclosed in absorbent gauze, attached to an open-wove bandage; the dressing is sterile.

Standard
Standard Dressing No. 14 is prepared from:

Absorbent Cotton Wool ..	approximately 12 g
Absorbent gauze	25 cm by 15 cm

or

Tubular absorbent gauze	23 cm in circumference by 15 cm
Open-wove Bandage	7·5 cm by 2·5 m

DESCRIPTION. A pad, measuring 15 cm by 10 cm, attached lengthwise, by continuous stitching across its narrow ends, to the outer surface of the rolled open-wove bandage, which complies with the standard for Open-wove Bandage, page 614, approximately 30 cm from one end.
The pad consists of the absorbent cotton wool, which complies with the standard for Absorbent Cotton Wool, page 618, enclosed in a piece of absorbent gauze, woven tubular or single width, which complies with the standard for Absorbent Cotton Gauze (13 Light), page 626, with the exception that the weft has an average of not less than 45 threads per 10 cm and weight per unit area has an average of 13 g per m².

STERILITY. It complies with the test for sterility described in Appendix 28, page 917.

Sterilisation. It is sterilised by one of the methods described for surgical dressings in Appendix 29 (page 926) or by any other suitable process.

Packaging. It is packed as described under Standard Dressing No. 13.

Labelling. It is labelled as described in the general monograph (page 611).

Uses. Standard dressing No. 14 is used as a sterile, absorbent, and protective dressing for wounds of medium area.

Standard Dressing No. 15

SYNONYM: Large Plain Wound Dressing

Standard Dressing No. 15 consists of an unmedicated pad, of absorbent cotton wool enclosed in absorbent gauze, attached to an open-wove bandage; the dressing is sterile.

Standard
Standard Dressing No. 15 is prepared from:

Absorbent Cotton Wool ..	approximately 25 g
Absorbent gauze	35 cm by 20 cm

or

Tubular absorbent gauze	33 cm in circumference by 20 cm
Open-wove Bandage	7·5 cm by 3·5 m

DESCRIPTION. A pad, measuring 15 cm by 20 cm, attached lengthwise, by continuous stitching across its narrow ends, to the outer surface of the rolled open-wove bandage, which complies with the standard for Open-wove Bandage, page 614, approximately 40 cm from one end.
The pad consists of the absorbent cotton wool, which complies with the standard for Absorbent Cotton Wool, page 618, enclosed in a piece of absorbent gauze, woven tubular or single width, which complies with the standard for Absorbent Cotton Gauze (13 Light), page 626, with the exception that the weft has an average of not less than 45 threads per 10 cm and the weight per unit area has an average of 13 g per m².

STERILITY. It complies with the test for sterility described in Appendix 28, page 917.

Sterilisation. It is sterilised by one of the methods described for surgical dressings in Appendix 29 (page 926) or by any other suitable process.

Packaging. It is packed as described under Standard Dressing No. 13.

Labelling. It is labelled as described in the general monograph (page 611).

Uses. Standard dressing No. 15 is used as a sterile, absorbent, and protective dressing for wounds of large area.

Standard Dressing No. 16

SYNONYM: Eye Pad with Bandage

Standard Dressing No. 16 consists of a pad of absorbent cotton wool, faced on both sides with absorbent muslin, attached to an open-wove bandage; the dressing is sterile.

Standard

Standard Dressing No. 16 is prepared from:

Absorbent Cotton Wool ..	approximately	1·25 g
Absorbent Muslin, two oval pieces,		
each		5 cm by 7·5 cm
Open-wove Bandage		5 cm by 1·5 m

DESCRIPTION. An oval pad, measuring 5 cm by 7·5 cm, attached lengthwise, by continuous stitching across its narrow ends, to the outer surface of the rolled open-wove bandage, which complies with the standard for Open-wove Bandage, page 614, approximately 20 cm from one end.

The pad consists of the absorbent cotton wool, which complies with the standard for Absorbent Cotton Wool, page 618, faced on both sides with the two pieces of absorbent muslin, which comply with the standard for Absorbent Muslin, page 635.

STERILITY. It complies with the test for sterility described in Appendix 28, page 917.

Sterilisation. It is sterilised by one of the methods described for surgical dressings in Appendix 29 (page 926) or by any other suitable process.

Packaging. The pad is folded in half across its length with the absorbent muslin facing inwards, the rolled bandage is placed on the outside of the folded pad, and the loose end of the bandage is wound round the rolled bandage and the pad.

The dressing is enclosed in an inner sealed wrapper, which will withstand the process of sterilisation and prevent access of micro-organisms, and in an outer sealed wrapper or carton fitted with a quick-tearing or quick-opening device.

Labelling. It is labelled as described in the general monograph (page 611).

Uses. Standard dressing No. 16 is used as a sterile protective covering for the eye.

GAUZES

Absorbent Cotton Gauze (13 Light)

SYNONYMS: Absorbent Gauze; Gauze; Tela Gossypii Absorbens; Unmedicated Gauze

Absorbent Cotton Gauze (13 Light) consists of cotton cloth of plain weave. It is usually supplied in pieces 90 cm wide, in various lengths, and folded longitudinally.

It absorbs water readily, but its absorbency may be reduced considerably by medication, by prolonged storage, or by exposure to heat. On sterilisation, the material may shrink slightly.

Eight types of gauze, differing in construction, are described in the European Pharmacopoeia. The other seven types are all heavier than type 13 (light).

Standard

Material which complies with this standard will meet the requirements of the European Pharmacopoeia for Absorbent Cotton Gauze, Type 13 Light.

DESCRIPTION. Cotton cloth of plain weave, bleached to a good white, clean, and reasonably free from weaving defects, cotton leaf and shell. It is odourless or almost odourless. It may be slightly off-white if it has been sterilised.

YARN. A uniform, good medium grade.

IDENTIFICATION TEST. Fibres freed from threads in the warp and weft comply with the microscopical description and identification test described under Absorbent Cotton Wool, page 618.

THREADS PER STATED LENGTH. Warp: average 73 per 10 cm; standard deviation 1·33.

Weft: average 57 per 10 cm; standard deviation 1·33.

WEIGHT PER UNIT AREA. Average 15 g per m²; standard deviation 0·33.

ABSORBENCY. Fold a piece weighing 1 g four times, i.e. into 16 folds, smooth it, and, by means of forceps, drop it lightly upon the surface of water at 20° contained in a beaker, 11 to 12 cm in diameter and filled to a depth of 10 cm. Measure with a stop-watch the time taken by the sample to sink below the surface of the water.

Repeat the test twice, and calculate the sinking time as the average of the three tests.

The sinking time is not more than 10 seconds.

ACIDITY OR ALKALINITY. To 10 g, add 100 ml of water, allow to stand for 2 hours in a closed vessel, decant, pressing the sample with a glass rod to express the residual liquid, and mix. Reserve 10 ml of the liquid for the test for Surface-active Substances.

Filter the remainder of the liquid.

To 25 ml of the filtrate add 0·15 ml of *phenolphthalein solution*; the solution does not show a pink colour.

To another 25 ml of the filtrate add 0·05 ml of *methyl orange solution*; the solution is yellow.

SURFACE-ACTIVE SUBSTANCES. Shake vigorously in a clean test tube the liquid reserved in the test for Acidity or Alkalinity and allow to stand for 10 minutes; not more than a ring of froth, in contact with the walls of the test tube, remains.

WATER-SOLUBLE SUBSTANCES. Not more than 0·50 per cent, determined by the following method:

Boil about 7 g, accurately weighed, with 700 ml of water for 30 minutes, stirring frequently, and replacing the water lost by evaporation. Decant the hot liquid, pressing the sample with a glass rod to express the residual liquid, and mix. Reserve 200 ml of the liquid for the test for Starch and Dextrins, and filter the remainder of the liquid while it is still hot.

Evaporate 400 ml of the filtrate (equivalent to four-sevenths of the weight of sample taken) to dryness and dry the residue to constant weight at 105°.

STARCH AND DEXTRINS. Cool the 200 ml of liquid reserved in the test for Water-soluble Substances and add 5 ml of *acetic acid* and 0·15 ml of 0·1N iodine; no blue, violet, reddish, or brown colour is produced.

ETHER-SOLUBLE SUBSTANCES. Not more than 0·50 per cent, determined by the following method:

Extract about 5 g, accurately weighed, with *solvent ether* for 4 hours in an apparatus for the continuous extraction of drugs or for intermittent extraction, with not less than four extractions per hour; evaporate the extract to dryness and dry the residue to constant weight at 105°.

COLOURING MATTER. Slowly extract 10 g, packed into a narrow percolator, with *alcohol (95 per cent)* until 50 ml of extract is obtained and examine a 20-cm layer of the extract against a white background.

The extract is not more than a very faint yellow and has no bluish or greenish tinge.

FLUORESCENCE. Examine a double layer under ultra-violet radiation, including radiation of wavelength 365 nm. The sample shows only a slight brownish-violet fluorescence and not more than an occasional yellow particle. It shows no intense blue fluorescence except that which may be shown by a few isolated fibres (absence of fluorescent brightening agents).

LOSS ON DRYING. Not more than 8·0 per cent, determined on 5 g, by drying to constant weight at 105°.

SULPHATED ASH. Not more than 0·75 per cent, determined on 5 g.

STERILITY. If the label on the package states that the material is sterile, the contents comply with the test for sterility described in Appendix 28, page 917.

Sterilisation. It may be sterilised by one of the methods described for surgical dressings in Appendix 29 (page 926) or by any other suitable process.

Packaging. It should be enclosed in either well-closed packages or sealed packages, according to the requirements of the user. Waxed paper should not be used for any wrapping in contact with the gauze, as it reduces the absorbency of the material.
If the material is sterile, it should be enclosed in a sealed package and the directions given in Appendix 29 (page 926) should be followed.

Labelling. If the material is supplied sterile, it is labelled as described in the general monograph (page 611).

Uses. Absorbent cotton gauze (13 light) is used externally as a direct wound dressing. Higher and lower grades are available, but the gauze complying with this standard represents a good average quality which gives a soft, highly absorbent pad suitable for most purposes.

Absorbent Gauze, X-ray-detectable

X-ray-detectable Absorbent Gauze consists of absorbent gauze to which is attached a non-toxic X-ray-detectable member, which may consist of a monofilament or multi-filament yarn.

Standard
DESCRIPTION. Absorbent gauze to which is securely attached, for example by heat-sealing or weaving, a distinctively coloured continuous X-ray-detectable member.
The absorbent gauze complies with the standard for Absorbent Cotton Gauze (13 Light), except that if the X-ray-detectable member is woven into the fabric and replaces one of the gauze threads, the minimum requirement for threads per 10 cm is reduced by 1 in the appropriate count in the region of the member.
The gauze may be dyed with a suitable non-toxic dye.

COLOUR FASTNESS. If the gauze is dyed, it complies with the test given in Appendix 27, page 913.

STERILITY. If the label on the package states that the material is sterile, the contents comply with the test for sterility described in Appendix 28, page 917.

Standard for the X-ray-detectable member
DESCRIPTION. The member is prepared from non-toxic materials and contains not less than 55 per cent of barium sulphate or a suitable percentage of any other non-toxic material which gives a comparable X-ray opacity.
It is distinctively coloured and reasonably free from loose fibres and particles; when attached it does not impair the softness or flexibility of the gauze.

TEX. If the member is a multifilament yarn, not less than 280 tex (2500 denier).

WEIGHT. If the member is a monofilament, not less than 0·50 g per m.

Sterilisation. It may be sterilised by one of the methods described for surgical dressings in Appendix 29 (page 926) or by any other suitable process.
Repeated autoclaving of products containing a mono-filament X-ray-detectable member may cause damage to that member unless the material is in a loosely packed form. Rolls of the absorbent gauze should be unrolled and cut to length before autoclaving.

Packaging. It should be packed as described under Absorbent Cotton Gauze (13 Light).

Labelling. If the material is supplied sterile, it is labelled as described in the general monograph (page 611).

Uses. X-ray-detectable absorbent gauze is used in the form of pads, the uses of which are described under X-ray-detectable Gauze Pad (page 628).
The X-ray image produced by a multifilament member is less bright than that produced by a monofilament member but, in certain instances, the former type may be preferred.

Absorbent Ribbon Gauze

SYNONYM: Unmedicated Ribbon Gauze

Absorbent Ribbon Gauze consists of cloth of plain weave, supplied in ribbons of various widths and lengths, in which the warp threads are of cotton and the weft threads are of cotton or rayon or of combined cotton and rayon yarn.
It absorbs water readily but its absorbency may be considerably reduced by medication; its absorbency may also be reduced by prolonged storage or by exposure to heat. On sterilisation the material may shrink slightly.

Standard
DESCRIPTION. Cloth of plain weave, bleached to a good white, clean, reasonably free from weaving defects, cotton leaf and shell, and having fast selvedge edges. It may be slightly off-white if it has been sterilised.

YARN. A uniform, good medium grade.

THREADS PER STATED LENGTH. Warp: average not less than 12 per cm.
Weft: average not less than 10 per cm.

WEIGHT PER UNIT AREA. Not less than 44 g per m^2.

ABSORBENCY. 1 g, compressed to a volume of about 20 ml, placed lightly by means of forceps on the surface of water at 20°, becomes saturated within 10 seconds.

WATER-SOLUBLE EXTRACTIVE. Not more than 0·5 per cent.

FOREIGN MATTER. Not more than 1·0 per cent; contains no added foreign matter.

FLUORESCENCE. Examine under ultraviolet radiation, including radiation of wavelength 365 nm; not more than an occasional point of fluorescence is visible (absence of fluorescent brightening agents).

STERILITY. If the label on the package states that the material is sterile, the contents comply with the test for sterility described in Appendix 28, page 917.

Sterilisation. It may be sterilised by one of the methods described for surgical dressings in Appendix 29 (page 926) or by any other suitable process.

Packaging. It should be packed as described under Absorbent Cotton Gauze (13 Light).

Labelling. If the material is supplied sterile, it is labelled as described in the general monograph (page 611).

Uses. Absorbent ribbon gauze is used to pack sinus, dental, and throat cavities, and to pack open infected wounds to assist healing.

Absorbent ribbon gauze swells in use and this should be taken into consideration when packing small cavities.

Absorbent Ribbon Gauze, X-ray-detectable

X-ray-detectable Absorbent Ribbon Gauze consists of absorbent ribbon gauze to which is attached a non-toxic X-ray-detectable member, which may consist of a monofilament or multifilament yarn.

Standard

DESCRIPTION. Absorbent ribbon gauze to which is securely attached, for example by heat-sealing or weaving, a distinctively coloured continuous X-ray-detectable member. The absorbent ribbon gauze complies with the standard for Absorbent Ribbon Gauze, except that if the X-ray-detectable member is woven into the fabric and replaces one of the gauze threads, the minimum requirement for threads per cm is reduced by 1 in the appropriate count in the region of the member.

STERILITY. If the label on the package states that the material is sterile, the contents comply with the test for sterility described in Appendix 28, page 917.

Standard for the X-ray-detectable member

It complies with the standard given for the X-ray-detectable member in X-ray-detectable Absorbent Gauze.

Sterilisation. It may be sterilised by one of the methods described for surgical dressings in Appendix 29 (page 926) or by any other suitable process.

Repeated autoclaving of products containing a mono-filament X-ray-detectable member may cause damage to that member unless the material is in a loosely packed form. Rolls of the absorbent gauze should be unrolled and cut before autoclaving.

Packaging. It should be packed as described under Absorbent Cotton Gauze (13 Light).

Labelling. If the material is supplied sterile, it is labelled as described in the general monograph (page 611).

Uses. X-ray-detectable absorbent ribbon gauze has the uses described under Absorbent Ribbon Gauze and, in addition, is used as a temporary absorbent in open surgery and for packing large cavities produced by abdominal surgery.

GAUZE PADS

Gauze Pad

SYNONYMS: Absorbent Gauze Pad; Gauze Sponge; Gauze Swab

Gauze Pad consists of folded absorbent gauze. The number of layers (ply) of gauze in the pad and its dimensions vary according to surgical requirements, the usual sizes being 5 cm, 7·5 cm, and 10 cm square, each of 8-, 12-, 16-, or 32-ply; larger sizes and other plies are also prepared.

Standard

DESCRIPTION. A cut piece of absorbent gauze, which complies with the standard for Absorbent Cotton Gauze (13 Light), page 626, folded into a square pad in such a manner that no cut edges are visible; the edges of the pad may be stitched.

The gauze may be dyed with a suitable non-toxic dye.

COLOUR FASTNESS. If the pad is dyed, it complies with the test given in Appendix 27, page 913.

Sterilisation. Gauze pads may be sterilised by one of the methods described for surgical dressings in Appendix 29 (page 926) or by any other suitable process.

Packaging. Gauze pads should be enclosed in either well-closed packages or sealed packages, according to the requirements of the user. The packages may contain more than one pad.

Waxed paper should not be used for any wrapping in contact with the pads, as it reduces the absorbency of the material.

If the pads are sterile, they should be enclosed in a sealed package and the directions given in Appendix 29 (page 926) should be followed; the inner wrapper may enclose up to five pads.

Labelling. The label on the package states the size of the pads and the ply and, if they are dyed, the colour. In addition, if the pads are supplied sterile, they are labelled as described in the general monograph (page 611).

Uses. Gauze pads are used for packing open wounds and swabbing procedures. They are also used as direct wound dressings.

Gauze Pad, X-ray-detectable

SYNONYMS: X-ray-detectable Gauze Sponge; X-ray-detectable Gauze Swab

X-ray-detectable Gauze Pad consists of folded X-ray-detectable absorbent gauze. The number of layers (ply) of the gauze in the pad and its dimensions vary according to surgical requirements, the usual sizes being 5 cm, 7·5 cm, and 10 cm square, each of 8-, 12-, 16-, or 32-ply; larger sizes and other plies are also prepared.

Standard

DESCRIPTION. A cut piece of X-ray-detectable absorbent gauze, which complies with the standard for X-ray-detectable Absorbent Gauze, page 627, folded into a square pad in such a manner that no cut edges are visible; the edges of the pad may be stitched.

The gauze may be dyed with a suitable non-toxic dye.

Sterilisation. The pads may be sterilised by one of the methods described for surgical dressings in Appendix 29 (page 926) or by any other suitable process.

Repeated autoclaving of pads containing a monofilament X-ray-detectable member may cause damage to that member, unless the pads are loosely packed.

Packaging. The pads should be packed as described under Gauze Pad.

Labelling. The label on the package states the size of the pads and the ply and, if they are dyed, the colour. In addition, if the pads are supplied sterile, they are labelled as described in the general monograph (page 611).

Uses. X-ray-detectable gauze pads are used

for packing open wounds and swabbing procedures during surgical operations.

The X-ray-detectable member enables any pad, accidentally left in the body after the wound has been closed, to be detected radiologically; the image produced by a multifilament member is less bright than that produced by a monofilament member, but, in certain instances, the former type may be preferred.

GAUZE TISSUES

Gauze and Capsicum Cotton Tissue

SYNONYM: Capsicum Tissue

Gauze and Capsicum Cotton Tissue consists of a thick layer of capsicum cotton wool enclosed in bleached gauze in tubular form, dyed orange-brown with a suitable non-toxic dye.

Standard
DESCRIPTION. A thick layer of capsicum cotton wool, which complies with the standard for Capsicum Cotton Wool, page 619, enclosed in gauze in tubular form.

AREA PER UNIT WEIGHT. 1 g has a superficial area of not less than 25 cm².

Standard for the gauze
DESCRIPTION. It complies with the requirement for Absorbent Cotton Gauze (13 Light), page 626, with the exception that it is dyed orange-brown.

COLOUR FASTNESS. It complies with the test given in Appendix 27, page 913.

YARN; WATER-SOLUBLE SUBSTANCES; FLUORESCENCE. It complies with the requirements described under Absorbent Cotton Gauze (13 Light), page 626.

THREADS PER STATED LENGTH. Warp: average 73 per 10 cm; standard deviation 1·5.
Weft: average 45 per 10 cm; standard deviation 1·5.

WEIGHT PER UNIT AREA. Average 13 g per m²; standard deviation 1·0. Any stitching thread used in making the tube is excluded.

Packaging. It should be enclosed in sealed packages, doubly wrapped to prevent loss of pungency.

Uses. Gauze and Capsicum Cotton Tissue has the uses described under Capsicum Cotton Wool (page 619); the gauze cover forms a more stable pad.

Gauze and Cellulose Wadding Tissue

SYNONYM: Cellulose Tissue

Gauze and Cellulose Wadding Tissue consists of a thick layer of cellulose wadding enclosed in gauze in tubular form.

Standard
DESCRIPTION. A thick layer of cellulose wadding, which complies with the standard for Cellulose Wadding, page 634, enclosed in gauze in tubular form.

AREA PER UNIT WEIGHT. 1 g has a superficial area of not less than 19 cm².

Standard for the gauze
DESCRIPTION; YARN; ABSORBENCY; WATER-SOLUBLE SUBSTANCES; FLUORESCENCE. It complies with the requirements described under Absorbent Cotton Gauze (13 Light), page 626.

THREADS PER STATED LENGTH. Warp: average 73 per 10 cm; standard deviation 1·5.
Weft: average 45 per 10 cm; standard deviation 1·5.

WEIGHT PER UNIT AREA. Average 13 g per m²; standard deviation 1·0. Any stitching thread used in making the tube is excluded.

Packaging. It should be packed as described under Absorbent Cotton Wool (page 618).

Uses. Gauze and Cellulose Wadding Tissue has the uses described under Gauze and Cotton Tissue.

Gauze and Cotton Tissue

SYNONYMS: Absorbent Gauze Tissue;
Gauze Tissue

Gauze and Cotton Tissue consists of a thick layer of absorbent cotton wool enclosed in gauze in tubular form.

Standard
DESCRIPTION. A thick layer of absorbent cotton wool, which complies with the standard for Absorbent Cotton Wool, page 618, enclosed in gauze in tubular form.

AREA PER UNIT WEIGHT. 1 g has a superficial area of not less than 25 cm².

Standard for the gauze
DESCRIPTION; YARN; ABSORBENCY; WATER-SOLUBLE SUBSTANCES; FLUORESCENCE. It complies with the requirements described under Absorbent Cotton Gauze (13 Light), page 626.

THREADS PER STATED LENGTH. Warp: average 73 per 10 cm; standard deviation 1·5.
Weft: average 45 per 10 cm; standard deviation 1·5.

WEIGHT PER UNIT AREA. Average 13 g per m²; standard deviation 1·0. Any stitching thread used in making the tube is excluded.

Packaging. It should be packed as described under Absorbent Cotton Wool (page 618).

Uses. Gauze and Cotton Tissue is used as an absorbent and protective pad, with or without an additional dressing.

LINTS

Absorbent Lint

SYNONYMS: Absorbent Cotton Lint; Cotton Lint; Lint; Plain Lint; White Lint

Absorbent Lint consists of cotton cloth of plain weave, on one side of which a nap has been raised from the warp yarns.

It absorbs water readily, but its absorbency may be considerably reduced by medication; its absorbency may also be reduced by prolonged storage or by exposure to heat.

Standard

DESCRIPTION. Cotton cloth of plain weave, having on one side a nap well raised from the warp yarns; it is bleached to a good white, clean, and reasonably free from weaving defects, neps, cotton leaf, shell and other foreign substances; it is readily tearable in both directions.

YARN. Reasonably free from slubs, snarls, and other defects.

THREADS PER STATED LENGTH. Warp: average 15·5 per cm; standard deviation 0·50.
Weft: average 96 per 10 cm; standard deviation 4·5.

AREA PER UNIT WEIGHT. 1 g has an average superficial area of 54 cm², standard deviation 2·0.

ABSORBENCY. A piece, 7·5 cm square, placed lightly by means of forceps, unraised side downwards, on the surface of water at 20°, becomes saturated within 10 seconds.

WATER-SOLUBLE EXTRACTIVE. Not more than 1·0 per cent.

FLUORESCENCE. Examine under ultraviolet radiation, including radiation of wavelength 365 nm; not more than an occasional point of fluorescence is visible (absence of fluorescent brightening agents).

Packaging. It should be enclosed in well-closed packages. Waxed paper should not be used for wrapping, as it reduces the absorbency of the material.

Uses. Absorbent lint is used as an external absorbent and protective dressing and for the application of ointments and lotions. Because of its ease of tearing, it is widely used in first-aid treatment and in the home.

Absorbent lint has a greater absorptive capacity, weight for weight, than any other woven dressing.

Euflavine Lint

Euflavine Lint consists of absorbent lint impregnated with euflavine. It may be prepared by immersing absorbent lint in an aqueous solution of euflavine, removing the material from the solution, pressing, and drying; it contains no additional dye.

Standard

DESCRIPTION. Cotton cloth of plain weave, having on one side a nap well raised from the warp yarns, impregnated as uniformly as possible with euflavine; it is clean, and reasonably free from weaving defects, neps, cotton leaf, shell and other foreign substances; it is readily tearable in both directions.

YARN; THREADS PER STATED LENGTH; AREA PER UNIT WEIGHT; WATER-SOLUBLE EXTRACTIVE. It complies with the requirements described under Absorbent Lint.

ABSORBENCY. A piece, 7·5 cm square, placed lightly by means of forceps, unraised side downwards, on the surface of water at 20°, becomes saturated within 12 seconds.

CONTENT OF EUFLAVINE. 0·08 to 0·20 per cent, calculated as $C_{14}H_{14}ClN_3$, determined by the method described in Appendix 27, page 917.

Packaging. It should be enclosed in sealed packages, doubly wrapped, with dark paper externally. Waxed paper should not be used for any wrapping in contact with the lint, as it reduces the absorbency of the material.

Uses. Euflavine lint is used as an antiseptic absorbent and protective dressing; it is used for the first-aid treatment of mild burns, and is a component of Standard Dressings No. 10, 11, and 12 (page 624).

SELF-ADHESIVE PLASTERS

Self-adhesive Plasters are prepared by spreading a self-adhesive mass on a supporting material which consists of plain or elastic cloths or plastic films. If the plaster is to be medicated, the medicament is normally incorporated in the mass before spreading. The constituents of the mass other than specific medicaments should be innocuous to the skin.

This monograph applies to the following self-adhesive plasters:

Belladonna Self-adhesive Plaster
Extension Plaster
Perforated Plastic Self-adhesive Plaster
Salicylic Acid Self-adhesive Plaster
Waterproof Microporous Plastic Self-adhesive Plaster

Waterproof Plastic Self-adhesive Plaster
Zinc Oxide Elastic Self-adhesive Plaster
Zinc Oxide Self-adhesive Plaster

Labelling. The label on the package states :
(1) "Apply to clean dry skin",
(2) "Store in a cool place", and
(3) whether the plaster is porous or perforated.
If the plaster-supporting material is dyed, the colour is also stated on the label.

Storage. Plasters should be stored in a dry place at a temperature between 15° and 20°, protected from light and from deleterious vapours and contaminants.

Belladonna Self-adhesive Plaster

SYNONYM: Belladonna Plaster

Belladonna Self-adhesive Plaster consists of a suitable cloth spread evenly with a self-adhesive plaster mass containing an extract of belladonna herb or root.

Standard
DESCRIPTION. Cotton or rayon or mixed cotton and rayon cloth spread with a self-adhesive plaster mass containing about 0·25 per cent of the total alkaloids of belladonna, calculated as hyoscyamine. It is spread evenly, except that the mass may be made porous or permeable to air.
The cloth is of plain weave, clean, and reasonably free from weaving defects, cotton leaf and shell. It is finished to a good white or dyed flesh colour with a suitable non-toxic dye.
The plaster may be perforated.
The adhesive surface is covered by a suitable protector.

YARN. A uniform, good medium grade.

THREADS PER STATED LENGTH. Warp: average not less than 28 per cm.
Weft: average not less than 27 per cm.

WEIGHT OF FABRIC. Not less than 125 g per m².

WEIGHT OF ADHESIVE MASS. Not less than 135 g per m².

TENSILE STRENGTH OF UNPERFORATED FABRIC. Not less than 20·4 kgf in the warp, the test being conducted on unperforated strips 2·5 cm wide.

PERFORATIONS. If the cloth is perforated, the perforations are 0·3 to 0·5 cm in diameter, are regularly distributed, and do not exceed in area 14 per cent of the total area of the fabric.

Labelling. It is labelled as described under Self-adhesive Plasters (above).

Storage. It should be stored as described under Self-adhesive Plasters (above).

Uses. Belladonna self-adhesive plaster is used as a counter-irritant in the treatment of rheumatism, lumbago, neuralgia, and similar conditions.

Extension Plaster

SYNONYMS: Extension Strapping;
Orthopaedic Strapping

Extension Plaster consists of elastic cloth which stretches in the direction of the weft, spread evenly with a self-adhesive plaster mass containing zinc oxide.

Standard
DESCRIPTION. Elastic cloth spread with a self-adhesive plaster mass, containing zinc oxide, which does not off-set when unrolled; it is spread evenly, except that the mass may be made porous or permeable to air.
The elastic cloth is in one continuous length containing no joins, clean, and reasonably free from weaving defects, cotton leaf and shell; it may be dyed flesh colour with a suitable non-toxic dye.

FABRIC. The warp threads consist of singles or twofold yarn of a count not finer than 59·0 tex (10's or 2/20's), each containing 4 to 8 turns per cm; they consist of cotton or rayon staple fibre, or cotton and rayon staple fibre spun together.
The weft threads consist of singles or twofold cotton yarn with a finished count, after crêpe-twisting, not finer than 28·2 tex (21's or 2/42's); the singles yarn contains not less than 12 turns per cm, and the twofold yarns not less than 16 folding turns per cm. They are arranged as follows: two threads S-twist and two threads Z-twist, repeated.

THREADS PER STATED LENGTH. Warp: average not less than 82 per 10 cm, determined on the fully stretched width.
Weft: average not less than 19 per cm, determined on the unstretched plaster.

WEIGHT OF FABRIC. Not less than 200 g per m², calculated on the unstretched plaster.

WEIGHT OF ADHESIVE MASS. Not less than 220 g per m², calculated on the unstretched plaster.

ELASTICITY. The regain length is not more than four-fifths of the fully stretched measurement.

CONTENT OF ZINC OXIDE IN THE ADHESIVE MASS. Not less than 10·0 per cent, calculated as ZnO, determined by the method for Zinc Oxide Self-adhesive Plaster, page 633.

Packaging. It should be wound in rolls suitably protected.

Labelling. It is labelled as described under Self-adhesive Plasters (above).

Storage. It should be stored as described under Self-adhesive Plasters (above).

Uses. Extension plaster is used for the support of slight sprains which are not immobilised, of joints and limbs after the removal of plaster casts, and of fractured ribs. It is used for traction bandaging, attachment of dressings, and for the preparation of Elastic Adhesive Dressing (page 620).

Perforated Plastic Self-adhesive Plaster

SYNONYM: Porous Plastic Plaster

Perforated Plastic Self-adhesive Plaster consists of an extensible perforated plastic film, permeable to air and water vapour, spread evenly with a self-adhesive plaster mass.

Standard
DESCRIPTION. Extensible plastic film perforated by suitable means and spread with a self-adhesive plaster mass which does not off-set when unrolled from the spool; it is spread evenly, except that the mass is made permeable to air and water vapour.
The film is in one continuous length containing no joins; it may be dyed flesh colour with a suitable non-toxic dye.

WEIGHT OF FILM. Not less than 60 g per m², calculated on the unstretched plaster.

WEIGHT OF ADHESIVE MASS. Not less than 25 g per m², calculated on the unstretched plaster.

PERFORATIONS. The perforations are not more than 1 mm in diameter, are regularly distributed, and do not exceed in area 20 per cent of the total area of the unstretched plaster.

WATER-VAPOUR PERMEABILITY. The weight of water vapour passing through the plaster in twenty-four hours at 37° is not less than 2000 g per m².

EXTENSIBILITY. It complies with the test described in Appendix 27, page 914.

Packaging. It should be wound on spools and suitably protected.

Labelling. It is labelled as described under Self-adhesive Plasters (page 631).

Storage. It should be stored as described under Self-adhesive Plasters (page 631).

Uses. Perforated plastic self-adhesive plaster is used to secure dressings and appliances and to cover sites of infection when a completely permeable plaster which will not lose its adhesive properties when immersed in water is required. It is also used to prepare Perforated Plastic Wound Dressing (page 621).

Salicylic Acid Self-adhesive Plaster

SYNONYM: Salicylic Acid Plaster

Salicylic Acid Self-adhesive Plaster consists of a suitable cloth spread evenly with a self-adhesive plaster mass containing up to 40 per cent of salicylic acid.

Standard
DESCRIPTION. Cotton or rayon or mixed cotton and rayon cloth spread with a self-adhesive plaster mass containing salicylic acid. It is spread evenly, except that the mass may be made porous or permeable to air.
The cloth is of plain weave, clean, reasonably free from weaving defects, cotton leaf and shell; it may be dyed green with a suitable non-toxic dye.
The plaster may be perforated.
The adhesive surface is covered by a suitable protector.

YARN; THREADS PER STATED LENGTH; WEIGHT OF FABRIC; TENSILE STRENGTH OF UNPERFORATED FABRIC; PERFORATIONS. It complies with the requirements described under Belladonna Self-adhesive Plaster, page 631.

WEIGHT OF ADHESIVE MASS. Not less than 100 g per m².

CONTENT OF SALICYLIC ACID IN THE ADHESIVE MASS. 90·0 to 110·0 per cent of the stated amount, calculated as C₇H₆O₃, determined by the following method:
Boil about 3 g of the plaster, accurately weighed and cut into strips, with 200 ml of water in a long-necked round-bottomed flask for 20 minutes and filter through glass wool; return the residue on the filter to the flask, boil with 100 ml of water for 10 minutes, and filter; continue the extraction process with further 50-ml portions of water, boiling each time for 10 minutes, until the salicylic acid is completely extracted.
Titrate the combined filtrates with 0·1N sodium hydroxide, using *phenolphthalein solution* as indicator; each ml of 0·1N sodium hydroxide is equivalent to 0·01381 g of C₇H₆O₃.
The weight of adhesive mass taken in the determination is calculated as described in Appendix 27, page 916, under "Weight of adhesive mass".

Labelling. It is labelled as described under Self-adhesive Plasters (page 631).
In addition, the proportion of salicylic acid in the plaster mass is stated on the label.

Storage. It should be stored as described under Self-adhesive Plasters (page 631).

Uses. Salicylic acid self-adhesive plaster is used as a keratolytic agent.

When the strength of the plaster is not specified, a plaster containing 20 per cent of salicylic acid in the plaster mass shall be supplied.

Waterproof Microporous Plastic Self-adhesive Plaster

SYNONYM: Semipermeable Waterproof Plaster

Waterproof Microporous Plastic Self-adhesive Plaster consists of an extensible water-impermeable plastic film, permeable to air and water vapour, spread with a self-adhesive plaster mass.

Standard
DESCRIPTION. Extensible plastic film made permeable to air and water vapour by suitable means, spread with a self-adhesive plaster mass which does not off-set when unrolled from the spool; it is spread evenly, except that the mass is made permeable to air and water vapour.
The film is in one continuous length containing no joins; it may be dyed flesh colour with a suitable non-toxic dye.

WEIGHT OF FILM. Not less than 65 g per m², calculated on the unstretched plaster.

WEIGHT OF ADHESIVE MASS. Not less than 25 g per m², calculated on the unstretched plaster.

WATERPROOFNESS. It complies with the test for waterproofness described in Appendix 27, page 915.

WATER-VAPOUR PERMEABILITY. The weight of water vapour passing through the plaster in 24 hours at 37° is not less than 1000 g per m².

EXTENSIBILITY. It complies with the test described in Appendix 27, page 914.

Packaging. It should be wound on spools and suitably protected.

Labelling. It is labelled as described under Self-adhesive Plasters (page 631).

Storage. It should be stored as described under Self-adhesive Plasters (page 631).

Uses. Waterproof microporous plastic self-adhesive plaster is used to cover dressings and sites of infection when free passage of air and water vapour but exclusion of water is required. It is also used to prepare Waterproof Microporous Plastic Wound Dressing (page 622).

Waterproof Plastic Self-adhesive Plaster

SYNONYMS: Plastic Adhesive Strapping; Waterproof Strapping

Waterproof Plastic Self-adhesive Plaster consists of an extensible water-impermeable plastic film spread evenly with a self-adhesive plaster mass.

Standard
DESCRIPTION. Extensible plastic film spread evenly with a self-adhesive plaster mass which does not off-set when unrolled from the spool.
The film is in one continuous length containing no joins; it may be dyed flesh colour with a suitable non-toxic dye.

WEIGHT OF FILM. Not less than 65 g per m², calculated on the unstretched plaster.

WEIGHT OF ADHESIVE MASS. Not less than 42 g per m², calculated on the unstretched plaster.

WATERPROOFNESS. It complies with the test for waterproofness described in Appendix 27, page 915.

EXTENSIBILITY. It complies with the test described in Appendix 27, page 914.

Packaging. It should be wound on spools and suitably protected.

Labelling. It is labelled as described under Self-adhesive Plasters (page 631).

Storage. It should be stored as described under Self-adhesive Plasters (page 631).

Uses. Waterproof plastic self-adhesive plaster is used to secure dressings and appliances and to cover sites of infection when total exclusion of water, water vapour, and air is required. It is also used to prepare Waterproof Plastic Wound Dressing (page 622).

Zinc Oxide Elastic Self-adhesive Plaster

SYNONYMS: Elastic Adhesive Plaster; Zinc Oxide Elastic Plaster

Zinc Oxide Elastic Self-adhesive Plaster consists of elastic cloth which stretches in the direction of the warp, spread evenly with a self-adhesive plaster mass containing zinc oxide.

Standard
DESCRIPTION. Elastic cloth spread with a self-adhesive plaster mass, containing zinc oxide, which does not off-set when unwound; it is spread evenly, except that the mass may be made porous or permeable to air.
The elastic cloth is in one continuous length containing no joins, clean, and reasonably free from weaving defects, cotton leaf and shell; it may be dyed flesh colour with a suitable non-toxic dye.

FABRIC. The warp threads consist of twofold, threefold, or fourfold cotton yarn with a finished count, after crêpe-twisting, not finer than 28·2 tex (2/42's or the equivalent in threefold and fourfold yarns), each containing not less than 19 folding turns per cm; they

are arranged as follows: two threads S-twist and two threads Z-twist, repeated.
The weft threads consist of cotton or rayon staple fibre, or cotton and rayon staple fibre spun together, of a count not finer than 59·0 tex (10's).

THREADS PER STATED LENGTH. Warp: average not less than 19 per cm, determined by counting the total number of warp threads in the plaster and dividing by the width, in cm, of the unstretched plaster.
Weft: average not less than 82 per 10 cm, determined on the fully stretched plaster.

WEIGHT OF FABRIC. Not less than 110 g per m², calculated from the unstretched width and the fully stretched length.

WEIGHT OF ADHESIVE MASS. Not less than 120 g per m², calculated from the unstretched width and the fully stretched length.

ELASTICITY. The regain length is not more than four-fifths of the fully stretched length.

CONTENT OF ZINC OXIDE IN THE ADHESIVE MASS. Not less than 10·0 per cent, calculated as ZnO, determined by the method for Zinc Oxide Self-adhesive Plaster (below).

Packaging. It should be wound in rolls suitably protected.

Labelling. It is labelled as described under Self-adhesive Plasters (page 631).

Storage. It should be stored as described under Self-adhesive Plasters (page 631).

Uses. Zinc oxide elastic self-adhesive plaster is used to secure dressings and appliances, to cover sites of infection, and for general support bandaging.

Zinc Oxide Self-adhesive Plaster

SYNONYMS: Zinc Oxide Plaster; Adhesive Plaster

Zinc Oxide Self-adhesive Plaster consists of a suitable cloth spread evenly with a self-adhesive plaster mass containing zinc oxide.

Standard
DESCRIPTION. Cotton or rayon or mixed cotton and rayon cloth spread with a self-adhesive plaster mass containing zinc oxide, which does not off-set when unrolled from the spool. It is evenly spread, except that the mass may be made porous or permeable to air.
The cloth is of plain weave, in one continuous length containing no joins, clean, and reasonably free from weaving defects, cotton leaf and shell. It is finished to a good white or dyed flesh colour with a suitable non-toxic dye.
The plaster may be perforated.

YARN; THREADS PER STATED LENGTH; WEIGHT OF FABRIC; TENSILE STRENGTH OF UNPERFORATED FABRIC; PERFORATIONS. It complies with the requirements described under Belladonna Self-adhesive Plaster, page 631.

ADHESIVENESS. It complies with the test described in Appendix 27, page 913.

WEIGHT OF ADHESIVE MASS. Not less than 115 g per m².

CONTENT OF ZINC OXIDE IN THE ADHESIVE MASS. Not less than 10·0 per cent, calculated as ZnO, determined by the following method:
Heat about 1 g of the plaster, accurately weighed and cut into strips, with 75 ml of *chloroform*, 6 ml of *acetic acid*, and 40 ml of water in a conical flask on a hot plate until the chloroform layer boils and continue the heating for 4 minutes, swirling the mixture frequently. Allow the mixture to cool slightly, stopper the flask, shake it vigorously for 2 minutes, and rinse the stopper

with water, collecting the rinsings in the flask. Add 10 ml of *ammonia buffer solution* and, while the mixture is still warm, titrate with 0·1M disodium edetate, with continuous swirling, using as indicator 0·2 ml of a solution containing 0·5 per cent w/v of *mordant black 11* and 4·5 per cent w/v of *hydroxylammonium chloride* in *methyl alcohol*; each ml of 0·1M disodium edetate is equivalent to 0·008137 g of ZnO.

Decant the titrated liquid through a fine sieve (No. 150) and return any collected fibres to the piece of fabric in the flask. Wash the material with several successive small portions of chloroform and dry at 105°. Condition the dried material as described in Appendix 27, page 913, under "Conditioning for testing" and weigh.

Calculate the weight of adhesive mass by subtracting the weight of the residual fabric from that of the plaster taken and hence the percentage of zinc oxide in the adhesive mass.

Packaging. It should be wound on spools and suitably protected.

Labelling. It is labelled as described under Self-adhesive Plasters (page 631).

Storage. It should be stored as described under Self-adhesive Plasters (page 631).

Uses. Zinc oxide self-adhesive plaster is used to secure dressings and to immobilise small areas.

WADDINGS

Absorbent Viscose Wadding

SYNONYM: Lanugo Cellulosi Absorbens

Absorbent Viscose Wadding consists of bleached new fibres of Regenerated Cellulose or of Delustred Regenerated Cellulose obtained by the viscose process and cut to a suitable staple length.

Standard
Material which complies with this standard will meet the requirements of the European Pharmacopoeia.

DESCRIPTION. It has the macroscopical and microscopical characteristics of Regenerated Cellulose, page 636, or of Delustred Regenerated Cellulose, page 637, with the addition that it consists of well-carded, crimped fibres, of average length 25 to 50 mm, with more or less straight ends. It consists exclusively of viscose rayon fibres. It may be slightly off-white if it has been sterilised.

IDENTIFICATION TESTS. 1. It complies with tests 1, 2, and 3 described under Regenerated Cellulose, page 636.

2. The lustrous material complies with test 4 described under Regenerated Cellulose, page 636, and the matt material complies with test 2 described under Delustred Regenerated Cellulose, page 637.

COLOUR OF AQUEOUS EXTRACT; ACIDITY OR ALKALINITY; WATER-SOLUBLE SUBSTANCES; ETHER-SOLUBLE SUBSTANCES; HYDROGEN SULPHIDE; COLOURING MATTER; LOSS ON DRYING. It complies with the tests described under Regenerated Cellulose, page 636.

ABSORBENCY. Carry out the test described under Absorbent Cotton Wool, page 618.
The sinking time is not more than 10 seconds and the water-holding capacity is not less than 18·0 g per gram of sample.

SURFACE-ACTIVE SUBSTANCES. To 2 g add 20 ml of water, allow to macerate for 2 hours, decant, pressing the sample with a glass rod to express the residual liquid, and mix; shake vigorously in a clean test tube 10 ml of the liquid and allow to stand for 10 minutes; not more than a ring of froth, in contact with the walls of the tube, remains.

FLUORESCENCE. Examine a layer, about 5 mm in thickness, under ultraviolet radiation, including radiation of wavelength 365 nm. The sample shows only a slight brownish-yellow fluorescence and no intense blue fluorescence, except that which may be shown by a few isolated fibres (absence of fluorescent brightening agents).

SULPHATED ASH. Not more than 0·45 per cent for the lustrous material or not more than 1·7 per cent for the matt material, both determined on 5 g.

STERILITY. If the label on the package states that the material is sterile, the contents comply with the test for sterility described in Appendix 28, page 917.

Sterilisation. It is sterilised by one of the methods described for surgical dressings in Appendix 29 (page 926) or by any other suitable process.

Uses. Absorbent viscose wadding is used for cleansing and swabbing wounds, for pre-operative skin preparation, and for the application of medicaments to wounds. It is not suitable for use in situations where it is necessary for absorbent material to be retained in place for any length of time.

Cellulose Wadding

Cellulose Wadding is made entirely from high-grade bleached wood pulp, which consists of delignified disintegrated timber. It consists almost entirely of pure cellulose and is reasonably free from lignified fibres.

Standard
DESCRIPTION. *Macroscopical:* Compressed sheets of felted fibres, bleached to a good white; somewhat harsh to the touch; quickly disintegrates when thrown into water; breaks off short when a wad is pulled.

Microscopical: The fibres of the pulp show the characters of the elements of the timber, usually coniferous, from which it has been prepared.
When treated with *ammoniacal copper oxide solution*, the fibres swell, some of them developing spherical swellings resembling those produced on raw cotton, and finally dissolve.
When soaked in *iodine water* for a few minutes on a microscope slide and the excess of reagent removed by filter paper, the fibres assume a blue colour on adding one or two drops of *sulphuric acid (66 per cent v/v)*.

AREA PER UNIT WEIGHT. 1 g has a superficial area of 18 to 24 cm².

ABSORBENCY. 1 g, compressed to a volume of about 20 ml, placed lightly by means of forceps on the surface of water at 20°, becomes saturated within 10 seconds.

MOISTURE. Not more than 10·0 per cent, determined by drying to constant weight at 105°.

CHLOROFORM-SOLUBLE EXTRACTIVE. Not more than 1·0 per cent, calculated with reference to the material dried at 105°, determined by extracting with *chloroform* for 6 hours in an apparatus for the continuous extraction of drugs, evaporating the extract to dryness, and drying the residue to constant weight at 105°.

SULPHATED ASH. Not more than 0·45 per cent, determined on 5 g.

LIGNIN. Place a portion of the wadding on a white porcelain tile, add 0·05 ml of *phloroglucinol solution*, followed by 0·05 ml of *hydrochloric acid*, allow to stand for two minutes, and examine with the aid of a magnifying lens.

The quantity of fibre stained deep red is not greater than that present in a similarly treated portion of the standard sample kept by the Manchester Chamber of Commerce Testing House.

Repeat the test on four further portions, each selected from different parts so as to be as representative of the wadding as possible.

FLUORESCENCE. Examine under ultraviolet radiation, including radiation of wavelength 365 nm; the material shows no general fluorescence and is reasonably free from fluorescent fibres (absence of fluorescent brightening agents).

Uses. Cellulose wadding is used as an absorbent and protective pad; it is used to prepare Gauze and Cellulose Wadding Tissue (page 629).

OTHER MATERIALS

Animal Wool for Chiropody

SYNONYMS: Animal Wool Long Strand; Lamb's Wool for Chiropody

Animal Wool for Chiropody is obtained from the sheep, *Ovis aries* L. (Fam. Bovidae).

When shorn from the sheep's body the wool contains animal grease and foreign substances. Most of the wool grease and a proportion of the foreign substances are removed by scouring and washing. The remainder of the foreign substances are removed by combing, which may be facilitated by the addition of a suitable vegetable oil.

Animal Wool for Chiropody is very hygroscopic, absorbing up to 50 per cent of moisture, but it has a recommended allowance for moisture regain of 18·25 per cent.

It chiefly consists of keratin.

Standard

DESCRIPTION. *Macroscopical:* A yellowish-white, continuous, slightly twisted, coherent sliver.

Microscopical: Each hair is composed of a cuticle of imbricated flattened epithelial scales, a wide cortex of nucleated spindle-shaped fibres, and may have a narrow medulla of polyhedral or rounded cells.

The free projecting edges of the epithelial scales are directed towards the apex of the hair and give rise to numerous irregular transverse markings upon the surface of the hair.

It is soluble, at 100°, in *dilute sodium hydroxide solution*; it is insoluble in, but coloured blue by, *ammoniacal copper oxide solution*, and is insoluble, at 20°, in *sulphuric acid (66 per cent v/v)*.

It is stained yellow by *trinitrophenol solution*.

QUALITY AND LENGTH OF STAPLE. The quality of the wool is 46's to 56's (Bradford classification), with an average length of not less than 12·5 cm, the longest fibres being not less than 23 cm.

ETHER-SOLUBLE MATTER. 2·0 to 5·0 per cent of the dry weight of wool, determined by the following method: Dry the sample at 35° for 30 minutes; extract about 15 g, accurately weighed, with dry redistilled *solvent ether* for 3 hours in an apparatus for the continuous extraction of drugs, evaporate off the ether, and dry the residue to constant weight at 90°.

Uses. Animal wool for chiropody is used mainly for protective purposes, for retaining dressings on toes, and occasionally as a substitute for felt or rubber padding when these are not well tolerated.

Calico, Unbleached

Unbleached Calico consists of unbleached cotton cloth of plain weave.

Standard

DESCRIPTION. Unbleached cotton cloth of plain weave, clean, and reasonably free from weaving defects, cotton leaf and shell.

YARN. A uniform, good medium grade.

THREADS PER STATED LENGTH. Warp: average 26·0 per cm; standard deviation 0·35.

Weft: average 24·1 per cm; standard deviation 0·50.

WEIGHT PER UNIT AREA. Average 91 g per m²; standard deviation 2·5.

FOREIGN MATTER. Not more than 10·0 per cent.

Uses. Unbleached calico is used in the preparation of Triangular Calico Bandage (page 611). It is occasionally used as a roller bandage where great strength is required.

If unbleached calico is used on an area where there is broken skin, the material should be sterilised by one of the methods described for surgical dressings in Appendix 29 (page 926).

Muslin, Absorbent

SYNONYM: Bleached Muslin

Absorbent Muslin consists of bleached cotton cloth of plain weave.

Standard

DESCRIPTION. Cotton cloth of plain weave, bleached to a good white, clean and reasonably free from weaving defects, cotton leaf and shell.

YARN. A uniform, good medium grade.

THREADS PER STATED LENGTH. Warp: average not less than 19 per cm.

Weft: average not less than 12 per cm.

WEIGHT PER UNIT AREA. Not less than 35 g per m².

ABSORBENCY. 1 g, compressed to a volume of about 20 ml, placed lightly by means of forceps on the surface of water at 20°, becomes saturated within 10 seconds.

FOREIGN MATTER. Not more than 1·0 per cent; contains no added foreign matter.

FLUORESCENCE. Examine under ultraviolet radiation, including radiation at wavelength 365 nm; not more than an occasional point of fluorescence is visible (absence of fluorescent brightening agents).

Uses. Absorbent muslin is used for the application of wet and dry dressings; it is also used in the treatment of extensive burns. It is a component of Standard Dressing No. 16 (page 626).

It is not suitable for the preparation of plaster slabs, for which purpose starched muslin is required.

Oiled Silk

Oiled Silk consists of silk fabric evenly proofed with drying oils or oil-modified synthetic resins so that the material is impervious to water.

Silk is prepared from the fibre obtained from the cocoons of *Bombyx mori* L. and other species of *Bombyx* (Fam. Bombycidae) and of *Antheraea paphia* L. and other species of *Antheraea* (Fam. Saturniidae). It is very hygroscopic and burns slowly with evolution of alkaline fumes which have the odour of burnt horn.

When examined under a microscope the fibres are seen to be homogeneous, hyaline, and solid, about 5 to 65 μm wide, rounded or rounded triangular in transverse section, externally smooth or finely striated longitudinally, and occasionally somewhat flattened and twisted round one another.

Silk is rapidly soluble in *hydrochloric acid*, in *sulphuric acid* (*66 per cent v/v*), and in *ammoniacal copper oxide solution*, but dissolves only slowly and with difficulty in *dilute sodium hydroxide solution*. It is coloured light brown with 0·02N iodine and red when warmed with *mercury nitrate solution*.

Standard

DESCRIPTION. Silk fabric made completely waterproof by treatment with suitable drying oils, or oil-modified synthetic resins, including alkyds; it is without added colour or it is dyed with a suitable green non-toxic dye.

The silk fabric is of regular plain weave and reasonably free from weaving defects.

THREADS PER STATED LENGTH. Warp: average not less than 47 per cm.

Weft: average not less than 33 per cm.

WEIGHT PER UNIT AREA. Not less than 84 g per m².

WEIGHT OF FABRIC. Not less than 11·3 g per m², determined by the following method:

Heat under a reflux condenser a piece of the dressing measuring 50 cm² with 125 ml of *sodium carbonate solution* diluted to 250 ml with water, until the proofing is removed from the fabric; in the case of resistant proofing the sodium carbonate solution is replaced by 250 ml of *alcoholic potassium hydroxide solution*.

Wash the fabric well with warm water and then with twelve successive 1000-ml portions of boiling water, wringing the fabric by hand after each washing and passing all the washings through a fine sieve; combine the residual fabric with any loose threads or fibres on the sieve and dry to constant weight at 105°.

To the weight of dry fabric add an allowance for moisture regain of 11·0 per cent and hence, from the area of the original sample, calculate the weight of fabric in g per m².

WATERPROOFNESS. It complies with the test described in Appendix 27, page 915.

Storage. It should be stored in a dry place at a temperature between 15° and 20°, protected from light and from deleterious vapours or contaminants.

Uses. Oiled silk is used to prevent wet dressings, such as fomentations or compresses, from drying out too rapidly and to protect adjacent clothing.

Regenerated Cellulose

SYNONYM: Rayon

Regenerated Cellulose is made from wood cellulose or cotton linters by solution in alkali and carbon disulphide, followed by reprecipitation of the cellulose in the form of a thread by forcing the solution of cellulose through fine holes in a metal plate into a coagulating fluid (viscose process).

Standard

DESCRIPTION: *Macroscopical:* White or slightly yellow, highly lustrous fibre, which burns without forming a bead or ash.

Tensile strength, not less than 1·35 g per dtex. Linear density, 1·7 to 3·3 dtex.

Microscopical: The fibres are solid and transparent with a diameter between about 10 and 20 μm and marked by longitudinal parallel lines distributed unequally over the width. Clearly visible in *chloral hydrate solution* and in *lactophenol*, almost invisible in *cresol*; transverse section rounded with an irregular crenate margin and invisible when viewed between crossed polars.

SOLUBILITY. Soluble in *sulphuric acid* (*66 per cent v/v*); swollen by *ammoniacal copper oxide solution* and ultimately dissolved; insoluble in *formic acid* and in *acetone*; almost insoluble in *dilute sodium hydroxide solution*.

IDENTIFICATION TESTS. 1. Soak in *iodine water* for a few minutes, remove the excess of reagent by filter paper, and add one or two drops of *sulphuric acid* (*66 per cent v/v*); it is stained blue.

2. Treat with *phloroglucinol solution*, followed by *hydrochloric acid*; no red colour is produced.

3. Treat with *iodinated zinc chloride solution*; a violet colour is produced.

4. Dissolve the sulphated ash in 5 ml of *sulphuric acid* by warming gently, cool, pour the solution into 4 ml of water, filter, and add 0·2 ml of *hydrogen peroxide solution*; no yellow colour is produced (absence of titanium dioxide).

COLOUR OF AQUEOUS EXTRACT. To 10 g add 100 ml of water, allow to stand for 2 hours in a closed vessel, and filter, pressing the sample with a glass rod to express the residual liquid; the filtrate does not differ in colour from the water used to prepare the extract. Reserve the filtrate for the tests for Acidity or Alkalinity and Hydrogen Sulphide.

ACIDITY OR ALKALINITY. To 25 ml of the filtrate reserved in the test for Colour of Aqueous Extract add 0·15 ml of *phenolphthalein solution*; the solution does not show a pink colour.

To another 25 ml of the filtrate add 0·05 ml of *methyl orange solution*; the solution is yellow.

WATER-SOLUBLE SUBSTANCES. Not more than 0·70 per cent, determined by the following method:

Boil about 5 g, accurately weighed, with 500 ml of water for 30 minutes, stirring frequently and replacing the water lost by evaporation. Decant the hot liquid, pressing the sample with a glass rod to express the residual liquid, mix, and filter the liquid while it is still hot.

Evaporate 400 ml of the filtrate (equivalent to four-fifths of the weight of sample taken) to dryness and dry the residue to constant weight at 105°.

ETHER-SOLUBLE SUBSTANCES. Not more than 0·30 per cent, determined by the following method:
Extract about 5 g, accurately weighed, with *solvent ether* for 4 hours in an apparatus for the continuous extraction of drugs or for intermittent extraction, with not less than four extractions per hour; evaporate the extract to dryness and dry the residue to constant weight at 105°.

HYDROGEN SULPHIDE. To 10 ml of the filtrate reserved in the test for Colour of Aqueous Extract add 1·9 ml of water, 0·3 ml of *dilute acetic acid*, and 1 ml of *lead acetate solution*, mix, and allow to stand for 2 minutes; the colour of the solution is not more intense than that of a solution prepared by adding to 10 ml of the filtrate 1·7 ml of *standard lead solution*, 0·3 ml of *dilute acetic acid*, and 1·2 ml of *thioacetamide reagent*.

COLOURING MATTER. Slowly extract 10 g with *alcohol (95 per cent)* in a narrow percolator until 50 ml of extract is obtained and examine a 20-cm layer of the extract against a white background. The extract is not more than a very faint yellow and has no bluish or greenish tinge.

LOSS ON DRYING. Not more than 13·0 per cent, determined on 5 g by drying to constant weight at 105°.

SULPHATED ASH. Not more than 0·45 per cent, determined on 5 g.

Uses. Regenerated cellulose is used for the preparation of rayon fabrics and of Absorbent Viscose Wadding (page 634).

Regenerated Cellulose, Delustred

SYNONYM: Delustred Rayon

Delustred Regenerated Cellulose is regenerated cellulose which has been deprived of its sheen by dispersing finely divided titanium dioxide throughout the material during manufacture.

Standard
DESCRIPTION. White matt fibre, having the tensile strength and microscopical characters of Regenerated Cellulose, with the addition of microscopic granular particles, of average diameter 0·25 to 1 μm, scattered throughout the material and appearing black by transmitted light.

IDENTIFICATION TESTS. 1. It complies with tests 1, 2, and 3 described under Regenerated Cellulose.
2. Carry out test 4 described under Regenerated Cellulose; a yellow colour is produced (presence of titanium dioxide).

COLOUR OF AQUEOUS EXTRACT; ACIDITY OR ALKALINITY; WATER-SOLUBLE SUBSTANCES; ETHER-SOLUBLE SUBSTANCES; HYDROGEN SULPHIDE; COLOURING MATTER; LOSS ON DRYING. It complies with the tests described under Regenerated Cellulose.

SULPHATED ASH. Not more than 1·7 per cent, determined on 5 g.

Uses. Delustred regenerated cellulose is used for the preparation of rayon fabrics and of Absorbent Viscose Wadding (page 634).

PART 6

Formulary

FORMULARY

The efficacy and safety of a medicinal product depend on a number of factors. These include the purity and chemical stability of its active constituents and the condition of the patient. There are also various other factors, such as variations in the physical form of the active constituents, the influence of other ingredients that are presumed to be pharmacologically inactive, and the method of preparation.

The specific surface area and size distribution of drug particles may be important for sparingly soluble drugs in tablets and other products that are administered by mouth. Some drugs, such as certain corticosteroids, may exist in various physical forms, and account must be taken of this in devising satisfactory methods of preparing products containing them and in storing the finished products.

The presence of pharmaceutical adjuvants in formulated products may influence the activity of the active medicaments. The presence of certain fillers in tablets may enhance or retard the rate of dissolution of a drug, while the presence of an excipient such as a surface-active agent may, in some instances, directly affect the rate of absorption of the drug. In a preparation intended for application to the skin, the nature of the basis may affect the rate of release of the drug and hence its penetration and absorption. Likewise, the chemical nature and physical properties of a suppository basis may affect the release of a drug in the rectum and, for certain enemas, the retention time in the colon may depend largely upon the chemical nature of the vehicle.

Processes of manufacture may also have important influences on the behaviour and effect of formulated products. The degree of compression of tablets, for example, may markedly affect their dissolution rate. Control both of the process of manufacture and of the ingredients is especially important for products that are formulated to provide release of drugs in the gastro-intestinal tract. The formulation and method of preparation of emulsions and suspensions also need to be carefully controlled.

In preparing products described in this Formulary, the possible influence of the various factors cited above must be considered in relation to the standards specified in the individual monographs. Where the complete formula is not given in a monograph, it must be recognised that while the chemical and physical standards detailed in that monograph provide a specification against which the product can be tested, compliance with these standards does not necessarily ensure that the product is satisfactory in all respects for the clinical purpose for which it is intended. In preparing such products, unspecified ingredients such as dispersing, suspending, flavouring, colouring, and stabilising agents, must be selected and incorporated in a way that ensures that the product is effective and safe in use.

Pharmaceutical problems in dispensing may arise from the mixing of one preparation with another and from the variation in composition of preparations complying with the same standard, as specified in a particular monograph, but originating from different sources of supply. Pharmacists are occasionally requested by prescribers to dispense mixtures of proprietary preparations with other drugs or preparations. The dilution or admixture of such preparations with others may yield an unstable product and affect its efficacy and safety. Where the pharmacist has reason to suspect that such mixtures, or other variation, may seriously affect the efficacy, safety, or stability of the final product, the prescriber should be appropriately informed.

Containers. To ensure maximum stability and safety, a medicinal product must be stored and supplied in a container which protects the preparation from adverse influences and is of an appropriate type. The container must withstand normal handling and transport. In addition, any legal requirements relating to containers must be complied with.

When selecting a container, various factors must be considered, such as the nature of the preparation, the required degree of protection from the atmosphere, from light, and from micro-organisms, the material of which the container is made, and the provision of a suitable closure. Where appropriate, recommendations on containers are given in the general monographs; these should be read in conjunction with any specific statements in monographs describing individual preparations.

Medicinal products for external use must not be supplied in types of container that are normally used for medicinal products taken internally. Liquid products for external use should preferably be dispensed in coloured fluted bottles but, where special considerations apply, other suitable containers may be used, provided that such containers are clearly distinguishable from types normally used for medicinal products taken internally.

Storage. The essential features of good storage are to prevent contamination of a product with extraneous materials and to minimise decomposition that may arise from chemical, physical, or microbiological changes.

In deciding on suitable storage conditions for a particular product, consideration must be given to (a) choice of container and closure and (b) environmental conditions. Definitions of containers suitable for different purposes are given under Containers in the General Notices.

These comments are intended for general guidance of the pharmacist and cannot replace the specific instructions for storage given in the appropriate monographs. In addition, it is desirable to avoid extremes of temperature fluctuation which may accelerate deterioration and also to avoid exposing the materials to direct sunlight even if light-resistant containers are used as these will not prevent temperature rise in the product within the container.

Where there is an indication of shelf-life given in the monograph, the information applies to the material stored, in accordance with the directions, in the original unopened container.

Freshly prepared. The direction that a preparation must be freshly prepared indicates that it must be made not more than twenty-four hours before it is issued for use.

Recently prepared. The direction that a preparation should be recently prepared indicates that deterioration is likely if the preparation is stored for longer than a few weeks under temperate room conditions.

Water. The term "water" used without qualification in recipes means potable water or freshly boiled and cooled Purified Water. Potable water is water freshly drawn direct from the public supply ("mains" water) and suitable for drinking. Water obtained from the supply via a local storage tank is unsuitable for this purpose. If such stored water is the only source of mains water, freshly boiled and cooled Purified Water should be used instead; this should also be used when the potable water in a district is unsuitable for a particular preparation.

AEROSOL INHALATIONS

An aerosol inhalation consists of a solution or suspension of a medicament in a mixture of inert propellents which is held under pressure in an aerosol dispenser, which consists of a suitable container fitted with a special metering valve. In the case of a solution, the medicament may be dissolved in a solvent (co-solvent) which is miscible with the propellents. The particle size of the medicament in a suspension and the droplet size of a solution must be controlled so that, when the aerosol is inhaled, the medicament reaches the region of the respiratory tract where it is intended to be deposited. Substances of low boiling-point suitable for use as propellents are described under Dichlorodifluoromethane (page 155). The preparation may also contain surface-active agents, stabilising agents, and other adjuvants.

For use, the aerosol dispenser is fitted with an adapter in order to facilitate the transfer of the preparation into the body through the mouth (an oral adapter being used) or through the nose (a nasal adapter being used). One form of oral adapter consists of a plastic tube, open at both ends, one of which fits over the valve mechanism, the other end being the mouthpiece; the tube is usually angled in the centre so that when the mouthpiece is correctly placed in the mouth, the aerosol dispenser is held vertically, either in an inverted position, which is the more usual, or in an upright position, in accordance with the manufacturer's instructions. The metering valve is actuated by finger pressure on the base of the container forcing the top of the valve stem against an inner wall of the adapter. Another form of oral adapter incorporates a mechanism which automatically applies pressure to the valve stem when actuated by the reduced pressure created when the patient inhales through the mouthpiece.

In use, actuation of the metering valve releases an appropriate quantity of the preparation in the form of an aerosol of appropriate droplet size, a portion of which becomes deposited on the inner surface of the adapter and the remainder issues from the open end of the adapter. The quantity of medicament available to the patient with each spray is therefore less than the quantity released by the valve.

To use the assembled unit, the patient exhales as fully as possible, inserts the open end of the adapter into his mouth or nostril as appropriate, and inhales, at the same time actuating the valve. The orally inhaled medicament is usually intended to be deposited in the bronchial or upper pulmonary regions.

Aerosol inhalations are potent preparations and care should be taken to ensure that the patient is fully aware of this. Any leaflet or card which is enclosed in the package and gives all the necessary instructions for using the unit should be issued with the appliance and the patient should be advised verbally to read all the directions before use.

Containers. They should be supplied in containers of metal or of glass protected with a plastic coating; this coating also serves to protect the user if the glass fractures. Aerosol dispensers should comply with the relevant part of British Standard 3914.

Labelling. The following directions should be followed:
A. The label on the pressurised container gives:
(1) the name of the preparation, with the B.P.C. title or the strength of the preparation expressed as the weight of active ingredient(s) per millilitre,
(2) the amount(s) of active ingredient(s) available to the patient each time the valve is actuated, and
(3) a warning indicating that the container is pressurised and must be kept away from heat, including the sun, and must not be punctured, broken, or incinerated even when apparently empty.
In addition, the label or marking on the container or the label or marking on the adapter gives, in a position such that the directions are visible when the unit is assembled for use:
(4) a direction to shake the container before use, if applicable,
(5) a warning that the patient should adhere strictly to and not exceed the prescribed dosage,
(6) a direction to read the instructions on the enclosed card or leaflet before use, and
(7) an indication of the correct aspect of the container in use.

B. A leaflet or card should be included in the package giving:
(1) the directions for the correct use of the preparation,
(2) the recommended dosage schedule,
(3) the maximum number of doses that may be taken in twenty-four hours,
(4) the directions for keeping the unit clean, and
(5) the directions for the disposal of the used, or partly used, container.

C. The label or wording on the carton gives:
(1) the name of the preparation,
(2) the amount(s) of active ingredient(s) available to the patient each time the valve is actuated,
(3) the expected number of times the valve can be actuated before the container becomes empty,
(4) the date after which the preparation is not intended to be used, if applicable,
(5) a direction to read the instructions enclosed before use, and
(6) sufficient space for the pharmacist to add any additional label without obscuring any directions that the patient needs to read.

Storage. Aerosol inhalations should be stored in a cool place but protected from frost. Aerosol dispensers must be protected from heat, including the sun, because they may explode, even when apparently empty.

Ergotamine Aerosol Inhalation

Ergotamine Aerosol Inhalation is a suspension of Ergotamine Tartrate, in sufficiently fine powder to meet the requirements of the standard, in a suitable mixture of aerosol propellents, which may contain a surface-active agent, stabilising agents, and other adjuvants. It is packed in a pressurised container fitted with a special metering valve and an oral adapter.

Standard
PRESENCE OF ERGOTAMINE. 1. Remove the oral adapter from the pressurised container, shake the container, place it inverted in a small beaker containing 10 ml of *tartaric acid solution*, and fire 5 sprays below the surface of the liquid, actuating the valve by pressing on the base of the container so that the valve stem is forced against the bottom of the beaker.
To 1 ml of the solution add 2 ml of *dimethylamino-benzaldehyde solution* and mix; a deep blue colour is produced.
2. It complies with the thin-layer chromatographic test given in Appendix 5A, page 863.

PARTICLE SIZE. With the oral adapter in position, fire 1 spray on to a clean dry microscope slide held about 5 cm from the end of the mouthpiece of the adapter and perpendicular to the direction of the spray. Rinse the slide with about 2 ml of *carbon tetrachloride*, taking care not to remove the deposit, allow to dry, and examine the residue under a microscope.
Most of the individual particles have a diameter not greater than 5 μm; no individual particle has a length, measured along its longest axis, greater than 20 μm.

RELATED ALKALOIDS. It complies with the thin-layer chromatographic test given in Appendix 5A, page 863 (not more than 10 per cent of the content of ergotamine tartrate).

CONTENT OF ERGOTAMINE TARTRATE PER SPRAY. 75·0 to 125·0 per cent of the amount stated on the label as being available to the patient, determined by subtracting the amount retained in the oral adapter from the amount delivered by the metering valve, these quantities being determined by the following methods:

Amount of ergotamine tartrate delivered by the metering valve. Remove the oral adapter from the pressurised container, gently shake the container, actuate the valve several times, wash the valve stem with *methyl alcohol*, and discard the washings; replace the oral adapter, invert the assembled unit, and place in a small beaker containing 40 ml of *carbon tetrachloride* and 20 ml of *tartaric acid solution*, ensuring that the mouth of the oral adapter is completely immersed below the surface of the carbon tetrachloride layer.
Fire 10 sprays by pressing on the base of the container, gently agitating the unit while keeping it in the liquids and swirling the contents of the beaker between each spray; remove the unit from the beaker, wash it with *tartaric acid solution*, and transfer the combined liquids and washings to a separating funnel; shake for 5 minutes, allow to separate, and transfer the upper aqueous layer to a 100-ml volumetric flask; extract the carbon tetrachloride layer with further successive 20-, 10-, and 10-ml portions of *tartaric acid solution*, dilute the combined aqueous extracts to 100 ml with *tartaric acid solution*, and measure the extinction of a 1-cm layer at the maximum at about 317 nm.
By reference to a calibration curve prepared with suitable quantities of a solution of *ergotamine tartrate* in *tartaric acid solution*, calculate the total quantity of ergotamine tartrate in the 10 sprays and divide by 10.

Amount of ergotamine tartrate retained in the oral adapter. Remove the oral adapter from the pressurised container, gently shake the container, actuate the valve several times, wash the valve stem with *methyl alcohol*, and discard the washings; replace the oral adapter, and fire 10 sprays into the air, gently shaking the assembled unit between each spray.
Remove the oral adapter, immerse it in 40 ml of *alcoholic tartaric acid solution* contained in a small beaker, swirl the contents of the beaker, remove the oral adapter from the beaker, wash it with *alcoholic tartaric acid solution*, dilute the combined solution and washings to 50 ml with *alcoholic tartaric acid solution*, and measure the extinction of a 2-cm layer at the maximum at about 317 nm.
By reference to a calibration curve prepared with suitable quantities of a solution of *ergotamine tartrate* in *alcoholic tartaric acid solution*, calculate the total quantity of ergotamine tartrate retained by the oral adapter from the 10 sprays and divide by 10.

Containers; Labelling; Storage. The directions given under Aerosol Inhalations (page 644) should be followed.

Dose. One inhalation of 360 micrograms of ergotamine tartrate, repeated, if required, at intervals of five minutes, up to a maximum of six inhalations in twenty-four hours. Not more than fifteen inhalations should be taken in any one week.

A preparation delivering 360 μg of ergotamine tartrate to the patient each time the valve is actuated is available.

Isoprenaline Aerosol Inhalation

Isoprenaline Aerosol Inhalation is a suspension of Isoprenaline Sulphate, in sufficiently fine powder to meet the requirements of the standard, in a suitable mixture of aerosol propellents, which may contain a surface-active agent, stabilising agents, and other adjuvants. It is packed in a pressurised container fitted with a special metering valve, delivering 80 micrograms of isoprenaline sulphate to the patient each time it is actuated, and an oral adapter.

Standard
PRESENCE OF ISOPRENALINE SULPHATE. 1. Remove the oral adapter from the pressurised container, shake the container, place it inverted in a small beaker containing 5 ml of water and 10 ml of *chloroform*, and fire 20 sprays below the surface of the chloroform layer, actuating the valve by pressing on the base of the container so that the valve stem is forced against the bottom of the beaker; remove the container from the beaker, transfer the liquids to a separating funnel, shake, and allow to separate; the upper aqueous layer complies with the following tests:
(i) to 2 ml add 0·1 ml of *ferric chloride test-solution*; an emerald green colour is produced, which, on the gradual addition of *sodium bicarbonate solution*, changes first to blue and then to red.
(ii) it gives the reactions characteristic of sulphates.
2. It complies with the paper chromatographic test given in Appendix 4, page 857.

PARTICLE SIZE. It complies with the test described under Ergotamine Aerosol Inhalation.

CONTENT OF ISOPRENALINE SULPHATE PER SPRAY. 75·0 to 125·0 per cent of the amount stated on the label as being available to the patient, determined by subtracting the amount retained in the oral adapter from the amount delivered by the metering valve, these quantities being determined by the following methods:

Amount of isoprenaline sulphate delivered by the metering valve. Remove the oral adapter from the pressurised container, gently shake the container, actuate the valve several times, wash the valve stem with *methyl alcohol*, and discard the washings; replace the oral adapter, invert the assembled unit, and place in a small beaker containing 25 ml of *carbon tetrachloride* and 25 ml of 0·01N sulphuric acid, ensuring that the mouth of the oral adapter is completely immersed below the surface of the carbon tetrachloride layer.

Fire 10 sprays by pressing on the base of the container, gently agitating the unit while keeping it in the liquids and swirling the contents of the beaker between each spray; remove the unit from the beaker, wash it with 0·01N sulphuric acid, and transfer the combined liquids and washings to a separating funnel; shake for 5 minutes, allow to separate, and transfer the upper aqueous layer to a 50-ml volumetric flask; extract the carbon tetrachloride layer with further successive 5-ml portions of 0·01N sulphuric acid until complete extraction of the isoprenaline sulphate is effected, and dilute the combined acid extracts to 50 ml with 0·01N sulphuric acid.

To 20 ml of this solution add 0·3 ml of *ferrous sulphate–citrate solution* and 3 ml of *aminoacetate buffer solution*, mix, allow to stand for 15 minutes, dilute to 25 ml with water, and measure the extinction of a 2-cm layer at 530 nm.

By reference to a calibration curve prepared with suitable quantities of a solution of *isoprenaline sulphate* in 0·01N sulphuric acid and treated as described above, beginning with the words "add 0·3 ml of *ferrous sulphate–citrate solution . . .*", calculate the total quantity of isoprenaline sulphate in the 10 sprays and divide by 10.

Amount of isoprenaline sulphate retained in the oral adapter. Remove the oral adapter from the pressurised container, gently shake the container, actuate the valve several times, wash the valve stem with *methyl alcohol*, and discard the washings; replace the oral adapter, and fire 20 sprays into the air, gently shaking the assembled unit between each spray.

Remove the oral adapter, immerse it in 25 ml of *carbon tetrachloride* and 25 ml of 0·01N sulphuric acid contained in a small beaker, swirl the contents of the beaker, remove the oral adapter from the beaker, wash it with 0·01N sulphuric acid, and continue by the method given above for the determination of the amount of isoprenaline sulphate delivered by the metering valve, beginning with the words "transfer the combined liquids and washings to a separating funnel . . .", measuring the extinction in a 4-cm cell instead of a 2-cm cell.

Calculate the total quantity of isoprenaline sulphate retained by the oral adapter from the 20 sprays and divide by 20.

Containers; Labelling; Storage. The directions given under Aerosol Inhalations (page 644) should be followed.

Dose. One to three inhalations of 80 micrograms of isoprenaline sulphate, repeated, if required, after thirty minutes, up to a maximum of eight inhalations in twenty-four hours. If more than one inhalation is taken at a time, at least one minute should elapse between any two inhalations.

Larger doses may be administered by means of Strong Isoprenaline Aerosol Inhalation.

Isoprenaline Aerosol Inhalation, Strong

Strong Isoprenaline Aerosol Inhalation is a suspension of Isoprenaline Sulphate, in sufficiently fine powder to meet the requirements of the standard, in a suitable mixture of aerosol propellents, which may contain a surface-active agent, stabilising agents, and other adjuvants.

It is packed in a pressurised container fitted with a special metering valve, delivering 400 micrograms of isoprenaline sulphate to the patient each time it is actuated, and an oral adapter.

Standard
PRESENCE OF ISOPRENALINE SULPHATE. It complies with the tests described under Isoprenaline Aerosol Inhalation.

PARTICLE SIZE. It complies with the test described under Ergotamine Aerosol Inhalation, page 645.

CONTENT OF ISOPRENALINE SULPHATE PER SPRAY. 75·0 to 125·0 per cent of the amount stated on the label as being available to the patient, determined by subtracting the amount retained in the oral adapter from the amount delivered by the metering valve, these quantities being determined by the following methods:

Amount of isoprenaline sulphate delivered by the metering valve. Carry out the method described for Isoprenaline Aerosol Inhalation, diluting the combined acid extracts to 250 ml instead of to 50 ml.

Amount of isoprenaline sulphate retained in the oral adapter. Carry out the method described for Isoprenaline Aerosol Inhalation, diluting the combined acid extracts to 200 ml instead of to 50 ml.

Containers; Labelling; Storage. The directions given under Aerosol Inhalations (page 644) should be followed.

Dose. One to three inhalations of 400 micrograms of isoprenaline sulphate, repeated, if required, after thirty minutes, up to a maximum of eight inhalations in twenty-four hours. If more than one inhalation is taken at a time, at least one minute should elapse between any two inhalations.

This preparation is approximately five times the strength of Isoprenaline Aerosol Inhalation.

Orciprenaline Aerosol Inhalation

Orciprenaline Aerosol Inhalation is a suspension of Orciprenaline Sulphate, in sufficiently fine powder to meet the requirements of the standard, in a suitable mixture of aerosol propellents, which may contain a surface-active agent, stabilising agents, and other adjuvants.

It is packed in a pressurised container fitted with a special metering valve and an oral adapter.

Standard
PRESENCE OF ORCIPRENALINE SULPHATE. 1. Remove the oral adapter from the pressurised container, shake the container, place it inverted in a small beaker containing 10 ml of water, and fire 10 sprays below the surface of the liquid, actuating the valve by pressing on the base of the container so that the valve stem is forced against the bottom of the beaker, remove the container from the beaker, and filter the solution. The filtrate complies with the following tests:

(i) To 2 ml add 0·1 ml of a saturated solution of *mercuric acetate* in water; a yellow colour is produced.

(ii) Dilute 5 ml to 100 ml with water. This solution exhibits a light absorption which has, in the range 230 to 360 nm, a maximum which remains almost constant from 276 to 280 nm.

(iii) It gives the reactions characteristic of sulphates.

2. It complies with the paper chromatographic test given in Appendix 4, page 857.

PARTICLE SIZE. It complies with the test described under Ergotamine Aerosol Inhalation, page 645.

CONTENT OF ORCIPRENALINE SULPHATE PER SPRAY. 75·0 to 125·0 per cent of the amount stated on the label as being available to the patient, determined by subtracting the amount retained in the oral adapter from the amount delivered by the metering valve, these quantities being determined by the following methods:

Amount of orciprenaline sulphate delivered by the metering valve. Remove the oral adapter from the pressurised container, gently shake the container, actuate the valve several times, wash the valve stem with water, and discard the washings; replace the oral adapter, invert the assembled unit, and place in a beaker containing 100 ml of 0·01N hydrochloric acid, ensuring that the mouth of the oral adapter is completely immersed below the surface of the liquid.

Fire 20 sprays by pressing on the base of the container, gently agitating the unit while keeping it in the liquid and swirling the contents of the beaker between each spray; remove the unit from the beaker, wash it with 0·01N hydrochloric acid, and transfer the combined solution and washings to a separating funnel; extract the aqueous liquid with 20 ml of *solvent ether*, allow to separate, wash the ethereal layer with 20 ml of 0·01N hydrochloric acid, and discard the ethereal extract. Dilute the combined aqueous solution and washings to 200 ml with 0·01N hydrochloric acid, and measure the extinction of a 1-cm layer at the maximum at about 276 nm.

For the purposes of calculation, use a value of 72·3 for the E(1 per cent, 1 cm) of orciprenaline sulphate. Calculate the total quantity in the 20 sprays and divide by 20.

Amount of orciprenaline sulphate retained in the oral adapter. Remove the oral adapter from the pressurised container, gently shake the container, actuate the valve several times, wash the valve stem with water, and discard the washings; replace the oral adapter, and fire 20 sprays into the air, gently shaking the assembled unit between each spray.

Remove the oral adapter, immerse it in 50 ml of 0·01N hydrochloric acid contained in a small beaker, swirl the contents of the beaker, remove the oral adapter from the beaker, wash it with 0·01N hydrochloric acid, and continue by the method given above for the determination of the amount of orciprenaline sulphate delivered by the metering valve, beginning with the words "transfer the combined solution and washings . . .", diluting the final solution to 100 ml instead of to 200 ml.

Calculate the total quantity of orciprenaline sulphate retained by the oral adapter from the 20 sprays and divide by 20.

Containers; Labelling; Storage. The directions given under Aerosol Inhalations (page 644) should be followed.

Dose. One or two inhalations of 670 micrograms of orciprenaline sulphate, repeated, if required, after thirty minutes, up to a maximum of twelve inhalations in twenty-four hours. If more than one inhalation is taken at a time, at least one minute should elapse between any two inhalations.

A preparation delivering 670 µg of orciprenaline sulphate to the patient each time the valve is actuated is available.

Salbutamol Aerosol Inhalation

Salbutamol Aerosol Inhalation is a suspension of Salbutamol, in sufficiently fine powder to meet the requirements of the standard, in a suitable mixture of aerosol propellents, which may contain a surface-active agent, stabilising agents, and other adjuvants.

It is packed in a pressurised container fitted with a special metering valve and an oral adapter.

Standard

PRESENCE OF SALBUTAMOL. 1. Remove the oral adapter from the pressurised container, shake the container, place it inverted in a small beaker containing 10 ml of *dehydrated alcohol*, and fire 10 sprays below the surface of the liquid, actuating the valve by pressing on the base of the container so that the valve stem is forced against the bottom of the beaker.

To 1 ml of the solution add 1 ml of a 0·04 per cent w/v solution of *2,6-dichloro-p-benzoquinone-4-chloroimine* in *dehydrated alcohol* and 0·1 ml of *dilute ammonia solution*; a bluish-green colour is produced.

2. It complies with the paper chromatographic test given in Appendix 4, page 857.

PARTICLE SIZE. It complies with the test described under Ergotamine Aerosol Inhalation, page 645.

CONTENT OF SALBUTAMOL PER SPRAY. 75·0 to 125·0 per cent of the amount stated on the label as being available to the patient, determined by subtracting the amount retained in the oral adapter from the amount delivered by the metering valve, these quantities being determined by the following methods:

Amount of salbutamol delivered by the metering valve. Remove the oral adapter from the pressurised container, gently shake the container, actuate the valve several times, wash the valve stem with *dehydrated alcohol*, and discard the washings; replace the oral adapter, invert the assembled unit, and place in a beaker containing 150 ml of *dehydrated alcohol*, ensuring that the mouth of the oral adapter is completely immersed below the surface of the liquid.

Fire 10 sprays by pressing on the base of the container, gently agitating the unit while keeping it in the liquid and swirling the contents of the beaker between each spray; remove the unit from the beaker, wash it with *dehydrated alcohol*, and dilute the combined alcoholic solution and washings to 200 ml with *dehydrated alcohol*.

Transfer 20 ml of this solution to a separating funnel, add 180 ml of water and then, in the following order, 4 ml of a 5 per cent w/v solution of *sodium bicarbonate* in water, 4 ml of *dimethyl-p-phenylenediamine reagent*, and 4 ml of an 8 per cent w/v solution of *potassium ferricyanide* in water; mix, allow to stand for 15 minutes in subdued light, extract the solution with two successive 10-ml portions of *chloroform*, filtering the extracts through a small pledget of cotton wool, and wash the filter with a small amount of *chloroform*; dilute the combined filtrate and washings to 25 ml with *chloroform*, and measure the extinction of a 1-cm layer of the solution at 605 nm.

By reference to a calibration curve, prepared with suitable quantities of a solution of *salbutamol sulphate A.S.* in *dehydrated alcohol* and treated as described above, beginning with the words "add 180 ml of water and then, . . .", calculate the total quantity of salbutamol in the 10 sprays and divide by 10.

Amount of salbutamol retained in the oral adapter. Remove the oral adapter from the pressurised container, gently shake the container, actuate the valve several times, wash the valve stem with *dehydrated alcohol*, and discard the washings; replace the oral adapter, and fire 10 sprays into the air, gently shaking the assembled unit before each spray.

Remove the oral adapter, immerse it in 40 ml of *dehydrated alcohol* contained in a small beaker, swirl the contents of the beaker, remove the oral adapter from the beaker, wash it with *dehydrated alcohol*, dilute the combined solution and washings to 50 ml with *dehydrated alcohol*, and continue by the method given above for the determination of the amount of salbutamol delivered by the metering valve, beginning with the words "Transfer 20 ml of this solution to a separating funnel, . . .".

Calculate the total quantity of salbutamol retained by the oral adapter from the 10 sprays and divide by 10.

Containers; Labelling; Storage. The directions given under Aerosol Inhalations (page 644) should be followed.

Dose. One or two inhalations of 100 micrograms of salbutamol every three or four hours up to a maximum of eight inhalations in twenty-four hours. If more than one inhalation is taken at a time, at least one minute should elapse between any two inhalations.

A preparation delivering 100 μg of salbutamol to the patient each time the valve is actuated is available.

APPLICATIONS

Applications are liquid or semi-liquid preparations for application to the skin.

Containers. Applications should preferably be dispensed in coloured fluted bottles, but other suitable containers may be used provided that such containers are clearly distinguishable from types normally used for medicinal products taken internally.

Labelling. The container should be labelled "For external use only".

Betamethasone Valerate Scalp Application

SYNONYMS: Betamethasone Application; Betamethasone Scalp Application; Betamethasone Valerate Application

Betamethasone Valerate Scalp Application is a solution of Betamethasone Valerate in aqueous Isopropyl Alcohol. It may contain a suitable thickening agent to render the preparation slightly viscous.

Standard
PRESENCE OF BETAMETHASONE. It complies with the thin-layer chromatographic test given in Appendix 5D, page 875.

CONTENT OF BETAMETHASONE. 90·0 to 115·0 per cent of the prescribed or stated amount, determined by the method given in Appendix 23A, page 904, for beta-methasone 17-valerate.

Containers. The directions given under Applications (above) should be followed.

Labelling. The directions given under Applications (above) should be followed; in addition, the container should be labelled "Caution. This preparation is inflammable. Keep away from a naked flame" and a warning should be given to keep the preparation away from the eyes.

Storage. It should be stored in a cool place, protected from light.

Note. When the strength of the application is not specified, a solution containing the equivalent of 0·1 per cent w/w of betamethasone shall be supplied.

Caution. *The application should not be diluted or mixed with any other preparation.*

Calamine Application, Compound

SYNONYMS: Compound Calamine Cream; Compound Calamine Liniment

Calamine, finely sifted	..	..		100 g
Zinc Oxide, finely sifted	..	..		50 g
Wool Fat	..	..	..	25 g
Zinc Stearate	..	..		25 g
Yellow Soft Paraffin	..	..		250 g
Liquid Paraffin	..	..		550 g

Triturate the calamine and the zinc oxide to a smooth paste with a portion of the liquid paraffin. Melt together the zinc stearate, the wool fat, and the yellow soft paraffin at a low temperature and mix with more of the liquid paraffin; incorporate this mixture with the calamine and zinc oxide paste, add the remainder of the liquid paraffin, and mix.

Standard
CONTENT OF ZINC. 8·3 to 10·8 per cent w/w, calculated as Zn, determined by the following method:
Heat gently about 0·5 g, accurately weighed, until the basis is completely volatilised or charred; increase the temperature until all the carbon is removed, and ignite the residue to constant weight; each g of residue is equivalent to 0·8034 g of Zn.

Containers; Labelling. The directions given under Applications (above) should be followed.

Dicophane Application

SYNONYM: DDT Application

Dicophane	..	..	..	20 g
Emulsifying Wax	..	..	..	40 g
Citronella Oil	..	..	..	5 ml
Xylene, of commerce		..	..	150 ml
Water (see page 642)		..	to 1000 ml

Dissolve the dicophane and the citronella oil in the xylene and mix the solution with the emulsifying wax, previously melted at a low temperature; pour the warm mixture into most of the water, previously warmed to the same temperature, stir thoroughly, add sufficient water to produce the required volume, and mix.

Standard
CONTENT OF DICOPHANE. 1·86 to 2·48 per cent w/w, calculated as $C_{14}H_9Cl_5$, determined by the following method:
Boil about 10 g, accurately weighed, under a reflux condenser for 30 minutes with 20 ml of *alcohol (95 per cent)* and 1 g of *sodium hydroxide*, cool, and complete the determination by the method given in Appendix 11, page 891; each ml of 0·1N silver nitrate is equivalent to 0·03545 g of $C_{14}H_9Cl_5$.

Containers; Labelling. The directions given under Applications (page 648) should be followed.

Caution. *This preparation should not be applied to the genital area.*

Gamma Benzene Hexachloride Application

Gamma Benzene Hexachloride	..		1 g
Emulsifying Wax	..	..	40 g
Lavender Oil ..	..	..	10 ml
Xylene, of commerce	..	..	150 ml
Water (see page 642)	..		to 1000 ml

Dissolve the gamma benzene hexachloride and the lavender oil in the xylene and mix the solution with the emulsifying wax, previously melted at a low temperature; pour the warm mixture into most of the water, previously warmed to the same temperature, stir thoroughly, add sufficient water to produce the required volume, and mix.

Standard

OTHER ISOMERS. Dilute 1 g to 100 ml with *acetone* and mix well; dilute 1 ml of this solution to 1000 ml with *toluene* which has been redistilled until it is free from impurities which would interfere with an electron-capture detector. Examine this solution in an apparatus for gas–liquid chromatography, as described in Appendix XIIC of the British Pharmacopoeia.
The chromatographic procedure may be carried out with a column, 60 cm in length and 4 mm in internal diameter, packed with 2 per cent w/w of butanediol succinate supported on white diatomaceous earth (100- to 120-mesh) maintained at 155°, nitrogen as the carrier gas, and an electron-capture detector.
Only one peak, due to gamma benzene hexachloride, is obtained.

CONTENT OF GAMMA BENZENE HEXACHLORIDE. 0·09 to 0·11 per cent w/w, calculated as $C_6H_6Cl_6$, determined by the following method:
To about 15 g, accurately weighed, add 50 ml of 0·5N alcoholic potassium hydroxide, boil under a reflux condenser for one hour, allow to cool, and complete the determination by the method given in Appendix 11, page 891, using 0·02N silver nitrate.
Repeat the procedure using as nearly as possible the same weight of sample, but neutralising the 0·5N alcoholic potassium hydroxide with *dilute nitric acid* before adding it to the sample.
The difference between the two titrations represents the amount of 0·02N silver nitrate required by the chlorine present in the sample; each ml of 0·02N silver nitrate is equivalent to 0·001939 g of $C_6H_6Cl_6$.

Containers; Labelling. The directions given under Applications (page 648) should be followed.

Selenium Sulphide Scalp Application

SYNONYM: Selenium Sulphide Application

Selenium Sulphide Scalp Application is a suspension of Selenium Sulphide in a suitable liquid basis.

Standard

PRESENCE OF SELENIUM SULPHIDE. 1. Digest a quantity, equivalent to 0·05 g of selenium sulphide, with 5 ml of *nitric acid* for 1 hour, dilute to 50 ml with water, and filter; to 5 ml of the filtrate add 10 ml of water and 5 g of *urea*, boil, cool, and add 2 ml of *potassium iodide solution*; a yellow to orange colour which darkens rapidly on standing is produced.
2. Allow the coloured solution obtained in test 1 to stand for 10 minutes and filter through a bed of *kieselguhr*; the filtrate gives the reactions characteristic of sulphates.

ACIDITY. pH, 4·0 to 5·5.

CONTENT OF SELENIUM SULPHIDE. 90·0 to 110·0 per cent of the prescribed or stated concentration, calculated as SeS_2, determined by the following method:
To an accurately weighed quantity, equivalent to about 0·15 g of selenium sulphide, add 25 ml of *fuming nitric acid*, digest on a water-bath for 2 hours, cool, and dilute to 250 ml with water; to 25 ml of this solution add 10 g of *urea* and 25 ml of water, boil, cool, add 10 ml of *potassium iodide solution* and 10 ml of *chloroform*, and titrate immediately with 0·05N sodium thiosulphate until the aqueous layer is a pale straw colour; stopper the flask, shake vigorously for 30 seconds, add 0·1 ml of *starch mucilage*, and continue the titration to the complete absence of blue colour in the aqueous layer; each ml of 0·05N sodium thiosulphate is equivalent to 0·001789 g of SeS_2.
Determine the weight per ml of the application and calculate the concentration of SeS_2, weight in volume.

Containers. The directions given under Applications (page 648) should be followed.

Labelling. The words "For external use only" and a direction to shake the bottle should be given on the label. In addition, the label states:
(1) the directions for using the preparation,
(2) that the preparation should be kept away from the eyes,
(3) that the preparation should not be used within two days of the application of hair tints or permanent waving solutions,
(4) that the preparation should not be allowed to come into contact with metals,
(5) that all silver jewellery, hairpins, and other metal objects should be removed whilst using the preparation, and
(6) that the hands should be carefully washed after using the preparation.

Note. When the strength of the application is not specified, a suspension containing 2·5 per cent w/v of selenium sulphide shall be supplied.

CACHETS

Cachets consist of a dry powder enclosed in a shell and form a convenient method of administering a medicament having an unpleasant taste. The shells are usually prepared from a mixture of rice flour and water by moulding into a suitable shape and drying. The shells thus made are available in two forms: the slip-over or dry-closing type, and the flanged type which is closed by moistening the edges and pressing the two halves together in a machine. Cachets are available in various sizes holding from 0·2 to 1·5 grams of a powder of medium density.

A medicament having a dose of less than 60 milligrams should be triturated with sufficient lactose to produce about 200 milligrams before filling into a cachet. Hygroscopic medicaments should not be enclosed in cachets.

For administration, the cachets are immersed in water for a few seconds, placed on the tongue, and swallowed with a draught of water.

Standard

UNIFORMITY OF WEIGHT AND COMPOSITION. *Method A.* Take a sample of 20 cachets, remove the contents of each cachet as completely as possible, and weigh the contents separately.

The mean weight does not deviate from the prescribed or stated weight by more than 2·5 per cent; the weight of the contents of not more than two cachets may deviate by more than 5 per cent from the mean weight and the weight of the contents of none of the cachets deviates by more than 10 per cent.

The mixed contents of the 20 cachets comply with the standard for the substance given in the British Pharmacopoeia.

Method B. Determine the weight of the contents of each of 20 cachets as described in Method A. The weight of the contents of not more than two cachets may deviate by more than 5 per cent from the mean weight and the weight of the contents of none of the cachets deviates by more than 10 per cent.

Mix the contents of the 20 cachets and determine the proportional amount of each active ingredient in the powder by the methods described in the appropriate monograph. From these figures, calculate the total amount of each active ingredient in the 20 cachets, and divide each weight by twenty.

The results lie within the ranges for the contents of the active ingredients stated in the monograph.

Containers and storage. Cachets should be stored and supplied in containers which provide adequate protection against moisture and crushing.

They should preferably be supplied in wide-mouthed glass or plastic containers, or aluminium containers internally coated with a suitable lacquer or lined with paper; lacquered or lined screw-cap closures or plastic caps should be used.

Labelling. When cachets are dispensed, directions should be given on the label regarding the method of administration.

Sodium Aminosalicylate Cachets

SYNONYM: P.A.S. Cachets

Sodium Aminosalicylate Cachets consist of Sodium Aminosalicylate, in powder, enclosed in a suitable cachet.

Standard
UNIFORMITY OF WEIGHT AND COMPOSITION. They comply with the standard under Cachets, above; Method A is used in the test.

Containers and storage. The directions given under Cachets (above) should be followed; containers should be light-resistant

Labelling. The directions given under Cachets (above) should be followed.

Dose. Sodium aminosalicylate, 10 to 20 grams daily, in divided doses.

When the quantity to be contained in the cachets is not specified, cachets each containing 1·5 g of sodium aminosalicylate shall be supplied.

Sodium Aminosalicylate and Isoniazid Cachets

SYNONYM: P.A.S. and Isoniazid Cachets

Sodium Aminosalicylate and Isoniazid Cachets consist of Sodium Aminosalicylate, in powder, and Isoniazid, in powder, enclosed in a suitable cachet.

Standard
UNIFORMITY OF WEIGHT AND COMPOSITION. They comply with the standard under Cachets, above; Method B is used in the test.

3-AMINOPHENOL. The contents comply with the thin-layer chromatographic test given in Appendix 5A, page 867 (not more than 0·03 per cent).

CONTENT OF ISONIAZID. 90·0 to 110·0 per cent of the prescribed or stated amount, determined by the following method:
Dissolve an accurately weighed quantity of the mixed contents of the cachets, equivalent to about 0·05 g of

isoniazid, in water, dilute to 1000 ml with water, and filter if necessary.

To three 20-ml graduated flasks add, respectively, 4 ml of this solution, 4 ml of *standard isoniazid solution*, and 4 ml of water; to each flask, commencing with the flask containing 4 ml of water, add, at 5-minute intervals, 5 ml of *potassium carbonate solution*, followed immediately by 5 ml of *2,3-dichloro-1,4-naphthaquinone solution*, allow the effervescence to subside, and dilute each solution to 20 ml with water; precautions should be taken to ensure that the final solutions are all at the same temperature, within the range 20° to 25°.

Allow the solutions to stand for 20 minutes and measure the extinction of a 1-cm layer of the sample solution and the standard solution at the maximum at about 605 nm, using as a blank the solution prepared using 4 ml of water; ensure that the time-interval between adding the reagents and measuring the extinction is exactly the same for each solution.

From the two extinctions, calculate the total weight of isoniazid in the 20 cachets and divide by 20.

CONTENT OF SODIUM AMINOSALICYLATE. 95·0 to 105·0 per cent of the prescribed or stated amount, calculated as $C_7H_6NNaO_3,2H_2O$, determined by the following method:

Dissolve an accurately weighed quantity of the mixed contents of the cachets, equivalent to about 0·5 g of sodium aminosalicylate, in water, and dilute to 250 ml with water.

To 25 ml of this solution in a glass-stoppered flask add 25 ml of 0·1N bromine and 5 ml of *hydrochloric acid*, shake the mixture repeatedly during 15 minutes,

allow to stand for 15 minutes, add 10 ml of *potassium iodide solution*, and titrate the liberated iodine with 0·1N sodium thiosulphate.

Repeat the procedure omitting the sample.

The difference between the two titrations, after the deduction of 0·029 ml for each milligram of isoniazid in the weight of sample taken, represents the amount of bromine required by the sodium aminosalicylate; each ml of 0·1N bromine is equivalent to 0·003519 g of $C_7H_6NNaO_3,2H_2O$.

Calculate the total weight of $C_7H_6NNaO_3,2H_2O$ in the 20 cachets and divide by 20.

Containers and storage. The directions given under Cachets (page 650) should be followed; containers should be light-resistant.

Labelling. The directions given under Cachets (page 650) should be followed.

Dose. Daily, in divided doses: sodium aminosalicylate, 10 to 20 grams, together with isoniazid, 200 to 300 milligrams.

When the quantities to be contained in the cachets are not specified, cachets each containing 1·5 g of sodium aminosalicylate and 33 mg of isoniazid shall be supplied.

Cachets containing the following are also available:
Sodium aminosalicylate 1·25 g; isoniazid 25 mg
Sodium aminosalicylate 1·5 g; isoniazid 25 mg, 33·3 mg, 37·5 mg, or 50 mg
Sodium aminosalicylate 1·67 g; isoniazid 33·3 mg
Sodium aminosalicylate 2·0 g; isoniazid 50 mg

CAPSULES

Capsules consist of a medicament enclosed in a shell and are convenient for administering medicaments which have an unpleasant taste. Hard capsules are cylindrical with hemispherical ends; the shell is composed mainly of gelatin. Flexible capsules are spherical, ovoid, or cylindrical with hemispherical ends and are made from gelatin and glycerol, in proportions varied to regulate the degree of hardness. Capsule shells may contain preservatives; coloured shells are available and may be used when so directed in the monograph. Capsule shells are made in various sizes and are usually filled by mechanical means. Hard-capsule shells are available which are designed to lock when fitted together so that they cannot later be pulled apart.

It is customary to issue capsules almost completely filled, and the monographs permit the use of inert diluents, which are essential when the dose of the medicament is small. Hard capsules are used for solid medicaments in powder or granule form; flexible capsules are used for solids, liquids, and semi-liquid substances.

Substances containing an appreciable amount of water or other solvent of gelatin are not suitable for filling directly into capsules; as much water as possible should be removed and the remaining material incorporated into liquid paraffin, soft paraffin, or a suitable fixed vegetable oil before filling.

Enteric-coated capsules are capsules treated or coated in such a manner that the active ingredient does not come into contact with the acid secretion of the stomach. The materials and methods used for enteric coating must prevent disintegration of the capsule in the stomach, but ensure disintegration when the capsule reaches the alkaline medium of the small intestine. Enteric-coated capsules have been largely superseded by enteric-coated tablets.

Sustained-release capsules consist of large numbers of small pellets contained in hard capsules. The pellets consist of a nucleus of sugar and starch to which firstly the active drug and then a special coating is applied. The coatings, which may be compounded of blends of special waxes, fats, or similar materials, vary in thickness and composition and allow ingress of fluids at different rates. Ingress of fluid results in the nucleus swelling faster than the coating and thus eventually rupturing the pellet and releasing the active medicament. A sustained release of drug is attained by mixing pellets which will rupture after different time intervals.

Another process, known as micro-encapsulation, can also be used to prepare sustained-release capsules. In this process, individual particles of the drug are coated with varying thicknesses of wax or gelatin.

The formulation of sustained release capsules carries with it the responsibility for demonstrating by tests *in vitro* and/or *in vivo* that the product performs in the manner intended; consequently the preparation of such products can only be properly carried out on a large scale.

Standard

COLOURING. Capsule shells may contain colouring agents only when specifically permitted in the individual monographs.

DISINTEGRATION TEST. Capsules comply with the requirements of the British Pharmacopoeia for the disintegration of Capsules.

UNIFORMITY OF WEIGHT AND COMPOSITION. *Hard capsules:* the contents of the capsules comply with the requirements of the British Pharmacopoeia for uniformity of weight of Capsules.

Mix the contents of the 20 capsules and determine the proportional amount of the active ingredient in the powder by the method described in the monograph on the capsules. From this figure, calculate the amount of the active ingredient in the 20 capsules and divide by 20.

The result lies within the range for the content of active ingredient stated in the monograph.

Soft capsules: the contents of the capsules comply with the requirements of the British Pharmacopoeia for uniformity of weight of Capsules, Method B being used; if it is so stated in the individual monograph, add the ethereal washings to the expressed contents instead of discarding them.

Mix the contents of the 10 capsules and determine the proportional amount of the active ingredient in the expressed contents by the method described in the monograph on the capsules. From this figure, calculate the amount of the active ingredient in the 10 capsules and divide by 10.

The result lies within the range for the content of active ingredient stated in the monograph.

Containers and storage. Capsules should be stored and supplied in containers that provide adequate protection against moisture and crushing. They should preferably be supplied in amber glass bottles, jars, or vials, in amber or opaque plastic containers, or in aluminium containers internally coated with a suitable lacquer or lined with paper; lacquered or lined screw-cap closures or plastic caps should be used. They should be stored in a cool place.

Paromomycin Capsules

SYNONYM: Paromomycin Sulphate Capsules

Paromomycin Capsules consist of Paromomycin Sulphate, in powder, which may be mixed with Lactose or other suitable inert diluent, enclosed in a hard capsule.

Standard
They comply with the standard under Capsules, page 652, with the following additions:

PRESENCE OF PAROMOMYCIN SULPHATE. 1. They comply with the thin-layer chromatographic test given in Appendix 5A, page 866.
2. They give the reactions characteristic of sulphates.

CONTENT OF PAROMOMYCIN SULPHATE. 95 to 110 per cent of the prescribed or stated number of Units, determined by the following method:
Dissolve an accurately weighed quantity of the mixed contents of 20 capsules, equivalent to about 175,000 Units, in 250 ml of water and carry out a microbiological assay of paromomycin; a suggested method is given in Appendix 18, page 897.
The precision of any assay must be such that the fiducial limits of error (P = 0·95) are not less than 95 per cent and not more than 105 per cent of the estimated potency. Calculate the upper and lower fiducial limits of the total number of Units in the 20 capsules and divide by 20.
The upper fiducial limit of the estimated number of Units is not less than 95 per cent and the lower fiducial limit is not more than 110 per cent of the prescribed or stated number of Units.

Containers and storage. The directions given under Capsules (page 652) should be followed.

Labelling. The label on the container states the directions for storage and the date after which the capsules are not intended to be used.

Dose. Paromomycin sulphate, 35,000 to 60,000 Units per kilogram body-weight daily in divided doses.

When the strength of the capsules is not specified, capsules each containing 250,000 Units shall be supplied.

Phensuximide Capsules

Phensuximide Capsules consist of Phensuximide, in powder, which may be mixed with an inert diluent, enclosed in a hard capsule. The capsule shells may be coloured.

Standard
They comply with the standard under Capsules, page 652, with the following additions:

PRESENCE OF PHENSUXIMIDE. Extract a suitable quantity of the mixed contents of the capsules with *solvent ether* and evaporate the extract to dryness; the residue complies with the following tests:
(i) Heat 0·1 g with 5 ml of *sodium hydroxide solution*; the odour of methylamine slowly develops.
(ii) The infra-red absorption spectrum exhibits maxima which are only at the same wavelengths as, and have similar relative intensities to, those in the spectrum of *phensuximide A.S.*

CONTENT OF PHENSUXIMIDE. 92·5 to 107·5 per cent of the prescribed or stated amount, calculated as $C_{11}H_{11}NO_2$, determined by the method given for Phensuximide, page 373, an accurately weighed quantity of the mixed contents of the capsules, equivalent to about 0·5 g of phensuximide, being used.
Calculate the total amount of $C_{11}H_{11}NO_2$ in the 20 capsules and divide by 20.

Containers and storage. The directions given under Capsules (page 652) should be followed.

Dose. Phensuximide:
ADULT. 0·5 to 1 gram daily, increased at intervals of two or three weeks by 0·5 gram to a total dose not exceeding 3 grams daily.
CHILD. Up to 5 years, 250 milligrams daily, increased at intervals of two to three weeks by 250 milligrams to a total not exceeding 1·5 grams daily; 6 to 12 years, 500 milligrams daily, increased at intervals of two to three weeks by 500 milligrams to a total not exceeding 3 grams daily.

When the strength of the capsules is not specified, capsules each containing 500 mg shall be supplied. Capsules containing 250 mg are also available.

Phenytoin Capsules

SYNONYM: Phenytoin Sodium Capsules

Phenytoin Capsules consist of Phenytoin Sodium, in powder, which may be mixed with a suitable inert diluent, enclosed in a hard capsule.
Calcium sulphate should not be used as a diluent as it is known to impair the absorption of phenytoin sodium.

Standard
They comply with the standard under Capsules, page 652, with the following additions:

PRESENCE OF PHENYTOIN. The residue obtained in the determination of the content of phenytoin sodium melts at about 295°.

CONTENT OF PHENYTOIN SODIUM. 92·5 to 107·5 per cent of the prescribed or stated amount, calculated as $C_{15}H_{11}N_2NaO_2$, determined by the following method: Dissolve as completely as possible an accurately weighed quantity of the mixed contents of the capsules, equivalent to about 1 g of phenytoin sodium, by stirring with 20 ml of water and 5 ml of 1N sodium hydroxide, allow to stand for 5 minutes, filter, and wash the filter with water; to the combined filtrate and washings add 10 ml of *dilute hydrochloric acid* and extract with successive 60-, 40-, and 20-ml portions of a mixture of 3 volumes of *chloroform* and 1 volume of *isopropyl alcohol*, washing each extract with the same 10 ml of water.
Evaporate off the solvent from the combined extracts, removing the last traces of solvent with care, and dry the residue to constant weight at 105°; each g of residue is equivalent to 1·087 g of $C_{15}H_{11}N_2NaO_2$.
Calculate the total amount of $C_{15}H_{11}N_2NaO_2$ in the 20 capsules and divide by 20.

Containers and storage. The directions given under Capsules (page 652) should be followed.

Dose. Phenytoin sodium, 50 to 100 milligrams three times daily, gradually increased to 200 milligrams three times daily in accordance with the needs of the patient.

When the strength of the capsules is not specified, capsules each containing 100 mg of phenytoin sodium shall be supplied. Capsules containing 50 mg are also available.

Vitamins A and D Capsules

For each capsule take:

Vitamin D	..	..	..	450 Units
Vitamin-A Activity	..	..	4500 Units

Mix the ingredients, with a suitable fixed vegetable oil if necessary, and enclose in a soft capsule.

Standard
They comply with the standard under Capsules, page 652, with the following additions:

CONTENT OF VITAMIN-A ACTIVITY. 3750 to 5250 Units, determined by the method given in Appendix 24, page 906.

CONTENT OF VITAMIN D. 375 to 525 Units, determined by the method given in Appendix 24, page 906.
The precision of any assay must be such that the fiducial limits of error (P = 0·95) are not less than 60 per cent and not more than 170 per cent of the estimated potency.

Containers and storage. The directions given under Capsules (page 652) should be followed; containers should be light-resistant.

Dose. 1 capsule daily.

Vitamins Capsules

For each capsule take:

Vitamin D	..	..	300 Units
Vitamin-A Activity	..	..	2500 Units
Riboflavine	..	..	0·5 mg
Thiamine Hydrochloride	..		1·0 mg
Nicotinamide	..	..	7·5 mg
Ascorbic Acid	..	..	15·0 mg

Mix the ingredients, with a suitable fixed vegetable oil if necessary, and enclose in a soft capsule.

Standard
They comply with the standard under Capsules, page 652, with the following additions:

CONTENT OF ASCORBIC ACID. 12·75 mg to 17·25 mg, determined by the method given in Appendix 24, page 906.

CONTENT OF NICOTINAMIDE. 6·375 mg to 8·625 mg, determined by the method given in Appendix 24, page 906.

CONTENT OF THIAMINE HYDROCHLORIDE. 0·85 mg to 1·15 mg, determined by the method given in Appendix 24, page 906.

CONTENT OF RIBOFLAVINE. 0·425 mg to 0·575 mg, determined by the method given in Appendix 24, page 906.

CONTENT OF VITAMIN-A ACTIVITY. 2100 to 2900 Units, determined by the method given in Appendix 24, page 906.

CONTENT OF VITAMIN D. 255 to 345 Units, determined by the method given in Appendix 24, page 906.
The precision of any assay must be such that the fiducial limits of error (P = 0·95) are not less than 60 per cent and not more than 170 per cent of the estimated potency.

Containers and storage. The directions given under Capsules (page 652) should be followed; containers should be light-resistant.

Dose. 1 or 2 capsules daily.

COLLODIONS

Collodions are liquid preparations consisting of a solution of pyroxylin in a mixture of organic solvents, usually ether and alcohol. They are intended for local external application and are applied by painting on the skin and allowing to dry. A flexible cellulose film is formed, covering the site of application.

Collodions may be used to seal off minor cuts and wounds or as a means of holding a dissolved medicament in contact with the skin for long periods.

Flexible Collodion (*Syn.* Collodion), a solution of pyroxylin, colophony, and castor oil in a mixture of alcohol and ether, is described in the British Pharmacopoeia.

Salicylic Acid Collodion

Salicylic Acid	..	..	.. 120 g
Flexible Collodion	..	..	to 1000 ml

Standard
CONTENT OF SALICYLIC ACID. 13·0 to 18·1 per cent w/w, determined by the following method:
Dilute about 2 g, accurately weighed, to 200 ml with *acetone*; to 2 ml of this solution add 35 ml of *acetate buffer solution pH 2·45* and 4 ml of a freshly prepared 0·5 per cent w/v solution of *ferric chloride* in water and dilute to 50 ml with *acetate buffer solution pH 2·45*;

filter, discarding the first 10 ml of filtrate, and measure the extinction of a 1-cm layer at the maximum at about 525 nm.
Repeat the procedure using 2 ml of a 0·12 per cent w/v solution of *salicylic acid* in *alcohol (95 per cent)* in place of the diluted sample solution.
From the two extinctions calculate the proportion of salicylic acid in the sample.

Containers and storage. It should be supplied in small coloured fluted glass bottles or jars with airtight closures and stored in a cool place.

Labelling. It should be labelled "For external use only".

CREAMS

Creams are viscous emulsions of semi-solid consistency and are either of an oil-in-water type (aqueous creams) or water-in-oil type (oily creams). The term "cream" should preferably be restricted to preparations for external use. Emulsifying agents for aqueous creams include anionic, cationic, and non-ionic emulsifying waxes, poly-sorbates, and sodium, potassium, ammonium, and triethanolamine soaps. Oily creams are usually prepared with emulsifying agents such as wool fat, wool alcohols, beeswax, calcium soaps, and certain sorbitan esters.

Physical stability of creams. Cracking of the emulsion or other undesirable changes, such as the development of a granular or "lumpy" appearance or a marked change in viscosity, may occur. Some of the factors which may produce these effects are: admixture of one cream with another which may be, for example, of the opposite type; incompatibilities, especially those which involve the emulsifying agent; tem-perature changes, particularly if these cause a change in the physical state of one of the phases; and addition of excess of one of the phases, especially if it is the disperse phase.

Avoidance of microbial contamination. Micro-organisms may grow if no pre-servative is included, particularly in aqueous creams. Even if a preservative is present, its efficacy may be reduced by an incompatibility with another ingredient or partition-ing of the preservative between the two phases. This may be overcome by raising the concentration of preservative but doing so may increase any undesirable side-effects of the preservative. It is better not to have to rely upon the preservative to kill or restrict growth of any organisms that are inadvertently introduced into the cream during manufacture, handling, or storage, but to adopt an aseptic technique, or as near to this standard of cleanliness as can be achieved, when preparing or handling creams. A con-tainer that minimises the risk of contamination should be chosen.

If heavy microbial contamination develops in a cream it may cause either deteriora-tion of the preparation or, if the cream is applied to broken, burnt, or inflamed skin, an infection in the patient; the number of micro-organisms in creams should therefore be kept as low as possible.

Preparation of creams. The apparatus used in the preparation of creams and the final containers should, before use, be thoroughly cleansed, rinsed with purified water which has been freshly boiled and cooled, and dried. Freshly boiled and cooled purified water should be used in the preparation of the creams and the highest hygienic standards should be observed during preparation and filling into containers.

Dilution of creams. For certain specified creams, when a strength lower than any available from a manufacturer is prescribed, a stronger cream should be diluted to the required strength with the diluent(s) specified in the monograph. Hygienic precau-tions must be taken and the diluted cream must be freshly prepared without the application of heat.

A diluent which does not contain a preservative or which contains a different pre-servative from the stronger cream may reduce the efficacy of the preservative system in the final cream with the consequent risk of microbial proliferation. If the diluent differs in pH from the original basis, chemical breakdown or inactivation of the medicament may result. It is inadvisable therefore to dilute creams for which information on a suit-able diluent is not available.

Containers and storage. Creams should be stored and supplied in well-closed containers which prevent evaporation and contamination and should be kept in a cool place. Collapsible tubes of metal or suitable plastics may be used.

If aluminium tubes are used, a phosphate buffer such as that provided by a mixture of 0·1 per cent of disodium hydrogen phosphate (anhydrous) and 0·02 per cent of sodium dihydrogen phosphate (dihydrate) may be included, if this is specified in the monograph, to inhibit corrosion of the aluminium and reduce the possibility of evolution of hydrogen. Alternatively, corrosion and hydrogen formation may be inhibited by using aluminium tubes having a lacquered inner surface. Aluminium tubes are not suitable for creams preserved with an organic mercury compound unless adequately protected by a suitable internal lacquer.

Alternatively, wide-mouthed glass or plastic jars should be used, fitted with plastic screw caps with impermeable liners or with close-fitting slip-on lids.

Labelling. The container should be labelled "For external use only". The label on the container of a diluted cream should also state that the contents should not be used later than one month after issue, unless otherwise stated in the individual monograph.

Betamethasone Valerate Cream

SYNONYM: Betamethasone Cream

Betamethasone Valerate Cream is a dispersion of Betamethasone Valerate in a suitable water-miscible basis containing a buffering agent and Chlorocresol as the preservative.

Standard
PRESENCE OF BETAMETHASONE. It complies with the thin-layer chromatographic test given in Appendix 5D, page 875.
CONTENT OF BETAMETHASONE. 90·0 to 115·0 per cent of the prescribed or stated amount, determined by the method given in Appendix 23A, page 904, for betamethasone 17-valerate.

Containers and storage; Labelling. The directions given under Creams (above) should be followed.

Note. When the strength of the cream is not specified, a cream containing the equivalent of 0·1 per cent of betamethasone shall be supplied.

When a strength less than that available from the manufacturer is prescribed, the stronger cream may be diluted, taking hygienic precautions, with Cetomacrogol Cream (Formula A) or with Buffered Cream. The diluted cream must be freshly prepared.

Diluents or medicaments which have an alkaline pH accelerate conversion of the active ingredient to the less active betamethasone 21-valerate. Coal Tar preparations are examples of medicaments which are strongly alkaline and Tar (that is, wood tar), which has an acid pH, is more suitable for mixing with betamethasone cream.

Buffered Cream

SYNONYM: Cremor Normalis

Citric Acid	5 g
Sodium Phosphate	25 g
Chlorocresol	1 g
Emulsifying Ointment	300 g
Purified Water, freshly boiled and cooled	669 g

Melt the emulsifying ointment with the aid of gentle heat, add the sodium phosphate, the citric acid, and the chlorocresol, previously dissolved in the water at the same temperature, and stir gently until cold.

Standard
ACIDITY. pH, 5·7 to 6·3, determined directly on the cream.

Containers and storage; Labelling. The directions give under Creams (above) should be followed. When aluminium tubes are used, they should be coated internally with a suitable lacquer.

Calamine Cream, Aqueous

SYNONYM: Calamine Cream

Calamine	40 g
Zinc Oxide	30 g
Emulsifying Wax	60 g
Arachis Oil	300 g
Purified Water, freshly boiled and cooled	570 g

Melt the emulsifying wax with the aid of gentle heat, add the arachis oil, and warm; add 400 g of the water at the same temperature and stir until cold. Triturate the calamine and the zinc oxide with the remainder of the water and incorporate in the cream.

Standard
CONTENT OF ZINC. 4·3 to 5·2 per cent w/w, calculated as Zn, determined by the following method:
Heat gently, taking precautions against loss caused by spitting, about 4 g, accurately weighed, until the basis is completely volatilised or charred; increase the temperature until all the carbon is removed and ignite the residue to constant weight; each g of residue is equivalent to 0·8034 g of Zn.

Containers and storage; Labelling. The directions given under Creams (above) should be followed.

Cetomacrogol Cream

Cetomacrogol Cream may be prepared according to one of the following formulae for use as a diluent as specified in the individual monographs:

Formula A

Cetomacrogol Emulsifying Ointment	300 g
Chlorocresol	1 g
Purified Water, freshly boiled and cooled	699 g

Formula B

Cetomacrogol Emulsifying Ointment	300·0 g
Thiomersal	0·02 g
Propyl Hydroxybenzoate ..	0·8 g
Methyl Hydroxybenzoate ..	1·5 g
Purified Water, freshly boiled and cooled	697·68 g

Dissolve the preservatives in the water with the aid of gentle heat; melt the cetomacrogol emulsifying ointment on a water-bath, add the solution containing the preservatives at the same temperature, and stir until cold.

To help to prevent production of a granular preparation, the temperature of the melted ingredients should not exceed 65°, and in the preparation of a cream according to Formula A, the chlorocresol should be dissolved in not less than 50 ml of warm water before adding to the melted emulsifying basis.

An improved product may also be obtained if, instead of using Cetomacrogol Emulsifying Ointment, the appropriate quantities of White Soft Paraffin, Cetomacrogol Emulsifying Wax, and Liquid Paraffin are melted together.

In view of the difficulty of achieving the highest hygienic standard, it is recommended that the cream should be freshly prepared, unless facilities are available for assessing the microbiological quality of the product.

Containers. If the cream is not freshly· prepared, it should preferably be packed in small collapsible tubes; aluminium tubes should not be used for cream prepared according to Formula B, unless adequately protected by a suitable internal lacquer. A readily breakable seal should cover the closure or the tube may be enclosed in a sealed plastic envelope or sealed carton. Alternatively, the cream may be supplied in jars.

Labelling. The directions given under Creams (page 656) should be followed.

Cetrimide Cream

Cetrimide	5 g
Cetostearyl Alcohol	50 g
Purified Water, freshly boiled and cooled	445 g
Liquid Paraffin	500 g

Melt the cetostearyl alcohol with the aid of gentle heat, add the liquid paraffin, and warm; dissolve the cetrimide in the water at the same temperature and add to the warm mixture, stirring gently until cold.

A phosphate buffer may be included.

Standard

CONTENT OF CETRIMIDE. 0·44 to 0·53 per cent w/w, calculated as $C_{17}H_{38}BrN$, determined by the following method:

To about 1 g, accurately weighed, in a stoppered cylinder, add 10 ml of hot water, and shake until the solid is dispersed; add 5 ml of *dilute sulphuric acid*, 20 ml of *chloroform*, and 1 ml of *dimethyl yellow solution* and titrate with 0·001M sodium lauryl sulphate; each ml of 0·001M sodium lauryl sulphate is equivalent to 0·0003364 g of $C_{17}H_{38}BrN$.

Containers and storage; Labelling. The directions given under Creams (page 656) should be followed.

Chlorhexidine Cream

Chlorhexidine Gluconate Solution	50 ml
Cetomacrogol Emulsifying Wax	250 g
Liquid Paraffin	100 g
Purified Water, freshly boiled and cooled	to 1000 g

Melt the cetomacrogol emulsifying wax in the liquid paraffin at 60° and add, with rapid stirring, to the chlorhexidine gluconate solution, previously diluted to 500 ml with the water, at the same temperature. Cool, add sufficient of the water to produce the required weight, and mix.

Standard

CONTENT OF CHLORHEXIDINE GLUCONATE. 0·90 to 1·10 per cent w/w, determined by the following method:

Shake about 3 g, accurately weighed, with 20 ml of water, add 10 ml of 1N hydrochloric acid, and extract with three successive 25-ml portions of *chloroform*; wash the combined extracts with two successive 10-ml portions of water, discard the chloroformic extracts, and dilute the combined aqueous solution and washings to 100 ml with water.

To 5 ml of this solution add 80 ml of water and 5 ml of *cetrimide solution*, neutralise to *litmus paper* with 1N sodium hydroxide and add a further 0·5 ml; add 1 ml of *isopropyl alcohol*, adjust the temperature to 18° to 22°, add 2 ml of *alkaline sodium hypobromite solution*, dilute to 100 ml with water, and allow to stand for exactly 25 minutes, maintaining the temperature at 18° to 22°; immediately measure the extinction of a 1-cm layer at 480 nm, using water as the blank.

At the same time, carry out the procedure, omitting the sample; the difference between the two extinctions represents the extinction due to the chlorhexidine gluconate.

For purposes of calculation, use a value of 214 for the E(1 per cent, 1 cm) of chlorhexidine gluconate. Calculate the percentage of chlorhexidine gluconate in the sample.

Containers and storage; Labelling. The directions given under Creams (page 656) should be followed.

Chlorphenesin Cream

Chlorphenesin	5 g
Sodium Lauryl Sulphate	9 g
Cetostearyl Alcohol	81 g
White Soft Paraffin	150 g
Purified Water, freshly boiled and cooled	755 g

Warm the cetostearyl alcohol and the white soft paraffin to 50° and mix. Add, with constant stirring, the sodium lauryl sulphate and the chlorphenesin dissolved in the water at the same temperature and stir until cold.

Standard
CONTENT OF CHLORPHENESIN. 0·45 to 0·55 per cent w/w, determined by the following method:
Disperse about 1 g, accurately weighed, in 20 ml of hot water, add 3 ml of *barium chloride solution*, mix well, and allow to cool; shake the mixture vigorously, extract with 20 ml of *light petroleum (boiling-range 40° to 60°)*, and allow to separate; wash the light-petroleum extract with 10 ml of water and discard the light petroleum.
To the combined aqueous solution and washings add 3 g of *sodium chloride* and extract with six successive 10-ml portions of *chloroform*; wash the combined chloroform extracts with two 5-ml portions of a 10 per cent w/v solution of *sodium chloride* in water and extract the combined washings with 5 ml of *chloroform*.
Filter the combined chloroform extracts through a filter containing a layer of *anhydrous sodium sulphate*, wash the filter with *chloroform*, dilute the combined filtrate and washings to 100 ml with *chloroform*, and measure the extinction of a 1-cm layer at the maximum at about 282 nm.
For purposes of calculation, use a value of 81 for the E(1 per cent, 1 cm) of chlorphenesin.
Calculate the concentration of chlorphenesin in the sample.

Containers and storage; Labelling. The directions given under Creams (page 656) should be followed.

Clioquinol Cream

Clioquinol, in very fine powder	..	30 g
Chlorocresol	.. .. ..	1 g
Cetomacrogol Emulsifying Ointment		300 g
Purified Water, freshly boiled and cooled	.. ..	669 g

Dissolve the chlorocresol in the water with the aid of gentle heat; melt the cetomacrogol emulsifying ointment on a water-bath, add the chlorocresol solution at the same temperature, stir until cold, and incorporate the clioquinol.
Clioquinol Cream may be prepared using any other suitable basis.

Standard
CONTENT OF CLIOQUINOL. 2·7 to 3·3 per cent w/w, determined by the following method:
Disperse an accurately weighed quantity, equivalent to about 0·015 g of clioquinol, in 25 ml of *chloroform* in a stoppered centrifuge tube, shake vigorously, and centrifuge; add sufficient *anhydrous sodium sulphate* to absorb all the aqueous phase and dilute 15 ml of the clear chloroform solution to 50 ml with *chloroform*.
Transfer 10 ml of this solution to a separating funnel, add 25 ml of *chloroform*, 10 ml of water, and 10 ml of *copper sulphate solution*, shake vigorously, allow to separate, dry the chloroform layer by shaking with *anhydrous sodium sulphate*, and measure the extinction of a 1-cm layer of the clear solution at 430 nm, using *chloroform* as the blank.
Calculate the concentration of clioquinol in the sample by comparing the extinction with that of a solution prepared by dissolving about 0·09 g of *clioquinol*, accurately weighed, in sufficient *chloroform* to produce 100 ml, diluting 10 ml of this solution to 50 ml with *chloroform* and continuing by the method given above beginning with the words "Transfer 10 ml of this solu-

tion to a separating funnel, add 25 ml of *chloroform* ...".

Containers; Labelling. The directions given under Creams (page 656) should be followed.
When collapsible tubes are used they should preferably be made of plastics. If made of aluminium, the inner surface of the tubes should be lacquered.

Storage. It should be protected from light.

Caution. *Clioquinol may stain clothing or discolour fair hair.*

Dimethicone Cream

SYNONYM: Silicone Cream

Dimethicone 350	..	..	..	100 g
Cetrimide	..	..	..	5 g
Chlorocresol	..	..	..	1 g
Cetostearyl Alcohol	..	..	50 g
Liquid Paraffin	..	..	..	400 g
Purified Water, freshly boiled and cooled	..	..	..	444 g

Warm and mix together the dimethicone 350, the liquid paraffin, and the cetostearyl alcohol until homogeneous; add, with mechanical stirring, the cetrimide and the chlorocresol dissolved in the water at the same temperature, and stir until cold.

Standard
CONTENT OF CETRIMIDE. 0·44 to 0·53 per cent w/w, calculated as $C_{17}H_{38}BrN$, determined by the method for Cetrimide Cream, page 657.

CONTENT OF DIMETHICONE. 9·0 to 11·0 per cent w/w, determined by the following method:
Mix about 5 g, accurately weighed, with 10 g of granular *anhydrous sodium sulphate*, extract the mixture with six successive 5-ml portions of *toluene*, filter the extracts, and dilute the combined filtrates to 50 ml with *toluene*.
Record the infra-red absorption spectrum of this solution in the region of the maximum at about 8 μm on a suitable instrument, using a 4 per cent w/w solution of *liquid paraffin* in *toluene* in the reference cell, and hence determine the extinction due to the dimethicone present.
Calculate the concentration of dimethicone in the sample by reference to a calibration curve prepared by determining, in the same manner, the extinctions of prepared solutions containing 0·2, 0·4, 0·6, 0·8, and 1·0 per cent of *dimethicone* in a 4 per cent w/w solution of *liquid paraffin* in *toluene*.

Containers and storage; Labelling. The directions given under Creams (page 656) should be followed.

Fluocinolone Cream

SYNONYM: Fluocinolone Acetonide Cream

Fluocinolone Cream is a dispersion of Fluocinolone Acetonide in a suitable water-miscible basis containing a mixture of thiomersal, methyl hydroxybenzoate, and propyl hydroxybenzoate as the preservative system.

Standard
CONTENT OF FLUOCINOLONE ACETONIDE. 90·0 to 110·0 per cent of the prescribed or stated amount, determined by the method given in Appendix 23B, page 905.

Containers and storage. The directions given under Creams (page 656) should be followed; aluminium tubes are not suitable for this cream, unless adequately protected by a suitable internal lacquer.

Labelling. The directions given under Creams (page 656) should be followed.

Note. The strength of the cream should be specified by the prescriber. Creams containing 0·2, 0·025 and 0·01 per cent of fluocinolone acetonide are available.

When a strength less than those available from a manufacturer is prescribed, the 0·025 per cent cream may be diluted, taking hygienic precautions, with Cetomacrogol Cream (Formula B). The diluted cream must be freshly prepared.

Diluents or medicaments which are strongly alkaline or acid, or which contain oxidising agents, accelerate the decomposition of fluocinolone acetonide. Diluents which contain ionic emulsifying compounds may be incompatible with the basis. Emulsifying Ointment and Aqueous Cream are examples of such diluents.

Hydrocortisone Cream

Hydrocortisone *or* Hydrocortisone
    Acetate in sufficiently fine powder
    to meet the requirements of the
    standard ..   ..   10 g
Chlorocresol   ..   ..   ..   1 g
Cetomacrogol Emulsifying Oint-
    ment .. ..   300 g
Purified Water, freshly boiled and
    cooled   ..   ..   689 g

Dissolve the chlorocresol in the water with the aid of gentle heat; melt the cetomacrogol emulsifying ointment on a water-bath, add the chlorocresol solution at the same temperature, stir until cold, and incorporate the hydrocortisone or hydrocortisone acetate.
A phosphate buffer may be included.

Standard
PRESENCE OF HYDROCORTISONE OR OF HYDROCORTISONE ACETATE. It complies with the thin-layer chromatographic test given in Appendix 5D, page 875.

PARTICLE SIZE. When determined by the method given in Appendix 25C, page 911, not less than 90 per cent of the particles have a maximum diameter less than 5 μm and no particle has a maximum diameter greater than 50 μm.

CONTENT OF HYDROCORTISONE OR OF HYDROCORTISONE ACETATE. 0·92 to 1·08 per cent w/w of hydrocortisone or of hydrocortisone acetate, determined by one of the following methods:

Creams containing hydrocortisone acetate. The following procedure should be carried out in subdued light or in low-actinic glassware.
Warm about 1 g, accurately weighed, with 20 ml of *aldehyde-free dehydrated alcohol* until the basis is melted, shake well, cool in ice, and decant through a pledget of cotton wool; repeat the extraction with three further 20-ml portions of *aldehyde-free dehydrated alcohol*, using a fresh pledget of cotton wool for each filtration, dilute the combined filtrates to 100 ml with the same solvent, and filter.
Dilute the filtrate with sufficient *aldehyde-free dehydrated alcohol* to produce a solution containing between 440 and 460 μg of hydrocortisone acetate in 10 ml and, using 10 ml of this solution, continue by the method given for Hydrocortisone and Neomycin Eardrops, page 665, beginning with the words "add 2·0 ml of *triphenyltetrazolium chloride solution* . . .".
Calculate the concentration of hydrocortisone acetate in the sample.

Creams containing hydrocortisone. Carry out the method described above for creams containing hydrocortisone acetate but dilute the filtrate with sufficient *aldehyde-free dehydrated alcohol* to produce a solution containing between 340 and 360 μg of hydrocortisone in 10 ml and use a solution containing between 340 and 360 μg of *hydrocortisone B.C.R.S.* in 10 ml of *aldehyde-free dehydrated alcohol* for the reference solution. Calculate the concentration of hydrocortisone in the sample.

Containers and storage. The directions given under Creams (page 656) should be followed.

Labelling. The directions given under Creams (page 656) should be followed. In addition, the label on the container should state whether the cream contains hydrocortisone or hydrocortisone acetate.

Hydrocortisone and Neomycin Cream

Hydrocortisone, in sufficiently fine
    powder to meet the requirements
    of the standard ..   ..   ..   5 g
Neomycin Cream ..   ..   ..   995 g

Incorporate the hydrocortisone in the neomycin cream.
A phosphate buffer may be included.

Standard
PRESENCE OF HYDROCORTISONE. It complies with the thin-layer chromatographic test given in Appendix 5D, page 875.

PARTICLE SIZE. When determined by the method given in Appendix 25C, page 911, not less than 75 per cent of the particles have a maximum diameter less than 10 μm and not less than 99 per cent of the particles have a maximum diameter less than 20 μm; no particle has a maximum diameter greater than 50 μm.

CONTENT OF HYDROCORTISONE. 0·45 to 0·55 per cent w/w, determined by the method for Hydrocortisone Cream (*Creams containing hydrocortisone*), about 2 g, accurately weighed, being used.

CONTENT OF NEOMYCIN. 2750 to 4000 Units per g, determined by the following method:
Mix about 1·2 g, accurately weighed, with 15 ml of *chloroform*, stir until the emulsion is completely broken, transfer to a separating funnel with the aid of 25 ml of *solution of standard pH 8·0* and 5 ml of *chloroform*, shake vigorously, and allow to separate; reserve the aqueous extract.
Extract the chloroform layer with two successive 25-ml portions of *solution of standard pH 8·0* and discard the chloroform solution; remove the dissolved chloroform in the combined aqueous extracts by passing *nitrogen* through the solution and carry out a microbiological assay of neomycin; a suggested method is given in Appendix 18, page 897.
The precision of any assay must be such that the fiducial limits of error (P = 0·95) are not less than 95 and not more than 105 per cent of the estimated potency.
Calculate the upper and lower fiducial limits of the concentration of neomycin in the cream.
The upper fiducial limit of the estimated concentration of neomycin is not less than 2750 Units per g and the lower fiducial limit is not more than 4000 Units per g.

Containers and storage; Labelling. The directions given under Creams (page 656) should be followed.

Mexenone Cream

Mexenone Cream is a dispersion of Mexenone in a suitable water-miscible base.

Standard
PRESENCE OF MEXENONE. Disperse 12 g in 50 ml of water, add 5 g of *sodium chloride*, extract with two successive 25-ml portions of *chloroform*, wash the combined chloroform extracts with 50 ml of water, discard the washings, and filter the chloroform solution through a bed of *kieselguhr*; evaporate the filtrate to dryness, dissolve the residue as completely as possible, with the aid of heat, in 10 ml of *alcohol (95 per cent)*,

cool, and filter through a bed of *kieselguhr*; to the filtrate slowly add *sodium hydroxide solution* until the solution is alkaline to *red litmus paper*, add a further 10 ml of *sodium hydroxide solution*, allow to stand for 5 minutes, and filter through a bed of *kieselguhr*; to the filtrate add *dilute hydrochloric acid* until the solution is acid to *blue litmus paper*, and filter.

The residue, after recrystallisation from a mixture of equal volumes of water and *alcohol (95 per cent)* and drying, has a melting-point of about 101°.

ACIDITY. pH of a dispersion prepared by mixing 4 g with 20 ml of *carbon dioxide-free water*, 4·0 to 5·0.

CONTENT OF MEXENONE. 95·0 to 105·0 per cent of the prescribed or stated amount, determined by the following method:

To an accurately weighed quantity, equivalent to about 0·02 g of mexenone, add 20 ml of *methyl alcohol*, warm to disperse the sample, dilute to 100 ml with *methyl alcohol*, and filter, rejecting the first portion of the filtrate; dilute 20 ml of the clear filtrate to 100 ml with *methyl alcohol*, further dilute 20 ml of this solution to 100 ml with the same solvent, and measure the extinction of a 1-cm layer at the maximum at about 287 nm. For purposes of calculation, use a value of 640 for the E(1 per cent, 1 cm) of mexenone.

Calculate the percentage of mexenone in the sample.

Containers and storage; Labelling. The directions given under Creams (page 656) should be followed.

Note. When the strength is not specified, a cream containing 4 per cent w/w of mexenone shall be supplied.

Neomycin Cream

Neomycin Sulphate	..	..	5·0 g
Disodium Edetate	..	..	0·1 g
Chlorocresol	..	..	1·0 g
Cetomacrogol Emulsifying Ointment	..	..	300·0 g
Purified Water, freshly boiled and cooled	..	..	693·9 g

Dissolve the disodium edetate and the chlorocresol in about 650 ml of the water with the aid of gentle heat; melt the cetomacrogol emulsifying ointment on a water-bath, add the aqueous solution at the same temperature, and stir until cold. Incorporate the neomycin sulphate dissolved in the remainder of the water. A phosphate buffer may be included.

Standard
CONTENT OF NEOMYCIN. 2750 to 4000 Units per g, determined by the method for neomycin in Hydrocortisone and Neomycin Cream, page 659.

The upper fiducial limit of the estimated concentration of neomycin is not less than 2750 Units per g and the lower fiducial limit is not more than 4000 Units per g.

Containers and storage; Labelling. The directions given under Creams (page 656) should be followed.

Proflavine Cream

SYNONYMS: Flavine Cream; Proflavine Emulsion

Proflavine Hemisulphate ..		..	1 g
Chlorocresol	..	..	1 g
Yellow Beeswax	..	..	25 g
Wool Fat ..	..	..	50 g
Purified Water, freshly boiled and cooled	..	..	250 g
Liquid Paraffin	..	..	673 g

Dissolve the chlorocresol in 600 g of the liquid paraffin with the aid of gentle heat and add to the yellow beeswax and the wool fat previously melted together; cool, add, with continuous stirring, the proflavine hemisulphate dissolved in the water, followed by the remainder of the liquid paraffin, and stir gently until cold.

Standard
CONTENT OF PROFLAVINE HEMISULPHATE. 0·09 to 0·11 per cent w/w, determined by the following method:

Dissolve about 1 g, accurately weighed, in a mixture of equal volumes of *chloroform* and *alcohol (95 per cent)* and dilute to 100 ml with the chloroform–alcohol mixture; dilute 5 ml of this solution to 25 ml with the chloroform–alcohol mixture, filter if necessary, and measure the extinction of a 1-cm layer of this solution at 458 nm.

For purposes of calculation, use a value of 1675 for the E(1 per cent, 1 cm) of proflavine hemisulphate.

Calculate the percentage of proflavine hemisulphate in the sample.

Containers and storage; Labelling. The directions given under Creams (page 656) should be followed.

Salicylic Acid and Sulphur Cream

SYNONYM: Salicylic Acid and Sulphur Application

Salicylic Acid, finely sifted	..		20 g
Precipitated Sulphur, finely sifted			20 g
Aqueous Cream	..	..	960 g

Triturate the salicylic acid and the sulphur with a portion of the aqueous cream until smooth and gradually add the remainder of the aqueous cream.

Standard
CONTENT OF SALICYLIC ACID. 1·80 to 2·20 per cent, calculated as $C_7H_6O_3$, determined by the following method:

To about 10 g, accurately weighed, add 80 ml of *alcohol (95 per cent)*, previously neutralised to *phenol red solution*, warm on a water-bath, shaking occasionally, until the sample is completely dispersed, and while still hot titrate with 0·1N sodium hydroxide, using *phenol red solution* as indicator; each ml of 0·1N sodium hydroxide is equivalent to 0·01381 g of $C_7H_6O_3$.

CONTENT OF SULPHUR. 1·80 to 2·20 per cent, calculated as S, determined by the following method:

Add about 5 g, accurately weighed, to a solution containing 2 g of *sodium sulphite* in 40 ml of water and boil under a reflux condenser until the sulphur is completely dissolved; cool, filter, wash the filter with hot water, cool the combined filtrate and washings, filter again, and wash the filter with hot water.

To the combined filtrate and washings add 10 ml of *formaldehyde solution* and 6 ml of *acetic acid*, dilute to 150 ml with water and titrate with 0·1N iodine, using *starch mucilage* as indicator; each ml of 0·1N iodine is equivalent to 0·003206 g of S.

Containers and storage; Labelling. The directions given under Creams (page 656) should be followed.

Triamcinolone Cream

SYNONYM: Triamcinolone Acetonide Cream

Triamcinolone Cream is a dispersion of Triamcinolone Acetonide in a suitable water-miscible basis containing a mixture of methyl hydroxybenzoate and propyl hydroxybenzoate as the preservative system. It may also contain potassium sorbate.

Standard

CONTENT OF TRIAMCINOLONE ACETONIDE. 90·0 to 110·0 per cent of the prescribed or stated amount, determined by one of the following methods:

If the cream contains 0·1 per cent of triamcinolone acetonide, determine the content by the following method: To an accurately weighed quantity, equivalent to about 2 mg of triamcinolone acetonide, add 30 ml of *chloroform* and 0·5 g of *anhydrous sodium sulphate*, shake for 10 minutes, filter, wash the filter with 10 ml of *chloroform*, dilute the combined filtrates to 50 ml with *chloroform*, and continue by the method for Triamcinolone Ointment, page 764, beginning with the words "To three 25-ml graduated flasks . . .".

If the cream contains 0·025 or 0·01 per cent of triamcinolone acetonide, determine the content by the following method:
Prepare a chromatographic column in the following manner: transfer 5 g of *Florisil* to a suitable chromatographic tube and pack it carefully with a glass plunger; mix intimately together 5 g of *Florisil* and 5 g of *washed Celite 545* and transfer this mixture, in portions, to the top of the column, packing each portion carefully with the glass plunger.
To an accurately weighed quantity of the sample, equivalent to about 1 mg of triamcinolone acetonide, add 10 g of *washed Celite 545*, mix well with a glass rod, and transfer the mixture to the top of the prepared chromatographic column, packing carefully with the glass plunger.
Pass through the column, successively, 200 ml of *chloroform*, 60 ml of a mixture of equal volumes of *chloroform* and *solvent ether*, and 100 ml of a 2·5 per cent v/v solution of *alcohol (95 per cent)* in *solvent ether*.
Evaporate the combined eluates to dryness on a water-bath, dissolve the residue in sufficient *chloroform* to produce 50 ml, and continue by the method given for Triamcinolone Ointment, page 764, beginning with the words "To three 25-ml graduated flasks . . .", and measuring the extinction of a 2-cm layer of the prepared solution, instead of a 1-cm layer.

Containers and storage; Labelling. The directions given under Creams (page 656) should be followed.

Note. When the strength of the cream is not specified, a cream containing 0·1 per cent of triamcinolone acetonide shall be supplied. Creams containing 0·025 and 0·01 per cent are also available.

When a strength less than those available from the manufacturer is prescribed, the 0·1 per cent cream may be diluted, taking hygienic precautions, with Aqueous Cream. The diluted cream must be freshly prepared.

Zinc and Ichthammol Cream

SYNONYM: Zinc Oxide and Ichthammol Cream

Zinc Cream	..	..	..	820 g
Ichthammol	..	..	..	50 g
Cetostearyl Alcohol		..	..	30 g
Wool Fat ..	..	..	..	100 g

Melt together the wool fat and the cetostearyl alcohol with the aid of gentle heat; triturate the warm mixture with the zinc cream until smooth and incorporate the ichthammol.

Standard

CONTENT OF ZINC OXIDE. 23·4 to 29·3 per cent w/w, calculated as ZnO, determined by the following method:
Heat gently, taking precautions against loss caused by spitting, about 0·4 g, accurately weighed, until the basis is completely volatilised or charred; cool, dissolve the residue in 10 ml of *dilute sulphuric acid*, and add 40 ml of water; adjust the solution to about pH 10 with *dilute ammonia solution*, add 10 ml of *ammonia buffer solution*, and titrate with 0·05M disodium edetate, using *mordant black 11 solution* as indicator; each ml of 0·05M disodium edetate is equivalent to 0·004068 g of ZnO.

Containers and storage; Labelling. The directions given under Creams (page 656) should be followed.

DRAUGHTS

Draughts are liquid preparations intended for administration by mouth and are usually formulated in single dose-volumes of 50 millilitres; Paediatric Ipecacuanha Emetic Draught is an exception.

Ipecacuanha Emetic Draught, Paediatric

Ipecacuanha Liquid Extract			70·0 ml
Hydrochloric Acid ..		..	2·5 ml
Glycerol	..	..	100·0 ml
Syrup	..	..	to 1000·0 ml

It has a weight per ml at 20° of about 1·29 g.

Standard

PRESENCE OF IPECACUANHA ALKALOIDS. It complies with the thin-layer chromatographic test given in Appendix 5B, page 871.

CONTENT OF TOTAL ALKALOIDS. 0·12 to 0·16 per cent w/v, calculated as emetine, $C_{29}H_{40}N_2O_4$, determined by the following method:
Transfer 25 ml to a separating funnel, add 20 ml of water and 5 ml of *dilute sulphuric acid*, and extract with

three successive 10-ml portions of *chloroform*, washing each extract with a mixture of 20 ml of 0·1N sulphuric acid and 4 ml of *alcohol (95 per cent)* contained in a second separating funnel.
Discard the chloroform extracts, transfer the acid–alcohol mixture from the second separating funnel to the first separating funnel, make the combined liquids distinctly alkaline with *dilute ammonia solution*, and extract with successive portions of *chloroform* until complete extraction of the alkaloids is effected, washing each chloroform extract with the same 10 ml of water. Combine the chloroform extracts, evaporate off the chloroform, add to the residue 2 ml of *alcohol (95 per cent)*, evaporate to dryness, and dry the residue at 80° in a current of air for 5 minutes.
Dissolve the residue in 2 ml of *alcohol (95 per cent)*, previously neutralised to *methyl red solution*, add 10 ml of 0·02N sulphuric acid, and titrate the excess of acid with 0·02N sodium hydroxide, using *methyl red solution* as indicator; each ml of 0·02N sulphuric acid is equivalent to 0·004806 g of $C_{29}H_{40}N_2O_4$.

Dose. CHILD. 6 months to 18 months, 10 millilitres; 18 months to 5 years, 15 millilitres.

The dose should be followed by a tumblerful of water and if there is no response after twenty minutes, a further dose and a tumblerful of water should be given.

Note. This preparation should only be given in the emergency treatment of poisoning under medical supervision. It should not be supplied for use in first-aid kits.

Male Fern Extract Draught

SYNONYMS: Haustus Filicis; Male Fern Draught

Male Fern Extract	..	..	..	4 g
Acacia, in powder	..	..	..	4 g
Water (see page 642)	..	..		to 50 ml

Triturate the male fern extract with the acacia, add in one quantity 10 ml of water, and stir briskly until emulsified. Add sufficient water to produce the required volume and mix. It should be recently prepared.

Dose. 50 millilitres.

Paraldehyde Draught

Paraldehyde	..	..	..	.. 4 ml
Liquorice Liquid Extract		..	.. 3 ml
Syrup	..	..	..	.. 8 ml
Water (see page 642)	..	..	to 50 ml

It should be freshly prepared.

Dose. 50 millilitres.

DUSTING-POWDERS

Dusting-powders are used externally and are usually mixtures of two or more substances in fine powder free from grittiness. They may be prepared as described under Powders (page 774).

Talc, kaolin, and other natural mineral ingredients are liable to be heavily contaminated with bacteria, including *Clostridium tetani*, *Cl. welchii*, and *Bacillus anthracis*. Such ingredients should be sterilised by heating for a sufficient length of time to ensure that the whole of the powder has been maintained at a temperature not lower than 160° for not less than one hour before mixing with the other ingredients. This procedure is not necessary when the final product is subjected to a sterilisation process, as indicated in the individual monograph, but must be carried out in all other cases.

Dusting-powders should not be applied to open wounds or to raw surfaces of large area.

Containers. Unless otherwise specified in the individual monograph, dusting-powders should be dispensed in suitable coloured glass or plastic jars, preferably fitted with a reclosable perforated lid.

Labelling. The container should be labelled "For external use only".

Chlorhexidine Dusting-powder

| Chlorhexidine Hydrochloride | .. | 5 g |
| Sterilisable Maize Starch | .. | 995 g |

Prepare as described under Powders (page 774). Distribute, in quantities of not more than 30 g, into suitable glass containers with reclosable perforated lids or into other suitable containers, and heat for a sufficient length of time to ensure that the whole of the powder is maintained at 150° to 155° for one hour.

Standard
PRESENCE OF STERILISABLE MAIZE STARCH. Boil 1 g with 15 ml of water and cool; a translucent viscous fluid or jelly is not produced. Add *iodine solution*; a purplish-blue or deep blue colour is produced.

STERILITY. It complies with the test for sterility, the powder being suspended in sterile *peptone water* or other suitable diluent to give a concentration of about 5 mg per ml and 1 ml of the suspension being inoculated into the media.

CONTENT OF CHLORHEXIDINE HYDROCHLORIDE. 0·45 to 0·55 per cent, determined by the following method: To about 5 g, accurately weighed, add 20 ml of *hydrochloric acid*, shake well, add 20 ml of water, and shake vigorously for 5 minutes; filter, with the aid of suction, through a hardened filter paper, wash the filter with two successive 10-ml portions of water, dilute the combined filtrate and washings to 1000 ml with water, and continue by the method given in Appendix 27, page 916, for the determination of chlorhexidine hydrochloride in surgical dressings, beginning with the words "To 40 ml of this solution . . .".

Labelling. The direction given under Dusting-powders (above) should be followed.

Chlorphenesin Dusting-powder

Chlorphenesin	..	..	..	10 g
Zinc Oxide ..	..	..	..	250 g
Purified Talc, sterilised	..	..	180 g
Starch	..	..	..	..	560 g

Prepare as described under Powders (page 774).

Standard
CONTENT OF ZINC OXIDE. 23·7 to 26·3 per cent, calculated as ZnO, determined by the following method: To about 5 g, accurately weighed, add 40 ml of 1N sulphuric acid and heat on a water-bath for 10 minutes; cool, add 2 g of *ammonium chloride*, and titrate the excess of acid with 1N sodium hydroxide, using *methyl orange solution* as indicator; each ml of 1N sulphuric acid is equivalent to 0·04068 g of ZnO.

CONTENT OF CHLORPHENESIN. 0·90 to 1·10 per cent, calculated as $C_9H_{11}ClO_3$, determined by the following method:
Extract about 0·5 g, accurately weighed, with 60 ml of *chloroform* in an apparatus for the continuous extraction of drugs for about 2 hours or until extraction is complete; dilute the chloroformic extract to 100 ml with *chloroform* and measure the extinction of a 1-cm layer at the maximum at about 282 nm.
For purposes of calculation, use a value of 81 for the E(1 per cent, 1 cm) of chlorphenesin.
Calculate the concentration of chlorphenesin in the sample.

Containers; Labelling. The directions given under Dusting-powders (page 662) should be followed.

Dicophane Dusting-powder

SYNONYM: DDT Dusting-powder

Dicophane, in powder	..	..	100 g
Calcium Carbonate	..	..	100 g
Light Kaolin, sterilised	..	..	800 g

Prepare as described under Powders (page 774).

Standard
PRESENCE OF DICOPHANE. 1. Strongly heat a small quantity; hydrogen chloride is produced.
2. Shake 1 g with 5 ml of *carbon tetrachloride*, filter, evaporate the filtrate to dryness, add to the residue 1 ml of a 0·5 per cent w/v solution of *hydroquinone* in *nitrogen-free sulphuric acid*, and heat the mixture; a wine-red colour is produced.

CONTENT OF DICOPHANE. 9·0 to 11·0 per cent, determined by the following method:
Extract about 5 g, accurately weighed, with *chloroform* in an apparatus for the continuous extraction of drugs for 3 hours, evaporate the extract to low bulk on a water-bath, dry the residue in a current of air at room temperature, and weigh.

CONTENT OF CALCIUM CARBONATE. 9·5 to 10·5 per cent, calculated as $CaCO_3$, determined by the following method:
Extract about 0·5 g, accurately weighed, by boiling with three 50-ml portions of 0·1N hydrochloric acid, allowing each extract to settle, filtering the decanted supernatant liquid, and washing the residue with water; evaporate the combined acid extracts and washings to low bulk, neutralise with *dilute sodium hydroxide solution*, using *methyl red solution* as indicator, add 10 ml of *triethanolamine*, 5 ml of 0·05M magnesium sulphate and 10 ml of *ammonia buffer solution*, and titrate with 0·05M disodium edetate, using *mordant black 11 solution* as indicator; each ml of 0·05M disodium edetate, after deducting the volume of 0·05M magnesium sulphate added, is equivalent to 0·005005 g of $CaCO_3$.

Containers; Labelling. The directions given under Dusting-powders (page 662) should be followed.

Hexachlorophane Dusting-powder

Hexachlorophane ..	..	..	3 g
Zinc Oxide	..	..	..	30 g
Sterilisable Maize Starch ..	..	967 g

Prepare as described under Powders (page 774). Distribute, in quantities of not more than 30 g, into suitable glass containers with reclosable perforated lids or into other suitable containers, and heat for a sufficient length of time to ensure that the whole of the powder is maintained at 150° to 155° for one hour.

Standard
PRESENCE OF STERILISABLE MAIZE STARCH. It complies with the test given under Chlorhexidine Dusting-powder, page 662.

STERILITY. It complies with the test for sterility, the powder being suspended in sterile *peptone water* or other suitable diluent to give a concentration of about 5 mg per ml and 1 ml of the suspension being inoculated into the media.

CONTENT OF HEXACHLOROPHANE. 0·27 to 0·33 per cent w/w, determined by the following method:
Shake about 5 g, accurately weighed, with 50 ml of *tris(hydroxymethyl)aminomethane solution* for 10 minutes, filter through a sintered-glass crucible (British Standard Grade No. 3), wash the filter with two successive 10-ml portions of *tris(hydroxymethyl)aminomethane solution*, and dilute the combined filtrate and washings to 100 ml with *tris(hydroxymethyl)aminomethane solution*.
Dilute 10 ml of this solution to 50 ml with *tris(hydroxymethyl)aminomethane solution* and measure the extinction of a 1-cm layer at the maximum at about 312 nm, using in the reference cell a 1-cm layer of a solution prepared by diluting 10 ml of the solution obtained from the sample to 50 ml with *acid methyl alcohol*.
For purposes of calculation, use a value of 144 for the ΔE(1 per cent, 1 cm) of hexachlorophane in these two solutions. Calculate the concentration of hexachlorophane in the sample.

CONTENT OF ZINC OXIDE. 2·70 to 3·30 per cent w/w, calculated as ZnO, determined by the following method:
To about 3 g, accurately weighed, add 10 ml of *dilute nitric acid* and 20 ml of water, boil for 2 minutes, cool, filter, and wash the filter with two 25-ml portions of water.
To the combined filtrate and washings add 3 g of *hexamine* and titrate with 0·05M disodium edetate using 2 ml of *xylenol orange solution* as indicator; each ml of 0·05M disodium edetate is equivalent to 0·004068 g of ZnO.

Labelling. The direction given under Dusting-powders (page 662) should be followed.
In addition, the label on the container states that the preparation should not be applied to infants or to large areas of skin except in accordance with medical advice.

Talc Dusting-powder

Purified Talc, sterilised	..	..	900 g
Starch, in powder ..	..	..	100 g

Prepare as described under Powders (page 774).

Standard
CONTENT OF ACID-INSOLUBLE MATTER. 86·0 to 91·0 per cent, determined by the following method:
Boil gently about 0·5 g, accurately weighed, for 5 minutes with 10 ml of *dilute hydrochloric acid*, cool,

filter through a tared sintered-glass crucible (British Standard Grade No. 4), wash the residue with water until the washings are free from acid, and dry to constant weight at 105°.

Containers; Labelling. The directions given under Dusting-powders (page 662) should be followed.

Zinc, Starch, and Talc Dusting-powder

SYNONYMS: Zinc Oxide and Starch Dusting-powder; Zinc Oxide, Starch, and Talc Dusting-powder

Zinc Oxide..	250 g
Starch, in powder	250 g
Purified Talc, sterilised	500 g

Prepare as described under Powders (page 774).

Standard
CONTENT OF ACID-INSOLUBLE MATTER. 46·1 to 52·5 per cent, determined by the method for Talc Dusting-powder, about 1 g, accurately weighed, being used.

CONTENT OF ZINC OXIDE. 23·3 to 26·4 per cent, calculated as ZnO, determined by the following method: Boil about 4 g, accurately weighed, for 2 minutes with 70 ml of *dilute nitric acid*, cool, filter, and dilute to 200 ml with water.
Dilute 20 ml of this solution to 100 ml with water, add 3 g of *hexamine*, and titrate with 0·05M disodium edetate using 2 ml of *xylenol orange solution* as indicator; each ml of 0·05M disodium edetate is equivalent to 0·004068 g of ZnO.

Containers; Labelling. The directions given under Dusting-powders (page 662) should be followed.

Zinc Undecenoate Dusting-powder

Zinc Undecenoate	100 g
Undecenoic Acid	20 g
Pumilio Pine Oil	5 ml
Starch, in powder	500 g
Light Kaolin, sterilised ..	to 1000 g

Triturate the pumilio pine oil and the undecenoic acid with most of the light kaolin, incorporate the starch, the zinc undecenoate, and the remainder of the light kaolin, sift, and mix.

Standard
CONTENT OF UNDECENOIC ACID. 1·6 to 2·2 per cent, calculated as $C_{11}H_{20}O_2$, determined by the following method:
Mix about 10 g, accurately weighed, with 100 ml of *light petroleum (boiling-range 60° to 80°)*, shake for 2 hours, and filter.
Add 50 ml of the filtrate to 200 ml of *alcohol (95 per cent)* which has previously been neutralised to *phenol-phthalein solution* and titrate with 0·1N sodium hydroxide, using *phenolphthalein solution* as indicator; each ml of 0·1N sodium hydroxide is equivalent to 0·01843 g of $C_{11}H_{20}O_2$.
CONTENT OF ZINC UNDECENOATE. 9·1 to 10·7 per cent, calculated as $C_{22}H_{38}O_4Zn$, determined by the following method:
Boil about 2 g, accurately weighed, with a mixture of 40 ml of water and 5 ml of *dilute hydrochloric acid*, cool, add 100 ml of water and 10 ml of *ammonia buffer solution*, and titrate with 0·05M disodium edetate, using *mordant black 11 solution* as indicator; each ml of 0·05M disodium edetate is equivalent to 0·02160 g of $C_{22}H_{38}O_4Zn$.

Containers; Labelling. The directions given under Dusting-powders (page 662) should be followed.

EAR-DROPS

Ear-drops are solutions or suspensions of medicaments in water, glycerol, diluted alcohol, propylene glycol, or other suitable solvent, for instillation into the ear.

Containers. Ear-drops should be supplied in coloured fluted glass bottles fitted with a plastic screw cap incorporating a glass dropper tube fitted with a rubber teat, or in plastic squeeze bottles fitted with a plastic cap incorporating a dropper device.

Labelling. The container should be labelled "For external use only".

Chloramphenicol Ear-drops

Chloramphenicol Ear-drops consist of a solution of Chloramphenicol in Propylene Glycol.

Standard
CONTENT OF CHLORAMPHENICOL. 90·0 to 110·0 per cent of the prescribed or stated concentration, calculated with reference to the substance free from 1-*p*-nitrophenyl-2-amino-1,3-propanediol, determined by the following method:
Dilute an accurately measured volume to give a final concentration of about 0·1 per cent w/v of chloramphenicol.
(i) To 25 ml of the prepared solution add 5 ml of 1N hydrochloric acid, extract with four successive 50-ml portions of *solvent ether*, and discard the extractions; dilute the apueous solution to 50 ml with water and measure the extinction of a 1-cm layer at the maximum at about 272 nm.
For purposes of calculation use a value of 474 for the E(1 per cent, 1 cm) of 1-*p*-nitrophenyl-2-amino-1,3-propanediol.
Calculate the concentration of 1-*p*-nitrophenyl-2-amino-1,3-propanediol in the sample.
(ii) Dilute 10 ml of the prepared solution to 100 ml with water, further dilute 10 ml of this solution to 100 ml with water, and measure the extinction of a 1-cm layer at the maximum at about 278 nm.
For purposes of calculation use a value of 298 for the E(1 per cent, 1 cm) of chloramphenicol.
From the result deduct the concentration of 1-*p*-nitrophenyl-2-amino-1,3-propanediol in the sample as determined in (i) above and hence calculate the concentration of chloramphenicol in the sample.

Containers; Labelling. The directions given under Ear-drops (above) should be followed.

Storage. It should be protected from light.

Note. When the strength of the ear-drops is not specified, ear-drops containing 5 per cent w/v of chloramphenicol shall be supplied. Ear-drops containing 10 per cent are also available.

Hydrocortisone and Neomycin Ear-drops

Hydrocortisone and Neomycin Ear-drops consist of a suspension of Hydrocortisone Acetate, in sufficiently fine powder to meet the requirements of the standard, with appropriate pharmaceutical adjuvants, in a solution of Neomycin Sulphate in freshly boiled and cooled Purified Water.

Standard
PRESENCE OF HYDROCORTISONE ACETATE. It complies with the thin-layer chromatographic test given in Appendix 5D, page 875.

ACIDITY OR ALKALINITY. pH, 6·5 to 8·0.

PARTICLE SIZE. When determined by the method given in Appendix 25C, page 911, not less than 75 per cent of the particles have a maximum diameter less than 10 µm and not less than 99 per cent of the particles have a maximum diameter less than 20 µm; no particle has a maximum diameter greater than 50 µm.

CONTENT OF HYDROCORTISONE ACETATE. 90·0 to 110·0 per cent of the prescribed or stated concentration, determined by the following method:
The following procedure should be carried out in subdued light or in low-actinic glassware.
To an accurately measured volume, equivalent to about 0·015 g of hydrocortisone acetate, add 15 ml of water and extract with three successive 30-ml portions of *chloroform*, filter the combined chloroform extracts through a pledget of cotton wool, and dilute the filtrate to 100 ml with *chloroform*.
Transfer a volume of this solution, equivalent to about 450 µg of hydrocortisone acetate, to a 25-ml graduated flask, evaporate off the chloroform in a current of air, dissolve the residue in 10 ml of *aldehyde-free dehydrated alcohol*, add 2·0 ml of *triphenyltetrazolium chloride solution*, displace the air in the flask with *oxygen-free nitrogen*, immediately add 2·0 ml of *dilute tetramethylammonium hydroxide solution*, again displace the air in the flask with *oxygen-free nitrogen*, stopper the flask, mix the contents by gentle swirling, and allow to stand in a water-bath at 30° for 1 hour.
Cool the solution rapidly, dilute to 25 ml with *aldehyde-free dehydrated alcohol*, mix, and measure the extinction of a 1-cm layer, in a closed cell, at the maximum at about 485 nm, using as the blank a solution prepared by treating 10 ml of *aldehyde-free dehydrated alcohol* in the same manner, beginning at the words "add 2·0 ml of *triphenyltetrazolium chloride solution . . .*".
Repeat the procedure using 10 ml of a solution of *hydrocortisone acetate B.C.R.S.* in *aldehyde-free dehydrated alcohol*, containing between 440 and 460 µg in 10 ml and beginning at the words "add 2·0 ml of *triphenyltetrazolium chloride solution . . .*", and hence calculate the concentation of hydrocortisone acetate in the sample.

CONTENT OF NEOMYCIN SULPHATE. 90 to 115 per cent of the prescribed or stated concentration, determined by the following method:
Carry out a microbiological assay of neomycin; a suggested method is given in Appendix 18, page 897. The precision of any assay must be such that the fiducial limits of error (P = 0·95) are not less than 95 per cent and not more than 105 per cent of the estimated potency.
Assuming that each 680 Units found is equivalent to 1 mg of neomycin sulphate, calculate the upper and

lower fiducial limits of the equivalent concentration of neomycin sulphate in the ear-drops.
The upper fiducial limit of the estimated equivalent concentration of neomycin sulphate is not less than 90 per cent and the lower fiducial limit is not more than 115 per cent of the prescribed or stated concentration.

Containers. The directions given under Ear-drops (page 664) should be followed.

Labelling. The label on the container or package should state the date after which the ear-drops should not be used. A direction should be given on the label to shake the bottle.

Storage. It should be stored in a cool place and protected from freezing.

Note. When the strength of the ear-drops is not specified, a suspension containing 1·5 per cent w/v of hydrocortisone acetate and 0·5 per cent w/v of neomycin sulphate shall be supplied.

Hydrogen Peroxide Ear-drops

Hydrogen Peroxide Solution	..	25 ml
Water (see page 642)	..	.. to 100 ml

Standard
CONTENT OF HYDROGEN PEROXIDE. 1·12 to 1·83 per cent w/v, calculated as H_2O_2, determined by the following method:
To 2 ml add 20 ml of water and 10 ml of *dilute sulphuric acid* and titrate with 0·1N potassium permanganate; each ml of 0·1N potassium permanganate is equivalent to 0·001701 g of H_2O_2.

Containers; Labelling. The directions given under Ear-drops (page 664) should be followed.

Phenol Ear-drops

Phenol Glycerin ..	..	..	40 ml
Glycerol ..	..	..	.. to 100 ml

Standard
CONTENT OF PHENOL. 5·4 to 7·3 per cent w/w, calculated as C_6H_6O, determined by the following method:
Mix about 0·5 g, accurately weighed, with 25 ml of water, in a glass-stoppered flask, add 30 ml of 0·1N bromine and 5 ml of *hydrochloric acid*, shake repeatedly during 15 minutes, and allow to stand for 15 minutes; add 10 ml of *potassium iodide solution* and titrate the liberated iodine with 0·1N sodium thiosulphate.
Repeat the procedure omitting the sample.
The difference between the two titrations represents the amount of bromine required by the sample; each ml of 0·1N bromine is equivalent to 0·001569 g of C_6H_6O.

Containers; Labelling. The directions given under Ear-drops (page 664) should be followed.

Caution. *Dilution with water renders Phenol Ear-drops caustic; the preparation may be diluted with glycerol, if desired.*

Sodium Bicarbonate Ear-drops

Sodium Bicarbonate	..	..	5 g
Glycerol ..	..	..	30 ml
Purified Water, freshly boiled and cooled ..	..	..	.. to 100 ml

Dissolve the sodium bicarbonate in about 60 ml of the water, add the glycerol and sufficient of the water to produce the required volume, and mix.

The ear-drops should be recently prepared.

Standard

WEIGHT PER ML. At 20°, 1·10 g to 1·12 g.

CONTENT OF SODIUM BICARBONATE. 4·75 to 5·25 per cent w/v, calculated as NaHCO₃, determined by the following method:

To 5 ml add 20 ml of water and titrate with 0·1N hydrochloric acid, using *methyl orange-xylene cyanol FF solution* as indicator; each ml of 0·1N hydrochloric acid is equivalent to 0·008401 g of NaHCO₃.

Containers; Labelling. The directions given under Ear-drops (page 664) should be followed.

Spirit Ear-drops

Alcohol (95 per cent)	..	..	50 ml
Water (see page 642)	..	..	to 100 ml

In making this preparation the alcohol (95 per cent) may be replaced by Industrial Methylated Spirit, provided that the law and the statutory regulations governing the use of industrial methylated spirit are observed.

Standard

SPECIFIC GRAVITY (20°/20°). 0·927 to 0·946.

Containers; Labelling. The directions given under Ear-drops (page 664) should be followed.

ELIXIRS

Elixirs are clear, pleasantly flavoured, liquid preparations of potent or nauseous medicaments. The vehicle frequently contains a high proportion of alcohol, sugar, glycerol, or propylene glycol together with adjuvants such as colouring matter, other sweetening or flavouring agents, and preservatives.

Synonyms. Because some of the elixirs described in the following monographs are available commercially under the title "syrup", this term has been used in synonyms to the titles of the relevant monographs; however, the products should not be confused with the medicated and flavoured syrups described on pages 798 to 801. Some elixirs were formerly classified as mixtures and this term likewise appears as a synonym in the relevant monographs.

Stability of elixirs. In general, elixirs are reasonably stable preparations provided they are stored in well-filled containers and are not diluted or mixed with other preparations. Any special precautions which may be necessary are indicated in the relevant monographs.

Some elixirs which cannot be kept for long periods are supplied in the form of granules or powder to which a specified quantity of water is added to prepare the elixir just before issue for use, and an appropriate warning regarding the limited shelf-life is given on the label.

Microbial contamination. Elixirs do not usually support the growth of micro-organisms but, as they are liable to contain a high proportion of syrup, dilution or admixture with other preparations may create an ideal growth medium for micro-organisms.

Dilution of elixirs. When a dose ordered or prescribed is less than or not a multiple of 5 millilitres, the elixir should be diluted with the vehicle recommended in the individual monograph, so that the dose to be measured for the patient is one 5-millilitre spoonful or multiple thereof. Instructions for dilution are given in the individual monographs.

Diluted elixirs must always be freshly prepared and not more than two weeks' supply should be issued at a time unless otherwise specified in the monograph.

Labelling. The following directions should be observed:

A. The label on a container of an elixir issued by the manufacturer states:

(1) for elixirs other than those for which a full recipe is given in the individual monograph, the name and concentration of the active ingredient; and

(2) directions for storage.

If the elixir is one which is to be prepared freshly before issue to the patient, the label on the container of granules or powder states:

(3) The name of the preparation in the form of "Granules (or Powder) for the Elixir", as specified in the individual monograph;

(4) the name and concentration of the active ingredient in the elixir when prepared according to the manufacturer's instructions;

(5) directions for storage; and

(6) the date after which the granules or powder should not be used.

The label on the container, or the package leaflet, or the label on the package states:

(1) the directions for preparing the elixir;

(2) the directions for storage of the elixir; and

(3) the period during which the elixir may be expected to retain its potency when stored under the stated conditions.

B. The label on the container of an elixir issued to the patient on a prescription states, in addition to the prescriber's directions:

(1) any special storage directions as directed in the monograph; and

(2) if such a recommendation is made by the manufacturer, the date after which the elixir should not be used; or, if the elixir has been diluted before issue "The contents to be discarded if not taken before . . . [a date two weeks, or other period specified by the manufacturer or in the individual monograph, after the date of issue]".

Caffeine Iodide Elixir

Caffeine	30 g
Sodium Iodide	90 g
Chloroform	2 ml
Liquorice Liquid Extract ..	60 ml

Decoction prepared from a sufficient quantity of recently ground roasted coffee of commerce and Water (see page 642) to 1000 ml

To make the decoction, add 100 g of the recently ground roasted coffee to 1000 ml of the boiling water, boil for one minute, strain, and pour sufficient water over the contents of the strainer to produce 1000 ml when cold.

Dissolve the caffeine and the sodium iodide in 500 ml of the decoction, add the liquorice liquid extract, the chloroform, and sufficient of the decoction to produce the required volume, and mix.

Standard

PRESENCE OF CAFFEINE. It complies with the thin-layer chromatographic test given in Appendix 5A, page 860.

PRESENCE OF SODIUM IODIDE. Shake 5 ml with 5 ml of *chloroform*, 1 ml of *potassium iodate solution*, and 5 ml of *acetic acid*, and allow to separate; the chloroform layer is purple.

Add 0·05 ml of the chloroform layer to 1 ml of *starch mucilage*; a deep blue colour is produced.

WEIGHT PER ML. At 20°, 1·08 g to 1·10 g.

CONTENT OF ANHYDROUS CAFFEINE. 2·85 to 3·25 per cent w/v, determined by the following method:
To 10 ml add 5 ml of *dilute hydrochloric acid* and 5 ml of water and extract with six successive 30-ml portions of *chloroform*; wash the combined extracts with 10 ml of 1N potassium hydroxide, followed by two successive 20-ml portions of water; evaporate off the chloroform from the washed extracts and dry the residue of anhydrous caffeine to constant weight at 105°.

CONTENT OF SODIUM IODIDE. 8·1 to 9·4 per cent w/v, calculated as NaI, determined by the method given in Appendix 11, page 891, 5 ml diluted with 20 ml of water being used and the pH being adjusted, if necessary, by the addition of *dilute sulphuric acid* instead of dilute nitric acid; each ml of 0·1N silver nitrate is equivalent to 0·01499 g of NaI.

Dose. 5 millilitres.

Cascara Elixir

Cascara, in coarse powder	..	1000.0 g
Saccharin Sodium	.. ..	1.0 g
Light Magnesium Oxide	..	50.0 g
Liquorice, unpeeled, in coarse powder		125.0 g
Coriander Oil	.. .. ..	0.15 ml
Anise Oil ..	.. .. ..	0.2 ml
Alcohol (90 per cent)	.. ..	12.5 ml
Glycerol ..	.. .. ..	300.0 ml
Water (see page 642)	..	to 1000.0 ml

Mix the cascara, the liquorice, and the light magnesium oxide and moisten with 1250 ml of boiling water, stirring thoroughly. Macerate for twenty-four hours in a well-covered vessel, pack moderately tightly in a percolator, and percolate with boiling water until exhausted.
Evaporate the percolate to about 650 ml on a water-bath.
Dissolve the saccharin sodium in 12 ml of water and the coriander oil and the anise oil in the alcohol. Mix both solutions with the glycerol and add the concentrated percolate and sufficient water to produce 1000 ml.
Shake thoroughly and allow to stand for not less than twelve hours; filter, if necessary.

Standard
PRESENCE OF CASCARA. Mix in a small flask 0.2 g with 5 ml of water, 1 ml of a 60 per cent w/v solution of *ferric chloride* in water, and 5 ml of *hydrochloric acid*, immerse the flask in a water-bath so that the level of the water is above the level of the liquid in the flask and heat for 30 minutes; cool, add 5 ml of water, transfer the solution to a separating funnel, add 20 ml of *carbon tetrachloride*, shake, allow to separate, discard the aqueous layer, add 10 ml of 1N sodium hydroxide, shake, and allow to separate; the aqueous layer is red and has a maximum absorbence at about 500 nm.

WEIGHT PER ML. At 20°, 1.16 g to 1.20 g.

Dose. 2 to 5 millilitres.

Chloral Elixir, Paediatric

Chloral Hydrate ..	..	..	40 g
Water (see page 642)	..	..	20 ml
Black Currant Syrup	..	..	200 ml
Syrup ..	..	..	to 1000 ml

Dissolve the chloral hydrate in the water, add the black currant syrup and sufficient syrup to produce the required volume, and mix.
It should be recently prepared.

Standard
PRESENCE OF CHLORAL HYDRATE. To 5 ml add 2 ml of *sodium hydroxide solution* and mix; a liquid having the odour of chloroform separates from the mixture.
Warm 0.05 ml of the separated liquid with 0.1 ml of *aniline*; the odour of phenyl isocyanide is produced.

WEIGHT PER ML. At 20°, 1.32 g to 1.33 g.

CONTENT OF CHLORAL HYDRATE. 3.80 to 4.20 per cent w/v, calculated as $C_2H_3Cl_3O_2$, determined by the following method:
To about 3 g, accurately weighed, add 2.5 g of *zinc powder*, 15 ml of *glacial acetic acid*, and 30 ml of water, boil under a reflux condenser for 30 minutes, cool, filter through cotton wool, and wash the residue with water.
Combine the filtrate and washings, add 20 ml of *dilute nitric acid* and 30 ml of 0.1N silver nitrate, shake vigorously, filter, wash the residue with water, and titrate the excess of silver nitrate in the combined filtrate and washings with 0.1N ammonium thiocyanate, using *ferric ammonium sulphate solution* as indicator; each ml of 0.1N silver nitrate is equivalent to 0.005513 g of $C_2H_3Cl_3O_2$.
Determine the weight per ml of the elixir and calculate the concentration of $C_2H_3Cl_3O_2$, weight in volume.

Dose. CHILD. Up to 1 year, 5 millilitres.

When a dose less than or not a multiple of 5 ml is prescribed, the elixir may be diluted, as described under Elixirs (page 666), with Syrup. The diluted elixir must be freshly prepared.

Chlorpheniramine Elixir

SYNONYM: Chlorpheniramine Syrup

Chlorpheniramine Elixir is a solution of Chlorpheniramine Maleate in a suitable, coloured, flavoured vehicle.

Standard
CONTENT OF CHLORPHENIRAMINE MALEATE. 90.0 to 110.0 per cent of the prescribed or stated concentration, determined by the following method:
Remove interfering substances from *anaesthetic ether* by extracting with 0.5N sodium hydroxide, washing with water, further extracting with 0.5N sulphuric acid, and finally washing with water until the washings are neutral to *litmus paper*.
To an accurately measured volume, equivalent to about 5 mg of chlorpheniramine maleate, add 10 g of *sodium chloride* and 25 ml of *sodium hydroxide solution*, and extract with five successive 30-ml portions of the washed anaesthetic ether; wash the combined ethereal extracts with 25 ml of water and discard the washings; extract with five successive 20-ml portions of 0.5N sulphuric acid, dilute the combined extracts to 200 ml with 0.5N sulphuric acid, and measure the extinction of a 1-cm layer at the maximum at about 265 nm.
For purposes of calculation, use a value of 212 for the E(1 per cent, 1 cm) of chlorpheniramine maleate.
Calculate the concentration of chlorpheniramine maleate in the sample.

Labelling. The directions given under Elixirs (page 667) should be followed.

Storage. It should be stored in a cool place, protected from light.

Dose. Chlorpheniramine maleate:
ADULT. 2 to 4 milligrams.
CHILD. Up to 1 year, 1 milligram twice daily; 1 to 5 years, 1 to 2 milligrams three times daily; 6 to 12 years, 4 milligrams three or four times daily.

When the strength of the elixir is not specified, a solution containing 2 mg of chlorpheniramine maleate in 5 ml shall be supplied.

When a dose less than or not a multiple of 5 ml is prescribed, the elixir may be diluted, as described under Elixirs (page 666), with Syrup. The diluted elixir must be freshly prepared.

Chlorpromazine Elixir

SYNONYM: Chlorpromazine Syrup

Chlorpromazine Elixir is a solution of Chlorpromazine Hydrochloride in a suitable, coloured, flavoured vehicle.

Standard
PRESENCE OF CHLORPROMAZINE. It complies with the thin-layer chromatographic test given in Appendix 5C, page 873.

CONTENT OF CHLORPROMAZINE HYDROCHLORIDE. 90·0 to 110·0 per cent of the prescribed or stated concentration, determined by the following method:
Dilute an accurately measured volume, equivalent to about 0·1 g of chlorpromazine hydrochloride, to 500 ml with *dilute hydrochloric acid* and mix.
To 10 ml of this solution add 20 ml of water, make distinctly alkaline to *litmus paper* by the addition of *strong ammonia solution*, extract with six successive 25-ml portions of *solvent ether*, and combine the extracts.
Extract the combined extracts with four successive 25-ml portions of a mixture containing 1 volume of *hydrochloric acid* and 99 volumes of water, discard the ether, remove any dissolved ether from the combined aqueous extracts with a current of air, dilute to 250 ml with the diluted hydrochloric acid, and measure the extinction of a 1-cm layer at the maximum at about 254 nm.
For purposes of calculation use a value of 914 for the $E(1$ per cent, 1 cm) of chlorpromazine hydrochloride.
Calculate the concentration of chlorpromazine hydrochloride in the sample.

Labelling. The directions given under Elixirs (page 667) should be followed.

Storage. It should be protected from light.

Dose. Chlorpromazine hydrochloride:
As an anti-emetic: 25 to 50 milligrams.
For psychiatric states: 75 to 800 milligrams daily in divided doses.

When the strength of the elixir is not specified, a solution containing 25 mg of chlorpromazine hydrochloride in 5 ml shall be supplied.

When a dose less than or not a multiple of 5 ml is prescribed, the elixir may be diluted, as described under Elixirs (page 666), with Syrup. The diluted elixir must be freshly prepared.

Caution. *Contact with the skin should be avoided to minimise the risk of dermatitis.*

Cloxacillin Elixir

SYNONYM: Cloxacillin Syrup

Cloxacillin Elixir is a solution of Cloxacillin Sodium in a suitable coloured flavoured vehicle. It is prepared freshly by dissolving a powder consisting of the dry mixed ingredients in the specified volume of Water (see page 642).

Standard
CONTENT OF CLOXACILLIN. 95·0 to 120·0 per cent of the prescribed or stated concentration, determined by the following method:
Prepare the elixir, as directed on the label, immediately before analysis, and reserve a portion for the test for stability.
Dilute an accurately weighed quantity of the elixir, equivalent to about 0·075 g of cloxacillin, to 50 ml with water and continue by the method given for Phenethicillin Elixir, page 674, beginning with the words "and transfer 2 ml of this solution . . .".

Calculate the amount of cloxacillin in the sample by reference to a calibration curve prepared at the same time, using suitable quantities of *cloxacillin sodium A.S.* treated in the same manner; each mg of cloxacillin sodium is equivalent to 0·9159 mg of cloxacillin.
Determine the weight per ml of the elixir and calculate the concentration of cloxacillin, weight in volume.

STABILITY OF ELIXIR. Store at $15° \pm 1°$ for 7 days the portion of the elixir reserved in the determination of content of cloxacillin and then repeat the determination on the stored elixir. The concentration of cloxacillin in the stored elixir is not less than 80 per cent of the concentration found in the freshly prepared elixir.

ACIDITY OF ELIXIR. pH, 5·0 to 6·0.

Labelling. The directions given under Elixirs (page 667) should be followed; the name on the label of the container of the dry powder is "Powder for Cloxacillin Elixir".

Storage. The elixir and the diluted elixir should be stored in a cool place and used within one week of preparation.

Dose. The equivalent of cloxacillin:
ADULT. 1·5 to 3 grams daily in divided doses.
CHILD. 25 milligrams per kilogram body-weight every six hours.

When the strength of the elixir is not specified, a solution containing the equivalent of 125 mg of cloxacillin in 5 ml shall be supplied.

When a dose less than or not a multiple of 5 ml is prescribed, the elixir may be diluted, as described under Elixirs (page 666), with Syrup. The diluted elixir must be freshly prepared.

Diamorphine and Cocaine Elixir

Diamorphine Hydrochloride	..		1 g
Cocaine Hydrochloride	..	..	1 g
Alcohol (90 per cent)	..	..	125 ml
Syrup	..	..	..	250 ml
Chloroform Water	..	..	to 1000 ml

It should be freshly prepared.

Dose. The dose is determined by the physician in accordance with the needs of the patient.

When *Diamorphine and Cocaine Elixir* is prescribed without qualification an elixir prepared in accordance with the formula above shall be supplied.

When *Morphine and Cocaine Elixir* is prescribed without qualification an elixir prepared in accordance with the formula above but containing 1 g of morphine hydrochloride instead of 1 g of diamorphine hydrochloride shall be supplied. It should be recently prepared.

When *Morphine, Cocaine, and Chlorpromazine Elixir* or *Diamorphine, Cocaine, and Chlorpromazine Elixir* is prescribed, the syrup in the above formulae is replaced by Chlorpromazine Elixir. These preparations should be protected from light.

When specified by the prescriber, the proportion of diamorphine hydrochloride or morphine hydrochloride in the above formulae may be altered.

Dichloralphenazone Elixir

Dichloralphenazone Elixir is a solution of Dichloralphenazone in a suitable, coloured, flavoured vehicle.

Standard
CONTENT OF DICHLORALPHENAZONE. 90·0 to 110·0 per

cent of the prescribed or stated concentration, determined by the following two methods:

(1) Dilute an accurately weighed quantity, equivalent to about 0·02 g of dichloralphenazone, to 250 ml with water.

To three 10-ml graduated flasks add, respectively, 1·0 ml of this solution, 1·0 ml of *standard chloral hydrate solution*, and 1·0 ml of water; to each flask add 6·0 ml of *isopropyl alcohol* and 1·0 ml of *quinaldine ethiodide solution*, mix thoroughly, add 0·5 ml of *ethanolamine solution*, dilute to 10 ml with water, mix well, and place in a water-bath at 60° for 1 hour; cool, and measure the extinction of a 1-cm layer of the sample solution and of the standard solution at the maximum at about 605 nm, using as a blank the solution prepared with the water.

From the two extinctions, calculate the amount of dichloralphenazone in the sample, assuming that 1 g of chloral hydrate is equivalent to 1·57 g of dichloralphenazone.

Determine the weight per ml of the elixir and calculate the concentration of dichloralphenazone, weight in volume.

(2) Mix an accurately weighed quantity, equivalent to about 0·5 g of dichloralphenazone, with 20 ml of a 10 per cent w/v solution of *sodium acetate* in water, add 25 ml of 0·1N iodine, and allow to stand for 20 minutes with occasional shaking; add 10 ml of *chloroform*, shake to dissolve the precipitate, and titrate the excess iodine with 0·1N sodium thiosulphate, using *starch mucilage*, added towards the end of the titration, as indicator.

Repeat the procedure omitting the sample.

The difference between the two titrations represents the amount of iodine required by the sample; each ml of 0·1N iodine is equivalent to 0·02595 g of $C_{15}H_{18}Cl_6N_2O_5$.

Determine the weight per ml of the elixir and calculate the concentration of dichloralphenazone, weight in volume.

Labelling. The directions given under Elixirs (page 667) should be followed.

Storage. It should be stored in well-filled airtight containers, in a cool place, protected from light.

Dose. Dichloralphenazone:
ADULT. See under Dichloralphenazone (page 155).

CHILD. Sedative dose: up to 1 year, 45 to 135 milligrams; 1 to 5 years, 135 to 225 milligrams; 6 to 12 years, 225 to 450 milligrams.

Hypnotic dose: up to 1 year, 90 to 270 milligrams; 1 to 5 years, 270 to 540 milligrams; 6 to 12 years, 540 to 675 milligrams.

When the strength of the elixir is not specified, a solution containing 225 mg of dichloralphenazone in 5 ml shall be supplied.

When a dose less than or not a multiple of 5 ml is prescribed, the elixir may be diluted, as described under Elixirs (page 666), with Syrup. The diluted elixir must be freshly prepared.

Dicyclomine Elixir

SYNONYM: Dicyclomine Syrup

Dicyclomine Elixir is a solution of Dicyclomine Hydrochloride in a suitable, coloured, flavoured vehicle.

Standard
PRESENCE OF DICYCLOMINE. It complies with the thin-layer chromatographic test given in Appendix 5A, page 862.

CONTENT OF DICYCLOMINE HYDROCHLORIDE. 90·0 to 110·0 per cent of the prescribed or stated concentra-

tion, calculated as $C_{19}H_{36}ClNO_2$, determined by the following method:

To an accurately weighed quantity, equivalent to about 5 mg of dicyclomine hydrochloride, add 5 ml of *sulphuric acid (10 per cent v/v)* and 2 ml of 0·1N potassium permanganate, mix, and allow to stand; to the decolorised solution add 20 ml of water, 20 ml of *chloroform*, and 1 ml of *dimethyl yellow solution* as indicator and titrate with 0·001M sodium lauryl sulphate; each ml of 0·001M sodium lauryl sulphate is equivalent to 0·0003460 g of $C_{19}H_{36}ClNO_2$.

Determine the weight per ml of the elixir and calculate the concentration of dicyclomine hydrochloride, weight in volume.

Labelling. The directions given under Elixirs (page 667) should be followed.

Storage. It should be protected from light.

Dose. Dicyclomine hydrochloride:
ADULT. 10 to 20 milligrams three times daily.
CHILD. Up to 1 year, 5 milligrams before feeds; 1 to 5 years, 5 to 10 milligrams three times daily.

When the strength of the elixir is not specified, a solution containing 10 mg of dicyclomine hydrochloride in 5 ml shall be supplied.

When a dose less than or not a multiple of 5 ml is prescribed, the elixir may be diluted, as described under Elixirs (page 666), with Syrup. The diluted elixir must be freshly prepared.

Digoxin Elixir, Paediatric

Paediatric Digoxin Elixir is a solution containing 0·005 per cent w/v of Digoxin, 10 per cent v/v of Alcohol, and Sodium Phosphate, with Methyl Hydroxybenzoate, or other suitable preservative, in a suitable, coloured, flavoured vehicle. The solution is adjusted to pH 7.

Standard
PRESENCE OF DIGOXIN. Extract 5 ml with four successive 20-ml portions of *chloroform*, washing each chloroform extract with the same 10 ml of water, evaporate the combined chloroform extracts to dryness, dissolve the residue in 1 ml of *glacial acetic acid* containing 0·01 per cent w/v of *ferric chloride*, and add 1 ml of *sulphuric acid* so as to form a subjacent layer; a pure brown ring free from red colour is formed at the junction of the liquids and, after a short time, the upper acetic acid layer acquires an indigo colour.

ACIDITY OR ALKALINITY. pH, 6·8 to 7·2.

ALCOHOL CONTENT. 9·2 to 10·8 per cent v/v of ethyl alcohol, determined by the method given in Appendix 10, page 888.

CONTENT OF DIGOXIN. 0·0045 to 0·0055 per cent w/v, determined by the following method:

Extract 20 ml with four successive 25-ml portions of *chloroform*, washing each extract with the same 5 ml of water, evaporate the combined chloroform extracts to dryness, add 3 ml of *dehydrated alcohol*, and evaporate to dryness in a current of air; add a further 3 ml of *dehydrated alcohol*, repeat the evaporation to dryness, and dissolve the cooled residue in 5 ml of a mixture of 65 volumes of *chloroform* and 35 volumes of *methyl alcohol*.

To this prepared sample solution add 20 ml of *glacial acetic acid* containing 0·005 per cent w/v of *ferric chloride* and 2 ml v/v of *sulphuric acid* and allow to stand for one and a half hours.

Compare the extinction of a 1-cm layer of this solution at the maximum at about 590 nm with that of a solution prepared at the same time and in the same manner with 5 ml of *standard digoxin solution* in place of the prepared sample solution; use the acetic acid reagent as the blank.

Calculate the concentration of digoxin in the sample.

Labelling. The directions given under Elixirs (page 667) should be followed.

Storage. It should be stored in a cool place, protected from light.

Dose. CHILD, up to 1 year, per kilogram body-weight: 0·5 millilitre, initially, followed by two doses of 0·2 millilitre with an interval of six hours between doses, and then 0·1 millilitre daily for maintenance.

This elixir should not be diluted. The general direction given under Elixirs that the preparation should be diluted so that the dose is contained in 5 ml does not apply to this elixir. The dose prescribed should be measured by means of a graduated pipette.

Paediatric Digoxin Elixir contains in 1 ml 50 µg of digoxin.

Diphenhydramine Elixir

Diphenhydramine Elixir is a solution of Diphenhydramine Hydrochloride in a suitable, coloured, flavoured vehicle.

Standard
PRESENCE OF DIPHENHYDRAMINE. It complies with the thin-layer chromatographic test given in Appendix 5A, page 862.

CONTENT OF DIPHENHYDRAMINE HYDROCHLORIDE. 90·0 to 110·0 per cent of the prescribed or stated concentration, calculated as $C_{17}H_{22}ClNO$, determined by the following method:
To an accurately measured volume, equivalent to about 0·1 g of diphenhydramine hydrochloride, add 2 ml of *dilute hydrochloric acid*, extract with two successive 15-ml portions of *solvent ether*, and discard the ether extracts; to the aqueous solution add 4 ml of *sodium hydroxide solution*, and extract with successive 15-ml portions of *solvent ether* until extraction is complete; wash the combined ethereal extracts with two successive 5-ml portions of water, and extract the combined washings with 15 ml of *solvent ether*; evaporate the combined ethereal extracts to dryness, dissolve the residue in 15 ml of 0·1N sulphuric acid, and titrate the excess of acid with 0·1N sodium hydroxide, using *methyl red solution* as indicator; each ml of 0·1N sulphuric acid is equivalent to 0·02918 g of $C_{17}H_{22}ClNO$.

Labelling. The directions given under Elixirs (page 667) should be followed.

Storage. It should be protected from light.

Dose. Diphenhydramine hydrochloride:
ADULT. 25 to 75 milligrams three times daily.
CHILD. Up to 1 year, 6·25 to 12·5 milligrams three or four times daily; 1 to 5 years, 12·5 to 25 milligrams three or four times daily; 6 to 12 years, 25 to 50 milligrams three times daily.

When the strength of the elixir is not specified, a solution containing 12·5 mg of diphenhydramine hydrochloride in 5 ml shall be supplied.

When a dose less than or not a multiple of 5 ml is prescribed, the elixir may be diluted, as described under Elixirs (page 666), with Syrup.
The diluted elixir must be freshly prepared, unless a preservative is added to the diluent; 0·2 per cent w/w of methyl hydroxybenzoate is a suitable preservative.

Ephedrine Elixir

SYNONYM: Ephedrine Hydrochloride Elixir

Ephedrine Hydrochloride	..	3·0 g
Lemon Spirit	.. ..	0·2 ml
Compound Tartrazine Solution..		10·0 ml
Chloroform Spirit	.. ..	40·0 ml
Water (see page 642)	.. ..	60·0 ml
Alcohol (90 per cent)	.. ..	100·0 ml
Invert Syrup	.. ..	200·0 ml
Glycerol ..	.. ..	200·0 ml
Syrup	.. .. ..	to 1000·0 ml

Dissolve the ephedrine hydrochloride in the water, add the glycerol, the compound tartrazine solution, the alcohol, the chloroform spirit, the lemon spirit, the invert syrup, and sufficient syrup to produce the required volume, and mix.

Standard
WEIGHT PER ML. At 20°, 1·23 g to 1·24 g.

ALCOHOL CONTENT. 11 to 13 per cent v/v of ethyl alcohol, determined by the method given in Appendix 10, page 888.

CONTENT OF EPHEDRINE HYDROCHLORIDE. 0·27 to 0·33 per cent w/v, determined by the following method:
Dilute about 12 g, accurately weighed, to 100 ml with water and further dilute 5 ml of this solution to 100 ml with water.
To 5 ml of this solution in a separating funnel add 1·25 ml of a saturated solution of *sodium bicarbonate* in water and 3 ml of *sodium periodate solution*, swirl to mix, and allow to stand for 15 minutes; add 10 ml of 0·1N hydrochloric acid and 15 ml of *cyclohexane*, shake for 3 minutes, allow to separate, discard the aqueous phase, filter the cyclohexane extract through a pledget of cotton wool and measure the extinction of a 1-cm layer of the filtrate at the maximum at about 241 nm, using as the blank a solution prepared in a similar manner but substituting 5 ml of water for the 5 ml of sample solution.
Calculate the concentration of ephedrine hydrochloride in the sample by reference to a calibration curve prepared by treating suitable aliquots of a solution of *ephedrine hydrochloride* in water in a similar manner.
Determine the weight per ml of the elixir and calculate the concentration of ephedrine hydrochloride, weight in volume.

Dose. ADULT. 5 to 10 millilitres.
CHILD. Up to 1 year, 2·5 millilitres; 1 to 5 years, 5 millilitres; 6 to 12 years, 10 millilitres.

When a dose less than or not a multiple of 5 ml is prescribed, the elixir may be diluted, as described under Elixirs (page 666), with Syrup. The diluted elixir must be freshly prepared.

Ethamivan Elixir

SYNONYMS: Ethamivan Oral Solution; Ethamivan Mixture

Ethamivan Elixir is a solution containing 5·0 per cent w/v of Ethamivan, 25·0 per cent v/v of Alcohol, and Glycerol in Purified Water.

Standard
ALCOHOL CONTENT. 24 to 26 per cent v/v of ethyl alcohol, determined by the method given in Appendix 10, page 888.

CONTENT OF ETHAMIVAN. 4·75 to 5·25 per cent w/v, determined by the following method:
Dilute 2 ml to 100 ml with water; to 2 ml of this solution add 10 ml of 0·1N hydrochloric acid, dilute to 100 ml with water, and measure the extinction of a 1-cm layer at the maximum at about 280 nm.
For the purposes of calculation, use a value of 155 for the E(1 per cent, 1 cm) of ethamivan.
Calculate the concentration of ethamivan in the sample.

Labelling. The directions given under Elixirs (page 667) should be followed.

Storage. It should be stored in a cool place.

Dose. PREMATURE INFANTS, 0·25 millilitre.
FULL-TERM INFANTS, 0·5 millilitre.

This elixir should not be diluted. The general direction given under Elixirs that the preparation should be diluted so that the dose is contained in 5 ml does not apply to this elixir; the dose prescribed should be measured by means of a graduated pipette.

Ethosuximide Elixir

SYNONYM: Ethosuximide Syrup

Ethosuximide Elixir is a solution of Ethosuximide in a suitable, coloured, flavoured vehicle.

Standard
CONTENT OF ETHOSUXIMIDE. 95·0 to 105·0 per cent of the prescribed or stated concentration, determined by the following method:
To an accurately measured volume, equivalent to about 0·5 g of ethosuximide, add 10 ml of water and 2 g of *sodium bicarbonate* and extract with five successive 30-ml portions of *chloroform*, washing each chloroform extract with the same 10 ml of water; evaporate the combined extracts to about 10 ml, and finally evaporate to dryness in a current of air at room temperature; the residue must not be subjected to heat.
Dissolve the residue in 80 ml of *alcohol (95 per cent)*, dilute to 100 ml with *alcohol (95 per cent)*, and mix; dilute 10 ml of this solution to 100 ml with *alcohol (95 per cent)* and measure the extinction of a 1-cm layer at the maximum at about 248 nm.
For the purposes of calculation, use a value of 8·5 for the E(1 per cent, 1 cm) of ethosuximide.
Calculate the concentration of ethosuximide in the sample.

Labelling. The directions given under Elixirs (page 667) should be followed.

Storage. It should be stored in a cool place.

Dose. Ethosuximide:
ADULT. 500 milligrams daily, in divided doses, increased to 2 grams in accordance with the needs of the patient.
CHILD. 1 to 5 years, 50 to 125 milligrams twice daily, increased to 250 milligrams three or four times daily.

When the strength of the elixir is not specified, a solution containing 250 mg of ethosuximide in 5 ml shall be supplied.

When a dose less than or not a multiple of 5 ml is prescribed, the elixir may be diluted, as described under Elixirs (page 666), with Syrup.
The diluted elixir must be freshly prepared, unless a preservative is added to the diluent; 0·1 per cent w/v of sodium benzoate is a suitable preservative.

Isoniazid Elixir

SYNONYM: Isoniazid Syrup

Isoniazid ..	..	..	..	10·0 g
Citric Acid	..	..	..	2·5 g
Sodium Citrate ..	..	..		12·0 g
Concentrated Anise Water		..		10·0 ml
Compound Tartrazine Solution				10·0 ml
Glycerol ..	..	..	..	200·0 ml
Chloroform Water, Double-strength		..	..	400·0 ml
Water (see page 642)		..		to 1000·0 ml

Dissolve the sodium citrate, the citric acid, and the isoniazid in 300 ml of the water, add the double-strength chloroform water, the glycerol, the compound tartrazine solution, and the concentrated anise water, mix, and add sufficient water to produce the required volume.
Alternatively, the double-strength chloroform water may be omitted and the preparation preserved with methyl hydroxybenzoate, 0·1 per cent w/v, together with propyl hydroxybenzoate, 0·02 per cent w/v. Dissolve these substances in 600 ml of the water with the aid of heat, cool, and dissolve the sodium citrate, the citric acid, and the isoniazid in the solution; add the glycerol, the compound tartrazine solution, and the concentrated anise water, mix, and add sufficient water to produce the required volume.
It has a weight per ml at 20° of about 1·07 g.

Standard
CONTENT OF ISONIAZID. 0·90 to 1·10 per cent w/v determined by the method given for isoniazid in Sodium Aminosalicylate and Isoniazid Cachets, page 650, using 5 ml and beginning with the words "dilute to 1000 ml with water . . .".
Calculate the concentration of isoniazid in the sample.

Labelling. The directions given under Elixirs (page 667) should be followed.

Storage. It should be protected from light. When stored in filled, unopened containers at a temperature not exceeding 25°, it may be expected to retain its potency for one year. When dispensed, each container should be filled and the contents should represent not more than one month's supply.

Dose. CHILD. Twice daily: up to 1 year, 2·5 to 5 millilitres; 1 to 5 years, 5 to 10 millilitres.

When a dose less than or not a multiple of 5 ml is prescribed, the elixir may be diluted, as described under Elixirs (page 666), with Chloroform Water. The diluted elixir must be freshly prepared.
Syrup must not be used as diluent as isoniazid is unstable in the presence of sugars.

Mepyramine Elixir

Mepyramine Elixir is a solution of Mepyramine Maleate in a suitable, coloured, flavoured vehicle.

Standard
PRESENCE OF MEPYRAMINE. It complies with the thin-layer chromatographic test given in Appendix 5A, page 865.

CONTENT OF MEPYRAMINE MALEATE. 90·0 to 110·0 per cent of the prescribed or stated concentration, calculated as $C_{21}H_{27}N_3O_5$, determined by the following method:

To an accurately measured volume, equivalent to about 0·1 g of mepyramine maleate, add 3 ml of *sodium hydroxide solution* and extract with successive 20-, 10-, 10-, and 10-ml portions of *chloroform*; wash the combined chloroformic extracts with five successive 10-ml portions of water, extract the combined washings with 10 ml of *chloroform*, and discard the aqueous washings; evaporate the combined chloroformic extracts to dryness on a water-bath, dissolve the residue in 20 ml of 0·02N hydrochloric acid, and titrate the excess of acid with 0·02N sodium hydroxide, using *methyl red solution* as indicator; each ml of 0·02N hydrochloric acid is equivalent to 0·008029 g of $C_{21}H_{27}N_3O_5$.

Labelling. The directions given under Elixirs (page 667) should be followed.

Storage. It should be protected from light.

Dose. Mepyramine maleate:

ADULT. 50 milligrams every four to six hours, gradually increased if necessary up to a total daily dose of 1 gram.

CHILD. For motion-sickness, three or four times daily: up to 1 year, 12·5 to 25 milligrams; 1 to 5 years, 25 to 50 milligrams; 6 to 12 years, 50 to 75 milligrams.

When the strength of the elixir is not specified, a solution containing 25 mg of mepyramine maleate in 5 ml shall be supplied.

When a dose less than or not a multiple of 5 ml is prescribed, the elixir may be diluted, as described under Elixirs (page 666), with Syrup. The diluted elixir must be freshly prepared.

Neomycin Elixir

SYNONYM: Neomycin Mixture

Neomycin Sulphate	..	..	20·0 g
Disodium Edetate	..	..	0·5 g
Saccharin Sodium	..	..	0·9 g
Benzoic Acid	..	..	..	2·0 g
Citric Acid	..	a sufficient quantity
Compound Tartrazine Solution	6·0 ml
Sorbitol Solution	..	..	385·0 ml
Purified Water, freshly boiled and			
cooled	..	..	..	to. 1000·0 ml

The mixture may be lime-flavoured. The compound tartrazine solution may be replaced by another suitable dye or mixture of dyes, provided that any dye used is of food grade of commerce and that its use for colouring food is permitted in the country concerned. If the mixture is recently prepared, the disodium edetate may be omitted.

Dissolve the benzoic acid, the saccharin sodium, and the disodium edetate in 500 ml of water with the aid of gentle heat, cool, and dissolve the neomycin sulphate in the solution. Add the sorbitol solution and mix; add the colouring, the flavouring, and sufficient of the water to produce the required volume, and mix. If necessary, add sufficient citric acid to adjust the pH to 4·0 to 5·0.

Standard
ACIDITY. pH, 4·0 to 5·0.

CONTENT OF NEOMYCIN. 11,000 to 16,100 Units per ml, determined by the following method:
Carry out a microbiological assay of neomycin; a suggested method is given in Appendix 18, page 897.
The precision of any assay must be such that the fiducial limits of error (P = 0·95) are not less than 95 per cent and not more than 105 per cent of the estimated potency.
Calculate the upper and lower fiducial limits of the concentration of neomycin in the elixir.
The upper fiducial limit of the estimated concentration of neomycin is not less than 11,000 Units per ml and the lower fiducial limit is not more than 16,100 Units per ml.

Storage. It should be stored in a cool place, protected from light.

Dose. CHILD. Every six hours: up to 1 year, 2·5 to 10 millilitres; 1 to 5 years, 10 to 20 millilitres.

When a dose less than or not a multiple of 5 ml is prescribed, the elixir may be diluted, as described under Elixirs (page 666), with Syrup. The diluted elixir must be freshly prepared.

Neomycin Elixir contains 400 mg (approximately 250,000 Units) of neomycin sulphate in 20 ml.

Nux Vomica Elixir

Nux Vomica Tincture	..	..	30 ml
Compound Cardamom Tincture		100 ml
Syrup	..	..	..	..	500 ml
Chloroform Water	..	.. to 1000 ml

Standard
PRESENCE OF NUX VOMICA ALKALOIDS. It complies with the thin-layer chromatographic test given in Appendix 5B, page 872.

WEIGHT PER ML. At 20°, 1·15 g to 1·17 g.

ALCOHOL CONTENT. 6 to 7·5 per cent v/v of ethyl alcohol, determined by the method given in Appendix 10, page 888.

Dose. 5 millilitres.

Orciprenaline Elixir

SYNONYMS: Orciprenaline Sulphate Elixir; Orciprenaline Syrup

Orciprenaline Elixir is a solution of Orciprenaline Sulphate in a suitable flavoured vehicle.

Standard
PRESENCE OF ORCIPRENALINE SULPHATE. It complies with the thin-layer chromatographic test given in Appendix 5A, page 866.

CONTENT OF ORCIPRENALINE SULPHATE. 90·0 to 110·0 per cent of the prescribed or stated amount, calculated as $C_{22}H_{36}N_2O_{10}S$, determined by the following method:
To an accurately weighed quantity, equivalent to about 0·02 g of orciprenaline sulphate, add 5 ml of water, extract with 15 ml of *solvent ether*, wash the ethereal extract with 20 ml of water, and discard the ether; to the combined aqueous solution and washings add 10 ml of 0·1N potassium bromate, 1 g of *potassium bromide*, and 5 ml of *hydrochloric acid*, gently shake for 1 minute, add 0·5 g of *potassium iodide*, and titrate with 0·1N sodium thiosulphate using *starch mucilage* as indicator.
Repeat the procedure omitting the sample.
The difference between the two titrations represents the amount of potassium bromate required by the

sample; each ml of 0·1N potassium bromate is equivalent to 0·004337 g of $C_{22}H_{36}N_2O_{10}S$. Determine the weight per ml of the elixir and calculate the concentration of $C_{22}H_{36}N_2O_{10}S$, weight in volume.

Labelling. The directions given under Elixirs (page 667) should be followed.

Storage. It should be stored in a cool place, protected from light.

Dose. Orciprenaline sulphate:
ADULT. 20 milligrams four times daily.
CHILD. Up to 1 year, 5 to 10 milligrams three times daily; 1 to 5 years, 5 to 10 milligrams four times daily.

When the strength of the elixir is not specified, a solution containing 10 mg in 5 ml shall be supplied.

When a dose less than or not a multiple of 5 ml is prescribed, the elixir may be diluted, as described under Elixirs (page 666), with Syrup. The diluted elixir must be freshly prepared.

Paracetamol Elixir, Paediatric

Paracetamol	..	..	..	24 g
Amaranth Solution	..	..		2 ml
Chloroform Spirit	..	..		20 ml
Concentrated Raspberry Juice	..			25 ml
Alcohol (95 per cent)	..	..		100 ml
Propylene Glycol..	..	..		100 ml
Invert Syrup	..	..	..	275 ml
Glycerol	..	..	..	.. to 1000 ml

Dissolve the paracetamol in a mixture of the alcohol, the propylene glycol, and the chloroform spirit, and add the concentrated raspberry juice diluted with the invert syrup, the amaranth solution, and sufficient glycerol to produce the required volume, and mix.

Standard
WEIGHT PER ML. At 20°, 1·21 g to 1·23 g.

ALCOHOL CONTENT. 10 to 12 per cent v/v of ethyl alcohol, determined by the method given in Appendix 10, page 888.

4-AMINOPHENOL. Not more than 0·5 per cent of the content of paracetamol, determined by the following method:
Dilute 1 ml to 20 ml with water, mix, and add 1 ml of a 1 per cent w/v solution of *phenol* in water and 3 ml of *sodium hyprobromite solution*; any blue colour which is produced is not more intense than that produced when a mixture of 1 ml of *standard 4-aminophenol solution* and 1 ml of *dilute amaranth solution* is used in place of the sample.

CONTENT OF PARACETAMOL. 2·28 to 2·52 per cent w/v, determined by the following method:
To about 1·5 g, accurately weighed, add 100 ml of water and 20 ml of 0·1N sodium hydroxide and dilute to 200 ml with water.
Add 5 ml of this solution to 9·5 ml of 0·1N sodium hydroxide, dilute to 100 ml with water, filter if necessary, and measure the extinction of a 1-cm layer at the maximum at about 257 nm.
For purposes of calculation, use a value of 715 for the E(1 per cent, 1 cm) of paracetamol.
Determine the weight per ml of the elixir and calculate the concentration of paracetamol, weight in volume.

Storage. It should be protected from light.

Dose. CHILD. Up to 1 year, 5 millilitres; 1 to 5 years, 10 millilitres.
This elixir should not be diluted. The general direction

given under Elixirs that the preparation should be diluted so that the dose is contained in 5 ml does not apply to this elixir; if necessary, the prescribed dose should be measured by means of a graduated pipette.

Phenethicillin Elixir

SYNONYM: Phenethicillin Syrup

Phenethicillin Elixir is a solution of Phenethicillin Potassium in a suitable, coloured, flavoured vehicle. It is prepared freshly by dissolving a powder consisting of the dry mixed ingredients in the specified volume of Water (see page 642).

Standard
CONTENT OF PHENETHICILLIN. 95·0 to 120·0 per cent of the prescribed or stated concentration, determined by the following method:
Prepare the elixir, as directed on the label, immediately before analysis, and reserve a portion for the test for stability.
Dilute an accurately weighed quantity of the elixir, equivalent to about 0·075 g of phenethicillin, to 50 ml with water, and transfer 2 ml of this solution to each of two tubes.
To the first tube add 1 ml of 2N sodium hydroxide, allow to stand for exactly 45 minutes, and add 1 ml of 2N sulphuric acid; to the second tube add 2 ml of water.
To each tube add 6 ml of *hydroxylammonium chloride reagent* and allow to stand for 40 minutes; add 2 ml of *ferric reagent*, allow to stand for 20 minutes, and measure the extinction of a 1-cm layer of the solution in the second tube at 490 nm, using as a blank the solution in the first tube.
Calculate the amount of phenethicillin in the sample by reference to a calibration curve prepared at the same time, using suitable quantities of *phenethicillin potassium A.S.* treated in the same manner; each mg of phenethicillin potassium is equivalent to 0·9054 mg of phenethicillin.
Determine the weight per ml of the elixir and calculate the concentration of phenethicillin, weight in volume.

STABILITY OF ELIXIR. Store at 15° ±1° for 7 days the portion of the elixir reserved in the determination of the content of phenethicillin and then repeat the determination on the stored elixir.
The concentration of phenethicillin in the stored elixir is not less than 90 per cent of the concentration found in the freshly prepared elixir.

ACIDITY OF ELIXIR. pH, 5·2 to 6·2.

Labelling. The directions given under Elixirs (page 667) should be followed; the name on the label of the container of the dry powder is "Powder for Phenethicillin Elixir".

Storage. The elixir and the diluted elixir should be stored in a cool place and used within one week of preparation.

Dose. The equivalent of phenethicillin:
ADULT. 125 to 250 milligrams every four to six hours.
CHILD. Every six hours: up to 1 year, 62·5 milligrams; 1 to 5 years, 125 milligrams; 6 to 12 years, 250 milligrams.

When the strength of the elixir is not specified, a solution containing the equivalent of 125 mg of phenethicillin in 5 ml shall be supplied.

When a dose less than or not a multiple of 5 ml is prescribed, the elixir may be diluted, as described under Elixirs (page 666), with Syrup. The diluted elixir must be freshly prepared and not more than one week's supply issued at a time.

Phenobarbitone Elixir

Phenobarbitone		3 g
Compound Tartrazine Solution		10 ml
Compound Orange Spirit	..	24 ml
Alcohol (90 per cent) ..	..	400 ml
Glycerol		400 ml
Water (see page 642) ..		.. to 1000 ml

Dissolve the phenobarbitone in the alcohol and add the glycerol, the compound orange spirit, the compound tartrazine solution, and sufficient water to produce the required volume. Add 25 g of sterilised Purified Talc, shake, allow to stand for a few hours, shaking occasionally, and filter.

Standard
PRESENCE OF PHENOBARBITONE. The melting-point of the residue obtained in the assay is about 175°.

WEIGHT PER ML. At 20°, 1·045 g to 1·055 g.

ALCOHOL CONTENT. 36 to 40 per cent v/v of ethyl alcohol, determined by the method given in Appendix 10, page 888.

CONTENT OF PHENOBARBITONE. 0·27 to 0·33 per cent w/v, determined by the following method:
Extract 50 ml with three successive 50-ml portions of *solvent ether*, wash the combined ethereal extracts with 20 ml of water, and discard the washings; extract the ethereal solution with a mixture of 5 ml of 2N sodium hydroxide and 25 ml of water, followed by two successive 5-ml portions of water; acidify the combined aqueous extracts to *litmus paper* with *dilute hydrochloric acid* and extract with four successive 25-ml portions of *solvent ether*; wash the combined ethereal extracts with two successive 2-ml portions of water and wash the combined aqueous washings with 10 ml of *solvent ether*; add the ethereal washings to the combined ethereal extracts, evaporate off the ether, and dry the residue of phenobarbitone to constant weight at 105°.

Storage. It should be protected from light.

Dose. ADULT. 5 to 10 millilitres.

CHILD. Up to 5 years, 5 millilitres three times daily, increased to 10 millilitres three times daily.

When a dose less than or not a multiple of 5 ml is prescribed, the elixir may be diluted, as described under Elixirs (page 666), with Syrup. The diluted elixir must be freshly prepared.

Phenoxymethylpenicillin Elixir

SYNONYMS: Phenoxymethylpenicillin Solution; Phenoxymethylpenicillin Syrup; Penicillin V Elixir

Phenoxymethylpenicillin Elixir is a solution of Phenoxymethylpenicillin Potassium in a suitable, coloured, flavoured vehicle. It is prepared freshly by dissolving granules consisting of the dry mixed ingredients in the specified volume of Water (see page 642).

Standard
CONTENT OF TOTAL PENICILLINS. 100·0 to 125·0 per cent of the prescribed or stated concentration of phenoxymethylpenicillin, calculated as $C_{16}H_{18}N_2O_5S$, determined by the following method:
Prepare the elixir, as directed on the label, immediately before analysis, and reserve a portion for the test for stability.

Dilute an accurately weighed quantity of the elixir, equivalent to about 0·06 g of phenoxymethylpenicillin, to 50 ml with water, transfer 10 ml to a stoppered flask, add 5 ml of 1N sodium hydroxide and allow to stand for 20 minutes; add 20 ml of a freshly prepared buffer solution containing 5·44 per cent w/v of *sodium acetate* and 2·40 per cent w/v of *glacial acetic acid*, 5 ml of 1N hydrochloric acid, and 25 ml of 0·02N iodine, close the flask with a wet stopper, and allow to stand for 20 minutes, protected from light.
Titrate the excess of iodine with 0·02N sodium thiosulphate, using *starch mucilage*, added towards the end of the titration, as indicator.
To a further 10 ml of the prepared solution add 20 ml of the buffer solution and 25 ml of 0·02N iodine, allow to stand for 20 minutes, and titrate with 0·02N sodium thiosulphate, using *starch mucilage*, added towards the end of the titration, as indicator.
The difference between the two titrations represents the volume of 0·02N iodine equivalent to the total penicillins present.
Calculate the content of total penicillins from the difference obtained by repeating the procedure with *phenoxymethylpenicillin potassium B.C.R.S.* in place of the sample; each mg of *phenoxymethylpenicillin potassium B.C.R.S.* is equivalent to 0·9019 mg of total penicillins, calculated as $C_{16}H_{18}N_2O_5S$.
Determine the weight per ml of the elixir and calculate the concentration of total penicillins, weight in volume.

STABILITY OF ELIXIR. Store at 15° ±1° for 7 days the portion of the elixir reserved in the determination of the content of total penicillins and then repeat the determination on the stored elixir.
The concentration of total penicillins in the stored elixir is not less than 80 per cent of the concentration found in the freshly prepared elixir.

Labelling. The directions given under Elixirs (page 667) should be followed; the name on the label of the container of the dry granules is "Granules for Phenoxymethylpenicillin Elixir".

Storage. The elixir and the diluted elixir should be stored in a cool place and used within one week of preparation.

Dose. The equivalent of phenoxymethylpenicillin:

ADULT. 125 to 250 milligrams every four hours.

CHILD. Every six hours: up to 1 year, 62·5 milligrams; 1 to 5 years, 125 milligrams; 6 to 12 years, 250 milligrams.

The strength of the elixir should be specified by the prescriber. Elixirs containing the equivalent of 62·5, 125, 150, and 250 mg of phenoxymethylpenicillin in 5 ml are available.

When a dose less than or not a multiple of 5 ml is prescribed, the elixir may be diluted, as described under Elixirs (page 666), with Syrup. The diluted elixir must be freshly prepared and not more than one week's supply issued at a time.

Piperazine Citrate Elixir

Piperazine Citrate	..	..	187·5 g
Peppermint Spirit	..	..	5·0 ml
Green S and Tartrazine Solution			15·0 ml
Glycerol ..	..	..	..	100·0 ml
Syrup ..	..	..	..	500·0 ml
Water (see page 642)	..		to 1000·0 ml

Dissolve the piperazine citrate in part of the water and add the green S and tartrazine solution, the glycerol, the syrup, the peppermint spirit, and sufficient water to produce the required volume, and mix.

Standard

PRESENCE OF PIPERAZINE CITRATE. 1. To 1 ml add 5 ml of *dilute hydrochloric acid* and, with stirring, 1 ml of a 50 per cent w/v solution of *sodium nitrite* in water, cool in ice for 15 minutes and induce crystallisation; the crystalline precipitate, after washing with water and drying at 105°, melts at about 159°.

2. Warm 10 ml with *decolorising charcoal* and filter. The filtrate complies with the following tests:

(i) Boil a portion of the filtrate with an excess of *mercuric sulphate solution*, filter, boil the filtrate, and add 0·25 ml of *potassium permanganate solution*; the potassium permanganate solution is decolorised and a white precipitate is produced.

(ii) Acidify a portion of the filtrate with *dilute sulphuric acid*, add 0·25 ml of *potassium permanganate solution*, warm until the colour due to potassium permanganate is discharged, and add an excess of *bromine solution*; a white precipitate is produced either immediately or on cooling.

WEIGHT PER ML. At 20°, 1·24 g to 1·26 g.

CONTENT OF PIPERAZINE CITRATE. 15·1 to 17·8 per cent w/v, calculated as $C_{24}H_{46}N_6O_{14}$, determined by the method given for Piperazine Hydrate, page 384, about 1·5 g, accurately weighed, being used; each g of residue is equivalent to 0·3935 g of $C_{24}H_{46}N_6O_{14}$. Determine the weight per ml of the elixir and calculate the concentration of $C_{24}H_{46}N_6O_{14}$, weight in volume.

Storage. It should be stored in a cool place, protected from light.

Dose. ADULT. For threadworm infections: 15 millilitres daily. As an ascaricide: 30 millilitres as a single dose.

CHILD. For threadworm infections: 9 months to 2 years, 2·5 millilitres daily; 2 to 3 years, 5 millilitres daily; 4 to 6 years, 7·5 millilitres daily; 7 to 12 years, 10 millilitres daily. As an ascaricide: up to 30 millilitres, according to the age of the patient, as a single dose.

When a dose less than or not a multiple of 5 ml is prescribed, the elixir may be diluted, as described under Elixirs (page 666), with Syrup. The diluted elixir must be freshly prepared.

Piperazine Citrate Elixir contains in 5 ml the equivalent of about 750 mg of piperazine hydrate.

Promethazine Elixir

Promethazine Elixir is a solution of Promethazine Hydrochloride in a suitable, coloured, flavoured vehicle.

Standard

PRESENCE OF PROMETHAZINE. It complies with the thin-layer chromatographic test given in Appendix 5C, page 873.

CONTENT OF PROMETHAZINE HYDROCHLORIDE. 90·0 to 110·0 per cent of the prescribed or stated concentration, determined by the following method:
Dilute an accurately weighed quantity, equivalent to about 0·02 g of promethazine hydrochloride, to 100 ml with water.
To 10 ml of this solution add 20 ml of *palladous chloride reagent*, dilute to 50 ml with water, and measure the extinction of a 2-cm layer at the maximum at about 472 nm, using as a blank a solution prepared by diluting 20 ml of *palladous chloride reagent* to 50 ml with water.
For purposes of calculation, use a value of 110 for the E(1 per cent, 1 cm) of promethazine hydrochloride under these conditions.
Determine the weight per ml of the elixir and calculate the concentration of promethazine hydrochloride, weight in volume.

Labelling. The directions given under Elixirs (page 667) should be followed.

Storage. It should be stored in a cool place, protected from light.

Dose. Promethazine hydrochloride:
ADULT. 20 to 50 milligrams daily, in divided doses.

CHILD. For motion-sickness: up to 1 year, 5 to 10 milligrams daily; 1 to 5 years, 10 to 15 milligrams daily; 6 to 12 years, 15 to 25 milligrams daily.
Sedative dose: up to 1 year, 2·5 to 5 milligrams three times daily; 1 to 5 years, 5 to 10 milligrams three times daily.
Hypnotic dose: up to 1 year, 5 to 10 milligrams, as a single dose; 1 to 5 years, 15 to 20 milligrams, as a single dose.

When the strength of the elixir is not specified, a solution containing 5 mg of promethazine hydrochloride in 5 ml shall be supplied.

When a dose less than or not a multiple of 5 ml is prescribed, the elixir may be diluted, as described under Elixirs (page 666), with Syrup. The diluted elixir must be freshly prepared.

Propicillin Elixir

SYNONYM: Propicillin Syrup

Propicillin Elixir is a solution of Propicillin Potassium in a suitable, coloured, flavoured vehicle. It is prepared freshly by dissolving a powder consisting of the dry mixed ingredients in the specified volume of Water (see page 642).

Standard

PRESENCE OF PROPICILLIN. It complies with the thin-layer chromatographic test given in Appendix 5A, page 867.

CONTENT OF PROPICILLIN. 95·0 to 120·0 per cent of the prescribed or stated concentration, determined by the method given for Phenethecillin Elixir, page 674, *propicillin potassium A.S.* being used in place of phenethicillin potassium A.S.

STABILITY OF ELIXIR. Store at 15° ±1° for 7 days the portion of elixir reserved in the determination of the content of propicillin and then repeat the determination on the stored elixir.
The concentration of propicillin in the stored elixir is not less than 85 per cent of the concentration found in the freshly prepared elixir.

ACIDITY OF ELIXIR. pH, 5·5 to 6·5.

Labelling. The directions given under Elixirs (page 667) should be followed; the name on the label of the container of the dry powder is "Powder for Propicillin Elixir".

Storage. The elixir and the diluted elixir should be stored in a cool place and used within one week of preparation.

Dose. The equivalent of propicillin:
ADULT. 125 to 250 milligrams every four to six hours, depending on the severity of the infection.
CHILD. 62·5 to 125 milligrams every four to six hours, depending on age and on the severity of the infection.

When the strength of the elixir is not specified, a solution containing the equivalent of 62·5 mg of propicillin in 5 ml shall be supplied.

When a dose less than or not a multiple of 5 ml is prescribed, the elixir may be diluted, as described under Elixirs (page 666), with Syrup. The diluted elixir must be freshly prepared and not more than one week's supply issued at a time.

Streptomycin Elixir, Paediatric

SYNONYM: Streptomycin Mixture, Paediatric

Streptomycin Sulphate	31·4 g
Citric Acid	1·0 g
Methyl Hydroxybenzoate ..	1·3 g
Sodium Citrate	9·0 g
Sucrose	750·0 g
Amaranth Solution	2·0 ml
Purified Water, freshly boiled and cooled	to 1000·0 ml

Dissolve the methyl hydroxybenzoate in 400 ml of the water with the aid of gentle heat, dissolve the sodium citrate, the citric acid, and the sucrose in the hot solution, and cool. Dissolve the streptomycin sulphate in 100 ml of the cold water and mix the two solutions. Add the amaranth solution and sufficient of the water to produce the required volume and mix.

Standard
CONTENT OF STREPTOMYCIN. 18,800 to 24,000 Units per ml, determined by the following method:
Carry out a microbiological assay of streptomycin; a suggested method is given in Appendix 18, page 897.
The precision of any assay must be such that the fiducial limits of error (P = 0·95) are not less than 95 per cent and not more than 105 per cent of the estimated potency.
Calculate the upper and lower fiducial limits of the concentration of streptomycin in the elixir.
The upper fiducial limit of the estimated concentration of streptomycin is not less than 18,800 Units per ml and the lower fiducial limit is not more than 24,000 Units per ml.

Dose. CHILD. 5 millilitres.

When a dose less than or not a multiple of 5 ml is prescribed, the elixir may be diluted, as described under Elixirs (page 666), with Syrup. The diluted elixir must be freshly prepared.

Paediatric Streptomycin Elixir contains in 5 ml the equivalent of about 125 mg of streptomycin base.

Triclofos Elixir

SYNONYM: Triclofos Syrup

Triclofos Elixir is a solution of Triclofos Sodium in a suitable, coloured, flavoured vehicle.

Standard
CONTENT OF TRICLOFOS SODIUM. 90·0 to 110·0 per cent of the prescribed or stated concentration, calculated as $C_2H_3Cl_3NaO_4P$, determined by the following method:
To an accurately weighed quantity, equivalent to about 0·13 g of triclofos sodium, add 15 ml of water, 1 ml of 1N sodium hydroxide, and 15 ml of *solvent ether*, shake for 1 minute, and allow to separate; wash the ethereal layer with 1 ml of water and discard the ethereal solution.

To the combined aqueous layer and washings add 2·5 ml of *dilute sulphuric acid* and extract with four successive 10-ml portions of *amyl alcohol*, allowing each extract to stand until a good separation has been achieved; combine the amyl alcohol extracts, remove any further water which separates, and dilute to 50 ml with *amyl alcohol*.
Transfer 10 ml of this solution to a 20-ml glass ampoule, add 10 ml of *alcoholic potassium hydroxide solution*, seal the ampoule, mix well, and autoclave at 120° for 2 hours; allow the ampoule to cool, transfer the contents to a flask with the aid of 20 ml of *dilute nitric acid*, add 25 ml of 0·02N silver nitrate, and titrate with 0·02N ammonium thiocyanate, using *ferric ammonium sulphate solution* as indicator.
Repeat the titration, using 10 ml of *alcoholic potassium hydroxide solution* in place of the contents of the ampoule.
The difference between the two titrations represents the volume of 0·02N silver nitrate required by the sample; each ml of 0·02N silver nitrate is equivalent to 0·001676 g of $C_2H_3Cl_3NaO_4P$.
Determine the weight per ml of the elixir and calculate the concentration of $C_2H_3Cl_3NaO_4P$, weight in volume.

Labelling. The directions given under Elixirs (page 667) should be followed.

Storage. It should be stored in a cool place.

Dose. Triclofos sodium:
ADULT. Sedative dose: 500 milligrams once or twice daily.
Hypnotic dose: 1 to 2 grams at bedtime.
CHILD. Sedative dose: up to 1 year, 100 milligrams; 1 to 5 years, 250 milligrams; 6 to 12 years, 500 milligrams.
Hypnotic dose: up to 1 year, 100 to 250 milligrams; 1 to 5 years, 250 to 500 milligrams; 6 to 12 years, 500 to 1000 milligrams.

When the strength of the elixir is not specified, a solution containing 500 mg of triclofos sodium in 5 ml shall be supplied.

When a dose less than or not a multiple of 5 ml is prescribed, the elixir may be diluted, as described under Elixirs (page 666), with Syrup. The diluted elixir must be freshly prepared.

Trimeprazine Elixir, Paediatric

SYNONYM: Trimeprazine Syrup

Paediatric Trimeprazine Elixir is a solution containing 0·15 per cent w/v of Trimeprazine Tartrate in a suitable, coloured, flavoured vehicle.

Standard
PRESENCE OF TRIMEPRAZINE. It complies with the thin-layer chromatographic test given in Appendix 5C, page 873.
CONTENT OF TRIMEPRAZINE TARTRATE. 0·13 to 0·16 per cent w/v, determined by the following method:
Dilute 10 ml to 100 ml with water; to 25 ml of this solution add 10 ml of 0·1N hydrochloric acid, dilute to 100 ml with water, and measure the extinction of a 1-cm layer at the maximum at about 301 nm.
For purposes of calculation, use a value of 96 for the E(1 per cent, 1 cm) of trimeprazine tartrate.
Calculate the concentration of trimeprazine tartrate in the sample.

Labelling. The directions given under Elixirs (page 667) should be followed.

Storage. It should be protected from light.

Dose. Trimeprazine tartrate:
CHILD. For the relief of pruritus: 2 months to

1 year, 5 to 7·5 milligrams three times daily; 1 to 5 years, 10 milligrams in the morning and up to 25 milligrams at night.

When a dose less than or not a multiple of 5 ml is prescribed, the elixir may be diluted, as described under Elixirs (page 666), with Syrup. The diluted elixir must be freshly prepared.

Paediatric Trimeprazine Elixir contains in 5 ml 7·5 mg of trimeprazine tartrate.

Trimeprazine Elixir, Paediatric, Strong

SYNONYM: Strong Trimeprazine Syrup

Strong Paediatric Trimeprazine Elixir is a solution containing 0·6 per cent w/v of Trimeprazine Tartrate in a suitable, coloured, flavoured vehicle.

Standard
PRESENCE OF TRIMEPRAZINE. It complies with the thin-layer chromatographic test given in Appendix 5C, page 873.

CONTENT OF TRIMEPRAZINE TARTRATE. 0·57 to 0·63 per cent w/v, determined by the method for Paediatric Trimeprazine Elixir, 5 ml being used and diluted to 200 ml for the first dilution.

Labelling. The directions given under Elixirs (page 667) should be followed.

Storage. It should be protected from light.

Dose. Trimeprazine tartrate:
CHILD. For pre-operative medication, 2 to 5 milligrams per kilogram body-weight.

Strong Paediatric Trimeprazine Elixir contains in 5 ml about 30 mg of trimeprazine tartrate.

EMULSIFYING WAXES

Emulsifying Waxes are wax-like solids with emulsifying properties. They are chiefly used in the preparation of ointments and creams. They include Emulsifying Wax B.P. (anionic), Cetomacrogol Emulsifying Wax B.P. (non-ionic), and Cetrimide Emulsifying Wax (cationic).

Cetrimide Emulsifying Wax

SYNONYM: Cationic Emulsifying Wax

Cetrimide	100 g
Cetostearyl Alcohol	900 g

Melt the cetostearyl alcohol on a water-bath, add the cetrimide, and stir until cold.

Standard
CONTENT OF CETRIMIDE. 8·8 to 10·5 per cent, calculated as $C_{17}H_{38}BrN$, determined by the method for Cetrimide Cream (page 657), about 0·1 g, accurately weighed, being used.

EMULSIONS

An emulsion consists of two liquid phases, one of which is finely subdivided and dispersed in the other, the system being stabilised by the presence of an emulsifying agent. In pharmaceutical practice, the term "emulsion" should be restricted to oil-in-water preparations intended for internal use.

The quantity of emulsifying agent stated in the formulae in the individual monographs is suitable for the preparation of emulsions by hand in a mortar. If emulsification is effected by mechanical means, the quantity of the emulsifying agent may be reduced at the discretion of the manufacturer, provided that the concentrations of the other ingredients are not changed and the viscosity of the resulting emulsion is the same.

Containers. Emulsions should be supplied in wide-mouthed bottles.

Labelling. A direction to shake the bottle should be given on the label.

Liquid Paraffin Emulsion

Liquid Paraffin	500·0 ml
Saccharin Sodium	0·05 g
Vanillin	0·5 g
Methylcellulose 20	20·0 g
Chloroform	2·5 ml
Benzoic Acid Solution	20·0 ml
Water (see page 642) ..	to 1000·0 ml

Mix the methylcellulose with 200 ml of boiling water, allow to stand for 2 hours with constant stirring, add sufficient water to produce 350 ml, and allow to stand for 16 hours. Alternatively, mix the methylcellulose with 120 ml of boiling water and, when the powder is thoroughly hydrated, add sufficient water in the form of ice to produce 350 ml, and stir until homogeneous.

Dissolve the vanillin in a mixture of the chloroform and the benzoic acid solution, and add, with vigorous stirring for 5 minutes, to the methylcellulose dispersion.

Add the saccharin sodium dissolved in water and sufficient water to produce 500 ml, and mix; add the liquid paraffin, with constant stirring, and pass through a homogeniser.

Standard
CONTENT OF LIQUID PARAFFIN. 44·0 to 49·0 per cent w/w, determined by the following method:
To about 5 g, accurately weighed, add 10 ml of water, extract with two successive portions, each a mixture of 10 ml of *alcohol (95 per cent)*, 15 ml of *light petroleum (boiling-range, 40° to 60°)*, and 15 ml of *solvent ether*, and then with a mixture of 15 ml each of *light petroleum (boiling-range, 40° to 60°)* and *solvent ether*.
Wash the combined extracts with 15 ml of 0·5N sodium hydroxide, followed by 15 ml of water, evaporate off the solvent, add 5 ml of *acetone*, and again evaporate; repeat the addition and evaporation of *acetone* until the residue is free from water, dry at 105° for 15 minutes, and weigh.

Containers; Labelling. The directions given under Emulsions (page 678) should be followed.

Dose. 10 to 30 millilitres.

Liquid Paraffin and Magnesium Hydroxide Emulsion

SYNONYM: Mixture of Magnesium Hydroxide and Liquid Paraffin

Liquid Paraffin	250 ml
Magnesium Hydroxide Mixture	700 ml
Chloroform Spirit	50 ml

Mix the chloroform spirit with the magnesium hydroxide mixture, add to the liquid paraffin, and pass through a homogeniser.

Standard
CONTENT OF MAGNESIUM HYDROXIDE. 4·9 to 6·7 per cent w/w, calculated as $Mg(OH)_2$, determined by the following method:
Dilute about 4 g, accurately weighed, with 50 ml of water, shake with 25 ml of 0·5N hydrochloric acid, and titrate the excess of acid with 0·5N sodium hydroxide, using *methyl orange solution* as indicator; each ml of 0·5N hydrochloric acid is equivalent to 0·01458 g of $Mg(OH)_2$.

CONTENT OF LIQUID PARAFFIN. 19·7 to 24·0 per cent w/w, determined by the following method:
Extract the neutralised liquid obtained in the determination of magnesium hydroxide with three successive 25-ml portions of a mixture of equal volumes of *light petroleum (boiling-range, 40° to 60°)* and *solvent ether*.
Wash the combined extracts with two successive 10-ml portions of water, discard the washings, and evaporate off the solvent; add 5 ml of *acetone* and again evaporate; repeat the addition and evaporation of acetone until the residue is free from water, dry at 105° for 15 minutes, and weigh.

Containers; Labelling. The directions given under Emulsions (page 678) should be followed.

Dose. 5 to 20 millilitres.

Liquid Paraffin and Phenolphthalein Emulsion

SYNONYM: Compound Liquid Paraffin Emulsion

Phenolphthalein, microcrystalline	3 g
Liquid Paraffin Emulsion ..	to 1000 ml

Triturate the phenolphthalein with the liquid paraffin emulsion.

It is essential to use phenolphthalein in which not more than an occasional particle has a diameter greater than 15 μm; larger particles tend to sediment in this emulsion on storage and may prove difficult to redisperse uniformly by shaking the product. If a suitable microcrystalline grade is not obtainable, it may be prepared in small batches from ordinary grades by the following method:

Dissolve the phenolphthalein, with the aid of gentle heat if necessary, in sufficient alcohol (95 per cent) to give a 5 per cent solution. Stir, by means of a high-speed stirrer, 25 times this volume of water in a suitable container, add slowly down the vortex the alcoholic phenolphthalein solution, and continue to stir for 5 minutes.

It is essential that an efficient stirrer is used in order to obtain particles of sufficiently small size.

Set the suspension aside for 1½ to 2 hours, collect the precipitated phenolphthalein on a suitable filter, such as a Whatman No. 42, and dry the phenolphthalein to constant weight at 80°. As phenolphthalein is slightly soluble in the diluted alcohol, a sufficient excess of phenolphthalein should be used and the quantity required for preparing the emulsion should be weighed from the final dry powder.

Standard
CONTENT OF LIQUID PARAFFIN. 44·0 to 49·0 per cent w/w, determined by the method for Liquid Paraffin Emulsion.

CONTENT OF PHENOLPHTHALEIN. 0·28 to 0·35 per cent w/w, determined by the following method:
Mix about 3 g, accurately weighed, with sufficient *Filtercel* (1 to 2 g) to form a stiff paste, add, in small portions, 20 ml of *alcohol (95 per cent)*, stirring to maintain a uniform paste, centrifuge, decant the supernatant liquid, and wash the residue by centrifuging with two successive 20-ml portions of *alcohol (95 per cent)*.
Combine the supernatant liquid and washings and dilute to 100 ml with *alcohol (95 per cent)*; evaporate 5 ml of this solution to dryness on a water-bath, dissolve the residue in *glycine buffer solution*, dilute to 100 ml with the buffer solution, and measure the extinction of a 1-cm layer at the maximum at about 555 nm, completing the measurement within 10 minutes of adding the first quantity of buffer solution to the residue.
For purposes of calculation, use a value of 1055 for the E(1 per cent, 1 cm) of phenolphthalein.
Calculate the percentage of phenolphthalein in the sample.

Containers; Labelling. The directions given under Emulsions (page 678) should be followed.

Dose. 5 to 20 millilitres.

Liquid Paraffin Emulsion with Cascara

Cascara Elixir	62·5 ml	
Liquid Paraffin Emulsion	to 1000·0 ml	

Standard
CONTENT OF LIQUID PARAFFIN. 41·1 to 46·1 per cent w/w, determined by the method for Liquid Paraffin Emulsion.

Containers; Labelling. The directions given under Emulsions (page 678) should be followed.

Dose. 10 to 30 millilitres.

Peppermint Emulsion, Concentrated

Peppermint Oil	20 ml
Quillaia Liquid Extract	1 ml
Chloroform Water, Double-strength..	500 ml

Purified Water, freshly boiled and
cooled .. .. to 1000 ml

Shake the peppermint oil with the quillaia liquid extract. Add gradually the double-strength chloroform water and sufficient of the purified water to produce the required volume, shaking well after each addition.

Containers. The general direction to supply emulsions in wide-mouthed bottles does not apply to Concentrated Peppermint Emulsion.

Labelling. The directions given under Emulsions (page 678) should be followed.

Dose. 0·25 to 1 millilitre

When diluted with thirty-nine times its volume of freshly boiled and cooled Purified Water, a preparation equivalent in strength to Peppermint Water B.P. is produced.

ENEMAS

Enemas are aqueous or oily solutions or suspensions for rectal administration. Any solid substances or oils contained in them should be uniformly dispersed.

Enemas are given for their anthelmintic, anti-inflammatory, nutritive, purgative, or sedative effects, or for X-ray examination of the lower bowel.

Large-volume enemas should be warmed to body temperature before administration.

Containers. Enemas should be supplied in coloured fluted glass bottles or in single-use plastic packs fitted with a rectal nozzle.

Paraldehyde Enema

Paraldehyde	100 ml	
Sodium Chloride Solution ..	to 1000 ml	

It must be freshly prepared.

Dose. 5 millilitres per kilogram body-weight, to a maximum of 300 millilitres, by rectal injection.

Paraldehyde Enema contains, in 5 ml, 0·5 ml of paraldehyde.

Phosphates Enema

SYNONYM: Sodium Phosphates Enema

Formula A

Sodium Acid Phosphate ..	160 g	
Sodium Phosphate	60 g	
Purified Water, freshly boiled and cooled	to 1000 ml	

A suitable preservative may be included.

Formula B

Sodium Acid Phosphate.. ..	100 g	
Sodium Phosphate	80 g	
Purified Water, freshly boiled and cooled	to 1000 ml	

A suitable preservative may be included.

Standard for formula A
PRESENCE OF SODIUM AND OF PHOSPHATE. It gives the reactions characteristic of sodium and of phosphates.

CONTENT OF SODIUM ACID PHOSPHATE. 15·2 to 16·8 per cent w/v, calculated as $NaH_2PO_4,2H_2O$, determined by the following method:
To 20 ml add 80 ml of water and 25 g of *sodium chloride* and titrate with 0·5N sodium hydroxide, using *phenolphthalein solution* as indicator; each ml of 0·5N sodium hydroxide is equivalent to 0·07800 g of $NaH_2PO_4,2H_2O$.

CONTENT OF SODIUM PHOSPHATE. 5·6 to 6·4 per cent w/v, calculated as $Na_2HPO_4,12H_2O$, determined by the following method:
Titrate 50 ml with 0·5N hydrochloric acid, using 2 ml of a mixture of 4 parts of *bromocresol green solution* and 1 part of *methyl red solution* as indicator, and titrating to the colour indicative of pH 4·4; each ml of 0·5N hydrochloric acid is equivalent to 0·1790 g of $Na_2HPO_4,12H_2O$.

Standard for formula B
PRESENCE OF SODIUM AND OF PHOSPHATE. It gives the reactions characteristic of sodium and of phosphates.

CONTENT OF SODIUM ACID PHOSPHATE. 9·5 to 10·5 per cent w/v, calculated as $NaH_2PO_4,2H_2O$, determined by the method for formula A.

CONTENT OF SODIUM PHOSPHATE. 7·5 to 8·5 per cent w/v, calculated as $Na_2HPO_4,12H_2O$, determined by the method for formula A.

Containers. Both enemas should be supplied in a suitable disposable plastic pack fitted with a rectal nozzle.

Dose. *Formula A*: 100 millilitres; *formula B*: 128 millilitres.

The prescription or order should state whether formula A or formula B is required.

Prednisolone Enema

SYNONYM: Prednisolone Sodium Phosphate Enema

Prednisolone Enema is an aqueous solution of Prednisolone Sodium Phosphate in a suitable buffered vehicle. It may contain stabilising agents and a preservative. The solution is adjusted to pH 7·0 to 7·5.

This preparation is required to be retained in the colon and the vehicle must be so formulated as to ensure that this requirement is fulfilled.

Standard
PRESENCE OF PREDNISOLONE SODIUM PHOSPHATE. Evaporate 5 ml to dryness on a water-bath, cool, and to the residue add 0·5 ml of *sulphuric acid*; a deep red colour is produced.

ACIDITY OR ALKALINITY. pH, 5·5 to 7·5.

CONTENT OF PREDNISOLONE. 90·0 to 115·0 per cent of the strength stated on the label, determined by the following method:

Dilute an accurately measured volume, equivalent to about 0·01 g of prednisolone, to 100 ml with water; to 25 ml of this solution add 2·5 g of *sodium chloride* and 1 ml of *hydrochloric acid*, extract with three successive 25-ml portions of *chloroform*, washing each extract with the same 1 ml of 0·1N hydrochloric acid, and discard the extracts.

Extract the combined aqueous liquid and washing with two successive 10-ml portions of *extracted tri-n-butyl phosphate* and dilute the combined extracts to 25 ml with *methyl alcohol*.

To 2 ml of this solution add 10 ml of *isoniazid solution*, heat in a stoppered tube at 50° for 3 hours, protecting the solution from light, cool, and measure the extinction of a 1-cm layer at the maximum at about 405 nm, using as the blank a solution prepared in the same manner but omitting the sample.

Repeat the procedure using 25 ml of a solution of *prednisolone sodium phosphate A.S.*, containing the equivalent of 0·01 per cent w/v of prednisolone, in place of the sample solution.

From the two extinctions calculate the concentration of prednisolone in the enema.

Containers. It should be supplied in a suitable disposable plastic pack fitted with a rectal nozzle.

Storage. It should be stored at a temperature not exceeding 25°, protected from light. Under these conditions, it may be expected to retain its potency for at least two years.

Dose. The equivalent of prednisolone, 20 milligrams once or twice daily as a retention enema.

A solution containing the equivalent of 20 mg of prednisolone in 100 ml is available.

EXTRACTS

Extracts are concentrated products containing the active principles of crude drugs.

Liquid extracts are prepared by maceration or percolation with suitable solvents, followed by concentration, and are usually of such a strength that one part by volume of the product is equivalent to one part by weight of the crude drug. If, however, the active principle is of a potent nature and permits of an assay, the liquid extract is adjusted to a definite strength.

Dry extracts are prepared by evaporating the extractive from the crude drug to dryness, usually under reduced pressure. If the active principle is of a potent nature and permits of an assay, the dried extractive is adjusted to a definite strength by dilution with an inert diluent. The strength of the adjusted dry extract bears no relation to the content of active principle in the crude drug, but is determined by the dose, its strength being so adjusted that the maximum dose is not less than 60 milligrams. Lactose and starch are suitable diluents for most dried extractives; if the dried extractive is deliquescent, however, an absorbent diluent, such as calcium phosphate, is used.

Soft extracts are prepared by evaporating the extractive from the crude drug until a soft mass is obtained.

Preparation of extracts. Extracts that are the subject of the following monographs are prepared on a small scale by the methods described in the specific monographs. When extracts are manufactured in larger quantities, the same method, appropriately scaled up, is used; for certain liquid extracts the following alternative method is permitted: the crude powdered drug is exhausted by percolating with a suitable solvent, the solvent is removed by evaporating the percolate to the consistence of a soft extract, and the extractive is subsequently mixed with an appropriate volume of a suitable mixture of alcohol and water to yield a product that complies with the standard given in the specific monograph.

Storage. Deliquescent dry and soft extracts should be stored in airtight containers.

Belladonna Liquid Extract

Small-scale preparation

Belladonna Root, in moderately
   coarse powder ..   ..   ..   1000 g
Alcohol (80 per cent)   a sufficient quantity

Exhaust the belladonna root with the alcohol by percolation and evaporate the percolate under reduced pressure to the consistence of a soft extract. Determine the proportion of total alkaloids in the soft extract and dissolve it in sufficient of the alcohol to produce an extract of the required strength; allow the extract to stand for not less than twelve hours and filter, if necessary.

Manufacture. Prepare the extract by the above method, appropriately scaled up, or by the alternative method described under Extracts (above).

Standard
WEIGHT PER ML. At 20°, 0·95 g to 1·02 g.

ALCOHOL CONTENT. 48 to 55 per cent v/v of ethyl alcohol, determined by the method given in Appendix 10, page 888.

CONTENT OF TOTAL ALKALOIDS. 0·70 to 0·80 per cent w/v, calculated as hyoscyamine, $C_{17}H_{23}NO_3$, determined by the following method:
To 10 ml add 10 ml of water and 10 ml of 0·2N sulphuric acid and extract with successive 10-ml portions of *chloroform* until an extract is obtained which is colourless; wash the combined extracts with 10 ml of 0·2N sulphuric acid, discard the extracts, add the washings to the aqueous solution, and continue by the method for Belladonna Root, page 43, beginning with the words "neutralise to *litmus paper* with *dilute ammonia solution* . . .".

Cocillana Liquid Extract

Small-scale preparation

Cocillana, in moderately coarse
   powder ..   ..   1000 g
Alcohol (60 per cent)   ..   .. to 1000 ml

Exhaust the cocillana with the alcohol by percolation, reserving the first 850 ml of percolate; evaporate the subsequent percolate to the consistence of a soft extract, dissolve it in the reserved portion, and add sufficient of the alcohol to produce 1000 ml.

Manufacture. Prepare the extract by the above method, appropriately scaled up, or by the alternative method described under Extracts (above).

Standard
WEIGHT PER ML. At 20°, 0·92 g to 0·96 g.

ALCOHOL CONTENT. 52 to 57 per cent v/v of ethyl alcohol, determined by the method given in Appendix 10, page 888.

TOTAL SOLIDS. 2·5 to 6·0 per cent w/v, determined on 5 g.

Dose. 0·5 to 1 millilitre.

Hamamelis Dry Extract

SYNONYM: Hamamelis Extract

Small-scale preparation

Hamamelis, in moderately coarse
   powder ..   ..   1000 g
Alcohol (45 per cent)   a sufficient quantity

Exhaust the hamamelis with the alcohol by percolation, remove the alcohol by evaporating to dryness at a low temperature, and reduce the residue to a fine powder.

Manufacture. Prepare the extract by the above method, appropriately scaled up.

In making this preparation the alcohol (45 per cent) may be replaced by Industrial Methylated Spirit diluted so as to be of equivalent alcoholic strength, provided that the law and the statutory regulations governing the use of industrial methylated spirit are observed.

Standard
ALCOHOL (45 PER CENT)-INSOLUBLE MATTER. Not more than 4·0 per cent, determined by the following method: Shake about 2 g, accurately weighed, with 50 ml of *alcohol (45 per cent)*, filter, wash the residue with *alcohol (45 per cent)* until all the soluble matter has been extracted, and dry the residue to constant weight at 105°.

Storage. It should be stored in airtight containers, in a cool place.

Hamamelis Liquid Extract

Small-scale preparation

Hamamelis, in moderately coarse
   powder ..   ..   1000 g
Alcohol (45 per cent)   ..   .. to 1000 ml

Exhaust the hamamelis with the alcohol by percolation, reserving the first 850 ml of percolate; evaporate the subsequent percolate to the consistence of a soft extract, dissolve it in the reserved portion, add sufficient of the alcohol to produce 1000 ml, allow to stand for not less than twelve hours, and filter.

Manufacture. Prepare the extract by the above method, appropriately scaled up, or by the alternative method described under Extracts (page 681).

Standard

WEIGHT PER ML. At 20°, 1·015 g to 1·045 g.

ALCOHOL CONTENT. 32 to 40 per cent v/v, determined by the method given in Appendix 10, page 888.

TOTAL SOLIDS. 18 to 25 per cent w/v, determined on 1 g.

Hyoscyamus Dry Extract

Small-scale preparation

Hyoscyamus, in moderately coarse powder	1000 g
Hyoscyamus, in fine powder, dried at 80°	of each a sufficient
Alcohol (70 per cent) ..	quantity

Percolate the hyoscyamus in moderately coarse powder with the alcohol until 4000 ml of percolate has been obtained. Determine the proportion of total solids in the percolate by evaporating 20 ml, drying the residue at 80°, and weighing. Determine also the proportion of alkaloids in the percolate by the assay described under Hyoscyamus Liquid Extract, using 100 ml, and the proportion of alkaloids present in the hyoscyamus in fine powder.

From the results of the three determinations, calculate the amount of hyoscyamus in fine powder that must be added to the percolate to produce a dry extract containing 0·3 per cent of alkaloids, calculated as hyoscyamine.

Add to the percolate a somewhat smaller amount of the hyoscyamus in fine powder than calculation has shown to be necessary, remove the alcohol by evaporating to dryness under reduced pressure at a temperature not exceeding 60°, and dry in a current of air at 80°.

Powder the residue, add the final necessary amount of hyoscyamus in fine powder, and triturate in a dry, slightly warmed mortar until thoroughly mixed.

Pass the powdered extract through a No. 710 sieve and mix.

Manufacture. Prepare the extract by the above method, appropriately scaled up.

In making this preparation, the alcohol (70 per cent) may be replaced by Industrial Methylated Spirit diluted so as to be of equivalent alcoholic strength, provided that the law and the statutory regulations governing the use of industrial methylated spirit are observed.

Standard

CONTENT OF TOTAL ALKALOIDS. 0·27 to 0·33 per cent, calculated as hyoscyamine, $C_{17}H_{23}NO_3$, determined by the following method:

Mix about 10 g, accurately weighed, with 50 ml of *alcohol (70 per cent)*, warm on a water-bath and allow to stand for 30 minutes with frequent shaking; transfer the mixture to a percolator and percolate slowly with successive portions of *alcohol (70 per cent)* until complete extraction of the alkaloids is effected. Evaporate the percolate at as low a temperature as possible to a volume of about 10 ml, transfer to a separating funnel with the aid of 40 ml of *chloroform*, add a mixture of 10 ml of water and 5 ml of *dilute ammonia solution*, shake well, allow to separate, and

filter the chloroform layer into a second separating funnel through a pledget of cotton wool previously moistened with *chloroform*; extract the aqueous solution in the first separator with successive 25-ml portions of *chloroform* until complete extraction of the alkaloids is effected, filtering each extract as before. Extract the combined chloroform extracts with successive portions of a mixture of 3 volumes of 0·2N sulphuric acid and 1 volume of *alcohol (95 per cent)* until complete extraction of the alkaloids is effected, and continue by the method for Belladonna Root, page 43, beginning with the words "wash the combined acid extractions . . .".

Storage. It should be stored in small, wide-mouthed, airtight containers, in a cool place.

Dose. 15 to 60 milligrams.

Hyoscyamus Dry Extract contains, in 60 mg, 0·18 mg of total alkaloids, calculated as hyoscyamine.

Hyoscyamus Liquid Extract

Small-scale preparation

Hyoscyamus, in moderately coarse powder	1000 g
Alcohol (70 per cent)	a sufficient quantity

Exhaust the hyoscyamus by percolation with the alcohol, reserving the first 850 ml of the percolate. Remove the alcohol from the remainder of the percolate by evaporation under reduced pressure at a temperature not exceeding 60°, evaporate the residue to a soft extract at a temperature not exceeding 60°, and dissolve this in the reserved portion.

Determine the proportion of alkaloids in the liquid thus obtained by the assay described below. To the remainder of the liquid add sufficient alcohol (70 per cent) to produce a hyoscyamus liquid extract of the required strength.

Allow to stand for not less than twenty-four hours; filter if necessary.

Manufacture. Prepare the extract by the above method, appropriately scaled up, or by the alternative method described under Extracts (page 681).

Standard

ALCOHOL CONTENT. 50 to 60 per cent v/v of ethyl alcohol, determined by the method given in Appendix 10, page 888.

CONTENT OF TOTAL ALKALOIDS. 0·045 to 0·055 per cent w/v, calculated as hyoscyamine, $C_{17}H_{23}NO_3$, determined by the following method:

Evaporate 50 ml at as low a temperature as possible to a volume of about 10 ml and continue by the method for Hyoscyamus Dry Extract, beginning with the words "transfer to a separating funnel . . .".

Dose. 0·2 to 0·5 millilitre.

Hyoscyamus Liquid Extract contains, in 0·5 ml, 0·25 mg of total alkaloids, calculated as hyoscyamine.

Liquorice Extract

SYNONYM: Extractum Glycyrrhizae

Small-scale preparation

Liquorice, unpeeled, in coarse powder	1000 g
Chloroform Water	a sufficient quantity

Exhaust the liquorice with the chloroform

water by percolation, boil the percolate for 5 minutes, and allow to stand for not less than 12 hours; decant the clear liquid and filter the remainder; mix the two liquids and evaporate to the consistence of a soft extract.

Manufacture. Prepare the extract by the above method, appropriately scaled up.

Storage. It should be stored in a cool place.

Dose. 0·6 to 2 grams.

Malt Extract with Cod-liver Oil

SYNONYM: Extractum Malti cum Oleo Morrhuae

Malt Extract	..	..	..	900 g
Cod-liver Oil	..	..	..	100 g

Mix thoroughly, with the aid of gentle heat. The extract may be flavoured.

Standard
CONTENT OF COD-LIVER OIL. 9·3 to 10·7 per cent w/w, determined by the following method:
Mix about 2·5 g, accurately weighed, with 8 ml of warm water and extract with a mixture of 5 ml of *alcohol (95 per cent)* and 15 ml of *solvent ether*; add to the aqueous solution 5 ml of *solvent ether* and, without shaking, remove the ethereal solution and add to the extract; add to the aqueous solution 3 ml of *alcohol (95 per cent)* and extract with two successive 15-ml portions of a mixture of equal volumes of *light petroleum (boiling-range, 40° to 60°)* and *solvent ether*.
Wash the combined extracts with three successive 3-ml portions of water, evaporate off the solvent, and add successive 2-ml portions of *acetone*, evaporating off the acetone between each addition, until the residue is clear; cool and weigh the residue of cod-liver oil.

ACID VALUE. Of the oil obtained in the determination of cod-liver oil, not more than 10.

CONTENT OF VITAMIN-A ACTIVITY. Not less than 60 Units per g, determined by the following method:
Mix about 2 g, accurately weighed, with 25 ml of warm water and cool; add 10 ml of *alcohol (95 per cent)*, 10 ml of 0·5N alcoholic potassium hydroxide, and 25 ml of *anaesthetic ether*, and shake vigorously; add 15 ml of *light petroleum (boiling-range, 40° to 60°)*, swirl gently, allow to separate, and reserve the ethereal extract.
Extract the aqueous solution with two successive portions, each of a mixture of 25 ml of *anaesthetic ether* and 15 ml of *light petroleum (boiling-range, 40° to 60°)*, wash the combined extracts with three successive 10-ml portions of water, filter, and evaporate off the solvent in a stream of *oxygen-free nitrogen*.
Add successive 2-ml portions of *dry acetone*, evaporating off the acetone in a stream of *oxygen-free nitrogen* between each addition, until all the water has been removed; add 15 ml of freshly prepared 0·5N alcoholic potassium hydroxide and 30 mg of *hydroquinone*, boil for 15 minutes, and continue by the method of Appendix XVIIA of the British Pharmacopoeia for the assay of vitamin A, beginning with the words "cool rapidly, and add 30 ml of water . . .", in the section headed "Other Vitamin A".

Storage. It should be stored in well-filled airtight containers, protected from light, in a cool place.

Dose. 10 to 30 millilitres daily.

Malt Extract with Cod-liver Oil contains in 30 ml about 4·5 ml of cod-liver oil.

Malt Extract with Halibut-liver Oil

SYNONYM: Extractum Malti cum Oleo Hippoglossi

Halibut-liver Oil	..	a sufficient quantity
Arachis Oil	..	a sufficient quantity
Malt Extract	.. .. ..	to 1000 g

Mix sufficient halibut-liver oil and arachis oil to give 25 ml of a vitamin-A solution of the appropriate strength and incorporate the mixture with sufficient malt extract to produce the required weight.

Standard
WEIGHT PER ML. At 20°, 1·38 g to 1·42 g.

CONTENT OF VITAMIN-A ACTIVITY. Not less than 60 Units per g, determined by the following method:
Mix about 2 g, accurately weighed, with 25 ml of warm water and cool; add 10 ml of *alcohol (95 per cent)*, 10 ml of 0·5N alcoholic potassium hydroxide, and 25 ml of *anaesthetic ether*, and shake vigorously; add 15 ml of *light petroleum (boiling-range, 40° to 60°)*, swirl gently, allow to separate, and reserve the ethereal extract.
Add to the aqueous solution 5 ml of *alcohol (95 per cent)* and repeat the extraction twice with 25 ml of *anaesthetic ether* and 15 ml of *light petroleum (boiling-range, 40° to 60°)*, as before; wash the combined extracts with 10 ml of water, evaporate off the solvent in a stream of *oxygen-free nitrogen*, add 5 ml of *dry acetone*, and evaporate again; add 15 ml of freshly prepared 0·5N alcoholic potassium hydroxide and 30 mg of *hydroquinone*, boil for 15 minutes, and continue by the method of Appendix XVIIA of the British Pharmacopoeia for the assay of vitamin A, beginning with the words "cool rapidly, and add 30 ml of water . . .", in the section headed "Other Vitamin A".

Storage. It should be stored in well-filled airtight containers, protected from light, in a cool place.

Dose. 5 to 30 millilitres daily.

Malt Extract with Halibut-liver Oil contains in 30 ml not less than 2500 Units of vitamin-A activity.

Quillaia Liquid Extract

Small-scale preparation

Quillaia, in moderately fine powder ..	..	..	..	1000 g
Alcohol (45 per cent)	..		..	to 1000 ml

Exhaust the quillaia with the alcohol by percolation, reserving the first 850 ml of percolate; evaporate the subsequent percolate to the consistence of a soft extract, dissolve it in the reserved portion, and add sufficient of the alcohol to produce 1000 ml; allow to stand for not less than twenty-four hours, and filter.

Manufacture. Prepare the extract by the above method, appropriately scaled up, or by the alternative method described under Extracts (page 681).

Standard
WEIGHT PER ML. At 20°, 1·02 g to 1·06 g.

ALCOHOL CONTENT. 28 to 34 per cent v/v of ethyl alcohol, determined by the method given in Appendix 10, page 888.

TOTAL SOLIDS. 20 to 30 per cent w/v, determined on 0·5 g.

Senega Liquid Extract

Small-scale preparation

Senega, in moderately coarse
  powder ..   ..   1000 g
Dilute Ammonia Solution a sufficient quantity
Alcohol (60 per cent)   ..   .. to 1000 ml

Exhaust the senega with the alcohol by percolation, reserving the first 800 ml of percolate; evaporate the subsequent percolate to
the consistence of a soft extract, dissolve it in
the reserved portion, and gradually add the
dilute ammonia solution until the product is
faintly alkaline; add sufficient of the alcohol
to produce 1000 ml, allow to stand for not
less than forty-eight hours, and filter.

Manufacture. Prepare the extract by the above
method, appropriately scaled up, or by the
alternative method described under Extracts
(page 681).

Standard
WEIGHT PER ML. At 20°, 1·03 g to 1·05 g.

ALCOHOL CONTENT. 38 to 42 per cent v/v of ethyl
alcohol, determined by the method given in Appendix
10, page 888.

TOTAL SOLIDS. 26 to 34 per cent w/v, determined on
0·5 g.

Dose. 0·3 to 1 millilitre.

Senna Liquid Extract

Small-scale preparation

Senna Fruit, crushed   ..   ..   1000 g
Coriander Oil   ..   ..   ..   6 ml
Alcohol (90 per cent)   ..   ..   250 ml
Chloroform Water   a sufficient quantity
Purified Water, freshly boiled and
  cooled   ..   ..   a sufficient quantity

Macerate the senna fruit in 5000 ml of the
chloroform water for eight hours, decant the
clear liquid, and strain; repeat the process
twice, using 2000 ml of the chloroform water
for each maceration. Lightly press the marc,
strain the expressed liquid, and mix it with
the previously decanted liquids. Heat the
liquid in a covered vessel for 3 minutes at
80°, allow to stand for twenty-four hours, and
filter.

Evaporate the filtrate to 750 ml under reduced
pressure at a temperature not exceeding 60°,
add the coriander oil dissolved in the alcohol
and sufficient of the water to produce 1000 ml,
allow to stand for not less than twenty-four
hours, and filter.

Manufacture. Prepare the extract by the
above method, appropriately scaled up.

Standard
WEIGHT PER ML. At 20°, 1·02 g to 1·09 g.

ALCOHOL CONTENT. 21 to 24 per cent v/v of ethyl
alcohol, determined by the method given in Appendix
10, page 888.

TOTAL SOLIDS. 17 to 25 per cent w/v, determined on 1 g.

Dose. 0·5 to 2 millilitres.

Squill Liquid Extract

Small-scale preparation

Squill, in coarse powder..   ..   1000 g
Alcohol (70 per cent)   ..   .. to 1000 ml

Exhaust the squill with the alcohol by percolation, reserving the first 850 ml of percolate; evaporate the subsequent percolate to
the consistence of a soft extract, dissolve it in
the reserved portion, add sufficient of the
alcohol to produce 1000 ml, and filter.

Manufacture. Prepare the extract by the above
method, appropriately scaled up, or by the
alternative method described under Extracts
(page 681).

Standard
WEIGHT PER ML. At 20°, 1·00 g to 1·14 g.

ALCOHOL CONTENT. 34 to 50 per cent v/v, of ethyl
alcohol, determined by the method given in Appendix
10, page 888.

TOTAL SOLIDS. 40 to 55 per cent w/v, determined on
0·5 g.

Dose. 0·06 to 0·2 millilitre.

EYE-DROPS

Eye-drops are sterile aqueous or oily solutions or suspensions for instillation into the
eye.

Aqueous eye-drops, unless in single-dose form, are prepared in a vehicle which is
bactericidal and fungicidal; for this purpose, phenylmercuric nitrate or acetate
(0·002 per cent), benzalkonium chloride (0·01 per cent), and chlorhexidine acetate
(0·01 per cent) are generally suitable, the choice being governed in certain circumstances by the compatibility of the antimicrobial substance with the other ingredients
and by the period of time during which the eye-drops are likely to be used. Benzal-

konium chloride is not suitable as a preservative for eye-drops containing local anaesthetics.

Single-dose forms consist of about 0·5 ml of the eye-drops in a flexible applicator pack enclosed in a sealed outer container; the applicator pack and its contents are sterile. The solution complies with the formula and standard given in the individual monograph except that the preservative is omitted.

It is known that some therapeutic agents and preservatives can be concentrated in soft, acrylic, hydrophilic contact lenses and that this may modify the intensity and/or duration of drug action and, in the case of preservatives, may lead to irritation. Where-ever possible, wearers of such lenses should remove them before administration of therapeutic preparations and if this is not practicable, single-dose units which do not contain preservatives are preferable. Wetting and storage solutions designed for use with hard contact lenses should never be used with hydrophilic lenses. The recom-mended procedure for maintenance of lens hygiene is heating in 0·9 per cent w/v sodium chloride solution, but storage solutions specially formulated for soft lenses are available.

When the eye-drops are dispensed for domiciliary use, the user should be warned of the need for hygiene to avoid contamination during use. In general, a container of eye-drops may be used for about one month for domiciliary purposes.

When the eye-drops are used in hospital wards, a separate container should be provided for each patient and, when both eyes are being treated, a separate container for each eye. They should be discarded not later than one week after first opening the container. In out-patient and casualty departments, opened containers should be discarded at the end of each day, but each patient who has undergone out-patient surgery should be treated with a separate supply of the drops. In operating theatres, single-dose containers should preferably be used, but if only multiple-dose contain-ers are available, a previously unopened container should be used for each patient.

Eye-drops of the British Pharmaceutical Codex are formulated for use in the conven-tional manner of instilling one or two drops into the conjunctival sac and they are not suitable for introduction into the anterior chamber of the eye during surgical procedures. Solutions for the latter purpose should likewise be sterile but should not contain any preservative.

Preparation of eye-drops. The apparatus used in the preparation of eye-drops and the containers must be thoroughly cleansed before use. The teats used on droppers must be cleansed, impregnated with the selected antimicrobial substance and any other preservative included in the eye-drops, and stored in the impregnating solution, as described for the pretreatment of rubber caps in Appendix 29, under "Rubber and Plastics" (page 925). It should be established by preliminary tests that rubber teats are compatible with the antimicrobial substance to be used; they should not yield a turbidity or precipitate when autoclaved in a solution of the selected antimicrobial substance after they have been subjected to this pretreatment.

Not more than 10 ml of solution should be supplied in each container. If more than 10 ml is dispensed at one time, the total quantity of solution should be distributed into an appropriate number of containers.

Unless otherwise indicated in the individual monographs, eye-drops of the British Pharmaceutical Codex are prepared by the following methods:

Method A. The medicament is dissolved in the aqueous vehicle containing one of the prescribed antimicrobial substances and any other preservative specified in the individual monograph and the solution is clarified by filtration, transferred to the final containers, which are then closed so as to exclude micro-organisms, and sterilised by autoclaving.

Method B. The medicament is dissolved in the aqueous vehicle containing one of the prescribed antimicrobial substances and any other preservative specified in the individual monograph and the solution is sterilised by filtration and transferred, by means of an aseptic technique, to sterile containers which are then closed so as to exclude micro-organisms.

Method C. The medicament is dissolved in the aqueous vehicle containing one of the prescribed antimicrobial substances and any other preservative specified in the individual monograph and the solution is clarified by filtration, transferred to the final containers which are then closed to exclude micro-organisms, and sterilised by maintaining at 98° to 100° for thirty minutes.

Eye-drops may be prepared by any other method provided that the final product is identical in appearance, quality, and composition with one prepared by the appropriate method described above or in the individual monograph.

Standard

STERILITY. Unless otherwise specified in the individual monograph, eye-drops comply with the test for sterility.

Containers. Eye-drops should be dispensed in amber-coloured fluted bottles of neutral or surface-treated glass complying with British Standard 1679:Part 5. These containers are fitted with a phenolic plastic screw cap which incorporates a neutral glass dropper tube fitted with a natural or synthetic rubber teat; alternatively, the complete dropper closure may be sterilised and supplied separately in a sealed package, the bottle being closed with a plain phenolic plastic screw cap fitted with a suitable liner. Applicator bottles made of a suitable plastic may also be used.

Rubber teats and bottles made of surface-treated glass should not be autoclaved more than once. Silicone rubber teats should be used in the presence of benzalkonium chloride unless the rubber teats have been shown to be suitable (as described under Preparation of Eye-drops, above).

The closure should be covered by a readily breakable seal unless the eye-drops have been prepared extemporaneously.

Labelling. The label on the container or the label or wrapper on the package, except when issued to the individual patient for domiciliary use, states:
(1) the name of the preparation and the concentration of the active ingredient if the strength of the eye-drops is permitted in the individual monograph to be varied; and
(2) the name and concentration of the antimicrobial substance used in the eye-drops.

Adrenaline Eye-drops, Neutral

Neutral Adrenaline Eye-drops consist of a sterile solution containing 1·0 per cent w/v of Adrenaline, with Sodium Metabisulphite, 8-hydroxyquinoline sulphate, and other adjuvants, in a borate buffer solution.

The pH of the solution is adjusted to 7·4 by the addition of sodium hydroxide.

The air in the container is replaced by nitrogen or other inert gas after filling.

Standard
It complies with the standard under Eye-drops, page 687, with the following additions:

PRESENCE OF ADRENALINE. To 0·05 ml add a 0·25 per cent w/v solution of *ferric chloride*; an emerald-green colour is produced which, on the gradual addition of *sodium bicarbonate solution*, changes first to blue and then to red.

ALKALINITY. pH, 7·2 to 7·6.

CONTENT OF ADRENALINE. 0·95 to 1·35 per cent w/v, calculated as $C_9H_{13}NO_3$, determined by the following method:
Dilute 0·5 ml to 100 ml with water; to 10 ml of this solution add 0·25 ml of *ferrous sulphate–citrate solution* and 1 ml of *aminoacetate buffer solution*, mix, allow to stand for 20 minutes, and measure the extinction of a 1-cm layer at the maximum at about 540 nm.
Calculate the concentration of adrenaline in the sample by reference to a calibration curve prepared using suitable quantities of a solution of *adrenaline acid tartrate* treated in a similar manner.

Containers; Labelling. The directions given under Eye-drops (page 687) should be followed.

Storage. It should be protected from light and stored in a cool place.

Amethocaine Eye-drops

Amethocaine Eye-drops consist of a sterile solution containing up to 1·0 per cent w/v of Amethocaine Hydrochloride, with 0·1 per cent w/v of Sodium Metabisulphite and 0·002 per cent w/v of Phenylmercuric Acetate or Nitrate, in Purified Water.
It is prepared by Method A, B, or C described under Eye-drops (page 687).

Standard
It complies with the standard under Eye-drops, page 687, with the following additions:

PRESENCE OF AMETHOCAINE. To a volume equivalent to about 0·01 g of amethocaine hydrochloride add 1 ml of a 5 per cent w/v solution of *sodium acetate* in water and 1 ml of a 25 per cent w/v solution of *ammonium thiocyanate* in water and mix; a white precipitate is produced which, after recrystallising from water and drying at 80°, melts at about 130°.

CONTENT OF AMETHOCAINE HYDROCHLORIDE. 90·0 to 110·0 per cent of the prescribed or stated concentration, calculated as $C_{15}H_{25}ClN_2O_2$, determined by the method given in Appendix 12, page 892; each ml of 0·01M sodium tetraphenylboron is equivalent to 0·003008 g of $C_{15}H_{25}ClN_2O_2$.

Containers. The directions given under Eye-drops (page 687) should be followed; this solution is adversely affected by alkali.

Labelling. The directions given under Eye-drops (page 687) should be followed.

Storage. It should be protected from light.

Note. When the strength of the eye-drops is not specified, a solution containing 0·25 per cent w/v of amethocaine hydrochloride shall be supplied.

Atropine Sulphate Eye-drops

Atropine Sulphate Eye-drops consist of a sterile solution containing up to 2·0 per cent w/v of Atropine Sulphate, with 0·002 per cent w/v of Phenylmercuric Acetate or Nitrate or 0·02 per cent v/v of Benzalkonium Chloride Solution, in Purified Water.
It is prepared by Method A, B, or C described under Eye-drops (page 687).

Standard
It complies with the standard under Eye-drops, page 687, with the following additions:

PRESENCE OF ATROPINE. To a volume equivalent to about 0·01 g of atropine sulphate add 0·5 ml of *trinitrophenol solution*; a yellow precipitate is produced which, after recrystallising from *dehydrated alcohol* and drying at 105°, melts at about 175°.

CONTENT OF ATROPINE SULPHATE. 90·0 to 110·0 per cent of the prescribed or stated concentration, calculated as $C_{34}H_{48}N_2O_{10}S,H_2O$, determined by the method given in Appendix 12, page 892; each ml of 0·01M sodium tetraphenylboron is equivalent to 0·003474 g of $C_{34}H_{48}N_2O_{10}S,H_2O$.

Containers. The directions given under Eye-drops (page 687) should be followed; this solution is adversely affected by alkali.

Labelling. The directions given under Eye-drops (page 687) should be followed.

Note. When the strength of the eye-drops is not specified, a solution containing 1·0 per cent w/v of atropine sulphate shall be supplied.

Betamethasone Eye-drops

SYNONYM: Betamethasone Sodium Phosphate Eye-drops

Betamethasone Eye-drops consist of a sterile solution containing Betamethasone Sodium Phosphate, with a suitable preservative and stabilising agent, in Purified Water.
It is prepared by Method B described under Eye-drops (page 687).

Standard
It complies with the standard under Eye-drops, page 687, with the following additions:

PRESENCE OF BETAMETHASONE. It complies with the thin-layer chromatographic test given in Appendix 5D, page 875.

CONTENT OF BETAMETHASONE SODIUM PHOSPHATE. 90·0 to 115·0 per cent of the prescribed or stated concentration, determined by the following method:
To an accurately measured volume, equivalent to about 2 mg of betamethasone sodium phosphate, add 20 ml of water, 2·5 g of *sodium chloride*, and 0·5 ml of *hydrochloric acid*, extract with three successive 25-ml portions of *chloroform*, washing each extract with the same 1 ml of 0·1N hydrochloric acid, and discard the extracts.
Extract the combined aqueous liquid and washing with two successive 10-ml portions of *extracted tri-n-butyl phosphate*, combine the extracts, and discard any further aqueous phase which separates.
Extract the organic liquid with successive 25- and 20-ml portions of a solution containing 10 per cent w/v of *sodium chloride* and 1·0 per cent w/v of *anhydrous sodium phosphate* in water, filter the combined extracts through a pledget of cotton wool, wash the filter with

3 ml of the sodium chloride–sodium phosphate solution, dilute the combined filtrate and washings to 100 ml with the sodium chloride–sodium phosphate solution, and measure the extinction of a 1-cm layer at the maximum at about 241 nm using the sodium chloride–sodium phosphate solution as the blank.

Repeat the procedure using 2 ml of water in place of the sample.

The difference between the two extinctions represents the extinction due to the sample.

For the purposes of calculation use a value of 297 for the E(1 per cent, 1 cm) of betamethasone sodium phosphate.

Calculate the percentage of betamethasone sodium phosphate in the eye-drops.

Containers; Labelling. The directions given under Eye-drops (page 687) should be followed.

Storage. It should be stored in a cool place, protected from light.

Note. When the strength of the eye-drops is not specified, a solution containing 0·1 per cent w/v of betamethasone sodium phosphate shall be supplied.

Carbachol Eye-drops

Carbachol Eye-drops consist of a sterile solution containing up to 3·0 per cent w/v of Carbachol, with 0·02 per cent v/v of Benzalkonium Chloride Solution, in Purified Water.

It is prepared by Method A, B, or C described under Eye-drops (page 687).

Standard
It complies with the standard under Eye-drops, page 687, with the following additions:

PRESENCE OF CARBACHOL. To a volume equivalent to about 0·01 g of carbachol add 1 ml of *gold chloride solution*; a yellow precipitate is produced which, after recrystallising from water and drying at 105°, melts at about 185°.

CONTENT OF CARBACHOL. 90·0 to 110·0 per cent of the prescribed or stated concentration, calculated as $C_6H_{15}ClN_2O_2$, determined by the method given in Appendix 12, page 892; each ml of 0·01M sodium tetraphenylboron is equivalent to 0·001826 g of $C_6H_{15}ClN_2O_2$.

Containers. The directions given under Eye-drops (page 687) should be followed; this solution is adversely affected by alkali.

Labelling. The directions given under Eye-drops (page 687) should be followed.

Note. The strength of the eye-drops should be specified by the prescriber.

Chloramphenicol Eye-drops

Chloramphenicol ..	..	..	0·5 g
Phenylmercuric Acetate or Nitrate			0·002 g
Borax ..	..	.. ..	0·3 g
Boric Acid	..	.. ..	1·5 g
Purified Water ..	..	..	to 100 ml

Dissolve the boric acid, the borax, and the phenylmercuric salt in 90 ml of the purified water with the aid of heat; adjust the temperature of the solution to 60°, add the chloramphenicol, and maintain the temperature at 60° until the chloramphenicol is dissolved. Cool the solution, add sufficient purified water to produce the required volume, and mix. Then, either (i) sterilise the solution

by filtration, and transfer by means of an aseptic technique to sterile containers, which are then closed so as to exclude micro-organisms (Method B) or (ii) clarify the solution by filtration, transfer it to the final containers, which are then closed to exclude micro-organisms, and sterilise it by maintaining at 98° to 100° for thirty minutes (Method C).

The eye-drops should not be issued for use later than three months from the date of preparation, when stored at room temperature in an unopened container.

The preparation is more stable at lower temperatures and provided that it is kept in an unopened container and maintained at a temperature of 2° to 8°, it may be stored for up to seventeen months from the date of preparation.

These storage times assume that the eye-drops will not usually be used for more than four weeks after the date of issue for use, so that the total times do not exceed those specified in the storage statement given below.

Alternatively, using an aseptic technique, dissolve a sterile dry powder, consisting of the chloramphenicol, the boric acid, the borax, and the phenylmercuric salt, in sterile Purified Water in the final sterile container. The eye-drops must be freshly prepared when this alternative method is used.

Standard
It complies with the standard under Eye-drops, page 687, with the following additions:

STERILITY. If the eye-drops are prepared by the alternative method described above, the solution is not required to comply with the test for sterility.

2-AMINO-1-*p*-NITROPHENYLPROPANE-1,3-DIOL.   Not more than 5·0 per cent of the content of chloramphenicol, determined by the following method:
To 5 ml add 2·5 ml of 1N hydrochloric acid, extract with four successive 10-ml portions of *solvent ether*, and discard the ethereal extracts; dilute the extracted aqueous solution to 25 ml with water and determine the extinction of a 1-cm layer at the maximum at about 272 nm.
For purposes of calculation, use a value of 474 for the E(1 per cent, 1 cm) of 2-amino-1-*p*-nitrophenylpropane-1,3-diol.
Calculate the percentage of 2-amino-1-*p*-nitrophenylpropane-1,3-diol in the chloramphenicol present.

CONTENT OF CHLORAMPHENICOL. 0·45 to 0·55 per cent w/v, determined by the following method:
Dilute 5 ml to 250 ml with water; dilute 10 ml of this solution to 100 ml with water and measure the extinction of a 1-cm layer at the maximum at about 278 nm.
For purposes of calculation, use a value of 298 for the E(1 per cent, 1 cm) of chloramphenicol.
Calculate the concentration of chloramphenicol in the sample.

Containers. The directions given under Eye-drops (page 687) should be followed.

Labelling. The label on the container of the eye-drops, except a container issued for an individual patient for domiciliary use, states:
(1) the name of the eye-drops,
(2) the directions for storage, and
(3) the date of preparation.

The label on the container of dry powder used for the

preparation of the eye-drops by the alternative method given above states:

(1) the name of the powder, indicating that it is for the preparation of Chloramphenicol Eye-drops, and

(2) the weight of chloramphenicol in the container or the volume of eye-drops prepared according to the manufacturer's instructions.

The label on the container or the label on the carton or the package leaflet states:

(3) the directions for preparing the eye-drops.

The label on a multiple-dose container issued for an individual patient for domiciliary use states:

(1) that the eye-drops should be kept in a cool place,

(2) if the eye-drops have been prepared by the alternative method given above, "The contents to be discarded if not used before . . ." [a date two weeks after the date of preparation], and

(3) if the eye-drops have been prepared by the other methods given above, the date after which the eye-drops should not be used.

Storage. It should be protected from light. When stored at a temperature of 2° to 8°, it may be expected to retain its potency for eighteen months from the date of preparation. When stored at a temperature not exceeding 25°, it may be expected to retain its potency for four months from the date of preparation.

Cocaine Eye-drops

Cocaine Eye-drops consist of a sterile solution containing up to 5·0 per cent w/v of Cocaine Hydrochloride, the usual strength being 4·0 per cent w/v, in Purified Water. The solution also contains 0·002 per cent w/v of Phenylmercuric Acetate or Nitrate or 0·01 per cent w/v of Chlorhexidine Acetate.

It is prepared by Method B or C described under Eye-drops (page 687).

Standard
It complies with the standard under Eye-drops, page 687, with the following additions:

PRESENCE OF COCAINE HYDROCHLORIDE. To a volume equivalent to about 0·025 g of cocaine hydrochloride add 1 ml of *trinitrophenol solution*; a yellow precipitate is produced which, after recrystallising from water and drying at 105°, melts at about 165°.

CONTENT OF COCAINE HYDROCHLORIDE. 90·0 to 110·0 per cent of the prescribed or stated concentration, calculated as $C_{17}H_{22}ClNO_4$, determined by the method given in Appendix 12, page 892; each ml of 0·01M sodium tetraphenylboron is equivalent to 0·003398 g of $C_{17}H_{22}ClNO_4$.

Containers. The directions given under Eye-drops (page 687) should be followed; this solution is adversely affected by alkali.

Labelling. The directions given under Eye-drops (page 687) should be followed.

Note. The strength of the eye-drops should be specified by the prescriber.

Cocaine and Homatropine Eye-drops

Cocaine and Homatropine Eye-drops consist of a sterile solution containing 2·0 per cent w/v of Cocaine Hydrochloride and 2·0 per cent w/v of Homatropine Hydrobromide, with 0·01 per cent w/v of Chlorhexidine Acetate, in Purified Water.

It is prepared by Method B or C described under Eye-drops (page 687).

Standard
It complies with the standard under Eye-drops, page 687, with the following additions:

PRESENCE OF COCAINE AND OF HOMATROPINE. It complies with the thin-layer chromatographic test given in Appendix 5A, page 861.

CONTENT OF ALKALOIDS. 3·50 to 4·30 per cent w/v, calculated as cocaine hydrochloride, $C_{17}H_{22}ClNO_4$, determined by the method given in Appendix 12, page 892; each ml of 0·01M sodium tetraphenylboron is equivalent to 0·003398 g of $C_{17}H_{22}ClNO_4$.

Containers. The directions given under Eye-drops (page 687) should be followed; this solution is adversely affected by alkali.

Labelling. The directions given under Eye-drops (page 687) should be followed.

Cyclopentolate Eye-drops

Cyclopentolate Eye-drops consist of a sterile solution containing up to 1·0 per cent w/v of Cyclopentolate Hydrochloride, with 0·02 per cent v/v of Benzalkonium Chloride Solution, in Purified Water. It may also contain Boric Acid and Potassium Chloride.

Standard
It complies with the standard under Eye-drops, page 687, with the following additions:

PRESENCE OF CYCLOPENTOLATE. To a volume equivalent to about 5 mg of cyclopentolate hydrochloride add 1 ml of *sodium hydroxide solution*, mix, warm on a water-bath for 1 minute, and add 0·25 ml of *nitric acid*; a sweet odour resembling that of phenylacetic acid is produced.

CONTENT OF CYCLOPENTOLATE HYDROCHLORIDE. 90·0 to 110·0 per cent of the prescribed or stated concentration, calculated as $C_{17}H_{26}ClNO_3$, determined by the following method:

To an accurately measured volume, equivalent to about 0·02 g of cyclopentolate hydrochloride, add sufficient *dilute ammonia solution* to make the solution distinctly alkaline to *litmus paper* and extract with successive 10-ml portions of *solvent ether* until extraction is complete; wash the combined ethereal extracts with two successive 10-ml portions of water, discard the washings, evaporate off the ether from the extracts, dissolve the residue in *alcohol (95 per cent)*, and dilute to 10 ml with *alcohol (95 per cent)*.

Determine the concentration of cyclopentolate hydrochloride, using Method II of Appendix 12, page 892, by evaporating to dryness, for each determination, 4 ml of the solution prepared above and dissolving the residue in the stated quantity of the appropriate buffer solution; each ml of 0·01M sodium tetraphenylboron is equivalent to 0·003279 g of $C_{17}H_{26}ClNO_3$.

Containers; Labelling. The directions given under Eye-drops (page 687) should be followed.

Storage. It should be stored in a cool place.

Note. When the strength of the eye-drops is not specified, a solution containing 0·5 per cent w/v of cyclopentolate hydrochloride shall be supplied.

Fluorescein Eye-drops

Fluorescein Eye-drops consist of a sterile solution containing up to 2·0 per cent w/v of Fluorescein Sodium in Purified Water.

It is prepared by Method A, B, or C described under Eye-drops (page 687). When prepared by Method C it contains 0·002 per cent w/v of Phenylmercuric Acetate or Nitrate.

Standard

It complies with the standard under Eye-drops, page 687, with the following addition:

CONTENT OF FLUORESCEIN SODIUM. 80·0 to 110·0 per cent of the prescribed or stated amount, calculated as $C_{20}H_{10}Na_2O_5$, determined by the following method:
To an accurately measured volume, equivalent to about 0·05 g of fluorescein sodium, add 15 ml of *dilute hydrochloric acid*, and extract with four successive 20-ml portions of a mixture containing equal volumes of *isobutyl alcohol* and *chloroform*.
Wash the combined extracts with 10 ml of water, extract the water with 5 ml of the same solvent mixture, add this to the combined extracts, and evaporate to dryness in a current of air.
Dissolve the residue in 10 ml of *alcohol (95 per cent)*, evaporate to dryness on a water-bath, and dry to constant weight at 105°; each g of residue is equivalent to 1·132 g of $C_{20}H_{10}Na_2O_5$.

Containers. The directions given under Eye-drops (page 687) should be followed. The eye-drops should preferably be supplied in single-dose containers.

Labelling. The directions given under Eye-drops (page 687) should be followed, except that when it is supplied in a multiple-dose container a direction should be given that the eye-drops should be discarded after use on one occasion.

Note. When the strength of the eye-drops is not specified, a solution containing 1·0 per cent w/v of fluorescein sodium shall be supplied.

Homatropine Eye-drops

Homatropine Eye-drops consist of a sterile solution containing up to 2·0 per cent w/v of Homatropine Hydrobromide, with 0·02 per cent v/v of Benzalkonium Chloride Solution or 0·01 per cent w/v of Chlorhexidine Acetate, in Purified Water.
It is prepared by Method A, B, or C described under Eye-drops (page 687).

Standard

It complies with the standard under Eye-drops, page 687, with the following additions:

PRESENCE OF HOMATROPINE. 1. To a volume equivalent to about 0·02 g of homatropine hydrobromide add an equal volume of *trinitrophenol solution*; a yellow precipitate is produced, which, after recrystallising from a mixture of equal parts of *alcohol (95 per cent)* and water and drying at 105°, melts at about 178°.
2. To 0·1 ml add 0·2 ml of *fuming nitric acid*, evaporate to dryness, cool, and add 2 ml of *acetone* and 0·2 ml of a 3 per cent w/v solution of *potassium hydroxide* in *methyl alcohol*; no violet colour is produced (distinction from atropine).

CONTENT OF HOMATROPINE HYDROBROMIDE. 90·0 to 110·0 per cent of the prescribed or stated concentration, calculated as $C_{16}H_{22}BrNO_3$, determined by the method given in Appendix 12, page 892; each ml of 0·01M sodium tetraphenylboron is equivalent to 0·003563 g of $C_{16}H_{22}BrNO_3$.

Containers. The directions given under Eye-drops (page 687) should be followed; this solution is adversely affected by alkali.

Labelling. The directions given under Eye-drops (page 687) should be followed.

Note. When the strength of the eye-drops is not specified, a solution containing 2·0 per cent w/v of homatropine hydrobromide shall be supplied.

Hydrocortisone Eye-drops

Hydrocortisone Eye-drops consist of a sterile suspension containing up to 1·0 per cent w/v of Hydrocortisone Acetate, in sufficiently fine powder to meet the requirements of the standard, with suitable preservatives, in Purified Water. It may also contain appropriate pharmaceutical adjuvants.
The Eye-drops are not generally suitable for extemporaneous preparation.

Adsorption: It is known that benzalkonium chloride can be adsorbed and partially inactivated by the hydrocortisone acetate in this preparation. The extent of adsorption of other preservatives is not known. These factors should be recognised in the selection of a suitable preservative system for the eye-drops.

Standard

It complies with the standard under Eye-drops, page 687, with the following additions:

PRESENCE OF HYDROCORTISONE. It complies with the thin-layer chromatographic test given in Appendix 5D, page 875.

ACIDITY OR ALKALINITY. pH, 6·0 to 8·0.

PARTICLE SIZE. When determined by the method given in Appendix 25C, page 911, not less than 75 per cent of the particles have a maximum diameter less than 10 µm and not less than 99 per cent of the particles have a maximum diameter less than 20 µm; no particle has a maximum diameter greater than 50 µm.

CONTENT OF HYDROCORTISONE ACETATE. 90·0 to 110·0 per cent of the prescribed or stated concentration, determined by the method for Hydrocortisone and Neomycin Ear-drops, page 665.

Containers. The directions given under Eye-drops (page 687) should be followed.

Labelling. The directions given under Eye-drops (page 687) should be followed. In addition, a direction to shake the bottle should be given on the label.

Storage. It should be stored in a cool place, but should not be allowed to freeze.

Note. When the strength of the eye-drops is not specified, a suspension containing 1·0 per cent w/v of hydrocortisone acetate shall be supplied.

Hydrocortisone and Neomycin Eye-drops

Hydrocortisone and Neomycin Eye-drops consist of a sterile suspension containing up to 1·5 per cent w/v of Hydrocortisone Acetate, in sufficiently fine powder to meet the requirements of the standard, in a solution containing 0·5 per cent w/v of Neomycin Sulphate, with 0·002 per cent w/v of Phenylmercuric Acetate or Nitrate or other suitable preservatives, in Purified Water.
It may also contain appropriate pharmaceutical adjuvants.

Standard

It complies with the standard under Eye-drops, page 687, and with the requirements described under Hydrocortisone and Neomycin Ear-drops, page 665, for presence of hydrocortisone, acidity or alkalinity, particle size, content of hydrocortisone acetate, and content of neomycin sulphate.

Containers. The directions given under Eye-drops (page 687) should be followed.

Labelling. The directions given under Eye-drops (page 687) should be followed. In addition, a direction to shake the bottle should be given on the label.

Storage. It should be stored in a cool place, but should not be allowed to freeze.

Note. When the strength of the eye-drops is not specified, a suspension containing 1·5 per cent w/v of hydrocortisone acetate and 0·5 per cent w/v of neomycin sulphate shall be supplied.

Hyoscine Eye-drops

Hyoscine Eye-drops consist of a sterile solution containing up to 0·5 per cent w/v of Hyoscine Hydrobromide, with 0·02 per cent v/v of Benzalkonium Chloride Solution or 0·01 per cent w/v of Chlorhexidine Acetate, in Purified Water.

It is prepared by Method A, B, or C described under Eye-drops (page 687).

Standard
It complies with the standard under Eye-drops, page 687, with the following additions:

PRESENCE OF HYOSCINE. To a volume equivalent to about 3 mg of hyoscine hydrobromide add an equal volume of *gold chloride solution*; a precipitate is produced which, after recrystallising from water and drying at 105°, melts at about 202°.

CONTENT OF HYOSCINE HYDROBROMIDE. 90·0 to 110·0 per cent of the prescribed or stated concentration, calculated as $C_{17}H_{22}BrNO_4,3H_2O$, determined by the method given in Appendix 12, page 892; each ml of sodium tetraphenylboron is equivalent to 0·004383 g of $C_{17}H_{22}BrNO_4,3H_2O$.

Containers. The directions given under Eye-drops (page 687) should be followed; this solution is adversely affected by alkali.

Labelling. The directions given under Eye-drops (page 687) should be followed.

Note. When the strength of the eye-drops is not specified, a solution containing 0·25 per cent w/v of hyoscine hydrobromide shall be supplied.

Hypromellose Eye-drops

SYNONYMS: Alkaline Eye-drops; Artificial Tears

Hypromellose 4500	..	..	0·30 g
Borax	..	..	0·19 g
Boric Acid	..	..	0·19 g
Potassium Chloride	..	..	0·37 g
Sodium Chloride	..	..	0·45 g
Benzalkonium Chloride Solution			0·02 ml
Purified Water	..	..	to 100 ml

Add the hypromellose to about 15 ml of the water at 80° to 90° and, when the powder is thoroughly hydrated, add a further 35 ml of the water, preferably in the form of ice, and stir until homogeneous. Dissolve the sodium chloride, the potassium chloride, the borax and the boric acid in 40 ml of the water, and add the benzalkonium chloride solution. Mix the two solutions, add sufficient of the water to produce the required volume, and mix.

Allow to stand overnight, and decant and filter the supernatant liquid.

Transfer the filtered solution to the final containers, close the containers so as to exclude micro-organisms, and sterilise by autoclaving or by maintaining at 98° to 100° for thirty minutes. Redisperse the coagulated hypromellose by shaking on cooling.

Alternatively, the filtered solution may be sterilised in bulk, the coagulated hypromellose redispersed by shaking on cooling, and the solution distributed, by an aseptic technique, into the final sterile containers, which are then closed so as to exclude micro-organisms.

Standard
It complies with the standard under Eye-drops, page 687, with the following addition:

ALKALINITY. pH, 8·4 to 8·6.

Containers. The directions given under Eye-drops (page 687) should be followed. If the eye-drops are transferred to the final container before sterilisation, the container should be closed with a screw cap, and a sterile dropper, suitably wrapped, supplied separately.

Labelling. The directions given under Eye-drops (page 687) should be followed.

Uses. Hypromellose Eye-drops may be used to replace lachrymal secretion where this is deficient. The solution is not intended as a vehicle for other drugs.

When Methylcellulose Eye-drops are ordered or prescribed, Hypromellose Eye-drops shall be supplied.

When the solution is supplied for use in gonioscopy procedures, the amount of hypromellose 4500 may be increased; a concentration between 0·7 and 1·5 per cent may be suitable.

Lachesine Eye-drops

Lachesine Eye-drops consist of a sterile solution containing up to 1·0 per cent w/v of Lachesine Chloride, with 0·002 per cent w/v of Phenylmercuric Acetate or Nitrate, in Purified Water.

It is prepared by Method A, B, or C described under Eye-drops (page 687).

Standard
It complies with the standard under Eye-drops, page 687, with the following additions:

PRESENCE OF LACHESINE. To a volume equivalent to about 0·5 mg of lachesine chloride add 1 ml of *sulphuric acid*; an orange-red colour is produced which quickly changes to rose-pink.

CONTENT OF LACHESINE CHLORIDE. 90·0 to 110·0 per cent of the prescribed or stated concentration, calculated as $C_{20}H_{26}ClNO_3$, determined by the method given in Appendix 12, page 892; each ml of 0·01M sodium tetraphenylboron is equivalent to 0·003639 g of $C_{20}H_{26}ClNO_3$.

Containers. The directions given under Eye-drops (page 687) should be followed; this solution is adversely affected by alkali.

Labelling. The directions given under Eye-drops (page 687) should be followed.

Note. When the strength of the eye-drops is not specified, a solution containing 1·0 per cent w/v of lachesine chloride shall be supplied.

Neomycin Eye-drops

Neomycin Eye-drops consist of a sterile solution containing up to 0·5 per cent w/v of Neomycin Sulphate, with 0·7 per cent w/v of Sodium Acid Phosphate, 0·7 per cent w/v of Sodium Phosphate, and 0·002 per cent w/v of Phenylmercuric Acetate or Nitrate, in Purified Water. It may also contain 0·01 per cent w/v of Disodium Edetate.

It is prepared by Method B or C described under Eye-drops (page 687).

Standard

It complies with the standard under Eye-drops, page 687, with the following addition:

CONTENT OF NEOMYCIN SULPHATE. 90 to 115 per cent of the prescribed or stated concentration, determined by the following method:

Carry out a microbiological assay of neomycin; a suggested method is given in Appendix 18, page 897.

The precision of any assay must be such that the fiducial limits of error (P = 0·95) are not less than 95 per cent and not more than 105 per cent of the estimated potency.

Assuming that each 680 Units found is equivalent to 1 mg of neomycin sulphate, calculate the upper and lower fiducial limits of the equivalent concentration of neomycin sulphate in the eye-drops.

The upper fiducial limit of the estimated equivalent concentration of neomycin sulphate is not less than 90 per cent and the lower fiducial limit is not more than 115 per cent of the prescribed or stated concentration.

Containers; Labelling. The directions given under Eye-drops (page 687) should be followed.

Storage. It should be protected from light.

Note. When the strength of the eye-drops is not specified, a solution containing 0·5 per cent w/v of neomycin sulphate shall be supplied.

Phenylephrine Eye-drops

Phenylephrine Hydrochloride	..		10·0 g
Sodium Citrate	..	..	0·3 g
Sodium Metabisulphite	..	..	0·5 g
Benzalkonium Chloride Solution			0·02 ml
Purified Water	..	..	to 100 ml

Prepare by Method B described under Eye-drops (page 687).

Standard

It complies with the standard under Eye-drops, page 687, with the following addition:

CONTENT OF PHENYLEPHRINE HYDROCHLORIDE. 9·00 to 10·50 per cent w/v, determined by the following method:

Using water as solvent, dilute 2 ml to 100 ml; dilute 10 ml of this solution to 1000 ml.

To 25 ml of this second dilution add 5 ml of a 0·5 per cent w/v solution of *4-aminophenazone* in water, 5 ml of a 2·0 per cent w/v solution of *potassium ferricyanide* in water, and 1 ml of an 8·4 per cent w/v solution of *sodium bicarbonate* in water, dilute to 100 ml with water, allow to stand for 30 minutes, and measure the extinction of a 1-cm layer at the maximum at about 500 nm, using as a blank a solution prepared in the same manner but with 25 ml of water in place of the diluted sample.

For the purposes of calculation, use a value of 690 for the E(1 per cent, 1 cm) of phenylephrine hydrochloride under these conditions.

Calculate the percentage of phenylephrine hydrochloride in the sample.

Containers; Labelling. The directions given under Eye-drops (page 687) should be followed.

Storage. It should be protected from light.

Physostigmine Eye-drops

SYNONYMS: Eserine Eye-drops; Physostigmine Sulphate Eye-drops

Physostigmine Eye-drops consist of a sterile solution containing up to 1·0 per cent w/v of Physostigmine Sulphate, with 0·2 per cent w/v of Sodium Metabisulphite and 0·02 per cent v/v of Benzalkonium Chloride Solution, in Purified Water.

It is prepared by Method B or C described under Eye-drops (page 687).

Standard

It complies with the standard under Eye-drops, page 687, with the following additions:

PRESENCE OF PHYSOSTIGMINE. A volume equivalent to about 5 mg of physostigmine sulphate complies with test 1 given under Physostigmine, page 380.

CONTENT OF PHYSOSTIGMINE SULPHATE. 90·0 to 110·0 per cent of the prescribed or stated concentration, calculated as $C_{30}H_{44}N_6O_8S$, determined by the method given in Appendix 12, page 892; each ml of 0·01M sodium tetraphenylboron is equivalent to 0·003244 g of $C_{30}H_{44}N_6O_8S$.

Containers. The directions given under Eye-drops (page 687) should be followed; this solution is adversely affected by alkali.

Labelling. The directions given under Eye-drops (page 687) should be followed.

Storage. It should be protected from light.

Note. When the strength of the eye-drops is not specified, a solution containing 0·25 per cent w/v of physostigmine sulphate shall be supplied.

Physostigmine and Pilocarpine Eye-drops

SYNONYM: Eserine and Pilocarpine Eye-drops

Physostigmine and Pilocarpine Eye-drops consist of a sterile solution containing up to 0·5 per cent w/v of Physostigmine Sulphate and up to 4·0 per cent w/v of Pilocarpine Hydrochloride, with 0·2 per cent w/v of Sodium Metabisulphite and 0·02 per cent v/v of Benzalkonium Chloride Solution, in Purified Water.

It is prepared by Method B or C described under Eye-drops (page 687).

Standard

It complies with the standard under Eye-drops, page 687, with the following additions:

PRESENCE OF PHYSOSTIGMINE AND OF PILOCARPINE. It complies with the test given in Appendix 4, page 857.

CONTENT OF PHYSOSTIGMINE SULPHATE. 90·0 to 110·0 per cent of the prescribed or stated concentration, determined by the following method:

Dilute 20 ml to 100 ml with water; further dilute 5 ml of this solution to 100 ml with 0·2N sulphuric acid, and measure the extinction of a 1-cm layer at the maximum at about 302 nm, using 0·2N sulphuric acid as the blank.

For purposes of calculation, use a value of 84 for the E(1 per cent, 1 cm) of physostigmine sulphate.

Calculate the percentage of physostigmine sulphate in the sample.

CONTENT OF PILOCARPINE HYDROCHLORIDE. 90·0 to 110·0 per cent of the prescribed or stated concentration, calculated as $C_{11}H_{17}ClN_2O_2$, determined by the following method:
Carry out the method given in Appendix 12, page 892, and calculate the number of millilitres of 0·01M sodium tetraphenylboron equivalent to the total nitrogenous bases present in 2 ml of the sample.
From the content of physostigmine sulphate found in the determination above, calculate the number of millilitres of 0·01M sodium tetraphenylboron equivalent to the amount of physostigmine sulphate, calculated as $C_{30}H_{44}N_6O_8S$, present in 2 ml of the sample, each ml of 0·01M sodium tetraphenylboron being equivalent to 0·003244 g of $C_{30}H_{44}N_6O_8S$; the difference between the two calculated volumes represents the volume of 0·01M sodium tetraphenylboron equivalent to the pilocarpine hydrochloride present; each ml of 0·01M sodium tetraphenylboron is equivalent to 0·002447 g of $C_{11}H_{17}ClN_2O_2$.

Containers. The directions given under Eye-drops (page 687) should be followed; this solution is adversely affected by alkali.

Storage. It should be protected from light.

Note. The strength of the eye-drops must be specified by the prescriber.
Strengths frequently prescribed are 0·25 per cent w/v of physostigmine sulphate with 2·0 per cent w/v of pilocarpine hydrochloride and 0·5 per cent w/v of physostigmine sulphate with 4·0 per cent w/v of pilocarpine hydrochloride.

Pilocarpine Eye-drops

SYNONYM: Pilocarpine Hydrochloride Eye-drops

Pilocarpine Eye-drops consist of a sterile solution containing up to 5·0 per cent w/v of Pilocarpine Hydrochloride, with 0·02 per cent v/v of Benzalkonium Chloride Solution, in Purified Water.
It is prepared by Method A, B, or C described under Eye-drops (page 687).

Standard
It complies with the standard under Eye-drops, page 687, with the following additions:

PRESENCE OF PILOCARPINE. To a volume equivalent to about 0·01 g add 0·1 ml of *dilute sulphuric acid*, 1 ml of *hydrogen peroxide solution*, 1 ml of *benzene*, and 0·05 ml of *potassium chromate solution*, shake well, and allow to separate; the benzene layer is coloured bluish-violet and the aqueous layer remains yellow.

CONTENT OF PILOCARPINE HYDROCHLORIDE. 90·0 to 110·0 per cent of the prescribed or stated concentration, calculated as $C_{11}H_{17}ClN_2O_2$, determined by the method given in Appendix 12, page 892; each ml of 0·01M sodium tetraphenylboron is equivalent to 0·002447 g of $C_{11}H_{17}ClN_2O_2$.

Containers. The directions given under Eye-drops (page 687) should be followed; this solution is adversely affected by alkali.

Labelling. The directions given under Eye-drops (page 687) should be followed.

Note. When the strength of the eye-drops is not specified, a solution containing 1·0 per cent w/v of pilocarpine hydrochloride shall be supplied.

Prednisolone Eye-drops

SYNONYM: Prednisolone Sodium Phosphate Eye-drops

Prednisolone Eye-drops consist of a sterile preparation containing Prednisolone Sodium Phosphate, with a suitable preservative and stabilising agents, in Purified Water.
A suitable solution may be prepared according to the following formula:

Prednisolone Sodium Phosphate		0·518 g
Disodium Edetate	.. ..	0·01 g
Sodium Acid Phosphate	..	0·30 g
Sodium Chloride..	..	0·50 g
Benzalkonium Chloride Solution		0·02 ml
Sodium Hydroxide	a sufficient quantity	
Purified Water	.. ..	.. to 100 ml

Dissolve the sodium acid phosphate, the prednisolone sodium phosphate, the disodium edetate, and the sodium chloride in 40 ml of the water and adjust to pH 8·0 by adding, dropwise, a 4 per cent w/v solution of the sodium hydroxide in the water.
Add the benzalkonium chloride solution mixed with 50 ml of the water, re-adjust, if necessary, to pH 8·0 with a further addition of the sodium hydroxide solution, add sufficient of the water to produce the required volume, and mix.
Transfer to the final containers, close the containers so as to exclude micro-organisms, and sterilise by maintaining at 98° to 100° for thirty minutes.

Standard
It complies with the standard under Eye-drops, page 687, with the following additions:

ALKALINITY. pH, 7·0 to 8·5.

CONTENT OF PREDNISOLONE SODIUM PHOSPHATE. 0·466 to 0·570 per cent w/v, determined by the following method:
Using water as solvent, dilute 5 ml to 100 ml; dilute 5 ml of this solution to 100 ml and measure the extinction of a 1-cm layer at the maximum at about 247 nm.
For purposes of calculation, use a value of 312 for the E(1 per cent, 1 cm) of prednisolone sodium phosphate.
Calculate the concentration of prednisolone sodium phosphate in the sample.

Containers; Labelling. The directions given under Eye-drops (page 687) should be followed.

Storage. It should be protected from light.

Proxymetacaine Eye-drops

Proxymetacaine Eye-drops consist of a sterile solution containing 0·52 per cent w/v of Proxymetacaine Hydrochloride, with suitable preservatives, in Purified Water. It may contain Glycerol.

Standard
It complies with the standard under Eye-drops, page 687, with the following addition:

CONTENT OF PROXYMETACAINE HYDROCHLORIDE. 0·47 to 0·57 per cent w/v, determined by the following method:

Dilute 2 ml to 500 ml with water and measure the extinction of a 1-cm layer of this solution at the maximum at about 269 nm.
For purposes of calculation, use a value of 290 for the E(1 per cent, 1 cm) of proxymetacaine hydrochloride.
Calculate the concentration of proxymetacaine hydrochloride in the sample.

Containers. The directions given under Eye-drops (page 687) should be followed. In addition, the air in the container should be replaced by nitrogen or other inert gas.

Labelling. The directions given under Eye-drops (page 687) should be followed. In addition, the label on the container states the conditions under which the eye-drops should be stored.

Storage. It should be protected from light. After opening the container, the eye-drops should be stored at a temperature between 2° and 10° but should not be allowed to freeze.

Sulphacetamide Eye-drops

Sulphacetamide Eye-drops consist of a sterile solution containing up to 30·0 per cent w/v of Sulphacetamide Sodium, with 0·1 per cent w/v of Sodium Metabisulphite and 0·002 per cent w/v of Phenylmercuric Acetate or Nitrate, or 0·01 per cent w/v of Thiomersal, in Purified Water.

It is prepared by Method A, B, or C described under Eye-drops (page 687).

In making this preparation, precautions should be taken to minimise oxidation of the active ingredient. The purified water used should be freshly boiled and cooled, or alternatively, if the water is prepared by distillation, freshly distilled water may be used, nitrogen or other inert gas being employed to remove dissolved oxygen. In addition, the air in the final container should be replaced by nitrogen or other inert gas.

A metal cap with a rubber liner should be used as the closure for the final container. A separate screw cap fitted with a teat and dropper, suitably wrapped and sterilised, should either be substituted for the metal cap by the pharmacist immediately before issue, care being taken to avoid contamination, or the wrapped sterile dropper assembly should be issued to the patient with instructions to exchange it for the metal cap on first using the eye-drops.

Standard
It complies with the standard under Eye-drops, page 687, with the following additions:

DESCRIPTION. A clear colourless to pale yellow liquid.

SULPHANILAMIDE. Not more than 1·5 per cent w/v, determined by the following method:
Prepare a chromatographic column by mixing 5 g of a neutral alumina, heated at 100° for 30 minutes before use, with sufficient of a mixture containing 70 volumes of *chloroform* and 30 volumes of *methyl alcohol* to form a slurry, transfer to a suitable chromatographic tube, allow the solvent mixture to drain, add a further 25 ml of solvent mixture, and allow to drain until the solvent just covers the alumina; cover the top of the column with a small pledget of glass wool and add sufficient of the solvent mixture to give a 1-cm layer above the glass wool.
Mix an accurately measured volume of the sample or of a dilution of the sample, equivalent to about 0·2 g of sulphacetamide sodium, with 30 ml of *methyl alcohol* and dilute to 100 ml with *chloroform*.
Add 5 ml of this solution to the top of the prepared column and elute with a mixture containing 30 volumes of *methyl alcohol* and 70 volumes of *chloroform* until 50 ml of the eluate has been collected; during the elution procedure maintain the solvent at a level of about 5 cm above the alumina in the column and allow the elution to proceed at a rate such that the 50 ml of eluate is collected in about 30 minutes.
Measure the extinction of a 1-cm layer of the eluate at the maximum at about 262 nm using as the blank 5 ml of the solvent mixture which has also been passed through the prepared column.
For purposes of calculation use a value of 1000 for the E(1 per cent, 1 cm) of sulphanilamide.

CONTENT OF SULPHACETAMIDE SODIUM. 92·5 to 107·5 per cent of the prescribed or stated concentration, calculated as $C_8H_9N_2NaO_3S,H_2O$, determined by the following method:
To an accurately measured volume, equivalent to about 0·5 g of sulphacetamide sodium, add 75 ml of water and 10 ml of *hydrochloric acid* and titrate with 0·1M sodium nitrite, determining the end-point electrometrically; each ml of 0·1M sodium nitrite is equivalent to 0·02542 g of $C_8H_9N_2NaO_3S,H_2O$.

Containers. The directions given under Eye-drops (page 687), as modified above, should be followed.

Labelling. The directions given under Eye-drops (page 687) should be followed. In addition, the label states:
(1) that the eye-drops should be stored at room temperature and should not be allowed to freeze, and
(2) that the contents should be discarded four weeks after first opening the container.

Storage. It should be protected from light. Chemical stability of the drug in aqueous solution after opening the container is limited and it deteriorates on storage. The eye-drops should therefore be used within four weeks of first opening the container.
It should be stored at room temperature. Storage at lower temperatures may result in formation of crystals. It should not be allowed to freeze.

Note. When the strength of the eye-drops is not specified or when Weak Sulphacetamide Eye-drops are ordered or prescribed, a solution containing 10·0 per cent w/v of sulphacetamide sodium shall be supplied.

When Strong Sulphacetamide Eye-drops are ordered or prescribed, a solution containing 30·0 per cent w/v of sulphacetamide sodium shall be supplied.

Zinc Sulphate Eye-drops

Zinc Sulphate Eye-drops consist of a sterile solution containing 0·25 per cent w/v of Zinc Sulphate, with 0·002 per cent w/v of Phenylmercuric Acetate or Nitrate, in Purified Water.

It is prepared by Method A, B, or C described under Eye-drops (page 687).

Standard
It complies with the standard under Eye-drops, page 687, with the following addition:

CONTENT OF ZINC SULPHATE. 0·22 to 0·28 per cent, calculated as $ZnSO_4,7H_2O$, determined by the following method:
To 5 ml add 50 ml of water and 5 ml of *ammonia buffer solution* and titrate with 0·01M disodium edetate, using *mordant black 11 solution* as indicator; each ml of 0·01M disodium edetate is equivalent to 0·002875 g of $ZnSO_4,7H_2O$.

Containers; Labelling. The directions given under Eye-drops (page 687) should be followed.

Zinc Sulphate and Adrenaline Eye-drops

Zinc Sulphate	0·25 g
Adrenaline Acid Tartrate ..	0·09 g
Phenylmercuric Acetate or Nitrate	0·002 g
Sodium Metabisulphite	0·05 g
Purified Water .. .. .. to 100 ml

Prepare by Method A, B, or C described under Eye-drops (page 687).

Standard
It complies with the standard under Eye-drops, page 687, with the following additions:

CONTENT OF ZINC SULPHATE. 0·22 to 0·28 per cent w/v calculated as $ZnSO_4,7H_2O$, determined by the method for Zinc Sulphate Eye-drops.

CONTENT OF ADRENALINE ACID TARTRATE. 0·079 to 0·099 per cent w/v, determined by the following method:
Dilute 2 ml to 50 ml with water; to 10 ml of this solution add 1 ml of *solution of standard pH 5·4* and 8 ml of 0·02N iodine, allow to stand for 10 minutes, and add 2 ml of 0·1N sodium thiosulphate; compare the colour intensity with that produced when 10 ml of a 0·00360 per cent w/v solution of *adrenaline acid tartrate* in water is similarly treated. Calculate the concentration of adrenaline acid tartrate in the sample.

Containers. The directions given under Eye-drops (page 687) should be followed; this solution is adversely affected by alkali.

Labelling. The directions given under Eye-drops (page 687) should be followed.

Storage. It should be stored in a cool place and protected from light.

Note. Zinc Sulphate and Adrenaline Eye-drops contain the equivalent of adrenaline, 1 in 2000.

EYE LOTIONS

Eye Lotions are solutions used for washing or bathing the eyes. There are two types of eye lotion:

(1) sterile aqueous solutions containing no added bactericide for first-aid or other purposes over a maximum period of twenty-four hours; and

(2) aqueous solutions containing a bactericide used for intermittent domiciliary administration for up to seven days.

When eye lotions are dispensed, a caution should be given to the user to avoid contamination of the solution after opening the container.

The information on the preparation of eye lotions and the standard given below applies to eye lotions of type (1).

Preparation of eye lotions. The apparatus used in the preparation of eye lotions and the containers must be thoroughly cleansed before use. The medicament is dissolved in the water and the solution is clarified by filtration, transferred to the final containers, which are then closed so as to exclude micro-organisms, and sterilised by autoclaving.

Alternatively, the solution is sterilised by filtration and transferred to the final sterile containers, which are then closed so as to exclude micro-organisms.

Standard

STERILITY. Eye lotions comply with the test for sterility.

Containers. Eye lotions should be supplied in coloured fluted glass bottles. The closure should be impermeable, must not contain cork, and must be covered with a readily breakable seal. If the preparation is sterilised by autoclaving, any closure must withstand the sterilisation process and prevent subsequent microbial contamination. If coloured fluted bottles are not available, an uncoloured container which meets the other requirements should be used.

Sodium Chloride Eye Lotion

Sodium Chloride..	..	..	9 g
Purified Water	..	..	.. to 1000 ml

Prepare as described under Eye Lotions (page 696).

Standard
It complies with the standard under Eye Lotions, page, 696 with the following addition:

CONTENT OF SODIUM CHLORIDE. 0·85 to 0·95 per cent w/v, determined by the following method: Titrate 25 ml by the method given in Appendix 11, page 891; each ml of 0·1N silver nitrate is equivalent to 0·005844 g of NaCl.

Containers; Labelling. The directions given under Eye Lotions (page 696) should be followed.

Note. Sodium Chloride Eye Lotion should be used undiluted.

EYE OINTMENTS

Eye ointments are sterile preparations for application to the conjunctival sac or lid margin. They usually contain substances with antiseptic, anti-inflammatory, anti-microbial, mydriatic, or miotic properties.

In using eye ointments, precautions should be taken to avoid contamination. The application is best made direct from the tube or with the aid of a clean glass rod. When used in hospital wards and out-patient departments, either single-dose containers should be used or a separate container reserved for each individual patient, the application being assisted by the use of a sterile glass rod.

Preparation of eye ointments. The apparatus used in the preparation of eye ointments must be thoroughly cleansed and sterilised. A suitable basis for eye ointments is given by the following formula:

EYE OINTMENT BASIS

Liquid Paraffin	..	..	..	100 g
Wool Fat	..	..	..	..	100 g
Yellow Soft Paraffin	..	..	..	800 g

Heat together the wool fat, the yellow soft paraffin, and the liquid paraffin, filter while hot through a coarse filter paper in a heated funnel, sterilise by heating for a sufficient time to ensure that the whole of the basis is maintained at a temperature of 150° for one hour, and allow to cool, taking precautions to avoid contamination with micro-organisms, before incorporating the sterile medicament.

For eye ointments intended to be used in tropical or subtropical climates, the proportions of the paraffins may be varied, or Hard Paraffin may be included, when prevailing high temperatures otherwise make the ointments too soft for convenience.

Eye ointments are prepared, by means of an aseptic technique, by either of the following methods:

Method A. If the medicament is readily soluble in water forming a stable solution, it is dissolved in the minimum quantity of water and the solution sterilised by auto-claving or by filtration and incorporated gradually in the melted sterile basis, the mixture being stirred continuously until it is cold. The eye ointment is then trans-ferred to the final sterile containers, which are closed so as to exclude micro-organisms.

Method B. If it is not readily soluble in water or if the aqueous solution is unstable, the medicament is finely powdered, thoroughly mixed with a small quantity of the melted sterile basis, and then incorporated with the remainder of the sterile basis.

The eye ointment is then transferred to the final sterile containers, which are closed so as to exclude micro-organisms.

If the medicament is insoluble in both water and the basis, it is essential that it be reduced to an extremely fine powder before incorporating with the basis, in order to avoid irritation to the eye.

Standard

STERILITY. Add 1 g of the sample to a mixture of 10 g of sterile arachis oil and 10 g of sterile polysorbate 80, previously warmed to between 40° and 45° in a water-bath, and swirl until uniformly mixed. The resulting mixture complies with the test for sterility, the whole of the mixture being used for the inoculation of the media.

Containers. Eye ointments should be packed in small collapsible tubes of suitable metal or plastic or in suitable single-dose containers. If metal tubes are used, they should comply with British Standard 4230: 1967.

All containers should be as free as possible, consistent with good manufacturing practice, from dirt and particles of the material used in their construction.

Tubes and screw caps, complete with wads if used, must be sterilised before use; the wads should not be of cork.

Unless the eye ointment has been prepared extemporaneously, the screw cap should be covered with a readily breakable seal or, alternatively, the whole tube should be enclosed in a sealed package from which the tube cannot be removed without breaking the seal; suitable outer packages include paperboard cartons with sealed flaps and sealed pouches of paper, plastic, or cellulose film.

Labelling. The label on the tube or outer sealed envelope, except one issued on medical prescription for an individual patient, should state that the contents are sterile provided that the container has not been opened.

Note. When Simple Eye Ointment or Non-medicated Eye Ointment is ordered or prescribed, sterile Eye Ointment Basis shall be supplied.

Chloramphenicol Eye Ointment

Chloramphenicol Eye Ointment is prepared by incorporating Chloramphenicol in Eye Ointment Basis, or any other suitable basis, by Method B described under Eye Ointments (above).

Standard
It complies with the standard under Eye Ointments, above, with the following addition:

CONTENT OF CHLORAMPHENICOL. 95·0 to 105·0 per cent of the prescribed or stated concentration, determined by the following method:
Dissolve an accurately weighed quantity, equivalent to about 10 mg of chloramphenicol, in 50 ml of *light petroleum (boiling-range 40° to 60°)* and extract with three successive 50-ml portions, followed by one 30-ml portion, of water, combine the extracts, dilute to 200 ml with water, mix well, and filter, discarding the first 20 ml of filtrate; dilute 10 ml of the filtrate to 50 ml with water and measure the extinction of a 1-cm layer at the maximum at about 278 nm.
For purposes of calculation, use a value of 298 for the E(1 per cent, 1 cm) of chloramphenicol.
Calculate the concentration of chloramphenicol in the sample.

Labelling. The directions given under Eye Ointments (above) should be followed.

Note. When the strength of the eye ointment is not specified, an eye ointment containing 1·0 per cent of chloramphenicol shall be supplied.

Chlortetracycline Eye Ointment

Chlortetracycline Eye Ointment is prepared by incorporating Chlortetracycline Hydrochloride in Eye Ointment Basis, or any other suitable basis, by Method B described under Eye Ointments (above).

Standard
It complies with the standard under Eye Ointments, above, with the following additions:

PRESENCE OF CHLORTETRACYCLINE. To an amount equivalent to about 0·5 mg of chlortetracycline hydrochloride add 2 ml of *sulphuric acid*; a deep blue colour is produced which changes to bluish-green.

CONTENT OF CHLORTETRACYCLINE HYDROCHLORIDE. 90 to 115 per cent of the prescribed or stated concentration, determined by the following method:
Disperse an accurately weighed quantity, equivalent

to about 0·03 g of chlortetracycline hydrochloride, in 200 ml of *acid acetone*, using a high-speed mixer, dilute to 250 ml with *acid acetone*, and carry out a microbiological assay of chlortetracycline; a suggested method is given in Appendix 18, page 897.

The precision of any assay must be such that the fiducial limits of error (P = 0·95) are not less than 95 per cent and not more than 105 per cent of the estimated potency.

Assuming that each 1000 Units found is equivalent to 1 mg of chlortetracycline hydrochloride, calculate the upper and lower fiducial limits of the equivalent concentration of chlortetracycline hydrochloride in the ointment.

The upper fiducial limit of the estimated equivalent concentration of chlortetracycline hydrochloride is not less than 90 per cent and the lower fiducial limit is not more than 115 per cent of the prescribed or stated concentration.

Labelling. The directions given under Eye Ointments (page 698) should be followed.

Storage. It should be protected from light.

Note. When the strength of the eye ointment is not specified, an eye ointment containing 1·0 per cent of chlortetracycline hydrochloride shall be supplied.

Hydrocortisone Eye Ointment

SYNONYM: Hydrocortisone Acetate Eye Ointment

Hydrocortisone Eye Ointment is prepared by incorporating Hydrocortisone Acetate, in sufficiently fine powder to meet the requirements of the standard, in Eye Ointment Basis, or any other suitable basis, by Method B described under Eye Ointments (page 697).

Standard
It complies with the standard under Eye Ointments, page 698, with the following additions:

PRESENCE OF HYDROCORTISONE. It complies with the thin-layer chromatographic test given in Appendix 5D, page 875.

PARTICLE SIZE. When determined by the method given in Appendix 25C, page 911, *liquid paraffin* being used as diluent, not less than 75 per cent of the particles have a maximum diameter less than 10 μm and not less than 99 per cent of the particles have a maximum diameter less than 20 μm; no particle has a maximum diameter greater than 50 μm.

CONTENT OF HYDROCORTISONE ACETATE. 92·5 to 107·5 per cent of the prescribed or stated concentration, determined by the method for Hydrocortisone Cream (*Creams containing hydrocortisone acetate*), page 659.

Labelling. The directions given under Eye Ointments (page 698) should be followed.

Note. When the strength of the eye ointment is not specified, an eye ointment containing 2·5 per cent of hydrocortisone acetate shall be supplied.

Hydrocortisone and Neomycin Eye Ointment

Hydrocortisone and Neomycin Eye Ointment is prepared by incorporating Hydrocortisone Acetate and Neomycin Sulphate, both in sufficiently fine powder to meet the requirements of the standard, in Eye Ointment Basis, or any other suitable basis, by Method B described under Eye Ointments (page 697).

Standard
It complies with the standard under Eye Ointments, page 698, with the following additions:

PRESENCE OF HYDROCORTISONE. It complies with the thin-layer chromatographic test given in Appendix 5D, page 875.

PARTICLE SIZE. When determined by the method given in Appendix 25C, page 911, *liquid paraffin* being used as the diluent, not less than 75 per cent of the particles have a maximum diameter less than 10 μm and not less than 99 per cent of the particles have a maximum diameter less than 20 μm; no particle has a maximum diameter greater than 50 μm.

CONTENT OF HYDROCORTISONE ACETATE. 92·5 to 107·5 per cent of the prescribed or stated concentration, determined by the method for Hydrocortisone Cream (*Creams containing hydrocortisone acetate*), page 659.

CONTENT OF NEOMYCIN SULPHATE. 90 to 115 per cent of the prescribed or stated amount, determined by the following method:

Dissolve an accurately weighed quantity, equivalent to about 0·005 g of neomycin sulphate, in 50 ml of *solvent ether*, extract the solution with three successive 30-ml portions of *solution of standard pH 8·0*, and discard the ethereal solution; remove the dissolved ether from the combined aqueous extracts by passing a stream of air through the solution, dilute to 100 ml with *solution of standard pH 8·0*, and carry out a microbiological assay of neomycin; a suggested method is given in Appendix 18, page 897.

The precision of any assay must be such that the fiducial limits of error (P = 0·95) are not less than 95 per cent and not more than 105 per cent of the estimated concentration.

Assuming that each 680 Units found is equivalent to 1 mg of neomycin sulphate, calculate the upper and lower fiducial limits of the equivalent concentration of neomycin sulphate in the sample.

The upper fiducial limit of the estimated equivalent concentration of neomycin sulphate is not less than 90 per cent and the lower fiducial limit is not more than 115 per cent of the prescribed or stated concentration.

Labelling. The directions given under Eye Ointments (page 698) should be followed.

Note. When the strength of the eye ointment is not specified, an eye ointment containing 1·5 per cent of hydrocortisone acetate and 0·5 per cent of neomycin sulphate shall be supplied.

Mercuric Oxide Eye Ointment

SYNONYM: Oculentum Hydrargyri Oxidi

Mercuric Oxide Eye Ointment is prepared by incorporating Yellow Mercuric Oxide in Eye Ointment Basis by Method B described under Eye Ointments (page 697).

Standard
It complies with the standard under Eye Ointments, page 698, with the following addition:

CONTENT OF MERCURIC OXIDE. 95·0 to 105·0 per cent of the prescribed or stated concentration, calculated as HgO, determined by the following method:

Shake an accurately weighed quantity, equivalent to about 0·1 g of yellow mercuric oxide, with 20 ml of *chloroform* and then with 10 ml of *dilute nitric acid* and 20 ml of water until solution is complete; add 50 ml of water and titrate with 0·1N ammonium thiocyanate at a temperature not exceeding 20°, using *ferric ammonium sulphate solution* as indicator; each ml of 0·1N ammonium thiocyanate is equivalent to 0·01083 g of HgO.

Labelling. The directions given under Eye Ointments (page 698) should be followed. In addition, a warning should be given on the label that prolonged use of the preparation may be injurious to the eyes.

Note. When the strength of the eye ointment is not specified, an eye ointment containing 1·0 per cent of yellow mercuric oxide shall be supplied.

Neomycin Eye Ointment

Neomycin Eye Ointment is prepared by incorporating Neomycin Sulphate in Eye Ointment Basis by Method B described under Eye Ointments (page 697).

Standard
It complies with the standard under Eye Ointments, page 698, with the following addition:

CONTENT OF NEOMYCIN SULPHATE. 90 to 115 per cent of the prescribed or stated concentration, determined by the following method:
Dissolve an accurately weighed quantity, equivalent to about 0·005 g of neomycin sulphate, in 50 ml of *solvent ether* and extract with successive 15-, 10-, 10-, and 10-ml portions of sterile *solution of standard pH 8·0*; combine the extracts, dilute to 50 ml with sterile *solution of standard pH 8·0*, and carry out a micro-biological assay of neomycin; a suggested method is given in Appendix 18, page 897.
The precision of any assay must be such that the fiducial limits of error (P = 0·95) are not less than 95 per cent and not more than 105 per cent of the estimated potency.
Assuming that each 680 Units found is equivalent to 1 mg of neomycin sulphate, calculate the upper and lower fiducial limits of the equivalent concentration of neomycin sulphate in the sample.
The upper fiducial limit of the estimated equivalent concentration of neomycin sulphate is not less than 90 per cent and the lower fiducial limit is not more than 115 per cent of the prescribed or stated concentration.

Labelling. The directions given under Eye Ointments (page 698) should be followed.

Note. When the strength of the eye ointment is not specified, an eye ointment containing 0·5 per cent of neomycin sulphate shall be supplied.

GARGLES

A gargle is an aqueous solution, usually in concentrated form, intended for use, after dilution, as a prophylactic or in the treatment of an infection of the throat. The particular method of using a gargle is intended to bring it into intimate contact with the membranous lining of the throat. It is not intended to act as a protective covering to the membrane and therefore oily substances requiring suspending agents, and drugs of a mucilaginous nature, should not be used.

Containers. Gargles should be dispensed in white fluted bottles and labelled in a manner which clearly distinguishes them from preparations intended for internal administration, except when directed to be swallowed after gargling, in which case they should be dispensed in bottles similar to those used for mixtures; if the gargle needs protection from light, the bottle should be coloured.

Labelling. Directions for diluting the gargle should be given on the label.

Phenol Gargle

SYNONYM: Carbolic Acid Gargle

Phenol Glycerin ..	..	..	50 ml
Amaranth Solution	..	..	10 ml
Water (see page 642)	..	.. to	1000 ml

Standard
CONTENT OF PHENOL. 0·84 to 1·13 per cent w/v, calculated as C_6H_6O, determined by the following method:
Dilute 5 ml with 25 ml of water in a glass-stoppered flask, add 50 ml of 0·1N bromine and 5 ml of *hydrochloric acid*, shake repeatedly during 15 minutes, allow to stand for 15 minutes, add 10 ml of *potassium iodide solution*, and immediately titrate the liberated iodine with 0·1N sodium thiosulphate until only a faint yellow colour remains; add a few drops of *starch mucilage* and 10 ml of *chloroform* and complete the titration with vigorous shaking.
Repeat the procedure omitting the sample.
The difference between the two titrations represents the amount of bromine required by the sample; each ml of 0·1N bromine is equivalent to 0·001569 g of C_6H_6O.

Containers; Labelling. The directions given under Gargles (above) should be followed.

Note. Phenol Gargle should be diluted with an equal volume of warm water before use.

Potassium Chlorate and Phenol Gargle

Potassium Chlorate	..	..	.. 30 g
Patent Blue V (Colour Index No. 42051), food grade of commerce			0·01 g
Liquefied Phenol..	..	..	15 ml
Water (see page 642)	..	.. to	1000 ml

Standard
CONTENT OF POTASSIUM CHLORATE. 2·85 to 3·15 per cent w/v, calculated as $KClO_3$, determined by the following method:
Evaporate 5 ml to dryness on a water-bath; dissolve the residue in 10 ml of water, add 10 ml of *dilute nitric acid* and 5 ml of *formaldehyde solution*, heat to boiling, cool, and complete the determination by the method given in Appendix 11, page 891.
Repeat the procedure omitting the sample.

The difference between the two titrations represents the amount of silver nitrate required by the sample; each ml of 0·1N silver nitrate is equivalent to 0·01226 g of $KClO_3$.

CONTENT OF PHENOL. 1·10 to 1·40 per cent w/v, calculated as C_6H_6O, determined by the following method:
Dilute 2 ml with 120 ml of water in a glass-stoppered flask, add 30 ml of 0·1N bromine and 15 ml of *hydrochloric acid* diluted with 20 ml of water, shake repeatedly during 15 minutes, allow to stand for 15 minutes, add 10 ml of *potassium iodide solution* and 10 ml of *chloroform*, and immediately titrate the liberated iodine with 0·1N sodium thiosulphate until only a faint yellow colour remains in the aqueous layer;

add a few drops of *starch mucilage* and complete the titration with vigorous shaking.
Repeat the procedure omitting the sample.
The difference between the two titrations represents the amount of bromine required by the sample; each ml of 0·1N bromine is equivalent to 0·001569 g of C_6H_6O.

Containers; Labelling. The directions given under Gargles (page 700) should be followed.

Storage. It should be protected from light.

Note. Potassium Chlorate and Phenol Gargle should be diluted with ten times its volume of warm water before use.

GELS

Gels are semi-solid aqueous preparations, prepared with the aid of a suitable gelling agent such as gelatin, tragacanth, gelatinised starch, or a cellulose derivative.

Lignocaine Gel

SYNONYM: Lignocaine Hydrochloride Gel

Lignocaine Gel is a solution of Lignocaine Hydrochloride in a suitable water-miscible basis containing chlorhexidine gluconate, or a mixture of the sodium salts of methyl hydroxybenzoate and propyl hydroxybenzoate, as the preservative. It is sterilised by autoclaving (see Appendix 29, page 921).

Standard
PRESENCE OF LIGNOCAINE HYDROCHLORIDE. 1. Disperse an amount equivalent to about 0·1 g in water, make alkaline with *sodium hydroxide solution*, filter, wash the filter with water, dissolve the residue on the filter in 1 ml of *alcohol (95 per cent)*, add 0·5 ml of a 10 per cent w/v solution of *cobalt chloride* in water, and shake for 2 minutes; a bluish-green precipitate is produced.
2. When dispersed in water it gives the reactions characteristic of chlorides.

STERILITY. It complies with the test for sterility.

CONTENT OF LIGNOCAINE HYDROCHLORIDE. 95·0 to 108·0 per cent of the prescribed or stated amount, calculated as $C_{14}H_{23}ClN_2O$ or $C_{14}H_{23}ClN_2O,H_2O$, determined by the following method:
Disperse an accurately weighed quantity, equivalent to about 0·01 g of lignocaine hydrochloride, in 20 ml of water, add 5 ml of *acetate buffer solution pH 2·8*, 120 ml of *chloroform*, and 5 ml of *dimethyl yellow–oracet blue B solution*, and titrate with 0·005M dioctyl sodium sulphosuccinate, with vigorous swirling, until near

the end-point; then add the titrant dropwise and, after each addition, swirl vigorously, allow to separate, and gently swirl for 5 seconds; the end-point is indicated when the colour of the chloroform layer changes from green to pinkish-grey.
Repeat the procedure omitting the sample.
The difference between the two titrations represents the amount of dioctyl sodium sulphosuccinate required by the sample; each ml of 0·005M dioctyl sodium sulphosuccinate is equivalent to 0·001354 g of $C_{14}H_{23}ClN_2O$ or 0·001444 g of $C_{14}H_{23}ClN_2O,H_2O$.
Assuming the weight per ml of the gel to be 1·02 g, calculate the concentration of $C_{14}H_{23}ClN_2O$ or $C_{14}H_{23}ClN_2O,H_2O$, weight in volume.

Containers. It should be packed in collapsible tubes of suitable metal or plastic material. If metal tubes of capacity 7·5 g or less are used they should comply with British Standard 4230:1967.
All containers should be as free as possible, consistent with good manufacturing practice, from dirt and particles of the material used in their construction.
Tubes and screw caps, complete with wads if used, must be sterilised before use; the wads should not be of cork.
The screw caps should be covered with a readily breakable seal or, alternatively, the tube should be enclosed in a sealed package from which the tube cannot be removed without breaking the seal; suitable outer packages include paperboard cartons with sealed flaps and sealed pouches of paper, plastic, or cellulose film.

Note. When the strength of the gel is not specified, a gel containing the equivalent of 2·0 per cent w/v of anhydrous lignocaine hydrochloride shall be supplied.

GLYCERINS

Glycerins consist of solutions of medicinal substances in glycerol, with or without the addition of water.

Ichthammol Glycerin

SYNONYM: Glycerin of Ammonium Ichthosulphonate

Ichthammol	..	..	..	100 g
Glycerol	..	..	..	900 g

Phenol Glycerin

Phenol	..	..	..	160 g
Glycerol	..	..	..	840 g

Dissolve the phenol in the glycerol, with the aid of gentle heat if necessary.

Standard

CONTENT OF PHENOL. 15·0 to 16·5 per cent w/w, calculated as C_6H_6O, determined by the following method:

To about 0·3 g, accurately weighed, in a glass-stoppered flask, add 25 ml of water and 50 ml of 0·1N bromine, followed by 5 ml of *hydrochloric acid*; shake repeatedly during 15 minutes, allow to stand for 15 minutes, add 10 ml of *potassium iodide solution*, and immediately titrate the liberated iodine with 0·1N sodium thiosulphate.

Repeat the procedure omitting the sample.

The difference between the two titrations represents the amount of bromine required by the sample; each ml of 0·1N bromine is equivalent to 0·001569 g of C_6H_6O.

Storage. It should be stored in airtight containers.

Caution. *Dilution with water renders Phenol Glycerin caustic; the preparation may be diluted with Glycerol, if desired.*

Thymol Glycerin, Compound

Thymol	0·5 g
Glycerol	100 ml
Carmine	0·3 g
Menthol	0·3 g
Sodium Metabisulphite	0·35 g
Sodium Salicylate	5·2 g
Sodium Benzoate	8·0 g
Sodium Bicarbonate	10·0 g
Borax	20·0 g
Methyl Salicylate	0·3 ml
Pumilio Pine Oil	0·5 ml
Dilute Ammonia Solution ..	0·75 ml
Cineole	1·3 ml
Alcohol (90 per cent) ..	25 ml
Water (see page 642) .. .. to	1000 ml

Dissolve the salts in 800 ml of the water and add the glycerol; dissolve the menthol, the thymol, the cineole, the methyl salicylate, and the pumilio pine oil in the alcohol, triturate with 25 g of sterilised Purified Talc or Kaolin, add the mixture gradually to the solution of the salts, and filter. Dissolve the carmine by stirring it into the dilute ammonia solution, warm gently to dissipate most of the ammonia, mix the two solutions, add sufficient water to produce the required volume, and mix.

In making this preparation the alcohol (90 per cent) may be replaced by Industrial Methylated Spirit diluted so as to be of equivalent alcoholic strength, provided that the law and the statutory regulations governing the use of industrial methylated spirit are observed.

Standard

WEIGHT PER ML. At 20°, 1·04 g to 1·05 g.

Storage. It should be protected from light.

Note. For use as a gargle or mouth-wash it should be diluted with about three times its volume of warm water. Diluted solutions should be used immediately and any unused portion discarded.

Tannic Acid Glycerin

Tannic Acid	150 g
Glycerol	850 g

Triturate the tannic acid with the glycerol and warm gently until solution is effected.

Standard

PRESENCE OF TANNIC ACID. Dilute with water and add *ferric chloride test-solution*; a bluish-black colour is produced. Add *dilute sulphuric acid*; the black colour disappears and a yellowish-brown precipitate is formed.

REFRACTIVE INDEX. At 20°, 1·487 to 1·498.

WEIGHT PER ML. At 20°, 1·288 g to 1·298 g.

Storage. It should be stored in airtight containers.

GRANULES

Granules are preparations of medicinal substances usually in the form of small irregular particles ranging from 2 to 4 millimetres in diameter.

Bephenium Granules

Bephenium Granules consist of Bephenium Hydroxynaphthoate with Starch and appropriate pharmaceutical adjuvants.

Standard

PRESENCE OF BEPHENIUM HYDROXYNAPHTHOATE. Shake an amount equivalent to about 0·2 of bephenium with 10 ml of warm *alcohol (95 per cent)*, cool, and filter; the filtrate complies with tests 1 and 2 given for Bephenium Hydroxynaphthoate, page 53.

SUSPENSION TEST. Stir 5 g with 50 ml of water; the granules are readily wetted and form a uniform suspension.

CONTENT OF BEPHENIUM. 97·5 to 107·5 per cent of the amount stated on the label, calculated as $C_{17}H_{22}NO$, determined by Method I of the British Pharmacopoeia for non-aqueous titration, about 1 g of the previously dried material, accurately weighed, being used; each ml of 0·1N perchloric acid is equivalent to 0·02564 g of $C_{17}H_{22}NO$.

Storage. They should be stored in well-filled airtight containers, in a cool place.

Dose. The equivalent of bephenium:

ADULT. 2·5 grams.

CHILD. Up to 2 years, 1·25 grams; 2 to 12 years, 2·5 grams.

When the quantity to be supplied is not specified, sachets each containing 5 g of granules, equivalent to 2·5 g of bephenium, shall be supplied.

Methylcellulose Granules

Methylcellulose 2500 or 4500, in powder	64·0 g
Amaranth, food grade of commerce	0·02 g
Saccharin Sodium	0·1 g
Vanillin	0·2 g
Acacia, powdered	4·0 g
Lactose	31·68 g

Mix the powdered ingredients, add sufficient Water (page 642) to form a coherent mass suitable for granulation, and pass through a No. 2·80 sieve; place the granules upon a No. 710 sieve and discard the powder which passes through. Dry the granules at a temperature not exceeding 60°.

Standard
VISCOSITY OF AQUEOUS SOLUTION. Not less than 2000 centistokes, determined by the following method:
Transfer 3·25 g to a wide-mouthed bottle, add 100 ml of water previously heated to 85° to 90°, close the bottle with a stopper fitted with a stirrer, and stir for 10 minutes; place the bottle in an ice-bath, continue stirring until the solution is of uniform consistence, remove the bottle from the ice-bath and allow the solution to attain room temperature.
Determine the viscosity of this solution by the method of the British Pharmacopoeia, Appendix IVH, for the determination of viscosity of Methylcellulose, using a suspended-level viscometer with capillary diameter of 3·70 ± 0·04 mm.

Containers and storage. They should be stored in airtight containers.
They should preferably be stored and supplied in wide-mouthed glass or plastic containers or in lined aluminium containers closed with lined screw caps or plastic caps.

Dose. As a laxative, 1·5 to 6 grams.

Sodium Aminosalicylate and Isoniazid Granules

Sodium Aminosalicylate and Isoniazid Granules are prepared by incorporating Sodium Aminosalicylate, with Isoniazid, in a suitable basis and granulating the product. The granules may be coated and the coating may be coloured.

Standard
3-AMINOPHENOL. It complies with the thin-layer chromatographic test given in Appendix 5A, page 868 (0·3 per cent).

CONTENT OF ISONIAZID. 90·0 to 110·0 per cent of the prescribed or stated amount, determined by the following method:
Shake an accurately weighed quantity of the powdered granules, equivalent to about 0·05 g of isoniazid, with 150 ml of water, dilute to 1000 ml with water, filter, rejecting the first 20 ml of the filtrate, and continue by the method for isoniazid in Sodium Aminosalicylate and Isoniazid Cachets, page 650, beginning with the words "To three 20-ml graduated flasks . . .".
Calculate the percentage of isoniazid in the sample.

CONTENT OF SODIUM AMINOSALICYLATE. 95·0 to 105·0 per cent of the prescribed or stated amount, calculated as $C_7H_6NNaO_3,2H_2O$, determined by the following method:
Shake an accurately weighed quantity of the powdered granules, equivalent to about 0·5 g of sodium aminosalicylate, with 150 ml of water, dilute to 250 ml with water, filter, rejecting the first 20 ml of filtrate, and continue by the method for sodium aminosalicylate in Sodium Aminosalicylate and Isoniazid Cachets, page 650, beginning with the words "To 25 ml of this solution . . .".
Calculate the percentage of sodium aminosalicylate in the sample.

Storage. They should be stored in airtight containers, protected from light, in a cool place.

Dose. Daily, in divided doses: sodium aminosalicylate, 10 to 20 grams; isoniazid, 200 to 300 milligrams.

When the quantity to be supplied is not specified, sachets each containing 6 g of sodium aminosalicylate with 150 mg of isoniazid shall be supplied.
Sachets containing 12 g of sodium aminosalicylate with 300 mg of isoniazid, and 2 g of sodium aminosalicylate with 50 mg of isoniazid, are also available.

INFUSIONS

Infusions are dilute solutions containing the readily soluble constituents of crude drugs. Formerly, fresh infusions, prepared by macerating the drug for a short period in cold or boiling water, were used. Now, infusions are usually prepared by diluting one volume of a concentrated infusion to ten volumes with water; concentrated infusions that were omitted from the B.P. and B.P.C. subsequent to 1963 are still diluted to eight volumes with water, because they were not reformulated for the 1968 editions.

Infusions are liable to fungous and bacterial growth, and it is necessary to dispense them within twelve hours of their preparation.

Preparation of infusions. *Concentrated infusions* that are the subjects of the following monographs are prepared on a small scale by the methods described in the specific monographs. When they are manufactured in larger quantities, the same method, appropriately scaled up, is used; alternatively, for certain concentrated infusions, they may be prepared by the alternative method described for liquid extracts (page 681).

Details of a method for preparing *fresh infusions* were given in the British Pharmaceutical Codex 1949.

Orange Peel Infusion, Concentrated

SYNONYM: Infusum Aurantii Concentratum

Dried Bitter-orange Peel, cut				
small	..	..	..	500 g
Alcohol (25 per cent)	..		..	1350 ml

Macerate the dried bitter-orange peel in 1000 ml of the alcohol in a covered vessel for forty-eight hours and press out the liquid. To the marc, add the remainder of the alcohol, macerate for twenty-four hours, press out the liquid, and add it to the product of the first pressing. Allow the mixed liquids to stand for not less than fourteen days and filter.

Standard

WEIGHT PER ML. At 20°, 1·01 g to 1·04 g.

ALCOHOL CONTENT. 18 to 23 per cent v/v of ethyl alcohol, determined by the method given in Appendix 10, page 888.

TOTAL SOLIDS. 10 to 15 per cent w/v, determined on 1 ml.

Dose. 2·5 to 5 millilitres.

Orange Peel Infusion is prepared by diluting one volume of Concentrated Orange Peel Infusion to ten volumes with water.

Senega Infusion, Concentrated

Small-scale preparation

Senega, in coarse powder	..	500 g
Dilute Ammonia Solution		
	a sufficient quantity	
Alcohol (25 per cent)	..	.. to 1000 ml

Extract the senega with the alcohol by percolation, reserving the first 750 ml of percolate. Continue percolation until a further 1000 ml has been collected, evaporate to a syrupy consistence, dissolve the residue in the reserved portion, gradually add dilute ammonia solution until the product is faintly alkaline, add sufficient of the alcohol to produce the required volume, and mix. Allow to stand for not less than fourteen days and filter.

Manufacture. Prepare the infusion by the above method, appropriately scaled up, or by the alternative method described for liquid extracts (page 681).

Standard

WEIGHT PER ML. At 20°, 1·01 g to 1·03 g.

ALCOHOL CONTENT. 19 to 23 per cent v/v of ethyl alcohol, determined by the method given in Appendix 10, page 888.

TOTAL SOLIDS. 10 to 13 per cent w/v, determined on 1 ml.

Dose. 2·5 to 5 millilitres.

Senega Infusion is prepared by diluting one volume of Concentrated Senega Infusion to ten volumes with water.

INHALATIONS

Inhalations are liquid preparations composed of or containing volatile ingredients which, when vaporised in a suitable manner, are intended to be brought into contact with the lining of the respiratory tract. The ingredients may be volatile at room temperature, in which case they may be inhaled from an absorbent pad on which they have been placed, or they may require to be added to water at about 65°, but not boiling water, and the vapour inhaled for five to ten minutes. Inhalations intended to be added to hot water may consist of alcoholic solutions or of mixtures with water to which a diffusing agent such as light magnesium carbonate has been added.

Containers. Inhalations should be dispensed in white fluted bottles.

Labelling. When an inhalation containing an insoluble diffusing agent is dispensed, a direction to shake the bottle before use should be given on the label.

Benzoin Inhalation

Benzoin, crushed..	..	..	100 g
Prepared Storax ..	..	..	50 g
Alcohol (95 per cent)	..	.. to 1000 ml

Macerate the benzoin and the prepared storax with 750 ml of the alcohol for twenty-four hours. Filter and pass sufficient of the alcohol through the filter to produce the required volume.

In making this preparation, the alcohol (95 per cent) may be replaced by Industrial Methylated Spirit, provided that the law and the statutory regulations governing the use of industrial methylated spirit are observed.

Standard
TOTAL SOLIDS. 9·0 to 12·0 per cent w/v, determined on 2 ml.

CONTENT OF TOTAL BALSAMIC ACIDS. Not less than 3·0 per cent w/v, calculated as cinnamic acid, $C_9H_8O_2$, determined by the following method:
Boil 10 ml with 25 ml of 0·5N alcoholic potassium hydroxide under a reflux condenser for $1\frac{1}{4}$ hours, evaporate off the alcohol, and diffuse the residue by warming with 50 ml of hot water; cool, add 80 ml of water and 50 ml of a 4·0 per cent w/v solution of *magnesium sulphate* in water, and continue by the method for Benzoin, page 49, beginning with the words "mix thoroughly . . .".

Menthol and Benzoin Inhalation

Menthol ..	..	..	..	20 g
Benzoin Inhalation	..	.. to 1000 ml

Standard
TOTAL SOLIDS. 9·0 to 12·0 per cent w/v, determined on 2 ml.

CONTENT OF TOTAL BALSAMIC ACIDS. Not less than 2·8 per cent w/v, calculated as cinnamic acid, $C_9H_8O_2$, determined by the method for Benzoin Inhalation.

Menthol and Eucalyptus Inhalation

Menthol ..	..	..	..	20 g
Eucalyptus Oil	..	..	..	100 ml
Light Magnesium Carbonate	..	70 g
Water (see page 642)	..	.. to 1000 ml

Dissolve the menthol in the eucalyptus oil and add the light magnesium carbonate and sufficient water to produce the required volume.

Standard
TOTAL OIL. 10·3 to 12·7 per cent v/v, determined by the method of the British Pharmacopoeia, Appendix IXE, for the determination of volatile oil in drugs, Method I, 25 ml, thoroughly mixed, being used.

Labelling. The directions given under Inhalations (page 704) should be followed.

INJECTIONS

Injections are sterile solutions or suspensions intended for parenteral administration. They are used to administer drugs which may be therapeutically inactive or not tolerated when given by mouth, to produce a rapid, localised, or prolonged action, or for diagnostic purposes.

Preparation of injections

Sterilisation of solutions and suspensions is described in Appendix 29 (page 925), where also are described methods for sterilising apparatus, containers, and closures. The methods suitable for a particular injection are given in the individual monograph.

> NOTE: *If an emergency precludes the application of a specified method of sterilisation to a substance or preparation, it is the duty of the pharmacist to obtain the prescriber's approval for any other course taken.*

Water for Injections may be replaced by unsterilised water prepared freshly by the method for preparing Water for Injections, provided that the injection is sterilised immediately after preparation. When an injection is required to be prepared with Water for Injections free from dissolved air or carbon dioxide, freshly prepared Water for Injections is used. It is boiled for ten minutes, cooled, and used to prepare the injection, precautions being taken to exclude air or carbon dioxide during preparation.

Addition of bactericides. Injections supplied in multiple-dose containers should contain a bactericide in a concentration sufficient to prevent the development of micro-organisms, unless the medicament itself is sufficiently bactericidal. Provided there is no therapeutic or chemical incompatibility with the ingredients of the injection, suitable bactericides and their concentrations for aqueous preparations are phenol 0·5 per cent w/v, cresol 0·3 per cent w/v, chlorbutol 0·5 per cent w/v, chlorocresol 0·1 per cent w/v, and phenylmercuric acetate or nitrate 0·001 per cent w/v; any other substance used must have a bactericidal activity at least equivalent to that of a 0·5 per cent w/v aqueous solution of phenol. Bactericides are included in oily preparations in multiple-dose containers and afford some protection against contamination with vegetative micro-organisms, but are ineffective against sporing organisms; suitable bactericides and their concentrations are phenol 0·5 per cent w/v, cresol 0·3 per cent w/v, and chlorocresol 0·1 per cent w/v.

Unstable injections. Injections of medicaments which are unstable in solution are prepared by dissolving or suspending the sterile drug in the required amount of vehicle by means of an aseptic technique. The volume of injection so prepared should be sufficient to ensure that the required volume of a solution of the correct strength can be withdrawn.

Isotonic solutions. Sodium chloride, or other suitable substance, should be added to an aqueous injection, if necessary, to make it isotonic and so decrease the discomfort for the patient. Methods for calculating the strengths of solutions of various substances isotonic with blood serum are given in Appendix 30 (page 927).

Classification of injections

Injections may be classified according to their route of administration.

GENERAL INJECTIONS

Intradermal or *intracutaneous injections* are usually aqueous solutions or suspensions used for diagnostic purposes; the volume injected is about 0·1 to 0·2 millilitre.

Subcutaneous or *hypodermic injections* are usually aqueous isotonic solutions of such a strength that the volume to be injected does not normally exceed 1 millilitre. Sometimes a vasoconstrictor such as adrenaline is added to localise the action of the drug, e.g., local anaesthetics. When intravenous infusion is contra-indicated, 3 to 4 litres of fluid per day may be given by the subcutaneous route if hyaluronidase is added to the injection, or given separately, to facilitate absorption; this procedure is known as hypodermoclysis.

Intramuscular injections are aqueous or oily solutions or suspensions. The volume injected at any one site should not exceed 4 millilitres. Intramuscular injections, unless of small volume, cause considerable pain if they are given rapidly.

Intravascular injections include both intravenous and intra-arterial injections.

Intravenous injections are usually aqueous solutions; they may contain a proportion of a non-irritant water-miscible liquid. Large volume injections are termed *intravenous infusions.* Oil-in-water emulsions may be administered intravenously if careful control is exercised over globule size. Preparations in which the continuous phase is an oil must not be given by this route. The injections are usually given in volumes of 1 to 10 millilitres, or in large volumes by infusion. If the single-dose volume is greater than 15 millilitres, the injections must not contain an added bactericide and, if greater than 10 millilitres, should be free from pyrogens.

Intra-arterial injections are similar to intravenous injections and may be used when an immediate action is required in a peripheral area. They must not contain an added bactericide.

Intracardiac injections are aqueous solutions for use in emergency treatment only and are injected into the cardiac muscle or ventricle. They must not contain an added bactericide.

Intrathecal or *subarachnoid, intracisternal,* and *peridural injections* are aqueous solutions; the volume injected does not normally exceed 20 millilitres. They must not contain a bactericide and must be dispensed in single-dose containers. The weight per ml may be adjusted by the addition of suitable substances to localise the action of the medicament.

Intra-articular injections are aqueous solutions or suspensions which are injected into the synovial fluid in a joint cavity.

Intrabursal injections are similar to intra-articular injections and are usually injected into the subacromial or the olecranon bursa.

OPHTHALMIC INJECTIONS

Subconjunctival injections are aqueous solutions or suspensions. The quantity of a soluble drug which can be administered by this route is limited by its solubility, as normally not more than 1 millilitre of solution can be injected.

Intracameral injections are made into the anterior chamber and are used in surgery to increase the volume of the chamber, to produce miosis, and for zonulysis. The injection of antibiotics by this route is rarely justified, as they can be given satisfactorily by the subconjunctival route.

Intravitreous injections are used to increase the volume of the vitreous chamber.

Retrobulbar injections are used to produce anaesthesia of the globe and akinesia of the extra-ocular muscles.

Standard

Dry Powders

UNIFORMITY OF WEIGHT AND COMPOSITION. The contents of the containers comply with the requirements of the British Pharmacopoeia for uniformity of weight for Injections; it is specified in the individual monographs whether Method A or Method B is to be used. When Method A is specified in the monograph, the mixed contents of the 10 containers also comply with the standard for the medicament given in the British Pharmacopoeia or in Part I of the British Pharmaceutical Codex.

STERILITY. The contents comply with the test for sterility.

Solvent

When the solvent to be used in the preparation of an injection from a dry powder is supplied, the contents of the solvent container comply with the following requirements:

VOLUME. 100 to 110 per cent of the volume stated on the label or on any leaflet, determined by the following method:

Check, by visual inspection, that the volume in each of 10 containers is approximately the same. Select a syringe with a capacity not exceeding twice the volume stated on the label of the container and fitted with an appropriate needle. Take up into the syringe a small quantity of water, and discharge it from the syringe with the needle pointing upwards so as to expel any air bubbles, leaving the needle full of water. Use this prepared syringe to transfer the solvent from each of the 10 containers to a graduated cylinder whose capacity is such that the total volume to be determined occupies not less than 50 per cent of its graduated volume. Measure the total volume of solvent collected from the 10 containers and divide by 10.

STERILITY. The contents comply with the test for sterility.

Liquids, Solutions, and Suspensions

VOLUME OF INJECTION. When the injection is supplied in single-dose containers, the volume in each container complies with the requirements of the British Pharmacopoeia for volume in single-dose containers for Injections.

For the purposes of this test, all injections of the British Pharmaceutical Codex are classified as mobile, with the exception of the viscous injection, Oily Phenol Injection, page 716.

PARTICULATE MATTER. Solutions to be injected should not contain particles of foreign matter that can readily be observed on visual inspection; in order to detect cellulosic material the solution should be examined in plane polarised light.

Where stated in the individual monograph, solutions for injection comply with the limit test for particulate matter given in the British Pharmacopoeia, Appendix XVIC.

STERILITY. The contents comply with the test for sterility.

Containers. Injections, or the sterile ingredients for the preparation of injections, should be supplied in single-dose or multiple-dose containers which are sealed to exclude micro-organisms. Containers are made of glass or suitable plastic material, and, where possible, single-dose containers sealed by fusion should be supplied. Multiple-dose containers usually consist of glass vials closed by rubber closures to permit the withdrawal of successive doses; they should not contain an excessive number of doses.

Glass containers comply with the requirements of the European Pharmacopoeia for Glass Containers for Injectable Preparations.

Plastic containers should be colourless and of sufficient clarity to permit inspection of the contents. The plastic material used should not yield more than a minimum of soluble matter. Additives in plastic materials such as stabilisers, antoxidants, plasticisers, and lubricants must not be toxic.

The rubber closures used with multiple-dose containers should be made from suitably compounded natural or synthetic rubber of good quality. They should be impregnated with any bactericide or preservative included in the injection, the procedure described in Appendix 29 (page 925) under the Sterilisation of Rubber and Plastics being used. The closures used for containers of oily injections should be made of oil-resistant material.

Large-volume injections are supplied in bottles complying with British Standard 2463: 1962, or in other appropriate glass or plastic bottles of a suitable standard.

Plastic containers of capacity 500 ml or more comply with the tests for metallic additives in plastic containers and the injections contained in them comply with the tests for toxicity and for ether-soluble extractive referred to in the British Pharmacopoeia under Injections.

Labelling. The label on the container states the strength of the injection as the amount of active ingredient in a suitable dose-volume.

The label on the container or the label on the package states:

(1) the name and proportion of any added bactericide;
(2) the name of any added buffering or stabilising agent;
(3) the date after which the preparation is not intended to be used; and
(4) the conditions under which it should be stored.

The label on the sealed container of a powdered medicament intended for the preparation of an injection states:

(1) the name of the medicament, followed by the words "for Injection";
(2) the nominal weight or number of units of medicament(s) in the container;
(3) the volume and composition of the solvent to be used;
(4) the concentration of medicament(s) in the solution when prepared as directed;
(5) the date after which the powder is not intended to be used; and
(6) the conditions under which the powder should be stored.

The label on the container of solvent to be used with the powdered medicament states the volume and composition of the solvent.

The label on the sealed container of powdered medicament or the label on the carton states:

(1) the name and proportion of any added bactericide;
(2) the name of any added buffering or stabilising agent;
(3) directions for preparing the injection;
(4) the conditions under which the injection should be stored; and
(5) the period during which the injection may be expected to be suitable for use when stored under the stated conditions.

Ascorbic Acid Injection

Ascorbic Acid	..	..	..	10·0 g
Sodium Bicarbonate	..	..	4·8 g
Water for Injections	..	..	to 100 ml

Dissolve, and sterilise the solution by filtration (see Appendix 29, page 923); distribute, by means of an aseptic technique, into sterile ampoules, replace the air in the ampoules by sterile nitrogen or other suitable gas, and seal.

Standard
It complies with the standard under Injections, above, with the following additions:

ACIDITY. pH, 5·0 to 6·5.

CONTENT OF ASCORBIC ACID. 8·8 to 10·5 per cent w/v, calculated as $C_6H_8O_6$, determined by the following method:
To 2 ml add 5 ml of *dilute sulphuric acid* and titrate with 0·1N iodine, using *starch mucilage* as indicator;

each ml of 0·1N iodine is equivalent to 0·008806 g of $C_6H_8O_6$.

Containers. The directions given under Injections (above) should be followed. The injection should be supplied in single-dose ampoules.

Labelling. The directions given under Injections (above) should be followed.

Storage. It should be protected from light.

Dose. Therapeutic, 2 to 6 millilitres daily.

Benethamine Penicillin Injection, Fortified

SYNONYMS: Benethamine Penicillin with Benzylpenicillin Sodium and Procaine Penicillin Injection; Triple Penicillin Injection

Fortified Benethamine Penicillin Injection is a sterile suspension of Benethamine Penicillin and Procaine Penicillin, with appropriate pharmaceutical adjuvants, in a solution of Benzylpenicillin Sodium in Water for Injections.

It is prepared by adding Water for Injections to the contents of a sealed container shortly before use.

Standard
The contents of the sealed container comply with the standard under Injections, page 707; Method B is used in the test for uniformity of weight and composition.

CONTENT OF BENZYLPENICILLIN SODIUM. 95.0 to 130.0 per cent of the amount stated on the label, calculated as $C_{16}H_{17}N_2NaO_4S$, determined by the following method:
To about 4 g, accurately weighed, add about 4 g of water, accurately weighed, mix, and centrifuge until a clear supernatant liquid is obtained; dilute about 0.6 g of the supernatant liquid, accurately weighed, to 100 ml with water, and continue by the method given for total penicillins in Phenoxymethylpenicillin Elixir, page 675, beginning with the words "transfer 10 ml to a stoppered flask...", and using *benzylpenicillin sodium B.C.R.S.* in place of phenoxymethylpenicillin potassium B.C.R.S.; each mg of *benzylpenicillin sodium B.C.R.S.* is equivalent to 1.000 mg of $C_{16}H_{17}N_2NaO_4S$.
The content of benzylpenicillin sodium is given by the formula:

$$\frac{100DH\left[A\left(\dfrac{100-X-Y}{100}\right)+B\right]}{ACK}$$

Where A = weight, in g, of sample taken,
B = weight, in g, of water added,
C = weight, in g, of the supernatant liquid taken for the determination,
D = weight, in g, of $C_{16}H_{17}N_2NaO_4S$ in 100 ml of the reference solution,
H = the volume, in ml, of 0.02N iodine equivalent to the total penicillins present in the sample solution,
K = the volume, in ml, of 0.02N iodine equivalent to the $C_{16}H_{17}N_2NaO_4S$ present in the reference solution,
X = the percentage of procaine penicillin in the sample as determined by the method given below, and
Y = the percentage of benethamine penicillin in the sample as determined by the method given below.

CONTENT OF PROCAINE PENICILLIN. 95.0 to 125.0 per cent of the amount stated on the label, determined by the following method:
Mix about 1 g, accurately weighed, with about 100 ml of water, dilute to 200 ml with water, mix well, and filter; dilute 5 ml of the filtrate to 250 ml with *phosphate buffer solution pH 7.0*, and measure the extinction of a 1-cm layer at the maximum at about 290 nm, using *phosphate buffer solution pH 7.0* as a blank.
For purposes of calculation, use a value of 310 for the E(1 per cent, 1 cm) of procaine penicillin.

CONTENT OF BENETHAMINE PENICILLIN. 95.0 to 125.0 per cent of the amount stated on the label, calculated as $C_{31}H_{35}N_3O_4S$, determined by the following method:
Determine the apparent content of $C_{31}H_{35}N_3O_4S$ by the method given for content of $C_{15}H_{17}N$ under Benethamine Penicillin, page 44; each ml of 0.01N sulphuric acid is equivalent to 0.005457 g of $C_{31}H_{35}N_3O_4S$.
Calculate the content of procaine penicillin, as determined by the method given above, in the weight of sample used in this assay, multiply this content by a factor of 0.926, and deduct the figure from the apparent content of benethamine penicillin; the result is the content of benethamine penicillin.

CONTENT OF TOTAL PENICILLINS. 95.0 to 125.0 per cent of the amount stated on the label, calculated as $C_{16}H_{17}N_2NaO_4S$, determined by the following method:

Dissolve about 0.17 g, accurately weighed, in a mixture of 80 ml of water and 50 ml of 1N sodium hydroxide, dilute to 150 ml with water, mix, and allow to stand for 30 minutes; transfer 15 ml of this solution to a stoppered flask, add 20 ml of a freshly prepared buffer solution containing 5.44 per cent w/v of *sodium acetate* and 2.40 per cent w/v of *glacial acetic acid*, 5 ml of 1N hydrochloric acid, and 25 ml of 0.02N iodine, close the flask with a wet stopper, and allow to stand for 20 minutes, protected from light.
Titrate the excess of iodine with 0.02N sodium thiosulphate, using *starch mucilage*, added towards the end of the titration, as indicator.
Repeat the procedure using 0.017 g of the sample suspended in 15 ml of water, and beginning at the words "add 20 ml of a freshly prepared buffer solution..." but omitting the 5 ml of 1N hydrochloric acid.
The difference between the two titrations represents the volume of 0.02N iodine equivalent to the total penicillins in the sample.
Calculate the content of total penicillins from the difference obtained by repeating the procedure with *benzylpenicillin sodium B.C.R.S.* in place of the sample; each mg of *benzylpenicillin sodium B.C.R.S.* is equivalent to 1.000 mg of total penicillins, calculated as $C_{16}H_{17}N_2NaO_4S$.

In addition, the injection complies with the following requirement:

STABILITY. Using an aseptic technique, prepare the injection, as directed on the label, in an individual unopened container immediately before analysis, and determine the concentration of benzylpenicillin sodium in the injection by the method described above, using an accurately measured volume, withdrawn aseptically from the container.
Store the remainder of the injection in the closed container at $15° \pm 1°$ for 7 days and then repeat the determination of benzylpenicillin sodium.
The concentration of benzylpenicillin sodium in the stored injection is not less than 80 per cent of the concentration found in the freshly prepared injection.

Containers. The directions given under Injections (page 708) should be followed.

Labelling. The directions given under Injections (page 709) should be followed; the name on the label should be "Fortified Benethamine Penicillin for Injection".
In addition, the label on the sealed container should state that the contents are to be used for intramuscular injection only.

Storage. The injection contains no bactericide and the aseptic precautions taken in its preparation should be such that the microbiological quality is maintained if it is stored.
Chemical stability of the drug in aqueous solution is limited. The injection should therefore be used within seven days of its preparation when stored in a cool place, or within fourteen days provided that it is stored during this period at 2° to 10°; at temperatures approaching 20°, it should be used within four days.

Dose. A single dose of 1.2 mega Units by intramuscular injection, repeated if necessary every three or four days.

When the strength of the injection is not specified, vials containing 500,000 Units of benethamine penicillin, 500,000 Units of benzylpenicillin (sodium salt), and 250,000 Units of procaine penicillin shall be supplied.

Benzathine Penicillin Injection, Fortified

SYNONYM: Benzathine Penicillin with Benzylpenicillin Potassium and Procaine Penicillin Injection

Fortified Benzathine Penicillin Injection is a sterile suspension of Benzathine Penicillin and

Procaine Penicillin, with appropriate pharmaceutical adjuvants, in a solution of Benzylpenicillin Potassium in Water for Injections.
It is prepared by adding Water for Injections to the contents of a sealed container shortly before use.

Standard
The contents of the sealed container comply with the standard under Injections, page 707; Method B is used in the test for uniformity of weight and composition.

CONTENT OF BENZYLPENICILLIN POTASSIUM. 95·0 to 130·0 per cent of the amount stated on the label, calculated as $C_{16}H_{17}KN_2O_4S$, determined by the method given for benzylpenicillin sodium in Fortified Benethamine Penicillin Injection.
In the formula, D = the weight, in g, of $C_{16}H_{17}KN_2O_4S$ in 100 ml of the reference solution, calculated by assuming that each mg of *benzylpenicillin sodium B.C.R.S.* is equivalent to 1·045 mg of $C_{16}H_{17}KN_2O_4S$, K = the volume, in ml, of 0·02N iodine equivalent to the $C_{16}H_{17}KN_2O_4S$ in the reference solution, and Y = the percentage of benzathine penicillin in the sample as determined by the method given below.

CONTENT OF PROCAINE PENICILLIN. It complies with the requirement described under Fortified Benethamine Penicillin Injection.

CONTENT OF BENZATHINE PENICILLIN. 95·0 to 125·0 per cent of the amount stated on the label, calculated as $C_{48}H_{56}N_6O_8S_2$, determined by the following method: Determine the apparent benzathine penicillin content in the following manner: to about 1 g, accurately weighed, add 30 ml of *brine* and 10 ml of *sodium hydroxide solution*, shake vigorously, and extract with four successive 50-ml portions of *anaesthetic ether*; wash the combined ethereal extracts with three successive 5-ml portions of water, extracting each aqueous washing with the same 25 ml of *anaesthetic ether*. Combine the ethereal extracts, evaporate to low bulk, add 2 ml of *dehydrated alcohol*, evaporate to dryness, dissolve the residue in 50 ml of *glacial acetic acid*, and titrate with 0·1N perchloric acid, using *1-naphtholbenzein solution* as indicator; each ml of 0·1N perchloric acid is equivalent to 0·04545 g of $C_{48}H_{56}N_6O_8S_2$. Calculate the apparent content of benzathine penicillin.
Calculate the content of procaine penicillin, as determined by the method given above, in the weight of sample used in this assay, multiply this content by a factor of 1·544, and deduct the figure from the apparent content of benzathine penicillin; the result is the content of benzathine penicillin.

CONTENT OF TOTAL PENICILLINS. It complies with the requirement described under Fortified Benethamine Penicillin Injection, each mg of *benzylpenicillin sodium B.C.R.S.* is equivalent to 1·045 g of total penicillins, calculated as $C_{16}H_{17}KN_2O_4S$.

In addition, the injection complies with the following requirement:

STABILITY. Using an aseptic technique, prepare the injection, as directed on the label, in an individual unopened container immediately before analysis, and determine the concentration of benzylpenicillin potassium in the injection by the method described above, using an accurately measured volume, withdrawn aseptically from the container.
Store the remainder of the injection in the closed container at 2° to 4° for 7 days and then repeat the determination of benzylpenicillin potassium.
The concentration of benzylpenicillin potassium in the stored injection is not less than 80 per cent of the concentration found in the freshly prepared injection.

Containers. The directions given under Injections (page 708) should be followed.

Labelling. The directions given under Injections (page 709) should be followed; the name on the label should be "Fortified Benzathine Penicillin for Injection".

In addition, the label on the sealed container should state that the contents are to be used for intramuscular injection only.

Storage. The injection contains no bactericide and the aseptic precautions taken in its preparation should be such that the microbiological quality is maintained if it is stored.
Chemical stability of the drug in aqueous solution is limited. The injection should therefore be used immediately after preparation, or within seven days of its preparation provided that it is stored during this period at 2° to 4°.

Dose. A single dose of 0·9 to 1·2 mega Units by deep intramuscular injection, repeated if necessary every two or three days.

When the strength of the injection is not specified, vials containing 600,000 Units of benzathine penicillin, 300,000 Units of benzylpenicillin potassium, and 300,000 Units of procaine penicillin shall be supplied.

Calciferol Injection

Calciferol ..	..	..	..	0·75 g
Ethyl Oleate, peroxide-free		..	to 100 ml

The ethyl oleate used should not require more than 0·15 ml of 0·01N sodium thiosulphate when subjected to the B.P. limit test for peroxides in ethyl oleate. In addition, it should not darken in colour significantly when heated at 150° for one hour.

Dissolve, and sterilise the solution by filtration (see Appendix 29, page 923). Alternatively, sterilise sufficient of the ethyl oleate by dry heat (see Appendix 29, page 921), and allow to cool; by means of an aseptic technique, dissolve the calciferol in the bulk of the cold sterile ethyl oleate and add sufficient of the ethyl oleate to produce the required volume.

By means of an aseptic technique, distribute the sterile solution into sterile ampoules, replace the air in the ampoules with sterile nitrogen or other suitable gas, and seal.

Standard
It complies with the standard under Injections, page 707, with the following additions:

DESCRIPTION. A pale yellow oily liquid.

CONTENT OF CALCIFEROL. 0·67 to 0·83 per cent w/v, determined by the following method:
Carry out the operations in subdued light. Dilute about 0·1 g, accurately weighed, to 50 ml with dry *ethylene chloride* which has been purified by passing it down a column of *anhydrous silica gel*.
To 1 ml of this solution add rapidly 9·0 ml of *antimony trichloride solution in ethylene chloride* and, $1\frac{1}{2}$ to 2 minutes after the addition of the reagent, measure the extinctions of a 1-cm layer at 500 and 550 nm.
Repeat the procedure using 1 ml of a 0·002 per cent w/v solution of *calciferol* in dry *ethylene chloride*, purified as described above, in place of the sample solution.
From the difference between the extinctions at 500 and 550 nm of the sample and of the standard, calculate the concentration of calciferol in the sample.
Assuming the weight per ml of the injection to be 0·87 g, calculate the concentration of calciferol, weight in volume.

Containers. The directions given under Injections (page 708) should be followed. The injection should be supplied in single-dose ampoules.

Labelling. The directions given under Injections (page 709) should be followed.

Storage. It should be stored in a cool place and protected from light.

Dose. In the treatment of vitamin-D-deficiency rickets 1 ml by intramuscular injection, as a single dose.

Calciferol Injection contains, in 1 ml, 300,000 Units of antirachitic activity (vitamin D).

Chloramphenicol Sodium Succinate Injection

Chloramphenicol Sodium Succinate Injection is a sterile solution of Chloramphenicol Sodium Succinate in Water for Injections, in Sodium Chloride Injection, or in Dextrose Injection (5 per cent).

It is prepared by dissolving the contents of a sealed container in the vehicle shortly before use.

Standard
UNIFORMITY OF WEIGHT AND COMPOSITION. The contents of the sealed container comply with the requirements for Chloramphenicol Sodium Succinate, page 95.

Determine the weight of the contents of 10 containers by Method A of the British Pharmacopoeia for uniformity of weight for Injections. From the result of the determination of the content of chloramphenicol sodium succinate, calculate the weight of chloramphenicol in each container; each g of chloramphenicol sodium succinate is equivalent to 0·7257 g of chloramphenicol.

The weight of chloramphenicol in each container complies with the standard for uniformity of weight, Method A, described in the British Pharmacopoeia.

STERILITY. It complies with the test for sterility.

Containers; Labelling. The directions given under Injections (page 708) should be followed.

Storage. It should be protected from light.

The injection contains no bactericide and the aseptic precautions taken in its preparation should be such that the microbiological quality is maintained if it is stored.

Chemical stability of the drug in aqueous solution is limited. The injection should therefore be used within one month of its preparation when stored at room temperature.

Dose. The equivalent of chloramphenicol, by subcutaneous, intramuscular, or intravenous injection:

ADULT. 1 gram every six to eight hours.

CHILD. 50 milligrams per kilogram bodyweight daily, in divided doses.

Higher doses may be necessary for severe infections.

PREMATURE INFANTS. 25 milligrams per kilogram body-weight daily in four equal doses at six-hourly intervals. These doses should not normally be exceeded.

Vials containing the equivalent of 250 mg and 1 g of chloramphenicol are available.

Corticotrophin Carboxymethylcellulose Injection

SYNONYM: Corticotrophin CMC Injection

Corticotrophin Carboxymethylcellulose Injection is a sterile solution of Corticotrophin as the carboxymethylcellulose complex in Water for Injections. The solution is rendered isotonic with blood serum by the addition of dextrose. It is sterilised by filtration.

Standard
It complies with the standard under Injections, page 707, with the following additions:

DESCRIPTION. A clear, colourless, slightly viscous liquid which does not solidify when cooled to a temperature between 0° and 10°.

ACIDITY. pH, 4·5 to 6·5.

UNDUE TOXICITY. Dilute a volume equivalent to 3 Units to 0·3 ml with *saline solution* and inject intravenously into each of five healthy mice, each weighing between 18 and 20 g; none of the mice dies within 48 hours.

If one of the five mice dies, the test is repeated and the sample complies with the test if none of the second group of five mice dies within 48 hours.

PROLONGATION OF CORTICOTROPHIN EFFECT. It complies with the test given in the British Pharmacopoeia, Appendix XIVC, a dose of 10 or 20 Units per 100 g of the rat's body-weight being used.

POTENCY. 80 to 125 per cent of the prescribed or stated concentration, determined by the biological assay of corticotrophin, subcutaneous method, of the British Pharmacopoeia, Appendix XIVC.

The precision of the assay must be such that the fiducial limits of error (P = 0·95) are between 64 and 156 per cent of the estimated potency.

The sample is diluted with *saline solution* and the Standard Preparation is dissolved in, and diluted to the same extent with, a 1·5 per cent w/v solution of *sodium carboxymethylcellulose* in water. Further dilutions of the sample and the Standard Preparation are made with *saline solution*. The rats are killed 1½ hours after the injection.

Containers; Labelling. The directions given under Injections (page 708) should be followed.

Storage. It should be protected from light and stored between 2° and 10°. Under these conditions, it may be expected to retain its potency for at least three years.

Dose. By subcutaneous injection, the dose is determined by the physician in accordance with the needs of the patient.

When the strength of the injection is not specified, a solution containing 40 Units of corticotrophin in 1 ml shall be supplied.

Vials containing 100 and 200 Units of corticotrophin in 5 ml are available.

Dextromoramide Injection

SYNONYM: Dextromoramide Tartrate Injection

Dextromoramide Injection is a sterile solution of Dextromoramide Tartrate, with Sodium Chloride, in Water for Injections. It is sterilised by autoclaving or by filtration (see Appendix 29, page 921).

Standard
It complies with the standard under Injections, page 707, with the following additions:

PRESENCE OF DEXTROMORAMIDE. It complies with the thin-layer chromatographic test given in Appendix 5A, page 862.

CONTENT OF DEXTROMORAMIDE. 95·0 to 105·0 per cent of the strength stated on the label, calculated as $C_{25}H_{32}N_2O_2$, determined by the following method:

Evaporate an accurately measured volume, equivalent

to about 0·05 g of dextromoramide, just to dryness on a water-bath, dissolve the residue, with the aid of gentle heat, in 30 ml of *glacial acetic acid*, cool, and titrate by Method I of the British Pharmacopoeia for non-aqueous titration, using 0·02N perchloric acid in place of 0·1N perchloric acid; each ml of 0·02N perchloric acid is equivalent to 0·007851 g of $C_{25}H_{32}N_2O_2$.

Containers; Labelling. The directions given under Injections (page 708) should be followed.

Dose. The equivalent of 5 milligrams of dextromoramide, increasing, if necessary, to 15 milligrams, by subcutaneous or intramuscular injection, repeated in accordance with the needs of the patient.

Ampoules containing the equivalent of 5 and 10 mg of dextromoramide in 1 ml are available.

Dextrose Injection, Strong

Anhydrous Dextrose	..	..	50 g
Water for Injections	..	..	to 100 ml

Dissolve and clarify by filtration. Sterilise, immediately after preparation, by autoclaving or by filtration (see Appendix 29, page 921).

Standard
It complies with the standard under Injections, page 707, with the following additions:

DESCRIPTION. A clear colourless to pale straw-coloured liquid.

ACIDITY. pH, 3·5 to 6·5.

WEIGHT PER ML. At 20°, 1·172 g to 1·195 g.

PARTICULATE MATTER. It complies with the limit test for particulate matter given in the British Pharmacopoeia, Appendix XVIC.

PYROGENS. Dilute 1 volume with 9 volumes of *water for injections*; the solution complies with the test for pyrogens, 10 ml per kg of the rabbit's body-weight being used.

CONTENT OF DEXTROSE. 47·5 to 52·5 per cent w/v, calculated as $C_6H_{12}O_6$, determined by the following method:
To 5 ml add 0·2 ml of *dilute ammonia solution*, dilute to 50 ml with water, allow to stand for 30 minutes, and measure the optical rotation in a 2-decimetre tube at 20°; the observed rotation, in degrees, multiplied by 0·9477 represents the weight in g of $C_6H_{12}O_6$ in the sample.
Calculate the concentration of $C_6H_{12}O_6$ in the sample.

Containers; Labelling. The directions given under Injections (page 708) should be followed.

Storage. It should be stored in a cool place.

Dose. The dose, determined by the physician in accordance with the needs of the patient, is administered by intravenous infusion at a rate not exceeding 500 millilitres per hour.

Ethanolamine Oleate Injection

Ethanolamine	..	..	..	0·91 g
Oleic Acid	..	..	..	4·23 g
Benzyl Alcohol	..	..	..	2 ml
Water for Injections	..	..	to 100 ml

Shake the oleic acid with 50 ml of the water in a closed container and gradually add the ethanolamine, shaking between each addition until combination is complete. Add the benzyl alcohol, shake, and add sufficient of the water to produce the required volume. Sterilise by autoclaving (see Appendix 29, page 921).

It is not necessary to add an additional bactericide when the injection is supplied in multiple-dose containers.

Standard
It complies with the standard under Injections, page 707, with the following additions:

ALKALINITY. pH, 8·0 to 9·2.

CONTENT OF OLEIC ACID. 3·9 to 4·5 per cent w/v, calculated as $C_{18}H_{34}O_2$, determined by the following method:
To 10 ml add 20 ml of 0·1N sulphuric acid and extract with three successive 25-ml portions of *chloroform*, washing each extract with the same 10 ml of water and reserving the aqueous solution and washings for the determination of ethanolamine; evaporate the combined extracts to dryness, dissolve the residue in *alcohol (95 per cent)*, previously neutralised to *phenolphthalein solution*, and titrate with 0·1N sodium hydroxide, using *phenolphthalein solution* as indicator; each ml of 0·1N sodium hydroxide is equivalent to 0·02825 g of $C_{18}H_{34}O_2$.

CONTENT OF ETHANOLAMINE. 0·85 to 0·95 per cent w/v, calculated as C_2H_7NO, determined by the following method:
Titrate the excess of acid in the combined aqueous solution and washings reserved in the determination of oleic acid with 0·1N sodium hydroxide, using *methyl orange solution* as indicator; each ml of 0·1N sulphuric acid is equivalent to 0·006108 g of C_2H_7NO.

Containers. The directions given under Injections (page 708) should be followed.

Labelling. The directions given under Injections (page 709) should be followed.
In addition, the label on the container and the label or wrapper on the package should state that the injection contains about 5 per cent of ethanolamine oleate and that the contents are to be used for intravenous injection only, as a sclerosing agent.

Storage. It should be protected from light.

Dose. As a sclerosing agent, 2 to 5 millilitres by intravenous injection, as a single dose, divided into three or four portions which are injected at different sites.

Hyaluronidase Injection

Hyaluronidase Injection is a sterile solution of Hyaluronidase in Water for Injections.
It is prepared by dissolving the contents of a sealed container in Water for Injections immediately before use.

Standard
The contents of the sealed container comply with the requirements of the British Pharmacopoeia for Hyaluronidase, with the following addition:

CONTENT OF HYALURONIDASE. Determine the weight of the contents of each of 10 containers by Method A of the British Pharmacopoeia for the determination of uniformity of weight for Injections.
Carry out the assay of hyaluronidase, British Pharmacopoeia, Appendix XVIIB, on the mixed contents of the 10 containers, and calculate the total number of Units in each container.
The number of Units in each container is not less than 90 per cent and not more than 130 per cent of the total number of Units stated on the label.

Containers. The directions given under Injections (page 708) should be followed.

Labelling. The directions given under Injections (page 709) should be followed.

In addition, the label on the container should state that the contents are not to be used for intravascular injection.

Storage. The sealed container should be stored in a cool place. The injection decomposes on storage and should be used immediately after preparation.

Dose. See **Actions and uses** under Hyaluronidase (page 223).

Hydrocortisone Sodium Phosphate Injection

Hydrocortisone Sodium Phosphate Injection is a sterile solution of Hydrocortisone Sodium Phosphate, with suitable buffering and stabilising agents, in Water for Injections. It is sterilised by filtration (see Appendix 29, page 923).

The injection must be so formulated that the product is clinically satisfactory.

Standard
It complies with the standard under Injections, page 707, with the following additions:

PRESENCE OF HYDROCORTISONE. It complies with the thin-layer chromatographic test given in Appendix 5D, page 876.

ALKALINITY. pH, 7·5 to 8·5.

CONTENT OF HYDROCORTISONE. 90·0 to 110·0 per cent of the strength stated on the label, determined by the following method:

Dilute an accurately measured volume, equivalent to about 0·1 g of hydrocortisone, to 500 ml with water; to 5 ml of this solution add 15 ml of water and continue by the method for Betamethasone Eye-drops, page 688, beginning with the words "[add] 2·5 g of *sodium chloride* . . .", the extinction of a 1-cm layer of the final solution being measured at the maximum at about 248 nm.

For purposes of calculation, use a value of 447 for the E(1 per cent, 1 cm) of hydrocortisone.

Calculate the concentration of hydrocortisone in the sample.

Containers. The directions given under Injections (page 708) should be followed.

Labelling. The directions given under Injections (page 709) should be followed.

In addition, the label on the container and the label or wrapper on the package should state that the injection should not be administered intrathecally.

Storage. It should be protected from light and stored in a cool place.

Dose. The equivalent of hydrocortisone, 100 to 300 milligrams by intravenous injection, in accordance with the needs of the patient.

When the strength of the injection is not specified, a solution containing the equivalent of 100 mg of hydrocortisone in each ml shall be supplied.

Isoniazid Injection

Isoniazid Injection is a sterile solution of Isoniazid in Water for Injections. The acidity of the solution is adjusted to pH 5·6 to 6·0 by the addition of 0·1N hydrochloric acid. The solution is sterilised by autoclaving or by filtration (see Appendix 29, page 921).

Standard
It complies with the standard under Injections, page 707, with the following additions:

PRESENCE OF ISONIAZID. To 0·1 ml add 5 ml of *alcohol* (*95 per cent*), 0·1 g of *borax*, and 5 ml of a 5·0 per cent w/v solution of *1-chloro-2,4-dinitrobenzene* in *alcohol* (*95 per cent*), evaporate to dryness on a water-bath, heat for a further 10 minutes, and dissolve the residue in 10 ml of *methyl alcohol*; a reddish-purple colour is produced.

CONTENT OF ISONIAZID. 95·0 to 105·0 per cent of the strength stated on the label, calculated as $C_6H_7N_3O$, determined by the following method:

Dilute an accurately measured volume, equivalent to about 0·4 g of isoniazid, to 250 ml with water; to 25 ml of this solution in a glass-stoppered flask add 25 ml of 0·1N bromine and 5 ml of *hydrochloric acid*, shake for 1 minute, allow to stand for 15 minutes, add 1 g of *potassium iodide*, and titrate the liberated iodine with 0·1N sodium thiosulphate, using *starch mucilage* as indicator.

Repeat the procedure omitting the sample.

The difference between the two titrations represents the amount of 0·1N bromine required by the sample; each ml of 0·1N bromine is equivalent to 0·003429 g of $C_6H_7N_3O$.

Containers; Labelling. The directions given under Injections (page 708) should be followed.

Dose. Isoniazid:

CHILD. By intramuscular injection: 10 milligrams per kilogram body-weight daily.

When the strength of the injection is not specified, a solution containing 50 mg of isoniazid in 2 ml shall be supplied.

Mannomustine Injection

SYNONYM: Mannomustine Hydrochloride Injection

Mannomustine Injection is a sterile solution of Mannomustine Hydrochloride in Sodium Chloride Injection.

It is prepared by dissolving the contents of a sealed container in Sodium Chloride Injection shortly before use.

Standard
The contents of the sealed container comply with the standard under Injections, page 707; Method A is used in the test for uniformity of weight and composition.

Containers; Labelling. The directions given under Injections (page 708) should be followed.

Storage. The injection decomposes on storage and should be used within twenty-four hours of preparation.

Dose. Mannomustine hydrochloride, initial dose 50 to 100 milligrams by intravenous injection; subsequent doses, determined by the physician in accordance with the haematological response.

Methoxamine Injection

SYNONYM: Methoxamine Hydrochloride Injection

Methoxamine Hydrochloride ..		2·0 g
Sodium Chloride..		0·43 g
Water for Injections		to 100 ml

Dissolve and filter. Distribute the solution

into ampoules, replace the air in the ampoules with nitrogen or other suitable gas, seal, and sterilise by autoclaving (see Appendix 29, page 921).

Standard
It complies with the standard under Injections, page 707, with the following additions:

DESCRIPTION. A clear colourless or almost colourless liquid.

PRESENCE OF METHOXAMINE. 1 ml diluted with 1 ml of water complies with identification test 1 given for Methoxamine Hydrochloride, page 303.

CONTENT OF METHOXAMINE HYDROCHLORIDE. 1·90 to 2·10 per cent w/v, determined by the following method: Dilute 1 ml to 100 ml with water; dilute 20 ml of this solution to 100 ml with water and measure the extinction of a 1-cm layer at the maximum at about 290 nm.
For purposes of calculation, use a value of 137 for the E(1 per cent, 1 cm) of methoxamine hydrochloride.
Calculate the concentration of methoxamine hydrochloride in the sample.

Containers. The directions given under Injections (page 708) should be followed.
The injection should be supplied in single-dose ampoules.

Labelling. The directions given under Injections (page 709) should be followed.

Dose. 0·25 to 1 millilitre by intramuscular injection; 0·25 to 0·5 millilitre by intravenous injection.

Morphine and Atropine Injection

Morphine Sulphate	..	..	1·0 g
Atropine Sulphate	..	..	0·06 g
Sodium Metabisulphite	..	..	0·1 g
Sodium Chloride	..	..	0·69 g
Water for Injections	..	..	to 100 ml

Dissolve, and clarify by filtration. Sterilise by heating with a bactericide or by filtration (see Appendix 29, pages 922–3).

Standard
It complies with the standard under Injections, page 707, with the following additions:

PRESENCE OF MORPHINE AND OF ATROPINE. It complies with the thin-layer chromatographic test given in Appendix 5A, page 865.

CONTENT OF ATROPINE SULPHATE. 0·054 to 0·066 per cent w/v, determined by the following method:
To 5 ml add 1 ml of *ferric chloride test-solution*, allow to stand for 2 minutes, add 2 g of *sodium citrate* and 10 ml of water, followed by 0·2 ml of *dilute ammonia solution*, and extract with successive 15-, 10-, and 10-ml portions of *chloroform*, washing each extract with the same 5 ml of water; evaporate off the solvent from the combined extracts, dissolve the residue in 1 ml of *dilute nitric acid*, and dilute the solution to 50 ml with water.
Evaporate 1 ml of this solution to dryness, add 0·25 ml of *fuming nitric acid*, and again evaporate to dryness; dissolve the residue in 1 ml of *dimethylformamide*, transfer the solution to a 10-ml graduated flask with the aid of small quantities of *dimethylformamide*, add 0·3 ml of *tetraethylammonium hydroxide solution*, and dilute to 10 ml with *dimethylformamide*; allow to stand for exactly 5 minutes after the addition of the tetraethylammonium hydroxide solution, and measure the extinction of a 1-cm layer at the maximum at about 550 nm.
Repeat the measurement, using 0·3 ml of *tetraethylammonium hydroxide solution* diluted to 10 ml with *dimethylformamide*.

The difference between the two extinctions represents the extinction due to the sample.
Calculate the quantity of atropine sulphate present by reference to a calibration curve prepared at the same time, using suitable quantities of a solution of *atropine sulphate* in water, evaporating to dryness, and continuing by the method described above, beginning with the words "add 0·25 ml of *fuming nitric acid* . . .".

CONTENT OF MORPHINE SULPHATE. 0·92 to 1·07 per cent w/v, calculated as $(C_{17}H_{19}NO_3)_2,H_2SO_4,5H_2O$, determined by the following method:
To 5 ml add 10 ml of water and 5 ml of 1N sodium hydroxide, extract with successive 15-, 10-, and 10-ml portions of *chloroform*, washing each extract with the same 5 ml of water, and discard the chloroform extracts.
To the combined aqueous solution and washings, add 1 g of *ammonium sulphate* and 25 ml of *alcohol (95 per cent)* and extract with successive 40-, 40-, 20-, and 20-ml portions of a mixture of 1 volume of *alcohol (95 per cent)* and 3 volumes of *chloroform*, washing each extract with the same two successive 5-ml portions of water; evaporate off the solvent from the combined extracts, dissolve the residue in 10 ml of 1N hydrochloric acid, add a further 40 ml of 1N hydrochloric acid, and dilute to 500 ml with water.
Dilute 25 ml of this solution to 100 ml with 0·1N hydrochloric acid and continue by the method for Aromatic Chalk with Opium Powder, page 776, beginning with the words "To 20 ml of this solution, add . . ."; each mg of anhydrous morphine is equivalent to 1·33 mg of $(C_{17}H_{19}NO_3)_2,H_2SO_4,5H_2O$.

Containers; Labelling. The directions given under Injections (page 708) should be followed.

Storage. It should be protected from light.

Dose. 0·5 to 1 millilitre by subcutaneous injection.

Noradrenaline Injection

Noradrenaline Injection is a sterile solution of Noradrenaline Acid Tartrate.
It is prepared immediately before use by diluting Sterile Strong Noradrenaline Solution (page 789) to 250 times its volume with Sodium Chloride and Dextrose Injection or Dextrose Injection (5 per cent w/v).

Dose. 0·25 to 2·5 millilitres per minute by intravenous infusion, according to the blood pressure of the patient.

Noradrenaline Injection contains, in 1 ml, 8 micrograms of noradrenaline acid tartrate, equivalent to approximately 4 micrograms of noradrenaline base.

Papaveretum Injection

Papaveretum	..	..	..	2·0 g
Glycerol	..	..	..	1·4 g
Water for Injections	..	..	to 100 ml

Dissolve the papaveretum in the bulk of the water, add the glycerol and sufficient of the water to produce the required volume, mix, and clarify the solution by filtration. Distribute the solution into the final containers, seal, and sterilise by heating with a bactericide (see Appendix 29, page 922); phenylmercuric nitrate is a suitable bactericide.
Alternatively, sterilise the solution by filtration (see Appendix 29, page 923); distribute,

by means of an aseptic technique, into sterile final containers, and seal.

Standard
It complies with the standard under Injections, page 707, with the following additions:

PRESENCE OF PAPAVERETUM. It complies with the thin-layer chromatographic test given in Appendix 5B, page 872.

CONTENT OF ANHYDROUS MORPHINE. 0·85 to 1·15 per cent w/v, determined by the following method: Dilute 0·5 ml to 250 ml with 0·1N hydrochloric acid; using 20 ml of this solution, continue by the method for Aromatic Chalk with Opium Powder, page 776, beginning with the words "add 8 ml of a freshly prepared 1·0 per cent w/v solution of *sodium nitrite . . .*".

Containers. The directions given under Injections (page 708) should be followed.
The injection should be supplied in single-dose containers.

Labelling. The directions given under Injections (page 709) should be followed.

Storage. It should be protected from light.

Dose. ADULT. 0·5 to 1 millilitre.
CHILD. By intramuscular injection: up to 1 month, 0·0075 millilitre per kilogram body-weight; 1 to 12 months, 0·01 millilitre per kilogram body-weight; 1 to 5 years, 0·125 to 0·25 millilitre; 6 to 12 years, 0·25 to 0·5 millilitre.

Papaveretum Injection contains in 1 ml approximately 10 mg of anhydrous morphine.

Paraldehyde Injection

Paraldehyde Injection consists of sterile Paraldehyde. It is sterilised by filtration (see Appendix 29, page 923). No bactericide should be added.

Standard
It complies with the standard under Injections, page 707.
In addition, the mixed contents of a sufficient number of containers comply with the requirements of the British Pharmacopoeia for Paraldehyde.

Containers. The directions given under Injections (page 708) should be followed.
The injection should be supplied in single-dose ampoules; contact with rubber and plastics should be avoided.

Labelling. The directions given under Injections (page 709) should be followed.
In addition, the label on the container and the label or wrapper on the package should state that plastic syringes should not be used for the administration of the injection.

Storage. It should be stored at 15° to 20° in complete darkness.

Dose. ADULT. 5 to 10 millilitres by intramuscular injection.
CHILD. By intramuscular injection: up to 1 year, 0·5 to 2 millilitres; 1 to 5 years, 2·5 to 5 millilitres; 6 to 12 years, 6 millilitres.

When the volume to be contained in the ampoule is not specified, ampoules each containing 10 ml shall be supplied.
Ampoules containing 2 and 5 ml are also available.

Phenol Injection, Oily

SYNONYM: 5 per cent Phenol in Oil Injection

Phenol	..	..	..	5 g
Almond Oil	..	..	..	to 100 ml

Dissolve the phenol in the bulk of the almond oil, previously warmed, add sufficient of the oil to produce the required volume, filter, distribute into the final containers, seal to give an airtight closure, and sterilise by dry heat (see Appendix 29, page 921).
Alternatively, sterilise sufficient of the almond oil by dry heat; by means of an aseptic technique, dissolve the phenol in the bulk of the warm sterile oil, add sufficient of the cold sterile oil to produce the required volume, distribute into the final sterile containers, and seal.

Standard
It complies with the standard under Injections, page 707, with the following addition:

CONTENT OF PHENOL. 4·75 to 5·25 per cent w/v, calculated as C_6H_6O, determined by the following method:
Dissolve about 10 g, accurately weighed, in 50 ml of *solvent ether* and extract with successive 10-ml portions of *dilute sodium hydroxide solution* until extraction is complete; boil the combined extracts for 2 minutes, cool, and dilute to 250 ml with water.
To 20 ml of this solution in a glass-stoppered flask, add 30 ml of 0·1N bromine and 6 ml of *hydrochloric acid*, shake repeatedly during 15 minutes, allow to stand for 15 minutes, add 30 ml of *potassium iodide solution*, and titrate the liberated iodine with 0·1N sodium thiosulphate; each ml of 0·1N bromine is equivalent to 0·001569 g of C_6H_6O.
Determine the weight per ml of the injection, and calculate the concentration of C_6H_6O, weight in volume.

Containers; Labelling. The directions given under Injections (page 708) should be followed.

Dose. 0·5 to 1·5 millilitres by injection into the submucous layer. Several injections may be given at different sites.

Phenytoin Injection

SYNONYMS: Phenytoin Sodium Injection; Soluble Phenytoin Injection

Phenytoin Injection is a sterile solution of Phenytoin Sodium, with 40 per cent v/v of Propylene Glycol and 10 per cent v/v of Alcohol, in Water for Injections.
It is prepared by dissolving the contents of a sealed container in the solvent shortly before use. As the phenytoin sodium is only slowly soluble, complete solution may take up to ten minutes.

Standard
The contents of the sealed container of the dry powder comply with the requirements of the British Pharmacopoeia for Phenytoin Sodium, with the following additions:

UNIFORMITY OF WEIGHT. Remove any paper labels from a sealed container, wash the outside with water, and thoroughly dry.
Weigh the container and its contents; open the container and remove the contents; wash all parts of the

container with water and then with *alcohol (95 per cent)*, dry at 105°, cool, and weigh. The difference between the two weights represents the weight of the contents.

Repeat the operation with a further 9 containers.

The weight of the contents of each container is within the limits 100 to 110 per cent of the weight stated on the label, with the exception that in one container the contents may be within the limits 95 to 115 per cent of the weight stated on the label.

STERILITY. The contents comply with the test for sterility.

The contents of the sealed container of the solvent comply with the general standard for Solvent under Injections, page 707, with the following additions:

ALKALINITY. pH, 11·8 to 12·3.

CONTENT OF ALCOHOL. 9·0 to 11·0 per cent v/v of ethyl alcohol, determined by the following method:

Carry out the method of Appendix XIIC of the British Pharmacopoeia for Gas-liquid Chromatography, using solutions containing (1) 2·0 per cent v/v of *propyl alcohol* (internal standard) and 2·0 per cent v/v of *dehydrated alcohol* in water, (2) the sample diluted with water so as to give an expected concentration of ethyl alcohol of about 2·0 per cent v/v, and (3) a solution prepared as for solution (2) but in which has been included 2·0 per cent v/v of *propyl alcohol*.

The chromatographic procedure may be carried out with a column 180 cm in length and 2 mm internal diameter, packed with *Chromosorb 102* (80- to 100-mesh) maintained at 120°, nitrogen as the carrier gas, and a flame ionisation detector.

Calculate the concentration of ethyl alcohol, volume in volume.

CONTENT OF PROPYLENE GLYCOL. 37·0 to 43·0 per cent v/v, determined by the following method:

Carry out the method of Appendix XIIC of the British Pharmacopoeia for Gas-liquid Chromatography, using solutions containing (1) 4·0 per cent w/v of *ethylene glycol* (internal standard) and 4·0 per cent w/v of *propylene glycol* in water, (2) the sample diluted with water, so as to given an expected concentration of about 4·0 per cent w/v of propylene glycol, and (3) a solution prepared as for solution (2) but in which has been included 4·0 per cent w/v of *ethylene glycol*.

The chromatographic procedure may be carried out using the same column and operating conditions as described in the determination of the content of alcohol, above, except that the column is maintained at 175° instead of 120°.

Assuming the weight per ml of propylene glycol to be 1·036 g, calculate the content of propylene glycol, volume in volume.

Containers; Labelling. The directions given under Injections (page 708) should be followed.

Storage. The injection contains no bactericide and the aseptic precautions taken in its preparation should be such that the microbiological quality is maintained if it is stored.

The chemical stability of the injection is limited. It should preferably be used immediately after preparation, but it may be stored for short periods. The solution is suitable for use as long as it remains free of haziness and precipitate. Haziness and precipitation develop in it gradually and only a clear solution should be used.

Dose. Phenytoin sodium:

ADULT. By slow intravenous injection at a rate not exceeding 50 milligrams per minute, 150 to 250 milligrams, followed, if necessary, after thirty minutes, by 100 to 150 milligrams.

By intramuscular injection, 100 to 200 milligrams every six to eight hours for a total of three or four injections.

CHILD. By intramuscular or slow intravenous injection: up to 5 milligrams per kilogram body-weight.

Vials containing 250 mg of phenytoin sodium, to which is to be added 5·2 ml of solvent to provide a solution containing 50 mg of phenytoin sodium in each ml, are available.

Polymyxin Injection

SYNONYM: Polymyxin B Sulphate Injection

Polymyxin Injection is a sterile solution of Polymyxin B Sulphate in Water for Injections or Sodium Chloride Injection.

It is prepared by dissolving the contents of a sealed container in Water for Injections or Sodium Chloride Injection shortly before use.

Standard

The contents of the sealed container comply with the standard under Injections, page 707; Method B is used in the test for uniformity of weight and composition.

CONTENT OF POLYMYXIN. 90 to 115 per cent of the amount stated on the label, determined by the following method:

Carry out a microbiological assay of polymyxin; a suggested method is given in Appendix 18, page 897.

The precision of any assay must be such that the fiducial limits of error (P = 0·95) are not less than 95 per cent and not more than 105 per cent of the estimated potency.

Calculate the upper and lower fiducial limits of the amount of polymyxin in each container.

The upper fiducial limit of the amount of polymyxin in each container is not less than 90 per cent and the lower fiducial limit is not more than 115 per cent of the amount stated on the label.

Containers; Labelling. The directions given under Injections (page 708) should be followed.

Storage. The injection decomposes on storage and should be used within twenty-four hours of preparation.

Dose. See **Actions and uses** under Polymyxin B Sulphate (page 388).

Vials containing 500,000 Units are available.

Procyclidine Injection

SYNONYM: Procyclidine Hydrochloride Injection

Procyclidine Injection is a sterile solution of Procyclidine Hydrochloride in Water for Injections. It is sterilised by autoclaving or by filtration (see Appendix 29, page 921).

Standard

It complies with the standard under Injections, page 707, with the following additions:

PRESENCE OF PROCYCLIDINE. The ultraviolet absorption spectrum of the injection, when diluted to the appropriate strength with water, exhibits the characteristics given for procyclidine hydrochloride in Appendix 3, page 856.

ACIDITY. pH, 4·5 to 7·0.

CONTENT OF PROCYCLIDINE HYDROCHLORIDE. 90·0 to 110·0 per cent of the amount stated on the label, determined by the following method:

Dilute 2 ml to 50 ml with water, mix, and further dilute 20 ml of this solution to 200 ml with water.

Transfer 10 ml of this solution to a separating funnel, add 25 ml, accurately measured, of *chloroform*, 10 ml of a solution containing 4·3 per cent w/v of *sodium dihydrogen phosphate* and 0·2 per cent w/v of *sodium phosphate* in water, and 10 ml of a solution prepared by dissolving 0·1 g of *bromocresol purple* in 10 ml of 0·1N sodium hydroxide and diluting to 100 ml with water; shake well, allow to separate, transfer the chloroform layer to a 50-ml stoppered flask containing 1 g of *anhydrous sodium sulphate*, shake, allow to stand, and measure the extinction of a 1-cm layer at 407 nm, using *chloroform* as the blank.

Repeat the procedure using 10 ml of *procyclidine hydrochloride standard solution* in place of the sample solution.

From the two extinctions calculate the amount of procyclidine hydrochloride in the injection.

Containers; Labelling. The directions given under Injections (page 708) should be followed.

Storage. It should be stored at a temperature not exceeding 25°; it should not be allowed to freeze.

Dose. Procyclidine hydrochloride, by intramuscular or intravenous injection, 5 to 10 milligrams.

When the strength of the injection is not specified, a solution containing 10 mg of procyclidine hydrochloride in 2 ml shall be supplied.

Pyridoxine Injection

SYNONYM: Pyridoxine Hydrochloride Injection

Pyridoxine Injection is a sterile solution of Pyridoxine Hydrochloride in Water for Injections. It is sterilised by autoclaving or by filtration (see Appendix 29, page 921).

Standard
It complies with the standard under Injections, page 707, with the following additions:

PRESENCE OF PYRIDOXINE. Dilute the injection to give a solution containing about 0·01 per cent w/v of pyridoxine hydrochloride; to 1 ml of this solution add 1 ml of a 0·04 per cent w/v solution of *dichloroquinonechloroimine* in *dehydrated alcohol* and 0·05 ml of *dilute ammonia solution*; a blue colour is produced.

To a further 1 ml of the solution add 1 ml of a saturated solution of *boric acid* in water, 1 ml of the solution of dichloroquinonechloroimine, and 0·05 ml of *dilute ammonia solution*; no blue colour is produced.

CONTENT OF PYRIDOXINE HYDROCHLORIDE. 95·0 to 105·0 per cent of the strength stated on the label, determined by the following method:

Dilute an accurately measured volume, equivalent to about 0·05 g of pyridoxine hydrochloride, to 100 ml with 0·1N hydrochloric acid; dilute 2 ml of this solution to 100 ml with 0·1N hydrochloric acid and measure the extinction of a 1-cm layer at the maximum at about 291 nm.

For purposes of calculation, use a value of 427 for the E(1 per cent, 1 cm) of pyridoxine hydrochloride.

Calculate the concentration of pyridoxine hydrochloride in the sample.

Containers; Labelling. The directions given under Injections (page 708) should be followed.

Storage. It should be protected from light.

Dose. Pyridoxine hydrochloride:
For pyridoxine-deficiency convulsions in infancy, 4 milligrams per kilogram body-weight daily for short periods.

For pyridoxine-deficiency anaemia of adults, 50 to 150 milligrams daily, in divided doses.

When the strength of the injection is not specified, a solution containing 50 mg of pyridoxine hydrochloride in 2 ml shall be supplied.

Sodium Nitrite Injection

| Sodium Nitrite | .. | .. | .. | 3 g |
| Water for Injections | | .. | .. | to 100 ml |

Dissolve, and clarify by filtration. Sterilise by autoclaving or by filtration (see Appendix 29, page 921).

Standard
It complies with the standard under Injections, page 707, with the following additions:

PRESENCE OF NITRITE. 1. Add 0·3 ml to a mixture of 0·5 ml of *aniline* and 5 ml of *glacial acetic acid*; a deep orange-red colour is produced.

2. To 2 ml add 5 ml of *ferrous sulphate solution*; a deep brown colour is produced.

CONTENT OF SODIUM NITRITE. 2·85 to 3·15 per cent w/v, calculated as $NaNO_2$, determined by the method for Sodium Nitrite, page 457, 20 ml being used.

Containers. The directions given under Injections (page 708) should be followed.
The injection should be supplied in single-dose ampoules.

Labelling. The directions given under Injections (page 709) should be followed.

Dose. In the treatment of cyanide poisoning, 10 millilitres by intravenous injection.

When the volume to be contained in each ampoule is not specified, ampoules each containing 10 ml shall be supplied.

Sodium Thiosulphate Injection

| Sodium Thiosulphate | .. | .. | 50 g |
| Water for Injections | | .. | .. | to 100 ml |

Dissolve, and filter. Distribute the solution into single-dose containers, replace the air in the containers with nitrogen or other suitable gas, seal, and sterilise by autoclaving (see Appendix 29, page 921).

Standard
It complies with the standard under Injections, page 707, with the following additions:

PRESENCE OF THIOSULPHATE. Dilute 0·5 ml to 5 ml with water and add 1 ml of *hydrochloric acid*; a white precipitate, which quickly changes to yellow, is produced, and sulphur dioxide is evolved.

CONTENT OF SODIUM THIOSULPHATE. 47·5 to 52·5 per cent w/v, calculated as $Na_2S_2O_3,5H_2O$, determined by the method for Sodium Thiosulphate, page 464, 2 ml being used.

Containers. The directions given under Injections (page 708) should be followed.
The injection should be supplied in single-dose containers.

Labelling. The directions given under Injections (page 709) should be followed.

Dose. In the treatment of cyanide poisoning, 50 millilitres by intravenous injection.

When the volume to be contained in each container is not specified, containers each containing 50 ml shall be supplied.

Suramin Injection

Suramin Injection is a sterile solution of Suramin in Water for Injections.
It is prepared by dissolving the contents of a

sealed container in Water for Injections immediately before use.

Standard
The contents of the sealed container comply with the standard under Injections, page 707; Method A is used in the test for uniformity of weight and composition.

Containers; Labelling. The directions given under Injections (page 708) should be followed.

Storage. The sealed container should be stored in a cool place and protected from light.
The injection decomposes on storage and should be used immediately after preparation.

Dose. Prophylactic, 2 grams as a single dose; therapeutic, initial dose 200 milligrams, followed by five weekly doses of 1 gram.

Tetracycline and Procaine Injection

Tetracycline and Procaine Injection is a sterile solution of Tetracycline Hydrochloride and Procaine Hydrochloride, with suitable buffering and stabilising agents, in Water for Injections.
It is prepared by dissolving the contents of a sealed container in Water for Injections shortly before use.

Standard
The contents of the sealed container comply with the standard under Injections, page 707, Method B being used in the test for uniformity of weight and composition (the proportionate amounts of tetracycline hydrochloride and of procaine hydrochloride being determined), with the following additions:

HYPOTENSIVE SUBSTANCES. Inject intravenously into a cat anaesthetised with chloralose or with a suitable barbiturate, a solution containing the equivalent of 3 mg of tetracycline hydrochloride per ml, corresponding to 1 ml per kg of the cat's weight.
The injection produces a smaller fall of arterial pressure than that produced by the injection of an equal volume of a solution of *histamine acid phosphate* in water containing 0·1 μg of histamine base per ml.

PYROGENS. It complies with the test for pyrogens, a quantity equivalent to not less than 5 mg of tetracycline hydrochloride per kg of the rabbit's weight dissolved in not more than 5 ml of *water for injections* being used.

CONTENT OF PROCAINE HYDROCHLORIDE. 92·5 to 107·5 per cent of the amount stated on the label, determined by the following method:
Dissolve an accurately weighed quantity of the powder, equivalent to about 0·025 g of procaine hydrochloride, in 50 ml of water and dilute to 100 ml with water; to 4 ml of this solution add 50 ml of a solution prepared by mixing 11·9 ml of 0·2N hydrochloric acid and 88·1 ml of 0·2M potassium chloride, followed by 5 ml of a freshly prepared 1·0 per cent w/v solution of *dimethylaminobenzaldehyde* in *alcohol (95 per cent)*, dilute to 100 ml with water, and measure the extinction of a 1-cm layer at the maximum at about 454 nm.
Repeat the procedure using 0·0250 g of *procaine hydrochloride* in place of the sample.
From the two extinctions calculate the amount of procaine hydrochloride in the sample.

CONTENT OF TETRACYCLINE HYDROCHLORIDE. 90 to 115 per cent of the amount stated on the label, determined by the following method:
Carry out a microbiological assay of tetracycline; a suggested method is given in Appendix 18 (page 897).
The precision of any assay must be such that the fiducial limits of error (P = 0·95) are not less than 95 per cent and not more than 105 per cent of the estimated potency.

Assuming that each 1000 Units found is equivalent to 1 mg of tetracycline hydrochloride, calculate the upper and lower fiducial limits of the amount of tetracycline hydrochloride in the dry powder.
The upper fiducial limit of the estimated equivalent amount of tetracycline hydrochloride in each container is not less than 90 per cent and the lower fiducial limit is not more than 115 per cent of the amount stated on the label.

Containers. The directions given under Injections (page 708) should be followed.

Labelling. The directions given under Injections (page 709) should be followed.
In addition, the label on the container should state that the contents are to be used for intramuscular injection only.

Storage. The injection decomposes on storage and should be used within twenty-four hours of preparation.

Dose. Tetracycline hydrochloride, in a concentration not exceeding 5 per cent w/v, 200 to 400 milligrams by intramuscular injection daily, in divided doses.

Vials containing 100 mg of tetracycline hydrochloride and 40 mg of procaine hydrochloride are available.

Trimeprazine Injection

Trimeprazine Injection is a sterile solution of Trimeprazine Tartrate, with suitable stabilising agents, in Water for Injections free from carbon dioxide. It is distributed into ampoules, the air being replaced by nitrogen or other suitable gas, and the ampoules are sealed and sterilised by autoclaving (see Appendix 29, page 921).

Standard
It complies with the standard under Injections, page 707, with the following additions:

DESCRIPTION. A clear colourless or almost colourless liquid.

PRESENCE OF TRIMEPRAZINE. It complies with the thin-layer chromatographic test given in Appendix 5C, page 873.

ACIDITY. pH, 4·5 to 5·5.

CONTENT OF TRIMEPRAZINE TARTRATE. 95·0 to 105·0 per cent of the strength stated on the label, determined by the following method:
Dilute an accurately measured volume, equivalent to about 0·05 g of trimeprazine tartrate, to 100 ml with water; to 10 ml of this solution add 10 ml of 0·1N hydrochloric acid, dilute to 100 ml with water, and measure the extinction of a 1-cm layer at the maximum at about 301 nm.
For purposes of calculation, use a value of 96 for the E(1 per cent, 1 cm) of trimeprazine tartrate.
Calculate the concentration of trimeprazine tartrate in the sample.

Containers; Labelling. The directions given under Injections (page 708) should be followed.

Storage. It should be protected from light.

Dose. Trimeprazine tartrate:
For pre-operative medication about 90 minutes before surgery, by deep intramuscular injection, 600 to 900 micrograms per kilogram body-weight.

When the strength of the injection is not specified, a solution containing 50 mg of trimeprazine tartrate in 2 ml shall be supplied.

Vitamins B and C Injection

Vitamins B and C Injection is a sterile solution of Thiamine Hydrochloride, Pyridoxine Hydrochloride, Riboflavine or the equivalent amount of Riboflavine Phosphate (Sodium Salt), Nicotinamide, and Ascorbic Acid (as the sodium salt), with Anhydrous Dextrose for the strong intravenous injection or Benzyl Alcohol for the intramuscular injections, in Water for Injections.

It is prepared immediately before use by mixing the contents of a pair of ampoules, one (No. 1) containing the thiamine hydrochloride, the pyridoxine hydrochloride, the riboflavine and, if present, the benzyl alcohol, and the other (No. 2) containing the ascorbic acid and, if present, the anhydrous dextrose. Either of the two ampoules contains the nicotinamide.

Sterilisation is effected by autoclaving, by heating with a bactericide, or by filtration. The air in the ampoules containing the ascorbic acid is replaced by nitrogen or other suitable gas.

Standard

The contents of the No. 1 ampoule comply with the standard under Injections, page 707, with the following additions:

CONTENT OF THIAMINE HYDROCHLORIDE. 92·0 to 106·0 per cent of the strength stated on the label, determined by the following method:
Dilute an accurately measured volume, equivalent to about 0·05 g of thiamine hydrochloride, to 50 ml with water, add 2 ml of *hydrochloric acid*, heat to boiling, rapidly add, dropwise, 4 ml of freshly filtered *silicotungstic acid solution* and boil for 4 minutes.
Filter through a sintered glass crucible (British Standard Grade No. 4), wash the filter with 50 ml of a boiling mixture containing 1 volume of *hydrochloric acid* and 19 volumes of a 0·2 per cent w/v solution of *silicotungstic acid* in water, followed by two successive 5-ml portions of *acetone*.
Dry the residue at 105° for 1 hour, allow to cool for 10 minutes, and then allow to stand in a desiccator over a solution of *sulphuric acid* containing 38 per cent w/w of H_2SO_4 for 2 hours and weigh; each g of residue is equivalent to 0·1929 g of $C_{12}H_{17}ClN_4OS,HCl$.

CONTENT OF PYRIDOXINE HYDROCHLORIDE. 90·0 to 110·0 per cent of the strength stated on the label, determined by the following method:
Dilute an accurately measured volume with water to give a solution containing 1 mg in 10 ml.
Dilute 10 ml of this aqueous solution to 100 ml with *glycerinated phosphate buffer pH 7·0* and measure the extinction of a 1-cm layer at the maximum at about 328 nm, using in the reference cell a 1-cm layer of a solution prepared by diluting 10 ml of the aqueous solution prepared from the sample to 100 ml with *glycerinated 0·1N hydrochloric acid*.
For purposes of calculation, use a value of 340 for the $\Delta E(1$ per cent, 1 cm) of pyridoxine hydrochloride in these two solutions.
Calculate the concentration of pyridoxine hydrochloride in the sample.

CONTENT OF RIBOFLAVINE. 90·0 to 110·0 per cent of the strength stated on the label, determined by the following method:
Dilute an accurately measured volume, equivalent to about 1 mg of riboflavine, to 50 ml with *solution of standard pH 4·0* and measure the extinction of a 1-cm layer at the maximum at about 444 nm.
For purposes of calculation, use a value of 323 for the E(1 per cent, 1 cm) of riboflavine.

Calculate the concentration of riboflavine in the sample.

CONTENT OF NICOTINAMIDE (if contained in this ampoule). 95·0 to 105·0 per cent of the strength stated on the label, determined by the following method:
Transfer an accurately measured volume, equivalent to about 0·15 g of nicotinamide, to an ammonia distillation apparatus, add 200 ml of water and 75 ml of *sodium hydroxide solution*, and boil gently for 20 minutes, collecting any distillate in 50 ml of 0·1N sulphuric acid; boil vigorously to complete the distillation of the ammonia and titrate the excess acid in the distillate with 0·1N sodium hydroxide, using *methyl red solution* as indicator.
Repeat the procedure omitting the sample.
The difference between the two titrations represents the amount of 0·1N sulphuric acid required to neutralise the ammonia formed from the nicotinamide; each ml of 0·1N sulphuric acid is equivalent to 0·01221 g of $C_6H_6N_2O$.

The contents of the No. 1 ampoule of both the Strong and the Weak Vitamins B and C Injection for intramuscular use also comply with the following requirement:

PRESENCE OF BENZYL ALCOHOL. Add 1 ml to a strong solution of *potassium permanganate* which has been acidified with *sulphuric acid*; the odour of benzaldehyde is produced.

The contents of the No. 2 ampoule comply with the standard under Injections, page 707, with the following additions:

CONTENT OF ASCORBIC ACID. 95·0 to 105·0 per cent of the strength stated on the label, calculated as $C_6H_8O_6$, determined by the following method:
To an accurately measured volume, equivalent to about 0·2 g of ascorbic acid, add 5 ml of *dilute sulphuric acid* and 50 ml of 0·1N iodine, and immediately titrate the excess of iodine with 0·1N sodium thiosulphate, using *starch mucilage* as indicator; each ml of 0·1N iodine is equivalent to 0·008806 g of $C_6H_8O_6$.

CONTENT OF NICOTINAMIDE (if contained in this ampoule). 95·0 to 105·0 per cent of the strength stated on the label, determined by the method given above for the No. 1 ampoule.

The contents of the No. 2 ampoule for the Strong Vitamins B and C Injection for intravenous use also comply with the following requirement:

CONTENT OF DEXTROSE, $C_6H_{12}O_6$. 90·0 to 110·0 per cent of the strength stated on the label, determined by the following method:
Dilute an accurately measured volume, equivalent to about 0·8 g of $C_6H_{12}O_6$, to 500 ml with water, and dilute 2 ml of this solution to 100 ml with water.
Transfer 3·0 ml of this second solution to a boiling-tube which has been previously cleaned with *chromic–sulphuric acid mixture* and rinsed with water; to two similar tubes add, respectively, 3·0 ml of *standard dextrose solution* and 3·0 ml of water.
To each tube add 6·0 ml of *anthrone reagent* in such a manner as to ensure rapid mixing, allow to stand for 10 minutes, cool quickly, and measure the extinction of a 1-cm layer of the sample solution and of the standard solution at the maximum at about 625 nm, using the solution prepared with water as the blank.
Calculate the concentration of $C_6H_{12}O_6$ in the sample.

Containers. The directions given under Injections (page 708) should be followed.

Labelling. The directions given under Injections (page 709) should be followed.
In addition, the label on each container should state whether the injection is for intravenous or intramuscular use.

Storage. It should be stored in a cool place and protected from light.

Dose. The dose is determined by the physician in accordance with the needs of the patient.

The potency and route of administration of the injection should be stated by the prescriber.

When *Strong Vitamins B and C Injection for intravenous use* is ordered or prescribed, a pair of ampoules, one containing a solution of 250 mg of thiamine hydrochloride, 50 mg of pyridoxine hydrochloride, and 4 mg of riboflavine or the equivalent amount of riboflavine phosphate (sodium salt) in 5 ml, the other containing a solution of 500 mg of ascorbic acid (as the sodium salt) and 1 g of anhydrous dextrose in 5 ml and either of the two ampoules containing 160 mg of nicotinamide, shall be supplied.

When *Weak Vitamins B and C Injection for intravenous use* is ordered or prescribed, a pair of ampoules, one containing a solution of 100 mg of thiamine hydrochloride, 50 mg of pyridoxine hydrochloride, and 4 mg of riboflavine or the equivalent amount of riboflavine phosphate (sodium salt) in 5 ml, the other containing a solution of 500 mg of ascorbic acid (as the sodium salt) in 5 ml and either of the two ampoules containing 160 mg of nicotinamide, shall be supplied.

When *Strong Vitamins B and C Injection for intramuscular use* is ordered or prescribed, a pair of ampoules, one containing a solution of 250 mg of thiamine hydrochloride, 50 mg of pyridoxine hydrochloride, 4 mg of riboflavine or the equivalent amount of riboflavine phosphate (sodium salt), and 0·14 ml of benzyl alcohol in 5 ml, the other containing a solution of 500 mg of ascorbic acid (as the sodium salt) in 2 ml and either of the two ampoules containing 160 mg of nicotinamide, shall be supplied.

When *Weak Vitamins B and C Injection for intramuscular use* is ordered or prescribed, a pair of ampoules, one containing a solution of 100 mg of thiamine hydrochloride, 50 mg of pyridoxine hydrochloride, 4 mg of riboflavine or the equivalent amount of riboflavine phosphate (sodium salt), and 0·08 ml of benzyl alcohol in 2 ml, the other containing a solution of 500 mg of ascorbic acid (as the sodium salt) in 2 ml and either of the two ampoules containing 160 mg of nicotinamide, shall be supplied.

INSUFFLATIONS

Insufflations are powders containing medicinal substances usually diluted with a suitable inert powder such as lactose. They are intended for introduction into the ear, nose, throat, body cavities, or wounds. They are administered by means of an insufflator or, when intended for the nose, they may be used in the same way as snuff.

Pituitary (Posterior Lobe) Insufflation is absorbed through the nasal mucous membrane and has a systemic action.

Pituitary (Posterior Lobe) Insufflation

SYNONYM: Pituitary Snuff

Powdered Pituitary
(Posterior Lobe) ..   a quantity containing 30,000 Units of antidiuretic activity

Lactose   ..   ..   to 100 g

Storage. It should be stored in airtight containers.

Dose. The dose is determined by the physician in accordance with the needs of the patient.

JUICES

Juices are liquids expressed from fruits and other parts of plants. They are usually clarified and a preservative may be added. Concentrated Raspberry Juice is used to prepare Raspberry Syrup.

Raspberry Juice, Concentrated

Concentrated Raspberry Juice is prepared from the clarified juice of raspberries, *Rubus idaeus* L. (Fam. Rosaceae).

Sufficient pectinase of commerce to destroy the pectin is stirred into pulped raspberries, the mixture allowed to stand for 12 hours, and the pulp pressed. The juice is clarified, sufficient sucrose added to adjust the weight per millilitre at 20° to 1·050 g to 1·060 g, and the juice concentrated to one-sixth of its original volume.

Sufficient sulphurous acid or sodium metabisulphite is added to preserve the product.

Standard

WEIGHT PER ML. At 20°, 1·30 g to 1·36 g.

SULPHUR DIOXIDE. Not more than 4700 parts per million w/w, determined by the method of the British Pharmacopoeia, Appendix XJ, for the determination of sulphur dioxide.

Storage. It should be stored in a cool place and protected from light.

Note. When 1 volume of Concentrated Raspberry Juice is diluted with 5 volumes of water, a product equivalent to natural raspberry juice is obtained.

LINCTUSES

Linctuses are viscous liquid preparations, usually containing sucrose and medicinal substances and possessing demulcent, expectorant, or sedative properties; they are usually used for the relief of cough. They are administered in doses of small volume and should be sipped and swallowed slowly without the addition of water.

Dilution of linctuses. When a dose ordered or prescribed is less than or not a multiple of 5 millilitres, the linctus should be diluted with the vehicle recommended in the individual monograph, so that the dose to be measured for the patient is one 5-ml spoonful or multiple thereof. Instructions for dilution are given in the individual monographs.

Diluted linctuses must always be freshly prepared and not more than two weeks' supply should be issued at a time unless otherwise specified in the monograph.

Codeine Linctus

Codeine Phosphate	3 g
Compound Tartrazine Solution	10 ml
Benzoic Acid Solution	20 ml
Chloroform Spirit	20 ml
Water (see page 642)	20 ml
Lemon Syrup	200 ml
Syrup .. .. to	1000 ml

Dissolve the codeine phosphate in the water, add 500 ml of the syrup, and mix; add the compound tartrazine solution, the benzoic acid solution, the chloroform spirit, the lemon syrup, and sufficient of the syrup to produce the required volume, and mix.

Standard
PRESENCE OF CODEINE. It complies with the test given for Codeine Phosphate Syrup, page 799, 0·5 ml being used.

WEIGHT PER ML. At 20°, 1·30 g to 1·32 g.

CONTENT OF CODEINE PHOSPHATE. 0·27 to 0·33 per cent w/v, calculated as $C_{18}H_{21}NO_3,H_3PO_4,\frac{1}{2}H_2O$, determined by the method for Codeine Phosphate Syrup, page 799, about 10 g, accurately weighed, being used.

Storage. It should be protected from light.

Dose. 5 millilitres.

When a dose less than or not a multiple of 5 ml is prescribed, the linctus may be diluted, as described under Linctuses (above), with Syrup.

Codeine Linctus contains, in 5 ml, 15 mg of codeine phosphate.

Codeine Linctus, Diabetic

Codeine Phosphate	3 g
Citric Acid	5 g
Lemon Spirit	1 ml
Compound Tartrazine Solution	10 ml
Benzoic Acid Solution	20 ml
Chloroform Spirit	20 ml
Water (see page 642)	20 ml
Sorbitol Solution, non-crystallising grade .. .. .. to	1000 ml

Dissolve the codeine phosphate and the citric acid in the water, add 750 ml of the sorbitol solution, and mix; add the lemon spirit, the compound tartrazine solution, the benzoic acid solution, the chloroform spirit, and sufficient of the sorbitol solution to produce the required volume, and mix.

It has a weight per ml at 20° of about 1·27 g.

Standard
PRESENCE OF CODEINE. It complies with the test given for Codeine Phosphate Syrup, page 799, 0·5 ml being used.

PRESENCE OF SORBITOL. To 0·1 ml add 3 ml of *catechol solution* and 6 ml *sulphuric acid* and warm on a water-bath for 30 seconds; a deep pink colour is produced.

ABSENCE OF SUGARS. To 1 ml add 5 ml of water and 2 ml of *dilute sulphuric acid*, warm on a water-bath for 5 minutes, cool, add 2·5 ml of *phenylhydrazine* and 2·5 ml of *glacial acetic acid*, warm on a water-bath for 15 minutes, and cool; no precipitate is produced immediately.

CONTENT OF CODEINE PHOSPHATE. 0·27 to 0·33 per cent w/v, calculated as $C_{18}H_{21}NO_3,H_3PO_4,\frac{1}{2}H_2O$, determined by the method for Codeine Phosphate Syrup, page 799, about 10 g, accurately weighed, being used.

Storage. It should be protected from light.

Dose. 5 millilitres.

When a dose less than or not a multiple of 5 ml is prescribed, the linctus may be diluted, as described under Linctuses (above), with Chloroform Water.

Diabetic Codeine Linctus contains, in 5 ml, 15 mg of codeine phosphate.

Each 5 ml contains about 4·2 g of carbohydrate and provides about 16 Calories.

Codeine Linctus, Paediatric

SYNONYM: Codeine Mixture, Paediatric

Codeine Linctus	200 ml
Syrup .. .. to	1000 ml

Standard
PRESENCE OF CODEINE. It complies with the test given for Codeine Phosphate Syrup, page 799, 2 ml being used.

CONTENT OF CODEINE PHOSPHATE. 0·051 to 0·069 per cent w/v, calculated as $C_{18}H_{21}NO_3,H_3PO_4,\frac{1}{2}H_2O$, determined by the method for Codeine Phosphate

Syrup, page 799, about 25 g, accurately weighed, being used.

Storage. It should be protected from light.

Dose. CHILD. Up to 1 year, 5 millilitres; 1 to 5 years, 10 millilitres.

When a dose less than or not a multiple of 5 ml is prescribed, the linctus may be diluted, as described under Linctuses (page 722), with Syrup.

Paediatric Codeine Linctus contains, in 5 ml, 3 mg of codeine phosphate.

Diamorphine Linctus

Diamorphine Hydrochloride ..	0·6 g
Compound Tartrazine Solution	12 ml
Glycerol	250 ml
Oxymel	250 ml
Syrup .. .. to	1000 ml

Dissolve the diamorphine hydrochloride in the compound tartrazine solution, add the oxymel, the glycerol, and sufficient syrup to produce the required volume, and mix. It should be recently prepared.

Standard
WEIGHT PER ML. At 20°, 1·29 g to 1·31 g.
CONTENT OF DIAMORPHINE HYDROCHLORIDE. 0·051 to 0·069 per cent w/v, calculated as $C_{21}H_{24}ClNO_5,H_2O$, determined by the following method:
To about 8 g, accurately weighed, add 25 ml of water and 2 ml of *dilute ammonia solution* and extract with 60 ml of a mixture of equal volumes of *alcohol (95 per cent)* and *chloroform* and then with two successive 45-ml portions of a mixture of one volume of *alcohol (95 per cent)* and two volumes of *chloroform*, washing each extract with the same 15 ml of a mixture of one volume of *alcohol (95 per cent)* and two volumes of water.
Combine the extracts, evaporate off the solvent, dissolve the residue in 10 ml of 2N hydrochloric acid, and boil under a reflux condenser for 10 minutes; cool, add 15 ml of water, extract with two successive 15-ml portions of *chloroform*, washing each extract with the same 10 ml of water, and discard the chloroform extracts; heat the combined aqueous solution and washings on a water-bath to remove the chloroform, cool, and dilute to 200 ml with water.
Using 20 ml of this solution, continue the determination by the method for Aromatic Chalk with Opium Powder, page 776, beginning with the words "add 8 ml of a freshly prepared 1·0 per cent w/v solution of *sodium nitrite, ...*"; each g of anhydrous morphine is equivalent to 1·486 g of $C_{21}H_{24}ClNO_5,H_2O$.
Determine the weight per ml of the linctus and calculate the concentration of $C_{21}H_{24}ClNO_5,H_2O$, weight in volume.

Dose. 2·5 to 10 millilitres.

When a dose less than or not a multiple of 5 ml is prescribed, the linctus may be diluted, as described under Linctuses (page 722), with Syrup.

Diamorphine Linctus contains, in 5 ml, 3 mg of diamorphine hydrochloride.

Ipecacuanha and Squill Linctus, Paediatric

Ipecacuanha Tincture	20·0 ml
Squill Tincture	30·0 ml
Compound Orange Spirit ..	1·5 ml
Black Currant Syrup	500·0 ml
Syrup .. .. .. to	1000·0 ml

Standard
WEIGHT PER ML. At 20°, 1·28 g to 1·30 g.
PRESENCE OF IPECACUANHA ALKALOIDS. It complies with the thin-layer chromatographic test given in Appendix 5B, page 871.

Storage. It should be stored in a cool place.

Dose. CHILD. 5 millilitres.

When a dose less than or not a multiple of 5 ml is prescribed, the linctus may be diluted, as described under Linctuses (page 722), with Syrup.

Methadone Linctus

SYNONYM: Amidone Linctus

Methadone Hydrochloride ..	0·4 g
Compound Tartrazine Solution	8 ml
Water (see page 642)	120 ml
Glycerol	250 ml
Tolu Syrup .. .. .. to	1000 ml

Dissolve the methadone hydrochloride in the water, add the compound tartrazine solution, the glycerol, and sufficient tolu syrup to produce the required volume, and mix.

Standard
WEIGHT PER ML. At 20°, 1·26 g to 1·28 g.
CONTENT OF METHADONE HYDROCHLORIDE. 0·036 to 0·044 per cent w/v, determined by the following method:
To about 20 g, accurately weighed, add 15 ml of water, acidify to *litmus paper* with *dilute sulphuric acid*, extract with 10 ml of *light petroleum (boiling-range, 40° to 60°)*, wash the extract with two successive 5-ml portions of water, add the washings to the aqueous solution, and discard the light-petroleum extract.
Make the aqueous solution just alkaline to *litmus paper* with *sodium hydroxide solution*, add 2 g of *sodium chloride*, and extract with successive 30-, 15-, and 15-ml portions of *anaesthetic ether*; wash the combined extracts with two successive 5-ml portions of water, and wash the combined aqueous washings with 5 ml of *anaesthetic ether*, adding the ethereal washings to the combined ethereal extracts.
Extract the ethereal solution with two successive 10-ml portions of 0·02N hydrochloric acid, warm the combined extracts with a small piece of porous pot to remove any dissolved ether, cool, dilute to 25 ml with water, and measure the extinction of a 1-cm layer at the maximum at about 293 nm.
For purposes of calculation, use a value of 15·4 for the E(1 per cent, 1 cm) of methadone hydrochloride.
Determine the weight per ml of the linctus and calculate the concentration of methadone hydrochloride, weight in volume.

Dose. 5 millilitres.

When a dose less than or not a multiple of 5 ml is prescribed, the linctus may be diluted, as described under Linctuses (page 722), with Syrup.

Methadone Linctus contains, in 5 ml, 2 mg of methadone hydrochloride.

Noscapine Linctus

Noscapine..	3 g
Citric Acid	10 g
Compound Tartrazine Solution	3 ml
Chloroform Spirit	75 ml
Purified Water, freshly boiled and cooled	100 ml
Syrup .. .. .. to	1000 ml

Add the noscapine and the citric acid to the water, previously heated to about 50°, and stir until dissolved; cool, add 800 ml of the syrup, followed by the compound tartrazine solution, the chloroform spirit, and sufficient syrup to produce the required volume, and mix.

Standard

WEIGHT PER ML. At 20°, 1·26 g to 1·28 g.

CONTENT OF NOSCAPINE. 0·270 to 0·330 per cent w/v, determined by the following method:
To about 20 g, accurately weighed, add 20 ml of water, 2 g of *sodium chloride*, and 2 ml of *sodium hydroxide solution* and extract with successive 50-, 50-, 25-, and 25-ml portions of *anaesthetic ether*.
Combine the extracts, wash with three successive 5-ml portions of water, evaporate to dryness, warm on a water-bath with 50 ml of 0·1N hydrochloric acid to dissolve the residue and to remove the last traces of ether, and dilute to 100 ml with water.
Dilute 3 ml of this solution to 50 ml with water, and measure the extinction of a 1-cm layer at the maximum at about 310 nm.
For purposes of calculation, use a value of 90·7 for the E(1 per cent, 1 cm) of noscapine.
Determine the weight per ml of the linctus and calculate the concentration of noscapine, weight in volume.

Storage. It should be stored in a cool place.

Dose. 5 to 10 millilitres.

When a dose less than or not a multiple of 5 ml is prescribed, the linctus may be diluted, as described under Linctuses (page 722), with Syrup.

Noscapine Linctus contains, in 5 ml, 15 mg of noscapine.

Pholcodine Linctus

Strong Pholcodine Linctus		..		500 ml
Syrup	..	..	..	500 ml

Standard

PRESENCE OF PHOLCODINE. To 20 ml add 20 ml of water, extract with 15-ml portions of *chloroform*, filter each extract through a layer of *anhydrous sodium sulphate*, and evaporate the combined filtrates to dryness. The residue complies with the following tests:
(i) To a portion of the residue add 0·05 ml of *nitric acid* and mix; a yellow colour is produced (distinction from morphine).
(ii) Dissolve the remainder of the residue in 1 ml of *sulphuric acid* and add 0·05 ml of *ammonium molybdate solution*; a pale blue colour is produced. Warm gently; the colour changes to deep blue. Add 0·05 ml of *dilute nitric acid*; the colour changes to brownish-red.

WEIGHT PER ML. At 20°, 1·29 g to 1·31 g.

CONTENT OF PHOLCODINE. 0·087 to 0·113 per cent w/v, calculated as $C_{23}H_{30}N_2O_4,H_2O$, determined by the following method:
Make about 50 g, accurately weighed, alkaline to *litmus paper* with *dilute ammonia solution* and extract with four successive 25-ml portions of *chloroform*, washing each extract with the same 5 ml of water.
Combine the extracts, evaporate off the chloroform until the volume is reduced to about 15 ml, and continue by Method I of the British Pharmacopoeia, Appendix XIB, for non-aqueous titration, titrating with 0·02N perchloric acid and using *quinaldine red solution* in place of crystal violet as indicator; each ml of 0·02N perchloric acid is equivalent to 0·004165 g of $C_{23}H_{30}N_2O_4,H_2O$.
Determine the weight per ml of the linctus and calculate the concentration of $C_{23}H_{30}N_2O_4,H_2O$, weight in volume.

Storage. It should be stored in a cool place.

Dose. 5 millilitres.

When a dose less than or not a multiple of 5 ml is prescribed, the linctus may be diluted, as described under Linctuses (page 722), with Syrup.

Pholcodine Linctus contains, in 5 ml, about 5 mg of pholcodine.

Pholcodine Linctus, Strong

Pholcodine	..	..	.. 2 g
Citric Acid	..	..	.. 20 g
Amaranth Solution	..	..	2 ml
Compound Tartrazine Solution			20 ml
Chloroform Spirit	..	..	150 ml
Syrup	..	..	.. to 1000 ml

Dissolve the citric acid and the pholcodine each in a separate 75-ml portion of the chloroform spirit, mix the two solutions, add the amaranth solution, the compound tartrazine solution, and sufficient syrup to produce the required volume, and mix.

Standard

PRESENCE OF PHOLCODINE. It complies with the test given for Pholcodine Linctus, 10 ml being used.

WEIGHT PER ML. At 20°, 1·26 g to 1·28 g.

CONTENT OF PHOLCODINE. 0·180 to 0·220 per cent w/v, calculated as $C_{23}H_{30}N_2O_4,H_2O$, determined by the method for Pholcodine Linctus, about 25 g, accurately weighed, being used.

Storage. It should be stored in a cool place.

Dose. 5 millilitres.

When a dose less than or not a multiple of 5 ml is prescribed, the linctus may be diluted, as described under Linctuses (page 722), with Syrup.

Strong Pholcodine Linctus contains, in 5 ml, 10 mg of pholcodine.

Simple Linctus

Citric Acid	..	..	.. 25 g
Concentrated Anise Water		..	10 ml
Amaranth Solution	..	..	15 ml
Chloroform Spirit	..	..	60 ml
Syrup	..	..	.. to 1000 ml

Standard

WEIGHT PER ML. At 20°, 1·27 g to 1·31 g.

CONTENT OF FREE ACID. 2·24 to 2·65 per cent w/v, calculated as citric acid, $C_6H_8O_7,H_2O$, determined by the following method:
Dilute about 15 g, accurately weighed, with 50 ml of water and titrate with 0·5N sodium hydroxide, using 2 ml of *thymol blue solution* as indicator; each ml of 0·5N sodium hydroxide is equivalent to 0·03502 g of $C_6H_8O_7,H_2O$.
Determine the weight per ml of the linctus and calculate the concentration of $C_6H_8O_7,H_2O$, weight in volume.

Storage. It should be stored in a cool place.

Dose. 5 millilitres.

When a dose less than or not a multiple of 5 ml is prescribed, the linctus may be diluted, as described under Linctuses (page 722), with Syrup.

Simple Linctus, Paediatric

Simple Linctus	..	..	..	250 ml
Syrup	..	..	..	to 1000 ml

Standard
WEIGHT PER ML. At 20°, 1·28 g to 1·33 g.

CONTENT OF FREE ACID. 0·53 to 0·69 per cent w/v, calculated as citric acid, $C_6H_8O_7,H_2O$, determined by the method for Simple Linctus, 0·1N sodium hydroxide being used in place of 0·5N sodium hydroxide; each ml of 0·1N sodium hydroxide is equivalent to 0·007005 g of $C_6H_8O_7,H_2O$.

Storage. It should be stored in a cool place.

Dose. CHILD. 5 to 10 millilitres.

When a dose less than or not a multiple of 5 ml is prescribed, the linctus may be diluted, as described under Linctuses (page 722), with Syrup.

Squill Linctus, Opiate

SYNONYMS: Compound Squill Linctus; Gee's Linctus

Squill Oxymel	..	..	..	300 ml
Camphorated Opium Tincture	..		300 ml
Tolu Syrup	..	..	..	300 ml

Mix. Alternatively, disperse 0·5 g of Powdered Tragacanth in the camphorated opium tincture, add the squill oxymel and the tolu syrup, and mix.

Standard
DESCRIPTION. A straw-coloured to light-brown opalescent or turbid liquid.

WEIGHT PER ML. At 20°, 1·16 g to 1·19 g.

ALCOHOL CONTENT. 17 to 20 per cent v/v of ethyl alcohol, determined by the method given in Appendix 10, page 888.

CONTENT OF ANHYDROUS MORPHINE. 0·013 to 0·020 per cent w/v, determined by the following method:
To about 12 g, accurately weighed, add 5 ml of water and 1 ml of *dilute ammonia solution* and extract with 30 ml of a mixture of equal volumes of *alcohol (95 per cent)* and *chloroform* and then with two successive 22·5-ml portions of a mixture of one volume of *alcohol (95 per cent)* and two volumes of *chloroform*, washing each extract with the same 20 ml of a mixture of equal volumes of *alcohol (95 per cent)* and water. Combine the extracts, evaporate off the solvent, extract the residue with 10 ml of *calcium hydroxide solution*, filter, and wash the filter with 10 ml of *calcium hydroxide solution*; to the combined filtrate and washings add 0·1 g of *ammonium sulphate*, extract with two successive 10-ml portions of *alcohol-free chloroform*, wash the combined extracts with 10 ml of water, and discard the chloroform solution.
To the combined alkaline liquid and aqueous washings add 10 ml of 1N hydrochloric acid, heat on a water-bath to remove any chloroform, cool, and dilute to 100 ml with water; using 20 ml of this solution, continue by the method for Aromatic Chalk with Opium Powder, page 776, beginning with the words "add 8 ml of a freshly prepared 1·0 per cent w/v solution of *sodium nitrite*, ...".

Determine the weight per ml of the linctus and calculate the concentration of anhydrous morphine, weight in volume.

Dose. 5 millilitres.

When a dose less than or not a multiple of 5 ml is prescribed, the linctus may be diluted, as described under Linctuses (page 722), with Syrup.

Opiate Squill Linctus contains, in 5 ml, about 800 µg of anhydrous morphine.

Squill Linctus, Opiate, Paediatric

SYNONYM: Opiate Linctus for Infants

Squill Oxymel	..	..	..	60 ml
Camphorated Opium Tincture	..		60 ml
Tolu Syrup	..	..	..	60 ml
Glycerol	..	..	..	200 ml
Syrup	..	..	..	to 1000 ml

Standard
WEIGHT PER ML. At 20°, 1·27 g to 1·30 g.

CONTENT OF ANHYDROUS MORPHINE. 0·0024 to 0·0036 per cent w/v, determined by the method for Opiate Squill Linctus, but use about 32 g, accurately weighed, use 5 ml of 1N hydrochloric acid instead of 10 ml, and, after cooling the acidified liquid and washings, dilute to 50 ml instead of to 100 ml with water.

Dose. CHILD. 5 to 10 millilitres.

When a dose less than or not a multiple of 5 ml is prescribed, the linctus may be diluted, as described under Linctuses (page 722), with Syrup.

Paediatric Opiate Squill Linctus contains, in 5 ml, about 150 µg of anhydrous morphine.

Tolu Linctus, Compound, Paediatric

Citric Acid	..	..	..	6 g
Benzaldehyde Spirit	..	..		2 ml
Compound Tartrazine Solution	..		10 ml
Glycerol	..	..	..	200 ml
Invert Syrup	..	..	..	200 ml
Tolu Syrup	..	..	..	to 1000 ml

Standard
WEIGHT PER ML. At 20°, 1·30 g to 1·32 g.

TOTAL ACIDITY. 0·57 to 0·70 per cent w/v, calculated as citric acid, $C_6H_8O_7,H_2O$, determined by the following method:
To about 15 g, accurately weighed, add 100 ml of water and titrate with 0·1N sodium hydroxide, using *phenolphthalein solution* as indicator; each ml of 0·1N sodium hydroxide is equivalent to 0·007005 g of $C_6H_8O_7,H_2O$.
Determine the weight per ml of the linctus and calculate the concentration of $C_6H_8O_7,H_2O$, weight in volume.

Storage. It should be stored in a cool place.

Dose. CHILD. 5 to 10 millilitres

When a dose less than or not a multiple of 5 ml is prescribed, the linctus may be diluted, as described under Linctuses (page 722), with Syrup.

LINIMENTS

Liniments are usually liquid or semi-liquid preparations which are intended for external application and may contain substances possessing analgesic, rubefacient, soothing, or stimulating properties. Analgesic and soothing liniments may be applied to the skin on warmed flannel or other suitable material, or by means of a camel-hair brush; stimulating liniments should be applied to the skin with considerable friction by massaging with the hand. Liniments should not be applied to broken skin.

Containers. Liniments should be dispensed in coloured fluted bottles.

Labelling. The container should be labelled "For external use only".

Methyl Salicylate Liniment

Methyl Salicylate	..	..	250 ml
Arachis Oil	..	..	.. to 1000 ml

Standard
WEIGHT PER ML. At 20°, 0·973 g to 0·989 g.

CONTENT OF METHYL SALICYLATE. 23·0 to 26·5 per cent v/v, determined by the method for Methyl Salicylate Ointment, page 762, 4·0 per cent w/v of the sample being used in the preparation of solutions (2) and (3).
Determine the weight per ml of the liniment and calculate the concentration of methyl salicylate, volume in volume.

Containers; Labelling. The directions given under Liniments (above) should be followed. Certain plastic containers, such as those made from polystyrene, are unsuitable for use with this liniment.

Storage. It should be stored in airtight containers, in a cool place.

Soap Liniment

SYNONYM: Linimentum Saponis

Camphor ..	..	..	..	40 g
Oleic Acid	..	..	..	40 g
Rosemary Oil	..	..	..	15 ml
Potassium Hydroxide Solution ..				140 ml
Alcohol (90 per cent)	..	..		700 ml
Purified Water, freshly boiled and cooled ..	..	..		.. to 1000 ml

Dissolve the oleic acid in 500 ml of the alcohol and add, with stirring, the potassium hydroxide solution. Dissolve the camphor and the rosemary oil in the remainder of the alcohol, mix the two solutions, add sufficient of the water to produce the required volume, mix, allow to stand for not less than seven days, and filter.

In making this preparation the alcohol (90 per cent) may be replaced by Industrial Methylated Spirit diluted so as to be of equivalent alcoholic strength, provided that the law and the statutory regulations governing the use of industrial methylated spirit are observed.

Standard
ALKALINITY. pH, 7·4 to 8·0.
WEIGHT PER ML. At 20°, 0·880 g to 0·900 g.

ALCOHOL CONTENT. 60 to 65 per cent v/v of ethyl alcohol, determined by the method given in Appendix 10, page 888.

CONTENT OF OLEIC ACID. Not less than 3·8 per cent w/v, determined by the following method:
To 25 ml add 5 ml of *sodium hydroxide solution*, extract with two successive 25-ml portions of *light petroleum (boiling-range, 40° to 60°)*, wash the combined extracts with 10 ml of water, and discard the extracts.
Acidify the combined aqueous solution and washings to *litmus paper* with *dilute sulphuric acid*, and extract with three successive 25-ml portions of *light petroleum (boiling-range 40° to 60°)*, combine the extracts, evaporate off the solvent, add 5 ml of *acetone*, evaporate to dryness, dry the residue of oleic acid for 2 hours at 80°, and weigh.

Containers; Labelling. The directions given under Liniments (above) should be followed.

White Liniment

SYNONYMS: Linimentum Album; White Embrocation

Ammonium Chloride	..	..	12·5 g
Dilute Ammonia Solution		..	45 ml
Oleic Acid	..	..	85 ml
Turpentine Oil	..	..	250 ml
Water (see page 642)	..	..	625 ml

Mix the oleic acid with the turpentine oil, add the dilute ammonia solution mixed with an equal volume of the water, previously warmed, and shake. Dissolve the ammonium chloride in the remainder of the water, add to the emulsion, and mix.

Standard
CONTENT OF VOLATILE OIL. 24·5 to 27·5 per cent v/w, determined by the following method:
Transfer about 100 g, accurately weighed, to an apparatus for steam distillation, acidify with *dilute sulphuric acid* using *methyl orange solution* as indicator, distil, and collect the distillate in a separating funnel; from time to time separate the aqueous portion of the distillate and return it to the flask.
When all the volatile matter has been distilled, discard the aqueous portion of the distillate and measure the volume of the oily liquid.
The refractive index of the oily distillate, determined at 20°, is 1·465 to 1·477.

Containers; Labelling. The directions given under Liniments (above) should be followed.

LOTIONS

Lotions are liquid preparations intended for application to the skin. The inclusion of alcohol in a lotion hastens its drying and accentuates its cooling effect, whilst the inclusion of glycerol keeps the skin moist for a considerable time.

Lotions are applied, without friction, on lint or other soft absorbent fabric and covered with waterproof material, or dabbed on the skin.

Avoidance of microbial contamination. Micro-organisms may grow in certain lotions if no preservative is included; even if a preservative is present, care should be taken to avoid contaminating the lotions during their preparation. If a lotion is likely to be applied to broken or inflamed skin, the directions given under Creams (page 655) for preparation and dilution should be followed.

Containers. Lotions should be dispensed in coloured fluted bottles or in suitable plastic containers.

Labelling. The container should be labelled "For external use only". The label on a diluted lotion should also state that the lotion should not be used later than one month after issue for use.

Aminobenzoic Acid Lotion

Aminobenzoic Acid	..	..		50 g
Glycerol ..	..	..	..	200 ml
Alcohol (95 per cent)	..	..		600 ml
Purified Water, freshly boiled and cooled ..	..	..	..	to 1000 ml

In making this preparation, the alcohol (95 per cent) may be replaced by Industrial Methylated Spirit, provided that the law and the statutory regulations governing the use of industrial methylated spirit are observed.

Standard
WEIGHT PER ML. At 20°, 0·930 g to 0·950 g.

ALCOHOL CONTENT. 54 to 58 per cent v/v of ethyl alcohol, determined by the method given in Appendix 10, page 888.

p-NITROBENZOIC ACID. It complies with the thin-layer chromatographic test given in Appendix 5A, page 858 (not more than 1·0 per cent of the content of aminobenzoic acid).

CONTENT OF AMINOBENZOIC ACID. 4·62 to 5·38 per cent w/v, determined by the following method:
Mix 2 ml with 20 ml of 1N sodium hydroxide, dilute to 200 ml with water, further dilute 2 ml of this solution to 200 ml with 0·1N sodium hydroxide, and measure the extinction of a 1-cm layer at the maximum at about 264 nm.
For purposes of calculation use a value of 1064 for the E(1 per cent, 1 cm) of aminobenzoic acid.
Calculate the percentage of aminobenzoic acid in the sample.

Labelling. A caution should be given on the label that the lotion may stain clothing. In addition, the label states that the preparation discolours slightly on storage.

Storage. It should be protected from light.

Betamethasone Valerate Lotion

SYNONYM: Betamethasone Lotion

Betamethasone Valerate Lotion is a dispersion of Betamethasone Valerate in a suitable lotion basis. It may contain a preservative.

Standard
PRESENCE OF BETAMETHASONE. It complies with the thin-layer chromatographic test given in Appendix 5D, page 875.

CONTENT OF BETAMETHASONE. 90·0 to 115·0 per cent of the prescribed or stated concentration, determined by the method given in Appendix 23A, page 904, for betamethasone 17-valerate.

Labelling. The container should be labelled "For external use only".

Storage. It should be stored in airtight containers at a temperature not exceeding 30°.

Note. When the strength of the lotion is not specified, a lotion containing the equivalent of 0·1 per cent w/v of betamethasone shall be supplied.

The lotion should not be diluted or mixed with any other preparation.

Calamine Lotion, Oily

SYNONYM: Calamine Liniment

Calamine ..	..	..	..	50 g
Wool Fat ..	..	..	..	10 g
Oleic Acid	..	..	..	5 ml
Arachis Oil	..	..	..	500 ml
Calcium Hydroxide Solution		..	to 1000 ml

Triturate the calamine with the wool fat, the arachis oil, and the oleic acid, previously melted together, transfer to a suitable container, add the calcium hydroxide solution, and shake vigorously.

Standard
CONTENT OF ZINC. 2·52 to 3·35 per cent w/w, calculated as Zn, determined by the method for Calamine and Coal Tar Ointment, page 760, using about 2 g, accurately weighed.

Containers; Labelling. The directions given under Lotions (above) should be followed.

Copper and Zinc Sulphates Lotion

SYNONYMS: Copper and Zinc Lotion; Dalibour Water

Copper Sulphate ..		..	..	10 g
Zinc Sulphate	..	..	..	15 g
Camphor Water, Concentrated ..			25 ml
Water (see page 642)	..		..	to 1000 ml

Dissolve the copper sulphate and the zinc

sulphate in 900 ml of the water, add the concentrated camphor water in small quantities, shaking vigorously after each addition, and add sufficient water to produce the required volume.

Standard

CONTENT OF ZINC SULPHATE. 1·43 to 1·57 per cent w/v, calculated as $ZnSO_4,7H_2O$, determined by the following method:
To 10 ml add 10 ml of a 10 per cent v/v solution of *thioglycerol* in water and allow to stand until precipitation has occurred; add 2 ml of *dilute hydrochloric acid* and 3 g of *hexamine*, allow to stand for 15 minutes, and titrate with 0·05M disodium edetate, using *xylenol orange solution* as indicator; each ml of 0·05M disodium edetate is equivalent to 0·01438 g of $ZnSO_4,7H_2O$.

CONTENT OF COPPER SULPHATE. 0·95 to 1·05 per cent w/v, calculated as $CuSO_4,5H_2O$, determined by the following method:
To 25 ml add 3 g of *potassium iodide* and 5 ml of *acetic acid* and titrate the liberated iodine with 0·1N sodium thiosulphate, using *starch mucilage* as indicator, until only a faint blue colour remains; add 2 g of *potassium thiocyanate* and continue the titration until the blue colour disappears; each ml of 0·1N sodium thiosulphate is equivalent to 0·02497 g of $CuSO_4,5H_2O$.

Containers; Labelling. The directions given under Lotions (page 727) should be followed.

Hydrocortisone Lotion

Hydrocortisone, in sufficiently fine powder to meet the requirements of the standard	10·0 g
Chlorocresol	0·5 g
Self-emulsifying Monostearin ..	40·0 g
Glycerol	63·0 g
Purified Water, freshly boiled and cooled	to 1000·0 g

Dissolve the chlorocresol in 850 ml of the water with the aid of gentle heat, add the self-emulsifying monostearin, heat to 60°, and stir until completely dispersed. Triturate the hydrocortisone with the glycerol, incorporate, with constant stirring, in the warm basis, allow to cool slowly, stirring until cold, add sufficient of the water to produce the required weight, and mix.
Hydrocortisone Lotion may be prepared using any other suitable basis.

Standard

DESCRIPTION. A white readily pourable liquid.

PRESENCE OF HYDROCORTISONE. It complies with the thin-layer chromatographic test given in Appendix 5D, page 876.

PARTICLE SIZE. When determined by the method given in Appendix 25C, page 911, not less than 75 per cent of the particles have a maximum diameter less than 10 μm and not less than 99 per cent of the particles have a maximum diameter less than 20 μm; no particle has a maximum diameter greater than 50 μm.

CONTENT OF HYDROCORTISONE. 0·90 to 1·10 per cent w/w, determined by the method for creams containing hydrocortisone given under Hydrocortisone Cream, page 659.

Containers; Labelling. The directions given under Lotions (page 727) should be followed.

Note. If prepared extemporaneously, the lotion should not be used later than one month after preparation.

Lead Lotion

SYNONYM: Lotio Plumbi

Strong Lead Subacetate Solution	20 ml
Purified Water, freshly boiled and cooled	to 1000 ml

It must be freshly prepared.

Containers; Labelling. The directions given under Lotions (page 727) should be followed.

Note. Lead Lotion should be used undiluted.

Lead Lotion, Evaporating

SYNONYM: Lead and Spirit Lotion

Strong Lead Subacetate Solution	25 ml
Alcohol (95 per cent)	125 ml
Purified Water, freshly boiled and cooled	to 1000 ml

It must be freshly prepared.

In making this preparation the alcohol (95 per cent) may be replaced by Industrial Methylated Spirit, provided that the law and the statutory regulations governing the use of industrial methylated spirit are observed.

Containers; Labelling. The directions given under Lotions (page 727) should be followed.

Note. Evaporating Lead Lotion should be used undiluted.

Salicylic Acid Lotion

Salicylic Acid	20 g
Castor Oil..	10 ml
Alcohol (95 per cent)	to 1000 ml

Dissolve the salicylic acid in a portion of the alcohol, add the castor oil and sufficient of the alcohol to produce the required volume, and mix.

In making this preparation the alcohol (95 per cent) may be replaced by Industrial Methylated Spirit, provided that the law and the statutory regulations governing the use of industrial methylated spirit are observed.

Standard

PRESENCE OF SALICYLIC ACID. To 5 ml of the solution obtained after titration in the determination of the content of salicylic acid add 1 ml of *ferric chloride test-solution*; an intense reddish-violet colour is produced.
Add *acetic acid*; the colour does not change.
Add *dilute hydrochloric acid*; the reddish-violet colour disappears and a slight white precipitate is produced.

ALCOHOL CONTENT. 90 to 93 per cent v/v of ethyl alcohol, determined by the method given in Appendix 10, page 888.

CONTENT OF SALICYLIC ACID. 1·90 to 2·10 per cent w/v, calculated as $C_7H_6O_3$, determined by the following method:
Dilute 10 ml with 10 ml of *carbon dioxide-free water* and titrate with 0·1N sodium hydroxide, using *phenol red solution* as indicator; each ml of 0·1N sodium hydroxide is equivalent to 0·01381 g of $C_7H_6O_3$.

Containers. The directions given under Lotions (page 727) should be followed.

Labelling. The directions given under Lotions (page 727) should be followed.
In addition, the container should be labelled "Caution. This preparation is inflammable. Do not use it or dry the hair near a fire or naked flame".

Salicylic Acid and Mercuric Chloride Lotion

SYNONYM: Lotio Acidi Salicylici et Hydrargyri Perchloridi

Salicylic Acid	..	..	..	20 g
Mercuric Chloride		..	..	1 g
Castor Oil..	..	..	..	10 ml
Acetone	..	..	..	125 ml
Alcohol (95 per cent)		..	.. to 1000 ml

Dissolve the mercuric chloride and the salicylic acid in 500 ml of the alcohol, add the castor oil, the acetone, and sufficient of the alcohol to produce the required volume, and mix.

In making this preparation the alcohol (95 per cent) may be replaced by Industrial Methylated Spirit, provided that the law and the statutory regulations governing the use of industrial methylated spirit are observed.

Standard
PRESENCE OF SALICYLIC ACID. It complies with the test given for Salicylic Acid Lotion.

CONTENT OF SALICYLIC ACID. 1·90 to 2·10 per cent w/v, calculated as $C_7H_6O_3$, determined by the following method:
Dilute 20 ml with 30 ml of water, make just alkaline to *litmus paper* with *sodium hydroxide solution*, extract with two successive 20-ml portions of *solvent ether*, washing each extract with the same 5 ml of water, and discard the ethereal extracts.
Combine the aqueous washings with the alkaline liquid, acidify to *litmus paper* with *dilute sulphuric acid*, and extract with successive 25-ml portions of *solvent ether* until extraction is complete.
Wash the combined extracts with two successive 5-ml portions of water and wash the combined aqueous washings with 20 ml of *solvent ether*; filter the combined ethereal solution and washings, wash the filter with *solvent ether*, and evaporate the combined filtrate and ethereal washings nearly to dryness at a temperature not exceeding 40° in a current of warm air.
Dissolve the residue in 15 ml of *alcohol (95 per cent)* previously neutralised to *phenol red solution*, add 20 ml of water, and titrate with 0·1N sodium hydroxide, using *phenol red solution* as indicator; each ml of 0·1N sodium hydroxide is equivalent to 0·01381 g of $C_7H_6O_3$.

CONTENT OF MERCURIC CHLORIDE. 0·09 to 0·11 per cent w/v, calculated as $HgCl_2$, determined by the following method:
Heat 100 ml with 5 ml of *glacial acetic acid* to a temperature not exceeding 55°, pass *hydrogen sulphide* through the hot solution for 10 minutes, and filter; wash the residue with *hydrogen sulphide solution*, then with *alcohol (95 per cent)*, and finally with *carbon disulphide*, and dry to constant weight at 105°; each g of residue is equivalent to 1·167 g of $HgCl_2$.

Containers. The directions given under Lotions (page 727) should be followed.

Labelling. The directions given under Lotions (page 727) should be followed.
In addition, the container should be labelled "Caution. This preparation is inflammable. Do not use it or dry the hair near a fire or naked flame".

Storage. It should be stored in airtight containers, in a cool place.

Sulphur Lotion, Compound

Precipitated Sulphur	..	..	40 g
Quillaia Tincture..	..	..	5 ml
Glycerol	..	..	20 ml
Alcohol (95 per cent)	..	..	60 ml
Calcium Hydroxide Solution		.. to 1000 ml

Disperse the precipitated sulphur in the alcohol and the glycerol previously mixed, add the quillaia tincture and sufficient of the calcium hydroxide solution to produce the required volume, and mix.

In making this preparation the alcohol (95 per cent) may be replaced by Industrial Methylated Spirit, provided that the law and the statutory regulations governing the use of industrial methylated spirit are observed.

Containers; Labelling. The directions given under Lotions (page 727) should be followed.

Triamcinolone Lotion

SYNONYM: Triamcinolone Acetonide Lotion

Triamcinolone Lotion is a dispersion of Triamcinolone Acetonide in a suitable lotion basis.

Standard
CONTENT OF TRIAMCINOLONE ACETONIDE. 90·0 to 110·0 per cent of the prescribed or stated amount, determined by the following method:
Evaporate to dryness on a water-bath, an accurately weighed quantity, equivalent to about 2 mg of triamcinolone acetonide, disperse the residue in 30 ml of *chloroform*, shake, dilute to 50 ml with *chloroform*, filter, and continue by the method for Triamcinolone Ointment, page 764, beginning with the words "To three 25-ml graduated flasks . . .".

Containers; Labelling. The directions given under Lotions (page 727) should be followed.

Note. When the strength of the lotion is not specified, a lotion containing 0·1 per cent w/w of triamcinolone acetonide shall be supplied.

When a strength less than that available from the manufacturer is prescribed, the 0·1 per cent lotion may be diluted, taking hygienic precautions, with a 3 per cent solution of sodium carboxymethylcellulose (medium-viscosity grade) in Water (see page 642) containing 0·2 per cent w/v of methyl hydroxybenzoate and 0·02 per cent w/v of propyl hydroxybenzoate.
The diluted lotion must be freshly prepared.

Zinc Sulphate Lotion

SYNONYM: Lotio Rubra

Zinc Sulphate	..	..	..	10 g
Amaranth Solution		..	..	10 ml
Water (see page 642)		..	.. to 1000 ml

Standard
CONTENT OF ZINC SULPHATE. 0·95 to 1·05 per cent w/v, calculated as $ZnSO_4,7H_2O$, determined by the following method:
To 20 ml add 150 ml of water and 5 ml of *ammonia buffer solution* and titrate with 0·05M disodium edetate, using *mordant black 11 solution* as indicator; each ml of 0·05M disodium edetate is equivalent to 0·01438 g of $ZnSO_4,7H_2O$.

Containers; Labelling. The directions given under Lotions (page 727) should be followed.

Zinc Sulphide Lotion

SYNONYMS: Sulphurated Potash and Zinc Lotion; Sulphurated Potash Lotion

Zinc Sulphate	50 g
Sulphurated Potash	50 g
Concentrated Camphor Water ..	25 ml
Water (see page 642)   ..   .. to 1000 ml

Dissolve the sulphurated potash and the zinc sulphate each in 450 ml of the water, add the solution of the sulphurated potash to the solution of the zinc sulphate, and stir; add sufficient water to produce almost the required volume, add gradually the concentrated camphor water, shaking thoroughly after each addition, and sufficient water to produce the required volume, and mix.

It should be freshly prepared.

Containers; Labelling. The directions given under Lotions (page 727) should be followed.

LOZENGES

Lozenges consist of medicaments incorporated in a flavoured basis and are intended to dissolve or disintegrate slowly in the mouth.

They are prepared either by moulding and cutting or by compression.

Moulded Lozenges

These are usually prepared by mixing the medicaments, in powder or solution, with the basis, usually sucrose and acacia or tragacanth, making the mixture into a uniform paste with water, acacia mucilage, and the other ingredients, cutting the mass into uniform shapes, and drying the lozenges in a hot-air chamber at a moderate temperature.

Lozenges with Simple Basis

For 100 lozenges take:

Acacia, in fine powder	7 g
Sucrose, in fine powder	100 g
Water (see page 642)	a sufficient quantity

Mix the medicaments intimately with the sucrose and the acacia, make the mixture into a paste with water, divide into 100 equal lozenges, and dry.

Standard for moulded lozenges

COLOURING AND FLAVOURING. Moulded lozenges may contain only colouring and flavouring agents specified in the individual monographs.

UNIFORMITY OF WEIGHT. Take a sample of 20 lozenges and determine the mean weight. When weighed singly, the weight of not more than two lozenges may deviate by more than 10 per cent from the mean weight and the weight of none of the lozenges deviates by more than 15 per cent.

If 20 lozenges are not available, 10 may be used for the determination; not more than one of the lozenges may deviate by more than 10 per cent from the mean weight and none of the lozenges deviates by more than 15 per cent.

CONTENT OF ACTIVE INGREDIENT. When limits for content of active ingredient are given in the monographs, all permissible allowances, including variations due to manufacturing methods and to purity of the active ingredient, are included. Unless otherwise specified, the limits are only applicable when the determination is carried out on a sample of 20 lozenges.

When it is not possible to obtain a sample of 20 lozenges, 10 are taken for the determination and the permitted tolerances are increased by ± 5 per cent. The methods and modified tolerances are not applicable when less than half the number of lozenges specified is available.

Compressed Lozenges

These are prepared by the method described under Tablets for compressed tablets (page 801). Heavy compression is necessary in order to ensure slow disintegration in the mouth. Each lozenge is made up to the weight specified in the individual monograph with an inert excipient which usually contains not less than 50 per cent of sucrose.

Standard for Compressed Lozenges

COLOURING AND FLAVOURING. Compressed lozenges may contain only the colouring and flavouring agents specified in the individual monographs.

UNIFORMITY OF DIAMETER. Circular compressed lozenges comply with the requirements given in Appendix 26, page 912.

UNIFORMITY OF WEIGHT; CONTENT OF ACTIVE INGREDIENT. They comply with the standard given under Tablets, page 804.

Containers. Lozenges should be stored in well-closed containers which provide adequate protection against moisture and crushing. They should be supplied in wide-mouthed glass jars or plastic containers, or aluminium containers, suitably protected; lined screw-cap closures or plastic caps should be used.

Amphotericin Lozenges

Amphotericin Lozenges are prepared by moist granulation and compression as described under Lozenges (above). The lozenges may contain suitable flavouring.
Each lozenge weighs about 1 gram.

Standard
They comply with the standard for compressed lozenges under Lozenges, above, with the following additions:

AMPHOTERICIN A. Not more than 15·0 per cent of the content of amphotericin, determined by the following method:
Shake an accurately weighed quantity of the powdered lozenges, equivalent to about 0·05 g of amphotericin, with 20 ml of *dimethyl sulphoxide*, dilute to 100 ml with *dehydrated methyl alcohol*, filter, dilute 10 ml of the filtrate to 50 ml with *dehydrated methyl alcohol*, and immediately measure the extinction of a 1-cm layer at 282 nm and at 304 nm, using as the blank a 0·8 per cent v/v solution of *dimethyl sulphoxide* in *dehydrated methyl alcohol*.
At the same time and in the same manner, measure the extinctions of reference solutions containing, respectively, 0·050 g of *amphotericin B A.S.* and 5·0 mg of *amphotericin A A.S.*, prepared by dissolving the stated quantity in 5 ml of *dimethyl sulphoxide*, diluting to 50 ml with *dehydrated methyl alcohol*, and further diluting 4 ml of each solution to 50 ml with *dehydrated methyl alcohol*.
Calculate the E(1 per cent, 1 cm) for the sample, with respect to the content of amphotericin as determined in the method given below, and for the two reference substances, at both wavelengths.
The content of amphotericin A in the amphotericin present is given by the formula:

$$F + \frac{100(BS_2 - bS_1)}{(aB - Ab)}$$

where F = the declared content of amphotericin A in *amphotericin B A.S.*,
A = the E(1 per cent, 1 cm) of *amphotericin A A.S.* at 282 nm,
a = the E(1 per cent, 1 cm) of *amphotericin A A.S.* at 304 nm,
B = the E(1 per cent, 1 cm) of *amphotericin B A.S.* at 282 nm,
b = the E(1 per cent, 1 cm) of *amphotericin B A.S.* at 304 nm,
S_1 = the E(1 per cent, 1 cm) of the sample at 282 nm, and
S_2 = the E(1 per cent, 1 cm) of the sample at 304 nm.

CONTENT OF AMPHOTERICIN. 90 to 120 per cent of the amount stated on the label, determined by the following method:
Weigh and powder 20 lozenges. Triturate an accurately weighed quantity of the powder, equivalent to about 0·01 g of amphotericin, with successive small portions of *dimethyl sulphoxide* to give a total volume of about 50 ml and shake the suspension vigorously for 10 minutes, suppressing the froth by the addition of a few drops of an antifoaming substance; dilute the suspension to 100 ml with *dimethyl sulphoxide*, filter, and carry out a turbidimetric assay of amphotericin; a suggested method is given in Appendix 18, page 898.
The precision of any assay must be such that the fiducial limits of error (P = 0·95) are not less than 95 per cent and not more than 105 per cent of the estimated content.
Assuming that each 1000 Units found is equivalent to 1 mg of amphotericin, calculate the upper and lower fiducial limits of the total weight of amphotericin in the 20 lozenges and divide by 20.
The upper fiducial limit is not less than 90 per cent and the lower fiducial limit is not more than 120 per cent of the stated amount.

Containers. The directions given under Lozenges (above) should be followed; the containers should be airtight.

Labelling. The label on the container states the date after which the lozenges are not intended to be used.

Storage. They should be stored in a cool dry place and protected from light.

Dose. Amphotericin, 10 milligrams (10,000 Units) four times daily.

When the strength of the lozenges is not specified, lozenges each containing 10 mg of amphotericin shall be supplied.

Benzalkonium Lozenges

SYNONYM: Benzalkonium Chloride Lozenges

For each lozenge take:

Benzalkonium Chloride Solution	0·001 ml
Menthol	0·6 mg
Thymol	0·6 mg
Eucalyptus Oil	0·002 ml
Lemon Oil	0·002 ml

Prepare by moist granulation and compression, as described under Lozenges (page 731). Each lozenge weighs about 1 gram.

Standard
They comply with the standard for compressed lozenges under Lozenges, page 731, with the following addition:

CONTENT OF BENZALKONIUM CHLORIDE. 0·00045 to 0·00055 g, determined by the following method:
Weigh and powder 20 lozenges. Transfer an accurately weighed quantity of the powder, equivalent to about 7 lozenges, to a separating funnel, add 50 ml of water, shake vigorously, add 5 ml of *dilute sulphuric acid* and 1 ml of a 0·01 per cent w/v solution of *dimethyl yellow* in *alcohol (90 per cent)*, shake, add 20 ml of *chloroform*, and shake vigorously until the chloroform layer is bright yellow.
Titrate the solution with *sodium lauryl sulphate solution (0·1 per cent)*, shaking vigorously and allowing to separate between additions, until the chloroform layer changes to a pinkish- or orange-yellow; the end-point may be detected by observing the colour of the droplets of chloroform which form on the surface of the aqueous phase.
Repeat the procedure omitting the sample.
The difference between the two titrations represents the amount of sodium lauryl sulphate required by the sample.
Determine the amount of benzalkonium chloride equivalent to each ml of the sodium lauryl sulphate solution by transferring 10 ml of *standard benzalkonium chloride solution* to a separating funnel, adding 40 ml of water, and carrying out the procedure described above, beginning with the words "add 5 ml of *dilute sulphuric acid . . .*".
Calculate the total weight of benzalkonium chloride in the 20 lozenges and divide by 20.

Containers. The directions given under Lozenges (page 731) should be followed.

Benzocaine Lozenges, Compound

For each lozenge take:

Benzocaine	100 mg
Menthol	3 mg

Prepare by moist granulation and compression, as described under Lozenges (page 731), adding the menthol dissolved in a little alcohol (95 per cent) to the dried granules. Each lozenge weighs about 1 gram.

Standard
They comply with the standard for compressed lozenges under Lozenges, page 731, with the following additions:
PRESENCE OF BENZOCAINE. Suspend a quantity of the powdered lozenges, equivalent to about 5 lozenges, in 50 ml of water, extract with two 25-ml portions of *light petroleum (boiling-range, 40° to 60°)*, discard the extracts, extract the aqueous suspension again with two 25-ml portions of *chloroform*, filter the combined chloroform extracts through a layer of *anhydrous*

sodium sulphate, and evaporate the filtrate to dryness; the residue melts at about 89°.
CONTENT OF BENZOCAINE. 0·095 g to 0·105 g, determined by the following method:
Weigh and powder 20 lozenges. Dissolve, as completely as possible, an accurately weighed quantity of the powder, equivalent to about 3 lozenges, in 75 ml of water and 10 ml of *hydrochloric acid* and titrate with 0·1M sodium nitrite, determining the end-point electrometrically; each ml of 0·1M sodium nitrite is equivalent to 0·01652 g of $C_9H_{11}NO_2$.
Calculate the total weight of $C_9H_{11}NO_2$ in the 20 lozenges and divide by 20.

Containers. The directions given under Lozenges (page 731) should be followed.

Bismuth Lozenges, Compound

For each lozenge take:

Bismuth Carbonate	0·15 g
Heavy Magnesium Carbonate ..	0·15 g
Calcium Carbonate	0·30 g
Rose Oil, of commerce	0·00006 ml

Prepare by the method for moulded lozenges using a sufficient quantity of Simple Basis, or by the method for compressed lozenges, as described under Lozenges (page 730). Each lozenge weighs about 1·6 grams.

Standard
They comply with the standard under Lozenges, page 730, with the following additions:

CONTENT OF CALCIUM CARBONATE. 0·278 g to 0·317 g, calculated as $CaCO_3$, determined by the following method:
Weigh and powder 20 lozenges. Determine the amount of calcium carbonate in an accurately weighed quantity of the powder by the method for calcium carbonate in Compound Bismuth Powder, page 775.
Calculate the total weight of $CaCO_3$ in the 20 lozenges and divide by 20.

CONTENT OF BISMUTH. 0·114 g to 0·130 g, calculated as Bi, determined by the following method:
Ignite about 2 g of the powdered lozenges, accurately weighed, at a temperature not exceeding 500°, until all the carbon is removed, cool, dissolve the residue by warming with 10 ml of water and 5 ml of *nitric acid*, and continue by the method for bismuth in Compound Bismuth Powder, page 775, beginning with the words "add 20 ml of *glycerol . . .*".
Calculate the total weight of Bi in the 20 lozenges and divide by 20.

CONTENT OF MAGNESIUM. 0·036 g to 0·043 g, calculated as Mg, determined by the following method:
Ignite about 1 g of the powdered lozenges, accurately weighed, at a temperature not exceeding 500°, until all the carbon is removed, cool, dissolve the residue in 6 ml of water and 3 ml of *nitric acid*, and continue by the method for magnesium in Compound Bismuth Powder, page 775, beginning with the words "add 2 ml of *dilute hydrochloric acid . . .*".
Calculate the total weight of Mg in the 20 lozenges and divide by 20.

Containers. The directions given under Lozenges (page 731) should be followed.

Storage. They should be protected from light.

Formaldehyde Lozenges

SYNONYMS: Formalin Throat Tablets; Formamint Tablets

The general use of the names "Formalin" and "Formamint" for Formaldehyde Lozenges is limited, and in any country in which the words "Formalin" and "Formamint" are trade marks they may be used only when applied to the products made by the owners of the trade marks.

For each lozenge take:

Paraformaldehyde	..	..		10·0 mg
Menthol ..	..	..	..	2·5 mg
Citric Acid	..	..	..	20·0 mg
Lemon Oil	..	..	..	0·0006 ml

Prepare by moist granulation and compression, as described under Lozenges (page 731), adding the paraformaldehyde, followed by the menthol and the lemon oil dissolved in a little alcohol (95 per cent), to the dried granules.
Each lozenge weighs about 1 gram.

Standard
They comply with the standard for compressed lozenges under Lozenges, page 731, with the following addition:

CONTENT OF FORMALDEHYDE. 0·0070 g to 0·0115 g, calculated as CH_2O, determined by the following method:
Weigh and powder 20 lozenges. Transfer an accurately weighed quantity of the powder, equivalent to about 5 lozenges, to a steam-distillation apparatus, add 50 ml of water and 5 ml of *dilute sulphuric acid*, and steam-distil into 100 ml of water until 650 ml of distillate has been collected.
Add to the distillate 50 ml of 0·1N iodine, followed by 20 ml of *sodium hydroxide solution*, allow to stand for 10 minutes, acidify with *hydrochloric acid*, and titrate the excess of iodine with 0·1N sodium thiosulphate; each ml of 0·1N iodine is equivalent to 0·001501 g of CH_2O.
Calculate the total weight of CH_2O in the 20 lozenges and divide by 20.

Containers. The directions given under Lozenges (page 731) should be followed; the containers should be airtight.

Storage. They should be stored in a cool dry place. They are liable to deteriorate on storage.

Hydrocortisone Lozenges

SYNONYM: Hydrocortisone Sodium Succinate Lozenges

Hydrocortisone Lozenges contain Hydrocortisone Sodium Succinate and may be prepared by moist granulation and compression, as described under Lozenges (page 731).
Each lozenge weighs about 100 milligrams.

Standard
They comply with the standard for compressed lozenges under Lozenges, page 731, with the following additions:

PRESENCE OF HYDROCORTISONE. They comply with the thin-layer chromatographic test given in Appendix 5D, page 876.

DISINTEGRATION TIME. Carry out the method of the British Pharmacopoeia for the Disintegration Test for Tablets, using 5 lozenges and water at 25°. None of the 5 lozenges disintegrates in less than 10 minutes, and not more than one lozenge disintegrates in less than 15 minutes.
If more than one lozenge disintegrates in less than 15 minutes repeat the test, but without using the guided disk; the sample passes the test if none of the lozenges disintegrates in less than 15 minutes.

CONTENT OF UNESTERIFIED HYDROCORTISONE. Not more than 15 per cent of the prescribed or stated amount of hydrocortisone, determined by the following method:
Weigh and powder 20 lozenges. Disperse an accurately weighed quantity of the powder, equivalent to about 5 mg of hydrocortisone, in 15 ml of *phosphate buffer solution pH 7·0*, extract with three successive 25-ml portions of *chloroform*, wash the combined extracts with 2 ml of water, discard the washings, and evaporate off the chloroform in a current of air.
Dissolve the residue in sufficient *aldehyde-free dehydrated alcohol* to produce 25 ml, transfer 10 ml to a 25-ml graduated flask, and continue by the method for Hydrocortisone and Neomycin Ear-drops, page 665, beginning with the words "add 2·0 ml of *triphenyltetrazolium chloride solution . . .*".
Calculate the total weight of unesterified hydrocortisone in the 20 lozenges and divide by 20.

CONTENT OF HYDROCORTISONE. 90·0 to 110·0 per cent of the prescribed or stated amount of hydrocortisone, determined by the following method:
Shake an accurately weighed quantity of the powdered lozenges, equivalent to about 0·02 mg of hydrocortisone, with 50 ml of water, dilute to 100 ml with water, filter, and discard the first part of the filtrate; dilute 3 ml of the filtrate to 50 ml with water, and measure the extinction of a 1-cm layer at the maximum at about 248 nm.
For purposes of calculation, use a value of 449 for the E(1 per cent, 1 cm) of hydrocortisone.
Calculate the total weight of hydrocortisone in the 20 lozenges and divide by 20.

Containers. The directions given under Lozenges (page 731) should be followed; the containers should be airtight.

Storage. They should be stored in a cool dry place.

Note. When the strength of the lozenges is not specified, lozenges each containing the equivalent of 2·5 mg of hydrocortisone shall be supplied.

Liquorice Lozenges

SYNONYMS: Trochisci Glycyrrhizae; Brompton Cough Lozenges

For each lozenge take:

Liquorice Extract	..	..	200·0 mg
Anise Oil ..	..	..	0·03 ml

Prepare by the method for moulded lozenges using a sufficient quantity of Simple Basis, or by the method for compressed lozenges, as described under Lozenges (page 730).
Each lozenge weighs about 1·5 grams.

Standard
They comply with the standard under Lozenges, page 730.

Containers. The directions given under Lozenges (page 731) should be followed.

Penicillin Lozenges

SYNONYM: Benzylpenicillin Lozenges

Penicillin Lozenges are prepared by compression of a mixture of Benzylpenicillin and previously prepared dry granules of Sucrose, Lactose, or a mixture of the two, and binding agents.
Each lozenge weighs about 1 gram.

Standard
They comply with the standard for compressed lozenges under Lozenges, page 731, with the following addition:

CONTENT OF BENZYLPENICILLIN. 90 to 120 per cent of the prescribed or stated number of Units of penicillin, determined by the following method:
Weigh and powder 20 lozenges. Mix an accurately weighed quantity of the powder, equivalent to about 1000 Units, with 3 ml of sterile *solution of standard pH 7·0*, dilute to 250 ml with sterile *solution of standard pH 7·0*, and carry out a microbiological assay of penicillin using *benzylpenicillin sodium B.C.R.S.* in place of the standard preparation; a suggested method is given in Appendix 18, page 897. For the purposes of the assay and calculations, each mg of benzylpenicillin sodium B.C.R.S. may be assumed to contain 1670 Units.
The precision of any assay must be such that the fiducial limits of error $(P = 0·95)$ are not less than 95 per cent and not more than 105 per cent of the estimated potency.
Calculate the upper and lower fiducial limits of the number of Units in the 20 lozenges and divide by 20. The upper fiducial limit of the estimated number of Units of penicillin is not less than 90 per cent and the lower fiducial limit is not more than 120 per cent of the prescribed or stated number of Units.

Containers. The directions given under Lozenges (page 731) should be followed; the containers should be airtight.

Storage. They should be stored in a cool dry place.

Note. When the strength of the lozenges is not specified, lozenges each containing 1000 Units of penicillin shall be supplied.

MIXTURES

Mixtures are liquid preparations intended for administration by mouth. They consist of one or more medicaments dissolved or suspended usually in an aqueous vehicle but occasionally in a suitable non-aqueous vehicle. Many of the mixtures included in this section are not formulated to keep for long periods and should be recently prepared or freshly prepared if this is indicated in the individual monographs.

Insoluble substances which do not diffuse evenly throughout the aqueous vehicle when shaken should be finely powdered and mixed with Compound Tragacanth Powder, sodium carboxymethylcellulose, or other suitable suspending agent; the vehicle is then added gradually with trituration to produce the required volume after any other ingredients have been incorporated. Suitable suspending agents have been included in the mixtures in this part of the Codex and it is not necessary to use additional substances.

Use of water. Care should be taken to prevent growth of micro-organisms in mixtures. Some of these organisms may originate from the water used to make the preparations. Potable water (see Water, page 642) may be used for preparing mixtures, but only in preparations that are adequately preserved.

The formulae of most of the monographs provide an adequate concentration of preservative. In cases where potable water is unsuitable, Purified Water is used and as it is liable to be heavily contaminated with micro-organisms, it must be freshly boiled and cooled.

In some districts, the water supply may be unsuitable for preparing certain B.P.C. mixtures because of chemical incompatibility. A footnote is included in the monograph where it is known that the preparation in question is liable to be affected in this manner.

Dilution of mixtures. Unless otherwise indicated in the individual monograph, when a dose prescribed or ordered is less than or not a multiple of 5 millilitres, the mixture should be diluted with the vehicle used in the preparation of the mixture or that specified in the individual monograph as a diluent, so that the dose to be measured for the patient is one 5-ml spoonful or multiple thereof.

Advice on the stability of diluted mixtures is given, if known, in the individual monographs. In the absence of such advice, it should be assumed that the diluted mixture is less stable than the undiluted preparation. Dilution should therefore be carried out immediately before the mixture is issued for use and not more than two weeks' supply should be issued at a time, unless otherwise indicated in the individual monograph.

Labelling. The following directions should be followed:

A. The label on the container of a mixture, other than one directed in an individual monograph to be recently prepared or freshly prepared, states:
(1) the name and concentration of the active ingredient for mixtures other than those for which a full recipe is given in the individual monograph; and
(2) directions for storage.

If the mixture is one which is to be prepared freshly before issue to the patient from dry powder or granules, the label on the container of powder or granules states:
(1) the name of the preparation in the form of "Granules (or Powder) for the Mixture", as specified in the individual monograph;
(2) the name and concentration of the active ingredient in the mixture when prepared according to the manufacturer's instructions;
(3) directions for storage; and
(4) the date after which the granules or powder should not be used.

The label on the container or on the package leaflet or the label on the carton states:
(1) the directions for preparing the mixture;
(2) the directions for storage of the mixture; and
(3) the period during which the mixture may be expected to retain its potency when stored under the stated conditions.

B. The label on the container of a mixture issued to the patient on a prescription states, in addition to the prescriber's directions:
(1) any special storage directions as directed in the monograph;
(2) for suspensions, a direction to shake the bottle;
(3) if such a recommendation is made by the manufacturer, the date after which the mixture should not be used; and
(4) if the mixture has been diluted before issue "The contents to be discarded if not taken before . . . [a date two weeks, or other period specified by the manufacturer or in the individual monograph, after the date of issue]".

Aluminium Hydroxide and Belladonna Mixture

Belladonna Tincture	.. ..	100 ml
Chloroform Spirit	.. ..	50 ml
Aluminium Hydroxide Gel	..	to 1000 ml

It should be recently prepared.

Standard

PRESENCE OF BELLADONNA ALKALOIDS. It complies with the thin-layer chromatographic test given in Appendix 5B, page 871.

CONTENT OF ALUMINIUM OXIDE. 3·21 to 4·08 per cent w/w, calculated as Al_2O_3, determined by the following method:

Dissolve about 5 g, accurately weighed, in 3 ml of *hydrochloric acid* by warming on a water-bath, cool to below 20°, and dilute to 100 ml with water. To 20 ml of this solution add 40 ml of 0·05M disodium edetate, 80 ml of water and 0·15 ml of *methyl red solution*, neutralise by the dropwise addition of 1N sodium hydroxide, warm on a water-bath for 30 minutes, add 3 g of *hexamine*, and titrate with 0·05M lead nitrate, using 0·5 ml of *xylenol orange solution* as indicator; each ml of 0·05M disodium edetate is equivalent to 0·002549 g of Al_2O_3.

Containers. It should be supplied in wide-mouthed containers.

Labelling. A direction to shake the bottle should be given on the label.

Dose. 5 millilitres suitably diluted.

Amitriptyline Mixture

SYNONYMS: Amitriptyline Embonate Mixture; Amitriptyline Syrup

Amitriptyline Mixture is a suspension of Amitriptyline Embonate in a suitable coloured flavoured vehicle.

Standard
PRESENCE OF AMITRIPTYLINE EMBONATE. 1. Evaporate to dryness 5 ml of the dichloromethane extract obtained in the determination of amitriptyline, dissolve the residue in 1 ml of *methyl alcohol*, add 1 ml of a 2·5 per cent w/v solution of *sodium bicarbonate* in water, 1 ml of a 2 per cent w/v solution of *sodium periodate* in water, and 1 ml of a 0·3 per cent w/v solution of *potassium permanganate* in water, and allow to stand for 15 minutes; acidify the solution with *dilute sulphuric acid* and extract with 10 ml of *trimethylpentane*.
The trimethylpentane extract exhibits a light absorption which has, in the range 230 to 350 nm, a well-defined maximum only at about 265 nm.
2. It complies with the thin-layer chromatographic test given in Appendix 5A, page 859.

ACIDITY. pH, 5·0 to 7·0.

CONTENT OF AMITRIPTYLINE. 90·0 to 110·0 per cent of the prescribed or stated amount, determined by the following method:
To an accurately weighed quantity, equivalent to about 4 mg of amitriptyline, add 20 ml of water, mix well, extract with four successive 20-ml portions, followed by one 15-ml portion, of *dichloromethane*, and dilute the combined extracts to 100 ml with *dichloromethane*; shake 20 ml of this solution with 10 ml of 1N sodium hydroxide, allow to separate, and filter the lower dichloromethane layer through a pledget of cotton wool, discarding the first portion of the filtrate.
Evaporate 10 ml of the clear filtrate to dryness on a water-bath in a stream of *nitrogen*, dissolve the residue in sufficient 0·1N hydrochloric acid to produce 50 ml, and measure the extinction of a 1-cm layer at the maximum at about 239 nm, using 0·1N hydrochloric acid as the blank.
For the purposes of calculation, use a value of 510 for the E(1 per cent, 1 cm) of amitriptyline.
Determine the weight per ml of the mixture and calculate the concentration of amitriptyline, weight in volume.

Labelling. The directions given under Mixtures (page 735) should be followed.

Dose. The equivalent of amitriptyline:

ADULT. 30 to 150 milligrams daily in divided doses, gradually reduced to a maintenance dosage of 20 to 100 milligrams daily in divided doses.

CHILD. For enuresis: 1 to 5 years, 10 milligrams; 6 to 12 years, up to 25 milligrams.

When the strength of the mixture is not specified, a suspension containing the equivalent of 10 mg of amitriptyline in 5 ml shall be supplied.

When a dose less than or not a multiple of 5 ml is prescribed, the mixture may be diluted, as described under Mixtures (page 734), with Syrup. The diluted mixture must be freshly prepared.

Ammonia and Ipecacuanha Mixture

SYNONYM: Mistura Expectorans

Ammonium Bicarbonate	..	20 g
Ipecacuanha Tincture	..	30 ml
Concentrated Anise Water	..	5 ml
Concentrated Camphor Water	..	10 ml

Liquorice Liquid Extract	..		50 ml
Chloroform Water, Double-strength	..	..	500 ml
Water (see page 642)	..	..	to 1000 ml

It should be recently prepared.

Standard
PRESENCE OF IPECACUANHA ALKALOIDS. It complies with the thin-layer chromatographic test given in Appendix 5B, page 871.

CONTENT OF AMMONIUM BICARBONATE. 1·90 to 2·12 per cent w/v, calculated as NH_4HCO_3, determined by the following method:
Transfer 10 ml to an ammonia-distillation apparatus, dilute to 200 ml with water, and add 1 g of *heavy magnesium oxide* suspended in 10 ml of water; distil into 50 ml of 0·1N sulphuric acid, boil to remove carbon dioxide, cool, and titrate the excess of acid with 0·1N sodium hydroxide, using *methyl red solution* as indicator.
Repeat the procedure omitting the sample.
The difference between the two titrations represents the amount of acid required by the sample; each ml of 0·1N sulphuric acid is equivalent to 0·007906 g of NH_4HCO_3.

Dose. 10 to 20 millilitres.

Ammonium Chloride Mixture

Ammonium Chloride	..	..	100 g
Aromatic Ammonia Solution	..		50 ml
Liquorice Liquid Extract	..		100 ml
Water (see page 642)	..	..	to 1000 ml

It should be recently prepared.

Standard
CONTENT OF AMMONIUM CHLORIDE. 9·50 to 10·66 per cent w/v, calculated as NH_4Cl, determined by the following method:
To 1 ml add 20 ml of water and continue by the method given in Appendix 11, page 891; each ml of 0·1N silver nitrate is equivalent to 0·005349 g of NH_4Cl.

Dose. 10 to 20 millilitres.

Ammonium Chloride and Morphine Mixture

SYNONYM: Mistura Tussi Sedativa

Ammonium Chloride	..	..		30 g
Chloroform and Morphine Tincture	..	..	..	30 ml
Ammonium Bicarbonate		..		20 g
Liquorice Liquid Extract		..		50 ml
Water (see page 642)		..		to 1000 ml

It should be recently prepared.

Standard
CONTENT OF AMMONIUM CHLORIDE. 2·81 to 3·28 per cent w/v, calculated as NH_4Cl, determined by the following method:
To 5 ml add 20 ml of water and continue by the method given in Appendix 11, page 891; each ml of 0·1N silver nitrate is equivalent to 0·005349 g of NH_4Cl.

CONTENT OF AMMONIUM BICARBONATE. 1·70 to 2·14 per cent w/v, calculated as NH_4HCO_3, determined by the method for Ammonia and Ipecacuanha Mixture, above, 5 ml being used; each ml of 0·1N sulphuric acid, after the volume of 0·1N silver nitrate required in the determination of ammonium chloride has been deducted, is equivalent to 0·007906 g of NH_4HCO_3.

CONTENT OF ANHYDROUS MORPHINE. 0·0040 to 0·0066 per cent w/v, determined by the following method: Transfer 100 ml to an apparatus for continuous liquid–liquid extraction, make alkaline to *litmus paper* with *strong ammonia solution*, add 0·05 g of *sodium meta-bisulphite*, and extract for 2 hours, or until extraction is complete, with a mixture of 3 volumes of *chloroform* and 1 volume of *isobutyl alcohol*; cool the extract, filter through cotton wool, wash the flask and filter with successive portions of the solvent mixture, and extract the combined filtrate and washings with three successive 10-ml portions of 0·5N sulphuric acid. Make the combined extracts alkaline to *litmus paper* with *dilute ammonia solution*, extract with three successive 30-ml portions of the chloroform–isobutyl alcohol mixture, washing each extract with the same 10 ml of water, filter, wash the filter with the solvent mixture, evaporate the combined filtrate and washings to dryness on a water-bath in a current of air, and allow to stand on the water-bath for a further 5 minutes; cool, dissolve the residue in 2·5 ml of 0·5N hydrochloric acid by warming gently, filter, wash the filter with successive portions of water, and dilute the combined filtrate and washings to 25 ml with water. To 10 ml of this solution add 2 ml of *iodic acid solution*, allow to stand for 2 minutes, add 10 ml of *nickel chloride–ammonia solution*, dilute to 25 ml, allow to stand for 90 minutes, and measure the extinction of a 1-cm layer at 670 nm, using as a blank a mixture of 5 ml of 0·1N hydrochloric acid and 10 ml of *nickel chloride–ammonia solution* diluted to 25 ml with water. Repeat the procedure using, in place of the sample, 10 ml of a solution of 4 mg of *anhydrous morphine* in 2·5 ml of 0·5N hydrochloric acid diluted to 25 ml with water, and beginning with the words "add 2 ml of *iodic acid solution*, . . .". Calculate the concentration of anhydrous morphine, weight in volume.

Dose. 10 to 20 millilitres.

Ampicillin Mixture

SYNONYM: Ampicillin Syrup

Ampicillin Mixture is a suspension of Ampicillin or Ampicillin Trihydrate in a suitable flavoured vehicle. It is prepared freshly by dispersing a powder consisting of the dry mixed ingredients in the specified volume of Water (see page 642).

Standard
PRESENCE OF AMPICILLIN. It complies with the thin-layer chromatographic test given in Appendix 5A, page 859.

CONTENT OF AMPICILLIN. 90·0 to 120·0 per cent of the prescribed or stated concentration, determined by the following method:
Prepare the mixture, as directed on the label, immediately before analysis, and reserve a portion for the test for stability.
Dissolve an accurately weighed quantity, equivalent to about 0·1 g of ampicillin, in *dilute sodium bicarbonate solution*, dilute to 100 ml with *dilute sodium bicarbonate solution*, and transfer 2 ml of this solution to each of two tubes.
To the first tube add 1 ml of 2N sodium hydroxide, allow to stand for exactly 30 minutes, and add 1 ml of 2N sulphuric acid; to the second tube add 2 ml of water. To each tube add 6 ml of *hydroxylammonium chloride reagent* and allow to stand for 10 minutes; add 2 ml of *ferric reagent*, again allow to stand for 10 minutes, and measure the extinction of a 1-cm layer of the solution in the second tube at 490 nm, using as a blank the solution in the first tube. Calculate the concentration of ampicillin in the sample by reference to a calibration curve prepared at the same time, using suitable quantities of *ampicillin A.S.*, treated in the same manner.

Determine the weight per ml of the mixture and calculate the concentration of ampicillin, weight in volume.

STABILITY OF MIXTURE. Store at 15° ± 1° for 7 days the portion of the mixture reserved in the determination of the content of ampicillin and then repeat the determination on the stored mixture.
The concentration of ampicillin in the stored mixture is not less than 90·0 per cent of the concentration found in the freshly prepared mixture.

ACIDITY OF MIXTURE. pH, 4·5 to 6·5.

Labelling. The directions given under Mixtures (page 735) should be followed; the name on the label of the container of the dry powder is "Powder for Ampicillin Mixture".

Storage. The mixture and the diluted mixture should be stored in a cool place and used within one week of preparation.

Dose. The equivalent of ampicillin:

ADULT. 1 to 6 grams daily, in divided doses.

CHILD. Every six hours: up to 1 year, 62·5 to 125 milligrams; 1 to 5 years, 125 milligrams; 6 to 12 years, 250 milligrams.

When the strength of the mixture is not specified, a suspension containing 125 mg of ampicillin, or the equivalent amount of ampicillin trihydrate, in 5 ml shall be supplied.

When Strong Ampicillin Mixture or Strong Ampicillin Syrup is ordered or prescribed, a suspension containing 250 mg of ampicillin, or the equivalent amount of ampicillin trihydrate, in 5 ml shall be supplied.

When a dose less than or not a multiple of 5 ml is prescribed, the mixture may be diluted, as described under Mixtures (page 734), with Syrup. The diluted mixture must be freshly prepared.

Belladonna Mixture, Paediatric

Belladonna Tincture	..	..	30 ml
Compound Orange Spirit		..	2 ml
Benzoic Acid Solution	..	..	20 ml
Glycerol ..	..	..	..	100 ml
Syrup	..	..	..	200 ml
Water (see page 642)	..	..	to 1000 ml

It should be recently prepared.

Standard
PRESENCE OF BELLADONNA ALKALOIDS. It complies with the thin-layer chromatographic test given in Appendix 5B, page 871.

Dose. CHILD. Up to 1 year, 5 millilitres; 1 to 5 years, 10 millilitres.

Belladonna and Ephedrine Mixture, Paediatric

Belladonna Tincture	..	30 ml
Ephedrine Hydrochloride	..	1·5 g
Potassium Iodide..	..	10·0 g
Concentrated Anise Water	..	20 ml
Benzoic Acid Solution	..	20 ml
Liquorice Liquid Extract	..	30 ml
Syrup	..	..	100 ml
Water (see page 642)	..	to 1000 ml

It should be recently prepared.

Standard

PRESENCE OF BELLADONNA ALKALOIDS. It complies with the thin-layer chromatographic test given in Appendix 5B, page 871.

CONTENT OF EPHEDRINE HYDROCHLORIDE. 0·135 to 0·165 per cent w/v, determined by the following method:

Pack a chromatographic tube, 25 cm in length and 1 cm in diameter, with sufficient Amberlite IRA 400 or other suitable strongly basic anion exchange resin to give a column 15 to 20 cm high; elute the column with 50 ml of a 10 per cent w/v solution of *sodium chloride* in water followed by 150 ml of water, finally retaining sufficient water in the column to give a depth of 1 cm of water above the resin.

Transfer to the top of the column 3 ml of the sample, allow it to run slowly into the resin and then elute the column with 200 ml of water, maintaining a level of 1 cm of water above the resin throughout the procedure; dilute the eluate to 250 ml with water and continue by the method given for Ephedrine Elixir, page 671, beginning with the words "To 5 ml of this solution . . .".

CONTENT OF POTASSIUM IODIDE. 0·95 to 1·05 per cent w/v, calculated as KI, determined by the following method:

To 15 ml add 10 ml of water and continue by the method given in Appendix 11, page 891, adjusting the pH, if necessary, with 0·5N sulphuric acid; each ml of 0·1N silver nitrate is equivalent to 0·01660 g of KI.

Dose. CHILD. Up to 1 year, 5 millilitres; 1 to 5 years, 10 millilitres.

Belladonna and Ipecacuanha Mixture, Paediatric

Belladonna Tincture	..	..	30 ml
Ipecacuanha Tincture	..	..	20 ml
Sodium Bicarbonate	..	..	20 g
Tolu Syrup	..	..	..	200 ml
Chloroform Water, Double-strength..	..	..	..	500 ml
Water (see page 642)	..	.. to 1000 ml

It should be recently prepared.

Standard

PRESENCE OF BELLADONNA AND IPECACUANHA ALKALOIDS. It complies with the thin-layer chromatographic test given in Appendix 5B, page 871.

CONTENT OF SODIUM BICARBONATE. 1·90 to 2·10 per cent w/v, calculated as NaHCO₃, determined by the method for Paediatric Ipecacuanha Mixture, page 744.

Dose. CHILD. Up to 1 year, 5 millilitres; 1 to 5 years, 10 millilitres.

Calcium Carbonate Mixture, Compound, Paediatric

Calcium Carbonate	..	..	10 g
Light Magnesium Carbonate	..	10 g
Sodium Bicarbonate	..	..	10 g
Aromatic Cardamom Tincture	..	10 ml
Syrup	..	..	..	..	100 ml
Chloroform Water, Double-strength..	..	..	..	500 ml
Water (see page 642)	..	.. to 1000 ml

It should be recently prepared.

Standard

CONTENT OF MAGNESIUM. 0·23 to 0·28 per cent w/w, calculated as Mg, determined by the following method:

Dissolve about 25 g, accurately weighed, in the minimum quantity of *dilute hydrochloric acid* and dilute to 100 ml with water.

To 20 ml of this solution, add 30 ml of water, 1 g of *ammonium chloride*, and 1 g of *ammonium oxalate*, neutralise to *litmus paper* with *dilute ammonia solution*, and add 5 ml in excess, boil for 5 minutes, allow to stand for 2 hours, filter, and wash the residue with hot water.

To the combined filtrate and washings add 5 ml of *ammonia buffer solution* and titrate with 0·05M disodium edetate, using *mordant black 11 solution* as indicator; each ml of 0·05M disodium edetate is equivalent to 0·001215 g of Mg.

CONTENT OF CALCIUM CARBONATE. 0·88 to 1·02 per cent w/w, calculated as CaCO₃, determined by the following method:

To 20 ml of the diluted solution prepared for the determination of magnesium add 30 ml of water, neutralise to *litmus paper* with *sodium hydroxide solution*, add 5 ml of *ammonia buffer solution*, and titrate with 0·05M disodium edetate, using *mordant black 11 solution* as indicator; each ml of 0·05M disodium edetate, after the volume required in the determination of magnesium has been deducted, is equivalent to 0·005005 g of CaCO₃.

CONTENT OF SODIUM BICARBONATE. 0·88 to 1·04 per cent w/w, calculated as NaHCO₃, determined by the following method:

Boil about 40 g, accurately weighed, for 5 minutes with 100 ml of water, and filter; boil the residue with 100 ml of water for 5 minutes, and filter.

Combine the filtrates, cool, and titrate with 0·5N hydrochloric acid, using *methyl orange–xylene cyanol FF solution* as indicator; add 10 ml of *ammonia buffer solution*, and titrate with 0·05M disodium edetate, using *mordant black 11 solution* as indicator; each ml of 0·5N hydrochloric acid, after one-fifth of the volume of 0·05M disodium edetate has been deducted, is equivalent to 0·04200 g of NaHCO₃.

Labelling. A direction to shake the bottle should be given on the label.

Dose. CHILD. Up to 1 year, 5 millilitres; 1 to 5 years, 10 millilitres.

Cascara and Belladonna Mixture

SYNONYM: Compound Cascara Mixture

Cascara Elixir	..	..	..	200 ml
Belladonna Tincture	..	..	50 ml
Chloroform Water, Double-strength..	..	..	..	500 ml
Water (see page 642)	..	.. to 1000 ml

It should be recently prepared.

Standard

PRESENCE OF BELLADONNA ALKALOIDS. It complies with the thin-layer chromatographic test given in Appendix 5B, page 871.

Dose. 10 to 20 millilitres.

Cephalexin Mixture

Cephalexin Mixture is a suspension of Cephalexin in a suitable flavoured vehicle which may be coloured. It is prepared freshly by dispersing granules consisting of the dry mixed ingredients in the specified volume of Water (see page 642).

Standard

PRESENCE OF CEPHALEXIN. The ultraviolet absorption spectrum of the mixture when diluted to the appropriate strength with water exhibits the characteristics given for cephalexin in Appendix 3, page 855.

CONTENT OF CEPHALEXIN. 90·0 to 120·0 per cent of the prescribed or stated concentration, calculated as $C_{16}H_{17}N_3O_4S$, determined by the following method:
Prepare the mixture, as directed on the label, immediately before analysis, and reserve a portion for the test for stability.
Dilute an accurately weighed quantity of the mixture, equivalent to about 0·25 g of cephalexin, to 250 ml with water and continue by the method given for total penicillins in Phenoxymethylpenicillin Elixir, page 675, beginning with the words "transfer 10 ml to a stoppered flask . . .".
The difference between the two titrations represents the volume of 0·02N iodine equivalent to the cephalexin in the sample.
Calculate the content of $C_{16}H_{17}N_3O_4S$ from the difference obtained by repeating the procedure using *cephalexin A.S.* in place of the sample and the declared content of $C_{16}H_{17}N_3O_4S$ in the cephalexin A.S.
Determine the weight per ml of the mixture and calculate the concentration of $C_{16}H_{17}N_3O_4S$, weight in volume.

STABILITY OF MIXTURE. Store at $15° \pm 1°$ for the number of days specified on the label the portion of the mixture reserved in the determination of the content of cephalexin and then repeat the determination on the stored mixture. The concentration of cephalexin in the stored mixture is not less than 90 per cent of the concentration found in the freshly prepared mixture.

ACIDITY OF MIXTURE. pH, 3·0 to 6·0.

Labelling. The directions given under Mixtures (page 735) should be followed; the name on the label of the container of the dry granules is "Granules for Cephalexin Mixture".

Storage. The mixture and the diluted mixture should be stored in a cool place and used within the period stated on the label.

Dose. Cephalexin:

ADULT. 1 to 4 grams daily, in divided doses.

CHILD. 25 to 50 milligrams per kilogram body-weight daily in divided doses.

Mixtures containing 125 mg, 250 mg, or 500 mg of cephalexin in 5 ml are available.

When a dose less than or not a multiple of 5 ml is prescribed, the mixture may be diluted, as described under Mixtures (page 734), with a suitable diluent*. The diluted mixture must be freshly prepared.

*Ceporex® may be diluted with Water and Keflex® may be diluted with Syrup.

Chalk Mixture, Paediatric

SYNONYM: Mistura Cretae pro Infantibus

Chalk	..	..	..	20 g
Tragacanth, in powder	..	..		2 g
Concentrated Cinnamon Water..				4 ml
Syrup	..	..	..	100 ml
Chloroform Water, Double-strength..	..	..	..	500 ml
Water (see page 642)	..	..	to 1000 ml

It should be recently prepared.

Standard

CONTENT OF CALCIUM CARBONATE. 1·67 to 1·97 per cent w/w, calculated as $CaCO_3$, determined by the following method:
Boil about 20 g, accurately weighed, for 5 minutes with

25 ml of 0·5N hydrochloric acid, cool, and titrate the excess of acid with 0·5N sodium hydroxide, using *methyl red solution* as indicator; each ml of 0·5N hydrochloric acid is equivalent to 0·02502 g of $CaCO_3$.

Labelling. A direction to shake the bottle should be given on the label.

Dose. CHILD. Up to 1 year, 5 millilitres; 1 to 5 years, 10 millilitres.

Chalk with Opium Mixture, Aromatic

SYNONYMS: Chalk and Opium Mixture; Mistura Cretae Aromatica cum Opio

Aromatic Chalk Powder..		..	130 g
Opium Tincture ..	..	..	50 ml
Aromatic Ammonia Solution	..		50 ml
Compound Cardamom Tincture			50 ml
Catechu Tincture	..	..	50 ml
Tragacanth, in powder	..	..	2 g
Chloroform Water, Double-strength	..	..	..	500 ml
Water (see page 642)	..	..	to 1000 ml

It should be recently prepared.

Standard

PRESENCE OF CHALK. Centrifuge 10 ml and reserve the supernatant liquid. To the residue add *dilute acetic acid*; the residue dissolves, with effervescence, and the solution gives the reactions characteristic of solutions of calcium salts.

PRESENCE OF OPIUM ALKALOIDS. The supernatant liquid obtained in the test for the presence of chalk complies with the thin-layer chromatographic test given in Appendix 5B, page 871.

Labelling. A direction to shake the bottle should be given on the label.

Dose. ADULT. 10 to 20 millilitres.

CHILD. Up to 1 year, 1 millilitre; 1 to 5 years, 2 to 5 millilitres.

Chloral Mixture

SYNONYM: Chloral Hydrate Mixture

Chloral Hydrate ..	..	..	100 g
Syrup	..	..	..	..	200 ml
Water (see page 642)	..	..	to 1000 ml

It should be recently prepared.

Standard

PRESENCE OF CHLORAL HYDRATE. It complies with the test given for Paediatric Chloral Elixir, page 668.

CONTENT OF CHLORAL HYDRATE. 9·40 to 10·55 per cent w/v, calculated as $C_2H_3Cl_3O_2$, determined by the method for Paediatric Chloral Elixir, page 668, about 1 g, accurately weighed, being used.
Determine the weight per ml of the mixture and calculate the content of $C_2H_3Cl_3O_2$, weight in volume.

Dose. ADULT. 5 to 20 millilitres, well diluted with water.

CHILD. Hypnotic dose, well diluted with water: 1 to 5 years, 2·5 to 5 millilitres; 6 to 12 years, 5 to 10 millilitres.

When a dose less than or not a multiple of 5 ml is prescribed, the mixture may be diluted, as described under Mixtures (page 734), with a mixture of one volume of Syrup with four volumes of Water (see page 642). The diluted mixture must be freshly prepared.

Chloramphenicol Mixture

SYNONYM: Chloramphenicol Palmitate Suspension

Chloramphenicol Mixture is a suspension of Chloramphenicol Palmitate in a suitable flavoured vehicle.
The method of manufacture must be such that the content of the biologically inactive chloramphenicol palmitate polymorph A is within the prescribed limit in the final product (see below).

Standard
CONTENT OF POLYMORPH A. It complies with the test given in Appendix 19, page 901.

CONTENT OF CHLORAMPHENICOL. 95·0 to 115·0 per cent of the prescribed or stated concentration, determined by the following method:
Dilute an accurately weighed quantity, equivalent to about 0·3 g of chloramphenicol, to 1000 ml with water, mix, and allow to stand for 10 minutes; mix again, immediately dilute 5 ml of the suspension to 100 ml with *alcohol (95 per cent)*, and measure the extinction of a 1-cm layer at the maximum at about 271 nm.
For purposes of calculation, use a value of 178 for the E(1 per cent, 1 cm) of chloramphenicol palmitate.
Determine the weight per ml of the mixture and, using a factor of 0·575, calculate the concentration of chloramphenicol, weight in volume.

Labelling. The directions given under Mixtures (page 735) should be followed.

Storage. It should be protected from light.

Dose. The equivalent of chloramphenicol:
ADULT. 1·5 to 3 grams daily, in divided doses.
CHILD. Premature infant, not more than 25 milligrams per kilogram body-weight daily, divided into six-hourly doses; full-term infant and up to 1 month, not more than 25 to 50 milligrams per kilogram body-weight daily, divided into six-hourly doses; 1 month to 1 year, 50 milligrams per kilogram body-weight daily, divided into six-hourly doses; 1 to 5 years, 125 to 250 milligrams every six hours; 6 to 12 years, 250 to 500 milligrams every six hours.

When the strength of the mixture is not specified, a suspension containing the equivalent of 125 mg of chloramphenicol in 5 ml shall be supplied.

When a dose less than or not a multiple of 5 ml is prescribed, the mixture may be diluted, as described under Mixtures (page 734), with Syrup. The diluted mixture must be freshly prepared.

Colchicum and Sodium Salicylate Mixture

Colchicum Tincture	..	..	100 ml
Sodium Salicylate	..	..	100 g
Potassium Bicarbonate	..	..	100 g
Liquorice Liquid Extract		..	30 ml
Chloroform Water, Double-strength..	..	..	..	500 ml
Water (see page 642)	..	..	to 1000 ml

It should be recently prepared.

Standard
PRESENCE OF COLCHICINE. It complies with the thin-layer chromatographic test given in Appendix 5B, page 871.

CONTENT OF POTASSIUM BICARBONATE. 9·50 to 10·50 per cent w/v, calculated as KHCO₃, determined by the following method:
To 5 ml add 150 ml of water and 25 ml of 0·5N hydrochloric acid and boil under a reflux condenser for 5 minutes; cool, and titrate the excess of acid with 0·5N sodium hydroxide, using *phenolphthalein solution* as indicator; each ml of 0·5N hydrochloric acid is equivalent to 0·05006 g of KHCO₃.

CONTENT OF SODIUM SALICYLATE. 9·50 to 10·50 per cent w/v, calculated as C₇H₅NaO₃, determined by the following method:
To 5 ml add 10 ml of *dilute hydrochloric acid* and extract with six successive 25-ml portions of *chloroform*, washing each extract with the same two 5-ml portions of water; dry the combined extracts by shaking with *anhydrous sodium sulphate*, filter through a dry filter paper, and evaporate at as low a temperature as possible in a current of warm air.
Dissolve the residue in 10 ml of *alcohol (95 per cent)*, previously neutralised to *phenol red solution*, and titrate with 0·1N sodium hydroxide, using *phenol red solution* as indicator; each ml of 0·1N sodium hydroxide is equivalent to 0·01601 g of C₇H₅NaO₃.

Dose. 10 to 20 millilitres.

Co-trimoxazole Mixture

SYNONYM: Trimethoprim and Sulphamethoxazole Mixture

Co-trimoxazole Mixture is a suspension containing 1·6 per cent w/v of Trimethoprim and 8 per cent w/v of Sulphamethoxazole in a suitable flavoured vehicle.

Standard
PRESENCE OF TRIMETHOPRIM AND SULPHAMETHOXAZOLE. It complies with the thin-layer chromatographic test given in Appendix 5A, page 861.

CONTENT OF SULPHAMETHOXAZOLE. 7·20 to 8·80 per cent w/v, determined by the following method:
To an accurately weighed quantity, equivalent to about 0·25 g of sulphamethoxazole, add 30 ml of 0·1N sodium hydroxide, mix, extract with four successive 50-ml portions of *chloroform*, washing each extract with the same two 10-ml portions of 0·1N sodium hydroxide, and reserve the combined chloroform extracts for the determination of trimethoprim; dilute the combined aqueous solution and washings to 250 ml with water, filter, discarding the first 5 ml of the filtrate, and dilute 5 ml of the clear filtrate to 200 ml with water.
The following procedure should be carried out in subdued light or in low-actinic glassware.
To 2 ml of the prepared sample solution add 0·5 ml of 4N hydrochloric acid and 1 ml of a 0·1 per cent w/v solution of *sodium nitrite* in water and allow to stand for 2 minutes; add 1 ml of a 0·5 per cent w/v solution of *ammonium sulphamate* in water and allow to stand for 3 minutes; add 1 ml of a 0·1 per cent w/v solution of *N-(1-naphthyl)-ethylenediamine hydrochloride* in water and allow to stand for 10 minutes; dilute the solution to 25 ml with water and compare the extinction of a 1-cm layer of the solution at 538 nm with that of a solution prepared at the same time and in the same manner with 2·0 ml of *standard sulphamethoxazole solution* in place of the prepared sample solution.
From the two extinctions, calculate the amount of sulphamethoxazole in the sample.
Determine the weight per ml of the mixture and calculate the concentration of sulphamethoxazole, weight in volume.

CONTENT OF TRIMETHOPRIM. 1·44 to 1·76 per cent w/v, determined by the following method:
Extract the chloroform solution reserved in the determination of sulphamethoxazole with four successive 50-ml portions of *dilute acetic acid*, wash the combined aqueous extracts with 5 ml of *chloroform*, and dilute the aqueous solution to 250 ml with *dilute acetic acid*.
To 10 ml of this solution add 10 ml of *dilute acetic acid*, dilute to 100 ml with water, and measure the extinction of a 1-cm layer at the maximum at about 271 nm, using as the blank a solution prepared by diluting 20 ml of *dilute acetic acid* to 100 ml with water.
For purposes of calculation, use a value of 204 for the E(1 per cent, 1 cm) of trimethoprim.
Determine the weight per ml of the mixture and calculate the concentration of trimethoprim, weight in volume.

Labelling. The directions given under Mixtures (page 735) should be followed.

Storage. It should be protected from light and stored in a cool place.

Dose. ADULT. 10 to 30 millilitres daily, divided into two or three doses.

When a dose less than or not a multiple of 5 ml is prescribed, the mixture may be diluted, as described under Mixtures (page 734), with Syrup. The diluted mixture must be freshly prepared.

Co-trimoxazole Mixture contains, in 5 ml, 80 mg of trimethoprim and 400 mg of sulphamethoxazole.

Co-trimoxazole Mixture, Paediatric

SYNONYM: Trimethoprim and Sulphamethoxazole Mixture, Paediatric

Paediatric Co-trimoxazole Mixture is a suspension containing 0·8 per cent w/v of Trimethoprim and 4 per cent w/v of Sulphamethoxazole in a suitable coloured flavoured vehicle.

Standard
PRESENCE OF TRIMETHOPRIM AND SULPHAMETHOXAZOLE. It complies with the thin-layer chromatographic test given in Appendix 5A, page 861.

CONTENT OF SULPHAMETHOXAZOLE. 3·60 to 4·40 per cent w/v, determined by the method for Co-trimoxazole Mixture.

CONTENT OF TRIMETHOPRIM. 0·72 to 0·88 per cent w/v, determined by the method for Co-trimoxazole Mixture.

Labelling. The directions given under Mixtures (page 735) should be followed.

Storage. It should be protected from light and stored in a cool place.

Dose. CHILD. Twice daily: up to 2 years, 2·5 millilitres; 2 to 5 years, 2·5 to 5 millilitres; 6 to 12 years, 5 to 10 millilitres.

When a dose less than or not a multiple of 5 ml is prescribed, the mixture may be diluted, as described under Mixtures (page 734), with Syrup. The diluted mixture must be freshly prepared.

Paediatric Co-trimoxazole Mixture contains, in 5 ml, 40 mg of trimethoprim and 200 mg of sulphamethoxazole.

Erythromycin Mixture

SYNONYM: Erythromycin Suspension

Erythromycin Mixture is a suspension of Erythromycin Stearate containing the equivalent of 2·0 per cent w/v of erythromycin in a suitable coloured flavoured vehicle.

Standard
CONTENT OF ERYTHROMYCIN. 90 to 110 per cent of the prescribed or stated concentration, determined by the following method:
To an accurately measured volume, equivalent to about 0·1 g of erythromycin, add 200 ml of *methyl alcohol* and mix well; add 100 ml of *solution of standard pH 7·0*, dilute to 500 ml with *water for injections*, maintain the solution at 60° for 3 hours and carry out a microbiological assay of erythromycin; a suggested method is given in Appendix 18, page 897.
The precision of any assay must be such that the fiducial limits of error (P = 0·95) are not less than 95 per cent and not more than 105 per cent of the estimated potency.
Assuming that each 1000 Units found is equivalent to 1 mg of erythromycin, calculate the upper and lower fiducial limits of the equivalent concentration of erythromycin in the mixture.
The upper fiducial limit of the estimated equivalent concentration of erythromycin is not less than 90 per cent and the lower fiducial limit is not more than 110 per cent of the prescribed or stated concentration.

Labelling. The directions given under Mixtures (page 735) should be followed.

Storage. The mixture and the diluted mixture should be stored in a cool place.

Dose. CHILD. Every six hours: up to 1 year, 2·5 millilitres; 1 to 5 years, 5 millilitres; 6 to 12 years, 10 millilitres.

When a dose less than or not a multiple of 5 ml is prescribed, the mixture may be diluted, as described under Mixtures (page 734), with Syrup. The diluted mixture must be freshly prepared.

Ferric Ammonium Citrate Mixture

SYNONYM: Iron and Ammonium Citrate Mixture

Ferric Ammonium Citrate	..	200 g
Chloroform Water, Double-strength..		500 ml
Water (see page 642) ..	.. to	1000 ml

It should be recently prepared.

Standard
CONTENT OF IRON. 3·89 to 4·72 per cent w/v, calculated as Fe, determined by the following method:
Dilute 3 ml to 12 ml with water, add 1 ml of *sulphuric acid*, warm until the dark brown colour becomes pale yellow, cool to below 20° and maintain the solution at this temperature throughout the procedure.
Add 0·1N potassium permanganate, dropwise, until a pink colour persists for 5 seconds, add 15 ml of *hydrochloric acid* and 2 g of *potassium iodide*, allow to stand for 3 minutes, add 60 ml of water, and titrate with 0·1N sodium thiosulphate, using *starch mucilage* as indicator; each ml of 0·1N sodium thiosulphate is equivalent to 0·005585 g of Fe.

Dose. 10 millilitres.

Ferric Ammonium Citrate Mixture, Paediatric

SYNONYM: Paediatric Iron and Ammonium Citrate Mixture

Ferric Ammonium Citrate	..	80 g
Compound Orange Spirit	..	2 ml
Syrup		100 ml
Chloroform Water, Double-strength..		500 ml
Water (see page 642) ..	.. to 1000 ml	

It should be recently prepared.

Standard
CONTENT OF IRON. 1·56 to 1·89 per cent w/v, calculated as Fe, determined by the following method:
To 5 ml add 45 ml of water, 0·2 ml of *hydrochloric acid* and *potassium permanganate solution*, dropwise, until a permanent pink colour is produced; add 10 ml of *hydrochloric acid* and 3 ml of *ammonium thiocyanate solution*, maintain a current of carbon dioxide through the flask, and titrate with 0·1N titanous chloride; each ml of 0·1N titanous chloride is equivalent to 0·005585 g of Fe.

Dose. CHILD. Well diluted with water: up to 1 year, 5 millilitres; 1 to 5 years, 10 millilitres.

Ferrous Fumarate Mixture

Ferrous Fumarate Mixture is a suspension of Ferrous Fumarate in a suitable coloured flavoured vehicle.

Standard
PRESENCE OF FUMARATE. Mix 20 ml with 10 ml of *hydrochloric acid*, warm on a water-bath for 15 minutes, cool, extract with two successive 50-ml portions of *solvent ether*, filter the combined extracts through a layer of *anhydrous sodium sulphate* and evaporate the filtrate to dryness.
The infra-red absorption spectrum of the residue exhibits maxima which are at the same wavelengths as, and have similar relative intensities to, those in the spectrum of *fumaric acid A.S.*
CONTENT OF FERROUS FUMARATE. 90·0 to 110·0 per cent of the prescribed or stated concentration, calculated as $C_4H_2FeO_4$, determined by the following method:
Mix an accurately weighed quantity, equivalent to about 0·35 g of ferrous fumarate, with 10 ml of water and 25 ml of *nitric acid* and warm carefully until the vigorous reaction has subsided; add a further 25 ml of *nitric acid*, evaporate to about 10 ml, and allow to cool; carefully add 10 ml of *sulphuric acid*, evaporate until white fumes are evolved, and allow to cool; add 10 ml of *nitric acid*, and again evaporate until white fumes are evolved; repeat the evaporation with 10-ml portions of *nitric acid* until all the organic matter is destroyed.
Add 10 ml of water and 0·5 g of *ammonium oxalate*, evaporate until white fumes are evolved, add 50 ml of water, boil until a clear solution is obtained, cool, dilute to 100 ml with water, and add 0·1N potassium permanganate, dropwise, until a faint pink colour persists for 10 seconds; add 10 ml of *hydrochloric acid* and 3 g of *potassium iodide*, allow to stand for 15 minutes in the dark, add 10 ml of *chloroform*, and titrate the liberated iodine with 0·1N sodium thiosulphate, with vigorous shaking, until the colour of the chloroform layer changes from purple to colourless.
Repeat the procedure omitting the sample.
The difference between the two titrations represents the amount of sodium thiosulphate required by the sample; each ml of 0·1N sodium thiosulphate is equivalent to 0·01699 g of $C_4H_2FeO_4$.

Determine the weight per ml of the mixture and calculate the concentration of $C_4H_2FeO_4$, weight in volume.

Labelling. The directions given under Mixtures (page 735) should be followed.

Storage. It should be protected from light.

Dose. Ferrous fumarate:
ADULT. Initial dose, 420 to 560 milligrams daily; maintenance dose 210 milligrams daily.
CHILD. Three times daily: up to 1 year, 35 milligrams; 1 to 5 years, 70 milligrams; 6 to 12 years, 140 milligrams.

When the strength of the mixture is not specified, a suspension containing 140 mg of ferrous fumarate in 5 ml shall be supplied.

When a dose less than or not a multiple of 5 ml is prescribed, the mixture may be diluted, as described under Mixtures (page 734), with Syrup. The diluted mixture must be freshly prepared.

Ferrous Sulphate Mixture

Ferrous Sulphate..	..	..	30 g
Ascorbic Acid	..	..	1 g
Orange Syrup	..	..	50 ml
Chloroform Water, Double-strength..	..	..	500 ml
Water (see page 642)	..	.. to 1000 ml	

It should be recently prepared.

The use of certain types of tap water, particularly those of temporary hardness, may lead to discoloration of this preparation. Freshly boiled and cooled Purified Water gives a satisfactory colourless or very pale yellow product.

Standard
CONTENT OF FERROUS SULPHATE. 2·76 to 3·24 per cent w/v, calculated as $FeSO_4,7H_2O$, determined by the method for iron in Paediatric Ferric Ammonium Citrate Mixture, 20 ml being used; each ml of 0·1N titanous chloride is equivalent to 0·02780 g of $FeSO_4,7H_2O$.

Dose. 10 millilitres, well diluted with water.

Ferrous Sulphate Mixture, Paediatric

Ferrous Sulphate..	..	..	12 g
Ascorbic Acid	..	..	1 g
Orange Syrup	..	..	100 ml
Chloroform Water, Double-strength..	..	..	500 ml
Water (see page 642)	..	.. to 1000 ml	

It should be recently prepared.

The use of certain types of tap water, particularly those of temporary hardness, may lead to discoloration of this preparation. Freshly boiled and cooled Purified Water gives a satisfactory colourless or pale yellow product.

Standard
CONTENT OF FERROUS SULPHATE. 1·10 to 1·30 per cent w/v, calculated as $FeSO_4,7H_2O$, determined by the method for iron in Paediatric Ferric Ammonium Citrate Mixture, 20 ml being used; each ml of

0·1N titanous chloride is equivalent to 0·02780 g of FeSO$_4$,7H$_2$O.

Dose. CHILD. Well diluted with water: up to 1 year, 5 millilitres; 1 to 5 years, 10 millilitres.

Fusidic Acid Mixture

SYNONYM: Fusidic Acid Suspension

Fusidic Acid Mixture is a suspension of Fusidic Acid in a suitable coloured flavoured aqueous vehicle.

Standard
ACIDITY. pH, 4·8 to 5·2.
PARTICLE SIZE. When determined by the method given in Appendix 25C, page 911, 95 per cent of the particles have a maximum diameter not greater than 5 μm and not more than a few have a maximum diameter greater than 15 μm.
CONTENT OF FUSIDIC ACID. 92·5 to 107·5 per cent of the prescribed or stated concentration, determined by the following method:
Mix an accurately weighed quantity, equivalent to about 0·25 g of fusidic acid, with 100 ml of *alcohol (95 per cent)* and dilute to 200 ml with water; to 10 ml of this solution add 100 ml of *alcohol (95 per cent)*, dilute to 200 ml with *citrate-phosphate buffer solution pH 6·0* and carry out a microbiological assay of fusidic acid; a suggested method is given in Appendix 18, page 897, *diethanolamine fusidate A.S.* being used in place of the standard preparation.
The precision of any assay must be such that the fiducial limits of error (P = 0·95) are not less than 95 per cent and not more than 105 per cent of the estimated potency.
Determine the weight per ml of the mixture and calculate the upper and lower fiducial limits of the estimated concentration of fusidic acid in the mixture, weight in volume.
The upper fiducial limit of fusidic acid is not less than 92·5 per cent and the lower fiducial limit is not more than 107·5 per cent of the prescribed or stated concentration.

Labelling. The directions given under Mixtures (page 735) should be followed.

Storage. It should be protected from light.

Dose. Fusidic acid:

ADULT. 1 to 2 grams daily, in divided doses.

CHILD. Three times daily: up to 1 year, 125 milligrams; 1 to 5 years, 250 milligrams; 6 to 12 years, 500 milligrams.

When the strength of the mixture is not specified, a suspension containing 250 mg of fusidic acid in 5 ml shall be supplied.

When a dose less than or not a multiple of 5 ml is prescribed, the mixture may be diluted, as described under Mixtures (page 734), with Water (see page 642). The diluted mixture must be freshly prepared.

When Fusidate Mixture is prescribed, Fusidic Acid Mixture shall be supplied.

Gelsemium and Hyoscyamus Mixture, Compound

Gelsemium Tincture	..	..		30 ml
Hyoscyamus Tincture	..	..		100 ml
Potassium Bromide	..	..		50 g
Chloroform Water, Double-strength..	..	..	..	500 ml
Water (see page 642)	..	.. to 1000 ml

It should be recently prepared.

Standard
PRESENCE OF HYOSCYAMUS AND GELSEMIUM ALKALOIDS. It complies with the thin-layer chromatographic test given in Appendix 5B, page 871.

CONTENT OF POTASSIUM BROMIDE. 4·75 to 5·25 per cent w/v, calculated as KBr, determined by the following method:
To 5 ml add 15 ml of water and continue by the method given in Appendix 11, page 891; each ml of 0·1N silver nitrate is equivalent to 0·01190 g of KBr.

Dose. 10 to 20 millilitres.

Gentian Mixture, Acid

Concentrated Compound Gentian Infusion..	..	..	..	100 ml
Dilute Hydrochloric Acid		..		50 ml
Chloroform Water, Double-strength..	..	..	..	500 ml
Water (see page 642)	..		.. to 1000 ml

It should be recently prepared.

Standard
CONTENT OF HYDROCHLORIC ACID. 0·48 to 0·56 per cent w/v, calculated as HCl, determined by the following method:
To 10 ml add 10 ml of water and continue by the method given in Appendix 11, page 891; each ml of 0·1N silver nitrate is equivalent to 0·003646 g of HCl.

Dose. 10 to 20 millilitres.

Gentian Mixture, Acid, with Nux Vomica

SYNONYM: Gentian, Nux Vomica, and Acid Mixture

Nux Vomica Tincture	..	..	50 ml
Acid Gentian Mixture	..	.. to 1000 ml

It should be recently prepared.

Standard
PRESENCE OF NUX VOMICA ALKALOIDS. It complies with the thin-layer chromatographic test given in Appendix 5B, page 871.

CONTENT OF HYDROCHLORIC ACID. 0·46 to 0·53 per cent w/v, calculated as HCl, determined by the following method:
To 10 ml add 10 ml of water and continue by the method given in Appendix 11, page 891; each ml of 0·1N silver nitrate is equivalent to 0·003646 g of HCl

Dose. 10 to 20 millilitres.

Gentian Mixture, Alkaline

SYNONYM: Mistura Gentianae cum Soda

Concentrated Compound Gentian Infusion..	..	..	..	100 ml
Sodium Bicarbonate	..	..		50 g
Chloroform Water, Double-strength..	..	..	..	500 ml
Water (see page 642)	..		.. to 1000 ml

It should be recently prepared.

Standard
CONTENT OF SODIUM BICARBONATE. 4·75 to 5·25 per cent w/v, calculated as NaHCO$_3$, determined by the following method:
To 10 ml add 100 ml of water and 25 ml of 0·5N

hydrochloric acid and boil for 10 minutes; cool, and titrate the excess of acid with 0·5N sodium hydroxide, using 0·5 ml of *methyl red solution* as indicator; each ml of 0·5N hydrochloric acid is equivalent to 0·04200 g of NaHCO₃.

Dose. 10 to 20 millilitres.

Gentian Mixture, Alkaline, with Nux Vomica

SYNONYM: Gentian, Nux Vomica, and Alkali Mixture

Nux Vomica Tincture	.. ..	50 ml
Alkaline Gentian Mixture	.. to 1000 ml	

It should be recently prepared.

Standard
PRESENCE OF NUX VOMICA ALKALOIDS. It complies with the thin-layer chromatographic test given in Appendix 5B, page 871.

CONTENT OF SODIUM BICARBONATE. 4·51 to 4·99 per cent w/v, calculated as NaHCO₃, determined by the method for Alkaline Gentian Mixture.

Dose. 10 to 20 millilitres.

Gentian Mixture, Alkaline, with Phenobarbitone

SYNONYM: Gentian and Alkali Mixture with Phenobarbitone

Phenobarbitone Sodium..	..	1·5 g
Alkaline Gentian Mixture	.. to 1000 ml	

It must be freshly prepared.

Dose. 10 to 20 millilitres.

Gentian and Rhubarb Mixture

SYNONYM: Mistura Gentianae cum Rheo

Concentrated Compound Gentian Infusion..	50 ml
Compound Rhubarb Tincture ..	100 ml
Sodium Bicarbonate	50 g
Peppermint Emulsion, Concentrated	25 ml
Chloroform Water, Double-strength..	500 ml
Water (see page 642) .. .. to 1000 ml	

It should be recently prepared

Standard
CONTENT OF SODIUM BICARBONATE. 4·75 to 5·25 per cent w/v, calculated as NaHCO₃, determined by the method for Alkaline Gentian Mixture (above).

Dose. 10 to 20 millilitres.

Indomethacin Mixture

SYNONYM: Indomethacin Suspension

Indomethacin Mixture is a suspension of Indomethacin in a suitable coloured flavoured vehicle. It may contain a suitable preservative.

Standard
PRESENCE OF INDOMETHACIN. The solution prepared in the determination of the content of indomethacin exhibits a light absorption which has, in the range 300 to 350 nm, a well-defined maximum only at about 318 nm.

ACIDITY. pH, 4·3 to 4·7.

CONTENT OF INDOMETHACIN. 90·0 to 110·0 per cent of the prescribed or stated concentration, determined by the following method:
Dilute an accurately measured volume, equivalent to about 0·015 g of indomethacin, to 25 ml with a mixture containing 1 volume of 1N hydrochloric acid and 9 volumes of *methyl alcohol*, mix, filter, dilute 5 ml of the filtrate to 100 ml with the same solvent mixture, and measure the extinction of a 1-cm layer at the maximum at about 318 nm.
For purposes of calculation, use a value of 180 for the E(1 per cent, 1 cm) of indomethacin.
Calculate the concentration of indomethacin in the sample.

Labelling. The directions given under Mixtures (page 735) should be followed.

Storage. It should be stored in a cool place, but should not be allowed to freeze.

Dose. Indomethacin, 50 to 150 milligrams daily, in divided doses, with food.

When the strength of the mixture is not specified, a suspension containing 25 mg of indomethacin in 5 ml shall be supplied.

This mixture should not be diluted. The general direction given under Mixtures that the preparation should be diluted so that the dose is contained in 5 ml does not apply to this mixture; where necessary, the dose should be measured by means of a graduated pipette.

Ipecacuanha Mixture, Paediatric

Ipecacuanha Tincture	.. ..	20 ml
Sodium Bicarbonate	.. ..	20 g
Tolu Syrup	.. .. ..	200 ml
Chloroform Water, Double-strength..		500 ml
Water (see page 642) ..	.. to 1000 ml	

It should be recently prepared.

Standard
PRESENCE OF IPECACUANHA ALKALOIDS. It complies with the thin-layer chromatographic test given in Appendix 5B, page 872.

CONTENT OF SODIUM BICARBONATE. 1·90 to 2·10 per cent w/v, calculated as NaHCO₃, determined by the following method:
To 20 ml add 20 ml of water and titrate with 0·5N hydrochloric acid, using *methyl orange–xylene cyanol FF solution* as indicator; each ml of 0·5N hydrochloric acid is equivalent to 0·04200 g of NaHCO₃.

Dose. CHILD. Up to 1 year, 5 millilitres; 1 to 5 years, 10 millilitres.

Ipecacuanha Mixture, Opiate, Paediatric

Ipecacuanha Tincture	.. ..	20 ml
Camphorated Opium Tincture ..		30 ml
Sodium Bicarbonate	.. ..	20 g
Tolu Syrup	.. .. ..	200 ml
Chloroform Water, Double-strength..		500 ml
Water (see page 642) ..	.. to 1000 ml	

It should be recently prepared.

Standard

PRESENCE OF IPECACUANHA AND OPIUM ALKALOIDS. It complies with the thin-layer chromatographic test given in Appendix 5B, page 872.

CONTENT OF SODIUM BICARBONATE. 1·90 to 2·10 per cent w/v, calculated as $NaHCO_3$, determined by the method for Paediatric Ipecacuanha Mixture.

Dose. CHILD. Up to 1 year, 5 millilitres; 1 to 5 years, 10 millilitres.

Ipecacuanha and Ammonia Mixture, Paediatric

Ipecacuanha Tincture	20 ml
Ammonium Bicarbonate ..	6 g
Sodium Bicarbonate	20 g
Tolu Syrup	100 ml
Chloroform Water, Double-strength..	500 ml
Water (see page 642) .. .. to 1000 ml	

It should be recently prepared.

Standard

PRESENCE OF IPECACUANHA ALKALOIDS. It complies with the thin-layer chromatographic test given in Appendix 5B, page 871.

CONTENT OF SODIUM BICARBONATE. 1·90 to 2·10 per cent w/v, calculated as $NaHCO_3$, determined by the following method:

Evaporate 10 ml to dryness on a water-bath, ignite the residue, cool, extract with hot water, and filter; wash the residue with hot water, cool the combined filtrate and washings, and titrate with 0·1N hydrochloric acid, using *methyl orange–xylene cyanol FF solution* as indicator; each ml of 0·1N hydrochloric acid is equivalent to 0·008401 g of $NaHCO_3$.

CONTENT OF AMMONIUM BICARBONATE. 0·57 to 0·63 per cent w/v, calculated as NH_4HCO_3, determined by the following method:

Transfer 25 ml to an ammonia-distillation apparatus, dilute to 200 ml with water, add 5 ml of *sodium hydroxide solution*, distil into 50 ml of 0·1N sulphuric acid, and titrate the excess of acid with 0·1N sodium hydroxide, using *methyl red solution* as indicator.

Repeat the procedure omitting the sample.

The difference between the two titrations represents the amount of acid required by the sample; each ml of 0·1N sulphuric acid is equivalent to 0·007906 g of NH_4HCO_3.

Dose. CHILD. Up to 1 year, 5 millilitres; 1 to 5 years, 10 millilitres.

Ipecacuanha and Morphine Mixture

SYNONYM: Mistura Tussi Nigra

Ipecacuanha Tincture	20 ml
Chloroform and Morphine Tincture	40 ml
Liquorice Liquid Extract ..	100 ml
Water (see page 642) .. .. to 1000 ml	

It should be recently prepared.

Standard

PRESENCE OF IPECACUANHA AND MORPHINE ALKALOIDS. It complies with the thin-layer chromatographic test given in Appendix 5B, page 871.

Dose. 10 millilitres.

Kaolin Mixture

SYNONYM: Mistura Kaolini Alkalina

Light Kaolin or Light Kaolin (Natural)	200 g
Light Magnesium Carbonate ..	50 g
Sodium Bicarbonate	50 g
Peppermint Emulsion, Concentrated	25 ml
Chloroform Water, Double-strength..	500 ml
Water (see page 642) .. .. to 1000 ml	

It should be recently prepared, unless the kaolin has been sterilised.

Standard

CONTENT OF ACID-INSOLUBLE MATTER. 13·8 to 18·4 per cent w/w, determined by the following method:

To about 3 g, accurately weighed, add 15 ml of water and make acid to *litmus paper* by the cautious addition of *dilute hydrochloric acid*; boil for 5 minutes, replacing water lost by evaporation, cool, and decant the supernatant liquid through a filter.

Boil the residue with 20 ml of water and 10 ml of *dilute hydrochloric acid*, cool, filter through the original filter, and wash the residue with water until the washings are free from chloride, reserving the filtrate and washings for the determination of magnesium.

Dry and ignite the residue of acid-insoluble matter to constant weight at red heat.

CONTENT OF MAGNESIUM. 1·04 to 1·25 per cent w/w, calculated as Mg, determined by the following method:

Dilute the combined filtrate and washings reserved in the determination of acid-insoluble matter to 100 ml with water; to 20 ml of this solution add 0·1 g of *ascorbic acid*, make slightly alkaline to *litmus paper* with *dilute ammonia solution*, add 10 ml of *triethanolamine*, 10 ml of *ammonia buffer solution*, 1 ml of *potassium cyanide solution*, and *mordant black 11 solution* as indicator, and titrate with 0·05M disodium edetate to a full blue colour; each ml of 0·05M disodium edetate is equivalent to 0·001215 g of Mg.

CONTENT OF SODIUM BICARBONATE. 4·05 to 4·65 per cent w/v, calculated as $NaHCO_3$, determined by the method for sodium bicarbonate in Paediatric Compound Calcium Carbonate Mixture, page 738, about 10 g, accurately weighed, being used.

Labelling. A direction to shake the bottle should be given on the label.

Dose. 10 to 20 millilitres.

Kaolin Mixture, Paediatric

Light Kaolin or Light Kaolin (Natural)	200 g
Amaranth Solution	10 ml
Benzoic Acid Solution	20 ml
Raspberry Syrup	200 ml
Chloroform Water, Double-strength..	500 ml
Water (see page 642) .. .. to 1000 ml	

It should be recently prepared, unless the kaolin has been sterilised.

Standard

RESIDUE ON IGNITION. 14·3 to 19·1 per cent w/w, determined by evaporating to dryness about 10 g, accurately weighed, and igniting the residue to constant weight at red heat.

Labelling. A direction to shake the bottle should be given on the label.

Dose. CHILD. Up to 1 year, 5 millilitres; 1 to 5 years, 10 millilitres.

Kaolin and Morphine Mixture

SYNONYM: Mistura Kaolini Sedativa

Light Kaolin or Light Kaolin (Natural)	200 g
Chloroform and Morphine Tincture	40 ml
Sodium Bicarbonate	50 g
Water (see page 642) .. .. to 1000 ml

It should be recently prepared, unless the kaolin has been sterilised.

Standard
PRESENCE OF MORPHINE. It complies with the thin-layer chromatographic test given in Appendix 5B, page 872.

CONTENT OF ACID-INSOLUBLE MATTER. 13·8 to 18·4 per cent w/w, determined by the method for acid-insoluble matter in Kaolin Mixture, page 745, the reservation of the filtrate and washings for the determination of magnesium being omitted.

CONTENT OF SODIUM BICARBONATE. 4·04 to 4·65 per cent w/w, calculated as $NaHCO_3$, determined by the following method:
Boil about 20 g, accurately weighed, with 40 ml of water for 5 minutes, cool, replace the water lost by evaporation, add 50 ml of *alcohol (95 per cent)*, previously neutralised to *methyl red solution*, and allow to stand for one hour; filter, and wash the residue with 100 ml of a mixture of equal volumes of the neutralised alcohol and water.
To the combined filtrate and washings add 50 ml of 0·5N hydrochloric acid, boil, cool, and titrate the excess of acid with 0·5N sodium hydroxide, using *methyl red solution* as indicator; each ml of 0·5N hydrochloric acid is equivalent to 0·04200 g of $NaHCO_3$.

Labelling. A direction to shake the bottle should be given on the label.

Dose. 10 millilitres.

Lobelia and Stramonium Mixture, Compound

SYNONYM: Mistura Lobeliae Composita

Lobelia Ethereal Tincture ..	50 ml
Stramonium Tincture	100 ml
Potassium Iodide..	20 g
Tragacanth Mucilage	100 ml
Chloroform Water, Double-strength..	500 ml
Water (see page 642) .. .. to 1000 ml

Dissolve the potassium iodide in the double-strength chloroform water and dilute to 700 ml with water, add the tragacanth mucilage, and mix; add the tinctures, with constant stirring, and sufficient water to produce the required volume.
It should be recently prepared.

Standard
PRESENCE OF LOBELIA AND STRAMONIUM ALKALOIDS. It complies with the thin-layer chromatographic test given in Appendix 5B, page 872.

CONTENT OF POTASSIUM IODIDE. 1·90 to 2·10 per cent w/v, calculated as KI, determined by the following method:
To 10 ml add 40 ml of water, 15 ml of *hydrochloric acid*, and 6 ml of *potassium cyanide solution*, and titrate with 0·05M potassium iodate, adding 5 ml of *starch mucilage* as indicator when the titration is almost complete; each ml of 0·05M potassium iodate is equivalent to 0·01660 g of KI.

Dose. 10 millilitres.

Magnesium Carbonate Mixture

Light Magnesium Carbonate ..	50 g
Sodium Bicarbonate	80 g
Peppermint Emulsion, Concentrated	25 ml
Chloroform Water, Double-strength	500 ml
Water (see page 642) .. .. to 1000 ml

It should be recently prepared.

Standard
CONTENT OF SODIUM BICARBONATE. 7·00 to 7·89 per cent w/w, calculated as $NaHCO_3$, determined by the method for sodium bicarbonate in Paediatric Compound Calcium Carbonate Mixture, page 738, about 10 g, accurately weighed, being used.

CONTENT OF MAGNESIUM. 1·09 to 1·34 per cent w/w, calculated as Mg, determined by the following method:
Dissolve about 15 g, accurately weighed, in the minimum quantity of *dilute hydrochloric acid* and dilute to 200 ml with water; to 20 ml of this solution add 200 ml of water and 10 ml of *ammonia buffer solution* and titrate with 0·05M disodium edetate, using *mordant black 11 solution* as indicator; each ml of 0·05M disodium edetate is equivalent to 0·001215 g of Mg.

Labelling. A direction to shake the bottle should be given on the label.

Dose. 10 to 20 millilitres.

Magnesium Carbonate Mixture, Aromatic

SYNONYM: Mistura Carminativa

Light Magnesium Carbonate ..	30 g
Aromatic Cardamom Tincture ..	30 ml
Sodium Bicarbonate	50 g
Chloroform Water, Double-strength	500 ml
Water (see page 642) .. .. to 1000 ml

It should be recently prepared.

Standard
CONTENT OF SODIUM BICARBONATE. 4·51 to 5·08 per cent w/w, calculated as $NaHCO_3$, determined by the method for sodium bicarbonate in Paediatric Compound Calcium Carbonate Mixture, page 738, about 10 g, accurately weighed, being used.

CONTENT OF MAGNESIUM. 0·68 to 0·83 per cent w/w, calculated as Mg, determined by the method for magnesium in Magnesium Carbonate Mixture, above, about 30 g, accurately weighed, being used.

Labelling. A direction to shake the bottle should be given on the label.

Dose. 10 to 20 millilitres.

Magnesium Sulphate Mixture

SYNONYM: Mistura Alba

Magnesium Sulphate	400 g
Light Magnesium Carbonate ..	50 g
Peppermint Emulsion, Concentrated	25 ml
Chloroform Water, Double-strength	300 ml
Water (see page 642) .. .. to 1000 ml	

It should be recently prepared.

Standard
CONTENT OF MAGNESIUM SULPHATE. 30·5 to 37·8 per cent w/w, calculated as MgSO₄,7H₂O, determined by the following method:
Boil about 0·7 g, accurately weighed, with 25 ml of water and 25 ml of *alcohol (95 per cent)*, cool, filter, and wash the residue with successive small portions of the diluted alcohol until the washings are free from sulphate, reserving the residue on the filter for the determination of magnesium carbonate.
To the combined filtrate and washings add 10 ml of *ammonia buffer solution* and titrate with 0·05M disodium edetate, using *mordant black 11 solution* as indicator; each ml of 0·05M disodium edetate is equivalent to 0·01232 g of MgSO₄,7H₂O.

CONTENT OF MAGNESIUM CARBONATE. 0·99 to 1·20 per cent w/w, calculated as Mg, determined by the following method:
Dissolve the residue reserved in the determination of magnesium sulphate in 10 ml of 1N hydrochloric acid and wash the filter with successive small portions of water until the washings are free from chloride.
To the combined filtrate and washings add 10 ml of *ammonia buffer solution* and titrate with 0·05M disodium edetate, using *mordant black 11 solution* as indicator; each ml of 0·05M disodium edetate is equivalent to 0·001215 g of Mg.

Labelling. A direction to shake the bottle should be given on the label.

Dose. 10 to 20 millilitres.

Magnesium Trisilicate Mixture

SYNONYM: Compound Magnesium Trisilicate Mixture

Magnesium Trisilicate	50 g
Light Magnesium Carbonate ..	50 g
Sodium Bicarbonate	50 g
Peppermint Emulsion, Concentrated	25 ml
Chloroform Water, Double-strength	500 ml
Water (see page 642) .. .. to 1000 ml	

It should be recently prepared

Standard
CONTENT OF SODIUM BICARBONATE. 4·35 to 5·10 per cent w/w, calculated as NaHCO₃, determined by the method for sodium bicarbonate in Paediatric Compound Calcium Carbonate Mixture, page 738, about 20 g, accurately weighed, being used.

Labelling. A direction to shake the bottle should be given on the label.

Dose. 10 to 20 millilitres.

Magnesium Trisilicate and Belladonna Mixture

Magnesium Trisilicate	50 g
Belladonna Tincture	50 ml
Light Magnesium Carbonate ..	50 g
Sodium Bicarbonate	50 g
Peppermint Emulsion, Concentrated	25 ml
Chloroform Water, Double-strength..	500 ml
Water (see page 642) .. .. to 1000 ml	

It should be recently prepared.

Standard
PRESENCE OF BELLADONNA ALKALOIDS. It complies with the thin-layer chromatographic test given in Appendix 5B, page 872.

CONTENT OF SODIUM BICARBONATE. 4·37 to 5·12 per cent w/w, calculated as NaHCO₃, determined by the method for sodium bicarbonate in Paediatric Compound Calcium Carbonate Mixture, page 738, about 20 g, accurately weighed, being used.

Labelling. A direction to shake the bottle should be given on the label.

Dose. 10 to 20 millilitres.

Nalidixic Acid Mixture

Nalidixic Acid Mixture is a suspension of Nalidixic Acid in a suitable coloured flavoured vehicle. It may contain a suitable preservative.

Standard
PRESENCE OF NALIDIXIC ACID. To 5 ml add 30 ml of water and 20 ml of *sodium carbonate solution*, mix, extract with two successive 30-ml portions of *chloroform*, and discard the chloroform extracts.
Acidify the aqueous solution with 5N hydrochloric acid, extract with 40 ml of *chloroform*, wash the chloroform extract with 10 ml of water which has been acidified with 0·5 ml of 5N hydrochloric acid, filter the chloroform solution through a pledget of cotton wool, and evaporate the filtrate to dryness.
The residue, after drying at 105°, melts at about 228°.

CONTENT OF NALIDIXIC ACID. 92·5 to 107·5 per cent of the prescribed or stated concentration, determined by the following method:
Dilute an accurately weighed quantity, equivalent to about 0·12 g of nalidixic acid, to 100 ml with 0·01N sodium hydroxide; dilute 2 ml of this solution to 250 ml with 0·01N sodium hydroxide, and measure the extinction of a 1-cm layer at the maximum at about 334 nm.
For purposes of calculation, use a value of 500 for the E(1 per cent, 1 cm) of nalidixic acid.
Determine the weight per ml of the mixture and calculate the concentration of nalidixic acid, weight in volume.

Labelling. The directions given under Mixtures (page 735) should be followed.

Dose. Nalidixic acid:

CHILD. 30 to 60 milligrams per kilogram body-weight daily in divided doses.

When the strength of the mixture is not specified, a suspension containing 300 mg of nalidixic acid in 5 ml shall be supplied.

When a dose less than or not a multiple of 5 ml is prescribed, the mixture may be diluted, as described under Mixtures (page 734), with Syrup. The diluted mixture must be freshly prepared.

Nitrofurantoin Mixture

SYNONYM: Nitrofurantoin Suspension

Nitrofurantoin Mixture is a homogeneous suspension of Nitrofurantoin in a suitable flavoured vehicle. It has a pH at 20° of about 5·4.

Standard
CONTENT OF NITROFURANTOIN. 90·0 to 110·0 per cent of the prescribed or stated concentration, determined by the following method:
Protect the solutions from light throughout the procedure by carrying out all operations in subdued light or by using low-actinic glassware.
To an accurately weighed quantity, equivalent to about 0·03 g of nitrofurantoin, add, in small portions, 50 ml of *dimethylformamide*, stirring well between each addition, and continue stirring until the sample is completely dissolved.
Dilute this solution to 500 ml with a solution containing 1·8 per cent w/v of *sodium acetate* and 0·14 per cent v/v of *glacial acetic acid* in water, further dilute 10 ml of this solution to 100 ml with the sodium acetate–glacial acetic acid solution, and measure the extinction of a 1-cm layer in a silica cell at the maximum at about 367 nm, using as the blank a 1 per cent v/v solution of *dimethylformamide* in the sodium acetate–glacial acetic acid solution.
For purposes of calculation, use a value of 765 for the E(1 per cent, 1 cm) of nitrofurantoin.
Determine the weight per ml of the mixture and calculate the concentration of nitrofurantoin, weight in volume.

Labelling. The directions given under Mixtures (page 735) should be followed.

Storage. It should be protected from light and stored in a cool place.

Dose. Nitrofurantoin:
ADULT. 50 to 150 milligrams four times daily.
CHILD. Every six hours: up to 1 year, 6·25 to 12·5 milligrams; 1 to 5 years, 12·5 to 25 milligrams; 6 to 12 years, 50 milligrams.

When the strength of the mixture is not specified, a suspension containing 25 mg of nitrofurantoin in 5 ml shall be supplied.

This mixture should not be diluted. The general direction given under Mixtures that the preparation should be diluted so that the dose is contained in 5 ml does not apply to this mixture; it may be necessary for a dose of 2·5 ml to be measured by the patient in a 5-ml spoon; if a dose smaller than 2·5 ml is required, the dose should be measured by means of a graduated pipette.

Novobiocin Mixture

SYNONYM: Novobiocin Syrup

Novobiocin Mixture is a suspension of Novobiocin Calcium, in sufficiently fine powder to meet the requirements of the standard, in a suitable flavoured vehicle, which may be coloured.

Standard
PRESENCE OF CALCIUM. Evaporate 2 ml to dryness, ignite, dissolve the residue as completely as possible in 10 ml of *dilute acetic acid*, filter, and to the filtrate add *ammonium oxalate solution*; a white precipitate is produced which is soluble in *hydrochloric acid*.

ACIDITY. pH, 6·5 to 7·5.

PARTICLE SIZE. When determined by the method given in Appendix 25C, page 911, not less than 75 per cent of the particles have a maximum diameter less than 10 μm and not less than 99 per cent of the particles have a maximum diameter less than 20 μm; no particle has a maximum diameter greater than 50 μm.

CONTENT OF NOVOBIOCIN. 90 to 120 per cent of the prescribed or stated concentration, determined by the following method:
To an accurately weighed quantity, equivalent to about 0·125 g of novobiocin, add 300 ml of a mixture containing equal volumes of *alcohol* (*90 per cent*) and *solution of standard pH 7·8*, mix well, and dilute to 500 ml with the same solvent mixture; dilute 4 ml of this solution to 100 ml with *solution of standard pH 6·0*, further dilute 3 ml of this solution to 10 ml with *solution of standard pH 6·0* and carry out a microbiological assay of novobiocin; a suggested method is given in Appendix 18, page 897.
The precision of any assay must be such that the fiducial limits of error (P = 0·95) are not less than 95 per cent and not more than 105 per cent of the estimated potency.
Determine the weight per ml and, assuming that each 970 Units found is equivalent to 1 mg of novobiocin, calculate the upper and lower fiducial limits of the equivalent concentration of novobiocin in the mixture, weight in volume.
The upper fiducial limit of the estimated equivalent concentration of novobiocin is not less than 90 per cent and the lower fiducial limit is not more than 120 per cent of the prescribed or stated concentration.

Labelling. The directions given under Mixtures (page 735) should be followed.

Storage. It should be protected from light and stored in a cool place.

Dose. The equivalent of novobiocin:
ADULT. 1 to 2 grams daily, in divided doses.
CHILD. Twice daily: 6 months to 1 year, 62·5 to 125 milligrams; 1 to 5 years, 125 to 250 milligrams; 6 to 12 years, 250 to 500 milligrams.

When the strength of the mixture is not specified, a suspension containing the equivalent of 125 mg of novobiocin in 5 ml shall be supplied.

When a dose less than or not a multiple of 5 ml is prescribed, the mixture may be diluted, as described under Mixtures (page 734), with Syrup. The diluted mixture must be freshly prepared.

Nux Vomica Mixture, Acid

SYNONYM: Nux Vomica and Acid Mixture

Nux Vomica Tincture	..	..	50 ml
Dilute Hydrochloric Acid		..	50 ml
Chloroform Water, Double-strength..	..	..	500 ml
Water (see page 642)	..	..	to 1000 ml

It should be recently prepared.

Standard
PRESENCE OF NUX VOMICA ALKALOIDS. It complies with the thin-layer chromatographic test given in Appendix 5B, page 872.

CONTENT OF HYDROCHLORIC ACID. 0·46 to 0·59 per cent w/v, calculated as HCl, determined by the following method:
To 10 ml add 10 ml of water and continue by the method given in Appendix 11, page 891; each ml of 0·1N silver nitrate is equivalent to 0·003646 g of HCl.

Dose. 10 to 20 millilitres.

Nux Vomica Mixture, Alkaline

SYNONYM: Nux Vomica and Alkali Mixture

Nux Vomica Tincture	50 ml
Sodium Bicarbonate	50 g
Chloroform Water, Double-strength..	500 ml
Water (see page 642) .. .. to	1000 ml

It should be recently prepared.

Standard
PRESENCE OF NUX VOMICA ALKALOIDS. It complies with the thin-layer chromatographic test given in Appendix 5B, page 872.

CONTENT OF SODIUM BICARBONATE. 4·70 to 5·30 per cent w/v, calculated as $NaHCO_3$, determined by the method for Alkaline Gentian Mixture, page 743.

Dose. 10 to 20 millilitres.

Nystatin Mixture

SYNONYM: Nystatin Suspension

Nystatin Mixture is a suspension of Nystatin in a suitable flavoured vehicle. It is prepared freshly by dispersing granules consisting of the dry mixed ingredients in the specified volume of Water (see page 642).

Standard
CONTENT OF NYSTATIN. 100 to 125 per cent of the prescribed or stated concentration, determined by the following method:
Prepare the mixture as directed on the label, immediately before analysis, and reserve a portion for the test for stability. Protect the solutions from light throughout the procedure.
Dissolve an accurately weighed quantity, equivalent to about 200,000 Units of nystatin, in *dimethylformamide* and dilute to 50 ml with *dimethylformamide*; dilute 10 ml of this solution to 200 ml with *phosphate buffer solution pH 6·0* and carry out a microbiological assay of nystatin; a suggested method is given in Appendix 18, page 897.
The precision of any assay must be such that the fiducial limits of error (P = 0·95) are not less than 95 per cent and not more than 105 per cent of the estimated potency.
Determine the weight per ml of the mixture and calculate the upper and lower fiducial limits of the concentration of nystatin in the mixture, weight in volume.
The upper fiducial limit of the estimated concentration of nystatin is not less than 100 per cent and the lower fiducial limit is not more than 125 per cent of the prescribed or stated concentration.
STABILITY. Store at 15° ± 1° for 7 days the portion of the mixture reserved in the determination of the content of nystatin and then repeat the determination on the stored mixture.
The concentration of nystatin in the stored mixture is not less than 80 per cent of the concentration found in the freshly prepared mixture.

Labelling. The directions given under Mixtures (page 735) should be followed; the name on the label of the container of the dry granules is "Granules for Nystatin Mixture".

Storage. The mixture should be stored in a cool place and used within one week of preparation.

Dose. Nystatin:
CHILD. Up to 5 years, 100,000 Units every six hours.
When the strength of the mixture is not specified, a suspension containing 100,000 Units in 1 ml shall be supplied.
This mixture should not be diluted. The general direction given under Mixtures that the preparation should be diluted so that the dose is contained in 5 ml does not apply to this mixture; the dose should be measured by means of a graduated pipette.

Opium Mixture, Camphorated, Compound

SYNONYM: Mist. Camph. Co.

Camphorated Opium Tincture ..	100 ml
Ammonium Bicarbonate ..	10 g
Strong Ammonium Acetate Solution	100 ml
Water (see page 642) .. .. to	1000 ml

It should be recently prepared.

Standard
PRESENCE OF OPIUM ALKALOIDS. It complies with the thin-layer chromatographic test given in Appendix 5B, page 872.

CONTENT OF AMMONIA. 1·35 to 1·62 per cent w/v, calculated as NH_3, determined by the method for ammonium bicarbonate in Ammonia and Ipecacuanha Mixture, page 736, 4 ml being used; each ml of 0·1N sulphuric acid is equivalent to 0·001703 g of NH_3.

Dose. 10 to 20 millilitres.

Phenoxymethylpenicillin Mixture

SYNONYM: Penicillin V Mixture

Phenoxymethylpenicillin Mixture is a suspension of Phenoxymethylpenicillin, of Phenoxymethylpenicillin Potassium, or of Phenoxymethylpenicillin Calcium, in a suitable flavoured oily vehicle, which may be coloured.

Standard
CONTENT OF PHENOXYMETHYLPENICILLIN. 92·5 to 107·5 per cent of the prescribed or stated concentration, calculated as $C_{16}H_{18}N_2O_5S$, determined by the following method:
To an accurately weighed quantity, equivalent to about 0·09 g of phenoxymethylpenicillin, add 10 ml of *methyl alcohol*, mix, add 50 ml of 1N sodium hydroxide, shake vigorously, add 50 ml of water, and continue shaking for 15 minutes; dilute to 150 ml with water, mix, and filter through a hardened filter paper.
Transfer 15 ml of the filtrate to a stoppered flask, add successively 20 ml of a freshly prepared buffer solution containing 5·44 per cent w/v of *sodium acetate* and 2·40 per cent w/v of *glacial acetic acid*, 5 ml of 1N hydrochloric acid, and 25 ml of 0·02N iodine, close the flask with a stopper moistened with water, allow to stand in the dark for 20 minutes, and titrate the excess of iodine with 0·02N sodium thiosulphate, using *starch mucilage*, added towards the end of the titration, as indicator.
To a similar accurately weighed quantity of the sample add 10 ml of *methyl alcohol*, mix, add 3 ml of a freshly prepared 3·3 per cent w/v solution of *sodium bicarbonate* in water, shake for 5 minutes, add 100 ml of water and 1 ml of 1N hydrochloric acid, dilute to 150 ml with water, and filter through a hardened filter paper.
Transfer 15 ml of the filtrate to a stoppered flask, add 20 ml of the buffer solution described above and 25 ml of 0·02N iodine, allow to stand for 20 minutes, and titrate with 0·02N sodium thiosulphate, using *starch mucilage*, added towards the end of the titration, as indicator.
From the volume of 0·02N iodine required in this second titration, calculate the volume that would be

required by the weight of sample taken for the first titration.

The difference between the actual volume required in the first titration and the calculated volume in the second titration represents the volume of the 0·02N iodine equivalent to the total penicillins, $C_{16}H_{18}N_2O_5S$, present.

Determine the exact equivalent of each ml of 0·02N iodine by the following method:

Dissolve about 0·1 g of *phenoxymethylpenicillin potassium B.C.R.S.*, accurately weighed, in sufficient water to produce 100 ml, transfer 10 ml to a stoppered flask, add 5 ml of 1N sodium hydroxide and allow to stand for 20 minutes.

Add 20 ml of a freshly prepared buffer solution containing 5·44 per cent w/v of *sodium acetate* and 2·40 per cent w/v of *glacial acetic acid*, 5 ml of 1N hydrochloric acid, and 25 ml of 0·02N iodine, close the flask with a wet stopper, and allow to stand for 20 minutes, protected from light.

Titrate the excess of iodine with 0·02N sodium thiosulphate, using *starch mucilage*, added towards the end of the titration, as indicator.

To a further 10 ml of the prepared solution add 20 ml of the buffer solution and 25 ml of 0·02N iodine, allow to stand for 20 minutes, and titrate with 0·02N sodium thiosulphate, using *starch mucilage*, added towards the end of the titration, as indicator.

The difference between the two titrations represents the volume of 0·02N iodine equivalent to the total penicillins present; each mg of phenoxymethylpenicillin potassium B.C.R.S. is equivalent to 0·9019 mg of total penicillins, calculated as $C_{16}H_{18}N_2O_5S$.

Calculate the concentration of $C_{16}H_{18}N_2O_5S$ in the sample.

Labelling. The directions given under Mixtures (page 735) should be followed.

Storage. The mixture should be stored in a cool place.

Dose. The equivalent of phenoxymethylpenicillin:

ADULT. 125 to 250 milligrams every four hours.

CHILD. Every six hours: up to 1 year, 62·5 milligrams; 1 to 5 years, 125 milligrams; 6 to 12 years, 250 milligrams.

When the strength of the mixture is not specified, a suspension containing 125 mg of phenoxymethylpenicillin, or an equivalent amount of the potassium or calcium salt, in 5 ml shall be supplied.

When a dose less than or not a multiple of 5 ml is prescribed, the mixture may be diluted, as described under Mixtures (page 734), with Fractionated Coconut Oil. The diluted mixture must be freshly prepared.

Phenytoin Mixture

SYNONYM: Phenytoin Suspension

Phenytoin Mixture is a suspension of Phenytoin in a suitable coloured flavoured vehicle.

Standard

PRESENCE OF PHENYTOIN. The infra-red absorption spectrum of the residue obtained in the determination of the content of phenytoin exhibits maxima which are at the same wavelengths as, and have similar relative intensities to, those in the spectrum of *phenytoin A.S.*

CONTENT OF PHENYTOIN. 90·0 to 110·0 per cent of the prescribed or stated concentration, determined by the following method:

To an accurately weighed quantity, equivalent to about 0·2 g of phenytoin, add 10 ml of *dilute hydrochloric acid* and 15 ml of water and extract with three successive 50-ml portions of a mixture of 3 volumes of *chloroform* and 1 volume of *isopropyl alcohol*, evaporate

the combined extracts to dryness, dry the residue at 105° for 1 hour, and cool.

To the residue add 3 ml of 1N sodium hydroxide and 50 ml of water, warm to dissolve, cool, pass a stream of *carbon dioxide* through the solution until the phenytoin is completely precipitated, filter through a sintered glass filter (British Standard Grade No. 4), wash the residue with two 10-ml portions of water, dry the residue of phenytoin for 2 hours at 105°, and weigh.

Determine the weight per ml of the mixture and calculate the concentration of phenytoin, weight in volume.

Labelling. The directions given under Mixtures (page 735) should be followed.

Dose. Phenytoin:

ADULT. 45 to 90 milligrams, three times daily, increased if necessary to 180 milligrams three times daily, in accordance with the needs of the patient.

CHILD. Up to 5 years, 30 to 60 milligrams three times daily; 6 to 12 years, 90 milligrams three or four times daily.

When the strength of the mixture is not specified, a suspension containing 30 mg of phenytoin in 5 ml shall be supplied.

When a dose less than or not a multiple of 5 ml is prescribed, the mixture may be diluted, as described under Mixtures (page 734), with Syrup. The diluted mixture must be freshly prepared.

Potassium Citrate Mixture

Potassium Citrate			300 g
Citric Acid	..	..	50 g
Lemon Spirit	..	..	5 ml
Quillaia Tincture..	..	..	10 ml
Syrup ..	..	..	250 ml
Chloroform Water, Double-strength..	..	..	300 ml
Water (see page 642)	..	.. to	1000 ml

It should be recently prepared.

Standard

PRESENCE OF POTASSIUM CITRATE. 1. Wet a loop of platinum wire with the sample and introduce into the flame of a Bunsen burner; the flame has a lilac colour which, when viewed through suitable blue glass, appears reddish-purple.

2. Boil a portion of the sample with an excess of *mercuric sulphate solution*, filter, boil the filtrate, and add 0·25 ml of *potassium permanganate solution*; the potassium permanganate solution is decolorised and a white precipitate is produced.

CONTENT OF POTASSIUM CITRATE. 28·5 to 31·5 per cent w/v, calculated as $C_6H_5K_3O_7,H_2O$, determined by the following method:

To about 1 g, accurately weighed, add 5 ml of *acetic anhydride* and 20 ml of *glacial acetic acid*, warm on a water-bath for 20 minutes, allow to cool, and continue by Method I of the British Pharmacopoeia for non-aqueous titration; each ml of 0·1N perchloric acid is equivalent to 0·01081 g of $C_6H_5K_3O_7,H_2O$.

Determine the weight per ml of the mixture and calculate the concentration of potassium citrate, weight in volume.

CONTENT OF CITRIC ACID. 4·75 to 5·25 per cent w/v calculated as $C_6H_8O_7,H_2O$, determined by the following method:

To 5 ml add 100 ml of water, boil, cool, and titrate with carbonate-free 0·1N sodium hydroxide, using *thymol blue solution* as indicator; each ml of 0·1N sodium hydroxide is equivalent to 0·007005 g of $C_6H_8O_7,H_2O$.

Labelling. Directions to shake the bottle and to dilute the dose well with water before administration should be given on the label.

Dose. ADULT. 10 millilitres, well diluted with water.

CHILD. Well diluted with water: up to 1 year, 2·5 millilitres; 1 to 5 years, 5 millilitres; 6 to 12 years, 10 millilitres.

When a dose less than or not a multiple of 5 ml is prescribed, the mixture may be diluted, as described under Mixtures (page 734), with Syrup.

Potassium Citrate and Hyoscyamus Mixture

Potassium Citrate	..	..	300 g
Hyoscyamus Tincture	..	..	200 ml
Citric Acid	..	..	50 g
Lemon Spirit	..	..	5 ml
Quillaia Tincture..	..	..	10 ml
Syrup	..	..	..	250 ml
Chloroform Water, Double-strength..	..	..	200 ml
Water (see page 642)	..	.. to 1000 ml

It should be recently prepared.

Standard
PRESENCE OF POTASSIUM CITRATE. It complies with the tests given for Potassium Citrate Mixture, above.

PRESENCE OF HYOSCYAMUS ALKALOIDS. It complies with the thin-layer chromatographic test given in Appendix 5B, page 872.

CONTENT OF POTASSIUM CITRATE. 28·5 to 31·5 per cent w/v, calculated as $C_6H_5K_3O_7,H_2O$, determined by the method for potassium citrate in Potassium Citrate Mixture.

CONTENT OF CITRIC ACID. 4·75 to 5·25 per cent w/v, calculated as $C_6H_8O_7,H_2O$, by the method for citric acid in Potassium Citrate Mixture, above.

Labelling. Directions to shake the bottle and to dilute the dose well with water before administration should be given on the label.

Dose. 10 millilitres, well diluted with water.

Potassium Iodide Mixture, Ammoniated

SYNONYM: Potassium Iodide and Ammonia Mixture

Potassium Iodide..	..	..	15 g
Ammonium Bicarbonate	..	15 g
Liquorice Liquid Extract	..	100 ml
Chloroform Water, Double-strength..	..	..	500 ml
Water (see page 642)	..	.. to 1000 ml

It should be recently prepared.

Standard
CONTENT OF AMMONIUM BICARBONATE. 1·42 to 1·62 per cent w/v, calculated as NH_4HCO_3, determined by the method for Ammonia and Ipecacuanha Mixture, page 736, the distillation being into 25 ml of 0·1N sulphuric acid.

CONTENT OF POTASSIUM IODIDE. 1·42 to 1·58 per cent w/v, calculated as KI, determined by the following method:
To 10 ml add 10 ml of water and continue by the method given in Appendix 11, page 891, adjusting the pH with 0·5N sulphuric acid; each ml of 0·1N silver nitrate is equivalent to 0·01660 g of KI.

Labelling. A direction to shake the bottle should be given on the label.

Dose. 10 to 20 millilitres.

Primidone Mixture

SYNONYM: Primidone Suspension

Primidone Mixture is a suspension of Primidone in a suitable flavoured vehicle.

Standard
CONTENT OF PRIMIDONE. 95·0 to 105·0 per cent of the prescribed or stated concentration, determined by the following method:
To an accurately weighed quantity, equivalent to about 0·4 g of primidone, add 75 ml of *methyl alcohol*, warm on a water-bath for 5 minutes with occasional shaking, cool, dilute to 100 ml with *methyl alcohol*, and allow any undissolved material to settle.
Examine the clear supernatant liquid in an apparatus for Gas–Liquid Chromatography, as described in the British Pharmacopoeia, Appendix XIIC, and determine the peak height due to primidone.
The chromatographic procedure may be carried out with a glass column, 1·5 m in length and 4 mm internal diameter, packed with 2 per cent w/w silicone gum rubber XE 60 supported on Gas Chrom Q (60- to 80-mesh), previously deactivated with dichloromethylsilane, maintained at 270°, nitrogen as the carrier gas, and a flame ionisation detector.
Calculate the concentration of primidone by reference to a calibration curve prepared by treating solutions containing, respectively, 0·375, 0·400, and 0·425 per cent w/v of *primidone A.S.* in *methyl alcohol* in the same manner.
Determine the weight per ml of the mixture and calculate the concentration of primidone, weight in volume.

Labelling. The directions given under Mixtures (page 735) should be followed.

Dose. Primidone:

ADULT. 500 milligrams daily, increasing to 1 to 2 grams daily in divided doses, in accordance with the needs of the patient.

CHILD. Up to 9 years, 250 milligrams daily, increased to 0·5 to 1 gram daily in divided doses, in accordance with the needs of the patient.

When the strength of the mixture is not specified, a suspension containing 250 mg of primidone in 5 ml shall be supplied.

When a dose less than or not a multiple of 5 ml is prescribed, the mixture may be diluted, as described under Mixtures (page 734), with Syrup. The diluted mixture must be freshly prepared.
If it is required to store a diluted mixture for more than two weeks, Syrup should not be used as the diluent.
A diluted mixture which is stable for three months may be prepared by using a diluent of the following composition:

Propyl Hydroxybenzoate ..	..	..	0·15 g
Methyl Hydroxybenzoate ..	..	..	1·5 g
Sodium Carboxymethylcellulose 50	..	10·0 g
Sucrose	..	..	..	..	200·0 g
Purified Water, freshly boiled and cooled, to 1000 ml

Rhubarb Mixture, Compound

SYNONYM: Mistura Rhei Composita

Compound Rhubarb Tincture ..		100 ml
Light Magnesium Carbonate ..		50 g
Sodium Bicarbonate		50 g
Strong Ginger Tincture		30 ml
Chloroform Water, Double-strength..		500 ml
Water (see page 642) .. .. to 1000 ml		

It should be recently prepared.

Standard
CONTENT OF SODIUM BICARBONATE. 4·48 to 5·05 per cent w/w, calculated as NaHCO₃, determined by the following method:
Evaporate about 10 g, accurately weighed, to dryness, ignite the residue, cool, boil for 5 minutes with 80 ml of water, filter, and continue by the method for sodium bicarbonate in Paediatric Compound Calcium Carbonate Mixture, page 738, beginning with the words "boil the residue . . .", reserving the residue, obtained after boiling with 100 ml of water and filtering, for the determination of magnesium.

CONTENT OF MAGNESIUM. 1·13 to 1·37 per cent w/w, calculated as Mg, determined by the following method:
Dissolve the residue reserved in the determination of sodium bicarbonate in the minimum quantity of *dilute hydrochloric acid* and dilute to 200 ml with water.
To 20 ml of this solution add 200 ml of water and 10 ml of *ammonia buffer solution* and titrate with 0·05M disodium edetate, using *mordant black 11 solution* as indicator; the sum of the volume of 0·05M disodium edetate used in this titration and one-tenth of the volume of 0·05M disodium edetate used in the determination of sodium bicarbonate represents the amount of Mg present; each ml of 0·05M disodium edetate is equivalent to 0·001215 g of Mg.

Labelling. A direction to shake the bottle should be given on the label.

Dose. 10 to 20 millilitres.

Rhubarb Mixture, Compound, Paediatric

SYNONYMS: Mistura Rhei Composita pro Infantibus; Rhubarb Mixture for Infants

Compound Rhubarb Tincture ..		60 ml
Light Magnesium Carbonate ..		15 g
Sodium Bicarbonate		15 g
Ginger Syrup		100 ml
Chloroform Water, Double-strength..		500 ml
Water (see page 642) .. .. to 1000 ml		

It should be recently prepared.

Standard
CONTENT OF SODIUM BICARBONATE. 1·35 to 1·52 per cent w/w, calculated as NaHCO₃, determined by the method for sodium bicarbonate in Compound Rhubarb Mixture, above, about 20 g, accurately weighed, being used.

CONTENT OF MAGNESIUM. 0·34 to 0·41 per cent w/w, calculated as Mg, determined by the method for magnesium in Compound Rhubarb Mixture, above.

Labelling. A direction to shake the bottle should be given on the label.

Dose. CHILD. Up to 1 year, 5 millilitres; 1 to 5 years, 10 millilitres.

Rhubarb and Soda Mixture, Ammoniated

SYNONYMS: Mistura Rhei Ammoniata et Sodae; Rhubarb, Ammonia, and Soda Mixture

Rhubarb, in powder		25 g
Sodium Bicarbonate		80 g
Ammonium Bicarbonate ..		20 g
Peppermint Emulsion, Concentrated		25 ml
Chloroform Water, Double-strength..		500 ml
Water (see page 642) .. .. to 1000 ml		

It should be recently prepared.

Standard
PRESENCE OF RHUBARB. Centrifuge 10 ml, separate off the supernatant liquid, wash the residue with two successive 10-ml portions of water, and examine the residue microscopically; the residue possesses the microscopical characters described under Rhubarb, page 429.

CONTENT OF SODIUM BICARBONATE. 7·08 to 8·00 per cent w/w, calculated as NaHCO₃, determined by the method for sodium bicarbonate in Paediatric Ipecacuanha and Ammonia Mixture, page 745, about 3 g, accurately weighed, being used.

CONTENT OF AMMONIUM BICARBONATE. 1·78 to 2·00 per cent w/w, calculated as NH₄HCO₃, determined by the method for ammonium bicarbonate in Paediatric Ipecacuanha and Ammonia Mixture, page 745, about 10 g, accurately weighed, being used.

Labelling. A direction to shake the bottle should be given on the label.

Dose. 10 to 20 millilitres.

Sodium Bicarbonate Mixture, Paediatric

SYNONYM: Mistura Carminativa pro Infantibus

Sodium Bicarbonate		10 g
Concentrated Dill Water ..		20 ml
Ginger Syrup		40 ml
Syrup		370 ml
Chloroform Water, Double-strength..		500 ml
Water (see page 642) .. .. to 1000 ml		

It should be recently prepared.

Standard
CONTENT OF SODIUM BICARBONATE. 0·95 to 1·05 per cent w/v, calculated as NaHCO₃, determined by the following method:
To 20 ml add 25 ml of water and titrate with 0·5N hydrochloric acid, using *methyl orange–xylene cyanol FF solution* as indicator; each ml of 0·5N hydrochloric acid is equivalent to 0·04200 g of NaHCO₃

Dose. CHILD. Up to 1 year, 5 millilitres; 1 to 5 years, 10 millilitres.

Sodium Chloride Mixture, Compound

Sodium Chloride..	..	..	20 g
Sodium Bicarbonate	..	.. .	50 g
Chloroform Water, Double-strength..	..	..	500 ml
Water (see page 642)	..	.. to 1000 ml

It should be recently prepared.

Standard
CONTENT OF SODIUM BICARBONATE. 4·75 to 5·25 per cent w/v, calculated as NaHCO₃, determined by the following method:
To 20 ml add 80 ml of water and titrate with 0·5N hydrochloric acid, using *methyl orange–xylene cyanol FF solution* as indicator; each ml of 0·5 N hydrochloric acid is equivalent to 0·04200 g of NaHCO₃.

CONTENT OF SODIUM CHLORIDE. 1·90 to 2·10 per cent w/v, calculated as NaCl, determined by the following method:
To 5 ml add 10 ml of water and continue by the method given in Appendix 11, page 891; each ml of 0·1N silver nitrate is equivalent to 0·005844 g of NaCl.

Dose. 10 to 20 millilitres in a tumblerful of hot water, sipped slowly.

Sodium Citrate Mixture

Sodium Citrate	..	..	..	300 g
Citric Acid	..	..	..	50 g
Lemon Spirit	..	..	..	5 ml
Quillaia Tincture..	..	..	10 ml
Syrup	..	..	..	..	250 ml
Chloroform Water, Double-strength..	..	..	..	300 ml
Water (see page 642)	..	.. to 1000 ml

It should be recently prepared.

Standard
PRESENCE OF SODIUM CITRATE. 1. Wet a loop of platinum wire with the sample and introduce into the flame of a Bunsen burner; the flame has a yellow colour.
2. Boil a portion of the sample with an excess of *mercuric sulphate solution*, filter, boil the filtrate, and add 0·25 ml of *potassium permanganate solution*; the potassium permanganate solution is decolorised and a white precipitate is produced.

CONTENT OF SODIUM CITRATE. 28·5 to 31·5 per cent w/v, calculated as C₆H₅Na₃O₇,2H₂O, determined by the following method:
To about 1 g, accurately weighed, add 5 ml of *acetic anhydride* and 20 ml of *glacial acetic acid*, warm on a water-bath for 20 minutes, allow to cool, and continue by Method I of the British Pharmacopoeia for non-aqueous titration; each ml of 0·1N perchloric acid is equivalent to 0·009803 g of C₆H₅Na₃O₇,2H₂O.
Determine the weight per ml of the mixture and calculate the content of sodium citrate, weight in volume.

CONTENT OF CITRIC ACID. 4·75 to 5·25 per cent w/v, calculated as C₆H₈O₇,H₂O, determined by the method for citric acid in Potassium Citrate Mixture, page 750.

Labelling. Directions to shake the bottle and to dilute the dose well with water before administration should be given on the label.

Dose. ADULT. 10 to 20 millilitres, well diluted with water.

CHILD. Well diluted with water: up to 1 year, 2·5 millilitres; 1 to 5 years, 5 millilitres; 6 to 12 years, 10 millilitres.

When a dose less than or not a multiple of 5 ml is prescribed, the mixture may be diluted, as described under Mixtures (page 734), with Syrup.

Sodium Salicylate Mixture

Sodium Salicylate	..	..	50 g
Sodium Metabisulphite ..	..	1 g
Concentrated Orange Peel Infusion	..	..	..	50 ml
Chloroform Water, Double-strength..	..	..	..	500 ml
Water (see page 642)	..	.. to 1000 ml

It should be recently prepared.

Standard
PRESENCE OF SALICYLATE. It complies with the test given for the presence of salicylic acid in Salicylic Acid Lotion, page 728.

CONTENT OF SODIUM SALICYLATE. 4·75 to 5·25 per cent w/v, calculated as C₇H₅NaO₃, determined by the method for Strong Sodium Salicylate Mixture, 25 ml being used.

Dose. 10 to 20 millilitres.

Sodium Salicylate Mixture, Strong

Sodium Salicylate	..	..	100 g
Sodium Metabisulphite ..	..	1 g
Peppermint Emulsion, Concentrated	..	..	..	25 ml
Chloroform Water, Double-strength..	..	..	..	500 ml
Water (see page 642)	..	.. to 1000 ml

It should be recently prepared.

Standard
PRESENCE OF SALICYLATE. It complies with the test given for the presence of salicylic acid in Salicylic Acid Lotion, page 728.

CONTENT OF SODIUM SALICYLATE. 9·50 to 10·50 per cent w/v, determined by the following method:
Dilute 20 ml with 25 ml of water, add 50 ml of *solvent ether* and a few drops of *bromophenol blue solution*, and titrate with 0·5N hydrochloric acid, with constant shaking, until the colour of the indicator begins to change; separate and reserve the lower aqueous layer; wash the ethereal layer with 10 ml of water, add the washings and a further 20 ml of *solvent ether* to the reserved aqueous layer, and complete the titration with 0·5N hydrochloric acid, shaking constantly; each ml of 0·5N hydrochloric acid is equivalent to 0·08005 g of C₇H₅NaO₃.

Dose. 10 to 20 millilitres.

Stramonium and Potassium Iodide Mixture

Stramonium Tincture	..	..	125 ml
Potassium Iodide..	..	..	20 g
Chloroform Water, Double-strength..	..	..	..	500 ml
Water (see page 642)	..	.. to 1000 ml

It should be recently prepared.

Standard
PRESENCE OF STRAMONIUM ALKALOIDS. It complies with the thin-layer chromatographic test given in Appendix 5B, page 873.

CONTENT OF POTASSIUM IODIDE. 1·90 to 2·10 per cent w/v, calculated as KI, determined by the method for Compound Lobelia and Stramonium Mixture, page 746.

Dose. 10 millilitres.

Succinylsulphathiazole Mixture, Paediatric

Succinylsulphathiazole, in fine powder	100 g
Light Kaolin or Light Kaolin (Natural)	60 g
Compound Tragacanth Powder	10 g
Amaranth Solution	10 ml
Benzoic Acid Solution	20 ml
Raspberry Syrup..	200 ml
Chloroform Water, Double-strength..	500 ml
Water (see page 642) .. .. to	1000 ml

Triturate the compound tragacanth powder, the succinylsulphathiazole, and the light kaolin with the raspberry syrup to form a smooth paste; add gradually, with constant stirring, the benzoic acid solution and the amaranth solution diluted with the double-strength chloroform water, and sufficient water to produce the required volume.

When prepared extemporaneously, it must be recently prepared, unless the kaolin has been sterilised.

When prepared other than extemporaneously, the compound tragacanth powder may be replaced by 1 per cent w/v of Sodium Carboxymethylcellulose 50. Maize Starch, 20 g, may be included; it should be incorporated in the form of a mucilage, which may be prepared by stirring a suspension of the starch in 125 ml of Water into 350 ml of boiling Water, maintaining the temperature until the mixture becomes translucent, and cooling rapidly. Chloroform Spirit, 50 ml, may be used in place of the double-strength chloroform water. Additional preservatives may be used.

Standard
PRESENCE OF SUCCINYLSULPHATHIAZOLE. 1. It complies with the thin-layer chromatographic test given in Appendix 5A, page 868.
2. Spot 5 μl of the sample solution prepared in the thin-layer chromatographic test on to a piece of filter paper and spray with *copper sulphate solution*; a grey-blue spot is produced (distinction from certain other sulphonamides).

CONTENT OF SUCCINYLSULPHATHIAZOLE. 7·82 to 8·96 per cent w/w, calculated as $C_{13}H_{13}N_3O_5S_2,H_2O$, determined by the following method:
Disperse about 6 g, accurately weighed, in 10 ml of *sodium hydroxide solution*, heat on a water-bath for 2 hours, cool, neutralise to *litmus paper* with *hydrochloric acid*, add 5 ml of 5N hydrochloric acid and 75 ml of water, and titrate with 0·1M sodium nitrite, determining the end-point electrometrically; each ml of 0·1M sodium nitrite is equivalent to 0·03734 g of $C_{13}H_{13}N_3O_5S_2,H_2O$.

Labelling. A direction to shake the bottle should be given on the label.

Dose. CHILD. Four times daily: 1 to 2 years, 10 millilitres; 3 to 5 years, 20 millilitres.

Sulphadimidine Mixture, Paediatric

Sulphadimidine, in fine powder..	100 g
Compound Tragacanth Powder	40 g
Amaranth Solution	10 ml
Benzoic Acid Solution	20 ml
Raspberry Syrup..	200 ml
Chloroform Water, Double-strength..	500 ml
Water (see page 642) .. .. to	1000 ml

Triturate the compound tragacanth powder and the sulphadimidine with the raspberry syrup to form a smooth paste; add gradually, with constant stirring, the benzoic acid solution and the amaranth solution diluted with the double-strength chloroform water, and sufficient water to produce the required volume.

When prepared extemporaneously it must be recently prepared.

When prepared other than extemporaneously, the compound tragacanth powder may be replaced by 1 per cent w/v of Sodium Carboxymethylcellulose 50. Maize Starch, 20 g, may be included; it should be incorporated in the form of a mucilage, which may be prepared by stirring a suspension of the starch in 125 ml of Water into 350 ml of boiling Water, maintaining the temperature until the mixture becomes translucent, and cooling rapidly. Chloroform Spirit, 50 ml, may be used in place of the double-strength chloroform water. Additional preservatives may be used.

Standard
PRESENCE OF SULPHADIMIDINE. It complies with the thin-layer chromatographic test given in Appendix 5A, page 868.

Standard
CONTENT OF SULPHADIMIDINE. 8·48 to 9·56 per cent w/w, calculated as $C_{12}H_{14}N_4O_2S$, determined by the following method:
Dissolve, by warming gently, about 6 g, accurately weighed, in 75 ml of water and 10 ml of *hydrochloric acid*, cool, and titrate with 0·1M sodium nitrite, determining the end-point electrometrically; each ml of 0·1M sodium nitrite is equivalent to 0·02783 g of $C_{12}H_{14}N_4O_2S$.

Labelling. A direction to shake the bottle should be given on the label.

Dose. CHILD. Initial dose: 6 months to 1 year, 5 millilitres; 1 to 5 years, 10 millilitres; 6 to 12 years, 15 millilitres.
Subsequent doses, in each case, one half the initial dose four times daily.

When a dose less than 5 ml is prescribed, the mixture may be diluted, as described under Mixtures (page 734), with Chloroform Water.

Tetracycline Mixture

SYNONYMS: Tetracycline Elixir; Tetracycline Syrup

Tetracycline Mixture is a suspension of

Tetracycline in a suitable coloured flavoured vehicle.

Standard
CONTENT OF TETRACYCLINE HYDROCHLORIDE. 90 to 115 per cent of the prescribed or stated concentration, determined by the following method:
Dilute an accurately weighed quantity, equivalent to about 0·25 g of tetracycline hydrochloride, to 500 ml with water and carry out a microbiological assay of tetracycline; a suggested method is given in Appendix 18, page 897.
The precision of any assay must be such that the fiducial limits of error (P = 0·95) are not less than 95 per cent and not more than 105 per cent of the estimated potency.
Determine the weight per ml of the mixture and, assuming that each 990 Units found is equivalent to 1 mg of tetracycline hydrochloride, calculate the upper and lower fiducial limits of the equivalent concentration of tetracycline hydrochloride in the mixture, weight in volume.
The upper fiducial limit of the estimated equivalent concentration of tetracycline hydrochloride is not less than 90 per cent and the lower fiducial limit is not more than 115 per cent of the prescribed or stated concentration.

Labelling. The directions given under Mixtures (page 735) should be followed.

Storage. It should be protected from light and stored in a cool place.

Dose. The equivalent of tetracycline hydrochloride:

ADULT. 1 to 4 grams daily, in divided doses.

CHILD. Every six hours: up to 1 year, 25 to 62·5 milligrams; 1 to 5 years, 62·5 to 125 milligrams; 6 to 12 years, 250 milligrams.

When the strength of the mixture is not specified, a suspension containing the equivalent of 125 mg of tetracycline hydrochloride in 5 ml shall be supplied.

When a dose less than or not a multiple of 5 ml is prescribed, the mixture may be diluted, as described under Mixtures (page 734), with Syrup. The diluted mixture must be freshly prepared.

Viprynium Mixture

SYNONYM: Viprynium Suspension

Viprynium Mixture is a suspension of Viprynium Embonate in a suitable flavoured vehicle.

Standard
CONTENT OF VIPRYNIUM. 90·0 to 110·0 per cent of the prescribed or stated concentration, determined by the following method:
Protect the solutions from light throughout the procedure by carrying out all operations in subdued light or by using low-actinic glassware.
To an accurately measured volume, equivalent to about 0·05 g of viprynium embonate, add 150 ml of *methoxyethanol*, heat on a water-bath with stirring for 5 minutes, cool, and dilute to 250 ml with *methoxyethanol*; dilute 5 ml of this solution to 200 ml with *methoxyethanol*, and measure the extinction of a 1-cm layer at the maximum at about 508 nm.
For purposes of calculation, use a value of 785 for the E(1 per cent, 1 cm) of viprynium embonate; each g of viprynium embonate is equivalent to 0·6644 g of viprynium.
Calculate the equivalent concentration of viprynium in the sample.

Labelling. The directions given under Mixtures (page 735) should be followed.

Storage. It should be protected from light.

Dose. Viprynium:

ADULT. 300 to 400 milligrams as a single dose.

CHILD. As a single dose: up to 1 year, 25 to 50 milligrams; 1 to 5 years, 50 to 100 milligrams; 6 to 12 years, 100 to 200 milligrams.

When the strength of the mixture is not specified, a suspension containing the equivalent of 50 mg of viprynium in 5 ml shall be supplied.

When a dose less than or not a multiple of 5 ml is prescribed, the mixture may be diluted, as described under Mixtures (page 734), with Syrup. The diluted mixture must be freshly prepared.

MOUTH-WASHES

Mouth-washes are usually aqueous solutions, in concentrated form, of substances with deodorant, antiseptic, local analgesic, or astringent properties.

Containers. Mouth-washes should be dispensed in white fluted bottles.

Labelling. When mouth-washes are dispensed, a direction should be given on the label, where appropriate, for diluting the mouth-wash before use. They should be labelled in a manner which clearly distinguishes them from preparations intended for internal administration.

Sodium Chloride Mouth-wash, Compound

Sodium Chloride..	.. ..	15 g
Sodium Bicarbonate	.. ..	10 g
Peppermint Emulsion, Concentrated ..	.. .. ..	25 ml
Chloroform Water, Double-strength..	.. .. ..	500 ml
Water (see page 642)	.. ..	to 1000 ml

Standard
CONTENT OF SODIUM CHLORIDE. 1·42 to 1·58 per cent w/v, calculated as NaCl, determined by the following method:
To 10 ml add 10 ml of water and continue by the method given in Appendix 11, page 891; each ml of 0·1N silver nitrate is equivalent to 0·005844 g of NaCl.

CONTENT OF SODIUM BICARBONATE. 0·95 to 1·05 per cent w/v, calculated as $NaHCO_3$, determined by the following method:
Titrate 20 ml with 0·1N hydrochloric acid, using *methyl orange–xylene cyanol FF solution* as indicator;

each ml of 0·1N hydrochloric acid is equivalent to 0·008401 g of NaHCO₃.

Containers; Labelling. The directions given under Mouth-washes (page 755) should be followed.

Note. Compound Sodium Chloride Mouth-wash should be diluted with an equal volume of warm water before use.

Zinc Sulphate and Zinc Chloride Mouth-wash

Zinc Sulphate	..	..	..	20 g
Zinc Chloride	..	..	..	10 g
Compound Tartrazine Solution				10 ml

Dilute Hydrochloric Acid		..		10 ml
Chloroform Water, Double-strength..	..	..	..	500 ml
Water (see page 642)		..		to 1000 ml

Standard

CONTENT OF ZINC. 0·89 to 0·98 per cent w/v, calculated as Zn, determined by the method for zinc sulphate in Zinc Sulphate Lotion, page 729, 10 ml being used; each ml of 0·05M disodium edetate is equivalent to 0·003269 g of Zn.

Containers; Labelling. The directions given under Mouth-washes (page 755) should be followed.

Note. Zinc Sulphate and Zinc Chloride Mouth-wash should be diluted with twenty times its volume of warm water before use.

MUCILAGES

Mucilages are viscous aqueous liquids prepared from gums, gelatinised starch, cellulose derivatives, or other thickening agents. They are used as thickening and suspending agents.

Starch Mucilage

SYNONYM: Mucilago Amyli

Starch	..	..	..	25 g
Water (see page 642)		..		to 1000 ml

Heat 800 ml of the water to boiling, add the starch previously triturated with the remainder of the water, again heat to boiling, and allow to cool. It should be freshly prepared.

Tragacanth Mucilage

Tragacanth, finely powdered	..		12·5 g
Alcohol (90 per cent)	..	..	25 ml
Chloroform Water	..	..	to 1000 ml

Mix the tragacanth with the alcohol in a dry bottle, add, as quickly as possible, sufficient of the chloroform water to produce the required volume, and shake vigorously.

Standard

PRESENCE OF TRAGACANTH. 1. To 2 ml add 0·5 ml of *hydrochloric acid* and heat in a water-bath for 30 minutes.

To half the liquid add 1·5 ml of *sodium hydroxide solution* and 3 ml of *potassium cupri-tartrate solution*, and warm; a red precipitate is formed.

To the other half of the liquid add *barium chloride solution*; no precipitate is formed (distinction from agar).

2. Dilute 4 ml to 20 ml with water and add 10 ml of a 20 per cent w/v solution of *lead acetate*; a voluminous, flocculent precipitate is produced. Filter, and to the filtrate add 10 ml of *strong lead subacetate solution*; the solution may become slightly cloudy but no precipitate is produced.

NASAL DROPS

Nasal drops are liquid preparations for instillation into the nostrils by means of a dropper. They may be aqueous or oily solutions and usually contain substances with antiseptic, local analgesic, or vasoconstrictor properties.

Oily nasal drops should not be used over long periods, as the oil retards the ciliary action of the nasal mucosa; drops of oil may enter the trachea and cause lipoid pneumonia.

Containers. Nasal drops should be supplied in coloured fluted glass bottles fitted with a plastic screw cap incorporating a glass dropper tube fitted with a rubber teat, or in a plastic squeeze bottle fitted with a plastic cap incorporating a dropper device.

Ephedrine Nasal Drops

Ephedrine Hydrochloride	..		0·5 g
Chlorbutol	..	..	..	0·5 g
Sodium Choride ..	..	..	0·5 g
Water (see page 642)	..	.. to 100 ml

Standard
CONTENT OF EPHEDRINE HYDROCHLORIDE. 0·45 to 0·55 per cent w/v, calculated as $C_{10}H_{15}NO,HCl$, determined by the following method:

Dilute 10 ml to 100 ml with water and further dilute 10 ml of this solution to 250 ml with water; transfer 5 ml of this solution to a separating funnel and continue by the method for Ephedrine Elixir, page 671, beginning with the words "add 1·25 ml of a saturated solution of *sodium bicarbonate* . . .".

Containers. The directions given under Nasal Drops (page 756) should be followed.

OINTMENTS

Ointments are semisolid preparations consisting usually of a medicament or mixture of medicaments dissolved or dispersed in a suitable basis which is often anhydrous. They are used as emollients, as protective preparations on the skin, or as a means for the local application of medicaments. Emollient and protective ointments may contain vegetable oils, synthetic esters of fatty acids, or wool fat, together with inert bases such as soft paraffin. A mildly antiseptic or astringent powder such as zinc oxide may be added. Suitable preservatives may be included when permitted in the monographs.

Oil-in-water emulsifying agents such as Emulsifying Wax, Cetrimide Emulsifying Wax, or Cetomacrogol Emulsifying Wax may be incorporated into anhydrous bases in order to render them miscible with exudate and more easily removable from the skin by washing. Water-miscible ointments may be prepared with a basis consisting of a mixture of macrogols. Such preparations are particularly suitable for application to the scalp.

The proportions of paraffins, oils, fats, and waxes may be varied in ointments intended to be used in tropical or subtropical climates to meet extremes of temperature, but the amounts of active ingredients must in all cases be maintained.

A number of preparations similar to ointments are described under Applications, Creams, and Pastes.

Dilution of ointments. For certain specific ointments, when a strength of ointment not available from a manufacturer is prescribed, a stronger ointment should be diluted to the required strength with the diluent suggested in the individual monograph. When the specified diluent is soft paraffin, a portion of it may be replaced by hard paraffin or liquid paraffin to obtain an ointment of suitable consistency.

Containers and storage. Ointments should be stored and supplied in glass or plastic jars fitted with screw caps with impermeable liners or with close-fitting slip-on lids so that absorption or diffusion of the contents is prevented. Alternatively, suitable collapsible tubes of metal or plastic may be used. Plastic containers normally available are unsuitable for ointments containing methyl salicylate, phthalate esters, or similar substances.

Ointments containing water or other volatile ingredients should be stored and supplied in well-closed containers which prevent evaporation.

Ointments should be stored in a cool place.

Labelling. When a preservative is included, the label on the container, except one issued on a medical prescription for an individual patient, should state the name and concentration of the preservative present.

Ammoniated Mercury and Coal Tar Ointment

SYNONYMS: Unguentum Hydrargyri Ammoniati et Picis Carbonis; Unguentum Picis Carbonis Compositum

Ammoniated Mercury	25 g
Strong Coal Tar Solution ..	25 g
Yellow Soft Paraffin	950 g

Triturate the ammoniated mercury with a portion of the yellow soft paraffin until smooth, mix with the remainder of the yellow soft paraffin, and incorporate the strong coal tar solution.

Standard
CONTENT OF AMMONIATED MERCURY. 2·30 to 2·68 per cent, calculated as NH_2HgCl, determined by the following method:
To about 5 g, accurately weighed, add 25 ml of *solvent ether*, 25 ml of *light petroleum (boiling-range, 40° to 60°)*, 2 g of *potassium iodide*, and 50 ml of water, shake frequently during 3 hours, and titrate with 0·1N hydrochloric acid, using *methyl orange solution* as indicator; each ml of 0·1N hydrochloric acid is equivalent to 0·01260 g of NH_2HgCl.

Containers and storage. The directions given under Ointments (page 757) should be followed; containers should prevent evaporation.

Ammoniated Mercury, Coal Tar, and Salicylic Acid Ointment

SYNONYM: Unguentum Hydrargyri Ammoniati et Picis Carbonis cum Acido Salicylico

Ammoniated Mercury and Coal Tar Ointment	980 g
Salicylic Acid, in fine powder ..	20 g

Triturate the salicylic acid with a portion of the ammoniated mercury and coal tar ointment until smooth and gradually incorporate the remainder of the ointment.

Standard
CONTENT OF SALICYLIC ACID. 1·90 to 2·10 per cent, calculated as $C_7H_6O_3$, determined by the method for salicylic acid in Salicylic Acid and Sulphur Ointment, page 763.

CONTENT OF AMMONIATED MERCURY. 2·25 to 2·63 per cent, calculated as NH_2HgCl, determined by the following method:
Disperse with the aid of gentle heat about 10 g, accurately weighed, in 80 ml of a mixture of equal volumes of *solvent ether* and *light petroleum (boiling-range, 60° to 80°)*, and extract with four successive 25-ml portions of warm *acetic acid*.
Combine the extracts in a flask, cool, add 50 ml of a 50 per cent w/v solution of *sodium hydroxide* in water and 2 g of *sodium thiosulphate*, immediately connect the flask to an ammonia-distillation apparatus, mix the contents, distil the liberated ammonia into 20 ml of 0·1N sulphuric acid, and titrate the excess of acid with

0·1N sodium hydroxide, using *methyl red solution* as indicator; each ml of 0·1N sulphuric acid is equivalent to 0·02521 g of NH_2HgCl.

Containers and storage. The directions given under Ointments (page 757) should be followed; containers should prevent evaporation.

Benzocaine Ointment, Compound

Benzocaine	100 g
Hamamelis Ointment	450 g
Zinc Ointment	450 g

Triturate the benzocaine with a portion of the hamamelis ointment until smooth and gradually incorporate the remainder of the hamamelis ointment and the zinc ointment.

Standard
PRESENCE OF BENZOCAINE. Warm 1 g with 5 ml of *dilute hydrochloric acid* until the ointment is melted, shake, and allow to cool. The aqueous layer complies with the following tests:
(i) To a portion of the solution add *iodine solution*; a precipitate is produced. To a further portion add *potassium mercuri-iodide solution*; there is no precipitate (distinction from procaine).
(ii) It gives the reaction characteristic of primary aromatic amines, producing an orange-red precipitate.

CONTENT OF ZINC OXIDE. 6·0 to 7·5 per cent, calculated as ZnO, determined by the following method:
Heat gently, taking precautions against loss caused by spitting, about 4 g, accurately weighed, until the basis is completely volatilised or charred; increase the temperature until all the carbon is removed and ignite the residue of ZnO to constant weight.

CONTENT OF BENZOCAINE. 9·5 to 10·5 per cent, calculated as $C_9H_{11}NO_2$, determined by the following method:
Dissolve about 4 g, accurately weighed, in 50 ml of *light petroleum (boiling-range, 40° to 60°)* and extract with four successive 20-ml portions of *dilute hydrochloric acid*; filter the combined extracts and titrate with 0·1M sodium nitrite, determining the end-point electrometrically; each ml of 0·1M sodium nitrite is equivalent to 0·01652 g of $C_9H_{11}NO_2$.

Containers and storage. The directions given under Ointments (page 757) should be followed; containers should prevent evaporation.

Benzoic Acid Ointment, Compound

SYNONYM: Whitfield's Ointment

Benzoic Acid, in fine powder ..	60 g
Salicylic Acid, in fine powder ..	30 g
Emulsifying Ointment	910 g

Triturate the benzoic acid and the salicylic acid with a portion of the emulsifying ointment until smooth and gradually incorporate the remainder of the ointment.

Standard
CONTENT OF BENZOIC ACID. 5·7 to 6·3 per cent, calculated as $C_7H_6O_2$, determined by the following method:
Dissolve as completely as possible, with the aid of

gentle heat, about 2·5 g, accurately weighed, in 50 ml of a mixture of equal volumes of *alcohol (95 per cent)* and *solvent ether*, previously neutralised to *phenolphthalein solution*, and titrate with 0·1N sodium hydroxide, using *phenolphthalein solution* as indicator; each ml of 0·1N sodium hydroxide, after deducting 1 ml for each 0·01381 g of salicylic acid in the weight of sample taken, is equivalent to 0·01221 g of $C_7H_6O_2$.

CONTENT OF SALICYLIC ACID. 2·7 to 3·3 per cent, calculated as $C_7H_6O_3$, determined by the following method:

Dissolve as completely as possible, with the aid of gentle heat, about 2·5 g, accurately weighed, in 50 ml of *solvent ether*; extract with five successive 10-ml portions of a saturated solution of *sodium bicarbonate* in water, washing each extract with the same 50 ml of *solvent ether*.

Combine the aqueous extracts, cautiously add *hydrochloric acid* until the solution is distinctly acid to *litmus paper*, and extract with four successive 25-ml portions of *solvent ether*; combine the extracts, evaporate off the ether at a temperature not exceeding 40°, dissolve the residue in 5 ml of 0·5N sodium hydroxide, add 50 ml of 0·1N bromine and 5 ml of *hydrochloric acid*, shake repeatedly during 15 minutes, and allow to stand for 15 minutes; add 10 ml of *potassium iodide solution* and titrate the liberated iodine with 0·1N sodium thiosulphate.

Repeat the procedure omitting the sample.

The difference between the two titrations represents the amount of bromine required by the sample; each ml of 0·1N bromine is equivalent to 0·002302 g of $C_7H_6O_3$.

Containers and storage. The directions given under Ointments (page 757) should be followed.

Betamethasone Valerate Ointment

SYNONYM: Betamethasone Ointment

Betamethasone Valerate Ointment is a dispersion of Betamethasone Valerate in a suitable anhydrous greasy basis.

Standard
PRESENCE OF BETAMETHASONE. It complies with the thin-layer chromatographic test given in Appendix 5D, page 875.

CONTENT OF BETAMETHASONE. 90·0 to 115·0 per cent of the prescribed or stated concentration, determined by the method given in Appendix 23A, page 904, for betamethasone 17-valerate.

Containers and storage; Labelling. The directions given under Ointments (page 757) should be followed.

Note. When the strength of the ointment is not specified, an ointment containing the equivalent of 0·1 per cent of betamethasone shall be supplied.

When a strength less than that available from the manufacturer is prescribed, the 0·1 per cent ointment may be diluted with White Soft Paraffin. Admixture with other materials may promote deterioration of the active ingredient, especially if water is present.

Betamethasone Valerate with Chlortetracycline Ointment

SYNONYM: Betamethasone with Chlortetracycline Ointment

Betamethasone Valerate with Chlortetracycline Ointment is a dispersion of Betamethasone Valerate and Chlortetracycline Hydrochloride in a suitable anhydrous greasy basis. It contains the equivalent of 0·1 per

cent w/w of betamethasone and 3·0 per cent w/w of chlortetracycline hydrochloride.

Standard
PRESENCE OF BETAMETHASONE. It complies with the thin-layer chromatographic test given in Appendix 5D, page 875.

PRESENCE OF CHLORTETRACYCLINE. To an amount equivalent to about 0·5 mg of chlortetracycline hydrochloride add 2 ml of *sulphuric acid*; a deep blue colour is produced which changes to bluish-green.

CONTENT OF BETAMETHASONE. 0·090 to 0·115 per cent, determined by the method given in Appendix 23A, page 904, for betamethasone 17-valerate.

CONTENT OF CHLORTETRACYCLINE HYDROCHLORIDE. 2·70 to 3·45 per cent, determined by the following method:

Mix about 1·2 g, accurately weighed, with 50 ml of *cyclohexane* and extract with two successive 50-ml portions of 0·01N hydrochloric acid, shaking each extract for 3 minutes, allowing to separate, and filtering each lower layer through a pledget of cotton wool previously washed with 0·01N hydrochloric acid; wash the cyclohexane solution with two further successive 10-ml portions of 0·01N hydrochloric acid, filter the washings through the same filter, and dilute the combined filtrates to 150 ml with 0·01N hydrochloric acid.

Dilute 10 ml of this solution to 500 ml with water, further dilute 2 ml of this solution to 50 ml with a 1·36 per cent w/v solution of *potassium dihydrogen phosphate* in water, and carry out a microbiological assay of chlortetracycline; a suggested method is given in Appendix 18, page 897.

The precision of any assay must be such that the fiducial limits of error (P = 0·95) are not less than 95 per cent and not more than 105 per cent of the estimated potency.

Assuming that each 1000 Units found is equivalent to 1 mg of chlortetracycline hydrochloride, calculate the upper and lower fiducial limits of the equivalent concentration of chlortetracycline hydrochloride in the ointment.

The upper fiducial limit of the estimated equivalent concentration of chlortetracycline hydrochloride is not less than 2·7 per cent and the lower fiducial limit is not more than 3·3 per cent.

Containers and storage; Labelling. The directions given under Ointments (page 757) should be followed.

Note. When an ointment containing a lower proportion of betamethasone valerate and chlortetracycline hydrochloride than that specified above is prescribed, the ointment may be diluted with White Soft Paraffin.

When an ointment containing a lower proportion of betamethasone valerate but the same proportion of chlortetracycline hydrochloride as that specified above is prescribed, the ointment may be diluted with Chlortetracycline Ointment. Admixture of the ointment with other materials may promote deterioration of the active ingredients, especially if water is present.

Calamine Ointment

Calamine, finely sifted	..	..	150 g
White Soft Paraffin	..	..	850 g

Triturate the calamine with a portion of the white soft paraffin until smooth and gradually incorporate the remainder of the paraffin.

Standard
CONTENT OF ZINC. 7·8 to 9·4 per cent, calculated as Zn, determined by the following method:
Heat gently about 1 g, accurately weighed, until the basis is completely volatilised or charred; increase the temperature until all the carbon is removed and ignite

the residue to constant weight; each g of residue is equivalent to 0·8034 g of Zn.

Containers and storage. The directions given under Ointments (page 757) should be followed.

Calamine and Coal Tar Ointment

SYNONYMS: Compound Calamine Ointment; Unguentum Sedativum

Calamine, finely sifted	..	..	125 g
Strong Coal Tar Solution		..	25 g
Zinc Oxide, finely sifted	..	..	125 g
Hydrous Wool Fat	..	..	250 g
White Soft Paraffin	..	..	475 g

Melt together the hydrous wool fat and the white soft paraffin, incorporate the calamine, the zinc oxide, and the strong coal tar solution, and stir until cold.

Standard
CONTENT OF ZINC. 15·9 to 18·3 per cent, calculated as Zn, determined by the following method:
Heat gently, taking precautions against loss caused by spitting, about 1 g, accurately weighed, until the basis is completely volatilised or charred; increase the temperature until all the carbon is removed and ignite the residue to constant weight; each g of residue is equivalent to 0·8034 g of Zn.

Containers and storage. The directions given under Ointments (page 757) should be followed; containers should prevent evaporation.

Capsicum Ointment

Capsicum Oleoresin	..	..	15 g
Emulsifying Wax	..	..	50 g
Simple Ointment	..	..	935 g

Melt together the simple ointment and the emulsifying wax, incorporate the capsicum oleoresin, and stir until cold.

Standard
CONTENT OF CAPSAICIN. 0·12 to 0·19 per cent, determined by the following method:
Heat on a water-bath about 3 g, accurately weighed, with 30 ml of water, add 10 ml of *barium hydroxide solution*, heat to boiling with constant stirring, cool, and filter through a moistened filter paper.
Transfer the residue and filter to the original vessel and repeat the extraction twice, washing the filter finally with 50 ml of water; combine the filtrates and washings, and continue by the method for Capsicum, page 73, beginning with the words "adjust the pH to 7·0 to 7·5 . . .".

Containers and storage. The directions given under Ointments (page 757) should be followed.

Chlortetracycline Ointment

Chlortetracycline Ointment is a dispersion containing up to 3 per cent of Chlortetracycline Hydrochloride, with 10 per cent of Wool Fat, in Yellow Soft Paraffin.
It is prepared by melting together the wool fat and the yellow soft paraffin, stirring until cold, and incorporating the chlortetracycline hydrochloride in the cold basis.
Chlortetracycline Ointment may be prepared with any other suitable basis.

Standard
PRESENCE OF CHLORTETRACYCLINE. To an amount equivalent to about 0·5 mg of chlortetracycline hydrochloride add 2 ml of *sulphuric acid*; a deep blue colour is produced which changes to bluish-green.

CONTENT OF CHLORTETRACYCLINE HYDROCHLORIDE. 90 to 115 per cent of the prescribed or stated concentration, determined by the method for Chlortetracycline Eye Ointment, page 698.

Containers and storage; Labelling. The directions given under Ointments (page 757) should be followed.

Note. When the strength of the ointment is not specified, an ointment containing 3·0 per cent of chlortetracycline hydrochloride shall be supplied.

When a strength less than that available from a manufacturer is prescribed, the 3·0 per cent ointment may be diluted with a basis consisting of 1 part of Wool Fat and 9 parts of Yellow Soft Paraffin.

Coal Tar and Salicylic Acid Ointment

Prepared Coal Tar	..	..	20 g
Salicylic Acid	..	..	20 g
Emulsifying Wax	..	..	114 g
White Soft Paraffin	..	..	190 g
Coconut Oil	..	..	540 g
Polysorbate 80	..	..	40 g
Liquid Paraffin	..	..	76 g

Disperse the prepared coal tar in the polysorbate 80, incorporate the salicylic acid, and mix with the emulsifying wax, previously melted. Separately melt the white soft paraffin and the coconut oil, incorporate the liquid paraffin, warmed to the same temperature, and add, with stirring, to the other mixed ingredients. Mix thoroughly and stir until cold.

Standard
PRESENCE OF SALICYLIC ACID. To the solution obtained after titration in the procedure for the determination of the content of salicylic acid add 1 ml of *ferric chloride test-solution*; an intense reddish-violet colour is produced.

CONTENT OF SALICYLIC ACID. 1·90 to 2·10 per cent w/w, calculated as $C_7H_6O_3$, determined by the following method:
Dissolve, with the aid of gentle heat, about 10 g, accurately weighed, in a mixture of equal volumes of *alcohol (95 per cent)* and *solvent ether*, previously neutralised to *phenol red solution*, add 10 g of *decolorising charcoal*, warm on a water-bath, filter, wash the filter with 25 ml of the neutralised alcohol–ether mixture, warm the combined filtrate and washings to dissolve the salicylic acid, if necessary, and titrate the hot solution with 0·1N sodium hydroxide, using *phenol red solution* as indicator; each ml of 0·1N sodium hydroxide is equivalent to 0·01381 g of $C_7H_6O_3$.

Containers and storage. The directions given under Ointments (page 757) should be followed.

Coal Tar and Zinc Ointment

Strong Coal Tar Solution	..	100 g
Zinc Oxide, finely sifted	..	300 g
Yellow Soft Paraffin	..	600 g

Mix the zinc oxide with the strong coal tar solution, triturate with a portion of the yellow soft paraffin until smooth, and gradually incorporate the remainder of the paraffin.

Standard

CONTENT OF ZINC OXIDE. 28·5 to 31·5 per cent, calculated as ZnO, determined by the following method: Heat gently about 1 g, accurately weighed, until the basis is completely volatilised or charred; increase the temperature until all the carbon is removed, and ignite the residue of ZnO to constant weight.

Containers and storage. The directions given under Ointments (page 757) should be followed; containers should prevent evaporation.

Fluocinolone Ointment

Fluocinolone Ointment is a dispersion of Fluocinolone Acetonide in a suitable anhydrous greasy basis.

Standard

CONTENT OF FLUOCINOLONE ACETONIDE. 90·0 to 110·0 per cent of the prescribed or stated concentration, determined by the method given in Appendix 23B, page 905, but 10 ml of water being added before the initial extraction with methyl alcohol.

Containers and storage; Labelling. The directions given under Ointments (page 757) should be followed.

Note. When the strength of the ointment is not specified, an ointment containing 0·025 per cent of fluocinolone acetonide shall be supplied.

An ointment containing 0·01 per cent is also available.

When a strength less than those available from the manufacturer is prescribed, the 0·025 per cent ointment may be diluted with White or Yellow Soft Paraffin or with Eye Ointment Basis.

Gentamicin Ointment

SYNONYM: Gentamicin Sulphate Ointment

Gentamicin Ointment is a dispersion of finely powdered Gentamicin Sulphate in a suitable anhydrous greasy basis.

Standard

CONTENT OF GENTAMICIN. 90 to 120 per cent of the prescribed or stated concentration, determined by the following method:

Dissolve, as completely as possible, an accurately weighed quantity, equivalent to about 0·004 g of gentamicin, in 20 ml of *chloroform*, extract with three successive 20-ml portions of *solution of standard pH 8·0*, dilute the combined extract to 100 ml with *solution of standard pH 8·0*, and carry out a microbiological assay of gentamicin; a suggested method is given in Appendix 18, page 897.

The precision of any assay must be such that the fiducial limits of error (P = 0·95) are not less than 90 per cent and not more than 110 per cent of the estimated potency.

Assuming that each 1000 Units found is equivalent to 1 mg of gentamicin, calculate the upper and lower fiducial limits of the equivalent estimated concentration of gentamicin in the ointment.

The upper fiducial limit of the estimated equivalent concentration is not less than 90 per cent and the lower fiducial limit is not more than 120 per cent of the prescribed or stated concentration.

Containers and storage; Labelling. The directions given under Ointments (page 757) should be followed.

Note. When the strength of the ointment is not specified, an ointment containing the equivalent of 0·3 per cent of gentamicin shall be supplied.

Hamamelis Ointment

Hamamelis Liquid Extract	..		100 g
Yellow Soft Paraffin	..	..	400 g
Wool Fat ..	..	..	500 g

Mix in a warm mortar.

In making this preparation, the hamamelis liquid extract may be replaced by hamamelis liquid extract prepared with Industrial Methylated Spirit suitably diluted, provided that the law and the statutory regulations governing the use of industrial methylated spirit are observed.

Containers and storage. The directions given under Ointments (page 757) should be followed; containers should prevent evaporation.

Hydrocortisone and Clioquinol Ointment

Hydrocortisone, or Hydrocortisone Acetate, in ultra-fine powder	10 g
Clioquinol, in very fine powder	30 g
Wool Fat	100 g
White Soft Paraffin	860 g

Melt together the wool fat and white soft paraffin and stir until cold. Incorporate the clioquinol and the hydrocortisone, or hydrocortisone acetate, in the cold basis.

The ointment may be prepared with any other suitable basis.

Standard

PRESENCE OF HYDROCORTISONE. It complies with the thin-layer chromatographic test given in Appendix 5D, page 875.

CONTENT OF CLIOQUINOL. 2·7 to 3·3 per cent, determined by the following method:

Dissolve, with the aid of gentle heat, about 0·3 g, accurately weighed, in sufficient *chloroform* to produce 50 ml and continue by the method for Clioquinol Cream, page 658, beginning at the words "Transfer 10 ml of this solution . . .".

CONTENT OF HYDROCORTISONE OR OF HYDROCORTISONE ACETATE. 0·925 to 1·075 per cent of hydrocortisone or of hydrocortisone acetate, determined by the appropriate method as described for Hydrocortisone Cream, page 659.

Containers and storage; Labelling. The directions given under Ointments (page 757) should be followed. The ointment should be protected from light.

When tubes are used they should preferably be made of plastic material. If aluminium tubes are used, their inner surfaces should be lacquered.

Caution. *Clioquinol may stain clothing or discolour fair hair.*

Hydrous Wool Fat Ointment

SYNONYM: Unguentum Adipis Lanae Hydrosi

Hydrous Wool Fat	..	..	500 g
Yellow Soft Paraffin	..	..	500 g

Melt together, and stir until cold.

Containers and storage. The directions given under Ointments (page 757) should be followed; containers should prevent evaporation.

Ichthammol Ointment

Ichthammol	..	..	..	100 g
Wool Fat ..	..	..	..	450 g
Yellow Soft Paraffin		..	..	450 g

Melt together the wool fat and the yellow soft paraffin, incorporate the ichthammol, and stir until cold.

Containers and storage. The directions given under Ointments (page 757) should be followed.

Macrogol Ointment

| Macrogol 4000 | .. | .. | .. | 350 g |
| Macrogol 300 | .. | .. | .. | 650 g |

Melt the macrogol 4000, add the macrogol 300, and stir continuously until cold.

Containers and storage. The directions given under Ointments (page 757) should be followed.

Methyl Salicylate Ointment

SYNONYM: Unguentum Methylis Salicylatis Forte

Methyl Salicylate	..	..	500 g
White Beeswax ..	..	..	250 g
Hydrous Wool Fat	..	..	250 g

Melt together the beeswax and the hydrous wool fat, add the methyl salicylate, and stir until cold.

Standard
CONTENT OF METHYL SALICYLATE. 45·0 to 52·5 per cent w/w, calculated as $C_8H_8O_3$, determined by the following method:
Carry out the method of Appendix XIIC of the British Pharmacopoeia for Gas–Liquid Chromatography, using solutions in *light petroleum* (*boiling-range, 80° to 100°*) containing (1) 1·0 per cent w/v of *benzyl alcohol* (internal standard) and 1·0 per cent w/v of *methyl salicylate*, (2) 2·0 per cent w/v of the sample, and (3) 2·0 per cent w/v of the sample and 1·0 per cent w/v of *benzyl alcohol*.
The chromatographic procedure may be carried out with a column, 60 cm in length and 6 mm in internal diameter, packed with 10 per cent w/w of macrogol 1540 supported on white diatomaceous earth (60- to 80-mesh) maintained at 110°, nitrogen as the carrier gas, and a flame-ionisation detector.
Calculate the concentration of methyl salicylate, weight in weight.

Containers and storage. The directions given under Ointments (page 757) should be followed; containers should prevent evaporation.
Certain plastic containers, such as those made from polystyrene, are unsuitable for use with this ointment.

Methyl Salicylate Ointment, Compound

SYNONYMS: Analgesic Balsam; Unguentum Methylis Salicylatis Compositum Forte

Methyl Salicylate	..	..	500 g
Cajuput Oil	..	..	..	25 g
Cineole	..	..	..	..	25 g
Water (see page 642)	..	..	45 g
Menthol	..	..	..	..	100 g
Wool Fat ..	..	..	..	105 g
White Beeswax ..	..	..	200 g

Melt together the white beeswax and the wool fat and add the menthol previously dissolved in the methyl salicylate, the cineole, and the cajuput oil. Incorporate the water at the same temperature, and stir until cold.

Standard
CONTENT OF METHYL SALICYLATE. 45·0 to 52·5 per cent w/w, calculated as $C_8H_8O_3$, determined by the method for Methyl Salicylate Ointment.
After carrying out this determination, adequate time must be allowed for other volatile ingredients to be eluted from the column before carrying out further determinations.

Containers and storage. The directions given under Ointments (page 757) should be followed; containers should prevent evaporation.
Certain plastic containers, such as those made from polystyrene, are unsuitable for use with this ointment.

Neomycin and Bacitracin Ointment

Neomycin Sulphate	..	..	5 g
Bacitracin Zinc ..	..	500,000 Units
Liquid Paraffin	..	..	..	100 g
White Soft Paraffin	..	..	to 1000 g

Melt the white soft paraffin, incorporate the liquid paraffin, and stir until cold. Triturate the neomycin sulphate and the bacitracin zinc with a portion of the basis and gradually incorporate the remainder of the basis.

Standard
CONTENT OF BACITRACIN. 450 to 575 Units per g, determined by the following method:
Disperse about 1 g, accurately weighed, in 10 ml of warm *chloroform*, cool, add 10 ml of *light petroleum* (*boiling-range, 40° to 60°*) and 25 ml of 0·1N hydrochloric acid, and shake vigorously for 30 minutes; add a further 10 ml of *chloroform*, allow to separate, discard the chloroform layer, and filter the aqueous solution, discarding the first 5 ml of filtrate.
Mix 10 ml of the filtrate with 50 ml of *solution of standard pH 7·6*, add 1·0 ml of 1N sodium hydroxide, dilute to 100 ml with *solution of standard pH 7·6*, and carry out a microbiological assay of bacitracin; a suggested method is given in Appendix 18, page 897.
The precision of any assay must be such that the fiducial limits of error (P = 0·95) are not less than 95 per cent and not more than 105 per cent of the estimated potency.
Calculate the upper and lower fiducial limits of the concentration of bacitracin in the ointment.
The upper fiducial limit of the estimated concentration of bacitracin is not less than 450 Units per g and the lower fiducial limit is not more than 575 Units per g.

CONTENT OF NEOMYCIN SULPHATE. 2750 to 4000 Units per g, determined by the following method:
Disperse about 1·5 g, accurately weighed, in 100 ml of a mixture containing equal volumes of *anaesthetic ether* and *light petroleum* (*boiling-range, 40° to 60°*), extract with five successive 40-ml portions of *solution of standard pH 7·8* and discard the organic solution; combine the extracts, remove any dissolved solvents by passing a current of *nitrogen* through the solution, dilute to 250 ml with *solution of standard pH 7·8* and carry out a microbiological assay of neomycin; a suggested method is given in Appendix 18, page 897.
The precision of any assay must be such that the fiducial limits of error (P = 0·95) are not less than 95 per cent and not more than 105 per cent of the estimated potency.
Calculate the upper and lower fiducial limits of the concentration of neomycin sulphate in the ointment.
The upper fiducial limit of the estimated concentration of neomycin sulphate is not less than 2750 Units per g

and the lower fiducial limit is not more than 4000 Units per g.

Containers and storage. The directions given under Ointments (page 757) should be followed; containers should be airtight.

The ointment may be expected to retain its potency for two years provided that the moisture content of the ointment does not exceed 0·2 per cent. When materials complying with the B.P.C. requirements are used, the moisture content may be expected to be below this figure.

Nystatin Ointment

Nystatin Ointment is a dispersion of Nystatin, in sufficiently fine powder to meet the requirements of the standard, in a polyethylene-mineral-oil gel or other suitable anhydrous basis.

Standard
PARTICLE SIZE. When determined by the method given in Appendix 25C, page 911, *liquid paraffin* being used as diluent, no particle has a maximum diameter greater than 75 μm.

CONTENT OF NYSTATIN. 90 to 115 per cent of the prescribed or stated concentration, determined by the following method:
Disperse an accurately weighed quantity, equivalent to about 400,000 Units of nystatin, in 20 ml of *solvent ether* in a stoppered flask, add 70 ml of *dimethylformamide*, shake for 15 minutes, add 10 ml of water, shake vigorously for 2 minutes, opening the stopper frequently to release the pressure of ether vapour, and filter.
Dilute 10 ml of the filtrate to 100 ml with *phosphate buffer solution pH 6·0* and carry out a microbiological assay of nystatin; a suggested method is given in Appendix 18, page 897.
The precision of any assay must be such that the fiducial limits of error (P = 0·95) are not less than 95 per cent and not more than 105 per cent of the estimated potency.
Calculate the upper and lower fiducial limits of the concentration of nystatin in the ointment.
The upper fiducial limit of the estimated concentration of nystatin is not less than 90 per cent and the lower fiducial limit is not more than 115 per cent of the prescribed or stated concentration.

Containers and storage; Labelling. The directions given under Ointments (page 757) should be followed.

Note. When the strength of the ointment is not specified, an ointment containing 100,000 Units of nystatin in 1 g shall be supplied.

Paraffin Ointment

Hard Paraffin	..	..	30 g
White Soft Paraffin	..	..	900 g
White Beeswax	..	..	20 g
Cetostearyl Alcohol	..	..	50 g

Melt together and stir until cold.

Containers and storage. The directions given under Ointments (page 757) should be followed.

Resorcinol Ointment, Compound

Resorcinol	..	..	40 g
Cade Oil ..	..	..	30 g
Zinc Oxide, finely sifted..	..	40 g
Bismuth Subnitrate, finely sifted	80 g

Starch, finely sifted	..	..	100 g
Sodium Metabisulphite ..	..	2 g
Hard Paraffin	..	..	..	20 g
Water (see page 642)	..	..	40 g
Wool Fat ..	..	..	..	100 g
Yellow Soft Paraffin	..	..	548 g

Triturate the bismuth subnitrate, the zinc oxide, and the starch with a portion of the yellow soft paraffin until smooth and incorporate the wool fat and the melted hard paraffin; add the resorcinol and the sodium metabisulphite previously dissolved in the water, the cade oil, and the remainder of the soft paraffin, and mix.

Standard
CONTENT OF BISMUTH. 5·4 to 6·1 per cent, calculated as Bi, determined by the following method:
Gently ignite about 6 g, accurately weighed, until the basis is completely volatilised or charred and continue the ignition at a temperature not exceeding 500°.
Dissolve the residue in a mixture of 5 ml of *nitric acid* and 10 ml of water, dilute to 50 ml with water, and reserve a portion of this solution for the determination of zinc oxide; to 20 ml add 30 ml of water, 20 ml of *glycerol*, and 0·2 g of *sulphamic acid*, allow to stand for one minute, and add 200 ml of water and 0·3 ml of *catechol violet solution*; if a violet colour is produced, add *dilute ammonia solution*, dropwise, until a blue colour is produced; titrate with 0·05M disodium edetate until a yellow colour is produced; each ml of 0·05M disodium edetate is equivalent to 0·01045 g of Bi.

CONTENT OF WATER-SOLUBLE PHENOLS. 3·8 to 4·4 per cent, calculated as resorcinol, $C_6H_6O_2$, determined by the following method:
Shake about 0·4 g, accurately weighed, with 20 ml of *light petroleum (boiling-range, 100° to 120°)* and extract with four successive 20-ml portions of warm water; filter the combined extracts and wash the filter with water.
To the combined filtrate and washings add 50 ml of 0·1N bromine and 5 ml of *hydrochloric acid*, shake vigorously for one minute, add 10 ml of *potassium iodide solution*, and titrate the liberated iodine with 0·1N sodium thiosulphate.
Repeat the procedure omitting the sample.
The difference between the two titrations represents the amount of bromine required by the sample; each ml of 0·1N bromine is equivalent to 0·001835 g of $C_6H_6O_2$.

CONTENT OF ZINC OXIDE. 3·8 to 4·2 per cent, calculated as ZnO, determined by the following method:
To 10 ml of the solution reserved in the determination of bismuth, add 2 ml of *dilute hydrochloric acid*, 150 ml of water, and then *dilute ammonia solution* until the solution is only slightly acid to *litmus solution*; boil for 2 minutes, cool to 15°, filter, wash the residue with water, and dilute the combined filtrate and washings to 250 ml with water.
To 50 ml of this solution add 50 ml of water and 10 ml of *ammonia buffer solution* and titrate with 0·05M disodium edetate, using *mordant black 11 solution* as indicator; each ml of 0·05M disodium edetate is equivalent to 0·004068 g of ZnO.

Containers and storage. The directions given under Ointments (page 757) should be followed; containers should prevent evaporation.

Salicylic Acid and Sulphur Ointment

Salicylic Acid, finely sifted	..	30 g
Precipitated Sulphur, finely sifted	30 g
Oily Cream	..	..	..	940 g

Triturate the salicylic acid and the precipitated sulphur with a portion of the oily cream until smooth and gradually incorporate the remainder of the cream.

Standard

CONTENT OF SALICYLIC ACID. 2·85 to 3·15 per cent, calculated as $C_7H_6O_3$, determined by the following method:
Dissolve about 2 g, accurately weighed, in 50 ml of *light petroleum (boiling-range, 40° to 60°)* and extract with four successive 10-ml portions of a 0·5 per cent w/v solution of *sodium carbonate* in water, filtering each extract successively into a glass-stoppered flask.
Cautiously add *hydrochloric acid* to the combined filtrates until effervescence ceases and the solution is just acid to *phenolphthalein solution* and then add 0·5N sodium hydroxide until the solution is just alkaline; add 50 ml of 0·1N bromine, 50 ml of water, and 5 ml of *hydrochloric acid*, shake repeatedly during 15 minutes, and allow to stand for 15 minutes; add 10 ml of *potassium iodide solution* and titrate the liberated iodine with 0·1N sodium thiosulphate.
Repeat the procedure omitting the sample.
The difference between the two titrations represents the amount of bromine required by the sample; each ml of 0·1N bromine is equivalent to 0·002302 g of $C_7H_6O_3$.

CONTENT OF SULPHUR. 2·85 to 3·15 per cent, calculated as S, determined by the method given for Salicylic Acid and Sulphur Cream, page 660, about 3 g, accurately weighed, being used.

Containers and storage. The directions given under Ointments (page 757) should be followed; containers should prevent evaporation.

OLEORESIN

Capsicum Oleoresin

SYNONYMS: Capsicin; Capsicum Extract

Capsicum, crushed	.. ..	1000 g
Acetone, if used ..	a sufficient quantity	
Alcohol (90 per cent)	a sufficient quantity	

Exhaust the capsicum by percolation with the acetone or, alternatively, with the alcohol (90 per cent) in an apparatus for the continuous extraction of drugs. Evaporate off the solvent and extract the residue with successive quantities of the cold alcohol until the insoluble material is free from pungency. Mix the alcoholic solutions and evaporate off the alcohol.

In making this preparation the alcohol (90 per cent) may be replaced by Industrial Methylated Spirit diluted so as to be of equivalent alcoholic strength,

OXYMELS

Oxymel

Acetic acid	..	..	..	150 ml
Purified Water, freshly boiled and				
cooled ..	..	..	..	150 ml
Purified Honey ..	..	..	to 1000 ml	

Mix thoroughly.

Triamcinolone Ointment

Triamcinolone Ointment is a dispersion of Triamcinolone Acetonide in a suitable anhydrous greasy basis.

Standard

CONTENT OF TRIAMCINOLONE ACETONIDE. 90·0 to 110·0 per cent of the prescribed or stated concentration, determined by the following method:
Disperse an accurately weighed quantity, equivalent to about 2 mg of triamcinolone acetonide, in 30 ml of *chloroform*, shake, dilute to 50 ml with *chloroform*, and filter.
To three 25-ml graduated flasks add, respectively, 5 ml of this solution, 5 ml of *standard triamcinolone acetonide solution*, and 5 ml of *chloroform*.
To each flask add 10 ml of *isoniazid solution*, heat in a water-bath at 55° for 45 minutes, cool, dilute each solution to 25 ml with *chloroform*, and measure the extinction of a 1-cm layer of the sample solution and of the standard solution at the maximum at about 415 nm, using as the blank the solution prepared with 5 ml of chloroform.
From the two extinctions, calculate the concentration of triamcinolone acetonide in the sample.

Containers and storage; Labelling. The directions given under Ointments (page 757) should be followed.

Note. When the strength of the ointment is not specified, an ointment containing 0·1 per cent of triamcinolone acetonide shall be supplied.
An ointment containing 0·025 per cent is also available.

When a strength less than those available from the manufacturer is prescribed, the 0·1 per cent ointment may be diluted with a basis consisting of 1 part of Wool Fat and 9 parts White Soft Paraffin.

provided that the law and statutory regulations governing the use of industrial methylated spirit are observed.

Solubility. Soluble in alcohol, in acetone, in chloroform, and in essential oils; soluble with opalescence in fixed oils.

Standard

CONTENT OF CAPSAICIN. Not less than 8·0 per cent w/w, determined by the following method:
Dissolve about 0·25 g, accurately weighed, in 2 ml of *anaesthetic ether*, dilute to 100 ml with *dehydrated methyl alcohol*, and continue by the method for Capsicum, page 73, beginning with the words "to 10 ml of this solution add 15 ml of *dehydrated methyl alcohol* . . .".

Storage. It should be stored in airtight containers. If separation occurs, the oleoresin should be warmed and mixed before use.

Caution. *Capsicum oleoresin is a powerful irritant and even a minute quantity produces an intense burning sensation in contact with the eyes and tender parts of the skin. A dilute solution of potassium permanganate for the skin, and cocaine eye-drops for the eyes, may be used to allay the irritation.*

Standard

OPTICAL ROTATION. +0·6° to −3·0°, determined, at 20°, in a 25 per cent w/v solution in water, decolorised if necessary by means of *decolorising charcoal*.

WEIGHT PER ML. At 20°, 1·250 g to 1·260 g.

CONTENT OF ACETIC ACID. 4·5 to 5·5 per cent w/v, calculated as $C_2H_4O_2$, determined by the following method:

Dilute 10 ml with 10 ml of *carbon dioxide-free water*, and titrate with 1N sodium hydroxide, using *phenolphthalein solution* as indicator; each ml of 1N sodium hydroxide is equivalent to 0·06005 g of $C_2H_4O_2$.

Dose. 2·5 to 10 millilitres.

Squill Oxymel

Squill, bruised	..	..	..	50 g
Acetic Acid	..	..	..	90 ml, or
			a sufficient quantity	
Purified Water, freshly boiled and cooled	..	..	..	250 ml
Purified Honey	..	a sufficient quantity		

Macerate the squill with the acetic acid and the water for seven days, with occasional agitation, strain, and press out the liquid. Heat the mixed liquids to boiling, filter while hot, cool, and determine the concentration of acetic acid present in the solution by the method given below. To the remainder of the solution add a sufficient quantity of the acetic acid to produce a solution containing approximately 8·5 per cent w/v of acetic acid and mix. To every 3 volumes of this solution, add 7 volumes of the honey and mix thoroughly.

Standard
OPTICAL ROTATION. +0·6° to −3·0°, determined, at 20°, in a 25 per cent w/v solution in water, decolorised if necessary by means of *decolorising charcoal*.

WEIGHT PER ML. At 20°, 1·260 g to 1·270 g.

CONTENT OF ACETIC ACID. 2·2 to 2·7 per cent w/v, calculated as $C_2H_4O_2$, determined by the following method:
Dilute 20 ml with 20 ml of *carbon dioxide-free water* and titrate with 1N sodium hydroxide, using *phenolphthalein solution* as indicator; each ml of 1N sodium hydroxide is equivalent to 0·06005 g of $C_2H_4O_2$.

Dose. 2·5 to 5 millilitres.

PAINTS

Paints are liquid preparations for application to the skin or mucous surfaces. They are usually medicated with substances possessing antiseptic, astringent, caustic, or analgesic properties. Resinous substances such as benzoin, prepared storax, or tolu balsam in ethereal solution are employed as bases of medicated varnishes.

Containers. They should be dispensed in coloured fluted bottles in order that they may be distinguished from preparations intended for internal administration; the bottles should be fitted with glass stoppers or other suitable closures.

Labelling. The container should be labelled "For external use only".

Storage. They should be stored in airtight containers, in a cool place.

Brilliant Green and Crystal Violet Paint

SYNONYMS: Liquor Tinctorium; Pigmentum Caeruleum; Pigmentum Tinctorium; Solution of Brilliant Green and Crystal Violet

Brilliant Green	..	..	..	5 g
Crystal Violet	..	..	..	5 g
Alcohol (90 per cent)	..	..	500 ml	
Water (see page 642)	..	.. to 1000 ml		

Dissolve the brilliant green and the crystal violet in the alcohol and add sufficient water to produce the required volume.

In making this preparation the alcohol (90 per cent) may be replaced by Industrial Methylated Spirit diluted so as to be of equivalent alcoholic strength, provided that the law and the statutory regulations governing the use of industrial methylated spirit are observed.

Standard
PRESENCE OF BRILLIANT GREEN AND OF CRYSTAL VIOLET. It complies with the paper chromatographic test given in Appendix 4, page 858.

WEIGHT PER ML. At 20°, 0·930 g to 0·950 g.

ALCOHOL CONTENT. 42 to 48 per cent v/v of ethyl alcohol, determined by the method given in Appendix 10, page 888.

Containers; Labelling; Storage. The directions given under Paints (above) should be followed.

Coal Tar Paint

SYNONYM: Pigmentum Picis Carbonis

Coal Tar ..	..	..	..	100 g
Acetone	..	} of each equal volumes	.. to 1000 ml	
Benzene, nitration grade of commerce	..			

Dissolve.

Benzene (nitration grade) complying with British Standard 135/2: 1963 is suitable for use in the above formula.

Standard
WEIGHT PER ML. At 20°, 0·850 g to 0·870 g.

Containers; Labelling; Storage. The directions given under Paints (above) should be followed. In addition, the label on the container states "This preparation is inflammable. Keep away from a naked flame".

Crystal Violet Paint

SYNONYM: Gentian Violet Paint

| Crystal Violet | .. | .. | .. | 5 g |
| Water (see page 642) | .. | .. to 1000 ml |

Dissolve.

Standard
LIGHT ABSORPTION. Dilute 5 ml to 250 ml with water. Dilute 5 ml of this solution to 250 ml with water and measure the extinction of a 1-cm layer at the maximum at about 585 nm; the extinction is not less than 0·32.

Containers; Labelling; Storage. The directions given under Paints (page 765) should be followed.

Magenta Paint

SYNONYMS: Castellani's Paint; Fuchsine Paint

Magenta	..	..	..	..	4 g
Boric Acid	..	..	..	8 g
Phenol	..	..	..	..	40 g
Resorcinol	..	..	..	80 g
Acetone	..	..	..	..	40 ml
Alcohol (90 per cent)	..	..	85 ml
Water (see page 642)	..	.. to 1000 ml

Dissolve the magenta in the alcohol and the acetone, previously mixed. Dissolve the boric acid in a portion of water; dissolve the phenol and the resorcinol in this solution, add the alcoholic magenta solution and sufficient water to produce the required volume, and mix.

In making this preparation the alcohol (90 per cent) may be replaced by Industrial Methylated Spirit diluted so as to be of equivalent alcoholic strength, provided that the law and the statutory regulations governing the use of industrial methylated spirit are observed.

Containers; Labelling. The directions given under Paints (page 765) should be followed.

Storage. It should be stored in airtight containers, protected from light, in a cool place.

Mastic Paint, Compound

SYNONYM: Benzo-mastic

Mastic	..	..	..	..	400 g
Castor Oil..	..	..	..	12·5 ml
Benzene, nitration grade of commerce	..	..	..	.. to 1000 ml

Dissolve and filter.

Benzene (nitration grade) complying with British Standard 135/2: 1963 is suitable for use in the above formula.

Standard
CONTENT OF NON-VOLATILE MATTER. 36·0 to 44·0 per cent w/v, determined by the following method:
Evaporate to dryness on a water-bath about 2 g, accurately weighed, dry the residue for 2 hours at 105°, and weigh.
Determine the weight per ml of the paint and calculate the concentration of non-volatile matter, weight in volume.

Containers; Labelling; Storage. The directions given under Paints (page 765) should be followed.
In addition, the label on the container states "This preparation is inflammable. Keep away from a naked flame".

Podophyllin Paint, Compound

| Podophyllum Resin | .. | .. | 150 g |
| Compound Benzoin Tincture | .. to 1000 ml |

The compound benzoin tincture used in making this preparation may be prepared with Industrial Methylated Spirit diluted so as to be of equivalent alcoholic strength, provided that the law and the statutory regulations governing the use of industrial methylated spirit are observed.

Standard
WEIGHT PER ML. At 20°, 0·925 g to 0·975 g.
TOTAL SOLIDS. 29·0 to 34·0 per cent w/v, determined on 0·5 g.
Determine the weight per ml and calculate the concentration of total solids, weight in volume.

Containers; Labelling; Storage. The directions given under Paints (page 765) should be followed.

Caution. Powdered podophyllin resin is strongly irritant and should be kept away from the eyes and tender parts of the skin.

PASTES

Pastes are semisolid preparations for external application. They usually consist of a high proportion of finely powdered medicaments mixed with soft or liquid paraffin or with a non-greasy basis made with glycerol, mucilage, or soap. They are used principally as antiseptic, protective, or soothing dressings which are often spread on lint before being applied.

Containers and storage. Pastes should be stored and supplied in glass or plastic jars fitted with screw caps with impermeable liners or with close-fitting slip-on lids so that absorption or diffusion of the contents is prevented. Alternatively, collapsible tubes of metal or suitable plastic material may be used.

Pastes containing water or other volatile ingredients should be stored and supplied in well-closed containers which prevent evaporation.

Aluminium Paste, Compound

SYNONYM: Baltimore Paste

Aluminium Powder	..	..	200 g
Zinc Oxide	..	..	400 g
Liquid Paraffin	..	..	400 g

Mix thoroughly the zinc oxide and the aluminium powder with the liquid paraffin until smooth.

Standard

CONTENT OF ZINC OXIDE. 37·0 to 42·0 per cent, calculated as ZnO, determined by the following method: Disperse about 1 g, accurately weighed, in a mixture of 20 ml of *hydrochloric acid* and 20 ml of water, by warming on a water-bath, filter through a wet filter paper, wash the filter with water, cool the combined filtrate and washings, and dilute to 100 ml with water; reserve a portion of this solution for the determination of aluminium.

To 20 ml of this solution add 1 g of *ammonium chloride* and sufficient *triethanolamine* to dissolve the precipitate which first forms, add 200 ml of water, 5 ml of *ammonia buffer solution*, and *mordant black 11 solution* as indicator, and titrate with 0·05M disodium edetate to a full blue colour; each ml of 0·05M disodium edetate is equivalent to 0·004068 g of ZnO.

CONTENT OF ALUMINIUM. 15·8 to 20·0 per cent, calculated as Al, determined by the following method: Neutralise to *congo red paper* 10 ml of the solution reserved in the determination of zinc oxide with *sodium hydroxide solution*, add 40 ml of 0·05M disodium edetate, warm on a water-bath for 30 minutes, cool, add 3 g of *hexamine* and *xylenol orange solution* as indicator, and titrate the excess of disodium edetate with 0·05M lead nitrate to a purple-red colour; each ml of 0·05M disodium edetate, after one half the volume required in the determination of zinc oxide has been deducted, is equivalent to 0·001349 g of Al.

Containers and storage. The directions given under Pastes (page 766) should be followed.

Coal Tar Paste

SYNONYM: Pasta Picis Carbonis

Strong Coal Tar Solution	..	75 g
Compound Zinc Paste	..	925 g

Triturate the strong coal tar solution with a portion of the compound zinc paste until smooth and gradually incorporate the remainder of the paste.

Standard

CONTENT OF ZINC OXIDE. 20·6 to 25·9 per cent w/w, determined by the method for Coal Tar and Zinc Ointment, page 760.

Containers and storage. The directions given under Pastes (page 766) should be followed; containers should prevent evaporation.

Dithranol Paste

Dithranol Paste consists of a dispersion containing up to 1 per cent w/w of Dithranol in Zinc and Salicylic Acid Paste.

It is prepared by mixing the dithranol thoroughly with a portion of the Zinc and Salicylic Acid Paste until smooth and then gradually incorporating the remainder of the paste.

Standard

CONTENT OF DITHRANOL. 80·0 to 120·0 per cent of the prescribed or stated concentration, determined by the following method:

Warm an accurately weighed quantity, equivalent to about 1 mg of dithranol, with 10 ml of *chloroform*, filter through a sintered-glass crucible (British Standard Grade No. 3) with the aid of suction, and wash the residue and the filter with three successive 10-ml portions of warm *chloroform*.

Extract the combined filtrate and washings with three successive 10-ml portions of a 1 per cent w/v solution of *sodium bicarbonate* in water; wash the combined aqueous extracts with 10 ml of *chloroform*, discard the aqueous solution, and add the chloroform washings to the extracted chloroform solution.

Evaporate off the solvent from the chloroform solution and extract the residue with four successive 5-ml portions of hot *glacial acetic acid*, cooling and filtering each extract through the same filter, and dilute the combined filtrates to 25 ml with *glacial acetic acid*.

To 5 ml of this solution add 1 ml of a 5 per cent solution of *sodium nitrite* in water, heat in a water-bath for 2 minutes, dilute to 25 ml with *glacial acetic acid*, filter if necessary, and measure the extinction of a 1-cm layer at the maximum at about 450 nm, ensuring that the measurement is made within 10 minutes of adding the sodium nitrite solution.

Calculate the concentration of dithranol by reference to a calibration curve prepared from 2-, 3-, 4- and 5-ml portions of an accurately prepared solution of *dithranol* in *glacial acetic acid* containing 0·05 mg of *dithranol* per ml, the method described above, beginning with the words "add 1 ml of a 5 per cent w/v solution of *sodium nitrite* . . .", being used.

CONTENT OF SALICYLIC ACID. 1·9 to 2·1 per cent, calculated as $C_7H_6O_3$, determined by the following method:

To about 5 g, accurately weighed, add 40 ml of *alcohol (95 per cent)*, previously neutralised to *phenol red solution*, warm on a water-bath for 5 minutes with frequent swirling, and titrate the hot solution with 0·1N sodium hydroxide, using *phenol red solution* as indicator; each ml of 0·1N sodium hydroxide is equivalent to 0·01381 g of $C_7H_6O_3$.

CONTENT OF ZINC OXIDE. 22·5 to 25·5 per cent, calculated as ZnO, determined by the method for Coal Tar and Zinc Ointment, page 760.

Containers and storage. The directions given under Pastes (page 766) should be followed. It should be protected from light.

Note. When the strength of the paste is not specified, or when Weak Dithranol Paste is ordered or prescribed, a paste containing 0·1 per cent of dithranol shall be supplied.

When Strong Dithranol Paste is ordered or prescribed, a paste containing 1 per cent of dithranol shall be supplied.

Caution. *Dithranol is a powerful irritant and should be kept away from the eyes and tender parts of the skin.*

Stains on the skin and clothing may be removed as described under Dithranol (page 173).

Magnesium Sulphate Paste

SYNONYM: Morison's Paste

Dried Magnesium Sulphate	a sufficient quantity
Phenol	0·5 g
Glycerol, previously heated at 120° for one hour and cooled..	55·0 g

Dry about 70 g of the dried magnesium sulphate for 1½ hours at 150° or for 4 hours at 130° and allow to cool in a desiccator; mix

45 g of this powder in a warm mortar with the phenol dissolved in the glycerol.

In preparing larger quantities of the paste the period of heating the dried magnesium sulphate should be increased, if necessary, to ensure that the dried powder contains at least 85 per cent of magnesium sulphate, calculated as $MgSO_4$.

Standard
CONTENT OF MAGNESIUM SULPHATE. 36·0 to 41·0 per cent, calculated as $MgSO_4$, determined by the following method:
Dissolve about 5 g, accurately weighed, in water, and dilute to 100 ml; to 10 ml of this solution add 150 ml of water, 10 ml of *ammonia buffer solution*, and *mordant black 11 solution* as indicator, and titrate with 0·05M disodium edetate to a full blue colour; each ml of 0·05M disodium edetate is equivalent to 0·006018 g of $MgSO_4$.

CONTENT OF PHENOL. 0·45 to 0·55 per cent, calculated as C_6H_6O, determined by the following method:
Dissolve about 5 g, accurately weighed, in 25 ml of water in a glass-stoppered flask, add 25 ml of 0·1N bromine and 5 ml of *hydrochloric acid*, insert the stopper, allow to stand for 30 minutes with occasional swirling, and then allow to stand for a further 15 minutes.
Add 5 ml of a 20 per cent w/v solution of *potassium iodide* in water, shake thoroughly, and titrate with 0·1N sodium thiosulphate until only a faint yellow colour remains, add 0·25 ml of *starch mucilage* and 10 ml of *chloroform*, and complete the titration with vigorous shaking.
Repeat the procedure omitting the sample.
The difference between the two titrations represents the amount of bromine required by the phenol; each ml of 0·1N bromine is equivalent to 0·001569 g of C_6H_6O.

Containers and storage. It should be stored and supplied in airtight glass jars or other suitable containers.

Labelling. The label on the container should state that the paste should be stirred before use.

Resorcinol and Sulphur Paste

Resorcinol, finely sifted ..	..	50 g
Precipitated Sulphur ..	..	50 g
Zinc Oxide, finely sifted..	..	400 g
Emulsifying Ointment ..	..	500 g

Triturate the zinc oxide, the resorcinol, and the precipitated sulphur with a portion of the emulsifying ointment until smooth and gradually incorporate the remainder of the emulsifying ointment.

Standard
PRESENCE OF RESORCINOL. Warm about 1 g with 1 ml of *sodium hydroxide solution* and 0·05 ml of *chloroform*; an intense red colour is produced.

CONTENT OF ZINC OXIDE. 38·0 to 42·0 per cent, calculated as ZnO, determined by the following method:
Warm about 2 g, accurately weighed, with 10 ml of *chloroform* until the fatty basis has dissolved, cool, add 25 ml of 1N sulphuric acid, and shake for 15 minutes; add 1 g of *ammonium chloride* and titrate the excess of acid with 1N sodium hydroxide, using *methyl orange solution* as indicator; each ml of 1N sulphuric acid is equivalent to 0·04068 g of ZnO.

CONTENT OF RESORCINOL. 4·75 to 5·25 per cent, calculated as $C_6H_6O_2$, determined by the following method:

Shake about 0·8 g, accurately weighed, with 20 ml of warm *light petroleum* (boiling-range, 60° to 80°) and extract with three successive 20-ml portions of warm water; filter the combined extracts and wash the filter with water.
To the combined filtrate and washings add 50 ml of 0·1N bromine and 5 ml of *hydrochloric acid*, shake vigorously for one minute, add 10 ml of *potassium iodide solution*, and titrate the liberated iodine with 0·1N sodium thiosulphate.
Repeat the procedure omitting the sample.
The difference between the two titrations represents the amount of bromine required by the sample; each ml of 0·1N bromine is equivalent to 0·001835 g of $C_6H_6O_2$.

CONTENT OF SULPHUR. 4·75 to 5·25 per cent, calculated as S, determined by the following method:
To about 1 g, accurately weighed, add a solution containing 2 g of *sodium sulphite* in 40 ml of water, boil under a reflux condenser until the sulphur has completely dissolved, cool, and filter; heat the residue of fat with hot water, cool, and filter.
To the combined filtrates add 10 ml of *formaldehyde solution* and 6 ml of *acetic acid*, dilute to 150 ml with water, and titrate with 0·1N iodine, using *starch mucilage* as indicator; each ml of 0·1N iodine is equivalent to 0·003206 g of S.

Containers and storage. The directions given under Pastes (page 766) should be followed. It should be protected from light.

Titanium Dioxide Paste

Titanium Dioxide	.. ..	200 g
Chlorocresol	..	1 g
Red Ferric Oxide, of commerce..		20 g
Light Kaolin or Light Kaolin (Natural), sterilised ..	..	100 g
Zinc Oxide, finely sifted..	..	250 g
Glycerol	..	150 g
Water (see page 642) ..	..	to 1000 g

Mix the ferric oxide, the light kaolin, the titanium dioxide, and the zinc oxide to form a homogeneous powder. Dissolve the chlorocresol in the glycerol, add the water, and gradually triturate the solution with the mixed powders to form a smooth paste.

Standard
PRESENCE OF TITANIUM DIOXIDE. To the residue obtained in the determination of residue on ignition, add 1 g of *potassium carbonate*, mix well, and ignite at 900°; allow to cool, extract the residue with 10 ml of *dilute sulphuric acid*, filter, and to the filtrate add 0·2 ml of *hydrogen peroxide solution*; an orange-red colour is produced.

RESIDUE ON IGNITION. 53·0 to 58·0 per cent, determined by the following method:
Heat gently about 1 g, accurately weighed, until the basis is completely volatilised or charred; increase the temperature until all the carbon is removed and ignite the residue to constant weight.

CONTENT OF ZINC OXIDE. 23·7 to 26·3 per cent, calculated as ZnO, determined by the following method:
Mix about 5 g, accurately weighed, with 50 ml of water, add 40 ml of 1N sulphuric acid, boil, cool, filter, and wash the filter with water.
To the combined filtrate and washings add 2 g of *ammonium chloride* and titrate the excess of acid with 1N sodium hydroxide, using *methyl orange solution* as

indicator; each ml of 1N sulphuric acid is equivalent to 0·04068 g of ZnO.

Containers and storage. The directions given under Pastes (page 766) should be followed. It should not be allowed to come into contact with aluminium.

Triamcinolone Dental Paste

Triamcinolone Dental Paste is a dispersion of Triamcinolone Acetonide in an adhesive gelatinous paste for application to oral surfaces.

Standard
CONTENT OF TRIAMCINOLONE ACETONIDE. 90·0 to 110·0 per cent of the prescribed or stated concentration, determined by the method for Triamcinolone Ointment, page 764.

Containers and storage. The directions given under Pastes (page 766) should be followed; it may be packed in small collapsible tubes.

Note. When the strength of the paste is not specified, a paste containing 0·1 per cent of triamcinolone acetonide shall be supplied.

Zinc and Coal Tar Paste

SYNONYMS: Zinc Oxide and Coal Tar Paste; White's Tar Paste

Zinc Oxide, finely sifted		..		60 g
Coal Tar ..	..	..	..	60 g
Emulsifying Wax..		..	..	50 g
Starch ..	..	..	..	380 g
Yellow Soft Paraffin		..	..	450 g

Melt the emulsifying wax at 70° and add the coal tar, followed by 225 g of the yellow soft paraffin; stir at 70° until completely melted and add the remainder of the yellow soft paraffin. When completely melted, cool to 30°, add the zinc oxide and the starch, with constant stirring, and mix until cold.

Standard
CONTENT OF ZINC OXIDE. 5·7 to 6·3 per cent, calculated as ZnO, determined by the method for Coal Tar and Zinc Ointment, page 760.

Containers and storage. The directions given under Pastes (page 766) should be followed.

PASTILLES

Pastilles consist of medicaments incorporated in an inert basis and are intended to dissolve slowly in the mouth. The basis is composed of a preparation containing gelatin and glycerol or a mixture of acacia and sucrose.

For extemporaneous preparation, a suitable basis may be prepared from the following formula:

Gelatin..	..	..	..	..	..	..	200 g
Sodium Benzoate	..	..	..	..	..		2 g
Citric Acid	..	..	..	..	..	..	20 g
Sucrose	..	..	..	..	..	..	50 g
Lemon Oil	..	..	..	..	..	..	1 ml
Amaranth Solution	..	..	..	..	..		20 ml
Glycerol	..	..	..	..	..	..	400 g
Purified Water, freshly boiled and cooled	..		..to 1000 g				

Soak the gelatin until softened in 300 g of the water at a temperature above 90°, add the glycerol, and heat on a water-bath until the gelatin is dissolved and the mass weighs 850 g; add the sucrose, the citric acid, and the sodium benzoate previously dissolved in 60 ml of the water, and add the lemon oil and the amaranth solution and sufficient water to produce the required weight. Strain and allow to cool.

Care should be taken to minimise microbial contamination by observing the highest standards of cleanliness during preparation. If a pastille which dissolves less rapidly is required, some of the gelatin in the above formula may be replaced by agar, but it should be noted that this will render the pastille basis opaque.

Standard

UNIFORMITY OF WEIGHT. Take a sample of 20 pastilles and determine the mean weight.

The weight of not more than one pastille may deviate by more than 10 per cent from the mean weight and the weight of none of the pastilles deviates by more than 15 per cent.

When testing crystallised pastilles, the loosely adhering sugar should be removed.

CONTENT OF ACTIVE INGREDIENT. When limits for content of active ingredient are given in a monograph, all permissible allowances, including variations due to manufacturing methods and to purity of the active ingredient, are included.

Unless otherwise stated, the limits are only applicable when the determination is carried out on a sample of 20 pastilles.

When it is not possible to obtain a sample of 20 pastilles, 10 are taken for the determination and the permitted tolerances increased by ± 5 per cent.

The methods and modified tolerances are not applicable when less than half the number of pastilles specified is available.

Containers and storage. Pastilles should be stored and supplied in containers that provide adequate protection against moisture and crushing. They should preferably be supplied in wide-mouthed glass or suitable plastic containers, or cylindrical aluminium containers internally coated with a suitable lacquer or lined with paper; lacquered or lined screw-cap closures or plastic caps should be used.

Squill Pastilles, Opiate

SYNONYMS: Gee's Linctus Pastilles; Gee's Pastilles

For each pastille take:

Squill Liquid Extract ..	..	0·03 ml
Concentrated Camphorated		
Opium Tincture ..	..	0·075 ml
Cinnamic Acid ..	.. ..	0·25 mg
Benzoic Acid ..	.. ..	0·60 mg
Glacial Acetic Acid ..	..	0·02 ml
Purified Honey ..	.. ..	0·2 ml

Standard
They comply with the standard under Pastilles, above, with the following addition:

CONTENT OF MORPHINE. 0·00024 g to 0·00036 g, calculated as anhydrous morphine determined by the following method:
Take a sample of 20 pastilles, remove any loosely adhering sugar if the pastilles are crystallised, and weigh.
Dissolve 2 of the pastilles, accurately weighed, in 20 ml of warm water, cool, add 0·5 g of *sodium bicar-*

bonate, and extract with four successive 30-ml portions of a mixture of 3 volumes of *chloroform* and 1 volume of *alcohol (95 per cent)*, shaking gently for 2 minutes at each extraction and washing each extract with the same 10 ml of water.

Evaporate the combined extracts to dryness, warm the residue on a water-bath with 20 ml of *calcium hydroxide solution*, filter, and wash the residue with two successive 10-ml portions of water.

Wash the combined filtrate and washings with two successive 5-ml portions of *solvent ether* and wash the combined ethereal washings with 5 ml of *calcium hydroxide solution*, adding the aqueous washings to the alkaline filtrate; add 0·25 g of *ammonium sulphate* and extract with four successive 20-ml portions of a mixture of 3 volumes of *chloroform* and 1 volume of *alcohol (95 per cent)*.

Evaporate the combined alcohol–chloroform extracts to dryness, dissolve the residue in 25 ml of warm 0·1N hydrochloric acid, cool, and dilute to 50 ml with 0·1N hydrochloric acid; using 20 ml of this solution, continue by the method for Aromatic Chalk with Opium Powder, page 776, beginning with the words "add 8 ml of a freshly prepared 1·0 per cent w/v solution of *sodium nitrite* . . .".

Calculate the total weight of anhydrous morphine in the 20 pastilles and divide by 20.

Note. Each pastille contains the approximate equivalent of 2 ml of Opiate Squill Linctus.

PESSARIES

Pessaries are solid bodies suitably shaped for vaginal administration and containing medicaments which are usually intended to act locally. They may be prepared by moulding, as described under Suppositories (page 795), or by compression, as described under Tablets (page 801).

Moulded pessaries are usually bluntly conical in shape. Theobroma Oil, Glycerol Suppositories mass of the British Pharmacopoeia, or other suitable basis, such as a hydrogenated vegetable oil, may be used. Bases containing gelatin should be maintained at 100° for one hour, replacing any water lost by evaporation, before incorporating the other ingredients. Bases should be formulated so that the pessaries melt at or slightly below 37°.

For pessaries intended to be used in tropical or subtropical climates, the amount of gelatin in the glycerol suppositories mass may be increased to an amount not exceeding 18 per cent w/w to meet conditions of temperature, but the amounts of active ingredients must in all cases be maintained.

Compressed pessaries are usually prepared in the form of a diamond, almond, wedge, disk, or other suitably shaped tablet. They may be manufactured by the moist-granulation or direct-compression techniques using similar diluents, disintegrating agents, moistening agents, and lubricants as described under Tablets (page 801).

Standard

Moulded Pessaries

UNIFORMITY OF WEIGHT. Moulded pessaries comply with the requirements of the British Pharmacopoeia for uniformity of weight given under Suppositories.

DISINTEGRATION TIME. Determine the disintegration time by the method of the British Pharmacopoeia for Suppositories. Moulded pessaries have a maximum disintegration time of 1 hour.

Compressed Pessaries

UNIFORMITY OF WEIGHT. Compressed pessaries comply with the requirements of the British Pharmacopoeia for the uniformity of weight of Tablets.

CONTENT OF ACTIVE INGREDIENT. When limits for content of active ingredient are given in the monographs, all permissible allowances, including variations due to manufacturing methods and to the purity of the active ingredient, are included.
Unless otherwise specified, the limits are only applicable when the determination is carried out on a sample of 20 compressed pessaries. When it is not possible to obtain a sample of 20 compressed pessaries, the wider limits given in the British Pharmacopoeia for Tablets for samples of 15, 10, or 5 tablets will apply.
When compressed pessaries containing relatively small amounts of active ingredient are assayed, 20 compressed pessaries may prove insufficient to give the specified amount of medicament; in these circumstances the number of compressed pessaries should be increased to enable that amount to be used for the determination.

DISINTEGRATION TIME. Determine the disintegration time by the method of the British Pharmacopoeia for Tablets. The maximum disintegration time for each compressed pessary is specified in the individual monograph.

Containers. Moulded pessaries should be dispensed in partitioned boxes, in shallow boxes lined with waxed paper, or in suitable plastic containers. When intended for use in tropical or subtropical climates or when containing volatile ingredients, pessaries should be wrapped separately in metal foil or enclosed in a suitable form of strip packing.

For compressed pessaries the directions given under Tablets (page 805) should be followed.

Storage. They should be stored in a cool place.

Acetarsol Pessaries

SYNONYM: Acetarsol Vaginal Tablets

For each pessary take:

Acetarsol ..	..	..	..	250 mg
Anhydrous Dextrose		..	..	320 mg
Starch ..	..	..	..	350 mg

Mix, and prepare by moist granulation and compression as described under Tablets (page 801).

Acetarsol Pessaries may be prepared using any other suitable basis, including an effervescent basis.

Standard

They comply with the standard for compressed pessaries under Pessaries, page 771, with the following additions:

DISINTEGRATION TIME. Maximum time, 15 minutes.

CONTENT OF ACETARSOL. 0·238 to 0·263 g, calculated as $C_8H_{10}AsNO_5$, determined by the following method:

Weigh and powder 20 pessaries. Transfer an accurately weighed quantity of the powder, equivalent to about 1 pessary, to a 600-ml conical flask, add 7·5 ml of *sulphuric acid* followed by 1·5 ml of *fuming nitric acid*, and heat at the boiling-point for 45 minutes; cool slightly, add 0·5 ml of *fuming nitric acid*, heat until brown fumes cease to be evolved, cool, gradually add 5 g of *ammonium sulphate*, and again heat gently, with occasional shaking, until the evolution of gas has ceased. The resulting solution should be colourless. Cool the solution, add sufficient water to produce 100 ml followed by 1 g of *potassium iodide*, boil gently until the volume is reduced to about 50 ml, cool, and add, dropwise, just sufficient 0·1N sodium sulphite to decolorise the solution; add 60 ml of water and 0·05 ml of *phenolphthalein solution*, make faintly alkaline by the addition of *sodium hydroxide solution*, add *dilute sulphuric acid* until the solution is faintly acid, cool, add sufficient *sodium bicarbonate* to neutralise the solution followed by 4 g in excess, and titrate with 0·1N iodine using *starch mucilage*, added towards the end of the titration, as indicator.

To 100 ml of water add 7·5 ml of *sulphuric acid*, cool, add 1 g of *potassium iodide* and 0·05 ml of *phenolphthalein solution*, and repeat the procedure above beginning at the words "make faintly alkaline . . .".

The difference between the two titrations represents the amount of iodine required by the sample; each ml of 0·1N iodine is equivalent to 0·01375 g of $C_8H_{10}AsNO_5$.

Calculate the total weight of $C_8H_{10}AsNO_5$ in the 20 pessaries and divide by 20.

Containers and storage. The directions given under Tablets (page 805) should be followed.

Note. Acetarsol Pessaries are intended to be inserted into the vagina without previously moistening them with water.

Crystal Violet Pessaries

Crystal Violet Pessaries are prepared as described under Pessaries (page 770) by dissolving Crystal Violet in melted Glycerol Suppositories mass.

Standard

They comply with the standard for moulded pessaries under Pessaries, page 771, with the following addition:

CONTENT OF CRYSTAL VIOLET. 87·5 to 112·5 per cent of the prescribed or stated amount, determined by the following method:

Weigh 5 pessaries, dissolve in 100 ml of water with the aid of gentle heat, and dilute to 500 ml with water; dilute an accurately measured volume of this solution, equivalent to about 5 mg of crystal violet, to 500 ml with water; further dilute 20 ml of this solution to 100 ml with water and measure the extinction of a 1-cm layer at the maximum at about 585 nm.

For purposes of calculation, use a value of 2250 for the E(1 per cent, 1 cm) of crystal violet.

Calculate the concentration of crystal violet in the sample.

Containers; Storage. The directions given under Pessaries (page 771) should be followed.

Note. When the strength of the pessaries is not specified, pessaries each containing 0·5 per cent w/w of crystal violet and prepared in a 4-g mould shall be supplied.

Di-iodohydroxyquinoline Pessaries

For each pessary take:

Di-iodohydroxyquinoline		..	100 mg
Phosphoric Acid ..	..	..	17 mg
Boric Acid	..	..	65 mg
Lactose ..	..	..	180 mg
Anhydrous Dextrose	..	..	300 mg

Mix, and prepare by moist granulation and compression as described under Tablets (page 801).

Standard

They comply with the standard, except for disintegration time, for compressed pessaries under Pessaries, page 771, with the following additions:

PRESENCE OF DI-IODOHYDROXYQUINOLINE. Warm a small portion of the powdered pessaries with 1 ml of *sulphuric acid*; the suspension darkens in colour and iodine vapour is evolved.

ACIDITY. pH of a suspension, prepared by triturating a quantity of the powdered pessaries, equivalent to 1 pessary, with 10 ml of water, 2·7 to 3·1.

CONTENT OF DI-IODOHYDROXYQUINOLINE. 0·095 g to 0·105 g, calculated as $C_9H_5I_2NO$, determined by the following method:

Weigh and powder 20 pessaries. Continue by the oxygen-flask method of the British Pharmacopoeia, Appendix XIC, for iodine, using an accurately weighed quantity of the powder equivalent to about 7 mg of di-iodohydroxyquinoline; each ml of 0·02N sodium thiosulphate is equivalent to 0·0006616 g of $C_9H_5I_2NO$.

Calculate the total weight of $C_9H_5I_2NO$ in the 20 pessaries and divide by 20.

Containers and storage. The directions given under Tablets (page 805) should be followed.

Note. Di-iodohydroxyquinoline Pessaries should be moistened with water before insertion into the vagina.

Lactic Acid Pessaries

Lactic Acid Pessaries are prepared as described under Pessaries (page 770) by incorporating Lactic Acid in melted Glycerol Suppositories mass.

Standard

They comply with the standard for moulded pessaries

under Pessaries, page 771, with the following addition:

CONTENT OF LACTIC ACID. 90·0 to 115·0 per cent of the prescribed or stated amount, calculated as $C_3H_6O_3$, determined by the following method:
Weigh 5 pessaries, melt together by warming, and allow to cool, stirring continuously; dissolve an accurately weighed quantity of the mass, equivalent to about 1 g of lactic acid, in 50 ml of water, add 50 ml of 0·5N sodium hydroxide, boil gently for 5 minutes, cool, and titrate the excess of alkali with 0·5N hydrochloric acid, using *phenolphthalein solution* as indicator; each ml of 0·5N sodium hydroxide is equivalent to 0·04504 g of $C_3H_6O_3$.
Calculate the concentration of lactic acid in the sample.

Containers; Storage. The directions given under Pessaries (page 771) should be followed.

Note. When the strength of the pessaries is not specified, pessaries each containing 5 per cent w/w of lactic acid and prepared in an 8-g mould shall be supplied.

Nystatin Pessaries

Nystatin Pessaries may be prepared by moist granulation and compression as described under Tablets (page 801).

Standard
They comply with the standard for compressed pessaries under Pessaries, page 771, with the following additions:

DISINTEGRATION TIME. Maximum time, 15 minutes.

CONTENT OF NYSTATIN. 90 to 120 per cent of the prescribed or stated number of Units, determined by the following method:
Weigh and powder 20 pessaries. Shake an accurately weighed quantity of the powder, equivalent to about 200,000 Units of nystatin, with 50 ml of *dimethylformamide* for 1 hour; centrifuge, dilute 10 ml of the clear supernatant liquid to 200 ml with *phosphate buffer solution pH 6·0* and carry out a microbiological assay of nystatin; a suggested method is given in Appendix 18, page 897.
The precision of any assay must be such that the fiducial limits of error (P = 0·95) are not less than 95 per cent and not more than 105 per cent of the estimated potency.
Calculate the upper and lower fiducial limits of the total number of Units of nystatin in the 20 pessaries and divide by 20.
The upper fiducial limit of the estimated number of Units of nystatin is not less than 90 per cent and the lower fiducial limit is not more than 120 per cent of the prescribed or stated number of Units.

Containers and storage. The directions given under Tablets (page 805) should be followed.

Note. When the strength of the pessaries is not specified, pessaries each containing 100,000 Units of nystatin shall be supplied.

Nystatin Pessaries should be moistened with water before insertion into the vagina.

Stilboestrol Pessaries

For each pessary take:

Stilboestrol	..	..	..	0·5 mg
Propylene Glycol..	..	..	0·07 ml

Glycerol Suppositories mass sufficient to fill a 4-g mould

Prepare as described under Pessaries (page 770), dissolving the stilboestrol in the propylene glycol, with the aid of gentle heat, before incorporating in the melted glycerol suppositories mass.

Standard
They comply with the standard for moulded pessaries under Pessaries, page 771, with the following addition:

CONTENT OF STILBOESTROL. 0·45 mg to 0·55 mg, determined by the following method:
Weigh 5 pessaries, melt together by warming, dissolve the mass in 10 ml of *dilute hydrochloric acid*, cool, and dilute to 50 ml with water.
Extract 10 ml of this solution with successive 100- and 25-ml portions of *solvent ether*, discard the aqueous layer, and extract the combined ethereal extracts with successive 20-, 10-, and 10-ml portions of 1N sodium hydroxide.
Discard the ethereal solution, wash the combined aqueous extracts with two successive 10-ml portions of *solvent ether*, discard the washings, adjust the pH of the aqueous solution to pH 9·5 by the addition of a 16 per cent v/v solution of *phosphoric acid* in water, and extract with four successive 20-ml portions of *solvent ether*.
Filter the combined extracts through a layer of *anhydrous sodium sulphate* in a sintered-glass filter (British Standard Grade No. 3), wash the filter with *solvent ether*, and evaporate the combined filtrates to dryness at room temperature with the aid of a current of air.
Dissolve the residue in a mixture of 5 ml of water and 5 ml of *alcohol (95 per cent)*, add 2 ml of *dilute hydrochloric acid*, 4 ml of *sodium molybdophosphotungstate solution*, and 50 ml of water, allow to stand for 10 minutes, add 10 ml of a 25 per cent w/v solution of *anhydrous sodium carbonate* in water, dilute to 100 ml with water, mix thoroughly, and allow to stand for 1 hour.
If the solution is hazy or contains a precipitate, transfer a suitable volume to a stoppered centrifuge tube, add a quarter of this volume of *solvent ether*, shake, centrifuge, and discard the upper layer including any precipitate which has collected at the interface.
Repeat the procedure using 10 ml of a solution prepared by dissolving 5 mg of *stilboestrol* in 50 ml of *alcohol (95 per cent)* and diluting to 100 ml with water and beginning at the words "add 2 ml of *dilute hydrochloric acid* . . .".
Determine the ratio of the colour intensities of the two solutions in a colorimeter, or by measuring the extinction at 750 nm, using as the blank a solution which has been prepared in the same manner but omitting the stilboestrol.
Calculate the total weight of stilboestrol in the 5 pessaries and divide by 5.

Containers; Storage. The directions given under Pessaries (page 771) should be followed.

PILLS

Pills are spherical or ovoid masses containing one or more medicaments. The active ingredients must be uniformly distributed throughout the mass, which should be of such a consistence that the pills retain their shape on keeping but are not so hard that they fail to disintegrate on ingestion. Very deliquescent substances should not be incorporated in pills.

Coatings may be applied to pills to mask the nauseous taste of medicaments and to improve their appearance and keeping properties. Pills may also be enteric coated. The materials and methods used for enteric coating must prevent disintegration of the pill in the stomach but ensure disintegration when the pill reaches the alkaline medium of the small intestine.

Standards are not imposed for total weight or diameter of pills, but the diameter should not normally be less than 3 millimetres for pills weighing up to 60 mg and not normally more than 8 millimetres for pills weighing about 300 mg.

Containers and storage. The directions given under Tablets (page 805) should be followed.

Phenolphthalein Pills, Compound

SYNONYM: Pilulae Phenaloini

For each pill take:

Phenolphthalein	30 mg
Belladonna Dry Extract ..	5 mg
Aloin	15 mg
Liquid glucose syrup	a sufficient quantity

Mix and form a mass of suitable shape and coat with a chocolate-coloured coating.
A suitable liquid glucose syrup may be prepared by mixing 2 parts by weight of Syrup with 1 part by weight of starch hydrolysate of commerce.

Standard
PRESENCE OF BELLADONNA ALKALOIDS. It complies with the thin-layer chromatographic test given in Appendix 5B, page 872.

CONTENT OF PHENOLPHTHALEIN. 0·027 to 0·033 g, determined by the following method:
Weigh and powder 20 pills. Dissolve, as completely as possible, an accurately weighed quantity of the powder, equivalent to about ¼ pill, in 100 ml of *alcohol* (*95 per cent*), allow to stand, and, using 5 ml of the clear supernatant liquid, continue by the method for phenolphthalein in Liquid Paraffin and Phenolphthalein Emulsion, page 679, beginning with the words "evaporate 5 ml of this solution to dryness . . .".
Calculate the total weight of phenolphthalein in the 20 pills and divide by 20.

Containers and storage. The directions given under Tablets (page 805) should be followed.

Dose. 1 or 2 pills.

POULTICES

Poultices are thick pasty preparations, usually intended to be made extemporaneously for application to the skin with the object of reducing inflammation and allaying pain.

Kaolin Poultice

SYNONYM: Cataplasma Kaolini

Heavy Kaolin, finely sifted, dried at 100°	527·0 g
Thymol	0·5 g
Boric Acid, finely sifted	45·0 g
Peppermint Oil	0·5 ml
Methyl Salicylate	2·0 ml
Glycerol	425·0 g

Mix the heavy kaolin and the boric acid with the glycerol, heat at 120° for one hour, stirring occasionally, and allow to cool. Add the thymol, previously dissolved in the methyl salicylate, and the peppermint oil, and mix thoroughly.

Standard
CONTENT OF BORIC ACID. 4·25 to 4·75 per cent, calculated as H_3BO_3, determined by the following method:
Mix about 20 g, accurately weighed, with a solution containing 10 g of *mannitol* in 40 ml of water, warm and stir until the sample is completely dispersed, and titrate with 1N sodium hydroxide, using *phenolphthalein solution* as indicator; each ml of 1N sodium hydroxide is equivalent to 0·06183 g of H_3BO_3.

Containers and storage. The directions given under Pastes (page 766) should be followed.

POWDERS

Powders are usually mixtures of two or more powdered medicaments intended for internal use. They may be prepared by mixing the medicament, or medicaments, specified in smallest quantity with gradually increasing quantities of the remaining material. After mixing, the product should be passed through a sieve of suitable mesh, usually No. 250, and triturated lightly, as partial separation of the ingredients may have occurred.

When the quantity of an ingredient is less than 60 milligrams or is such that it cannot be weighed conveniently on a dispensing balance, a suitable trituration is prepared by admixture with lactose or other suitable inert diluent, and a proportionately larger quantity of the triturate is weighed.

When a small quantity of a potent medicament is ordered by itself as a powder, it should be diluted by trituration with an amount of an inert diluent such as lactose so that the weight of the triturate to be taken as a dose is 120 milligrams; the triturate should then be supplied, suitably wrapped, as single doses.

Containers and storage. Powders should preferably be stored and supplied in white plain glass powder-jars with close-fitting lids. Deliquescent or volatile powders supplied as single doses should be doubly wrapped, the inner wrapper consisting of waxed or parchment paper; in exceptional cases, the wrapped powder should be enclosed in metal foil.

Individually wrapped powders should be enclosed in cartons or rigid slide boxes of paperboard or plastic material.

Bismuth Powder, Compound

Bismuth Carbonate	.. ..	125 g
Sodium Bicarbonate	.. ..	125 g
Calcium Carbonate	.. ..	375 g
Heavy Magnesium Carbonate ..		375 g

Mix, as described under Powders (above).

Standard
CONTENT OF BISMUTH. 9·50 to 10·83 per cent, calculated as Bi, determined by the following method:
Dissolve about 2 g, accurately weighed, by warming with 10 ml of water and 5 ml of *nitric acid*, add 20 ml of *glycerol* and 0·2 g of *sulphamic acid*, allow to stand for one minute, and add 200 ml of water and 0·3 ml of *catechol violet solution*; if a violet colour is produced add *dilute ammonia solution*, dropwise, until a blue colour is produced.
Titrate with 0·05M disodium edetate until a yellow colour is produced; each ml of 0·05M disodium edetate is equivalent to 0·01045 g of Bi.

CONTENT OF MAGNESIUM. 8·96 to 10·69 per cent, calculated as Mg, determined by the following method:
Dissolve about 1 g, accurately weighed, in 6 ml of water and 3 ml of *nitric acid*, add 2 ml of *dilute hydrochloric acid* and 150 ml of water, followed by *dilute ammonia solution* until the solution remains just acid to *litmus paper*, boil for 2 minutes, cool to 15°, filter, dilute the filtrate to 250 ml with water, and reserve a portion of the solution for the determination of calcium carbonate.
To 50 ml of this solution add 1 g of *ammonium chloride* and 1 g of *ammonium oxalate*, neutralise to *litmus paper* with *dilute ammonia solution* and add 5 ml in excess, boil for 5 minutes, allow to stand for 2 hours, and filter, washing the residue with hot water.
To the combined filtrate and washings add 5 ml of *ammonia buffer solution* and titrate with 0·05M disodium edetate, using *mordant black 11 solution* as indicator; each ml of 0·05M disodium edetate is equivalent to 0·001216 g of Mg.

CONTENT OF CALCIUM CARBONATE. 34·7 to 39·8 per cent, calculated as $CaCO_3$, determined by the following method:
To 50 ml of the solution reserved in the determination of magnesium add 5 ml of *ammonia buffer solution* and titrate with 0·05M disodium edetate, using *mordant black 11 solution* as indicator; each ml of 0·05M disodium edetate, after the volume required in the determination of magnesium has been deducted, is equivalent to 0·005005 g of $CaCO_3$.

CONTENT OF SODIUM BICARBONATE. 11·8 to 13·3 per cent, calculated as $NaHCO_3$, determined by the method for sodium bicarbonate in Paediatric Compound Calcium Carbonate Mixture, page 738, about 5 g, accurately weighed, being used.

Containers and storage. The directions given under Powders (above) should be followed.

Dose. 1 to 5 grams.

Calcium Carbonate Powder, Compound

Calcium Carbonate	.. ..	375 g
Light Kaolin or Light Kaolin (Natural)	.. .. ..	125 g
Heavy Magnesium Carbonate ..		125 g
Sodium Bicarbonate	.. ..	375 g

Mix, as described under Powders (above).

Standard
CONTENT OF ACID-INSOLUBLE MATTER. 11·7 to 13·1 per cent, determined by the following method:
To about 2 g, accurately weighed, in a 50-ml centrifuge tube, add 5 ml of water and an excess of *dilute hydrochloric acid*, fill the tube with water, mix thoroughly, and centrifuge; decant the supernatant liquid, disperse the residue in water, and centrifuge again; repeat the washing with water and dry the residue to constant weight at 105°.

CONTENT OF MAGNESIUM. 2·99 to 3·56 per cent, calculated as Mg, determined by the following method:
Dissolve as completely as possible about 3 g, accurately weighed, in 20 ml of *dilute hydrochloric acid*, filter, and dilute to 250 ml with water; to 50 ml of this solution add 1 g of *ammonium chloride* and 1 g of *ammonium oxalate* and continue by the method for magnesium in Paediatric Compound Calcium Carbonate Mixture, page 738, beginning with the words "neutralise to *litmus paper* . . .".

CONTENT OF CALCIUM CARBONATE. 34·7 to 39·6 per cent, calculated as CaCO₃, determined by the method for calcium carbonate in Paediatric Compound Calcium Carbonate Mixture, page 738, 10 ml of the solution prepared in the assay for magnesium being used; each ml of 0·05M disodium edetate, after one-fifth of the volume required in the determination of magnesium has been deducted, is equivalent to 0·005005 g of CaCO₃.

CONTENT OF SODIUM BICARBONATE. 35·3 to 39·8 per cent, calculated as NaHCO₃, determined by the method for sodium bicarbonate in Paediatric Compound Calcium Carbonate Mixture, page 738, about 2 g, accurately weighed, being used.

Containers and storage. The directions given under Powders (page 775) should be followed.

Dose. 1 to 5 grams.

Chalk Powder, Aromatic

SYNONYM: Pulvis Cretae Aromaticus

Chalk, in powder	250 g
Cardamom seed, freshly removed from the fruit, powdered, and used at once	30 g
Clove, in powder	40 g
Nutmeg, in powder	80 g
Cinnamon, in powder	100 g
Sucrose, in powder	500 g

Mix, as described under Powders (page 774).

Standard
CONTENT OF CHALK. 22·8 to 26·4 per cent, calculated as CaCO₃, determined by the following method:
Ignite about 5 g, accurately weighed, dissolve the residue in a mixture of 50 ml of 1N hydrochloric acid and 100 ml of water, filter, wash the filter with water, and titrate the excess of acid in the combined filtrate and washings with 1N sodium hydroxide, using *methyl orange–xylene cyanol FF* as indicator; each ml of 1N hydrochloric acid is equivalent to 0·05005 g of CaCO₃.

Containers and storage. The directions given under Powders (page 775) should be followed; containers should be airtight.

Dose. 0·5 to 5 grams.

Chalk with Opium Powder, Aromatic

SYNONYM: Pulvis Cretae Aromaticus cum Opio

Aromatic Chalk Powder	975 g
Powdered Opium	25 g

Mix, as described under Powders (page 774).

Standard
CONTENT OF CHALK. 22·3 to 25·8 per cent, calculated as CaCO₃, determined by the method for Aromatic Chalk Powder.

CONTENT OF ANHYDROUS MORPHINE. 0·226 to 0·276 per cent, determined by the following method:
Mix intimately about 4 g, accurately weighed, with 0·25 g of *calcium hydroxide* in a glass mortar, triturate with a little water, and transfer to a 100-ml graduated flask, rinsing in with further small quantities of water, using about 90 ml in all. Shake frequently during 30 minutes, dilute to 100 ml with water, mix, and filter.
To 10 ml of the filtrate add 0·15 g of *ammonium sulphate*, extract with two successive 10-ml portions of *alcohol-free chloroform*, washing each extract with the same 10 ml of water, and discard the chloroform.
Extract the combined aqueous layer and washings first with 60 ml of a mixture of equal volumes of *alcohol* (*95 per cent*) and *chloroform* and then with two successive 45-ml portions of a mixture of 1 volume of *alcohol* (*95 per cent*) and 2 volumes of *chloroform*, washing each alcohol–chloroform extract with the same mixture of 5 ml of *alcohol* (*95 per cent*) and 10 ml of water.
Evaporate the combined alcohol–chloroform extracts to dryness, dissolve the residue in 5 ml of 1N hydrochloric acid, and dilute to 50 ml with water.
To 20 ml of this solution, add 8 ml of a freshly prepared 1·0 per cent w/v solution of *sodium nitrite* in water, allow to stand for 15 minutes, add 12 ml of *dilute ammonia solution*, dilute to 50 ml with water, and measure the extinction of a 4-cm layer at the maximum at about 442 nm, using as a blank a solution prepared in the same manner and at the same time with 20 ml of 0·1N hydrochloric acid in place of the 20 ml of sample solution.
Calculate the content of anhydrous morphine by reference to a calibration curve prepared from 2-, 4-, 6-, and 8-ml portions of an accurately prepared 0·008 per cent w/v solution of *anhydrous morphine* in 0·1N hydrochloric acid, each diluted to 20 ml with 0·1N hydrochloric acid, and using the method described above beginning with the words "add 8 ml of a freshly prepared 1·0 per cent w/v solution of *sodium nitrite* . . .".

Containers and storage. The directions given under Powders (page 775) should be followed; containers should be airtight.

Dose. 0·5 to 5 grams.

Effervescent Powder, Compound

SYNONYM: Seidlitz Powder

No. 1 Powder

Sodium Bicarbonate, in powder	2·5 g
Sodium Potassium Tartrate, in powder	7·5 g

Mix, and wrap in blue paper.

No. 2 Powder

Tartaric Acid, in powder . .	2·5 g

Wrap in white paper.

Standard for No. 1 Powder
WEIGHT. 9·5 g to 10·5 g.

CONTENT OF SODIUM POTASSIUM TARTRATE. 73·0 to 77·0 per cent, calculated as C₄H₄KNaO₆,4H₂O, determined by the following method:
Gently ignite about 2 g, accurately weighed, digest the residue with hot water, filter, wash the residue with hot water, adding the washings to the filtrate, and reserve the combined liquids.
Ignite the filter paper and residue, cool, dissolve the white ash in water, combine with the reserved liquid, add 50 ml of 0·5N hydrochloric acid, boil to remove carbon dioxide, cool, and titrate the excess of acid with 0·5N sodium hydroxide, using *methyl red solution* as indicator; each ml of 0·5N hydrochloric acid, after the volume equivalent to the sodium bicarbonate in the

weight of sample taken has been deducted, is equivalent to 0·07056 g of $C_4H_4KNaO_6,4H_2O$.

CONTENT OF SODIUM BICARBONATE. 24·0 to 26·0 per cent, calculated as $NaHCO_3$, determined by the following method:
Dissolve about 2 g, accurately weighed, in 25 ml of water, add 25 ml of 0·5N hydrochloric acid, boil to remove carbon dioxide, cool, and titrate the excess of acid with 0·5N sodium hydroxide, using *phenolphthalein solution* as indicator; each ml of 0·5N hydrochloric acid is equivalent to 0·04200 g of $NaHCO_3$.

Standard for No. 2 Powder
PRESENCE OF TARTARIC ACID. 1. A solution in water is strongly acid and dextrorotatory.
2. A solution in water, after neutralisation, gives the reactions characteristic of tartrates.

WEIGHT. 2·25 g to 2·75 g.

Labelling. The label on the container gives the directions for taking the powder.

Dose. One of each powder.

The No. 1 powder should be dissolved in a tumblerful ($\frac{1}{2}$ pint) of cold or warm water, the No. 2 powder added, the mixture stirred, and the liquid taken while it is effervescing.

Effervescent Powder, Compound, Double-strength

SYNONYM: Double-strength Seidlitz Powder

No. 1 Powder

Sodium Bicarbonate, in powder	2·5 g
Sodium Potassium Tartrate, in powder	15·0 g

Mix, and wrap in blue paper.

No. 2 Powder

Tartaric Acid, in powder ..	2·5 g

Wrap in white paper.

Standard for No. 1 Powder
WEIGHT. 16·6 g to 18·4 g.

CONTENT OF SODIUM POTASSIUM TARTRATE. 83·4 to 90·6 per cent, calculated as $C_4H_4KNaO_6,4H_2O$, determined by the method for sodium potassium tartrate in Compound Effervescent Powder.

CONTENT OF SODIUM BICARBONATE. 12·7 to 15·9 per cent, calculated as $NaHCO_3$, determined by the method for sodium bicarbonate in Compound Effervescent Powder.

Standard for No. 2 Powder
PRESENCE OF TARTARIC ACID. It complies with the tests given in the standard for the No. 2 powder under Compound Effervescent Powder.

WEIGHT. 2·25 g to 2·75 g.

Labelling. The label on the container gives the directions for taking the powder.

Dose. One of each powder.

The No. 1 powder should be dissolved in a tumblerful ($\frac{1}{2}$ pint) of cold or warm water, the No. 2 powder added, the mixture stirred, and the liquid taken while it is effervescing.

Ipecacuanha and Opium Powder

SYNONYMS: Compound Ipecacuanha Powder; Dover's Powder

Prepared Ipecacuanha ..	..	100 g
Powdered Opium ..	..	100 g
Lactose, finely powdered	..	800 g

Mix, as described under Powders (page 774).

Standard
PRESENCE OF IPECACUANHA AND OF OPIUM. It possesses the microscopical characters described under Ipecacuanha, page 249, and under Opium, page 337.

CONTENT OF ANHYDROUS MORPHINE. 0·90 to 1·10 per cent, determined by the following method:
Triturate about 5 g, accurately weighed, for 3 minutes in a porcelain dish with a mixture of 3 ml of *alcohol (95 per cent)* and 1 ml of *dilute ammonia solution* and add gradually, with stirring, sufficient *anhydrous alumina* (about 10 to 15 g) to produce a free-flowing powder; transfer the powder to a dry chromatography tube, previously lightly plugged with cotton wool immediately above the plug; wipe the dish and stirring rod with a piece of cotton wool moistened with *alcohol (95 per cent)* and place the cotton wool on the top of the column.
Fit the lower end of the tube into a separating funnel fitted with a side-arm assembly which enables gentle suction to be applied to the column and elute the column with a mixture of 3 volumes of *chloroform* and 1 volume of *isopropyl alcohol*, using about 10 ml of the mixture for each g of anhydrous alumina used and adjusting the rate of flow to about 1·5 ml per minute by applying gentle suction.
Extract the eluate with successive 20-, 15-, and 15-ml portions of 0·1N sodium hydroxide, filter the extracts through the same plug of moistened cotton wool, wash the separating funnel and filter with 5 ml of water, neutralise the combined extracts and washings to *litmus paper* with 1N hydrochloric acid and add 0·05 ml in excess, and heat on a water-bath until the volume is reduced to about 30 ml; cool, add 30 ml of *1-fluoro-2,4-dinitrobenzene solution* and 5 ml of *dilute ammonia solution*, stir gently, and allow to stand for 4 hours at a temperature between 15° and 20°.
Filter through a sintered glass crucible (British Standard Grade No. 3), using the filtrate to transfer the precipitate to the crucible, wash the residue and filter with four successive 2-ml portions of *acetone*, allowing each portion to remain in contact with the filter for several seconds before applying suction, dry the residue for 1 hour at 85°, cool, and weigh; each g of residue is equivalent to 0·6321 g of anhydrous morphine.

Containers and storage. The directions given under Powders (page 775) should be followed; containers should be airtight.

Dose. 300 to 600 milligrams.

Ipecacuanha and Opium Powder contains, in 600 milligrams, 6 milligrams of anhydrous morphine.

Liquorice Powder, Compound

SYNONYM: Pulvis Glycyrrhizae Compositus

Liquorice, peeled, in powder	..	160 g
Sublimed Sulphur	..	..	80 g
Senna Leaf, in powder	..	..	160 g
Fennel, in powder	..	..	80 g
Sucrose, in powder	..	..	520 g

Mix, as described under Powders (page 774).

Standard
CONTENT OF SULPHUR. 7·6 to 8·4 per cent, calculated as S, determined by the following method:

To about 1 g, accurately weighed, add 40 ml of a 5·0 per cent w/v solution of *sodium sulphite* in water, boil under a reflux condenser for 1½ hours or until the sulphur has completely dissolved, cool, add 10 ml of *formaldehyde solution* and 6 ml of *acetic acid*, dilute to 100 ml with water, and titrate with 0·1N iodine, using *starch mucilage* as indicator; each ml of 0·1N iodine is equivalent to 0·003206 g of S.

Containers and storage. The directions given under Powders (page 775) should be followed.

Dose. 5 to 10 grams.

Magnesium Carbonate Powder, Compound

Heavy Magnesium Carbonate ..		400 g
Light Kaolin or Light Kaolin (Natural)		100 g
Sodium Bicarbonate		300 g
Calcium Carbonate		400 g

Mix, as described under Powders (page 774).

Standard
CONTENT OF ACID-INSOLUBLE MATTER. 7·5 to 9·0 per cent, determined by the method for acid-insoluble matter in Compound Calcium Carbonate Powder, page 775.

CONTENT OF MAGNESIUM. 7·97 to 9·50 per cent, calculated as Mg, determined by the following method: Dissolve as completely as possible about 1 g, accurately weighed, in 10 ml of *dilute hydrochloric acid*, filter, and dilute to 250 ml with water; to 50 ml of this solution add 1 g of *ammonium chloride* and 1 g of *ammonium oxalate* and continue by the method for magnesium in Paediatric Compound Calcium Carbonate Mixture, page 738, beginning with the words "neutralise to *litmus paper* . . .".

CONTENT OF CALCIUM CARBONATE. 30·9 to 35·3 per cent, calculated as CaCO₃, determined by the method for calcium carbonate in Paediatric Compound Calcium Carbonate Mixture, page 738.

CONTENT OF SODIUM BICARBONATE. 23·5 to 26·5 per cent, calculated as NaHCO₃, determined by the method for sodium bicarbonate in Paediatric Compound Calcium Carbonate Mixture, page 738, about 1·5 g, accurately weighed, being used.

Containers and storage. The directions given under Powders (page 775) should be followed.

Dose. 1 to 5 grams.

Magnesium Trisilicate Powder, Compound

Magnesium Trisilicate		250 g
Chalk, in powder..		250 g
Heavy Magnesium Carbonate ..		250 g
Sodium Bicarbonate		250 g

Mix, as described under Powders (page 774).

Standard
PRESENCE OF CALCIUM. Shake 0·5 g with 5 ml of *dilute hydrochloric acid*, filter, and reserve part of the filtrate for the test for the presence of magnesium.
To 0·05 ml of the filtrate add 0·2 ml of a 1 per cent w/v solution of *glyoxal bis(2-hydroxyanil)* in *alcohol (95*

per cent) and 0·05 ml of a 10 per cent w/v solution of *sodium hydroxide* in water; a reddish-brown precipitate is produced which, on the addition of *chloroform*, dissolves to give a red solution.

PRESENCE OF MAGNESIUM. To the portion of the filtrate reserved in the test for the presence of calcium add an excess of *ammonium oxalate solution*, filter, and to the filtrate add *sodium hydroxide solution* followed by *diphenylcarbazide solution*; a violet-red precipitate is produced.

CONTENT OF SILICA. 11·0 to 15·2 per cent, calculated as SiO₂, determined by the following method:
Mix about 1·5 g, accurately weighed, with 5 ml of water and 10 ml of *perchloric acid (60 per cent w/w)* in a beaker, heat until dense white fumes are evolved, cover the beaker with a watch-glass and continue heating for a further 3 hours; allow to cool, add 30 ml of water, filter, wash the filter with 200 ml of hot water and discard the filtrate and washings.
Dry the filter paper and its contents and ignite at 1000° until, after further ignition, two successive weighings do not differ by more than 0·2 per cent of the weight of the residue of crude silica.
To the crude silica add 0·25 ml of *sulphuric acid* followed by 15 ml of *hydrofluoric acid*, heat cautiously on a sandbath until all the acid has evaporated, ignite at 1000°, cool, and weigh; deduct the weight of any residue so obtained from the weight of crude silica obtained above and hence calculate the percentage of SiO₂ in the sample.

CONTENT OF SODIUM BICARBONATE. 23·7 to 26·3 per cent, calculated as NaHCO₃, determined by the method for sodium bicarbonate in Paediatric Compound Calcium Carbonate Mixture, page 738, about 2·5 g, accurately weighed, being used.

Containers and storage. The directions given under Powders (page 775) should be followed.

Dose. 1 to 5 grams.

Rhubarb Powder, Compound

SYNONYMS: Gregory's Powder; Pulvis Rhei Compositus

Rhubarb, in powder		250 g
Ginger, in powder		100 g
Heavy Magnesium Carbonate ..		325 g
Light Magnesium Carbonate ..		325 g

Mix, as described under Powders (page 774).

Standard
PRESENCE OF MAGNESIUM CARBONATE. The powder, mounted in *dilute glycerol* and examined microscopically, shows crystals similar to those described under Heavy Magnesium Carbonate, page 275, and Light Magnesium Carbonate, page 276, respectively.

PRESENCE OF RHUBARB AND OF GINGER. To 1 g add 30 ml of *acetic acid*, allow to settle after effervescence ceases, and examine the insoluble matter microscopically.
The insoluble matter possesses the microscopical characters described under Rhubarb, page 429, and Ginger, page 211, respectively; the cluster crystals rarely exceed 100 μm in diameter; lignified elements are absent.

CONTENT OF MAGNESIUM. 15·6 to 19·3 per cent, calculated as Mg, determined by the following method:
Ignite about 2 g, accurately weighed, dissolve the residue in the minimum quantity of *hydrochloric acid*, and dilute to 100 ml with water; to 10 ml of this solution add 200 ml of water, neutralise to *methyl orange–xylene cyanol FF solution* with *dilute ammonia*

solution, add 10 ml of *ammonia buffer solution*, and titrate with 0·05M disodium edetate, using *mordant black 11 solution* as indicator; each ml of 0·05M disodium edetate is equivalent to 0·001215 g of Mg.

Containers and storage. The directions given under Powders (page 775) should be followed.

Dose. 0·5 to 5 grams.

SOLUTIONS

Solutions are liquid preparations containing one or more soluble ingredients usually dissolved in water. They are intended for internal or external use or for instillation into body cavities. They are issued sterile or unsterilised, depending on the purpose for which they are intended.

Aqueous solutions of antiseptics are liable to become contaminated with resistant micro-organisms, and the following precautions should be taken.

Solutions should be prepared with freshly distilled or freshly boiled water and transferred to thoroughly cleansed containers (preferably sterile); closures of cork or containing cork liners must not be used; the contents should preferably not be used later than one week after the container has first been opened.

Solutions of antiseptics for application to broken skin or to the eyes or for introduction into body cavities should be sterilised and supplied in a sterile condition (see below).

Sterile solutions. These include solutions for external application to wounds and abraded surfaces, anticoagulant solutions, bladder irrigations, intraperitoneal dialysis solutions, and concentrated solutions for the preparation of injections.

Preparation of sterile solutions. The apparatus used in the preparation of sterile solutions and the containers should be thoroughly cleansed before use. The medicament is dissolved in the solvent and the solution clarified by filtration, transferred to the final containers, which are then closed, and sterilised by autoclaving or by heating with a bactericide (see Appendix 29, page 921). Alternatively, the solution is sterilised by filtration (see Appendix 29, page 923), and transferred by means of an aseptic technique to the final sterile containers, which are then closed to exclude micro-organisms.

Standard

STERILITY. Sterile solutions comply with the test for sterility.

Containers. Containers of sterile solutions should be readily distinguishable from containers used for intravenous fluids and should be closed so as to exclude micro-organisms. A readily breakable seal should cover the closure.

Labelling. The label on the sealed container of a sterile solution states that the solution is sterile and that it is not to be used for injection.

Unsterilised solutions. These include solutions for internal administration, either alone or as ingredients of other preparations, solutions for external application to unabraded surfaces, and haemodialysis solutions. Precautions should be taken to minimise any microbial contamination during preparation.

Aluminium Acetate Solution

SYNONYMS: Burow's Solution; Aluminium Acetate Ear-drops

Aluminium Sulphate	..	..	225 g
Acetic Acid	..	..	250 ml
Tartaric Acid	..	..	45 g
Calcium Carbonate	..	..	100 g
Water (see page 642)	..	..	750 ml

Dissolve the aluminium sulphate in 600 ml of the water, add the acetic acid and then the calcium carbonate mixed with the remainder of the water, and allow to stand for not less than twenty-four hours in a cool place, stirring occasionally; filter, add the tartaric acid to the filtered solution, and mix.

Standard
DESCRIPTION. A clear liquid.
WEIGHT PER ML. At 20°, 1·06 g to 1·08 g.
SULPHATE. Dilute 4 ml to 100 ml with water; 1 ml of this solution complies with the limit test for sulphates.
CONTENT OF ALUMINIUM. 1·7 to 1·9 per cent w/v, calculated as Al, determined by the following method: Dilute 10 ml to 100 ml with water; to 10 ml of this solution add 40 ml of 0·05M disodium edetate, 90 ml of water, and 0·15 ml of *methyl red solution*, neutralise by the dropwise addition of 1N sodium hydroxide, and warm on a water-bath for 30 minutes; cool, add 1 ml of *dilute nitric acid* and 5 g of *hexamine*, and titrate with 0·05M lead nitrate, using 0·5 ml of a 0·1 per cent w/v solution of *xylenol orange* in water as indicator; each ml of 0·05M disodium edetate is equivalent to 0·001349 g of Al.

Storage. It should be stored in well-filled containers, in a cool place.

Note. Aluminium Acetate Solution contains about 13 per cent w/v of aluminium acetate.

Amaranth Solution

Amaranth, food grade of commerce	..	..	..	10 g
Chloroform Water	..	..	to 1000 ml	

Standard
LIGHT ABSORPTION. Dilute 10 ml to 500 ml with water. Dilute 5 ml of this solution to 100 ml with water and measure the extinction of a 1-cm layer at the maximum at about 525 nm; the extinction is not less than 0·360 and not more than 0·440.

Ammonia Solution, Aromatic

SYNONYM: Sal Volatile Solution

Ammonium Bicarbonate	..	25 g
Strong Ammonia Solution	..	67·5 ml
Nutmeg Oil ..	..	0·3 ml
Lemon Oil ..	..	0·5 ml
Alcohol (90 per cent)	..	37·5 ml
Purified Water, freshly boiled and cooled		to 1000 ml

Dissolve the ammonium bicarbonate in 800 ml of the water and add the lemon oil and the nutmeg oil previously dissolved in the alcohol, the strong ammonia solution, and

sufficient water to produce the required volume. Add 25 g of Purified Talc, previously sterilised, shake, allow to stand for a few hours, shaking occasionally, and filter.

Standard
WEIGHT PER ML. At 20°, 0·980 g to 1·005 g.
ALCOHOL CONTENT. 2·6 to 3·5 per cent v/v of ethyl alcohol, determined by the method given in Appendix 10, page 888.
CONTENT OF AMMONIUM CARBONATE. 2·76 to 3·24 per cent w/v, calculated as $(NH_4)_2CO_3$, determined by the following method:
To 20 ml add 25 ml of 1N sodium hydroxide and 40 ml of *barium chloride solution*, heat on a water-bath for 15 minutes, cool, add 10 ml of *formaldehyde solution*, previously neutralised to *thymol blue solution*, and titrate the excess of alkali with 1N hydrochloric acid to the grey colour indicative of pH 8·8, using *thymol blue solution* as indicator; each ml of 1N sodium hydroxide is equivalent to 0·04804 g of $(NH_4)_2CO_3$.
CONTENT OF FREE AMMONIA. 1·12 to 1·25 per cent w/v, calculated as NH_3, determined by the following method:
To 20 ml add 50 ml of 1N hydrochloric acid, boil, cool, and titrate the excess of acid with 1N sodium hydroxide, using *methyl red solution* as indicator; each ml of 1N hydrochloric acid, after the volume of 1N sodium hydroxide required in the determination of ammonium carbonate has been deducted, is equivalent to 0·01703 g of NH_3.

Storage. It should be stored in airtight containers, in a cool place.

Dose. 1 to 5 millilitres, diluted with water.

Ammonia Solution, Dilute

Strong Ammonia Solution	..	375 ml
Purified Water, freshly boiled and cooled		to 1000 ml

Standard
WEIGHT PER ML. At 20°, 0·955 g to 0·959 g.
CONTENT OF AMMONIA. 9·5 to 10·5 per cent w/w, calculated as NH_3, determined by the following method:
Weigh accurately about 6 g into 50 ml of 1N hydrochloric acid and titrate the excess of acid with 1N sodium hydroxide, using *methyl red solution* as indicator; each ml of 1N hydrochloric acid is equivalent to 0·01703 g of NH_3.

Storage. It should be stored in airtight containers, in a cool place.

Note. When Ammonia Solution or Liquor Ammoniae is prescribed or demanded, Dilute Ammonia Solution shall be supplied.

Ammonium Acetate Solution, Strong

It may be prepared as follows:

Ammonium Bicarbonate	..	470 g
Glacial Acetic Acid	..	453 g
Strong Ammonia Solution	a sufficient quantity	
Purified Water, freshly boiled and cooled		to 1000 ml

Dissolve the ammonium bicarbonate by adding gradually to the glacial acetic acid diluted with 350 ml of the water and add the strong ammonia solution until one drop of the resulting solution diluted with ten drops of purified water gives a full blue colour with one drop of *bromothymol blue solution* and a full yellow colour with one drop of *thymol blue solution*; about 100 ml of the strong ammonia solution is required. Add sufficient of the water to produce the required volume.

Standard

ACIDITY OR ALKALINITY. pH of a 10·0 per cent v/v solution in *carbon dioxide-free water*, 7·0 to 8·0.

WEIGHT PER ML. At 20°, 1·085 g to 1·095 g.

CONTENT OF AMMONIUM ACETATE. 55·0 to 60·0 per cent w/v, calculated as $C_2H_7NO_2$, determined by the following method:
To 5 ml add 50 ml of water and 12 ml of *formaldehyde solution*, previously neutralised to *phenolphthalein solution*, and titrate with 1N sodium hydroxide, using *phenolphthalein solution* as indicator; each ml of 1N sodium hydroxide is equivalent to 0·07708 g of $C_2H_7NO_2$.

Storage. It should be stored in lead-free glass bottles.

Dose. 1 to 5 millilitres.

When Ammonium Acetate Solution, Liquor Ammonii Acetatis, Dilute Ammonium Acetate Solution, or Liquor Ammonii Acetatis Dilutus is prescribed or demanded, Strong Ammonium Acetate Solution diluted to eight times its volume with freshly boiled and cooled Purified Water shall be supplied.

Benzoic Acid Solution

Benzoic Acid	..	..	50 g
Propylene Glycol..	..	..	750 ml
Purified Water, freshly boiled and cooled	..	..	1000 ml

Dissolve the benzoic acid in the propylene glycol and add sufficient water, in small quantities and with constant stirring, to produce the required volume.

Standard

WEIGHT PER ML. At 20°, 1·045 g to 1·055 g.

CONTENT OF BENZOIC ACID. 4·75 to 5·25 per cent w/v, calculated as $C_7H_6O_2$, determined by the following method:
To 10 ml add 20 ml of *alcohol (95 per cent)*, previously neutralised to *phenolphthalein solution*, and titrate with 0·1N sodium hydroxide, using *phenolphthalein solution* as indicator; each ml of 0·1N sodium hydroxide is equivalent to 0·01221 g of $C_7H_6O_2$.

Calcium Hydroxide Solution

SYNONYM: Lime Water

Calcium Hydroxide	.. ..	10 g
Purified Water, freshly boiled and cooled	.. ..	1000 ml

Shake together thoroughly and repeatedly; allow to stand until clear. The clear solution may be drawn off with a siphon, as required.

Standard

DESCRIPTION. A clear colourless liquid. It absorbs carbon dioxide from the air, a film of calcium carbonate being formed on the surface of the liquid. It becomes turbid when boiled and clear again after cooling.

PRESENCE OF CALCIUM. It gives the reactions characteristic of calcium.

CONTENT OF CALCIUM HYDROXIDE. Not less than 0·15 per cent w/v, calculated as $Ca(OH)_2$, determined by the following method:
Titrate 25 ml with 0·1N hydrochloric acid, using *phenolphthalein solution* as indicator; each ml of 0·1N hydrochloric acid is equivalent to 0·003705 g of $Ca(OH)_2$.

Storage. It should be stored in well-filled airtight containers.

Cetrimide Solution

Strong Cetrimide Solution	..	25 ml
Purified Water, freshly boiled and cooled	.. .. ..	to 1000 ml

It must be freshly prepared unless it is issued as sterile in sealed containers.

Standard

CONTENT OF CETRIMIDE. 0·90 to 1·10 per cent w/v, calculated as $C_{17}H_{38}BrN$, determined by the method for Cetrimide Cream, page 657, using 1 ml diluted to 10 ml with water and beginning with the words "add 5 ml of *dilute sulphuric acid* . . .".

Sterilisation. The solution may be sterilised by autoclaving or by filtration (see Appendix 29, page 921).

Containers. Containers should be thoroughly cleansed before being filled. Closures should be such that the solution does not come into contact with cork. In addition, if the solution is issued as sterile, the directions given under Solutions (page 779) should be followed.

Labelling. The label on the container of a non-sterilised solution states that the solution should not be used later than one week after issue for use.

The label on the sealed container of a solution issued as sterile states:
(1) the name of the solution as "Sterile Cetrimide Solution",
(2) the words "Not for Injection", and
(3) that the solution should not be used later than one week after the container is first opened.

Cetrimide Solution, Strong

Strong Cetrimide Solution is a 40 per cent w/v aqueous solution of Cetrimide, containing 7·5 per cent v/v of Alcohol (95 per cent) and 0·0075 per cent w/v of tartrazine (food grade of commerce). It may be perfumed.

In making this preparation the alcohol (95 per cent) may be replaced by Industrial Methylated Spirit, provided that the law and the statutory regulations governing the use of industrial methylated spirit are observed.

Standard

ALCOHOL CONTENT. 6·5 to 7·5 per cent v/v of ethyl alcohol, determined by the method given in Appendix 10, page 888.

CONTENT OF CETRIMIDE. 38·0 to 42·0 per cent w/v, calculated as $C_{17}H_{38}BrN$, determined by the following method:
Dilute 5 ml to 100 ml with water and to 25 ml of this solution add 10 ml of 0·1N sodium hydroxide and 10·0 ml of a freshly prepared 5 per cent w/v solution of *potassium iodide* in water and extract with 25 ml of *chloroform* followed by three successive 10-ml portions of *chloroform*, shaking well and discarding each chloroform extract.
To the aqueous solution add 40 ml of *hydrochloric acid*, cool, titrate with 0·05M potassium iodate until the solution is pale brown, add 2 ml of *chloroform*, and

continue the titration, shaking well between each addition, until the chloroform layer is colourless.

Titrate a mixture of 20 ml of water, 10·0 ml of the potassium iodide solution, and 40 ml of *hydrochloric acid* with 0·05M potassium iodate in a similar manner. The difference between the titrations represents the amount of 0·05M potassium iodate required by the sample; each ml of 0·05M potassium iodate is equivalent to 0·03364 g of $C_{17}H_{38}BrN$.

Containers. Containers should be thoroughly cleansed before being filled. Closures should be such that the solution does not come into contact with cork.

Chlorhexidine Solution, Dilute

SYNONYM: Alcoholic Chlorhexidine Solution

Chlorhexidine Gluconate Solution	25 ml
Carmoisine, food grade of commerce	0·5 g
Alcohol (95 per cent)	700 ml
Purified Water, freshly boiled and cooled	to 1000 ml

In making this preparation, the alcohol (95 per cent) may be replaced by Industrial Methylated Spirit, provided that the law and the statutory regulations governing the use of industrial methylated spirit are observed; alternatively, if specified by the prescriber, the alcohol (95 per cent) may be replaced by Isopropyl Alcohol.

Standard

PRESENCE OF CHLORHEXIDINE GLUCONATE. 1. Warm 10 ml on a water-bath until the alcohol has evaporated, cool, add 1 ml of *ferric chloride solution*, and heat gently to boiling; a deep orange colour is produced. Add 1 ml of *hydrochloric acid*; the colour changes to yellow.

2. To 20 ml add 5 mg of *sodium dithionite* to decolorise the solution, warm on a water-bath until the alcohol has evaporated, cool, add *sodium hydroxide solution*, dropwise, until the solution is alkaline to *titan yellow paper*, and add 1 ml in excess; a precipitate is produced which, after washing with water and recrystallising from *alcohol (70 per cent)*, melts at about 132°.

CONTENT OF CHLORHEXIDINE GLUCONATE. 0·45 to 0·55 per cent w/v, determined by the following method:

Dilute 5 ml to 100 ml with *methyl alcohol*, mix, and continue the method given for Chlorhexidine Cream, page 657, beginning with the words "To 5 ml of this solution add . . .".

Containers. Containers should be thoroughly cleansed before being filled. Closures should be such that the solution does not come into contact with cork.

Note. When prepared with alcohol (95 per cent) or industrial methylated spirit the solution should be used within one year, and when prepared with isopropyl alcohol the solution should be used within three years of the date of preparation.

Chlorinated Lime and Boric Acid Solution

SYNONYM: Eusol

Chlorinated Lime	12·5 g
Boric Acid, in powder	12·5 g
Water (see page 642) ..	to 1000 ml

Reduce the chlorinated lime to fine powder, triturate it with sufficient of the water to form a paste, and add a further portion of the water; add the boric acid, shake well, add

sufficient water to produce the required volume, allow to stand, and filter.

It should be recently prepared.

Standard

CONTENT OF AVAILABLE CHLORINE. Not less than 0·25 per cent w/v, calculated as Cl, determined by the following method:

Add 20 ml to 5 ml of a 20 per cent w/v solution of *potassium iodide* in water; add 4 ml of *acetic acid* and titrate the liberated iodine with 0·1N sodium thiosulphate; each ml of 0·1N sodium thiosulphate is equivalent to 0·003545 g of available chlorine, Cl.

Storage. It should be stored in well-filled airtight bottles, protected from light, in a cool place.

It deteriorates on storage and should be used within two weeks of its preparation.

Labelling. The label on the container states the date after which the solution is not intended to be used.

Chlorinated Soda Solution, Surgical

SYNONYM: Dakin's Solution

Boric Acid ..	a sufficient quantity
Chlorinated Lime	a sufficient quantity
Sodium Carbonate	a sufficient quantity
Purified Water, freshly boiled and cooled	1000 ml

Determine the proportion of available chlorine in the chlorinated lime by the assay described under Chlorinated Lime (page 99) and prepare the solution by the following method, using the quantities of ingredients indicated in the table.

Available Chlorine in Chlorinated Lime per cent w/w	Chlorinated Lime g	Sodium Carbonate g	Boric Acid g
30	18·8	37·6	4·00
31	18·2	36·4	3·87
32	17·6	35·2	3·75
33	17·1	34·2	3·64
34	16·6	33·2	3·53
35	16·1	32·2	3·43
36	15·7	31·4	3·33
37	15·3	30·6	3·24
38	14·9	29·8	3·16
39	14·5	29·0	3·08
40	14·1	28·2	3·00

Dissolve the sodium carbonate in the water and add the solution, gradually and with constant trituration, to the chlorinated lime, previously powdered; shake occasionally during twenty minutes, allow to stand for a further ten minutes, decant, and filter through a bleached filter; dissolve the boric acid in the filtrate.

It should be recently prepared.

Standard

CONTENT OF AVAILABLE CHLORINE. 0·50 to 0·55 per cent w/v, calculated as Cl, determined by the following method:

Add 10 ml to 5 ml of a 20 per cent w/v solution of *potassium iodide* in water; add 4 ml of *acetic acid* and titrate the liberated iodine with 0·1N sodium thiosulphate; each ml of 0·1N sodium thiosulphate is equivalent to 0·003545 g of available chlorine, Cl.

Storage. It should be stored in well-filled airtight bottles, protected from light, in a cool place.

Chloroxylenol Solution

SYNONYM: Roxenol

Chloroxylenol	..	..	..	50·0 g
Potassium Hydroxide	..	..		13·6 g
Oleic Acid	..	..	..	7·5 ml
Castor Oil..	..	..	..	63·0 g
Terpineol ..	..	..	..	100 ml
Alcohol (95 per cent)	..	..		200 ml
Purified Water, freshly boiled and cooled	..	..	..	to 1000 ml

Dissolve the potassium hydroxide in 15 ml of the water, add a solution of the castor oil in 63 ml of the alcohol, mix, allow to stand for one hour or until a small portion of the mixture remains clear when diluted with nineteen times its volume of purified water, and then add the oleic acid. Mix the terpineol with a solution of the chloroxylenol in the remainder of the alcohol, pour into the soap solution, and add sufficient of the water to produce the required volume.

In making this preparation the alcohol (95 per cent) may be replaced by Industrial Methylated Spirit, provided that the law and the statutory regulations governing the use of industrial methylated spirit are observed.

Standard
ALCOHOL CONTENT. 16 to 20 per cent v/v of ethyl alcohol, determined by the method given in Appendix 10, page 888.

CONTENT OF CHLOROXYLENOL. 4·5 to 5·5 per cent w/v, calculated as C_8H_9ClO, determined by the following method:
To 5 ml add 5 ml of *sodium hydroxide solution*, evaporate to dryness, mix the residue with 2 g of *anhydrous sodium carbonate* in a platinum crucible, fill the crucible with *anhydrous sodium carbonate*, place 3 pellets of *sodium hydroxide* on the top of the sodium carbonate, and invert the crucible in a larger crucible containing *anhydrous sodium carbonate*; add sufficient *anhydrous sodium carbonate* to seal the junction of the crucibles, heat gently for 10 minutes, then heat strongly for 30 minutes, and allow to cool.
Dissolve the residue in water, filter, wash the filter with water, combine the filtrate and washings, and continue by the method given in Appendix 11, page 891; each ml of 0·1N silver nitrate is equivalent to 0·01566 g of C_8H_9ClO.

Containers. Containers should be thoroughly cleansed before being filled. Closures should be such that the solution does not come into contact with cork.

Coal Tar Solution, Strong

SYNONYM: Liquor Picis Carbonis Fortis

Prepared Coal Tar	..	..	400 g
Quillaia, in moderately coarse powder ..	..	..	.. 100 g
Alcohol (95 per cent)	..	..	to 1000 ml

Macerate the prepared coal tar and the quillaia with 800 ml of the alcohol in a closed vessel for seven days, shaking occasionally; filter,

pass through the filter sufficient of the alcohol to produce the required volume, and mix.

In making this preparation, the alcohol (95 per cent) may be replaced by Industrial Methylated Spirit, provided that the law and the statutory regulations governing the use of industrial methylated spirit are observed.

Standard
ALCOHOL CONTENT. 77 to 83 per cent v/v of ethyl alcohol, determined by the method given in Appendix 10, page 888.

Note. This preparation cannot be mixed with alcohol to prepare Coal Tar Solution, as precipitation occurs on dilution.

Ferric Chloride Solution

SYNONYM: Liquor Ferri Perchloridi

Strong Ferric Chloride Solution..		250 ml
Water (see page 642)	..	.. to 1000 ml

Standard
CONTENT OF FERRIC CHLORIDE. 13·9 to 16·1 per cent w/v, calculated as $FeCl_3$, determined by the following method:
Dilute 25 ml to 250 ml with water; to 20 ml of this solution add 1 ml of *sulphuric acid* and 0·1N potassium permanganate, dropwise, until the pink colour persists for 5 seconds, and continue by the method for Strong Ferric Chloride Solution, below, beginning with the words "Add 15 ml of *hydrochloric acid* . . .".

Dose. 0·3 to 1 millilitre.

Ferric Chloride Solution is incompatible with alkalis, iodides, astringent infusions, and acacia mucilages.

Ferric Chloride Solution, Strong

SYNONYM: Liquor Ferri Perchloridi Fortis

It may be prepared as follows:

Iron	..	..	..	210 g
Nitric Acid	..	..	..	90 ml
Hydrochloric Acid		..	..	1230 ml
Water (see page 642)		a sufficient quantity		

Place the iron in a flask, add a mixture of 750 ml of the hydrochloric acid and 420 ml of the water, heat at a moderate temperature until effervescence ceases, boil, and filter from undissolved iron, washing the flask and contents with a little water and pouring the washings over the filter.

To the combined filtrate and washings add 420 ml of the hydrochloric acid, mix, and pour the solution in a slow continuous stream into the nitric acid, chemical action being promoted, if necessary, by gently warming.

Evaporate the product until a precipitate begins to form and add 60 ml of the hydrochloric acid and sufficient water to produce 1050 ml or to make the resulting solution correspond to the following standard.

Standard
WEIGHT PER ML. At 20°, 1·42 g to 1·46 g.

ARSENIC. It complies with the test given in Appendix 6, page 878 (8 parts per million).

COPPER. To 2·5 ml add 7·5 ml of water, 18 ml of *hydrochloric acid*, and 0·2 ml of *hydrogen peroxide solution*, boil gently for 5 minutes, cool, extract with four successive 20-ml portions of *solvent ether*, and discard the extracts; evaporate the acid layer to dryness, and dissolve the residue in 10 ml of 1N hydrochloric acid. Reserve a portion of the solution for the test for zinc.

To 1 ml of this solution add 25 ml of water·and 1 g of *copper-free citric acid*, make alkaline to *litmus paper* with *dilute ammonia solution*, dilute to 50 ml with water, add 1 ml of *sodium diethyldithiocarbamate solution*, and allow to stand for 5 minutes.

Any colour which develops is not deeper than that produced by 6 ml of *dilute copper sulphate solution* and 1 ml of 1N hydrochloric acid when similarly treated.

FERROUS IRON. In the determination of ferric chloride below, not more than 0·3 ml of 0·1N potassium permanganate is required.

LEAD. It complies with the test given in Appendix 7, page 882 (60 parts per million).

ZINC. To 5 ml of the solution prepared for the test for copper, add 15 ml of 1N sodium hydroxide, boil, filter, wash the residue with water, and dilute the combined filtrate and washings to 25 ml with water.

To 5 ml of this solution add 5 ml of 1N hydrochloric acid and 2 g of *ammonium chloride*, dilute to 50 ml with water, add 1 ml of *potassium ferrocyanide solution*, and allow to stand for 5 minutes.

Any opalescence is not greater than that produced when 1 ml of *potassium ferrocyanide solution* is added to a solution prepared from 5 ml of *dilute zinc sulphate solution*, 3 ml of 1N sodium hydroxide, 6 ml of 1N hydrochloric acid, and 2 g of *ammonium chloride*, diluted to 50 ml with water, and allowed to stand for 5 minutes.

HYDROCHLORIC ACID. Not more than 4·0 per cent w/v, calculated as HCl, determined by the method given in Appendix 11, page 891, 5 ml of the dilution prepared in the determination of ferric chloride being used; deduct from twice the volume of 0·1N silver nitrate used three times the volume of 0·1N sodium thiosulphate required in the determination of ferric chloride; each ml of 0·1N silver nitrate is equivalent to 0·003646 g of HCl.

CONTENT OF FERRIC CHLORIDE. 58·5 to 61·5 per cent w/v, calculated as $FeCl_3$, determined by the following method:

Dilute 10 ml to 200 ml with water; to 10 ml of this solution add 10 ml of water, 1 ml of *sulphuric acid*, and 0·1N potassium permanganate, dropwise, until the pink colour persists for 5 seconds.

Add 15 ml of *hydrochloric acid* and 2 g of *potassium iodide*, allow to stand for 3 minutes, and titrate the liberated iodine with 0·1N sodium thiosulphate; each ml of 0·1N sodium thiosulphate is equivalent to 0·01622 g of $FeCl_3$.

Note. Strong Ferric Chloride Solution is incompatible with alkalis, iodides, astringent infusions, and acacia mucilages.

Green S and Tartrazine Solution

Green S, food grade of commerce	..	5 g
Tartrazine, food grade of commerce ..	.. .. ..	5 g
Chloroform Water	..	to 1000 ml

Standard
PRESENCE OF GREEN S AND OF TARTRAZINE. It complies with the thin-layer chromatographic test given in Appendix 5A, page 864.

Haemodialysis Solutions

SYNONYMS: Haemodialysis Fluids; Dialysing Solutions for Artificial Kidney

Haemodialysis solutions are aqueous solutions of electrolytes and dextrose approximating in composition to a normal extracellular body fluid.

Although there is no necessity for haemodialysis solutions to be sterile, precautions should be taken to prevent heavy bacterial contamination during their preparation and use, as some metabolic products of bacteria can pass through the membrane of the artificial kidney.

Preparation of haemodialysis solutions. These are prepared for use in a kidney machine by diluting a concentrated solution with an appropriate type of water (see below). There are three methods of dilution that may be used: batch blending, fixed proportioning, and flexible proportioning.

Batch blending involves the dilution of the requisite volume of concentrate to the stated volume in a large tank, which may or may not be part of the kidney machine.

Fixed proportioning pumps are fitted to some kidney machines. With these pumps a fixed ratio of concentrate is added to the diluting water flowing into the kidney machine, but there is no means whereby this ratio may be changed if it becomes necessary to adjust the strength of the diluted solution.

Flexible proportioning pumps on kidney machines allow the ratio of concentrate to diluent to be adjusted to a limited extent.

Concentrated solutions. A number of concentrated solutions, each differing in composition and in the extent to which they must be diluted, are in use. They usually contain sodium acetate as a source of bicarbonate, because this salt is more soluble in water than sodium bicarbonate.

The quantities of the salts in the concentrated haemodialysis solutions are such that when the solutions are diluted to an appropriate extent, usually 35 or 40 times, the final concentrations of the ions, per litre, are usually in the ranges:

sodium, 130 to 140 mmol (mEq); potassium, 0 to 4 mmol (mEq); calcium, 1·5 to 2 mmol (3 to 4 mEq); magnesium, 0·45 to 0·75 mmol (0·9 to 1·5 mEq); bicarbonate (or its equivalent as acetate or lactate), 25 to 35 mmol (mEq); and chloride, 101 to 112 mmol (mEq). The final concentration of dextrose is usually 0·1 to 0·2 per cent.

Suitable concentrated solutions may be prepared according to the following formulae:

Concentrated Haemodialysis Solution (35 ×)

Potassium Chloride	..	..	2·6 g
Dextrose (monohydrate)..		..	70·0 g
Sodium Acetate ..	..	..	166·6 g
Sodium Chloride..	..	..	194·5 g
Purified Water, freshly boiled and cooled ..	..	..	to 1000 ml

For each 35 litres of haemodialysis solution required in the artificial kidney, dilute 1 litre of Concentrated Haemodialysis Solution (35 ×) with 34 litres of the appropriate type of water (see below).

The diluted solution, when prepared with Purified Water, contains in 1 litre the following concentrations of ions: 130 mmol (mEq) of Na^+, 1·0 mmol (mEq) of K^+, the equivalent of 35 mmol (mEq) of HCO_3^-, and 96 mmol (mEq) of Cl^-.

Concentrated Haemodialysis Solution (40 ×)

Potassium Chloride	.. ..	4·0 g
Dextrose (monohydrate)..	..	80·0 g
Sodium Acetate ..	.. ..	190·4 g
Sodium Chloride..	.. ..	222·4 g
Lactic Acid	.. .. ..	4 ml
Purified Water, freshly boiled and		
cooled ..	.. .. ..	to 1000 ml

For each 40 litres of haemodialysis solution required in the artificial kidney, dilute 1 litre of Concentrated Haemodialysis Solution (40 ×) with 39 litres of the appropriate type of water (see below).

The diluted solution, when prepared with Purified Water, contains in 1 litre the following concentrations of ions: 130 mmol (mEq) of Na^+, 1·3 mmol (mEq) of K^+, the equivalent to 36 mmol (mEq) of HCO_3^-, and 96 mmol (mEq) of Cl^-.

Water for diluting concentrated haemodialysis solutions. Mains water, mains water softened by base exchange, or Purified Water is used.

Where Purified Water is used, the formulae given above are suitable for use without modification in respect of the sodium content of the diluted solution.

In hard water areas, if mains water is to be used, it is usual to pass it first through a base-exchange water softener, but in removing the calcium and magnesium salts responsible for the hardness, equivalent amounts of sodium ions are introduced into the softened water. These amounts vary from 5 to 7 mmol per litre in the London area, but will differ in other places and, in addition, might be subject to seasonal variation in any given area.

In soft water areas where the natural calcium content of mains water is less than 1·5 mmol per litre, softening may or may not be carried out and the ordinary mains water may be used, allowance again being made, if necessary, for the sodium present. Whichever type of water is used for diluting the concentrate, it should be de-gassed and filtered to remove particles larger than 25 micrometres.

Inclusion of calcium and magnesium ions. The calcium and magnesium ions required in the diluted haemodialysis solution may be obtained in some areas simply by using the unsoftened mains water to dilute the concentrate. In other areas, supplementary additions of Calcium Acetate or Calcium Chloride and Magnesium Acetate or Magnesium Chloride may need to be made.

If Purified Water or softened mains water is used as the diluent, the whole of the required calcium and magnesium ions in the form of the salts must either be added to the dilute artificial kidney solution or included in the concentrated solution.

Standard for Concentrated Haemodialysis Solutions

DESCRIPTION. A colourless to pale straw-coloured liquid.

CONTENT OF DEXTROSE. 95·0 to 105·0 per cent of the concentration stated on the label, calculated as $C_6H_{12}O_6$, determined by the method given in Appendix 15, page 894.

CONTENT OF TOTAL CHLORIDE. 95·0 to 105·0 per cent of the concentration stated on the label, calculated as Cl, determined by the method given in Appendix 11, page 891, an accurately weighed quantity, equivalent to about 2 mmol of sodium chloride, diluted with 50 ml of water, being used; each ml of 0·1N silver nitrate is equivalent to 0·1 mmol of Cl. Determine the weight per ml of the sample and calculate the concentration of Cl in mmol per litre.

CONTENT OF SODIUM. 97·0 to 103·0 per cent of the concentration stated on the label, calculated as Na, determined by the method of the British Pharmacopoeia, Appendix XIA, for flame photometry, an accurately weighed quantity, diluted to a suitable volume with water, being used; use *sodium solution FP*, diluted if necessary with water, for the standard solutions.
Determine the weight per ml of the sample and calculate the concentration of Na in mmol per litre.

CONTENT OF POTASSIUM. 95·0 to 105·0 per cent of the concentration stated on the label, calculated as K, determined by the method of the British Pharmacopoeia, Appendix XIA, for flame photometry, an accurately weighed quantity, diluted to a suitable volume with water, being used; use *potassium solution FP*, diluted if necessary with water, for the standard solutions.
Determine the weight per ml of the sample and calculate the concentration of K in mmol per litre.

If the concentrated haemodialysis solution contains calcium and magnesium ions, it complies with the following additional requirements:

CONTENT OF CALCIUM. 95·0 to 105·0 per cent of the concentration stated on the label, calculated as Ca, determined by the method for Intraperitoneal Dialysis Solutions, page 787, an accurately measured volume, equivalent to about 1 mmol of calcium being used and the titration being with 0·05M disodium edetate; each ml of 0·05M disodium edetate is equivalent to 0·05 mmol of Ca.
Calculate the concentration of Ca in mmol per litre.

CONTENT OF MAGNESIUM. 95·0 to 105·0 per cent of the concentration stated on the label, calculated as Mg, determined by the method for Intraperitoneal Dialysis Solutions, page 787, an accurately measured volume, equivalent to about 1 mmol of magnesium, being used and the titration being with 0·05M disodium edetate; each ml of 0·05M disodium edetate is equivalent to 0·05 mmol of Mg.
Calculate the concentration of Mg in mmol per litre.

Containers. Concentrated haemodialysis solutions are supplied in suitable glass or plastic containers which do not release ions or harmful substances into the solution. Separation of solid particles from the glass containers may occur on storage; solutions containing such particles must not be used.

Labelling. The label on the container of the concentrated solution states:
(1) the strength of the solution stated as a percentage or weight per litre for each ingredient, the quantity of dextrose being expressed in terms of anhydrous dextrose, $C_6H_{12}O_6$;
(2) the number of millimoles of each ion present per litre;
(3) that the solution must be diluted before use; and
(4) the directions for diluting the solution.
The label may state, in addition, the number of milli-equivalents of each ion present per litre.

Storage. Concentrated Haemodialysis Solution ($40 \times$) should be kept in a warm place as it is liable to deposit crystals on keeping.

Uses. Haemodialysis solutions are employed, in cases of temporary or permanent renal failure, in the artificial kidney to remove the excess of water and accumulated waste products normally excreted from the body by the kidney, and to correct electrolyte imbalance.

In the treatment of poisoning, elimination of poisons which diffuse across the dialyser membrane may be hastened by haemodialysis and elimination may sometimes be assisted by adjustment of the pH of the dialysis solution. Substances that are strongly bound to body protein are not effectively removed by dialysis.

Haemodialysis has been shown to be of value in the treatment of renal failure occurring with *P. falciparum* infections (malignant tertian malaria). In this condition renal damage associated with tubular necrosis may give rise to oliguria or anuria with uraemia. Dialysis may prolong life until the renal lesion has healed and should be considered in all patients with *P. falciparum* infections who have oliguria and a rising blood urea.

In patients with a severe degree of renal damage, dialysis may need to be continued for several weeks and for such patients haemodialysis is the only practicable method. For those with less severe degrees of renal damage intraperitoneal dialysis may be satisfactory.

Cholera, severe dysentery, and gastro-enteritis, particularly in infants and young children, may similarly give rise to renal damage necessitating haemodialysis or peritoneal dialysis.

Concentrated Haemodialysis Solution ($35 \times$) contains in 1 litre approximately 4500 mmol (mEq) of Na^+, 35 mmol (mEq) of K^+, the equivalent of 1225 mmol (mEq) of HCO_3^-, and 3360 mmol (mEq) of Cl^-.

Concentrated Haemodialysis Solution ($40 \times$) contains in 1 litre approximately 5200 mmol (mEq) of Na^+, 54 mmol (mEq) of K^+, the equivalent of 1445 mmol (mEq) of HCO_3^-, and 3855 mmol (mEq) of Cl^-.

Hexachlorophane Solution, Concentrated

Hexachlorophane..	..	..	100 g
Sodium Hydroxide	..	..	10 g
Alcohol (95 per cent)	..	..	400 ml
Purified Water, freshly boiled and cooled ..	..	..	.. to 1000 ml

Dissolve the hexachlorophane in the alcohol. Dissolve the sodium hydroxide in 500 ml of the water, mix the two solutions, add sufficient of the water to produce the required volume, and mix.

In making this preparation the alcohol (95 per cent) may be replaced by Industrial Methylated Spirit, provided that the law and the statutory regulations governing the use of industrial methylated spirit are observed.

Standard
PRESENCE OF HEXACHLOROPHANE. To 5 ml add 5 ml of *dilute hydrochloric acid*, extract with two successive 15-ml portions of *solvent ether*, and evaporate the combined extracts to dryness on a water-bath.
The residue complies with the following tests:
(i) Heat 0·1 g in a dry tube; a colourless to amber liquid is produced which, on further heating, becomes green, then blue, and finally purple.
(ii) Dissolve 5 mg in 5 ml of *alcohol (95 per cent)* and add 0·05 ml of *ferric chloride solution*; a transient purple colour is produced.
(iii) Dissolve 0·1 g in 0·5 ml of *acetone*, add *titanous chloride solution*, and shake; a yellowish-orange oil separates, which is soluble in *benzene*, in *chloroform*, and in *solvent ether*.
(iv) It melts at about 164°.

CONTENT OF HEXACHLOROPHANE. 9·5 to 10·5 per cent w/v, determined by the following method:
Evaporate 10 ml to dryness on a water-bath; dissolve the residue in 7·5 ml of 1N sodium hydroxide and dilute to 100 ml with water.
Dilute 5 ml of this solution to 500 ml with 0·1N sodium hydroxide, further dilute 10 ml of this solution to 100 ml with 0·1N sodium hydroxide, and measure the extinction of a 1-cm layer at the maximum at about 321 nm, using 0·1N sodium hydroxide as the blank.
For purposes of calculation, use a value of 300 for the E(1 per cent, 1 cm) of hexachlorophane.
Calculate the percentage of hexachlorophane in the sample.

Containers. It should not be dispensed in types of containers that are normally used for medicinal products taken internally. Containers should be thoroughly cleansed before being filled.
Closures should be such that the solution does not come into contact with cork.

Labelling. The container should be labelled "30 ml (1 fl. oz.) to be added to a bath of about 100 to 150 litres (20 to 30 gallons) of water". In addition, if the preparation is to be used in a hard water area, the label should state that a suitable water softener should be added to the water before adding the solution.
The label also states that this preparation should only be used in accordance with medical advice.

Storage. It should be protected from light.

Intraperitoneal Dialysis Solutions

SYNONYMS: Intraperitoneal Dialysis Fluids; Peritoneal Dialysis Solutions

Intraperitoneal dialysis solutions are sterile aqueous solutions of electrolytes and dextrose approximating in composition to a normal extracellular body fluid. They contain sodium ions, calcium ions, and magnesium ions, in association with chloride ions and bicarbonate ions. Either lactate or acetate is used as the source of the bicarbonate ions.

The solutions are rendered slightly hypertonic by the inclusion of dextrose, which is usually present in a concentration of about

1·4 per cent, but when a more rapid removal of water is required, the tonicity is increased by including higher concentrations of dextrose, which can be up to 7 per cent.

Potassium chloride is usually administered separately in accordance with the needs of the patient.

Preparation of intraperitoneal dialysis solutions. Suitable solutions may be prepared according to the following formulae:

Intraperitoneal Dialysis Solution (Lactate)

Magnesium Chloride	..	..	0·15 g
Calcium Chloride	..	..	0·26 g
Lactic Acid ⎤ equivalent to			
Sodium Hydroxide ⎦ sodium lactate	..		5·00 g
Sodium Chloride..	..	..	5·60 g
Anhydrous Dextrose	..	..	13·60 g
Sodium Metabisulphite ..	..		0·05 g
Water for Injections	..	.. to 1000 ml	

The quantity of sodium lactate required may be obtained from 3·8 ml of the lactic acid and 1·8 g of the sodium hydroxide and the procedure described in the British Pharmacopoeia for the preparation of Sodium Lactate Injection followed; if the sodium lactate is prepared in this way, a small quantity of sodium chloride is formed and consequently the amount of sodium chloride in the recipe should be reduced by an amount corresponding to the volume of hydrochloric acid used in the preparation of the solution.

Dissolve the other ingredients in a portion of the water, mix with the sodium lactate solution, filter, and sterilise by autoclaving (see Appendix 29, page 921); the type of autoclave used should be such that rapid cooling of the solution may be effected, in order to prevent caramelisation of the dextrose.

Intraperitoneal Dialysis Solution (Acetate)

Magnesium Chloride	..	..	0·152 g
Calcium Chloride	..	..	0·220 g
Sodium Acetate ..	..	..	4·760 g
Sodium Chloride..	..	..	5·560 g
Anhydrous Dextrose	..	..	17·000 g
Sodium Metabisulphite ..	..		0·150 g
Water for Injections	..	.. to 1000 ml	

Dissolve, filter, and sterilise by autoclaving (see Appendix 29, page 921); the type of autoclave used should be such that rapid cooling of the solution may be effected, in order to prevent caramelisation of the dextrose.

Standard

It complies with the standard under Solutions, page 779, with the following additions:

PYROGENS. It complies with the test for pyrogens, a volume of not less than 10 ml per kg of the rabbit's weight being used.

CONTENT OF DEXTROSE. 92·5 to 107·5 per cent of the concentration stated on the label, calculated as $C_6H_{12}O_6$, determined by the method given in Appendix 15, page 894.

CONTENT OF TOTAL CHLORIDE. 95·0 to 105·0 per cent of the concentration stated on the label, calculated as Cl, determined by the method given in Appendix 11, page 891, an accurately measured volume, equivalent to about 2 mmol of sodium chloride, diluted to 50 ml with water, being used; each ml of 0·1N silver nitrate is equivalent to 0·1 mmol of Cl.
Calculate the concentration of Cl in mmol per litre.

CONTENT OF SODIUM. 95·0 to 105·0 per cent of the concentration stated on the label, calculated as Na, determined by the method of the British Pharmacopoeia, Appendix XIA, for flame photometry, an accurately measured volume, diluted to a suitable volume with water, being used; use *sodium solution FP*, diluted if necessary with water, for the standard solutions.
Calculate the concentration of Na in mmol per litre.

CONTENT OF CALCIUM. 90·0 to 110·0 per cent of the concentration stated on the label, calculated as Ca, determined by the following method:
To an accurately measured volume, equivalent to about 0·1 mmol of calcium, add 40 ml of water and 10 ml of a 40 per cent w/v solution of *potassium hydroxide* in water, mix well, allow to stand for 3 minutes, and titrate with 0·02M disodium edetate, using *calcon carboxylic acid mixture* as indicator; each ml of 0·02M disodium edetate is equivalent to 0·02 mmol of Ca.
Calculate the concentration of Ca in mmol per litre.

CONTENT OF MAGNESIUM. 87·0 to 113·0 per cent of the concentration stated on the label, calculated as Mg, determined by the following method:
To an accurately measured volume, equivalent to about 0·05 mmol of magnesium, add 40 ml of water and 20 ml of *ammonia buffer solution* and titrate with 0·02M disodium edetate, using *mordant black 11 solution* as indicator; each ml of 0·02M disodium edetate, after a volume equivalent to the calcium present in the sample has been deducted, is equivalent to 0·02 mmol of Mg.
Calculate the concentration of Mg in mmol per litre.

If the intraperitoneal dialysis solution contains lactate, it complies with the following additional requirement:

CONTENT OF LACTATE. 90·0 to 110·0 per cent of the concentration stated on the label, calculated as the equivalent number of millimoles of HCO_3^-, determined by the following method:
Evaporate an accurately measured volume, equivalent to about 0·05 g of sodium lactate, almost to dryness on a water-bath, add 5 ml of *acetone*, and again evaporate almost to dryness; repeat the evaporation with two further 5-ml portions of *acetone*.
Dissolve the residue as completely as possible in 50 ml of *glacial acetic acid*, with the aid of heat, cool, and titrate by Method I of the British Pharmacopoeia for non-aqueous titration; each ml of 0·01N perchloric acid is equivalent to 0·1 mmol of HCO_3^-.
Calculate the equivalent concentration of HCO_3^- in mmol per litre.

Containers. Intraperitoneal dialysis solutions are supplied in suitable glass or plastic containers which do not release ions or harmful substances into the solution. Separation of solid particles from the glass containers may occur on storage; solutions containing such particles must not be used.

Labelling. The label on the container states:
(1) the strength of the solution, stated as a percentage or weight per litre for each ingredient, the quantity of dextrose being expressed in terms of anhydrous dextrose, $C_6H_{12}O_6$;
(2) the number of millimoles of each ion present per litre;
(3) the volume of solution in the container;

(4) that the solution is not for intravenous administration; and

(5) that any portion of the solution remaining after the contents are first used should be discarded.

The label may state, in addition, the number of milli-equivalents of each ion per litre.

Uses. Intraperitoneal dialysis solutions are employed, in cases of temporary or permanent renal failure, to remove the excess of water and accumulated waste products normally excreted from the body by the kidney and to correct electrolyte imbalance without the use of an artificial kidney.

The elimination of poisons of low molecular weight, e.g. aspirin and certain barbiturates, as well as substances of higher molecular weight, may also be hastened by this technique but substances that are strongly bound to body protein are not effectively removed by dialysis.

Intraperitoneal dialysis may also be used in the treatment of malaria, cholera, dysentery, and gastro-enteritis with renal involvement, as described under Haemodialysis Solutions (page 786).

The solutions are infused into the peritoneal cavity through a catheter under aseptic conditions, allowed to remain in the body for about one hour, and then drained from the cavity through the catheter. During the time the solution is in the body, the removal of water and accumulated waste products from the extracellular fluid and the exchange of ions between the solution and the extracellular fluid occur across the peritoneal membrane.

Intraperitoneal Dialysis Solution (Lactate) contains in 1 litre approximately 140 mmol (mEq) of Na^+, 1·8 mmol (3·6 mEq) of Ca^{2+}, 0·75 mmol (1·5 mEq) of Mg^{2+}, 100 mmol (mEq) of Cl^-, and the equivalent of 45 mmol (mEq) of HCO_3^- (as lactate).

Intraperitoneal Dialysis Solution (Acetate) contains in 1 litre approximately 130 mmol (mEq) of Na^+, 1·5 mmol (3·0 mEq) of Ca^{2+}, 0·75 mmol (1·5 mEq) of Mg^{2+}, 100 mmol (mEq) of Cl^-, and the equivalent of 35·0 mmol (mEq) of HCO_3^- (as lactate).

Lead Subacetate Solution, Dilute

SYNONYM: Liquor Plumbi Subacetatis Dilutus

Strong Lead Subacetate Solution	12·5 ml
Purified Water, freshly boiled and cooled	to 1000 ml

It must be freshly prepared.

Lead Subacetate Solution, Strong

SYNONYM: Liquor Plumbi Subacetatis Fortis

Lead Monoxide, in powder ..	175 g
Lead Acetate	250 g
Purified Water, freshly boiled and cooled	to 1000 ml

Dissolve the lead acetate in 750 ml of the water, add the lead monoxide, and allow to stand for forty-eight hours, shaking occasionally; filter, pass through the filter sufficient of the water to produce the required volume, and mix.

Standard

DESCRIPTION. A clear, colourless, alkaline liquid, which becomes turbid from absorption of carbon dioxide on exposure to air.

ALKALINITY. 10·5 to 12·5 per cent w/w, calculated as PbO, determined by the following method:
Dilute about 2 g, accurately weighed, with 20 ml of *carbon dioxide-free water*, add 50 ml of 0·1N oxalic acid, shake thoroughly, filter, wash the flask and filter with *carbon dioxide-free water*, and titrate the combined filtrate and washings with 0·1N sodium hydroxide, using *phenolphthalein solution* as indicator.
Repeat the procedure omitting the sample.
The difference between the two titrations represents the amount of oxalic acid required by the sample; each ml of 0·1N oxalic acid is equivalent to 0·01116 g of PbO.

CONTENT OF TOTAL LEAD. 19·0 to 21·5 per cent w/w, calculated as Pb, determined by the following method:
To about 2 g, accurately weighed, add 2 ml of *acetic acid*, 100 ml of water, 5 g of *hexamine*, and 0·2 ml of *xylenol orange solution* as indicator, and titrate with 0·05M disodium edetate until the solution becomes pale bright yellow; each ml of 0·05M disodium edetate is equivalent to 0·01036 g of Pb.

Storage. It should be stored in airtight containers.

Morphine Hydrochloride Solution

Morphine Hydrochloride	..	10 g
Dilute Hydrochloric Acid	..	20 ml
Alcohol (90 per cent) ..	..	250 ml
Purified Water, freshly boiled and cooled		to 1000 ml

Mix the alcohol with an equal volume of the water, add the dilute hydrochloric acid, dissolve the morphine hydrochloride in the mixture, add sufficient of the water to produce the required volume, and mix.

Standard

PRESENCE OF MORPHINE. Evaporate 0·5 ml to dryness on a water-bath; the residue complies with the following tests:
(i) Add a portion of the residue to 0·05 ml of *nitric acid*; an orange-red colour is produced.
(ii) Add a portion of the residue to 1 ml of *sulphuric acid* containing 0·05 ml of *formaldehyde solution*; a purple colour is produced.

ALCOHOL CONTENT. 21 to 24 per cent v/v of ethyl alcohol, determined by the method given in Appendix 10, page 888.

CONTENT OF MORPHINE HYDROCHLORIDE. 0·95 to 1·05 per cent w/v, determined by the following method:
Dilute 2 ml to 200 ml with water and measure the extinction of a 1-cm layer at the maximum at about 285 nm.
For purposes of calculation use a value of 41 for the E(1 per cent, 1 cm) of morphine hydrochloride.
Calculate the concentration of morphine hydrochloride in the sample.

Storage. It should be protected from light.

Dose. 0·5 to 2 millilitres.

Morphine Hydrochloride Solution contains, in 2 ml, 20 mg of morphine hydrochloride.

Noradrenaline Solution, Strong, Sterile

Noradrenaline Acid Tartrate	..	0·2 g
Sodium Metabisulphite ..	..	0·1 g
Sodium Chloride..	.. ..	0·8 g
Water for Injections	.. ..	to 100 ml

It is prepared as described under Solutions (page 779). Sterilise by autoclaving or by filtration (see Appendix 29, page 921).

Standard
It complies with the standard under Solutions, page 779, with the following additions:

ACIDITY. pH, 3·0 to 4·6.

PRESENCE OF NORADRENALINE. Mix 0·5 ml with 10 ml of *solution of standard pH 3·6*, add 1 ml of 0·1N iodine, allow to stand for 5 minutes, and add 2 ml of 0·1N sodium thiosulphate; not more than a very faint red colour is produced.
Repeat the test using *solution of standard pH 6·6*; a strong reddish-violet colour is produced (distinction from adrenaline and isoprenaline).

CONTENT OF NORADRENALINE ACID TARTRATE. 0·18 to 0·23 per cent w/v, determined by the following method: Dilute 5 ml to 200 ml with water, and measure the extinction of a 1-cm layer at the maximum at about 279 nm.
For purposes of calculation, use a value of 80 for the E(1 per cent, 1 cm) of noradrenaline acid tartrate. Calculate the percentage of noradrenaline acid tartrate in the sample.

Containers. The directions given under Injections (page 708) should be followed. The solution must be supplied in single-dose ampoules which comply with the requirements of the European Pharmacopoeia for Glass Containers for Injectable Preparations.

Labelling. The label on the container states:
(1) "Sterile Strong Noradrenaline Solution"; and
(2) "This solution must be diluted before use".
The label on the container or the label or wrapper on the package states:
(1) "Sterile Strong Noradrenaline Solution for the preparation of Noradrenaline Injection", and
(2) "One volume of this solution diluted to 250 volumes with Sodium Chloride and Dextrose Injection or with Dextrose Injection (5 per cent w/v) produces Noradrenaline Injection, which must be used immediately after preparation".

Storage. It should be protected from light; it should not be used if it is brown in colour.

Soap Solution, Ethereal

SYNONYMS: Ether Soap; Liquor Saponis Aethereus; Solutio Saponis Aetherea

Potassium Hydroxide		a sufficient quantity
Oleic Acid	.. ..	350·0 ml
Lavender Oil	.. ..	2·1 ml
Alcohol (90 per cent)	.. ..	150·0 ml
Water (see page 642)		a sufficient quantity
Solvent Ether	.. ..	to 1000 ml

Mix the oleic acid with the alcohol and neutralise with a saturated solution of potassium hydroxide in water (1 in 1), using *phenolphthalein solution* as indicator; about 75 ml of the potassium hydroxide solution will be required. Allow the neutralised product to cool, add the lavender oil and sufficient of the solvent ether to produce the required volume, and mix.

In making this preparation the alcohol (90 per cent) may be replaced by Industrial Methylated Spirit diluted so as to be of equivalent alcoholic strength, provided that the law and the statutory regulations governing the use of industrial methylated spirit are observed.

Standard
ACIDITY OR ALKALINITY. 10 ml requires for neutralisation not more than 1·0 ml of 0·1N sodium hydroxide or 0·2 ml of 0·1N hydrochloric acid, using *phenolphthalein solution* as indicator.

WEIGHT PER ML. At 20°, 0·860 g to 0·900 g.

ALCOHOL CONTENT. 13 to 15 per cent v/v of ethyl alcohol, determined by the method given in Appendix 10, page 888.

CONTENT OF OLEIC ACID. Not less than 33·0 per cent v/v, determined by the following method:
To 10 ml add 20 ml of water and 20 ml of 1N hydrochloric acid and extract with two successive 20-ml portions of *light petroleum* (boiling-range, 40° to 60°); wash the combined extracts with two 10-ml portions of water, evaporate off the light petroleum, add 5 ml of *acetone*, again evaporate, and dry the residue of oleic acid to constant weight at 80°.
Assuming a weight per ml of 0·892 g for oleic acid, calculate the concentration, volume in volume.

Containers and storage. It should be stored in airtight containers, in a cool place.

Labelling. The label on the container states "Caution. This preparation is inflammable. Keep away from a naked flame".

Sodium Chloride Solution

SYNONYM: Normal Saline

Sodium Chloride..	.. ..	9 g
Purified Water, freshly boiled and cooled	.. .. ..	to 1000 ml

Dissolve, and filter.

Standard
PRESENCE OF SODIUM CHLORIDE. Wet a loop of platinum wire with the solution and introduce into the flame of a Bunsen burner; the flame has a yellow colour.

CONTENT OF SODIUM CHLORIDE. 0·85 to 0·95 per cent w/v, calculated as NaCl, determined by the method given in Appendix 11, page 891, 25 ml being used; each ml of 0·1N silver nitrate is equivalent to 0·005844 g of NaCl.

If the solution is issued as sterile, it complies, in addition, with the standard under Solutions, page 779.

Sterilisation. The solution may be sterilised by autoclaving or by filtration (see Appendix 29, page 921).

Containers; Labelling. The directions given under Solutions (page 779) should be followed.

Sodium Citrate Solution for Bladder Irrigation, Sterile

Sodium Citrate	.. ..	30 g
Dilute Hydrochloric Acid	..	2 ml
Purified Water, freshly boiled and cooled	.. .. ..	to 1000 ml

It is prepared as described under Solutions (page 779). Sterilise by autoclaving or by filtration (see Appendix 29, page 921).

Standard

It complies with the standard under Solutions, page 779, with the following additions:

PRESENCE OF SODIUM CITRATE. It complies with the tests given for Sodium Citrate Mixture, page 753.

CONTENT OF SODIUM CITRATE. 2·85 to 3·15 per cent w/v, calculated as $C_6H_5Na_3O_7,2H_2O$, determined by the following method:

Evaporate 50 ml to dryness and heat the residue until carbonised; cool, boil the residue with 50 ml of water and 50 ml of 0·5N hydrochloric acid, and filter; wash the filter with water, cool, and titrate the excess of acid in the combined filtrate and washings with 0·5N sodium hydroxide, using *methyl orange–xylene cyanol FF solution* as indicator; each ml of 0·5N hydrochloric acid is equivalent to 0·04902 g of $C_6H_5Na_3O_7,2H_2O$.

Containers; Labelling. The directions given under Solutions (page 779) should be followed.

Storage. Separation of solid particles from the glass containers may occur on storage; solutions containing such particles must not be used.

Sodium Hypochlorite Solution, Dilute

Dilute Sodium Hypochlorite Solution is a solution containing about 1 per cent w/w of available chlorine.

It may be prepared by dilution of a strong sodium hypochlorite solution of known available chlorine content or by the electrolysis of a strong solution of sodium chloride.

It may contain stabilising agents and sodium chloride.

Standard

CONTENT OF AVAILABLE CHLORINE. 0·90 to 1·10 per cent w/w, calculated as Cl, determined by the method for Strong Sodium Hypochlorite Solution, 10 ml being used and the initial dilution omitted.

Determine the weight per ml of the solution and calculate the concentration of available chlorine, weight in weight.

Storage. It should be stored in well-filled airtight bottles, protected from light, in a cool place.

Uses. The uses of Dilute Sodium Hypochlorite Solution are described under Chlorinated Lime (page 99).

Sodium Hypochlorite Solution, Strong

Strong Sodium Hypochlorite Solution is prepared, in strengths of up to about 18 per cent w/w of available chlorine, by absorption of chlorine in sodium hydroxide solution.

It is often supplied as solutions of lower available-chlorine contents. The solutions decrease in strength fairly rapidly and should be used as soon as possible. They may contain stabilising agents.

Standard

TOTAL ALKALINITY. Not more than 1·8 per cent w/w, calculated as NaOH, determined by the following method:

Mix 25 ml with 50 ml of water, add 35 ml of *hydrogen peroxide solution*, and titrate with 0·5N hydrochloric acid, using *methyl orange solution* as indicator; each ml of 0·5N hydrochloric acid is equivalent to 0·0200 g of NaOH.

Determine the weight per ml of the solution and calculate the total alkalinity, weight in weight.

CONTENT OF AVAILABLE CHLORINE. Not less than 8·0 per cent w/w, determined by the following method: Dilute 10 ml to 250 ml with water; to 10 ml of this solution add 50 ml of 0·1N sodium arsenite followed by 5 g of *sodium bicarbonate*, swirl to dissolve, and titrate the excess sodium arsenite with 0·1N iodine, using freshly prepared *starch mucilage* as indicator; each ml of 0·1N sodium arsenite is equivalent to 0·003545 g of Cl.

Determine the weight per ml of the solution and calculate the concentration of available chlorine, weight in weight.

Containers and storage. It should be stored in well-filled airtight bottles, closed with glass stoppers or suitable plastic caps, and protected from light, in a cool place away from acids.

It should not be stored for longer than a few months.

Labelling. The label on the container states:

(1) that the solution must be diluted before use, and

(2) the date after which the solution is not expected to comply with the standard.

Sorbitol Solution

SYNONYM: Sorbitol Liquid

Sorbitol Solution is an aqueous solution containing 70 per cent w/w of total solids, consisting mainly of D-sorbitol, $CH_2OH\cdot[CH\cdot OH]_4\cdot CH_2OH$, and may be prepared by the catalytic hydrogenation of glucose.

Sorbitol Solution is commonly available in two grades, a "crystallising" grade and a "non-crystallising" grade. The latter usually contains a small proportion of related products which help to retard crystallisation of the sorbitol under normal conditions of storage.

Solubility. Miscible with water.

Standard

DESCRIPTION. A clear, colourless, syrupy liquid; odourless; taste sweet.

IDENTIFICATION TESTS. 1. Dilute 1 ml to 75 ml with water; to 3 ml of this solution add 3 ml of *catechol solution*, mix, add 6 ml of *sulphuric acid*, mix, and heat gently for about 30 seconds; a deep pink colour is produced.

2. To 12 ml add 14 ml of *methyl alcohol*, 2 ml of *benzaldehyde*, and 2 ml of *hydrochloric acid*, and shake until crystals are formed.

Collect the crystals by filtering with the aid of suction, dissolve the residue in 20 ml of boiling *sodium bicarbonate solution*, filter while hot, cool the filtrate, and again filter with the aid of suction.

The residue, after washing with 5 ml of a mixture of equal volumes of *methyl alcohol* and water and drying in air, melts at about 175°.

WEIGHT PER ML. At 20°, not less than 1·290 g.

ACIDITY. pH of a 10·0 per cent v/v solution in water, 6·0 to 7·0, using *bromothymol blue solution* as indicator.

REFRACTIVE INDEX. At 20°, 1·457 to 1·462.

ARSENIC. It complies with the test given in Appendix 6, page 880 (1 part per million).

IRON. 8 g complies with the limit test for iron (5 parts per million).

LEAD. It complies with the test given in Appendix 7, page 884 (1 part per million).

NICKEL. To 10 g add 20 ml of water, 2 ml of a 20 per cent w/v solution of *citric acid* in water, and 3 ml of *bromine solution*, mix, and add 10 ml of *dilute ammonia solution* and 1 ml of a 1 per cent w/v solution of *dimethylglyoxime* in *alcohol (95 per cent)*, mix well, dilute to 50 ml with water, and allow to stand for 5 minutes.

Any colour which develops is not deeper than that produced by 1 ml of *dilute nickel chloride solution* when similarly treated.

REDUCING SUGARS. Not more than 0·15 per cent w/w, calculated as $C_6H_{12}O_6$, determined by the following method:

Add about 13 g, accurately weighed, to 20·0 ml of *copper reagent* in a 300-ml conical flask carrying a small funnel inserted loosely in the neck and add a few small pieces of clean porous pot or *pumice powder*.

Heat the solution in such a manner that it boils in 4 minutes and continue boiling for a further 3 minutes. Cool rapidly, add 100 ml of a 2·4 per cent v/v solution of *glacial acetic acid* in water, followed by 20·0 ml of 0·04N iodine.

Add, with continuous swirling, 25 ml of a 6·0 per cent v/v solution of *hydrochloric acid* in water, ensuring that any precipitate has redissolved, and titrate the excess of iodine with 0·04N sodium thiosulphate, using *starch mucilage*, added towards the end of the titration, as indicator; each ml of 0·04N iodine is equivalent to 0·00112 g of $C_6H_{12}O_6$.

SULPHATED ASH. Not more than 0·1 per cent w/w.

TOTAL SOLIDS. 68 to 72 per cent w/w, determined by drying about 1 g, accurately weighed, for 6 hours at 80° in vacuo.

Labelling. The label on the container states whether the solution is the "crystallising" or "non-crystallising" grade.

Storage. It should be stored in airtight containers.

Uses. Sorbitol Solution is used as a sweetening agent and vehicle in elixirs, linctuses, and mixtures; it has about half the sweetening power of Syrup. When added to syrups containing sucrose it reduces their tendency to deposit crystals on storage; for this purpose, about 20 to 30 per cent of Sorbitol Solution is usually sufficient.

Although the solubility of sorbitol is decreased in the presence of alcohol, Sorbitol Solution can usually be employed in elixirs and other preparations containing up to 40 per cent v/v of alcohol.

It is used as a humectant in pharmaceutical and cosmetic creams and is an ingredient of some toothpastes. It is also employed as a plasticiser in the manufacture of gelatin capsules.

It is used in place of sugar in diabetic diets, as it does not produce a rise in the blood-sugar level when taken by mouth.

Tartrazine Solution, Compound

SYNONYM: Liquor Flavus

Tartrazine, food grade of commerce	7·5 g
Orange G, food grade of commerce	2·5 g
Glycerol	250 ml
Chloroform Water	to 1000 ml

Dissolve the tartrazine and the orange G in about 700 ml of the chloroform water, add the glycerol and sufficient chloroform water to produce the required volume, and mix.

Standard

PRESENCE OF TARTRAZINE AND OF ORANGE G. It complies with the thin-layer chromatographic test given in Appendix 5A, page 868.

WEIGHT PER ML. At 20°, 1·070 g to 1·085 g.

Tolu Solution

Tolu Balsam	50 g
Sucrose	500 g
Alcohol (90 per cent)	300 ml
Water (see page 642) ..	to 1000 ml

Dissolve the tolu balsam in 200 ml of the alcohol, add sterilised Purified Talc and 350 ml of the water heated to 70°, shake vigorously, and allow to stand for twenty-four hours.

Filter, dissolve the sucrose in the filtrate with the aid of gentle heat, cool, add the remainder of the alcohol and sufficient water to produce the required volume, and mix.

Standard

WEIGHT PER ML. At 20°, 1·140 g to 1·175 g.

ALCOHOL CONTENT. 23 to 25 per cent v/v of ethyl alcohol, determined by the method given in Appendix 10, page 888.

SOLUTION-TABLETS

Solution-tablets are compact products containing a medicament or a mixture of medicaments in compressed form and are intended, after being dissolved in water, to be used externally or on mucous surfaces. They are usually circular in shape with slightly convex surfaces, but solution-tablets containing poisons may be of a distinctive shape and coloured by the addition of a suitable dye.

Solution-tablets may be prepared by the methods described under Tablets (page 801), but any lubricant or diluent used should be readily soluble in water. Boric acid is frequently used as a lubricant, but the proportion present should not exceed 5 per cent; by careful manipulation it is possible to prepare most solution-tablets without boric acid, which may react with other ingredients. Sodium chloride is normally used as a diluent, but solution-tablets containing this substance become less readily soluble on storage. Solution-tablets should be completely soluble in water.

Content of active ingredient. When solution-tablets include a substance that has a standard permitting a relatively high proportion of moisture, or where the content of pure drug may vary within relatively wide limits, a sufficient quantity of the substance must be used to ensure that the solution-tablets comply with any requirements for content of active ingredient.

Containers and storage. All solution-tablets should be stored and supplied in containers which provide adequate protection against crushing. In addition, solution-tablets which deteriorate if exposed to a moist atmosphere or to light should be stored and supplied in containers which are airtight or light resistant, or both.

They should preferably be stored and supplied in amber glass bottles, jars, or vials, in amber or opaque plastic containers, or in cylindrical aluminium containers, suitably protected internally; lined screw-cap closures or plastic caps should be used.

Solution-tablets may also be packaged in strip foil, each tablet being hermetically sealed in a pocket of foil. This method gives good protection against ingress of moisture but effervescent solution-tablets so packed must have an exceedingly low initial moisture content.

Mouth-wash Solution-tablets

SYNONYMS: Effervescing Mouth-wash Tablets; Solvellae pro Collutorio

For each solution-tablet take:

Menthol	0·81 mg	
Thymol	0·81 mg	
Sodium Benzoate, in powder ..	32·4 mg	
Tartaric Acid, in powder ..	259·2 mg	
Sodium Bicarbonate	324·0 mg	
Saccharin	0·65 mg	
Amaranth, food grade of commerce	2·62 mg	
Eucalyptus Oil	.. 0·00296 ml	
Lemon Oil	.. 0·00296 ml	
Alcohol (95 per cent)	a sufficient quantity	
Water (see page 642)	a sufficient quantity	

Dissolve the amaranth in a sufficient quantity of a mixture of equal parts of the alcohol and water. Prepare sodium bicarbonate granules by the moist granulation process described under Tablets (page 801), using a sufficient quantity of the amaranth solution as the liquid excipient. Mix the tartaric acid and the saccharin, and prepare granules by the moist granulation process, using the remainder of the amaranth solution as the liquid excipient. Dry the granules, and mix. Dissolve the menthol, the thymol, the eucalyptus oil, and the lemon oil in a sufficient quantity of the alcohol, mix with the dried granules, add the sodium benzoate, and compress.

Standard

UNIFORMITY OF WEIGHT. They comply with the requirements of the British Pharmacopoeia for uniformity of weight given under Tablets.

DISINTEGRATION TIME. Maximum time, 5 minutes, determined by the method of the British Pharmacopoeia for Tablets.

CONTENT OF AVAILABLE CARBON DIOXIDE. Not less than 0·05 g, calculated as CO_2, determined by the following method:
Weigh and powder 20 solution-tablets. Transfer an accurately weighed quantity of the powder, equivalent to about two-thirds of a solution-tablet, to a dry test-tube, 150 mm in length and 20 mm in diameter, and insert a loose plug of glass wool about half way down the tube; place the test-tube in a 750-ml filtering flask containing 50 ml of 0·1N barium hydroxide, close the neck of the flask with a stopper through which passes the stem of a 50-ml separating funnel in such a manner that the stem of the funnel enters the test-tube; exhaust the flask rapidly until the pressure is reduced to 20 mm of mercury, and close the exit-tube; through the funnel add gradually 10 ml of freshly boiled and cooled water, allow to stand for 16 hours, and titrate the excess of barium hydroxide with 0·1N oxalic acid, using *phenolphthalein solution* as indicator. Repeat the procedure omitting the sample.
The difference between the two titrations represents the amount of barium hydroxide required by the sample; each ml of 0·1N barium hydroxide is equivalent to 0·002201 g of CO_2. Calculate the total weight of available CO_2 in the 20 solution-tablets, and divide by 20.

Containers and storage. The directions given under Solution-tablets (above) should be followed.

Note. For use, one solution-tablet should be dissolved in a tumblerful (¼ pint) of warm water.

SPIRITS

Spirits consist of medicinal substances or flavouring agents, usually of a volatile nature, dissolved in alcohol. Aromatic Ammonia Spirit is prepared by a process of distillation but most other spirits in current use are prepared by simple solution in alcohol.

Ammonia Spirit, Aromatic

SYNONYM: Spirit of Sal Volatile

Ammonium Bicarbonate	..	25·0 g
Strong Ammonia Solution	..	67·5 ml
Nutmeg Oil ..	.. ..	3·0 ml
Lemon Oil ..	.. ..	5·0 ml
Alcohol (90 per cent) ..	..	750·0 ml
Purified Water ..	..	to 1000·0 ml

Distil the lemon oil, the nutmeg oil, the alcohol, and 375 ml of the water, reserving the first 875 ml. Distil a further 55 ml, add the ammonium bicarbonate and the strong ammonia solution, and heat on a water-bath to 60° in a sealed bottle of not less than 120-ml capacity, shaking occasionally, until solution is complete; cool, filter through cotton wool, mix the filtrate with the reserved portion of the distillate, add sufficient of the water to produce the required volume, and mix.

Standard
WEIGHT PER ML. At 20°, 0·880 g to 0·893 g.

ALCOHOL CONTENT. 64 to 70 per cent v/v of ethyl alcohol, determined by the method given in Appendix 10, page 888.

CONTENT OF AMMONIUM CARBONATE. 2·76 to 3·24 per cent w/v, calculated as $(NH_4)_2CO_3$, determined by the method for ammonium carbonate in Aromatic Ammonia Solution, page 780.

CONTENT OF FREE AMMONIA. 1·12 to 1·25 per cent w/v, calculated as NH_3, determined by the method for free ammonia in Aromatic Ammonia Solution, page 780.

Storage. It should be stored in well-filled airtight containers, in a cool place.

Dose. 1 to 5 millilitres, diluted with water.

Benzaldehyde Spirit

Benzaldehyde ..	.. ..	10 ml
Alcohol (90 per cent) ..	..	800 ml
Purified Water ..	..	to 1000 ml

Dissolve the benzaldehyde in the alcohol and add sufficient of the water to produce the required volume.

Standard
WEIGHT PER ML. At 20°, 0·870 g to 0·885 g.

ALCOHOL CONTENT. 69 to 72 per cent v/v of ethyl alcohol, determined by the method given in Appendix 10, page 888.

CONTENT OF BENZALDEHYDE. 0·85 to 1·05 per cent v/v, calculated as C_7H_6O, determined by the method given in Appendix 14, page 893, for the determination of aldehydes in volatile oils; use 10 ml of the sample and titrate with 0·1N potassium hydroxide in alcohol (95 per cent); each ml of 0·1N potassium hydroxide in alcohol (95 per cent) is equivalent to 0·01061 g of C_7H_6O.

Assuming the weight per ml of benzaldehyde to be 1·046 g, calculate the concentration of benzaldehyde, volume in volume.

Storage. It should be stored in well-filled airtight containers, protected from light, in a cool place.

Ether Spirit

Anaesthetic Ether	.. ..	330 ml
Alcohol (90 per cent)	..	.. to 1000 ml

Standard
WEIGHT PER ML. At 20°, 0·790 g to 0·805 g.

ALCOHOL CONTENT. 59 to 65 per cent v/v of ethyl alcohol, determined by the method given in Appendix 10, page 888.

Storage. It should be stored in airtight containers, protected from light, in a cool place.

Labelling. The label on the container states "Caution. This preparation is inflammable. Keep away from a naked flame".

Lemon Spirit

Terpeneless Lemon Oil ..	..	100 ml
Alcohol (95 per cent) ..	..	to 1000 ml

Standard
WEIGHT PER ML. At 20°, 0·814 g to 0·823 g.

ALCOHOL CONTENT. 84 to 87 per cent v/v of ethyl alcohol, determined by the method given in Appendix 10, page 888.

CONTENT OF ALDEHYDES. 3·45 to 4·60 per cent w/v, calculated as citral, $C_{10}H_{16}O$, determined by the method for Lemon Oil, page 264, 10 ml being used.

Orange Spirit, Compound

SYNONYM: Spiritus Aurantii Compositus

Terpeneless Orange Oil ..	..	2·5 ml
Terpeneless Lemon Oil ..	..	1·3 ml
Anise Oil ..	.. ..	.. 4·25 ml
Coriander Oil ..	.. ..	6·25 ml
Alcohol (90 per cent) ..	..	.. to 1000 ml

Standard
WEIGHT PER ML. At 20°, 0·828 g to 0·841 g.

ALCOHOL CONTENT. 86 to 90 per cent v/v of ethyl alcohol, determined by the method given in Appendix 10, page 888.

Peppermint Spirit

SYNONYMS: Essence of Peppermint; Spiritus Menthae Piperitae

Peppermint Oil ..	.. ..	100 ml
Alcohol (90 per cent) ..	..	to 1000 ml

Dissolve; if the solution is not clear, shake with sterilised Purified Talc, and filter.

Standard
WEIGHT PER ML. At 20°, 0·830 g to 0·840 g.

ALCOHOL CONTENT. 78 to 82 per cent v/v of ethyl alcohol, determined by the method given in Appendix 10, page 888.

CONTENT OF OIL. 9·0 to 11·0 per cent v/v, determined by the following method:
Add 25 ml, together with 5 ml of *xylene*, to 90 ml of a 10 per cent w/v solution of *sodium chloride* in water, to which has been added 1·0 per cent v/v of *hydrochloric acid*, in a flask of about 150-ml capacity with a long neck which is graduated in tenths of a millilitre and is of such a diameter that not less than 15 cm in length has a capacity of 10 ml.
Shake the mixture for about 30 minutes, allow to separate, and raise the undissolved oily layer into the graduated part of the neck of the flask by the gradual addition of a further quantity of the acid sodium chloride solution; allow to stand for 2 hours, or until there is no further change in the volume of the oily layer, and measure the volume of the oily layer.
The volume of the oily layer, after 5 ml has been deducted, represents the volume of oil in the sample.
Calculate the concentration of oil, volume in volume.

Dose. 0·3 to 2 millilitres.

Soap Spirit

SYNONYM: Spiritus Saponatus

Soft Soap ..	..	..	..	650 g
Alcohol (90 per cent)	..		..	to 1000 ml

Dissolve, and decant.

In making this preparation the alcohol (90 per cent) may be replaced by Industrial Methylated Spirit diluted so as to be of equivalent alcoholic strength, provided that the law and the statutory regulations governing the use of industrial methylated spirit are observed.

Standard
WEIGHT PER ML. At 20°, 0·945 g to 0·970 g.

ALCOHOL CONTENT. 28 to 32 per cent v/v of ethyl alcohol, determined by the method given in Appendix 10, page 888.

CONTENT OF FATTY ACIDS. Not less than 27·0 per cent w/v, determined by the following method:
To 10 ml add 20 ml of water and 20 ml of 1N hydrochloric acid and extract with two successive 20-ml portions of *light petroleum (boiling-range, 40° to 60°)*; wash the combined extracts with two 10-ml portions of water, evaporate off the light petroleum, add 5 ml of *acetone*, again evaporate, and dry the residue of fatty acids for 2 hours at 80°.

Surgical Spirit

SYNONYMS: Spiritus Chirurgicalis; Surgical Spirit No. 1

Methyl Salicylate	..	..	5 ml
Diethyl Phthalate	..	..	20 ml
Castor Oil..	..	..	25 ml
Industrial Methylated Spirit		..	to 1000 ml

Standard
CONTENT OF METHYL SALICYLATE. 0·45 to 0·55 per cent v/v, determined by the following method:
Using *dehydrated alcohol* as solvent, dilute 5 ml to 100 ml; dilute 5 ml of this solution to 100 ml and measure the extinction of a 1-cm layer at the maximum at about 306 nm.
For purposes of calculation, use a value of 335 for the E(1 per cent, 1 cm) of methyl salicylate.
Calculate the concentration of methyl salicylate in the sample.

CONTENT OF DIETHYL PHTHALATE. 1·80 to 2·20 per cent v/v, determined by the following method:
Dilute 10 ml of the final dilution used in the determination of methyl salicylate to 50 ml with *dehydrated alcohol* and measure the extinction of a 1-cm layer at 227 nm.
From the observed extinction, subtract the extinction due to the methyl salicylate present, as determined above, using a value of 432 for the E(1 per cent, 1 cm) at 227 nm of methyl salicylate.
For purposes of calculation, use a value of 419 for the E(1 per cent, 1 cm) of diethyl phthalate.
Calculate the concentration of diethyl phthalate in the sample.

Labelling. The container should be labelled "Caution. This preparation is inflammable. Keep away from a naked flame".

SPRAYS

Sprays are preparations of medicaments in aqueous, alcoholic, or glycerol-containing media to be applied to the nose or throat by means of an atomiser. The choice of atomiser depends on the viscosity of the liquid; the more viscous the liquid, the more powerful the atomiser required.

Oily sprays have been used, but the oil retards the ciliary action of the nasal mucosa; drops of oil may enter the trachea and cause lipoid pneumonia.

Containers. Sprays should be supplied in small, coloured, fluted, glass bottles.

Adrenaline and Atropine Spray, Compound

Adrenaline Acid Tartrate	..		8 g
Atropine Methonitrate ..		..	1 g
Papaverine Hydrochloride		..	8 g
Sodium Metabisulphite ..		..	1 g
Chlorbutol	..	..	5 g
Propylene Glycol..	..	..	50 ml
Purified Water, freshly boiled and cooled	..	..	to 1000 ml

Standard
CONTENT OF ADRENALINE ACID TARTRATE. 0·72 to 0·88 per cent w/v, determined by the following method:
Dilute 5 ml to 250 ml with water; to 15 ml of this solution add 3 ml of 0·5N hydrochloric acid and 1 ml of *solution of standard pH 5·4*, followed by 12 ml of 0·1N sodium hydroxide, and dilute to 50 ml with water.
To 10 ml of this solution add 8 ml of 0·02N iodine, allow to stand for 10 minutes, add 2 ml of 0·1N sodium thiosulphate, and mix well; compare the colour intensity with that produced when 15 ml of a freshly prepared 0·0167 per cent w/v solution of *adrenaline acid tartrate* in water is similarly treated, and calculate

the concentration of adrenaline acid tartrate, weight in volume.

CONTENT OF PAPAVERINE HYDROCHLORIDE. 0·72 to 0·88 per cent w/v, calculated as $C_{20}H_{22}ClNO_4$, determined by the following method:
To 20 ml add 1 ml of *dilute sulphuric acid* and extract with five successive 8-ml portions of *chloroform*, washing each extract with the same mixture of 10 ml of water and 0·05 ml of *dilute sulphuric acid* and reserving the acid solution and washings.
Filter the chloroform extracts through cotton wool covered with a layer of *anhydrous sodium sulphate*, wash the residue with *chloroform*, combine the filtrate and washings, wash with a mixture of 2 ml of *dilute ammonia solution* and 8 ml of water, and reserve the washings.
Repeat the washing with 10 ml of water, and reserve the washings.
Extract the ammoniacal washings and then the water washings with three successive 25-ml portions of *chloroform*, combine the chloroform solution and extracts, evaporate off the chloroform, dry the residue

at 105° for 30 minutes, and weigh; each g of residue is equivalent to 1·107 g of $C_{20}H_{22}ClNO_4$.

CONTENT OF ATROPINE METHONITRATE. 0·09 to 0·11 per cent w/v, calculated as $C_{18}H_{26}N_2O_6$, determined by the following method:
Combine the acid solution and washings reserved in the determination of papaverine hydrochloride, filter, and wash the filter with three successive 5-ml portions of water.
Combine the filtrate and washings, add 20 ml of *dilute sulphuric acid* and 30 ml of *ammonium reineckate solution*, mix well, and allow to stand for 30 minutes.
Filter, wash the residue first with *atropine metho-reineckate solution* until the washings are free from sulphate, then with 3 ml of water, and finally with 2 ml of *alcohol (95 per cent)*, dry in vacuo over *phosphorus pentoxide* for 2 hours, and weigh; each g of residue is equivalent to 0·5884 g of $C_{18}H_{26}N_2O_6$.

Containers. The directions given under Sprays (page 794) should be followed.

Storage. It should be stored in well-filled airtight containers, protected from light.

SUPPOSITORIES

Suppositories are solid bodies suitably shaped for rectal administration and usually containing medicaments.

Suppositories are prepared by incorporating the requisite quantity of the finely powdered medicament in the melted basis and pouring the mixture at a suitable temperature into previously lubricated moulds. Alternatively, the medicaments may be distributed evenly throughout the basis and the mass shaped by cold compression in the moulds or by means of a machine.

Where theobroma oil is specified in the following monographs it may be replaced by any other suitable basis, such as Fractionated Palm Kernel Oil or other suitable hydrogenated vegetable oil, provided that the melting-point of the suppositories is not more than 37°. If suppositories are intended for use in tropical or subtropical countries, the melting-point of the basis may be raised by the addition of White Beeswax or an alternative basis of higher melting-point may be used. For suppositories containing substances such as a volatile oil, phenol, or chloral hydrate, similar changes may be made, provided that the melting-point of the suppositories is not higher than 37°.

Glycerol Suppositories mass of the British Pharmacopoeia is sometimes employed as a basis, but its use is limited, as the gelatin is incompatible with several substances, including tannins. When made with Glycerol Suppositories mass, suppositories should be very slightly greased with a fixed vegetable oil or liquid paraffin.

Suppository moulds generally hold 1 g or 2 g of theobroma oil; a 1-g mould will hold about 1·2 g of Glycerol Suppositories mass.

Standard

UNIFORMITY OF WEIGHT. Suppositories comply with the requirements of the British Pharmacopoeia for uniformity of weight of Suppositories.

DISINTEGRATION TIME. Determine the disintegration time by the method of the British Pharmacopoeia for Suppositories. Suppositories have a maximum disintegration time of 30 minutes.

Containers. Suppositories should be supplied in shallow boxes of rigid paperboard, metal, or plastic material. The boxes should be partitioned or lined with waxed paper. When intended for use in tropical or subtropical climates or when containing volatile ingredients, suppositories should be wrapped separately in metal foil or enclosed in a suitable form of strip packing.

Storage. They should be stored in a cool place.

Bismuth Subgallate Suppositories

Bismuth Subgallate Suppositories are prepared as described under Suppositories (page 795) by incorporating Bismuth Subgallate in Theobroma Oil or other suitable fatty basis.

Approximately 3 g of bismuth subgallate displaces 1 g of theobroma oil.

Standard

They comply with the standard under Suppositories, page 795, with the following addition:

CONTENT OF BISMUTH. 38·2 to 57·2 per cent of the prescribed or stated amount of bismuth subgallate, determined by the method for bismuth in Compound Bismuth Subgallate Suppositories, below, an accurately weighed quantity of the melted mass, equivalent to about 0·6 g of bismuth subgallate, being used.

Containers; Storage. The directions given under Suppositories (above) should be followed.

Note. When the strength of the suppositories is not specified, suppositories each containing 300 mg of bismuth subgallate shall be supplied.

Bismuth Subgallate Suppositories, Compound

SYNONYM: Compound Bismuth and Resorcin Suppositories

For each suppository take:

Bismuth Subgallate	..	..	200 mg
Resorcinol	..	..	60 mg
Zinc Oxide	..	..	120 mg
Castor Oil..	..	..	60 mg

Theobroma Oil, or other suitable fatty basis   sufficient to fill a 1-g mould

Powder the bismuth subgallate and the resorcinol, mix with the zinc oxide and the castor oil, and make into a smooth paste with part of the melted basis; gradually incorporate the remainder of the melted basis and pour into the mould.

The following quantities approximately displace 1 g of theobroma oil: bismuth subgallate 3 g; zinc oxide 5 g; castor oil 1 g; resorcinol 1·5 g.

Standard

They comply with the standard under Suppositories, page 795, with the following additions:

PRESENCE OF RESORCINOL. Dissolve 1 suppository, as completely as possible, by heating with 50 ml of *solvent ether* on a water-bath, filter, evaporate the filtrate to dryness, add to the residue 1 ml of *sodium hydroxide*

solution followed by 0·05 ml of *chloroform* and warm on a water-bath for half a minute; an intense crimson colour is produced which changes to pale yellow on the addition of excess *dilute hydrochloric acid*.

CONTENT OF BISMUTH. 0·07 g to 0·11 g, calculated as Bi, determined by the following method:

Weigh 5 suppositories, melt together by warming, and allow to cool, stirring continuously until the mass is set.

Extract about 3 g of the mass, accurately weighed, with *solvent ether* in an apparatus for the continuous extraction of drugs and discard the ether extract.

Moisten the extraction thimble with 1 ml of *sulphuric acid* and ignite at a temperature not exceeding 500° until all the organic matter is destroyed; dissolve the residue, with the aid of heat, in a mixture of 5 ml of *nitric acid* and 10 ml of water, filter, wash the filter with water, and dilute the combined filtrate and washings to 50 ml with water.

To 20 ml of this solution add 30 ml of water, 20 ml of *glycerol*, and 0·2 g of *sulphamic acid*, allow to stand for one minute, and add 200 ml of water and 0·3 ml of *catechol violet solution*; if a violet colour is produced add *dilute ammonia solution*, dropwise, until a blue colour is produced.

Titrate with 0·05M disodium edetate until a yellow colour is produced; each ml of 0·05M disodium edetate is equivalent to 0·01045 g of Bi.

Calculate the amount of Bi in the 5 suppositories, and divide by 5.

CONTENT OF ZINC OXIDE. 0·11 g to 0·13 g, calculated as ZnO, determined by the following method:

To 10 ml of the solution prepared in the determination of bismuth add 2 ml of *dilute hydrochloric acid*, followed by 200 ml of water; add *dilute ammonia solution* until the solution is only just acid to *litmus paper*, boil for 2 minutes, cool, filter, and wash the filter with water.

To the combined filtrate and washings add 10 ml of *ammonia buffer solution* and titrate with 0·05M disodium edetate, using *mordant black 11 solution* as indicator; each ml of 0·05M disodium edetate is equivalent to 0·004068 g of ZnO.

Calculate the amount of ZnO in the 5 suppositories and divide by 5.

Containers; Storage. The directions given under Suppositories (above) should be followed.

Chlorpromazine Suppositories

Chlorpromazine Suppositories are prepared as described under Suppositories (page 795) by incorporating Chlorpromazine in a hydrogenated vegetable oil or other suitable basis.

Standard

They comply with the standard under Suppositories, page 795, with the following additions:

PRESENCE OF CHLORPROMAZINE. They comply with the thin-layer chromatographic test given in Appendix 5C, page 873.

CONTENT OF CHLORPROMAZINE. 90·0 to 110·0 per cent of the prescribed or stated amount, determined by the following method:

Weigh 5 suppositories, dissolve them in sufficient *chloroform* to produce 100 ml, and dilute 20 ml of this solution to 100 ml with *alcohol (95 per cent)*.

Dilute 10 ml of this solution to 100 ml with *alcohol (95 per cent)*, further dilute 5 ml of this solution to 100 ml with *alcohol (95 per cent)*, and measure the extinction of a 1-cm layer at the maximum at about 258 nm, using *alcohol (95 per cent)* as the blank.

For purposes of calculation use a value of 1150 for the E(1 per cent, 1 cm) of chlorpromazine.

Calculate the total weight of chlorpromazine in the 5 suppositories and divide by 5.

Containers; Storage. The directions given under Suppositories (page 796) should be followed; containers should be light-resistant.

Note. When the strength of the suppositories is not specified, suppositories each containing 100 mg of chlorpromazine shall be supplied.

Cinchocaine Suppositories

Cinchocaine Suppositories are prepared as described under Suppositories (page 795) by incorporating Cinchocaine Hydrochloride in Theobroma Oil or other suitable fatty basis.

Approximately 1·5 g of cinchocaine hydrochloride displaces 1 g of theobroma oil.

Standard

They comply with the standard under Suppositories, page 795, with the following addition:

CONTENT OF CINCHOCAINE HYDROCHLORIDE. 90·0 to 110·0 per cent of the prescribed or stated amount, determined by the following method:

Weigh 5 suppositories, melt together by warming, and allow to cool, stirring continuously until the mass is set.

To an accurately weighed quantity of the mass, equivalent to about 10 mg of cinchocaine hydrochloride, add 20 ml of water and 25 ml of *solvent ether*, shake to dissolve, add 5 ml of 0·1N sodium hydroxide, shake for one minute, and allow to separate; extract the aqueous layer with a further 25-ml portion of *solvent ether*, discard the aqueous solutions, combine the ethereal extracts, wash with 2 ml of water, and discard the washings.

Shake the ethereal solution with a mixture of 20 ml of water and 5 ml of 1N hydrochloric acid, allow to separate, wash the ethereal layer with 2 ml of water, dilute the combined aqueous extract and washings to 500 ml with water, and measure the extinction of a 1-cm layer at the maximum at about 242 nm.

For purposes of calculation, use a value of 494 for the E(1 per cent, 1 cm) of cinchocaine hydrochloride. Calculate the total amount of cinchocaine hydrochloride in the 5 suppositories and divide by 5.

Containers; Storage. The directions given under Suppositories (page 796) should be followed.

Note. When the strength of the suppositories is not specified, suppositories each containing 11 mg of cinchocaine hydrochloride shall be supplied.

Hamamelis Suppositories

Hamamelis Suppositories are prepared as described under Suppositories (page 795) by incorporating Hamamelis Dry Extract in Theobroma Oil or other suitable fatty basis.

Approximately 1·5 g of hamamelis dry extract displaces 1 g of theobroma oil.

Containers; Storage. The directions given under Suppositories (page 796) should be followed.

Note. When the strength of the suppositories is not specified, suppositories each containing 200 mg of Hamamelis Dry Extract shall be supplied.

Hamamelis and Zinc Oxide Suppositories

Hamamelis and Zinc Oxide Suppositories are prepared as described under Suppositories (page 795) by incorporating Hamamelis Dry Extract and Zinc Oxide in Theobroma Oil or other suitable fatty basis.

The following quantities approximately displace 1 g of theobroma oil: hamamelis dry extract 1·5 g; zinc oxide 5 g.

Standard

They comply with the standard under Suppositories, page 795, with the following addition:

CONTENT OF ZINC OXIDE. 90·0 to 110·0 per cent of the prescribed or stated amount, calculated as ZnO, determined by the following method:

Weigh 5 suppositories, melt together by warming, and allow to cool, stirring continuously until the mass is set.

Ignite an accurately weighed quantity of the mass, equivalent to about 0·3 g of ZnO, gently at first and then more strongly until all the organic matter is destroyed, cool, dissolve the residue in 10 ml of *dilute hydrochloric acid*, and dilute to 100 ml with water.

To 25 ml of this solution add 10 ml of *ammonia buffer solution* and 100 ml of water and titrate with 0·05M disodium edetate, using *mordant black 11 solution* as indicator; each ml of 0·05M disodium edetate is equivalent to 0·004068 g of ZnO.

Calculate the amount of ZnO in the 5 suppositories and divide by 5.

Containers; Storage. The directions given under Suppositories (page 796) should be followed.

Note. When the size and strength of the suppositories are not specified, suppositories each containing 600 mg of zinc oxide and 200 mg of Hamamelis Dry Extract, and prepared in a 2-g mould, shall be supplied.

Hydrocortisone Suppositories

Hydrocortisone Suppositories are prepared as described under Suppositories (page 795) by incorporating Hydrocortisone or Hydrocortisone Acetate, in sufficiently fine powder to meet the requirements of the standard, in Theobroma Oil or other suitable fatty basis.

Approximately 1·5 g of hydrocortisone or hydrocortisone acetate displaces 1 g of theobroma oil.

Standard

They comply with the standard under Suppositories, page 795, with the following additions:

PRESENCE OF HYDROCORTISONE. They comply with the thin-layer chromatographic test given in Appendix 5D, page 876.

PARTICLE SIZE. Melt one suppository with the aid of gentle heat, dilute with a suitable volume of *liquid paraffin*, and determine the particle size in the resultant suspension by the method given in Appendix 25C, page 911.

Not less than 90 per cent of the particles have a maximum diameter less than 5 μm and no particle has a maximum diameter greater than 50 μm.

CONTENT OF HYDROCORTISONE OR OF HYDROCORTISONE ACETATE. 90·0 to 110·0 per cent of the prescribed or stated amount of hydrocortisone or of hydrocortisone acetate, determined by the following method:

Weigh 5 suppositories, melt together by warming, and allow to cool, stirring continuously until the mass is set, and, using an accurately weighed quantity of the mass, equivalent to about 0·01 g of hydrocortisone or of

hydrocortisone acetate, carry out the appropriate method as described for Hydrocortisone Cream, page 659.
Calculate the amount of hydrocortisone or of hydrocortisone acetate in the 5 suppositories and divide by 5.

Containers; Storage. The directions given under Suppositories (page 796) should be followed.

Note. When the strength of the suppositories is not specified, suppositories each containing 25 mg of hydrocortisone or of hydrocortisone acetate shall be supplied.

Morphine Suppositories

Morphine Suppositories are prepared as described under Suppositories (page 795) by incorporating Morphine Hydrochloride or Morphine Sulphate in Theobroma Oil or other suitable fatty basis.
Approximately 1·5 g of morphine hydrochloride or of morphine sulphate displaces 1 g of theobroma oil.

Standard
They comply with the standard under Suppositories, page 795, with the following additions:

PRESENCE OF MORPHINE. Extract 2 suppositories with three successive 25-ml portions of *solvent ether*, filtering each extract through a sintered glass filter (British Standard Grade No. 4); dissolve the residue on the filter in 10 ml of warm *alcohol (95 per cent)* and evaporate the solution to dryness on a water-bath. The residue complies with the following tests:

(i) Add a small portion of the residue to 0·05 ml of *nitric acid*; an orange-red colour is produced.
(ii) Add a small portion of the residue to 1 ml of *sulphuric acid* containing 0·05 ml of *formaldehyde solution*; a purple colour is produced.

CONTENT OF MORPHINE HYDROCHLORIDE OR OF MORPHINE SULPHATE. 90·0 to 110·0 per cent of the prescribed or stated amount, determined by the following method:
Weigh 5 suppositories, melt together by warming and allow to cool, stirring continuously until the mass is set.
Dissolve an accurately weighed quantity of the mass, equivalent to about 0·015 g of morphine hydrochloride or of morphine sulphate, in 20 ml of *chloroform* and extract with four successive 30-ml portions of 0·1N hydrochloric acid, washing each extract with the same 10 ml of *chloroform*; combine the acidic extracts and dilute to 200 ml with 0·1N hydrochloric acid.
Dilute 20 ml of this solution to 50 ml with 0·1N hydrochloric acid and, using 20 ml of this further dilution, continue by the method for anhydrous morphine in Aromatic Chalk with Opium Powder, page 776, beginning with the words "add 8 ml of a freshly prepared 1·0 per cent w/v solution of *sodium nitrite* . . ."; each g of anhydrous morphine is equivalent to 1·317 g of morphine hydrochloride, or to 1·330 g of morphine sulphate.
Calculate the amount of morphine hydrochloride or of morphine sulphate in the 5 suppositories and divide by 5.

Containers; Storage. The directions given under Suppositories (page 796) should be followed.

Note. When the strength of the suppositories is not specified, suppositories each containing 15 mg of morphine hydrochloride or of morphine sulphate, as specified by the prescriber, shall be supplied.
Suppositories containing 30 and 60 mg of either salt are also available.

SYRUPS

Syrups are concentrated aqueous solutions of sucrose or other sugars to which medicaments or flavourings may be added. Glycerol, sorbitol, or other polyhydric alcohols are sometimes added in small amounts to medicated syrups to retard crystallisation of sucrose or to increase the solubility of other ingredients.

Medicated syrups provide a convenient form of stock solution of certain drugs for use in extemporaneous preparations.

Flavouring syrups are not usually medicated but contain various aromatic or pleasantly flavoured substances and are intended to be used as vehicles or flavours for extemporaneous preparations. They are of particular use in masking the disagreeable taste of bitter or saline drugs.

Dilute solutions of sucrose will support the growth of moulds, yeasts, and other micro-organisms. The apparatus used in the preparation of syrups should therefore be thoroughly cleansed before use. Freshly distilled water should be used and care should be taken to avoid contamination during preparation. Growth of micro-organisms is usually retarded when the concentration of sucrose is higher than 65 per cent w/w, but at this strength crystallisation of the sucrose may occur.

Dilution of syrups. Unless otherwise indicated in the individual monograph, when a dose ordered or prescribed is less than or not a multiple of 5 millilitres, the syrup should be diluted appropriately with Syrup, so that the dose to be measured by the patient is one 5-ml spoonful or multiple thereof.

Storage. Syrups should be recently prepared unless special precautions have been taken to prevent their contamination. Fruit syrups may be stored for longer periods if they have been heated to boiling point and filled into sterile bottles, which are then sealed to exclude micro-organisms.

Black Currant Syrup

SYNONYM: Syrupus Ribis Nigri

Black Currant Syrup may be prepared from the clarified juice of fresh black currants, *Ribes nigrum* L. (Fam. Grossulariaceae), or from the concentrated black currant juice of commerce.

To obtain the clarified juice, pulp a sufficient quantity of black currants, stir in sufficient pectinase of commerce to destroy the pectin, allow to stand for 24 hours, press, clarify the juice, and, if necessary, adjust the weight per ml at 20° to not less than 1·045 g by the addition of water.

To prepare the syrup add 700 g of sucrose to 560 ml of the clarified juice or to a suitable quantity of concentrated juice diluted with water to the same weight per ml at 20°, stir until dissolved, and add sufficient benzoic acid to produce a final content of not more than 800 parts per million, or sufficient sulphurous acid or sodium metabisulphite to produce a final content of not more than 350 parts per million w/w of sulphur dioxide.

A dye, or a mixture of dyes, may be added, provided that any dye used is of food grade of commerce and that its use for colouring food is permitted in the country concerned.

Standard
WEIGHT PER ML. At 20°, 1·27 g to 1·30 g.

SULPHUR DIOXIDE. Not more than 350 parts per million w/w, determined by the method of the British Pharmacopoeia, Appendix XJ, for the determination of sulphur dioxide.

CONTENT OF ASCORBIC ACID. Not less than 0·055 per cent w/w, calculated as $C_6H_8O_6$, determined by the following method:

Mix about 5 g, accurately weighed, with 25 ml of *metaphosphoric acid solution*, add 20 ml of *acetone*, and dilute to 100 ml with water.

To four 3-ml portions of this solution, add 0·4, 0·5, 0·6, and 0·7 ml, respectively, of *double-strength standard 2,6-dichlorophenolindophenol solution*, mix well by agitation with a fine stream of *carbon dioxide*, add 3 ml of *chloroform*, and agitate for a further 15 seconds; view the solutions against a white background and select the two which are on either side of the end-point, that is, one colourless and one pink.

Prepare a further six solutions as before, but adding to the first an amount of dye solution equal to the amount added to the selected colourless solution, to the second, third, fourth and fifth solutions this amount increased by successive increments of 0·02 ml, and to the sixth solution an amount equal to that added to the selected pink solution.

Select the solution showing the faintest pink colour; each ml of *double-strength standard 2,6-dichlorophenolindophenol solution* added to this solution is equivalent to 0·0002 g of $C_6H_8O_6$.

When the syrup is used for dispensing purposes as a flavouring agent, the standard for content of ascorbic acid does not apply.

Storage. It should be stored in well-filled airtight containers, protected from light, in a cool place.

Dose. 5 to 10 millilitres.

Black Currant Syrup contains in 10 ml about 7·5 mg of ascorbic acid.

Codeine Phosphate Syrup

SYNONYM: Codeine Syrup

Codeine Phosphate	..	..		5 g
Purified Water, freshly boiled and cooled	..	..	..	15 ml
Chloroform Spirit	..	..		25 ml
Syrup	..	..	..	to 1000 ml

Dissolve the codeine phosphate in the water, add 750 ml of the syrup, and mix; add the chloroform spirit and sufficient of the syrup to produce the required volume, and mix.

Standard
WEIGHT PER ML. At 20°, 1·30 g to 1·33 g.

PRESENCE OF CODEINE. To 0·3 ml add 15 ml of water, make alkaline with *dilute ammonia solution*, extract with two successive 15-ml portions of *chloroform*, filter the extracts through a layer of *anhydrous sodium sulphate*, evaporate to dryness, and to the residue add 1 ml of *sulphuric acid and formaldehyde reagent*; a deep blue-violet colour is produced immediately.

CONTENT OF CODEINE PHOSPHATE. 0·45 to 0·55 per cent w/v, calculated as $C_{18}H_{21}NO_3,H_3PO_4,\frac{1}{2}H_2O$, determined by the following method:

To about 7·5 g, accurately weighed, add 20 ml of water, 5 ml of *acetate buffer solution pH 2·8*, 120 ml of *chloroform*, and 5 ml of *dimethyl yellow-oracet blue B solution*, and titrate with 0·01M dioctyl sodium sulphosuccinate solution, with vigorous swirling, until near the end-point; then add the titrant dropwise and, after each addition, swirl vigorously, allow to separate, and gently swirl for 5 seconds; the end-point is indicated when the colour of the chloroform layer changes from green to pinkish-grey.

Repeat the procedure omitting the sample.

The difference between the two titrations represents the amount of dioctyl sodium sulphosuccinate required by the sample; each ml of 0·01M dioctyl sodium sulphosuccinate is equivalent to 0·004064 g of $C_{18}H_{21}NO_3,H_3PO_4,\frac{1}{2}H_2O$.

Determine the weight per ml of the syrup and calculate the concentration of $C_{18}H_{21}NO_3,H_3PO_4,\frac{1}{2}H_2O$, weight in volume

Storage. It should be protected from light.

Dose. 2·5 to 10 millilitres.

Codeine Phosphate Syrup contains, in 10 ml, 50 mg of codeine phosphate.

Figs Syrup, Compound

SYNONYM: Aromatic Syrup of Figs

Fig, cut small	..	..	..	320 g
Cascara Elixir	..	..	..	50 ·ml
Compound Rhubarb Tincture	..			50 ml
Senna Liquid Extract	..		..	100 ml
Sucrose	..	..	..	..	540 g
Water	..	..	..	.. to 1000 ml

Add the fig to 800 ml of boiling water, digest at a gentle heat for one hour, strain, express, and wash the pulp with sufficient warm water to produce 800 ml; evaporate the liquid to one half its volume, dissolve the sucrose in the concentrated liquid, add the compound rhubarb tincture, the senna liquid extract, the cascara elixir, and sufficient water to produce the required volume, and mix.

Standard
WEIGHT PER ML. At 20°, 1·25 g to 1·29 g.

ALCOHOL CONTENT. 4·5 to 5·5 per cent v/v of ethyl alcohol, determined by the method given in Appendix 10, page 888.

Dose. 2·5 to 10 millilitres.

Ginger Syrup

SYNONYM: Syrupus Zingiberis

Strong Ginger Tincture	..		..	50 ml
Syrup	..	..	..	.. to 1000 ml

Mix.

Standard
WEIGHT PER ML. At 20°, 1·29 g to 1·31 g.

ALCOHOL CONTENT. 4·0 to 4·5 per cent v/v of ethyl alcohol, determined by the method given in Appendix 10, page 888.

Dose. 2·5 to 5 millilitres.

Invert Syrup

Invert Syrup contains a mixture of glucose and fructose and may be prepared by hydrolysing sucrose with a mineral acid, such as hydrochloric acid, and neutralising the solution with, for example, calcium carbonate or sodium carbonate.

Syrups are available commercially at strengths corresponding to up to 84 per cent w/w of sugars and to various degrees of inversion; the standard in this monograph refers to a syrup corresponding to at least 95 per cent inversion of a 66·7 per cent w/w solution of sucrose.

Solubility. Miscible with water, forming a clear solution; partly soluble in alcohol.

Standard
DESCRIPTION. A clear colourless to pale straw-coloured syrupy liquid; odourless; taste sweet.

IDENTIFICATION TESTS. 1. Heat 1 g with 10 ml of water and 5 ml of *potassium cupri-tartrate solution*; a red precipitate is formed.

2. A solution in water is laevorotatory.

ACIDITY. pH, 5·0 to 6·0.

REFRACTIVE INDEX. At 20°, 1·4608 to 1·4630.

WEIGHT PER ML. At 20°, 1·338 g to 1·344 g.

ARSENIC. It complies with the test given in Appendix 6, page 880 (1 part per million).

LEAD. It complies with the test given in Appendix 7, page 884 (2 parts per million).

SULPHUR DIOXIDE. Not more than 70 parts per million, determined by the method of the British Pharmacopoeia, Appendix XJ, for the determination of sulphur dioxide.

SULPHATED ASH. Not more than 0·1 per cent.

CONTENT OF INVERT SUGARS. Not less than 67·0 per cent w/w, determined by the method for reducing sugars given in Appendix 15, page 894.

Storage. It should be stored at a temperature between 35° and 45°.

Uses. Invert syrup, when mixed in suitable proportions with syrup, prevents the deposition of crystals of sucrose under most conditions of storage.

Lemon Syrup

Lemon Spirit	..	..	..	5 ml
Citric Acid	..	..	..	25 g
Invert Syrup	..	..	..	100 ml
Syrup	..	..	..	.. to 1000 ml

Dissolve the citric acid in a portion of the syrup, add the invert syrup, the lemon spirit, and sufficient syrup to produce the required volume, and mix. It has a weight per ml at 20° of about 1·33 g.

Standard
CONTENT OF CITRIC ACID. 2·37 to 2·63 per cent w/v, calculated as $C_6H_8O_7,H_2O$, determined by the following method:
Mix about 8 g, accurately weighed, with 100 ml of water and titrate with 0·1N sodium hydroxide, using *phenolphthalein solution* as indicator; each ml of 0·1N sodium hydroxide is equivalent to 0·007005 g of $C_6H_8O_7,H_2O$.
Determine the weight per ml of the syrup and calculate the concentration of $C_6H_8O_7,H_2O$, weight in volume.

Storage. It should be stored in a cool place.

Dose. 2·5 to 5 millilitres.

Orange Syrup

SYNONYM: Syrupus Aurantii

Orange Tincture	..	..	..	60 ml
Syrup	..	..	..	.. to 1000 ml

Mix.

Standard
WEIGHT PER ML. At 20°, 1·29 g to 1·31 g.

Dose. 2·5 to 5 millilitres.

Raspberry Syrup

SYNONYM: Syrupus Rubi Idaei

Raspberry Syrup may be prepared by diluting one volume of Concentrated Raspberry Juice with eleven volumes of Syrup.

If it is prepared with precautions which will prevent fermentation and packed in such a manner as to preserve it in this condition, it need not be freshly prepared; once the container has been opened, however, it should be used within a few weeks.

If it is made without taking precautions to prevent fermentation, it must be freshly prepared.

A dye, or a mixture of dyes, may be added, provided that any dye used is of food grade of commerce and that its use for colouring food is permitted in the country concerned.

Standard
WEIGHT PER ML. At 20°, 1·31 g to 1·34 g.

SULPHUR DIOXIDE. Not more than 420 parts per million w/w, determined by the method of the British Pharmacopoeia, Appendix XJ, for the determination of sulphur dioxide.

Storage. It should be stored in a cool place, protected from light.

Note. Raspberry Syrup is intended only for flavouring pharmaceutical products. If it is used for other purposes, it may not comply with the Preservatives in Food Regulations in respect of sulphur dioxide content.

Squill Syrup

Squill Vinegar	..	..	..	450 ml
Sucrose	..	..	..	..	800 g
Water (see page 642)		..	.. to 1000 ml

Dissolve the sucrose in the squill vinegar with the aid of gentle heat, strain, cool, add sufficient water to produce the required volume, and mix.

Standard
WEIGHT PER ML. At 20°, 1·30 g to 1·33 g.

CONTENT OF ACETIC ACID. 2·0 to 3·0 per cent w/v, calculated as $C_2H_4O_2$, determined by the following method:
Dilute 20 ml with 20 ml of water and titrate with 1N sodium hydroxide, using *phenolphthalein solution* as indicator; each ml of 1N sodium hydroxide is equivalent to 0·06005 g of $C_2H_4O_2$.

Dose. 2·5 to 5 millilitres.

Tolu Syrup

Tolu Solution	..	..	..	100 ml
Syrup	..	..	..	.. to 1000 ml

Mix.

Standard
WEIGHT PER ML. At 20°, 1·29 g to 1·32 g.

Wild Cherry Syrup

SYNONYMS: Syrupus Pruni Serotinae; Virginian Prune Syrup

Wild Cherry Bark, in moderately coarse powder ..		..	..	150 g
Sucrose	..	..	..	..	800 g
Glycerol	..	..	..	..	50 ml
Water (see page 642)		..	.. to 1000 ml

Percolate the wild cherry bark with water, collecting the percolate in a vessel containing the sucrose and the glycerol; continue the percolation until the total volume is 1000 ml, shake to dissolve the sucrose, without the aid of heat, and add sufficient water to produce the required volume.

Standard
WEIGHT PER ML. At 20°, 1·30 g to 1·33 g.

Storage. It should be stored in a cool place.

Dose. 2·5 to 10 millilitres.

TABLETS

Tablets are compact products containing medicaments in compressed or moulded form.

Compressed tablets are usually circular in shape with either flat or convex surfaces. They are prepared by compressing a granulated preparation of the medicament, or mixture of medicaments, by means of punches in suitable dies. The material may be prepared for compression in a dry granular form by one of the following processes.

Dry granulation may be used for materials which can be made into tablets by direct compression. Certain substances can be produced in the form of crystals or granules for compression. It may be necessary to remove larger particles with a suitable sieve and to dry before compressing. The addition of suitable excipients and lubricants may be necessary.

Alternatively, the medicament, or mixture of medicaments, may be mixed with a readily compressible diluent to produce a free-flowing material suitable for direct compression. The addition of suitable excipients and lubricants may be necessary.

When this method is used, especial care is necessary in mixing to ensure uniformity of content in the tablets.

Moist granulation. The medicament, or mixture of medicaments, in powder, is mixed when necessary with an inert substance to act as diluent, absorbent, or adhesive; lactose, sucrose, dextrose, starch, sodium chloride, and acacia, all in powder, are examples of such substances. The material is moistened with a suitable liquid excipient until the powder becomes just coherent but will not adhere to the mesh when pressed through a sieve; moistening agents include water, alcohol of suitable strength, isopropyl alcohol, acacia mucilage, starch mucilage, and solutions of dextrose, sucrose, or gelatin in varying strengths or mixtures.

The moistened material is pressed through a sieve, the granules so formed are dried at a temperature not exceeding 60°, and sieved to remove powder and small granules. A disintegrating agent may be required and for this purpose starch or some other suitable substance may be lightly mixed with the dried granules; lubricants such as stearic acid, stearates, and talc in fine powder, and liquid paraffin are added to prevent the material from sticking to the punches and dies during compression.

Diluents, disintegrating agents, moistening agents, lubricants, and any other added materials must of themselves have no therapeutic action in the quantities present and must be compatible with other ingredients of the tablets.

Granulation by preliminary compression is effected by first compressing the material into large tablets and then breaking these into granules of a suitable size, which are sieved to remove powder and small particles. If necessary, a disintegrating agent and a lubricant are added before final compression.

Moulded tablets, or tablet triturates, are flat disks usually containing a potent medicament diluted with lactose, dextrose, or other suitable diluent. They are prepared by finely powdering the medicament and triturating with the appropriate amount of diluent. The powder is moistened with alcohol (60 per cent), or other suitable liquid, and pressed into holes in a plate. The moulded tablets are ejected from the plate and dried at room temperature.

Chocolate-base tablets are prepared by the above methods with the chocolate basis of the British Pharmacopoeia. The cocoa powder, sucrose, and lactose are added to the medicament before granulation.

Coated tablets. Tablets may be coated to improve their appearance and stability, to mask an unpleasant taste, or to protect the medicament from the acid of the stomach. The coat is usually composed of inert materials and may contain colouring matter only when this is permitted in the individual monograph. A coat generally influences the size and disintegration rate of a tablet, usually the smallest effect being produced by film coats and the greatest by sugar coats. The cores of tablets intended for coating should comply with the requirements of the British Pharmacopoeia for uniformity of weight given under Tablets.

COATING PROCESSES. The following processes are used for coating tablets.

Pan coating. The process consists of rotating the tablet cores and applying either an aqueous solution or suspension of the coating composition or a solution of the composition in a volatile solvent.

Compression coating. The coating composition in the form of granules is applied by means of compression around the tablet cores.

Air-suspension coating. The tablet cores are placed in a cylinder and kept in a state of motion by an upward current of air while the coating composition, consisting of a suspension or solution in a suitable volatile solvent, is sprayed into the cylinder.

COATING COMPOSITIONS. The following types of coat are applied to tablets.

Sugar coat. The coat contains a high proportion of sucrose, with purified talc, starch, or other suitable substances, and is applied either by the pan-coating or compression-coating process.

Compression coat. The coat consists of lactose, calcium phosphate, or other suitable substances; in certain compound tablets, medicaments intended for quick release may be included in the coat.

Film coat. The coat contains water-soluble, dispersible, or permeable substances of natural or synthetic origin, such as cellacephate, methylcellulose, or povidone, and is applied by the pan-coating or air-suspension-coating process.

Enteric coat. The coat consists of substances which are relatively insoluble in the acid medium of the stomach but which disintegrate in the alkaline medium of the small intestine. It is applied by the pan-coating, compression-coating, or air-suspension-coating process.

Slow tablets, or sustained-release tablets, are formulated to release the medicament slowly in the gastro-intestinal tract over a period of hours, thus prolonging the period during which an effective concentration is maintained in the tissues. Slow tablets may be used to secure a reduction in the frequency of administration of a drug and may also be formulated to prevent a rapid release of an irritant medicament in the gastro-intestinal tract.

Numerous methods are adopted in order to depress the release of a medicament; for example, the tablet can be very firmly compacted or the medicament in fine particles may be imbedded in fatty alcohols or in a glyceride so that slow leaching from the core takes place. Other techniques involve the use of inert porous carriers or the coating of particles of medicament with a relatively resistant film or coat. Ion-exchange resins are also used for acidic and basic drugs. The formulation of slow tablets carries with it the responsibility of demonstrating that the products perform in the manner intended.

Extemporaneous preparation of tablets. Small batches of special tablet formulations may sometimes be prepared by compression or moulding but this is usually impracticable and it may be preferable, with the prescriber's permission, to dispense the medicaments in the form of capsules, provided that this does not significantly alter their therapeutic efficacy.

Administration of tablets. Tablets may be swallowed, chewed, or crushed and administered with water or other liquid. Sublingual tablets are intended to be dissolved slowly under the tongue. Some tablets are intended to be dissolved in water before administration. Unless otherwise specified, tablets are intended to be swallowed whole.

Weight of tablets. Tablets may be made up with an inert substance to a weight which is suitable for the specified diameter. Owing to unavoidable variation in size of granules and to slight variation in the filling of the die, tablets are subject to some variation in weight. This variation, however, should be kept within reasonable limits and will depend upon the size of the tablets, so that the limits for deviation from the mean weight are wider in the case of small tablets. Limits are specified in the British Pharmacopoeia for tablets weighing 80 milligrams or less, tablets weighing between 80 and 250 milligrams, and tablets weighing 250 milligrams or more.

Content of active ingredient. When tablets include substances that have a standard permitting a relatively high proportion of moisture or where the content of pure drug may vary within relatively wide limits, a sufficient quantity of the substance must be used to ensure that the tablets comply with the requirements given in the monograph.

Standard

COATING. Tablets may be coated only when coating is specifically permitted in the individual monographs.

COLOURING AND FLAVOURING. Tablets, and tablet coatings other than enteric coatings or compression coatings, may contain colouring and flavouring agents only when these are specifically permitted in the individual monographs.

UNIFORMITY OF DIAMETER. Unless otherwise specified, tablets are circular in shape; uncoated and compression-coated tablets comply with the requirements given in Appendix 26, page 912.

UNIFORMITY OF WEIGHT. Tablets which are not sugar coated or enteric coated comply with the requirements of the British Pharmacopoeia for uniformity of weight given under Tablets.

CONTENT OF ACTIVE INGREDIENT. When limits for content of active ingredient are given in the monographs, all permissible allowances, including variations due to manufacturing methods and to the purity of the active ingredient, are included. Unless otherwise specified, the limits are only applicable when the determination is carried out on a sample of at least 20 tablets.
When it is not possible to obtain a sample of 20 tablets, the wider limits given in the British Pharmacopoeia for samples of 15, 10, or 5 tablets will apply.
When tablets containing relatively small doses of active ingredient are assayed, 20 tablets may prove insufficient to give the specified amount of medicament; in these circumstances, the number of tablets taken should be increased to enable that amount to be used for the determination.

DISINTEGRATION TIME. Determine the disintegration time by the method of the British Pharmacopoeia. Uncoated tablets have a maximum disintegration time of 15 minutes. Sugar-coated tablets have a maximum disintegration time of 1 hour.

The maximum disintegration times of compression-coated and film-coated tablets are given in the individual monographs concerned.

Enteric-coated tablets comply with the specific disintegration test given in the British Pharmacopoeia.

Containers and storage. All tablets should be stored and supplied in containers which provide adequate protection against crushing. In addition, tablets which deteriorate if exposed to a moist atmosphere or to light should be stored and supplied in containers which are airtight or light-resistant, or both, as specified in the individual monographs. Sugar coating generally prevents this deterioration to a large extent, and, if the tablets are coated, or if a patient is being supplied with a quantity sufficient for use over a short period, it may not be necessary to follow the directions in individual monographs that the containers should be airtight or light-resistant.

Tablets should preferably be stored and supplied in amber glass bottles, jars, or vials, in amber or opaque plastic containers, or in aluminium containers, suitably protected internally; lined screw-cap closures or plastic caps should be used. Tablets may also be packaged in strip foil, each tablet being hermetically sealed in a pocket of foil. This method gives good protection against ingress of moisture but effervescent tablets so packed must have an exceedingly low initial moisture content.

Acetarsol Tablets

SYNONYM: Acetarsone Tablets

Acetarsol Tablets may be prepared by moist granulation and compression as described under Tablets (page 801).

Standard
They comply with the standard under Tablets, above, with the following additions:

PRESENCE OF ACETARSOL. To 1 tablet, finely powdered, add 10 ml of 1N sodium hydroxide, shake, filter, using an apparatus for vacuum filtration, and carefully acidify the filtrate with *dilute hydrochloric acid*; a white precipitate is produced.
Wash the precipitate with water, dissolve it in 2 ml of 1N sodium hydroxide, add 2 ml of *sulphuric acid* and 2 ml of *alcohol (95 per cent)*, and heat the solution; the odour of ethyl acetate is produced.

INORGANIC ARSENATES. Dissolve, as completely as possible, an accurately weighed quantity of the powdered tablets, equivalent to 1 g of acetarsol, in a mixture of 2 ml of *dilute ammonia solution* and 8 ml of water and filter; to 5 ml of the filtrate add 5 ml of *magnesium ammonio-sulphate solution*, shake, and allow to stand for 30 minutes; no precipitate is produced.

CONTENT OF ACETARSOL. 92·5 to 107·5 per cent of the prescribed or stated amount, calculated as $C_8H_{10}AsNO_5$, determined by the following method:
Weigh and powder 20 tablets. Determine by the method for Acetarsol Pessaries, page 772, an accurately weighed quantity of the powder, equivalent to about 0·2 g of acetarsol, being used.
Calculate the total weight of $C_8H_{10}AsNO_5$ in the 20 tablets and divide by 20.

Containers and storage. The directions given under Tablets (above) should be followed.

Dose. Acetarsol, 250 to 500 milligrams.

When the strength of the tablets is not specified, tablets each containing 250 mg of acetarsol shall be supplied.

Ammonium Chloride Tablets

Ammonium Chloride Tablets may be prepared by moist granulation and compression as described under Tablets (page 801). They may be enteric coated and the coating may be coloured.

Standard
They comply with the standard under Tablets, above, with the following addition:

CONTENT OF AMMONIUM CHLORIDE. 95·0 to 105·0 per cent of the prescribed or stated amount, calculated as NH_4Cl, determined by the following method:
Weigh and powder 20 tablets. Transfer to an ammonia-distillation apparatus an accurately weighed quantity of the powder, equivalent to about 0·15 g of ammonium chloride, add 5 ml of *sodium hydroxide solution*, distil into 50 ml of 0·1N sulphuric acid, and titrate the excess of acid with 0·1N sodium hydroxide, using *methyl red solution* as indicator.
Repeat the procedure omitting the sample.
The difference between the two titrations represents the amount of acid required by the sample; each ml of 0·1N sulphuric acid is equivalent to 0·005349 g of NH_4Cl.
Calculate the total weight of NH_4Cl in the 20 tablets and divide by 20.

Containers and storage. The directions given under Tablets (above) should be followed.

Dose. Ammonium chloride, 0·3 to 2 grams; before the administration of mersalyl injection, 3 to 6 grams daily, in divided doses.

When the strength of the tablets is not specified, enteric-coated tablets each containing 450 mg of ammonium chloride shall be supplied.
Enteric-coated tablets containing 500 mg are also available.

Ampicillin Tablets, Paediatric

Paediatric Ampicillin Tablets contain Ampicillin or Ampicillin Trihydrate and may be prepared by the process of granulation by preliminary compression followed by compression as described under Tablets (page 801).

Standard

They comply with the standard under Tablets, page 804, with the following additions:

PRESENCE OF AMPICILLIN. They comply with the thin-layer chromatographic test given in Appendix 5A, page 859.

CONTENT OF AMPICILLIN. 90·0 to 110·0 per cent of the prescribed or stated amount, determined by the following method:

Weigh and powder 20 tablets. To an accurately weighed quantity of the powder, equivalent to about 0·1 g of ampicillin, add 70 ml of *dilute sodium bicarbonate solution*, shake vigorously for 10 minutes, dilute to 100 ml with *dilute sodium bicarbonate solution*, filter, discarding the first 20 ml of the filtrate, transfer 2 ml of the filtrate to each of two tubes, and continue by the method for Ampicillin Mixture, page 737, beginning with the words "To the first tube add . . .".
Calculate the total weight of ampicillin in the 20 tablets and divide by 20.

Containers and storage. The directions given under Tablets (page 805) should be followed; containers should be airtight. The tablets should be stored in a cool place.

Dose. The equivalent of ampicillin, every six hours:

CHILD. 1 to 5 years, 125 to 187·5 milligrams; 6 to 12 years, 187·5 to 250 milligrams.

When the strength of the tablets is not specified, tablets each containing the equivalent of 125 mg of ampicillin shall be supplied.

Aspirin Tablets, Compound

SYNONYMS: Compound Tablets of Acetylsalicylic Acid; A.P.C. Tablets

For each tablet take:

Aspirin, in crystals	..	..	225 mg
Caffeine ..	..	..	30 mg
Phenacetin	..	..	150 mg

Mix the phenacetin with the caffeine and granulate by moist granulation as described under Tablets (page 801); dry, mix with the aspirin, and prepare by compression.

Standard

They comply with the standard under Tablets, page 804, with the following additions:

PRESENCE OF CAFFEINE. Dissolve 0·01 g of the residue obtained in the determination of anhydrous caffeine in 1 ml of *hydrochloric acid*, add 0·1 g of *potassium chlorate*, and evaporate to dryness in a porcelain dish; a reddish residue is obtained which becomes purple on exposure to the vapour of *dilute ammonia solution*.

PRESENCE OF PHENACETIN. Boil 0·1 g of the residue obtained in the determination of phenacetin with 1 ml of *hydrochloric acid* for 3 minutes, dilute to 10 ml with water, cool, filter, and to the filtrate add 0·05 ml of 0·1N potassium dichromate; a violet colour is produced which rapidly changes to ruby-red.

4-CHLOROACETANILIDE. They comply with the thin-layer chromatographic test given in Appendix 5A, page 860 (100 parts per million with respect to the phenacetin present).

SALICYLIC ACID. To a quantity of the powdered tablets, equivalent to 0·25 g of aspirin, add 50 ml of *chloroform* and 10 ml of water, shake well, allow to separate, filter the chloroform layer through a dry filter paper, and evaporate 10 ml of the filtrate to dryness in a current of air at room temperature.

Dissolve the residue in 4 ml of *alcohol (95 per cent)*, dilute to 100 ml with water, filter, and to 50 ml of the filtrate add 1 ml of *acid ferric ammonium sulphate solution* and allow to stand for 1 minute.

Any violet colour produced is not more intense than that produced when 1 ml of *acid ferric ammonium sulphate solution* is added to a solution prepared by diluting a mixture containing 1 ml of a freshly prepared 0·01 per cent w/v solution of *salicylic acid* in water and 2 ml of *alcohol (95 per cent)* to 50 ml with water (0·4 per cent with respect to the aspirin present).

CONTENT OF ASPIRIN. 0·214 g to 0·236 g, calculated as $C_9H_8O_4$, determined by the following method:

Weigh and powder 20 tablets. Boil an accurately weighed quantity of the powder, equivalent to about 4 tablets, under a reflux condenser for 30 minutes with 20 ml of water and 2 g of *sodium citrate*, wash the condenser with 30 ml of warm water, add the washings to the contents of the flask, and titrate with 0·5N sodium hydroxide, using *phenolphthalein solution* as indicator; each ml of 0·5N sodium hydroxide is equivalent to 0·04504 g of $C_9H_8O_4$.
Calculate the total weight of $C_9H_8O_4$ in the 20 tablets and divide by 20.

CONTENT OF ANHYDROUS CAFFEINE. 0·028 g to 0·032 g, determined by the following method:

Boil an accurately weighed quantity of the powder, equivalent to about 1 tablet, under a reflux condenser for one hour with 10 ml of *dilute sulphuric acid*, cool, add 10 ml of water, and extract with successive 30-ml portions of *chloroform* until extraction is complete, reserving the aqueous solution for the determination of phenacetin.

Extract the combined extracts with three successive 20-ml portions of 1N sodium hydroxide and then with 20 ml of water, discard the aqueous extracts, evaporate off the chloroform, and dry the residue of anhydrous caffeine to constant weight at 105°.
Calculate the total weight of anhydrous caffeine in the 20 tablets and divide by 20.

CONTENT OF PHENACETIN. 0·142 g to 0·158 g, determined by the following method:

Make alkaline to *litmus paper* the aqueous solution reserved in the determination of anhydrous caffeine by the addition of *sodium bicarbonate*, add 0·5 ml of *acetic anhydride*, and shake vigorously.

Extract with four successive 25-ml portions of *chloroform*, evaporate the combined extracts to dryness, repeatedly treat the residue with small portions of *alcohol (95 per cent)*, evaporating off the solvent each time, until the residue is free from the odour of acetic acid, and dry the residue of phenacetin to constant weight at 105°.
Calculate the total weight of phenacetin in the 20 tablets and divide by 20.

Containers and storage. The directions given under Tablets (page 805) should be followed; containers should be airtight. The tablets should be stored in a cool place.

Dose. 1 or 2 tablets.

Aspirin Tablets, Soluble, Paediatric

SYNONYM: Soluble Tablets of Acetylsalicylic Acid, Paediatric

For each tablet take:

Aspirin, in fine powder ..	..	75·0 mg
Saccharin Sodium	..	..	0·75 mg
Anhydrous Citric Acid ..	..	7·5 mg
Calcium Carbonate	..	..	25·0 mg

Mix, and prepare by preliminary compression, or moist granulation using a non-aqueous liquid excipient, and compression as described under Tablets (page 801).

Standard

They comply with the standard, except for disintegration time, under Tablets, page 804, with the following additions:

DISINTEGRATION TIME. Maximum time, 3 minutes.

SALICYLIC ACID. To a quantity of the powdered tablets, equivalent to 0·50 g of aspirin, add 20 ml of *chloroform*, shake vigorously for 2 minutes, filter through a dry filter paper, and evaporate 5 ml of the filtrate to dryness in a current of air at room temperature.
Transfer the residue, with the aid of a total of 3 ml of *alcohol (95 per cent)*, to a suitable tube, dilute to 50 ml with water, add 1 ml of *acid ferric ammonium sulphate solution*, mix, and allow to stand for 1 minute.
Any violet colour produced is not more intense than that produced when 1 ml of *acid ferric ammonium sulphate solution* is added to a solution prepared by diluting a mixture containing 2 ml of a freshly prepared 0·01 per cent w/v solution of *salicylic acid* in water and 3 ml of *alcohol (95 per cent)* to 50 ml with water (0·16 per cent with respect to the aspirin present).

CONTENT OF ASPIRIN. 0·069 g to 0·081 g, calculated as $C_9H_8O_4$, determined by the following method:
Weigh and powder 20 tablets. Boil an accurately weighed quantity of the powder, equivalent to about 4 tablets, under a reflux condenser for 1 hour with 10 ml of *dilute sulphuric acid*.
Cool, transfer the solution to a separating funnel with the aid of small quantities of water, extract with four successive 20-ml portions of *solvent ether*, wash the combined extracts with two successive 5-ml portions of water, and evaporate off the ether in a current of air at a temperature not exceeding 30°.
Dissolve the residue in 20 ml of 0·5N sodium hydroxide and dilute to 200 ml with water.
To 50 ml of this solution in a stoppered flask add 50 ml of 0·1N bromine and 5 ml of *hydrochloric acid*, shake repeatedly during 15 minutes, allow to stand for 15 minutes, add 20 ml of *potassium iodide solution*, shake thoroughly, and titrate with 0·1N sodium thiosulphate; each ml of 0·1N bromine is equivalent to 0·003003 g of $C_9H_8O_4$.
Calculate the total weight of aspirin in the 20 tablets and divide by 20.

Containers and storage. The directions given under Tablets (page 805) should be followed; containers should be airtight. The tablets should be stored in a cool place.

Dose. CHILD. 1 to 2 years, 1 to 2 tablets not more than four times daily; 3 to 5 years, 3 to 4 tablets not more than three times daily; 6 to 12 years, 4 tablets not more than three or four times daily.
These doses are to be given for not more than two days, except under medical supervision.

Belladonna and Phenobarbitone Tablets

For each tablet take:

Belladonna Dry Extract ..	..	12·5 mg
Phenobarbitone ..	.. ..	25·0 mg

Mix, and prepare by moist granulation and compression as described under Tablets (page 801).

Standard

They comply with the standard under Tablets, page 804, with the following additions:

PRESENCE OF PHENOBARBITONE. The residue obtained in the determination of phenobarbitone complies with the following tests:
Dissolve 1 mg of the residue in 2 ml of *chloroform*, add 0·6 ml of a 5 per cent v/v solution of *isopropylamine* in *methyl alcohol*, mix, and add 0·1 ml of a 1 per cent w/v solution of *cobalt chloride* in *methyl alcohol*; a reddish-purple colour slowly develops.
Crystallise the remainder of the residue, using 6 ml of *toluene* as the solvent; the crystals, after washing with *toluene* and drying, melt at about 176°.

PRESENCE OF BELLADONNA ALKALOIDS. They comply with the thin-layer chromatographic test given in Appendix 5B, page 871.

CONTENT OF PHENOBARBITONE. 0·023 g to 0·027 g, determined by the following method:
Weigh and powder 20 tablets. Dissolve an accurately weighed quantity of the powder, equivalent to about half a tablet, in 10 ml of 0·1N sodium hydroxide, saturate the solution with *sodium chloride*, acidify to *litmus paper* with *hydrochloric acid*, and extract with successive 15-ml portions of *solvent ether* until extraction is complete.
Extract the combined extracts with four successive 20-ml portions of a mixture of 6 ml of *sodium hydroxide solution* and 76 ml of *brine*; acidify the combined aqueous extracts to *litmus paper* with *hydrochloric acid*, and extract with successive 15-ml portions of *solvent ether* until extraction is complete.
Wash the combined ethereal extracts with two successive 2-ml portions of water, discard the washings, filter the extracts, and wash the filter with *solvent ether*.
Evaporate off the ether from the combined extracts and washings, and dry the residue of phenobarbitone to constant weight at 105°.
Calculate the total weight of phenobarbitone in the 20 tablets and divide by 20.

Containers and storage. The directions given under Tablets (page 805) should be followed; containers should be airtight and light resistant.

Dose. 1 tablet.

Calcium Aminosalicylate Tablets

Calcium Aminosalicylate Tablets may be prepared by moist granulation and compression as described under Tablets (page 801). They are sugar coated and the coat may be coloured.

Standard

They comply with the standard, except for disintegration time, under Tablets, page 804, with the following additions:

DISINTEGRATION TIME. Maximum time, 2 hours.

PRESENCE OF CALCIUM. Remove the sugar coating from one tablet by washing with water, cut the tablet in half, remove any remaining coating by hand, dissolve as much of the core as possible in 10 ml of water, and filter; the filtrate gives the reactions characteristic of calcium.

3-AMINOPHENOL. Dissolve a quantity of the powdered tablets, equivalent to 0·30 g of calcium aminosalicylate, in 20 ml of water, add 1 ml of *alcohol (95 per cent)*, shake, dilute to 25 ml with water, and filter.
To 5 ml of the filtrate add 2 ml of *4-amino-NN-diethylaniline sulphate solution*, 0·35 ml of *dilute ammonia solution*, 10 ml of *toluene*, and 4 ml of *potassium ferricyanide solution*, shake for 20 seconds, discard the aqueous layer, wash the toluene layer with two successive quantities each consisting of a mixture of 0·35 ml of *dilute ammonia solution* and 4·5 ml of water, shaking each wash for 20 seconds.
Dry the toluene layer over *anhydrous sodium sulphate* and dilute to 50 ml with *toluene*; any colour in the toluene solution is not more intense than that produced when 4 ml of *3-aminophenol solution* is treated in

the same manner (0·1 per cent with respect to the calcium aminosalicylate present).

CONTENT OF CALCIUM AMINOSALICYLATE. 90·0 to 110·0 per cent of the prescribed or stated amount, calculated as $C_{14}H_{12}CaN_2O_6,3H_2O$, determined by the following method:
Weigh and powder 20 tablets. To an accurately weighed quantity of the powder, equivalent to about 0·6 g of calcium aminosalicylate, add 75 ml of water, shake until the calcium aminosalicylate is completely dissolved, dilute to 100 ml with water and filter, rejecting the first 20 ml of the filtrate.
To 50 ml of the filtrate add 150 ml of cold water, 25 g of ice, and 10 ml of *hydrochloric acid*, and titrate slowly with 0·1M sodium nitrite, with vigorous stirring, until a drop of the solution on a glass rod immediately gives a blue colour when drawn quickly across the surface of a film of *starch-iodide paste*, the titration being complete when the end-point is reproduced after the titrated solution has been allowed to stand for 2 minutes; each ml of 0·1M sodium nitrite is equivalent to 0·01992 g of $C_{14}H_{12}CaN_2O_6,3H_2O$.
Calculate the total weight of $C_{14}H_{12}CaN_2O_6,3H_2O$ in the 20 tablets and divide by 20.

Containers and storage. The directions given under Tablets (page 805) should be followed; containers should be airtight. The tablets should be stored in a cool place.

Dose. Calcium aminosalicylate, 10 to 15 grams daily, in divided doses.

When the strength of the tablets is not specified, sugar-coated tablets each containing 500 mg of calcium aminosalicylate shall be supplied.

Calcium Gluconate Tablets

For each tablet take:

Calcium Gluconate	..	..	600·0 mg
Vanillin ..	..	..	0·5 mg
Prepared Theobroma	..	..	150·0 mg
Sucrose ..	..	..	450·0 mg

Mix, and prepare by moist granulation and compression as described under Tablets (page 801).

Standard
They comply with the standard, except for disintegration time, under Tablets, page 804, with the following additions:

PRESENCE OF GLUCONATE. Extract 5 tablets, finely powdered, with two successive 25-ml portions of *light petroleum (boiling-range, 40° to 60°)*, discard the extracts, and repeat the extraction with three 10-ml portions of water, again discarding the extracts.
Dissolve the residue as completely as possible in 30 ml of hot water and filter; the filtrate complies with the following tests:
(i) To 0·5 ml add 0·05 ml of *ferric chloride test-solution*; an intense yellow colour is produced.
(ii) To 5 ml add 0·65 ml of *glacial acetic acid* and 1 ml of *phenylhydrazine*, heat on a water-bath for 30 minutes, cool, and induce crystallisation; filter, dissolve the residue on the filter in 10 ml of hot water, add a suitable quantity of *decolorising charcoal*, shake, filter, allow the filtrate to cool and induce crystallisation; a white crystalline precipitate is produced which melts with decomposition at about 201°.

CONTENT OF CALCIUM GLUCONATE. 0·57 g to 0·63 g, calculated as $C_{12}H_{22}CaO_{14},H_2O$, determined by the following method:
Weigh and powder 20 tablets. Ignite an accurately weighed quantity of the powder, equivalent to about 1 tablet, cool, dissolve the residue in the minimum quantity of *dilute hydrochloric acid*, filter, wash the residue on the filter with water, and dilute the combined filtrate and washings to 50 ml.

Add 0·1 g of *ascorbic acid*, neutralise to *litmus paper* with *dilute ammonia solution*, add 5 ml of 0·05M magnesium sulphate, 10 ml of *ammonia buffer solution*, and 1 ml of *potassium cyanide solution*, and titrate with 0·05M disodium edetate, using *mordant black 11 solution* as indicator; each ml of 0·05M disodium edetate, after deducting the volume of 0·05M magnesium sulphate added, is equivalent to 0·02242 g of $C_{12}H_{22}CaO_{14},H_2O$.
Calculate the total weight of $C_{12}H_{22}CaO_{14},H_2O$ in the 20 tablets and divide by 20.

Containers and storage. The directions given under Tablets (page 805) should be followed; containers should be airtight.

Labelling. A direction to chew the tablets before they are swallowed should be given on the label.

Dose. 1 to 10 tablets, repeated in accordance with the needs of the patient.

Calcium Gluconate Tablets, Effervescent

For each tablet take:

Calcium Gluconate	..	..	1 g
Saccharin Sodium	..	..	1 mg
Anhydrous Citric Acid	..	..	150 mg
Tartaric Acid	..	..	300 mg
Sodium Bicarbonate	..	..	375 mg

Mix, and prepare by moist granulation, using a non-aqueous liquid excipient, and compression as described under Tablets (page 801).

Standard
They comply with the standard, except for disintegration time, under Tablets, page 804, with the following additions:

PRESENCE OF GLUCONATE. Dissolve 1 tablet, finely powdered, in 20 ml of hot water, cool, and filter; the filtrate complies with tests (i) and (ii) for the presence of gluconate described under Calcium Gluconate Tablets, 10 ml being used for test (ii).

SOLUBILITY. When placed in water at 20°, they dissolve almost completely within 5 minutes.

CONTENT OF AVAILABLE CARBON DIOXIDE. Not less than 0·07 g, calculated as CO_2, determined by the method for Mouth-wash Solution-tablets, page 792, about 0·3 g of the powdered tablets, accurately weighed, being used.

CONTENT OF CALCIUM GLUCONATE. 0·95 g to 1·05 g, calculated as $C_{12}H_{22}CaO_{14},H_2O$, determined by the method for Calcium Gluconate Tablets, an accurately weighed quantity of the powdered tablets, equivalent to about 0·5 g of calcium gluconate, being used.

Containers and storage. The directions given under Tablets (page 805) should be followed; containers should be well filled and airtight. The tablets should be stored in a cool place.

Labelling. A direction to dissolve the tablets in water and take the solution as soon as the tablets have dissolved should be given on the label.

Dose. 1 to 6 tablets, repeated in accordance with the needs of the patient.

Calcium Sodium Lactate Tablets

Calcium Sodium Lactate Tablets may be prepared by moist granulation and compression as described under Tablets (page 801).

Standard
They comply with the standard, except for disintegration time, under Tablets, page 804, with the following additions:

DISINTEGRATION TIME. Maximum time, 30 minutes.

PRESENCE OF LACTATE. To one tablet, finely powdered, add 5 ml of *dilute sulphuric acid* and 0·1 g of *potassium permanganate* and heat; the potassium permanganate is decolorised and the odour of acetaldehyde is produced.

CONTENT OF CALCIUM. 7·1 to 8·9 per cent of the prescribed or stated amount of calcium sodium lactate, calculated as Ca, determined by the following method: Weigh and powder 20 tablets. Dissolve, as completely as possible, an accurately weighed quantity of the powder, equivalent to about 0·05 g of Ca, in 50 ml of water and continue by the method for Ca in Calcium Sodium Lactate, page 70, beginning with the words "add 5 ml of 0·05M magnesium sulphate . . .".
Calculate the total weight of Ca in the 20 tablets and divide by 20.

CONTENT OF SODIUM. 8·0 to 10·5 per cent of the prescribed or stated amount of calcium sodium lactate, calculated as Na, determined by the following method: Weigh and powder 20 tablets and determine by the method for Na in Calcium Sodium Lactate, page 70, using an accurately weighed quantity of the powder, equivalent to about 2 g of calcium sodium lactate. Calculate the total weight of Na in the 20 tablets and divide by 20.

Containers and storage. The directions given under Tablets (page 805) should be followed; containers should be airtight.

Dose. Calcium sodium lactate, 0·3 to 2 grams.

When the strength of the tablets is not specified, tablets each containing 450 mg of calcium sodium lactate shall be supplied.

Calcium with Vitamin D Tablets

For each tablet take:

Calcium Sodium Lactate	..	..	450·0 mg
Calcium Phosphate	..	..	150·0 mg
Calciferol ..	..	..	0·0125 mg

Mix the calcium sodium lactate with the calcium phosphate and granulate by moist granulation as described under Tablets (page 801); dry the granules, add the calciferol, either dissolved in a suitable quantity of a fixed oil, as a pre-granulated dispersion, or as a triturate with calcium phosphate, and prepare by compression.

Standard
They comply with the standard, except for disintegration time, under Tablets, page 804, with the following additions:

PRESENCE OF LACTATE. Warm one tablet, finely powdered, with 5 ml of *dilute sulphuric acid* and 5 ml of 0·1N potassium permanganate; the potassium permanganate is decolorised and the odour of acetaldehyde is produced.

PRESENCE OF PHOSPHATE. Warm one tablet, finely powdered, with 10 ml of *dilute nitric acid*, cool, filter, and to the filtrate add an equal volume of *ammonium molybdate solution* and warm; a bright canary-yellow precipitate is produced.

CONTENT OF CALCIUM. Not less than 0·079 g, calculated as Ca, determined by the following method: Weigh and powder 20 tablets. Dissolve as completely as possible an accurately weighed quantity of the powder, equivalent to about half a tablet, in 5 ml of *hydrochloric acid* and dilute to 100 ml with water. Add 40 ml of 0·05M disodium edetate, neutralise to *litmus paper* with *sodium hydroxide solution*, add 10 ml of *ammonia buffer solution*, and titrate with 0·05M zinc chloride, using *mordant black 11 solution* as indicator; each ml of 0·05M disodium edetate is equivalent to 0·002004 g of Ca. Calculate the total weight of Ca in the 20 tablets and divide by 20.

CONTENT OF CALCIFEROL. 0·0122 mg to 0·0169 mg, determined by the following method, all operations being carried out in subdued light:
To about 3·5 g, accurately weighed, of the powdered tablets add 50 ml of *aldehyde-free alcohol (95 per cent)*, 14 ml of *glycerol*, and 20 ml of a 50 per cent w/v solution of *potassium hydroxide* in water, and boil under a reflux condenser for 30 minutes with occasional swirling.
Add 110 ml of water, allow to stand for 10 minutes with occasional stirring, cool, dilute to 250 ml with *aldehyde-free alcohol (95 per cent)*, and allow to stand until the insoluble matter has settled.
Extract 50 ml of the supernatant liquid with three successive 30-ml portions of *light petroleum (boiling-range, 40° to 60°)*, wash the combined extracts with successive 50-ml portions of water until the washings are no longer alkaline to *phenolphthalein solution*, and evaporate to dryness while maintaining an atmosphere of *oxygen-free nitrogen*.
Continue by the method given for Calciferol Injection, page 711, dissolving the residue in 1 ml of the dry purified ethylene chloride and beginning with the words "add rapidly 9 0 ml of *antimony trichloride solution in ethylene chloride* . . .". Calculate the total amount of calciferol in the 20 tablets and divide by 20.

Containers and storage. The directions given under Tablets (page 805) should be followed; containers should be airtight. The tablets should be stored in a cool place.

Labelling. A direction to crush the tablets before administration should be given on the label.

Dose. 1 tablet.

Each tablet contains 500 Units of antirachitic activity (vitamin D).

Carbromal Tablets

Carbromal Tablets may be prepared by moist granulation and compression as described under Tablets (page 801).

Standard
They comply with the standard under Tablets, page 804, with the following additions:

PRESENCE OF CARBROMAL. The residue obtained in the determination of carbromal melts at about 117°.

CONTENT OF CARBROMAL. 95·0 to 105·0 per cent of the prescribed or stated amount, determined by the following method:
Weigh and powder 20 tablets. Extract an accurately weighed quantity of the powder, equivalent to about 0·25 g of carbromal, with *acetone* in an apparatus for continuous extraction until complete extraction is effected; evaporate off the acetone and dry the residue to constant weight at 80°.
Calculate the total weight of carbromal in the 20 tablets and divide by 20.

Containers and storage. The directions given under Tablets (page 805) should be followed.

Dose. Carbromal, 0·3 to 1 gram.

When the strength of the tablets is not specified, tablets each containing 300 mg of carbromal shall be supplied.

Clefamide Tablets

Clefamide Tablets may be prepared by moist granulation and compression as described under Tablets (page 801).

Standard
They comply with the standard under Tablets, page 804, with the following addition:
CONTENT OF CLEFAMIDE. 95·0 to 105·0 per cent of the prescribed or stated amount, determined by the following method:
Weigh and powder 20 tablets. Dissolve as completely as possible an accurately weighed quantity of the powder, equivalent to about 0·25 g of clefamide, by warming with 50 ml of *alcohol (95 per cent)*, cool, dilute to 250 ml with *alcohol (95 per cent)*, and filter.
Dilute 2 ml of the filtrate to 100 ml with *alcohol (95 per cent)* and measure the extinction of a 1-cm layer at the maximum at about 303 nm.
For purposes of calculation, use a value of 308 for the E(1 per cent, 1 cm) of clefamide.
Calculate the total weight of clefamide in the 20 tablets and divide by 20.

Containers and storage. The directions given under Tablets (page 805) should be followed.

Dose. Clefamide:

ADULT. 1·5 grams daily for ten days.

CHILD. The dose is reduced in proportion to body-weight.

When the strength of the tablets is not specified, tablets each containing 250 mg of clefamide shall be supplied.

Co-trimoxazole Tablets, Paediatric

SYNONYM: Trimethoprim and Sulphamethoxazole Tablets, Paediatric

For each tablet take:

Trimethoprim	..	..	20 mg
Sulphamethoxazole	..	..	100 mg

Mix, and prepare by moist granulation and compression as described under Tablets (page 801).

Standard
They comply with the standard under Tablets, page 804, with the following additions:
PRESENCE OF TRIMETHOPRIM AND SULPHAMETHOXAZOLE. They comply with the test given for Co-trimoxazole Mixture in Appendix 5A, page 861, solution (1) being prepared by shaking a quantity of powdered tablets equivalent to 0·4 g of sulphamethoxazole with 10 ml of *methyl alcohol* and filtering.

CONTENT OF SULPHAMETHOXAZOLE. 0·093 g to 0·107 g, determined by the following method:
Weigh and powder 20 tablets and determine by the method for Co-trimoxazole Mixture, page 740, an accurately weighed quantity of the powdered tablets, equivalent to about 0·25 g of sulphamethoxazole, being used.
Calculate the total weight of sulphamethoxazole in the 20 tablets and divide by 20.

CONTENT OF TRIMETHOPRIM. 0·0185 g to 0·0215 g, determined by the method given for Co-trimoxazole Mixture, page 740.
Calculate the total weight of trimethoprim in the 20 tablets and divide by 20.

Containers and storage. The directions given under Tablets (page 805) should be followed; containers should be light resistant.

Dose. CHILD. Twice daily: up to 2 years, 1 tablet; 2 to 5 years, 1 or 2 tablets; 6 to 12 years, 2 to 4 tablets.

Ferrous Phosphate, Quinine, and Strychnine Tablets

SYNONYM: Easton's Tablets

Ferrous Phosphate, Quinine, and Strychnine Tablets are prepared in two strengths.

Formula A

For each tablet take:

Iron Phosphate	..	..	200·0 mg
Quinine Sulphate	..	..	50·0 mg
Strychnine Hydrochloride		..	0·1 mg

Formula B

For each tablet take:

Iron Phosphate	..	..	100·0 mg
Quinine Sulphate		..	25·0 mg
Strychnine Hydrochloride		..	0·05 mg

Mix, and prepare by moist granulation and compression as described under Tablets (page 801). The tablets may be coated with sugar or other suitable material.

Standard
They comply with the standard under Tablets, page 804, with the following additions:
Formula A

CONTENT OF IRON. Not less than 0·030 g, calculated as Fe, determined by the following method:
Weigh and powder 20 tablets. Digest the powder with 30 ml of *dilute sulphuric acid* until it is completely disintegrated and only a white residue remains, filter, and wash the residue with *dilute sulphuric acid* until the washings are free from iron and from alkaloids.
Dilute the combined filtrate and washings to 150 ml with water and to 25 ml of the solution add 0·2 ml of *hydrochloric acid* and a 2 per cent w/v solution of *potassium permanganate* in water, dropwise, until a permanent pink colour is produced; add 10 ml of *hydrochloric acid* and 3 ml of *ammonium thiocyanate solution*, maintain a current of *carbon dioxide* through the flask, and titrate with 0·1N *titanous chloride*; each ml of 0·1N titanous chloride is equivalent to 0·005585 g of Fe.
Calculate the total weight of Fe in the 20 tablets and divide by 20.

CONTENT OF ANHYDROUS QUININE. 0·039 g to 0·045 g, determined by the following method:
Weigh and powder 20 tablets. To an accurately weighed quantity of the powder, equivalent to about one-fifth of a tablet, add 50 ml of 0·1N sulphuric acid, shake for 30 minutes, dilute to 100 ml with 0·1N sulphuric acid, and allow to stand until the insoluble matter has deposited.
Dilute 10 ml of the clear solution to 100 ml with 0·1N sulphuric acid; dilute 5 ml of this solution to 100 ml with 0·1N sulphuric acid and measure the secondary radiation at about 450 nm in a fluorimeter, using a primary light source with a wavelength of about 366 nm.
Compare the fluorescence with that of a solution containing 0·5 μg of *quinine sulphate* in 0·1N sulphuric acid.
Each g of quinine sulphate is equivalent to 0·8287 g of anhydrous quinine.
Calculate the total weight of anhydrous quinine in the 20 tablets and divide by 20.
The dilutions used for this assay may be varied to suit the fluorimeter in use.

CONTENT OF STRYCHNINE. They comply with the test for strychnine given in Appendix 5A, page 863.

Formula B

CONTENT OF IRON. Not less than 0·015 g, calculated as Fe, determined by the method for tablets of formula A, 50 ml of the solution being used in place of 25 ml.

CONTENT OF ANHYDROUS QUININE. 0·019 g to 0·022 g, determined by the method for tablets of formula A, a quantity of the powder equivalent to about two-fifths of a tablet being used.

CONTENT OF STRYCHNINE. They comply with the test for strychnine given in Appendix 5A, page 863.

Containers and storage. The directions given under Tablets (page 805) should be followed.

Dose. 1 tablet.

When the strength of the tablets is not specified, tablets prepared according to formula A shall be supplied.

Ferrous Sulphate Tablets, Compound

For each tablet take:

Dried Ferrous Sulphate ..	.. ..	a quantity equivalent to 170 mg of FeSO$_4$
Copper Sulphate ..	.. ..	2·5 mg
Manganese Sulphate	.. ..	2·5 mg

Mix, and prepare by moist granulation and compression as described under Tablets (page 801). The tablets may be coated with sugar or other suitable material and the coat may be coloured.

The manufacturing techniques used in the preparation of these tablets should ensure that increases in the disintegration time on prolonged storage do not exceed the limit. Alternatively, an appropriate expiry date should be specified on the label.

Standard

They comply with the standard under Tablets, page 804, with the following additions:

CONTENT OF COPPER SULPHATE. 2·25 mg to 3·00 mg, determined by the following method:

Weigh and powder 20 tablets. Ignite an accurately weighed quantity of the powder, equivalent to about 2 tablets, at a temperature not exceeding 450°; to the residue add 10 ml of *hydrochloric acid*, evaporate to dryness, add 5 ml of *nitric acid*, and again evaporate to dryness.

Extract the residue with three successive 10-ml portions of hot *dilute hydrochloric acid*, combine the extracts, dilute to 50 ml with water, and reserve a portion of this solution for the determination of manganese sulphate.

To 1 ml of this solution add 10 ml of *edetate–citrate solution*, 0·1 ml of *thymol blue solution*, and sufficient *dilute ammonia solution* to give a green or blue-green solution, add 10 ml of *sodium diethyldithiocarbamate solution*, and extract with three or more successive 5-ml portions of *carbon tetrachloride* until an extract is obtained which is colourless, filtering each extract through a small plug of cotton wool.

Combine the extracts, dilute to 20 ml with *carbon tetrachloride*, taking care to avoid undue exposure to light, and measure the extinction of a 1-cm layer at the maximum at about 435 nm.

Calculate the concentration of copper sulphate in the sample by reference to a calibration curve prepared

with suitable aliquots of *dilute copper sulphate solution* treated in the manner described above, beginning with the words "add 10 ml of *edetate–citrate solution . . .*".

Calculate the total weight of copper sulphate in the 20 tablets and divide by 20.

CONTENT OF MANGANESE SULPHATE. 2·25 mg to 3·25 mg, calculated as MnSO$_4$,4H$_2$O, determined by the following method:

To 2 ml of the solution reserved in the determination of copper sulphate, add 2·5 ml of *dilute sulphuric acid*, and evaporate to dryness.

Dissolve the residue, with the aid of heat, in 3 ml of *phosphoric acid*, add 6 ml of water and 0·5 g of *sodium periodate*, heat in a water-bath for 30 minutes, cool, dilute to 10 ml with water, and measure the extinction of a 1-cm layer at the maximum at about 526 nm.

Calculate the proportion of manganese sulphate in the sample by reference to a calibration curve prepared from the extinctions, at the same maximum, of solutions prepared by diluting 1-, 2-, 3-, 4-, and 5-ml aliquots of a 0·005 per cent w/v solution of *potassium permanganate* in water to 10 ml with water; each mg of potassium permanganate is equivalent to 1·4114 mg of MnSO$_4$,4H$_2$O.

Calculate the total weight of manganese sulphate in the 20 tablets and divide by 20.

CONTENT OF FERROUS SULPHATE. 0·161 g to 0·178 g, calculated as FeSO$_4$, determined by the following method:

Dissolve as completely as possible an accurately weighed quantity of the powder, equivalent to about 3 tablets, in a mixture of 30 ml of water and 20 ml of *dilute sulphuric acid* and titrate with 0·1N ceric ammonium sulphate, using *ferroin sulphate solution* as indicator; each ml of 0·1N ceric ammonium sulphate is equivalent to 0·01519 g of FeSO$_4$.

Calculate the total weight of FeSO$_4$ in the 20 tablets and divide by 20.

Containers and storage. The directions given under Tablets (page 805) should be followed; containers should be airtight and light resistant.

Dose. 1 or 2 tablets.

Each tablet contains about 60 mg of iron.

Ipecacuanha and Opium Tablets

SYNONYM: Dover's Powder Tablets

Ipecacuanha and Opium Tablets contain Ipecacuanha and Opium Powder and may be prepared by moist granulation and compression as described under Tablets (page 801).

Standard

They comply with the standard under Tablets, page 804, with the following additions:

PRESENCE OF IPECACUANHA AND OF OPIUM. The powdered tablets possess the microscopical characters described under Ipecacuanha, page 249, and under Opium, page 337.

CONTENT OF ANHYDROUS MORPHINE. 0·90 to 1·10 per cent of the prescribed or stated amount of Ipecacuanha and Opium Powder, determined by the following method:

Weigh and powder 20 tablets and determine by the method for Ipecacuanha and Opium Powder, page 777, using an accurately weighed quantity of the powder, equivalent to about 5 g of Ipecacuanha and Opium Powder.

Calculate the total weight of anhydrous morphine in the 20 tablets and divide by 20.

Containers and storage. The directions given under Tablets (page 805) should be followed; containers should be airtight. The tablets should be stored in a cool place.

Dose. Ipecacuanha and Opium Powder, 300 to 600 milligrams.

When the strength of the tablets is not specified, tablets each containing 300 mg of Ipecacuanha and Opium Powder shall be supplied.

Isothipendyl Tablets

SYNONYM: Isothipendyl Hydrochloride Tablets

Isothipendyl Tablets contain Isothipendyl Hydrochloride and may be prepared by moist granulation and compression as described under Tablets (page 801). They may be sugar coated and the coat may be coloured.

Standard
They comply with the standard under Tablets, page 804, with the following additions:

PRESENCE OF ISOTHIPENDYL. They comply with the thin-layer chromatographic test given in Appendix 5C, page 873.

CONTENT OF ISOTHIPENDYL HYDROCHLORIDE. 90·0 to 110·0 per cent of the prescribed or stated amount, determined by the following method:
Weigh and powder 20 tablets. Mix an accurately weighed quantity of the powder, equivalent to about 2 mg of isothipendyl hydrochloride, with 20 ml of 0·1N hydrochloric acid, shake vigorously for 15 minutes, dilute to 100 ml with 0·1N hydrochloric acid, further dilute 10 ml of this solution to 50 ml with 0·1N hydrochloric acid and filter.
Measure the extinction of a 1-cm layer of the filtrate at 234 nm, at 244 nm, and at 254 nm, using 0·1N hydrochloric acid as the blank, and calculate the corrected extinction at 244 nm from the formula:

$$e_2 - \tfrac{1}{2}(e_1 + e_3)$$

where e_1 = the extinction at 234 nm,
e_2 = the extinction at 244 nm, and
e_3 = the extinction at 254 nm.

Repeat the procedure using a solution of *isothipendyl hydrochloride A.S.* and hence calculate the amount of isothipendyl hydrochloride present in the sample solution.
Calculate the total weight of isothipendyl hydrochloride in the 20 tablets and divide by 20.

Containers and storage. The directions given under Tablets (page 805) should be followed.

Dose. Isothipendyl hydrochloride, 12 to 32 milligrams daily.

When the strength of the tablets is not specified, sugar-coated tablets each containing 4 mg of isothipendyl hydrochloride shall be supplied.

Magnesium Carbonate Tablets, Compound

For each tablet take:

Heavy Magnesium Carbonate ..	200 mg
Light Kaolin or Light Kaolin (Natural)	60 mg
Ginger, in powder	60 mg
Sodium Bicarbonate	120 mg
Calcium Carbonate	200 mg
Peppermint Oil	0·006 ml

Mix the solid ingredients and granulate by the moist-granulation process as described

under Tablets (page 801); to the dried granules add the peppermint oil previously dissolved in a small quantity of Alcohol (95 per cent), mix, and compress.

Standard
They comply with the standard, except for disintegration time, under Tablets, page 804, with the following additions:

CONTENT OF SODIUM BICARBONATE. 0·113 g to 0·127 g, calculated as $NaHCO_3$, determined by the following method:
Weigh and powder 20 tablets. Heat an accurately weighed quantity of the powder, equivalent to about 2 tablets, with 100 ml of water at 50° for 5 minutes, and filter.
Heat the residue with a further 100 ml of water at 50° for 5 minutes and filter.
Cool the combined filtrates and titrate with 0·5N hydrochloric acid, using *methyl orange–xylene cyanol FF solution* as indicator; add 10 ml of *ammonia buffer solution*, and titrate with 0·05M disodium edetate, using *mordant black 11 solution* as indicator; each ml of 0·5N hydrochloric acid, after one-fifth of the volume of 0·05M disodium edetate has been deducted, is equivalent to 0·04200 g of $NaHCO_3$.
Calculate the total weight of $NaHCO_3$ in the 20 tablets, and divide by 20.

CONTENT OF MAGNESIUM. 0·048 to 0·057 g, calculated as Mg, determined by the following method:
Dissolve as completely as possible an accurately weighed quantity of the powder, equivalent to about 2 tablets, in 10 ml of *dilute hydrochloric acid*, filter, and dilute to 250 ml with water.
To 50 ml of this solution add 1 g of *ammonium chloride* and 1 g of *ammonium oxalate* and continue by the method for magnesium in Paediatric Compound Calcium Carbonate Mixture, page 738, beginning with the words "neutralise to *litmus paper* . . .".
Calculate the total weight of Mg in the 20 tablets and divide by 20.

CONTENT OF CALCIUM CARBONATE. 0·185 to 0·212 g, calculated as $CaCO_3$, determined by the method for calcium carbonate in Paediatric Compound Calcium Carbonate Mixture, page 738, an accurately weighed quantity of the powdered tablets, equivalent to about 2 tablets, being used.
Calculate the total weight of $CaCO_3$ in the 20 tablets and divide by 20.

Containers and storage. The directions given under Tablets (page 805) should be followed.

Labelling. A direction to chew the tablets before they are swallowed should be given on the label.

Dose. 1 or 2 tablets.

Magnesium Trisilicate Tablets, Compound

SYNONYM: Aluminium Hydroxide and Magnesium Trisilicate Tablets

For each tablet take:

Magnesium Trisilicate ..	..	250 mg
Dried Aluminium Hydroxide Gel	120 mg
Peppermint Oil	..	0·003 ml

Mix the solid ingredients and granulate by moist granulation as described under Tablets (page 801); dry the granules at a temperature not exceeding 30°, mix with the peppermint oil previously dissolved in a small quantity of Alcohol (95 per cent), and prepare by compression.

Standard

They comply with the standard, except for disintegration time, under Tablets, page 804, with the following additions:

CONTENT OF ALUMINIUM. 0·028 g to 0·040 g, calculated as Al, determined by the following method:
Weigh and powder 20 tablets. To an accurately weighed quantity of the powder, equivalent to about 4 tablets, add 7 ml of *hydrochloric acid*, and dissolve as completely as possible by heating on a water-bath for about 5 minutes, avoiding excessive charring; add 50 ml of water, filter, wash the residue with hot water, and dilute the combined filtrate and washings to 100 ml with water.
Neutralise 25 ml of this solution to *congo red paper* with *sodium hydroxide solution*, add 75 ml of water and 50 ml of 0·05M disodium edetate, heat on a water-bath for 30 minutes, cool, add 3 g of *hexamine*, and titrate the excess of disodium edetate with 0·05M lead nitrate, using *xylenol orange solution* as indicator; each ml of 0·05M disodium edetate is equivalent to 0·001349 g of Al.
Calculate the total weight of Al in the 20 tablets and divide by 20.

CONTENT OF MAGNESIUM. 0·030 g to 0·041 g, calculated as Mg, determined by the following method:
To 25 ml of the solution prepared for the determination of aluminium add 1g of *ammonium chloride* and 10 ml of *triethanolamine*, or a sufficient quantity to redissolve the precipitate which first forms; add 160 ml of water, 5 ml of *ammonia buffer solution*, and *mordant black 11 solution* as indicator, and titrate immediately with 0·05M disodium edetate to the full blue colour; each ml of 0·05M disodium edetate is equivalent to 0·001215 g of Mg.
Calculate the total weight of Mg in the 20 tablets and divide by 20.

Containers and storage. The directions given under Tablets (page 805) should be followed.

Labelling. A direction to chew the tablets before they are swallowed should be given on the label.

Dose. 1 or 2 tablets.

Methallenoestril Tablets

Methallenoestril Tablets may be prepared by moist granulation and compression as described under Tablets (page 801).

Standard
They comply with the standard under Tablets, page 804, with the following additions:

PRESENCE OF METHALLENOESTRIL. The ultraviolet absorption spectrum of a solution prepared as directed in the determination of methallenoestril, exhibits the characteristics given for methallenoestril in Appendix 3, page 855.

CONTENT OF METHALLENOESTRIL. 90·0 to 110·0 per cent of the prescribed or stated amount, determined by the following method:
Weigh and powder 20 tablets. To an accurately weighed quantity of the powder, equivalent to about 0·018 g of methallenoestril, add 100 ml of *methyl alcohol*, boil on a water-bath for one minute, cool, dilute to 200 ml with *methyl alcohol*, and filter, discarding the first portion of the filtrate.
Measure the extinction of a 1-cm layer of the filtrate at the maximum at about 332 nm.
For purposes of calculation, use a value of 67·5 for the E(1 per cent, 1 cm) of methallenoestril.
Calculate the total weight of methallenoestril in the 20 tablets and divide by 20.

Containers and storage. The directions given under Tablets (page 805) should be followed.

Dose. See under Methallenoestril (page 298).

When the strength of the tablets is not specified, tablets

each containing 3 mg of methallenoestril shall be supplied.

Nalidixic Acid Tablets

Nalidixic Acid Tablets may be prepared by moist granulation and compression as described under Tablets (page 801). They may be coloured.

Standard
They comply with the standard under Tablets, page 804, with the following additions:

PRESENCE OF NALIDIXIC ACID. To a quantity of the powdered tablets, equivalent to about 0·1 g of nalidixic acid, add 50 ml of *chloroform*, shake for 15 minutes, filter, and evaporate off the chloroform; the residue, after drying, melts at about 228°.

CONTENT OF NALIDIXIC ACID. 95·0 to 105·0 per cent of the prescribed or stated amount, calculated as $C_{12}H_{12}N_2O_3$, determined by the following method:
Weigh and powder 20 tablets. To an accurately weighed quantity of the powder, equivalent to about 0·1 g of nalidixic acid, add 150 ml of 1N sodium hydroxide, shake for 3 minutes, dilute to 200 ml with 1N sodium hydroxide, mix well, and allow to stand for 15 minutes.
Dilute 2 ml of this solution to 200 ml with water and measure the extinction of a 1-cm layer at the maximum at about 258 nm, using 0·01N sodium hydroxide as the blank.
For purposes of calculation, use a value of 1120 for the E(1 per cent, 1 cm) of nalidixic acid.
Calculate the total weight of nalidixic acid in the 20 tablets and divide by 20.

Containers and storage. The directions given under Tablets (page 805) should be followed; containers should be airtight and light resistant.

Dose. Nalidixic acid:

ADULT. 0·5 to 1 gram four times daily.

CHILD. 30 to 60 milligrams per kilogram body-weight daily, in divided doses.

When the strength of the tablets is not specified, tablets each containing 500 mg of nalidixic acid shall be supplied.

Nicotinamide Tablets

SYNONYM: Niacinamide Tablets

Nicotinamide Tablets may be prepared by moist granulation and compression as described under Tablets (page 801).

Standard
They comply with the standard under Tablets, page 804, with the following additions:

PRESENCE OF NICOTINAMIDE. 1. Shake an amount of powdered tablet, equivalent to about 0·1 g of nicotinamide, with 50 ml of *alcohol (95 per cent)* for 15 minutes, dilute to 100 ml with *alcohol (95 per cent)*, filter, and dilute 2 ml of the filtrate to 100 ml with *alcohol (95 per cent)*.
The ultraviolet absorption spectrum of this solution exhibits the characteristics given for nicotinamide in Appendix 3, page 855.
2. Mix an amount of powdered tablet, equivalent to about 0·15 g of nicotinamide, with 5 ml of *sodium hydroxide solution* and heat; ammonia is evolved.

CONTENT OF NICOTINAMIDE. 92·5 to 107·5 per cent of the prescribed or stated amount, calculated as $C_6H_6N_2O$, determined by the following method:
Weigh and powder 20 tablets, and determine by the method given for Nicotinamide in Vitamins B and C Injection, page 720, using an accurately weighed

quantity of the powder equivalent to about 0·3 g of nicotinamide.
Calculate the total weight of $C_6H_6N_2O$ in the 20 tablets and divide by 20.

Containers and storage. The directions given under Tablets (page 805) should be followed; containers should be airtight and light resistant.

Dose. Nicotinamide, prophylactic, 15 to 30 milligrams daily; therapeutic, 50 to 250 milligrams daily.

When the strength of the tablets is not specified, tablets each containing 50 mg of nicotinamide shall be supplied.
Tablets containing 500 mg are also available.

Papaveretum Tablets

Papaveretum Tablets may be prepared by moist granulation and compression as described under Tablets (page 801).

Standard
They comply with the standard under Tablets, page 804, with the following additions:

PRESENCE OF PAPAVERETUM. They comply with the thin-layer chromatographic test given in Appendix 5B, page 872.

CONTENT OF ANHYDROUS MORPHINE. 45·0 to 55·0 per cent of the prescribed or stated amount of papaveretum, determined by the following method:
Weigh and powder 20 tablets. Dissolve as completely as possible an accurately weighed quantity of the powder, equivalent to about 0·01 g of papaveretum, in warm 0·1N hydrochloric acid, cool, and dilute to 250 ml with 0·1N hydrochloric acid; using 20 ml of this solution, continue by the method for Aromatic Chalk with Opium Powder, page 776, beginning with the words "add 8 ml of a freshly prepared 1·0 per cent w/v solution of *sodium nitrite* . . .".
Calculate the total weight of anhydrous morphine in the 20 tablets and divide by 20.

Containers and storage. The directions given under Tablets (page 805) should be followed.

Dose. Papaveretum, 10 to 20 milligrams.

The quantity of papaveretum in each tablet should be specified by the prescriber.
Tablets containing 10 mg are available.

Phenobarbitone and Theobromine Tablets

For each tablet take:

Phenobarbitone	..	..	..	30 mg
Theobromine	..	..	..	300 mg

Mix, and prepare by moist granulation and compression as described under Tablets (page 801).

Standard
They comply with the standard, except for disintegration time, under Tablets, page 804, with the following additions:

DISINTEGRATION TIME. Maximum time, 30 minutes.

PRESENCE OF PHENOBARBITONE. They comply with the test given under Belladonna and Phenobarbitone Tablets, page 807.

PRESENCE OF THEOBROMINE. They comply with the thin-layer chromatographic test given in Appendix 5A, page 866.

CONTENT OF THEOBROMINE. 0·285 g to 0·315 g, calculated as $C_7H_8N_4O_2$, determined by the following method:

Weigh and powder 20 tablets. Shake an accurately weighed quantity of the powder, equivalent to about 2 tablets, with 50 ml of *solvent ether*, filter, and wash the residue with four successive 12-ml portions of *solvent ether*, reserving the ethereal solutions for the determination of phenobarbitone.
Dissolve the residue in 150 ml of water and 25 ml, or a sufficient quantity, of 0·1N sulphuric acid, boil vigorously for 2 minutes, cool to 40°, and add 1·5 ml of *phenol red solution*; make distinctly alkaline with 0·2N sodium hydroxide, add 0·1N sulphuric acid, dropwise, until the bluish-red colour just becomes distinctly yellow, add 50 ml of 0·1N silver nitrate, and titrate the liberated acid slowly with 0·2N sodium hydroxide until a deep red-violet colour is obtained; each ml of 0·2N sodium hydroxide is equivalent to 0·03603 g of $C_7H_8N_4O_2$.
To the weight of theobromine found add 0·006 g to correct for its solubility in solvent ether.
Calculate the total weight of $C_7H_8N_4O_2$ in the 20 tablets and divide by 20.

CONTENT OF PHENOBARBITONE. 0·027 g to 0·033 g, determined by the following method:
Extract the combined ethereal solutions reserved in the determination of theobromine with successive 20-ml portions of a 1 per cent w/v solution of *sodium hydroxide in brine* until extraction is complete.
Wash the combined extracts with two successive 15-ml portions of *solvent ether* and wash the combined ethereal washings with the same 3-ml portion of water, adding the aqueous washing to the alkaline solution, and discard the ethereal washings; acidify to *litmus paper* with *hydrochloric acid* and extract with successive 15-ml portions of *solvent ether* until extraction is complete.
Wash the combined extracts with two successive 2-ml portions of water and wash the combined aqueous washings with 10 ml of *solvent ether*, filter the combined ethereal extracts and washings, wash the filter with *solvent ether*, combine the filtrate and washings, evaporate off the ether, and dry the residue of phenobarbitone to constant weight at 105°.
Calculate the total weight of phenobarbitone in the 20 tablets and divide by 20.

Containers and storage. The directions given under Tablets (page 805) should be followed; containers should be airtight and light resistant.

Dose. 1 or 2 tablets.

Prothionamide Tablets

Prothionamide Tablets may be prepared by moist granulation and compression as described under Tablets (page 801). They may be coated with sugar or other suitable material.

Standard
They comply with the standard under Tablets, page 804, with the following additions:

PRESENCE OF PROTHIONAMIDE. 1. They comply with identification tests 1 and 2 described under Prothionamide, page 415, a quantity of the powdered tablets equivalent to 0·1 g of prothionamide being used.

2. Shake a quantity of the powdered tablets, equivalent to 0·10 g of prothionamide, with 80 ml of *alcohol* (95 per cent), filter, dilute the filtrate to 100 ml with *alcohol* (95 per cent), and further dilute 0·1 ml of this solution to 100 ml with the same solvent. The ultraviolet absorption spectrum of this solution exhibits the characteristics given for prothionamide in Appendix 3, page 856.

CONTENT OF PROTHIONAMIDE. 92·5 to 107·5 per cent of the prescribed or stated amount, calculated as $C_9H_{12}N_2S$, determined by the following method:
Weigh and powder 20 tablets. Stir an accurately weighed quantity of the powder, equivalent to about

0·2 g of prothionamide, with four successive 10-ml portions of *methyl alcohol* in a small beaker, filtering each portion through a sintered-glass filter (British Standard Grade No. 3), wash the beaker and filter with a further 20 ml of *methyl alcohol*, and evaporate the combined filtrate and washings to dryness.

Dissolve the residue in 50 ml of *glacial acetic acid* and continue by Method I of the British Pharmacopoeia for non-aqueous titration; each ml of 0·1N perchloric acid is equivalent to 0·01803 g of $C_9H_{12}N_2S$.

Calculate the total weight of $C_9H_{12}N_2S$ in the 20 tablets and divide by 20.

Containers and storage. The directions given under Tablets (page 805) should be followed.

Dose. Prothionamide:

ADULT. 0·75 to 1 gram daily in single or divided doses.

CHILD. 10 milligrams per kilogram body-weight, gradually increased, if tolerated, to 20 milligrams per kilogram body-weight, daily.

When the strength of the tablets is not specified, tablets each containing 125 mg of prothionamide shall be supplied.

Pyridoxine Tablets

SYNONYMS: Pyridoxine Hydrochloride Tablets; Vitamin B_6 Tablets

Pyridoxine Tablets contain Pyridoxine Hydrochloride and may be prepared by moist granulation and compression as described under Tablets (page 801).

Standard
They comply with the standard under Tablets, page 804, with the following additions:

PRESENCE OF PYRIDOXINE. Triturate a quantity of the powdered tablets, equivalent to about 0·02 g of pyridoxine hydrochloride, with 50 ml of water, dilute to 200 ml with water, and allow to stand; 1 ml of this solution complies with the test given for the presence of pyridoxine in Pyridoxine Injection, page 718.

CONTENT OF PYRIDOXINE HYDROCHLORIDE. 90·0 to 110·0 per cent of the prescribed or stated amount, determined by the following method:
Weigh and powder 20 tablets. To an accurately weighed quantity of the powder, equivalent to about 0·025 g of pyridoxine hydrochloride, add 50 ml of 0·1N hydrochloric acid and heat on a water-bath for 15 minutes, swirling occasionally and taking precautions to prevent loss by evaporation; cool, dilute to 100 ml with 0·1N hydrochloric acid, and filter, discarding the first 20 ml of the filtrate.
Dilute 5 ml of the filtrate to 100 ml with 0·1N hydrochloric acid and measure the extinction of a 1-cm layer at the maximum at about 291 nm.
For purposes of calculation, use a value of 430 for the E(1 per cent, 1 cm) of pyridoxine hydrochloride.
Calculate the total weight of pyridoxine hydrochloride in the 20 tablets and divide by 20.

Containers and storage. The directions given under Tablets (page 805) should be followed; containers should be light resistant.

Dose. Pyridoxine hydrochloride:

For pyridoxine-deficiency convulsions in infancy: 4 milligrams per kilogram body-weight daily for short periods.

For pyridoxine-deficiency anaemia of adults: 50 to 150 milligrams daily, in divided doses.

When the strength of the tablets is not specified, tablets

each containing 50 mg of pyridoxine hydrochloride shall be supplied.
Tablets containing 10 and 20 mg are also available.

Quinine Dihydrochloride Tablets

SYNONYM: Quinine Acid Hydrochloride Tablets

Quinine Dihydrochloride Tablets may be prepared by moist granulation and compression as described under Tablets (page 801). They may be sugar coated.

Standard
They comply with the standard under Tablets, page 804, with the following addition:

CONTENT OF QUININE DIHYDROCHLORIDE. 95·0 to 105·0 per cent of the prescribed or stated amount, calculated as $C_{20}H_{24}N_2O_2,2HCl$, determined by the following method:
Digest 20 tablets with a mixture of 100 ml of water and 10 ml of *dilute hydrochloric acid* until the tablets are completely disintegrated and not more than a small residue remains; filter, wash the residue with a mixture containing 10 volumes of water and 1 volume of *dilute hydrochloric acid* until complete extraction of the alkaloid is effected, and dilute the combined filtrate and washings to 200 ml with the acidified water.
Shake an accurately measured volume of the solution, equivalent to about 0·5 g of quinine dihydrochloride, with two successive 20-ml portions of *chloroform*, washing each chloroform extract with the same 10 ml of water; discard the chloroform, combine the aqueous solution and washing, make just alkaline by the addition of *dilute ammonia solution*, and extract with successive portions of *chloroform* until complete extraction of the alkaloid is effected, washing each extraction with the same 10 ml of water.
Combine the chloroform extracts, filter, wash the filter with *chloroform*, evaporate the filtrate to dryness, add to the residue 3 ml of *alcohol* (95 per cent), again evaporate to dryness and dry the residue to constant weight at 105°; each g of residue is equivalent to 1·225 g of $C_{20}H_{24}N_2O_2,2HCl$.
Calculate the total weight of $C_{20}H_{24}N_2O_2,2HCl$ in the 20 tablets and divide by 20.

Containers and storage. The directions given under Tablets (page 805) should be followed; containers should be airtight and light resistant.

Dose. Quinine dihydrochloride:

For suppression of malaria: 300 to 600 milligrams daily.

For treatment of an attack: 600 milligrams three times daily for four days.

When the strength of the tablets is not specified, sugar-coated tablets each containing 300 mg of quinine dihydrochloride shall be supplied.

Riboflavine Tablets

Riboflavine Tablets may be prepared by moist granulation and compression as described under Tablets (page 801). They may be coated with sugar or other suitable material and the coat may be coloured.

Standard
They comply with the standard under Tablets, page 804, with the following addition:

CONTENT OF RIBOFLAVINE. 90·0 to 115·0 per cent of the prescribed or stated amount, determined by the following method, all operations being carried out in subdued light:
Weigh and powder 20 tablets. To an accurately weighed

quantity of the powder, equivalent to about 10 mg of riboflavine, add a mixture of 5 ml of *glacial acetic acid* and 100 ml of water and heat on a water-bath for one hour with occasional shaking; dilute with water, cool, add 30 ml of 1N sodium hydroxide, with constant stirring, dilute to 1000 ml with water, mix, and filter, discarding the first portion of the filtrate.

Measure the extinction of a 1-cm layer of the filtrate at the maximum at about 444 nm.

For purposes of calculation, use a value of 320 for the E(1 per cent, 1 cm) of riboflavine.

Calculate the total weight of riboflavine in the 20 tablets and divide by 20.

Containers and storage. The directions given under Tablets (page 805) should be followed; containers should be airtight and light resistant.

Dose. Riboflavine, 2 to 10 milligrams daily.

When the strength of the tablets is not specified, tablets each containing 3 mg of riboflavine shall be supplied. Unless the contrary is indicated, uncoated tablets shall be supplied.

Tablets containing 10 mg are also available.

Saccharin Tablets

Saccharin Tablets may be prepared by moist granulation of a mixture of saccharin and sodium bicarbonate, or of saccharin sodium, followed by compression as described under Tablets (page 801).

Standard

They comply with the standard, except for disintegration time, under Tablets, page 804, with the following additions:

SOLUBILITY. When placed in water at 80° and gently stirred, they dissolve almost completely within one minute.

CONTENT OF SACCHARIN. 90·0 to 110·0 per cent of the prescribed or stated amount, calculated as $C_7H_5NO_3S$, determined by the following method:

Weigh and powder a sufficient number of tablets. Transfer an accurately weighed quantity of the powder, equivalent to about 0·5 g of saccharin, to a long-necked 200-ml flask, add 10 ml of a 30 per cent w/v solution of *sodium hydroxide* in water, boil gently for 2 minutes, avoiding loss by evaporation, cool, add 15 ml of *hydrochloric acid*, and boil for 50 minutes under a reflux condenser.

Allow the solution to cool, rinse the condenser with 50 ml of water, pass a current of air through the flask to remove acid vapour, add 20 ml of a 30 per cent w/v solution of *sodium hydroxide* in water, connect the flask to an ammonia distillation apparatus, and distil, collecting the distillate in 40 ml of 0·1N sulphuric acid.

Titrate the excess acid in the distillate with 0·1N sodium hydroxide, using *methyl red solution* as indicator; each ml of 0·1N sulphuric acid is equivalent to 0·01832 g of $C_7H_5NO_3S$.

Calculate the total weight of $C_7H_5NO_3S$ in the tablets taken and divide by the number of tablets.

Containers and storage. The directions given under Tablets (page 805) should be followed.

Note. When the strength of the tablets is not specified, tablets each containing 12·5 mg of saccharin shall be supplied.

Sulphaguanidine Tablets

Sulphaguanidine Tablets may be prepared by moist granulation and compression as described under Tablets (page 801).

Standard

They comply with the standard under Tablets, page 804, with the following additions:

PRESENCE OF SULPHAGUANIDINE. Triturate a quantity of the powdered tablets, equivalent to about 0·5 g of sulphaguanidine, with 5 ml of 0·1N hydrochloric acid, filter, and neutralise the filtrate to *litmus paper* with 0·1N sodium hydroxide; a precipitate is formed which, after washing with water and drying at 105°, complies with the identification tests given for Sulphaguanidine, page 480.

CONTENT OF SULPHAGUANIDINE. 95·0 to 105·0 per cent of the prescribed or stated amount, calculated as $C_7H_{10}N_4O_2S,H_2O$, determined by the following method:

Weigh and powder 20 tablets. Dissolve, as completely as possible, an accurately weighed quantity of the powder, equivalent to about 0·5 g of sulphaguanidine, in 75 ml of water and 10 ml of *hydrochloric acid*, and titrate with 0·1M sodium nitrite, determining the end-point electrometrically; each ml of 0·1M sodium nitrite is equivalent to 0·02323 g of $C_7H_{10}N_4O_2S,H_2O$.

Calculate the total weight of $C_7H_{10}N_4O_2S,H_2O$ in the 20 tablets and divide by 20.

Containers and storage. The directions given under Tablets (page 805) should be followed; containers should be airtight and light resistant.

Dose. Sulphaguanidine, initial dose, 9 to 12 grams daily in divided doses for three days; subsequent doses, 6 to 10 grams daily in divided doses.

When the strength of the tablets is not specified, tablets each containing 500 mg of sulphaguanidine shall be supplied.

Sulphathiazole Tablets

Sulphathiazole Tablets may be prepared by moist granulation and compression as described under Tablets (page 801).

Standard

They comply with the standard under Tablets, page 804, with the following additions:

PRESENCE OF SULPHATHIAZOLE. Triturate a quantity of the powdered tablets, equivalent to about 0·5 g of sulphathiazole, with two successive 5-ml portions of *chloroform*, decanting and discarding each chloroform extract; triturate the residue with 10 ml of *dilute ammonia solution*, add 10 ml of water, and filter.

Warm the filtrate to expel most of the ammonia, cool, and acidify with *acetic acid*; a precipitate is formed which, after washing with water and drying at 105°, complies with the identification tests given for Sulphathiazole, page 484.

CONTENT OF SULPHATHIAZOLE. 95·0 to 105·0 per cent of the prescribed or stated amount, calculated as $C_9H_9N_3O_2S_2$, determined by the following method:

Weigh and powder 20 tablets. Dissolve, as completely as possible, an accurately weighed quantity of the powder, equivalent to about 0·5 g of sulphathiazole, in 75 ml of water and 10 ml of *hydrochloric acid* and titrate with 0·1M sodium nitrite, determining the end-point electrometrically; each ml of 0·1M sodium nitrite is equivalent to 0·02553 g of $C_9H_9N_3O_2S_2$.

Calculate the total weight of $C_9H_9N_3O_2S_2$ in the 20 tablets and divide by 20.

Containers and storage. The directions given under Tablets (page 805) should be followed; containers should be airtight and light resistant.

Dose. Sulphathiazole, initial dose, 3 grams; subsequent doses, 1 gram every four hours.

When the strength of the tablets is not specified, tablets each containing 500 mg of sulphathiazole shall be supplied.

Thiabendazole Tablets

Thiabendazole Tablets may be prepared by moist granulation and compression as described under Tablets (page 801). They may contain suitable colouring and flavouring.

Standard
They comply with the standard, except for disintegration time, under Tablets, page 804, with the following additions:

PRESENCE OF THIABENDAZOLE. They comply with identification test 1 described under Thiabendazole, page 502, a quantity of the powdered tablets equivalent to 0·02 g of thiabendazole being used.

CONTENT OF THIABENDAZOLE. 95·0 to 105·0 per cent of the prescribed or stated amount, determined by the following method:
Weigh and powder 20 tablets. To an accurately weighed quantity of the powdered tablets, equivalent to about 0·1 g of thiabendazole, add 75 ml of 0·1N hydrochloric acid, warm on a water-bath for 15 minutes with occasional shaking, cool, dilute to 100 ml with 0·1N hydrochloric acid, and filter, rejecting the first 20 ml of the filtrate.
Dilute 5 ml of the clear filtrate to 1000 ml with 0·1N hydrochloric acid and measure the extinction of a 1-cm layer at the maximum at about 302 nm.
For purposes of calculation, use a value of 1230 for the E(1 per cent, 1 cm) of thiabendazole.
Calculate the total weight of thiabendazole in the 20 tablets and divide by 20.

Containers and storage. The directions given under Tablets (page 805) should be followed.

Labelling. A direction to chew the tablets before they are swallowed should be given on the label.

Dose. Thiabendazole, 25 milligrams per kilogram body-weight twice daily for two to three days, or for mass therapy 50 milligrams per kilogram body-weight as a single dose.

When the strength of the tablets is not specified, tablets each containing 500 mg of thiabendazole shall be supplied.

Thiacetazone Tablets

Thiacetazone Tablets may be prepared by moist granulation and compression as described under Tablets (page 801).

Standard
They comply with the standard under Tablets, page 804, with the following additions:

PRESENCE OF THIACETAZONE AND LIMIT OF *p*-ACETAMIDO-BENZALAZINE. They comply with the thin-layer chromatographic test given in Appendix 5A, page 869.

CONTENT OF THIACETAZONE. 90·0 to 110·0 per cent of the prescribed or stated amount, determined by the following method:
Weigh and powder 20 tablets. To an accurately weighed quantity of the powdered tablets, equivalent to about 0·012 g of thiacetazone, add 100 ml of *dehydrated alcohol*, boil on a water-bath for 10 minutes with occasional stirring, cool, dilute to 200 ml with *dehydrated alcohol*, and filter.
Dilute 5 ml of the filtrate to 100 ml with *dehydrated alcohol* and measure the extinction of a 1-cm layer at the maximum at about 328 nm, using *dehydrated alcohol* as the blank solution.
For purposes of calculation use a value of 1930 for the E(1 per cent, 1 cm) of thiacetazone.
Calculate the total weight of thiacetazone in the 20 tablets and divide by 20.

Containers and storage. The directions given under Tablets (page 805) should be followed; containers should be light resistant.

Dose. See under Thiacetazone (page 503).

When the strength of the tablets is not specified, tablets each containing 50 mg of thiacetazone shall be supplied.
Tablets containing 25 and 75 mg are also available.

Thiopropazate Tablets

SYNONYM: Thiopropazate Hydrochoride Tablets

Thiopropazate Tablets contain Thiopropazate Hydrochloride and may be prepared by moist granulation and compression as described under Tablets (page 801). They may be coated with sugar or other suitable material and the coat may be coloured.

Standard
They comply with the standard, except for disintegration time, under Tablets, page 804, with the following additions:

DISINTEGRATION TIME. Maximum time, 30 minutes.

PRESENCE OF THIOPROPAZATE. They comply with the thin-layer chromatographic test given in Appendix 5C, page 873.

CONTENT OF THIOPROPAZATE HYDROCHLORIDE. 90·0 to 110·0 per cent of the prescribed or stated amount, determined by the following method:
Weigh and powder 20 tablets. To an accurately weighed quantity of the powder, equivalent to about 10 mg of thiopropazate hydrochloride, add 20 ml of *methyl alcohol*, boil, cool, filter, wash the residue with *methyl alcohol*, and dilute the combined filtrate and washings to 100 ml with *methyl alcohol*.
To 10 ml of this solution, add 0·2 ml of 5N hydrochloric acid, dilute to 100 ml with *methyl alcohol*, and measure the extinction of a 1-cm layer at the maximum at about 256 nm.
For purposes of calculation, use a value of 662 for the E(1 per cent, 1 cm) of thiopropazate hydrochloride.
Calculate the total weight of thiopropazate hydrochloride in the 20 tablets and divide by 20.

Containers and storage. The directions given under Tablets (page 805) should be followed.

Dose. Thiopropazate hydrochloride, 5 to 10 milligrams three times daily.

When the strength of the tablets is not specified, tablets each containing 5 mg of thiopropazate hydrochloride shall be supplied.
Tablets containing 10 mg are also available.

Triamcinolone Tablets

Triamcinolone Tablets may be prepared by moist granulation and compression as described under Tablets (page 801).

Standard
They comply with the standard under Tablets, page 804, with the following additions:

PRESENCE OF TRIAMCINOLONE. Evaporate to dryness 20 ml of the solution in alcohol (95 per cent) obtained in the determination of triamcinolone; the residue complies with Identification Test 1 given under Triamcinolone, page 515.

CONTENT OF TRIAMCINOLONE. 90·0 to 110·0 per cent of the prescribed or stated amount, determined by the following method:
Weigh and powder 20 tablets. Shake an accurately weighed quantity of the powder, equivalent to about 0·015 g of triamcinolone, with 50 ml of *alcohol (95 per cent)* for 2 hours, filter, wash the residue with *alcohol*

(95 per cent), and dilute the combined filtrate and washings to 250 ml with *alcohol (95 per cent)*.
Carefully evaporate 30 ml of this solution to dryness and dissolve the residue in sufficient *aldehyde-free dehydrated alcohol* to produce a solution containing between 140 and 160 µg of triamcinolone in 10 ml.
To 10 ml of this solution in a 25-ml graduated flask add 2·0 ml of *triphenyltetrazolium chloride solution*, displace the air in the flask with *oxygen-free nitrogen*, immediately add 2·0 ml of *dilute tetramethylammonium hydroxide solution*, again displace the air in the flask with *oxygen-free nitrogen*, stopper the flask, mix by gentle swirling, and allow to stand in a water-bath at 30° for one hour; cool rapidly, dilute to 25 ml with *aldehyde-free dehydrated alcohol*, mix, and immediately measure the extinction of a 1-cm layer at the maximum at about 485 nm.
Repeat the procedure using 10 ml of *aldehyde-free dehydrated alcohol* in place of the sample solution; the difference between the extinctions of the two solutions represents the extinction due to the sample.
Calculate the quantity of triamcinolone present by reference to a calibration curve prepared with a solution of *triamcinolone A.S.* in *aldehyde-free dehydrated alcohol* containing between 140 and 160 µg of triamcinolone in 10 ml.
Calculate the total weight of triamcinolone in the 20 tablets and divide by 20.

Containers and storage. The directions given under Tablets (page 805) should be followed.

Dose. Triamcinolone, initially, 4 to 48 milligrams daily, in divided doses; maintenance dose, up to 6 milligrams daily.

The quantity of triamcinolone in each tablet should be specified by the prescriber.
Tablets containing 1, 2, 4, and 8 mg are available.

Trimeprazine Tablets

SYNONYM: Trimeprazine Tartrate Tablets

Trimeprazine Tablets contain Trimeprazine Tartrate and may be prepared by moist granulation and compression as described under Tablets (page 801). They may be sugar coated and the coat may be coloured. A sealing coat of polyvinyl acetate may be applied before the sugar coat.

Standard
They comply with the standard under Tablets, page 804, with the following additions:

PRESENCE OF TRIMEPRAZINE. They comply with the thin-layer chromatographic test given in Appendix 5C, page 873.

CONTENT OF TRIMEPRAZINE TARTRATE. 90·0 to 110·0 per cent of the prescribed or stated amount, determined by the following method:
Weigh and finely powder 20 tablets. Immediately mix an accurately weighed quantity of the powder, equivalent to about 0·06 g of trimeprazine tartrate, with 50 ml of *ammoniacal methyl alcohol*, stir well for 3 minutes, filter through a sintered-glass filter (British Standard Grade No. 3), and wash the filter with successive small quantities of *ammoniacal methyl alcohol*.
Dilute the combined filtrate and washings to 100 ml with *ammoniacal methyl alcohol* and dilute 10 ml of this solution to 100 ml with *methyl alcohol*; dilute 10 ml of this second solution to 100 ml with *methyl alcohol* and measure the extinction of a 1-cm layer at the maximum at about 255 nm.
For purposes of calculation, use a value of 870 for the E(1 per cent, 1 cm) of trimeprazine tartrate.
Calculate the total weight of trimeprazine tartrate in the 20 tablets and divide by 20.

Containers and storage. The directions given under Tablets (page 805) should be followed.

Dose. Trimeprazine tartrate, 10 to 40 milligrams daily in divided doses.

When the strength of the tablets is not specified, tablets each containing 10 mg of trimeprazine tartrate shall be supplied.

Troxidone Tablets, Paediatric

Paediatric Troxidone Tablets may be prepared by moist granulation and compression as described under Tablets (page 801). They may be cuboid in shape and contain suitable flavouring.

Standard
They comply with the standard, except for uniformity of diameter and disintegration, under Tablets, page 804, with the following additions:

PRESENCE OF TROXIDONE. To an amount of the powdered tablets equivalent to 1 g of troxidone add 25 ml of *solvent ether*, allow to stand for 20 minutes, decant through a filter, and, if an insoluble residue remains, add 10 ml of *solvent ether*, allow to stand for 20 minutes and filter.
Evaporate the combined ethereal solutions to dryness and dry the residue under reduced pressure for 2 hours; the residue melts at about 46°.

CONTENT OF TROXIDONE. 95·0 to 105·0 per cent of the prescribed or stated amount, calculated as $C_6H_9NO_3$, determined by the following method:
Weigh and powder 20 tablets. Boil under a reflux condenser an accurately weighed quantity of the powdered tablets, equivalent to about 3 g of troxidone, with 100 ml of *alcohol (95 per cent)* for 1 hour; filter, wash the filter with three successive 20-ml portions of hot *alcohol (95 per cent)*, cool the filtrate, and dilute to 200 ml with *alcohol (95 per cent)*.
Transfer an accurately measured volume of this solution, equivalent to about 0·3 g of troxidone, to an ammonia distillation apparatus, add 150 ml of water and 100 ml of *sodium hydroxide solution*, and boil gently for 6 hours, collecting any distillate in 40 ml of a 4 per cent w/v solution of *boric acid* in water.
Increase the distillation rate, collect about 200 ml of distillate, cool the distillation flask, add 75 ml of water, distil again, collecting a further 70 ml of distillate, and titrate the combined distillates with 0·1N hydrochloric acid, using *methyl red solution* as indicator.
Repeat the distillation and titration omitting the sample solution.
The difference between the two titrations represents the amount of acid required by the methylamine formed from the troxidone; each ml of 0·1N hydrochloric acid is equivalent to 0·01431 g of $C_6H_9NO_3$.
Calculate the total weight of $C_6H_9NO_3$ in the 20 tablets and divide by 20.

Containers and storage. The directions given under Tablets (page 805) should be followed; containers should be light resistant.

Labelling. A direction to crush or chew the tablets before they are swallowed should be given on the label.

Dose. Troxidone, daily in divided doses:
CHILD: Up to 2 years, 300 milligrams, gradually increased if necessary to 600 milligrams; 2 to 6 years, 600 milligrams, gradually increased if necessary to 1·2 grams.

When the strength of the tablets is not specified, tablets each containing 150 mg of troxidone shall be supplied.

Vitamin B Tablets, Compound

SYNONYMS: Compound Aneurine Tablets;
Compound Thiamine Tablets

For each tablet take:

Nicotinamide	15 mg
Riboflavine	1 mg
Thiamine Hydrochloride ..	1 mg

Mix, and prepare by moist granulation and
compression as described under Tablets (page
801).

Standard
They comply with the standard under Tablets, page
804, with the following additions:
CONTENT OF NICOTINAMIDE. 13·5 mg to 16·5 mg,
determined by the following method:
Weigh and powder 20 tablets. Determine by the
method for nicotinamide in Strong Compound
Vitamin B Tablets, below, using 50 ml of a 0·5 per
cent v/v solution of *acetic acid* in water in place of
100 ml, and omitting the measurement of the extinction
at 291 nm.
For purposes of calculation, use a value of 411 for the
E(1 per cent, 1 cm) of nicotinamide.
Calculate the total weight of nicotinamide in the
20 tablets and divide by 20.

CONTENT OF THIAMINE HYDROCHLORIDE. 0·9 mg to
1·1 mg, determined by the method for thiamine
hydrochloride in Strong Compound Vitamin B Tablets,
below, 150 ml of 2N hydrochloric acid in place of
250 ml being used to elute the column.

CONTENT OF RIBOFLAVINE. 0·9 mg to 1·1 mg, determined
by the method for riboflavine in Strong Compound
Vitamin B Tablets, below, an accurately weighed
quantity of the powdered tablets, equivalent to about
5 tablets, being used.

Containers and storage. The directions given under
Tablets (page 805) should be followed; containers
should be airtight and light resistant and the tablets
should not be in contact with metal.

Labelling. The label on the container states the date
after which the tablets are not intended to be used.

Dose. Prophylactic, 1 or 2 tablets daily.

Vitamin B Tablets, Compound, Strong

SYNONYMS: Strong Compound Aneurine
Tablets; Strong Compound Thiamine
Tablets

For each tablet take:

Nicotinamide	20 mg
Pyridoxine Hydrochloride ..	2 mg
Riboflavine	2 mg
Thiamine Hydrochloride ..	5 mg

Mix, and prepare by moist granulation and
compression as described under Tablets
(page 801). The tablets may be coated with a
chocolate-coloured coating of sugar or other
suitable material.

Standard
They comply with the standard under Tablets, page
804, with the following additions:
CONTENT OF NICOTINAMIDE. 18 mg to 22 mg, determined
by the following method:
Prepare an adsorption column by the following method:
soak 4 g of *alginic acid* in water until swelling is complete,
transfer the mixture to an adsorption tube,

15 cm long, 2 cm in diameter, and plugged with a
small piece of glass wool, and allow the alginic acid to
settle; place a small piece of glass wool on the top of
the column and wash the column with successive portions
of 2N hydrochloric acid until the extinction of a
1-cm layer of the washings at 245, 261, and 291 nm
is less than 0·005; then pass water through the column
until the washings are neutral to *litmus solution*.
Weigh and powder 20 tablets. Shake an accurately
weighed quantity of the powder, equivalent to about
7 tablets, for 30 minutes with 100 ml of a 0·5 per cent
v/v solution of *acetic acid* in water, filter, and discard
the first 10 ml of filtrate.
Transfer 10 ml of the filtrate to the top of the column
and pass it through the column at the rate of 1 ml per
minute.
When nearly all the solution has passed through, pass
200 ml of water through the adsorption column and
discard the eluate.
Elute the column with 0·005N hydrochloric acid,
collect 500 ml of eluate, and measure the extinction
of a 4-cm layer of the eluate at 291 nm; dilute 25 ml of
this solution to 50 ml with 0·005N hydrochloric acid
and measure the extinction of a 1-cm layer at 261 nm.
The weight of nicotinamide is given by the formula:

$$0·243 \, A - 0·00344 \, B,$$

where A = the extinction of the 1-cm layer at 261 nm,
and
B = the extinction of the 4-cm layer at 291 nm.

Calculate the total weight of nicotinamide in the
20 tablets and divide by 20.

CONTENT OF PYRIDOXINE HYDROCHLORIDE. 1·8 mg to
2·2 mg, determined by the method given above for
nicotinamide; the weight of pyridoxine is given by the
formula:

$$0·02925 \, B - 0·00128 \, A.$$

Calculate the total weight of pyridoxine hydrochloride
in the 20 tablets and divide by 20.

CONTENT OF THIAMINE HYDROCHLORIDE. 4·5 mg to
6·5 mg, determined by the following method:
Elute the column after the determination of nicotinamide
and pyridoxine hydrochloride with 250 ml
of 2N hydrochloric acid and measure the extinction
of a 1-cm layer at the maximum at about 246 nm.
For purposes of calculation, use a value of 416 for the
E(1 per cent, 1 cm) of thiamine hydrochloride.
Calculate the total weight of thiamine hydrochloride in
the 20 tablets and divide by 20.

CONTENT OF RIBOFLAVINE. 1·8 mg to 2·2 mg, determined
by the following method:
Weigh and powder 20 tablets. To an accurately weighed
quantity of the powder, equivalent to about 3 tablets,
add 50 ml of *solution of standard pH 4·0*, and dissolve
as completely as possible by heating on a water-bath
for about 15 minutes; cool, filter, and dilute the filtrate
to 100 ml with *solution of standard pH 4·0*.
Dilute 25 ml of this solution to 100 ml with *solution
of standard pH 4·0* and measure the extinction of a
1-cm layer at the maximum at about 445 nm.
For purposes of calculation, use a value of 308 for the
E(1 per cent, 1 cm) of riboflavine.
Calculate the total weight of riboflavine in the 20
tablets and divide by 20.

Containers and storage. The directions given under
Tablets (page 805) should be followed; containers
should be airtight and light resistant and the tablets
should not be in contact with metal.

Labelling. The label on the container states the date
after which the tablets are not intended to be used.

Dose. Therapeutic, 1 or 2 tablets three times
daily.

Yeast Tablets

SYNONYMS: Dried Yeast Tablets; Tabellae Cerevisiae Fermenti

Yeast Tablets contain Dried Yeast and may be prepared by moist granulation and compression as described under Tablets (page 801).

Standard
They comply with the standard, except for disintegration time, under Tablets, page 804, with the following additions:

CONTENT OF NICOTINIC ACID. Not less than 0·285 mg per g of the prescribed or stated amount of dried yeast, determined by the method given in Appendix 24, page 907.

CONTENT OF RIBOFLAVINE. Not less than 0·038 mg per g of the prescribed or stated amount of dried yeast, determined by the method given in Appendix 24, page 908.

CONTENT OF THIAMINE. Not less than 0·095 mg per g of the prescribed or stated amount of dried yeast, determined by the method given in Appendix 24, page 909.

Containers and storage. The directions given under Tablets (page 805) should be followed; containers should be airtight.

Dose. Dried Yeast, 1 to 8 grams.

When the strength of the tablets is not specified, tablets each containing 300 mg of Dried Yeast shall be supplied.

TINCTURES

Tinctures are alcoholic liquids usually containing, in comparatively low concentration, the active principles of crude drugs. They are generally prepared by maceration or percolation or obtained by dilution of the corresponding liquid or soft extract.

Maceration process. The solid ingredient(s) are placed in a closed vessel with the whole of the solvent and allowed to stand for seven days with occasional stirring. The mixture is strained, the marc is pressed, and the combined liquids are clarified by filtration or by allowing them to stand and decanting.

Percolation process. The solid ingredient(s) are moistened evenly with a sufficient quantity of the solvent and allowed to stand for four hours in a well-closed vessel. The damp mass is packed firmly in a suitable percolator, sufficient solvent is added to saturate the mass, and the top of the percolator is closed. When the liquid is about to drip, the lower outlet of the percolator is closed, sufficient additional solvent is added to give a shallow layer above the mass, and the mixture is allowed to macerate in the closed percolator for twenty-four hours. The percolation is then allowed to proceed slowly until the percolate measures about three-quarters of the required volume of the finished tincture. The marc is pressed, the expressed liquid mixed with the percolate, and sufficient solvent added to produce the required volume. The combined liquids are mixed and clarified by filtration or by allowing them to stand and decanting.

Benzoin Tincture

SYNONYM: Simple Tincture of Benzoin

Benzoin, crushed..	..	..	100 g
Alcohol (90 per cent)	..	.. to 1000 ml	

Macerate the benzoin with 800 ml of the alcohol for one hour, with frequent agitation; filter and pass sufficient alcohol through the filter to produce the required volume.

Standard
WEIGHT PER ML. At 20°, 0·845 g to 0·860 g.

ALCOHOL CONTENT. 81 to 85 per cent v/v of ethyl alcohol, determined by the method given in Appendix 10, page 888.

CONTENT OF BALSAMIC ACIDS. Not less than 1·65 per cent w/v, calculated as cinnamic acid, $C_9H_8O_2$, determined by the method for Compound Benzoin Tincture, below, 30 ml being used.

Dose. 2·5 to 5 millilitres.

Benzoin Tincture, Compound

SYNONYM: Friars' Balsam

Benzoin, crushed..	..	..	100 g
Aloes	.. ..	..	20 g
Tolu Balsam	..	..	25 g
Prepared Storax	..	..	75 g
Alcohol (90 per cent)	..	.. to 1000 ml	

Macerate the solid materials with 800 ml of the alcohol in a closed vessel for not less than two days, shaking occasionally; filter and pass sufficient of the alcohol through the filter to produce the required volume.

Standard
WEIGHT PER ML. At 20°, 0·890 g to 0·910 g.

ALCOHOL CONTENT. 70 to 76 per cent v/v of ethyl alcohol, determined by the method given in Appendix 10, page 888.

TOTAL SOLIDS. 15 to 19 per cent w/v, determined by evaporating 1 ml to dryness on a water-bath and drying the residue at 105° for 4 hours.

CONTENT OF BALSAMIC ACIDS. Not less than 4·5 per cent w/v, calculated as cinnamic acid, $C_9H_8O_2$, determined by the following method:
Boil 10 ml with 25 ml of 0·5N alcoholic potassium hydroxide under a reflux condenser for 1½ hours, evaporate off the alcohol, and diffuse the residue by warming with 50 ml of hot water; cool, add 80 ml of water and 50 ml of a 4·0 per cent w/v solution of *magnesium sulphate* in water, and continue by the method for Benzoin, page 49, beginning with the words "mix thoroughly . . .".

Capsicum Tincture

| Capsicum Oleoresin | .. | .. | 3·2 g |
| Alcohol (90 per cent) | .. | .. | to 1000 ml |

Prepare by the maceration process.

Standard
ALCOHOL CONTENT. 83 to 88 per cent v/v of ethyl alcohol, determined by the method given in Appendix 10, page 888.

CONTENT OF CAPSAICIN. Not less than 0·025 per cent w/v, determined by the method for Capsicum, page 73; use 10 ml and begin at the words "add 15 ml of *dehydrated methyl alcohol* . . .".

Dose. 0·3 to 1 millilitre.

Cardamom Tincture, Aromatic

SYNONYM: Tinctura Carminativa

Cardamom Oil	..	..	..	3 ml
Caraway Oil	..	..	..	10 ml
Cinnamon Oil	..	..	..	10 ml
Clove Oil ..	..	..	..	10 ml
Strong Ginger Tincture..		..	60 ml
Alcohol (90 per cent)	..	..	to 1000 ml

Mix.

Standard
WEIGHT PER ML. At 20°, 0·825 g to 0·845 g.

ALCOHOL CONTENT. 84 to 87 per cent v/v of ethyl alcohol, determined by the method given in Appendix 10, page 888.

Dose. 0·12 to 0·6 millilitre.

Catechu Tincture

Catechu, crushed..	..	..	200 g
Cinnamon, bruised	..	..	50 g
Alcohol (45 per cent)	..	..	1000 ml

Prepare by the maceration process.

Standard
WEIGHT PER ML. At 20°, 0·990 g to 1·010 g.

ALCOHOL CONTENT. 36 to 40 per cent v/v of ethyl alcohol, determined by the method given in Appendix 10, page 888.

TOTAL SOLIDS. 12 to 17 per cent w/v, determined on 1 ml.

Dose. 2·5 to 5 millilitres.

Chloroform and Morphine Tincture

SYNONYMS: Chlorodyne; Tinct. Chlorof. et Morph., B.P. '85

Chloroform ..	..	..	..	125 ml
Morphine Hydrochloride ..		..	2·29 g
Peppermint Oil	..	..	..	1 ml
Anaesthetic Ether	..	..	..	30 ml
Water (see page 642)	..	..	50 ml
Alcohol (90 per cent)	..	..	125 ml
Liquorice Liquid Extract ..		..	125 ml
Treacle, of commerce	..	..	125 ml
Syrup	..	..	..	to 1000 ml

Dissolve the peppermint oil in the alcohol, add the water, dissolve the morphine hydrochloride in the mixture, and add the chloroform and the anaesthetic ether. Mix the liquorice extract and the treacle with 400 ml of the syrup, add to the previously formed solution, mix thoroughly, add sufficient syrup to produce the required volume, and mix.

Standard
WEIGHT PER ML. At 20°, 1·22 g to 1·26 g.

ALCOHOL CONTENT. 12 to 15 per cent v/v of ethyl alcohol, determined by the method given in Appendix 10, page 888.

CONTENT OF CHLOROFORM. 11·25 to 13·75 per cent v/v, calculated as $CHCl_3$, determined by the following method:
Add about 0·4 g, accurately weighed, to 30 ml of 0·5N alcoholic potassium hydroxide contained in a stoppered flask, shake vigorously, and allow to stand for 12 hours.
Heat on a water-bath under a reflux condenser for one hour, cool, evaporate off the alcohol in a current of air, add 20 ml of water, and complete the determination by the method given in Appendix 11, page 891; each ml of 0·1N silver nitrate is equivalent to 0·002695 ml of $CHCl_3$.
Determine the weight per ml of the tincture and calculate the concentration of $CHCl_3$, volume in volume.

CONTENT OF ANHYDROUS MORPHINE. 0·157 to 0·191 per cent w/v, determined by the following method:
To about 13 g, accurately weighed, add 1 ml of *dilute ammonia solution* and 4 ml of water and extract with 30 ml of a mixture of equal volumes of *alcohol (95 per cent)* and *chloroform*; continue the extraction with two successive 22·5-ml portions of a mixture of 2 volumes of *chloroform* and 1 volume of *alcohol (95 per cent)*, washing each extract with the same 20 ml of a mixture of equal volumes of *alcohol (95 per cent)* and water.
Evaporate the combined extracts to dryness, dissolve the residue in 100 ml of 1N hydrochloric acid, and dilute to 500 ml with water.
To 10 ml of this solution add 10 ml of water and continue by the method for Aromatic Chalk with Opium Powder, page 776, beginning with the words "add 8 ml of a freshly prepared 1·0 per cent w/v solution of *sodium nitrite* . . .".
Determine the weight per ml of the tincture and calculate the concentration of anhydrous morphine, weight in volume.

Storage. It should be stored in airtight containers.

Labelling. A direction to shake the bottle well before use should be given on the label.

Dose. 0·3 to 0·6 millilitre.

Gelsemium Tincture

Gelsemium, in moderately fine
  powder ..   ..   100 g
Alcohol (60 per cent)   a sufficient quantity

Prepare 1000 ml of tincture by the percolation process and determine the proportion of total alkaloids present in 25 ml of the percolate; dilute the remainder of the percolate with sufficient of the alcohol to produce a tincture of the specified strength.

Standard
WEIGHT PER ML. At 20°, 0·910 g to 0·925 g.

ALCOHOL CONTENT. 56 to 59 per cent v/v of ethyl alcohol, determined by the method given in Appendix 10, page 888.

CONTENT OF TOTAL ALKALOIDS. 0·030 to 0·034 per cent w/v, calculated as gelsemine, $C_{20}H_{22}N_2O_2$, determined by the following method:
Evaporate 100 ml to about 20 ml, transfer to a separator with the aid of successive small portions of 1N sulphuric acid and *chloroform*, shake, and allow to separate.
Continue by the method for Gelsemium, page 209, beginning with the words "transfer the washings to a second separator containing 20 ml of 0·1N sulphuric acid, . . .".

Dose. 0·3 to 1 millilitre.

Gentian Tincture, Compound

Gentian, cut small and bruised ..   100·0 g
Cardamom Seed, freshly removed
  from the Fruit, immediately
  bruised, and used at once   ..   12·5 g
Dried Bitter-orange Peel, cut
  small   ..   ..   37·5 g
Alcohol (45 per cent)   ..   ..   1000 ml

Prepare by the maceration process.

Standard
WEIGHT PER ML. At 20°, 0·955 g to 0·970 g.

ALCOHOL CONTENT. 40 to 45 per cent v/v of ethyl alcohol, determined by the method given in Appendix 10, page 888.

Dose. 2 to 5 millilitres.

Lobelia Tincture, Ethereal

Lobelia, in moderately coarse
  powder ..   ..   200 g
Ether Spirit   ..   a sufficient quantity

Prepare 1000 ml of tincture by the percolation process and determine the proportion of total alkaloids present in 25 ml of the percolate; dilute the remainder of the percolate with sufficient of the ether spirit to produce a tincture of the specified strength.

Standard
WEIGHT PER ML. At 20°, 0·800 g to 0·825 g.

ALCOHOL CONTENT. 55 to 63 per cent v/v of ethyl alcohol, determined by the method given in Appendix 10, page 888.

CONTENT OF TOTAL ALKALOIDS. 0·050 to 0·075 per cent w/v, calculated as lobeline, $C_{22}H_{27}NO_2$, determined by the following method:
To 50 ml add 100 ml of *solvent ether* and extract with 20 ml of 0·5N sulphuric acid; repeat the extraction with successive 15-ml portions of a mixture of 3 volumes of 0·1N sulphuric acid and 1 volume of *alcohol (95 per cent)* until extraction is complete.
Wash the combined extracts with successive 10-, 5-, and 5-ml portions of *chloroform*, washing each chloroform extract with the same 20 ml of 0·1N sulphuric acid, and discard the chloroform extracts.
Neutralise the combined acid extract and washings to *litmus paper* with *dilute ammonia solution* and add a further 5 ml; extract with successive 10-ml portions of *chloroform* until extraction is complete, wash the combined extracts with 3 ml of water, discard the washings, filter, and wash the filter with *chloroform*.
Evaporate the combined filtrate and washings to about 2 ml on a water-bath, add three successive 2-ml portions of *dehydrated alcohol*, evaporating to dryness on a water-bath after each addition, and dry the residue for one hour at 80°.
Dissolve the residue in 2 ml of warm *alcohol (95 per cent)*, previously neutralised to *methyl red and methylene blue solution*, add 5 ml of 0·05N hydrochloric acid and 10 ml of water, cool, and titrate the excess of acid with 0·05N sodium hydroxide, using *methyl red and methylene blue solution* as indicator; each ml of 0·05N hydrochloric acid is equivalent to 0·01687 g of $C_{22}H_{27}NO_2$.

Storage. It should be stored in airtight containers, in a cool place.

Dose. 0·3 to 1 millilitre.

Myrrh Tincture

Myrrh, crushed ..   ..   ..   200 g
Alcohol (90 per cent)   ..   .. to 1000 ml

Macerate the myrrh with 800 ml of the alcohol in a closed vessel for seven days, with frequent shaking; filter, and pass sufficient of the alcohol through the filter to produce the required volume.

Standard
WEIGHT PER ML. At 20°, 0·840 g to 0·860 g.

ALCOHOL CONTENT. 81 to 87 per cent v/v of ethyl alcohol, determined by the method given in Appendix 10, page 888.

TOTAL SOLIDS. 4·5 to 6·5 per cent w/v, determined on 5 ml.

Dose. 2·5 to 5 millilitres.

Opium Tincture, Camphorated, Concentrated

SYNONYM: Liquor Opii Camphoratus Concentratus

Opium Tincture ..   ..   ..   400 ml
Camphor ..   ..   24 g
Benzoic Acid   ..   ..   ..   40 g
Anise Oil ..   ..   24 ml
Alcohol (95 per cent)   ..   ..   400 ml
Water (see page 642)   ..   .. to 1000 ml

Dissolve the benzoic acid, the camphor, and the anise oil in the alcohol, add the opium tincture and sufficient water to produce the required volume, mix, and filter if necessary.

Standard

WEIGHT PER ML. At 20°, 0·910 g to 0·930 g.

ALCOHOL CONTENT. 54 to 59 per cent v/v of ethyl alcohol, determined by the method given in Appendix 10, page 888.

CONTENT OF ANHYDROUS MORPHINE. 0·36 to 0·44 per cent w/v, determined by the following method:
Dilute 10 ml to 80 ml with *alcohol (60 per cent)*.
Evaporate 5 ml of this solution to dryness, extract the residue with 10 ml of *calcium hydroxide solution*, filter, wash the dish and the filter with a further 10 ml of *calcium hydroxide solution*, and to the combined filtrate and washings add 0·1 g of *ammonium sulphate* and extract with two successive 10-ml portions of *alcohol-free chloroform*, washing each extract with the same 10 ml of water.
Discard the chloroform extracts and extract the combined aqueous solution and washing with 60 ml of a mixture containing equal volumes of *alcohol (95 per cent)* and *chloroform*, followed by two successive 45-ml portions of a mixture containing 1 volume of *alcohol (95 per cent)* and 2 volumes of *chloroform*, washing each extract with the same mixture of 5 ml of *alcohol (95 per cent)* and 10 ml of water.
Evaporate the combined extracts to dryness, dissolve the residue in 10 ml of 1N hydrochloric acid, filter, and wash the filter with sufficient water to dilute the filtrate to 50 ml.
To 10 ml of the filtrate add 10 ml of water and 8 ml of a freshly prepared 1·0 per cent w/v solution of *sodium nitrite* in water, allow to stand for 15 minutes, and add 12 ml of *dilute ammonia solution*.
To a further 10 ml of the filtrate add 10 ml of water and 5 ml of *dilute ammonia solution*.
Compare the colours of the two solutions and determine the volume of *morphine and nitrite reagent* which must be added to the second solution to produce an equal depth of colour when both solutions are diluted to the same volume; each ml of *morphine and nitrite reagent* is equivalent to 0·02 mg of anhydrous morphine.

Dose. 0·25 to 1·25 millilitres.

Concentrated Camphorated Opium Tincture is approximately eight times as strong as camphorated opium tincture.

Orange Tincture

SYNONYM: Tinctura Aurantii

Dried Bitter-orange Peel, in moderately fine powder		110 g
Alcohol (70 per cent)	a sufficient quantity	

Prepare 1000 ml of tincture by the percolation process.

Standard

WEIGHT PER ML. At 20°, 0·895 g to 0·920 g.

ALCOHOL CONTENT. 62 to 69 per cent v/v of ethyl alcohol, determined by the method given in Appendix 10, page 888.

TOTAL SOLIDS. 3·5 to 4·5 per cent w/v, determined on 5 ml.

Dose. 1 to 2 millilitres.

Quillaia Tincture

Quillaia Liquid Extract ..	..	50 ml
Alcohol (45 per cent)	..	.. to 1000 ml

Mix, allow to stand for not less than twelve hours, and filter.

Standard

WEIGHT PER ML. At 20°, 0·940 g to 0·955 g.

ALCOHOL CONTENT. 43 to 45 per cent v/v of ethyl alcohol, determined by the method given in Appendix 10, page 888.

TOTAL SOLIDS. 1·0 to 1·5 per cent w/v, determined on 20 ml.

Dose. 2·5 to 5 millilitres.

Senega Tincture

Senega Liquid Extract ..	..	200 ml
Alcohol (60 per cent)	..	.. to 1000 ml

Mix, allow to stand for not less than twelve hours, and filter.

Standard

WEIGHT PER ML. At 20°, 0·930 g to 0·940 g.

ALCOHOL CONTENT. 54 to 58 per cent v/v of ethyl alcohol, determined by the method given in Appendix 10, page 888.

TOTAL SOLIDS. 4·9 to 7·0 per cent w/v, determined on 5 ml.

Dose. 2·5 to 5 millilitres.

Squill Tincture

Squill, bruised ..	..	..	100 g
Alcohol (60 per cent)	..	..	1000 ml

Prepare by the maceration process.

Standard

WEIGHT PER ML. At 20°, 0·925 g to 0·945 g.

ALCOHOL CONTENT. 52 to 57 per cent v/v of ethyl alcohol, determined by the method given in Appendix 10, page 888.

TOTAL SOLIDS. 4·5 to 6·5 per cent w/v, determined on 5 ml.

Dose. 0·3 to 2 millilitres.

VINEGAR

Squill Vinegar

SYNONYM: Acetum Scillae

Squill, bruised ..	..	..	100 g
Dilute Acetic Acid	..	..	1000 ml

Macerate the squill with the dilute acetic acid in a closed vessel for seven days, shaking occasionally, strain, press the marc, and heat the combined liquids to boiling; allow to stand for not less than seven days and filter.

Standard

WEIGHT PER ML. At 20°, 1·025 g to 1·045 g.

TOTAL SOLIDS. Not less than 4·5 per cent w/v, determined on 5 ml.

CONTENT OF ACETIC ACID. 5·4 to 6·3 per cent w/v,

calculated as $C_2H_4O_2$, determined by the following method:
To 10 ml add 10 ml of water and titrate with 1N sodium hydroxide, using *phenolphthalein solution* as indicator; each ml of 1N sodium hydroxide is equivalent to 0·06005 g of $C_2H_4O_2$.

Dose. 0·6 to 2 millilitres.

VITRELLAE

Vitrellae consist of thin-walled glass capsules containing a volatile medicament; they are protected by a wrapping of fabric or other suitable material. They are intended for use by crushing the glass and inhaling the vapour of the medicament.

The crushable glass capsule should be completely enclosed in absorbent cotton wool, ensuring that no glass is exposed, a label placed on the cotton wool, and the whole fitted into a silk sleeve, the ends of which are tied with silk thread and trimmed. Alternatively, the glass capsule may be placed in a suitable tube, plugged at both ends, or enclosed completely in other suitable material which will not permit the escape of fragments of glass and will allow complete volatilisation of the medicament.

Amyl Nitrite Vitrellae

Amyl Nitrite Vitrellae consist of Amyl Nitrite enclosed in crushable glass capsules, as described under Vitrellae (above).

Amyl nitrite is liable to decompose with evolution of nitrogen, particularly if it has become acid in reaction. In preparing the vitrellae, the amyl nitrite should be tested immediately before filling to ensure that it complies with the test for acidity (see page 28).

Standard
Take a sample of 10 vitrellae and determine the pressure required to break each by applying a gradually and evenly increasing pressure by the following method:
Remove the glass capsule from its protective covering and place transversely across a horizontal metal bar, 12·5 mm in thickness, in a V-shaped notch, 3·0 mm in depth and 9·0 mm in width, so that the bar supports the central portion of the body of the capsule.

Place a round-ended metal rod, 12·5 mm in diameter, against the upper surface of the capsule so that the rod is vertical and the point of contact is opposite the centre of the notch.
Apply the pressure to the capsule by compression between the rod and the bar, and record the applied pressure at which the capsule breaks.
The pressure required to break each glass capsule is not greater than 5 kgf.

Containers. They should be supplied in shallow paperboard, metal, or plastic boxes.

Storage. They should be stored at a temperature not exceeding 15°, as decomposition of the contents may occur at higher temperatures, resulting in loss of activity and development of high pressure.

Dose. Amyl nitrite, 0·12 to 0·3 millilitre by inhalation.

When the quantity to be contained in the vitrellae is not specified, vitrellae each containing 0·2 ml of amyl nitrite shall be supplied.

AROMATIC WATERS

Aromatic waters are solutions, usually saturated, of volatile oils or other aromatic substances in water. Some of them have a mild therapeutic action, but they are mainly used for their flavouring properties as vehicles for the internal administration of medicaments. Hamamelis Water is only used externally.

Preparation of aromatic waters. Aromatic waters are prepared by diluting the concentrated water with thirty-nine times its volume of freshly boiled and cooled Purified Water. The aromatic waters thus prepared contain a small proportion, usually about 1·5 per cent v/v, of alcohol (90 per cent).

Anise Water, Concentrated

Anise Oil ..	..	..	..	20 ml
Alcohol (90 per cent)	..	..		700 ml
Water (see page 642)	..	..	to	1000 ml

Dissolve the anise oil in the alcohol and add sufficient water, in successive small portions, to produce 1000 ml, shaking vigorously after each addition; add 50 g of sterilised Purified Talc or other suitable filtering aid, shake occasionally during a few hours, and filter.

Standard
WEIGHT PER ML. At 20°, 0·898 g to 0·908 g.

ALCOHOL CONTENT. 60 to 64 per cent v/v of ethyl alcohol, determined by the method given in Appendix 10, page 888.

Dose. 0·3 to 1 millilitre.

Camphor Water, Concentrated

Camphor ..	..	..	..	40 g
Alcohol (90 per cent)	..	..		600 ml
Water (see page 642)	..		.. to 1000 ml

Dissolve the camphor in the alcohol and add sufficient water in successive small portions to produce the required volume, shaking vigorously after each addition.

Standard
ALCOHOL CONTENT. 51 to 55 per cent v/v of ethyl alcohol, determined by the method given in Appendix 10, page 888.

Dose. 0·3 to 1 millilitre.

Caraway Water, Concentrated

Caraway Oil	..	..	..	20 ml
Alcohol (90 per cent)	..	..		600 ml
Water (see page 642)	..		.. to 1000 ml

Dissolve the caraway oil in the alcohol and add sufficient water in successive small portions to produce 1000 ml, shaking vigorously after each addition; add 50 g of sterilised Purified Talc or other suitable filtering aid, shake occasionally during a few hours, and filter.

Standard
WEIGHT PER ML. At 20°, 0·915 g to 0·923 g.

ALCOHOL CONTENT. 51 to 55 per cent v/v of ethyl alcohol, determined by the method given in Appendix 10, page 888.

Dose. 0·3 to 1 millilitre.

Chloroform Water, Double-strength

| Chloroform | .. | .. | .. | 5 ml |
| Purified Water, freshly boiled and |
| cooled .. | .. | .. | .. to 1000 ml |

Shake frequently until solution is effected.

Dose. 5 to 15 millilitres.

Cinnamon Water, Concentrated

Cinnamon Oil	..	..	..	20 ml
Alcohol (90 per cent)	..	..		600 ml
Water (see page 642)	..		.. to 1000 ml

Dissolve the cinnamon oil in the alcohol and add sufficient water, in successive small portions, to produce 1000 ml, shaking vigorously after each addition; add 50 g of sterilised

Purified Talc or other suitable filtering aid, shake occasionally during a few hours, and filter.

Standard
WEIGHT PER ML. At 20°, 0·914 g to 0·922 g.

ALCOHOL CONTENT. 52 to 56 per cent v/v of ethyl alcohol, determined by the method given in Appendix 10, page 888.

Dose. 0·3 to 1 millilitre.

Dill Water, Concentrated

SYNONYM: Aqua Anethi Concentrata

Dill Oil	..	..	..	..	20 ml
Alcohol (90 per cent)	..	..		600 ml
Water (see page 642)	..		.. to 1000 ml

Dissolve the dill oil in the alcohol and add sufficient water, in successive small portions, to produce 1000 ml, shaking vigorously after each addition; add 50 g of sterilised Purified Talc or other suitable filtering aid, shake occasionally during a few hours, and filter.

Standard
WEIGHT PER ML. At 20°, 0·914 g to 0·922 g.

ALCOHOL CONTENT. 52 to 56 per cent v/v of ethyl alcohol, determined by the method given in Appendix 10, page 888.

Dose. 0·3 to 1 millilitre.

Hamamelis Water

SYNONYMS: Aqua Hamamelidis; Distilled Witch Hazel; Liquor Hamamelidis

Hamamelis Water is prepared by macerating recently cut and partially dried dormant twigs of *Hamamelis virginiana* L. (Fam. Hamamelidaceae) in water, distilling, and adding the requisite quantity of alcohol to the distillate.

Standard
DESCRIPTION. A clear colourless liquid; odour characteristic.

ACIDITY OR ALKALINITY. It is neutral or slightly acid to *litmus solution.*

WEIGHT PER ML. At 20°, 0·976 g to 0·982 g.

FORMALDEHYDE. Add 2 ml to a mixture of 2 ml of a 1 per cent w/v solution of *phloroglucinol* in water and 5 ml of *sodium hydroxide solution*; no red colour is produced.

RESIDUE ON EVAPORATION. Not more than 0·025 per cent w/v, the residue being dried to constant weight at 105°.

ALCOHOL CONTENT. 13 to 15 per cent v/v of ethyl alcohol, determined by the method given in Appendix 10, page 888.

Uses. Hamamelis water is used to alleviate minor affections of the skin such as irritation, roughness, or soreness. It has also been employed, well diluted, as a constituent of eye lotions.

APPENDIXES

Appendix 1

Reagents and Solutions

Most of the reagents and solutions required for testing substances of the British Pharmaceutical Codex are listed below; details of certain other reagents and solutions that are required only for specific tests described in other appendixes are given in the appropriate appendix. The standards for the reagents and the strengths of the solutions are suitable for the purposes for which they are required in the British Pharmaceutical Codex.

The list is divided into

    A. General Reagents and Solutions (pages 829–851)
    B. Volumetric Solutions (page 851)
    C. Authentic Specimens and British Chemical Reference Substances (page 852)

Alcohols. Unless expressly stated otherwise, dehydrated alcohol, alcohol (95 per cent), or the dilute alcohols, when required in any tests, or in the preparation of reagent solutions, may be replaced by Industrial Methylated Spirit of equivalent alcoholic strength, provided that the legal requirements relating to the use of industrial methylated spirit are observed. Industrial Methylated Spirit must not be used for solubility tests or for any other tests which would thereby be vitiated.

Water. As elsewhere in the British Pharmaceutical Codex, except in Part 6, "water" without qualification means Purified Water of the British Pharmacopoeia.

Note. Names of reagents preceded by an asterisk (★) are Registered Trade Marks.

A. GENERAL REAGENTS AND SOLUTIONS

Acacia: of the European Pharmacopoeia.

Acacia Solution: a freshly prepared filtered 0·5 per cent w/v solution of *acacia* in cold water.

Acetate Buffer Solution pH 2·45: mix 200 ml of 1N hydrochloric acid with 200 ml of *1M sodium acetate* and dilute to 1000 ml with water; adjust the pH to 2·45 by the addition of 1N hydrochloric acid or *1M sodium acetate*, as required.

Acetate Buffer Solution pH 2·8: dissolve 4 g of *anhydrous sodium acetate* in water, add 155 ml of *glacial acetic acid*, and dilute to 1000 ml with water.

Acetate Buffer Solution pH 3·7: dissolve 10 g of *anhydrous sodium acetate* in about 300 ml of water, add 1 ml of *bromophenol blue solution* and *glacial acetic acid* until the indicator changes from blue to a pure green, and dilute to 1000 ml with water.

Acetate Buffer Solution pH 5·0: dissolve 13·6 g of *sodium acetate* and 6 ml of *glacial acetic acid* in water and dilute to 1000 ml.

Acetic Acid: dilute *glacial acetic acid* with sufficient water to produce a solution containing 33·0 per cent w/w of $C_2H_4O_2$.

Acetic Acid, Dilute: dilute *glacial acetic acid* with sufficient water to produce a solution containing 6·0 per cent w/w of $C_2H_4O_2$.

Acetic Acid, Glacial: of the British Pharmacopoeia, Appendix I.

Acetic Anhydride: of the British Pharmacopoeia, Appendix I.

Acetone: of the British Pharmacopoeia, Appendix I.

Acetone (50 per cent): mix 1 volume of water with 1 volume of *acetone*.

Acetone, Acid: to 650 ml of *acetone* add 50 ml of 4N hydrochloric acid and dilute to 1000 ml with water. It should be freshly prepared.

Acetone, Dry: of the British Pharmacopoeia, Appendix I: contains not more than 0·3 per cent w/v of water.

Acetonitrile: of the British Pharmacopoeia, Appendix I.

Acetonitrile, Purified: mix 1000 ml of *acetonitrile* with 75 g of Amberlite resin I.R.C. 50, allow to stand for 24 hours with occasional shaking, and filter.

Acetyl Chloride: of the British Pharmacopoeia, Appendix I.

Adrenaline Acid Tartrate: Adrenaline Tartrate of the European Pharmacopoeia.

Alcohol (95 per cent): of the British Pharmacopoeia.

Alcohol (90 per cent): of the British Pharmacopoeia.

Alcohol (80 per cent): of the British Pharmacopoeia.

Alcohol (70 per cent): of the British Pharmacopoeia.

Alcohol (60 per cent): of the British Pharmacopoeia.

Alcohol (50 per cent): of the British Pharmacopoeia.

Alcohol (45 per cent): of the British Pharmacopoeia.

Alcohol (20 per cent): of the British Pharmacopoeia.

Alcohol (95 per cent), Aldehyde-free: of the British Pharmacopoeia, Appendix I.

Alcohol, Dehydrated: of the British Pharmacopoeia, Appendix I.

Alcohol, Dehydrated, Aldehyde-free: of the British Pharmacopoeia, Appendix I.

Alginic Acid: of the British Pharmaceutical Codex.

Alizarin Fluorine Blue: of the British Pharmacopoeia, Appendix I.

Alizarin Fluorine Blue Solution: dissolve 0·38 g of *alizarin fluorine blue* in a solution of 0·3 g of *sodium hydroxide* in 25 ml of water, dilute to about 1500 ml with water, add 0·5 g of *sodium acetate*, and then add *dilute hydrochloric acid* until a thin layer of the solution is pale pink in colour; finally dilute to 2000 ml with water.

Alkaline Tetrazolium Blue Solution: mix 1 volume of a 0·2 per cent w/v solution of *tetrazolium blue* in *methyl alcohol* with 3 volumes of a 12 per cent w/v solution of *sodium hydroxide* in *methyl alcohol*; the solution should be prepared immediately before use.

Alumina: of the British Pharmacopoeia, Appendix I.

Alumina, Anhydrous: an aluminium oxide, dehydrated and activated by heat treatment and consisting of γ-Al_2O_3. The particle size is such that all the aluminium oxide passes through a No. 150 sieve but is retained on a No. 75 sieve.

Aluminium Hydroxide Gel: of the British Pharmacopoeia.

Amaranth: the trisodium salt of 3-hydroxy-4-(4 - sulpho - 1 - naphthylazo)naphthalene - 2, 7 - disulphonic acid.
When used for the titration of iodine and iodides with potassium iodate, the colour changes from orange-red to yellow.

Amaranth Solution, Dilute: a 0·02 per cent w/v solution of *amaranth* in water.

Aminoacetate Buffer Solution: mix 42 g of *sodium bicarbonate* and 50 g of *potassium bicarbonate* with 180 ml of water, add a solution containing 37·5 g of *aminoacetic acid* and 15 ml of *strong ammonia solution* in 180 ml of water, dilute to 500 ml with water, and stir until solution is complete.

Aminoacetic Acid: of the British Pharmacopoeia, Appendix I.

4-Amino-*NN*-diethylaniline Sulphate: of the British Pharmacopoeia, Appendix I.

4-Amino-*NN*-diethylaniline Sulphate Solution: a 0·2 per cent w/v solution of *4-amino-*NN-*diethylaniline sulphate* in water; it should be freshly prepared and protected from light.

1-Amino-2-naphthol-4-sulphonic Acid: $NH_2 \cdot C_{10}H_5(OH) \cdot SO_3H$
DESCRIPTION. A pinkish-white powder which tends to darken on storage.

SOLUBILITY. Very slightly soluble in water; insoluble in alcohol and in ether; soluble in solutions of alkali hydroxides.

SULPHATED ASH. Not more than 0·5 per cent.

CONTENT OF $C_{10}H_9NO_4S$. Not less than 97·0 per cent, determined by the following method: Dissolve, without the aid of heat, about 0·6 g, accurately weighed, in 50 ml of 0·1N sodium hydroxide and titrate the excess of sodium hydroxide with 0·1N sulphuric acid to a potentiometric end-point; each ml of 0·1N sodium hydroxide is equivalent to 0·02393 g of $C_{10}H_9NO_4S$.

1-Amino-2-naphthol-4-sulphonic Acid Solution: dissolve 2·4 g of *sodium sulphite*, 12 g of *sodium metabisulphite*, and 0·2 g of *1-amino-2-naphthol-4-sulphonic acid* in 100 ml of water.

4-Aminophenazone: of the British Pharmacopoeia, Appendix I.

3-Aminophenol: of the British Pharmacopoeia, Appendix I.

3-Aminophenol Solution: dissolve 7·5 mg of *3-aminophenol* in 20 ml of *alcohol (95 per cent)* and dilute to 500 ml with water.

4-Aminophenol: of the British Pharmacopoeia, Appendix I.

4-Aminophenol Solution, Standard: dissolve 0·120 g of *4-aminophenol* in 100 ml of water and dilute 10 ml of this solution to 100 ml with water.

Ammonia Buffer Solution: Strong Ammonia-ammonium Chloride Solution of the British Pharmacopoeia, Appendix I: dissolve 67·5 g of *ammonium chloride* in 650 ml of *strong ammonia solution* and dilute to 1000 ml with water.

Ammonia Solution, Dilute: dilute 375 ml of *strong ammonia solution* to 1000 ml with water: contains about 10 per cent w/w of NH_3.

Ammonia Solution, Strong: of the British Pharmacopoeia, Appendix I: contains 27·0 to 30·0 per cent w/w of NH_3 and has a weight per ml of about 0·896 g.

Ammonia-ammonium Chloride Solution: dissolve 5·4 g of *ammonium chloride* in 70 ml of *dilute ammonia solution* and add sufficient water to produce 100 ml.

Ammonium Acetate: of the British Pharmacopoeia, Appendix I.

Ammonium Bicarbonate: of the British Pharmaceutical Codex.

Ammonium Carbonate: of the British Pharmacopoeia, Appendix I.

Ammonium Carbonate Solution: dissolve 5 g of *ammonium carbonate* in a mixture of 7·5 ml of *dilute ammonia solution* and 50 ml of water, dilute to 100 ml with water, and filter if necessary.

Ammonium Chloride: of the European Pharmacopoeia.

Ammonium Citrate: triammonium citrate, $(NH_4)_3C_6H_5O_7$
DESCRIPTION. White crystals or a white crystalline powder.

SOLUBILITY. Soluble in water.

CHLORIDE. 0·5 g complies with the limit test for chlorides (700 parts per million).

SULPHATED ASH. Not more than 0·05 per cent.

CONTENT OF $(NH_4)_3C_6H_5O_7$. Not less than 97·0 per cent, determined by the following method:
Dissolve 3·5 g, accurately weighed, in 50 ml of water, add 50 ml of 1N sodium hydroxide, boil for 15 minutes, or until ammonia ceases to be evolved, add sufficient 1N sulphuric acid to make the solution acid to *phenolphthalein solution*, boil for 5 minutes, cool, and titrate with 1N sodium hydroxide, using *phenolphthalein solution* as indicator; each ml of 1N sodium hydroxide is equivalent to 0·08107 g of $(NH_4)_3C_6H_5O_7$.

Ammonium Cobaltothiocyanate Solution: dissolve 37·5 g of *cobalt nitrate* and 150 g of *ammonium thiocyanate* in sufficient water to produce 100 ml. It should be freshly prepared.

Ammonium Molybdate: of the British Pharmacopoeia, Appendix I.

Ammonium Molybdate Solution: a 10·0 per cent w/v solution of *ammonium molybdate* in water.

Ammonium Molybdate with Sulphuric Acid Solution: add 100 ml of a 10 per cent w/v solution of *ammonium molybdate* in water to a cooled mixture of 150 ml of *sulphuric acid* and 100 ml of water. It should be stored in a bottle made of resistance glass and protected from light.

Ammonium Oxalate: of the British Pharmacopoeia, Appendix I.

Ammonium Oxalate Solution: a 2·5 per cent w/v solution of *ammonium oxalate* in water.

Ammonium Persulphate: of the British Pharmacopoeia, Appendix I.

Ammonium Phosphate: $(NH_4)_2HPO_4$
DESCRIPTION. White crystals or granules.
SOLUBILITY. Very soluble in water; insoluble in alcohol.
ALKALINITY. Dissolve 1·0 g in 100 ml of *carbon dioxide-free water* and add *cresol red solution*; a pink colour, indicative of about pH 8·0, is produced.
IRON. 2·0 g complies with the limit test for iron (20 parts per million).
LEAD. It complies with the test given in Appendix 7, page 881 (20 parts per million).
CHLORIDE. 3·5 g, with an additional 35 ml of *dilute nitric acid*, complies with the limit test for chlorides (100 parts per million).
SULPHATE. 1·0 g, with an additional 7 ml of *dilute hydrochloric acid*, complies with the limit test for sulphates (600 parts per million).

Ammonium Reineckate: of the British Pharmacopoeia, Appendix I.

Ammonium Reineckate Solution: a freshly prepared 1·0 per cent w/v solution of *ammonium reineckate* in water.

Ammonium Sulphamate: of the British Pharmacopoeia, Appendix I.

Ammonium Sulphate: of the British Pharmacopoeia, Appendix I.

Ammonium Sulphide Solution: saturate 120 ml of *dilute ammonia solution* with washed *hydrogen sulphide* and add 80 ml of *dilute ammonia solution*. It must be recently prepared.

Ammonium Thiocyanate: of the British Pharmacopoeia, Appendix I.

Ammonium Thiocyanate Solution: a 10·0 per cent w/v solution of *ammonium thiocyanate* in water.

Ammonium Vanadate: of the British Pharmacopoeia, Appendix I.

Ammonium Vanadate Solution: dissolve, with the aid of heat, 5 g of *ammonium vanadate* in a mixture of 10 ml of *sodium hydroxide solution* and 90 ml of water, cool, and, if necessary, filter through glass wool.

Amyl Acetate: of the British Pharmacopoeia, Appendix I.

Amyl Alcohol: of the British Pharmacopoeia, Appendix I.

Aniline: of the British Pharmacopoeia, Appendix I.

Aniline Acetate Solution: a freshly prepared 25·0 per cent w/w solution of *aniline* in *glacial acetic acid*.

Anthrone: of the British Pharmacopoeia, Appendix I.

Anthrone Reagent: a 0·2 per cent w/v solution of *anthrone* in *nitrogen-free sulphuric acid*; the solution should be allowed to stand for 4 hours before use and should be discarded after 7 days.

Antimony Potassium Tartrate: of the British Pharmaceutical Codex.

Antimony Solution, Standard: dissolve 2·669 g of *antimony potassium tartrate* in water and dilute to 100 ml with water; dilute 5 ml of this solution to 500 ml with water. Dilute 5 ml of this second dilution to 500 ml with water; 1 ml of this solution contains 0·001 mg of Sb.

Antimony Trichloride: of the British Pharmacopoeia, Appendix I.

Antimony Trichloride Solution in Ethylene Chloride: prepare a 22·0 per cent w/v solution of *antimony trichloride* in dry *ethylene chloride* which has been purified by passing it down a column of silica gel and allow the solution to stand for 24 hours; to 100 ml add 2·5 ml of *acetyl chloride* and allow to stand for a further 24 hours before use.

Arsenic Trioxide: of the British Pharmacopoeia, Appendix I.

Arsenic Trioxide Solution: dissolve 2·0 g of *arsenic trioxide* in hot water to which has been added 5 ml of *sodium hydroxide solution*, cool, make slightly acid by the addition of *hydrochloric acid*, and dilute to 100 ml with water.

Ascorbic Acid: of the European Pharmacopoeia.

Atropine Methonitrate: of the British Pharmacopoeia.

Atropine Methoreineckate Solution: mix equal volumes of a 1 per cent w/v solution of *atropine methonitrate* and a 1 per cent w/v solution of *ammonium reineckate* and acidify with *dilute sulphuric acid*; wash the precipitate with water until the washings are free from sulphate, shake the precipitate with water to produce a saturated solution, and filter.

Atropine Sulphate: of the British Pharmacopoeia.

Azo Violet: 4-(*p*-nitrophenylazo)resorcinol.

Azo Violet Solution: a 0·2 per cent w/v solution of *azo violet* in *benzene*.

Barbituric Acid: of the British Pharmacopoeia, Appendix I.

Barbituric Acid and Pyridine Solution: to 55 ml of *pyridine* add, with cooling, a mixture of 7 ml of *hydrochloric acid* and 14 ml of water, mix, and add 30 ml of a 0·8 per cent w/v solution of *barbituric acid* in *dilute hydrochloric acid*.

Barium Chloride: of the British Pharmacopoeia, Appendix I.

Barium Chloride, 0·25M: a 6·1 per cent w/v solution of *barium chloride* in water.

Barium Chloride Solution: a 10·0 per cent w/v solution of *barium chloride* in water.

Barium Hydroxide: of the British Pharmacopoeia, Appendix I.

Barium Hydroxide Solution: a 3·0 per cent w/v solution of *barium hydroxide* in water.

Barium Solution FP: dissolve 1·7785 g of *barium chloride* in sufficient water to produce 1000 ml; 1 ml contains 1 mg of Ba.

Benzaldehyde: of the British Pharmaceutical Codex.

Benzalkonium Chloride Solution: of the British Pharmacopoeia.

Benzalkonium Chloride Solution, Standard: determine the benzalkonium chloride content of *benzalkonium chloride solution* by the method given for the content of cetrimide in Strong Cetrimide Solution (page 781), using about 4 g, accurately weighed; each ml of 0·05M potassium iodate is equivalent to 0·03540 g of $C_{22}H_{40}ClN$. Determine the weight per ml, calculate the concentration of $C_{22}H_{40}ClN$, weight in volume, and accurately dilute the solution with water to give a solution containing about 0·1 per cent w/v of $C_{22}H_{40}ClN$.

Benzene: of the British Pharmacopoeia, Appendix I.

Benzilic Acid: $(C_6H_5)_2 \cdot C(OH) \cdot CO_2H$

DESCRIPTION. A white or almost white crystalline powder.

SOLUBILITY. Slightly soluble in water; soluble in alcohol and in ether.

MELTING-POINT. 152° to 155°.

SULPHATED ASH. Not more than 0·1 per cent.

CONTENT OF $C_{14}H_{12}O_3$. Not less than 99·5 per cent, determined by the following method:

Dissolve about 1 g, accurately weighed, in 20 ml of *alcohol (95 per cent)*, previously neutralised to *phenolphthalein solution*, and titrate with 0·1N sodium hydroxide, using *phenolphthalein solution* as indicator; each ml of 0·1N sodium hydroxide is equivalent to 0·02282 g of $C_{14}H_{12}O_3$.

Benzoic Acid: of the British Pharmacopoeia, Appendix I.

Benzoyl Chloride: of the British Pharmacopoeia, Appendix I.

Benzyl Alcohol: of the British Pharmacopoeia.

Bismuth Oxide Nitrate: bismuth oxynitrate: of the British Pharmacopoeia, Appendix I.

Bismuth Sulphite Medium (Wilson and Blair): a selective medium, for the isolation and preliminary identification of salmonellae, containing bismuth sulphite and brilliant green together with appropriate nutrient and buffering substances.

Details of the preparation of the medium are given in "Medical Microbiology" (Ed., Robert Cruickshank), 11th Edn., 1965. Suitable material may be obtained from Oxoid Ltd., Southwark Bridge Road, London, S.E.1.

Borax: of the British Pharmacopoeia.

Boric Acid: of the European Pharmacopoeia.

Brilliant Green Solution: a freshly prepared 0·05 per cent w/v solution of brilliant green (Colour Index No. 42040) in water.

Brilliant Yellow: sodium 4,4'-di(*p*-hydroxyphenylazo)stilbene-2,2'-disulphonate, $C_{26}H_{18}N_4Na_2O_8S_2$

DESCRIPTION. A reddish-brown powder.

SOLUBILITY. 0·1 g dissolves in 100 ml of *alcohol (20 per cent)* forming an orange solution.

Brine: a saturated solution of *sodium chloride* in water.

Bromine: of the British Pharmacopoeia, Appendix I.

Bromine Solution: a saturated solution of *bromine* in water; it should be freshly prepared.

Bromine Solution AsT: of the British Pharmacopoeia, Appendix VIA.

Bromocresol Green: 4,4'-(3*H*-2,1-benzoxathiol-3-ylidene)bis(2,6-dibromo-*m*-cresol) *SS*-dioxide.

A solution changes in colour over the pH range 3·6 to 5·2 from yellow through green to blue.

Bromocresol Green Paper: soak white unglazed paper in *bromocresol green solution* and allow to dry.

Bromocresol Green Solution: dissolve 0·1 g of *bromocresol green* in a mixture of 2·9 ml of 0·05N sodium hydroxide and 5 ml of *alcohol (90 per cent)*, warming if necessary, and dilute to 250 ml with *alcohol (20 per cent)*.

Bromocresol Purple: 4,4'-(3*H*-2,1-benzoxathiol-3-ylidene)bis(2,6-dibromo-*o*-cresol) *SS*-dioxide.

A solution changes in colour over the pH range 5·2 to 6·8 from yellow through grey to blue-violet.

Bromocresol Purple Solution: dissolve 0·1 g of *bromocresol purple* in 5 ml of *alcohol (90 per cent)*, warming if necessary, add 100 ml of *alcohol (20 per cent)* and 3·7 ml of 0·05N sodium hydroxide, and dilute to 250 ml with *alcohol (20 per cent)*.

Bromocresol Purple Solution (0·1 per cent): dissolve 0·25 g of *bromocresol purple* in 20 ml of 0·05N sodium hydroxide and dilute to 250 ml with water.

Bromophenol Blue: 4,4'-(3*H*-2,1-benzoxathiol-3-ylidene)bis(2,6-dibromophenol) *SS*-dioxide.

A solution changes in colour over the pH range 2·8 to 4·6 from yellow through grey to blue-violet.

Bromophenol Blue Solution: dissolve 0·1 g of *bromophenol blue* in a mixture of 5 ml of *alcohol*

(*90 per cent*) and 3·0 ml of 0·05N sodium hydroxide, warming if necessary, and dilute to 250 ml with *alcohol* (*20 per cent*).

Bromophenol Blue Solution (0·5 per cent): dissolve 0·5 g of *bromophenol blue* in 20 ml of *alcohol* (*20 per cent*) and dilute to 100 ml with water.

Bromophenol Blue Solution, Alcoholic: a 0·5 per cent w/v solution of *bromophenol blue* in *alcohol* (*95 per cent*).

Bromothymol Blue: 6,6′-(3*H*-2,1-benzoxathiol-3-ylidene)bis(2-bromothymol) *S S*-dioxide.
A solution changes in colour over the pH range 6·0 to 7·6 from yellow through green to blue.

Bromothymol Blue Solution: dissolve 0·1 g of *bromothymol blue* in a mixture of 5 ml of *alcohol* (*90 per cent*) and 3·2 ml of 0·05N sodium hydroxide, warming if necessary, and dilute to 250 ml with *alcohol* (*20 per cent*).

Brown Standard Solution: standard solution B for colour measurement of the European Pharmacopoeia; 100 ml of brown standard solution contains 1·350 g of FeCl₃,6H₂O, 1·785 g of CoCl₂,6H₂O, 1·4976 g of CuSO₄,5H₂O, and the equivalent of 2·5 ml of *hydrochloric acid*.

Brownish-yellow Standard Solution: standard solution BY for colour measurement of the European Pharmacopoeia; 100 ml of brownish-yellow standard solution contains 1·080 g of FeCl₃,6H₂O, 0·595 g of CoCl₂,6H₂O, 0·2496 g of CuSO₄,5H₂O, and the equivalent of 2·5 ml of *hydrochloric acid*.

Buffer Solution pH 4·3: dissolve 63 g of *anhydrous sodium acetate* in 500 ml of water, add 100 ml of *glacial acetic acid*, and dilute to 1000 ml with water.

Buffer Solution pH 9: dissolve 3·092 g of *boric acid* and 3·728 g of *potassium chloride* in water, add 21·3 ml of 1N sodium hydroxide, and dilute to 1000 ml with water.

Buffer Solution pH 10: to 100 ml of *0·2M sodium phosphate* add 6 ml of *0·25M trisodium phosphate*.

Butyl Alcohol: n-Butyl Alcohol of the British Pharmacopoeia, Appendix I.

Calciferol: of the British Pharmacopoeia.

Calcium Acetate, Dried: of the British Pharmacopoeia, Appendix I.

Calcium Carbonate: of the European Pharmacopoeia.

Calcium Chloride: of the European Pharmacopoeia.

Calcium Chloride, Anhydrous: of the British Pharmacopoeia, Appendix I.

Calcium Chloride Solution: a 10·0 per cent w/v solution of *calcium chloride* in water.

Calcium Hydroxide: of the British Pharmacopoeia.

Calcium Hydroxide Solution: of the British Pharmaceutical Codex: contains about 0·15 per cent w/v of Ca(OH)₂.

Calcium Solution FP: of the British Pharmacopoeia, Appendix XIA.

Calcium Solution, Standard: dissolve 2·497 g of *calcium carbonate* in 12 ml of *acetic acid*, dilute

to 1000 ml with water and further dilute 10 ml of this solution to 1000 ml with water; 1 ml contains 0·01 mg of Ca.

Calcium Sulphate: CaSO₄,2H₂O
DESCRIPTION. A white powder.
SOLUBILITY. Slightly soluble in water.
ALKALINITY. Boil 1·0 with 50 ml of water, cool, and titrate with 0·1N hydrochloric acid, using *bromothymol blue solution* as indicator; not more than 0·3 ml of 0·1N hydrochloric acid is required.
CARBONATE. Boil 1·0 g with 10 ml of water and add 1 ml of *hydrochloric acid*; no carbon dioxide is evolved.
CHLORIDE. Boil 5·0 g with 50 ml of water and filter while hot; the filtrate, after cooling, complies with the limit test for chlorides (70 parts per million).
ACID-INSOLUBLE MATTER. Boil 2·0 g with 100 ml of 1N hydrochloric acid, filter, wash the residue with hot *dilute hydrochloric acid* and then with water, dry, and ignite to constant weight; the residue weighs not more than 2 mg.
RESIDUE ON IGNITION. 78·5 to 80·0 per cent.

Calcon Carboxylic Acid: 2-hydroxy-1-(2-hydroxy - 4 - sulpho - 1 - naphthylazo) - 3 - naphthoic acid.
In the presence of calcium ions in alkaline solution, it gives a pink colour; when an excess of disodium edetate is added the colour changes to blue or reddish-blue.

Calcon Carboxylic Acid Mixture: grind thoroughly together 0·5 g of *calcon carboxylic acid*, 2·5 g of *ascorbic acid*, and 5 g of *anhydrous sodium sulphate*; add a further 40 g of *anhydrous sodium sulphate*, mix well, and store in an airtight container protected from light.

Carbon Dioxide: of the European Pharmacopoeia.

Carbon Disulphide: of the British Pharmacopoeia, Appendix I.

Carbon Tetrachloride: of the British Pharmacopoeia, Appendix I.

Catechol: *o*-dihydroxybenzene, C₆H₄(OH)₂
DESCRIPTION. A white crystalline powder, becoming tinted on exposure to light or air.
SOLUBILITY. Soluble in water, in alcohol, and in ether.
MELTING-POINT. 101° to 105°.
SULPHATED ASH. Not more than 0·05 per cent.

Catechol Solution: a freshly prepared 10·0 per cent w/v solution of *catechol* in water.

Catechol Violet: 4,4′-(3*H*-2,1-benzoxathiol-3-ylidene)dipyrocatechol *S S*-dioxide.
It gives a blue colour with bismuth ions in moderately acid solution; when an excess of disodium edetate is added the solution changes to yellow.

Catechol Violet Solution: a 0·1 per cent w/v solution of *catechol violet* in water.

*Celite 545: a flux-calcined diatomaceous earth obtainable from Johns-Manville Company Ltd., 20 Albert Embankment, London, S.E.1.

Celite 545, Washed: to 500 g of *Celite 545* add 2000 ml of *hydrochloric acid*, mix, allow to stand, with occasional stirring, for 12 hours, filter, and wash the residue with water until the washings are neutral to *litmus paper*; continue washing the residue on the filter, using 500 ml of *methyl alcohol*, followed by 1000 ml of a mixture of equal volumes of *methyl alcohol* and *ethyl acetate*; finally dry the washed residue at 100° until it no longer smells of solvent. It should be stored in airtight containers.

Ceric Ammonium Sulphate:
$Ce(SO_4)_2,2(NH_4)_2SO_4,2H_2O$
DESCRIPTION. Yellow or orange-yellow crystals or crystalline powder.
SOLUBILITY. Slowly soluble in water; insoluble in alcohol.
CONTENT OF $Ce(SO_4)_2,2(NH_4)_2SO_4,2H_2O$. Not less than 95·0 per cent, determined by the following method:
Dissolve about 1 g, accurately weighed, in *dilute sulphuric acid*, add 3 g of *potassium iodide*, and titrate the liberated iodine with 0·1N sodium thiosulphate; each ml of 0·1N sodium thiosulphate is equivalent to 0·06325 g of $Ce(SO_4)_2,2(NH_4)_2SO_4,2H_2O$.

Cerous Nitrate: of the British Pharmacopoeia, Appendix I.

Cerous Nitrate Solution: dissolve 0·217 g of *cerous nitrate* in sufficient water to produce 1000 ml.

Cetrimide: of the British Pharmacopoeia.

Cetrimide Solution: dissolve 20 g of *cetrimide* in 80 ml of warm water, cool, and dilute to 100 ml with water.

Cetylpyridinium Chloride: of the British Pharmacopoeia.

Charcoal, Decolorising: of the British Pharmacopoeia, Appendix I.

Chloral Hydrate: of the European Pharmacopoeia.

Chloral Hydrate Solution: dissolve 50 g of *chloral hydrate* in 20 ml of water.

Chloral Hydrate Solution, Standard: a 0·0050 per cent w/v solution of *chloral hydrate* in water.

Chlorhexidine Acetate: of the British Pharmaceutical Codex.

Chlorhexidine Hydrochloride: of the British Pharmacopoeia.

Chloride Solution, Standard: dissolve 0·824 g of *sodium chloride* in sufficient water to produce 1000 ml and further dilute 10 ml of this solution to 1000 ml with water; 1 ml contains 0·5 μg of Cl.

4-Chloroacetanilide: of the British Pharmacopoeia, Appendix I.

4-Chloroaniline: of the British Pharmacopoeia, Appendix I.

1-Chloro-2,4-dinitrobenzene: of the British Pharmacopoeia, Appendix I.

Chloroform: of the British Pharmacopoeia.

Chloroform, Alcohol-free: of the British Pharmacopoeia, Appendix I.

Chloroform Water: of the British Pharmacopoeia.

Chromic-Sulphuric Acid Mixture: a saturated solution of *chromium trioxide* in *sulphuric acid*.

Chromium Trioxide: of the British Pharmacopoeia, Appendix I.

Chromium Trioxide Solution: a 30 per cent w/w solution of *chromium trioxide* in water.

*Chromosorb 102: a porous styrene divinyl-benzene copolymer obtainable from Perkin Elmer, Beaconsfield, Buckinghamshire.

Cineole–o-Cresol Compound: the equimolecular compound of o-*cresol* and cineole purified by recrystallisation from *light petroleum (boiling-range, 40° to 60°)*.
FREEZING-POINT. Not below 55·2°, determined by the method of the British Pharmacopoeia for the determination of cineole, about 5 g being used. It should be stored in airtight containers, protected from light.

Citrate-Phosphate Buffer Solution pH 6·0: dissolve 15·3 g of *anhydrous sodium phosphate* and 6·59 g of *citric acid* in sufficient water to produce 1000 ml.

Citric Acid: of the British Pharmacopoeia.

Citric Acid, Copper-free: of the British Pharmacopoeia, Appendix I.

Citric Acid FeT: of the British Pharmacopoeia, Appendix VIB.

Citric Acid 0·5M: dissolve 10·50 g of *citric acid* in sufficient water to produce 100 ml.

Clioquinol: of the British Pharmacopoeia.

Cobalt Chloride: of the British Pharmacopoeia, Appendix I.

Cobalt Nitrate: of the British Pharmacopoeia, Appendix I.

Codeine Phosphate: of the European Pharmacopoeia.

Congo Red: a solution changes in colour over the pH range 3·0 to 5·0 from blue through violet to red.

Congo Red Paper: impregnate unglazed white paper with a solution of *congo red* and allow to dry.

Copper: Cu: the pure metal known commercially as "electrolytic".

Copper Acetate: of the British Pharmacopoeia, Appendix I.

Copper Acetate Solution, Dilute: a 0·5 per cent w/v solution of *copper acetate* in water.

Copper Acetate Solution, Strong: a 5·0 per cent w/v solution of *copper acetate* in water.

Copper Carbonate: a basic carbonate.
DESCRIPTION. A blue or greenish-blue powder.
SOLUBILITY. Insoluble in water; soluble with effervescence in dilute acids; soluble in dilute ammonia solution forming a deep blue solution.
CHLORIDE. 1·0 g complies with the limit test for chlorides (350 parts per million).
SULPHATE. 0·5 g complies with the limit test for sulphates (0·12 per cent).
IRON. Dissolve 5·0 g in an excess of *dilute ammonia solution*, filter, wash the residue with *dilute ammonia solution*, dissolve in *dilute hydrochloric acid*, add an excess of *dilute ammonia solution*, again filter, and wash the residue with *dilute ammonia solution*, dry, and ignite to constant

weight; the residue weighs not more than 0·01 g (400 parts per million).

Copper Chloride: Copper (II) chloride dihydrate: of the British Pharmacopoeia, Appendix I.

Copper Chloride Solution, Ammoniacal: dissolve 22·5 g of *copper chloride* in 200 ml of water, add 100 ml of *strong ammonia solution*, and mix.

Copper Nitrate: of the British Pharmacopoeia, Appendix I.

Copper Oxide Solution, Ammoniacal: triturate 0·5 g of *copper carbonate* with 10 ml of water and gradually add 10 ml of *strong ammonia solution*.

Copper Reagent: Benedict's Qualitative Reagent: dissolve, with the aid of heat, 150 g of *sodium citrate*, 130 g of *anhydrous sodium carbonate*, and 10 g of *sodium bicarbonate* in about 650 ml of water, cool, add a solution containing 16 g of *copper sulphate* in 150 ml of water, dilute to 1000 ml with water, and filter.

Copper Sulphate: of the British Pharmacopoeia, Appendix I.

Copper Sulphate Solution: a 10·0 per cent w/v solution of *copper sulphate* in water.

Copper Sulphate Solution, Dilute: a 0·00393 per cent w/v solution of *copper sulphate* in water: 1 ml contains 0·01 mg of Cu.

Copper Sulphate with Pyridine Solution: dissolve 4 g of *copper sulphate* in 90 ml of water and add 30 ml of *pyridine*. It should be freshly prepared.

Corallin: the sodium salt of aurine (rosolic acid).
DESCRIPTION. Hard dull-red masses with a faint phenolic odour.
SOLUBILITY. Soluble in water and in alcohol (90 per cent), forming red solutions.
IDENTIFICATION TESTS. 1. A 0·1 per cent w/v solution in water gives a flocculent orange precipitate with *dilute hydrochloric acid* and the supernatant liquid is yellow.
2. A 0·1 per cent w/v solution in water gives the following colours when added to solutions of standard pH: pH 6·0, orange-yellow; pH 7·0, orange; pH 8·0, orange-red.

Corallin Solution, Alkaline: dissolve 5 g of *corallin* in 100 ml of *alcohol (90 per cent)*. Dissolve 25 g of *sodium carbonate* in 100 ml of water. When required, add 1 ml of the corallin solution to 20 ml of the sodium carbonate solution. The mixed solution must be freshly prepared.

Cresol: of the British Pharmacopoeia.

o-**Cresol:** C_7H_8O: pure dry recrystallised *o*-cresol with a freezing-point not below 30°.

Cresol Red: 4,4'-(3*H*-2,1-benzoxathiol-3-ylidene)di-*o*-cresol *SS*-dioxide.
A solution changes in colour over the pH range 0·2 to 1·8 from red through orange to yellow, and over the pH range 7·2 to 8·8 from yellow through pink to red.

Cresol Red Solution: dissolve 0·05 g of *cresol red* in a mixture of 5 ml of *alcohol (90 per cent)* and 2·65 ml of 0·05N sodium hydroxide, warming if

necessary, and dilute to 250 ml with *alcohol (20 per cent)*.

Crystal Violet: 4-[bis(*p*-dimethylaminophenyl) methylene]cyclohexa - 2,5 - dien - 1 - ylidenedimethylammonium chloride.
When used for titration in non-aqueous media, it changes from violet (basic) through blue-green (neutral) to yellowish-green (acidic).

Crystal Violet Solution: a 0·5 per cent w/v solution of *crystal violet* in *glacial acetic acid*.

Cyclohexane: of the British Pharmacopoeia, Appendix I.

Desoxycholate Citrate Agar: a selective medium, for the isolation and recovery of intestinal pathogens, containing sodium desoxycholate and neutral red together with appropriate nutrient and buffering substances.
Details of the preparation of the medium are given in "Medical Microbiology" (Ed., Robert Cruickshank), 11th Edn., 1965. Suitable material may be obtained from Oxoid Ltd., Southwark Bridge Rd., London, S.E.1.

Dextrose: of the British Pharmacopoeia.

Dextrose, Anhydrous: of the European Pharmacopoeia.

Dextrose Solution, Standard: dissolve 0·100 g of *anhydrous dextrose* in a saturated solution of *benzoic acid* in water, dilute to 100 ml with the saturated benzoic acid solution, and further dilute 2 ml of this solution to 100 ml with water; each ml contains 20 μg of dextrose.

3,3'-Diaminobenzidine Tetrahydrochloride: $(NH_2)_2 \cdot C_6H_3 \cdot C_6H_3 \cdot (NH_2)_2, 4HCl, 2H_2O$
DESCRIPTION. An almost white or slightly pink powder.
SOLUBILITY. Soluble in water.
MELTING-POINT. 342° to 345°, with decomposition.
CONTENT OF $C_{12}H_{18}Cl_4N_4, 2H_2O$. Not less than 98·0 per cent, determined by the method of the British Pharmacopoeia, Appendix XL, for the determination of nitrogen, about 0·4 g, accurately weighed, and 10 ml of *nitrogen-free sulphuric acid*, being used; each ml of 0·1N sulphuric acid is equivalent to 0·009904 g of $C_{12}H_{18}Cl_4N_4, 2H_2O$.

Dichlorobenzene: 1,2-dichlorobenzene: $C_6H_4Cl_2$.
A colourless, oily liquid; almost insoluble in water; soluble in alcohol, in ether, and in chloroform. It has a weight per ml of about 1·31 g and boils at about 180°.

2,6-Dichloro-*p*-benzoquinone-4-chloroimine: $O:C_6H_2Cl_2:NCl$
DESCRIPTION. A yellow or brownish-yellow crystalline powder.
SOLUBILITY. Very slightly soluble in water; soluble in chloroform, in ether, and in hot alcohol.
MELTING-POINT. 64° to 67°.
SULPHATED ASH. Not more than 0·1 per cent.
CONTENT OF $C_6H_2Cl_3NO$. Not less than 97·0 per cent, determined by the following method:
Burn about 0·015 g, accurately weighed, by the oxygen-flask method of the British Pharmacopoeia, Appendix XIC, using as the absorbing liquid a mixture of 10 ml of 0·1N sodium hydroxide and 2 ml of *hydrogen peroxide solution*; boil the

resulting solution gently for 10 minutes, cool, add 5 ml of *dilute nitric acid* and 25 ml of 0·02N silver nitrate, and allow to stand until precipitation is complete.

Filter, wash the precipitate with water, and titrate the excess of silver nitrate in the combined filtrate and washings with 0·02N ammonium thiocyanate, using *ferric ammonium sulphate solution* as indicator; each ml of 0·02N silver nitrate is equivalent to 0·001403 g of $C_6H_2Cl_3NO$.

Dichloromethane: Methylene Chloride: CH_2Cl_2

DESCRIPTION. A colourless volatile liquid with a characteristic odour.

SOLUBILITY. Soluble in 50 parts of water; miscible with most organic solvents.

WEIGHT PER ML. At 20°, 1·323 g to 1·325 g.

REFRACTIVE INDEX. At 20°, 1·4235 to 1·4250.

DISTILLATION RANGE. Not less than 95 per cent distils between 39° and 41°.

NON-VOLATILE MATTER. Not more than 0·01 per cent, determined by evaporating to dryness and drying to constant weight at 105°.

2,3-Dichloro-1,4-naphthaquinone: $C_{10}H_4Cl_2O_2$

DESCRIPTION. A yellow crystalline powder.

SOLUBILITY. Soluble in water; slightly soluble in hot alcohol and in ether.

MELTING-POINT. 195° to 197°.

2,3-Dichloro-1,4-naphthaquinone Solution: a 0·03 per cent w/v solution of *2,3-dichloro-1,4-naphthaquinone* in *dehydrated alcohol*.

2,6-Dichlorophenolindophenol Sodium Salt: of the British Pharmacopoeia, Appendix I.

2,6-Dichlorophenolindophenol Solution, Standard, Double-strength: dissolve 0·1 g of *2,6-dichlorophenolindophenol sodium salt* in 100 ml of water and filter. Standardise, immediately before use, by the method given in the British Pharmacopoeia, Appendix IIA, for Standard 2,6-Dichlorophenolindophenol Solution, and dilute the solution so that 1 ml is equivalent to 0·0002 g of ascorbic acid, $C_6H_8O_6$.

Dichloroquinonechloroimine: of the British Pharmacopoeia, Appendix I.

Dicyclomine Hydrochloride: of the British Pharmacopoeia.

Diethylamine: of the British Pharmacopoeia, Appendix I.

Diethylammonium Diethyldithiocarbamate: $(C_2H_5)_2N \cdot CS \cdot S \cdot NH_2(C_2H_5)_2$

DESCRIPTION. A white crystalline powder.

SOLUBILITY. Soluble in water.

MELTING-POINT. 79° to 81°.

SENSITIVITY. Dissolve 1 g of *copper sulphate* in sufficient water to produce 1000 ml and dilute 1 ml of this solution to 1000 ml with water; to 1 ml of this solution add 15 ml of *strong ammonia solution* and 2 g of *ammonium citrate* and dilute to 50 ml with water; to this solution add 10 ml of a 0·1 per cent w/v solution of the sample to be examined in *carbon tetrachloride*, shake, and allow to separate; the lower layer exhibits a yellow colour compared with a solution obtained in a similar experiment, omitting the diluted copper sulphate solution.

Digoxin Solution, Standard: dissolve 0·010 g of *digoxin B.C.R.S.*, previously dried over *phosphorus pentoxide* at a pressure not exceeding 5 mm of mercury for twenty-four hours, in sufficient of a mixture containing 65 volumes of *chloroform* and 35 volumes of *methyl alcohol* to give 50 ml; each ml contains 0·2 mg of digoxin.

Dimethicone: of the British Pharmaceutical Codex.

Dimethyl Sulphoxide: of the British Pharmacopoeia, Appendix I.

Dimethyl Yellow: 4-dimethylaminoazobenzene. A solution changes in colour over the pH range 2·8 to 4·0 from red through orange to yellow.

Dimethyl Yellow Solution: a 0·2 per cent w/v solution of *dimethyl yellow* in *alcohol (90 per cent)*.

Dimethyl Yellow–Oracet Blue B Solution: dissolve 0·015 g of *dimethyl yellow* and 0·015 g of *oracet blue B* in *chloroform* and dilute to 500 ml with *chloroform*.

Dimethylaminobenzaldehyde: of the British Pharmacopoeia, Appendix I.

Dimethylaminobenzaldehyde Solution: dissolve 0·125 g of *dimethylaminobenzaldehyde* in a cooled mixture of 65 ml of *sulphuric acid* and 35 ml of water and add 0·1 ml of *ferric chloride testsolution*.

This solution must be allowed to stand for 24 hours before use; it must be discarded when a yellow colour develops.

Dimethylaniline: of the British Pharmacopoeia, Appendix I.

Dimethylformamide: of the British Pharmacopoeia, Appendix I.

Dimethylglyoxime: $CH_3 \cdot C(N \cdot OH) \cdot C(N \cdot OH) \cdot CH_3$

DESCRIPTION. A white crystalline powder.

SOLUBILITY. Soluble in alcohol.

MELTING-POINT. 238° to 240° with decomposition.

SULPHATED ASH. Not more than 0·05 per cent.

SUITABILITY FOR NICKEL DETERMINATIONS. Dissolve 0·6 g of *nickel chloride* in water and dilute to 50 ml; dilute 20 ml of this solution with water to 100 ml, heat to boiling, add 0·25 g of the dimethylglyoxime under test dissolved in 25 ml of *alcohol (95 per cent)*, make alkaline to *litmus paper* by the dropwise addition of a mixture of 1 volume of *dilute ammonia solution* and 4 volumes of water, cool, and filter; to the filtrate add 1 ml of the nickel chloride solution and heat to boiling; a substantial precipitate is formed.

***NN*-Dimethyl-*p*-nitrosoaniline:** $(CH_3)_2N \cdot C_6H_4 \cdot NO$

DESCRIPTION. A green granular powder.

SOLUBILITY. Insoluble in water; soluble in alcohol and in ether.

MELTING-POINT. 85° to 87°.

SULPHATED ASH. Not more than 0·1 per cent.

Dimethyl-*p*-phenylenediamine Reagent: dissolve 0·1 g of NN-*dimethyl-p-nitrosoaniline* in 100 ml of hot water, cool, and filter. Store in an amber bottle; this solution is stable for 1 week.

Prepare the reagent, immediately before use, by adding to 10 ml of the above solution, 0·05 ml of *copper sulphate solution* and an excess of *zinc powder*, shaking until the solution is decolorised, and filtering.

Dinitrobenzene: of the British Pharmacopoeia, Appendix I.

Dioctyl Sodium Sulphosuccinate: of the British Pharmaceutical Codex.

Dioctyl Sodium Sulphosuccinate Solution, Standard: dissolve 0·45 g of *dioctyl sodium sulphosuccinate* in 15 ml of warm water, cool, and dilute to 100 ml with water.
Standardise by carrying out the determination of codeine phosphate described under Codeine Phosphate Syrup, page 799, using 5 ml of an accurately prepared solution of *codeine phosphate* containing approximately 5 mg per ml.
Determine the percentage purity of the codeine phosphate by the method of the British Pharmacopoeia and calculate the equivalent, in terms of the mg of $C_{18}H_{21}NO_3,H_3PO_4,\frac{1}{2}H_2O$ per ml, of the standard dioctyl sodium sulphosuccinate solution.

Dioxan: of the British Pharmacopoeia, Appendix I.

Diphenylamine: of the British Pharmacopoeia, Appendix I.

Diphenylamine Solution: a 0·10 per cent w/v solution of *diphenylamine* in *sulphuric acid*.

Diphenylcarbazide: of the British Pharmacopoeia, Appendix I.

Diphenylcarbazide Solution: a 0·2 per cent w/v solution of *diphenylcarbazide* in a mixture of 10 ml of *glacial acetic acid* and 90 ml of *alcohol* (*90 per cent*).

Dipotassium Hydrogen Phosphate: of the British Pharmacopoeia, Appendix I.

Disodium Edetate: of the British Pharmacopoeia.

Di-t-butyl-*p*-cresol: Butylated Hydroxytoluene of the British Pharmacopoeia.

Dithiocarbamate Solution: a 0·1 per cent w/v solution of *diethylammonium diethyldithiocarbamate* in *carbon tetrachloride*.

Dithranol: of the British Pharmacopoeia.

Domiphen Bromide: of the British Pharmacopoeia.

Domiphen Bromide Solution, Standard: a 0·200 per cent w/v solution of *domiphen bromide* in *methyl alcohol*.

Edetate–Citrate Solution: dissolve 20 g of *ammonium citrate* and 5 g of *disodium edetate* in sufficient water to produce 100 ml and extract with successive 15-ml portions of *dithiocarbamate solution* until a colourless extract is obtained.

Eosin: of the British Pharmacopoeia, Appendix I.

Eosin Solution: a 0·5 per cent w/v solution of *eosin* in water.

Ephedrine Hydrochloride: of the British Pharmacopoeia.

Ergotamine Tartrate: of the British Pharmacopoeia.

Ethanolamine: of the British Pharmaceutical Codex.

Ethanolamine Solution: dissolve 0·61 g of *ethanolamine* in water and dilute to 100 ml with water.

Ether, Anaesthetic: of the British Pharmacopoeia.

Ether, Solvent: of the British Pharmacopoeia.

Ethyl Acetate: of the British Pharmacopoeia, Appendix I.

Ethyl Methyl Ketone: of the British Pharmacopoeia, Appendix I.

Ethylene Chloride: of the British Pharmacopoeia, Appendix I.

Ethylene Glycol: $CH_2(OH)\cdot CH_2(OH)$
DESCRIPTION. A clear, colourless, viscous liquid.
SOLUBILITY. Miscible with water, with alcohol, and with chloroform.
ACIDITY OR ALKALINITY. 20 ml diluted with 50 ml of *carbon dioxide-free water* requires for neutralisation not more than 0·2 ml of 0·1N hydrochloric acid or of 0·1N sodium hydroxide, *bromothymol blue solution* being used as indicator.
WEIGHT PER ML. At 20°, 1·112 g to 1·114 g.
PROPYLENE GLYCOL. Not more than 1 per cent w/w, determined by the method of the British Pharmacopoeia for Gas-Liquid Chromatography. The chromatographic procedure may be carried out with a column, 50 cm in length, packed with Porapak Q and maintained at 150°, nitrogen as the carrier gas, and a flame-ionisation detector.

Ferric Ammonium Sulphate: of the British Pharmacopoeia, Appendix I.

Ferric Ammonium Sulphate Solution: a 10·0 per cent w/v solution of *ferric ammonium sulphate* in water.

Ferric Ammonium Sulphate Solution, Acid: dissolve 0·2 g of *ferric ammonium sulphate* in 50 ml of water, add 6 ml of *dilute nitric acid*, and dilute to 100 ml with water.

Ferric Chloride: of the British Pharmacopoeia, Appendix I.

Ferric Chloride Solution: of the British Pharmacopoeia, Appendix I.

Ferric Chloride Test-solution: a 5·0 per cent w/v solution of *ferric chloride* in water.

Ferric Reagent: dissolve 300 g of *ferric ammonium sulphate* in a mixture of 700 ml of water and 93 ml of *sulphuric acid*, allow to cool, and dilute to 1000 ml with water.

Ferroin Sulphate Solution: Phenanthroline Ferrous Complex Solution: dissolve 0·7 g of *ferrous sulphate* in about 70 ml of water, add 1·5 g of *1,10-phenanthroline*, and dilute to 100 ml with water.

Ferrous Ammonium Sulphate: of the British Pharmacopoeia, Appendix I.

Ferrous Sulphate: of the European Pharmacopoeia.

Ferrous Sulphate Solution: a freshly prepared 2·0 per cent w/v solution of *ferrous sulphate* in freshly boiled and cooled water.

Ferrous Sulphate-citrate Solution: dissolve 1 g of *sodium metabisulphite* in 200 ml of water, add 1 ml of 1N hydrochloric acid, 1·5 g of *ferrous* *sulphate*, and 10 g of *sodium citrate* and shake to dissolve; it should be freshly prepared.

*Filtercel: a natural diatomaceous earth obtainable from Johns-Manville Company Ltd., 20, Albert Embankment, London, S.E.1.

*Florisil: a synthetic magnesia–silica gel absorbent obtainable from Hermadex Ltd., 43, Berners St., London, W.1.

Fluorine Solution, Standard: dissolve 1·105 g of *sodium fluoride* in sufficient water to produce 1000 ml and dilute 5 ml of this solution to 500 ml with water; 1 ml contains 0·5 µg of F.

1-Fluoro-2,4-dinitrobenzene: of the British Pharmacopoeia, Appendix I.

1-Fluoro-2,4-dinitrobenzene Solution: a 0·8 per cent w/v solution of *1-fluoro-2,4-dinitrobenzene* in *acetone*.

Formaldehyde Solution: of the British Pharmacopoeia.

Formaldehyde Solution, Standard: dilute 5·0 ml of *formaldehyde solution* to 1000 ml with water and further dilute 5·0 ml of this solution to 1000 ml with water; 1 ml contains 10 µg of HCHO. It should be freshly prepared.

Formamide: of the British Pharmacopoeia, Appendix I.

Formic Acid: of the British Pharmacopoeia, Appendix I.

Formic Acid 2·5M: a solution of *formic acid* in water, containing in 1000 ml 115·06 g of CH_2O_2.

Glycerin: dilute *glycerol* with water to give a solution containing 84 to 87 per cent w/w of $C_3H_8O_3$. It has a weight per ml of about 1·23 g.

Glycerol: of the British Pharmacopoeia.

Glycerol, Dilute: a 33 per cent v/v solution of *glycerol* in water.

Glycine Buffer Solution: dissolve 0·3755 g of *aminoacetic acid* and 0·2925 g of *sodium chloride* in water, dilute to 50 ml with water, and add 50 ml of 0·1N sodium hydroxide; the pH of this solution should be measured electrometrically and, if necessary, adjusted to 11·1.

Glyoxal Bis(2-hydroxyanil): of the British Pharmacopoeia, Appendix I.

Gold Chloride: of the British Pharmacopoeia, Appendix I.

Gold Chloride Solution: a 2·0 per cent w/v solution of *gold chloride* in water.

Guaiacol: *o*-methoxyphenol, *o*-$(CH_3O)C_6H_4OH$

DESCRIPTION. White or yellowish crystalline mass or colourless to yellowish liquid; odour characteristic.

SOLUBILITY. Soluble in 60 parts of water; readily soluble in alcohol and in ether; slightly soluble in light petroleum.

FREEZING-POINT. 27·5° to 28·3°.

NON-VOLATILE MATTER. Not more than 0·05 per cent.

Guaiacum Resin: resin obtained from the heartwood of *Guaiacum officinale* L. and *Guaiacum sanctum* L.

DESCRIPTION. Reddish-brown or greenish-brown, hard, glassy fragments.

Guaiacum Tincture: macerate 20 g of *guaiacum resin* with 100 g of *alcohol (80 per cent v/v)* for 10 days, with occasional shaking, and filter; it should be recently prepared.

Hexamine: of the British Pharmacopoeia, Appendix I.

Hexane: of the British Pharmacopoeia, Appendix I.

Histamine Acid Phosphate: of the British Pharmacopoeia.

Hydrazine Hydrate: of the British Pharmacopoeia, Appendix I.

Hydrochloric Acid: Concentrated Hydrochloric Acid of the European Pharmacopoeia: contains 35·0 to 38·0 per cent w/w of HCl.

Hydrochloric Acid (25 per cent w/w): dilute *hydrochloric acid* with sufficient water to give a solution containing 25 per cent w/w of HCl.

Hydrochloric Acid, Dilute: of the European Pharmacopoeia: contains about 10 per cent w/w of HCl.

Hydrochloric Acid, Diluted (1 per cent w/v): dilute 24 ml of *hydrochloric acid* to 1000 ml with water.

Hydrochloric Acid FeT: of the British Pharmacopoeia, Appendix VIB.

Hydrochloric Acid, Gaseous: Hydrogen Chloride, HCl.
Prepared by the action of *sulphuric acid* on *sodium chloride*.

Hydrochloric Acid, Methanolic: a solution of gaseous hydrochloric acid (prepared by the action of *sulphuric acid* on *sodium chloride*) in *methyl alcohol*, adjusted to approximately 1N, as determined by titration with 1N sodium hydroxide.

Hydrochloric Acid, 0·1N, Glycerinated: mix 100 ml of 1N hydrochloric acid with 10 ml of *glycerol* and dilute to 1000 ml with water.

Hydrofluoric Acid: of the British Pharmacopoeia, Appendix I.

Hydrogen Peroxide Solution: of the British Pharmacopoeia, Appendix I: contains about 6 per cent w/v of H_2O_2.

Hydrogen Peroxide Solution, Diluted: a solution prepared by diluting *hydrogen peroxide solution* and containing 3·0 per cent w/v of H_2O_2. The content of H_2O_2 should be determined, immediately before use, by the method of the British Pharmacopoeia for Hydrogen Peroxide Solution, 5 ml being used for the determination, and the strength adjusted, if necessary.

Hydrogen Peroxide Solution, Strong: of the European Pharmacopoeia.

Hydrogen Sulphide: of the British Pharmacopoeia, Appendix I.

Hydrogen Sulphide Solution: a recently prepared solution of *hydrogen sulphide* in water.

Hydroquinone: Quinol: of the British Pharmacopoeia, Appendix I.

Hydroxylammonium Chloride: Hydroxylamine Hydrochloride: of the British Pharmacopoeia, Appendix I.

Hydroxylammonium Chloride Reagent
A. Dissolve 357·6 g of *hydroxylammonium chloride*

in water and dilute to 1000 ml with water. This solution should not be kept for more than one month.

B. Dissolve 173 g of *sodium hydroxide* and 31·8 g of *sodium acetate* in water and dilute to 1000 ml with water.

To prepare the reagent, mix equal volumes of solutions A and B, adjust the pH to 7·0 by the addition of solution B or of *hydrochloric acid*, and dilute this mixture to three times its volume with *alcohol (90 per cent)*. The reagent must be freshly prepared.

Hydroxylammonium Chloride Reagent in Alcohol (90 per cent): dissolve 70 g of *hydroxylammonium chloride* in 900 ml of *alcohol (90 per cent)*, add 4 ml of *dimethyl yellow solution*, followed by sufficient 1N *potassium hydroxide in alcohol (90 per cent)* to produce the full yellow colour of the indicator, and dilute to 1000 ml with *alcohol (90 per cent)*.

Hydroxylammonium Chloride Reagent in Alcohol (60 per cent): dissolve 34·75 g of *hydroxylammonium chloride* in 950 ml of *alcohol (60 per cent)*, add 5 ml of a 0·2 per cent w/v solution of *methyl orange in alcohol (60 per cent)*, followed by sufficient 0·5N *potassium hydroxide in alcohol (60 per cent)* to produce the full yellow colour of the indicator, and dilute to 1000 ml with *alcohol (60 per cent)*.
The reagent complies with the following test:
To 10 ml add 0·05 ml of 0·5N *potassium hydroxide in alcohol (60 per cent)*; no change in colour is produced. To a further 10 ml add 0·05 ml of 0·5N *hydrochloric acid*; the colour changes slightly towards orange.

Indigo Carmine: of the British Pharmacopoeia, which may not necessarily comply with the test for pyrogens.

Indigo Carmine Solution: to a mixture of 10 ml of *hydrochloric acid* and 990 ml of a 20·0 per cent w/v solution of *nitrogen-free sulphuric acid* in water add sufficient *indigo carmine* to produce a solution which complies with the following test:
Add 10 ml to a solution of 1·0 mg of *potassium nitrate* in 10 ml of water, add rapidly 20 ml of *nitrogen-free sulphuric acid*, and heat to boiling; the blue colour is just discharged in 1 minute.

Industrial Methylated Spirit: of the British Pharmacopoeia.

Iodic Acid: of the British Pharmacopoeia, Appendix I.

Iodic Acid Solution: a 4·5 per cent w/v solution of *iodic acid* in water.

Iodine: of the European Pharmacopoeia.

Iodine Solution: dissolve 2 g of *iodine* and 3 g of *potassium iodide* in water and dilute to 100 ml with water.

Iodine Solution, Alcoholic: a solution containing 1·0 per cent w/v of *potassium iodide* and 1·0 per cent w/v of *iodine* in *alcohol (95 per cent)*.

Iodine Water: mix 1 volume of 0·1N iodine and 4 volumes of water.

Iodoplatinate Solution: a solution containing 0·25 per cent w/v of *platinic chloride* and 5 per cent w/v of *potassium iodide* in water.

Iodoplatinate Solution, Acidified: add 2 ml of *hydrochloric acid* to 100 ml of *iodoplatinate solution*.

Iron Solution FeT, Standard: of the British Pharmacopoeia, Appendix VIB.

Iron Standard Solution, Weak: dissolve 1·727 g of *ferric ammonium sulphate* in water, add 50 ml of *dilute sulphuric acid*, dilute to 1000 ml with water, and further dilute 5 ml of this solution to 1000 ml with water; each ml contains 1 μg of Fe.

Isobutyl Alcohol: of the British Pharmacopoeia, Appendix I.

Isoniazid: of the European Pharmacopoeia.

Isoniazid Solution: dissolve 0·5 g of *isoniazid* in 250 ml of *methyl alcohol*, add 0·63 ml of *hydrochloric acid*, and dilute to 500 ml with *methyl alcohol*.

Isoniazid Solution, Standard: dissolve 0·0500 g of *isoniazid* in water and dilute to 1000 ml with water.

Isoprenaline Sulphate: of the British Pharmacopoeia.

Isopropyl Alcohol: of the British Pharmacopoeia.

Isopropyl Alcohol (90 per cent v/v): dilute 90 ml of *isopropyl alcohol* to 100 ml with water.

Isopropyl Ether: of the British Pharmacopoeia, Appendix I.

Isopropylamine: $(CH_3)_2CH \cdot NH_2$
DESCRIPTION. A colourless liquid with a strong ammoniacal odour.
SOLUBILITY. Miscible with water, with alcohol, and with ether.
WEIGHT PER ML. At 20°, 0·685 g to 0·690 g.
CONTENT OF C_3H_9N. Not less than 99·2 per cent, determined by the following method:
Taking care to avoid loss by evaporation, dissolve about 2 g, accurately weighed, in 50 ml of 1N hydrochloric acid and titrate the excess acid with 1N sodium hydroxide, using *methyl red solution* as indicator; each ml of 1N hydrochloric acid is equivalent to 0·05911 g of C_3H_9N.

Kieselguhr: a natural diatomaceous earth, purified by treating it with *dilute hydrochloric acid*, washing it with water, and drying.
Microscopical description. It consists of the frustules of fossil diatoms, both pennate and discoid forms, with a few sponge spicules and very occasional grains of sand; the diatoms vary in length or diameter from 5 to **50** to **100** to 500 μm and the surface of the valves often exhibits a characteristic and graceful design; mounted in *chloral hydrate solution* they are almost invisible, but are easily seen in *cresol*; when examined between crossed polars, diatoms and sponge spicules are invisible but grains of sand shine brightly.

Lactic Acid: of the British Pharmacopoeia.

Lactophenol: dissolve 20 g of *phenol* in a mixture of 20 g of *lactic acid*, 40 g of *glycerol*, and 20 ml of water.

Lead Acetate: of the British Pharmacopoeia, Appendix I.

Lead Acetate Solution: a 10·0 per cent w/v solution of *lead acetate* in *carbon dioxide-free water*.

Lead Acetate Suspension, Basic: suspend 20 g of *lead monoxide* and 10 g of *lead acetate* in sufficient *methyl alcohol* to produce 100 ml.

Lead Dioxide: of the British Pharmacopoeia, Appendix I.

Lead Monoxide: of the British Pharmacopoeia, Appendix I.

Lead Nitrate: of the British Pharmacopoeia, Appendix I.

Lead Paper: impregnate thin white filter paper, 100 × 50 mm, with *lead acetate solution* and allow to dry.

Lead Solution, Standard: dissolve 1·598 g of *lead nitrate* in sufficient water to produce 1000 ml and dilute 10 ml of this solution to 1000 ml with water.

Lead Subacetate Solution, Strong: of the British Pharmaceutical Codex.

Lithium and Sodium Molybdophospho-tungstate Solution: dissolve 100 g of *sodium tungstate* and 25 g of *sodium molybdate* in 800 ml of water in a 1500-ml flask, add 50 ml of *phosphoric acid* and 100 ml of *hydrochloric acid*, and heat for 10 hours under a reflux condenser. Cool, add 150 g of *lithium sulphate*, 50 ml of water, and 0·2 to 0·3 ml of *bromine*, allow to stand for 2 hours, remove the excess bromine by boiling for 15 minutes without the condenser, cool, filter, and dilute to 1000 ml with water.

It should be stored at a temperature not exceeding 4° and must not be used later than 4 months after preparation. It is golden yellow in colour and must not be used if any trace of green colour is present.

Lithium Sulphate: of the British Pharmacopoeia, Appendix I.

Litmus: a blue pigment prepared from various lichens, chiefly from species of *Roccella* DC. It gives a red colour with acids and a blue colour with alkalis (pH range, 5 to 8).

DESCRIPTION. Small dark-blue or bluish-violet friable cubical or brick-shaped cakes, containing a considerable proportion of chalk or gypsum in addition to the extract from the lichens.

Litmus Paper, Blue: impregnate unglazed white paper with a solution of *litmus* and allow to dry.

Litmus Paper, Red: impregnate unglazed white paper with a solution of *litmus* reddened by the previous addition of a minute quantity of *sulphuric acid* and allow to dry.

Litmus Solution: boil 25 g of *litmus* with 100 ml of *alcohol (90 per cent)* under a reflux condenser for 1 hour, discard the clear liquid, and repeat the operation with two further 75-ml portions of *alcohol (90 per cent)*; digest the washed litmus with 250 ml of water and filter.

Macrogol 300: Polyethylene glycol 300: of the British Pharmacopoeia.

Macrogol 400: Polyethylene glycol 400: of the British Pharmacopoeia, Appendix I.

Macrogol 600: Polyethylene glycol 600.

Magenta Solution, Decolorised: of the British Pharmacopoeia, Appendix I.

Magnesium Ammonio-sulphate Solution: dissolve 10 g of *magnesium sulphate* and 20 g of *ammonium chloride* in 80 ml of water, add 42 ml of *dilute ammonia solution*, and allow to stand for a few days; decant and filter.

Magnesium Chloride: of the British Pharmacopoeia.

Magnesium Nitrate: of the British Pharmacopoeia, Appendix I.

Magnesium Oxide, Heavy: MgO

DESCRIPTION. A white powder; odourless; taste slightly alkaline.

SOLUBILITY. Very slightly soluble in water; insoluble in alcohol; soluble in dilute acids.

IDENTIFICATION TEST. A solution in *acetic acid* gives the reactions characteristic of magnesium.

LOSS ON IGNITION. Not more than 5·0 per cent, determined by igniting to constant weight at a temperature not lower than 900°.

Magnesium Solution FP: dissolve 9 g of *magnesium chloride* in sufficient water to produce 500 ml. Determine the content of Mg in the solution by the following method:

To 25 ml add 25 ml of water and 10 ml of *ammonia buffer solution* and titrate with 0·05M disodium edetate, using 0·1 g of *mordant black 11 mixture* as indicator; each ml of 0·05M disodium edetate is equivalent to 0·001215 g of Mg.

Dilute the remainder of the prepared solution with water so that 1 ml contains 1 mg of Mg.

Magnesium Solution, Standard: dissolve 10·14 g of *magnesium sulphate* in 1000 ml of water and dilute 10 ml of this solution to 1000 ml with water; each ml contains 10 μg of Mg.

Magnesium Sulphate: of the European Pharmacopoeia.

Magnesium Sulphate, Anhydrous: heat *dried magnesium sulphate* for 1½ hours at 150° or for 4 hours at 130° and allow to cool in a desiccator.

Magnesium Sulphate, Dried: of the British Pharmacopoeia.

Manganese Sulphate: of the British Pharmaceutical Codex.

Mannitol: of the British Pharmacopoeia.

Mercuric Acetate: of the British Pharmacopoeia, Appendix I.

Mercuric Acetate Solution: a 5·0 per cent w/v solution of *mercuric acetate* in *glacial acetic acid* which has been neutralised, if necessary, to *crystal violet solution* by the addition of 0·1N perchloric acid.

Mercuric Bromide: $HgBr_2$

DESCRIPTION. White or faintly yellow crystals or crystalline powder.

SOLUBILITY. Slightly soluble in water; soluble in alcohol.

Mercuric Chloride: of the British Pharmacopoeia, Appendix I.

Mercuric Chloride Test-solution: a 5·0 per cent w/v solution of *mercuric chloride* in water.

Mercuric Oxide, Yellow: of the British Pharmacopoeia, Appendix I.

Mercuric Sulphate Solution: mix 5 g of *yellow mercuric oxide* with 40 ml of water and, with stirring, add 20 ml of *sulphuric acid*; add 40 ml of water and stir until completely dissolved.

Mercury: of the British Pharmacopoeia, Appendix I.

Mercury Nitrate Solution: Millon's Reagent: dissolve 3 ml of *mercury* in 27 ml of cold *fuming nitric acid* and dilute with an equal quantity of water. It must be recently prepared.

Metaphosphoric Acid: of the British Pharmacopoeia, Appendix I.

Metaphosphoric Acid Solution: a freshly prepared 20·0 per cent w/v solution of *metaphosphoric acid* in water.

Methoxyethanol: of the British Pharmacopoeia, Appendix I.

Methyl Alcohol: Methanol: of the British Pharmacopoeia, Appendix I.

Methyl Alcohol (80 per cent v/v): dilute 800 ml of *methyl alcohol* to 1000 ml with water.

Methyl Alcohol (60 per cent v/v): dilute 3 volumes of *methyl alcohol* with 2 volumes of water.

Methyl Alcohol, Acid: to 900 ml of *methyl alcohol* add 18 ml of *glacial acetic acid* and 3 ml of *hydrochloric acid* and dilute to 1000 ml with water.

Methyl Alcohol, Ammoniacal: mix 10 ml of *dilute ammonia solution* with 990 ml of *methyl alcohol*.

Methyl Alcohol, Dehydrated: *methyl alcohol* which complies with the following additional requirement:
WATER. Not more than 0·1 per cent w/w, determined by the method given in Appendix 16, page 895.

Methyl Carbonate: of the British Pharmacopoeia, Appendix I.

Methyl Orange: the sodium salt of 4′-dimethylaminoazobenzene-4-sulphonic acid.
A solution changes in colour over the pH range 2·8 to 4·0 from red through orange to yellow.

Methyl Orange Solution: a 0·04 per cent w/v solution of *methyl orange* in *alcohol (20 per cent)*.

Methyl Orange–Xylene Cyanol FF Solution: dissolve 0·1 g of *methyl orange* and 0·26 g of *xylene cyanol FF* in 50 ml of *alcohol (95 per cent)* and dilute to 100 ml with water.

Methyl Red: 4′-dimethylaminoazobenzene-2-carboxylic acid.
A solution changes in colour over the pH range 4·2 to 6·3 from red through orange to yellow.

Methyl Red and Methylene Blue Solution: mix 20 ml of a 0·05 per cent w/v solution of *methyl red* in *alcohol (80 per cent)* with 0·4 ml of a 2·0 per cent w/v solution of *methylene blue* in water. It must be recently prepared.

Methyl Red Solution: dissolve 0·025 g of *methyl red* in a mixture of 5 ml of *alcohol (90 per cent)* and 0·95 ml of 0·05N sodium hydroxide, warming if necessary, and dilute to 250 ml with *alcohol (50 per cent)*.

Methyl Salicylate: of the European Pharmacopoeia.

Methyl Thymol Blue: [3*H*-2,1-benzoxathiol-3-ylidenebis(6-hydroxy-5-isopropyl-2-methyl-*m*-phenylene)methylenenitrilo]tetra-acetic acid *SS*-dioxide.
It gives a blue colour with calcium in alkaline solution; in the presence of an excess of disodium edetate the solution is grey.

Methyl Thymol Blue Mixture: Mix 1 part of *methyl thymol blue* with 100 parts of *potassium nitrate*.

Methylaminophenol: of the British Pharmacopoeia, Appendix I.

Methylaminophenol with Sulphite Solution: dissolve 0·1 g of *methylaminophenol*, 20 g of *sodium metabisulphite*, and 1 g of *sodium sulphite* in sufficient water to produce 100 ml.

Methylene Blue: of the British Pharmacopoeia.

Methylene Blue Solution: a 1·0 per cent w/v solution of *methylene blue* in water.

Methylene Blue Solution, Alcoholic: a 0·1 per cent w/v solution of *methylene blue* in *alcohol (95 per cent)*.

Mordant Black 11: Colour Index No. 14645: the sodium salt of 2-(2-hydroxy-6-nitro-4-sulpho-1-naphthylazo)-1-naphthol.
It gives a wine-red colour in the presence of calcium, magnesium, zinc, and certain other metals in alkaline solution; in the presence of an excess of disodium edetate the solution is blue.

Mordant Black 11 Mixture: mix 0·2 part of *mordant black 11* with 100 parts of *sodium chloride*. It should be recently prepared.

Mordant Black 11 Solution: a freshly prepared 0·1 per cent w/v solution of *mordant black 11* in *alcohol (95 per cent)*.

Morphinated Water: shake *morphine* with *chloroform water* and allow to stand for not less than 7 days at room temperature, shaking occasionally; filter the solution immediately before use.

Morphine: add a slight excess of *dilute ammonia solution* to a solution of *morphine sulphate* in water and wash the precipitated morphine with water until the washings are free from ammonium salts.

Morphine and Nitrite Reagent: dissolve 0·01 g of *anhydrous morphine* in sufficient 0·2N hydrochloric acid to produce 100 ml; to 10 ml of this solution add 10 ml of water and 8 ml of a 1·0 per cent w/v solution of *sodium nitrite* in water, allow to stand for 15 minutes, add 12 ml of *dilute ammonia solution*, and dilute to 50 ml with water; it should be freshly prepared.

Morphine, Anhydrous: dry *morphine* at 110° and allow to cool.

Morphine Hydrochloride: of the European Pharmacopoeia.

Morphine Sulphate: of the British Pharmacopoeia.

β-Naphthol: 2-Naphthol of the British Pharmacopoeia, Appendix I.

β-Naphthol Solution: dissolve 5 g of freshly recrystallised *β-naphthol* in 8 ml of *sodium hydroxide solution* and 20 ml of water and dilute to 100 ml with water. It must be freshly prepared.

1-Naphtholbenzein: when used for titration in non-aqueous media, it changes from blue or green-blue (basic) through orange (neutral) to dark green (acidic).

1-Naphtholbenzein Solution: a 0·2 per cent w/v solution of *1-naphtholbenzein* in *glacial acetic acid.*

Naphthoresorcinol: 1,3-dihydroxynaphthalene, 1,3-$C_{10}H_6(OH)_2$
DESCRIPTION. A pale grey-brown crystalline powder.
SOLUBILITY. Soluble in water, in alcohol, and in ether.
MELTING-POINT. 122° to 125°.

N - (1 - Naphthyl)ethylenediamine Hydrochloride: of the British Pharmacopoeia, Appendix I.

N-(1-Naphthyl)ethylenediamine Hydrochloride Solution: a 0·2 per cent w/v solution of N-*(1-naphthyl)ethylenediamine hydrochloride* in *methyl alcohol.*

Nickel Chloride: $NiCl_2,6H_2O$
DESCRIPTION. Apple-green crystals or crystalline powder.
SOLUBILITY. Soluble in water.
SULPHATE. 0·5 g complies with the limit test for sulphates (0·12 per cent).

Nickel Chloride Solution, Dilute: a 0·00405 per cent w/v solution of *nickel chloride* in water: 1 ml contains 0·01 mg of Ni.

Nickel Chloride–Ammonia Solution: dissolve 0·1 g of *nickel chloride* in 10 ml of water, add a solution containing 5·4 g of *ammonium chloride*, 8 g of *ammonium bicarbonate*, and 1·5 ml of *strong ammonia solution* in 80 ml of water, and dilute to 100 ml with water.

Ninhydrin: Indanetrione Hydrate: of the British Pharmacopoeia, Appendix I.

Nitrate Solution, Standard: dissolve 1·631 g of *potassium nitrate* in sufficient water to produce 1000 ml and dilute 10 ml of this solution to 1000 ml with water; 1 ml contains 10 μg of NO_3.

Nitric Acid: of the British Pharmacopoeia, Appendix I: contains 70 per cent w/w of HNO_3.

Nitric Acid, Dilute: mix 106 ml of *nitric acid* with sufficient water to produce 1000 ml: contains about 10 per cent w/w of HNO_3.

Nitric Acid, Fuming: of the British Pharmacopoeia, Appendix I: contains not less than 95·0 per cent w/w of HNO_3.

Nitric Acid, 2M: dilute 143 ml of *nitric acid* to 1000 ml with water: contains 12·6 per cent w/v of HNO_3.

4-Nitroaniline: of the British Pharmacopoeia, Appendix I.

Nitroaniline Solution: dissolve, with the aid of heat, 0·5 g of *4-nitroaniline* in a mixture of 10 ml of 2N hydrochloric acid and 90 ml of water, cool, and filter.

Nitroaniline Solution, Diazotised: dissolve 0·4 g of *4-nitroaniline* in 60 ml of 1N hydrochloric acid, cool to 15°, and add a 10 per cent w/v solution of *sodium nitrite* in water until 0·05 ml of the mixture turns *starch-iodide paper* blue; it should be freshly prepared.

2-Nitrobenzaldehyde: of the British Pharmacopoeia, Appendix I.

2-Nitrobenzaldehyde Solution: a 1·0 per cent w/v solution of *2-nitrobenzaldehyde* in *alcohol (50 per cent).*

Nitrobenzene: $C_6H_5NO_2$
DESCRIPTION. A pale yellow liquid with a characteristic odour.
SOLUBILITY. Insoluble in water.
DISTILLATION RANGE. Not less than 95 per cent distils between 209° and 211°.
FREEZING-POINT. Not lower than 5·3°.
REFRACTIVE INDEX. At 20°, 1·5520 to 1·5530.
WEIGHT PER ML. At 20°, 1·201 g to 1·203 g.
ACIDITY. Shake 20 g with 50 ml of water, allow to separate, and titrate the aqueous layer with 0·02N sodium hydroxide, using *bromophenol blue solution* as indicator; not more than 0·5 ml of 0·02N sodium hydroxide is required.

Nitrogen: N_2, washed and dried.

Nitrogen, Oxygen-free: *nitrogen* which has been freed from oxygen by passing it through *alkaline pyrogallol solution.*

★Oracet Blue B: Solvent Blue 19: when used for titration in non-aqueous media, its colour changes from blue in basic solutions, through purple in neutral solutions, to pink in acidic solutions.

Oxalic Acid: of the British Pharmacopoeia, Appendix I.

Oxalic Acid and Sulphuric Acid Solution: a 5·0 per cent w/v solution of *oxalic acid* in a cooled mixture of equal volumes of *sulphuric acid* and water.

Palladous Chloride: $PdCl_2$
DESCRIPTION. A brown powder.
SOLUBILITY. Soluble in water, in alcohol, and in acetone.

Palladous Chloride Reagent: dissolve, with the aid of gentle heat, 0·2 g of *palladous chloride* in 116 ml of 1N hydrochloric acid, cool, add 13·6 g of *sodium acetate*, and dilute to 1000 ml with water.

Paraffin, Liquid: of the British Pharmacopoeia.

Penicillinase Solution: of the British Pharmacopoeia, Appendix I.

Peptone Water: mix 10 g of peptone and 5 g of *sodium chloride* to a smooth paste with 250 ml of water at 60°, dilute to 1000 ml with cold water, heat at 98° to 100° for 30 minutes, and filter. Sterilise by heating in an autoclave.

Perchloric Acid (60 per cent w/w): of the British Pharmacopoeia, Appendix I.

Periodic Acid: $HIO_4,2H_2O$
DESCRIPTION. A white or cream-coloured powder.
SOLUBILITY. Soluble in water.
SULPHATED ASH. Not more than 0·5 per cent.
CONTENT OF $HIO_4,2H_2O$. Not less than 98·0 per cent, determined by the following method:
Dissolve about 0·3 g, accurately weighed, in 50 ml of water, add 3 g of *sodium bicarbonate* and 3 g of *potassium iodide*, and titrate the liberated iodine with 0·1N sodium arsenite, using *starch mucilage* as indicator; each ml of 0·1N sodium arsenite is equivalent to 0·01140 g of $HIO_4,2H_2O$.

Periodic–Acetic Acid Solution: dissolve 5 g of *periodic acid* in 200 ml of water and dilute to 1000 ml with *glacial acetic acid*. It should be stored in dark-coloured glass-stoppered bottles.

Petroleum, Light, (boiling-range, 40° to 60°): of the British Pharmacopoeia, Appendix I.

Petroleum, Light, (boiling-range, 60° to 80°): of the British Pharmacopoeia, Appendix I.

Petroleum, Light, (boiling-range, 80° to 100°): of the British Pharmacopoeia, Appendix I.

Petroleum, Light, (boiling-range, 100° to 120°): of the British Pharmacopoeia, Appendix I.

1,10-Phenanthroline: of the British Pharmacopoeia, Appendix I.

Phenazone: of the British Pharmaceutical Codex.

Phenol: of the British Pharmacopoeia.

Phenol Red: 4,4′-(3*H*-2,1-benzoxathiol-3-ylidene)diphenol *SS*-dioxide.
A solution changes in colour over the pH range 6·8 to 8·4 from yellow through pink to red.

Phenol Red Solution: dissolve 0·05 g of *phenol red* in a mixture of 5 ml of *alcohol (90 per cent)* and 2·85 ml of 0·05N sodium hydroxide, warming if necessary, and dilute to 250 ml with *alcohol (20 per cent)*.

Phenolphthalein: a solution changes in colour over the pH range 8·3 to 10·0 from colourless through pink to red.

Phenolphthalein Solution: a 1·0 per cent w/v solution of *phenolphthalein* in *alcohol (95 per cent)*.

Phenoxyethanol: of the British Pharmaceutical Codex.

***p*-Phenylenediamine Dihydrochloride:** $C_6H_4(NH_2)_2,2HCl$
DESCRIPTION. A white or pink powder.
SOLUBILITY. Soluble in water.
SULPHATED ASH. Not more than 0·1 per cent.

Phenylhydrazine: of the British Pharmacopoeia, Appendix I.

Phenylhydrazine Hydrochloride: of the British Pharmacopoeia, Appendix I.

Phloroglucinol: of the British Pharmacopoeia, Appendix I.

Phloroglucinol Solution: a 1·0 per cent w/v solution of *phloroglucinol* in *alcohol (90 per cent)*.

Phosphate Buffer Solution pH 6·0: dissolve 20 g of *dipotassium hydrogen phosphate* and 80 g of *potassium dihydrogen phosphate* in sufficient water to produce 1000 ml.

Phosphate Buffer Solution pH 7·0: dissolve 3·63 g of *potassium dihydrogen phosphate* and 5·68 g of *anhydrous sodium phosphate* in sufficient water to produce 1000 ml.

Phosphate Buffer pH 7·0, Glycerinated: to 50 ml of 0·02M potassium dihydrogen phosphate add 29·63 ml of 0·02N sodium hydroxide and 2 ml of *glycerol* and dilute to 200 ml with water.

Phosphomolybdic Acid: of the British Pharmacopoeia, Appendix I.

Phosphoric Acid: of the European Pharmacopoeia: contains 85·0 to 90·0 per cent w/w of H_3PO_4.

Phosphoric Acid Solution, Standard: dissolve 2·777 g of *potassium dihydrogen phosphate* in sufficient water to produce 1000 ml and dilute 10 ml of this solution to 100 ml with water; each ml is equivalent to 0·02 mg of H_3PO_4.

Phosphorus Pentoxide: of the British Pharmacopoeia, Appendix I.

Phosphotungstic Acid: $H_3PO_4,12WO_3,xH_2O$
DESCRIPTION. A white or cream-coloured crystalline powder.
SOLUBILITY. Soluble in warm water, forming an almost clear colourless solution.
AMMONIA. Dissolve 1·0 g in 45 ml of water and add 5 ml of *sodium hydroxide solution* and 2 ml of *potassium mercuri-iodide solution*; any colour which develops is not deeper than that produced by 1 ml of a solution of *ammonium chloride* in water, containing the equivalent of 1 mg of NH_3, when similarly treated.
CHLORIDE. 1·0 g complies with the limit test for chlorides.
NITRATE. Dissolve 1·0 g in 10 ml of warm water, add 1 ml of *indigo carmine solution* and 10 ml of *sulphuric acid*, and heat to boiling; the blue colour is not discharged.

Phosphotungstic Acid Solution: dissolve 20 g of *phosphotungstic acid* and 5 g of *sulphuric acid* in water and dilute to 100 ml with water.

Picrolonic Acid: of the British Pharmacopoeia, Appendix I.

Platinic Chloride: of the British Pharmacopoeia, Appendix I.

Platinic Chloride Solution: a solution of *platinic chloride* in water, containing the equivalent of 5·0 per cent w/v of $H_2PtCl_6,6H_2O$.

Potassium Antimonate: of the British Pharmacopoeia, Appendix I.

Potassium Antimonate Solution: mix 2 g of *potassium antimonate* with 95 ml of water, boil to dissolve, cool rapidly, add 50 ml of *potassium hydroxide solution* and 5 ml of 1N sodium hydroxide, and allow to stand for 24 hours; filter and dilute the filtrate to 150 ml with water. It should be freshly prepared.
SENSITIVITY. To 10 ml add 7 ml of 0·1N sodium hydroxide; a white crystalline precipitate is produced within 15 minutes.

Potassium Bicarbonate: of the British Pharmaceutical Codex.

Potassium Bisulphate: $KHSO_4$
DESCRIPTION. White fused hygroscopic lumps.
SOLUBILITY. Very soluble in water, giving an acid solution.
CONTENT OF $KHSO_4$. Not less than 98·0 and not more than the equivalent of 102·0 per cent, determined by the following method:
Dissolve about 4·5 g, accurately weighed, in 50 ml of water and titrate with 1N sodium hydroxide, using *phenolphthalein solution* as indicator; each ml of 1N sodium hydroxide is equivalent to 0·1362 g of $KHSO_4$.

Potassium Bromide: of the European Pharmacopoeia.

Potassium Carbonate: of the British Pharmacopoeia, Appendix I.

Potassium Carbonate Solution: a 0·1 per cent w/v solution of *potassium carbonate* in water.

Potassium Chlorate: of the British Pharmacopoeia, Appendix I.

Potassium Chloride: of the European Pharmacopoeia.

Potassium Chromate: of the British Pharmacopoeia, Appendix I.

Potassium Chromate Solution: a 5·0 per cent w/v solution of *potassium chromate* in water.

Potassium Citrate: of the British Pharmacopoeia.

Potassium Cupri-tartrate Solution: Fehling's Solution:
SOLUTION NO. 1: dissolve 34·64 g of *copper sulphate* in 400 ml of water containing 0·50 ml of *sulphuric acid* and dilute to 500 ml with water.
SOLUTION NO. 2: dissolve 176 g of *potassium sodium tartrate* and 77 g of *sodium hydroxide* in sufficient water to produce 500 ml.
Mix equal volumes of the two solutions immediately before use.

Potassium Cyanide: of the British Pharmacopoeia, Appendix I.

Potassium Cyanide Solution: a 10·0 per cent w/v solution of *potassium cyanide* in water.

Potassium Cyanide Solution PbT: of the British Pharmacopoeia, Appendix VIC.

Potassium Dichromate: of the British Pharmacopoeia, Appendix I.

Potassium Dichromate Solution: a 7·0 per cent w/v solution of *potassium dichromate* in water.

Potassium Dihydrogen Phosphate: of the British Pharmacopoeia, Appendix I.

Potassium Dihydrogen Phosphate 0·2M: dissolve 27·218 g of *potassium dihydrogen phosphate* in sufficient *carbon dioxide-free water* to produce 1000 ml.

Potassium Ferricyanide: of the British Pharmacopoeia, Appendix I.

Potassium Ferricyanide Solution: wash about 1 g of *potassium ferricyanide*, in crystals, with water and dissolve the washed crystals in 100 ml of water. It must be freshly prepared.

Potassium Ferrocyanide: of the British Pharmacopoeia, Appendix I.

Potassium Ferrocyanide Solution: a 5·0 per cent w/v solution of *potassium ferrocyanide* in water.

Potassium Hydroxide: of the British Pharmacopoeia.

Potassium Hydroxide Solution: of the British Pharmacopoeia: contains about 5 per cent w/v of KOH.

Potassium Hydroxide Solution, Alcoholic: a recently prepared 10·0 per cent w/v solution of *potassium hydroxide* in *alcohol (95 per cent)*.

Potassium Hydroxide Solution in Aldehyde-free Alcohol: dissolve 40 g of *potassium hydroxide* in about 900 ml of *aldehyde-free alcohol (95 per cent)* maintained at a temperature not exceeding 15°; when solution is complete, warm to 20° and dilute to 1000 ml with *aldehyde-free alcohol (95 per cent)*.

Potassium Iodate: of the British Pharmacopoeia, Appendix I.

Potassium Iodate Solution: a 1·0 per cent w/v solution of *potassium iodate* in water.

Potassium Iodide: of the European Pharmacopoeia.

Potassium Iodide Solution: a 10·0 per cent w/v solution of *potassium iodide* in water.

Potassium Iodide Solution, Iodinated: dissolve 4 g of *potassium iodide* and 2 g of *iodine* in 10 ml of water and dilute to 100 ml with water.

Potassium Iodobismuthate Solution: dissolve 100 g of *tartaric acid* in 400 ml of water, add 8·5 g of *bismuth oxide nitrate*, shake for 1 hour, add 200 ml of a 40 per cent w/v solution of *potassium iodide* in water, shake well, and allow to stand for 24 hours; filter.

Potassium Iodobismuthate Solution, Dilute: dissolve 100 g of *tartaric acid* in 500 ml of water and add 50 ml of *potassium iodobismuthate solution*.

Potassium Mercuri-iodide Solution: Mayer's Reagent: add 1·36 g of *mercuric chloride* dissolved in 60 ml of water to a solution of 5 g of *potassium iodide* in 20 ml of water, mix, and dilute to 100 ml with water.

Potassium Nitrate: of the British Pharmacopoeia.

Potassium Perchlorate: of the British Pharmacopoeia, Appendix I.

Potassium Permanganate: of the European Pharmacopoeia.

Potassium Permanganate and Phosphoric Acid Solution: dissolve 3 g of *potassium permanganate* in a mixture of 15 ml of *phosphoric acid* and 70 ml of water and dilute to 100 ml with water.

Potassium Permanganate Solution: a 1·0 per cent w/v solution of *potassium permanganate* in water.

Potassium Plumbite Solution: dissolve 1·7 g of *lead acetate*, 3·4 g of *potassium citrate*, and 50 g of *potassium hydroxide* in water and dilute to 100 ml with water.

Potassium Sodium Tartrate: of the British Pharmacopoeia, Appendix I.

Potassium Solution FP: of the British Pharmacopoeia, Appendix XIA.

Potassium Sulphate: of the British Pharmacopoeia, Appendix I.

Potassium Thiocyanate: of the British Pharmacopoeia, Appendix I.

Procaine Hydrochloride: of the European Pharmacopoeia.

Procyclidine Hydrochloride: of the British Pharmacopoeia.

Procyclidine Hydrochloride Solution, Standard: dissolve about 0·05 g, accurately weighed, of *procyclidine hydrochloride* in sufficient water to produce 100 ml and dilute 10 ml of this solution to 250 ml with water.

Propyl Alcohol: of the British Pharmacopoeia, Appendix I.

Propylene Glycol: of the British Pharmacopoeia.

Pumice Powder: pumice of commerce, powdered and sifted, which passes through a No. 710 sieve, but is retained by a No. 250 sieve.

Pyridine: of the British Pharmacopoeia, Appendix I.

Pyridine, Dehydrated: *pyridine* containing not more than 0·1 per cent w/w of water.

Pyridine–Acetic Anhydride Reagent: a freshly prepared mixture of 25 ml of *acetic anhydride* with 75 ml of *pyridine*.

Pyrogallol: of the British Pharmacopoeia, Appendix I.

Pyrogallol Solution, Alkaline: dissolve 0·5 g of *pyrogallol* in 2 ml of water; dissolve 12 g of *potassium hydroxide* in 8 ml of water; mix the two solutions immediately before use.

Quassin: crystalline quassin of commerce.

Quinaldine Ethiodide:
$C_6H_4CH:CH\cdot C(CH_3):N,C_2H_5I$
DESCRIPTION. A yellow to orange crystalline powder.
SOLUBILITY. Soluble in water; very slightly soluble in alcohol; insoluble in ether.
MELTING-POINT. 238° to 241°.
SULPHATED ASH. Not more than 0·1 per cent.
CONTENT OF $C_{12}H_{14}NI$. Not less than 98·5 per cent, determined by the following method:
Dissolve about 0·8 g, accurately weighed, in water, acidify with *dilute nitric acid*, add 50 ml of 0·1N silver nitrate, shake, filter, wash the filter with water, and titrate the combined filtrate and washings with 0·1N ammonium thiocyanate, using *ferric ammonium sulphate solution* as indicator; each ml of 0·1N ammonium thiocyanate is equivalent to 0·02991 g of $C_{12}H_{14}NI$.

Quinaldine Ethiodide Solution: a 1·5 per cent w/v solution of *quinaldine ethiodide* in water.

Quinaldine Red: 2-(4-dimethylaminostyryl)-quinoline ethiodide.
When used for the titration of bases with perchloric acid in glacial acetic acid, it changes from magenta to almost colourless.

Quinaldine Red Solution: a 0·1 per cent w/v solution of *quinaldine red* in *methyl alcohol*.

Quinine Sulphate: of the British Pharmacopoeia.

Rappaport's Medium, Double-strength: an enrichment medium, for the isolation of certain salmonellae, containing magnesium chloride and malachite green together with appropriate nutrient and buffering substances. Details of the preparation of the single-strength medium are given by Rappaport, Konforti, and Navon (*J. clin. Path.*, 1956, **9**, 261).

Reserpine: of the British Pharmacopoeia, which complies with the following additional requirement:
Dissolve 0·002 g in 100 ml of *alcohol (95 per cent)*; to 10 ml add 2 ml of 0·5N sulphuric acid and 2 ml of a 0·3 per cent w/v solution of *sodium nitrite* in water, maintain at 55° for 30 minutes, cool, add 1 ml of a 5 per cent w/v solution of *sulphamic acid* in water, dilute to 20 ml with *alcohol (95 per cent)*, and measure the extinction of a 1-cm layer at 390 nm, using as a blank a solution prepared by the above procedure, using 10 ml of *alcohol (95*

per cent) in place of the reserpine solution; the extinction is not less than 0·390.

Resorcinol: of the British Pharmacopoeia.

Resorcinol and Hydrochloric Acid Solution: a 1·0 per cent w/v solution of *resorcinol* in *hydrochloric acid*.

Ruthenium Red
DESCRIPTION. A dark brown powder.
SOLUBILITY. Completely soluble in water, yielding a bright crimson solution; soluble in *lead acetate solution*.

Ruthenium Red Solution: a freshly prepared solution of 8 mg of *ruthenium red* in 10 ml of *lead acetate solution*.

Safranine: of the British Pharmacopoeia, Appendix I.

Safranine Solution: a saturated solution of *safranine* in *alcohol (70 per cent)*.

Salicylic Acid: of the British Pharmacopoeia.

Saline Solution: a 0·9 per cent w/v solution of *sodium chloride* in freshly purified water, sterilised by heating in an autoclave.

Selenite F Broth, Double-strength: an enrichment medium, for the isolation of salmonellae, containing sodium acid selenite together with appropriate nutrient and buffering substances. Details of the preparation of the single-strength medium are given in "Medical Microbiology" (Ed., Robert Cruickshank), 11th Edn., 1965. Suitable material may be obtained from Oxoid Ltd., Southwark Bridge Rd., London, S.E.1.

Selenium Solution, Standard: dissolve 0·0654 g of *selenous acid* in sufficient water to produce 1000 ml, and dilute 25 ml of this solution to 1000 ml with water; each ml contains 1·0 µg of Se.

Selenous Acid: H_2SeO_3
DESCRIPTION. Colourless hygroscopic crystals.
SOLUBILITY. Soluble in water and in alcohol.
SULPHATED ASH. Not more than 0·1 per cent.
CONTENT OF H_2SeO_3. Not less than 98·0 per cent, determined by the following method:
Dissolve about 0·12 g, accurately weighed, in 100 ml of water, add 5 ml of *dilute hydrochloric acid*, 5 g of *potassium iodide*, and 50 ml of *chloroform*, shake vigorously for 1 minute, and titrate the liberated iodine with 0·1N sodium thiosulphate until the yellow colour of the aqueous layer has almost disappeared; add 0·1 ml of *starch mucilage* and continue the titration, with gentle swirling, until the aqueous layer is colourless; each ml of 0·1N sodium thiosulphate is equivalent to 0·003224 g of H_2SeO_3.

Sennoside A: $C_{42}H_{38}O_{20}$
DESCRIPTION. Yellow crystals.
SOLUBILITY. Almost insoluble in water and in ether; slightly soluble in alcohol; soluble in solutions of alkali hydroxides.
MELTING-POINT. 200° to 240° with decomposition.
SPECIFIC ROTATION. About −147°, determined, at 20°, in a 0·1 per cent w/v solution in acetone (70 per cent v/v).

Sennoside B: $C_{42}H_{38}O_{20}$
DESCRIPTION. Pale yellow crystals.

SOLUBILITY. Almost insoluble in water and in ether; slighly soluble in alcohol; soluble in solutions of alkali hydroxides.

MELTING-POINT. 180° to 186° with decomposition.

SPECIFIC ROTATION. About −100°, determined, at 20°, in a 0·2 per cent w/v solution in acetone (70 per cent v/v).

Silica Gel, Anhydrous: partially dehydrated, polymerised, colloidal silicic acid containing cobalt chloride as indicator. It is almost insoluble in water and partially soluble in sodium hydroxide solutions. It adsorbs, at 20°, about 30 per cent of its weight of water.

Silicotungstic Acid: of the British Pharmacopoeia, Appendix I.

Silicotungstic Acid Solution: a 10·0 per cent w/v solution of *silicotungstic acid* in water.

Silver Nitrate: of the European Pharmacopoeia.

Silver Nitrate Solution: a freshly prepared 5·0 per cent w/v solution of *silver nitrate* in water.

Silver Nitrate Solution, Dilute: a freshly prepared 1·7 per cent w/v solution of *silver nitrate* in water.

Silver Nitrate Solution, Methanolic: boil, until dissolved, 5 g of *silver nitrate* with 60 ml of *methyl alcohol* under reflux on a water-bath. Use the solution whilst still hot.

Sodium: of the British Pharmacopoeia, Appendix I.

Sodium Acetate: of the British Pharmacopoeia.

Sodium Acetate, Anhydrous: of the British Pharmacopoeia, Appendix I.

Sodium Acetate, 2M: a solution of *sodium acetate* in water, containing in 1000 ml 272·2 g of $C_2H_3NaO_2,3H_2O$.

Sodium Acetate, 1M: a solution of *sodium acetate* in water, containing in 1000 ml 136·1 g of $C_2H_3NaO_2,3H_2O$.

Sodium Bicarbonate: of the European Pharmacopoeia.

Sodium Bicarbonate Solution: a 5·0 per cent w/v solution of *sodium bicarbonate* in water.

Sodium Bicarbonate Solution, Dilute: a 2·0 per cent w/v solution of *sodium bicarbonate* in water.

Sodium Bismuthate: $NaBiO_3$

DESCRIPTION. A yellow or brown amorphous powder.

MANGANESE. Dissolve 2·0 g in 15 ml of *nitric acid* and 35 ml of water by boiling gently, cool, add a further 0·5 g of sample, shake for 5 minutes, and allow to stand until clear; any pink colour which develops is not deeper than that of 50 ml of a solution containing 0·1 ml of 0·01N potassium permanganate.

CONTENT OF $NaBiO_3$. Not less than 85·0 per cent, determined by the following method:
To about 0·5 g, accurately weighed, add 10 ml of water, 5 g of *potassium iodide*, and 40 ml of *dilute hydrochloric acid*, allow to stand for 30 minutes, and titrate the liberated iodine with 0·1N sodium thiosulphate, using *starch mucilage* as indicator; each ml of 0·1N sodium thiosulphate is equivalent to 0·01400 g of $NaBiO_3$.

Sodium Carbonate: of the British Pharmacopoeia, Appendix I.

Sodium Carbonate, Anhydrous: of the British Pharmacopoeia, Appendix I.

Sodium Carbonate Solution: a 10·0 per cent w/v solution of *sodium carbonate* in water.

Sodium Carboxymethylcellulose: of the British Pharmaceutical Codex, the grade used being such that a 1·0 per cent w/v solution in water has a viscosity at 20° of 6 to 8 centipoises.

Sodium Chloride: of the European Pharmacopoeia.

Sodium Chloride 0·0004M: dissolve 11·7 g of *sodium chloride* in water and dilute to 1000 ml with water; dilute 20 ml of this solution to 100 ml with water; contains 14·2 mg of Cl per litre.

Sodium Chloride 0·00002M: dissolve 11·7 g of *sodium chloride* in water and dilute to 1000 ml with water; dilute 1·0 ml of this solution to 100 ml with water and further dilute 1·0 ml of this second dilution to 100 ml with water; contains 0·71 mg of Cl per litre.

Sodium Chloride Solution: a 20 per cent w/v solution of *sodium chloride* in water.

Sodium Citrate: of the British Pharmacopoeia.

Sodium Diethyldithiocarbamate: of the British Pharmacopoeia, Appendix I.

Sodium Diethyldithiocarbamate Solution: a 0·1 per cent w/v solution of *sodium diethyldithiocarbamate* in water.

Sodium Dihydrogen Citrate: $C_6H_7NaO_7$

DESCRIPTION. A fine white powder.

SOLUBILITY. Soluble in water.

CHLORIDE. 1 g dissolved in water, with the addition of 2 ml of *nitric acid*, complies with the limit test for chlorides (350 parts per million).

SULPHATE. 1 g dissolved in water, with the addition of 2·5 ml of *dilute hydrochloric acid*, complies with the limit test for sulphates (600 parts per million).

LOSS ON DRYING. Not more than 5·0 per cent, determined by drying to constant weight at 105°.

CONTENT OF $C_6H_7NaO_7$. Not less than 98·0 per cent, calculated with reference to the substance dried under the prescribed conditions, determined by the following method:
Dissolve about 4 g, accurately weighed, in 100 ml of water and titrate with 1N sodium hydroxide, using *thymol blue solution* as indicator; each ml of 1N sodium hydroxide is equivalent to 0·1071 g of $C_6H_7NaO_7$.

Sodium Dihydrogen Phosphate: Sodium Acid Phosphate of the British Pharmacopoeia.

Sodium Dithionite: of the British Pharmacopoeia, Appendix I.

Sodium Fluoride: of the British Pharmacopoeia.

Sodium Formate: $H·COONa$

DESCRIPTION. A white crystalline powder.

SOLUBILITY. Soluble in water; slightly soluble in alcohol.

CALCIUM. Not more than 0·01 per cent, determined by the following method:
Dissolve 1·0 g in sufficient water to produce 100 ml and determine by atomic absorption spectroscopy

at a wavelength of 422·7 nm, using Method II of the British Pharmacopoeia, Appendix XIA; use *calcium solution FP*, diluted if necessary with water, for the standard solution.

CHLORIDE. 2 g complies with the limit test for chlorides (175 parts per million).

SULPHATE. Dissolve 1 g in 10 ml of a 25 per cent v/v solution of *hydrochloric acid* in water and evaporate to dryness. Dissolve the residue in a further 10 ml of the diluted hydrochloric acid, again evaporate to dryness, and repeat the solution and evaporation once more; the residue complies with the limit test for sulphates (600 parts per million).

LOSS ON DRYING. Not more than 1·0 per cent, determined by drying to constant weight at 130°.

CONTENT OF CHNaO₂. Not less than 99·0 per cent, calculated with reference to the substance dried under the prescribed conditions, determined by the following method :
Dissolve about 5 g, accurately weighed, in sufficient water to produce 50 ml. To 10 ml of this solution add 1·5 ml of *sodium hydroxide solution* and 50 ml of 0·1N potassium permanganate, heat for 20 minutes on a water-bath, cool, add 4 g of *potassium iodide* and 25 ml of *dilute sulphuric acid*, and titrate the liberated iodine with 0·1N sodium thiosulphate, using *starch mucilage* as indicator; each ml of 0·1N potassium permanganate is equivalent to 0·0034004 g of CHNaO₂.

Sodium Hexametaphosphate: of the British Pharmacopoeia, Appendix I.

Sodium Hexametaphosphate Solution: a 10·0 per cent w/v solution of *sodium hexametaphosphate* in water.

Sodium Hydroxide: of the British Pharmacopoeia.

Sodium Hydroxide Solution: a 20·0 per cent w/v solution of *sodium hydroxide* in water.

Sodium Hydroxide Solution, Dilute: a 5·0 per cent w/v solution of *sodium hydroxide* in water.

Sodium Hydroxide Solution, Strong: a 40·0 per cent w/v solution of *sodium hydroxide* in water.

Sodium Hypobromite Solution: add 1 ml of *bromine solution* to 20 ml of 1N sodium carbonate and mix; it should be freshly prepared.

Sodium Hypobromite Solution, Alkaline: dissolve 10 g of *sodium hydroxide* in 400 ml of water, add 5·5 ml of *bromine*, stirring to dissolve, and dilute to 500 ml with water; ascertain the strength by adding to 10 ml 25 ml of water, 2 g of *potassium iodide*, and 10 ml of *glacial acetic acid*, and titrating the liberated iodine with 0·1N sodium thiosulphate; each ml of 0·1N sodium thiosulphate is equivalent to 0·008 g of available bromine; dilute the remainder to contain 1·5 per cent w/v of available bromine. To 66 ml of this solution add 20 ml of *sodium hydroxide solution* and dilute to 100 ml with water.

Sodium Lauryl Sulphate, Purified: of the British Pharmacopoeia, Appendix I.

Sodium Lauryl Sulphate Solution (0·1 per cent): a 0·1 per cent w/v solution of *purified sodium lauryl sulphate* in water.

Sodium Metabisulphite: of the British Pharmacopoeia.

Sodium Molybdate: of the British Pharmacopoeia, Appendix I.

Sodium Molybdophosphotungstate Solution: add 50 g of *sodium tungstate*, 12 g of *phosphomolybdic acid*, and 25 ml of *phosphoric acid* to 350 ml of water, boil under a reflux condenser for 2 hours, cool, and dilute to 500 ml with water.

Sodium Nitrite: of the British Pharmacopoeia, Appendix I.

Sodium Nitrite Solution: a freshly prepared 10·0 per cent w/v solution of *sodium nitrite* in water.

Sodium Nitroprusside: of the British Pharmacopoeia, Appendix I.

Sodium Nitroprusside Solution: a recently prepared 1·0 per cent w/v solution of *sodium nitroprusside* in water.

Sodium Perchlorate Solution: neutralise 50 ml of *perchloric acid* (*60 per cent w/w*) to *litmus paper* with *sodium hydroxide solution* and dilute to 300 ml with water.

Sodium Periodate: of the British Pharmacopoeia, Appendix I.

Sodium Periodate Solution: a 5·0 per cent w/v solution of *sodium periodate* in water.

Sodium Phosphate: of the European Pharmacopoeia.

Sodium Phosphate, Anhydrous: Na₂HPO₄
DESCRIPTION. A white hygroscopic powder.
SOLUBILITY. Soluble, at 20°, in 12 parts of water; insoluble in alcohol.
ALKALINITY. pH of a 2·0 per cent w/v solution in *carbon dioxide-free water*, 9·0 to 9·2.
IRON. Boil 0·50 g with 5 ml of water and 2 ml of *hydrochloric acid FeT*, cool, add 0·05 ml of 0·1N potassium permanganate, and mix; add 10 ml of *ammonium thiocyanate solution* and 10 ml of a mixture of equal volumes of *amyl alcohol* and *amyl acetate*, shake vigorously, and allow to separate.
Any red colour produced in the upper layer is not more intense than that produced by treating 1 ml of *standard iron solution FeT* in a similar manner.
CHLORIDE. 0·50 g, dissolved in water with the addition of 2 ml of *nitric acid*, complies with the limit test for chlorides (700 parts per million).
SULPHATE. 0·10 g, dissolved in water with the addition of 3 ml of *dilute hydrochloric acid*, complies with the limit test for sulphates (0·6 per cent).
LOSS ON DRYING. Not more than 0·4 per cent, determined by drying at 120° for 1 hour.
CONTENT OF Na₂HPO₄. Not less than 99·5 per cent, calculated with reference to the substance dried under the prescribed conditions, determined by the following method:
Dissolve about 2·5 g, accurately weighed, in 100 ml of water and titrate with 0·5N hydrochloric acid, using 1 ml of a mixture containing 4 volumes of *bromocresol green solution* and 1 volume of *methyl red solution*, and titrating to the colour indicative of pH 4·4; each ml of 0·5N hydrochloric acid is equivalent to 0·07098 g of Na₂HPO₄.

Sodium Phosphate, 0·2M: dissolve 71·62 g of *sodium phosphate* in sufficient water to produce 1000 ml.

Sodium Phosphate Solution: a 10·0 per cent w/v solution of *sodium phosphate* in water.

Sodium Potassium Tartrate: $C_4H_4KNaO_6$, $4H_2O$

DESCRIPTION. Colourless crystals or a white crystalline powder; odourless.

SOLUBILITY. Soluble in water; almost insoluble in alcohol.

ACIDITY OR ALKALINITY. Dissolve 1·0 g in 10 ml of *carbon dioxide-free water* and titrate with 0·1N sodium hydroxide and with 0·1N hydrochloric acid, using *phenolphthalein solution* as indicator; not more than 0·1 ml of either titrant is required.

IRON. 0·50 g complies with the limit test for iron (80 parts per million).

CHLORIDE. 0·50 g complies with the limit test for chlorides (700 parts per million).

SULPHATE. 0·50 g complies with the limit test for sulphates (0·12 per cent).

CONTENT OF $C_4H_4KNaO_6,4H_2O$. Not less than 99·0 and not more than 104·0 per cent, determined by the following method:

Heat, until carbonised, about 2 g, accurately weighed, cool, boil the residue with 50 ml of water and 50 ml of 0·5N hydrochloric acid, filter, wash the filter with water, and titrate the excess acid in the combined filtrate and washings with 0·5N sodium hydroxide, using *methyl orange solution* as indicator; each ml of 0·5N hydrochloric acid is equivalent to 0·07056 g of $C_4H_4KNaO_6,4H_2O$.

Sodium Solution FP: of the British Pharmacopoeia, Appendix XIA.

Sodium Starch Glycollate

DESCRIPTION. A white or creamy-white powder.

SOLUBILITY. Soluble in 200 parts of water.

SENSITIVITY. Dissolve 10 mg in 7 ml of water and add 0·2 ml of 0·01N iodine; a distinct blue colour is produced.

Sodium Sulphate: of the European Pharmacopoeia.

Sodium Sulphate, Anhydrous: of the British Pharmacopoeia, Appendix I.

Sodium Sulphide: of the British Pharmacopoeia, Appendix I.

Sodium Sulphide and Glycerin Solution: dissolve 12 g of *sodium sulphide* in a mixture of 10 ml of water and 29 ml of *glycerin* and dilute to 100 ml with water.

Sodium Sulphide Solution: a 10·0 per cent w/v solution of *sodium sulphide* in water.

Sodium Sulphide Solution PbT: dissolve 10 g of *sodium sulphide* in water, dilute to 100 ml with water, and filter.

Sodium Sulphite: of the British Pharmacopoeia, Appendix I.

Sodium Tetraphenylboron: $[(C_6H_5)_4B]Na$

DESCRIPTION. A white crystalline powder.

SOLUBILITY. Soluble in water.

CONTENT OF $C_{24}H_{20}BNa$. Not less than 96·0 per cent, determined by method (i), and not less than 85·0 per cent, determined by method (ii).

(i) Ignite gently about 1 g, accurately weighed, to a white residue in a platinum dish, dissolve the residue in hot water, boil for 5 minutes, and titrate with 0·1N sulphuric acid, using *methyl red solution* as indicator; each ml of 0·1N sulphuric acid is equivalent to 0·03422 g of $C_{24}H_{20}BNa$.

(ii) Proceed by method (i) as far as the words ". . . boil for 5 minutes", then add 50 ml of *glycerol*, and titrate with 0·1N sodium hydroxide, using *phenolphthalein solution* as indicator; each ml of 0·1N sodium hydroxide is equivalent to 0·3422 g of $C_{24}H_{20}BNa$.

Sodium Thiosulphate: of the British Pharmacopoeia, Appendix I.

Sodium Tungstate: of the British Pharmacopoeia, Appendix I.

Standard pH, Solutions of: of the British Pharmacopoeia, Appendix IIIA.

Stannous Chloride: of the British Pharmacopoeia, Appendix I.

Stannous Chloride Solution: dissolve 330 g of *stannous chloride* in 100 ml of *hydrochloric acid* and sufficient water to give a final volume of 1000 ml.

Starch: potato starch of the European Pharmacopoeia.

Starch Mucilage: triturate 0·5 g of *starch* with 5 ml of water, and add this, with constant stirring, to sufficient water to produce 100 ml; boil for a few minutes, cool, and filter. It should be recently prepared.

It gives a blue colour with free iodine in the presence of a soluble iodide.

Starch-iodide Paper: impregnate unglazed white paper with *starch mucilage* which has been diluted with an equal volume of a 0·4 per cent w/v solution of *potassium iodide* in water.

Starch-iodide Paste: dissolve 0·75 g of *potassium iodide* in 5 ml of water and dissolve 2 g of *zinc chloride* in 10 ml of water; mix the two solutions, add 100 ml of water, boil, and add, with constant stirring, a suspension of 5 g of *starch* in 35 ml of water; boil for a further 2 minutes and cool.

It should be stored in a well-closed container, in a cool place.

Starch-iodide Reagent: mix 40 ml of *starch mucilage* with 60 ml of water, add 1 ml of *iodine solution* and 6 ml of *glacial acetic acid*, and mix.

Stilboestrol: of the British Pharmacopoeia.

Strontium Carbonate: $SrCO_3$: the reagent grade of commerce.

Strontium Solution FP: dissolve 1·685 g of *strontium carbonate* in a mixture of 5 ml of *hydrochloric acid* and 5 ml of water and dilute to 1000 ml with water; 1 ml contains 1 mg of Sr.

Sucrose: of the European Pharmacopoeia.

Sulphamethoxazole Solution, Standard: dissolve 0·050 g of *sulphamethoxazole A.S.* in 10 ml of 0·1N sodium hydroxide, dilute to 50 ml with water, and further dilute 5 ml of this solution to 200 ml with water; each ml contains 25 µg of sulphamethoxazole.

Sulphamic Acid: of the British Pharmacopoeia, Appendix I.

Sulphanilic Acid: of the British Pharmacopoeia, Appendix I.

Sulphanilic Acid, Diazotised: dissolve, with the aid of heat, 0·2 g of *sulphanilic acid* in 20 ml of 1N hydrochloric acid, cool to about 4°, add dropwise, with constant stirring, 2·2 ml of a 4 per cent w/v solution of *sodium nitrite* in water, allow to stand in ice for 10 minutes, and then add 1 ml of a 5 per cent w/v solution of *sulphamic acid* in water.

Sulphanilic Acid, Diazotised, Alkaline: heat 0·2 g of *sulphanilic acid* with 20 ml of 1N hydrochloric acid until dissolved, cool to about 4°, add dropwise, with constant swirling, 2·2 ml of a 4 per cent w/v solution of *sodium nitrite* in water, allow to stand in ice for 10 minutes, and add 20 ml of 1N sodium hydroxide.

Sulphate Solution, Standard: dissolve 1·814 g of *potassium sulphate* in water, dilute to 1000 ml with water, and dilute 10 ml of this solution to 1000 ml with water; each ml contains 10 μg of SO_4.

Sulphomolybdic Acid Solution: a 1·0 per cent w/v solution of *ammonium molybdate* in *sulphuric acid*.

Sulphur Dioxide: of the British Pharmacopoeia, Appendix I.

Sulphuric Acid: of the British Pharmacopoeia, Appendix I: contains not less than 97·0 per cent w/w of H_2SO_4.

Sulphuric Acid (80 per cent v/v): mix carefully 4 volumes of *sulphuric acid* with 1 volume of water and cool.

Sulphuric Acid (66 per cent v/v): mix carefully 2 volumes of *sulphuric acid* with 1 volume of water and cool.

Sulphuric Acid (60 per cent v/v): mix carefully 3 volumes of *sulphuric acid* with 2 volumes of water and cool.

Sulphuric Acid (50 per cent v/v): mix carefully equal volumes of *sulphuric acid* and water and cool.

Sulphuric Acid (25 per cent v/v): mix carefully 1 volume of *sulphuric acid* with 3 volumes of water and cool.

Sulphuric Acid (20 per cent v/v): mix carefully 1 volume of *sulphuric acid* with 4 volumes of water and cool.

Sulphuric Acid (14 per cent v/v): mix carefully 14·0 ml of *sulphuric acid* with 86·0 ml of water and cool.

Sulphuric Acid (10 per cent v/v): mix carefully 1 volume of *sulphuric acid* with 9 volumes of water and cool.

Sulphuric Acid and Formaldehyde Reagent: mix 0·1 ml of *formaldehyde solution* with 1 ml of *sulphuric acid*.

Sulphuric Acid, Dilute: mix carefully 104 g of *sulphuric acid* with 896 g of water and cool.

Sulphuric Acid, Nitrogen-free: of the British Pharmacopoeia, Appendix I.

Sulphurous Acid: of the British Pharmacopoeia, Appendix I.

Tannic Acid: of the British Pharmacopoeia.

Tannic Acid Solution: a 10·0 per cent w/v solution of *tannic acid* in water.

Tartaric Acid: of the British Pharmacopoeia.

Tartaric Acid Solution: a 1·0 per cent w/v solution of *tartaric acid* in water.

Tartaric Acid Solution, Alcoholic: a 1·0 per cent w/v solution of *tartaric acid* in *alcohol (95 per cent)*.

Tetrabutylammonium Iodide: of the British Pharmacopoeia, Appendix I.

Tetraethylammonium Hydroxide Solution: a 25 per cent w/w solution of tetraethylammonium hydroxide, $(C_2H_5)_4N \cdot OH$, in water.

DESCRIPTION. A clear very pale yellow liquid.

WEIGHT PER ML. At 20°, about 1·01 g.

TOTAL HALIDES. Not more than 0·15 per cent w/w, calculated as bromide, determined by the following method:
Mix 10 g with 30 ml of water and 5 ml of *nitric acid*, add 5 ml of 0·1N silver nitrate, and titrate with 0·1N ammonium thiocyanate, using *ferric ammonium sulphate solution* as indicator; not less than 3·1 ml of 0·1N ammonium thiocyanate is required.

SULPHATED ASH. Not more than 0·1 per cent w/w.

TOTAL BASES. 24·5 to 26·0 per cent w/w, calculated as $C_8H_{21}NO$, determined by the following method:
Mix about 12 g, accurately weighed, with 25 ml of water and titrate with 1N hydrochloric acid, using *phenolphthalein solution* as indicator; each ml of 1N hydrochloric acid is equivalent to 0·1473 g of $C_8H_{21}NO$.

Tetramethylammonium Hydroxide Solution: of the British Pharmacopoeia, Appendix I.

Tetramethylammonium Hydroxide Solution, Dilute: a freshly prepared 4·0 per cent v/v solution of *tetramethylammonium hydroxide solution* in *aldehyde-free dehydrated alcohol*.

Tetrazolium Blue: of the British Pharmacopoeia, Appendix I.

Thiamine Hydrochloride: of the European Pharmacopoeia.

Thioacetamide: of the British Pharmacopoeia, Appendix I.

Thioacetamide Reagent: to 0·2 ml of a 0·4 per cent w/v solution of *thioacetamide* in water add 1 ml of a mixture containing 15 ml of 1N sodium hydroxide, 5 ml of water, and 20 ml of *glycerin* and heat on a water-bath for 20 seconds. It should be prepared immediately before use.

Thioglycerol: α-Thioglycerol: 3-mercaptopropane-1,2-diol, $CH_2(SH) \cdot CH(OH) \cdot CH_2OH$

DESCRIPTION. A colourless, slightly viscous liquid with a strong odour of mercaptan.

WEIGHT PER ML. At 20°, about 1·23 g.

CONTENT OF $C_3H_8O_2S$. Not less than 90·0 per cent w/w, determined by the following method:
Dissolve about 0·5 g, accurately weighed, in about 30 ml of *glacial acetic acid* and titrate with 0·1N iodine to a permanent pale yellow colour; each ml of 0·1N iodine is equivalent to 0·01082 g of $C_3H_8O_2S$.

Thioglycollic Acid: of the British Pharmacopoeia, Appendix I.

Thiourea: of the British Pharmacopoeia, Appendix I.

Thymol Blue: 6,6'-(3*H*-2,1-benzoxathiol-3-ylidene)dithymol *SS*-dioxide.
A solution changes in colour over the pH range 1·2 to 2·8 from red through orange to yellow, and over the pH range 8·0 to 9·6 from yellow through grey to violet-blue.

Thymol Blue Solution: warm 0·1 g of *thymol blue* with 4·3 ml of 0·05N sodium hydroxide and 5 ml of *alcohol (90 per cent)*; when dissolved, dilute to 250 ml with *alcohol (20 per cent)*.

Thymolphthalein: a solution changes in colour over the pH range 9·3 to 10·5 from colourless through pale blue to blue.

Titan Yellow: the sodium salt of 2,2'-[(diazoamino)di-*p*-phenylene]bis(6-methylbenzothiazole-7-sulphonic acid).
A solution changes in colour over the pH range 12·0 to 13·0 from yellow through orange to red.

Titan Yellow Paper: impregnate unglazed white paper with a solution of *titan yellow* and allow to dry.

Titan Yellow Solution: a 0·05 per cent w/v solution of *titan yellow* in water.
TEST FOR SENSITIVITY. To 0·1 ml add 10 ml of water, 0·2 ml of *standard magnesium solution*, and 1·0 ml of 1N sodium hydroxide; a pronounced pink colour is produced when compared with a reference solution prepared in a similar manner omitting the standard magnesium solution.

Titanous Chloride Solution: a 15 per cent w/v solution of titanous chloride, $TiCl_3$, in *dilute hydrochloric acid*.
DESCRIPTION. A dull purplish-brown liquid; strongly acidic.
CONTENT OF $TiCl_3$. When diluted and titrated according to the directions given under 0·1N titanous chloride in Appendix IIA of the British Pharmacopoeia, the strength of the diluted solution is not less than 0·1N.
Titanous Chloride Solution must be protected from the atmosphere to avoid oxidation.

Toluene: of the British Pharmacopoeia, Appendix I.

Triacetin: of the British Pharmacopoeia, Appendix I.

Triamcinolone Acetonide Solution, Standard: dissolve 0·050 g of *triamcinolone acetonide A.S.* in *chloroform*, dilute to 100 ml with *chloroform*, and further dilute 10 ml of this solution to 100 ml with *chloroform*; 1 ml contains 50 µg of triamcinolone acetonide.

Trichloroacetic Acid: of the British Pharmacopoeia.

1,1,1-Trichloroethane: Methylchloroform, $CH_3 \cdot CCl_3$
DESCRIPTION. A clear colourless liquid.
SOLUBILITY. Insoluble in water; miscible with alcohol, with ether, and with chloroform.
DISTILLATION-RANGE. Not less than 95·0 per cent distils between 73° and 77°.
REFRACTIVE INDEX. At 20°, 1·4350 to 1·4370.
WEIGHT PER ML. At 20°, 1·29 g to 1·32 g.

Trichloroethylene: of the British Pharmacopoeia.

Triethanolamine: of the British Pharmaceutical Codex.

Trimethylpentane: of the British Pharmacopoeia, Appendix I.

Tri-n-butyl Phosphate: $[CH_3(CH_2)_3]_3PO_4$
DESCRIPTION. A colourless liquid; odourless.
SOLUBILITY. Slightly soluble in water; miscible with alcohol and with ether.
WEIGHT PER ML. At 20°, 0·975 g to 0·976 g.
REFRACTIVE INDEX. At 20°, 1·424 to 1·425.
FREE ACID. Mix 5 ml with 20 ml of *alcohol (90 per cent)*, previously neutralised to *phenolphthalein solution*, and titrate with 0·1N sodium hydroxide, using *phenolphthalein solution* as indicator; not more than 0·25 ml of 0·1N sodium hydroxide is required.

Tri-n-butyl Phosphate, Extracted: extract 150 ml of *tri-n-butyl phosphate* with three 25-ml portions of a solution containing 10·0 per cent w/v of *sodium chloride* and 1·0 per cent of *anhydrous sodium phosphate*, discard the aqueous extractions, and filter the extracted tri-n-butyl phosphate through a plug of dry cotton wool, discarding the first 10 ml of the filtrate.

Trinitrophenol: Picric Acid: of the British Pharmacopoeia, Appendix I.

Trinitrophenol Solution: Sodium Picrate–Picric Acid Solution: add 0·5 ml of *sodium hydroxide solution* to 100 ml of a saturated solution of *trinitrophenol* in water.

Trinitrophenol Solution, Dilute: dilute 5 ml of a saturated solution of *trinitrophenol* in water to 100 ml with water.

2,3,5-Triphenyltetrazolium Chloride: of the British Pharmacopoeia, Appendix I.

Triphenyltetrazolium Chloride Solution: a 0·5 per cent w/v solution of *2,3,5-triphenyltetrazolium chloride* in *aldehyde-free dehydrated alcohol*.

Tris(hydroxymethyl)aminomethane:
2-amino-2-(hydroxymethyl)propane-1,3-diol, $NH_2 \cdot C(CH_2OH)_3$
DESCRIPTION. White crystals or a white crystalline powder.
MELTING-POINT. 168° to 172°.
SULPHATED ASH. Not more than 0·15 per cent.
CONTENT OF $C_4H_{11}NO_3$. Not less than 99·0 per cent, determined by the following method: Dissolve about 0·1 g, accurately weighed, in 30 ml of *glacial acetic acid*, previously neutralised to *oracet blue B* with 0·1N perchloric acid, and titrate with 0·1N perchloric acid, using *oracet blue B* as indicator; each ml of 0·1N perchloric acid is equivalent to 0·01211 g of $C_4H_{11}NO_3$.

Tris(hydroxymethyl)aminomethane Solution: dissolve 6·07 g of *tris(hydroxymethyl)-aminomethane* in 900 ml of *methyl alcohol*, add 50 ml of 0·5N hydrochloric acid, and dilute to 1000 ml with water.

Trisodium Phosphate: trisodium orthophosphate: $Na_3PO_4,12H_2O$

Trisodium Phosphate 0·25M: dissolve 95·03 g of *trisodium phosphate* in sufficient water to produce 1000 ml.

Urea: of the British Pharmacopoeia.

Vanillic Acid: $C_6H_3(OH)(OCH_3) \cdot CO_2H$

DESCRIPTION. A white or almost white crystalline powder.

SOLUBILITY. Slightly soluble in water; soluble in alcohol.

MELTING-POINT. 210° to 213°.

CONTENT OF $C_8H_8O_4$. Not less than 98·0 per cent, determined by the following method:
Dissolve about 0·5 g, accurately weighed, in 20 ml of *alcohol* (*90 per cent*), previously neutralised to *phenolphthalein solution*, and titrate with 0·1N sodium hydroxide, using *phenolphthalein solution* as indicator; each ml of 0·1N sodium hydroxide is equivalent to 0·01681 g of $C_8H_8O_4$.

Water, Carbon Dioxide-free: water which has been boiled vigorously for a few minutes and protected from absorption of carbon dioxide from the atmosphere during cooling and storage.

Water for Injections: of the British Pharmacopoeia.

Xylene: of the British Pharmacopoeia, Appendix I.

Xylene Cyanol FF: Colour Index No. 42135: the sodium salt of 4′,4″-bis(ethylamino)-3′,3″-dimethyltriphenylmethano-2,4-disulphonic anhydride.
It is a blue alcohol-soluble dye used as a screening agent in *methyl orange–xylene cyanol FF solution*.

Xylenol Orange: [3*H*-2,1-benzoxathiol-3-ylidenebis(6 - hydroxy - 5 - methyl - *m* - phenylene)-methylenenitrilo]tetra-acetic acid *SS*-dioxide.
It gives a reddish-purple colour with mercury, lead, zinc, and certain other metal ions in acid solution; in the presence of an excess of disodium edetate the solution is yellow.

Xylenol Orange Solution: shake 0·1 g of *xylenol orange* with 100 ml of water and filter if necessary.

Xylenol Orange Mixture: mix 1 part of *xylenol orange* with 99 parts of *potassium nitrate*.

Yeast Nutrient: mix 2 parts of *calcium sulphate*, 1 part of *ammonium phosphate*, and 16 parts of *sucrose*.

Yellow Standard Solution: standard solution Y for colour measurement of the European Pharmacopoeia: 100 ml of *yellow standard solution* contains 1·08 g of $FeCl_3,6H_2O$, 0·357 g of $CoCl_2,6H_2O$, and the equivalent of 2·5 ml of *hydrochloric acid*.

Zinc Chloride: of the British Pharmacopoeia, Appendix I.

Zinc Chloride Solution, Iodinated: dissolve 20 g of *zinc chloride* and 6·5 g of *potassium iodide* in 10·5 ml of water, add 0·5 g of *iodine*, shake for 15 minutes, and filter, if necessary. It should be protected from light.

Zinc, Granulated: of the British Pharmacopoeia, Appendix I.

Zinc Powder: of the British Pharmacopoeia, Appendix I.

Zinc Solution, Standard: dissolve 4·398 g of *zinc sulphate* in water, add 1 ml of *acetic acid*, dilute to 1000 ml with water, and dilute 10 ml of this solution to 1000 ml with water; 1 ml contains 10 µg of Zn.

Zinc Sulphate: of the European Pharmacopoeia.

Zinc Sulphate Solution, Dilute: a 0·011 per cent w/v solution of *zinc sulphate* in water; 1 ml contains 0·025 mg of Zn.

B. VOLUMETRIC SOLUTIONS

Solutions employed in volumetric determinations, in addition to those given in the British Pharmacopoeia.

Barium Hydroxide, 0·1N: a solution of *barium hydroxide* in *carbon dioxide-free water*, containing in 1000 ml 15·78 g of $Ba(OH)_2,8H_2O$.

Borax, 0·01N: a solution of *borax* in water, containing in 1000 ml 1·9072 g of $Na_2B_4O_7,10H_2O$.

Calcium Acetate, 0·25M: a solution of *dried calcium acetate* in water, containing in 1000 ml 39·542 g of $(CH_3 \cdot CO_2)_2Ca$.

Ceric Ammonium Sulphate, 0·1N: a solution of *ceric ammonium sulphate* in a mixture of *sulphuric acid* and water, containing in 1000 ml 63·25 g of $Ce(SO_4)_2,2(NH_4)_2SO_4,2H_2O$.
Dissolve 66 g of *ceric ammonium sulphate*, with the aid of gentle heat, in a mixture of 30 ml of *sulphuric acid* and 500 ml of water; cool, filter the solution if turbid, and dilute to 1000 ml with water. Determine the exact strength of the solution by titrating it with 0·1N ferrous sulphate using *ferroin sulphate solution* as indicator.

Cetylpyridinium Chloride, 0·005M: dissolve 1·80 g of *cetylpyridinium chloride* in 10 ml of *alcohol* (*95 per cent*) and dilute to 1000 ml with water. Store in an amber-coloured flask.

Dicyclomine Hydrochloride, 0·001M: a solution of *dicyclomine hydrochloride* in water, containing in 1000 ml 0·346 g of $C_{19}H_{36}ClNO_2$.

Dioctyl Sodium Sulphosuccinate, 0·005M: dissolve 0·225 g of *dioctyl sodium sulphosuccinate* in 15 ml of warm water, cool, and dilute to 1000 ml with water.
Standardise by carrying out a titration as described under content of codeine phosphate in Codeine Phosphate Syrup, page 799, using an accurately prepared solution of *codeine phosphate* in water, containing approximately 2·5 mg per ml. Determine the percentage purity of the codeine phosphate by the method of the British Pharmacopoeia and calculate the molarity of the dioctyl sodium sulphosuccinate solution; 1 ml of 0·005M dioctyl sodium sulphosuccinate is equivalent to 0·002032 g of $C_{18}H_{21}NO_3,H_3PO_4,\frac{1}{2}H_2O$.

Ferrous Ammonium Sulphate, 0·01N: a solution of *ferrous ammonium sulphate* in water, containing in 1000 ml ferrous iron equivalent to 5·585 g of Fe.

Hydroxylammonium Chloride, 1N: a solution of *hydroxylammonium chloride* in water, containing in 1000 ml 69·491 g of $NH_2 \cdot OH,HCl$.

Perchloric Acid in Dioxan, 0·02N: shake 1000 ml of *dioxan* with suitable asbestos for one hour and filter; add sufficient *perchloric acid* (*72 per cent w/w*) to produce a solution containing in 1000 ml 2·010 g of $HClO_4$.

Periodic Acid, 0·1M: a solution of *periodic acid* in water, containing in 1000 ml 22·79 g of $HIO_4,2H_2O$.
Standardise by the following method:
To 25 ml add 30 ml of *potassium iodide solution*, allow to stand for one minute, and titrate with 0·1N sodium thiosulphate, using *starch mucilage* as indicator.

Potassium Chloride, 0·2M: a solution of *potassium chloride* in water, containing in 1000 ml 14·911 g of KCl.

Potassium Ferricyanide, 0·04M: a solution of *potassium ferricyanide* in water, containing in 1000 ml 13·17 g of $K_3Fe(CN)_6$.

Potassium Hydroxide in Alcohol (90 per cent), 1N: a solution of *potassium hydroxide* in *alcohol (90 per cent)*, containing in 1000 ml 56·11 g of KOH.

Potassium Hydroxide in Dehydrated Alcohol, 1N: a solution of *potassium hydroxide* in *dehydrated alcohol*, containing in 1000 ml 56·11 g of KOH.

Sodium Lauryl Sulphate, 0·001M: a 0·03 per cent w/v solution of *purified sodium lauryl sulphate* in water.
Standardise by the following method:
To 10 ml of 0·001M dicyclomine hydrochloride add 5 ml of *dilute sulphuric acid*, 20 ml of *chloroform*, and 1 ml of *dimethyl yellow solution* and titrate with the 0·001M sodium lauryl sulphate.

Sodium Tetraphenylboron, 0·01M: a solution of *sodium tetraphenylboron* in water, containing in 1000 ml 3·422 g of $[(C_6H_5)_4B]Na$, prepared by the following method:

Dissolve 3·422 g of *sodium tetraphenylboron* in 50 ml of water, shake for 20 minutes with 0·5 g of *aluminium hydroxide gel*, add 250 ml of water and 16·6 g of *sodium chloride*, and allow to stand for 30 minutes. Filter, add 600 ml of water, adjust the pH to 8·0 to 9·0 with 0·1N sodium hydroxide, and dilute to 1000 ml with water.
Standardise by the following method:
Dissolve about 7 mg, accurately weighed, of *potassium chloride*, previously dried at 150° for one hour, in 5 ml of *acetate buffer solution pH 3·7* and 5 ml of water, add 15 ml of the sodium tetraphenylboron solution, allow to stand for 5 minutes, and filter through a dry sintered-glass filter; to 20 ml of the filtrate add 0·5 ml of *bromophenol blue solution* as indicator, and titrate the excess of sodium tetraphenylboron with 0·005M cetylpyridinium chloride to the blue colour of the indicator.
Repeat the procedure omitting the potassium chloride.
The molarity of the solution is given by the formula:

$$\frac{A \times W}{15(A - B) \times 0.07456}$$

where A = volume of 0·005M cetylpyridinium chloride required when the potassium chloride is omitted,
B = volume of 0·005M cetylpyridinium chloride required when the potassium chloride is present, and
W = weight, in grams, of the potassium chloride taken.

Sodium Thiosulphate, 0·04M: a solution of *sodium thiosulphate* in water, containing in 1000 ml 9·928 g of $Na_2S_2O_3,5H_2O$.

Tetrabutylammonium Iodide, 0·01M: a solution of *tetrabutylammonium iodide* in water, containing in 1000 ml 3·694 g of $(C_4H_9)_4NI$.

C. AUTHENTIC SPECIMENS AND BRITISH CHEMICAL REFERENCE SUBSTANCES

Where Authentic Specimens or British Chemical Reference Substances are referred to in the assays and tests of the British Pharmaceutical Codex, they are printed in *italic* type, followed respectively by the letters *A.S.* or *B.C.R.S.*

1. Authentic Specimens
(a) The following Authentic Specimens (*see* General Notices) may be obtained from the Director, Department of Pharmaceutical Sciences, 36 York Place, Edinburgh EH1 3HU.

p-Acetamidobenzalazine
Aminobenzoic Acid
Amitriptyline Embonate
Atropine Sulphate
Bephenium Hydroxynaphthoate
Brucine Sulphate
Caffeine
Chloramphenicol Palmitate
Chloramphenicol Palmitate (Polymorph A)
Chlorhexidine Acetate
Chlorpromazine
Clefamide

Codeine Phosphate
Deoxycortone Pivalate
Diethanolamine Fusidate
Dimethicone
2,4-Dimethoxy-4′-methylbenzophenone
Dioctyl Sodium Sulphosuccinate
Diphenhydramine Hydrochloride
Emetine Hydrochloride
Ethamivan
Fumaric Acid
Fusidic Acid
Gelsemine
Green S
Guaiphenesin
Homatropine Hydrobromide
Hydrocortisone Sodium Phosphate
Hyoscine Hydrobromide

Hyoscyamine Sulphate
Isothipendyl Hydrochloride
Lobeline Hydrochloride
Mexenone
Morphine Sulphate
Nalidixic Acid
p-Nitrobenzoic Acid
Noscapine Hydrochloride
Orange G
Orciprenaline Sulphate
Papaverine Hydrochloride
Phensuximide
Phenytoin
Physostigmine Sulphate
Pilocarpine Hydrochloride
Potassium Sorbate
Propicillin
Propylhexedrine
Prothionamide
Riboflavine
Sorbic Acid
Strychnine Hydrochloride
Sulphaguanidine
Sulphathiazole
Tartrazine
Theobromine
Theophylline
Thiabendazole
Thiacetazone
Thiopropazate Hydrochloride
Triamcinolone
Trimeprazine Tartrate

(b) The following Authentic Specimens (see General Notices) may be obtained from the Scientific Director, British Pharmacopoeia Commission, 8 Bulstrode Street, London W1M 5FT.

Amphotericin A
Amphotericin B
Ampicillin
Betamethasone Sodium Phosphate
Betamethasone Valerate

Cephaëline Hydrochloride
Cephalexin
Chlorpromazine Hydrochloride
Clioquinol
Cloxacillin Sodium
Colchicine
1,2:4,5-Dibenzocyclohepta-1,4-dien-3-one
Ergotamine Tartrate
Fluocinolone Acetonide
Hydrocortisone Sodium Succinate
Mepyramine Maleate
Methaqualone
Phenethecillin Potassium
Prednisolone Sodium Phosphate
Primidone
Promethazine Hydrochloride
Propicillin Potassium
Salbutamol Sulphate
Succinylsulphathiazole
Sulphadimidine
Sulphamethoxazole
Sulphanilamide
Tetracycline Hydrochloride
Triamcinolone Acetonide
Trimethoprim

2. British Chemical Reference Substances

The following British Chemical Reference Substances (see General Notices) may be obtained from the Scientific Director, British Pharmacopoeia Commission, 8 Bulstrode Street, London W1M 5FT.

Benzylpenicillin Sodium
Cortisone Acetate
Deoxycortone Acetate
Digoxin
Hydrocortisone
Hydrocortisone Acetate
Phenacetin
Phenoxymethylpenicillin Potassium
Prednisolone
Prednisone

Appendix 2

Qualitative Reactions

A. Bismuth

1. Solutions of bismuth salts yield with *hydrogen sulphide* a brownish-black precipitate insoluble in *sodium hydroxide solution*, in *dilute hydrochloric acid*, and in *ammonium sulphide solution*, but soluble in warm *nitric acid*.

2. Solutions of bismuth salts in the minimum quantity of a mixture of one volume of *nitric acid* and three volumes of water, when treated with *potassium iodide solution*, yield a black precipitate soluble in an excess of the reagent to give a yellowish-brown or orange-coloured solution. When the black precipitate or, after considerable dilution, the yellowish-brown or orange-coloured solution is heated with water, an orange or copper-coloured precipitate is obtained.

3. Solutions of bismuth salts, when acidified with *dilute nitric acid* and treated with a 10 per cent w/v solution of *thiourea*, become deep yellow.

B. Lead

1. Solutions of lead salts, in the absence of very strong acid, yield with *hydrogen sulphide* a black precipitate which is insoluble in *dilute hydrochloric acid* and *ammonium sulphide solution* but is soluble in hot *dilute nitric acid*.

2. Solutions of lead salts, when treated with *dilute sulphuric acid*, yield a white precipitate which is almost insoluble in water but soluble in *ammonium acetate solution*.

3. Solutions of lead salts, when treated with *potassium iodide solution*, yield a yellow precipitate which dissolves when the mixture is boiled and is reprecipitated as glistening plates when the solution is cooled.

4. Solutions of lead salts, when treated with *potassium chromate solution*, yield a yellow precipitate which is readily soluble in *sodium hydroxide solution* and in hot *nitric acid*.

5. Solutions of lead salts, when treated with *potassium cyanide solution*, made alkaline with *dilute ammonia solution*, and shaken with *diphenylthiocarbazone solution PbT*, yield a brick-red-coloured lower layer.

C. Mercuric Salts

1. Solutions of mercuric salts yield with *hydrogen sulphide* a black precipitate which is insoluble in *ammonium sulphide solution* and in boiling *dilute nitric acid*.

2. Solutions of mercuric salts which are free from an excess of nitric acid deposit a coating of mercury on bright *copper* foil; the deposit becomes bright when it is rubbed and may be volatilised from the foil by heat and obtained in globules.

3. Solutions of mercuric salts, when treated with *stannous chloride solution*, yield a white precipitate which rapidly becomes grey with an excess of the reagent.

4. Neutral solutions of mercuric salts, when treated with *potassium iodide solution*, yield a scarlet precipitate which is soluble in an excess of the reagent and in a considerable excess of the solution of the mercuric salt.

5. Solutions of mercuric salts, when treated with *sodium hydroxide solution*, yield a yellow precipitate.

Appendix 3

Ultraviolet Absorption for Identification

This Appendix gives details of the ultraviolet absorption characteristics of certain substances in Part 1 and of certain substances used in preparations in Part 6. The information is used, in conjunction with the other tests and quantitative determinations in the individual monograph, to establish the identity of the substance or to establish the presence of the substance in the preparation. The apparatus and general methods used are those of Appendix IV(I) of the British Pharmacopoeia.

The absorption maxima quoted are the only maxima which can usually be observed at wavelengths in the range 230 to 360 nm for the particular substance when the solution used is of a strength suitable for carrying out absorption measurements at the principal maxima. In order to allow for instrumental variations, the wavelength at which a maximum occurs is given a tolerance which varies according to the relative sharpness of the maximum.

Extinction values relate to a 2-cm layer of the solution at the stated concentration when using a recording instrument and, again because of instrumental variations, should be considered to be approximate only.

If a value quoted is not in the optimum working range for a particular instrument, the path length should be varied, not the concentration, in a way that will bring the value into the optimum range.

Substance	Solvent	Maxima nm	Concentration % w/v	Extinction (approx.)
Aminobenzoic Acid	alcohol (95 per cent)	280 ± 5	0·00025	0·48
	0·1N sodium hydroxide	265 ± 5	0·00025	0·53
Amitriptyline Embonate	0·1N sodium hydroxide*	236 ± 3	0·00025	0·97
		277 ± 3	0·0025	0·90
		288 ± 3	0·0025	1·00
		363 ± 5	0·0025	0·67
Antazoline Mesylate	water	242 ± 3	0·001	0·82
		292 ± 3	0·005	0·58
Cephalexin	water	262 ± 3	0·002	0·94
Chloramphenicol Palmitate	dehydrated alcohol	271 ± 3	0·0025	0·89
Chloramphenicol Sodium Succinate	water	276 ± 5	0·002	0·86
Chlorhexidine Acetate	methyl alcohol	259 ± 5	0·0005	0·62
Chlorpromazine	alcohol (95 per cent)	258 ± 3	0·0005	1·15
		312 ± 5	—	—
Clefamide	alcohol (95 per cent)	303 ± 5	0·001	0·62
Ethamivan	0·01N hydrochloric acid	280 ± 3	0·003	0·92
Guaiphenesin	water	272 ± 3	0·004	0·96
Isoprenaline Hydrochloride	water	280 ± 3	0·004	0·88
Isothipendyl Hydrochloride	0·1N hydrochloric acid	245 ± 3	0·0005	0·77
Mephenesin	water	270 ± 3	0·005	0·80
Methallenoestril	methyl alcohol	232 ± 3	0·0001	0·61
		253 ± 3	0·0025	0·74
		264 ± 3	0·0025	0·90
		273 ± 3	0·0025	0·90
		317 ± 3	0·005	0·52
		332 ± 3	0·005	0·68
Methoxamine Hydrochloride	water	290 ± 3	0·003	0·80
Mexenone	methyl alcohol	287 ± 3	0·00075	0·90
Nalidixic Acid	0·1N sodium hydroxide	258 ± 3	0·0004	0·90
		334 ± 5	0·0006	0·59
Nicotinamide	alcohol (95 per cent)	262 ± 3	0·002	1·00

Substance	Solvent	Maxima nm	Concentration % w/v	Extinction (approx.)
Phensuximide	*alcohol (95 per cent)*	247 ± 3	0·02	0·69
		252 ± 3	0·02	0·65
		258 ± 3	0·02	0·58
		264 ± 3	0·04	0·77
Potassium Sorbate	0·01N hydrochloric acid	264 ± 3	0·00025	0·72
Procyclidine Hydrochloride	water	251 ± 3	0·08	0·84
		257 ± 3	0·08	0·98
		263 ± 3	0·08	0·74
Prothionamide	*alcohol (95 per cent)*	290 ± 5	0·001	0·78
Proxymetacaine Hydrochloride	water	269 ± 3	0·001	0·29
		310 ± 5	0·001	0·16
Riboflavine Phosphate (Sodium Salt)	*solution of standard pH 7·0*	266 ± 3	0·0005	0·61
Sorbic Acid	0·1N hydrochloric acid	264 ± 3	0·00025	0·94
Thiabendazole	0·1N hydrochloric acid	243 ± 5	0·0004	0·47
		302 ± 3	0·0004	0·98
Thiacetazone	*dehydrated alcohol*	328 ± 3	0·0003	1·16
Thiopropazate Hydrochloride	*methyl alcohol†*	256 ± 3	0·0005	0·66
		309 ± 5	0·005	0·72
Triamcinolone	*methyl alcohol*	238 ± 5	0·001	0·78
Trimeprazine Tartrate	*ammoniacal methyl alcohol*	255 ± 3	0·0004	0·70
		301 ± 5	0·002	0·52

* Solution prepared by dissolving 0·020 g in 20 ml of *dichloromethane*, adding 20 ml of 0·5N sodium hydroxide, shaking for 2 minutes, centrifuging for 2 minutes, and diluting 5 ml of the upper aqueous layer to 100 ml with 0·1N sodium hydroxide.

† Containing 0·2 ml of 5N hydrochloric acid in 100 ml.

Appendix 4

Ascending Paper Chromatography

This Appendix describes methods for detecting the presence of and distinguishing between isoprenaline, orciprenaline, and salbutamol in the aerosol inhalations described on pages 645–648.

Methods for detecting the presence of the active ingredients in Physostigmine and Pilocarpine Eye-drops and in Brilliant Green and Crystal Violet Paint are also described.

Apparatus

The apparatus consists of a rectangular glass tank about 60 cm high and 30 cm by 16 cm in cross-section, ground at the top to take a closely fitting glass lid which has a hole in its centre about 1·5 cm in diameter closed by a heavy ground-glass plate; it is essential that the closed tank should be completely airtight.

Near the top of the tank is a device which will suspend the strip of paper and is capable of being lowered without opening the chamber. In the bottom of the tank is a dish to contain the mobile phase into which the paper may be lowered.

The chromatographic paper consists of a suitable filter paper such as Whatman No. 1 (chromatographic use), cut in strips 55 cm long and not less than 2·5 cm wide; the paper is cut so that the chromatograms run in the direction of the grain of the paper. Care should be taken to avoid contaminating the paper.

General Method

Transfer to the dish in the bottom of the tank sufficient of the specified mobile phase to give a layer 2·5 cm deep; close the tank and allow to stand for 24 hours at 20° to 25°. The tank should be maintained at this temperature throughout the subsequent procedure.

Draw a fine pencil line horizontally across the paper 3 cm from one end and, using a micro-pipette, apply to a spot on the pencil line the volume of solution (1) specified for the individual preparation and similarly apply, at spots along the pencil line not less than 3 cm apart, the specified volume of solution (2) and, where stated, of solution (3). If the total volume to be applied would produce a spot greater than 10 mm in diameter, the solution should be applied in portions, allowing each portion to dry before making the next application.

Insert the paper into the tank, close the lid, and allow to stand for $1\frac{1}{2}$ hours; lower the paper into the mobile phase and allow elution to proceed for the prescribed distance or time. The paper should be protected from bright light during the elution process.

Aerosol Inhalations

SOLUTIONS

Isoprenaline Aerosol Inhalation. (1) Remove the oral adapter from the pressurised container, shake the container, place it inverted in a small beaker containing 2 ml of *methyl alcohol (80 per cent v/v),* and fire 20 sprays below the surface of the liquid, actuating the valve by pressing on the base of the container so that the valve stem is forced against the bottom of the beaker.

Remove the container from the beaker and use the methyl alcohol solution for the test.

(2) A reference solution containing 0·1 per cent w/v of *isoprenaline sulphate* in *methyl alcohol (80 per cent v/v).*

Isoprenaline Aerosol Inhalation, Strong. (1) A solution prepared as described for solution (1) under Isoprenaline Aerosol Inhalation, above, except that 4 sprays are fired instead of 20.

(2) A reference solution prepared as described for solution (2) under Isoprenaline Aerosol Inhalation.

Orciprenaline Aerosol Inhalation. (1) A solution prepared as described for solution (1) under Isoprenaline Aerosol Inhalation, above, except that 5 sprays are fired instead of 20.

(2) A reference solution containing 0·2 per cent w/v of *orciprenaline sulphate A.S.* in *methyl alcohol (80 per cent v/v).*

Salbutamol Aerosol Inhalation. (1) A solution prepared as described for solution (1) under Isoprenaline Aerosol Inhalation, above, except that 40 sprays are fired instead of 20.

(2) A reference solution containing 0·2 per cent w/v of *salbutamol sulphate A.S.* in *methyl alcohol (80 per cent v/v).*

MOBILE PHASE

A 0·48 per cent w/v solution of *citric acid* in a mixture containing 87 volumes of *butyl alcohol* and 13 volumes of water.

PROCEDURE

Saturate the chromatographic paper with a 5 per cent w/v solution of *sodium dihydrogen citrate* in water and allow to dry in air at 25°.

Apply separately to the paper a 10-μl portion of the solution (1) and of the solution (2) appropriate to the preparation(s) being tested. Develop the chromatograms by the general method, using the mobile phase stated above and allowing the development to proceed for 18 hours.

Remove the paper from the tank, allow to dry in a current of air, spray with a 20 per cent w/v solution of *sodium carbonate* in water, allow to dry in a current of air, and spray with *lithium and sodium molybdophosphotungstate solution.*

For each preparation the spot revealed in the chromatogram obtained with solution (1) corresponds in position and colour to the spot revealed in the chromatogram obtained with the reference solution (2).

Physostigmine and Pilocarpine Eye-drops

SOLUTIONS

Prepare the following solutions: (1) The undiluted sample.

(2) A reference solution containing 0·5 per cent w/v of *physostigmine sulphate A.S.* in *alcohol (95 per cent).*

(3) A reference solution containing 4 per cent w/v of *pilocarpine hydrochloride A.S.* in *alcohol (95 per cent).*

MOBILE PHASE

A 0·48 per cent w/v solution of *citric acid* in a mixture containing 87 volumes of *butyl alcohol* and 13 volumes of water.

PROCEDURE

Saturate the chromatographic paper with a 5 per cent w/v solution of *sodium dihydrogen citrate* in water and allow to dry in air at 25°.

Apply separately to the paper a 5-μl portion of solution (1), of solution (2), and of solution (3).

Develop the chromatograms by the general method, using the mobile phase stated above and allowing the development to proceed for 5 hours.

Remove the paper from the tank, allow to dry in a current of air, and spray with *iodoplatinate solution*.

The two spots revealed in the chromatogram obtained with solution (1) correspond, respectively, in position and colour with the spots revealed in the chromatograms obtained with reference solutions (2) and (3).

Brilliant Green and Crystal Violet Paint

SOLUTION
Use the sample, undiluted.

MOBILE PHASE
Ethyl acetate, 55 volumes + *pyridine*, 5 volumes + water, 40 volumes; shake together for 2 minutes and use the upper layer.

PROCEDURE
Apply to the chromatographic paper a 5-μl portion of the sample.

Develop the chromatogram by the general method, using the mobile phase stated above and allowing the chromatogram to develop for 20 cm.

Remove the paper from the tank and allow to dry in a current of air.

Two spots with colours characteristic, respectively, of brilliant green and of crystal violet are revealed.

Appendix 5
Thin-layer Chromatography

This Appendix describes methods for the examination by thin-layer chromatography of certain substances and preparations of the British Pharmaceutical Codex.

Section A gives details of identification tests and limit tests for certain impurities applicable to certain specified substances and preparations.

Section B (page 870) describes the procedures to be used for testing for the presence of certain alkaloids in specified preparations.

Section C (page 873) describes the procedures to be used for the identification of those phenothiazines, and their preparations, which are included in the British Pharmaceutical Codex.

Section D (page 874) describes the procedures to be used for testing for the presence of certain steroids in specified preparations.

The apparatus and general method of testing are those of Appendix XIIB of the British Pharmacopoeia. The coating substance of the chromatoplate and the mobile phase to be used are stated in the individual procedures given below. Other coating substances, similar to those specified, may also be used, providing that the analyst is satisfied that similar results can be achieved with them.

A. METHODS FOR SPECIFIED SUBSTANCES AND PREPARATIONS

Aminobenzoic Acid

Identification Test
Limit Test for p-*Nitrobenzoic Acid*

SOLUTIONS
Prepare the following solutions in *alcohol (95 per cent)*:
(1) A 1 per cent w/v solution of the sample.
(2) A 10·0 per cent w/v solution of the sample.
(3) A reference solution containing 1 per cent w/v of *aminobenzoic acid A.S.*
(4) A reference solution containing 0·1 per cent w/v of p-*nitrobenzoic acid A.S.*

MOBILE PHASE
Isobutyl alcohol, 7 volumes + *dilute ammonia solution*, 1·5 volumes + water, 3 volumes.

PROCEDURE
Apply separately to a chromatoplate, prepared with Cellulose MN 300 as the coating substance, a 1-μl portion of solution (1), a 5-μl portion of solution (2), and a 1-μl portion of solution (3) and of solution (4).

Develop the chromatograms by the general method for thin-layer chromatography, using the mobile phase stated above, allow the plate to dry in a current of air, and examine the plate under ultraviolet radiation, including radiation of wavelength 254 nm.

Identification. The main spot revealed in the chromatogram obtained with solution (1) corresponds in position and colour to the main spot revealed in the chromatogram obtained with reference solution (3).

Limit of p-*nitrobenzoic acid.* Any spot revealed in the chromatogram obtained with solution (2) which corresponds in position to the spot revealed in the chromatogram obtained with reference solution (4) is not more intense than this reference spot.

Aminobenzoic Acid Lotion

Limit Test for p-*Nitrobenzoic Acid*

SOLUTIONS
Prepare the following solutions:
(1) Use the sample, undiluted.

(2) A reference solution containing 0·05 per cent w/v of p-*nitrobenzoic acid A.S.* in *alcohol (95 per cent)*.

MOBILE PHASE
Isobutyl alcohol, 7 volumes + *dilute ammonia solution,* 1·5 volumes + water, 3 volumes.

PROCEDURE
Apply separately to a chromatoplate, prepared with Cellulose MN 300 as the coating substance, a 1-μl portion of solution (1) and of solution (2).
Develop the chromatograms by the general method for thin-layer chromatography, using the mobile phase stated above, allow the plate to dry in a current of air, and examine the plate under ultra-violet radiation, including radiation of wavelength 254 nm.
Any spot revealed in the chromatogram obtained with solution (1) which corresponds in position to the spot revealed in the chromatogram obtained with reference solution (2) is not more intense than this reference spot.

Amitriptyline Embonate

Identification Test

SOLUTIONS
Prepare the following solutions in *dichloromethane*:
(1) A 2 per cent w/v solution of the sample.
(2) A reference solution containing 2 per cent w/v of *amitriptyline embonate A.S.*

MOBILE PHASE
Methyl alcohol, 100 volumes + *strong ammonia solution,* 1·5 volumes.

PROCEDURE
Apply separately to a chromatoplate, prepared with Silica Gel GF254 as the coating substance, a 5-μl portion of solution (1) and of solution (2).
Develop the chromatograms by the general method for thin-layer chromatography, using the mobile phase stated above, allow the plate to dry in a current of air, and examine under ultraviolet radiation, including radiation of wavelength 254 nm.
The two main spots revealed in the chromatogram obtained with solution (1) correspond in position and colour to the two main spots revealed in the chromatogram obtained with solution (2).

Limit Test for Ketone

SOLUTIONS
Prepare the following solutions:
(1) A 2·0 per cent w/v solution of the sample in *dichloromethane*.
(2) A reference solution containing 0·001 per cent w/v of *1,2:4,5-dibenzocyclohepta-1,4-dien-3-one A.S.* in *alcohol (95 per cent)*.

MOBILE PHASE
Benzene, 7 volumes + *carbon tetrachloride,* 3 volumes.

PROCEDURE
Apply separately to a chromatoplate, prepared with Silica Gel GF254 as the coating substance, a 5-μl portion of solution (1) and of solution (2).
Develop the chromatograms by the general method for thin-layer chromatography, using the mobile phase stated above, but allowing the solvent front to travel 12 cm beyond the line of application instead of 15 cm, allow the plate to dry in a current of air, spray with *sulphuric acid*

containing 4 per cent v/v of *formaldehyde solution,* and immediately examine the plate under ultra-violet radiation, including radiation of wavelength 366 nm.
Any spot revealed in the chromatogram obtained with solution (1) which corresponds in position to the spot revealed in the chromatogram obtained with reference solution (2) is not more intense than this reference spot.

Amitriptyline Mixture

Test for the Presence of Amitriptyline Embonate

SOLUTIONS
Prepare the following solutions:
(1) Shake a volume of the sample, equivalent to 0·02 g of amitriptyline embonate, with 10 ml of *chloroform* for 2 minutes, allow to separate, and use the chloroform layer.
(2) A reference solution containing 0·2 per cent w/v of *amitriptyline embonate A.S.* in *chloroform*.

MOBILE PHASE; PROCEDURE
Using the above solutions, proceed as described in the identification test for Amitriptyline Embonate, above.
The chromatogram obtained with solution (1) includes two main spots which correspond in position and colour to the two main spots revealed in the chromatogram obtained with solution (2); any other spots in the chromatogram should be ignored.

Ampicillin Mixture

Test for the Presence of Ampicillin

SOLUTIONS
Prepare the following solutions:
(1) Dilute the sample with water to give a solution containing 0·1 per cent w/v of ampicillin.
(2) A reference solution containing 0·1 per cent w/v of *ampicillin A.S.* in water.

MOBILE PHASE
To 100 ml of *0·5M citric acid* add 20 ml of *butyl alcohol,* shake, allow to separate, and use the aqueous layer.

PROCEDURE
Apply separately to a chromatoplate, prepared with Cellulose MN 300 as the coating substance, a 2-μl portion of solution (1) and of solution (2).
Develop the chromatograms by the general method for thin-layer chromatography, using the mobile phase stated above, allow the plate to dry in a current of air, and spray with *starch-iodide reagent*.
The main spot revealed in the chromatogram obtained with solution (1) corresponds in position and colour to the main spot revealed in the chromatogram obtained with reference solution (2).

Ampicillin Tablets, Paediatric

Test for the Presence of Ampicillin

SOLUTIONS
Prepare the following solutions:
(1) Shake a quantity of the powdered tablets, equivalent to 0·05 g of ampicillin, with 30 ml of water for 5 minutes, filter, wash the residue on the filter with 10 ml of water, followed by two 10-ml portions of *alcohol (95 per cent)*, and finally with

two 10-ml portions of *solvent ether*; discard the filtrate and washings and dissolve the residue in 50 ml of warm water.

(2) A reference solution containing 0·1 per cent w/v of *ampicillin A.S.*

MOBILE PHASE; PROCEDURE
Using the above solutions, proceed as described in the test for the presence of ampicillin in Ampicillin Mixture, above.
The main spot revealed in the chromatogram obtained with solution (1) corresponds in position and colour to the main spot revealed in the chromatogram obtained with reference solution (2).

Aspirin Tablets, Compound

Limit Test for 4-Chloroacetanilide

SOLUTIONS
Prepare the following solutions:
(1) Mix an accurately weighed quantity of the powdered tablets, equivalent to 0·4 g of phenacetin, with 6 ml of *alcohol (95 per cent)* and 10 ml of *dilute hydrochloric acid*, boil under a reflux condenser for 15 minutes, allow to cool, transfer the solution to a stoppered cylinder, add 4 ml of *strong ammonia solution*, mix, again allow to cool, add 5·0 ml of *cyclohexane*, shake for 2 minutes, allow to separate, centrifuge if necessary, and use the cyclohexane layer.

(2) Proceed as directed for solution (1), above, but use 0·4 g, accurately weighed, of *phenacetin B.C.R.S.* and 0·04 mg, accurately weighed, of *4-chloroacetanilide* in place of the sample.

MOBILE PHASE
Dichloromethane

PROCEDURE
Apply separately to a chromatoplate, prepared with Silica Gel G as the coating substance, a 5-μl portion of solution (1) and of solution (2).
Develop the chromatograms by the general method for thin-layer chromatography, using the mobile phase stated above, but allowing the solvent front to travel 10 cm beyond the line of application, and allow the plate to dry in a current of air.
Immediately expose the plate to nitrous fumes [which may be generated by adding *sulphuric acid (50 per cent w/w)*, dropwise, to a solution containing 10 per cent w/v of *sodium nitrite* and 3 per cent w/v of *potassium iodide*] in a closed glass tank for 15 minutes; place the plate in a current of warm air for 15 minutes and spray with a 0·5 per cent w/v solution of N-(1-naphthyl)ethylene-diamine hydrochloride in *alcohol (95 per cent)*; if necessary, allow the plate to dry and spray again.
Any spot revealed in the chromatogram obtained with solution (1) which corresponds in position with the leading spot revealed in the chromatogram obtained with reference solution (2) is not more intense than this reference spot.

Bephenium Hydroxynaphthoate

Limit Test for Related Compounds

SOLUTIONS
Prepare the following solutions in *methyl alcohol*:
(1) A 4·0 per cent w/v solution of the sample.

(2) A reference solution containing 0·04 per cent of the sample.

MOBILE PHASE
Butyl alcohol, 5 volumes + water, 4 volumes + *acetic acid*, 1 volume.

PROCEDURE
Apply separately to a chromatoplate, prepared with Silica Gel GF254 as the coating substance, a 5-μl portion of solution (1) and of solution (2).
Develop the chromatograms by the general method for thin-layer chromatography using the mobile phase stated above and allow the plate to dry in a current of air.
(i) Examine the plate under ultraviolet radiation, including radiation of wavelength 254 nm. In the chromatograms obtained with solutions (1) and (2), two main spots are revealed, one of which absorbs the ultraviolet radiation and the other of which fluoresces. Any subsidiary absorbing spot revealed in the chromatogram obtained with solution (1) is not greater in intensity than the main absorbing spot revealed in the chromatogram obtained with reference solution (2).
(ii) Spray the plate with *sodium molybdophospho-tungstate solution* and then with a 20 per cent w/v solution of *sodium carbonate* in water and examine the plate immediately. In the chromatograms obtained with solutions (1) and (2), two main spots are revealed one of which is yellowish-blue in colour and the other of which is grey-blue in colour and is the faster running of the two. Any subsidiary spot revealed in the chromatogram obtained with solution (1), other than any subsidiary spot which may have been compared in (i), above, is not greater in intensity than the faster running of the two main spots revealed in the chromatogram obtained with reference solution (2).

Caffeine Iodide Elixir

Test for the Presence of Caffeine

SOLUTIONS
Prepare the following solutions:
(1) A 0·1 per cent w/v solution in *chloroform* of the residue obtained in the determination of caffeine.

(2), (3), and (4) The reference solutions (2), (3), and (4) described in the Test for the Presence of Theobromine in Phenobarbitone and Theobromine Tablets, page 866.

MOBILE PHASE; PROCEDURE
Using the above solutions, proceed as described in the Test for the Presence of Theobromine in Phenobarbitone and Theobromine Tablets, page 866.
The main spot revealed in the chromatogram obtained with solution (1) corresponds in position and colour with the main spot revealed in the chromatogram obtained with reference solution (4).

Chlorhexidine Acetate

Test for Related Compounds

SOLUTIONS
Prepare the following solutions in a mixture of equal volumes of *acetic acid* and water:
(1) A 20·0 per cent w/v solution of the sample.

(2) A 0·4 per cent w/v solution of *chlorhexidine acetate A.S.*

MOBILE PHASE
Chloroform, 50 volumes + *alcohol (95 per cent),* 50 volumes + *formic acid,* 7 volumes.

PROCEDURE
Prepare a chromatoplate using Silica Gel GF254 as the coating substance, the slurry being prepared by using, for each 8 g of the silica gel, 16 ml of water in which has been dissolved 1 g of *sodium formate.*
Apply separately to the chromatoplate, in the form of bands 4·0 cm wide, a 20-µl portion of solution (1) and of solution (2).
Develop the chromatograms by the general method for thin-layer chromatography, using the mobile phase stated above, allow the plate to dry in a current of air, and examine the plate under ultraviolet radiation, including radiation of wavelength 254 nm.
Score a rectangular area around each spot, other than the main spot, revealed in the chromatogram obtained with solution (1), quantitatively transfer the enclosed areas of silica gel to a glass-stoppered tube, add 5 ml of *methyl alcohol,* shake for 15 minutes, centrifuge, and measure the extinction of a 1-cm layer of the clear supernatant liquid at 257 nm, using as the blank a solution obtained by treating in the same manner equivalent sized areas of silica gel removed from the coating adjacent to the areas previously removed.
Repeat the procedure by measuring the extinction of a solution prepared by treating in the same manner the area of silica gel corresponding to the main spot revealed in the chromatogram obtained with solution (2) and using as the blank an equivalent adjacent area.
The extinction due to the solution prepared from the chromatogram obtained with solution (1) is not greater than the extinction due to the solution prepared from the chromatogram obtained with solution (2).

Chlorpromazine

Test for Related Compounds
(For the identification test *see* Section C of this Appendix, page 873).

SOLUTIONS
Prepare the following solutions:
(1) A 2·0 per cent w/v solution of the sample in *chloroform.*
(2) Dilute 1 ml of solution (1) to 200 ml with *chloroform.*

MOBILE PHASE
Acetone, 50 volumes + *strong ammonia solution,* 1 volume.

PROCEDURE
Apply separately to a chromatoplate, prepared with Silica Gel GF254 as the coating substance, a 5-µl portion of solution (1) and of solution (2).
Develop the chromatograms by the general method for thin-layer chromatography, using the mobile phase stated above, allow the plate to dry in a current of air, and examine the plate under ultraviolet radiation, including radiation of wavelength 254 nm.
Any spots, other than the main spot, which are revealed in the chromatogram obtained with solution (1) are not, individually, more intense than the main spot revealed in the chromatogram obtained with solution (2).

Cocaine and Homatropine Eye-drops

Test for the Presence of Cocaine and Homatropine
SOLUTIONS
Prepare the following solutions:
(1) Use the sample, undiluted.
(2) A reference solution containing 2 per cent w/v of *homatropine hydrobromide A.S.* in water.

MOBILE PHASE
Methyl alcohol, 100 volumes + *strong ammonia solution,* 1·5 volumes.

PROCEDURE
Apply separately to a chromatoplate, prepared with Silica Gel G as the coating substance, a 1-µl portion of solution (1) and of solution (2).
Develop the chromatograms by the general method for thin-layer chromatography, using the mobile phase stated above, allow the plate to dry in a current of air, and spray with *acidified iodoplatinate solution.*
Two main spots are revealed in the chromatogram obtained with solution (1). The slower-running of the two spots corresponds in position and colour to the spot revealed in the chromatogram obtained with reference solution (2); the second, faster-running, spot has an Rf value relative to the first spot of about 3.

Co-trimoxazole Mixture
Co-trimoxazole Mixture, Paediatric

Test for the Presence of Trimethoprim and Sulphamethoxazole
SOLUTIONS
Prepare the following solutions:
(1) Dilute 5 ml of the sample to 20 ml with *methyl alcohol,* pass the solution through a column packed with 20 g of granular *anhydrous sodium sulphate,* and evaporate the resulting solution to a volume of 10 ml.
(2) A reference solution containing 0·4 per cent w/v of *trimethoprim A.S.* in *methyl alcohol.*
(3) A reference solution containing 2·0 per cent w/v of *sulphamethoxazole A.S.* in *methyl alcohol.*

MOBILE PHASE
Chloroform, 9 volumes + *methyl alcohol,* 1 volume.

PROCEDURE
Apply separately to a chromatoplate, prepared with Silica Gel G as the coating substance, a 5-µl portion of solution (1), of solution (2), and of solution (3).
Develop the chromatograms by the general method for thin-layer chromatography, using the mobile phase stated above, allow the plate to dry in a current of air, and spray with *dilute potassium iodobismuthate solution.*
The two main spots revealed in the chromatogram obtained with solution (1) correspond, respectively, in position and colour to the main spots revealed in the chromatograms obtained with reference solutions (2) and (3).

Deoxycortone Pivalate

Identification Test
SOLUTIONS
Prepare the following solutions in a mixture containing 9 volumes of *chloroform* and 1 volume of *methyl alcohol:*
(1) A 0·25 per cent w/v solution of the sample.

(2) A reference solution containing 0·25 per cent w/v of *deoxycortone pivalate A.S.*

MOBILE PHASE

A mixture containing equal volumes of *cyclohexane* and *light petroleum (boiling-range, 40° to 60°)*.

PROCEDURE

Prepare a chromatoplate using Kieselguhr G as the coating substance.

Impregnate the prepared plate by immersing it to a depth of 5 mm in a closed chamber containing a suitable volume of a mixture containing 9 volumes of *acetone* and 1 volume of *propylene glycol*, until the solvent front has risen at least 17 cm.

Remove the plate from the impregnation liquid, allow the plate to dry in a current of air, and use within 2 hours.

Apply separately to the chromatoplate a 2-µl portion of solution (1) and of solution (2).

Develop the chromatograms by the general method for thin-layer chromatography, using the mobile phase stated above, allow the plate to dry in a current of air, heat the plate at 120° for 15 minutes, spray the hot plate with a 10 per cent v/v solution of *sulphuric acid* in *alcohol (95 per cent)*, again heat the plate at 120° for a further 10 minutes, and examine the plate under ultraviolet radiation, including radiation of wavelength 366 nm.

The main spot revealed in the chromatogram obtained with solution (1) corresponds in position and colour to the main spot revealed in the chromatogram obtained with reference solution (2).

Limit Test for Related Foreign Steroids

SOLUTIONS

Prepare the following solutions in a mixture containing 9 volumes of *chloroform* and 1 volume of *methyl alcohol*:

(1) A 1·5 per cent w/v solution of the sample.

(2) A reference solution containing 0·03 per cent w/v of each of *prednisolone B.C.R.S.*, *prednisone B.C.R.S.*, *cortisone acetate B.C.R.S.*, and *deoxycortone acetate B.C.R.S.*

MOBILE PHASE

Ethylene chloride, 95 volumes + *methyl alcohol*, 5 volumes + water, 0·2 volume.

PROCEDURE

Apply separately to a chromatoplate, prepared with Silica Gel G as the coating substance, a 1-µl portion of solution (1) and of solution (2).

Develop the chromatograms by the general method for thin-layer chromatography, using the mobile phase stated above, allow the plate to dry in a current of air, heat the plate at 105° for 10 minutes, allow to cool, and spray with *alkaline tetrazolium blue solution*.

Any spot, other than the main spot, revealed in the chromatogram obtained with solution (1) which corresponds in position with a spot revealed in the chromatogram obtained with reference solution (2) is not more intense than this reference spot.

Dextromoramide Injection

Test for the Presence of Dextromoramide

SOLUTIONS

Prepare the following solutions:

(1) Use the sample, undiluted.

(2) A reference solution containing 0·1 per cent w/v of *methaqualone A.S.* in *methyl alcohol*.

MOBILE PHASE

Methyl alcohol, 100 volumes + *strong ammonia solution*, 1·5 volumes.

PROCEDURE

Apply separately to a chromatoplate, prepared with Silica Gel G as the coating substance, a 10-µl portion of solution (1) and of solution (2).

Develop the chromatograms by the general method for thin-layer chromatography, using the mobile phase stated above, allow the plate to dry in a current of air, and spray it with *dilute potassium iodobismuthate solution*.

The main spot revealed in the chromatogram obtained with solution (1) corresponds in position (but not in colour) with the main spot revealed in the chromatogram obtained with reference solution (2).

Dicyclomine Elixir

Test for the Presence of Dicyclomine

SOLUTIONS

Prepare the following solutions:

(1) Shake a volume of the sample, equivalent to 0·04 g of dicyclomine hydrochloride, with 25 ml of *solvent ether*, allow to separate, and discard the ethereal extract; extract the aqueous solution with two successive 15-ml portions of *chloroform*; dry the combined chloroform extracts over *anhydrous sodium sulphate*, evaporate off the chloroform, and dissolve the cooled residue in 1 ml of *chloroform*.

(2) A reference solution containing 4 per cent w/v of *dicyclomine hydrochloride* in *chloroform*.

MOBILE PHASE

Methyl alcohol, 100 volumes + *strong ammonia solution*, 1·5 volumes.

PROCEDURE

Apply separately to a chromatoplate, prepared with Silica Gel G as the coating substance, a 5-µl portion of solution (1) and of solution (2).

Develop the chromatograms by the general method for thin-layer chromatography, using the mobile phase stated above, allow the plate to dry in a current of air, and spray with *acidified iodoplatinate solution*.

The main spot revealed in the chromatogram obtained with solution (1) corresponds in position and colour to the main spot revealed in the chromatogram obtained with reference solution (2).

Diphenhydramine Elixir

Test for the Presence of Diphenhydramine

SOLUTIONS

(1) Shake a volume of the sample, equivalent to 0·05 g of diphenhydramine hydrochloride, with two successive 20-ml portions of *solvent ether* and discard the ethereal extracts; extract the aqueous solution with two successive 20-ml portions of *chloroform*, dry the combined chloroform extracts over *anhydrous sodium sulphate*, evaporate off the chloroform, and dissolve the cooled residue in 5 ml of *chloroform*.

(2) A reference solution containing 1 per cent w/v of *diphenhydramine hydrochloride A.S.* in *chloroform*.

MOBILE PHASE

Alcohol (95 per cent), 5 volumes + *glacial acetic acid*, 3 volumes + *water*, 2 volumes.

PROCEDURE

Apply separately to a chromatoplate, prepared with Silica Gel G as the coating substance, a 5-μl portion of solution (1) and of solution (2). Develop the chromatograms by the general method for thin-layer chromatography, using the mobile phase stated above, allow the plate to dry in a current of air, and spray with *iodoplatinate solution*.

The main spot revealed in the chromatogram obtained with solution (1) corresponds in position and colour to the main spot revealed in the chromatogram obtained with reference solution (2).

Ergotamine Aerosol Inhalation

Test for the Presence of Ergotamine
Limit Test for Related Alkaloids

SOLUTIONS

Prepare the following solutions:
(1) Remove the oral adapter from the pressurised container, gently shake the container, actuate the valve several times, wash the valve stem with *methyl alcohol*, discarding the washings, and replace the oral adapter.

The following procedure should be carried out in subdued light.

Invert the assembled unit and place it in a small beaker containing 40 ml of *light petroleum (boiling-range, 40° to 60°)*, ensuring that the mouth of the oral adapter is completely immersed below the surface of the liquid.

Fire 20 sprays by pressing on the base of the container, gently agitating the unit while keeping it in the liquid and swirling the contents of the beaker between each spray; remove the unit from the beaker, wash it with *light petroleum (boiling-range, 40° to 60°)*, and filter the combined solution and washings through a suitable filter having a pore diameter not greater than 0·45 μm.

Wash the filter with *light petroleum (boiling-range, 40° to 60°)*, and dissolve the residue on the filter in 4·5 ml of a mixture containing equal volumes of *chloroform* and *methyl alcohol*.

(2) A reference solution containing 0·02 per cent w/v of *ergotamine tartrate A.S.* in a mixture containing equal volumes of *chloroform* and *methyl alcohol*.

MOBILE PHASE

Chloroform, 9 volumes + *methyl alcohol*, 1 volume.

PROCEDURE

The following procedure should be carried out in subdued light.

Apply separately to a chromatoplate, prepared with Silica Gel G as the coating substance, a 10-μl portion of solution (1) and of solution (2). Develop the chromatograms by the general method for thin-layer chromatography, using the mobile phase stated above, allow the plate to dry in a current of air, spray with a 0·5 per cent w/v solution of *dimethylaminobenzaldehyde* in *cyclohexane*, and expose it to *gaseous hydrochloric acid* for 1 or 2 seconds.

Presence of ergotamine. The main spot revealed in the chromatogram obtained with solution (1) corresponds in position and colour to the main spot revealed in the chromatogram obtained with reference solution (2).

Limit of related alkaloids. Any spot other than the main spot revealed in the chromatogram obtained with solution (1), is not more intense than the spot revealed in the chromatogram obtained with reference solution (2).

Ethamivan

Identification Test
Limit Test for Related Compounds

SOLUTIONS

Prepare the following solutions in *alcohol (95 per cent)*:
(1) A 0·5 per cent w/v solution of the sample.
(2) A reference solution containing 0·5 per cent w/v of *ethamivan A.S.*
(3) A 2·0 per cent w/v solution of the sample.
(4) A reference solution containing 0·01 per cent w/v of *vanillic acid*.

MOBILE PHASE

Chloroform, 8 volumes + *methyl alcohol*, 2 volumes.

PROCEDURE

Apply separately to a chromatoplate, prepared with Silica Gel G as the coating substance, a 5-μl portion of solution (1) and of solution (2) and a 10-μl portion of solution (3) and of solution (4). Develop the chromatograms by the general method for thin-layer chromatography, using the mobile phase stated above, allow the plate to dry in a current of air, spray with *diazotised sulphanilic acid*, allow to dry, and spray with *sodium carbonate solution*.

Identification. The main spot revealed in the chromatogram obtained with solution (1) corresponds in position and colour to the main spot revealed in the chromatogram obtained with reference solution (2).

Limit of related compounds. Any spot, other than the main spot, revealed in the chromatogram obtained with solution (3) is not more intense than the spot revealed in the chromatogram obtained with reference solution (4).

Ferrous Phosphate, Quinine, and Strychnine Tablets

Test for Strychnine

SOLUTIONS

Prepare the following solutions:
(1) Prepare a chromatographic column by the following method:
Mix 1 g of *Celite 545* with 1 ml of water, transfer the suspension to a chromatographic tube which is fitted at its lower end with a sintered-glass disk (British Standard Grade No. 3), and pack the material firmly with the aid of a suitable plunger.
Mix 3 g of *Celite 545* with 3 ml of 1N hydrochloric acid, transfer the suspension to the top of the column, and again pack the material firmly.
Mix a quantity of the powdered tablets, equivalent to 1 mg of strychnine hydrochloride, with 5 g of *Celite 545* and 3 ml of 4N hydrochloric acid, transfer the suspension to the top of the chromatographic column, add a further 1 g of *Celite 545*, pack firmly, clean the container in which the sample was mixed with a small piece of cotton

wool and place the cotton wool on the top of the chromatographic column.

Wash the column with successive 50-, 25-, 25-, 25-, and 25-ml portions of water-saturated *anaesthetic ether* by applying a slight pressure and discard the washings.

Elute the column with six successive 25-ml portions of water-saturated *chloroform*, combine the eluates, evaporate off the chloroform in a current of air, dissolve the residue in 0·5 ml of *alcohol (95 per cent)*, warming if necessary, and dilute to 2 ml with *alcohol (95 per cent)*.

(2) A reference solution containing 0·05 per cent w/v of *strychnine hydrochloride A.S.* in *alcohol (95 per cent)*.

MOBILE PHASE
Methyl alcohol

PROCEDURE
Apply separately to a chromatoplate, prepared with Silica Gel G as the coating substance, a 10-μl portion of solution (1) and 8-, 10-, and 12-μl portions of solution (2). Develop the chromatograms by the general method for thin-layer chromatography, using the mobile phase stated above, allow the plate to dry in a current of air, and spray with *dilute potassium iodobismuthate solution*.

A spot is revealed in the chromatogram obtained with solution (1) which corresponds in position to the spots revealed in the chromatograms obtained with reference solution (2). The colour intensity of the spot revealed in the chromatogram obtained with solution (1) is not less than that of the spot revealed in the chromatogram obtained from 8-μl of reference solution (2) and not greater than that of the spot revealed in the chromatogram obtained from 12-μl of reference solution (2).

Fusidic Acid

Identification Test
Limit Test for Related Compounds

SOLUTIONS
Prepare the following solutions in *dehydrated alcohol*:
(1) A 2·0 per cent w/v solution of the sample.
(2) A reference solution containing 0·04 per cent w/v of the sample.
(3) A reference solution containing 0·02 per cent w/v of the sample.
(4) A reference solution containing 2 per cent w/v of *fusidic acid A.S.*

MOBILE PHASE
Chloroform, 8 volumes + *cyclohexane*, 1 volume + *glacial acetic acid*, 1 volume + *methyl alcohol*, 0·25 volume.

PROCEDURE
Apply separately to a chromatoplate, prepared with Silica Gel GF254 as the coating substance, a 5-μl portion of solution (1), of solution (2), of solution (3), and of solution (4).
Develop the chromatograms by the general method for thin-layer chromatography, using the mobile phase stated above, allow the plate to dry in a current of air, spray with a saturated solution of *antimony trichloride* in *chloroform*, heat at 105° for 20 minutes, and examine the plate under ultraviolet radiation, including radiation of wavelength 366 nm.

Identification. The main spot revealed in the chromatogram obtained with solution (1) corresponds in position and colour to the main spot revealed in the chromatogram obtained with reference solution (4).

Limit of related compounds. Any one spot, other than the main spot, revealed in the chromatogram obtained with solution (1) is not more intense than the spot revealed in the chromatogram obtained with reference solution (2), and any subsidiary spots revealed in the chromatogram obtained with solution (1) are not more intense than the spot revealed in the chromatogram obtained with reference solution (3).

Green S and Tartrazine Solution

Test for the Presence of Green S and of Tartrazine

SOLUTIONS
Prepare the following solutions:
(1) Use the sample, undiluted.
(2) A reference solution containing 0·5 per cent w/v of *green S A.S.* in water.
(3) A reference solution containing 0·5 per cent w/v of *tartrazine A.S.* in water.

MOBILE PHASE
Alcohol (95 per cent), 2 volumes + *isobutyl alcohol*, 1 volume + water, 1 volume.

PROCEDURE
Apply separately to a chromatoplate, prepared with Cellulose MN 300 as the coating substance, a 1-μl portion of solution (1), of solution (2), and of solution (3).
Develop the chromatograms by the general method for thin-layer chromatography, using the mobile phase stated above, and allow the plate to dry in a current of air.
Spots are present in the chromatogram obtained with solution (1) which correspond in position and colour to the spots in the chromatograms obtained with reference solutions (2) and (3).

Hydrocortisone Sodium Phosphate

Identification Test

SOLUTIONS
Prepare the following solutions:
(1) A 0·25 per cent w/v solution of the sample in *methyl alcohol*.
(2) A reference solution containing 0·25 per cent w/v of *hydrocortisone sodium phosphate A.S.* in *methyl alcohol*.

MOBILE PHASE
Butyl alcohol, 3 volumes + *acetic anhydride*, 1 volume + water, 1 volume; it should be freshly prepared.

PROCEDURE
Apply separately to a chromatoplate, prepared with Silica Gel G as the coating substance, a 5-μl portion of solution (1) and of solution (2).
Develop the chromatograms by the general method for thin-layer chromatography, using the mobile phase stated above, allow the plate to dry in a current of air, spray with a 10 per cent v/v solution of *sulphuric acid* in *alcohol (95 per cent)*, heat at 120° for 10 minutes, and examine under ultraviolet radiation, including radiation of wavelength 366 nm.
The main spot revealed in the chromatogram

obtained with solution (1) corresponds in position and colour to the main spot revealed in the chromatogram obtained with solution (2).

Limit Test for Free Hydrocortisone and other Derivatives

SOLUTIONS

Prepare the following solutions in *methyl alcohol*:
(1) A 1·0 per cent w/v solution of the sample calculated with reference to the anhydrous substance.
(2) A reference solution containing 1·0 per cent w/v of *hydrocortisone sodium phosphate A.S.*
(3) A reference solution containing 0·02 per cent w/v of *hydrocortisone B.C.R.S.*

MOBILE PHASE
Methyl alcohol

PROCEDURE

Apply separately to a chromatoplate, prepared with Silica Gel G as the coating substance, a 2-μl portion of solution (1), of solution (2), and of solution (3).
Develop the chromatograms by the general method for thin-layer chromatography, using the mobile phase stated above, allow the plate to dry in a current of air, spray with a 30 per cent w/v solution of *zinc chloride* in *methyl alcohol*, heat the plate at about 125° for 1 hour, and examine under ultraviolet radiation, including radiation of wavelength 366 nm.
Any spot revealed in the chromatogram obtained with solution (1), other than the spot corresponding to that revealed in the chromatogram obtained with solution (2), is not more intense than the spot revealed in the chromatogram obtained with reference solution (3).

Mepyramine Elixir

Test for the Presence of Mepyramine

SOLUTIONS

Prepare the following solutions:
(1) Dilute a volume of the sample, equivalent to 0·1 g of mepyramine maleate, with an equal volume of water, shake with 25 ml of *solvent ether*, allow to separate, and discard the ethereal extract.
Extract the aqueous solution with two successive 15-ml portions of *chloroform*, dry the combined chloroform extracts over *anhydrous sodium sulphate*, evaporate off the chloroform, and dissolve the cooled residue in 5 ml of *chloroform*.
(2) A reference solution containing 2 per cent w/v of *mepyramine maleate A.S.* in *chloroform*.

MOBILE PHASE
Methyl alcohol, 100 volumes + *strong ammonia solution*, 1·5 volumes.

PROCEDURE

Apply separately to a chromatoplate, prepared with Silica Gel G as the coating substance, a 2-μl portion of solution (1) and of solution (2).
Develop the chromatograms by the general method for thin-layer chromatography, using the mobile phase stated above, allow the plate to dry in a current of air, and spray with *acidified iodoplatinate solution*.
The main spot revealed in the chromatogram obtained with solution (1) corresponds in position and colour to the spot revealed in the chromatogram obtained with reference solution (2).

Mexenone

Identification Test
Limit Test for Related Compounds

SOLUTIONS

Prepare the following solutions in *ethyl methyl ketone*:
(1) A 1 per cent w/v solution of the sample.
(2) A reference solution containing 1 per cent w/v of *mexenone A.S.*
(3) A 10·0 per cent w/v solution of the sample.
(4) A reference solution containing 0·05 per cent w/v of *2,4-dimethoxy-4'-methylbenzophenone A.S.*

MOBILE PHASE
Toluene, 10 volumes + *ethyl methyl ketone*, 1 volume.

PROCEDURE

Apply separately to a chromatoplate, prepared with Silica Gel GF254 as the coating substance, a 5-μl portion of solution (1), of solution (2), of solution (3), and of solution (4).
Develop the chromatograms by the general method for thin-layer chromatography, using the mobile phase stated above, allow the plate to dry in a current of air, spray with *sulphuric acid (20 per cent v/v)*, heat the plate at 120° for 5 minutes, and examine under ultraviolet radiation, including radiation of wavelength 254 nm.

Identification. The main spot revealed in the chromatogram obtained with solution (1) corresponds in position and colour to the main spot revealed in the chromatogram obtained with reference solution (2).

Limit of related compounds. Any spot revealed in the chromatogram obtained with solution (3) which corresponds in position to the spot revealed in the chromatogram obtained with reference solution (4) is not more intense than this reference spot.

Morphine and Atropine Injection

Test for the Presence of Morphine and of Atropine

SOLUTIONS

Prepare the following solutions:
(1) To 1 ml of the sample add 1 ml of *dilute ammonia solution* and extract with two 5-ml portions of *chloroform*, filtering each extract through a layer of *anhydrous sodium sulphate*; evaporate the combined extracts to dryness with the aid of a current of warm air and dissolve the residue in 0·5 ml of *chloroform*.
(2) A reference solution prepared by treating 1 ml of a 0·06 per cent w/v solution of *atropine sulphate A.S.* in water by the method given for solution (1).
(3) A reference solution prepared by treating 1 ml of a 1 per cent w/v solution of *morphine sulphate A.S.* in water by the method given for solution (1).

MOBILE PHASE
Methyl alcohol, 100 volumes + *strong ammonia solution*, 1·5 volumes.

PROCEDURE

Apply separately to a chromatoplate, prepared with Silica Gel G as the coating substance, a 10-μl portion of solution (1), of solution (2), and of solution (3).
Develop the chromatograms by the general method for thin-layer chromatography, using the mobile phase stated above, allow the plate to dry

in a current of air, and spray with *dilute potassium iodobismuthate solution*.

Spots are revealed in the chromatogram obtained with solution (1) which correspond in position and colour with the spots revealed in the chromatograms obtained with reference solutions (2) and (3).

Orciprenaline Elixir

Test for the Presence of Orciprenaline Sulphate

SOLUTIONS

Prepare the following solutions:
(1) The sample, diluted, if necessary, with water so as to give a solution containing 0·1 per cent w/v of orciprenaline sulphate.
(2) A reference solution containing 0·1 per cent w/v of *orciprenaline sulphate A.S.* in water.

MOBILE PHASE

Butyl alcohol, 10 volumes + *formic acid*, 1 volume + water, 5 volumes; shake together, allow to separate, and use the upper layer.

PROCEDURE

Apply separately to a chromatoplate, prepared with Silica Gel G as the coating substance, a 5-μl portion of solution (1) and of solution (2).

Develop the chromatograms by the general method for thin-layer chromatography, using the mobile phase stated above, allow the plate to dry in a current of air, and spray with *alkaline diazotised sulphanilic acid*.

The main spot revealed in the chromatogram obtained with solution (1) corresponds in position and colour to the main spot revealed in the chromatogram obtained with reference solution (2).

Paromomycin Capsules

Test for the Presence of Paromomycin

Carry out the test described below for the identification of Paromomycin Sulphate, but prepare solution (1) by dissolving a quantity of the contents of the capsules, equivalent to 150,000 Units, in 10 ml of water and filtering if necessary.

Paromomycin Sulphate

Identification Test

SOLUTIONS

Prepare the following solutions in water:
(1) A 2 per cent w/v solution of the sample.
(2) A reference solution containing 2 per cent w/v of the Standard Preparation of paromomycin.
(3) A reference solution containing 2 per cent w/v of the Standard Preparation of neomycin.

MOBILE PHASE

A 3·85 per cent w/v solution of *ammonium acetate* in water; it should be freshly prepared.

PROCEDURE

Apply separately to a chromatoplate, prepared with a suitable silica gel (free from binder) as the coating substance, a 1-μl portion of solution (1), of solution (2), and of solution (3).

Develop the chromatoplate by the general method for thin-layer chromatography, using the mobile phase stated above, allow the plate to dry in a current of air for 10 minutes, heat at 105° for 1 hour, spray with a 0·1 per cent w/v solution of *ninhydrin* in *butyl alcohol* saturated with water, and heat at 105° for 5 minutes.

The main spot revealed in the chromatogram obtained with solution (1) corresponds in position and colour with the spot revealed in the chromatogram obtained with reference solution (2) (distinction from neomycin sulphate).

Phenobarbitone and Theobromine Tablets

Test for the Presence of Theobromine

SOLUTIONS

Prepare the following solutions:
(1) Dissolve, as completely as possible, a quantity of the powdered tablets, equivalent to 0·1 g of theobromine, in 100 ml of *dilute sodium hydroxide solution*.
(2) A reference solution containing 0·1 per cent w/v of *theobromine A.S.* in *dilute sodium hydroxide solution*.
(3) A reference solution containing 0·1 per cent w/v of *theophylline A.S.* in *dilute sodium hydroxide solution*.
(4) A reference solution containing 0·1 per cent w/v of *caffeine A.S.* in *dilute sodium hydroxide solution*.

MOBILE PHASE

Chloroform, 9 volumes + *alcohol (95 per cent)*, 1 volume.

PROCEDURE

Apply separately to a chromatoplate, prepared with Silica Gel GF254 as the coating substance and using *solution of standard pH 6·8* to prepare the slurry instead of water, a 10-μl portion of solution (1), of solution (2), of solution (3), and of solution (4).

Develop the chromatograms by the general method for thin-layer chromatography, using the mobile phase stated above, allow the plate to dry in a current of air, and expose the plate to ultraviolet radiation, including radiation of wavelength 254 nm.

A spot is revealed in the chromatogram obtained with solution (1) which corresponds in position and colour to the spot revealed in the chromatogram obtained with reference solution (2).

Pilocarpine Hydrochloride

Test for the Presence of Certain Other Alkaloids

SOLUTION

Prepare a solution containing 5 per cent w/v of the sample in water.

MOBILE PHASE.

Chloroform, 25 volumes + *acetone*, 20 volumes + *strong ammonia solution*, 0·4 volume.

PROCEDURE

Apply to a chromatoplate, prepared with Silica Gel G as the coating substance, a 5-μl portion of the prepared solution.

Develop the chromatogram by the general method for thin-layer chromatography, using the mobile phase stated above, allow the plate to dry in a current of air, and spray with *dilute potassium iodobismuthate solution*.

No spot, other than the main spot, is revealed in the chromatogram.

Propicillin Elixir

Test for the Presence of Propicillin

Proceed by the method given for Ampicillin Mixture (page 859), using *propicillin A.S.* in place of ampicillin A.S. in the preparation of solution (2).

Propylhexedrine

Limit Test for Related Compounds

SOLUTIONS

Prepare the following solutions in *alcohol (95 per cent)*:
(1) A 10·0 per cent w/v solution of the sample.
(2) A reference solution containing 0·1 per cent w/v of the sample.
(3) A reference solution containing 0·05 per cent w/v of the sample.

MOBILE PHASE
Methyl alcohol, 20 volumes + *strong ammonia solution*, 1 volume.

PROCEDURE
Apply separately to a chromatoplate, prepared with Silica Gel G as the coating substance, a 1-µl portion of solution (1), of solution (2), and of solution (3).
Develop the chromatograms by the general method for thin-layer chromatography, using the mobile phase stated above, allow the plate to dry in a current of air, and expose the plate to *iodine vapour* in a closed glass tank for 10 minutes.
Any one spot, other than the main spot, revealed in the chromatogram obtained with solution (1) is not more intense than the spot revealed in the chromatogram obtained with reference solution (2); any subsidiary spots revealed with solution (1) are not more intense than the spot revealed in the chromatogram obtained with reference solution (3).

Prothionamide

Limit Test for Related Compounds

SOLUTIONS

Prepare the following solutions in *methyl alcohol*:
(1) A 5·0 per cent w/v solution of the sample.
(2) A reference solution containing 0·025 per cent w/v of *prothionamide A.S.*

MOBILE PHASE
Chloroform, 9 volumes + *methyl alcohol*, 1 volume.

PROCEDURE
Apply separately to a chromatoplate, prepared with Silica Gel G as the coating substance, a 5-µl portion of solution (1) and of solution (2).
Develop the chromatograms by the general method for thin-layer chromatography, using the mobile phase stated above, allow the plate to dry in a current of air, and spray with *dilute potassium iodobismuthate solution*.
Any spot, other than the main spot, revealed in the chromatogram obtained with solution (1) is not more intense than the spot revealed in the reference solution (2).

Senna Leaf

Chromatographic Test

SOLUTIONS

Prepare the following solutions:
(1) Mix 0·50 g of the sample, in fine powder, with 5 ml of a mixture containing equal volumes of alcohol (*95 per cent*) and water, heat to boiling, centrifuge, and use the clear supernatant liquid.
(2) A reference solution prepared by dissolving 0·01 g of *sennoside A* and 0·01 g of *sennoside B* in 10 ml of the mobile phase, warming, if necessary, to aid dissolution.

MOBILE PHASE
Propyl alcohol, 4 volumes + *ethyl acetate*, 4 volumes + water, 3 volumes.

PROCEDURE
Apply separately to a chromatoplate, prepared with Silica Gel GF254 as the coating substance, a 10-µl portion of solution (1) and of solution (2).
Develop the chromatograms by the general method for thin-layer chromatography, using the mobile phase stated above, but allowing the solvent front to travel 10 cm beyond the line of application instead of 15 cm, allow the plate to dry in a current of air, spray with a 25 per cent w/v solution of *nitric acid* in water, and heat at 120° for 10 minutes; allow the plate to cool and spray with a 5 per cent w/v solution of *potassium hydroxide* in *alcohol (50 per cent)*.
The two main purplish-brown spots revealed in the chromatogram obtained with solution (1) correspond in position and colour with the two spots revealed in the chromatogram obtained with reference solution (2).
In addition, in the chromatogram obtained with solution (1), two minor purplish-brown spots, situated on either side of a red spot, are revealed immediately in front of the main spots.

Sodium Aminosalicylate and Isoniazid Cachets

Limit Test for 3-Aminophenol

SOLUTIONS

Prepare the following solutions:
(1) Dissolve an accurately weighed quantity of the mixed contents of the cachets, equivalent to 1 g of sodium aminosalicylate, in sufficient *methyl alcohol* to produce 5 ml.
(2) A reference solution containing 0·006 per cent w/v of *3-aminophenol* in *methyl alcohol*.

MOBILE PHASE
Solvent ether

PROCEDURE
Apply separately to a chromatoplate, prepared with Silica Gel G as the coating substance, a 5-µl portion of solution (1) and of solution (2).
Develop the chromatograms by the general method for thin-layer chromatography, using the mobile phase stated above, and allow the plate to dry in a current of air.
Expose the plate to nitrogen dioxide gas (which may be generated by adding 10 ml of *nitric acid* to 10 g of *sodium nitrite*) in a closed glass tank for 30 minutes; place the plate in a current of air for 3 minutes and spray with N-(*1-naphthyl*)ethylenediamine hydrochloride solution.
Any spot revealed in the chromatogram obtained with solution (1) which corresponds in position with the spot revealed in the chromatogram obtained with reference solution (2) is not more intense than this reference spot.

Sodium Aminosalicylate and Isoniazid Granules

Limit Test for 3-Aminophenol

Proceed by the method given for Sodium Amino-salicylate and Isoniazid Cachets, above, but using a reference solution containing 0·06 per cent w/v of *3-aminophenol* in *methyl alcohol* as solution (2).

Succinylsulphathiazole Mixture, Paediatric

Test for the Presence of Succinylsulphthathiazole

SOLUTIONS

Prepare the following solutions:

(1) Mix 10 ml of the sample with 10 ml of 1N sodium hydroxide, stir until the suspended material is dissolved as completely as possible, filter, and dilute the filtrate to 100 ml with water.

(2) A reference solution containing 1 per cent w/v of *succinylsulphthathiazole A.S.* in 0·1N sodium hydroxide.

MOBILE PHASE

Acetone, 4 volumes + *methyl alcohol*, 1 volume.

PROCEDURE

Apply separately to a chromatoplate, prepared with Silica Gel G as the coating substance and using 0·1N sodium hydroxide to prepare the slurry instead of water, a 1-μl portion of solution (1) and of solution (2).

Develop the chromatograms by the general method for thin-layer chromatography, using the mobile phase stated above, allow the plate to dry in a current of air, and spray with a 0·5 per cent w/v solution of *bromocresol purple* in *alcohol (95 per cent)*.

A spot is revealed in the chromatogram obtained with solution (1) which corresponds in position and colour with the spot revealed in the chromatogram obtained with reference solution (2).

Sulphadimidine Mixture, Paediatric

Test for the Presence of Sulphadimidine

SOLUTIONS

Prepare the following solutions:

(1) Mix 10 ml of the sample with 10 ml of 1N sodium hydroxide, stir until the suspended material is dissolved as completely as possible, filter, and dilute the filtrate to 100 ml with water.

(2) A reference solution containing 1 per cent w/v of *sulphadimidine A.S.* in 0·1N sodium hydroxide.

MOBILE PHASE

Chloroform, 4 volumes + *methyl alcohol*, 1 volume.

PROCEDURE

Apply separately to a chromatoplate, prepared with Silica Gel G as the coating substance and using 0·1N sodium hydroxide to prepare the slurry instead of water, a 2-μl portion of solution (1) and of solution (2).

Develop the chromatograms by the general method for thin-layer chromatography, using the mobile phase stated above, allow the plate to dry in a current of air, and spray with a 5 per cent w/v solution of *copper sulphate* in water.

A spot is revealed in the chromatogram obtained with solution (1) which corresponds in position and colour with the spot revealed in the chromatogram obtained with reference solution (2).

Sulphaguanidine

Limit Test for Related Compounds

SOLUTIONS

Prepare the following solutions in *methyl alcohol*:

(1) A 1·0 per cent w/v solution of the sample.

(2) A reference solution containing 0·005 per cent w/v of *sulphanilamide A.S.*

MOBILE PHASE

Chloroform, 4 volumes + *methyl alcohol*, 1 volume.

PROCEDURE

Apply separately to a chromatoplate, prepared with Silica Gel G as the coating substance, a 5-μl portion of solution (1) and of solution (2).

Develop the chromatograms by the general method for thin-layer chromatography, using the mobile phase stated above, allow the plate to dry in a current of air, and spray with a solution prepared by dissolving 1 g of *dimethylaminobenzaldehyde* in 25 ml of *hydrochloric acid* and diluting to 100 ml with *methyl alcohol*.

Any spot, other than the main spot, revealed in the chromatogram obtained with solution (1), is not more intense than the spot revealed in the chromatogram obtained with reference solution (2).

Sulphathiazole

Limit Test for Related Compounds

SOLUTIONS

Prepare the following solutions in a mixture containing 9 volumes of *alcohol (95 per cent)* and 1 volume of *strong ammonia solution*:

(1) A 2 per cent w/v solution of the sample.

(2) A reference solution containing 0·01 per cent w/v of *sulphanilamide A.S.*

MOBILE PHASE

Butyl alcohol, 5 volumes + 1N ammonia, 1 volume.

PROCEDURE

Apply separately to a chromatoplate, prepared with Silica Gel G as the coating substance, a 5-μl portion of solution (1) and of solution (2).

Develop the chromatograms by the general method for thin-layer chromatography, using the mobile phase stated above, and spray with a solution prepared by dissolving 1 g of *dimethyl-aminobenzaldehyde* in 25 ml of *hydrochloric acid* and diluting to 100 ml with *methyl alcohol*.

Any spot, other than the main spot, revealed in the chromatogram obtained with solution (1) is not more intense than the spot revealed in the chromatogram obtained with reference solution (2).

Tartrazine Solution, Compound

Test for the Presence of Tartrazine and of Orange G

SOLUTIONS

Prepare the following solutions:

(1) Use the sample, undiluted.

(2) A reference solution containing 0·75 per cent w/v of *tartrazine A.S.*

(3) A reference solution containing 0·25 per cent w/v of *orange G A.S.*

MOBILE PHASE; PROCEDURE

Using the above solutions, proceed as directed for Green S and Tartrazine Solution, page 864.

Tetracycline

Identification Test

SOLUTIONS
Prepare the following solutions in *methyl alcohol*:
(1) A 0·05 per cent w/v solution of the sample.
(2) A reference solution containing 0·05 per cent w/v of *tetracycline hydrochloride A.S.*

MOBILE PHASE
Ethyl acetate which has been saturated with 0·1M disodium edetate previously adjusted to pH 7 with *dilute ammonia solution.*

PROCEDURE
Prepare a chromatoplate in the following manner:
Boil 50 g of Kieselguhr G with a mixture of 250 ml of *hydrochloric acid* and 250 ml of water for 10 minutes, filter, and wash the filter with water until the washings are alkaline to *congo red*; dry the residue at 105° and spread the plate with a slurry prepared by mixing 25 g of the dried residue with a mixture containing 2·5 ml of a 20 per cent v/v solution of *macrogol 400* in *glycerol* and 47·5 ml of 0·1M disodium edetate previously adjusted to pH 7 with *dilute ammonia solution.*
Allow the prepared chromatoplate to dry at room temperature until the surface acquires a uniform matt appearance, usually after about 1 to 2 hours. Transfer the plate to a tank, the atmosphere of which has been allowed to equilibrate with a saturated solution of *ammonium chloride* for at least 24 hours previously. Allow the plate to remain in the tank for 24 hours and use immediately after removal.
Apply separately to the prepared chromatoplate, a 1-μl portion of solution (1) and of solution (2).
Develop the chromatograms by the general method for thin-layer chromatography, using the mobile phase stated above, allow the plate to dry in air, expose the plate to the vapour of *strong ammonia solution*, and examine under ultraviolet radiation, including radiation of wavelength 366 nm.
The main spot revealed in the chromatogram obtained with solution (1) corresponds to the main spot revealed in the chromatogram obtained with solution (2).

Thiacetazone

Identification Test
Limit Test for p-*Acetamidobenzalazine*

SOLUTIONS
Prepare the following solutions:
(1) A 0·4 per cent w/v solution of the sample in *methyl alcohol*, the mixture being warmed to facilitate solution.
(2) A reference solution prepared by dissolving, with the aid of heat, 0·016 g of p-*acetamido-benzalazine A.S.* in 150 ml of *methyl alcohol*, cooling, diluting to 200 ml with *methyl alcohol*, and further diluting 5 ml of this solution to 100 ml with *methyl alcohol.*
(3) A reference solution containing 0·4 per cent w/v of *thiacetazone A.S.* in *methyl alcohol*, the mixture being warmed to facilitate solution.

MOBILE PHASE
Ethyl acetate

PROCEDURE
Apply separately to a chromatoplate, prepared with Silica Gel GF254 as the coating substance, a 5-μl portion of solution (1), a 10-μl portion of solution (2), and a 5-μl portion of solution (3).
Develop the chromatograms by the general method for thin-layer chromatography, using the mobile phase stated above, allow the plate to dry in a current of air, spray with 2N nitric acid, and, within 2 minutes, examine the plate under ultraviolet radiation, including radiation of wavelength 366 nm.
Identification. The main spot revealed in the chromatogram obtained with solution (1) corresponds in position and colour to the main spot revealed in the chromatogram obtained with reference solution (3).
Limit of p-*acetamidobenzalazine.* Any spot revealed in the chromatogram obtained with solution (1) which corresponds in position to the spot revealed in the chromatogram obtained with reference solution (2) is not more intense than this reference spot.

Thiacetazone Tablets

Test for the Presence of Thiacetazone
Limit Test for p-*Acetamidobenzalazine*

SOLUTIONS
Prepare the following solutions:
(1) Disperse a quantity of the powdered tablets, equivalent to 0·04 g of thiacetazone, in 10 ml of *methyl alcohol*, heat to boiling, filter whilst hot, and allow the filtrate to cool.
(2) and (3) The reference solutions (2) and (3) described in the Identification Test and Limit Test for p-Acetamidobenzalazine in Thiacetazone, above.

MOBILE PHASE; PROCEDURE
Using the above solutions, proceed as described in the Identification Test and Limit Test for p-Acetamidobenzalazine in Thiacetazone, above.

Triamcinolone

Identification Test
Limit Test for Related Foreign Steroids

SOLUTIONS
Prepare the following solutions in a mixture containing 9 volumes of *chloroform* and 1 volume of *methyl alcohol*:
(1) A 1·5 per cent w/v solution of the sample.
(2) A reference solution containing 1·5 per cent w/v of *triamcinolone A.S.*
(3) A reference solution containing 0·03 per cent w/v of each of *prednisolone B.C.R.S.*, *prednisone B.C.R.S.*, and *cortisone acetate B.C.R.S.*

MOBILE PHASE
Dichloromethane, 77 volumes + *solvent ether*, 15 volumes + *methyl alcohol*, 8 volumes + water, 1·2 volumes.

PROCEDURE
Apply separately to a chromatoplate, prepared with Silica Gel G as the coating substance, a 1-μl portion of solution (1), of solution (2), and of solution (3).
Develop the chromatograms by the general

method for thin-layer chromatography, using the mobile phase stated above, allow the plate to dry in a current of air, heat the plate at 105° for 10 minutes, allow to cool, and spray with *alkaline tetrazolium blue solution*.

Identification. The main spot revealed in the chromatogram obtained with solution (1) corresponds in position and colour to the main spot

revealed in the chromatogram obtained with solution (2).

Limit of related foreign steroids. Any spot, other than the main spot, revealed in the chromatogram obtained with solution (1) which corresponds to a spot revealed in the chromatogram obtained with reference solution (3) is not more intense than this reference spot.

B. TESTS FOR THE PRESENCE OF CERTAIN ALKALOIDS IN SPECIFIED PREPARATIONS

General Method for the Preparation of the Sample Solution. Unless otherwise directed, mix 10 ml of the sample with 10 ml of *dilute sulphuric acid*, extract with two successive 10-ml portions of *chloroform*, and discard the chloroform extracts; make the aqueous solution distinctly alkaline to *litmus paper* by the addition of *dilute ammonia solution*, extract with four successive 10-ml portions of *chloroform*, evaporate the combined extracts to dryness, cool the residue, and dissolve it in 0·5 ml of *alcohol (95 per cent)*.

Reference Solutions

The reference solutions are solutions in *alcohol (95 per cent)* containing, individually, 0·1 per cent w/v of the specified reference substance:

a. *Brucine sulphate A.S.*	g. *Hyoscyamine sulphate A.S.*
b. *Cephaëline hydrochloride A.S.*	h. *Lobeline hydrochloride A.S.*
c. *Codeine phosphate*	i. *Morphine sulphate*
d. *Colchicine A.S.*	j. *Noscapine hydrochloride A.S.*
e. *Emetine hydrochloride A.S.*	k. *Papaverine hydrochloride*
f. *Gelsemine A.S.*	l. *Strychnine hydrochloride A.S.*

Mobile Phases

A. *Benzene*, 7 volumes + *ethyl acetate*, 2 volumes + *diethylamine*, 1 volume.

B. *Benzene*, 16 volumes + *ethyl acetate*, 4 volumes + *diethylamine*, 1 volume.

C. *Chloroform*, 9 volumes + *diethylamine*, 1 volume.

D. *Methyl alcohol*.

Procedures

METHOD I. Apply separately to a chromatoplate, prepared with Silica Gel G as the coating substance, the specified volume of the sample solution and a 10-μl portion of the specified reference solution(s).

Develop the chromatograms by the general method for thin-layer chromatography, using the mobile phase specified, heat the chromatoplate at 105° to 110° for 30 minutes, allow to cool, and spray with *dilute potassium iodobismuthate solution*.

A spot is revealed in the chromatogram obtained with the sample solution which corresponds in position and colour to the spot revealed in the chromatogram(s) obtained with the reference solution(s).

In addition to the main spot(s), other subsidiary spots may be revealed in the chromatogram obtained with certain preparations, but these should be ignored.

METHOD II. Proceed as directed in Method I but use Silica Gel GF254 as the coating substance for the chromatoplate.

After drying and allowing to cool, expose the chromatoplate to ultraviolet radiation, including radiation of wavelength 254 nm.

A spot is revealed in the chromatogram obtained with the sample solution which corresponds in position to the spot revealed in the chromatogram obtained with reference solution *b*.

Spray the plate with *dilute potassium iodobismuthate solution*. A spot is revealed in the chromatogram obtained with the sample solution which corresponds in position and colour to the spot revealed in the chromatogram(s) obtained with the reference solution(s), other than reference solution *b*. In addition to the main spot(s), other subsidiary spots may be revealed in the chromatogram of certain preparations, but these should be ignored.

METHOD III. Proceed as directed in Method I but prepare the chromatoplate by mixing the Silica Gel G with 0·1N sodium hydroxide instead of with water, and allow the chromatoplate to dry without the aid of heat.

PROCEDURE FOR INDIVIDUAL PREPARATIONS

Aluminium Hydroxide and Belladonna Mixture
SAMPLE SOLUTION: prepare by the General Method, page 870.

VOLUME APPLIED: 20 μl

REFERENCE SOLUTION: *g*

MOBILE PHASE: *C*

PROCEDURE: Method I

Ammonia and Ipecacuanha Mixture
Proceed as described for Ipecacuanha and Squill Linctus, Paediatric.

Belladonna and Ephedrine Mixture, Paediatric
Proceed as described for Aluminium Hydroxide and Belladonna Mixture.

Belladonna and Ipecacuanha Mixture, Paediatric
SAMPLE SOLUTION: prepare by the General Method, page 870.

VOLUME APPLIED: 20 μl

REFERENCE SOLUTIONS: *b*, *e*, and *g*

MOBILE PHASE: *C*

PROCEDURE: Method II

Belladonna and Phenobarbitone Tablets
Proceed as described for Phenolphthalein Pills, Compound, using 4 tablets, finely powdered.

Belladonna Mixture, Paediatric
Proceed as described for Aluminium Hydroxide and Belladonna Mixture.

Cascara and Belladonna Mixture
SAMPLE SOLUTION: prepare by the General Method, page 870.

VOLUME APPLIED: 10 μl

REFERENCE SOLUTION: *g*

MOBILE PHASE: *C*

PROCEDURE: Method I

Chalk with Opium Mixture, Aromatic
SAMPLE SOLUTION: treat the supernatant liquid obtained in the test for the presence of chalk by the General Method, page 870 for preparing the sample solution, but use four successive 10-ml portions of a mixture containing equal volumes of *chloroform* and *alcohol (95 per cent)*, in place of chloroform, for the alkaline extraction.

VOLUME APPLIED: 10 μl

REFERENCE SOLUTIONS: *c*, *i*, *j*, and *k*

MOBILE PHASE: *B*

PROCEDURE: Method I

Colchicum and Sodium Salicylate Mixture
SAMPLE SOLUTION: shake 20 ml with 25 ml of *solvent ether* and discard the ethereal layer; add 3 ml of 1N sodium hydroxide, extract with three successive 15-ml portions of *chloroform*, evaporate the combined extracts to dryness, and dissolve the residue in 0·5 ml of *alcohol (95 per cent)*.

VOLUME APPLIED: 10 μl

REFERENCE SOLUTION: *d*

MOBILE PHASE: *C*

PROCEDURE: Method I

Gelsemium and Hyoscyamus Mixture, Compound
SAMPLE SOLUTION: prepare by the General Method, page 870, but use 25 ml of the sample instead of 10 ml.

VOLUME APPLIED: 20 μl

REFERENCE SOLUTIONS: *f* and *g*

MOBILE PHASE: *D*

PROCEDURE: Method III

Gentian Mixture, Acid, with Nux Vomica
Proceed as described for Nux Vomica Elixir.

Gentian Mixture, Alkaline, with Nux Vomica
Proceed as described for Nux Vomica Elixir.

Ipecacuanha and Ammonia Mixture, Paediatric
Proceed as described for Ipecacuanha and Squill Linctus, Paediatric.

Ipecacuanha and Morphine Mixture
SAMPLE SOLUTION: prepare by the General Method, page 870, but use four successive 10-ml portions of a mixture containing equal volumes of *chloroform* and *alcohol (95 per cent)*, in place of chloroform, for the alkaline extraction.

VOLUME APPLIED: 10 μl

REFERENCE SOLUTIONS: *b*, *e*, and *i*

MOBILE PHASE: *B*

PROCEDURE: Method II

Ipecacuanha and Squill Linctus, Paediatric
SAMPLE SOLUTION: prepare by the General Method, page 870.

VOLUME APPLIED: 10 μl

REFERENCE SOLUTIONS: *b* and *e*

MOBILE PHASE: *C*

PROCEDURE: Method I

Ipecacuanha Emetic Draught, Paediatric
SAMPLE SOLUTION: prepare by the General Method, page 870, but use 5 ml of the sample instead of 10 ml.

VOLUME APPLIED: 2 μl

REFERENCE SOLUTIONS: *b* and *e*

MOBILE PHASE: *C*

PROCEDURE: Method I

Ipecacuanha Mixture, Paediatric

Proceed as described for Ipecacuanha and Squill Linctus, Paediatric.

Ipecacuanha Mixture, Opiate, Paediatric

SAMPLE SOLUTION: prepare by the General Method, page 870, but use four successive 10-ml portions of a mixture containing equal volumes of *chloroform* and *alcohol* (*95 per cent*) in place of chloroform for the alkaline extraction.

VOLUME APPLIED: 10 μl

REFERENCE SOLUTIONS: *b, e, i, j,* and *k*

MOBILE PHASE: *B*

PROCEDURE: Method II

Kaolin and Morphine Mixture

SAMPLE SOLUTION: centrifuge 10 ml of the sample and reserve the supernatant liquid; extract the residue by shaking with four successive 10-ml portions of a mixture of 38 ml of *acetone* and 2 ml of *dilute ammonia solution*, centrifuging after each extraction.

Combine the extracts, evaporate on a water-bath to about 5 ml, add to the reserved supernatant liquid, mix, add 10 ml of *dilute sulphuric acid*, extract with two successive 10-ml portions of *chloroform*, and discard the extracts.

Make the aqueous solution distinctly alkaline to *litmus paper* with *dilute ammonia solution*, extract with three successive 10-ml portions of a mixture of *chloroform* and *alcohol* (*95 per cent*), evaporate the combined extracts to dryness, cool the residue, and dissolve it in 0·5 ml of *alcohol* (*95 per cent*).

VOLUME APPLIED: 10 μl

REFERENCE SOLUTION: *i*

MOBILE PHASE: *A*

PROCEDURE: Method I

Lobelia and Stramonium Mixture, Compound

SAMPLE SOLUTION: prepare by the General Method, page 870.

VOLUME APPLIED: 10 μl

REFERENCE SOLUTIONS: *g* and *h*

MOBILE PHASE: *C*

PROCEDURE: Method I

Magnesium Trisilicate and Belladonna Mixture

SAMPLE SOLUTION: centrifuge 10 ml of the sample and reserve the supernatant liquid; extract the residue by shaking with successive 10-, 5-, and 5-ml portions of a mixture of 20 ml of *acetone* and 2 ml of *dilute ammonia solution*, centrifuging after each extraction.

Combine the extracts, evaporate on a water-bath to about 5 ml, add to the reserved supernatant liquid, mix, add 10 ml of *dilute sulphuric acid*, and continue by the General Method, page 870, beginning with the words "extract with two successive 10-ml portions . . .".

VOLUME APPLIED: 10 μl

REFERENCE SOLUTION: *g*

MOBILE PHASE: *C*

PROCEDURE: Method I

Nux Vomica Elixir

SAMPLE SOLUTION: prepare by the General Method, page 870.

VOLUME APPLIED: 10 μl

REFERENCE SOLUTIONS: *a* and *l*

MOBILE PHASE: *A*

PROCEDURE: Method I

Nux Vomica Mixture, Acid

Proceed as described for Nux Vomica Elixir.

Nux Vomica Mixture, Alkaline

Proceed as described for Nux Vomica Elixir.

Opium Mixture, Camphorated, Compound

SAMPLE SOLUTION: prepare by the General Method, page 870, but use four successive 10-ml portions of a mixture containing equal volumes of *chloroform* and *alcohol* (*95 per cent*) in place of chloroform for the alkaline extraction.

VOLUME APPLIED: 10 μl

REFERENCE SOLUTIONS: *c, i, j,* and *k*

MOBILE PHASE: *B*

PROCEDURE: Method I

Papaveretum Injection

SAMPLE SOLUTION: dilute 1 ml to 10 ml with water.

VOLUME APPLIED: 10 μl

REFERENCE SOLUTIONS: *c, i, j,* and *k*

MOBILE PHASE: *B*

PROCEDURE: Method I

Papaveretum Tablets

SAMPLE SOLUTION: triturate a quantity of the powdered tablets, equivalent to about 0·01 g of papaveretum, with 2 ml of water, dilute to 10 ml with water, shake well, allow to stand, and use the supernatant liquid.

VOLUME APPLIED: 10 μl

REFERENCE SOLUTIONS: *c, i, j,* and *k*

MOBILE PHASE: *B*

PROCEDURE: Method I

Phenolphthalein Pills, Compound

SAMPLE SOLUTION: disperse 10 pills, finely powdered, in 10 ml of water, add 10 ml of *dilute sulphuric acid*, and continue by the General Method, page 870, beginning with the words "extract with two successive 10-ml portions of *chloroform* . . .".

VOLUME APPLIED: 10 μl

REFERENCE SOLUTION: *g*

MOBILE PHASE: *C*

PROCEDURE: Method I

Potassium Citrate and Hyoscyamus Mixture

SAMPLE SOLUTION: prepare by the General Method, page 870, but use 50 ml of the sample instead of 10 ml.

VOLUME APPLIED: 10 μl

REFERENCE SOLUTION: *g*

MOBILE PHASE: *C*

PROCEDURE: Method I

Stramonium and Potassium Iodide Mixture
Proceed as described for Cascara and Belladonna Mixture.

C. IDENTIFICATION OF PHENOTHIAZINES

Solutions

CHLORPROMAZINE
(1) A 0·2 per cent w/v solution of the sample in *chloroform*.
(2) A reference solution containing 0·2 per cent w/v of *chlorpromazine A.S.* in *chloroform*.

CHLORPROMAZINE ELIXIR
(1) Dilute an appropriate volume of the sample with water to give a solution containing 0·2 per cent w/v of chlorpromazine hydrochloride.
(2) A reference solution containing 0·2 per cent w/v of *chlorpromazine hydrochloride A.S.* in *chloroform*.

CHLORPROMAZINE SUPPOSITORIES
(1) Disperse one suppository by warming with 40 ml of *alcohol* (*95 per cent*), cool at 0° for 30 minutes, and filter.
(2) A reference solution containing 0·2 per cent w/v of *chlorpromazine A.S.* in *chloroform*.

ISOTHIPENDYL HYDROCHLORIDE
(1) A 0·2 per cent w/v solution of the sample in *chloroform*.
(2) A reference solution containing 0·2 per cent w/v of *isothipendyl hydrochloride A.S.* in *chloroform*.

ISOTHIPENDYL TABLETS
(1) Shake a quantity of the powdered tablets, equivalent to about 0·02 g of isothipendyl hydrochloride, with 10 ml of *chloroform*, filter, and use the filtrate.
(2) A reference solution containing 0·2 per cent w/v of *isothipendyl hydrochloride A.S.* in *chloroform*.

PROMETHAZINE ELIXIR
(1) Dilute an appropriate volume of the sample with water to give a solution containing 0·08 per cent w/v of promethazine hydrochloride.
(2) A reference solution containing 0·2 per cent w/v of *promethazine hydrochloride A.S.* in *chloroform*.

THIOPROPAZATE HYDROCHLORIDE
(1) A 0·2 per cent w/v solution of the sample in *chloroform*.
(2) A reference solution containing 0·2 per cent w/v of *thiopropazate hydrochloride A.S.* in *chloroform*.

THIOPROPAZATE TABLETS
(1) Shake a quantity of the powdered tablets, equivalent to about 0·05 g of thiopropazate hydrochloride, with 25 ml of *chloroform*, filter, and use the filtrate.
(2) A reference solution containing 0·2 per cent w/v of *thiopropazate hydrochloride A.S.* in *chloroform*.

TRIMEPRAZINE TARTRATE
(1) A 0·2 per cent w/v solution of the sample in *chloroform*.
(2) A reference solution containing 0·2 per cent w/v of *trimeprazine tartrate A.S.* in *chloroform*.

TRIMEPRAZINE ELIXIR, PAEDIATRIC
(1) Dilute 4 ml of the sample to 10 ml with water.
(2) A reference solution containing 0·2 per cent w/v of *trimeprazine tartrate A.S.* in *chloroform*.

TRIMEPRAZINE ELIXIR, PAEDIATRIC, STRONG
(1) Dilute 3 ml of the sample to 9 ml with water.
(2) A reference solution containing 0·2 per cent w/v of *trimeprazine tartrate A.S.* in *chloroform*.

TRIMEPRAZINE INJECTION
(1) Dilute an appropriate volume of the sample with *alcohol* (*95 per cent*) to give a solution containing 0·2 per cent w/v of trimeprazine tartrate.
(2) A reference solution containing 0·2 per cent w/v of *trimeprazine tartrate A.S.* in *chloroform*.

TRIMEPRAZINE TABLETS
(1) Shake a quantity of the powdered tablets, equivalent to 0·04 g of trimeprazine tartrate, with 20 ml of *chloroform*, filter, and use the filtrate.
(2) A reference solution containing 0·2 per cent w/v of *trimeprazine tartrate A.S.* in *chloroform*.

Chromatoplate Impregnation Liquids
A. Mix 10 ml of *phenoxyethanol* with 5 ml of *macrogol 300* and dilute to 100 ml with *acetone*.

B. Mix 2·5 ml of *phenoxyethanol* with 7·5 ml of *formamide* and dilute to 100 ml with *acetone*.

Mobile Phase
To 100 ml of *light petroleum* (*boiling-range, 40° to 60°*), add 2 ml of *diethylamine*, mix, add 8 ml of *phenoxyethanol*, shake, allow to separate, and use the cloudy upper layer.

Procedure
(i) *For chlorpromazine, isothipendyl hydrochloride, promethazine, and trimeprazine tartrate.* Prepare a chromatoplate using Kieselguhr G as the coating substance. Impregnate the prepared plate by immersing it to a depth of 5 mm in a closed chamber containing a suitable volume of impregnation liquid A, described above, until the solvent front has risen at least 17 cm.
Remove the plate from the impregnation liquid, allow the plate to dry in a current of air, and apply, separately, a 2-µl portion of the solution (1) and of the solution (2) appropriate to the substance or preparation being tested, except that in the case of Promethazine Elixir and of Paediatric Trimeprazine Elixir, a 5-µl portion of solution (1) should be applied.
Develop the chromatograms, in the same direction in which the impregnation of the plate was carried out, by the general method for thin-layer chromatography, page 858, using the mobile phase stated above; the chromatoplate should be protected from light during the development.
Examine the plate under ultraviolet radiation, including radiation of wavelength 366 nm, and observe the fluorescence after exposure to the radiation for 2 minutes; spray the plate with a 10 per cent v/v solution of *sulphuric acid* in *alcohol* (*95 per cent*) and observe the colour of the spots.

Allow the plate to stand for 20 minutes, note the stability of the spots, and again examine the plate under ultraviolet radiation, including radiation of wavelength 366 nm.

The main spot revealed in the chromatogram obtained with solution (1) corresponds in position to the main spot revealed in the chromatogram obtained with reference solution (2) and has the characteristics given in the table, below.

(ii) *For thiopropazate hydrochloride.* Prepare a chromatoplate using Kieselguhr G as the coating substance. Impregnate the prepared plate by immersing to a depth of 5 mm in a closed chamber containing a suitable volume of impregnation liquid B, described above, until the solvent front has risen at least 17 cm.

Remove the plate from the impregnation liquid, allow to dry in a current of air, and apply, separately, a 2-μl portion of the solution (1) and

of the solution (2) appropriate to the substance or preparation being tested.

Develop the chromatograms in the same direction in which impregnation of the plate was carried out, by the general method for thin-layer chromatography, using the mobile phase stated above; the chromatoplate should be protected from light during development.

Examine the plate under ultraviolet radiation, including radiation of wavelength 366 nm, and observe the fluorescence after exposure to the radiation for 2 minutes; dry the plate at 120° for 20 minutes, allow to cool, and spray with a 10 per cent v/v solution of *sulphuric acid* in *alcohol (95 per cent)*.

The main spot revealed in the chromatogram obtained with solution (1) corresponds in position with the main spot revealed in the chromatogram obtained with reference solution (2) and has the characteristics shown in the table, below.

Substance	Fluorescence	Colour with *sulphuric acid*	Stability of spot	Fluorescence after 20 minutes
Chlorpromazine	green-blue	violet	stable	weak
Isothipendyl	blue	yellow	stable	very strong
Promethazine	blue	red-violet	fades	insignificant
Trimeprazine	blue	pink	stable	insignificant
Thiopropazate	green-blue	violet	—	—

D. TESTS FOR THE PRESENCE OF CERTAIN STEROIDS IN SPECIFIED PREPARATIONS

Reference Solutions

The reference solutions are 0·25 per cent w/v solutions of the following substances in the specified solvent:

a. Betamethasone valerate A.S. in *alcohol (95 per cent)*.

b. Betamethasone sodium phosphate A.S. in *alcohol (95 per cent)*.

c. Hydrocortisone B.C.R.S. in *alcohol (95 per cent)*.

d. Hydrocortisone acetate B.C.R.S. in *chloroform*.

e. Hydrocortisone sodium phosphate A.S. in *methyl alcohol*.

f. Hydrocortisone sodium succinate A.S. in *methyl alcohol*.

Mobile Phase

A. *Butyl alcohol*, 3 volumes + *acetic anhydride*, 1 volume + water, 1 volume; it should be freshly prepared.

B. *Dichloromethane*, 77 volumes + *solvent ether*, 15 volumes + *methyl alcohol*, 8 volumes + water, 1·2 volumes.

Visualisation Methods

I. Spray with a 10 per cent v/v solution of *sulphuric acid* in *alcohol (95 per cent)*, heat at 120° for 10 minutes, and examine under ultraviolet radiation, including radiation of wavelength 366 nm.

II. Spray with *alkaline tetrazolium blue solution*.

Procedure

Apply separately to a chromatoplate, prepared with Silica Gel G as the coating substance, the specified volume of the prepared sample solution and a 5-µl portion of the specified reference solution.

Develop the chromatograms by the general method for thin-layer chromatography, page 858, using the mobile phase specified, allow the plate to dry in a current of air, and carry out the specified visualisation procedure.

The main spot revealed in the chromatogram obtained with the sample solution corresponds in position and colour to the main spot revealed in the chromatogram obtained with the reference solution. In addition to the main spot, other subsidiary spots may be revealed in the chromatogram obtained with certain preparations, but these should be ignored.

PROCEDURE FOR INDIVIDUAL PREPARATIONS

Betamethasone Eye-drops
SAMPLE SOLUTION: use the sample, undiluted.

VOLUME APPLIED: 10 µl

REFERENCE SOLUTION: *b*

MOBILE PHASE: *A*

VISUALISATION METHOD: I

Betamethasone Valerate Cream
SAMPLE SOLUTION: mix 2·5 g of the sample with 10 ml of *alcohol (95 per cent)*, heat to boiling, cool, allow to stand at 0° for 30 minutes, filter, and use the filtrate.

VOLUME APPLIED: 5 µl

REFERENCE SOLUTION: *a*

MOBILE PHASE: *A*

VISUALISATION METHOD: I

Betamethasone Valerate Lotion
SAMPLE SOLUTION: disperse, by warming and shaking, a volume of the sample, equivalent to 0·0025 g of betamethasone valerate, in 20 ml of *alcohol (95 per cent)*, cool, allow to stand at 0° for 30 minutes, filter, and evaporate the filtrate to 1 ml.

VOLUME APPLIED: 5 µl

REFERENCE SOLUTION: *a*

MOBILE PHASE: *A*

VISUALISATION METHOD: I

Betamethasone Valerate Ointment
Proceed as described for Betamethasone Valerate Cream.

Betamethasone Valerate Scalp Application
SAMPLE SOLUTION: use the sample, undiluted.

VOLUME APPLIED: 10 µl

REFERENCE SOLUTION: *a*

MOBILE PHASE: *A*

VISUALISATION METHOD: I

Betamethasone Valerate with Chlortetracycline Ointment
Proceed as described for Betamethasone Valerate Cream.

Hydrocortisone and Clioquinol Ointment
Proceed as described for Hydrocortisone Cream.

Hydrocortisone and Neomycin Cream
SAMPLE SOLUTION: prepare as directed for Hydrocortisone Cream, using 5 g of the sample.

VOLUME APPLIED: 5 µl

REFERENCE SOLUTION: *c*

MOBILE PHASE: *B*

VISUALISATION METHOD: II

Hydrocortisone and Neomycin Ear-drops
SAMPLE SOLUTION: the sample, diluted if necessary with *alcohol (95 per cent)* to give a solution containing 0·25 per cent w/v of hydrocortisone acetate.

VOLUME APPLIED: 5 µl

REFERENCE SOLUTION: *d*

MOBILE PHASE: *B*

VISUALISATION METHOD: II

Hydrocortisone and Neomycin Eye-drops
Proceed as directed for Hydrocortisone and Neomycin Ear-drops.

Hydrocortisone and Neomycin Eye Ointment
SAMPLE SOLUTION: prepare as directed for Hydrocortisone Cream, using 1·67 g of the sample.

VOLUME APPLIED: 5 µl

REFERENCE SOLUTION: *d*

MOBILE PHASE: *B*

VISUALISATION METHOD: II

Hydrocortisone Cream
SAMPLE SOLUTION: disperse, by warming and shaking, 2·5 g of the sample in 10 ml of *alcohol (95 per cent)*, cool, allow to stand at 0° for 30 minutes, filter, and use the filtrate.

VOLUME APPLIED: 5 µl

REFERENCE SOLUTION: *c* or *d*, as appropriate

MOBILE PHASE: *B*

VISUALISATION METHOD: II

Hydrocortisone Eye-drops
Proceed as directed for Hydrocortisone and Neomycin Ear-drops.

Hydrocortisone Eye Ointment
SAMPLE SOLUTION: prepare as directed for Hydrocortisone Cream.

VOLUME APPLIED: 5 µl

REFERENCE SOLUTION: *d*

MOBILE PHASE: *B*

VISUALISATION METHOD: II

Hydrocortisone Lotion
SAMPLE SOLUTION: prepare as directed for Hydrocortisone Cream but evaporate the filtrate to a volume of 1 ml.

VOLUME APPLIED: 5 µl

REFERENCE SOLUTION: *c*

MOBILE PHASE: *B*

VISUALISATION METHOD: II

Hydrocortisone Lozenges
SAMPLE SOLUTION: shake a quantity of the powdered lozenges, equivalent to 0·025 g of hydrocortisone, with 10 ml of *alcohol (95 per cent)*, filter, and use the filtrate.

VOLUME APPLIED: 5 µl

REFERENCE SOLUTION: *f*

MOBILE PHASE: *A*

VISUALISATION METHOD: I

Hydrocortisone Sodium Phosphate Injection
SAMPLE SOLUTION: dilute a volume of the sample, equivalent to about 0·2 g of hydrocortisone sodium phosphate, to 100 ml with water.

VOLUME APPLIED: 5 µl

REFERENCE SOLUTION: *e*

MOBILE PHASE: *A*

VISUALISATION METHOD: I

Hydrocortisone Suppositories
Proceed as directed for Hydrocortisone Cream, using one suppository.

Appendix 6

Quantitative Test for Arsenic

The apparatus, reagents, and solutions and the general method of testing to be used for the quantitative test for arsenic in the substances of the British Pharmaceutical Codex are, unless otherwise specified, those of Appendix VIA of the British Pharmacopoeia.

This Appendix gives the method of preparing the solution from the substance to be examined, together with the quantity of the substance to be taken when the test is used as a limit test, in which, unless otherwise directed, the stain produced is not deeper than the 1-ml Standard Stain, corresponding to the arsenic limit stated in the monograph.

When the solution to be examined is prepared for use in both the quantitative test for arsenic and for lead, the reagents and solutions used in the preparation of the solution to be examined must also comply with the requirements for reagents and solutions in the quantitative test for lead.

ADDITIONAL REAGENTS

Arsenic Solution, Standard, Dilute: dilute 10 ml of *strong standard arsenic solution* to 100 ml with water; 1 ml contains 1 µg of As.

Arsenic Solution, Standard, Strong: dissolve a quantity of *arsenic trioxide*, equivalent to 1·320 g of As_2O_3, in 20 ml of 2N sodium hydroxide and dilute to 2000 ml with water; further dilute 20 ml of this solution to 1000 ml with water; 1 ml contains 10 µg of As.

Calcium Hydroxide AsT: *Calcium hydroxide* which complies with the following additional test:

Dissolve 5 g in 25 ml of *brominated hydrochloric acid AsT* and 35 ml of water, remove the excess of bromine with a few drops of *stannous chloride solution AsT*, and apply the general test; no visible stain is produced.

Hydrochloric Acid (constant-boiling composition) AsT: boil *hydrochloric acid AsT* to constant boiling composition in the presence of *hydrazine hydrate*, using 1 ml of a 10 per cent w/v solution in water per litre of the acid.

Mercuric Bromide Paper: prepare a 5 per cent w/v solution of *mercuric bromide* in *alcohol (95 per cent)* and immerse in it pieces, each measuring 15 mm by 20 cm, of white filter paper weighing 80 g per m² and having a speed of filtration of 40 to 60 seconds per 100 ml of water at 20° with a filter surface of 10 cm² and a constant pressure of 50 mmHg.

Decant the excess liquid, allow the paper to dry, protected from light, by suspending it over a non-metallic thread, cut off the folded edge to a width of 1 cm, and similarly remove the outer edges; it should be stored in a stoppered bottle, protected from light.

Zinc, Activated: cover a suitable quantity of *zinc AsT* with sufficient of a 0·005 per cent w/v solution of *platinic chloride* in water, allow to stand for 10 minutes, decant, wash the metal with water, and dry immediately.

ACTIVITY. To 5 g add 15 ml of *hydrochloric acid* and 25 ml of water; add 0·1 ml of *stannous chloride solution*, 5 ml of *potassium iodide solution*, and 1 ml of *dilute standard arsenic solution* and apply the general test; an appreciable stain is produced.

ARSENIC. Transfer 5 g to an apparatus for the determination of arsenic prepared with *mercuric bromide paper* instead of mercuric chloride paper, add 15 ml of *hydrochloric acid AsT*, 25 ml of water, 0·1 ml of *stannous chloride solution AsT* and 5 ml of *potassium iodide solution*, and allow the reaction to proceed for 2 hours; no stain is produced on the mercuric bromide paper.

METHODS OF PREPARING THE SOLUTIONS TO BE EXAMINED AND THE LIMITS OF ARSENIC IN PARTS PER MILLION (*p.p.m.*)

Acetic Acid, Glacial   *2 p.p.m.*
Mix 5 g with 50 ml of water and 10 ml of *stannated hydrochloric acid AsT*.

Alginic Acid   *3 p.p.m.*
Mix 3·3 g with 3 g of *anhydrous sodium carbonate AsT*, add 10 ml of *bromine solution AsT*, mix thoroughly, and evaporate to dryness on a waterbath; gently ignite the residue in a porcelain dish, cool, add 16 ml of *brominated hydrochloric acid AsT* and 45 ml of water, and remove the excess bromine by the addition of 2 ml of *stannous chloride solution AsT*.

Aluminium Magnesium Silicate   *3 p.p.m.*
Disperse 1·25 g in 50 ml of water and add 10 ml of *stannated hydrochloric acid AsT*.

Ammonia Solution, Strong   *0·4 p.p.m.*
Evaporate 22·5 g on a water-bath until reduced to 5 ml, add 40 ml of water and 15 ml of *brominated hydrochloric acid AsT*, and remove the excess of bromine with a few drops of *stannous chloride solution AsT*.

Ammonium Bicarbonate   *2 p.p.m.*
Boil 5 g with 50 ml of water until the greater part of the ammonia is volatilised, then add 15 ml of *brominated hydrochloric acid AsT*, and remove the excess of bromine with a few drops of *stannous chloride solution AsT*.

Antimony Potassium Tartrate   *8 p.p.m.*
Dissolve 1·25 g in 10 ml of water and 16 ml of *stannated hydrochloric acid AsT* in a flask, connect to a condenser, and distil 20 ml; wash the flask and condenser, return the distillate to the flask, add 1 drop of *stannous chloride solution AsT*, and redistil 16 ml; to the distillate add 45 ml of water and 2 drops of *stannous chloride solution AsT*.

Bismuth Carbonate   *5 p.p.m.*
Mix 0·2 g with 2 ml of water, add 2 ml of *hydrochloric acid AsT*, and warm, if necessary, until dissolved.
The stain produced by this solution should be compared with the stain produced by 1 ml of *standard arsenic solution*, both stains being prepared using *mercuric bromide paper* in the apparatus, adding 5 g of *activated zinc* instead of 10 g

of zinc AsT, and allowing the reaction to proceed for at least 2 hours.

Bismuth Subgallate   *2 p.p.m.*
Mix 5 g with 1 g of *calcium hydroxide AsT* and 5 ml of water in a porcelain dish, dry, and ignite gently.
Dissolve the residue in 20 ml of *brominated hydrochloric acid AsT* and 10 ml of water, transfer to a small flask, remove the excess of bromine with a few drops of *stannous chloride solution AsT*, connect to a condenser, and distil 22 ml; to the distillate add 40 ml of water and 3 drops of *stannous chloride solution AsT*.

Bismuth Subnitrate   *2 p.p.m.*
Mix 5 g with 5 ml of water, add 2 ml of *sulphuric acid AsT*, and heat until white fumes are evolved; cool, add 5 ml of water, again heat until white fumes are evolved, and cool.
Dissolve the residue in 20 ml of water and 10 ml of *stannated hydrochloric acid AsT*, connect to a condenser, and distil 20 ml; add to the distillate sufficient *bromine solution AsT* to oxidise any sulphurous acid, remove the excess of bromine with *stannous chloride solution AsT*, and add 40 ml of hot water.

Calcium Acetate   *2 p.p.m.*
Dissolve 5 g in 50 ml of water and add 10 ml of *stannated hydrochloric acid AsT*.

Calcium Alginate   *3 p.p.m.*
Mix 3·3 g with 10 ml of *bromine solution AsT*, evaporate to dryness on a water-bath, ignite gently, cool, dissolve the residue, ignoring any carbon, in a mixture of 50 ml of water and 14 ml of *brominated hydrochloric acid AsT*, and remove the excess bromine by the addition of *stannous chloride solution AsT*.

Calcium Phosphate   *4 p.p.m.*
Dissolve 2·5 g in 50 ml of water and 12 ml of *stannated hydrochloric acid AsT*.

Calcium Sodium Lactate   *2 p.p.m.*
Dissolve 5 g in 50 ml of water and 12 ml of *stannated hydrochloric acid AsT*.

Caramel   *5 p.p.m.*
Heat gently 4 g with 25 ml of water and 10 ml of
nitric acid AsT in a long-necked flask until frothing has subsided, cool, add gradually 10 ml of
sulphuric acid AsT, and heat until the mixture
becomes perceptibly darker; then add *nitric acid
AsT*, dropwise, and continue heating until white
fumes are evolved and the liquid is almost colourless; cool, dilute with water to 30 ml, and reserve
15 ml of this solution for the quantitative test for
lead.
To the remainder of the solution add 15 ml of a
saturated solution of *ammonium oxalate AsT* in
water, boil until white fumes are evolved, cool,
dilute to 50 ml with water, and add 10 ml of
stannated hydrochloric acid AsT and 0·1 ml of
stannous chloride solution AsT.

Carmine   *5 p.p.m.*
Heat gently 5 g with 15 ml of *nitric acid AsT* in
a long-necked flask until the first reaction has
subsided, cool, add gradually 5 ml of *sulphuric
acid AsT*, and continue heating until the solution
is colourless, adding, dropwise, more of the nitric
acid if necessary; cool, add 10 ml of water,
evaporate to low bulk, cool, dilute to 50 ml with
water, and reserve 25 ml of this solution for the
quantitative test for lead.
To the remainder of the solution add 10 ml of
hydrochloric acid AsT, 0·2 ml of *stannous chloride
solution AsT*, and 20 ml of water.

Cellulose, Microcrystalline   *2 p.p.m.*
Prepare the solution by the method given for
Alginic Acid, above, using 5 g.

Charcoal   *2 p.p.m.*
Mix 5 g with 2 g of *calcium hydroxide AsT* and
5 ml of water in a porcelain dish, gently heat to
dryness, and ignite until the organic matter has
been destroyed; cool, add a mixture of 16 ml of
brominated hydrochloric acid AsT and 5 ml of
bromine solution AsT followed by 40 ml of water,
boil gently, adding sufficient *bromine solution AsT*
from time to time to maintain a slight excess,
filter, and remove the excess of bromine with
stannous chloride solution AsT.

Congo Red   *1 p.p.m.*
Heat gently 12·5 g with 20 ml of water and 15 ml
of *nitric acid AsT* in a long-necked flask until the
first reaction has subsided, cool, add gradually
10 ml of *sulphuric acid AsT*, and continue heating
until the solution is colourless, adding, dropwise,
more of the nitric acid if necessary; add 7 ml of
water, evaporate to low bulk, cool, dilute to 25 ml
with water, and reserve 5 ml of this solution for
the quantitative test for lead.
To the remainder of the solution, add 4 ml of
water and 10 ml of *stannated hydrochloric acid AsT*,
connect to a condenser, and distil 20 ml; to the
distillate add 40 ml of water.

Copper Sulphate   *8 p.p.m.*
Dissolve 1·25 g in 10 ml of water, add 15 ml of
hydrochloric acid AsT and sufficient *stannous
chloride solution AsT* to decolorise the solution,
connect to a condenser, and distil 20 ml; to the
distillate add a few drops of *bromine solution AsT*,
remove the excess of bromine with a few drops
of *stannous chloride solution AsT*, and add 40 ml
of water.

Ferric Chloride Solution, Strong   *8 p.p.m.*
Heat 1·25 g in a porcelain dish with 1 ml of
sulphuric acid AsT until white fumes are evolved;
cool, add an equal volume of water, and again
heat until white fumes are evolved; cool, dissolve
the residue in 10 ml of water and 15 ml of *hydrochloric acid AsT*, transfer to a small flask, add
stannous chloride solution AsT until the yellow
colour disappears, connect to a condenser, and
distil 20 ml.
To the distillate add a few drops of *bromine
solution AsT*, remove the excess of bromine with
a few drops of *stannous chloride solution AsT*, and
add 40 ml of water.

Hypromellose   *2 p.p.m.*
To 5 g in a dry Kjeldahl flask add 20 ml of *nitric
acid AsT*, warm cautiously until the reaction
begins, allow the reaction to subside without
further heating, add a mixture of 20 ml of *nitric
acid AsT* and 5 ml of *sulphuric acid AsT*, and heat
until brown fumes cease to be evolved; add 0·5 ml
of *perchloric acid (60 per cent w/w)*, heat until
white fumes appear, and, if the liquid is still dark
in colour, add further small portions of *nitric
acid AsT* and heat until the liquid is pale yellow.
Heat again until white fumes appear, continue
the heating for a further 15 minutes, add 0·5 ml
of *perchloric acid (60 per cent w/w)*, heat for
5 minutes, cool, add 10 ml of water, heat until
white fumes appear, cool, add a further 5 ml of
water, and again heat until white fumes appear;
allow to cool and add 40 ml of water and 10 ml of
stannated hydrochloric acid AsT.

Iron   *100 p.p.m.*
Mix 1 g with 1 g of *potassium chlorate AsT* and
10 ml of water and add 15 ml of *hydrochloric acid
AsT*.
When the reaction has ceased and all the iron is
dissolved, boil gently to expel the chlorine, removing the last traces with *stannous chloride
solution AsT*, connect to a condenser, and distil
16 ml; dilute the distillate to 50 ml with water;
to 5 ml of this solution add 10 ml of *stannated
hydrochloric acid AsT* and 45 ml of water.

Iron Phosphate   *4 p.p.m.*
Mix 2·5 g with 1·5 g of *anhydrous sodium carbonate AsT*, add 10 ml of *bromine solution AsT*, mix
thoroughly, evaporate to dryness on a water-bath,
gently ignite, cool, and dissolve the residue in
20 ml of *brominated hydrochloric acid AsT* and
10 ml of water.
Transfer the solution to a small flask, add sufficient *stannous chloride solution AsT* to remove the
yellow colour, connect to a condenser, and distil
22 ml; to the distillate add 40 ml of water and
0·15 ml of *stannous chloride solution AsT*.

Kaolin, Heavy   *2 p.p.m*
Disperse 5 g in 50 ml of water and add 10 ml of
stannated hydrochloric acid AsT.

Magnesium Acetate   *2 p.p.m.*
Dissolve 5 g in 50 ml of water and add 10 ml of
stannated hydrochloric acid AsT.

Magnesium Hydroxide   *2 p.p.m.*
Dissolve 5 g in 20 ml of *brominated hydrochloric
acid AsT* and 40 ml of water and remove the excess bromine by the addition of *stannous chloride
solution AsT*.

Malt Extract   *1 p.p.m.*
Dissolve 10 g in 30 ml of water in a 500-ml flat-bottomed flask with ground-glass neck, add 10 ml of *hydrochloric acid AsT* and about 0·1 g of a suitable antifoaming agent, such as antifoam A (suspension of silica in dimethicone), boil under a reflux condenser for 2 hours, cool, transfer to the apparatus for the general test with the aid of 20 ml of water, add 0·1 ml of *bromine solution AsT*, and remove the excess of bromine with *stannous chloride solution AsT*.

Manganese Sulphate   *4 p.p.m.*
Dissolve 2·5 g in 50 ml of water and add 10 ml of *stannated hydrochloric acid AsT*.

Methylcellulose   *1 p.p.m.*
As for Hypromellose, page 878, but use a 0·5-ml standard stain.

Nitric Acid   *1 p.p.m.*
Heat 10 g in a porcelain dish with 2 ml of *sulphuric acid AsT* until white fumes are evolved; cool, add 2 ml of water, and again heat until white fumes are evolved; cool and add 50 ml of water and 10 ml of *stannated hydrochloric acid AsT*.

Polysorbate 20   *3 p.p.m.*
Heat gently 3·3 g with 2 ml of *nitric acid AsT* and 0·5 ml of *sulphuric acid AsT*, in a long-necked flask, until the first reaction has subsided, cool, add carefully and in small portions, 15 ml of *nitric acid AsT* and 6 ml of *sulphuric acid AsT*, taking care to avoid excessive foaming, and continue heating, adding further small portions of *nitric acid AsT*, if necessary, until white fumes are evolved and the solution becomes colourless or nearly colourless.
Cool, carefully add 10 ml of water, evaporate until white fumes are evolved, and repeat the addition of water and evaporation until all the nitric acid has been removed.
Cool, dilute to 50 ml with water, and add 10 ml of *stannated hydrochloric acid AsT*.

Polysorbate 60   *3 p.p.m.*
As for Polysorbate 20.

Polysorbate 80   *3 p.p.m.*
As for Polysorbate 20.

Potassium Acetate   *2 p.p.m.*
Dissolve 5 g in 50 ml of water and add 15 ml of *stannated hydrochloric acid AsT*.

Potassium Acid Tartrate   *1 p.p.m.*
Dissolve 10 g in 50 ml of water and 13 ml of *brominated hydrochloric acid AsT* and remove the excess of bromine with a few drops of *stannous chloride solution AsT*.

Potassium Bicarbonate   *2 p.p.m.*
Dissolve 5 g in 50 ml of water, add 15 ml of *brominated hydrochloric acid AsT*, and remove the excess of bromine with a few drops of *stannous chloride solution AsT*.

Potassium Chlorate   *2 p.p.m.*
Mix 5 g with 20 ml of water and 22 ml of *hydrochloric acid AsT*; when the first reaction has subsided, warm to expel the chlorine, removing the last traces with *stannous chloride solution AsT*, and add 20 ml of water.

Potassium Gluconate   *2 p.p.m.*
Dissolve 5 g in 50 ml of water and 12 ml of *stannated hydrochloric acid AsT*.

Potassium Sorbate   *2 p.p.m.*
As for Calcium Alginate, page 877, but use 5 g.

Povidone   *2 p.p.m.*
As for Alginic Acid, page 877, but use 5 g.

Sodium Alginate   *3 p.p.m.*
As for Calcium Alginate, page 877.

Sodium Carbonate   *2 p.p.m.*
Dissolve 5 g in a mixture of 25 ml of water and 5 ml of *hydrochloric acid AsT*, boil, cool, neutralise to *litmus paper* by the addition of 2N sodium hydroxide solution, and dilute to 50 ml with water; use 5 ml of this solution for the test.
The stain produced by this solution should be compared with the stain produced by 1 ml of *dilute standard arsenic solution*, both stains being prepared by using *mercuric bromide paper* in the apparatus, adding 5 g of *activated zinc* instead of 10 g of zinc AsT, and allowing the reaction to proceed for at least 2 hours.

Sodium Carboxymethylcellulose   *1 p.p.m.*
As for Hypromellose, page 878, but use a 0·5 ml standard stain.

Sodium Nitrite   *2 p.p.m.*
Heat 5 g in a porcelain dish with 2 ml of *sulphuric acid AsT* and 5 ml of water until white fumes are evolved, cool, add 5 ml of water, and again heat until white fumes are evolved; cool and add 50 ml of water and 5 ml of *stannated hydrochloric acid AsT*.

Sodium Perborate   *8 p.p.m.*
Heat 1·25 g in a porcelain dish with 5 ml of *sulphuric acid AsT* and 5 ml of water until white fumes are evolved, cool, add 5 ml of water, and again heat until white fumes are evolved; cool and add 50 ml of water and 5 ml of *stannated hydrochloric acid AsT*.

Sodium Polymetaphosphate   *2 p.p.m.*
Dissolve 5 g in 50 ml of water and add 15 ml of *stannated hydrochloric acid AsT*.

Sodium Potassium Tartrate   *2 p.p.m.*
As for Sodium Polymetaphosphate, above.

Sodium Sulphate, Anhydrous   *3·3 p.p.m.*
Dissolve 3 g in 50 ml of water and add 10 ml of *stannated hydrochloric acid AsT*.

Sodium Sulphite   *2 p.p.m.*
Mix 5 g in a porcelain dish with 10 ml of water, 1·25 g of *potassium chlorate AsT*, and 16 ml of *hydrochloric acid AsT*, allow to stand for 1 hour, and heat to expel chlorine; remove the last traces of chlorine by the addition of *stannous chloride solution AsT* and add 35 ml of water.

Sorbic Acid   *2 p.p.m.*
As for Alginic Acid, page 877, but use 5 g.

Sorbitan Monolaurate   *3 p.p.m.*
As for Polysorbate 20.

Sorbitan Mono-oleate   *3 p.p.m.*
As for Polysorbate 20.

Sorbitan Monostearate   *3 p.p.m.*
As for Polysorbate 20, page 879.

Sorbitol Solution   *1 p.p.m.*
Dissolve 10 g in 50 ml of water, add 10 ml of *brominated hydrochloric acid AsT*, allow to stand for 5 minutes, and remove the excess of bromine by the addition of *stannous chloride solution AsT*.

Sulphur, Sublimed   *2 p.p.m.*
Heat 5 g with 50 ml of water and 5 ml of *dilute ammonia solution* on a water-bath for 1 hour, filter, and evaporate the filtrate to dryness.
Boil the residue with 1 g of *anhydrous sodium carbonate AsT* and 10 ml of water and add, dropwise, while boiling, *bromine solution AsT* until the mixture is yellow, add 5 ml of *hydrochloric acid AsT*, and boil gently to expel the bromine.
Remove the last traces of bromine by the addition of *stannous chloride solution AsT* and add 50 ml of water and 8 ml of *stannated hydrochloric acid AsT*.

Sulphuric Acid   *2 p.p.m.*
Mix 5 g carefully with 10 ml of water and add 40 ml of water and 8 ml of *stannated hydrochloric acid AsT*.

Syrup, Invert   *1 p.p.m.*
As for Sorbitol Solution, above.

Titanium Dioxide   *5 p.p.m.*
Mix 1 g intimately with 2 g of *potassium carbonate* and ignite in a furnace at about 950° for 30 minutes.
Allow to cool, break up the mass, transfer to a flask, add 0·1 ml of *stannous chloride solution AsT*

and 30 ml of *hydrochloric acid (constant-boiling composition) AsT*, attach a condenser to the flask, heat at just below the boiling-point for 1 hour, and then distil 16 ml; to the distillate add 45 ml of water and 0·1 ml of *stannous chloride solution AsT*.
Use the 0·5-ml standard stain for comparison.

Yeast, Dried   *2 p.p.m.*
Heat gently 5 g with 25 ml of water and 10 ml of *nitric acid AsT* in a long-necked flask until frothing has subsided, cool, add gradually 10 ml of *sulphuric acid AsT*, and heat until the mixture begins to darken; then add *nitric acid AsT*, drop-wise, and continue heating until white fumes are evolved and the liquid is almost colourless.
Cool, add 25 ml of a saturated solution of *ammonium oxalate AsT* in water, and boil until white fumes are evolved; cool, dilute to 50 ml with water, and add 10 ml of *stannated hydrochloric acid AsT* and 0·1 ml of *stannous chloride solution AsT*.

Zinc Chloride   *10 p.p.m.*
Dissolve, as completely as possible, 2·0 g in 38 ml of *carbon dioxide-free water* and then add *dilute hydrochloric acid*, dropwise, until solution is complete; use 2 ml of this solution for the test.
The stain produced by this solution should be compared with the stain produced by 1 ml of *dilute standard arsenic solution*, both stains being prepared using *mercuric bromide paper* in the apparatus, adding 5 g of *activated zinc* instead of 10 g of zinc AsT, and allowing the reaction to proceed for at least 2 hours.

Appendix 7

Quantitative Test for Lead

The apparatus, reagents, and solutions and the general methods of testing to be used for the quantitative test for lead in the substances of the British Pharmaceutical Codex are those of Appendix VIC of the British Pharmacopoeia.

This Appendix gives the methods for the preparation of the primary and the auxiliary solutions and the quantities of *dilute lead solution PbT* corresponding to the lead limits stated in the monograph.

When the solution to be examined is prepared for use in both the quantitative test for arsenic and for lead, the reagents and solutions used in the preparation of the solution to be examined must also comply with the requirements for reagents and solutions used in the quantitative test for arsenic.

ADDITIONAL REAGENTS

Ammonium Citrate Solution PbT: dissolve 400 g of *citric acid PbT* in water, add gradually about 340 ml of *strong ammonia solution* until alkaline to *litmus paper*, and dilute to 1000 ml with water. The resulting solution complies with the following test:

To 25 ml add 1 ml of *potassium cyanide solution PbT*, dilute to 50 ml with water, and add two drops of *sodium sulphide solution PbT*; no darkening is produced.

Potassium Hydroxide Solution PbT: dissolve 33 g of *potassium hydroxide* in sufficient water to produce 100 ml.

The solution complies with the quantitative test for lead, 25 ml being used in the primary solution, 5 ml together with 0·5 ml of *dilute lead solution PbT* in the auxiliary solution, and the addition of *acetic acid PbT* and *ammonia solution PbT* being omitted.

METHODS OF PREPARING PRIMARY AND AUXILIARY SOLUTIONS AND THE LIMITS OF LEAD IN PARTS PER MILLION (*p.p.m.*)

Acetic Acid, Glacial   *3 p.p.m.*
PRIMARY SOLUTION. Use 7 g of the sample.

AUXILIARY SOLUTION. Use 2 g of the sample; 1·5 ml of *dilute lead solution PbT* is used in the test.

Alginic Acid   *10 p.p.m.*
PRIMARY SOLUTION. Ignite 2 g with *sulphuric acid PbT* and dissolve the residue in 5 ml of *acetic acid PbT* and 5 ml of water.

AUXILIARY SOLUTION. Prepare as described for the primary solution but omit the sample; 2 ml of *dilute lead solution PbT* is used in the test.

Aluminium Powder   *100 p.p.m.*
PRIMARY SOLUTION. Boil 0·4 g with 20 ml of *dilute hydrochloric acid PbT* and 10 ml of water until effervescence ceases, add 0·5 ml of *nitric acid PbT*, boil for 30 seconds, and cool; add 2 g of *ammonium chloride PbT* and 2 g of *ammonium thiocyanate*, extract with three successive 10-ml portions of a mixture of equal volumes of *amyl alcohol* and *solvent ether*, reject the extracts, and add 2 g of *citric acid PbT*.

AUXILIARY SOLUTION. Dissolve 2 g of *citric acid PbT* in 10 ml of *dilute hydrochloric acid PbT*; 4 ml of *dilute lead solution PbT* is used in the test.

Amitriptyline Embonate   *20 p.p.m.*
PRIMARY SOLUTION. Ignite 1 g until thoroughly charred, add 2 ml of *nitric acid PbT* and 0·1 ml of *sulphuric acid PbT*, heat gently until white fumes are evolved, and ignite until free from carbon; cool, add 2 ml of *hydrochloric acid PbT* and evaporate to dryness on a water-bath. Moisten the residue with *hydrochloric acid PbT*, add 10 ml of hot water, heat for two minutes, add, dropwise, *ammonia solution PbT* until just alkaline, make slightly acid with *dilute acetic acid PbT* and add a further 2 ml, filter, and dilute to 25 ml with water.

AUXILIARY SOLUTION. Use 2 ml of *acetic acid PbT*; 2 ml of *dilute lead solution PbT* is used in the test.

Ammonia Solution, Strong   *1 p.p.m.*
PRIMARY SOLUTION. Use 12 g of the sample.

AUXILIARY SOLUTION. Use 2 g of the sample; 1 ml of *dilute lead solution PbT* is used in the test.

Ammonium Bicarbonate   *5 p.p.m.*
PRIMARY SOLUTION. Use 7 g of the sample and 25 ml of *acetic acid PbT*.

AUXILIARY SOLUTION. Use 2 g of the sample and 10 ml of *acetic acid PbT*; 2·5 ml of *dilute lead solution PbT* is used in the test.

Ammonium Phosphate   *20 p.p.m.*
PRIMARY SOLUTION. Use 7 g of the sample and 5 ml of *acetic acid PbT*.

AUXILIARY SOLUTION. Use 2 g of the sample and 5 ml of *acetic acid PbT*; 10 ml of *dilute lead solution PbT* is used in the test.

Antimony Potassium Tartrate   *20 p.p.m.*
PRIMARY SOLUTION. Dissolve 2 g in a solution of 1 g of *sodium potassium tartrate* in water and add 7 ml of *sodium hydroxide solution PbT*. No *ammonia solution PbT* is used subsequently in the test.

AUXILIARY SOLUTION. Follow the directions given for the primary solution, using 1 g; 2 ml of *dilute lead solution PbT* is used in the test.

Calcium Acetate   *10 p.p.m.*
PRIMARY SOLUTION. Use 12 g of the sample and 5 ml of *acetic acid PbT*.

AUXILIARY SOLUTION. Use 2 g of the sample and 5 ml of *acetic acid PbT*; 10 ml of *dilute lead solution PbT* is used in the test.

Calcium Alginate   *10 p.p.m.*
PRIMARY and AUXILIARY SOLUTIONS. Prepare as described for Alginic Acid; 2 ml of *dilute lead solution PbT* is used in the test.

Calcium Phosphate   *5 p.p.m.*
PRIMARY SOLUTION. Dissolve 4 g in 25 ml of *dilute hydrochloric acid PbT*, add 0·1 ml of *copper sulphate solution*, and pass a current of *hydrogen sulphide* through the solution to saturation. Filter, wash the precipitate with 50 ml of *hydrogen sulphide solution*, transfer the precipitate to a 100-ml flask, add 1 ml of *sulphuric acid PbT* and 2 ml of *nitric acid PbT*, and heat gently until oxidation begins.
Remove from the source of heat until the reaction subsides and then continue heating until the liquid becomes dark brown.
Complete the oxidation by adding *nitric acid PbT*, dropwise, and heat until white fumes are evolved. Cool, add 5 ml of water, and heat until white fumes are again evolved. Cool, add 20 ml of water and 5 g of *ammonium acetate PbT*, allow to dissolve, and make alkaline with *ammonia solution PbT*.

AUXILIARY SOLUTION. Dissolve 5 g of *ammonium acetate PbT* in 20 ml of water and make alkaline with *ammonia solution PbT*; 2 ml of *dilute lead solution PbT* is used in the test.

Calcium Sodium Lactate   *10 p.p.m.*
PRIMARY SOLUTION. Use 3 g of the sample and 5 ml of *acetic acid PbT*.

AUXILIARY SOLUTION. Use 1 g of the sample and 2 ml of *acetic acid PbT*; 2 ml of *dilute lead solution PbT* is used in the test.

Caramel   *5 p.p.m.*
PRIMARY SOLUTION. To 15 ml of the solution prepared in the quantitative test for arsenic, page 878, add 10 ml of water and 2 g of *citric acid PbT*, shake to dissolve, make alkaline with *ammonia solution PbT*, add 1 ml of *potassium cyanide solution PbT*, and extract with 10 ml of *diphenylthiocarbazone solution PbT*, shaking vigorously; separate off the lower layer and extract again with

two further successive 5-ml portions of *diphenyl-thiocarbazone solution PbT*.

If, after the third extraction, the lower layer is bright red, continue the extraction with 5-ml portions of *diphenylthiocarbazone solution PbT* until the colour of the reagent no longer changes to bright red.

Wash the combined extracts by shaking with 10 ml of water, discard the washing, and extract with two successive 10-ml portions of *dilute hydrochloric acid PbT*; wash the combined acid extracts with 10 ml of *chloroform* and discard the washing.

AUXILIARY SOLUTION. Mix 2 ml of *acetic acid PbT* with 20 ml of *dilute hydrochloric acid PbT*; 1 ml of *dilute lead solution PbT* is used in the test.

Carmine   10 p.p.m.
PRIMARY SOLUTION. Add 12 ml of *potassium hydroxide solution PbT* to 10 ml of the solution prepared in the quantitative test for arsenic, page 878.

AUXILIARY SOLUTION. Use 12 ml of *potassium hydroxide solution PbT*; 1·7 ml of *dilute lead solution PbT* is used in the test.

Cellulose, Microcrystalline   10 p.p.m.
PRIMARY SOLUTION. Mix 5 g with 10 ml of a 10 per cent w/v solution of *magnesium nitrate* in water, evaporate to dryness, heat to char the organic matter, and then ignite at a temperature of 450° to 500° until a white ash is obtained.

Moisten the residue with 10 ml of water, add 10 ml of 5N hydrochloric acid, cover the dish, and heat for 20 minutes, replacing any water lost by evaporation.

Filter, wash the filter with hot water, cool the combined filtrate and washings, dilute to 50 ml with water, and, using 20 ml of this solution, continue by the method given for the preparation of the primary solution under Caramel, above, beginning with the words "add 10 ml of water . . .".

AUXILIARY SOLUTION. Mix 2 ml of *acetic acid PbT* with 20 ml of *dilute hydrochloric acid PbT*; 2 ml of *dilute lead solution PbT* is used in the test.

Clefamide   10 p.p.m.
PRIMARY SOLUTION. Ignite 1 g in a silica basin until completely ashed, at a temperature not exceeding 450°, dissolve the residue in a mixture of 0·5 ml of *nitric acid PbT* and 5 ml of water, dilute to 40 ml with water, add 5 ml of *ammonium thiocyanate solution*, and extract with successive portions of a mixture of equal volumes of *amyl alcohol* and *solvent ether* until no further colour is removed.

AUXILIARY SOLUTION. Dilute 0·5 ml of *nitric acid PbT* to 40 ml with water and continue by the method given for the primary solution, beginning with the words "add 5 ml of *ammonium thiocyanate solution* . . ."; 1 ml of *dilute lead solution PbT* is used in the test.

Congo Red   10 p.p.m.
PRIMARY SOLUTION. Carry out the method given for the preparation of the primary solution under Caramel, above, using 4 ml of the solution prepared in the quantitative test for arsenic, page 878.

AUXILIARY SOLUTION. Mix 2 ml of *acetic acid PbT* with 20 ml of *dilute hydrochloric acid PbT*; 2 ml of *dilute lead solution PbT* is used in the test.

Ferric Chloride Solution, Strong   60 p.p.m.
PRIMARY SOLUTION. Mix 1·67 g with 12 ml of *hydrochloric acid PbT*, add 0·5 ml of *nitric acid PbT*, boil very gently for five minutes, cool, and extract the iron with three successive 20-ml portions of *solvent ether*; make a fourth extraction with a further 20 ml of *solvent ether* if the acid solution is more than faintly yellow.

Wash the fourth ether extract with 5 ml of a mixture of 2 volumes of *hydrochloric acid PbT* and 1 volume of water, reject the extracts, transfer the acid solution and washings to a narrow-necked flask, boil to remove part of the hydrochloric acid, and make alkaline with *ammonia solution PbT*.

AUXILIARY SOLUTION. Mix 10 ml of *hydrochloric acid PbT* and 0·5 ml of *nitric acid PbT* and make alkaline with *ammonia solution PbT*; 10 ml of *dilute lead solution PbT* is used in the test.

Hypromellose   5 p.p.m.
PRIMARY and AUXILIARY SOLUTIONS. Prepare as described for Microcrystalline Cellulose, but use 10 g of the sample; 2 ml of *dilute lead solution PbT* is used in the test.

Iron   100 p.p.m.
PRIMARY SOLUTION. Dissolve 0·4 g, as completely as possible, by warming with 2 ml of *hydrochloric acid PbT*, 1 ml of water, and 0·25 ml of *nitric acid PbT*; add 1 ml of *nitric acid PbT*, evaporate almost to dryness, dissolve the residue by warming with 6 ml of *hydrochloric acid PbT*, add 2 ml of water, cool, extract with four successive 5-ml portions of *solvent ether*, reject the extracts, and evaporate to dryness.

Dissolve the residue in 1 ml of *dilute hydrochloric acid PbT* and add 20 ml of water.

AUXILIARY SOLUTION. Use 1 ml of *dilute hydrochloric acid PbT*; 4 ml of *dilute lead solution PbT* is used in the test.

Iron Phosphate   50 p.p.m.
PRIMARY SOLUTION. Dissolve 0·5 g in 5 ml of *hydrochloric acid PbT* and 7 ml of water, add 6 ml of *ammonium citrate solution PbT* and 10 ml of *potassium cyanide solution PbT*, and extract with successive portions of 10 ml, 5 ml, and 5 ml of *diphenylthiocarbazone solution PbT*.

Wash the combined extracts with 5 ml of water, evaporate to dryness on a water-bath, add 2 ml of *sulphuric acid PbT*, and heat until white fumes are evolved; add, dropwise, *nitric acid PbT* until the liquid is almost colourless and continue heating until white fumes are again evolved; cool, dilute to 25 ml with water, boil, cool, and add 2 g of *ammonium acetate PbT*.

AUXILIARY SOLUTION. Dissolve 2 g of *ammonium acetate PbT* in 2 ml of *sulphuric acid PbT* diluted with water; 2·5 ml of *dilute lead solution PbT* is used in the test.

Kaolin, Heavy   10 p.p.m.
PRIMARY SOLUTION. Mix 10 g with 70 ml of water and 10 ml *hydrochloric acid PbT*, heat under a reflux condenser on a water-bath for 15 minutes, and filter.

To 40 ml of the filtrate add 0·5 ml of *nitric acid PbT*, evaporate to small volume, add 20 ml of water, 2 g of *ammonium chloride PbT*, and 2 g of *ammonium thiocyanate*, and extract with two successive 10-ml portions of a mixture containing equal parts of *amyl alcohol* and *solvent ether*.

Discard the extracts and to the aqueous solution add 2 g of *citric acid PbT*.

AUXILIARY SOLUTION. Mix 5 ml of *hydrochloric acid PbT* and 30 ml of water and continue by the method given above for the primary solution beginning with the words "[add] 2 g of *ammonium chloride PbT* . . ."; 5 ml of *dilute lead solution PbT* is used in the test.

Magnesium Acetate   *20 p.p.m.*
PRIMARY and AUXILIARY SOLUTIONS. Prepare as described for Calcium Acetate, page 881; 2 g of *ammonium chloride PbT* is added to each solution before making alkaline and 10 ml of *dilute lead solution PbT* is used in the test.

Magnesium Hydroxide   *20 p.p.m.*
PRIMARY SOLUTION. Use 3 g of the sample and 25 ml of *acetic acid PbT*.

AUXILIARY SOLUTION. Use 1 g of the sample and 10 ml of *acetic acid PbT*; 4 ml of *dilute lead solution PbT* is used in the test.

Manganese Sulphate   *20 p.p.m.*
PRIMARY SOLUTION. Dissolve 1·5 g in 20 ml of water and add 2 ml of *acetic acid PbT* and 2 g of *ammonium chloride PbT*.
Carry out the test by adding 1 ml of *potassium cyanide solution PbT*, making strongly alkaline with *ammonia solution PbT*, adjusting the volume to 35 ml with water, and adding 15 ml of *hydrogen sulphide solution*.

AUXILIARY SOLUTION. Prepare as described for the primary solution but use 0·5 g of the sample; 2 ml of *dilute lead solution PbT* is used in the test.

Methylcellulose   *5 p.p.m.*
PRIMARY and AUXILIARY SOLUTIONS. Prepare as described for Microcrystalline Cellulose, page 882, but use 10 g of the sample; 2 ml of *dilute lead solution PbT* is used in the test.

Nitric Acid   *2 p.p.m.*
PRIMARY SOLUTION. Use 7 g of the sample.

AUXILIARY SOLUTION. Use 2 g of the sample; 1 ml of *dilute lead solution PbT* is used in the test.

Piperazine Hydrate   *10 p.p.m.*
PRIMARY SOLUTION. Dissolve 4 g in 30 ml of water and add 1 g of *citric acid PbT*.

AUXILIARY SOLUTION. Dissolve 2 g in 30 ml of water and add 1 g of *citric acid PbT* in 30 ml of water; 2 ml of *dilute lead solution PbT* is used in the test.

Potassium Acetate   *2 p.p.m.*
PRIMARY SOLUTION. Use 12 g of the sample and 5 ml of *acetic acid PbT*.

AUXILIARY SOLUTION. Use 2 g of the sample and 5 ml of *acetic acid PbT*; 2 ml of *dilute lead solution PbT* is used in the test.

Potassium Acid Tartrate   *10 p.p.m.*
PRIMARY SOLUTION. Dissolve 7 g in *ammonia solution PbT*, warming if necessary, and add 5 ml of *acetic acid PbT*.

AUXILIARY SOLUTION. Dissolve 2 g in *ammonia solution PbT*, warming if necessary, and add 5 ml of *acetic acid PbT*; 5 ml of *dilute lead solution PbT* is used in the test.

Potassium Bicarbonate   *5 p.p.m.*
PRIMARY SOLUTION. Use 7 g of the sample and 20 ml of *acetic acid PbT*.

AUXILIARY SOLUTION. Use 2 g of the sample and 10 ml of *acetic acid PbT*; 2·5 ml of *dilute lead solution PbT* is used in the test.

Potassium Chlorate   *10 p.p.m.*
PRIMARY SOLUTION. Use 2 g of the sample and 5 ml of *acetic acid PbT*.

AUXILIARY SOLUTION. Use 1 g of the sample and 5 ml of *acetic acid PbT*; 1 ml of *dilute lead solution PbT* is used in the test.

Potassium Gluconate   *10 p.p.m.*
PRIMARY SOLUTION. Use 7 g of the sample and 5 ml of *acetic acid PbT*.

AUXILIARY SOLUTION. Use 2 g of the sample and 5 ml of *acetic acid PbT*; 5 ml of *dilute lead solution PbT* is used in the test.

Potassium Sorbate   *10 p.p.m.*
PRIMARY SOLUTION. Use 12 g of the sample and 5 ml of *acetic acid PbT*.

AUXILIARY SOLUTION. Use 2 g of the sample and 5 ml of *acetic acid PbT*; 10 ml of *dilute lead solution PbT* is used in the test.

Povidone   *10 p.p.m.*
PRIMARY and AUXILIARY SOLUTIONS. Prepare as described for Potassium Chlorate, above; 1 ml of *dilute lead solution PbT* is used in the test.

Prothionamide   *10 p.p.m.*
PRIMARY SOLUTION. Ignite 1 g gently until thoroughly charred, cool, add 2 ml of *nitric acid PbT* and five drops of *sulphuric acid PbT*, heat cautiously until white fumes are evolved, and ignite until the residue is free from carbon.
Cool, add 2 ml of *hydrochloric acid PbT*, evaporate to dryness on a water-bath, and dissolve the residue in a mixture of 2 ml of *acetic acid PbT* and 10 ml of hot water.

AUXILIARY SOLUTION. Use 2 ml of *acetic acid PbT*; 1 ml of *dilute lead solution PbT* is used in the test.

Sodium Alginate   *10 p.p.m.*
PRIMARY and AUXILIARY SOLUTIONS. Prepare as described for Alginic Acid, page 881; 2 ml of *dilute lead solution PbT* is used in the test.

Sodium Carboxymethylcellulose   *10 p.p.m.*
PRIMARY and AUXILIARY SOLUTIONS. Prepare as described for Microcrystalline Cellulose, page 882, but use 10 g of the sample; 4 ml of *dilute lead solution PbT* is used in the test.

Sodium Nitrite   *10 p.p.m.*
PRIMARY SOLUTION. Use 7 g of the sample and 5 ml of *acetic acid PbT*.

AUXILIARY SOLUTION. Use 2 g of the sample and 5 ml of *acetic acid PbT*; 5 ml of *dilute lead solution PbT* is used in the test.

Sodium Perborate   *10 p.p.m.*
PRIMARY SOLUTION. Dissolve 4 g by warming with 20 ml of *dilute hydrochloric acid PbT*, evaporate to dryness, with stirring, and dissolve the residue in 5 ml of *acetic acid PbT* diluted with 35 ml of hot water.

AUXILIARY SOLUTION. Prepare as described for the primary solution but using 2 g of the sample; 2 ml of *dilute lead solution PbT* is used in the test.

Sodium Polymetaphosphate   25 p.p.m.
PRIMARY SOLUTION. Use 7 g of the sample and 5 ml of *acetic acid PbT*.

AUXILIARY SOLUTION. Use 2 g of the sample and 5 ml of *acetic acid PbT*; 12·5 ml of *dilute lead solution PbT* is used in the test.

Sodium Potassium Tartrate   10 p.p.m.
PRIMARY SOLUTION. Dissolve 7 g in 30 ml of water and add 1 g of *citric acid PbT* and 10 ml of *acetic acid PbT*.

AUXILIARY SOLUTION. Dissolve 2 g in 30 ml of water and add 1 g of *citric acid PbT* and 7 ml of *acetic acid PbT*; 5 ml of *dilute lead solution PbT* is used in the test.

Sodium Sulphite   10 p.p.m.
PRIMARY SOLUTION. Use 7 g of the sample and 10 ml of *acetic acid PbT*.

AUXILIARY SOLUTION. Use 2 g of the sample and 5 ml of *acetic acid PbT*; 5 ml of *dilute lead solution PbT* is used in the test.

Sorbic Acid   10 p.p.m.
PRIMARY and AUXILIARY SOLUTIONS. Prepare as described for Potassium Acid Tartrate, page 883; 5 ml of *dilute lead solution PbT* is used in the test.

Sorbitol Solution   1 p.p.m.
PRIMARY SOLUTION. Use 12 g of the sample and 5 ml of *acetic acid PbT*.

AUXILIARY SOLUTION. Use 2 g of the sample and 5 ml of *acetic acid PbT*; 1 ml of *dilute lead solution PbT* is used in the test.

Sulphaguanidine   10 p.p.m.
PRIMARY SOLUTION. Boil 2 g with a solution of 2 g of *ammonium acetate PbT* in a mixture of 5 ml of *acetic acid PbT* and 40 ml of water until a clear solution is obtained, cool, and filter by suction.

AUXILIARY SOLUTION. Dissolve 2 g of *ammonium acetate PbT* in a mixture of 5 ml of *acetic acid PbT* and 40 ml of water; 2 ml of *dilute lead solution PbT* is used in the test.

Sulphathiazole   10 p.p.m.
PRIMARY SOLUTION. Dissolve 2 g in 7 ml of *sodium hydroxide solution PbT*.

AUXILIARY SOLUTION. Dissolve 1 g in 7 ml of *sodium hydroxide solution PbT*; 1 ml of *dilute lead solution PbT* is used in the test.

Sulphuric Acid   10 p.p.m.
PRIMARY SOLUTION. Use 4 g of the sample.

AUXILIARY SOLUTION. Use 2 g of the sample; 2 ml of *dilute lead solution PbT* is used in the test.

Suramin   10 p.p.m.
PRIMARY SOLUTION. Mix 2 g with 10 ml of *fuming nitric acid PbT* in a large, round-bottomed, long-necked flask and, when the initial reaction has subsided, heat very gently until the volume is reduced to one-half, controlling the frothing by removing the flask from the source of heat; cool, add dropwise and at intervals 5 ml of *sulphuric acid PbT*, allowing the mixture to cool between each addition, then add, dropwise, 5 ml of *fuming nitric acid PbT*.
When carbonisation is complete and frothing has subsided, heat until white fumes are evolved and the mixture is colourless, cool, add 10 ml of water, heat again until white fumes are evolved, cool, add 5 ml of water, and again heat until white fumes are evolved; cool, dilute to 20 ml with water, and continue by the method given for the preparation of the primary solution under Caramel, page 881, beginning with the words "add 10 ml of water . . .".

AUXILIARY SOLUTION. Mix 2 ml of *acetic acid PbT* with 20 ml of *dilute hydrochloric acid PbT*; 2 ml of *dilute lead solution PbT* is used in the test.

Syrup, Invert   2 p.p.m.
PRIMARY SOLUTION. Use 12 g of the sample and 5 ml of *acetic acid PbT*.

AUXILIARY SOLUTION. Use 2 g of the sample and 5 ml of *acetic acid PbT*; 2 ml of *dilute lead solution PbT* is used in the test.

Thiacetazone   10 p.p.m.
PRIMARY and AUXILIARY SOLUTIONS. Prepare as described for Amitriptyline Embonate, page 881; 1 ml of *dilute lead solution PbT* is used in the test.

Titanium Dioxide   10 p.p.m.
PRIMARY SOLUTION. Dissolve 3 g of *citric acid PbT* in 20 ml of the solution reserved in the determination of acid-soluble antimony, page 511.

AUXILIARY SOLUTION. Dissolve 3 g of *citric acid PbT* in 18 ml of 0·5N hydrochloric acid; 2 ml of *dilute lead solution PbT* is used in the test.

Appendix 8

Quantitative Tests for Copper, Lead, Zinc, and Heavy Metals

This appendix describes methods for the determination of copper, lead, and zinc in charcoal, of copper and lead in dried yeast, of lead in bismuth carbonate, in bismuth subgallate and bismuth subnitrate, in polysorbates 20, 60, and 80, and in sorbitan monolaurate, sorbitan mono-oleate, and sorbitan monostearate, and of heavy metals in aluminium sulphate, in sodium carbonate, and in anhydrous sodium sulphate.

ADDITIONAL REAGENTS

Most of the reagents required in these determinations are described in Appendix VIC of the British Pharmacopoeia or in Appendix 1 of the British Pharmaceutical Codex. The following additional reagents are required:

Ammoniacal Potassium Cyanide Solution, Lead-free: dissolve 0·5 g of *potassium cyanide* in 8 ml of *dilute ammonia solution* and dilute to 100 ml with water. The solution complies with the following test:

To 10 ml add 2 ml of *sodium sulphide solution*; the solution does not darken in colour.

Ammonium Citrate Solution, Lead-free: dissolve 21 g of *citric acid* in 62·5 ml of *dilute ammonia solution*, dilute to 100 ml with water, and shake with successive portions of a mixture containing 0·2 ml of *diphenylthiocarbazone solution PbT* and 5 ml of *chloroform* until the colour of the chloroform layer remains constant.

Discard the chloroform layer and wash the aqueous solution with successive 10-ml portions of *chloroform* until the chloroform layer remains colourless.

Borax Buffer Solution: dissolve 3·0 g of *borax* in 90 ml of water and extract with successive 5-ml portions of a mixture of 1 volume of *diphenylthiocarbazone solution PbT* and 4 volumes of *chloroform*, with vigorous shaking, until a blue or purple extract is obtained; continue the extraction with successive 10-ml portions of *chloroform* until a colourless extract is obtained; discard the extracts and dilute the extracted solution to 100 ml with water.

Buffer Solution pH 3·5: dissolve 5·0 g of *ammonium acetate* in 5·5 ml of *hydrochloric acid* and dilute to 20 ml with water.

Citric Acid Solution: a 10 per cent w/v solution of *citric acid PbT* in water.

Copper Solution, Standard: dissolve 0·630 g of *copper sulphate* in sufficient water to produce 1000 ml; dilute 25 ml of this solution to 1000 ml with water; 1 ml contains 4 µg of Cu.

Diphenylthiocarbazone Solution, Standard: extract 15 ml of *diphenylthiocarbazone solution PbT* with two successive 50-ml portions of water containing 5 ml of *dilute ammonia solution*; acidify the combined extracts with *dilute hydrochloric acid PbT* and extract with 100 ml of *chloroform*; wash the extract with two successive 10-ml portions of water and filter through a dry filter.

Determine the approximate strength of this solution by the method for determination of zinc in charcoal (page 886), using 5 ml of *standard zinc solution (A)* diluted to 25 ml with water in place of the 25 ml of reserved acid solution, and dilute with *chloroform* so that 3 ml is approximately equivalent to 1 ml of *standard zinc solution (A)*.

The solution must be freshly prepared.

Hydroxylammonium Hydrochloride Solution, Lead-free: dissolve 10 g of *hydroxylammonium hydrochloride* in 30 ml of water in a separating funnel, add 0·05 ml of *phenol red solution*, make just alkaline by the addition of *dilute ammonia solution*, and shake with successive portions of a mixture containing 0·2 ml of *diphenylthiocarbazone solution PbT* and 5 ml of *chloroform* until the colour of the chloroform layer remains constant.

Discard the chloroform layer and wash the aqueous layer with successive portions of *chloroform* until the chloroform remains colourless.

Discard the chloroform, add 0·05 ml of *methyl red solution*, make just acid by the addition of *hydrochloric acid*, and shake with 10-ml portions of *chloroform* until the chloroform layer remains colourless.

Lead Solution FP, Dilute: dissolve 0·4 g of *lead nitrate* in sufficient water to produce 500 ml and dilute 5 ml of this solution to 100 ml with water.

Lead Solution (A), Standard: dissolve a quantity of *lead nitrate* equivalent to 1·598 g of Pb(NO$_3$)$_2$ in sufficient water to produce 1000 ml; dilute 20 ml of this solution to 100 ml with water; 1 ml contains 2 µg of Pb.

Lead Solution (A), Standard, Dilute: dilute *standard lead solution (A)* with an equal volume of water; 1 ml contains 1 µg of Pb.

Nitric Acid FP, Dilute: dilute 37 ml of *nitric acid PbT* to 100 ml with water.

Sulphurous Acid PbT: *sulphurous acid* which complies with the following test:

Boil 50 ml until most of the sulphur dioxide is removed, make alkaline with *ammonia solution PbT*, add 1 ml of *potassium cyanide solution PbT*, dilute to 50 ml with water, and add two drops of *sodium sulphide solution PbT*. No darkening is produced.

Zinc Solution (A), Standard: dissolve 0·440 g of *zinc sulphate* in sufficient water to produce 1000 ml; dilute 50 ml of this solution to 1000 ml with water; 1 ml contains 5 µg of Zn.

Copper, Lead, and Zinc in Charcoal

Heat 2·0 g with 10 ml of *sulphuric acid PbT* and 5 ml of *nitric acid PbT* in a long-necked flask, adding more of the nitric acid, dropwise, until the mixture is clear and pale yellow in colour.

Cool, add 5 ml of water, evaporate to low bulk, cool, add 5 ml of water, again evaporate to low bulk, cool, and dilute to 100 ml with water; add 10 ml of *citric acid solution*, 5 ml of *sulphurous acid PbT*, and 0·2 ml of *thymol blue solution*, make just alkaline with *ammonia solution PbT*, and extract with successive 5-ml portions of *diphenylthiocarbazone solution PbT* until an extract which is not bright red in colour is obtained.

Wash the combined extracts with 5 ml of water and reject the washings; extract the chloroformic solution with two successive 5-ml portions of 0·1N hydrochloric acid, dilute the combined extracts to 100 ml with water, and reserve this acid solution. Reserve also the chloroformic solution.

Prepare a control by repeating the above procedure, replacing the sample with a mixture of 25 ml of *standard copper solution*, 6 ml of *dilute lead solution PbT*, and 20 ml of *standard zinc solution (A)*, and using a total volume of *nitric acid PbT* equal to that required for the digestion of the sample.

TEST FOR COPPER. Transfer the reserved chloroformic solution to a long-necked flask, evaporate off the chloroform, cool, add 5 ml of *sulphuric acid PbT*, heat gently, and add *strong hydrogen peroxide solution*, dropwise, until the mixture is colourless.

Cool, dilute to 100 ml with water, add 10 ml of *citric acid solution* and 0·2 ml of *thymol blue solution*, and make just alkaline with *dilute ammonia solution*; add 5 ml of *sodium diethyldithiocarbamate solution*, extract with four successive 5-ml portions of *chloroform*, and dilute the combined extracts to 25 ml with *chloroform*.

The colour of the solution is not deeper than that of the chloroformic solution derived from the control when similarly treated.

TEST FOR LEAD. To 50 ml of the reserved acid solution add 0·1 ml of *thymol blue solution* and make just alkaline with *ammonia solution PbT*; add 5 ml of *potassium cyanide solution PbT* and 10 ml of *borax buffer solution* and titrate with *standard diphenylthiocarbazone solution* by adding the reagent in small portions and, after each addition,

shaking vigorously, allowing to separate, and withdrawing the lower chloroformic layer; the end-point is reached when the chloroformic layer remains purple.

The amount of *standard diphenylthiocarbazone solution* used is not more than that required when 50 ml of the reserved acid solution derived from the control is similarly treated.

TEST FOR ZINC. To 25 ml of the reserved acid solution add 0·1 ml of *thymol blue solution* and make just alkaline with *ammonia solution PbT*; add 10 ml of *borax buffer solution* and titrate with *standard diphenylthiocarbazone solution* as described in the test for lead.

From the amount of reagent used subtract half the amount used in the test for lead; the amount of *standard diphenylthiocarbazone solution* is not more than that required when 25 ml of the reserved acid solution derived from the control is similarly treated and half the amount used in the test for lead in the control has been deducted.

Copper and Lead in Dried Yeast

Proceed by the methods given above, using 4·0 g of sample and diluting the combined chloroformic extracts in the test for copper to 100 ml with *chloroform*.

Prepare a control by repeating the procedure, replacing the sample with a mixture of 120 ml of *standard copper solution* and 2·8 ml of *dilute lead solution PbT*, and using a total volume of *nitric acid PbT* equal to that required for the digestion of the sample.

For the test for lead use the whole of the reserved acid solutions derived from the sample and from the control.

Lead in Bismuth Carbonate

Dissolve 0·5 g in a mixture of 2 ml of *nitric acid* and 3 ml of water, evaporate the solution to dryness on a water-bath, ignite the residue gently until brown fumes are evolved and allow to cool; triturate the residue with 9 ml of boiling water, allow to cool, add 1 ml of *strong sodium hydroxide solution*, mix and filter.

Transfer 0·5 ml of the filtrate to a separating funnel containing 2 ml of *lead-free hydroxyl-ammonium hydrochloride solution* and 5 ml of *sodium diethyldithiocarbamate solution*, shake for 2 minutes, and allow to stand for 15 minutes.

Extract with two 5-ml portions of a mixture containing equal volumes of *amyl alcohol* and *toluene*, shaking each extract for 2 minutes; discard the aqueous solution and extract the combined solvent extracts with two successive 2·5-ml portions of 0·1N hydrochloric acid, shaking each extract for 2 minutes; discard the solvent solution and combine the acid extracts.

To the combined acid extracts add 0·05 ml of *phenol red solution*, make just alkaline by the addition of *dilute ammonia solution*, then add 2 ml in excess followed by 2 ml of *lead-free ammonium citrate solution*, 2 ml of *lead-free hydroxylammonium hydrochloride solution* and 10 ml of *lead-free ammonium cyanide solution*, allow to stand for 1 minute, add 0·5 ml of *diphenylthiocarbazone solution PbT* and 9 ml of *chloroform*, shake, allow to separate, transfer the chloroform layer to a second separator, and wash with two successive 10-ml portions of *lead-free ammoniacal potassium cyanide solution*, shaking each washing for 1 minute.

Discard the aqueous solution and washings and dry the chloroform solution by shaking with 0·5 g of *anhydrous sodium sulphate*; any colour in the chloroform solution is not more intense than that produced when a mixture of 2·0 ml of *standard lead solution (A)* and 3·0 ml of water is treated by the method given above, beginning at the words "add 0·05 ml of *phenol red solution . . .*".

Lead in Bismuth Subgallate and Bismuth Subnitrate

The apparatus and general method of testing are those of Method II of the British Pharmacopoeia, Appendix XIA, for atomic absorption spectrophotometry, the measurements being made at a wavelength of 284 nm. The preparation of the sample solutions is described below. *Dilute lead solution FP* is used for the standard solution and *dilute nitric acid FP* is used, instead of water, for making the dilutions and for the initial setting of the spectrophotometer.

PREPARATION OF SAMPLE SOLUTIONS
Bismuth Subgallate. Gently ignite 12·5 g until no carbon remains, dissolve the residue in 75 ml of a mixture containing equal volumes of *nitric acid PbT* and water, cool, and dilute to 100 ml with water.

Bismuth Subnitrate. Dissolve 12·5 g in 75 ml of a mixture containing equal volumes of *nitric acid PbT* and water, heat to boiling, boil gently for 1 minute, cool, and dilute to 100 ml with water.

Lead in Polysorbates and Sorbitan Derivatives

Prepare a solution as directed in the quantitative test for arsenic, but using 3 g and omitting the addition of the stannated hydrochloric acid AsT.

To this solution add 0·1 ml of *thymol blue solution*, make just alkaline by the addition of *ammonia solution PbT*, add 5 ml of *ammonium citrate solution PbT* and 5 ml of *potassium cyanide solution PbT*, and titrate with *standard diphenylthiocarbazone solution*, adding the reagent in small portions and, after each addition, shaking vigorously, allowing to separate, and withdrawing the chloroformic layer; the end-point is reached when the chloroformic layer remains purple.

The volume of standard diphenylthiocarbazone solution used is no more than that required by a solution prepared in the same manner but using 3 ml of *dilute lead solution PbT* in place of the sample and using a total volume of *nitric acid PbT* and *sulphuric acid PbT* equal to that required for the digestion of the sample.

Heavy Metals in Aluminium Sulphate, Sodium Carbonate, and Anhydrous Sodium Sulphate

Add 12 ml of the sample solution, prepared as described below, to 1·2 ml of *thioacetamide reagent*, add 2 ml of *buffer solution pH 3·5*, mix immediately, and allow to stand for 2 minutes.

Any brown colour which develops is not more intense than that which develops in a reference solution prepared at the same time and in the same manner, using 10 ml of the standard lead solution specified below for the individual substance and 2 ml of the prepared sample solution in place of 12 ml.

PREPARATION OF SOLUTIONS
Aluminium Sulphate. Dissolve 2·5 g in sufficient water to produce 50 ml and further dilute 6 ml of this solution to 15 ml with water.
The reference solution is prepared using *dilute standard lead solution (A)*.

Sodium Carbonate. Dissolve 5·0 g, in portions, in a mixture of 25 ml of water and 5 ml of *hydrochloric acid*, boil, cool, neutralise the solution to *litmus paper* with 2N sodium hydroxide, and dilute to 50 ml with water.
The reference solution is prepared using *standard lead solution (A)*.

Sodium Sulphate, Anhydrous. Dissolve 2·2 g in sufficient water to produce 100 ml.
The reference solution is prepared using *dilute standard lead solution (A)*.

Appendix 9

Determination of Distillation Range and Boiling-point

A. DISTILLATION RANGE
The distillation range of a substance is the range of temperature, corrected to standard pressure, within which a specified portion distils.

Apparatus. The apparatus to be used and the mode of assembly comply with the specifications

given in British Standard 658:1962. The apparatus consists of the following items:

DISTILLATION FLASK. A flask having a nominal distillation capacity of 100 ml.

THERMOMETER. An accurately standardised thermometer having a range suitable for the substance being examined and complying with British Standard 593:1954.

DRAUGHT SCREEN. A draught screen which complies with the specification for Type 1 of British Standard 658:1962.

ASBESTOS ADAPTOR BOARD. An asbestos board 150 mm square and 6 mm thick with a central circular hole. The hole is 30 mm in diameter for the distillation of liquids boiling below 60° and 50 mm in diameter for the distillation of other liquids.

SOURCE OF HEAT. A Bunsen burner or other source of heat which can be controlled to give the required rate of distillation.

CONDENSER. A condenser complying with the specification for Type 1 of British Standard 658:1962 is used for liquids boiling below 150° and an unjacketed condenser complying with the specification for Type 2 is used for liquids boiling above 150°.

RECEIVER. A 100-ml Crow receiver which complies with the specification for Type 1 of British Standard 658:1962.

Method. Using the receiver to be used for collecting the distillate, measure 100 ml of the sample, transfer it as completely as possible to the distillation flask, and add a few small pieces of clean porous pot or pumice. Place the receiver, without rinsing or drying it, below the outlet of the condenser so that the end of the tube extends about 2·5 cm below the rim of the receiver.

Read the barometer immediately before distillation and correct the reading to standard conditions as described in British Standard 658:1962.

If the corrected pressure deviates from normal, i.e. 760 mm at 0°, and standard gravity, adjust the temperatures specified in the individual monograph by adding or subtracting, for every 10 mm that the corrected pressure is above or below 760 mm, an amount "k" as indicated in the following table:

Specified temperature	"k"
Below 100°	0·4
100° to 140°	0·45
141° to 190°	0·5
191° to 240°	0·55
Above 240°	0·6

Heat the flask and, when the first drop of distillate falls from the condenser, move the receiver so that the end of the condenser touches the side of the receiver.

Control the rate of distillation so that it is between 4 and 6 ml per minute for liquids boiling below 150° or between 2 and 4 ml per minute for liquids boiling above 150°.

Record the temperatures and volumes of distillate in accordance with the requirements stated in the individual monograph, adjusting the temperature of the distillate to about 20°, if necessary, before measuring the volume.

B. BOILING-POINT

Apparatus. The apparatus consists of the following items:

HEATING BATH. A glass heating vessel of suitable construction and capacity containing a suitable liquid to a depth of not less than 14 cm. Suitable liquids are water, a liquid paraffin of sufficiently high boiling-point, or a silicone fluid of sufficiently high boiling-point.

STIRRING DEVICE. A stirring device capable of rapidly mixing the liquid.

THERMOMETER. An accurately standardised thermometer having a range suitable for the substance being examined and complying with British Standard 1365:1951.

GLASS TUBE. A thin-walled tube of soft soda glass, 12 to 25 cm in length and 2·5 to 3·5 mm in internal diameter and closed at one end.

CAPILLARY TUBE. A thin-walled capillary tube of soft soda glass, 15 to 18 cm in length and about 0·5 mm in external diameter and sealed about 3 to 5 mm from one end.

Method. Introduce about 0·1 ml of the sample into the glass tube and attach the tube to the thermometer by means of a rubber band or piece of wire so that the closed end of the tube is near the middle of the bulb of the thermometer. Insert the capillary tube into the glass tube, with the shorter open end immersed in the liquid.

Place the thermometer assembly in the heating bath so that the immersion mark of the thermometer is at the level of the surface of the liquid.

Heat the bath, with constant stirring and regulating the rate of rise of temperature to 2° to 3° per minute, until the single air bubbles which rise from the capillary tube are replaced by an apparently uninterrupted thread of vapour bubbles.

Remove or diminish the source of heat so that the bath cools at a rate not exceeding 3° per minute until the stream of bubbles ceases and the liquid recedes into the capillary tube.

The temperature at which the liquid recedes into the capillary tube is the boiling-point of the liquid.

Appendix 10

Determination of Alcohol Content

The alcohol content of a preparation in the British Pharmaceutical Codex is determined by Method I, II, or III, described below, as indicated in Table 2. Any special directions needed are indicated by footnotes to the table.

Alternatively, a gas-liquid chromatographic method may be used provided that the analyst is satisfied that the results obtained are of equivalent accuracy.

Method I

Measure 25 ml of the preparation, at 20·0°, in a graduated flask. Transfer the measured volume to a distillation flask of 500- to 800-ml capacity, wash

TABLE 1

ETHYL ALCOHOL (QUADRUPLE BULK)

Specific gravity at 20°/20° of the distillate obtained by distillation to quadruple bulk	Percentage v/v of ethyl alcohol in the original preparation at 20°	Refractive index at 20° of the distillate obtained by distillation to quadruple bulk	Immersion refractometer readings*
0·9710	95·93	1·34661	50·3
0·9720	92·32	1·34605	48·8
0·9730	88·66	1·34549	47·3
0·9740	84·96	1·34493	45·8
0·9750	81·26	1·34437	44·3
0·9760	77·53	1·34380	42·8
0·9770	73·82	1·34324	41·3
0·9780	70·10	1·34267	39·8
0·9790	66·38	1·34211	38·3
0·9800	62·72	1·34154	36·8
0·9810	59·09	1·34098	35·3
0·9820	55·48	1·34044	33·9
0·9830	51·94	1·33991	32·5
0·9840	48·45	1·33942	31·2
0·9850	45·02	1·33892	29·9
0·9860	41·62	1·33842	28·6
0·9870	38·28	1·33796	27·4
0·9880	34·99	1·33751	26·2
0·9890	31·76	1·33705	25·0
0·9900	28·62	1·33663	23·9
0·9910	25·53	1·33620	22·8
0·9920	22·49	1·33578	21·7
0·9930	19·50	1·33540	20·7
0·9940	16·59	1·33501	19·7
0·9950	13·71	1·33466	18·8
0·9960	10·89	1·33432	17·9
0·9970	8·10	1·33397	17·0
0·9980	5·38	1·33362	16·1
0·9990	2·68	1·33331	15·3
1·0000	0·00	1·33300	14·5

* The readings refer to the scale proposed by Pulfrich and are applicable only to instruments calibrated in units corresponding to 14·5 = 1·33300; 50·0 = 1·34650; and 100 = 1·36464.

the graduated flask with 100 to 150 ml of water, add the washings to the distillation flask, add a little *pumice powder*, connect the flask to a condenser by means of a suitable still-head, and distil, collecting at least 90 ml of distillate in a 100-ml graduated flask.
Adjust the temperature of the distillate to 20·0° and dilute to 100 ml with water at the same temperature. Determine the specific gravity at 20·0° and the refractive index at 20·0° of this diluted distillate and if, by reference to the Ethyl Alcohol (Quadruple Bulk) Table (Table 1), the refractive index does not differ by more than

0·00007 (equivalent to 0·2 on the immersion refractometer scale) from that corresponding to the specific gravity, read off the percentage of ethyl alcohol corresponding to the specific gravity.
If the refractive index differs by more than the stated amount, transfer 75 ml of the diluted distillate to a separating funnel, add sufficient *sodium chloride* to saturate the liquid, add 100 ml of *light petroleum (boiling-range, 40° to 60°)*, shake vigorously for 2 to 3 minutes, allow to stand for 15 to 30 minutes, and transfer the lower layer into a distillation flask; wash the light petroleum in the

TABLE 2

Preparation	Method of determination	Preparation	Method of determination
Aminobenzoic Acid Lotion	I	Hamamelis Liquid Extract	I
Ammonia Solution, Aromatic	III[d]	Hamamelis Water	I
Ammonia Spirit, Aromatic	III[d]	Hyoscyamus Liquid Extract	I
Anise Water, Concentrated	II	Lemon Spirit	II
Belladonna Liquid Extract	I	Lobelia Tincture, Ethereal	III[f]
Benzaldehyde Spirit	II	Morphine Hydrochloride Solution	I[b]
Benzoin Tincture	III		
Benzoin Tincture, Compound	III	Myrrh Tincture	III
Brilliant Green and Crystal Violet Paint	I	Nux Vomica Elixir	I
		Opium Tincture, Concentrated Camphorated	III
Camphor Water, Concentrated	II		
Capsicum Tincture	III	Orange Peel Infusion, Concentrated	III
Caraway Water, Concentrated	II		
Cardamom Tincture, Aromatic	III	Orange Spirit, Compound	II
Catechu Tincture	I	Orange Tincture	III
Cetrimide Solution, Strong	I[e]	Paracetamol Elixir, Paediatric	II
Chloroform and Morphine Tincture	III	Peppermint Spirit	II
		Phenobarbitone Elixir	III
Chloroxylenol Solution	II[c]	Quillaia Liquid Extract	I
Cinnamon Water, Concentrated	II[f]	Quillaia Tincture	I
Coal Tar Solution, Strong	III	Salicylic Acid Lotion	III
Cocillana Liquid Extract	I	Senega Infusion, Concentrated	I[a]
Digoxin Elixir, Paediatric	I	Senega Liquid Extract	I[a]
Dill Water, Concentrated	II	Senega Tincture	I[a]
Ephedrine Elixir	III	Senna Liquid Extract	I
Ethamivan Elixir	I	Soap Liniment	I[c]
Ether Spirit	II[f]	Soap Solution, Ethereal	III[d]
Fig Syrup, Compound	III	Soap Spirit	III[d]
Gelsemium Tincture	I	Squill Linctus, Opiate	III[b]
Gentian Tincture, Compound	I	Squill Liquid Extract	I
Ginger Syrup	III	Squill Tincture	I
Glyceryl Trinitrate Solution	II	Tolu Solution	III

[a] After distillation wash the distillate into a 500- to 800-ml flask with about 50 ml of water, acidify with *dilute sulphuric acid*, add a little *pumice powder*, redistil at least 90 ml into a 100-ml graduated flask, and continue by Method I, commencing with the words "Adjust the temperature of the distillate . . .".
[b] Neutralise with *sodium hydroxide solution* before the first distillation.
[c] Acidify with *dilute sulphuric acid* before extraction.
[d] Acidify with *dilute sulphuric acid* before the first distillation.
[e] Before distillation add a few small pieces of clean porous pot or a little *pumice powder* and a sufficient quantity of a silicone antifoaming agent.
[f] With double separation.

separating funnel by shaking vigorously with 25 ml of *brine*, allow to separate, transfer the lower layer to the distillation flask, and distil, collecting about 70 ml of distillate.

Dilute the distillate to 75 ml with water and determine the specific gravity and the refractive index as before.

If the refractive index still does not correspond with the specific gravity, the distillate contains some impurity, and the specific gravity does not indicate the true proportion of ethyl alcohol.

When the distillate contains steam-volatile substances other than alcohol (it will then usually be turbid or contain oily drops), proceed by Method III. When steam-volatile acids are present, make the solution just alkaline by the addition of 1N sodium hydroxide, using solid *phenolphthalein* as indicator, before the final distillation.

Method II

Measure 25 ml of the preparation, at 20·0°, in a graduated flask. Transfer the measured volume to a separating funnel, wash the flask with 100 ml of water, transfer the washings to the separating funnel, add sufficient *sodium chloride* to saturate the liquid, add 100 ml of *light petroleum* (*boiling-range, 40° to 60°*), shake vigorously for 2 to 3 minutes, allow to stand for 15 to 30 minutes, and transfer the lower layer into a distillation flask, wash the light petroleum in the separating funnel by shaking vigorously with 25 ml of *brine*, allow to separate, and transfer the lower layer to the distillation flask.

Where the method stated in Table 2 directs a double separation, transfer the lower layer obtained after the first extraction with light petroleum to a second separating funnel, shake it with a further 100-ml portion of *light petroleum* (*boiling-range, 40° to 60°*), allow to separate, transfer the aqueous solution to a distillation flask, and wash both of the light petroleum extracts with the same 25 ml of *brine*.

Make the combined aqueous solutions just alkaline by the addition of 1N sodium hydroxide, using solid *phenolphthalein* as indicator, add a little *pumice powder* and 100 ml of water, distil, collecting at least 90 ml of distillate, and determine the amount of ethyl alcohol as described in Method I, beginning at the words "Adjust the temperature of the distillate . . .".

Method III

Measure 25 ml of the preparation, at 20·0°, in a graduated flask. Transfer the measured volume to a distillation flask of 500- to 800-ml capacity, wash the graduated flask with 100 to 150 ml of water, add the washings to the distillation flask, add a little *pumice powder*, connect the flask to a condenser by means of a suitable still-head, and distil, collecting 100 ml of distillate.

Transfer the distillate to a separating funnel and continue by Method II, beginning at the words "add sufficient *sodium chloride* . . .".

Tests on the Final Distillate

A. The final distillate obtained by Method I, II, or III complies with the following tests (except where Industrial Methylated Spirit has been used in the formulation of the preparation—see B, below):

1. The refractive index corresponds to the specific gravity. When Method I or Method II, although directed to be used in Table 2, gives a distillate which does not comply with this requirement, Method III is used.

2. Adjust the final distillate to contain approximately 10 per cent v/v of ethyl alcohol, either by dilution with water or by the addition of *alcohol* (*90 per cent*).

To 5 ml of this solution add 2·0 ml of *potassium permanganate and phosphoric acid solution* and allow to stand for 10 minutes; add 2·0 ml of *oxalic acid and sulphuric acid solution* and, to the colourless solution, add 5 ml of *decolorised magenta solution* and allow to stand at a temperature between 15° and 30° for 30 minutes; no colour is produced (absence of Industrial Methylated Spirit).

When industrial methylated spirit has been used for certain preparations, this test will show the presence of methyl alcohol. With certain preparations, the colour in the test, characteristic of the presence of formaldehyde, may be due to the presence in the original preparation of methyl compounds occurring naturally or produced during manufacture, and in this case does not necessarily denote the presence of industrial methylated spirit.

3. Mix 1 ml with 2 ml of *mercuric sulphate solution* and heat just to boiling-point; no precipitate is produced (absence of isopropyl alcohol).

B. For preparations in which, in accordance with the authority given in the individual monographs, Industrial Methylated Spirit has been used, proceed by the method given in Table 2, but omit the determination of the refractive index of the distillate. The final distillate complies with the following tests:

1. Proceed as directed for test 2 under A, above; a violet colour is produced which is similar in intensity to that produced when 0·5 ml of *industrial methylated spirit*, diluted to 5 ml with water, is similarly treated.

2. It complies with test 3 under A, above.

Appendix 11

Electrometric Determination of Bromide, Chloride, and Iodide

Apparatus. A titration vessel, of about 250-ml capacity, is fitted with a stirrer and two electrodes. One of the electrodes, the reference electrode, may be either a mercury/mercurous sulphate half-cell, with a saturated solution of *potassium sulphate* as a bridge, or, preferably, a glass electrode.

The other electrode, the indicator electrode, should be a piece of silver wire, about 3 cm in length and 1 mm in diameter, formed into an open spiral.

Before each determination, the indicator elec-

trode should be washed with *strong ammonia solution* and rinsed with purified water. Any convenient potentiometer may be used, but, if a glass electrode is used as reference electrode, the potentiometer must have a high impedance input through a shielded socket; most commercial pH meters are equipped with a millivolt scale and are suitable for this purpose.

Method. Prepare a solution as directed in the monograph; if necessary, adjust the pH to 5·0 to 6·0 by the addition of *dilute nitric acid* or *sodium* *hydroxide solution* and dilute to 25 ml with water. Add 75 ml of *acetate buffer solution pH 5·0* and, unless otherwise specified, titrate with 0·1N silver nitrate, with constant stirring.

Determine the end-point graphically either by plotting the electromotive force (e.m.f.) against volume of titrant or, preferably, by plotting the rate of change of e.m.f. against volume of titrant

(*d*E/*d*V). In certain cases, the change of e.m.f. is so great that it is unnecessary to titrate beyond the equivalence point.

If the use of 0·02N silver nitrate is specified, satisfactory results may be obtained either by the addition of a suitable colloid, such as a de-ionised gelatin solution, or by diluting the solution to 200 ml with water after adding the buffer solution.

Appendix 12

Assays for Eye-drops

This appendix describes methods for the determination of nitrogenous bases in eye-drops. The methods are designed to take account of the interference due to the use of relatively high concentrations of the basic preservatives, benzalkonium chloride and chlorhexidine acetate, and also the difficulties which may be caused by the wide range of strengths in which the eye-drops are available.

Method I describes the direct determination of the medicament and is to be used when interference from the preservative is negligible, for example when the concentration of the medicament is above 1 per cent or when a phenylmercuric salt is present.

Method II should be used for eye-drops containing less than 1 per cent of medicament when the preservative is benzalkonium chloride and, similarly, Method III when the preservative is chlorhexidine acetate.

With eye-drops containing very low concentrations of medicament it may be found convenient when applying Method I, to reduce the volume of the sodium tetraphenylboron solution added.

Method I

If necessary, dilute the sample with water to produce a solution containing 1 per cent of the medicament.

To 2 ml of the sample or of the dilution add 5 ml of *acetate buffer solution pH 3·7* and 15 ml of 0·01M sodium tetraphenylboron, mix well, allow to stand for 10 minutes, filter through a sintered-glass filter (British Standard Grade No. 4), wash the filter with 5 ml of water, and titrate the excess of sodium tetraphenylboron in the combined filtrate and washings with 0·005M cetylpyridinium chloride, using 0·5 ml of *bromophenol blue solution* as indicator.

Repeat the procedure omitting the sample and the filtration.

From the difference between the two titrations, expressed in terms of 0·01M sodium tetraphenyl-

boron, calculate the concentration of medicament in the sample.

Method II

To 2 ml of the sample in a stoppered flask add 5 ml of *buffer solution pH 10*, 5 ml of *chloroform*, and 0·1 ml of *bromophenol blue solution* and titrate slowly with 0·01M sodium tetraphenylboron, shaking well between successive small additions, until the chloroform layer changes from blue to colourless; the chloroform layer may not become blue until the first drop of titrant is added. The volume of 0·01M sodium tetraphenylboron required is equivalent to the benzalkonium chloride present.

Using a further 2 ml of the sample, carry out the procedure described under Method I to obtain the volume of 0·01M sodium tetraphenylboron equivalent to the total amount of medicament and benzalkonium chloride in the sample.

From the difference between the titrations at pH 3·7 and pH 10, expressed in terms of 0·01M sodium tetraphenylboron, calculate the concentration of medicament in the sample.

Method III

To 2 ml of the sample add 0·4 g of *anhydrous sodium sulphate*, swirl to dissolve, allow to stand for 10 minutes, add 5 ml of *acetate buffer solution pH 3·7* and 5 ml of 0·01M sodium tetraphenyl-boron, allow to stand for 6 minutes, transfer the solution to a sintered-glass filter (British Standard Grade No. 4), wash the beaker with two 1-ml portions of water, adding the washings to the solution in the filter, filter the combined solution and washings, and titrate the excess of sodium tetraphenylboron in the filtrate with 0·005M cetyl-pyridinium chloride, using 0·5 ml of *bromophenol blue solution* as indicator.

Repeat the procedure omitting the sample and the filtration.

From the difference between the two titrations, expressed in terms of 0·01M sodium tetraphenyl-boron, calculate the concentration of medicament in the sample.

Appendix 13

Determination of Volatile Oil in Drugs

The apparatus and general methods used for the determination of volatile oil in a crude drug included in the British Pharmaceutical Codex are those of Appendix IXE of the British Pharmacopoeia, any special directions being indicated in the table below.

Drug	Weight of drug used (grams)	Condition when distilled	Method	Approximate time of distillation (hours)
Clove	4	coarsely crushed	II[a]	4
Fennel	25	whole	II[a]	4
Myrrh	15	No. 710 powder	II	4
Nutmeg	15	No. 710 powder	I	3

[a] Use 150 ml each of *glycerol* and of water in place of 300 ml of water in the distillation flask.

Appendix 14

Examination of Volatile Oils

This appendix describes methods for the determination of aldehydes and carvone in volatile oils and preparations and for the determination of the ester value after acetylation of volatile oils containing linalol.

Determination of Aldehydes

Transfer about 1 g of the sample, accurately weighed, to a glass-stoppered tube, approximately 25 mm in diameter and 150 mm in length, add 5 ml of *toluene* and 15 ml of *hydroxylammonium chloride reagent in alcohol (60 per cent)*, shake vigorously, and titrate immediately with 0·5N potassium hydroxide in alcohol (60 per cent) until the red colour changes to yellow; continue the shaking and neutralising until the full yellow colour of the indicator is permanent in the lower layer after shaking vigorously for 2 minutes and allowing to separate; the reaction is complete in about 15 minutes.

This procedure gives an approximate value for the aldehyde content of the sample.

Obtain an accurate value by carrying out a second determination in exactly the same manner, using, as the colour standard for the end-point of the titration, the titrated liquid of the first determination with the addition of 0·5 ml of 0·5N potassium hydroxide in alcohol (60 per cent).

Calculate the aldehyde content of the sample from this second determination.

Determination of Carvone

Transfer about 1·5 g of the sample, accurately weighed, to a glass-stoppered tube, approximately 25 mm in diameter and 150 mm in length, add 10 ml of *hydroxylammonium chloride reagent in alcohol (90 per cent)*, and titrate with 1N potassium hydroxide in alcohol (90 per cent) until the red colour changes to yellow.

Place the tube in a water-bath at 75° to 80° and, at 5-minute intervals, neutralise the liberated acid with 1N potassium hydroxide in alcohol (90 per cent); after 40 minutes complete the titration to the full yellow colour of the indicator; each ml of 1N potassium hydroxide in alcohol (90 per cent) is equivalent to 0·1514 g (i.e. 0·1502 × 1·008) of carvone.

This procedure gives an approximate value for the carvone content of the oil.

Obtain an accurate value by carrying out a second determination in exactly the same manner, using, as the colour standard for the end-point of the titration, the titrated liquid of the first determination with the addition of 0·5 ml of 1N potassium hydroxide in alcohol (90 per cent).

Calculate the carvone content of the oil from this second determination.

Determination of Ester Value after Acetylation of Volatile Oils containing Linalol

Cool in ice 10 ml of the sample, previously dried with *anhydrous magnesium sulphate* and filtered, mix with 20 ml of *dimethylaniline*, add 8 ml of *acetyl chloride* and 5 ml of *acetic anhydride*, and allow to stand in ice for 5 minutes, then at room temperature for 30 minutes, and finally at 39° to 41° for 3 hours.

Wash the mixture by shaking for 30 seconds with the following solutions: two successive 75-ml portions of a 20 per cent w/v solution of *sodium sulphate* in water; successive 50-ml portions of a 2·5 per cent w/v solution of *sulphuric acid* in the sodium sulphate solution until the last washing produces no turbidity on being made alkaline to *litmus paper* with *sodium hydroxide solution*; two successive 25-ml portions of a 5 per cent w/v solution of *sodium bicarbonate* in the sodium sulphate solution; and finally, two successive 25-ml portions of the sodium sulphate solution. Dry the washed acetylated oil with 3 g of *anhy-* *drous magnesium sulphate*, filter, and determine the ester value of the acetylated oil by the method of Appendix IXB of the British Pharmacopoeia.

Appendix 15

Determination of Reducing Sugars

Prepare a solution of the sample of such concentration that more than 15 ml and less than 50 ml will be required for the titration.

For a preliminary titration, measure 10·0 ml of *potassium cupri-tartrate solution* into a conical flask of about 300-ml capacity. From a burette, add 15 ml of the prepared solution, and heat to boiling over an asbestos-covered wire gauze. Continue adding the prepared solution in fairly large portions at 15-second intervals, until, from the colour of the mixture, the reduction appears to be nearly complete, then boil for 2 minutes, add 0·2 ml of *methylene blue solution*, and continue the titration until the blue colour is discharged.

Carry out an accurate determination by repeating the preliminary titration, but adding, before heating, almost the full amount of the prepared solution required to reduce all the copper; after boiling has commenced, maintain a moderate degree of ebullition for 2 minutes, and, without removing the flame, add 0·2 ml of *methylene blue solution*.

Continue the titration so that it is just complete in a total boiling time of exactly 3 minutes; the end-point is clearly indicated by the disappearance of the blue colour, the solution becoming orange. The flask must not be removed from the gauze at any stage of the titration.

Method for Invert Syrup. Using Table A, below, calculate, as invert sugars, the reducing sugars present in 100 ml of the prepared solution and hence the percentage, weight in weight, in the sample.

Method for Haemodialysis and Intraperitoneal Dialysis Solutions. Using Table B, calculate, as anhydrous dextrose, the reducing sugars present in 100 ml of the prepared solution and hence the percentage, weight in volume, in the sample.

TABLE A

Quantity of prepared solution required (millilitres)	Invert sugar factor*	Quantity of invert sugar per 100 ml (milligrams)	Quantity of prepared solution required (millilitres)	Invert sugar factor*	Quantity of invert sugar per 100 ml (milligrams)
15	50·5	336·0	33	51·7	156·6
16	50·6	316·0	34	51·7	152·2
17	50·7	298·0	35	51·8	147·9
18	50·8	282·0	36	51·8	143·9
19	50·8	267·0	37	51·9	140·2
20	50·9	254·5	38	51·9	136·6
21	51·0	242·9	39	52·0	133·3
22	51·0	231·8	40	52·0	130·1
23	51·1	222·2	41	52·1	127·1
24	51·2	213·3	42	52·1	124·2
25	51·2	204·8	43	52·2	121·4
26	51·3	197·4	44	52·2	118·7
27	51·4	190·4	45	52·3	116·1
28	51·4	183·7	46	52·3	113·7
29	51·5	177·6	47	52·4	111·4
30	51·5	171·7	48	52·4	109·2
31	51·6	166·3	49	52·5	107·1
32	51·6	161·2	50	52·5	105·1

* Milligrams of invert sugar corresponding to 10 millilitres of *potassium cupri-tartrate solution*.

TABLE B

Quantity of prepared solution required (millilitres)	Dextrose factor*	Quantity of anhydrous dextrose per 100 ml (milligrams)	Quantity of prepared solution required (millilitres)	Dextrose factor*	Quantity of anhydrous dextrose per 100 ml (milligrams)
15	49·1	327	33	50·3	152·4
16	49·2	307	34	50·3	148·0
17	49·3	289	35	50·4	143·9
18	49·3	274	36	50·4	140·0
19	49·4	260	37	50·5	136·4
20	49·5	247·4	38	50·5	132·9
21	49·5	235·8	39	50·6	129·6
22	49·6	225·5	40	50·6	126·5
23	49·7	216·1	41	50·7	123·6
24	49·8	207·4	42	50·7	120·8
25	49·8	199·3	43	50·8	118·1
26	49·9	191·8	44	50·8	115·5
27	49·9	184·9	45	50·9	113·0
28	50·0	178·5	46	50·9	110·6
29	50·0	172·5	47	51·0	108·4
30	50·1	167·0	48	51·0	106·2
31	50·2	161·8	49	51·0	104·1
32	50·2	156·9	50	51·1	102·2

* Milligrams of anhydrous dextrose corresponding to 10 millilitres of *potassium cupri-tartrate solution*.

Appendix 16

Determination of Water

REAGENTS
The reagents required for this determination are included in Appendix 1, except for the following special reagent:

Karl Fischer Reagent: dissolve 63 g of *iodine* in 100 ml of *dehydrated pyridine*, cool in ice, and pass *sulphur dioxide* into the solution until a gain in weight of 32·3 g has occurred, taking care to avoid absorption of atmospheric moisture. Add sufficient *dehydrated methyl alcohol* to produce 500 ml and allow to stand for 24 hours.
The reagent is stored in a bottle into which is fitted an automatic burette and a device for pumping the reagent into the burette when required; the access of moisture to the reagent is prevented by a suitable arrangement of desiccant tubes.
Standardise the reagent by the following method: titrate about 20 ml of *dehydrated methyl alcohol* with the prepared *Karl Fischer reagent*, using the apparatus described below, without recording the volume required. Introduce in an appropriate form a suitable amount of water, accurately weighed, and titrate again with the *Karl Fischer reagent*. Calculate the water equivalent of the reagent in mg of water per ml.
Karl Fischer reagent deteriorates continuously and should be standardised immediately before use or

daily, as required. When freshly prepared, 1 ml is equivalent to about 5 mg of water.

APPARATUS
The reagents and solutions used in the determination are sensitive to water and precautions must be taken to prevent exposure to atmospheric moisture.
The titration vessel is of about 60-ml capacity and is fitted with two platinum electrodes, a nitrogen inlet tube, a stopper into which is fitted the tip of the automatic burette, and a vent tube protected by a desiccant; the sample is introduced through a side-arm fitted with a ground-glass stopper.
The titration liquid is stirred either by passing a stream of suitably dried *nitrogen* through the liquid or with a magnetic stirrer.
The dead-stop end-point is obtained by the use of a 1·5- or 2-volt dry battery connected across a variable resistance of about 2000 ohms.
The resistance is arranged so that a suitable initial current passes through the platinum electrodes which are connected in series with a micro-ammeter.
After each addition of *Karl Fischer reagent* the pointer of the micro-ammeter is deflected but quickly returns to its original position; at the end-point a deflection is obtained which persists for a longer period.

METHOD

Unless otherwise directed in the individual monograph, add about 20 ml of *methyl alcohol* to the titration vessel and titrate to the end-point with *Karl Fischer reagent*.

Transfer quickly a suitable amount of the sample,

accurately weighed, stir for one minute, and titrate again with *Karl Fischer reagent*.

Note. Any similar apparatus or method may be used, provided that the analyst is satisfied that the results obtained are of equivalent accuracy.

Appendix 17

Examination of Aerosol Propellents

This appendix describes methods for the determination of the distillation range and water content in dichlorodifluoromethane, dichlorotetrafluoroethane, and trichlorofluoromethane.

A. DETERMINATION OF DISTILLATION RANGE

Apparatus. *Boiling-tube:* A thick-walled tube of resistance glass of the dimensions shown in the diagram.

Thermometer: An accurately standardised thermometer of the mercury-in-glass solid-stem type with a short bulb and the stem graduated in tenths of a degree. The bulb of the thermometer is covered with a piece of muslin, a small wick of

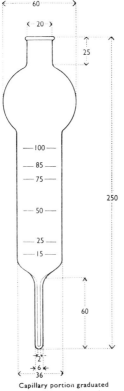

Capillary portion graduated
in 0.01 ml up to 0.2 ml

Dimensions in mm
Graduations in ml

which is allowed to hang 10 to 15 mm below the bulb.

Method. Fill the boiling-tube to the 100-ml mark with the liquid sample; for dichlorodifluoromethane and dichlorotetrafluoroethane the sample is transferred from a sample container, a small metal cylinder fitted with a fine-control needle valve which must be cooled, for example, in a solid carbon dioxide–alcohol mixture, in order to deliver a liquid sample of the propellent, but with trichlorofluoromethane a liquid sample may be obtained direct from the supply cylinder.

Add a few small pieces of carborundum, or other suitable material, and insert the thermometer into the boiling-tube. Support the thermometer so that the bulb is just above the surface of the sample and the wick of muslin dips into the liquid.

Place the capillary section of the boiling-tube in a water-bath, maintained at a temperature which varies with the propellent being tested; for dichlorodifluoromethane, the temperature is 20°, for dichlorotetrafluoroethane, 34°, and for trichlorofluoromethane, 54°.

As the sample evaporates, the position of the thermometer is altered continually so that its position relative to the surface of the liquid remains constant throughout the test.

Read the temperature when 15 ml and 85 ml of the sample have evaporated.

Read the barometer immediately before distillation and correct the thermometer reading to standard conditions by adding or subtracting, for every mm that the barometric pressure is below or above 760 mm, the following amount:

dichlorodifluoromethane .. .. .. 0·031°
dichlorotetrafluoroethane .. .. 0·034°
trichlorofluoromethane .. .. .. 0·035°

The distillation range is the difference between the temperature when 15 per cent and that when 85 per cent of the sample has evaporated.

B. DETERMINATION OF WATER CONTENT

Reagents. *Karl Fischer reagent* is described in Appendix 16, page 895, and *dehydrated methyl alcohol* is described in Appendix 1, page 841. The following special reagent is also required:

Water–Methyl Alcohol Solution: a 0·3 per cent w/w solution of water in *dehydrated methyl alcohol,* standardised by titration with *Karl Fischer reagent.*

Method. Determine by the method of Appendix 16 with the following modifications:

Place 100 ml of *dehydrated methyl alcohol* in the titration vessel, titrate with *Karl Fischer reagent*, and add 2·0 ml in excess.

Weigh the sample container containing the sample, transfer about 200 g of sample, in liquid form, to the titration vessel by means of a copper tube fitted with a fine-control valve, and again weigh the sample container; the difference between the two weighings represents the weight of sample transferred to the titration vessel.

Titrate the excess of *Karl Fischer reagent* with *water–methyl alcohol solution* and from the volume of *Karl Fischer reagent* required by the sample calculate the water content, weight in weight.

Appendix 18

Biological Assays and Tests

DESIGN AND PRECISION

Details of the design and precision of biological assays are given in the European Pharmacopoeia. Guidance to manufacturers on the minimum precision of an acceptable assay is given in the British Pharmacopoeia, Appendix XIVA.

STANDARD PREPARATIONS AND UNITS

Standard Preparations for Great Britain and Northern Ireland are kept at the National Institute for Medical Research, Hampstead, London, and may be obtained therefrom for biological assays and tests. Standard Preparations for other countries are the same as those for Great Britain and Northern Ireland, except for those countries in which similar standard preparations, kept at a different institute, have been defined by law; in those countries the standard preparations so defined are used.

Information on the use and storage of Standard Preparations and on the use of local laboratory standards is given in the British Pharmacopoeia, Appendix XIV.

The *Unit* for a particular substance is, for Great Britain and Northern Ireland, the specific biological activity contained in such an amount of the respective Standard Preparation as the Medical Research Council may from time to time indicate. The Unit for other countries is the same, except for those countries in which a similar unit has been defined by law; in those countries the unit so defined is used.

Where an international standard preparation has been set up, the Unit is the same as the unit, defined by the World Health Organisation, which is accepted for international use.

Details of Standard Preparations and Units required for use in biological assays of the British Pharmaceutical Codex are given in Table A (page 898). They are supplied as dry powders in sealed ampoules containing the approximate quantity stated in the last column of the Table. In the first column, the name of the Preparation is followed by the number of the International (Int.) Standard Preparation and the year in which it was established.

Biological Assay of Antibiotics

The potency of an antibiotic, or of a preparation containing an antibiotic, is determined by comparing the amount of the sample which inhibits the growth of a suitable susceptible micro-organism with the amount of the Standard Preparation of that antibiotic which produces the same degree of inhibition.

This comparison may be made either by means of an agar-gel diffusion method (plate assay) or by a turbidimetric method (tube assay). The agar-gel diffusion method is suggested for all antibiotics and antibiotic preparations of the British Pharmaceutical Codex except for Amphotericin Lozenges, for which the turbidimetric method is suggested.

SUGGESTED METHOD FOR THE DETERMINATION OF POTENCY

(i) *Agar-gel diffusion method.* A suggested procedure for this method is given in the British Pharmacopoeia, Appendix XIVA.

Determine the potency of the substance or, in the case of preparations, of the solution prepared as described in the individual monograph, by this method, using the appropriate organism, medium, solution of standard pH, solution concentration, and incubation temperature indicated in Table B (page 899) for the particular antibiotic.

(ii) *Turbidimetric method.* This method depends upon the growth of a suitable micro-organism in a solution of the antibiotic in a fluid medium that encourages rapid growth in the absence of the antibiotic. The degree of inhibition of growth caused by the presence of the antibiotic is assessed by measuring the difference in the turbidity of the solutions spectrophotometrically.

Prepare, as required by the assay design, in a sterile solution of standard pH, solutions of the Standard Preparation of known concentrations which increase stepwise in a logarithmic manner within the range of concentrations specified for the particular antibiotic.

Similarly prepare solutions, presumed to be of the same concentrations as those of the solutions of the Standard Preparation, of the sample being tested. If directions are given in an individual monograph for the preparation of a solution of the sample, the solution so prepared is diluted as necessary with the sterile solution of standard pH to produce solutions of the required concentrations.

To an appropriate number of suitable test-tubes add the appropriate volume of the specified assay medium which has previously been inoculated with a suitable volume of an inoculum of the specified susceptible test micro-organism.

To an appropriate number of the prepared tubes add the specified volume of each of the prepared dilutions of the Standard Preparation, and to another series of tubes add the same volume of the prepared dilutions of the sample being tested, mix well, and immediately place the tubes in a water-bath at the specified incubation temperature.

When suitable growth has occurred, add one drop of a 1 per cent solution of formaldehyde to stop

TABLE A
STANDARD PREPARATIONS AND UNITS

Standard Preparation	Nature of the Preparation	Units contained in 1 mg	mg containing 1 Unit	Approximate quantity supplied
Amphotericin B 1st Int., 1963	Amphotericin B	940	0·001064	100 mg
Bacitracin 2nd Int., 1964	Bacitracin Zinc	74	0·01351	100 mg
Chlortetracycline 2nd Int., 1969	Chlortetracycline Hydrochloride	1000	0·001	75 mg
Erythromycin 1st Int., 1957	Erythromycin Dihydrate	950	0·001053	200 mg
Gentamicin 1st Int., 1968	Gentamicin Sulphate	641	0·00156	50 mg
Neomycin 1st Int., 1958	Neomycin Sulphate	680	0·00147	100 mg
Novobiocin 1st Int., 1965	Novobiocin	970	0·001031	100 mg
Nystatin 1st Int., 1963	Nystatin	3000	0·000333	75 mg
Paromomycin 1st Int., 1965	Paromomycin Sulphate	750	0·001333	75 mg
Polymyxin B 2nd Int., 1969	Polymyxin B Sulphate	8403	0·000119	75 mg
Streptomycin 2nd Int., 1958	Streptomycin Sulphate	780	0·001282	175 mg
Tetracycline 2nd Int., 1970	Tetracycline Hydrochloride	982	0·00101833	75 mg

the growth, and measure the turbidity of each tube in turn at 530 nm in a suitable spectrophotometer. From the results, calculate by methods described under the design and precision of biological assays given in the European Pharmacopoeia the potency of the sample being tested.

Repeat the assay a sufficient number of times to obtain a statistically satisfactory result.

Amphotericin Lozenges
The content of amphotericin in these lozenges may be determined by the following method:
Carry out the turbidimetric assay described above, using the micro-organism, medium, solution concentrations, and incubation temperature indicated for amphotericin in Table B; the final dilutions of the Standard Preparation and sample solution are made, instead of with a sterile solution of standard pH, with a solvent consisting of a mixture of 4 volumes of *methyl alcohol*, 3 volumes of *dimethyl sulphoxide*, and 3 volumes of water.
All solutions of amphotericin must be kept out of direct sunlight and the assay should be carried out in subdued light or in low-actinic glassware.
To prepare the solutions of the Standard Preparation of known concentration, first prepare a solution in *dimethyl sulphoxide* to contain 100 μg, of the Standard Preparation per ml, dilute suitable aliquots of this solution to 4 ml with *dimethyl*

sulphoxide if necessary, and then further dilute to 100 ml with the solvent mixture given above.
Likewise dilute suitable aliquots of the sample solution, prepared as directed in the monograph, to 4 ml with *dimethyl sulphoxide* and then further dilute to 100 ml with the same solvent mixture.
The medium specified in Table B is inoculated with a suitable volume of an inoculum of the specified test micro-organism and, just before use, sufficient penicillin is added to give 1000 Units per ml and sufficient streptomycin to give 1000 μg per ml; 10 ml portions of this inoculated assay medium are added to 60-μl portions of the prepared dilutions of the Standard Preparation and of the sample in two series of test-tubes.

MEDIA
Formulae for the media referred to in Table B are as follows. In each case, the final pH is adjusted to that stated in the table. Media A, B, and D are the same as media A, B, and D of the British Pharmacopoeia, Appendix XIVA.
Medium A

Peptone	6 g
Pancreatic digest of casein	4 g
Yeast extract	3 g
Beef extract	1·5 g
Anhydrous dextrose	1 g
Agar	15 g
Water	.. to 1000 ml

TABLE B

MICRO-ORGANISMS AND ASSAY CONDITIONS

Antibiotic	Organism	Medium; final pH	Solution of standard pH	Potency of solutions (Units per ml)	Incubation temperature
Amphotericin	*Candida tropicalis*[1] (N.C.Y.C. 470)	W:pH 6·8	—	1 to 4	37°
Bacitracin	*Micrococcus flavus* (N.C.I.B. 8994)	X:pH 7·5	pH 7·6	1 to 2	37° to 39°
Chlortetracycline	*Bacillus pumilus* (N.C.T.C. 8241)	A:pH 6·6	pH 5·8	2 to 20	37° to 39°
Erythromycin	*Bacillus pumilus* (N.C.T.C. 8241)	A:pH 7·8	pH 8·0	5 to 25	37° to 39°
Fusidic Acid	*Corynebacterium xerosis* (N.C.T.C. 9755)	V:pH 7·6	see below[2]	see below[2]	30° to 37°
Gentamicin	*Bacillus pumilus* (N.C.T.C. 8241)	A:pH 7·2	pH 8·0	2 to 20	37° to 39°
Neomycin	*Bacillus pumilus* (N.C.T.C. 8241)	A:pH 7·8	pH 8·0	2 to 14	37° to 39°
	Escherichia coli[3] (N.C.I.B. 10072)	Y:pH 7·9	pH 7·8	5 to 20	37° to 39°
Novobiocin	*Sarcina lutea*[4] (N.C.I.B. 8553)	A:pH 6·6	pH 6·0	1 to 5	32° to 35°
Nystatin	*Saccharomyces cerevisiae* (N.C.Y.C. 87)	D:pH 6·1	see below[5]	25 to 100	35° to 37°
Paromomycin	*Bacillus subtilis* (N.C.T.C. 10,400)	A:pH 8·0	pH 7·8	1 to 4	37° to 39°
Penicillin	*Bacillus subtilis* (N.C.I.B. 8739)	A:pH 6·0	pH 7·0	0·5 to 8	37° to 39°
Polymyxin B	*Bordetella bronchiseptica* (N.C.T.C. 8344)	B:pH 7·3	pH 6·0	20 to 200	35° to 37°
Streptomycin	*Bacillus subtilis* (N.C.I.B. 8739)	Z:pH 7·8	pH 8·0	5 to 20	37° to 39°
Tetracycline	*Bacillus pumilus* (N.C.T.C. 8241)	A:pH 6·6	pH 5·8	2 to 20	37° to 39°

N.C.I.B.—National Collection of Industrial Bacteria, Torry Research Station, Aberdeen, Scotland.

N.C.T.C.—National Collection of Type Cultures, Central Public Health Laboratory, Colindale, London, England.

N.C.Y.C.—National Collection of Yeast Cultures, Brewing Industry Research Foundation, Nutfield, Surrey, England.

[1] This micro-organism is potentially pathogenic and should be handled with caution.

[2] Use *citrate-phosphate buffer solution pH 6·0* and solution concentrations in the range 0·05 to 0·15 µg of fusidic acid per ml.

[3] This micro-organism and the associated assay conditions are used when determining the potency of the neomycin in Neomycin and Bacitracin Ointment.

[4] Also known as *Micrococcus luteus*.

[5] Solution prepared by adding 5 ml of *dimethylformamide* to 95 ml of a solution containing 9·56 per cent w/v of *potassium dihydrogen phosphate* and 11·5 per cent v/v of 1N potassium hydroxide.

Medium B

Pancreatic digest of casein	..	..		17 g
Papaic digest of soya bean	..	..		3 g
Sodium chloride	..	..	..	5 g
Dipotassium hydrogen phosphate		..		2·5 g
Anhydrous dextrose	..	..	..	2·5 g
Agar	..	..	..	..	15 g
Polysorbate 80	..	..	..	10 g
Water	..	..	..	.. to 1000 ml

The polysorbate 80 is added to a hot solution of the other ingredients immediately before diluting to volume.

Medium D

Peptone	..	..	..	9·4 g
Yeast extract	..	..	..	4·7 g
Beef extract	..	..	..	2·4 g
Sodium chloride	..	..	..	10 g
Anhydrous dextrose	..	..	..	10 g
Agar	..	..	..	..	23·5 g
Water	..	..	..	.. to 1000 ml

Medium V

Casein acid hydrolysate (vitamin-free)*	..	..	15 g
Yeast extract	..	..	..	5 g
L-Cystine	..	..	..	0·05 g
Sodium chloride	..	..	..	2·5 g
Anhydrous dextrose	..	..	..	1 g
Water	..	..	..	.. to 1000 ml

* Suitable material may be obtained from Difco Laboratories, P.O. Box 14B, Central Avenue, West Molesey, Surrey, England.

Medium W

Casein hydrolysate	..	..	9 g
Dextrose (monohydrate)	..	..	20 g
Yeast extract	..	..	..	5 g
Trisodium citrate	..	..	10 g
Dipotassium hydrogen phosphate	..	0·25 g
Potassium dihydrogen phosphate	..	0·25 g
Water	..	..	..	.. to 1000 ml

Medium X

Peptone	..	..	..	10 g
Beef extract	..	..	..	3 g
Sodium chloride	..	..	..	3 g
Yeast extract	..	..	..	1·5 g
Brown sugar	..	..	..	1 g
Agar	..	..	..	..	15 g
Water	..	..	..	.. to 1000 ml

Medium Y

Peptone	..	..	..	5 g
Beef extract	..	..	..	3 g
Yeast extract	..	..	..	1·5 g
Sodium chloride	..	..	..	3·5 g
Disodium hydrogen phosphate	..	..	0·5 g
Potassium dihydrogen phosphate	..	0·4 g
Agar	..	..	..	..	15 g
Water	..	..	..	.. to 1000 ml

Medium Z

Medium A with the addition of 0·4 per cent w/v of *anhydrous dextrose*.

Biological Determination of Antidiuretic Activity of Powdered Pituitary (Posterior Lobe)

The antidiuretic activity of a sample of powdered pituitary (posterior lobe) is determined by comparing its activity with that of a standard preparation of pituitary (posterior lobe) by a biological method. For this purpose an extract of the Standard Preparation, or of an equivalent laboratory standard preparation, is required.

As the amount of the Standard Preparation which will be supplied on request is limited, each worker should prepare for use as a laboratory standard preparation a quantity of dry pituitary powder, the strength of which must be determined in relation to that of the Standard Preparation.

Methods for the preparation of a laboratory standard preparation of dry pituitary (posterior lobe) powder and of an extract of this or the Standard Preparation are described in Appendix XIVC of the British Pharmacopoeia under the Biological Assay of Oxytocin Injection.

Standard Preparation and Unit

The Standard Preparation is a quantity of acetone-dried powder obtained from the posterior lobes of fresh pituitary bodies of oxen.

The Unit is that defined in the Regulations made under the Therapeutic Substances Act, 1956. The Unit is the specific antidiuretic activity corresponding to that yielded by 0·5 mg of the Standard Preparation when extracted by the prescribed method. The Unit is the same as the international unit.

Suggested Method

A male rat weighing about 200 g is deprived of food but not water overnight. Next morning it is given by stomach tube 3 ml of water per 100 g body-weight and, one hour later, 5 ml of a 12 per cent v/v solution of ethyl alcohol per 100 g body-weight.

One hour after the dose of ethyl alcohol, a cannula is inserted in one of the jugular veins and a catheter in the bladder and a volume of water equal to the volume of urine excreted from the time the water was administered to the completion of the insertion of the catheter is given by stomach tube, which is left in position.

The rat is placed on the pan of a balance and the urine excreted is replaced by administering a 2·5 per cent v/v solution of ethyl alcohol so as to maintain a constant water load throughout the assay.

When the flow of urine has become steady, a dose of the Standard Preparation is injected into the jugular vein and the antidiuretic effect is calculated from the expression $100 (a - b)/a$, where a is the volume of urine excreted in the 10 minutes lasting from the eighth minute before injection to the second minute after injection, and b is the volume excreted in the ten minutes lasting from the second to the twelfth minute after injection.

The injection of the Standard Preparation is repeated several times if necessary until similar antidiuretic effects are obtained for equal doses. The rat is then ready for the assay.

Two dose levels of the Standard Preparation and two of the sample being tested are used, the ratio of the high dose to the low dose being the same for each. Suggested doses are 0·01 and 0·02 milli-unit per 100 g body-weight.

A (2 and 2) dose assay of up to three groups may be conveniently run on the same animal, provided that the volumes injected do not exceed 0·1 ml per 100 g body-weight. The result is calculated by standard statistical methods as described in the European Pharmacopoeia.

Absence of Undue Toxicity and Therapeutic Potency of Suramin

SUGGESTED METHOD FOR ABSENCE OF UNDUE TOXICITY

Inject intravenously each of a group of 10 mice with a dose of 0·0125 ml per g of body-weight with a 2·5 per cent w/v solution of the sample in freshly distilled water.

If not more than 5 mice die within three days, the sample passes the test. If more than 5 mice die, a second group of 20 mice are similarly injected. If the total number of mice which have died in the two groups within three days is not greater than 15, the sample passes the test.

SUGGESTED METHOD FOR THERAPEUTIC POTENCY

Mice are inoculated with a strain of *Trypanosoma equiperdum* and, after 48 hours, the blood of each mouse is examined microscopically and the number of trypanosomes per ml in the blood of each mouse is estimated; this number should lie between 1000 and 20,000. The estimate may be made by examining a thin film of the blood in the form of a cover-slip preparation and counting the trypanosomes in at least ten microscopical fields having an area of 0·12 mm². The presence of 1 to 20 trypanosomes in each of two fields corresponds approximately to a content of 1000 to 20,000 trypanosomes per ml.

Inject into a vein of each of a group of ten of the infected mice 0·016 ml per g body-weight of a 0·005 per cent w/v solution of the sample in freshly distilled water and examine the blood of each mouse on the first and third days following the injection by the method given above, observing 20 fields.

If no trypanosomes are found in the blood of five or more of the mice after the third day, the sample passes the test. If trypanosomes are found in the blood of five or more of the mice the test may be repeated. The sample passes the test if no trypanosomes are found under these conditions in the blood of not less than 50 per cent of the total number of mice treated.

Appendix 19

Limit Test for Chloramphenicol Palmitate Polymorph A in Chloramphenicol Mixture

This Appendix describes the method for testing Chloramphenicol Mixture in order to ensure that the content of the biologically inactive polymorphic form of chloramphenicol palmitate is within the prescribed limit. The method involves comparison of the infra-red spectrum of the sample with that of a standard.

Preparation of Standards

(i) STANDARD CONTAINING 20 PER CENT W/W OF POLYMORPH A. Mix thoroughly together one part by weight of *chloramphenicol palmitate (polymorph A) A.S.* and four parts by weight of *chloramphenicol palmitate A.S.*

(ii) STANDARD CONTAINING 10 PER CENT W/W OF POLYMORPH A. Mix thoroughly together one part by weight of *chloramphenicol palmitate (polymorph A) A.S.* and nine parts by weight of *chloramphenicol palmitate A.S.*

Preparation of Sample

Mix 20 ml of the well-mixed sample of Chloramphenicol Mixture with 20 ml of water, centrifuge for 15 minutes at a speed of not less than 18,000 revolutions per minute, and discard the supernatant liquid.

Wash the residue by adding 2 ml of water, triturating to form a paste, adding 18 ml of water, mixing thoroughly, centrifuging, and discarding the supernatant liquid; wash the residue twice more in a similar manner.

Dry the residue at 20° for 14 hours in vacuo and grind to a fine powder.

Procedure

Prepare a mull of the residue obtained in the preparation of the sample by triturating a small quantity of the solid with about twice its weight of *liquid paraffin* until uniformly dispersed.

Place a drop of the mull in the centre of a rock-salt plate, place another similar plate gently on top of the drop, and slowly squeeze the plates together to spread the mull uniformly. Similarly mount between plates mulls of the two standard mixtures.

Record the infra-red spectrum of each mull over the range 11·0 μm to 13·0 μm, using identical instrumental conditions which should be such that 20 to 30 per cent transmittance occurs at 12·3 μm.

Calculation

Inspect the recorded spectrum of the standard containing 20 per cent of polymorph A and determine the exact wavelengths of minimum absorption at about 11·3 μm and 12·65 μm and the exact wavelengths of maximum absorption at about 11·65 μm and 11·86 μm.

Using these exact wavelengths, draw, on the recorded spectrum of the standard containing 10 per cent of polymorph A, a straight baseline between the minima occurring at about 11·3 μm and 12·65 μm.

Draw straight lines, at the maxima occurring at about 11·65 μm and 11·86 μm, intersecting both the recorded spectrum and the baseline, and hence obtain the corrected extinctions at these maxima.

Calculate the ratio of the corrected extinction at the maximum at about 11·65 μm to that at the maximum at about 11·86 μm.

Carry out the same procedure on the recorded spectrum of the sample.

The extinction ratio of the sample is greater than the extinction ratio of the standard containing 10 per cent w/w of polymorph A.

Appendix 20

Determination of Fluorine in Calcium Phosphate

APPARATUS

The apparatus consists of a 250-ml round-bottomed flask having 3 necks; one of the necks is connected to a steam generator in which the water has been made alkaline to *phenolphthalein solution* by the addition of *sodium hydroxide solution*; a second neck is fitted with a suitable thermometer and the third is fitted with a vertical column, wrapped with asbestos lagging and having a side-arm at the top leading to a vertical condenser and a receiver.

METHOD

Add to the flask 40 ml of a 35 per cent v/v solution of *sulphuric acid* in water, heat the solution to $150° \pm 3°$, pass steam through the apparatus, maintaining the temperature of the solution within the stated limits throughout, and collect 70 ml of distillate; reserve this distillate (1st distillate).

Allow the flask to cool, add about 1 g of the sample, accurately weighed, again heat the solution to $150° \pm 3°$, and steam-distil as before, again collecting 70 ml of distillate; reserve this distillate (2nd distillate) and continue the steam distillation until a further 70 ml of distillate has been collected (3rd distillate).

Transfer the three distillates, separately, to 100-ml graduated flasks and to a fourth 100-ml graduated flask add 50 ml of water; to each flask add 10 ml of *alizarin fluorine blue solution*, 2 ml of *buffer solution pH 4·3*, and 10 ml of *cerous nitrate solution*, dilute each solution to 100 ml with water, allow to stand for 1 hour and measure the extinction at 610 nm of a 4-cm layer of each of the solutions prepared from the three distillates, using the solution prepared from 50 ml of water as the blank. (*Note:* the extinction of the reagent blank tends to rise as the reagents age; if it rises by more than 0·02 then fresh reagents should be prepared.)

Calculate the amount of fluorine in each solution by reference to a calibration curve prepared by treating 2-, 4-, 6-, 8-, and 10-ml portions of *standard fluorine solution*, each diluted with 50 ml of water, by the method given above beginning at the words "add 10 ml of *alizarin fluorine blue solution . . .*", using a solution similarly prepared, but omitting the standard fluorine solution as the blank.

The content of fluorine in the sample, expressed as parts per million, is given by the formula:

$$\frac{S - \frac{1}{2}B_1 - \frac{1}{2}B_2}{W}$$

where B_1 = the weight, in µg, of fluorine in the 1st distillate,
B_2 = the weight, in µg, of fluorine in the 3rd distillate,
S = the weight, in µg, of fluorine in the 2nd distillate, and
W = the weight, in g, of sample taken.

If the value of B_2 is significantly greater than B_1, the recovery of fluorine in the second distillate is incomplete. In this case, the content of fluorine in the sample is given by the formula:

$$\frac{S_1 - B_1}{W}$$

where $S_1 = S + (B_2 - B_1)$.

Appendix 21

Determination of Hydroxyl Value of Polysorbates and Sorbitan Derivatives

This Appendix describes the method for the determination of the hydroxyl value of Polysorbate 20, Polysorbate 60, Polysorbate 80, Sorbitan Monolaurate, Sorbitan Mono-oleate, and Sorbitan Monostearate.

PROCEDURE

Weigh accurately the amount of sample indicated in the individual monograph and transfer to a 250-ml flask; add 5 ml of *pyridine–acetic anhydride reagent*, mix, attach a reflux condenser to the flask, and heat on a water-bath for 1 hour; add 10 ml of water, heat for a further 10 minutes, and allow to cool.

Rinse the inside of the condenser with 25 ml of *butyl alcohol*, previously neutralised to *phenol-phthalein solution*, and titrate the combined solution and washings with 0·5N alcoholic potassium hydroxide, using *phenolphthalein solution* as indicator.

Repeat the procedure omitting the sample.

Determine the acidity of the sample by dissolving about 10 g, accurately weighed, in 10 ml of *pyridine*, previously neutralised to *phenolphthalein solution*, and titrating with 0·5N alcoholic potassium hydroxide, using *phenolphthalein solution* as indicator.

The hydroxyl value of the sample is given by the expression:

$$\frac{28·05[B + (WA/w) - C]}{W}$$

where A = volume, in ml, of 0·5N alcoholic potassium hydroxide required in the acidity titration,
B = volume, in ml, of 0·5N alcoholic potassium hydroxide required in the blank titration,
C = volume, in ml, of 0·5N alcoholic potassium

hydroxide required in the titration of the acetylated sample,
W = weight, in g, of sample taken for the acetylation, and
w = weight, in g, of sample taken for the acidity titration.

Appendix 22

Examination of Hypromellose

This Appendix describes methods for the determination of the hydroxypropoxyl content and the methoxyl content of hypromellose.

Determination of Hydroxypropoxyl Content

Using the apparatus shown in the diagram, carry out the following method:
Transfer about 0·05 g of the sample, accurately weighed, to the flask, add 10 ml of *chromium trioxide solution*, assemble the apparatus, and

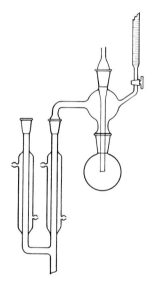

immerse the flask in an oil-bath fitted with a stirrer and thermometer. Connect a supply of *nitrogen* to the inlet tube, and pass a slow stream of the gas through the apparatus; pass a stream of water through the condensers, and raise the temperature of the oil-bath to 155°, heating slowly at first but attaining this temperature within 30 minutes. Maintain this temperature throughout the remainder of the determination.
Collect the distillate in a 50-ml measuring cylin-

der, and as successive 5-ml volumes of distillate are collected, add 5-ml volumes of water to the flask from the burette. Continue the distillation until 55 ml of water has been added and 50 ml of a faintly yellow distillate has been collected.
Wash down the condensers with water, transfer the distillate and washings to a glass-stoppered flask, add *phenolphthalein solution* as indicator, and titrate with 0·02N sodium hydroxide, until a pink coloration just begins to fade; boil, cool, and continue the titration until the pink coloration remains for 10 seconds.
Add 0·5 g of *sodium bicarbonate* and 10 ml of *dilute sulphuric acid*, and, when effervescence has ceased, add 1 g of *potassium iodide*, mix, and titrate the liberated iodine with 0·02N sodium thiosulphate, using *starch mucilage* as indicator.
Repeat the procedure omitting the sample.
The hydroxypropoxyl content is given by the expression:

$$\frac{0·15(X - KY)}{W}$$

where X = volume, in ml, of 0·02N sodium hydroxide used in the titration of the sample,
Y = volume, in ml, of 0·02N sodium thiosulphate used in the titration of the sample,
W = weight, in grams, of sample taken, corrected for moisture content, and
$K = \dfrac{a}{b}$, where a and b are the volumes, in ml, of
0·02N sodium hydroxide, and of 0·02N sodium thiosulphate, respectively, used in the titration of the blank.

Determination of Methoxyl Content
Determine the total alkoxyl content, expressed as methoxyl, OCH_3, by the method for the determination of methoxyl given in the British Pharmacopoeia, Appendix X(I).
Determine the hydroxypropoxyl content by the method given above, correct the value so found for the propylene produced in the determination of total alkoxyl content by multiplying by a factor of 0·93, express the result in terms of methoxyl by multiplying by a factor of 0·413, subtract the figure so obtained from the total alkoxyl content, and hence obtain the methoxyl content.

Appendix 23

Determination of Certain Steroids in Specified Preparations

This Appendix describes the methods to be used for the determination of betamethasone 17-valerate and of fluocinolone acetonide in certain specified preparations.

A. DETERMINATION OF BETAMETHASONE 17-VALERATE

REAGENTS
Some of the reagents are included in Appendix 1; the following special reagents are required:

Betamethasone Valerate Solution, Standard: a 0·10 per cent w/v solution of *betamethasone valerate A.S.* in *chloroform*.

Chloroform, Redistilled: *chloroform* of the British Pharmacopoeia, Appendix I, which has been redistilled, the first and last 10 per cent of the distillate being discarded. It should be freshly prepared.

Dioxan (low in peroxides): *dioxan* of the British Pharmacopoeia, Appendix I, which has been stored in unopened bottles in a refrigerator; if the whole content of the bottle has not been used, the bottle should be flushed out with *nitrogen* before returning to storage, in order to minimise the formation of peroxides.

Hexane (low in aromatic hydrocarbons): *hexane* of the British Pharmacopoeia, Appendix I, which complies with the following additional test: the extinction of a 1-cm layer at 235 nm measured against air, is less than 0·7.

Stationary Phase and **Eluent Phase:** mix 2000 ml of *hexane (low in aromatic hydrocarbons)*, 600 ml of *dioxan (low in peroxides)*, 100 ml of *methyl alcohol*, and 100 ml of water, shake well, and allow to separate. Reserve the upper layer for use as the *eluent phase* and the lower layer for use as the *stationary phase*. They should be freshly prepared and the same batch should be used throughout the determination.

PREPARATION OF SAMPLE

Betamethasone Valerate Scalp Application. Mix an accurately weighed quantity, equivalent to about 2 mg of betamethasone, with 20 ml of water and 2 ml of 0·1N hydrochloric acid in a 100-ml separating funnel and extract with successive 40-, 40-, 40-, 5-, and 5-ml portions of *redistilled chloroform*, shaking each extraction vigorously, allowing to separate, and transferring each lower layer to a 250-ml separating funnel; discard the contents of the 100-ml separating funnel.

Shake the combined chloroform extracts with 5 ml of a 1 per cent w/v solution of *sodium bicarbonate* in water, allow to separate, and immediately transfer the lower layer to a second 250-ml separating funnel with two successive 10-ml portions of *redistilled chloroform*, transfer these washings to the second separating funnel, and discard the contents of the first separating funnel.

Wash the combined chloroform extracts in the second separating funnel with 5 ml of water, allow to separate, filter the chloroform solution through a pledget of cotton wool which has previously been washed with *redistilled chloroform*, wash the aqueous solution in the separating funnel with two successive 10-ml portions of *redistilled chloroform*, and filter the washing through the same filter.

Evaporate the combined filtrates to dryness at a temperature not exceeding 35°, transfer the residue to a small beaker with the aid of four successive 5-ml portions of *acetone*, and evaporate the solution to dryness at a temperature not exceeding 35° in a current of *nitrogen*.

The residue should be protected from light and stored in a desiccator over *phosphorus pentoxide* until required for the chromatographic procedure.

Betamethasone Valerate Cream. Transfer an accurately weighed quantity, equivalent to about 1·5 mg of betamethasone, to a dry 250-ml separating funnel, add 100 ml of *cyclohexane* and 50 ml of *methyl alcohol*, shake vigorously until the materials are uniformly dispersed and then for a further 3 minutes, allow to separate, and transfer the lower layer to a 500-ml separating funnel containing 215 ml of water and 1 g of *sodium chloride*.

Continue the extraction of the solution in the first separating funnel with successive 25-, 5- and 5-ml portions of a mixture of 4 volumes of *methyl alcohol* and 1 volume of water, shaking vigorously for each extraction, allowing to separate, and transferring each lower layer to the second separating funnel containing the first extract.

Discard the contents of the first separating funnel and extract the combined solutions in the second separating funnel with successive 100-, 50-, 10-, and 10-ml portions of *redistilled chloroform*, shaking each extract vigorously, combine the extracts and continue by the method given above for Betamethasone Valerate Scalp Application, beginning with the words "Shake the combined chloroform extracts with 5 ml . . .".

Betamethasone Valerate Lotion. Prepare the sample by the method given above for Betamethasone Valerate Cream.

Betamethasone Valerate Ointment. Transfer an accurately weighed quantity, equivalent to about 1·5 mg of betamethasone, to a dry 250-ml separating funnel, add 100 ml of *cyclohexane* which has been previously warmed to 80°, shake gently until the materials are dissolved, cool, add 10 ml of water and 50 ml of *methyl alcohol*, shake vigorously for 3 minutes, allow to separate and continue by the method given above for Betamethasone Valerate Cream beginning with the words "transfer the lower layer to a 500-ml separating funnel . . .".

Betamethasone Valerate with Chlortetracycline Ointment. Prepare the sample by the method given above for Betamethasone Valerate Ointment.

PREPARATION OF CHROMATOGRAPHIC COLUMNS

Mix 16·5 g of *washed Celite 545* with 8·25 ml of *stationary phase* and transfer the suspension, in successive small portions, to a chromatographic tube, 80 cm in length and 1·0 cm in diameter, fitted at its lower end with a sintered-glass disk (British Standard Grade No. 1) and a tap; carefully pack each portion with the aid of a plunger having a diameter almost the same as the internal diameter of the chromatographic tube. The column should be prepared immediately before use. Repeat the process for two more columns.

CHROMATOGRAPHIC PROCEDURE

The chromatographic procedure should be carried out at a temperature between 25° and 28°.

Dissolve the residue obtained in the preparation of the sample in 0·25 ml of *stationary phase*, add 0·5 g of *washed Celite 545*, mix thoroughly, pack the mixture on to the top of the prepared chromatographic column, and finally transfer any of the mixture remaining in the beaker to the top of the column with the aid of small portions of *eluent phase*; add more *eluent phase* carefully to the top of the column, taking care not to disturb the column, and adjust the rate of flow from the bottom of the column to about 3 ml per minute, maintaining the level of liquid above the column by the addition of *eluent phase* to the top of the column.

Collect successive 10-ml fractions of the eluate until a total of 450 ml has been collected and discard the first five fractions.

Repeat the procedure twice, using a freshly prepared chromatographic column each time, but (i) using the residue obtained by evaporating 2 ml of *standard betamethasone valerate solution* to dryness in a current of *nitrogen* in the first instance, and (ii) omitting the residue obtained from the sample in the second instance.

Measure the extinction of a 1-cm layer of each fraction obtained from the sample and from the standard betamethasone valerate solution at the maximum at about 235 nm, in each case using as the blank the corresponding fraction obtained in the procedure in which the residue from the sample was omitted.

From the extinctions so obtained, construct a graph relating extinctions and volumes of eluate for the sample solution and for the standard solution. Then, ignoring any small peak which occurs on the graph before the main peak, summate the area under the main peak due to the sample and the area under the main peak due to the standard.

The percentage of betamethasone 17-valerate in the sample is given by the expression:

$$\frac{200A_1W}{A_2w}$$

where A_1 = area under sample peak,
A_2 = area under standard peak,
W = concentration of betamethasone valerate, in mg per ml, in the standard solution, and
w = weight of sample, in mg.

Hence calculate the equivalent concentration of betamethasone valerate in the sample; each mg of betamethasone valerate is equivalent to 0·8235 mg of betamethasone.

The recovery of betamethasone valerate from the column may be checked by evaporating 2 ml of *standard betamethasone valerate solution* to dryness in a current of *nitrogen*, dissolving the residue in sufficient *eluent phase* to give 100 ml, measuring the extinction of a 1-cm layer of this solution at the maximum at about 235 nm and comparing the extinction so obtained with the total extinction obtained, by the method above, with the standard betamethasone valerate solution.

NOTE. After experience with the above method has been gained, the necessity for collecting and measuring the extinctions of large numbers of fractions obtained with each chromatographic run may be avoided by carrying out the following procedure with each fresh 500-g batch of *washed Celite 545*, care being taken to ensure that standardised operating conditions are maintained, especially with regard to temperatures.

Determine the elution characteristics of prepared columns by carrying out the column chromatography described above under Chromatographic Procedure, using, on one column, the residue obtained by evaporating 2 ml of *standard betamethasone valerate solution* and, on a second column, the residue obtained by evaporating 2 ml of *redistilled chloroform*.

Then, measure the extinction of a 1-cm layer of each fraction obtained in the chromatography of the residue from the standard betamethasone valerate solution at the maximum at about 235 nm, in each case using as the blank the corresponding solvent blank fraction.

Construct a graph by plotting the extinctions against volume of eluate and hence determine with which fractions the elution of betamethasone 17-valerate begins and ends.

The chromatographic procedure on the sample, the standard solution, and the blank may now be carried out, as described above, on freshly prepared columns in each case, but instead of collecting successive 10-ml fractions, make use of the known elution characteristics and discard the first fractions of the eluate, collect two 10-ml fractions immediately prior to the expected elution of the betamethasone 17-valerate, the fraction estimated to contain the whole of the betamethasone 17-valerate, and an immediate further two 10-ml fractions.

To the extinction due to the fraction (volume = x ml) estimated to contain the whole of the betamethasone 17-valerate add $10/x$ times the total of the extinctions, if any, due to the four 10-ml fractions, for the sample solution and for the standard solution; by comparison, calculate the quantity of betamethasone 17-valerate in the weight of sample taken and hence calculate the concentration of betamethasone 17-valerate in the sample; each mg of betamethasone valerate is equivalent to 0·8235 mg of betamethasone.

B. DETERMINATION OF FLUOCINOLONE ACETONIDE

The following method is based on that of Bailey, Holbrook, and Miller (*J. Pharm. Pharmacol.*, 1966, **18**, 12S).

REAGENTS

Most of the reagents are included in Appendix 1 or described under the determination of betamethasone 17-valerate, page 904; the following special reagents are required:

Fluocinolone Acetonide Solution, Standard: a 0·10 per cent w/v solution of *fluocinolone acetonide A.S.* in *stationary phase*.

Stationary Phase and **Eluent Phase:** mix 2000 ml of *hexane (low in aromatic hydrocarbons)*, 800 ml of *dioxan (low in peroxides)*, and 100 ml of water, shake well, and allow to separate. Reserve the upper layer for use as the *eluent phase* and the lower layer for use as the *stationary phase*.

PREPARATION OF SAMPLE

Fluocinolone Cream and **Fluocinolone Ointment.** Transfer an accurately weighed sample, equivalent to about 2 mg of fluocinolone acetonide, to a separating funnel with the aid of 100 ml of *cyclohexane*; add 50 ml of *methyl alcohol*, shake vigorously for 3 minutes, allow to separate, and transfer the lower layer to a second separating funnel containing 140 ml of water; to the second separating funnel add 100 ml of *redistilled chloroform*, shake vigorously for 3 minutes, and allow to separate; filter the lower layer and evaporate 50 ml of the filtrate to dryness in a small beaker on a water-bath.

PREPARATION OF CHROMATOGRAPHIC COLUMN

Mix 15 g of *washed Celite 545* with 7·5 ml of *stationary phase* and transfer the mixture, in successive small portions, to a chromatographic tube, 70 cm in length and 2 cm in diameter, fitted at its lower end with a sintered-glass disk (British Standard Grade No. 1) and a tap; carefully pack each portion with the aid of a suitable plunger.

CHROMATOGRAPHIC PROCEDURE

Dissolve the residue obtained in the preparation of the sample in 1 ml of *stationary phase*, add 2 g of *washed Celite 545*, mix thoroughly, pack the mixture on to the top of the prepared chromatographic column, and finally transfer any of the mixture remaining in the beaker to the top of the column with the aid of small portions of *eluent phase*; add carefully to the top of the column more *eluent phase* sufficient to give a layer of liquid about 45 cm in depth on top of the column and adjust the rate of flow from the bottom of the column to 8 to 10 ml per minute, maintaining the level of liquid by the addition of *eluent phase* to the top of the column.

Collect successive 10-ml fractions of the eluate until a total of 650 ml has been collected.

Discard the first nine fractions and measure the extinction of a 1-cm layer of each of the remaining fractions at the maximum at about 238 nm, using *eluent phase* as the blank.

Repeat the entire procedure using 1·0 ml of *standard fluocinolone acetonide solution* in place of the prepared sample solution.

From the extinctions so obtained, construct a graph relating extinctions and volumes of eluate for the sample solution and for the standard solution and summate the area under the peak due to the sample and the area under the peak due to the standard.

The percentage of fluocinolone acetonide in the sample is given by the expression:

$$\frac{200\,A_1 W}{A_2 w}$$

where A_1 = area under sample peak,
A_2 = area under standard peak,
W = concentration of fluocinolone acetonide, in mg per ml, of the standard solution, and
w = weight of sample, in mg.

Appendix 24

Determination of Vitamins

This appendix describes methods for the determination of vitamins in Vitamins Capsules, Vitamins A and D Capsules, Dried Yeast, and Yeast Tablets. Methods are described for the determination of ascorbic acid, nicotinic acid, nicotinamide, riboflavine, and thiamine hydrochloride. Although the requirements for the content of vitamins stated in the monographs have been based on these methods, other suitable methods of at least equivalent accuracy may be used.

Vitamins Capsules

DETERMINATION OF VITAMIN A ACTIVITY, OF VITAMIN D, AND OF ASCORBIC ACID. Weigh not less than 10 capsules; open the capsules carefully without loss of shell material and express as much of the contents as possible. Examine the expressed liquid by the following methods:

(i) Determine the amount of vitamin A activity by the method of the British Pharmacopoeia, Appendix XVIIA, for the assay of vitamin A.

(ii) Determine the amount of vitamin D by the

method of the British Pharmacopoeia, Appendix XIVG. If it is known that the vitamin D is derived from synthetic material, the method given on page 910 is also applicable.

(iii) Determine the ascorbic acid by the method given below.

Wash the shells with *solvent ether*, allow to stand until the odour of ether is no longer perceptible, and weigh; the difference between the two weighings is equivalent to the weight of the total contents. Calculate the total amount of the vitamins in the capsules taken and divide by the number of capsules.

DETERMINATION OF NICOTINAMIDE, RIBOFLAVINE, AND THIAMINE HYDROCHLORIDE. Determine by the methods described below. Calculate the total amount of the vitamins in the capsules taken and divide by the number of capsules.

Vitamins A and D Capsules

DETERMINATION OF VITAMIN A ACTIVITY AND OF VITAMIN D. Weigh not less than 10 capsules; open the capsules carefully without loss of shell material and express as much of the contents as possible. Examine the expressed liquid by the following methods:

(i) Determine the amount of vitamin A activity by the method of the British Pharmacopoeia, Appendix XVIIA, for the assay of vitamin A.

(ii) Determine the amount of vitamin D by the method of the British Pharmacopoeia, Appendix XIVG. If it is known that the vitamin D is derived from synthetic material, the method given on page 910 is also applicable.

Wash the shells with *solvent ether*, allow to stand until the odour of ether is no longer perceptible, and weigh; the difference between the two weighings is equivalent to the weight of the total contents. Calculate the total amount of the vitamins in the capsules taken and divide by the number of capsules.

Dried Yeast

DETERMINATION OF NICOTINIC ACID, RIBOFLAVINE, AND THIAMINE HYDROCHLORIDE. Determine the amounts of nicotinic acid, riboflavine, and thiamine hydrochloride in each gram by the methods described below.

Yeast Tablets

DETERMINATION OF NICOTINIC ACID, RIBOFLAVINE, AND THIAMINE HYDROCHLORIDE. Weigh and powder 20 tablets. Determine the amounts of nicotinic acid, riboflavine, and thiamine hydrochloride in the powdered tablets by the methods described below. Calculate the total amounts of the vitamins in the tablets taken and divide by 20.

A. DETERMINATION OF ASCORBIC ACID

Reagents. These are included in Appendix 1.

Method for Vitamins Capsules. Shake an accurately weighed quantity of the liquid expressed from the capsules, containing about 75 mg of ascorbic acid, with 25 ml of *metaphosphoric acid solution* until completely dispersed, centrifuge, and filter.

Wash the residue with successive portions of a 5 per cent w/v solution of *trichloroacetic acid* in water until the combined filtrate and washings measure 100 ml; titrate 2·5 ml with *double-strength standard 2,6-dichlorophenolindophenol solution*, avoiding oxidation by air, and calculate the amount of ascorbic acid present.

B. DETERMINATION OF NICOTINIC ACID AND NICOTINAMIDE

The following microbiological assay is described in fuller detail in the *Analyst*, 1946, **71**, 401.

Reagents. Most of the reagents are included in Appendix 1 or described under the determination of riboflavine below; the following additional special reagents are required:

BIOTIN SOLUTION: dissolve 25 micrograms of biotin in *water*, add 1 ml of *potassium phosphates solution,* and dilute to 250 ml with *water*. Store under *toluene* or *chloroform* and use within 3 months of preparation.

NICOTINIC ACID SOLUTION, STANDARD: dilute 1 ml of *nicotinic acid stock solution* to 1000 ml with *water* immediately before use; 1 ml contains 0·1 microgram of nicotinic acid.

THIAMINE SOLUTION: dissolve 0·1 g of *thiamine*

hydrochloride in a 2 per cent w/v solution of *hydrochloric acid* and dilute to 1000 ml with *water.* Store under *toluene* or *chloroform.*

MEDIUM FOR THE ASSAY OF NICOTINIC ACID:

Sodium Acetate	33 g
Dextrose (monohydrate)	20 g
Casein Acid Hydrolysate (Vitamin-free)★	10 g
Sodium Chloride	5 g
Ammonium Sulphate	3 g
Xylose	1 g
Cystine Solution	50 ml
Tryptophan Solution	50 ml
Adenine–Guanine–Uracil Solution ..	10 ml
Xanthine Solution	10 ml
Riboflavine Stock Solution	8 ml
Inorganic Salt Solution	5 ml
Potassium Phosphates Solution ..	5 ml
Biotin Solution	4 ml
p-Aminobenzoic Acid Solution ..	1 ml
Calcium Pantothenate Solution ..	1 ml
Pyridoxine Solution	1 ml
Thiamine Solution	1 ml
Water	to 500 ml

★ Suitable material may be obtained from Difco Laboratories, P.O. Box 14B, Central Avenue, West Molesey, Surrey, England.

Mix and adjust the medium to pH 6·8 by the addition of *sodium hydroxide solution.* Store at a temperature not exceeding 4° and use within 48 hours of preparation. The medium is sterilised after the addition of the nicotinic acid or the test solution, as described in the method, by heating in an autoclave at 115° for exactly 10 minutes.

Preparation of Inoculum. To 5 ml of *medium for the assay of nicotinic acid* add 2 micrograms of nicotinic acid and 5 ml of *water,* and sterilise by heating in an autoclave at 115° for 10 minutes; cool, inoculate with a culture of a suitable strain of *Lactobacillus arabinosus,* and incubate for 18 hours at 37°; centrifuge, reject the supernatant liquid, and suspend the bacterial cells in 10 ml of *saline solution;* add 1 ml of this suspension to 10 or 20 ml of *saline solution.* This suspension must be prepared freshly for each assay.

Method for Vitamins Capsules, Dried Yeast, and Yeast Tablets. Autoclave 5 capsules or about 1 g of dried yeast or of powdered tablets, accurately weighed, with 50 ml of 1N hydrochloric acid at 15 lb per sq in. pressure for 15 minutes; cool, add 2 ml of *2·5M sodium acetate,* adjust the pH to 4·5, using *bromophenol blue solution* as an external indicator, dilute to 100 ml with *water,* add 20 ml of *anaesthetic ether,* extract, filter, extract with 20 ml of *anaesthetic ether,* and reject the extract; adjust the pH of 20 ml of the solution to 6·8, using *bromothymol blue solution* as an external indicator, and dilute to 100 ml with *water.*

To 5-ml quantities of *medium for the assay of nicotinic acid,* contained in bacteriological test-tubes, add graded doses of *standard nicotinic acid solution,* and to a further series add similar graded doses of the test solution; dilute each mixture to 10 ml with *water.* A suitable range of doses contains 0·05 to 0·3 microgram of nicotinic acid; at least three replicate series should be prepared for the standard and for the sample. Sterilise the contents of the tubes by heating in an autoclave at 115° for exactly 10 minutes, cool, inoculate each of the tubes with one drop of the freshly prepared inoculum, and incubate at 37° for 3 to 4 days.

Titrate the lactic acid produced in each tube with 0·1N sodium hydroxide, using *bromothymol blue solution* as indicator and titrating to pH 6·8. Prepare a standard curve for the mean results obtained in the three series of tubes containing the standard nicotinic acid solution. From the mean amounts of lactic acid produced in the tubes containing the material derived from the sample and by reference to the standard curve, obtain the amount of nicotinic acid or nicotinamide present.

C. DETERMINATION OF RIBOFLAVINE

The following microbiological assay is described in fuller detail in the *Analyst*, 1946, **71**, 398.

Reagents. Some of the reagents are included in Appendix 1; the following special reagents are required:

ADENINE–GUANINE–URACIL SOLUTION: warm 0·1 g of adenine, 0·1 g of guanine, and 0·1 g of uracil with *water*, add *hydrochloric acid*, dropwise, to effect solution, cool, and dilute to 100 ml with *water*.

Store under *toluene* or with *chloroform* at a temperature not exceeding 4°, and use within 14 days of preparation.

p-AMINOBENZOIC ACID SOLUTION: dissolve 0·1 g of *p*-aminobenzoic acid in 2 ml of *glacial acetic acid* and dilute to 1000 ml with *water*.

Store under *toluene* or with *chloroform* at a temperature not exceeding 4° and use within 7 days of preparation.

CALCIUM PANTOTHENATE SOLUTION: dissolve 0·1 g of calcium (+)-pantothenate or 0·2 g of calcium (±)-pantothenate in 1000 ml of *water*.

Store under *toluene* or with *chloroform* at a temperature not exceeding 4° and use within 7 days of preparation.

CYSTINE SOLUTION: boil 2 g of L-cystine with 50 ml of *water*, add gradually 5 ml of *hydrochloric acid* to the boiling solution, cool, and dilute to 500 ml with *water*.

Store under *toluene* or with *chloroform* at a temperature not exceeding 4°.

INORGANIC SALT SOLUTION: dissolve 10 g of *magnesium sulphate*, 0·5 g of *manganese sulphate*, 0·1 g of *ferric chloride*, and 0·3 ml of *hydrochloric acid* in 250 ml of *water*.

Store under *toluene* or with *chloroform*.

MEDIUM FOR THE ASSAY OF RIBOFLAVINE:

Dextrose (monohydrate)	20 g
Sodium Chloride	5 g
Ammonium Sulphate	3 g
Xylose	1 g
Photolysed Peptone Solution	100 ml
Cystine Solution	25 ml
Tryptophan Solution	25 ml
Yeast Supplement	20 ml
Adenine–Guanine–Uracil Solution ..	10 ml
Nicotinic Acid Stock Solution ..	10 ml
Xanthine Solution	10 ml
Inorganic Salt Solution	5 ml
Potassium Phosphates Solution ..	5 ml
p-Aminobenzoic Acid Solution ..	4 ml
Calcium Pantothenate Solution ..	1 ml
Pyridoxine Solution	1 ml
Water	to 500 ml

Mix and adjust the medium to pH 6·8 by the addition of *sodium hydroxide solution*. Store at a temperature not exceeding 4° and use within 24 hours of preparation. The medium is sterilised, after the addition of the riboflavine or the test solution, as described in the method, by heating in an autoclave at 115° for exactly 10 minutes.

NICOTINIC ACID STOCK SOLUTION: dissolve 0·1 g, accurately weighed, of nicotinic acid in 1000 ml of *water*.

Store under *toluene* or with *chloroform* and use within 7 days of preparation.

PHOTOLYSED PEPTONE SOLUTION: dissolve 40 g of a suitable peptone in 250 ml of *water*, add 20 g of *sodium hydroxide* dissolved in 250 ml of *water*, allow the mixture to stand in the light at room temperature for 24 hours, during at least 12 hours of which it is exposed to strong light; neutralise the solution with *glacial acetic acid*, add 11·6 g of *sodium acetate*, and dilute to 800 ml with *water*.

Store under *toluene* or with *chloroform* at a temperature not exceeding 4° and use within 14 days of preparation; the solution should not be used if a precipitate forms.

POTASSIUM PHOSPHATES SOLUTION: dissolve 25 g of *potassium dihydrogen phosphate* and 25 g of *dipotassium hydrogen phosphate* in 250 ml of *water*.

Store under *toluene* or with *chloroform*.

PYRIDOXINE SOLUTION: dissolve 0·1 g of pyridoxine hydrochloride in 1000 ml of *water*.

Store under *toluene* or with *chloroform* at a temperature not exceeding 4° and use within 7 days of preparation. It should be protected from light.

RIBOFLAVINE SOLUTION, STANDARD: dilute 4·0 ml of *riboflavine stock solution* to 1000 ml with *water* immediately before use; 1 ml contains 0·1 microgram of riboflavine. During the preparation and storage of the solution it should be protected from light.

RIBOFLAVINE STOCK SOLUTION: dissolve 25 mg of riboflavine, accurately weighed, in 1 ml of *glacial acetic acid*, and dilute to 1000 ml with *water*.

Store under *toluene* or with *chloroform* at a temperature not exceeding 4° and use within 14 days of preparation. During the preparation and storage of the solution it should be protected from light.

SODIUM ACETATE, 2·5M: a solution of *sodium acetate* in *water*, containing in 1000 ml 340·3 g of $C_2H_3NaO_2,3H_2O$.

TRYPTOPHAN SOLUTION: boil 2 g of DL-tryptophan with a little *water*, add *hydrochloric acid*, dropwise, to effect solution, cool, and dilute to 500 ml with *water*.

Store under *toluene* or with *chloroform* at a temperature not exceeding 4°.

WATER: glass-distilled water must be used throughout the assay and in the preparation of the reagents.

XANTHINE SOLUTION: dissolve 0·1 g of xanthine in a small quantity of *strong ammonia solution* and dilute to 100 ml with *water*.

Store under sulphur-free *toluene* or with *chloroform* at a temperature not exceeding 4° and use within 14 days of preparation.

YEAST SUPPLEMENT: dissolve 100 g of a suitable yeast extract in 500 ml of *water*, add 150 g of basic lead acetate dissolved in 500 ml of *water*, adjust to pH 10 with *dilute ammonia solution*, and filter; make the filtrate acid to *litmus paper* with *glacial acetic acid*, pass *hydrogen sulphide* through the solution until all the lead has been precipitated, filter, and dilute to 1000 ml with *water*.

Store under *toluene* or with *chloroform* at a temperature not exceeding 4° and use within 3 months of preparation.

Preparation of Inoculum. To 5 ml of *medium for the assay of riboflavine* add 2·5 ml of *standard riboflavine solution* and 2·5 ml of *water* and sterilise by heating in an autoclave at 115° for 10 minutes; cool, inoculate with a culture of a suitable strain of *Lactobacillus helveticus*, and incubate for 18 hours at 37°; centrifuge, reject the supernatant liquid, and suspend the bacterial cells in 10 ml of *saline solution*; add 1 ml of this suspension to 10 or 20 ml of *saline solution*. This suspension must be prepared freshly for each assay.

Method for Vitamins Capsules, Dried Yeast, and Yeast Tablets. Autoclave 5 capsules or about 1 g of dried yeast or of powdered tablets, accurately weighed, with 50 ml of 0·1N hydrochloric acid at 15 lb per sq in. pressure for 15 minutes; cool, add 2 ml of *2·5M sodium acetate*, adjust the pH to 4·5, using *bromophenol blue solution* as an external indicator, dilute to 100 ml with *water*, filter, extract with 20 ml of *anaesthetic ether*, and reject the extract; adjust the pH of 20 ml of the solution to 6·8, using *bromothymol blue solution* as an external indicator, and dilute to 100 ml with *water*.

This part of the procedure must be carried out in a dim light. To 5-ml quantities of *medium for the assay of riboflavine*, contained in bacteriological test-tubes, add graded doses of *standard riboflavine solution* and to a further series add similar graded doses of the test solution; dilute each mixture to 10 ml with *water*. A suitable range of doses contains 0·05 to 0·2 microgram of riboflavine; at least three replicate series should be prepared for the standard and for the sample. Sterilise the contents of the tubes by heating in an autoclave at 115° for exactly 10 minutes, cool, inoculate each of the tubes with one drop of the freshly prepared inoculum, and incubate at 37° for 3 to 4 days.

Titrate the lactic acid produced in each tube with 0·1N sodium hydroxide, using *bromothymol blue solution* as indicator and titrating to pH 6·8. Prepare a standard curve from the mean results obtained in the three series of tubes containing the standard riboflavine solution. From the mean amounts of lactic acid produced in the tubes containing the material derived from the sample and by reference to the standard curve, obtain the amount of riboflavine present.

D. DETERMINATION OF THIAMINE HYDROCHLORIDE

Reagents. Most of the reagents are included in Appendix 1; the following special reagents are required:

POTASSIUM CHLORIDE SOLUTION: a 25 per cent w/v solution of *potassium chloride* in 0·1N hydrochloric acid.

POTASSIUM FERRICYANIDE SOLUTION, ALKALINE: dilute 4 ml of *potassium ferricyanide solution* to 100 ml with a 15 per cent w/v solution of *sodium hydroxide* in water. The solution must be used within 4 hours of preparation.

THIAMINE HYDROCHLORIDE SOLUTION: a 0·020 per cent w/v solution of *thiamine hydrochloride* in 0·005N hydrochloric acid; 1 ml contains 0·2 mg of thiamine hydrochloride.

Method for Vitamins Capsules. Dilute 5 ml of *thiamine hydrochloride solution* to 100 ml with 0·1N hydrochloric acid and dilute 10 ml of this solution to 100 ml with *potassium chloride solution*; dilute 1, 2, and 4 ml of this solution (equivalent to 1, 2, and 4 micrograms of thiamine hydrochloride) with sufficient *potassium chloride solution* to produce three solutions, each of 5 ml; to each solution, contained in a small grease-free separator, add 3 ml of *alkaline potassium ferricyanide solution*, shake for 1 minute, add 25 ml of *isobutyl alcohol* saturated with water, shake vigorously for 1½ minutes, and allow to separate; to the alcoholic layer add 1 ml of *dehydrated alcohol* and measure the fluorescence in a suitable fluorimeter fitted with filters having maximum transmission between 400 nm and 450 nm, using a 0·0001 per cent w/v solution of *quinine sulphate* in 0·1N sulphuric acid for comparison, if necessary.

Prepare a calibration curve from the figures obtained, or use a previously prepared calibration curve after it has been checked by carrying out a determination on 5 ml of a solution containing 2·5 micrograms of thiamine hydrochloride, prepared by diluting 5 ml of *thiamine hydrochloride solution* to 100 ml with 0·1N hydrochloric acid and diluting 5 ml of this solution to 100 ml with *potassium chloride solution*.

Digest 2 capsules on a water-bath for 30 minutes with 60 ml of 0·1N hydrochloric acid, cool, and dilute the aqueous solution to 200 ml with water; dilute 5 ml of this solution to 100 ml with *potassium chloride solution* and transfer 5 ml to a small grease-free separator and continue by the method used for the preparation of the calibration curve, beginning with the words "add 3 ml of *alkaline potassium ferricyanide solution* . . .". Obtain the amount of thiamine hydrochloride present by reference to the calibration curve.

Digest 1 capsule and 5 ml of *thiamine hydrochloride solution*, as before, and repeat the determination. The amount of thiamine hydrochloride found is not less than 85 and not more than 105 per cent of the amount of added thiamine hydrochloride together with the amount of thiamine hydrochloride calculated from the result of the first determination to be present in the contents of the 2 capsules.

Method for Dried Yeast and Yeast Tablets. Prepare a calibration curve as described in the method for vitamins capsules. Digest about 0·5 g of the sample, accurately weighed, on a water-bath for 30 minutes with 60 ml of 0·1N sulphuric acid, keeping the liquid distinctly acid to *thymol blue solution* by adding more acid if necessary, cool, and adjust the pH to 4·0 to 4·5 with *2M sodium acetate*, using *bromocresol green solution* as an external indicator; add 0·2 g of a suitable source of phosphatase, such as Taka-diastase or Clarase, and allow to stand at 38° for 16 hours. Cool, dilute to 100 ml with water, centrifuge, and pass 10 ml of the clear solution through a column containing a base-exchange silicate prepared and used as described in the *Analyst*, 1951, **76**, 127.

Wash the column with three 5-ml portions of boiling water and reject all the eluates; then, elute with three 5-ml portions of boiling *potassium chloride solution*, cool the combined eluates, dilute to 25 ml with *potassium chloride solution*, and continue by the method for vitamins capsules, beginning with the words "transfer 5 ml to a small grease-free separator, . . .". Obtain the amount of thiamine hydrochloride present by reference to the calibration curve.

Mix about 0·5 g of the sample, accurately weighed, with 0·05 mg of *thiamine hydrochloride* and repeat the determination, but diluting the digest to 200 ml with water, in place of 100 ml, before centrifuging. The amount of thiamine hydrochloride found is not less than 85 and not more than 105 per cent of the amount of added thiamine hydrochloride together with the amount of thiamine hydrochloride calculated from the result of the first determination to be present in the sample.

E. DETERMINATION OF VITAMIN D

Reagents. Most of the reagents are included in Appendix 1; the following special reagents are required:

CALCIFEROL SOLUTION, STANDARD: dissolve 0·010 g of *calciferol* in sufficient *ethylene chloride* to produce 100 ml and dilute 10 ml of this solution to 100 ml with *ethylene chloride*; 1 ml contains 10 micrograms of calciferol.

*FLOREX XXS: a chromatographic grade of kaolin obtainable from Hermadex Ltd., 43, Berners St., London, W.1.

The following procedures should all be carried out in subdued light or in low actinic glasssware.

Preparation of Chromatographic Columns

COLUMN NO. 1. Shake 200 ml of *trimethylpentane* with sufficient *macrogol 600* so that, on separation, two layers are obtained; to 100 ml of the supernatant liquid add 25 g of *Celite 545*, shake vigorously to form a thin slurry, add, in small portions and with vigorous stirring, 10 ml of *macrogol 600*, and continue to stir for a further 2 minutes to produce a uniform suspension.

Transfer the suspension, in small portions, to a chromatographic tube 28 cm in length and 22 mm in diameter, fitted at its lower end with a sintered-glass disk and a tap, and pack carefully with the aid of a glass plunger; add sufficient of the suspension to produce a column 15 cm in length and discard any eluate.

Standardisation of column. Determine the volume in which calciferol is recovered from the column by the following method:

Transfer 2 ml of a 0·03 per cent w/v solution of *calciferol* in *trimethylpentane* to the top of the column and rinse it into the column with not more than 5 ml of *trimethylpentane*; elute the column with *trimethylpentane*, adjusting the rate of flow from the bottom of the column to 2 to 3 ml per minute, and collect successive 5-ml fractions of the eluate.

Measure the extinction of a 1-cm layer of each fraction at the maximum at about 263 nm, and hence determine the position, relative to volume of eluate, at which the elution of calciferol begins and finishes.

COLUMN NO. 2. Mix 5 g of *Florex XXS* with sufficient *trimethylpentane* to form a slurry and transfer the slurry to a chromatographic tube 20 cm in length and 6 mm in diameter, fitted at its lower end with a sintered-glass disk and a tap, packing it carefully with the aid of a glass plunger, and discarding the eluate.

Method for Vitamins Capsules and Vitamins A and D Capsules. To an accurately weighed quantity of the expressed contents, equivalent to about one capsule, add 15 ml of a 50 per cent w/v solution of *potassium hydroxide* in water and 15 ml of *alcohol (90 per cent)* and reflux on a water-bath for 30 minutes; cool, transfer the solution to a separator with the aid of 50 ml of water, add 75 ml of *solvent ether*, shake vigorously, allow to separate, transfer the aqueous layer to a second separator, and extract with three successive 30-ml portions of *solvent ether*, adding each ethereal extract to the liquid in the first separator and finally discarding the aqueous solution.

Pour two successive 100-ml portions of water through the ethereal solution, without shaking, and discard the aqueous layers; add successive 10-ml portions of water to the ethereal solution, agitating gently each time, and discarding the aqueous extracts, continuing the process until the aqueous extracts are neutral to *phenolphthalein solution*.

Dry the ethereal solution by stirring with *anhydrous sodium sulphate*, decant the ethereal solution, wash the residue with successive small portions of *solvent ether*, and evaporate the combined solution and washings on a water-bath to a volume of about 5 ml; cool, and evaporate to dryness in a current of *nitrogen*.

Dissolve the residue in 5 ml of *trimethylpentane* and transfer the solution to the top of chromatographic column No. 1 with the aid of 5 ml of *trimethylpentane*; elute the column with *trimethylpentane*, adjusting the rate of flow of eluate from the bottom of the column to 2 to 3 ml per minute, and collect the fraction of eluate estimated to contain the calciferol, as indicated by the standardisation of the column.

Transfer the eluate collected from chromatographic column No. 1 to the top of chromatographic column No. 2, allow the liquid to flow, add to the top of the column 10 ml of *trimethylpentane*, and discard the eluate. Elute the column with 50 ml of *benzene*, evaporate the eluate on a water-bath to a volume of about 5 ml, cool, evaporate to dryness in a current of *nitrogen*, and dissolve the residue in 4 ml of *ethylene chloride*.

Add 1 ml of the prepared solution to each of three tubes; to the first tube add 1 ml of *ethylene chloride* and 10 ml of *antimony trichloride solution in ethylene chloride*, to the second tube add 1 ml of a mixture of equal volumes of *ethylene chloride* and *acetic anhydride* and 10 ml of *antimony trichloride solution in ethylene chloride*, and to the third tube add 1 ml of *standard calciferol solution* and 10 ml of *antimony trichloride solution in ethylene chloride*.

Measure the extinction of a 1-cm layer of each solution, exactly 1 minute after the addition of the antimony trichloride solution, at the maximum at about 500 nm, using *ethylene chloride* as the blank.

The amount of calciferol, in mg, in the weight of sample taken is given by the formula:

$$\frac{0.04(e_1 - e_2)}{(e_3 - e_1)}$$

where e_1 = the extinction due to the solution in the first tube,

e_2 = the extinction due to the solution in the second tube, and

e_3 = the extinction due to the solution in the third tube.

Each mg of calciferol is equivalent to 40,000 Units of vitamin D.

Appendix 25

Powders and Suspensions

A. Classification of Powders

The descriptive term used to indicate the degree of comminution of substances employed in the manufacture of preparations in the British Pharmaceutical Codex can usually be related to the size of the mesh of the sieve or sieves through which the whole or a portion of the powder is able to pass. The wire sieves used in sifting powders are distinguished by numbers and should comply with the requirements of British Standard 410:1969. In the British Pharmacopoeia and the British Pharmaceutical Codex, sieves were formerly designated by the mesh count or mesh number which was the number of meshes per inch. Sieves are now designated by aperture size and the numbers indicate the nominal aperture size, measured in millimetres for aperture sizes of 1 mm or greater and in micrometers (μm) for aperture sizes of less than 1 mm.

The table below relates the sieve numbers now used to the mesh numbers formerly used. The relationship of the mesh number to the actual number of meshes per inch depends on the wire diameter and should be taken as an approximation.

Sieve Number	Mesh Number	Sieve Number	Mesh Number
mm		μm	
4·00	4	355	44
3·35	5	250	60
2·80	6	180	85
1·70	10	150	100
μm		125	120
710	22	106	150
500	30	75	200

The following terms are used in the description of powders:

COARSE POWDER. A powder of which all the particles pass through a No. 1·70 sieve and not more than 40·0 per cent pass through a No. 355 sieve.

MODERATELY COARSE POWDER. A powder of which all the particles pass through a No. 710 sieve and not more than 40·0 per cent pass through a No. 250 sieve.

MODERATELY FINE POWDER. A powder of which all the particles pass through a No. 355 sieve and not more than 40·0 per cent pass through a No. 180 sieve.

FINE POWDER. A powder of which all the particles pass through a No. 180 sieve.

VERY FINE POWDER. A powder of which all the particles pass through a No. 125 sieve.

ULTRA-FINE POWDER. A powder of which the maximum diameter of 90 per cent of the particles is not greater than 5 μm and of which the diameter of none of the particles is greater than 50 μm.

When the degree of comminution of a powder is defined by means of a number, the whole of the powder passes through the sieve described by that number.

B. Determination of the Surface Area of Bephenium Hydroxynaphthoate

Determine by the air-permeability method described by F. M. Lea and R. W. Nurse, *J. Soc. Chem. Ind., Lond.* (Transactions), 1939, **58**, 277–283, using a compact 2·54 cm in diameter, 1·00 cm in height, and having a porosity within the range 0·475 to 0·525.

For the purpose of the calculations, the density of the particles may be assumed to be 1·298 g per cm³.

C. Determination of Particle Size in Suspensions

The following method is to be used, when directed, to determine the particle size of a suspended solid in a preparation:

Dilute a suitable quantity of the preparation with an equal volume of *glycerol* and further dilute, if necessary, with a mixture of equal volumes of *glycerol* and water; alternatively, where specified in the individual monograph, use *liquid paraffin* as the diluent.

Mount the diluted preparation on a slide and examine random fields microscopically using a microscope providing adequate resolution for the observation of small particles.

Observe that there are no particles (or, if stated, not more than a few particles) above the maximum size permitted in the individual monograph.

Count the numbers of particles having maximum diameters above and/or below the limiting sizes permitted in the individual monographs and hence calculate the percentages of particles having maximum diameters within the stated limits.

The percentages should be calculated from observations on at least 1000 particles.

Appendix 26

Uniformity of Diameter of Tablets and Lozenges

TABLETS which are not sugar coated, film coated, or enteric coated, comply with the requirements for diameter stated in the following table. A deviation of ±5 per cent from the stated diameter is allowed, except that when the stated diameter exceeds 12·5 mm the permissible deviation is ±3 per cent.

Tablet	Strength (mg)	Diameter (mm)
Acetarsol	60	6·5
	250	10·5
Ammonium chloride	300	9·5
Ampicillin	125	10·5
Aspirin, compound	—	10·5
Aspirin, soluble, paediatric	—	8·0
Belladonna and phenobarbitone	—	5·5
Calcium gluconate	—	16·0
Calcium gluconate, effervescent	—	19·0
Calcium sodium lactate	300	10·5
	450	11·0
Calcium with vitamin D	—	12·5
Carbromal	300	10·5
Clefamide	250	8·5
Co-trimoxazole, paediatric	—	8·0 or 8·5
Ipecacuanha and opium	60	5·5
	300	9·5
	600	12·5
Magnesium carbonate, compound	—	12·5
Magnesium trisilicate, compound	—	16·0
Methallenoestril	3	8·5
Nalidixic acid	500	12·5
Nicotinamide	50	6·5
Papaveretum	10	5·0
Phenobarbitone and theobromine	—	10·5
Prothionamide	125	12·5*

Tablet	Strength (mg)	Diameter (mm)
Pyridoxine	10	5·5
	20	7·0
	50	9·0
Riboflavine	1	5·5
	3	6·5
Sulphaguanidine	500	12·5
Sulphathiazole	500	12·5
Thiabendazole	500	19·0
Thiacetazone	25	6·5
	50	8·0
	75	9·0
Thiopropazate	5	8·0*
	10	8·5*
Triamcinolone	1	8·0
	2	8·0
	4	9·5
Vitamin B, compound	—	8·0
Yeast	300	9·5

* When compression coated.

COMPRESSED LOZENGES that are circular in shape comply with the requirements for diameter stated below. A deviation of ±5 per cent from the stated diameter is allowed, except that when the stated diameter exceeds 12·5 mm the permissible deviation is ±3 per cent.

Lozenge	Strength	Diameter (mm)
Amphotericin	10 mg	16·0
Benzalkonium	—	16·0
Benzocaine, compound	—	12·5
Bismuth, compound	—	19·0
Formaldehyde	—	14·0
Hydrocortisone	2·5 mg	5·5
Liquorice	—	16·0
Penicillin	1000 Units	16·0

Appendix 27

Examination of Surgical Dressings

Requirements for adhesiveness, area per unit weight, colour fastness, elasticity, extensibility, foreign matter, sterility, sulphated ash, tensile strength, threads per stated length, water-soluble extractive, water-vapour permeability, water-proofness, weight per unit area, weight of fabric, weight of film, weight of adhesive mass, and content of antiseptic are included in a number of monographs on surgical dressings in Part 5.

When specific methods for determining these

requirements are not described in the monograph, the methods given in this appendix are used. Additional details of some of the procedures and descriptions of suitable apparatus are given in British Standards Handbook No. 11, 1963: Methods of Test for Textiles.

Physical and Chemical Testing
STANDARD ATMOSPHERIC CONDITIONS FOR TESTING. Unless otherwise stated, the atmosphere in which physical tests on surgical dressings are carried out shall be controlled at 63 to 67 per cent relative humidity and 18° to 22°.

CONDITIONING FOR TESTING. When weights, areas, counts, tensile strength, and absorbency are to be determined, the surgical dressing shall first be unwrapped, opened out, and conditioned by exposure to standard atmospheric conditions for not less than 12 hours before testing.

FULLY STRETCHED CONDITION. A surgical dressing is considered to be fully stretched when the full load has been applied, as described under Elasticity, below.

PERFORATED AND SHAPED DRESSINGS. In the determination of the weight per unit area, weight of fabric, weight of film, and weight of adhesive mass of self-adhesive bandages and plasters prepared with perforated cloth or perforated plastic film, allowance is made for the area of the perforations in calculating the results. In the case of a dressing whose corners have been cut to a radius, the actual area of the dressing is used for calculating these weights.

DRYING TEMPERATURES. When a drying temperature of 105° is specified in this section, the temperature shall be between 102° and 108°.

REAGENTS. The reagents used in the following tests are described in Appendix 1, page 829.

METHODS OF TESTING

Adhesiveness. The steel plate and the roller used in this test are described in British Standard 2J 10 (Pressure-sensitive adhesive waterproof P.V.C. tape for aeronautical purposes).
Clean the steel plate as described in B.S.2J 10. Bring the adhesive side of one end of a length of the plaster into contact with the cleaned surface of the plate in such a manner that the whole of the width of the strip for a distance of 2·5 cm from the end is attached to the plate with the sides of the strip parallel to those of the plate and the unattached portion of the strip overhanging the edge of the plate. In attaching the strip, ensure that no air bubbles are trapped between the plaster and the plate.
Pass the roller over the attached portion of the plaster three times, ensuring that the roller travels in the exact line of the strip. Mark the line of the end of the strip.
Select a weight, equivalent to 200 g for each 2·5 cm width of the plaster, and attach it to the free end of the strip by means of a stirrup which distributes the load evenly.
Suspend the plate for 30 minutes in a hot-air oven, fitted with a means of circulating air at a temperature of 36° to 38°, in such a manner that the plate is inclined at an angle of 2° to the vertical

in a direction which prevents the plaster peeling from the plate and the weight is hanging freely. Under these conditions, the top edge of the plaster attached to the plate does not slip by more than 2·5 mm during the period in the oven.

Area per unit weight. Determine this as described for Weight per Unit Area, page 915, but calculate from the measurements made the average value for the area, in cm², of 1 g of the sample.

In the case of absorbent lint, the dressing complies with the standard in respect of this requirement if the average found does not deviate from the average value stated in the monograph on this dressing by more than 3 times the standard deviation stated in the same monograph—see also the advice to manufacturers given in the test for Threads per Stated Length, page 914.

In the case of other dressings, the dressing complies with the standard in respect of this requirement if the average found is not lower than the average value stated in the appropriate monograph.

Colour fastness. Make an 8-ply square pad of the dyed gauze to be tested, measuring 5 cm by 5 cm, place it between two pieces of undyed bleached cotton cloth* of the same size, and sew the three pieces together along one edge. Prepare two such composite pads and carry out the following tests:

(i) Saturate one of the composite pads with *alcohol (70 per cent v/v)*, lay it smoothly in a flat-bottomed dish of a suitable size, add sufficient *alcohol (70 per cent v/v)* to cover the pad completely, place centrally on top of the pad a rectangular smooth glass plate, measuring approximately 5 cm by 5 cm and weighing about 50 g, press lightly on the glass plate to remove air bubbles, and keep at 36° to 38° for 15 minutes; without removing the glass plate, pour off the alcohol, and keep the pad at 36° to 38° for 4 hours. Remove the glass plate, separate the three pieces of cloth forming the composite pad, allow them to dry separately at a temperature not exceeding 60°, and examine the two outer pieces of undyed cotton cloth for staining.

(ii) Autoclave the other composite pad at 134° to 138° for 3 minutes, separate the three pieces of cloth forming the pad, and compare the two outer pieces of undyed cotton cloth with a piece of the same material autoclaved at the same time without being in contact with the gauze under test.

In both of these tests, the undyed cloth is virtually unstained.

* The standard bleached cotton cloth available from The Society of Dyers and Colourists, 19 Piccadilly, Bradford 1, Yorkshire, is suitable.

Elasticity. Measure the length of the material in the unstretched condition (*L* cm). Place one end of the material in a fixed grip and the other in a movable grip in such a way that the material stretches in the elastic direction. Ensure that the ends of the material are securely gripped, e.g. by means of pins in the grips, to minimise any slip while the material is under tension. Mark the material at the points where it enters the grips. Adjust the movable grip so that the material is under the minimum tension necessary to eliminate any wrinkles present and measure the length of material between the marks (l cm).

Apply gradually to the movable grip a force of 1·07 kgf per cm width, ensuring that the full load is applied within 5 seconds from starting to stretch.

Measure the length of material between the marks to the nearest cm as soon as the full load is applied (s cm).

Maintain this load for a total stretching time of 60 ± 5 seconds, ensuring that at no time is the load exceeded, and then release the tension as rapidly as possible without tangling the material.

Remove the material from the grips, loosely fold the whole length in a zig-zag with folds of 15 to 20 cm, and allow the material to relax for 5 ± ¼ minutes from the time of release of the tension; in the case of adhesive material, fold it edge to edge along its length with the adhesive side innermost before removing the material from the grips. Unfold the zig-zag, and measure the length of material between the marks to the nearest cm (r cm).

Then the *fully stretched length* $= L \times s/l$, and *regain length* $= L \times r/l$.

Extensibility. Carry out the test on a constant-rate-of-traverse machine. Test six specimens of the material, as representative of the sample as possible, and take the average figure as the result.

The load required to produce 20 per cent extension of the material at a rate of extension of 30 cm per minute is not more than 1·4 kgf per cm width. The permanent set after elongation of the material by 20 per cent, maintenance of the stretching for 60 ± 5 seconds, and a recovery time of 5 ± ¼ minutes is not greater than 5 per cent of the original unstretched length of the specimen.

Foreign matter. Dry about 5 g of the sample to constant weight at 105° and weigh the dried sample accurately while it is contained in a stoppered bottle. Extract the dried sample with *chloroform* for one hour in an apparatus for the continuous extraction of drugs. Remove the sample from the apparatus and allow the residual chloroform to evaporate.

Transfer the extracted sample to a suitable vessel, add 400 ml of water, heat it slowly, and boil for about 1 minute. Cool by adding an approximately equal volume of water and decant the liquid through a fine sieve (No. 150), wringing the material by hand to remove as much of the liquid as possible. Return the material to the vessel and repeat the washing process with five further 400-ml portions of water.

Place the washed material and any loose threads or fibres from the sieve in a beaker, cover with a 0·5 per cent solution of diastase, and maintain at 70° until free from any starch.

Decant the liquid through the sieve, return any loose threads or fibres on the sieve to the material in the beaker, and repeat the washing process with boiling water. Dry the material to constant weight at 105°, and determine the loss in weight.

To allow for the loss of natural soluble matter in grey (unscoured and unbleached) cotton in cotton crêpe, cotton stretch, cotton and rubber elastic, and elastic net bandages and unbleached calico that have not been dyed pink, subtract from the loss in weight 3 per cent of the weight of the final dry sample.

With the corresponding bandages that have been dyed, deduct 1 per cent; with crêpe bandage and domette bandage, deduct 2 per cent; and with flannel bandage, deduct 1 per cent. The loss in weight, corrected if necessary, is foreign matter.

Calculate the percentage of foreign matter with reference to the sample dried to constant weight at 105°.

When a sample is known to be free from starch, the treatment with solution of diastase and the second series of washings with boiling water may be omitted.

When the dressing consists of wool or union fabric, the temperature of the wash waters should be 45° to 50°.

With materials containing insoluble matter, indicated by pronounced milkiness in the first wash waters, complete removal of the insoluble matter can be assisted by repeated hand wringing and checked by carrying out an ash determination on the final dry residue. The ash should be not more than 0·2 per cent, calculated with reference to the final weight of the sample after drying at 105°.

Sterility. See Appendix 28, page 917.

Sulphated ash. Place the amount of material specified in the individual monograph, compressed if necessary and accurately weighed, in a silica or platinum dish, and moisten it with 2 ml of *dilute sulphuric acid*. Heat at first on a water-bath, then carefully over a small flame, and finally incinerate at dull red heat (600°).

Continue the incineration until all the black particles have disappeared and allow to cool. Add a few more drops of *dilute sulphuric acid* and repeat the heating and cooling procedures. Add a few drops of *ammonium carbonate solution*, again repeat the heating and cooling procedures, and weigh. Repeat the incineration for 5 minutes, cool, and weigh.

Repeat the incineration and cooling until two successive weighings do not differ by more than 0·5 mg.

Tensile strength. Carry out the test on a constant-rate-of-traverse machine having a movable jaw with a speed of 30 ± 3 cm per minute and a capacity such that when the specimen breaks the reading obtained is between 15 and 85 per cent of the complete scale.

Test six specimens of the material, as representative of the sample as possible and having the specified width.

Place one end of the material in the fixed grip and the other in the movable grip in such a way that the distance between the grips is 17·5 cm; in the case of plastic films, this distance may be reduced to 10 cm. If any specimen under test slips in the grips or breaks within 1 cm of the grips, exclude it from the test and replace it by another specimen.

Record the tensile strength as the average breaking load of the six test specimens.

Threads per stated length. With materials containing not less than 10 threads per cm, count the number of threads in 1 in. (2·54 cm) separately in both the warp and the weft by means of a suitable instrument, and calculate the number of threads per cm.

With materials of more open texture, count the number of threads in lengths of 10 cm; if it is impracticable to use 10 cm, use the greatest lengths of the warp and the weft allowed by the sample and calculate the number of threads in 10 cm.

If the size of the sample permits, make counts at not less than five independent positions selected so as to be as representative of the sample as possible and calculate the average number of threads per cm (or per 10 cm).

With those elastic materials on which thread counts must be calculated on the fully stretched material, use the following method:

Apply a force of 1·07 kgf per cm width of the sample (or other appropriate force indicated in an individual monograph), measure the number of threads in 1 in. separately in both the warp and the weft by means of a suitable instrument, and calculate the number of threads per cm.

If the size of the sample permits, make counts at eight independent positions selected so as to be as representative of the sample as possible, and calculate the average number of threads per cm or per 10 cm.

In the case of open-wove bandage, unbleached calico, absorbent gauze, gauze and capsicum cotton tissue, gauze and cellulose wadding tissue, gauze and cotton tissue, and absorbent lint, the dressing complies with the standard in respect of this requirement if the average found does not deviate from the average value stated in the appropriate monograph on the dressing by more than 3 times the standard deviation stated in the same monograph.

In order to increase the likelihood that any isolated sample of a dressing will meet the requirements for threads per stated length, it is necessary for the manufacturer to work within narrower limits than those stated above.

To assist the manufacturers of open-wove bandages etc., who will have more than one random sample available for testing, the following table shows the factor *x* by which the standard deviation should be multiplied to give the limits within which the average number of threads, determined on the indicated number of random samples, should fall in order to ensure that in 99 cases out of 100 any isolated sample of that batch of the dressing will comply with the requirement of the standard.

Number of random samples	Value of factor *x*	Number of random samples	Value of factor *x*
1	3	8	1·1
2	2·2	9 and 10	1·0
3	1·8	11 to 13	0·9
4	1·5	14 to 17	0·8
5	1·4	18 to 22	0·7
6	1·3	23 to 25	0·6
7	1·2		

In the case of other dressings, the dressing complies with the standard in respect of this requirement

if the average found is not lower than the average value stated in the appropriate monograph.

Water-soluble extractive. Dry about 5 g of the sample to constant weight at 105° and weigh the dried sample accurately while it is contained in a stoppered bottle.

Wash the dried sample thoroughly 12 times with hot water, using about 1000 ml for each washing and wringing the material by hand after each washing; pass all wash waters through a fine sieve (No. 150). Combine the washed material with any loose threads or fibres from the sieve and dry to constant weight at 105°.

The loss in weight, expressed as a percentage of the weight of sample dried to constant weight at 105°, is water-soluble extractive.

Water-vapour permeability. Place a tray containing approximately 1 kg of anhydrous calcium chloride on the floor of an electrically heated humidity cabinet fitted with an efficient means of circulating the air and maintained at 36° to 38°.

Place about 20 ml of water in each of five unlacquered metal boxes, complying with the description in Appendix D of British Standard 2 J 10 (Pressure-sensitive adhesive waterproof P.V.C. tape for aeronautical purposes), and cover the opening in the top of each box with a length of the plaster, pressed down without stretching the plaster, so that the opening is completely sealed. Weigh the sealed boxes, and place them in the humidity cabinet for 16 to 20 hours, noting the time to the nearest quarter-hour.

Remove the boxes from the oven, allow to cool (not in a desiccator), and weigh immediately.

From the mean loss in weight and the area of the opening in the top of each box, calculate the water-vapour permeability, in g per m² per 24 hours.

Waterproofness. This test can be applied to a product only if the sample is at least 7·5 cm square. If the width of a plaster is less than 7·5 cm, the test should be applied by the manufacturer to the sheet of material from which the product is prepared before the sheet is cut.

Carry out the test, using the apparatus and method described in the Hydrostatic Head Test given in British Standards Handbook No. 11, 1963, page 324, with the following modifications.

Slip the test specimens on to the completely filled cylinders from the side, with a sliding movement, so that air is excluded from between the undersides of the specimens and the upper surfaces of the water in the cylinders.

The hydrostatic head, indicated by the manometer reading when the first drop of water penetrates the specimen, is not less than 50 cm. For extensible plastic films each specimen is covered with a dry filter-paper, 7 cm in diameter, to prevent distortion of the specimen under pressure.

Weight per unit area. Cut a conveniently shaped specimen, preferably not less than 100 cm² in area, from the sample and determine its area and its weight. When the test does not give it directly, calculate the weight, in g per m² of the specimen; if the test has been carried out on a dried sample, correct the weight for percentage moisture regain.

If the size of the sample permits, repeat the

determination on further specimens and calculate the average value for the weight per m².

In the case of open-wove bandage, unbleached calico, and absorbent gauze, the dressing complies with the standard with respect to this requirement if the average found does not deviate from the average value stated in the appropriate monograph on the dressing by more than 3 times the standard deviation stated in the same monograph—see also the advice to manufacturers given under the test for Threads per Stated Length, page 914.

In the case of other dressings, the dressing complies with the standard in respect of this requirement if the average found is not lower than the average value stated in the appropriate monograph.

Weight of fabric. Weigh accurately the whole adhesive bandage or plaster (*W*g). Measure the width and length (or in the case of elastic products, the fully stretched length (*FSL*), measured as described under Elasticity, page 913, and calculate the total area (*A* m²).
Cut out rectangular full-width samples, each weighing about 3 to 4 g, from three positions approximately equidistant along the length, combine the samples, and weigh accurately (*w* g).
Macerate the combined samples with successive 250-ml portions of *chloroform*, or other suitable solvent, until the adhesive mass appears to be completely removed, decanting each extract through a fine sieve (No. 150). Return any fibres collected on the sieve to the extracted fabric, cover with an approximately 50 per cent v/v solution of *acetic acid* in water, and allow to stand until all the zinc oxide retained in the cloth is dissolved. Decant the liquid, and wash the material with successive portions of water until free from acidity, passing the washings through the sieve. Return any fibres collected on the sieve to the extracted material and dry the material to constant weight at 105°. Condition the dried material as described under Conditioning for Testing, page 913, and reweigh (*f* g).
Calculate the weight of fabric, in g per m², from the expression: $(f \times W)/(A \times w)$.

Weight of film. Take about 10 g, accurately weighed, of the plastic self-adhesive plaster and measure the area of the sample.
Macerate the sample with successive portions of *light petroleum (boiling-range, 40° to 60°)* until the adhesive mass appears to be completely removed, and dry the residual film to constant weight in a current of warm air.
From the area of the unextracted sample, calculate the weight of film, in g per m².

Weight of adhesive mass. Carry out the procedure described under Weight of Fabric, above, but measure the spread width of adhesive if this is different from the width of fabric.
Calculate the weight of adhesive mass, in g per m², from the expression:

$$\frac{(w - f) \times W}{B \times w}$$

where *B* = total area, in m², of adhesive mass, and *w*, *f*, and *W* = the quantities indicated above under Weight of Fabric.

In the case of plastic self-adhesive plasters, carry out the procedure described under Weight of Film, above, and calculate the weight of adhesive mass from the expression:

$$\frac{W - f}{A}$$

where *W* = the weight, in g, of the sample, *f* = the weight, in g, of the dry residual film, and *A* = the area, in m², of the sample.

Content of antiseptic
Those surgical dressings that are permitted or required in a particular monograph to be impregnated with an antiseptic specified in the general monograph, page 609, shall contain the stated content of one of the following antiseptics.

CONTENT OF AMINACRINE HYDROCHLORIDE. 0·07 to 0·13 per cent, calculated as $C_{13}H_{11}ClN_2,H_2O$, determined by the following method:
Extract about 25 g of the material, accurately weighed, in small pieces, with *solvent ether* in an apparatus for the continuous extraction of drugs until extraction of fatty matter is complete; shake the ether extract with 20 ml of water, allow to separate, reserve the lower aqueous layer, and discard the upper ether layer.
Dry the extracted material in a current of warm air and re-extract with *methyl alcohol*, containing 1 ml of *dilute hydrochloric acid*, until extraction of the antiseptic is complete.
Evaporate the extract to about 10 ml on a water-bath, add the reserved aqueous washings and 100 ml of water, boil until the volume is reduced to about 60 ml, and adjust the pH to 5·0 with a 10 per cent w/v solution of *sodium acetate* in water; add, with stirring, 5 ml of 0·04M potassium ferricyanide, allow to stand for 30 minutes, filter, and wash the residue with 50 ml of water.
To the combined filtrate and washings add successively, mixing after each addition, 1 ml of *hydrochloric acid*, 1 g of *sodium chloride* and 0·1 g of *potassium iodide* dissolved in 5 ml of water, and 0·3 g of *zinc sulphate* dissolved in 2 ml of water, allow to stand for 3 minutes, and titrate the liberated iodine with 0·04M sodium thiosulphate, using a 1 per cent w/v solution of *sodium starch glycollate* in water as indicator.
Repeat the procedure omitting the sample.
The difference between the two titrations represents the amount of 0·04M sodium thiosulphate required by the sample; each ml of 0·04M sodium thiosulphate is equivalent to 0·02985 g of $C_{13}H_{11}ClN_2,H_2O$.

CONTENT OF CHLORHEXIDINE HYDROCHLORIDE. 0·07 to 0·13 per cent, determined by the following method:
To about 30 g of the material, accurately weighed, in small pieces, add 140 ml of water and 60 ml of 1N hydrochloric acid, shake for 30 minutes, and decant the extract; shake the residue for 15 minutes with two successive 100-ml portions of a mixture of 7 volumes of water and 3 volumes of 1N hydrochloric acid and again decant each extract; dilute the combined extracts to 1000 ml with water.
To 40 ml of this solution add 45 ml of water and 5 ml of a 20 per cent w/v solution of *cetrimide* in water, make slightly alkaline to *litmus paper*

with *sodium hydroxide solution*, add 2 ml of *alkaline sodium hypobromite solution*, and shake; add 1 ml of *isopropyl alcohol* to suppress the froth, dilute to 100 ml with water, and maintain at 20° for 25 minutes.

Measure the extinction of a 1-cm layer of the solution at the maximum at about 480 nm and calculate the amount of antiseptic in the sample by reference to a calibration curve prepared using solutions containing 0·001 to 0·005 per cent w/v of *chlorhexidine hydrochloride* in a mixture of 5 volumes of 1N hydrochloric acid and 95 volumes of water and proceeding by the method described above, beginning with the words "To 40 ml of this solution . . .", and plotting the extinctions against the concentrations of antiseptic.

CONTENT OF CHLORHEXIDINE GLUCONATE. 0·11 to 0·20 per cent, determined by the method for chlorhexidine hydrochloride, using a solution of chlorhexidine gluconate for the preparation of the calibration curve.

CONTENT OF DOMIPHEN BROMIDE. 0·08 to 0·20 per cent, determined by Method I or Method II, given below. Method I will usually be found suitable. However, certain dye systems used in dressings containing domiphen bromide may interfere with the normal blue colour of the chloroform layer in the titration, with consequent difficulty in determining the end-point, and, in these circumstances, Method II may be used.

Method I. Dry about 5 g of the material, accurately weighed, in small pieces, to constant weight at 105°; immerse the dried material in 100 ml of *methanolic hydrochloric acid* and shake the mixture for 30 minutes; decant the solution, transfer 50 ml of the decanted solution to a round flat-bottomed flask, evaporate on a water-bath to a volume of 5 to 10 ml, and allow to cool.

Add 35 ml of water and 0·2 ml of *bromophenol blue solution* and titrate with 2N sodium hydroxide until a blue or green colour is produced; add 5 ml of a 60 per cent w/v solution of *anhydrous sodium acetate* in water and 10 ml of *chloroform*, shake the mixture and titrate with a 0·014 per cent w/v solution of *purified sodium lauryl sulphate* in water until the chloroform layer changes to colourless or yellow.

Repeat the procedure using, in place of the sample, 5 g of undyed non-impregnated cotton fabric on which 5·0 ml of *standard domiphen bromide solution* has been dispersed and which has been subsequently dried at 105°.

Calculate the percentage of domiphen bromide in the sample from the formula:

$$\text{Percentage of domiphen bromide} = \frac{V \times 0.007 \times 100}{S \times W}$$

where W = weight, in g, of the sample taken, V = volume, in ml, of the sodium lauryl sulphate solution used in the titration with the sample, and S = volume, in ml, of the sodium lauryl sulphate solution used in the titration with the domiphen bromide solution.

Method II. Prepare a chromatographic column in the following manner:

Suspend a suitable quantity of De-acidite FF-1P in 2N hydrochloric acid, allow to stand for 10 minutes, transfer sufficient of the suspension to a suitable chromatographic tube, fitted with a glass wool plug at its tapered end, to give a column height of about 15 cm, wash the column with water until the eluate has a pH of 6 to 7, and finally wash with several volumes of *methyl alcohol*.

Dry about 5 g of the material, accurately weighed, in small pieces, to constant weight at 105°; immerse the dried material in 100 ml of *methyl alcohol*, and shake the mixture for 30 minutes.

Decant the solution, transfer 50 ml of the decanted solution to a separating funnel arranged so that its stem is above the top of the prepared column, and allow the solution to flow through the column at a rate of about 3 ml per minute, collecting the eluate in a round flat-bottomed flask; wash the column with 40 ml of *methyl alcohol*, evaporate the combined eluate and washings on a water-bath to a volume of 5 to 10 ml, allow to cool, and continue as described in Method I, above, beginning with the words "Add 35 ml of water . . .".

CONTENT OF EUFLAVINE. 0·08 to 0·20 per cent, calculated as $C_{14}H_{14}ClN_3$, determined by the following method:

Dry about 20 g of the material, accurately weighed, in small pieces, to constant weight at 105°, and extract the dried material with *alcohol (95 per cent)* containing 2 ml of *dilute hydrochloric acid* in each 250 ml in an apparatus for the continuous extraction of drugs which is screened from light by impervious material.

Extract for 3 hours, or until extraction of the antiseptic is complete; to the extract add 50 ml of water, evaporate to low bulk, add a further 50 ml of water, again evaporate to low bulk, cool, filter through a sintered-glass or asbestos-packed Gooch crucible, which should not be allowed to run dry, and wash the residue with water.

To the combined filtrate and washings, which should not exceed 100 ml, add an excess (about 10 ml) of a saturated solution of *trinitrophenol* in water, allow to stand in ice for at least one hour, filter through a sintered-glass crucible, wash the residue with ice-cold *dilute trinitrophenol solution*, followed by 15 ml of ice-water, and dry to constant weight at 105°; each g of residue is equivalent to 0·5729 g of $C_{14}H_{14}ClN_3$.

Appendix 28

Test for Sterility of Surgical Dressings and Sutures

A surgical dressing or suture which is issued as sterile must have been subjected to a properly applied and monitored sterilisation process.

Presumptive evidence that the product is sterile may be derived from two sources; first, from a knowledge that good manufacturing procedures were followed throughout the manufacture of the product and that a wrapping material or container has been used which under normal conditions will prevent subsequent contamination of the product with micro-organisms, and, second, from an examination of the control records of the sterilisation process applied.

Such evidence will be readily available to the manufacturer of the product and from it the microbial quality of the product can be assessed. Usually, however, this information is not readily available to an independent analyst who has to examine for compliance with official requirements a sample of a dressing or suture labelled as sterile and in this circumstance application of a test for sterility is the only means available for assessing whether or not the sample might be regarded as sterile.

It must be emphasised that if the sample consists of only one homogeneous item, i.e. homogeneous with respect to risk of contamination—and it should be noted that a package which contains several dressings must be regarded as only one homogeneous item if the enclosed dressings are not individually wrapped—an analyst has no justification for assuming that the microbial quality of the remainder of the batch from which the sample was derived is the same as that of the sample.

Thus, if the test for sterility does not show the presence of any micro-organisms, it does not necessarily indicate that all the other items in the batch are sterile.

On the other hand, if micro-organisms are shown to be present in the sample and there is no reason to suspect either the integrity of the wrapping or container or the testing technique itself, the effectiveness of the sterilisation process that was applied to the batch shall be in doubt, but more reliable information should be sought, either by testing further samples if these are available or, preferably, by examining the manufacturer's control records if that is possible, before judging the microbial quality of the rest of the batch.

The probability that the result of a test for sterility truthfully reflects the microbial quality of the batch from which the sample was drawn increases as the number of homogeneous items in the sample increases; an indication of the quality can be obtained by examination of a sample of at least twenty homogenous items.

It is essential that a test for sterility is controlled by frequent and regular checks on the adequacy of the analyst's aseptic technique and of the nutritive properties (fertility) of the culture medium used. Under properly controlled conditions, experienced personnel testing familiar items should be able to carry out a test for sterility with an accidental contamination rate not greater than 0·1 per cent. However, when an unfamiliar item is tested, the accidental contamination rate may rise to as high as 5 per cent. The statistical inadequacy of the test for sterility is obvious in the latter instance and controls must be designed accordingly.

It is recognised that a well-established culture medium, under favourable conditions, will support the vigorous growth of the more common micro-organisms but it is still advisable to check the nutritive properties of a new batch of a medium. Of greater importance, however, are the nutritive properties of the medium when it has been inoculated with the dressing or suture under test and these must be checked.

The directions given in this Appendix for carrying out a test for sterility on a surgical dressing or suture are framed to enable an independent analyst to assess whether or not a sample consisting of a limited number of homogeneous items meets the requirements of the British Pharmaceutical Codex in respect of sterility.

A manufacturer who performs a test for sterility on a batch of a product in order to judge the microbial quality of the batch should test a sufficient number of items to ensure that the results have a statistically satisfactory basis to give him an acceptable degree of confidence in his assessment—see Advice to Manufacturers, page 921.

METHOD OF TESTING

Testing Area
The test for sterility must be carried out under aseptic conditions so that the items in the sample can be manipulated without becoming contaminated. These conditions may be achieved by using a laminar-airflow module specially designed for this purpose. In no circumstances may any sterilising agent, e.g. ultraviolet radiation, be used to maintain sterility in the area during testing.

Sample
A. If the sample consists of a number of homogeneous items, e.g. individually wrapped dressings or sealed containers of sutures, the items should be divided into three approximately equal groups, so that each necessary repeat test (see Test Procedure, below) can be carried out on a previously unopened item. If more than three items are available, it may be possible to carry out more than one complete test for sterility (including the permitted repeat tests) on the sample; consideration should be given, however, to reserving a sufficient number of unopened items to enable the test to be repeated on another occasion or by another independent analyst.

If the sample consists of less than three homogeneous items, it is not possible to conclude that it fails to meet the requirements of the Codex with respect to sterility, because the analyst cannot carry out on previously unopened items the two repeat tests that are permitted before a sample may be deemed to have failed; it is possible, however, for such a sample to pass the test if no micro-organisms are detected on the first re-test or on the original test.

Once the wrapping on a dressing or the sealed container of a suture has been opened it is not possible to store the item with a certainty that its microbial status will remain unchanged and therefore in no circumstances should the unused portion of an opened item be retained for the purpose of a re-test or for carrying out another test for sterility.

B. *In the case of dressings*, if a homogeneous item is too small to allow the full test portions to be taken for the test, the whole of the item should be used, undivided if it is less than 1 gram or less than 10 cm², or, if it is larger, divided into an appropriate number of approximately equal portions sufficient for the test and control procedures.

In the case of sutures, the whole of the strand in the container should be used for the test.

Culture Media

Recently prepared tryptone-soya broth is recommended for use in the test; it has the following composition:

Tryptone	17·0 g
Soya peptone	3·0 g
Anhydrous dextrose	2·5 g
Sodium chloride	5·0 g
Dipotassium hydrogen phosphate ..	2·5 g
Distilled water .. .. .. to 1000 ml

Dissolve the solids in the water by heating if necessary on a water-bath. The pH of the solution should be adjusted, if necessary, to pH 7·3 ± 0·1. If the solution is not clear when it is cold, heat it without boiling and filter it while it is hot through a filter paper. Transfer 50-ml, 100-ml, or 150-ml portions, as appropriate, of the clear filtrate to suitable containers, close the containers, and sterilise them by autoclaving at 121° to 123° for 15 minutes.

A suitable anaerobic medium is prepared by incorporating 0·1 to 0·2 per cent of agar in the tryptone-soya broth. This semi-solid medium should either be used soon after sterilisation or be heated and cooled just before inoculation. Conditions of low oxygen tension will only exist deep in this medium and therefore test portions should be immersed well below the surface.

Any other culture medium suitable for aerobic or anaerobic bacteria, or both, may be used provided that it has been recently prepared and its nutritive properties have been demonstrated in a fertility test to be at least as good as the recommended medium—see under Controls, below.

Test Procedure for Dressings other than Paraffin Gauze Dressing

QUANTITIES TO BE USED IN THE TEST. 1. *Culture medium:* use the volume prescribed in the individual monograph.

2. *Test items:* take three test portions, each of about 1 g if the dressing is made of unwoven material or of about 10 cm^2 if the dressing is made of woven material, from three different places in a freshly opened item including those areas where contamination is most likely to be present, i.e. the outer layers and the centre.

If a re-test is necessary (see Interpretation of Results, page 920) repeat the procedure, using six portions from another freshly opened item. If a second re-test is necessary, repeat the procedure again, using twelve portions from a third freshly opened item.

INOCULATION OF MEDIUM. Inoculate the appropriate number of containers of the selected medium with the test portions, each portion in a different container.

INCUBATION. After inoculation with the test portions, incubate the containers of medium at 32° ± 2° for 10 days and examine them at intervals for growth of micro-organisms.

CONTROLS. 1. *Establishment of the adequacy of the aseptic transfer techniques:* at the same time that the test is applied to the sample items, carry out the test for sterility on an equal number of control items which are similar, or preferably identical, in construction to the sample items. These control items must have been recently sterilised by a recognised effective sterilisation process so that they can be regarded with confidence as "known sterile" controls.

No growth of micro-organisms should occur in any of the containers of medium inoculated with the control items.

2. *Establishment of the effectiveness of the culture medium in the absence and presence of the sample items (fertility test):* take at least four containers with the same volume of the culture medium as is used in the test for sterility on the sample items and inoculate half the containers with a test portion of the sample item. Inoculate all the containers with 0·1 ml of a culture of a suitable strain either of *Bacillus subtilis* var. *niger* if an aerobic medium is being tested or of *Clostridium sphenoides* (*Plectridium sphenoides*) if an anaerobic medium is being tested, the appropriate culture having been diluted to contain about 100 viable spores per ml (i.e. an inoculation of about 10 spores). Incubate all the containers at 32° ± 2° for 10 days.

A profuse growth of the test micro-organisms occurs which is similar in the presence and absence of the test portions of the sample items.

ELIMINATION OF ANTIMICROBIAL PROPERTIES. The presence of antimicrobial properties in the item under test is shown when, in the fertility test of the medium (see under Controls, above), there is retardation in the growth of micro-organisms in the containers inoculated with the test portions.

If the sample is found or is known to have antimicrobial properties, these must be counteracted (a) by including a specific inactivator in the culture medium, or (b) preferably by using a membrane-filtration technique to remove the antimicrobial agent.

The use of an inactivator is restricted in its application because the number of inactivators which can be used is limited. Thus, apart from penicillinase (specific for penicillin preparations) and *p*-aminobenzoic acid (specific for the sulpha drugs), there is no satisfactory inactivator for any other antibiotic, and for other antimicrobial agents, inactivators are only partially effective. The inclusion of ox serum (5 or 10 per cent v/v) in the medium has some inactivating effect, as does also lecithin (0·07 per cent) with polysorbate 80 (Tween 80) (0·5 per cent). If this method is used, a fertility test should still be carried out to ensure that the antimicrobial agent has been sufficiently inactivated to allow growth should contaminating micro-organisms be present in the sample.

Membrane filtration is the method of choice for counteracting antimicrobial properties:

Shake each test portion for about 10 minutes with 50 ml of Letheen broth [a suitable nutrient broth containing 0·07 per cent of lecithin and 0·5 per cent of polysorbate 80 (Tween 80)]. Without delay, filter as much of the Letheen broth as can be poured off through a sterilised membrane filter which has previously been moistened with Letheen broth. Wash the membrane filter with three or four successive 50-ml portions of Letheen broth and then transfer it to a container of the selected medium in place of the test portion.

Test procedure for Paraffin Gauze Dressing

Carry out the procedure described above for other dressings with the following modifications:

Take three test portions from, if possible, different levels in a freshly opened item and inoculate three containers of the selected culture medium, previously warmed to 52°, each with a test portion. Close the containers tightly, and shake them on a reciprocating shaker for 10 minutes.

Allow the containers to cool until the paraffin forms a solid seal on the surface of the medium, break the seal with a quick shake, and incubate the containers at 32° ± 2° for 7 days.

Shake the containers on a reciprocating shaker for 10 minutes and transfer aseptically a 0·5-ml portion of the fluid in each container, separately, to another three containers with 15 ml of the same medium in each. Incubate this second set of containers at 32° ± 2° for 4 days and examine them for growth of micro-organisms.

If a re-test is necessary (see Interpretation of Results, below), repeat the above procedure as described on page 919 for re-testing dressings other than Paraffin Gauze Dressing.

Test procedure for non-absorbable sutures

Carry out the procedure described on page 919 for dressings other than Paraffin Gauze Dressing with the following modifications:

QUANTITIES TO BE USED IN THE TEST. 1. *Culture medium:* use 50-ml portions of the medium.

2. *Test items:* use a whole strand from a freshly opened container as a test portion.

If a re-test or second re-test is necessary, repeat the procedure, using the same number of test portions as were used in the original test, each taken from a freshly opened container.

INCUBATION. Incubate the inoculated containers of medium for 12 days.

CONTROLS. *Establishment of the effectiveness of the culture medium:* use 2 strands as the test portion in each container of medium inoculated with the sample item and incubate all the containers for 24 to 48 hours.

If the test indicates the presence of inhibitory effects due to the sterilisation method or to the constituents of the tubing fluid, repeat the test after removal or appropriate neutralisation of the inhibiting substances.

Interpretation of Results

If at the end of the incubation period in the initial test no growth of micro-organisms is observed in any of the cultures, the sample complies with the test; if growth has occurred in more than one culture, the sample does not comply with the test. If growth has occurred in not more than one culture, the test is repeated.

If at the end of the incubation period in the re-test, no growth of micro-organisms is observed in any of the cultures, the sample complies with the test; if growth has occurred in more than one culture or if growth of the same micro-organism has occurred in only one culture, the sample does not comply with the test. If growth of a different micro-organism has occurred in not more than one culture, the test is repeated a second time.

Number of packages or containers in the batch	Number to be taken
Surgical dressings	
Not more than 100 packages	10 per cent or 4 packages whichever is the greater
More than 100 but not more than 500 packages	10
More than 500 packages	2 per cent or 20 packages whichever is the greater
Sutures	
Not more than 1000 strands	2 per cent or 5 strands whichever is the greater
For each additional 1000 strands	An additional 2 strands up to a maximum total of 40

GROWTH OF MICRO-ORGANISMS IN CONTAINERS INOCULATED WITH TEST PORTIONS

1st Test	1st Re-test	2nd Re-test	Decision
no growth	—	—	Pass
growth in 1 container	no growth	—	Pass
	growth in more than 1 container	—	Fail
	growth of same micro-organism in 1 container	—	Fail
	growth of different micro-organism in 1 container	no growth	Pass
		growth in 1 or more containers	Fail
growth in 2 containers	no growth	—	Pass
	growth in 1 or more containers	—	Fail
growth in more than 2 containers	—	—	Fail

If at the end of the incubation period in the second re-test, growth is observed in any of the cultures, the sample does not comply with the test.

It should be noted that if, in the first test or either re-test, there is growth of micro-organisms in any of the containers of medium inoculated with the control item, the results of that test or re-test may be rejected and that stage of the procedure repeated; if, in this circumstance, there is no growth in the containers inoculated with the test portions, the results may be accepted.

ADVICE TO MANUFACTURERS

The following information is intended for guidance to manufacturers in producing sterile dressings and sutures that are required to comply with the test for sterility.

A batch is a collection of sealed items prepared in such a manner that they are homogeneous with respect to the risk of contamination. In testing for sterility a sample of items is selected at random from a single batch. The number of items

to be taken is set out in the upper table on page 920.

Although the items should be selected at random, care should be taken to ensure that some come from those positions in the load which are most inaccessible to the sterilising agent, e.g. steam in autoclaving, during the sterilisation process.

Interpretation of results. The lower table on page 920 indicates a suitable interpretation of the results of a test for sterility carried out by a manufacturer. If there is failure to comply with the requirements of the test, the batch should be rejected.

It should be noted that if, in the first test or either re-test, there is growth of micro-organisms in any of the containers of medium inoculated with the control item, the results of that test or re-test may be rejected and that stage of the procedure repeated; if, in this circumstance, there is no growth in the containers inoculated with the test portions, the results may be accepted.

Appendix 29

Sterilisation

Sterilisation is the process of killing or removing micro-organisms. It may be effected by killing the micro-organisms by physical or chemical methods or by removing them by filtration.

Medicaments to be used for the preparation of sterile products should be stored in containers fitted with the type of stopper which prevents dust falling between the stopper and the neck and should be kept apart from materials used for normal manufacturing or dispensing purposes.

The method of sterilisation chosen must not cause any important undesirable change in the materials (medicaments, vehicles, fabrics, apparatus, containers, wrappings) so that they remain suitable for their purpose. Failure to follow a recommended process meticulously, involves the risk of producing either a non-sterile product or some deterioration of the material.

Processes employing heat are the most reliable and are recommended whenever possible. Whichever method is chosen, the product should, if possible, be sterilised in its final container, thereby obviating the risk of contamination associated with the aseptic transference of a sterile material.

A product is accepted as sterile if, after it has been subjected to a properly applied sterilisation process, it complies with the test for sterility described in the European Pharmacopoeia or, in the case of surgical dressings and non-absorbable surgical sutures, in the British Pharmaceutical Codex.

The term "sterilised" is applied in the Codex to a product which has been subjected to a process of sterilisation and is sterile immediately on completion of the process; the term does not necessarily imply that the product is sterile subsequent to this.

In this appendix, methods of sterilisation and the techniques employed in aseptic processing are described first, followed by information on the application of these methods to the sterilisation of various types of material.

A. METHODS OF STERILISATION

Method 1. Dry Heat

The material is heated in a hot-air oven so that the whole of the load is kept at a specified minimum temperature for a stated time. In order to meet the required conditions, it is essential that the oven be provided with an efficient mechanical means for circulating the heated air; full details of the performance requirements of such ovens operating at temperatures between 140° and 180° are specified in British Standard 3421:1961.

Various combinations of temperature and time are recommended depending on the material being sterilised; for example, the usual recommended minimum holding times and temperatures are: 150° for one hour for fixed oils, ethyl oleate, liquid paraffin, and glycerol; 160° for one hour or 180° for 11 minutes for glassware and other apparatus. The heating-up time of the material is not included in the periods stated.

Method 2. Autoclaving

The material is exposed to saturated steam at a selected temperature above 100° for an appropriate time in a suitable pressure apparatus (autoclave).

Full details of the construction and performance requirements of automatically controlled autoclaves suitable for sterilising different types of loads are given in British Standard 3970:1966; similar considerations should be applied to non-automatic autoclaves.

In order to meet any performance requirements, regular inspection and maintenance of an autoclave are essential.

The temperature–time combination used is selected having regard to the stability of the material being sterilised. Provided that the steam in the autoclave is saturated and free from air, the different temperatures may be attained by de-

TABLE A

| Temperature | Corresponding nominal pressure in excess of atmospheric | | Recommended minimum holding time |
°C	kgf/cm²	lbf/in.²	minutes
115° to 116°	0·70	10	30
121° to 123°	1·05	15	15
126° to 129°	1·40	20	10
134° to 138°	2·25	32	3

TABLE B

BACTERICIDES RECOMMENDED FOR METHOD 3

Name of bactericide	Concentration per cent w/v	Recommended by B.P. and B.P.C. for parenteral use	by B.P.C. for ophthalmic use
Benzalkonium chloride	0·01	No	Yes
Chlorhexidine acetate	0·01	No	Yes
Chlorocresol	0·2	Yes	No
Phenylmercuric acetate	0·002	No	Yes
Phenylmercuric nitrate	0·002	Yes	Yes

veloping various specified pressures in the autoclave. It is preferable, however, to control the process by the temperature attained rather than by the pressure, as the presence of air in the autoclave results in a lower temperature than that expected under the correct conditions from the indicated pressure; in the case of porous materials, the air must be abstracted or displaced from the interstices in order to achieve sterilising conditions, as the presence of residual pockets of air within material may prevent contact between the steam and parts of the load.

Corresponding temperatures and steam pressures attained under the correct conditions, together with the recommended minimum holding times required to effect sterilisation, are given in Table A.

The period of heating must be sufficiently long to ensure that the whole of the material is maintained at the selected temperature for the appropriate recommended holding time. The time taken for the material to attain the sterilising temperature or to cool at the end of the holding time can vary considerably; it is dependent on a number of factors, including the size of the container and the thickness of its walls and the design, loading, and operation of the autoclave. It is necessary, therefore, that adequate tests be conducted to ensure that the procedure adopted is capable of sterilising the material and that the latter can withstand the treatment.

The process can be monitored by temperature-sensitive elements at different positions within the load.

Some indication that the heat treatment has been adequate can be gained by placing indicators at positions within the load where the required conditions are least likely to be attained. One such indicator is a Browne's tube which changes colour after the specified temperature has been maintained for a given time. Reliance should not be placed, however, on chemical indicators except when they suggest failure to attain sterilising conditions.

When it is inconvenient or impossible to use such means, the bactericidal efficiency of the process may be assessed by enclosing in different parts of the load small packets of material containing suitable heat-resistant spores, such as those of a suitable strain of *Bacillus stearothermophilus*; these are checked subsequently for the absence of viable test organisms.

Method 3. Heating with a Bactericide

This process is used for sterilising aqueous solutions and suspensions of medicaments that are unstable at the higher temperatures attained in the autoclaving process. It must not be used, however, if the preparation is to be administered parenterally by any route which contra-indicates the presence of a bactericide.

In this process, one of the bactericides listed in Table B is included in the preparation to give the concentration recommended, and the solution or suspension, in the final sealed container, is maintained at 98° to 100° for 30 minutes; this temperature can be conveniently attained by supporting the container in an atmosphere of steam produced above vigorously boiling water in a suitable container covered with a loose-fitting lid. The bactericide chosen must not interfere with the therapeutic efficacy of the medicament nor be the cause of any physical or chemical incompatibility in the preparation. For ophthalmic use, the choice is also governed by other considerations which are detailed in the General Monograph on Eye-drops, page 685.

Method 4. Filtration

Liquids may be freed from vegetative organisms and spores by passage through a bacteria-proof filter.

This process has the advantage that the use of heat is avoided. It has the disadvantage, however, that there is always a risk that there may be an undetected fault in the apparatus or technique used, and because of this each batch of liquid sterilised by filtration must be tested for compliance with the test for sterility described in the European Pharmacopoeia.

The filters are made of cellulose derivatives or other suitable plastics, asbestos, porous ceramics, or sintered glass. The maximum pore size consistent with effective filtration varies with the material of which the filter is made and ranges from about 2 μm for ceramic filters to about 0·2 μm for plastic membrane filters. Methods of determining maximum pore diameter and uniformity of pore diameter are described in British Standard 1752:1963.

All filters must comply with the following test:

> Assemble the filter into a filtering unit and sterilise the whole unit. Dilute an adequately large volume of a 24- to 48-hour culture of *Serratia marcescens* (*Chromobacterium prodigiosum*) in nutrient broth to 25 times its volume with nutrient broth and filter through the sterile apparatus, using a pressure of not less than 400 mm of mercury. By means of an aseptic technique, transfer 50 ml of the filtrate to a sterile container, close the container so as to exclude bacteria, and maintain at 25° for 5 days; no growth of *S. marcescens* or other micro-organism is visible in the sealed container.

Non-disposable filters should be tested periodically before use to ensure that their efficiency has not become impaired. An additional safeguard can be introduced by passing, after the filtration of a particular batch is finished, a test culture through the filter used and establishing that this filtrate is sterile.

Provided that a preparation is not to be administered parenterally by any route which contra-indicates the presence of a bactericide, a bactericide may be included in a concentration that prevents the growth of micro-organisms.

When required for use, the selected filter is attached to a filter flask, or other suitable receiver, having a bacteria-proof air-filter incorporated in the air exit. The receiver should preferably be fitted with a device to assist the aseptic transference (see Aseptic Technique, page 924) of the filtrate to the final sterile containers. All joints in the filtration system are made completely airtight and the assembled apparatus, suitably protected from recontamination, is sterilised.

Filtration is best carried out with the aid of positive pressure, as this reduces the possibility of airborne contamination of the sterile filtered solution through leaks in the system; if the filtration is likely to take a long time and the preparation is susceptible to oxidation, nitrogen or other inert gas under pressure should be used rather than compressed air.

On completion of the filtration, the filtrate is transferred with aseptic precautions to the final sterile containers. Alternatively, the filtrate can be collected in the final sterile containers.

Small volumes of liquids, such as eye-drops, can be conveniently sterilised by this method by passage through a small filter disk which is either incorporated in a special filter-syringe or is enclosed in a suitable holder which can be attached to an ordinary hypodermic syringe.

Method 5. Exposure to Gaseous Ethylene Oxide

Some materials which cannot be sterilised by dry heat or autoclaving may be sterilised by exposure to gaseous ethylene oxide. The method can be carried out at low temperatures and damages relatively few materials. It is, however, difficult to control, and the use of ethylene oxide should be considered only where the process is under the supervision of staff skilled in the method and having adequate facilities for bacteriological testing available.

Compared to other methods of sterilisation, the bactericidal efficiency of ethylene oxide is low and consequently particular attention should be paid to keeping microbial contamination of materials to be sterilised at a minimum.

Ethylene oxide forms explosive mixtures with air. This disadvantage can be overcome, either by using mixtures containing 10 per cent of ethylene oxide in carbon dioxide or halogenated hydrocarbons, or by removing at least 95 per cent of the air from the apparatus before admitting either ethylene oxide or a mixture of 90 per cent ethylene oxide in carbon dioxide.

A suitable apparatus consists of a sterilising chamber capable of withstanding the necessary changes of pressure, fitted with an efficient vacuum pump and with a control system incorporating valves to regulate the introduction of the gas mixture and to maintain the desired gas pressure, a device to adjust the humidity within the chamber to the desired level, and, if required, a heating element with temperature controls.

The sterilising efficiency of the process depends upon

(1) the partial pressure of ethylene oxide within the load,

(2) the temperature of the load,

(3) the state of hydration of the micro-organisms on the surfaces to be sterilised, and

(4) the time of exposure to the gas.

All these factors must be closely controlled for successful sterilisation. The sensitivity of micro-organisms to ethylene oxide is dependent on their state of hydration. Organisms which have been dried are not only resistant to the process but are also slow to rehydrate. Because of this, it is not sufficient to rely solely on humidification of the atmosphere within the chamber during the sterilising cycle.

It has been found in practice that hydration and heating of the load can be more reliably achieved by conditioning it in a suitable atmosphere prior to commencing the sterilisation.

The bactericidal efficiency of the process is not assured simply by relying on physical monitoring of the above factors. Therefore, in addition, each sterilising cycle must be monitored by:

(1) the insertion of a minimum of 10 bacteriological test pieces into different parts of the load most inaccessible to the ethylene oxide, and

(2) sterility testing of random samples taken from the load.

Any failure in these tests indicates the need for reprocessing the load. The test pieces should consist of aluminium foil on which has been dried a suspension of at least 10^6 spores of *Bacillus subtilis* Camp Detrick strain NCTC 10073 (*B. subtilis* var. *globigii*).

Ethylene oxide is absorbed by some materials and, because of its toxic nature, great care must be taken to remove all traces of it after the sterilisation is finished; this can be achieved by drawing sterile air through the load.

Method 6. Exposure to Ionising Radiation

Sterilisation may be effected by exposure to high-energy electrons from a particle accelerator or to gamma radiation from a source such as cobalt-60.

These types of radiation in a dosage of 2·5 megarads have been shown to be satisfactory for sterilising certain surgical materials and equipment, provided that precautions have been taken to keep microbial contamination of the articles to a minimum.

This method can also be used for some materials which will not withstand the other sterilisation methods.

The method has the advantage over other "cold" methods of sterilisation in that bacteriological testing is not an essential part of the routine control procedure, as the process may be accurately monitored by physical and chemical methods. It also allows the use of a wider range of packaging materials.

B. ASEPTIC TECHNIQUE

Aseptic processing is a method of handling sterile materials by employing techniques which minimise the chances of microbial contamination. It is used in preparing products which, because of their instability, cannot be subjected to a final sterilisation process.

This technique is not easy to perform successfully and there is no certainty that the final product will, in fact, be sterile. Sterility in the final product can only be assumed if the material complies with the test for sterility described in the European Pharmacopoeia.

In the preparation of a sterile solution by this process, the medicament, preferably sterile, is dissolved or dispersed in the sterile vehicle and the product transferred to the final sterile containers, which are then sealed to exclude micro-organisms.

Aseptic techniques are especially important when carrying out the process of sterilisation by filtration (Method 4) and during the transference of sterile materials to the final sterile containers.

In the particular case of the aseptic transference of liquids it is possible to assess whether or not asepsis is being achieved in the technique em-ployed by transferring sterile bacteriological medium instead of the pharmaceutical liquid. The filled containers are closed and incubated at 32° for 7 days. Evidence of microbial growth in the incubated medium indicates that contamination has occurred during the transference. This type of process control should be used when setting up new aseptic liquid-filling processes and also as a periodic check that asepsis is being maintained.

For success in aseptic processing, scrupulous care should be taken to reduce the risk of contamination of the materials being processed. If practicable, a room should be set aside for this work and a positive pressure maintained in it by introducing air which has been passed through a bacteria-proof filter. In addition, all manipulations should be carried out under a protective screen or in a current of sterile filtered air.

Likely sources of contamination include the hair, hands, clothing, and breath of the operator and the air impinging on exposed surfaces. The risk of contamination from these sources should be countered by accepted methods of cleansing and disinfection and by the use of protective clothing.

All working surfaces and the interior surfaces of screens should be disinfected; pressurised alcoholic sprays are convenient and effective for this purpose. If the screen is a sealed-cabinet type, gaseous ethylene oxide can be used; the air in the sealed cabinet is replaced by nitrogen or carbon dioxide and an effective concentration of ethylene oxide is introduced, allowed to remain for a specified period, and then removed by flushing the cabinet thoroughly with a sterile gas, initially either nitrogen or carbon dioxide and subsequently air. A minimum gaseous concentration of ethylene oxide of 10 per cent v/v at normal pressure (equivalent to 200 mg per litre) maintained for at least 16 hours at 20° is recommended.

Sterile containers and equipment should be available in adequate quantity.

C. APPLICATION OF STERILISATION METHODS

Glass and Metal Apparatus

Apparatus should be freed from dirt and grease by washing with hot soapy water or other suitable detergent and thoroughly rinsed with purified water. New glass apparatus should be given a preliminary treatment with a mixture of sulphuric acid (46 parts by volume), sodium nitrate (6 parts), and water (46 parts). The apparatus is then wrapped in a suitable grade of paper or cloth and sterilised; it is not unwrapped until required for use.

Syringes are enclosed in glass or metal tubes.

Bottles or flasks should be closed with paper or metal foil caps or with some other suitable closure; if they are to be autoclaved, a small quantity of water should be placed in the vessels, or alternatively they should be closed with a steam-permeable closure.

Sterilisation is effected by autoclaving (Method 2), by heating at a temperature not lower than 160° for 1 hour or 180° for 11 minutes (Method 1), or by exposing to ionising radiation (Method 6).

Glass is likely to discolour and darken when sterilised by exposure to ionising radiation.

Rubber and Plastics

Natural rubber articles should be sterilised by autoclaving (Method 2); they must not be subjected to dry heat. If a long length of tubing is to be autoclaved, some water should be placed in it beforehand. Some synthetic rubbers, e.g. silicone rubber, have good heat resistance and may be sterilised by dry heat (Method 1) as well as by autoclaving (Method 2).

Rubber teats and closures should be made of high-quality materials which release negligible amounts of undesirable substances and absorb the minimum of materials from solutions in contact with them.

Before use, teats and closures should be washed with a suitable detergent, rinsed with purified water, and boiled in several changes of purified water. If they are to be used to close containers of a preparation which contains a bactericide, the teats or closures should first be placed in a closed container with a solution of the bactericide in Purified Water; the concentration of bactericide in the solution should be at least twice that used in the preparation and the volume of the solution sufficient to cover the articles and equivalent to not less than 2 millilitres for each gram of rubber. The closed container is then autoclaved at 115° to 116° for a time sufficient to ensure that the contents are maintained at this temperature for 30 minutes. The teats and closures are then stored in this autoclaved solution until required for use.

If the preparation with which the teats or closures are to be used also contains an antoxidant, the antoxidant is included, at double the concentration used in the preparation, in the bactericidal solution in which the teats and closures are heated and stored.

Rubber closures used for containers of oily injections should be made of oil-resistant material or should be prevented from coming into contact with the oil by the use of protective material.

Plastic containers and other items of medical and surgical equipment that are not thermostable may be sterilised by exposure to gaseous ethylene oxide (Method 5) or to ionising radiation (Method 6). With the latter method, degradation, discoloration, and darkening of some plastics may occur.

Pharmaceutical Containers

The methods of cleansing and sterilisation described for glass, rubber, and plastics are generally applicable to containers made of these materials, but the particular properties of each type of container should be established so that possible detrimental effects of sterilisation procedures can be minimised.

Glass containers for sterile products should not react with the medicament or affect its therapeutic properties, nor should they yield small solid particles. Soda-glass eye-drop bottles which have been specially treated to reduce the amount of alkali released when in contact with aqueous liquids should not be autoclaved more than once.

All containers should be capable of being sealed effectively to exclude micro-organisms. Tests for efficiency of closure of eye-drop bottles by rubber teats are described in British Standard 1679: Part 5:1973.

SUBSTANCES AFFECTED BY ALKALI. The following are examples of substances that may, when in aqueous solution, be adversly affected by small amounts of alkali released by untreated soda-glass containers:

adrenaline acid tartrate	hyoscine hydrobromide
apomorphine	isoniazid
hydrochloride	lachesine chloride
ascorbic acid	levallorphan tartrate
atropine sulphate	levorphanol tartrate
calcium gluconate	mephenesin
carbachol	methoxamine
chlorhexidine acetate	hydrochloride
chlorhexidine gluconate	morphine sulphate
cocaine hydrochloride	nalorphine
corticotrophin	hydrobromide
cyanobalamin	neostigmine
digoxin	methylsulphate
diphenhydramine	noradrenaline acid
hydrochloride	tartrate
dipipanone	papaveretum
hydrochloride	physostigmine sulphate
emetine hydrochloride	phytomenadione
ergometrine maleate	pilocarpine
ergotamine tartrate	hydrochloride
ethylmorphine	pyridostigmine bromide
hydrochloride	pyridoxine
heparin	hydrochloride
histamine acid phosphate	quinine dihydrochloride
homatropine	strychnine hydrochloride
hydrobromide	suxamethonium chloride
hydroxocobalamin	thiamine hydrochloride

Aqueous Solutions and Suspensions

Scrupulous attention should be paid to clean preparative methods and to the achievement of minimal contamination during preparation. The process of sterilisation by heating with a bactericide may fail if these precautions are not observed.

Solutions should be clarified by filtration before the preparation is filled into final containers, which are then sealed and sterilised by autoclaving (Method 2), by heating with a bactericide (Method 3), or by exposure to ionising radiation (Method 6).

The sterilisation method selected must take into account the stability of the preparation. The process of heating with a bactericide is used for aqueous preparations which are unstable at the higher temperatures attained in the process of autoclaving, but it must not be used for the sterilisation of preparations to be administered by intrathecal, intracisternal, peridural, intra-ocular or, if the volume of a single dose exceeds 15 millilitres, intravenous injection. Vehicles for suspensions should be filtered before making the preparation.

Solutions may also be sterilised by filtration (Method 4) and then transferred aseptically to previously sterilised final containers which are then sealed to exclude micro-organisms.

Non-aqueous Liquids, Solutions, and Suspensions

Non-aqueous substances and preparations capable of withstanding fairly high temperatures may be sterilised in their final sealed containers, or in containers temporarily closed so as to exclude micro-organisms, by heating in a hot-air oven for a time sufficient to ensure that the whole of the contents is maintained at not less than 150° for one hour (Method 1).

This process is suitable for sterilising liquids, soft and hard paraffins, fixed oils, ethyl oleate, glycerol, waxes, and solutions or suspensions of stable substances in fixed oils or ethyl oleate. It must be emphasised, however, than when certain suspensions are sterilised in this way, the suspended substances may partly dissolve on heating and crystallise in large aggregates on cooling.

Sterile oily solutions or suspensions of substances which are incapable of withstanding the conditions of Method 1 are prepared aseptically, previously sterilised and cooled vehicle being used and the preparation being transferred aseptically to sterile final containers, which are then sealed to exclude micro-organisms.

Powders

Included among the procedures which may be satisfactory for the sterilisation of powdered substances are heating in a hot-air oven (Method 1), exposure to ethylene oxide (Method 5) or to ionising radiation (Method 6), and, if a suitable solvent is available, bacterial filtration (Method 4). The method selected must not cause decomposition or deterioration of the substance.

When dry heat is employed, the substance is spread in a thin layer in a suitable container, heated in a hot-air oven until the whole of the powder is at 150°, and then maintained at at least this temperature for one hour. Provided that it is not necessary to maintain asepsis, some substances may be heated to red heat in a muffle furnace.

If ionising radiation is used, the substance is exposed to gamma rays or accelerated electrons so that it is subjected to a dose of at least 2·5 megarads.

When filtration is used, the solution of the substance in a suitable inert solvent is filtered through a sterile bacteria-proof filter into previously sterilised containers and the solvent removed by an appropriate method to leave the residue in a suitable crystalline form or as a solid, which should, if necessary, be powdered. Aseptic precautions should be observed throughout.

Surgical Dressings

Surgical dressings are sterilised by autoclaving, dry heat, or exposure to ethylene oxide or ionising radiation, the choice depending on the nature of the dressing, with suitable modifications described below; any other method may be used provided that the finished sterilised dressing complies with the standard given in the individual monograph in Part 5, pages 609–637.

Sterilisation by any method may cause some deterioration in quality, and a dressing which complies with the appropriate standard before sterilisation may not do so afterwards; it may therefore be necessary to ensure that the sterile dressing is prepared from materials that are not too close to the minimum standard.

PACKAGING

Packaging suitable for sterile surgical dressings falls into two main categories depending upon the manner in which the dressing is intended to be used:

(1) that suitable for dressings which are handled and applied with aseptic precautions, and

(2) that suitable for dressings which, although not applied with aseptic precautions, are required to reach the user in a sterile condition.

The first category covers sterile dressings for use in operating theatres, hospital wards, clinics, etc., while the second category covers those intended, for example, for domestic use.

In both instances, the packaging must be adequate to maintain sterility of the dressing at least up to the time of opening the package. Dressings packed in such a manner may be labelled as "Sterile", and any dressing so labelled complies with the test for sterility described in Appendix 28, page 917.

The sterilisation process chosen governs both the choice of the wrapping material and the design of the pack. Double wrapping affords a distinct advantage over the use of a single wrapper for presenting a product in an aseptic manner, and when a surgical dressing or a composite pack (that is, a pack containing a variety of articles used in a single procedure) is to be used with aseptic precautions, double wrapping is essential. Both wrappers should be applied and the outer wrapper sealed before the package is sterilised. For such products, a packing carton or case is not a suitable outer wrapper.

Packaging which maintains sterility of its contents during normal conditions may not do so if it becomes wet. It is important, therefore, that the outer wrapper chosen should, when wet, be as impervious as possible to the passage of micro-organisms in case the package is wetted inadvertently.

METHODS

AUTOCLAVING (Method 2, page 921). Surgical dressings composed chiefly of cotton, rayon, or other cellulose material may be sterilised by the following method, which is designed to achieve efficient sterilisation and to deliver the sterilised dressings dry and ready for use.

A suitable apparatus consists of a sterilising chamber capable of withstanding the necessary changes in pressure and either insulated or surrounded by a steam jacket maintained at the sterilising temperature.

The chamber is provided with a suitable supply of steam under pressure which is dry but not superheated, a condensate discharge drain fitted with a near-to-steam trap, a thermometer to indicate the lowest temperature in the chamber during the process, a pressure gauge, a pump capable of removing sufficient air from the load to ensure almost instantaneous penetration of the steam into the dressing, and a filter to allow sterile air to be admitted at the end of the process. A device is fitted which will detect the presence of sufficient residual air in the chamber to delay penetration of the steam and thereby interfere with the sterilising process. There must be no leaks in the valves or door seal of the chamber, and the chamber door must be adequately insulated. Full details of the construction and performance requirements of automatically controlled autoclaves suitable for sterilising porous loads are given in British Standard 3970: Part 1 : 1966.

Steam is first admitted to the jacket, if one is provided. The dressings are placed in the sterilising chamber and so arranged by suitable packing that they can be permeated by steam. The chamber is closed, and air removed from the chamber by reducing the pressure. The removal of air during this part of the process may be assisted by the admission of steam, either as a series of pulses or a continuous flush.

Steam is then admitted until the chamber temperature reaches the chosen value, which is then maintained for the appropriate period, after which the steam is removed from the chamber and drying accomplished by reducing the pressure in the chamber.

Sterile air is then admitted through the filter, the chamber opened, and the dressings are removed. The whole process is usually automatically controlled.

The sterilisation conditions used must be chosen with regard to the stability of the dressing. For materials which can withstand exposure to a temperature of 134° to 138° for 3 minutes, these conditions are usually chosen if suitable apparatus which can be carefully controlled is available. Most fabrics can be autoclaved at a temperature of 121° to 122° for 15 minutes. However, dressings containing boric acid become tender at this temperature, but they may be sterilised by using a temperature of 115° to 116° for 30 minutes; at this temperature the damage caused at the higher temperature is largely avoided.

Sterilisation can also be accomplished without the use of high vacuum by using steam to displace the air by the normal "downward displacement" method, but it requires extreme care and skill in packing the load and in carrying out the sterilisation process in order to effect the complete removal of air from all parts of the load and adequate penetration of the steam.

DRY HEAT (Method 1, page 921). Dressings impregnated with soft paraffin may be sterilised by maintaining at a temperature not lower than 150° for one hour. It is essential that all parts of the dressing are maintained at this temperature.

EXPOSURE TO ETHYLENE OXIDE (Method 5, page 923). Wrappers enclosing the material must permit access of ethylene oxide, water vapour, and air, but prevent access of micro-organisms, and be able to withstand the changes of pressure in the chamber during sterilisation. After the sterilisation process, complete removal of ethylene oxide from the dressings by ventilation before final packing must be ensured, as prolonged contact with the skin, even in very low concentrations, may cause dermatitis or blistering.

EXPOSURE TO IONISING RADIATION (Method 6, page 924). This method is suitable for sterilising certain surgical dressings.

Some natural and synthetic fibres and plastics are likely to be degraded to a significant extent by repeated exposure to ionising radiation. With some materials, for example, cellulosic materials, major degradation occurs if they are autoclaved after they have been exposed to a sterilising dose of gamma radiation. There is also the possibility of toxicity developing in certain products if they are exposed to ethylene oxide after previous irradiation. Therefore no attempt should be made to resterilise a dressing which has been previously sterilised by exposure to ionising radiation.

Appendix 30

Isotonic and Isosmotic Solutions

The following table lists the freezing-point depression values for 1 per cent w/v aqueous solutions of various substances described in the British Pharmaceutical Codex for use in calculating the quantity of an adjusting substance to be added to an aqueous solution to render it isosmotic with a 0·9 per cent w/v solution of sodium chloride and thus, in most cases, isotonic with blood serum and lachrymal secretion.

The amount of adjusting substance required may be calculated from the equation:

$$W = \frac{0.52 - a}{b}$$

where W = the weight, in g, of the added substance in 100 millilitres of the final solution,
a = the depression of the freezing-point of water produced by the medicament already in solution, calculated by multiplying the value for b for the medicament by the strength of the solution expressed as a percentage w/v, and
b = the depression of the freezing-point of water produced by 1 per cent w/v of the added substance.

Substance	b
Adrenaline Acid Tartrate	0·098
Amethocaine Hydrochloride	0·109
Aminophylline	0·098
Amitriptyline Hydrochloride	0·100
Amphetamine Sulphate	0·129
Amylobarbitone Sodium	0·143
Antazoline Hydrochloride	0·132
Antimony Sodium Tartrate	0·075
Apomorphine Hydrochloride	0·080
Ascorbic Acid	0·105
Atropine Methonitrate	0·100
Atropine Sulphate	0·074
Barbitone Sodium	0·171
Benzalkonium Chloride Solution	0·046
Benzyl Alcohol	0·094
Benzylpenicillin (Potassium Salt)	0·102
Benzylpenicillin (Sodium Salt)	0·100
Borax	0·241

Substance	b	Substance	b
Boric Acid	0·288	Oxytetracycline Hydrochloride	0·075
Calcium Chloride ($2H_2O$)	0·298	Papaverine Hydrochloride	0·061
Calcium Gluconate	0·091	Pentobarbitone Sodium	0·145
Carbachol	0·205	Pentolinium Tartrate	0·098
Cetrimide	0·051	Pethidine Hydrochloride	0·125
Chloramphenicol Sodium Succinate	0·080	Phenazone	0·093
Chlorpheniramine Maleate	0·085	Phenobarbitone Sodium	0·135
Chlorpromazine Hydrochloride	0·058	Phenylephrine Hydrochloride	0·184
Cinchocaine Hydrochloride	0·074	Phenylpropanolamine Hydrochloride	0·219
Cocaine Hydrochloride	0·090	Physostigmine Salicylate	0·090
Codeine Phosphate	0·080	Physostigmine Sulphate	0·074
Copper Sulphate	0·100	Pilocarpine Hydrochloride	0·138
Cyclopentolate Hydrochloride	0·115	Pilocarpine Nitrate	0·132
Dextrose, Anhydrous	0·101	Polymyxin B Sulphate	0·052
Dextrose (monohydrate)	0·091	Potassium Chloride	0·439
Diphenhydramine Hydrochloride	0·161	Potassium Iodide	0·196
Edrophonium Chloride	0·179	Potassium Nitrate	0·324
Emetine Hydrochloride	0·058	Potassium Permanganate	0·223
Ephedrine Hydrochloride	0·165	Prilocaine Hydrochloride	0·125
Ergometrine Maleate	0·089	Procainamide Hydrochloride	0·127
Ethanolamine	0·306	Procaine Hydrochloride	0·122
Ethylenediamine Hydrate	0·253	Promethazine Hydrochloride	0·104
Ethylmorphine Hydrochloride	0·088	Pyridoxine Hydrochloride	0·213
Fluorescein Sodium	0·181	Quinine Dihydrochloride	0·130
Gallamine Triethiodide	0·046	Quinine Hydrochloride	0·077
Glycerol	0·203	Resorcinol	0·161
Histamine Acid Phosphate	0·149	Silver Nitrate	0·190
Homatropine Hydrobromide	0·097	Sodium Acetate ($3H_2O$)	0·265
Hyoscine Hydrobromide	0·068	Sodium Acid Phosphate	0·207
Isoniazid	0·144	Sodium Aminosalicylate	0·170
Lactic Acid	0·239	Sodium Benzoate	0·230
Lactose	0·040	Sodium Bicarbonate	0·380
Lignocaine Hydrochloride	0·130	Sodium Chloride	0·576
Magnesium Chloride ($6H_2O$)	0·259	Sodium Citrate	0·178
Magnesium Sulphate	0·094	Sodium Iodide	0·222
Mannitol	0·098	Sodium Metabisulphite	0·386
Menaphthone Sodium Bisulphite	0·115	Sodium Nitrite	0·480
Mephenesin	0·109	Sodium Salicylate	0·210
Mepyramine Maleate	0·108	Sodium Sulphate	0·148
Mersalyl Acid	0·069	Sodium Thiosulphate	0·181
Methacholine Chloride	0·184	Streptomycin Sulphate	0·036
Methadone Hydrochloride	0·101	Strychnine Hydrochloride	0·104
Methoxamine Hydrochloride	0·150	Sucrose	0·047
Methylamphetamine Hydrochloride	0·213	Sulphacetamide Sodium	0·132
Morphine Hydrochloride	0·086	Suxamethonium Chloride	0·115
Morphine Sulphate	0·079	Tartaric Acid	0·143
Neomycin Sulphate	0·063	Tetracycline Hydrochloride	0·081
Neostigmine Bromide	0·127	Thiamine Hydrochloride	0·139
Neostigmine Methylsulphate	0·115	Thiopentone Sodium	0·155
Nicotinamide	0·148	Tolazoline Hydrochloride	0·196
Nicotinic Acid	0·144	Tropicamide	0·050
Nikethamide	0·100	Tubocurarine Chloride	0·076
Noscapine Hydrochloride ($C_{22}H_{24}ClNO_7$)	0·058	Zinc Chloride	0·351
		Zinc Sulphate	0·086

Appendix 31

Millimoles and Milliequivalents

The strengths of intravenous transfusion fluids are sometimes expressed in terms of the number of millimoles or milliequivalents.

A mole is the basic unit of amount of substance of a specified chemical formula, containing the same number of formula units (atoms, molecules, ions, electrons, quanta, or other entities) as there are in 12 g of the pure nuclide ^{12}C. A millimole is one thousandth of this amount and for ions it is the ionic weight, that is, the sum of the atomic weights of the elements of an ion, expressed in milligrams. A milliequivalent is this quantity divided by the valency of the ion.

Ion	Millimole (mmol) mg	Milliequivalent (mEq) mg	Salt	Milligrams of salt containing 1 mmol = W_1*	1 mEq = W_2* of specified ion
Ca^{2+}	40·0	20·0	Calcium Acetate, $C_4H_6CaO_4$	158	79
			Calcium Chloride, $CaCl_2,2H_2O$	147	73·5
			Calcium Gluconate, $C_{12}H_{22}CaO_{14},H_2O$	448	224
			Calcium Lactate, $C_6H_{10}CaO_6,5H_2O$	308	154
K^+	39·1	39·1	Potassium Acetate, $C_2H_3KO_2$	98	98
			Potassium Bicarbonate, $KHCO_3$	100	100
			Potassium Bromide, KBr	119	119
			Potassium Chloride, KCl	74·5	74·5
			Potassium Citrate, $C_6H_5K_3O_7,H_2O$	108	108
			Potassium Gluconate, $C_6H_{11}KO_7$	234	234
Mg^{2+}	24·3	12·15	Magnesium Acetate, $C_4H_6MgO_4,4H_2O$	214	107
			Magnesium Chloride, $MgCl_2,6H_2O$	203	101·5
			Magnesium Sulphate, $MgSO_4,7H_2O$	246	123
Na^+	23·0	23·0	Sodium Acetate, $C_2H_3O_2Na,3H_2O$	136	136
			Sodium Acid Citrate, $C_6H_6Na_2O_7,1\frac{1}{2}H_2O$	131	131
			Sodium Acid Phosphate, $NaH_2PO_4,2H_2O$	156	156
			Sodium Bicarbonate, $NaHCO_3$	84	84
			Sodium Chloride, $NaCl$	58·5	58·5
			Sodium Citrate, $C_6H_5Na_3O_7,2H_2O$	98	98
			Sodium Hydroxide, $NaOH$	40	40
			Sodium Lactate†	112	112
			Sodium Phosphate, $Na_2HPO_4,12H_2O$	179	179
			Sodium Salicylate, $C_7H_5NaO_3$	160	160
			Sodium Sulphate, $Na_2SO_4,10H_2O$	161	161
NH_4^+	18·0	18·0	Ammonium Chloride, NH_4Cl	53·5	53·5
Cl^-	35·5	35·5	Ammonium Chloride, NH_4Cl	53·5	53·5
			Calcium Chloride, $CaCl_2,2H_2O$	73·5	73·5
			Magnesium Chloride, $MgCl_2,6H_2O$	101·5	101·5
			Potassium Chloride, KCl	74·5	74·5
			Sodium Chloride, $NaCl$	58·5	58·5
$C_2H_3O_2^-$ (Acetate)	59·0	59·0	Calcium Acetate, $C_4H_6CaO_4$	79	79
			Magnesium Acetate, $C_4H_6MgO_4,4H_2O$	107	107
			Potassium Acetate, $C_2H_3KO_2$	98	98
			Sodium Acetate, $C_2H_3O_2Na,3H_2O$	136	136

Ion	Millimole (mmol) mg	Milliequi- valent (mEq) mg	Salt	Milligrams of salt containing 1 mmol $= W_1{}^*$ of specified ion	1 mEq $= W_2{}^*$
$C_3H_5O_3{}^-$ (Lactate)	89·0	89·0	Calcium Lactate, $C_6H_{10}CaO_6,5H_2O$	154	154
$HCO_3{}^-$	61·0	61·0	Sodium Lactate†	112	112
			Potassium Bicarbonate, $KHCO_3$	100	100
			Sodium Bicarbonate, $NaHCO_3$	84	84
$HPO_4{}^{2-}$	96·0	48·0	Sodium Phosphate, $Na_2HPO_4,12H_2O$	358	179
$H_2PO_4{}^-$	97·0	97·0	Sodium Acid Phosphate, $NaH_2PO_4,2H_2O$	156	156

* W_1 may be calculated by dividing the molecular weight of the salt used by the number of the specified ions in a molecule of the salt. W_2 may be obtained by dividing W_1 by the valency of the specified ion.

† Prepared in solution by neutralising lactic acid with sodium hydroxide; 1·0 ml of 1M sodium lactate contains the equivalent of 112 mg.

Use of Table of Millimoles and Milliequivalents

EXAMPLE. To prepare a solution containing 67 mmol sodium, 6 mmol potassium, 2 mmol calcium, and 77 mmol chloride.

Millimoles required				Salts and quantities used
Ca^{2+}	K^+	Na^+	Cl^-	
2			4	Calcium Chloride 2×147 mg $= 0·294$ g
	6		6	Potassium Chloride $6 \times 74·5$ mg $= 0·447$ g
		67	67	Sodium Chloride $67 \times 58·5$ mg $= 3·92$ g

Conversion Equations

To convert percentage strength w/v of a solution of a salt to millimoles or milliequivalents per litre of the specified ion the following equations may be used:

$$\text{Millimoles per litre} = \frac{C \times 10,000}{W_1}$$

$$\text{Milliequivalents per litre} = \frac{C \times 10,000}{W_2}$$

and to convert millimoles or milliequivalents per litre to percentage strength w/v, the following equations:

$$\text{Percentage strength w/v} = \frac{W_1 \times M}{10,000} \text{ or } \frac{W_2 \times E}{10,000}$$

where C = percentage strength w/v,
W_1 = milligrams of salt containing 1 mmol of the specified ion,
W_2 = milligrams of salt containing 1 mEq of specified ion,
E = milliequivalents per litre, and
M = millimoles per litre.

Concentration of Ions in Intravenous Fluids

Intravenous fluid	Approximate number of millimoles per litre					
	Ca^{2+}	K^+	Na^+	H^+ equivalent	Cl^-	HCO_3^- (or equivalent)
Sodium Bicarbonate Injection (1·4 per cent)			167			167
Sodium Chloride Injection (0·9 per cent)			154		154	
Sodium Chloride (0·18 per cent) and Dextrose (4·3 per cent) Injection			31		31	
Compound Sodium Lactate Injection	2	5	131		112	29
M/6 Ammonium Chloride				167	167	
M/6 Sodium Lactate			167			167

Appendix 32

Weights and Measures

A. Metric System

MASS (WEIGHTS)

1 kilogram (kg) is the mass of the International Prototype Kilogram

1 gram (g)	= the 1000th part of 1 kilogram
1 milligram (mg)	= the 1000th part of 1 gram
1 microgram (μg)	= the 1000th part of 1 milligram

For the purpose of writing prescriptions the word "microgram" should be written in full; when an abbreviation is essential, the British Pharmacopoeia recommends that "mcg" should be used as the contraction. This divergence from international practice is recommended to avoid the possibility of confusion between "μg" and "mg".

CAPACITY (VOLUMES)

1 litre (l)* is the volume occupied at its temperature of maximum density by a quantity of water having a mass of 1 kilogram.

1 millilitre (ml) = the 1000th part of 1 litre

1 microlitre (μl) = the 1000th part of 1 millilitre

* The accepted relation between the litre and the cubic centimetre is 1 litre = 1000·028 cubic centimetres. The principal unit of volume recommended by the General Congress on Weights and Measures held in 1964 is the cubic decimetre (dm^3), which it is intended shall in due course replace the litre for scientific and technological purposes. The litre will then be regarded as equivalent to the cubic decimetre, and the millilitre as the equivalent of the cubic centimetre, and these units may continue to be used for purposes where a high degree of precision is not required as in pharmacy and medicine.

PREFIXES DENOTING DECIMAL MULTIPLES AND SUBMULTIPLES

Prefix	Symbol	Multiple or Submultiple
tera	T	$10^{12} = 1\ 000\ 000\ 000\ 000$
giga	G	$10^9 = 1\ 000\ 000\ 000$
mega	M	$10^6 = 1\ 000\ 000$
kilo	k	$10^3 = 1\ 000$
hecto	h	$10^2 = 100$
deca	da	$10^1 = 10$
deci	d	$10^{-1} = 0·1$
centi	c	$10^{-2} = 0·01$
milli	m	$10^{-3} = 0·001$
micro	μ	$10^{-6} = 0·000\ 001$
nano	n	$10^{-9} = 0·000\ 000\ 001$
pico	p	$10^{-12} = 0·000\ 000\ 000\ 001$
femto	f	$10^{-15} = 0·000\ 000\ 000\ 000\ 001$
atto	a	$10^{-18} = 0·000\ 000\ 000\ 000\ 000\ 001$

LENGTH

1 metre (m) is the Metre as defined in the Weights and Measures (International Definitions) Order 1963

1 decimetre (dm)	= the 10th part of 1 metre
1 centimetre (cm)	= the 100th part of 1 metre
1 millimetre (mm)	= the 1000th part of 1 metre
1 micrometre (μm)	= the 1000th part of 1 millimetre
1 nanometre (nm)	= the 1000th part of 1 micrometre

RADIOACTIVITY

The curie (Ci) is the unit of activity of radio-nuclides

1 curie (Ci) = $3 \cdot 7 \times 10^{10}$ disintegrations per second

1 millicurie (mCi) = $3 \cdot 7 \times 10^{7}$ disintegrations per second

1 microcurie (μCi) = $3 \cdot 7 \times 10^{4}$ disintegrations per second

B. Imperial System

MASS (WEIGHTS)

1 pound (avoirdupois) (lb) is the Imperial Pound as defined in the Weights and Measures Act, 1963, Schedule 1

1 ounce (avoirdupois) (oz)	= the 16th part of 1 pound
	= 437·5 grains
1 grain (gr)	= the 7000th part of 1 pound

CAPACITY (VOLUMES)

1 pint (pt) is the Imperial Pint as defined in the Weights and Measures Act, 1963, Schedule 1

1 fluid Ounce (fl oz)	= the 20th part of 1 pint
	= 8 fluid drachms
1 fluid Drachm (fl dr)	= the 8th part of 1 fluid ounce
	= 60 minims
1 minim (min)	= the 60th part of 1 fluid drachm

RELATION OF CAPACITY TO WEIGHT

The following equivalents are stated to five significant figures:

1 minim	= the volume at $16 \cdot 7°$ ($62°$ F) of 0·91146 grain of water
1 fluid drachm	= the volume at $16 \cdot 7°$ ($62°$ F) of 54·688 grains of water
1 fluid ounce	= the volume at $16 \cdot 7°$ ($62°$ F) of 1 ounce (avoirdupois) or 437·5 grains of water
109·71 Minims*	= the volume at $16 \cdot 7°$ ($62°$ F) of 100 grains of water

* Usually taken as 110 minims

LENGTH

1 yard (yd) is the Imperial Yard as defined in the Weights and Measures Act, 1963, Schedule 1

1 foot (ft)	= the 3rd part of 1 yard
1 inch (in.)	= the 12th part of 1 foot

C. Imperial Equivalents of Metric Weights and Measures

The following equivalents are stated to five significant figures.

WEIGHTS OR MEASURES OF MASS

1 microgram (μg)	= $15 \cdot 432 \times 10^{-6}$ grain
1 milligram (mg)	= 0·015432 grain
1 gram (g)	= 15·432 grains
	= 0·03215 ounce (apothecaries')
	= 0·03527 ounce (avoirdupois)
1 kilogram (kg)	= 2·2046 pounds

MEASURES OF CAPACITY

1 millilitre (ml)	= 16·894 minims
1 litre (l)	= 0·21997 gallon
	= 1·7598 pints
	= 35·196 fluid ounces

MEASURES OF LENGTH

1 ångström (Å)	= $3 \cdot 9370 \times 10^{-9}$ inch
1 nanometre (nm)	= $3 \cdot 9370 \times 10^{-8}$ inch
1 micrometre (μm)	= $3 \cdot 9370 \times 10^{-5}$ inch
1 millimetre (mm)	= 0·039370 inch
1 centimetre (cm)	= 0·39370 inch
1 decimetre (dm)	= 3·9370 inches
1 metre (m)	= 39·370 inches

D. Metric Equivalents of Imperial Weights and Measures

The following equivalents are stated to five significant figures.

WEIGHTS OR MEASURES OF MASS

1 grain (gr)	= 0·064799 gram
1 ounce (avoirdupois) (437·5 gr) (oz)	= 28·350 grams
1 ounce (apothecaries') (480 gr)	= 31·104 grams
1 pound (lb)	= 453·59 grams

MEASURES OF CAPACITY

1 minim (min)	= 0·059192 millilitre
1 fluid drachm (fl dr)	= 3·5515 millilitres
1 fluid ounce (fl oz)	= 28·412 millilitres
	= 0·028412 litre
1 pint (pt)	= 568·25 millilitres
	= 0·56825 litre
1 gallon (gal)	= 4·5460 litres

MEASURES OF LENGTH

1 inch (in.)	= $25 \cdot 400 \times 10^{7}$ ångströms
	= $25 \cdot 400 \times 10^{6}$ nanometres
	= $25 \cdot 400 \times 10^{3}$ micrometres
	= 25·400 millimetres
1 foot (ft)	= 304·80 millimetres
1 yard (yd)	= 914·40 millimetres

E. Atomic Weights of Elements

$^{12}C = 12$

Element	Atomic Number	Symbol	Atomic Weight
Aluminium	13	Al	26·98154
Antimony	51	Sb	121·75
Arsenic	33	As	74·9216
Barium	56	Ba	137·34
Bismuth	83	Bi	208·9804
Boron	5	B	10·81
Bromine	35	Br	79·904
Cadmium	48	Cd	112·40
Calcium	20	Ca	40·08
Carbon	6	C	12·011
Cerium	58	Ce	140·12
Chlorine	17	Cl	35·453
Chromium	24	Cr	51·996
Cobalt	27	Co	58·9332
Copper	29	Cu	63·546

Element	Atomic Number	Symbol	Atomic Weight	Element	Atomic Number	Symbol	Atomic Weight
Fluorine	9	F	18·99840	Potassium	19	K	39·098
Gold	79	Au	196·9665	Ruthenium	44	Ru	101·07
Helium	2	He	4·00260	Selenium	34	Se	78·96
Hydrogen	1	H	1·0079	Silicon	14	Si	28·086
Indium	49	In	114·82	Silver	47	Ag	107·868
Iodine	53	I	126·9045	Sodium	11	Na	22·98977
Iron	26	Fe	55·847	Strontium	38	Sr	87·62
Lead	82	Pb	207·2	Sulphur	16	S	32·06
Lithium	3	Li	6·941	Technetium	43	Tc	98·9062
Magnesium	12	Mg	24·305	Thallium	81	Tl	204·37
Manganese	25	Mn	54·9380	Thorium	90	Th	232·0381
Mercury	80	Hg	200·59	Tin	50	Sn	118·69
Molybdenum	42	Mo	95·94	Titanium	22	Ti	47·90
Nickel	28	Ni	58·71	Tungsten	74	W	183·85
Nitrogen	7	N	14·0067	Uranium	92	U	238·029
Oxygen	8	O	15·9994	Vanadium	23	V	50·9414
Palladium	46	Pd	106·4	Xenon	54	Xe	131·30
Phosphorus	15	P	30·97376	Zinc	30	Zn	65·38
Platinum	78	Pt	195·09	Zirconium	40	Zr	91·22

INDEX

Entries are arranged alphabetically in word-by-word order; entries consisting of abbreviations represented by initial letters, e.g. ACTH, are treated as single words.

When an entry is followed by more than one page reference, the principal reference is printed in **bold** type.

935

Adrenaline (*continued*)—
    injection, procaine and, strong,
        10, 404
    solution, 10
Adrenaline acid tartrate, xxiv, **9**, 829
Adrenaline tartrate, 9, 829
    injection, 9
    solution, 10
Adrenalinii tartras, 9
Adrenocorticotrophic hormone,
    130
Adreson, 133
Adulterants of crude drugs, xxxiv
Aerosol inhalations, xx, 643–648
    containers for, 644
    labelling of, 644
    storage of, 644
    —*for individual products see
        under names of substances*
Aerosol propellents, examination
    of, 896
Aerosporin, 389
Aethinyloestradiolum, 187
African bdellium, 317
African ginger, 211
African rauwolfia, 427
Ailanthus altissima, 42
Air-suspension coating of tablets,
    803
Ajmalicine, 426
Ajmaline, 426, 427
Ajmalinine, 426
Albamycin, 332, 333
Albaspidin, 280, 281
Albucid, 476
Albumin fraction (saline), human,
    xxiii, 585
    dried, xxiii, 585
Albumin, human, xix, 584
    dried, xix, 584
Albumin injection, iodinated (^{125}I)
    human, xx, xxiii, 244
Albumin injection, iodinated (^{131}I)
    human, 245
    macroaggregated, 273
Alcohol, 10
    (20 per cent), **10**, 830
    (25 per cent), 10
    (45 per cent), **10**, 830
    (50 per cent), **10**, 830
    (60 per cent), **10**, 829
    (70 per cent), **10**, 829
    (80 per cent), **10**, 829
    (90 per cent), **10**, 829
    (95 per cent), **10**, 829
        aldehyde-free, 830
    absolute, 11
    amyl, 831
    benzyl, **50**, 832
    butyl, 833
    cetostearyl, 88
    cetyl, 88
    dehydrated, **11**, 830
        aldehyde-free, 830
    ethyl, 10
    isobutyl, 839
    isopropyl, **255**, 839
        (90 per cent v/v), 839
    methyl, 841
        (60 per cent), 841
        (80 per cent), 841
        acid, 841

Alcohol (*continued*)—
    methyl
        ammoniacal, 841
        dehydrated, 841
    myristyl, 88
    stearyl, 88
Alcohol content, determination of,
    888–891
Alcohols, dilute, 10
Alcohols for reagents, 829
Alcohols, wool, 535
    ointment, 536
Alcohols, wool wax, 535
Alcohol-soluble extractive, xxxiii
Alcopar, 53
Aldactone-A, 467
Aldehydes in volatile oils, deter-
    mination of, 893
Aldobionic acid, 3
Aldomet, 309
Aleudrin, 255
Alexandrian senna, 437, 438
    leaflets, 438
    pods, 437
Alginic acid, **11**, 830
Alizarin fluorine blue, 830
    solution, 830
Alkali, substances affected by, 925
Alkaline eye-drops, 692
Alkaloids, complete extraction of,
    xxxiii
Alkeran, 288
Alkyldimethyl-2-phenoxyethylam-
    monium bromides, 174
Allegron, 331
Alleppey cardamoms, 79
Allopurinol, xx, 12
    tablets, 12
(−)-*N*-Allyl-3-hydroxymorphinan
    hydrogen tartrate, 265
4-Allyl-2-methoxyphenol, 193
N-Allylnormorphine hydrobro-
    mide, 318
Almond, bitter, 13
Almond oil, 13
Almond, sweet, 13
Alocol-P, 15
Aloe, 13
Aloë barbadensis, 13
Aloë ferox, 13
Aloë perryi, 14
Aloë spectabilis, 14
Aloe-emodin, 13, 81, 429, 437,
    438
Aloe-emodin anthrone, 13, 14, 81
Aloe-emodin anthrone diglucoside,
    437, 438
Aloe-emodin 8-glucoside, 437, 438
Aloes, 13
    Barbados, 13
    Cape, 13, 14
    Curaçao, 13, 14
    Natal, 14
    Socotrine, 14
    Zanzibar, 14
Aloin, 13, **14**
    amorphous, 13, 14
Aloinoside A, 13
Aloinoside B, 13
Alprenolol hydrochloride, xiv
Alstonine, 427
Aludrox, 15

Alum, xxiv, 14
    and zinc dusting-powder, pae-
        diatric, xxii
    potash, 14
Alum. hydrox. gel, 15
    dried, 15
Alum. phosph. gel, 16
    dried, 17
Alumen, 14
Alumina, 830
    anhydrous, 830
Aluminii sulfas, 18
Aluminium
    paste, compound, 18, 539, **767**
    powder, 17
    reactions characteristic of,
        xxxiii
Aluminium acetate
    ear-drops, 780
    solution, 18, **780**
Aluminium carbonate, basic, 15
Aluminium hydroxide
    and belladonna mixture, 15,
        42, **735**
    and magnesium trisilicate tab-
        lets, 812
    gel, **15**, 830
        dried, 15
    mixture, 15
    powder, 15
    tablets, 15
Aluminium magnesium silicate, 16
Aluminium orthophosphate, 16
    hydrated, 17
Aluminium oxide, 15
    hydrated, 17
Aluminium phosphate gel, xviii,
    16
    dried, xviii, 17
Aluminium phosphate tablets, 17
Aluminium silicate, hydrated, 258,
    259
Aluminium sulphate, xxvi, 18
Alupent, 340
Aluphos, 17
Aluphos gel, 16
Amaranth, 830
    solution, 780
        dilute, 830
American mandrake, 386
American peppermint oil, 357
American storax, 472
American turpentine oil, 524
Amethocaine eye-drops, 19, **688**
Amethocaine hydrochloride, xxiv,
    19
Amidone hydrochloride, 297
Amidone linctus, 723
Aminacrine hydrochloride, xxi
    in surgical dressings, 609
        determination of, 916
Aminacyl sodium, 442
Amines, primary aromatic, reac-
    tions characteristic of, xxxiii
Aminoacetate buffer solution, 830
Aminoacetic acid, 830
4-*p*-Aminobenzenesulphonamido-
    2,6-dimethoxypyrimidine, 478
5-*p*-Aminobenzenesulphonamido-
    3, 4-dimethylisoxazole, 480
2-*p*-Aminobenzenesulphonamido-
    4,6-dimethylpyrimidine, 478

Durabolin, 319
Durenate, 483
Dusting-powder, absorbable, xxiii, 280
Dusting-powders, 662–664
  containers for, 662
  labelling of, 662
  —*for individual dusting-powders see under names of substances*
Dydrogesterone, xx, 175
  tablets, 175
Dyes in surgical dressings, 609
Dyflos, xxi
Dytac, 516

EACA, 20
Ear-drops, 664–666
  containers for, 664
  labelling of, 664
  —*for individual ear-drops see under names of substances*
East African capsicums, 73
East Indian arrowroot, 34
East Indian dill oil, 166
East Indian mastic, 284
East Indian rhubarb, 429
Easton's tablets, 810
Ecgonine, 120
Economycin, 499
Econopen V, 372
Ecothiopate iodide, xx, 176
Edecrin, 183
Edetate-citrate solution, 837
Edifas B, 447
Edrophonium chloride, 176
Edrophonium injection, 176
Efcortelan, 225
Efcortelan Soluble, 227
Efcortesol, 226
Effervescent calcium gluconate tablets, 69, **808**
Effervescent potassium tablets, xxii
Effervescent powder, compound, 461, 494, **776**
  double-strength, 461, 494, **777**
Effervescing mouth-wash tablets, 792
Egyptian henbane, 231
El Tor biotype of *Vibrio cholerae*, 558
Elaeis guineensis, 346
Elapine snakes, 570
Elastic adhesive bandage, 617
  diachylon, 616
  diachylon, ventilated, 617
  half-spread, 618
  semi-spread, 618
  ventilated, 618
Elastic adhesive dressing, 620
Elastic adhesive plaster, 633
Elastic bandage
  cotton, 611
  cotton and rubber, 611
  rayon and rubber, xxii
Elastic diachylon bandage, 616
  ventilated, 617
Elastic net bandage
  cotton and, 612
  cotton and rubber, 612
Elastic plaster, zinc oxide, 633

Elastic self-adhesive bandage
  zinc oxide, 617
  zinc oxide, half-spread, 618
  zinc oxide, ventilated, 618
Elastic self-adhesive plaster, zinc oxide, 633
Elasticity of surgical dressings, test for, 913
Elemicin, 333
Elettaria cardamomum var. *major*, 80
Elettaria cardamomum var. *minuscula*, 79
Elixirs, 666–678
  dilution of, 666
  labelling of, 667
  microbial contamination of, 666
  stability of, 666
  synonyms for, 666
  —*for individual elixirs see under names of substances*
Eltor/Vac, 558
Eltor vaccine, xix, 558
Eltroxin, 510
Embequin, 165
Embrocation, white, 726
Emeside, 190
Emet. bism. iod., 177
Emet. hydrochlor., 177
Emetamine, 249
Emetic draught, ipecacuanha, paediatric, xix, 250, **661**
Emetine, 249
Emetine and bismuth iodide, 177
  tablets, 177
Emetine hydrochloride, 177
Emetine hydrochloride A.S., 852
Emetine injection, 178
Emodin, 81, 429
Emodin, monomethyl ether of, 208
Emodin oxanthrone, 81
Empiquat BAC, 47
Emulsifying ointment, 350
  cetomacrogol, xxii, 87
  cetrimide, xxii, 89
  hydrous, 350
Emulsifying wax, 88, 455
  anionic, 88, 455
  cationic, 678
  cetomacrogol, xxii, 87, 88
  cetrimide, 88, 89, **678**
  non-ionic, 87, 88
Emulsifying waxes, 678
Emulsin, 210, 537
Emulsio, xxix
Emulsions, 678–680
  containers for, 678
  feeding, 207
  labelling of, 678
  —*for individual emulsions see under names of substances*
Endografin, 247
Endoxana, 139
Enemas, 680–681
  containers for, 680
  —*for individual enemas see under names of substances*
English arrowroot, 33, **469**
English coriander, 129
English lavender oil, 262
English peppermint oil, 357

Entacyl, 383
Enteric coat for tablets, 803
Eosin, 837
  solution, 837
Epanutin, 377, 378
Ephed. hydrochlor., 179
Ephedra species, 178, 417
Ephedrine, 178
  elixir, 179, **671**
  hydrated, 178
  mixture, belladonna and, paediatric, 42, 179, 396, **737**
  nasal drops, 179, **757**
(−)-Ephedrine, 7
Ephedrine hydrochloride, **179**, 837
  elixir, 671
  tablets, 179
Ephedrinum hydratum, 178
(+)-Epicatechin, 83
Epinephrine, 8
Epinephrine bitartrate, 9
Epiphen, 378
Epontol, 411
Epsikapron, 20
Epsilon aminocaproic acid, 20
Epsom salts, 278
  dried, 278
Equanil, 291
Eraldin, 398
Ergocalciferol, 65
Ergometrine injection, 180
Ergometrine maleate, xxiv, 180
Ergometrine tablets, 180
Ergometrinii maleas, 180
Ergonovine maleate, 180
  injection, 180
  tablets, 180
Ergosterol, 537
Ergot, xxi, 180
  prepared, xxi
  tablets, xxii
Ergotamine aerosol inhalation, xx, 181, **645**
Ergotamine injection, 181
Ergotamine tablets, 181
Ergotamine tartrate, xxiv, **180**, 837
Ergotamine tartrate A.S., 853
Ergotaminii tartras, 180
Eriodictyol glycoside, 339
Erycen, 182
Erythrocin, 182
Erythromid, 182
Erythromycin, xxiv, 181
  mixture, 182, **741**
  standard preparation of, 898
  suspension, 741
  tablets, 182
  unit of, 898
Erythromycin estolate, 182
  capsules, 182
Erythromycin ethyl carbonate, xxi
Erythromycin propionyl ester, lauryl sulphate salt of, 182
Erythromycin stearate, 182
  tablets, 182
Erythromycinum, 181
Erythroxylum coca, 120
Erythroxylum truxillense, 120
Esbatal, 56
Eserine, 380
  and pilocarpine eye-drops, 693
  eye-drops, 693